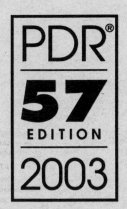

PHYSICIANS' DESK REFERENCE®

Supplement A

For important errata, turn the page.

IMPORTANT NOTICE

Supplements to PHYSICIANS' DESK REFERENCE are published twice yearly to provide readers with significant revisions of existing product listings as well as comprehensive information on new drugs and other products not included in the current annual edition. Before prescribing or administering any product described in PHYSICIANS' DESK REFERENCE, be sure to consult this supplement to determine whether revisions have occurred since the 2003 edition of PDR went to press.

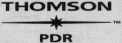

Copyright © 2003 and published by Thomson PDR at Montvale, NJ 07645-1742. All rights reserved. None of the content of this publication may be reproduced, stored in a retrieval system, resold, redistributed, or transmitted in any form or by any means (electronic, mechanical, photocopying, recording, or otherwise) without the prior written permission of the publisher. PHYSICIANS' DESK REFERENCE®, PDR®, Pocket PDR®, The PDR® Family Guide to Prescription Drugs®, The PDR® Family Guide to Women's Health and Prescription Drugs®, and The PDR® Family Guide to Nutrition and Health®, are registered trademarks used herein under license. PDR for Nonprescription Drugs and Dietary Supplements™, PDR For Ophthalmic Medicines™, PDR® Medical Dictionary™, PDR® Nurse's Drug Handbook™, PDR® Nurse's Dictionary™, PDR Companion Guide™, PDR® for Herbal Medicines™, PDR® for Nutritional Supplements™, PDR Pharmacopoeia™ Pocket Dosing Guide, PDR® Monthly Prescribing Guide™, PDR® Electronic Library™, The PDR Family Guide Encyclopedia of Medical Care™, The PDR® Family Guide to Over-the-Counter Drugs™, The PDR® Family Guide to Common Ailments™, The PDR® Family Guide to Nutritional Supplements™, and The PDR® Family Guide to Natural Medicines and Healing Therapies™ are trademarks used herein under license.

This supplement is a compilation of information submitted by the products' manufacturers. Each entry has been prepared, edited, and approved by the manufacturer's medical department, medical director, and/or medical consultant. The publisher does not warrant or guarantee any of the products described herein nor is the publisher responsible for misuse of a product due to typographical error. The publisher does not perform any independent analysis in connection with the product information contained herein.

Officers of Thomson Healthcare, Inc.: *President and Chief Executive Officer:* Richard Noble; *Chief Financial Officer:* Paul Hilger; *Executive Vice President, Clinical Trials:* Tom Kelly; *Executive Vice President, Medical Education:* Jeff MacDonald; *Executive Vice President, Clinical Solutions:* Jeff Reihl; *Executive Vice President, Medical Education & Communications:* Terry Meacock; *Executive Vice President, Physicians' Desk Reference:* Paul Walsh; *Senior Vice President, Business Development:* William Gole; *Vice President, Human Resources:* Pamela M. Bilash; *President, Physician's World:* Marty Cearnal

ERRATA

Product Identification Guide

1. Under the photo of Kineret (Amgen) on page 305 of the 2003 PDR, the strength should be listed as "100 mg/0.67 mL," not "100 mg/mL."

2. Under the photos of Avita Cream and Avita Gel (Bertek) on page 309 of the 2003 PDR, the size of the tubes shown should be listed as 45 g, not 20 g.

3. Under the photo of Curosurf (Dey) on page 311 of the 2003 PDR, the generic name should be listed as "poractant alfa," not "poractant alpha."

4. Under the photos of Diovan HCT (Novartis) on page 324 of the 2003 PDR, the "160 mg/25 mg" tablet (brown orange, debossed HXH) was incorrectly marked as "160 mg/12.5 mg," and the "160 mg/12.5 mg" tablet (dark red, debossed HHH) was incorrectly marked as "160 mg/25 mg."

5. Under the photo of Cormax Scalp Application (Oclassen) on page 326 of the 2003 PDR, the strength should be listed as "0.05%," not "0.5%."

6. In the Medicis, the Dermatology Company listing is the Manufacturers' Index on page 10 of the 2003 PDR, the contact information for Medical Information should be: Medical Affairs Department, (602) 808-8800, fax (602) 808-0822 for General information; and (602) 808-8800 for Emergencies.

NEW PRODUCT LISTINGS INDEX

Listed below are new *PDR* listings first appearing in 2003 *PDR Supplement A*. These listings include comprehensive descriptions of new pharmaceutical products introduced since publication of the 2003 *PDR*, new dosage forms of products already described, and existing pharmaceutical products not described in the 2003 *PDR*.

Brand or Generic Name	Supplement Page

A
Abbokinase (Abbott)..A3
Abilify Tablets (Bristol-Myers Squibb)......................A16
ACYCLOVIR
Zovirax Cream 5% (Biovail).....................................A15
ADALIMUMAB
Humira Injection (Abbott)..A5
ADEFOVIR DIPIVOXIL
Hepsera Tablets (Gilead)...A31
ALBUTEROL SULFATE
VoSpire ER Extended-Release Tablets (Odyssey).................A62
ALEFACEPT
Amevive for Injection (Biogen).................................A13
Alinia for Oral Suspension (Romark)..........................A88
ALPRAZOLAM
Xanax XR Tablets (Pharmacia & Upjohn)....................A74
Amevive for Injection (Biogen).................................A13
AMMONIUM LACTATE
Ammonium Lactate Cream 12% (Clay-Park).....................A25
Ammonium Lactate Cream 12% (Clay-Park).....................A25
AMOXICILLIN
Augmentin XR Tablets (GlaxoSmithKline)...................A34
ANTIPYRINE
Antipyrine/Benzocaine Otic Drops (Clay-Park)................A25
Antipyrine/Benzocaine Otic Drops (Clay-Park)................A25
ARIPIPRAZOLE
Abilify Tablets (Bristol-Myers Squibb)......................A16
ATOMEXETINE HYDROCHLORIDE
Strattera Capsules (Lilly)......................................A53
Augmentin XR Tablets (GlaxoSmithKline)...................A34
Avandamet Tablets (GlaxoSmithKline).......................A36
Avodart Capsules (GlaxoSmithKline).........................A41
Azasan Tablets (AAI Pharma).....................................A1
AZATHIOPRINE
Azasan Tablets (AAI Pharma).....................................A1
AZELAIC ACID
Finacea Gel, 15% (Berlex)..A11

B
BENZOCAINE
Antipyrine/Benzocaine Otic Drops (Clay-Park)................A25
BENZOYL PEROXIDE
Duac Topical Gel (Stiefel).......................................A96
Erythromycin-Benzoyl Peroxide Topical Gel (Clay-Park)........A25
BETAMETHASONE DIPROPIONATE
Betamethasone Dipropionate Lotion USP,
0.05% (Clay-Park)..A25
Betamethasone Dipropionate Lotion USP,
0.05% (Clay-Park)..A25

C
Cardene I.V. (ESP Pharma).......................................A26
CLAVULANATE POTASSIUM
Augmentin XR Tablets (GlaxoSmithKline)...................A34
CLINDAMYCIN
Duac Topical Gel (Stiefel).......................................A96
CLINDAMYCIN PHOSPHATE
Clindamycin Phosphate Pledgets, 1% (Clay-Park)...............A25
Clindamycin Phosphate Pledgets, 1% (Clay-Park)...............A25

CLONAZEPAM
Klonopin Wafers (Roche Labs)..................................A280
Copegus Tablets (Roche Labs)..................................A77

D
DESONIDE
Desonide Cream 0.05% (Clay-Park)............................A25
Desonide Ointment 0.05% (Clay-Park)........................A25
Tridesilon 0.05% Cream (Clay-Park)..........................A25
Tridesilon 0.05% Ointment (Clay-Park)......................A25
Desonide Cream 0.05% (Clay-Park)............................A25
Desonide Ointment 0.05% (Clay-Park)........................A25
DIPHTHERIA & TETANUS TOXOIDS AND ACELLULAR PERTUSSIS VACCINE ADSORBED
Pediarix Vaccine (GlaxoSmithKline)..........................A44
Duac Topical Gel (Stiefel).......................................A96
DUTASTERIDE
Avodart Capsules (GlaxoSmithKline).........................A41

E
ELETRIPTAN HYDROBROMIDE
Relpax Tablets (Pfizer)...A67
ENFUVIRTIDE
Fuzeon for Injection (Roche Labs)..............................A80
ERYTHROMYCIN
Erythromycin Topical Solution USP, 2% (Clay-Park)...........A25
Erythromycin-Benzoyl Peroxide Topical Gel (Clay-Park)........A25
Erythromycin Topical Solution USP, 2% (Clay-Park)...........A25
Erythromycin-Benzoyl Peroxide Topical Gel (Clay-Park)........A25
ESCITALOPRAM OXALATE
Lexapro Oral Solution (Forest)................................A153
EZETIMIBE
Zetia Tablets (Merck/Schering Plough).......................A57
Zetia Tablets (Schering)...A91

F
FENOFIBRATE
Lofibra Capsules (Gate)...A28
Finacea Gel, 15% (Berlex)..A11
Forteo Injection (Lilly)..A49
Fuzeon for Injection (Roche Labs)..............................A80

G
GENTAMICIN SULFATE
Gentamicin Sulfate Cream, USP (Clay-Park)..................A25
Gentamicin Sulfate Ointment, USP (Clay-Park)...............A25
Gentamicin Sulfate Cream, USP (Clay-Park)..................A25
Gentamicin Sulfate Ointment, USP (Clay-Park)...............A25
GLIPIZIDE
Metaglip Tablets (Bristol-Myers Squibb)....................A20

H
HEPATITIS B VACCINE, RECOMBINANT
Pediarix Vaccine (GlaxoSmithKline)..........................A44
Hepsera Tablets (Gilead)...A31
Humira Injection (Abbott)..A5
HYDROCORTISONE
Hydrocortisone Cream USP, 2.5% (Clay-Park)................A25
Hydrocortisone Ointment USP, 2.5% (Clay-Park)..............A25
HYDROCORTISONE ACETATE
Hydrocortisone Acetate Suppositories, 25 mg (Clay-Park)...A25

Brand or Generic Name	Supplement Page
Hydrocortisone Acetate Suppositories, 25 mg (Clay-Park)	A25
Hydrocortisone Cream USP, 2.5% (Clay-Park)	A25
Hydrocortisone Ointment USP, 2.5% (Clay-Park)	A25

HYDROCORTISONE VALERATE
- Hydrocortisone Valerate Cream USP, 0.2% (Clay-Park) A25
- Hydrocortisone Valerate Cream USP, 0.2% (Clay-Park) A25

I
- Imdur Tablets (Schering) A90

INTERFERON BETA-1A
- Rebif Injection (Pfizer) A64
- Ismo (ESP) A26

ISOSORBIDE MONONITRATE
- Imdur Tablets (Schering) A90

K
- Klonopin Wafers (Roche Labs) A28

L
- Levaquin in 5% Dextrose Injection (Ortho-McNeil) A201

LEVOFLOXACIN
- Levaquin in 5% Dextrose Injection (Ortho-McNeil) A201
- Lexapro Oral Solution (Forest) A153
- Lofibra Capsules (Gate) A28

M
- Metaglip Tablets (Bristol-Myers Squibb) A20

METFORMIN HYDROCHLORIDE
- Avandamet Tablets (GlaxoSmithKline) A36
- Metaglip Tablets (Bristol-Myers Squibb) A20

MOMETASONE FUROATE
- Mometasone Furoate Ointment USP, 0.1% (Clay-Park) A25
- Mometasone Furoate Ointment USP, 0.1% (Clay-Park) A25
- M.V.I. Pediatric for Injection (AAI Pharma) A2

N

NICARDIPINE HYDROCHLORIDE
- Cardene I.V. (ESP Pharma) A26

NITAZOXANIDE
- Alinia for Oral Suspension (Romark) A88

NYSTATIN
- Nystatin Cream, USP (Clay-Park) A25
- Nystatin Ointment, USP (Clay-Park) A25
- Nystatin Cream, USP (Clay-Park) A25
- Nystatin Ointment, USP (Clay-Park) A25

O

OXYBUTYNIN
- Oxytrol Transdermal System (Watson) A97
- Oxytrol Transdermal System (Watson) A97

P
- Pediarix Vaccine (GlaxoSmithKline) A44
- Pegasys (Roche Labs) A84

PEGINTERFERON ALFA-2A
- Pegasys (Roche Labs) A84

PEGVISOMANT
- Somavert Injection (Pharmacia & Upjohn) A71

PERMETHRIN
- Permethrin Cream, 5% (Clay-Park) A25
- Permethrin Cream, 5% (Clay-Park) A25

POLIOVIRUS VACCINE INACTIVATED
- Pediarix Vaccine (GlaxoSmithKline) A44

Brand or Generic Name	Supplement Page

R
- Rebif Injection (Pfizer) A64
- Relpax Tablets (Pfizer) A67

RIBAVIRIN
- Copegus Tablets (Roche Labs) A77

ROSIGLITAZONE MALEATE
- Avandamet Tablets (GlaxoSmithKline) A36

S
- Sectal (ESP) A26

SELENIUM SULFIDE
- Selenium Sulfide Lotion USP, 2.5% (Clay-Park) A25
- Selenium Sulfide Lotion USP, 2.5% (Clay-Park) A25
- Somavert for Injection (Pharmacia & Upjohn) A71
- Strattera Capsules (Lilly) A53

T
- Tenex (ESP) A26

TERIPARATIDE
- Forteo Injection (Lilly) A49
- Testim 1% Gel (Auxilium) A9

TESTOSTERONE
- Testim 1% Gel (Auxilium) A9

TRIAMCINOLONE ACETONIDE
- Triamcinolone Acetonide Cream USP, 0.025% (Clay-Park) A25
- Triamcinolone Acetonide Cream USP, 0.1% (Clay-Park) A25
- Triamcinolone Acetonide Cream USP, 0.5% (Clay-Park) A25
- Triamcinolone Acetonide Ointment USP, 0.025% (Clay-Park) A25
- Triamcinolone Acetonide Ointment USP, 0.1% (Clay-Park) A25
- Triamcinolone Acetonide Ointment USP, 0.5% (Clay-Park) A25
- Triamcinolone Acetonide Cream USP, 0.025% (Clay-Park) A25
- Triamcinolone Acetonide Cream USP, 0.1% (Clay-Park) A25
- Triamcinolone Acetonide Cream USP, 0.5% (Clay-Park) A25
- Triamcinolone Acetonide Ointment USP, 0.025% (Clay-Park) A25
- Triamcinolone Acetonide Ointment USP, 0.1% (Clay-Park) A25
- Triamcinolone Acetonide Ointment USP, 0.5% (Clay-Park) A25
- Tridesilon Cream 0.05% (Clay-Park) A25
- Tridesilon Ointment 0.05% (Clay-Park) A25

TRIMETHOBENZAMIDE
- Trimethobenzamide Suppositories, 100 mg (Clay-Park) A25
- Trimethobenzamide Suppositories, 200 mg (Clay-Park) A25
- Trimethobenzamide Suppositories, 100 mg (Clay-Park) A25
- Trimethobenzamide Suppositories, 200 mg (Clay-Park) A25

U

UROKINASE
- Abbokinase (Abbott) A3

V

VITAMINS, MULTIPLE
- M.V.I. Pediatric for Injection (AAI Pharma) A2
- VoSpire ER Extended-Release Tablets (Odyssey) A62

X
- Xanax XR Tablets (Pharmacia & Upjohn) A74

Z
- Zetia Tablets (Merck/Schering Plough) A57
- Zetia Tablets (Schering) A91

REVISED PRODUCT INFORMATION INDEX

As new research data and clinical findings become available, the product information in PDR is revised accordingly. Revisions submitted since the 2003 edition went to press can be found below. To remind yourself of a revision, write "See Supplement A" next to the product's heading in the book.

Brand or Generic Name (Manufacturer, PDR Page No.)	Supplement Page

A

ABACAVIR SULFATE
Trizivir Tablets (GlaxoSmithKline, 1664)..............A178
Ziagen Oral Solution (GlaxoSmithKline, 1690).........A180
Ziagen Tablets (GlaxoSmithKline, 1690)..............A180
Advair Diskus 100/50 (GlaxoSmithKline, 1433).........A157
Advair Diskus 250/50 (GlaxoSmithKline, 1433).........A157
Advair Diskus 500/50 (GlaxoSmithKline, 1433).........A157
Agenerase Capsules (GlaxoSmithKline, 1439)...........A157
Agenerase Oral Solution (GlaxoSmithKline, 1444)......A158

ALENDRONATE SODIUM
Fosamax Tablets (Merck, 1996)........................A189

AMIODARONE HYDROCHLORIDE
Cordarone Intravenous (Wyeth, 3387)..................A325
Cordarone Tablets (Wyeth, 3384)......................A321

AMOXICILLIN
Augmentin Powder for Oral Suspension
  (GlaxoSmithKline, 1464)............................A158
Augmentin Chewable Tablets (GlaxoSmithKline, 1464)...A158

AMPRENAVIR
Agenerase Capsules (GlaxoSmithKline, 1439)...........A157
Agenerase Oral Solution (GlaxoSmithKline, 1444)......A158

ANASTROZOLE
Arimidex Tablets (AstraZeneca, 653)..................A127

ANTIHEMOPHILIC FACTOR (RECOMBINANT)
Refacto Vials (Wyeth, 3474)..........................A359
AquaMEPHYTON Injection (Merck, 1944).................A181
Aricept Tablets (Pfizer, 2574).......................A210
Arimidex Tablets (AstraZeneca, 653)..................A127

ASPARAGINASE
Elspar for Injection (Merck, 1993)...................A189
Astramorph/PF Injection, USP (Preservative-Free)
  (AstraZeneca LP, 593)..............................A107
Atacand Tablets (AstraZeneca LP, 594)................A109

ATORVASTATIN CALCIUM
Lipitor Tablets (Pfizer, 2610).......................A230
Augmentin Powder for Oral Suspension
  (GlaxoSmithKline, 1464)............................A158
Augmentin Chewable Tablets (GlaxoSmithKline, 1464)...A158
Avandia Tablets (GlaxoSmithKline, 1473)..............A158
Avonex (Biogen, 1006)................................A144

AZITHROMYCIN DIHYDRATE
Zithromax Capsules, 250mg (Pfizer, 2667).............A256
Zithromax for IV Infusion (Pfizer, 2672).............A261
Zithromax for Oral Suspension, 1g (Pfizer, 2667).....A256
Zithromax for Oral Suspension, 300 mg, 600 mg,
  900 mg, 1200 mg (Pfizer, 2661).....................A249
Zithromax Tablets, 250 mg, 500 mg (Pfizer, 2661).....A249
Zithromax Tablets, 600 mg (Pfizer, 2667).............A256

B

BECLOMETHASONE DIPROPIONATE MONOHYDRATE
Beconase AQ Nasal Spray (GlaxoSmithKline, 1481)......A159
Beconase AQ Nasal Spray (GlaxoSmithKline, 1481)......A159
Bextra Tablets (Pfizer, 2577)........................A213

BISOPROLOL FUMARATE
Zebeta Tablets (Wyeth, 3493).........................A361
Ziac Tablets (Wyeth, 3495)...........................A362

BUDESONIDE
Pulmicort Respules (AstraZeneca LP, 632).............A120

BUPROPION HYDROCHLORIDE
Zyban Sustained-Release Tablets
  (GlaxoSmithKline, 1708)............................A181

C

Cancidas for Injection (Merck, 1950).................A181

CANDESARTAN CILEXETIL
Atacand Tablets (AstraZeneca LP, 594)................A109

CARBEDILOL
Coreg Tablets (GlaxoSmithKline, 1491)................A164
Cardura Tablets (Pfizer, 2581).......................A216

CASPOFUNGIN ACETATE
Cancidas for Injection (Merck, 1950).................A181
Cefobid Intravenous/Intramuscular (Pfizer, 2584).....A219
Cefobid Pharmacy Bulk Package (Pfizer, 2586).........A219

CEFOPERAZONE
Cefobid Intravenous/Intramuscular (Pfizer, 2584).....A219

CEFOPERAZONE SODIUM
Cefobid Pharmacy Bulk Package (Pfizer, 2586).........A219

CEFOXITIN SODIUM
Mefoxin for Injection (Merck, 2029)..................A190
Mefoxin Premixed Intravenous Solution (Merck, 2031)..A191
Ceftin for Oral Suspension (GlaxoSmithKline, 1482)...A164
Ceftin Tablets (GlaxoSmithKline, 1482)...............A164

CEFUROXIME AXETIL
Ceftin for Oral Suspension (GlaxoSmithKline, 1482)...A164
Ceftin Tablets (GlaxoSmithKline, 1482)...............A164
Celebrex Capsules (Pfizer, 2589).....................A224

CELECOXIB
Celebrex Capsules (Pfizer, 2589).....................A224
Celexa Oral Solution (Forest, 1344)..................A153
Celexa Tablets (Forest, 1344)........................A153
Cellcept Capsules (Roche Labs, 2875).................A273
Cellcept Intravenous (Roche Labs, 2875)..............A173
Cellcept Oral Suspension (Roche Labs, 2875)..........A273
Cellcept Tablets (Roche Labs, 2875)..................A273
Cenestin Tablets, 0.3 mg (Duramed, 1237).............A149
Cenestin Tablets, 0.625 mg, 0.9 mg, 1.25 mg
  (Duramed, 1237)....................................A149

CETIRIZINE HYDROCHLORIDE
Zyrtec Syrup (Pfizer, 2681)..........................A270
Zyrtec Tablets (Pfizer, 2681)........................A270

CHLORPROMAZINE
Thorazine Suppositories (GlaxoSmithKline, 1651)......A177

CHLORPROMAZINE HYDROCHLORIDE
Thorazine Ampuls (GlaxoSmithKline, 1651).............A177
Thorazine Multi-dose Vials (GlaxoSmithKline, 1651)...A177
Thorazine Syrup (GlaxoSmithKline, 1651)..............A177
Thorazine Tablets (GlaxoSmithKline, 1651)............A177

CITALOPRAM HYDROBROMIDE
Celexa Oral Solution (Forest, 1344)..................A153
Celexa Tablets (Forest, 1344)........................A153

Brand or Generic Name (Manufacturer, PDR Page No.)	Supplement Page
CLAVULANATE POTASSIUM	
Augmentin Powder for Oral Suspension (GlaxoSmithKline, 1464)	A158
Augmentin Chewable Tablets (GlaxoSmithKline, 1464)	A158
CLONAZEPAM	
Klonopin Tablets (Roche Labs, 2905)	A280
Combivir Tablets (GlaxoSmithKline, 1486)	A164
Cordarone Intravenous (Wyeth, 3387)	A325
Cordarone Tablets (Wyeth, 3384)	A321
Coreg Tablets (GlaxoSmithKline, 1491)	A164
Cozaar Tablets (Merck, 1968)	A185
Crixivan Capsules (Merck, 1970)	A189
Cutivate Ointment (GlaxoSmithKline, 1498)	A169
D	
Daraprim Tablets (GlaxoSmithKline, 1499)	A169
Depakote ER Tablets (Abbott, 437)	A101
DIPHTHERIA & TETANUS TOXOIDS AND ACELLULAR PERTUSSIS VACCINE ADSORBED	
Infanrix Vaccine (GlaxoSmithKline, 1554)	A170
DIVALPROEX SODIUM	
Depakote ER Tablets (Abbott, 437)	A101
DONEPEZIL HYDROCHLORIDE	
Aricept Tablets (Pfizer, 2574)	A210
DOXAZOSIN MESYLATE	
Cardura Tablets (Pfizer, 2581)	A216
DOXYCYCLINE CALCIUM	
Vibramycin Calcium Oral Suspension Syrup (Pfizer, 2656)	A247
DOXYCYCLINE HYCLATE	
Vibramycin Hyclate Capsules (Pfizer, 2656)	A247
Vibra-Tabs Film Coated Tablets (Pfizer, 2656)	A247
DOXYCYCLINE MONOHYDRATE	
Vibramycin Monohydrate for Oral Suspension (Pfizer, 2656)	A247
E	
Effexor Tablets (Wyeth, 3392)	A328
Effexor XR Capsules (Wyeth, 3397)	A328
Elidel Cream 1% (Novartis, 2257)	A198
Elocon Cream 0.1% (Schering, 3030)	A288
Elocon Lotion 0.1% (Schering, 3031)	A290
Elocon Ointment 0.1% (Schering, 3031)	A291
Elspar for Injection (Merck, 1993)	A189
ENALAPRIL MALEATE	
Lexxel Tablets (AstraZeneca LP, 608)	A111
ENOXAPARIN SODIUM	
Lovenox Injection (Aventis, 739)	A138
Epivir Oral Solution (GlaxoSmithKline, 1508)	A169
Epivir Tablets (GlaxoSmithKline, 1508)	A169
ESCITALOPRAM OXALATE	
Lexapro Tablets (Forest, 3532)	A153
ESOMEPRAZOLE MAGNESIUM	
Nexium Delayed-Release Capsules (AstraZeneca LP, 619)	A115
ESTROGENS, CONJUGATED	
Premarin Tablets (Wyeth, 3444)	A338
Premphase Tablets (Wyeth, 3450)	A342
Prempro Tablets (Wyeth, 3450)	A342
ESTROGENS, CONJUGATED, SYNTHETIC A	
Cenestin Tablets, 0.3 mg (Duramed, 1237)	A149
Cenestin Tablets, 0.625 mg, 0.9 mg, 1.25 mg (Duramed, 1237)	A149
F	
FAMOTIDINE	
Pepcid Injection (Merck, 2057)	A194
Pepcid Injection Premixed (Merck, 2057)	A194
Pepcid for Oral Suspension (Merck, 2055)	A193
Pepcid Tablets (Merck, 2055)	A193
Pepcid RPD Orally Disintegrating Tablets (Merck, 2055)	A193
Faslodex Injection (AstraZeneca, 668)	A131
FELODIPINE	
Lexxel Tablets (AstraZeneca LP, 608)	A111
FINASTERIDE	
Proscar Tablets (Merck, 2080)	A195
Flovent 44mcg Inhalation Aerosol (GlaxoSmithKline, 1523)	A169
Flovent 110mcg Inhalation Aerosol (GlaxoSmithKline, 1523)	A169
Flovent 220mcg Inhalation Aerosol (GlaxoSmithKline, 1523)	A169
Flovent Rotadisk 50mcg (GlaxoSmithKline, 1529)	A169
Flovent Rotadisk 100mcg (GlaxoSmithKline, 1529)	A169
Flovent Rotadisk 250mcg (GlaxoSmithKline, 1529)	A169
FLUTICASONE PROPIONATE	
Advair Diskus 100/50 (GlaxoSmithKline, 1433)	A157
Advair Diskus 250/50 (GlaxoSmithKline, 1433)	A157
Advair Diskus 500/50 (GlaxoSmithKline, 1433)	A157
Cutivate Ointment (GlaxoSmithKline, 1498)	A169
Flovent 44mcg Inhalation Aerosol (GlaxoSmithKline, 1523)	A169
Flovent 110mcg Inhalation Aerosol (GlaxoSmithKline, 1523)	A169
Flovent 220mcg Inhalation Aerosol (GlaxoSmithKline, 1523)	A169
Flovent Rotadisk 50mcg (GlaxoSmithKline, 1529)	A169
Flovent Rotadisk 100mcg (GlaxoSmithKline, 1529)	A169
Flovent Rotadisk 250mcg (GlaxoSmithKline, 1529)	A169
Fosamax Tablets (Merck, 1996)	A189
FULVESTRANT	
Faslodex Injection (AstraZeneca, 668)	A131
G	
GEMFIBROZIL	
Lopid Tablets (Parke-Davis, 2559)	A207
GEMTUZUMAB OZOGAMICIN	
Mylotarg for Injection (Wyeth, 3424)	A335
GLIPIZIDE	
Glucotrol XL Extended-Release Tablets (Pfizer, 2608)	A228
Glucotrol XL Extended-Release Tablets (Pfizer, 2608)	A228
GRANISETRON HYDROCHLORIDE	
Kytril Injection (Roche Labs, 2908)	A283
H	
Havrix Vaccine (GlaxoSmithKline, 1536)	A170
HEPATITIS A VACCINE, INACTIVATED	
Havrix Vaccine (GlaxoSmithKline, 1536)	A170
Vaqta (Merck, 2105)	A197
Hivid Tablets (Roche Labs, 2898)	A280
Hycamtin for Injection (GlaxoSmithKline, 1538)	A170
HYDROCHLOROTHIAZIDE	
Ziac Tablets (Wyeth, 3495)	A362
HYDROXYPROPYL CELLULOSE	
Lacrisert Sterile Ophthalmic Insert (Merck, 2021)	A190

Brand or Generic Name (Manufacturer, PDR Page No.)	Supplement Page
I	
Imitrex Injection (GlaxoSmithKline, 1542)	A170
Imitrex Nasal Spray (GlaxoSmithKline, 1546)	A170
Imitrex Tablets (GlaxoSmithKline, 1550)	A170
Inderal LA Long-Acting Capsules (Wyeth, 3404)	A334
INDINAVIR SULFATE	
Crixivan Capsules (Merck, 1970)	A189
Infanrix Vaccine (GlaxoSmithKline, 1554)	A170
INTERFERON ALFA-2B, RECOMBINANT	
Intron A for Injection (Schering, 3038)	A292
Rebetron Combination Therapy (Schering, 3076)	A315
INTERFERON BETA-1A	
Avonex (Biogen, 1006)	A144
Intron A for Injection (Schering, 3038)	A292
IVERMECTIN	
Stromectol Tablets (Merck, 2090)	A197
K	
Klonopin Tablets (Roche Labs, 2905)	A280
Kytril Injection (Roche Labs, 2908)	A283
L	
LABETALOL HYDROCHLORIDE	
Normodyne Tablets (Schering, 3057)	A304
Lacrisert Sterile Ophthalmic Insert (Merck, 2021)	A190
Lamictal Tablets (GlaxoSmithKline, 1559)	A170
Lamictal Chewable Dispersible Tablets (GlaxoSmithKline, 1559)	A170
LAMIVUDINE	
Combivir Tablets (GlaxoSmithKline, 1486)	A164
Epivir Oral Solution (GlaxoSmithKline, 1508)	A169
Epivir Tablets (GlaxoSmithKline, 1508)	A169
Trizivir Tablets (GlaxoSmithKline, 1664)	A178
LAMOTRIGINE	
Lamictal Tablets (GlaxoSmithKline, 1559)	A170
Lamictal Chewable Dispersible Tablets (GlaxoSmithKline, 1559)	A170
Lariam Tablets (Roche Labs, 2912)	A286
Levaquin Injection (Ortho-McNeil, 2466)	A201
Levaquin Tablets (Ortho-McNeil, 2466)	A201
LEVOFLOXACIN	
Levaquin Injection (Ortho-McNeil, 2466)	A201
Levaquin Tablets (Ortho-McNeil, 2466)	A201
Lexapro Tablets (Forest, 3532)	A153
Lexxel Tablets (AstraZeneca LP, 608)	A111
LIDOCAINE HYDROCHLORIDE	
Xylocaine Injection for Ventricular Arrhythmias (AstraZeneca LP, 650)	A127
Lipitor Tablets (Pfizer, 2610)	A230
LITHIUM CARBONATE	
Lithobid Slow-Release Tablets (Solvay, 3165)	A320
Lithobid Slow-Release Tablets (Solvay, 3165)	A320
Lopid Tablets (Parke-Davis, 2559)	A207
LOSARTAN POTASSIUM	
Cozaar Tablets (Merck, 1968)	A185
LOVASTATIN	
Mevacor Tablets (Merck, 2036)	A192
Lovenox Injection (Aventis, 739)	A138
M	
MEDROXYPROGESTERONE ACETATE	
Premphase Tablets (Wyeth, 3450)	A342
Prempro Tablets (Wyeth, 3450)	A342
MEFLOQUINE HYDROCHLORIDE	
Lariam Tablets (Roche Labs, 2912)	A286
Mefoxin for Injection (Merck, 2029)	A190
Mefoxin Premixed Intravenous Solution (Merck, 2031)	A191
Mephyton Tablets (Merck, 2034)	A192
MERCAPTOPURINE	
Purinethol Tablets (GlaxoSmithKline, 1615)	A177
METHOTREXATE SODIUM	
Methotrexate Sodium Injection (Wyeth, 3415)	A334
Methotrexate Sodium Injection (Wyeth, 3415)	A334
METOPROLOL SUCCINATE	
Toprol-XL Tablets (AstraZeneca LP, 645)	A124
Mevacor Tablets (Merck, 2036)	A192
MOMETASONE FUROATE	
Elocon Cream 0.1% (Schering, 3030)	A288
Elocon Lotion 0.1% (Schering, 3031)	A290
Elocon Ointment 0.1% (Schering, 3031)	A291
MOMETASONE FUROATE MONOHYDRATE	
Nasonex Nasal Spray, 50 mcg (Schering, 3052)	A300
MONTELUKAST SODIUM	
Singulair Tablets (Merck, 2086)	A195
Singulair Chewable Tablets (Merck, 2086)	A195
MORPHINE SULFATE	
Astramorph/PF Injection, USP (Preservative-Free) (AstraZeneca LP, 593)	A107
MYCOPHENOLATE MOFETIL	
Cellcept Capsules (Roche Labs, 2875)	A273
Cellcept Oral Suspension (Roche Labs, 2875)	A273
Cellcept Tablets (Roche Labs, 2875)	A273
MYCOPHENOLATE MOFETIL HYDROCHLORIDE	
Cellcept Intravenous (Roche Labs, 2875)	A273
Mylotarg for Injection (Wyeth, 3424)	A335
N	
Nasonex Nasal Spray, 50 mcg (Schering, 3052)	A300
Navane Capsules (Pfizer, 2616)	A234
Navane Concentrate (Pfizer, 2616)	A234
Navane Intramuscular (Pfizer, 2617)	A235
Navelbine Injection (GlaxoSmithKline, 1597)	A177
Neumega for Injection (Wyeth, 3427)	A335
Nexium Delayed-Release Capsules (AstraZeneca LP, 619)	A115
Nitro-Dur Transdermal Infusion System (Schering, 3055)	A302
NITROGLYCERIN	
Nitro-Dur Transdermal Infusion System (Schering, 3055)	A302
NORFLOXACIN	
Noroxin Tablets (Merck, 2050)	A193
NORGESTREL	
Ovrette Tablets (Wyeth, 3431)	A337
Normodyne Tablets (Schering, 3057)	A304
Noroxin Tablets (Merck, 2050)	A193
O	
OMEPRAZOLE	
Prilosec Delayed-Release Capsules (AstraZeneca LP, 627)	A115
OPRELVEKIN	
Neumega for Injection (Wyeth, 3427)	A335
Ovrette Tablets (Wyeth, 3431)	A337

Brand or Generic Name (Manufacturer, PDR Page No.)	Supplement Page

P
PAROXETINE HYDROCHLORIDE
- Paxil Oral Suspension (GlaxoSmithKline, 1603) A177
- Paxil Tablets (GlaxoSmithKline, 1603) A177
- Paxil Oral Suspension (GlaxoSmithKline, 1603) A177
- Paxil Tablets (GlaxoSmithKline, 1603) A177

PEGINTERFERON ALFA-2B
- PEG-Intron Powder for Injection (Schering, 3059) A306
- PEG-Intron Powder for Injection (Schering, 3059) A306
- Pepcid Injection (Merck, 2057) A194
- Pepcid Injection Premixed (Merck, 2057) A194
- Pepcid for Oral Suspension (Merck, 2055) A193
- Pepcid Tablets (Merck, 2055) A193
- Pepcid RPD Orally Disintegrating Tablets (Merck, 2055) A193

PIMECROLIMUS
- Elidel Cream 1% (Novartis, 2257) A198
- Pipracil (Wyeth, 3434) A337

PNEUMOCOCCAL VACCINE, DIPHTHERIA CONJUGATE
- Prevnar for Injection (Wyeth, 3455) A347

PIPERACILLIN SODIUM
- Pipracil (Wyeth, 3434) A337
- Zosyn (Wyeth, 3498) A365
- Zosyn in Galaxy Containers (Wyeth, 3498) A365
- Premarin Tablets (Wyeth, 3444) A338
- Premphase Tablets (Wyeth, 3450) A342
- Prempro Tablets (Wyeth, 3450) A342
- Prevnar for Injection (Wyeth, 3455) A347
- Prilosec Delayed-Release Capsules (AstraZeneca LP, 627) A115

PROPRANOLOL HYDROCHLORIDE
- Inderal LA Long-Acting Capsules (Wyeth, 3404) A334
- Proscar Tablets (Merck, 2080) A195
- Pulmicort Respules (AstraZeneca LP, 632) A120
- Purinethol Tablets (GlaxoSmithKline, 1615) A177

PYRIMETHAMINE
- Daraprim Tablets (GlaxoSmithKline, 1499) A169

R
- Rapamune Oral Solution and Tablets (Wyeth, 3469) A353
- Rebetol Capsules (Schering, 3072) A310
- Rebetron Combination Therapy (Schering, 3076) A315
- Refacto Vials (Wyeth, 3474) A359
- Relenza Rotadisk (GlaxoSmithKline, 1619) A177

RIBAVIRIN
- Rebetol Capsules (Schering, 3072) A310
- Rebetron Combination Therapy (Schering, 3076) A315

ROFECOXIB
- Vioxx Oral Suspension (Merck, 2120) A198
- Vioxx Tablets (Merck, 2120) A198

ROSIGLITAZONE MALEATE
- Avandia Tablets (GlaxoSmithKline, 1473) A158

S
SALMETEROL XINAFOATE
- Advair Diskus 100/50 (GlaxoSmithKline, 1433) A157
- Advair Diskus 250/50 (GlaxoSmithKline, 1433) A157
- Advair Diskus 500/50 (GlaxoSmithKline, 1433) A157
- Serevent Diskus (GlaxoSmithKline, 1636) A177
- Serevent Inhalation Aerosol (GlaxoSmithKline, 1632) A177
- Serevent Diskus (GlaxoSmithKline, 1636) A177
- Serevent Inhalation Aerosol (GlaxoSmithKline, 1632) A177

SERTRALINE HYDROCHLORIDE
- Zoloft Oral Concentrate (Pfizer, 2675) A264
- Zoloft Tablets (Pfizer, 2675) A264

SILDENAFIL CITRATE
- Viagra Tablets (Pfizer, 2653) A244
- Singulair Tablets (Merck, 2086) A195
- Singulair Chewable Tablets (Merck, 2086) A195

SIROLIMUS
- Rapamune Oral Solution and Tablets (Wyeth, 3469) A353
- Stromectol Tablets (Merck, 2090) A197

SUMATRIPTAN
- Imitrex Nasal Spray (GlaxoSmithKline, 1546) A170

SUMATRIPTAN SUCCINATE
- Imitrex Injection (GlaxoSmithKline, 1542) A170
- Imitrex Tablets (GlaxoSmithKline, 1550) A170

T
TAZOBACTAM SODIUM
- Zosyn (Wyeth, 3498) A365
- Zosyn in Galaxy Containers (Wyeth, 3498) A365

THEOPHYLLINE
- Uniphyl 400mg and 600mg Tablets (Purdue Frederick, 2842) A273

THIOTHIXENE
- Navane Capsules (Pfizer, 2616) A234

THIOTHIXENE HYDROCHLORIDE
- Navane Concentrate (Pfizer, 2616) A234
- Navane Intramuscular (Pfizer, 2617) A235
- Thorazine Ampuls (GlaxoSmithKline, 1651) A177
- Thorazine Multi-dose Vials (GlaxoSmithKline, 1651) A177
- Thorazine Suppositories (GlaxoSmithKline, 1651) A177
- Thorazine Syrup (GlaxoSmithKline, 1651) A177
- Thorazine Tablets (GlaxoSmithKline, 1651) A177

TOPOTECAN HYDROCHLORIDE
- Hycamtin for Injection (GlaxoSmithKline, 1538) A170
- Toprol-XL Tablets (AstraZeneca LP, 645) A124
- Trizivir Tablets (GlaxoSmithKline, 1664) A178

U
- Uniphyl 400mg and 600mg Tablets (Purdue Frederick, 2842) A273

V
VALACYCLOVIR HYDROCHLORIDE
- Valtrex Caplets, (GlaxoSmithKline, 1672) A178

VALDECOXIB
- Bextra Tablets (Pfizer, 2577) A213
- Valtrex Caplets (GlaxoSmithKline, 1672) A178
- Vaqta (Merck, 2105) A197

VENLAFAXINE HYDROCHLORIDE
- Effexor Tablets (Wyeth, 3392) A328
- Effexor XR Capsules (Wyeth, 3397) A328
- VFEND I.V. (Pfizer, 2645) A236
- VFEND Tablets (Pfizer, 2645) A236
- Viagra Tablets (Pfizer, 2653) A244
- Vibramycin Calcium Oral Suspension Syrup (Pfizer, 2656) A247
- Vibramycin Hyclate Capsules (Pfizer, 2656) A247
- Vibramycin Monohydrate for Oral Suspension (Pfizer, 2656) A247
- Vibra-Tabs Film Coated Tablets (Pfizer, 2656) A247

Brand or Generic Name (Manufacturer, PDR Page No.)	Supplement Page
VINORELBINE TARTRATE	
Navelbine Injection (GlaxoSmithKline, 1597)	A177
VITAMIN K1	
AquaMEPHYTON Injection (Merck, 1944)	A181
Mephyton Tablets (Merck, 2034)	A192
Vioxx Oral Suspension (Merck, 2120)	A198
Vioxx Tablets (Merck, 2120)	A198
VORICONAZOLE	
VFEND I.V. (Pfizer, 2645)	A236
VFEND Tablets (Pfizer, 2645)	A236
X	
Xylocaine Injection for Ventricular Arrhythmias (AstraZeneca LP, 650)	A127
Z	
ZALCITABINE	
Hivid Tablets (Roche Labs, 2898)	A280
ZANAMIVIR	
Relenza Rotadisk (GlaxoSmithKline, 1619)	A177
Zebeta Tablets (Wyeth, 3493)	A361
Ziac Tablets (Wyeth, 3495)	A362
Ziagen Oral Solution (GlaxoSmithKline, 1690)	A180
Ziagen Tablets (GlaxoSmithKline, 1690)	A180
ZIDOVUDINE	
Combivir Tablets (GlaxoSmithKline, 1486)	A164
Trizivir Tablets (GlaxoSmithKline, 1664)	A178
Zithromax Capsules, 250mg (Pfizer, 2667)	A256
Zithromax for IV Infusion (Pfizer, 2672)	A261
Zithromax for Oral Suspension, 1g (Pfizer, 2667)	A256
Zithromax for Oral Suspension, 300 mg, 600 mg, 900 mg, 1200 mg (Pfizer, 2661)	A249
Zithromax Tablets, 250 mg, 500 mg (Pfizer, 2661)	A249
Zithromax Tablets, 600 mg (Pfizer, 2667)	A256
Zoloft Oral Concentrate (Pfizer, 2675)	A264
Zoloft Tablets (Pfizer, 2675)	A264
ZOLMITRIPTAN	
Zomig Tablets (AstraZeneca, 701)	A134
Zomig-ZMT Tablets (Astrazeneca, 701)	A134
Zomig Tablets (AstraZeneca, 701)	A134
Zomig-ZMT Tablets (Astrazeneca, 701)	A134
Zosyn (Wyeth, 3498)	A365
Zosyn in Galaxy Containers (Wyeth, 3498)	A365
Zyban Sustained-Release Tablets (GlaxoSmithKline, 1708)	A181
Zyrtec Syrup (Pfizer, 2681)	A270
Zyrtec Tablets (Pfizer, 2681)	A270

NEW PRODUCT LISTINGS

This section contains comprehensive descriptions of new pharmaceutical products introduced since publication of the 2003 PDR, new dosage forms of products already described, and existing pharmaceutical products not described in the 2003 PDR.

---

aaiPharma
2320 SCIENTIFIC PARK DRIVE
WILMINGTON NC 28405

Direct Inquiries to:
Phone: 1-877-263-6726
Fax 1 (910) 815-2300

AZASAN™ ℞
(Azathioprine Tablets, USP)
25 mg Scored Tablets
50 mg Scored Tablets
75 mg Scored Tablets
100 mg Scored Tablets

> **WARNING**
> Chronic immunosuppression with this purine antimetabolite increases *risk of neoplasia* in humans. Physicians using this drug should be very familiar with this risk as well as with the mutagenic potential to both men and women and with possible hematologic toxicities. See WARNINGS.

DESCRIPTION
AZASAN™, an immunosuppressive antimetabolite, is available in tablet form for oral administration. Each scored tablet contains 25 mg, 50 mg, 75 mg or 100 mg azathioprine and the inactive ingredients lactose monohydrate, pregelatinized starch, povidone, corn starch, magnesium stearate, and stearic acid.
Azathioprine is chemically 1H-purine, 6-[(1-methyl-4-nitro-1H-imidazol-5-yl)thio]-. The structural formula of azathioprine is:

$C_9H_7N_7O_2S$ M.W. 277.27

It is an imidazolyl derivative of 6-mercaptopurine (PURINETHOL®) and many of its biological effects are similar to those of the parent compound.
Azathioprine is insoluble in water, but may be dissolved with addition of one molar equivalent of alkali. The sodium salt of azathioprine is sufficiently soluble to make a 10 mg/mL water solution which is stable for 24 hours at 59° to 77°F (15° to 25°C). Azathioprine is stable in solution at neutral or acid pH but hydrolysis to mercaptopurine occurs in excess sodium hydroxide (0.1N), especially on warming. Conversion to mercaptopurine also occurs in the presence of sulfhydryl compounds such as cysteine, glutathione, and hydrogen sulfide.

CLINICAL PHARMACOLOGY
Metabolism: Azathioprine is well absorbed following oral administration. Maximum serum radioactivity occurs at 1 to 2 hours after oral ^{35}S-azathioprine and decays with a half-life of 5 hours. This is not an estimate of the half-life of azathioprine itself but is the decay rate for all ^{35}S-containing metabolites of the drug. Because of extensive metabolism, only a fraction of the radioactivity is present as azathioprine. Usual doses produce blood levels of azathioprine, and of mercaptopurine derived from it, which are low (<1 mcg/mL). Blood levels are of little predictive value for therapy since the magnitude and duration of clinical effects correlate with thiopurine nucleotide levels in tissues rather than with plasma drug levels. Azathioprine and mercaptopurine are moderately bound to serum proteins (30%) and are partially dialyzable.
Azathioprine is cleaved *in vivo* to mercaptopurine. Both compounds are rapidly eliminated from blood and are oxidized or methylated in erythrocytes and liver; no azathioprine or mercaptopurine is detectable in urine after 8 hours. Conversion to inactive 6-thiouric acid by xanthine oxidase is an important degradative pathway, and the inhibition of this pathway in patients receiving allopurinol is the basis for the azathioprine dosage reduction required in these patients (see PRECAUTIONS: Drug Interactions). Proportions of metabolites are different in individual patients, and this presumably accounts for variable magnitude and duration of drug effects. Renal clearance is probably not important in predicting biological effectiveness or toxicities, although dose reduction is practiced in patients with poor renal function.
Homograft Survival: Summary information from transplant centers and registries indicates relatively universal use of AZASAN™ with or without other immunosuppressive agents. Although the use of azathioprine for inhibition of renal homograft rejection is well established, the mechanism(s) for this action are somewhat obscure. The drug suppresses hypersensitivities of the cell-mediated type and causes variable alterations in antibody production. Suppression of T-cell effects, including ablation of T-cell suppression, is dependent on the temporal relationship to antigenic stimulus or engraftment. This agent has little effect on established graft rejections or secondary responses.
Alterations in specific immune responses or immunologic functions in transplant recipients are difficult to relate specifically to immunosuppression by azathioprine. These patients have subnormal responses to vaccines, low numbers of T-cells, and abnormal phagocytosis by peripheral blood cells, but their mitogenic responses, serum immunoglobulins, and secondary antibody responses are usually normal.
Immunoinflammatory Response: Azathioprine suppresses disease manifestations as well as underlying pathology in animal models of autoimmune disease. For example, the severity of adjuvant arthritis is reduced by azathioprine.
The mechanisms whereby azathioprine affects autoimmune diseases are not known. Azathioprine is immunosuppressive, delayed hypersensitivity and cellular cytotoxicity tests being suppressed to a greater degree than are antibody responses. In the rat model of adjuvant arthritis, azathioprine has been shown to inhibit the lymph node hyperplasia which precedes the onset of the signs of the disease. Both the immunosuppressive and therapeutic effects in animal models are dose-related. Azathioprine is considered a slow-acting drug and effects may persist after the drug has been discontinued.

INDICATIONS AND USAGE
AZASAN™ is indicated as an adjunct for the prevention of rejection in renal homotransplantation. It is also indicated for the management of severe, active rheumatoid arthritis unresponsive to rest, aspirin, or other nonsteroidal anti-inflammatory drugs, or to agents in the class of which gold is an example.
Renal Homotransplantation: AZASAN™ is indicated as an adjunct for the prevention of rejection in renal homotransplantation. Experience with over 16,000 transplants shows a 5-year patient survival of 35% to 55%, but this is dependent on donor, match for HLA antigens, anti-donor and anti B-cell alloantigen antibody, and other variables. The effect of azathioprine on these variables has not been tested in controlled trials.
Rheumatoid Arthritis: AZASAN™ is indicated only in adult patients meeting criteria for classic or definite rheumatoid arthritis as specified by the American Rheumatism Association. AZASAN™ should be restricted to patients with severe, active and erosive disease not responsive to conventional management including rest, aspirin, or other nonsteroidal drugs or to agents in the class of which gold is an example. Rest, physiotherapy, and salicylates should be continued while AZASAN™ is given, but it may be possible to reduce the dose of corticosteroids in patients on AZASAN™. The combined use of AZASAN™ with gold, antimalarials, or penicillamine has not been studied for either added benefit or unexpected adverse effects. The use of AZASAN™ with these agents cannot be recommended.

CONTRAINDICATIONS
AZASAN™ should not be given to patients who have shown hypersensitivity to the drug.
AZASAN™ should not be used for treating rheumatoid arthritis in pregnant women.
Patients with rheumatoid arthritis previously treated with alkylating agents (cyclophosphamide, chlorambucil, melphalan, or others) may have a prohibitive risk of neoplasia if treated with AZASAN™.

WARNINGS
Severe *leukopenia and/or thrombocytopenia* may occur in patients on AZASAN™. Macrocytic anemia and severe bone marrow depression may also occur. Hematologic toxicities are dose related and may be more severe in renal transplant patients whose homograft is undergoing rejection. It is suggested that patients on AZASAN™ have complete blood counts, including platelet counts, weekly during the first month, twice monthly for the second and third months of treatment, then monthly or more frequently if dosage alterations or other therapy changes are necessary. Delayed hematologic suppression may occur. Prompt reduction in dosage or temporary withdrawal of the drug may be necessary if there is a rapid fall in, or persistently low leukocyte count, or other evidence of bone marrow depression. Leukopenia does not correlate with therapeutic effect; therefore, the dose should not be increased intentionally to lower the white blood cell count.
Serious infections are a constant hazard for patients receiving chronic immunosuppression, especially for homograft recipients. Fungal, viral, bacterial, and protozoal infections may be fatal and should be treated vigorously. Reduction of azathioprine dosage and/or use of other drugs should be considered.
AZASAN™ is mutagenic in animals and humans, carcinogenic in animals, and may increase the patient's *risk of neoplasia*. Renal transplant patients are known to have an increased risk of malignancy, predominantly skin cancer and reticulum cell or lymphomatous tumors. The risk of post-transplant lymphomas may be increased in patients who receive aggressive treatment with immunosuppressive drugs. The degree of immunosuppression is determined not only by the immunosuppressive regimen but also by a number of other patient factors. The number of immunosuppressive agents may not necessarily increase the risk of post-transplant lymphomas. However, transplant patients who receive multiple immunosuppressive agents may be at risk for over-immunosuppression; therefore, immunosuppressive drug therapy should be maintained at the lowest effective levels. Information is available on the spontaneous neoplasia risk in rheumatoid arthritis, and on neoplasia following immunosuppressive therapy of other autoimmune disease. It has not been possible to define the precise risk of neoplasia due to AZASAN™. The data suggest the risk may be elevated in patients with rheumatoid arthritis, though lower than for renal transplant patients. However, acute myelogenous leukemia as well as solid tumors have been reported in patients with rheumatoid arthritis who have received azathioprine. Data on neoplasia in patients receiving AZASAN™ can be found under ADVERSE REACTIONS.
AZASAN™ has been reported to cause temporary depression in spermatogenesis and reduction in sperm viability

Continued on next page

Azasan—Cont.

and sperm count in mice at doses 10 times the human therapeutic dose; a reduced percentage of fertile matings occurred when animals received 5 mg/kg.

Pregnancy: Pregnancy Category D. AZASAN™ can cause fetal harm when administered to a pregnant woman. AZASAN™ should not be given during pregnancy without careful weighing of risk versus benefit. Whenever possible, use of AZASAN™ in pregnant patients should be avoided. This drug should not be used for treating rheumatoid arthritis in pregnant women.

AZASAN™ is teratogenic in rabbits and mice when given in doses equivalent to the human dose (5 mg/kg daily). Abnormalities included skeletal malformations and visceral anomalies.

Limited immunologic and other abnormalities have occurred in a few infants born of renal allograft recipients on AZASAN™. In a detailed case report, documented lymphopenia, diminished IgG and IgM levels, CMV infection, and a decreased thymic shadow were noted in an infant born to a mother receiving 150 mg azathioprine and 30 mg prednisone daily throughout pregnancy. At 10 weeks most features were normalized. DeWitte et al reported pancytopenia and severe immune deficiency in a preterm infant whose mother received 125 mg azathioprine and 12.5 mg prednisone daily. There have been two published reports of abnormal physical findings. Williamson and Karp described an infant born with preaxial polydactyly whose mother received azathioprine 200 mg daily and prednisone 20 mg every other day during pregnancy. Tallent et al described an infant with a large myelomeningocele in the upper lumbar region, bilateral dislocated hips, and bilateral talipes equinovarus. The father was on long-term azathioprine therapy. Benefit versus risk must be weighed carefully before use of AZASAN™ in patients of reproductive potential. There are no adequate and well-controlled studies in pregnant women. If this drug is used during pregnancy or if the patient becomes pregnant while taking this drug, the patient should be apprised of the potential hazard to the fetus. Women of childbearing age should be advised to avoid becoming pregnant.

PRECAUTIONS

General: A gastrointestinal hypersensitivity reaction characterized by severe nausea and vomiting has been reported. These symptoms may also be accompanied by diarrhea, rash, fever, malaise, myalgias, elevations in liver enzymes, and occasionally, hypotension. Symptoms of gastrointestinal toxicity most often develop within the first several weeks of AZASAN™ therapy and are reversible upon discontinuation of the drug. The reaction can recur within hours after rechallenge with a single dose of AZASAN™.

Information for Patients: Patients being started on AZASAN™ should be informed of the necessity of periodic blood counts while they are receiving the drug and should be encouraged to report any unusual bleeding or bruising to their physician. They should be informed of the danger of infection while receiving AZASAN™ and asked to report signs and symptoms of infection to their physician. Careful dosage instructions should be given to the patient, especially when AZASAN™ is being administered in the presence of impaired renal function or concomitantly with allopurinol (see PRECAUTIONS - Drug Interactions subsection and DOSAGE AND ADMINISTRATION). Patients should be advised of the potential risks of the use of AZASAN™ during pregnancy and during the nursing period. The increased risk of neoplasia following therapy with AZASAN™ should be explained to the patient.

Laboratory Tests: See WARNINGS and ADVERSE REACTIONS sections.

Drug Interactions:

Use with Allopurinol: The principal pathway for detoxification of AZASAN™ is inhibited by allopurinol. Patients receiving AZASAN™ and allopurinol concomitantly should have a dose reduction of AZASAN™, to approximately 1/3 to 1/4 the usual dose.

Use with Other Agents Affecting Myelopoiesis: Drugs which may affect leukocyte production, including co-trimoxazole, may lead to exaggerated leukopenia, especially in renal transplant recipients.

Use with Angiotensin-Converting Enzyme Inhibitors: The use of angiotensin-converting enzyme inhibitors to control hypertension in patients on azathioprine has been reported to induce severe leukopenia.

Carcinogenesis, Mutagenesis, Impairment of Fertility: See WARNINGS section.

Pregnancy: *Teratogenic Effects:* Pregnancy Category D. See WARNINGS section.

Nursing Mothers: The use of AZASAN™ in nursing mothers is not recommended. Azathioprine or its metabolites are transferred at low levels both transplacentally and in breast milk. Because of the potential for tumorgenicity shown for azathioprine, a decision should be made whether to discontinue nursing or discontinue the drug, taking into account the importance of the drug to the mother.

Pediatric Use: Safety and efficacy of azathioprine in pediatric patients have not been established.

ADVERSE REACTIONS

The principal and potentially serious toxic effects of AZASAN™ are hematologic and gastrointestinal. The risks of secondary infection and neoplasia are also significant (see WARNINGS). The frequency and severity of adverse reactions depend on the dose and duration of AZASAN™ as well as on the patient's underlying disease or concomitant therapies. The incidence of hematologic toxicities and neoplasia encountered in groups of renal homograft recipients is significantly higher than that in studies employing AZASAN™ for rheumatoid arthritis. The relative incidences in clinical studies are summarized below:

Toxicity	Renal Homograft	Rheumatoid Arthritis
Leukopenia		
Any Degree	>50%	28%
<2500/mm³	16%	5.3%
Infections	20%	<1%
Neoplasia		*
Lymphoma	0.5%	
Others	2.8%	

*Data on the rate and risk of neoplasia among persons with rheumatoid arthritis treated with azathioprine are limited. The incidence of lymphoproliferative disease in patients with RA appears to be significantly higher than that in the general population. In one completed study, the rate of lymphoproliferative disease in RA patients receiving higher than recommended doses of azathioprine (5 mg/kg/day) was 1.8 cases per 1000 patient years of follow-up, compared with 0.8 cases per 1000 patient years of follow-up in those not receiving azathioprine. However, the proportion of the increased risk attributable to the azathioprine dosage or to other therapies (i.e., alkylating agents) received by azathioprine-treated patients cannot be determined.

Hematologic: Leukopenia and/or thrombocytopenia are dose dependent and may occur late in the course of therapy with AZASAN™. Dose reduction or temporary withdrawal allows reversal of these toxicities. Infection may occur as a secondary manifestation of bone marrow suppression or leukopenia, but the incidence of infection in renal homotransplantation is 30 to 60 times that in rheumatoid arthritis. Macrocytic anemia and/or bleeding have been reported in two patients on azathioprine.

Gastrointestinal: Nausea and vomiting may occur within the first few months of AZASAN™ therapy, and occurred in approximately 12% of 676 rheumatoid arthritis patients. The frequency of gastric disturbance often can be reduced by administration of the drug in divided doses and/or after meals. However, in some patients, nausea and vomiting may be severe and may be accompanied by symptoms such as diarrhea, fever, malaise, and myalgias (see PRECAUTIONS). Vomiting with abdominal pain may occur rarely with a hypersensitivity pancreatitis. Hepatotoxicity manifest by elevation of serum alkaline phosphatase, bilirubin, and/or serum transaminases is known to occur following azathioprine use, primarily in allograft recipients. Hepatotoxicity has been uncommon (less than 1%) in rheumatoid arthritis patients. Hepatotoxicity following transplantation most often occurs within 6 months of transplantation and is generally reversible after interruption of AZASAN™. A rare, but life-threatening hepatic veno-occlusive disease associated with chronic administration of azathioprine has been described in transplant patients and in one patient receiving AZASAN™ for panuveitis. Periodic measurement of serum transaminases, alkaline phosphatase, and bilirubin is indicated for early detection of hepatotoxicity. If hepatic veno-occlusive disease is clinically suspected, AZASAN™ should be permanently withdrawn.

Others: Additional side effects of low frequency have been reported. These include skin rashes (approximately 2%), alopecia, fever, arthralgias, diarrhea, steatorrhea and negative nitrogen balance (all less than 1%).

OVERDOSAGE

The oral LD$_{50}$s for single doses of AZASAN™ in mice and rats are 2500 mg/kg and 400 mg/kg, respectively. Very large doses of this antimetabolite may lead to marrow hypoplasia, bleeding, infection, and death. About 30% of AZASAN™ is bound to serum proteins, but approximately 45% is removed during an 8-hour hemodialysis. A single case has been reported of a renal transplant patient who ingested a single dose of 7500 mg AZASAN™. The immediate toxic reactions were nausea, vomiting, and diarrhea, followed by mild leukopenia and mild abnormalities in liver function. The white blood cell count, SGOT, and bilirubin returned to normal 6 days after the overdose.

DOSAGE AND ADMINISTRATION

Renal Homotransplantation: The dose of AZASAN™ required to prevent rejection and minimize toxicity will vary with individual patients; this necessitates careful management. The initial dose is usually 3 to 5 mg/kg daily, beginning at the time of transplant. AZASAN™ is usually given as a single daily dose on the day of, and in a minority of cases 1 to 3 days before, transplantation. AZASAN™ is often initiated with the intravenous administration of the sodium salt, with subsequent use of tablets (at the same dose level) after the postoperative period. Intravenous administration of the sodium salt is indicated only in patients unable to tolerate oral medications. Dose reduction to maintenance levels of 1 to 3 mg/kg daily is usually possible. The dose of AZASAN™ should not be increased to toxic levels because of threatened rejection. Discontinuation may be necessary for severe hematologic or other toxicity, even if rejection of the homograft may be a consequence of drug withdrawal.

Rheumatoid Arthritis: AZASAN™ is usually given on a daily basis. The initial dose should be approximately 1 mg/kg (50 to 100.mg) given as a single dose or on a twice daily schedule. The dose may be increased, beginning at 6 to 8 weeks and thereafter by steps at 4-week intervals, if there are no serious toxicities and if initial response is unsatisfactory. Dose increments should be 0.5 mg/kg daily, up to a maximum dose of 2.5 mg/kg/day. Therapeutic response occurs after several weeks of treatment, usually 6 to 8; an adequate trial should be a minimum of 12 weeks. Patients not improved after 12 weeks can be considered refractory. AZASAN™ may be continued long-term in patients with clinical response, but patients should be monitored carefully, and gradual dosage reduction should be attempted to reduce risk of toxicities.

Maintenance therapy should be at the lowest effective dose, and the dose given can be lowered decrementally with changes of 0.5 mg/kg or approximately 25 mg daily every 4 weeks while other therapy is kept constant. The optimum duration of maintenance AZASAN™ has not been determined. AZASAN™ can be discontinued abruptly, but delayed effects are possible.

Use in Renal Dysfunction: Relatively oliguric patients, especially those with tubular necrosis in the immediate postcadaveric transplant period, may have delayed clearance of AZASAN™ or its metabolites, may be particularly sensitive to this drug, and are usually given lower doses.

Procedures for proper handling and disposal of this immunosuppressive antimetabolite drug should be considered. Several guidelines on this subject have been published.[1-7] There is no general agreement that all of the procedures recommended in the guideline are necessary or appropriate.

HOW SUPPLIED

AZASAN™ Tablets, USP, 25 mg are oval-shaped, yellow, scored tablets, bottles of 100 (NDC 66591-211-41).
AZASAN™ Tablets, USP, 50 mg are capsule-shaped, yellow, scored tablets, bottles of 100 (NDC 66591-221-41).
AZASAN™ Tablets, USP, 75 mg are triangle-shaped, yellow, scored tablets, bottles of 100 (NDC 66591-231-41).
AZASAN™ Tablets, USP, 100 mg are diamond-shaped, yellow, scored tablets, bottles of 100 (NDC 66591-241-41).
Rx only.
Store at 15° to 25°C (59° to 77°F) in a dry place and protect from light.
Dispense in a tight, light-resistant container as defined in the USP.

1. Recommendations for the Safe Handling of Parenteral Antineoplastic Drugs, NIH Publication No. 83-2621. For sale by the Superintendent of Documents, U.S. Government Printing Office, Washington, DC 20402.
2. AMA Council Report, Guidelines for Handling Parenteral Antineoplastics. *JAMA*, 1985;253(11):1590–1592.
3. National Study Commission on Cytotoxic Exposure - Recommendations for Handling Cytotoxic Agents. Available from Louis P. Jeffrey, ScD., Chairman, National Study Commission on Cytotoxic Exposure, Massachusetts College of Pharmacy and Allied Health Sciences, 179 Longwood Avenue, Boston, Massachusetts 02115.
4. Clinical Oncological Society of Australia, Guidelines and Recommendations for Safe Handling of Antineoplastic Agents. *Med J Australia*, 1983;1:426–428.
5. Jones RB, et al: Safe Handling of Chemotherapeutic Agents: A Report from the Mount Sinai Medical Center. *CA-A Cancer Journal for Clinicians*, 1983;(Sept/Oct) 258–263.
6. American Society of Hospital Pharmacists Technical Assistance Bulletin on Handling Cytotoxic and Hazardous Drugs. *Am J Hosp Pharm*, 1990;47:1033–1049.
7. OSHA Work-Practice Guidelines for Personnel Dealing with Cytotoxic (Antineoplastic) Drugs. *Am J Hosp Pharm*, 1986;43:1193–1204.

AZASAN is a trademark of aaiPharma LLC.
© 2002 aaiPharma LLC
Manufactured by:
AAI International
An aaiPharma™ Company
1726 North 23rd St.
Wilmington, NC 28405
Manufactured for:
aaiPharma™
aaiPharma
Wilmington, NC 28405

Rev 08/02

M.V.I. PEDIATRIC™ ℞
Multi-Vitamins for Infusion
For dilution in intravenous infusions only
Rx only

DESCRIPTION

M.V.I. Pediatric™ is a lyophilized, sterile powder intended for reconstitution and dilution in intravenous infusions. Each 5 mL of reconstituted product provides:

Ascorbic acid (vitamin C) .... 80 mg
Vitamin A* (retinol) .... 0.7 mg(a)
Ergocalciferol* (vitamin D) .... 10 mcg(b)
Thiamine (vitamin B$_1$)
 (as the hydrochloride) .... 1.2 mg
Riboflavin (vitamin B$_2$) (as riboflavin-
 5-phosphate sodium) .... 1.4 mg
Pyridoxine (vitamin B$_6$)
 (as the hydrochloride) .... 1 mg

Niacinamide	17 mg
Dexpanthenol (d-pantothenyl alcohol)	5 mg
Vitamin E* (dl-alpha tocopheryl acetate)	7 mg(c)
Biotin	20 mcg
Folic acid	140 mcg
Cyanocobalamin (vitamin B_{12})	1 mcg
Phytonadione* (vitamin K_1)	200 mcg

with 375 mg mannitol; sodium hydroxide for pH adjustment; 50 mg polysorbate 80; 0.8 mg polysorbate 20; 58 mg butylated hydroxytoluene; 14 mcg butylated hydroxyanisole.

*Oil-soluble vitamins A, D, E and K_1 water-solubilized with polysorbate 80.
(a) 0.7 mg vitamin A equals 2,300 USP units.
(b) 10 mcg ergocalciferol equals 400 USP units.
(c) 7 mg vitamin E equals 7 USP units.

Multivitamin Formula for Intravenous Infusion: M.V.I. Pediatric™ (Multi-Vitamins for Infusion) provides a combination of important oil-soluble and water-soluble vitamins, formulated especially for incorporation into intravenous infusions after reconstitution. Through special processing techniques, the liposoluble vitamins A, D, E and K_1 have been water solubilized with polysorbate 80, permitting intravenous administration of these vitamins.

INDICATIONS AND USAGE
This formulation is indicated as daily multivitamin maintenance dosage for infants and children up to 11 years of age receiving parenteral nutrition.

It is also indicated in other situations where administration by the intravenous route is required. Such situations include surgery, extensive burns, fractures and other trauma, severe infectious diseases, and comatose states, which may provoke a "stress" situation with profound alterations in the body's metabolic demands and consequent tissue depletion of nutrients.

The physician should not await the development of clinical signs of vitamin deficiency before initiating vitamin therapy.

M.V.I. Pediatric™ (reconstituted and administered in intravenous fluids under proper dilution) contributes intake of these necessary vitamins toward maintaining the body's normal resistance and repair processes.

Patients with multiple vitamin deficiencies or with markedly increased requirements may be given multiples of the daily dosage for two or more days as indicated by the clinical status. Blood vitamin concentrations should be monitored to ensure maintenance of adequate levels, particularly in patients receiving parenteral multivitamins as their sole source of vitamins for long periods of time.

CONTRAINDICATIONS
Known hypersensitivity to any of the vitamins or excipients in this product or a pre-existing hypervitaminosis.

Allergic reaction has been known to occur following intravenous administration of thiamine and vitamin K. The formulation is contraindicated prior to blood sampling for detection of megaloblastic anemia, as the folic acid and cyanocobalamin in the vitamin solution can mask serum deficits.

WARNINGS
WARNING: This product contains aluminum that may be toxic. Aluminum may reach toxic levels with prolonged parenteral administration if kidney function is impaired. Premature neonates are particularly at risk because their kidneys are immature, and they require large amounts of calcium and phosphate solutions, which contain aluminum. Research indicates that patients with impaired kidney function, including premature neonates, who receive parenteral levels of aluminum at greater than 4 to 5 μg/kg/day accumulate aluminum at levels associated with central nervous system and bone toxicity. Tissue loading may occur at even lower rates of administration.

PRECAUTIONS
General: Caution should be exercised when administering this multivitamin formulation to patients on warfarin sodium-type anticoagulant therapy. In such patients, vitamin K may antagonize the hypoprothrombinemic response to anticoagulant drugs. Therefore, periodic monitoring of prothrombin time is essential in determining the appropriate dosage of anticoagulant therapy.

Adequate blood levels of vitamin E are achieved when M.V.I. Pediatric™ is given to infants at the recommended dosage. Larger doses or supplementation with oral or parenteral vitamin E are not recommended because elevated blood levels of vitamin E may result.

Studies have shown that vitamin A may adhere to plastic, resulting in inadequate vitamin A administration in the doses recommended with M.V.I. Pediatric™. Additional vitamin A supplementation may be required, especially in low birth weight infants.

Where long-standing specific vitamin deficiencies exist, it may be necessary to add therapeutic amounts of specific vitamins to supplement the maintenance vitamins provided in M.V.I. Pediatric™.

In patients receiving parenteral multivitamins, blood vitamin concentrations should be periodically monitored to determine if vitamin deficiencies or excesses are developing.

Polysorbates have been associated with the E-Ferol syndrome (thrombocytopenia, renal dysfunction, hepatomegaly, cholestasis, ascites, hypotension, and metabolic acidosis) in low birth weight infants.

M.V.I. Pediatric™ should be aseptically transferred to the infusion fluid.

Drug – Drug Interactions
Physical Incompatibilities: M.V.I. Pediatric™ is not physically compatible with alkaline solutions or moderately alkaline drugs such as Diamox (Acetazolamide), Diuril Intravenous Sodium (Chlorothiazide sodium), Aminophylline or sodium bicarbonate. M.V.I. Pediatric™ is not physically compatible with ampicillin and it may not be physically compatible with ACHROMYCIN (tetracycline HCl). It has also been reported that folic acid is unstable in the presence of calcium salts such as calcium gluconate. Direct addition of M.V.I. Pediatric™ to intravenous fat emulsions is not recommended. Consult appropriate references for listings of physical compatibility of solutions and drugs with the vitamin infusion. In such circumstances, admixture or Y-site administration with vitamin solutions should be avoided.

Several vitamins have been reported to decrease the activity of certain antibiotics. Thiamine, riboflavin, pyridoxine, niacinamide, and ascorbic acid have been reported to decrease the antibiotic activity of erythromycin, kanamycin, streptomycin, doxycycline, and lincomycin. Bleomycin is inactivated *in vitro* by ascorbic acid and riboflavin.

Some of the vitamins in M.V.I. Pediatric™ may react with vitamin K bisulfite or sodium bisulfite; if bisulfite solutions are necessary, patients should be monitored for vitamin A and thiamine deficiencies.

Clinical Interactions: A number of interactions between vitamins and drugs have been reported which may affect the metabolism of either agent. The following are examples of these types of interactions.

Folic acid may lower the serum concentration of phenytoin resulting in increased seizure frequency. Conversely, phenytoin may decrease serum folic acid concentrations and, therefore, should be avoided in pregnancy. Folic acid may decrease the patient's response to methotrexate therapy.

Pyridoxine may decrease the efficacy of levodopa by increasing its metabolism. Concomitant administration of hydralazine or isoniazid may increase pyridoxine requirements.

In patients with pernicious anemia, the hematologic response to vitamin B_{12} therapy may be inhibited by concomitant administration of chloramphenicol.

Vitamin K may antagonize the hypoprothrombinemic effect of oral anticoagulants (see bolded statement).

Consult appropriate references for additional specific vitamin-drug interactions.

Drug-Laboratory Test Interactions: Ascorbic acid in the urine may cause false negative urine glucose determinations.

Carcinogenesis, Mutagenesis, and Impairment of Fertility: Carcinogenicity studies have not been performed.

ADVERSE REACTIONS
There have been rare reports of anaphylactic reactions following parenteral multivitamin administration. Rare reports of anaphylactoid reactions have also been reported after large intravenous doses of thiamine. The risk, however, is negligible if thiamine is coadministered with other vitamins in the B group. There have been no reports of fatal anaphylactoid reactions associated with M.V.I. Pediatric™. There have been rare reports of the following types of reactions:

Dermatologic—rash, erythema, pruritus
CNS—headache, dizziness, agitation, anxiety
Ophthalmic—diplopia
Allergic—urticaria, shortness of breath, wheezing, and angioedema

OVERDOSAGE
The possibility of hypervitaminosis A or D should be borne in mind. Clinical manifestations of hypervitaminosis A have been reported in patients with renal failure receiving 1.5 mg/day retinol. Therefore, vitamin A supplementation of renal failure patients should be undertaken with caution.

DOSAGE AND ADMINISTRATION
The single dose vial of M.V.I. Pediatric™ is reconstituted by adding 5 mL of Sterile Water for Injection USP, Dextrose Injection USP 5%, or Sodium Chloride Injection to the 10 mL vial.

The vial may be swirled gently after the addition of the water to hasten reconstitution. Use of this product is restricted to a suitable work area, such as a laminar flow hood. The reconstituted solution is ready within three minutes for immediate use. The withdrawal of container contents should be accomplished without delay. However, should this not be possible, a maximum time of 4 hours from initial closure entry is permitted to complete fluid transfer operations. The amount to be administered should be added to appropriate intravenous infusion fluids (see below).

The reconstituted M.V.I. Pediatric™ should not be given as a direct, undiluted intravenous injection as it may give rise to dizziness, faintness and possible tissue irritation.

For a single dose, 5 mL of reconstituted M.V.I. Pediatric™ should be added directly to not less than 100 mL of intravenous dextrose, saline or similar infusion solutions.

Infants weighing less than 1 kg: The daily dose is 30% (1.5 mL) of a single full dose (5 mL). Do not exceed this daily dose.

Infants weighing 1 to 3 kg: The daily dose is 65% (3.25 mL) of a single full dose (5 mL). Multiples of this recommended dose should not be given to infants weighing less than 3 kg. A supplemental vitamin A may be required for low birth weight infants.

Infants and children weighing 3 kg or more up to 11 years of age: The daily dose is 5 mL unless there is clinical or laboratory evidence for increasing or decreasing the dosage.

DISCARD ANY UNUSED PORTION.

Parenteral drug products should be inspected visually for particulate matter and discoloration prior to administration, whenever solution and container permit.

After M.V.I. Pediatric™ is reconstituted it should be immediately diluted into the intravenous solution. The resulting solution should be administered immediately. Some of the vitamins in this product, particularly vitamins A and D and riboflavin, are light-sensitive and exposure to light should be minimized.

HOW SUPPLIED
M.V.I. Pediatric™ is available as:
NDC 66591-839-31, Single Dose Vial, Boxes of 10.
Store under refrigeration, 2–8°C (36–46°F).
M.V.I. Pediatric is a trademark of aaiPharma LLC.
© 2002 aaiPharma LLC
Manufactured by: DSM Pharmaceuticals, Inc., Greenville, NC 27834
Manufactured for:
aaiPharma
Wilmington, NC 28405
Rev. 8/02
646650

Abbott Laboratories
Pharmaceutical Products Division
NORTH CHICAGO, IL 60064, U.S.A.

Pharmaceutical Products Division—
Direct Inquiries to:
Customer Service:
(800) 255-5162
Technical Services:
(800) 441-4987
For Medical Information Contact:
Generally:
(800) 633-9110
Adverse Drug Experiences:
(800) 633-9110
Sales and Ordering:
(800) 255-5162
Hospital Products Division—
Direct Inquiries to:
Customer Service
(800) 222-6883
For Medical Information Contact:
(800) 633-9110
Sales and Ordering:
(800) 222-6883

ABBOKINASE® ℞
[ă bō kī'nās]
UROKINASE

DESCRIPTION
Abbokinase® (urokinase) is a thrombolytic agent obtained from human neonatal kidney cells grown in tissue culture. The principle active ingredient of Abbokinase® is the low molecular weight form of urokinase, and consists of an A chain of 2,000 daltons linked by a sulfhydryl bond to a B chain of 30,400 daltons. Abbokinase® is supplied as a sterile lyophilized white powder containing 250,000 IU urokinase per vial, mannitol (25 mg/vial), Albumin (Human) (250 mg/vial), and sodium chloride (50 mg/vial).

Following reconstitution with 5 mL of Sterile Water for Injection, USP, Abbokinase® is a clear, slightly straw-colored solution; each mL contains 50,000 IU of urokinase activity, 0.5% mannitol, 5% Albumin (Human), and 1% sodium chloride (pH range 6.0 to 7.5).

Thin translucent filaments may occasionally occur in reconstituted Abbokinase® vials (see **DOSAGE AND ADMINISTRATION**).

Abbokinase® is for intravenous infusion only.

Abbokinase® is produced from human neonatal kidney cells (see **WARNINGS**). No fetal tissue is used in the production of Abbokinase®. Kidney donations are obtained exclusively in the United States from neonates (birth to 28 days) for whom death has not been attributed to infectious causes and that have exhibited no evidence of an infectious disease based in part, on an examination of the maternal and neonatal donor medical records. The maternal and neonatal donor screening process also identifies specific risk factors for known infectious diseases and includes testing of sera for HBV, HCV, HIV-1, HIV-2, HTLV-I, HTLV-II, CMV, and EBV. Donors with sera testing positive or associated with other risk factors are excluded. During the manufacturing process, cells are tested at multiple stages for the presence of viruses using *in vitro* and *in vivo* tests that are capable of detecting a wide range of viruses. Cells are also screened for HPV using a DNA detection-based test and for reovirus using a polymerase chain reaction-based test. The manufacturing process used for this product has been validated in laboratory studies to inactivate and/or remove a diverse panel of spiked model enveloped and non-enveloped viruses, and includes purification steps and a heat treatment step (10 hours at 60°C in 2% sodium chloride). A single vial of Abbokinase® contains urokinase produced using cells derived from one or two donors.

Continued on next page

Abbokinase—Cont.

CLINICAL PHARMACOLOGY

Urokinase is an enzyme (protein) produced by the kidney, and found in the urine. There are two forms of urokinase which differ in molecular weight but have similar clinical effects. Abbokinase® is the low molecular weight form. Abbokinase® acts on the endogenous fibrinolytic system. It converts plasminogen to the enzyme plasmin. Plasmin degrades fibrin clots as well as fibrinogen and some other plasma proteins.

Information about the pharmacokinetic properties in man is limited. Urokinase administered by intravenous infusion is rapidly cleared by the liver with an elimination half-life for biologic activity of 12.6 +/− 6.2 minutes and a distribution volume of 11.5 L. Small fractions of the administered dose are excreted in bile and urine. Although the pharmacokinetics of exogenously administered urokinase have not been characterized in patients with hepatic impairment, endogenous urokinase-type plasminogen activator plasma levels are elevated 2- to 4-fold in patients with moderate to severe cirrhosis.[1] Thus, reduced urokinase clearance in patients with hepatic impairment might be expected.

Intravenous infusion of Abbokinase® in doses recommended for lysis of pulmonary embolism is followed by increased fibrinolytic activity in the circulation. This effect disappears within a few hours after discontinuation, but a decrease in plasma levels of fibrinogen and plasminogen and an increase in the amount of circulating fibrin and fibrinogen degradation products may persist for 12-24 hours.[2] There is a lack of correlation between embolus resolution and changes in coagulation and fibrinolytic assay results.

Treatment with urokinase demonstrated more improvement on pulmonary angiography, lung perfusion scanning, and hemodynamic measurements within 24 hours than did treatment with heparin. Lung perfusion scanning showed no significant treatment-associated difference by day 7.[3]

Information based on patients treated with fibrinolytics for pulmonary embolus suggests that improvement in angiographic and lung perfusion scans is lessened when treatment is instituted more than several days (e.g., 4 to 6 days) after onset.[4]

INDICATIONS AND USAGE

Abbokinase® is indicated in adults:
- For the lysis of acute massive pulmonary emboli, defined as obstruction of blood flow to a lobe or multiple segments.
- For the lysis of pulmonary emboli accompanied by unstable hemodynamics, i.e., failure to maintain blood pressure without supportive measures.

The diagnosis should be confirmed by objective means, such as pulmonary angiography or non-invasive procedures such as lung scanning.

CONTRAINDICATIONS

The use of Abbokinase® is contraindicated in patients with a history of hypersensitivity to the product (see **WARNINGS** and **ADVERSE REACTIONS**).

Because thrombolytic therapy increases the risk of bleeding, Abbokinase® is contraindicated in the situations listed below (see **WARNINGS**).
- Active internal bleeding
- Recent (e.g., within two months) cerebrovascular accident
- Recent (e.g., within two months) intracranial or intraspinal surgery
- Recent trauma including cardiopulmonary resuscitation
- Intracranial neoplasm, arteriovenous malformation, or aneurysm
- Known bleeding diatheses
- Severe uncontrolled arterial hypertension

WARNINGS

Bleeding

The risk of serious bleeding is increased with use of Abbokinase®. Fatalities due to hemorrhage, including intracranial and retroperitoneal, have been reported in association with urokinase therapy.

Concurrent administration of Abbokinase® with other thrombolytic agents, anticoagulants, or agents inhibiting platelet function may further increase the risk of serious bleeding.

Abbokinase® therapy requires careful attention to all potential bleeding sites (including catheter insertion sites, arterial and venous puncture sites, cutdown sites, and other needle puncture sites).

Intramuscular injections and nonessential handling of the patient must be avoided during treatment with Abbokinase®. Venipunctures should be performed as infrequently as possible and with care to minimize bleeding. Should an arterial puncture be necessary, upper extremity vessels are preferable. Direct pressure should be applied for at least 30 minutes, a pressure dressing applied, and the puncture site checked frequently for evidence of bleeding.

In the following conditions, the risk of bleeding may be increased and should be weighed against the anticipated benefits:
- Recent (within 10 days) major surgery, obstetrical delivery, organ biopsy, previous puncture of non-compressible vessels
- Recent (within 10 days) serious gastrointestinal bleeding
- High likelihood of a left heart thrombus, for example, mitral stenosis with atrial fibrillation
- Subacute bacterial endocarditis
- Hemostatic defects including those secondary to severe hepatic or renal disease
- Pregnancy
- Cerebrovascular disease
- Diabetic hemorrhagic retinopathy
- Any other condition in which bleeding might constitute a significant hazard or be particularly difficult to manage because of its location

When internal bleeding occurs, it may be more difficult to manage than that which occurs with conventional anticoagulant therapy. Should potentially serious spontaneous bleeding (not controllable by direct pressure) occur, the infusion of Abbokinase® should be terminated immediately, and measures to manage the bleeding implemented. Serious blood loss may be managed with volume replacement, including packed red blood cells. Dextran should not be used. When appropriate, fresh frozen plasma and/or cryoprecipitate may be considered to reverse the bleeding tendency.

Anaphylaxis and Other Infusion Reactions

Post-marketing reports of hypersensitivity reactions have included anaphylaxis (with rare reports of fatal anaphylaxis), bronchospasm, orolingual edema and urticaria (see **ADVERSE REACTIONS: Allergic Reactions**). There have also been reports of other infusion reactions which have included one or more of the following: fever and/or chills/rigors, hypoxia, cyanosis, dyspnea, tachycardia, hypotension, hypertension, acidosis, back pain, vomiting, and nausea. Reactions generally occurred within one hour of beginning Abbokinase® infusion. Patients who exhibit reactions should be closely monitored and appropriate therapy instituted.

Infusion reactions generally respond to discontinuation of the infusion and/or administration of intravenous antihistamines, corticosteroids, or adrenergic agents.

Antipyretics which inhibit platelet function (aspirin and other non-steroidal anti-inflammatory agents) may increase the risk of bleeding and should not be used for treatment of fever.

Cholesterol Embolization

Cholesterol embolism has been reported rarely in patients treated with all types of thrombolytic agents; the true incidence is unknown. This serious condition, which can be lethal, is also associated with invasive vascular procedures (e.g., cardiac catheterization, angiography, vascular surgery) and/or anticoagulant therapy. Clinical features of cholesterol embolism may include livedo reticularis, "purple toe" syndrome, acute renal failure, gangrenous digits, hypertension, pancreatitis, myocardial infarction, cerebral infarction, spinal cord infarction, retinal artery occlusion, bowel infarction and rhabdomyolysis.

Product Source and Formulation with Albumin

Abbokinase® is made from human neonatal kidney cells grown in tissue culture. Products made from human source material may contain infectious agents, such as viruses, that can cause disease. The risk that Abbokinase® will transmit an infectious agent has been reduced by screening donors for prior exposure to certain viruses, by testing donors for the presence of certain current virus infections, by testing for certain viruses during manufacturing, and by inactivating and/or removing certain viruses during manufacturing (see **DESCRIPTION**). Despite these measures, Abbokinase® may carry a risk of transmitting infectious agents, including those that cause the Creutzfeldt-Jakob disease (CJD) or other diseases not yet known or identified; thus, the risk of transmission of infectious agents cannot be totally eliminated. A theoretical risk for transmission of Creutzfeldt-Jakob disease (CJD) is considered extremely remote.

This product is formulated in 5% albumin, a derivative of human blood. Based on effective donor screening and product manufacturing processes, albumin carries an extremely remote risk for transmission of viral diseases. A theoretical risk for transmission of Creutzfeldt-Jakob disease (CJD) also is considered extremely remote. No cases of transmission of viral diseases or CJD have ever been identified for albumin.

All infections thought by a physician possibly to have been transmitted by this product should be reported by the physician or other healthcare provider to Abbott Laboratories [1-800-441-4100].

PRECAUTIONS

General

Abbokinase® should be used in hospitals where the recommended diagnostic and monitoring techniques are available.

The clinical response and vital signs should be observed frequently during and following Abbokinase® infusion. Blood pressure should not be taken in the lower extremities to avoid dislodgement of possible deep vein thrombi.

Laboratory Tests

Before beginning thrombolytic therapy, obtain a hematocrit, platelet count, and an activated partial thromboplastin time (aPTT). If heparin has been given, it should be discontinued and the aPTT should be less than the normal control value before thrombolytic therapy is started.

Following the intravenous infusion of Abbokinase®, before (re)instituting anticoagulants, the aPTT should be less than twice the normal control value.

Results of coagulation tests and measures of fibrinolytic activity do not reliably predict either efficacy or risk of bleeding for patients receiving Abbokinase®.

Drug Interactions

Anticoagulants and agents that alter platelet function (such as aspirin, other non-steroidal anti-inflammatory agents, dipyridamole, and GP IIb/IIIa inhibitors) may increase the risk of serious bleeding.

Administration of Abbokinase® prior to, during, or after other thrombolytic agents may increase the risk of serious bleeding.

Dose Preparation-Pulmonary Embolism

Patient Weight (pounds)	Total Dose[a] Abbokinase® (IU)	Number of Vials of Abbokinase®	Volume of Abbokinase® After Reconstitution (mL)[b]	+	Volume of Diluent (mL)	=	Final Volume (mL)
81-90	2,250,000	9	45		150		195
91-100	2,500,000	10	50		145		195
101-110	2,750,000	11	55		140		195
111-120	3,000,000	12	60		135		195
121-130	3,250,000	13	65		130		195
131-140	3,500,000	14	70		125		195
141-150	3,750,000	15	75		120		195
151-160	4,000,000	16	80		115		195
161-170	4,250,000	17	85		110		195
171-180	4,500,000	18	90		105		195
181-190	4,750,000	19	95		100		195
191-200	5,000,000	20	100		95		195
201-210	5,250,000	21	105		90		195
211-220	5,500,000	22	110		85		195
221-230	5,750,000	23	115		80		195
231-240	6,000,000	24	120		75		195
241-250	6,250,000	25	125		70		195

Infusion Rate: Loading Dose 15 mL/10 min[c] Dose for 12-Hour Period 15 mL/hr for 12 hrs

[a] Loading dose + dose administered during 12-hour period.
[b] After addition of 5 mL of Sterile Water for Injection, USP, per vial. (See Preparation.)
[c] Pump rate = 90 mL/hr

Because concomitant use of Abbokinase® with agents that alter coagulation, inhibit platelet function, or are thrombolytic may further increase the potential for bleeding complications, careful monitoring for bleeding is recommended. The interaction of Abbokinase® with other drugs has not been studied and is not known.

Carcinogenicity
Adequate data are not available on the long-term potential for carcinogenicity in animals or humans.

Pregnancy
Pregnancy Category B: Reproduction studies have been performed in mice and rats at doses up to 1,000 times the human dose and have revealed no evidence of impaired fertility or harm to the fetus due to Abbokinase®. There are, however, no adequate and well-controlled studies in pregnant women. Because animal reproduction studies are not always predictive of human response, this drug should be used during pregnancy only if clearly needed.

Nursing Mothers
It is not known whether this drug is excreted in human milk. Because many drugs are excreted in human milk, caution should be exercised when Abbokinase® is administered to a nursing woman.

Pediatric Use
Safety and effectiveness in pediatric patients have not been established.

Geriatric Use
Clinical studies of Abbokinase® did not include sufficient numbers of subjects aged 65 and over to determine whether they respond differently from younger subjects. Abbokinase® should be used with caution in elderly patients.

ADVERSE REACTIONS
The most serious adverse reactions reported with Abbokinase® administration include fatal hemorrhage and anaphylaxis (see **WARNINGS**).

Bleeding
Bleeding is the most frequent adverse reaction associated with Abbokinase® and can be fatal (see **WARNINGS**).

In controlled clinical studies using a 12-hour infusion of urokinase for the treatment of pulmonary embolism (UPET and USPET),[3,5,6] bleeding resulting in at least a 5% decrease in hematocrit was reported in 52 of 141 urokinase-treated patients. Significant bleeding events requiring transfusion of greater than 2 units of blood were observed during the 14-day study period in 3 of 141 urokinase-treated patients in these studies. Multiple bleeding events may have occurred in an individual patient. Most bleeding occurred at sites of external incisions and vascular puncture, with lesser frequency in gastrointestinal, genitourinary, intracranial, retroperitoneal, and intramuscular sites.

Sources of Information on Adverse Reactions
There are limited well-controlled clinical studies performed using urokinase. The adverse reactions described in the following sections reflect both the clinical use of Abbokinase® in the general population and limited controlled study data. Because post-marketing reports of adverse reactions are voluntary and the population is of uncertain size, it is not always possible to reliably estimate the frequency of the reaction or establish a causal relationship to drug exposure.

Allergic Reactions
Rare cases of fatal anaphylaxis have been reported (see **WARNINGS**). In controlled clinical trials, allergic reaction was reported in 1 of 141 patients (<1%).

The following allergic-type reactions have been observed in clinical trials and/or post-marketing experience: bronchospasm, orolingual edema, urticaria, skin rash, and pruritus (see **WARNINGS**).

Infusion reaction symptoms include hypoxia, cyanosis, dyspnea, tachycardia, hypotension, hypertension, acidosis, fever and/or chills/rigors, back pain, vomiting, and nausea (see **WARNINGS**).

Other Adverse Reactions
Other adverse events occurring in patients receiving Abbokinase® therapy in clinical studies, regardless of causality, include myocardial infarction, recurrent pulmonary embolism, hemiplegia, stroke, decreased hematocrit, substernal pain, thrombocytopenia, and diaphoresis.

Additional adverse reactions reported from post-marketing experience include cardiac arrest, vascular embolization (cerebral and distal) including cholesterol emboli (see **WARNINGS**), cerebral vascular accident, pulmonary edema, reperfusion ventricular arrhythmias and chest pain. A cause and effect relationship has not been established.

Immunogenicity
The immunogenicity of Abbokinase® has not been studied.

DOSAGE AND ADMINISTRATION
ABBOKINASE® IS INTENDED FOR INTRAVENOUS INFUSION ONLY.

Abbokinase® treatment should be instituted soon after onset of pulmonary embolism. Delay in instituting therapy may decrease the potential for optimal efficacy (see **CLINICAL PHARMACOLOGY**).

Preparation
Abbokinase® contains no preservatives. Do not reconstitute until immediately before use. Any unused portion of the reconstituted material should be discarded.

Reconstitute Abbokinase® by aseptically adding 5 mL of Sterile Water for Injection, USP, to the vial. Abbokinase® should be reconstituted with Sterile Water for Injection, USP, without preservatives. Do not use Bacteriostatic Water for Injection, USP. After reconstituting, visually inspect each vial of Abbokinase® for discoloration and for the presence of particulate material. The solution should be pale and straw-colored; highly colored solutions should not be used.

Thin translucent filaments may occasionally occur in reconstituted Abbokinase® vials, but do not indicate any decrease in potency of this product. To minimize formation of filaments, avoid shaking the vial during reconstitution. Roll and tilt the vial to enhance reconstitution. The solution may be terminally filtered, for example through a 0.45 micron or smaller cellulose membrane filter. No other medication should be added to this solution.

Administration
Prior to infusing, dilute the reconstituted Abbokinase® with 0.9% Sodium Chloride Injection, USP or 5% Dextrose Injection, USP. The following table may be used as an aid in the preparation of Abbokinase® for administration.
[See table at top of previous page]

Abbokinase® is administered using a constant infusion pump that is capable of delivering a total volume of 195 mL. A loading dose of 2,000 IU/lb (4,400 IU/kg) of Abbokinase® is given as the Abbokinase® 0.9% Sodium Chloride Injection, USP, or 5% Dextrose Injection, USP, admixture at a rate of 90 mL/hour over a period of 10 minutes. This is followed by a continuous infusion of 2,000 IU/lb/hr (4,400 IU/kg/hr) of Abbokinase® at a rate of 15 mL/hour for 12 hours. Since some Abbokinase® admixture will remain in the tubing at the end of an infusion pump delivery cycle, the following flush procedure should be performed to insure that the total dose of Abbokinase® is administered. A solution of 0.9% Sodium Chloride Injection, USP, or 5% Dextrose Injection, USP, approximately equal in amount to the volume of the tubing in the infusion set should be administered via the pump to flush the Abbokinase® admixture from the entire length of the infusion set. The pump should be set to administer the flush solution at the continuous rate of 15 mL/hour.

Anticoagulation After Terminating Abbokinase® Treatment
After infusing Abbokinase®, anticoagulation treatment is recommended to prevent recurrent thrombosis. Do not begin anticoagulation until the aPTT has decreased to *less than twice* the normal control value. If heparin is used, do not administer a loading dose of heparin. Treatment should be followed by oral anticoagulants.

HOW SUPPLIED
Abbokinase® is supplied as a sterile lyophilized preparation (NDC 0074-6109-05). Each vial contains 250,000 IU urokinase activity, 25 mg mannitol, 250 mg Albumin (Human), and 50 mg sodium chloride. Refrigerate Abbokinase® powder at 2° to 8°C (36° to 46°F) (see USP).

REFERENCES
1. Sato S, et al. Elevated Urokinase-Type Plasminogen Activator Plasma Levels Are Associated With Deterioration of Liver Function But Not With Hepatocellular Carcinoma. *J Gastroenterology*. 1994; 29: 745-750.
2. Bell WR. Thrombolytic Therapy: A Comparison Between Urokinase and Streptokinase. *Sem Thromb Hemost*. 1975; 2:1-13.
3. Sasahara AA, Hyers TM, Cole CM, et al. The Urokinase Pulmonary Embolism Trial. *Circulation*. 1973; 47 (suppl. 2): 1-108.
4. Daniels LB, Parker JA, Patel SR, Grodstein F, Goldhaber SZ. Relation of Duration of Symptoms With Response to Thrombolytic Therapy in Pulmonary Embolism. *Am J Cardiol*. 1997; 80:184-188.
5. Urokinase Pulmonary Embolism Trial Study Group: Urokinase-Streptokinase Embolism Trial. *JAMA*. 1974; 229:1606-1613.
6. Sasahara AA, Bell WR, Simon TL, et al. The Phase II Urokinase-Streptokinase Pulmonary Embolism Trial. *Thrombos Diathes Haemorrh* (Stuttg). 1975; 33:464-476.

©Abbott 2002
ABBOTT LABORATORIES, NORTH CHICAGO, IL 60064, USA
Reference 58-6978-R4-Rev. October, 2002

HUMIRA™ ℞
(adalimumab)
Rx only

> **WARNING**
> **RISK OF INFECTIONS**
> Cases of tuberculosis (frequently disseminated or extrapulmonary at clinical presentation) have been observed in patients receiving HUMIRA.
> Patients should be evaluated for latent tuberculosis infection with a tuberculin skin test. Treatment of latent tuberculosis infection should be initiated prior to therapy with HUMIRA.

DESCRIPTION
HUMIRA (adalimumab) is a recombinant human IgG1 monoclonal antibody specific for human tumor necrosis factor (TNF). HUMIRA was created using phage display technology resulting in an antibody with human derived heavy and light chain variable regions and human IgG1:κ constant regions. HUMIRA is produced by recombinant DNA technology in a mammalian cell expression system and is purified by a process that includes specific viral inactivation and removal steps. It consists of 1330 amino acids and has a molecular weight of approximately 148 kilodaltons.

HUMIRA is supplied in single-use, 1 mL pre-filled glass syringes as a sterile, preservative-free solution for subcutaneous administration. The solution of HUMIRA is clear and colorless, with a pH of about 5.2. Each syringe delivers 0.8 mL (40 mg) of drug product. Each 0.8 mL HUMIRA contains 40 mg adalimumab, 4.93 mg sodium chloride, 0.69 mg monobasic sodium phosphate dihydrate, 1.22 mg dibasic sodium phosphate dihydrate, 0.24 mg sodium citrate, 1.04 mg citric acid monohydrate, 9.6 mg mannitol, 0.8 mg polysorbate 80 and Water for Injection, USP. Sodium hydroxide added as necessary to adjust pH.

CLINICAL PHARMACOLOGY
General
Adalimumab binds specifically to TNF-alpha and blocks its interaction with the p55 and p75 cell surface TNF receptors. Adalimumab also lyses surface TNF expressing cells *in vitro* in the presence of complement. Adalimumab does not bind or inactivate lymphotoxin (TNF-beta). TNF is a naturally occurring cytokine that is involved in normal inflammatory and immune responses. Elevated levels of TNF are found in the synovial fluid of rheumatoid arthritis patients and play an important role in both the pathologic inflammation and the joint destruction that are hallmarks of rheumatoid arthritis.

Adalimumab also modulates biological responses that are induced or regulated by TNF, including changes in the levels of adhesion molecules responsible for leukocyte migration (ELAM-1, VCAM-1, and ICAM-1 with an IC_{50} of $1-2 \times 10^{-10}$M).

Pharmacodynamics
After treatment with HUMIRA, a rapid decrease in levels of acute phase reactants of inflammation (C-reactive protein (CRP) and erythrocyte sedimentation rate (ESR)) and serum cytokines (IL-6) was observed compared to baseline in patients with rheumatoid arthritis. Serum levels of matrix metalloproteinases (MMP-1 and MMP-3) that produce tissue remodeling responsible for cartilage destruction were also decreased after HUMIRA administration.

Pharmacokinetics
The maximum serum concentration (C_{max}) and the time to reach the maximum concentration (T_{max}) were 4.7 ± 1.6 μg/mL and 131 ± 56 hours respectively, following a single 40 mg subcutaneous administration of HUMIRA to healthy adult subjects. The average absolute bioavailability of adalimumab estimated from three studies following a single 40 mg subcutaneous dose was 64%. The pharmacokinetics of adalimumab were linear over the dose range of 0.5 to 10.0 mg/kg following a single intravenous dose.

The single dose pharmacokinetics of adalimumab were determined in several studies with intravenous doses ranging from 0.25 to 10 mg/kg. The distribution volume (V_{ss}) ranged from 4.7 to 6.0 L. The systemic clearance of adalimumab is approximately 12 mL/hr. The mean terminal half-life was approximately 2 weeks, ranging from 10 to 20 days across studies. Adalimumab concentrations in the synovial fluid from five rheumatoid arthritis patients ranged from 31–96% of those in serum.

Adalimumab mean steady-state trough concentrations of approximately 5 μg/mL and 8 to 9 μg/mL, were observed without and with methotrexate (MTX) respectively. The serum adalimumab trough levels at steady increased approximately proportionally with dose following 20, 40 and 80 mg every other week and every week subcutaneous dosing. In long-term studies with dosing more than two years, there was no evidence of changes in clearance over time.

Population pharmacokinetic analyses revealed that there was a trend toward higher apparent clearance of adalimumab in the presence of anti-adalimumab antibodies, and lower clearance with increasing age in patients aged 40 to >75 years.

Minor increases in apparent clearance were also predicted in patients receiving doses lower than the recommended dose and in patients with high rheumatoid factor or CRP concentrations. These increases are not likely to be clinically important.

No gender-related pharmacokinetic differences were observed after correction for a patient's body weight. Healthy volunteers and patients with rheumatoid arthritis displayed similar adalimumab pharmacokinetics.

No pharmacokinetic data are available in patients with hepatic or renal impairment

HUMIRA has not been studied in children.

Drug Interactions
MTX reduced adalimumab apparent clearance after single and multiple dosing by 29% and 44% respectively.

CLINICAL STUDIES
The efficacy and safety of HUMIRA were assessed in four randomized, double-blind studies in patients ≥ age 18 with active rheumatoid arthritis diagnosed according to American College of Rheumatology (ACR) criteria. Patients had at least 6 swollen and 9 tender joints. HUMIRA was administered subcutaneously in combination with MTX (12.5 to 25 mg, Studies I and III) or as monotherapy (Study II) or with other disease-modifying anti-rheumatic drugs (DMARDs) (Study IV).

Study I evaluated 271 patients who had failed therapy with at least one but no more than four DMARDs and had inadequate response to MTX. Doses of 20, 40 or 80 mg of HUMIRA or placebo were given every other week for 24 weeks.

Continued on next page

Humira—Cont.

Study II evaluated 544 patients who had failed therapy with at least one DMARD. Doses of placebo, 20 or 40 mg of HUMIRA were given as monotherapy every other week or weekly for 26 weeks.

Study III evaluated 619 patients who had an inadequate response to MTX. Patients received placebo, 40 mg of HUMIRA every other week with placebo injections on alternate weeks, or 20 mg of HUMIRA weekly for up to 52 weeks. Study III had an additional primary endpoint at 52 weeks of inhibition of disease progression (as detected by X-ray results).

Study IV assessed safety in 636 patients who were either DMARD-naive or were permitted to remain on their pre-existing rheumatologic therapy provided that therapy was stable for a minimum of 28 days. Patients were randomized to 40 mg of HUMIRA or placebo every other week for 24 weeks.

The percent of HUMIRA treated patients achieving ACR 20, 50 and 70 responses in Studies II and III are shown in Table 1.

[See table 1 above]

The results of Study I were similar to Study III; patients receiving HUMIRA 40 mg every other week in Study I also achieved ACR 20, 50 and 70 response rates of 65%, 52% and 24%, respectively, compared to placebo responses of 13%, 7% and 3% respectively, at 6 months (p<0.01).

The results of the components of the ACR response criteria for Studies II and III are shown in Table 2. Improvement was seen in all components and was maintained to week 52.

[See table 2 above]

The time course of ACR 20 response for Study III is shown in Figure 1. In Study III, 85% of patients with ACR 20 responses at week 24 maintained the response at 52 weeks. The time course of ACR 20 response for Study I and Study II were similar.

Figure 1: Study III ACR 20 Responses over 52 Weeks

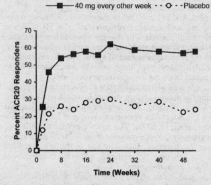

In Study IV, 53% of patients treated with HUMIRA 40 mg every other week plus standard of care had an ACR 20 response at week 24 compared to 35% on placebo plus standard of care (p<0.001). No unique adverse reactions related to the combination of HUMIRA and other DMARDs were observed.

In all four studies, HUMIRA showed significantly greater improvement than placebo in the disability index of Health Assessment Questionnaire (HAQ) from baseline to the end of study, and significantly greater improvement than placebo in the health-outcomes as assessed by The Short Form Health Survey (SF 36). Improvement was seen in both the Physical Component Summary (PCS) and the Mental Component Summary (MCS).

Radiographic Response

In Study III, structural joint damage was assessed radiographically and expressed as change in Total Sharp Score (TSS) and its components, the erosion score and Joint Space Narrowing (JSN) score, at month 12 compared to baseline. At baseline, the median TSS was approximately 55 in the placebo and 40 mg every other week groups. The results are shown in Table 3. HUMIRA/MTX treated patients demonstrated less radiographic progression than patients receiving MTX alone.

[See table 3 at right]

INDICATIONS AND USAGE

HUMIRA is indicated for reducing signs and symptoms and inhibiting the progression of structural damage in adult patients with moderately to severely active rheumatoid arthritis who have had an inadequate response to one or more DMARDs. HUMIRA can be used alone or in combination with MTX or other DMARDs.

CONTRAINDICATIONS

HUMIRA should not be administered to patients with known hypersensitivity to HUMIRA or any of its components.

WARNINGS

SERIOUS INFECTIONS AND SEPSIS, INCLUDING FATALITIES, HAVE BEEN REPORTED WITH THE USE OF TNF BLOCKING AGENTS INCLUDING HUMIRA. MANY OF THE SERIOUS INFECTIONS HAVE OCCURRED IN PATIENTS ON CONCOMITANT IMMUNOSUPPRESSIVE THERAPY THAT, IN ADDITION TO THEIR RHEUMATOID ARTHRITIS, COULD PREDISPOSE THEM TO INFECTIONS. TUBERCULOSIS AND INVASIVE OPPORTUNISTIC FUNGAL INFECTIONS HAVE BEEN OBSERVED IN PATIENTS TREATED WITH TNF BLOCKING AGENTS INCLUDING HUMIRA.

TREATMENT WITH HUMIRA SHOULD NOT BE INITIATED IN PATIENTS WITH ACTIVE INFECTIONS INCLUDING CHRONIC OR LOCALIZED INFECTIONS. PATIENTS WHO DEVELOP A NEW INFECTION WHILE UNDERGOING TREATMENT WITH HUMIRA SHOULD BE MONITORED CLOSELY. ADMINISTRATION OF HUMIRA SHOULD BE DISCONTINUED IF A PATIENT DEVEVLOPS A SERIOUS INFECTION. PHYSICIANS SHOULD EXERCISE CAUTION WHEN CONSIDERING THE USE OF HUMIRA IN PATIENTS WITH A HISTORY OF RECURRENT INFECTION OR UNDERLYING CONDITIONS WHICH MAY PREDISPOSE THEM TO INFECTIONS, OR PATIENTS WHO HAVE RESIDED IN REGIONS WHERE TUBERCULOSIS AND HISTOPLASMOSIS ARE ENDEMIC (see PRECAUTIONS - Tuberculosis and ADVERSE REACTIONS - Infections). THE BENEFITS AND RISKS OF HUMIRA TREATMENT SHOULD BE CAREFULLY CONSIDERED BEFORE INITIATION OF HUMIRA THERAPY.

Neurologic Events

Use of TNF blocking agents, including HUMIRA, has been associated with rare cases of exacerbation of clinical symptoms and/or radiographic evidence of demyelinating disease. Prescribers should exercise caution in considering the use of HUMIRA in patients with preexisting or recent-onset central nervous system demyelinating disorders.

Malignancies

Lymphomas have been observed in patients treated with TNF blocking agents including HUMIRA. In clinical trials, patients treated with HUMIRA had a higher incidence of lymphoma than the expected rate in the general population (see **ADVERSE REACTIONS-Malignancies**). While patients with rheumatoid arthritis, particularly those with highly active disease, may be at a higher risk (up to several fold) for the development of lymphoma, the role of TNF blockers in the development of malignancy is not known[4,5].

PRECAUTIONS

General

Allergic reactions have been observed in approximately 1% of patients receiving HUMIRA. If an anaphylactic reaction or other serious allergic reaction occurs, administration of HUMIRA should be discontinued immediately and appropriate therapy initiated.

Information to Patients

The first injection should be performed under the supervision of a qualified health care professional. If a patient or caregiver is to administer HUMIRA, he/she should be instructed in injection techniques and their ability to inject subcutaneously should be assessed to ensure the proper administration of HUMIRA (see **HUMIRA, PATIENT INFORMATION LEAFLET**). A puncture-resistant container for disposal of needles and syringes should be used. Patients or caregivers should be instructed in the technique as well as proper syringe and needle disposal, and be cautioned against reuse of these items.

Tuberculosis

As observed with other TNF blocking agents, tuberculosis associated with the administration of HUMIRA in clinical trials has been reported (see **WARNINGS**). While cases were observed at all doses, the incidence of tuberculosis reactivations was particularly increased at doses of HUMIRA that were higher than the recommended dose. All patients recovered after standard antimicrobial therapy. No deaths due to tuberculosis occurred during the clinical trials.

Table 1: ACR Responses in Placebo-Controlled Trials (Percent of Patients)

Response	Study II Monotherapy (26 weeks)			Study III Methotrexate Combination (24 and 52 weeks)	
	Placebo N=110	HUMIRA 40 mg every other week N=113	HUMIRA 40 mg weekly N=103	Placebo/MTX N=200	HUMIRA/MTX 40 mg every other week N=207
ACR20					
Month 6	19%	46%*	53%*	30%	63%*
Month 12	NA	NA	NA	24%	59%*
ACR50					
Month 6	8%	22%*	35%*	10%	39%*
Month 12	NA	NA	NA	10%	42%*
ACR70					
Month 6	2%	12%*	18%*	3%	21%*
Month 12	NA	NA	NA	5%	23%*

*p<0.01, HUMIRA vs. placebo

Table 2: Components of ACR Response in Studies II and III

Parameter (median)	Study II				Study III			
	Placebo N=110		HUMIRA[a] N=113		Placebo/MTX N=200		HUMIRA[a]/MTX N=207	
	Baseline	Wk 26	Baseline	Wk 26	Baseline	Wk 24	Baseline	Wk 24
Number of tender joints (0–68)	35	26	31	16*	26	15	24	8*
Number of swollen joints (0–66)	19	16	18	10*	17	11	18	5*
Physician global assessment[b]	7.0	6.1	6.6	3.7*	6.3	3.5	6.5	2.0*
Patient global assessment[b]	7.5	6.3	7.5	4.5*	5.4	3.9	5.2	2.0*
Pain[b]	7.3	6.1	7.3	4.1*	6.0	3.8	5.8	2.1*
Disability index (HAQ)[c]	2.0	1.9	1.9	1.5*	1.5	1.3	1.5	0.8*
CRP (mg/dL)	3.9	4.3	4.6	1.8*	1.0	0.9	1.0	0.4*

[a] 40 mg HUMIRA administered every other week
[b] Visual analogue scale; 0 = best, 10 = worst
[c] Disability Index of the Health Assessment Questionnaire[2]; 0 = best, 3 = worst, measures the patient's ability to perform the following: dress/groom, arise, eat, walk, reach, grip, maintain hygiene, and maintain daily activity
*p<0.001, HUMIRA vs. placebo, based on mean change from baseline

Table 3: Radiographic Mean Changes Over 12 Months in Study III

	Placebo/MTX	HUMIRA/MTX 40 mg every other week	Placebo/MTX-HUMIRA/MTX (95% Confidence Interval*)	P-value**
Total Sharp score	2.7	0.1	2.6 (1.4, 3.8)	<0.001
Erosion score	1.6	0.0	1.6 (0.9, 2.2)	<0.001
JSN score	1.0	0.1	0.9 (0.3, 1.4)	0.002

*95% confidence intervals for the differences in change scores between MTX and HUMIRA.
**Based on rank analysis

Before initiation of therapy with HUMIRA, patients should be evaluated for active or latent tuberculosis infection with a tuberculin skin test. If latent infection is diagnosed, appropriate prophylaxis in accordance with the Centers for Disease Control and Prevention guidelines[6] should be instituted. Patients should be instructed to seek medical advice if signs/symptoms (e.g., persistent cough, wasting/weight loss, low grade fever) suggestive of a tuberculosis infection occur.

Immunosuppression
The possibility exists for TNF blocking agents, including HUMIRA, to affect host defenses against infections and malignancies since TNF mediates inflammation and modulates cellular immune responses. In a study of 64 patients with rheumatoid arthritis treated with HUMIRA, there was no evidence of depression of delayed-type hypersensitivity, depression of immunoglobulin levels, or change in enumeration of effector T- and B-cells and NK-cells, monocyte/macrophages, and neutrophils. The impact of treatment with HUMIRA on the development and course of malignancies, as well as active and/or chronic infections is not fully understood (see **WARNINGS, ADVERSE REACTIONS, Infections and Malignancies**). The safety and efficacy of HUMIRA in patients with immunosuppression have not been evaluated.

Immunizations
No data are available on the effects of vaccination in patients receiving HUMIRA. Live vaccines should not be given concurrently with HUMIRA. No data are available on the secondary transmission of infection by live vaccines in patients receiving HUMIRA.

Autoimmunity
Treatment with HUMIRA may result in the formation of autoantibodies and, rarely, in the development of a lupus-like syndrome. If a patient develops symptoms suggestive of a lupus-like syndrome following treatment with HUMIRA, treatment should be discontinued (see **ADVERSE REACTIONS, Autoantibodies**).

Drug Interactions
HUMIRA has been studied in rheumatoid arthritis patients taking concomitant MTX (see **CLINICAL PHARMACOLOGY: Drug Interactions**). The data do not suggest the need for dose adjustment of either HUMIRA or MTX.

Carcinogenesis, Mutagenesis, and Impairment of Fertility
Long-term animal studies of HUMIRA have not been conducted to evaluate the carcinogenic potential or its effect on fertility. No clastogenic or mutagenic effects of HUMIRA were observed in the *in vivo* mouse micronucleus test or the *Salmonella-Escherichia coli* (Ames) assay, respectively.

Pregnancy
Pregnancy Category B—An embryo-fetal perinatal development toxicity study has been performed in cynomolgus monkeys at dosages up to 100 mg/kg (266 times human AUC when given 40 mg subcutaneous with MTX every week or 373 times human AUC when given 40 mg subcutaneous without MTX) and has revealed no evidence of harm to the fetuses due to adalimumab. There are, however, no adequate and well-controlled studies in pregnant women. Because animal reproduction and developmental studies are not always predictive of human response, HUMIRA (adalimumab) should be used during pregnancy only if clearly needed.

Nursing Mothers
It is not known whether adalimumab is excreted in human milk or absorbed systemically after ingestion. Because many drugs and immunoglobulins are excreted in human milk, and because of the potential for serious adverse reactions in nursing infants from HUMIRA, a decision should be made whether to discontinue nursing or to discontinue the drug, taking into account the importance of the drug to the mother.

Pediatric Use
Safety and effectiveness of HUMIRA in pediatric patients have not been established.

Geriatric Use
A total of 519 patients 65 years of age and older, including 107 patients 75 years and older, received HUMIRA in clinical studies. No overall difference in effectiveness was observed between these subjects and younger subjects. The frequency of serious infection and malignancy among HUMIRA treated subjects over age 65 was higher than for those under age 65. Because there is a higher incidence of infections and malignancies in the elderly population in general, caution should be used when treating the elderly.

ADVERSE REACTIONS
General
The most serious adverse reactions were (see **WARNINGS**):
• Serious Infections
• Neurologic Events
• Malignancies

The most common adverse reaction with HUMIRA was injection site reactions. In placebo-controlled trials, 20% of patients treated with HUMIRA developed injection site reactions (erythema and/or itching, hemorrhage, pain or swelling), compared to 14% of patients receiving placebo. Most injection site reactions were described as mild and generally did not necessitate drug discontinuation.

The proportion of patients who discontinued treatment due to adverse events during the double-blind, placebo-controlled portion of Studies I, II, III and IV was 7% for patients taking HUMIRA and 4% for placebo-treated patients.

The most common adverse events leading to discontinuation of HUMIRA were clinical flare reaction (0.7%), rash (0.3%) and pneumonia (0.3%).
Because clinical trials are conducted under widely varying and controlled conditions, adverse reaction rates observed in clinical trials of a drug cannot be directly compared to rates in the clinical trials of another drug and may not predict the rates observed in a broader patient population in clinical practice.

Infections
In placebo-controlled trials, the rate of infection was 1 per patient year in the HUMIRA treated patients and 0.9 per patient year in the placebo-treated patients. The infections consisted primarily of upper respiratory tract infections, bronchitis and urinary tract infections. Most patients continued on HUMIRA after the infection resolved. The incidence of serious infections was 0.04 per patient year in HUMIRA treated patients and 0.02 per patient year in placebo-treated patients. Serious infections observed included pneumonia, septic arthritis, prosthetic and post-surgical infections, erysipelas, cellulitis, diverticulitis, and pyelonephritis (see **WARNINGS**).
Thirteen cases of tuberculosis, including miliary, lymphatic, peritoneal, and pulmonary were reported in clinical trials. Most of the cases of tuberculosis occurred within the first eight months after initiation of therapy and may reflect recrudescence of latent disease. Six cases of invasive opportunistic infections caused by histoplasma, aspergillus, and nocardia were also reported in clinical trials (see **WARNINGS**).

Malignancies
Among 2468 rheumatoid arthritis patients treated in clinical trials with HUMIRA for a median of 24 months, 48 malignancies of various types were observed, including 10 patients with lymphoma. The Standardized Incidence Ratio (SIR) (ratio of observed rate to age-adjusted expected frequency in the general population) for malignancies was 1.0 (95% CI, 0.7, 1.3) and for lymphomas was 5.4 (95% CI, 2.6, 10.0). An increase of up to several fold in the rate of lymphomas has been reported in the rheumatoid arthritis patient population[4], and may be further increased in patients with more severe disease activity[5] (see **WARNINGS-Malignancies**). The other malignancies observed during use of HUMIRA were breast, colon-rectum, uterine-cervical, prostate, melanoma, gallbladder-bile ducts, and other carcinomas.

Autoantibodies
In the controlled trials, 12% of patients treated with HUMIRA and 7% of placebo-treated patients that had negative baseline ANA titers developed positive titers at week 24. One patient out of 2334 treated with HUMIRA developed clinical signs suggestive of new-onset lupus-like syndrome. The patient improved following discontinuation of therapy. No patients developed lupus nephritis or central nervous system symptoms. The impact of long-term treatment with HUMIRA on the development of autoimmune diseases is unknown.

Immunogenicity
Patients in Studies I, II, and III were tested at multiple time points for antibodies to adalimumab during the 6 to 12 month period. Approximately 5% (58 of 1,062) of adult rheumatoid arthritis patients receiving HUMIRA developed low-titer antibodies to adalimumab at least once during treatment, which were neutralizing *in vitro*. Patients treated with concomitant MTX had a lower rate of antibody development than patients on HUMIRA monotherapy (1% versus 12%). No apparent correlation of antibody development to adverse events was observed. With monotherapy, patients receiving every other week dosing may develop antibodies more frequently than those receiving weekly dosing. In patients receiving the recommended dosage of 40 mg every other week as monotherapy, the ACR 20 response was lower among antibody-positive patients than among antibody-negative patients. The long-term immunogenicity of HUMIRA is unknown.
The data reflect the percentage of patients whose test results were considered positive for antibodies to adalimumab in an ELISA assay, and are highly dependent on the sensitivity and specificity of the assay. Additionally the observed incidence of antibody positivity in an assay may be influenced by several factors including sample handling, timing of sample collection, concomitant medications, and underlying disease. For these reasons, comparison of the incidence of antibodies to adalimumab with the incidence of antibodies to other products may be misleading.

Other Adverse Reactions
The data described below reflect exposure to HUMIRA in 2334 patients, including 2073 exposed for 6 months, 1497 exposed for greater than one year and 1380 in adequate and well-controlled studies (Studies I, II, III, and IV). HUMIRA was studied primarily in placebo-controlled trials and in long-term follow up studies for up to 36 months duration. The population had a mean age of 54 years, 77% were female, 91% were Caucasian and had moderately to severely active rheumatoid arthritis. Most patients received 40 mg HUMIRA every other week.
Table 4 summarizes events reported at a rate of at least 5% in patients treated with HUMIRA 40 mg every other week compared to placebo and with an incidence higher than placebo. Adverse event rates in patients treated with HUMIRA 40 mg weekly were similar to rates in patients treated with HUMIRA 40 mg every other week.

Table 4: Adverse Events Reported by ≥5% of Patients Treated with HUMIRA During Placebo-Controlled Period of Rheumatoid Arthritis Studies

Adverse Event (Preferred Term)	HUMIRA 40 mg subcutaneous Every Other Week (N=705) Percentage	Placebo (N=690) Percentage
Respiratory		
Upper respiratory infection	17	13
Sinusitis	11	9
Flu syndrome	7	6
Gastrointestinal		
Nausea	9	8
Abdominal pain	7	4
Laboratory Tests*		
Laboratory test abnormal	8	7
Hypercholesterolemia	6	4
Hyperlipidemia	7	5
Hematuria	5	4
Alkaline phosphatase increased	5	3
Other		
Injection site pain	12	12
Headache	12	8
Rash	12	6
Accidental injury	10	8
Injection site reaction**	8	1
Back pain	6	4
Urinary tract infection	8	5
Hypertension	5	3

* Laboratory test abnormalities were reported as adverse events in European trials
** Does not include erythema and/or itching, hemorrhage, pain or swelling

Other Adverse Events
Other infrequent serious adverse events occurring at an incidence of less than 5% in patients treated with HUMIRA were:
Body As A Whole: Fever, infection, pain in extremity, pelvic pain, sepsis, surgery, thorax pain, tuberculosis reactivated
Cardiovascular System: Arrhythmia, atrial fibrillation, cardiovascular disorder, chest pain, congestive heart failure, coronary artery disorder, heart arrest, hypertensive encephalopathy, myocardial infarct, palpitation, pericardial effusion, pericarditis, syncope, tachycardia, vascular disorder
Collagen Disorder: Lupus erythematosus syndrome
Digestive System: Cholecystitis, cholelithiasis, esophagitis, gastroenteritis, gastrointestinal disorder, gastrointestinal hemorrhage, hepatic necrosis, vomiting
Endocrine System: Parathyroid disorder
Hemic And Lymphatic System: Agranulocytosis, granulocytopenia, leukopenia, lymphoma like reaction, pancytopenia, polycythemia
Metabolic And Nutritional Disorders: Dehydration, healing abnormal, ketosis, paraproteinemia, peripheral edema
Musculo—Skeletal System: Arthritis, bone disorder, bone fracture (not spontaneous), bone necrosis, joint disorder, muscle cramps, myasthenia, pyogenic arthritis, synovitis, tendon disorder
Neoplasia: Adenoma, carcinomas such as breast, gastrointestinal, skin, urogenital, and others; lymphoma, and melanoma.
Nervous System: Confusion, multiple sclerosis, paresthesia, subdural hematoma, tremor
Respiratory System: Asthma, bronchospasm, dyspnea, lung disorder, lung function decreased, pleural effusion, pneumonia
Skin And Appendages: Cellulitis, erysipelas, herpes zoster
Special Senses: Cataract
Thrombosis: Thrombosis leg
Urogenital System: Cystitis, kidney calculus, menstrual disorder, pyelonephritis

OVERDOSAGE
The maximum tolerated dose of HUMIRA has not been established in humans. Multiple doses up to 10 mg/kg have been administered to patients in clinical trials without evidence of dose-limiting toxicities. In case of overdosage, it is

Continued on next page

Humira—Cont.

recommended that the patient be monitored for any signs or symptoms of adverse reactions or effects and appropriate symptomatic treatment instituted immediately.

DOSAGE AND ADMINISTRATION

The recommended dose of HUMIRA for adult patients with rheumatoid arthritis is 40 mg administered every other week as a subcutaneous injection. MTX, glucocorticoids, salicylates, nonsteroidal anti-inflammatory drugs (NSAIDs), analgesics or other DMARDs may be continued during treatment with HUMIRA. Some patients not taking concomitant MTX may derive additional benefit from increasing the dosing frequency of HUMIRA to 40 mg every week.
HUMIRA is intended for use under the guidance and supervision of a physician. Patients may self-inject HUMIRA if their physician determines that it is appropriate and with medical follow-up, as necessary, after proper training in injection technique.
The solution in the syringe should be carefully inspected visually for particulate matter and discoloration prior to subcutaneous administration. If particulates and discolorations are noted, the product should not be used. HUMIRA does not contain preservatives; therefore, unused portions of drug remaining from the syringe should be discarded. NOTE: The needle cover of the syringe contains dry rubber (latex), which should not be handled by persons sensitive to this substance.
Patients using the pre-filled syringes should be instructed to inject the full amount in the syringe (0.8 mL), which provides 40 mg of HUMIRA, according to the directions provided in the Patient Information Leaflet.
Injection sites should be rotated and injections should never be given into areas where the skin is tender, bruised, red or hard (see **PATIENT INFORMATION LEAFLET**).
Instructions For Activating the Needle Stick Device: Cartons for institutional use contain a syringe and needle with a needle protection device (see **HOW SUPPLIED**). To activate the needle stick protection device after injection, hold the syringe in one hand and, with the other hand, slide the outer protective shield over the exposed needle until it locks into place.
Storage and Stability
Do not use beyond the expiration date on the container. HUMIRA must be refrigerated at 2–8° C (36–46° F). DO NOT FREEZE. Protect the pre-filled syringe from exposure to light. Store in original carton until time of administration.

HOW SUPPLIED

HUMIRA™ (adalimumab) is supplied in pre-filled syringes as a preservative-free, sterile solution for subcutaneous administration. The following packaging configurations are available:
Patient Use Syringe Carton
HUMIRA is dispensed in a carton containing two alcohol preps and two dose trays. Each dose tray consists of a single-use, 1 mL pre-filled glass syringe with a fixed 27 gauge ½ inch needle, providing 40 mg (0.8 mL) of HUMIRA. **The NDC number is 0074-3799-02.**
Institutional Use Syringe Carton
Each carton contains two alcohol preps and one tray. Each dose tray consists of a single use, 1 mL pre-filled glass syringe with a fixed 27 gauge ½ inch needle (with a needle stick protection device) providing 40 mg (0.8 mL) of HUMIRA. **The NDC number is 0074-3799-01.**

REFERENCES

1. Arnett FC, Edworthy SM, Bloch DA, et. al. The American Rheumatology Association 1987 Revised Criteria for the Classification of Rheumatoid Arthritis. Arthritis Rheum 1988; 31:315–24.
2. Ramey DR, Fries JF, Singh G. The Health Assessment Questionnaire 1995 - Status and Review. In: Spilker B, ed. "Quality of Life and Pharmacoeconomics in Clinical Trials." 2nd ed. Philadelphia, PA. Lippincott-Raven 1996.
3. Ware JE, Gandek B. Overview of the SF-36 Health Survey and the International Quality of Life Assessment (IQOLA) Project. J Clin Epidemiol 1998; 51(11):903–12.
4. Mellemkjaer L, Linet MS, Gridley G, et al. Rheumatoid Arthritis and Cancer Risk, European Journal of Cancer 1996; 32A (10): 1753–1757.
5. Baecklund E, Ekbom A, Sparen P, et al. Disease Activity and Risk of Lymphoma in Patients With Rheumatoid Arthritis: Nested Case-Control Study, BMJ 1998; 317: 180–181.
6. Centers for Disease Control and Prevention. Targeted Tuberculin Testing and Treatment of Latent Tuberculosis Infection. MMWR 2000; 49(No. RR-6):26–38.

Revised: January, 2003

ABBOTT LABORATORIES
NORTH CHICAGO, IL 60064, U.S.A.
U.S. Govt. Lic. No. 0043

HUMIRA™
(adalimumab)
Patient Information

Read this leaflet carefully before you start taking HUMIRA (**hu-mare-ah**). You should also read this leaflet each time you get your prescription refilled, in case something has changed. The information in this leaflet does not take the placebo of talking with your doctor before you start taking this medicine and at check ups. Talk to your doctor if you have any questions about your treatment with HUMIRA.

What is HUMIRA?
HUMIRA is a medicine that is used in people with moderate to severe rheumatoid arthritis (RA). RA is an inflammatory disease of the joints. People with RA are usually given other medicines for their disease before they are given HUMIRA. HUMIRA is for people with RA who have not responded well enough to these other medicines.
How does HUMIRA work?
HUMIRA is a medicine called a *TNF blocker*, that is a type of protein that blocks the action of a substance your body makes called TNF-alpha. TNF-alpha (tumor necrosis factor alpha) is made by your body's immune system. People with RA have too much of it in their bodies. The extra TNF-alpha in your body can attack normal healthy body tissues and cause inflammation especially in the tissues in your bones, cartilage, and joints. HUMIRA helps reduce the signs and symptoms of RA (such as pain and swollen joints) and may help prevent further damage to your bones and joints.
HUMIRA can block the damage that too much TNF-alpha can cause, and it can also lower your body's ability to fight infections. Taking HUMIRA can make your more prone to getting infections or make any infection you have worse.
Who should not take HUMIRA?
You should not take HUMIRA if you have an allergy to any of the ingredients in HUMIRA (sodium phosphate, sodium citrate, citric acid, mannitol, and polysorbate 80). The needle cover on the pre-filled syringe contains dry natural rubber. Tell your doctor if you have any allergies to rubber or latex.
Before you start taking HUMIRA you should tell your doctor if you have or have had any of the following:
- Any kind of infection including an infection that is in only one place in your body (such as an open cut or sore), or an infection that is in your whole body (such as the flu). Having an infection could put you at risk for serious side effects from HUMIRA. If you are unsure, please ask your doctor.
- A history of infections that keep coming back or other conditions that might increase your risk of infections.
- If you have ever had tuberculosis (TB), or if you have been in close contact with someone who has had tuberculosis. If you develop any of the symptoms of tuberculosis (a dry cough that doesn't go away, weight loss, fever, night sweats) call your doctor right away. Your doctor will need to examine you for TB and perform a skin test.
- If you experience any numbness or tingling or have or have ever had a disease that affects your nervous system like multiple sclerosis.
- If you are scheduled to have major surgery.
- If you are scheduled to be vaccinated for anything.

If you are not sure or have any questions about any of this information, ask your doctor.
What important information do I need to know about side effects with HUMIRA?
Any medicine can have side effects. Like all medicines that affect your immune system, HUMIRA can cause serious side effects. The possible serious side effects include:
Serious infections: There have been rare cases where patients taking HUMIRA or other TNF-blocking agents have developed serious infections, including tuberculosis (TB) and infections caused by bacteria or fungi. Some patients have died when the bacteria that cause infections have spread throughout their body (sepsis).
Nervous system diseases: There have been rare cases of disorders that affect the nervous system of people taking HUMIRA or other TNF blockers. Signs that you could be experiencing a problem affecting your nervous system include: numbness or tingling, problems with your vision, weakness in your legs and dizziness.
Malignancies: There have been very rare cases of certain kinds of cancer in patients taking HUMIRA or other TNF blockers. People with more serious RA that have had the disease for a long time may have a higher than average risk of getting a kind of cancer that affects the lymph system, called lymphoma. If you take HUMIRA or other TNF blockers, your risk may increase.
Lupus-like symptoms: Some patients have developed lupus-like symptoms that got better after their treatment was stopped. If you have chest pains that do not go away, shortness of breath, joint pain or a rash on your cheeks or arms that is sensitive to the sun, call your doctor right away. Your doctor may decide to stop your treatment.
Allergic reactions: If you develop a severe rash, swollen face or difficulty breathing while taking HUMIRA, call your doctor right away.
What are the other more common side effects with HUMIRA?
Many patients experience a reaction where the injection was given. These reactions are usually mild and include redness, rash, swelling, itching or bruising. Usually, the rash will go away within a few days. If the skin around the area where you injected HUMIRA still hurts or is swollen, try using a towel soaked with cold water on the injection site. If you have pain, redness or swelling around the injection site that doesn't go away within a few days or gets worse, call your doctor right away. Other side effects are upper respiratory infections (sinus infections), headache and nausea.
Can I take HUMIRA if I am pregnant or breast-feeding?
HUMIRA has not been studied in pregnant women or nursing mothers, so we don't know what the effects are on pregnant women or nursing babies. You should tell your doctor if you are pregnant, become pregnant or are thinking about becoming pregnant.

Can I take HUMIRA if I am taking other medicines for my RA or other conditions?
Yes, you can take other medicines provided your doctor has prescribed them, or has told you it is ok to take them while you are taking HUMIRA. It is important that you tell your doctor about any other medicines you are taking for other conditions (for example, high blood pressure medicine) before you start taking HUMIRA.
You should also tell your doctor about any over-the-counter drugs, herbal medicines and vitamin and mineral supplements you are taking.
You should not take HUMIRA with other TNF blockers. If you have questions, ask your doctor.
How do I take HUMIRA?
You take HUMIRA by giving yourself an injection under the skin once every other week, or more frequently (every week) if your doctor tells you to. If you accidentally take more HUMIRA than you were told to take, you should call your doctor. Make sure you have been shown how to inject HUMIRA before you do it yourself. You can call your doctor or the HUMIRA Patient Resource Center at 1-800 4HUMIRA (448-6472) if you have any questions about giving yourself an injection. Someone you know can also help you with your injection. Remember to take this medicine just as your doctor has told you and do not miss any doses.
What should I do if I miss a dose of HUMIRA?
If you forgot to take HUMIRA when you are supposed to, inject the next dose right away. Then, take your next dose when your next scheduled dose is due. This will put you back on schedule.
Is one time better than another for taking HUMIRA?
Always follow your doctor's instructions about when and how often to take HUMIRA. To help you remember when to take HUMIRA, you can mark your calendar ahead of time with the stickers provided in the back of the patient information booklet. For other information and ideas you can enroll in a patient support program by calling the HUMIRA Patient Resource Center at 1-800-4HUMIRA (448-6472).
What do I need to do to prepare and give an injection of HUMIRA?
1) Setting up for an injection
- Find a clean flat working surface.
- Remove one dose tray containing a pre-filled syringe of HUMIRA from the refrigerator. Do not use a pre-filled syringe that is frozen or if it has been left in direct sunlight. You will need the following items for each dose:
  - A dose tray containing a pre-filled syringe of HUMIRA with a fixed needle
  - 1 alcohol prep
  - The card with the drawing of the pre-filled syringe

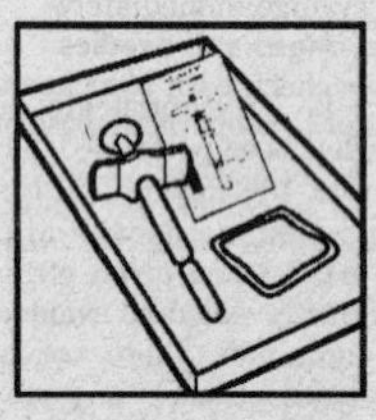

If you do not have all of the pieces you need to give yourself an injection, call your pharmacist. Use only the items provided in the box your HUMIRA comes in.
- Check and make sure the name HUMIRA appears on the dose tray and pre-filled syringe label.
- Check the expiration date on the dose tray label and pre-filled syringe to make sure the date has not passed. Do not use a pre-filled syringe if the date has passed.
- Make sure the liquid in the pre-filled syringe is clear and colorless. Do not use a pre-filled syringe if the liquid is cloudy or discolored or has flakes or particles in it.
- Have a puncture proof container nearby for disposing of used needles and syringes.

FOR YOUR PROTECTION, IT IS IMPORTANT THAT YOU FOLLOW THESE INSTRUCTIONS.
2) Choosing and preparing an injection site
- Wash your hands thoroughly
- Choose a site on the front of your thighs or your abdomen. If you choose your abdomen, you should avoid the area 2 inches around your navel.
  - Choose a different site each time you give yourself an injection. Each new injection should be given at least one inch from a site you used before. Do **NOT** inject into areas where the skin is tender, bruised, red or hard or where you have scars or stretch marks.
  - You may find it helpful to keep notes on the location of previous injections.

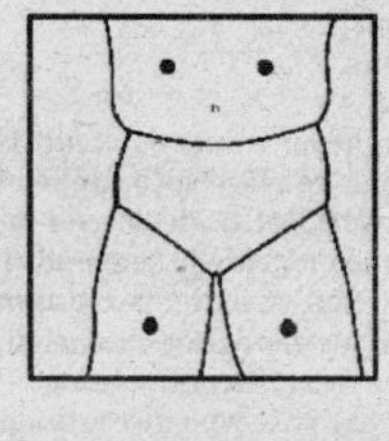

- Wipe the site where HUMIRA is to be injected with an alcohol prep, using a circular motion. Do NOT touch this area again until you are ready to inject.

3) How to prepare your HUMIRA dose for injection with a Pre-filled Syringe

- Hold the syringe upright with the needle facing down. Take the card with the drawing of the syringe and hold it next to the syringe so the drawing and the real syringe are side-by-side. Check to make sure that the amount of liquid in the syringe is the same or very close to the 0.8 mL arrow shown on the card with the drawing of the pre-filled syringe. The top of the liquid may be curved as shown in the drawing. The 0.8 mL arrow should point near the middle of the curved liquid. If the real syringe does not have the correct amount of liquid, DO NOT USE THAT SYRINGE. Call your pharmacist.
- Remove the needle cover taking care not to touch the needle with your fingers or allow it to touch any surface.
- Turn the syringe so the needle is facing up and slowly push the plunger in to push the air in the syringe out through the needle. If a small drop of liquid comes out of the needle that is ok.

4) Injecting HUMIRA

- With your other hand, gently pinch the cleaned area of skin and hold it firmly. Hold the syringe like a pencil at about a 45° angle to the skin.

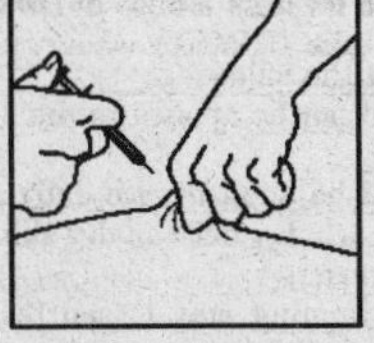

- With a quick, short, "dart-like" motion, push the needle into the skin.
- After the needle is in, let go of the skin. Pull back slightly on the plunger, if blood appears in the syringe it means that you have entered a blood vessel. Do not inject HUMIRA. Withdraw the needle and repeat the steps to choose and clean a new injection site. DO NOT use the same syringe; discard it in your puncture proof container. If no blood appears, slowly push the plunger all the way in until all of the HUMIRA is injected.
- When the syringe is empty, remove the needle from the skin keeping it at the same angle it was when it was inserted.
- Press a cotton ball over the injection site and hold it for 10 seconds. Do **NOT** rub the injection site. If you have slight bleeding, do not be alarmed.
- Dispose of the syringe immediately.

5) Disposing of syringes and needles

You should always check with your healthcare provider for instructions on how to properly dispose of used needles and syringes. You should follow any special state or local laws regarding the proper disposal of needles and syringes. **DO NOT throw the needle or syringe in the household trash or recycle.**

- Place the used needles and syringes in a container made specially for disposing of used syringes and needles (called a "Sharps" container), or a hard plastic container with a screw-on cap or metal container with a plastic lid labeled *"Used Syringes"*. Do not use glass or clear plastic containers.
- Always keep the container out of the reach of children.
- When the container is about two-thirds full, tape the cap or lid down so it does not come off and dispose of it as instructed by your doctor, nurse or pharmacist. DO NOT THROW THE CONTAINER IN THE HOUSEHOLD TRASH OR RECYCLE.
- Used preps may be placed in the trash, unless otherwise instructed by your doctor, nurse or pharmacist. The dose tray and cover may be recycled.

HOW DO I STORE HUMIRA?

Store at 2°C–8°C/36–46°F (in a refrigerator) in the original container until it is used. Protect from light. DO NOT FREEZE HUMIRA. Refrigerated HUMIRA remains stable until the expiration date printed on the pre-filled syringe. If you need to take it with you, such as when traveling, store it in a cool carrier with an ice pack and protect it from light. Keep HUMIRA, injection supplies, and all other medicines out of the reach of children.

Revised: January, 2003

Ref: 03-5236-R2

ABBOTT LABORATORIES
NORTH CHICAGO, IL 60064, U.S.A.

To keep your **PDR** up to date throughout the year, note these revisions on the corresponding pages of the annual volume. Simply write **"See Supplement A"** next to the product heading.

Auxilium Pharmaceuticals, Inc.

160 WEST GERMANTOWN PIKE
NORRISTOWN, PA 19401

Direct Inquiries to:
610-239-1499

TESTIM™ 1% Ⓒ℞

[tĕs-tĭm]
(testosterone gel)
Rx only

DESCRIPTION

Testim™ (testosterone gel) is a clear to translucent hydroalcoholic topical gel containing 1% testosterone. Testim™ provides continuous transdermal delivery of testosterone for 24 hours, following a single application to intact, clean, dry skin of the shoulders and upper arms.

One 5 g or two 5 g tubes of Testim™ contains 50 mg or 100 mg of testosterone, respectively, to be applied daily to the skin's surface. Approximately 10% of the applied testosterone dose is absorbed across skin of average permeability during a 24-hour period.

The active pharmacological ingredient in Testim™ is testosterone.

Testosterone ($C_{19}H_{28}O_2$) MW: 288.42

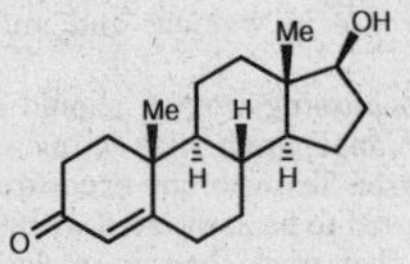

Testosterone

Testosterone USP is a white to practically white crystalline powder chemically described as 17-β hydroxyandrost-4-en-3-one. Inactive ingredients in Testim™ are purified water, pentadecalactone, carbopol, acrylates, propylene glycol, glycerin, polyethylene glycol, ethanol (74%), and tromethamine.

CLINICAL PHARMACOLOGY

Testim™ 1% (testosterone gel) delivers physiologic amounts of testosterone, producing circulating testosterone levels that approximate normal levels (e.g., 300 – 1000 ng/dL) seen in healthy men.

Testosterone – General Androgen Effects:

Testosterone and dihydrotestosterone (DHT), endogenous androgens, are responsible for normal growth and development of the male sex organs and for maintenance of secondary sex characteristics. These effects include the growth and maturation of the prostate, seminal vesicles, penis, and scrotum; the development of male hair distribution, such as facial, pubic, chest, and axillary hair; laryngeal enlargement; vocal cord thickening; alterations in body musculature; and fat distribution.

Male hypogonadism results from insufficient secretion of testosterone and is characterized by low serum testosterone concentrations. Symptoms associated with male hypogonadism include decreased sexual desire with or without impotence, fatigue and loss of energy, mood depression, regression of secondary sexual characteristics, and osteoporosis. Hypogonadism is a risk factor for osteoporosis in men.

Drugs in the androgen class also promote retention of nitrogen, sodium, potassium, phosphorus, and decreased urinary excretion of calcium.

Androgens have been reported to increase protein anabolism and decrease protein catabolism. Nitrogen balance is improved only when there is sufficient intake of calories and protein. Androgens have been reported to stimulate the production of red blood cells by enhancing erythropoietin production.

Androgens are responsible for the growth spurt of adolescence and for the eventual termination of linear growth brought about by fusion of the epiphyseal growth centers. In children, exogenous androgens accelerate linear growth rates but may cause a disproportionate advancement in bone maturation. Use over long periods may result in fusion of the epiphyseal growth centers and termination of the growth process.

During exogenous administration of androgens, endogenous testosterone release may be inhibited through feedback inhibition of pituitary luteinizing hormone (LH). At large doses of exogenous androgens, spermatogenesis may also be suppressed through feedback inhibition of pituitary follicle-stimulating hormone (FSH).

There is a lack of substantial evidence that androgens are effective in accelerating fracture healing or in shortening post-surgical convalescence.

Pharmacokinetics

The pharmacokinetics of Testim™ have been evaluated with administration of doses containing 50 mg and 100 mg of testosterone to adult males with morning testosterone levels ≤300 ng/dL.

Absorption

Testim™ is a topical formulation that dries quickly when applied to the skin surface. The skin serves as a reservoir for the sustained release of testosterone into the systemic circulation. Approximately 10% of the testosterone applied on the skin surface is absorbed into the systemic circulation during a 24-hour period.

Single Dose

In single dose studies, when either Testim™ 50 mg or 100 mg was administered, absorption of testosterone into the blood continued for the entire 24 hour dosing period. Also, mean peak and average serum concentrations within the normal range were achieved within 24 hours.

Multiple Dose

With single daily applications of Testim™ 50 mg and 100 mg, follow-up measurements at 30 and 90 days after starting treatment have confirmed that serum testosterone and DHT concentrations are generally maintained within the normal range.

Figure 1 summarizes the 24-hour pharmacokinetic profile of testosterone for patients maintained on Testim™ 50 mg or Testim™ 100 mg for 30 days.

Figure 1
Mean Steady-State Serum Testosterone (±SD) (ng/dL) Concentrations on Day 30 in Patients Applying Testim™ Once Daily

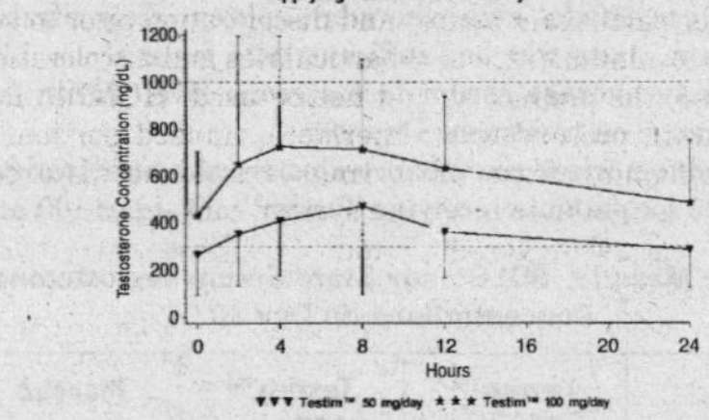

The average daily testosterone concentration produced by Testim™ 100 mg at Day 30 was 612 (± 286) ng/dL and by Testim™ 50 mg at Day 30 was 365 (± 187) ng/dL.

Figure 2 summarizes the 24-hour pharmacokinetic profile of DHT for patients maintained on Testim™ 50 mg or Testim™ 100 mg for 30 days.

Figure 2
Mean Steady-State Serum Dihydrotestosterone (±SD) (pg/mL) Concentrations on Day 30 in Patients Applying Testim™ Once Daily

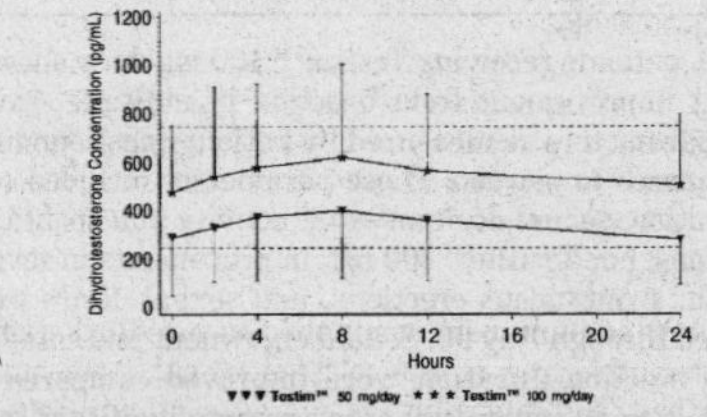

The average daily DHT concentration produced by Testim™ 100 mg at Day 30 was 555 (± 293) pg/mL and by Testim™ 50 mg at Day 30 was 346 (± 212) pg/mL.

Washing

The effect of showering (with mild soap) at 1, 2 and 6 hours post application of Testim™ 100 mg was evaluated in a clinical trial in 12 men. The study demonstrated that the overall effect of washing was to lessen testosterone levels; however, when washing occurred two or more hours post drug application, serum testosterone levels remained within the normal range.

Distribution

Circulating testosterone is chiefly bound in the serum to sex hormone-binding globulin (SHBG) and albumin. The albumin-bound fraction of testosterone easily dissociates from albumin and is presumed to be bioactive. The portion of testosterone bound to SHBG is not considered biologically active. Approximately 40% of testosterone in plasma is bound to SHBG, 2% remains unbound (free) and the rest is bound to albumin and other proteins. The amount of SHBG in the serum and the total testosterone level will determine the distribution of bioactive and nonbioactive androgen.

Metabolism

There is considerable variation in the half-life of testosterone as reported in the literature, ranging from ten to 100 minutes.

Testosterone is metabolized to various 17-keto steroids through two different pathways. The major active metabolites of testosterone are estradiol and DHT. Testosterone is metabolized to DHT by steroid 5α-reductase located in the skin, liver, and the urogenital tract of the male. DHT binds with greater affinity to SHBG than does testosterone. In many tissues, the activity of testosterone depends on its reduction to DHT, which binds to cytosol receptor proteins. The steroid-receptor complex is transported to the nucleus where it initiates transcription and cellular changes related to androgen action. In reproductive tissues, DHT is further metabolized to 3α and 3ß androstanediol. Inactivation of testosterone occurs primarily in the liver.

DHT concentrations increased in parallel with testosterone concentrations during Testim™ treatment. After 90 days of treatment, mean DHT concentrations remained generally within the normal range for Testim™-treated subjects.

Excretion

About 90% of a testosterone dose given intramuscularly is excreted in the urine as glucuronic and sulfuric acid conjugates of testosterone and metabolites; about 6% of a dose is excreted in the feces, mostly in the unconjugated form.

Continued on next page

Testim—Cont.

Special Population

In patients treated with Testim™ there are no observed differences in the average daily serum testosterone concentration at steady-state based on age or cause of hypogonadism. No formal studies were conducted in a pediatric age population or in patients with renal or hepatic insufficiencies.

Clinical Studies

Testim™ was evaluated in a randomized multicenter, multidose, active and placebo controlled 90-day study in 406 adult males with morning testosterone levels ≤300 ng/dL. The study was double-blind for the doses of Testim™ and placebo, but open label for the non-scrotal testosterone transdermal system. During the first 60 days, patients were evenly randomized to Testim™ 50 mg, Testim™ 100 mg, placebo gel, or testosterone transdermal system. At Day 60, patients receiving Testim™ were maintained at the same dose, or were titrated up or down within their treatment group, based on 24-hour averaged serum testosterone concentration levels obtained on Day 30.

Of 192 hypogonadal men who were appropriately titrated with Testim™ and who had sufficient data for analysis, 74% achieved an average serum testosterone level within the normal range on treatment Day 90.

Table 1 summarizes the mean testosterone concentrations on Day 30 for patients receiving Testim™ 50 mg or 100 mg.

Table 1: Mean (± SD) Steady-State Serum Testosterone Concentrations on Day 30

	Testim™ 50 mg n=94	Testim™ 100 mg n=95	Placebo n=93
C_{avg} (ng/dL)	365 ± 187	612 ± 286	216 ± 79
C_{max} (ng/dL)	538 ± 371	897 ± 565	271 ± 110
C_{min} (ng/dL)	223 ± 126	394 ± 189	164 ± 64

At Day 30, patients receiving Testim™ 100 mg daily showed significant improvement from baseline in multiple sexual function parameters as measured by patient questionnaires when compared to placebo. These parameters included sexual motivation, sexual desire, sexual activity and spontaneous erections. For Testim™ 100 mg, improvements in sexual motivation, spontaneous erections, and sexual desire were maintained through Day 90. Sexual enjoyment and satisfaction with erection duration were improved compared to baseline but these improvements were not significant compared to the placebo group.

In Testim™-treated patients, the number of days in which sexual activity was reported to occur increased by 123% from baseline at Day 30 and was still increased from baseline by 59% at Day 90. The number of days with spontaneous erections increased by 137% at Day 30 and was maintained at 78% at Day 90 for Testim™-treated patients compared to baseline.

Table 2 summarizes the changes in body composition at Day 90 for patients receiving Testim™ 50 mg or 100 mg as measured by standardized whole body DEXA (Dual Energy X-ray Absorptiometry) scanning.

[See table 2 below]

At Day 90, mean increases from baseline in lean body mass and mean decreases from baseline in total fat mass and percent body fat in Testim™-treated patients were significant when compared to placebo-treated patients.

Potential for Testosterone Transfer

The potential for dermal testosterone transfer following Testim™ use was evaluated in two clinical trials with males dosed with Testim™ and their untreated female partners.

In the first trial (AUX-TG-206), 30 couples were evenly randomized to five groups. In the first four groups, 100 mg of Testim™ was applied to the male abdomen and the couples were then asked to rub abdomen-to-abdomen for 15 minutes at 1 hour, 4 hours, 8 hours or 12 hours after dose application, respectively. In these couples, serum testosterone concentrations in female partners increased from baseline by at least 4 times and potential for transfer was seen at all timepoints.

When 6 males used a shirt to cover the abdomen at 15 minutes post-application and partners again rubbed abdomens for 15 minutes at the 1 hour timepoint, the potential for transfer was markedly reduced.

In the second trial (AUX-TG-209), 24 couples were evenly randomized to four groups. Testim™ 100 mg was applied to the male arms and shoulders. In one group, 15 minutes of direct skin-to-skin rubbing began at 4 hours after application. In these six women, all of whom showered immediately after the rubbing activity, mean maximum serum testosterone concentrations increased from baseline by approximately 4 times. When males wore a long-sleeved T-shirt and rubbing was started at 1 and at 4 hours after application, the transfer of testosterone from male to female partners was prevented.

Table 2: Effect of Testim™ on Lean Body Mass, Total Fat Mass and % Body Fat

Days of Treatment	Lean Body Mass (Muscle) (kg)	Total Fat Mass (kg)	% Body Fat
Baseline	61.6	29.4	30.9
Day 90	63.3	28.6	29.8
Change from Baseline	↑1.6	↓0.8	↓1.1

INDICATIONS AND USAGE

Testim™ is indicated for testosterone replacement therapy in adult males for conditions associated with a deficiency or absence of endogenous testosterone:

1. Primary hypogonadism (congenital or acquired): testicular failure due to cryptorchidism, bilateral torsion, orchitis, vanishing testis syndrome, orchiectomy, Klinefelter's syndrome, chemotherapy, or toxic damage from alcohol or heavy metals. These men usually have low serum testosterone levels and gonadotropins (FSH, LH) above the normal range.
2. Hypogonadotropic hypogonadism (congenital or acquired): idiopathic gonadotropin or luteinizing hormone-releasing hormone (LHRH) deficiency or pituitary-hypothalamic injury from tumors, trauma, or radiation. These men have low testosterone serum levels but have gonadotropins in the normal or low range.

Testim™ has not been clinically evaluated in males under 18 years of age.

CONTRAINDICATIONS

Androgens are contraindicated in men with carcinoma of the breast or known or suspected carcinoma of the prostate. Testim™ is not indicated for use in women, has not been evaluated for use in women, and must not be used in women.

Pregnant and nursing women should avoid skin contact with Testim™ application sites on men. Testosterone may cause fetal harm. Testosterone exposure during pregnancy has been reported to be associated with fetal abnormalities. In the event that unwashed or unclothed skin to which Testim™ has been applied comes in direct contact with the skin of a pregnant or nursing woman, the general area of contact on the woman should be immediately washed with soap and water.

Testim™ should not be used in patients with known hypersensitivity to any of its ingredients, including testosterone USP that is chemically synthesized from soy.

WARNINGS

1. Testim™ should not be applied to the abdomen.
2. Prolonged use of high doses of orally active 17-alpha-alkyl androgens (e.g., methyltestosterone) has been associated with serious hepatic adverse effects (peliosis hepatitis, hepatic neoplasms, cholestatic hepatitis, and jaundice). Peliosis hepatitis can be a life-threatening or fatal complication. Long-term therapy with testosterone enanthate, which elevates blood levels for prolonged periods has produced multiple hepatic adenomas. Transdermal testosterone is not known to produce these adverse effects.
3. Geriatric patients treated with androgens may be at an increased risk for the development of prostatic hyperplasia and prostatic carcinoma.
4. Geriatric patients and other patients with clinical or demographic characteristics that are recognized to be associated with an increased risk of prostate cancer should be evaluated for the presence of prostate cancer prior to initiation of testosterone replacement therapy. In men receiving testosterone replacement therapy, surveillance for prostate cancer should be consistent with current practices for eugonadal men (see PRECAUTIONS: Carcinogenesis, Mutagenesis, Impairment of Fertility and Laboratory Tests).
5. Edema, with or without congestive heart failure, may be a serious complication in patients with preexisting cardiac, renal, or hepatic disease. In addition to discontinuation of the drug, diuretic therapy may be required.
6. Gynecomastia occasionally develops and occasionally persists in patients being treated for hypogonadism.
7. The treatment of hypogonadal men with testosterone may potentiate sleep apnea in some patients, especially those with risk factors such as obesity or chronic lung diseases.

PRECAUTIONS

Transfer of testosterone to another person can occur when vigorous skin-to-skin contact is made with the application site (See Clinical Studies).

The following precautions are recommended to minimize potential transfer of testosterone from Testim™-treated skin to another person:

- Patients should wash their hands thoroughly and immediately with soap and water after application of Testim™. Studies of hand-washing show that Testim™ is effectively removed from the skin surface by thorough washing with soap and water.
- Patients should cover the application site(s) with clothing after the gel has dried (e.g. a shirt).
- Prior to any situation in which direct skin-to-skin contact is anticipated, patients should wash the application sites thoroughly with soap and water so as to remove drug residue.
- In the event that unwashed or unclothed skin to which Testim™ has been applied does come in direct contact with the skin of another person, the general area of contact on the other person should be washed thoroughly with soap and water as soon as possible.

Changes in body hair distribution, significant increase in acne, or other signs of virilization of the female partner should be brought to the attention of a physician.

General

The physician should instruct patients to report any of the following:

- Too frequent or persistent erections of the penis.
- Any changes in skin color, ankle swelling or unexplained nausea and vomiting.
- Breathing disturbances, including those associated with sleep.

Information for Patients

Advise patients to carefully read the information brochure that accompanies each carton of 30 Testim™ single-use tubes.

Advise patients of the following:

- Testim™ should not be applied to the scrotum, penis, or abdomen.
- Testim™ should be applied once daily at approximately the same time each day to clean dry skin of the shoulders and/or upper arms.
- Washing or swimming may lessen testosterone levels; however, when washing occurs two or more hours post drug application, serum testosterone levels remain within the normal range.
- Testim™ may be transferred to another person by vigorous contact with the application site. Potential for transfer may be reduced by washing hands thoroughly after application, by wearing clothing to cover the sites, and by washing the application sites thoroughly with soap and water prior to any direct skin-to-skin contact.

Laboratory Tests

1. Hemoglobin and hematocrit levels should be checked periodically (to detect polycythemia) in patients on long-term androgen therapy.
2. Liver function, prostate specific antigen (PSA), cholesterol, and high-density lipoprotein (HDL) should be checked periodically.
3. To ensure proper dosing, serum testosterone concentrations should be measured (see DOSAGE AND ADMINISTRATION).

Drug Interactions

Oxyphenbutazone: Concurrent administration of oxyphenbutazone and androgens may result in elevated serum levels of oxyphenbutazone.

Insulin: In diabetic patients, the metabolic effects of androgens may decrease blood glucose and, therefore, insulin requirements.

Propranolol: In a published pharmacokinetic study of an injectable testosterone product, administration of testosterone cypionate led to an increased clearance of propranolol in the majority of men tested. It is unknown if this would apply to Testim™.

Corticosteroids: The concurrent administration of testosterone with ACTH or corticosteroids may enhance edema formation; thus these drugs should be administered cautiously, particularly in patients with cardiac or hepatic disease.

Drug/Laboratory Test Interactions

Androgens may decrease levels of thyroxin-binding globulin, resulting in decreased total T4 serum levels and increased resin uptake of T3 and T4. Free thyroid hormone levels remain unchanged, however, and there is no clinical evidence of thyroid dysfunction.

Carcinogenesis, Mutagenesis, Impairment of Fertility

Animal Data: Testosterone has been tested by subcutaneous injection and implantation in mice and rats. In mice, the implant induced cervical-uterine tumors, which metastasized in some cases. There is suggestive evidence that injection of testosterone into some strains of female mice increases their susceptibility to hepatoma. Testosterone is also known to increase the number of tumors and decrease the degree of differentiation of chemically induced carcinomas of the liver in rats.

Human Data: There are rare reports of hepatocellular carcinoma in patients receiving long-term oral therapy with androgens in high doses. Withdrawal of the drugs did not lead to regression of the tumors in all cases.

Geriatric patients treated with androgens may be at an increased risk for the development of prostatic hyperplasia and prostatic carcinoma. Geriatric patients and other patients with clinical or demographic characteristics that are recognized to be associated with an increased risk of prostate cancer should be evaluated for the presence of prostate cancer prior to initiation of testosterone replacement therapy.

In men receiving testosterone replacement therapy, surveillance for prostate cancer should be consistent with current practices for eugonadal men.

Pregnancy Category X (see Contraindications) – Teratogenic Effects: Testim™ is not indicated for women and must not be used in women. Testosterone may cause fetal harm.

Table 3: Incidence of Adverse Events Judged Possibly, Probably or Definitely Related to Use of Testim™ in the Controlled Clinical Trial

Event	Testim™ 50 mg	Testim™ 100 mg	Placebo
Application Site Reactions	2%	4%	3%
Benign Prostatic Hyperplasia	0%	1%	1%
Blood Pressure Diastolic Decreased	1%	0%	0%
Blood Pressure Increased	1%	1%	0%
Gynecomastia	1%	0%	0%
Headache	1%	1%	0%
Hematocrit/hemoglobin Increased	1%	2%	0%
Hot Flushes	1%	0%	0%
Insomnia	1%	0%	0%
Lacrimation Increased	1%	0%	0%
Mood Swings	1%	0%	0%
Smell Disorder	1%	0%	0%
Spontaneous Penile Erection	1%	0%	0%
Taste Disorder	1%	1%	0%

Nursing Mothers: Testim™ is not indicated for women and must not be used in nursing mothers.

Pediatric Use: Safety and efficacy of Testim™ in patients <18 years old has not been established.

ADVERSE REACTIONS

In a controlled clinical study, 304 patients were treated with Testim™ 50 mg or 100 mg or placebo gel for up to 90 days. Two hundred-five (205) patients received Testim™ 50 mg or 100 mg daily and 99 patients received placebo. Patients with adverse events that were possibly or probably related to study drug and reported by ≥1% of the Testim™ patients and greater than placebo are listed in Table 3. [See table 3 above]

The following adverse events possibly or probably related to Testim™ occurred in fewer than 1% of patients but were greater in Testim™ groups compared to the placebo group: activated partial thromboplastin time prolonged, blood creatinine increased, prothrombin time prolonged, appetite increased, sensitive nipples, and acne.

In this clinical trial of Testim™, six patients had adverse events that led to their discontinuation. These events included: vertigo, coronary artery disease, depression with suicidal ideation, urinary tract infection/pneumonia (none of which were considered related to Testim™ administration), mood swings and hypertension. No Testim™ patients discontinued due to skin reaction.

In one foreign Phase 3 trial, one subject discontinued due to a skin-related adverse event. In the pivotal U.S. and European Phase 3 trials combined, at the 50 mg dosage strength, the percentage of subjects reporting clinically notable increases in hematocrit or hemoglobin were similar to placebo. However, in the 100 mg dose group, 2.3% and 2.8% of patients had a clinically notable increase in hemoglobin (≥ 19 gm/dL) or hematocrit (≥ 58%), respectively.

In the combined ongoing U.S. and European open label extension studies, approximately 140 patients received Testim™ for at least 6 months. The preliminary results from these studies are consistent with those reported for the U.S. controlled clinical trial.

DRUG ABUSE AND DEPENDENCE

Testim™ contains testosterone, a Schedule III controlled substance as defined by the Anabolic Steroids Control Act. Oral ingestion of Testim™ will not result in clinically significant serum testosterone concentrations due to extensive first-pass metabolism.

OVERDOSAGE

There were no reports of overdose in the Testim™ clinical trials. There is one report of acute overdosage by injection of testosterone enanthate: testosterone levels of up to 11,400 ng/dL were implicated in a cerebrovascular accident.

DOSAGE AND ADMINISTRATION

The recommended starting dose of Testim™ is 5 g of gel (one tube) containing 50 mg of testosterone applied once daily (preferably in the morning) to clean, dry intact skin of the shoulders and/or upper arms. Morning serum testosterone levels should then be measured approximately 14 days after initiation of therapy to ensure proper serum testosterone levels are achieved. If the serum testosterone concentration is below the normal range, or if the desired clinical response is not achieved, the daily Testim™ dose may be increased from 5 g (one tube) to 10 g (two tubes) as instructed by the physician.

Upon opening the tube the entire contents should be squeezed into the palm of the hand and immediately applied to the shoulders and/or upper arms. Application sites should be allowed to dry for a few minutes prior to dressing. Hands should be washed thoroughly with soap and water after Testim™ has been applied.

In order to prevent transfer to another person, clothing should be worn to cover the application sites. If direct skin-to-skin contact with another person is anticipated, the application sites must be washed thoroughly with soap and water.

In order to maintain serum testosterone levels in the normal range, the sites of application should not be washed for at least two hours after application of Testim™.

Do not apply Testim™ to the genitals or to the abdomen.

HOW SUPPLIED

Testim™ contains testosterone, a Schedule III controlled substance as defined by the Anabolic Steroids Control Act. Testim™ is supplied in unit-dose tubes in cartons of 30. Each tube contains 50 mg testosterone in 5 g of gel, and is supplied as follows:

NDC Number	Strength	Package Size
66887-001-05	1% (50 mg)	30 tubes: 5 g per tube

Storage
Store at room temperature 25°C (77°F); Excursions permitted to 15°-30°C (59°-86°F) [See USP Controlled Room Temperature].

Disposal
Used Testim™ tubes should be discarded in household trash in a manner that prevents accidental application or ingestion by children or pets; contents flammable.

Manufactured for:
Auxilium Pharmaceuticals, Inc.
Norristown, PA, 19401 USA
By: DPT Laboratories, Ltd.
San Antonio, TX 78215
Labeling Code: AA2500.07
Issued: February, 2003
0206-04
127933

Berlex Laboratories
6 WEST BELT
WAYNE, NJ 07470
www.Berlex.com

Direct Inquiries to:
(973) 694-4100

For Medical Information and to report adverse drug events Contact:
Global Medical Safety-USA
6 West Belt
Wayne, NJ 07470-6806
(888) BERLEX-4, Option 3

FINACEA™ ℞
For Dermatologic Use Only—Not for Ophthalmic, Oral, or Intravaginal Use

Rx only

DESCRIPTION

FINACEA™ (azelaic acid) Gel, 15%, contains azelaic acid, a naturally occurring saturated dicarboxylic acid. Chemically, azelaic acid is 1,7-heptanedicarboxylic acid, with the molecular formula $C_9H_{16}O_4$, a molecular weight of 188.22, and the structural formula:

[HOOC-(CH$_2$)$_7$-COOH]

Azelaic acid is a white, odorless crystalline solid that is poorly soluble in water at 20°C (0.24%), but freely soluble in boiling water and in ethanol.

Each gram of FINACEA™ Gel, 15%, contains 0.15 gm azelaic acid (15% w/w) as the active ingredient in an aqueous gel base containing benzoic acid (as a preservative), disodium-EDTA, lecithin, medium-chain triglycerides, polyacrylic acid, polysorbate 80, propylene glycol, purified water, and sodium hydroxide to adjust pH.

CLINICAL PHARMACOLOGY

The mechanism(s) by which azelaic acid interferes with the pathogenic events in rosacea are unknown.

Pharmacokinetics: The percutaneous absorption of azelaic acid after topical application of FINACEA™ Gel, 15%, could not be reliably determined. Mean plasma azelaic acid concentrations in rosacea patients treated with FINACEA™ Gel, 15%, twice daily for at least 8 weeks are in the range of 42 to 63.1 ng/mL. These values are within the maximum concentration range of 24.0 to 90.5 ng/mL observed in rosacea patients treated with vehicle only. This indicates that FINACEA™ Gel, 15%, does not increase plasma azelaic acid concentration beyond the range derived from nutrition and endogenous metabolism.

In vitro and human data suggest negligible cutaneous metabolism of ^{3}H-azelaic acid 20% cream after topical application. Azelaic acid is mainly excreted unchanged in the urine, but undergoes some β-oxidation to shorter chain dicarboxylic acids.

CLINICAL STUDIES

FINACEA™ Gel, 15%, was evaluated for the treatment of mild to moderate papulopustular rosacea in 2 clinical trials comprising a total of 664 (333 active to 331 vehicle). Both trials were multicenter, randomized, double-blind, vehicle-controlled 12-week studies with identical protocols. Overall, 92.5% of patients were Caucasian and 73% of patients were women, and the mean age was 49 (range 21 to 86) years. Enrolled patients had mild to moderate rosacea with a mean lesion count of 18 (range 8 to 60) inflammatory papules and pustules. Subjects without papules and pustules, with nodules, rhinophyma, or ocular involvement, and a history of hypersensitivity to propylene glycol or to any other ingredients of the study drug were excluded. FINACEA™ Gel, 15%, or its vehicle were to be applied twice daily for 12 weeks; no other topical or systemic medication affecting the course of rosacea and/or evaluability was to be used during the studies. Patients were instructed to avoid spicy foods, thermally hot foods and drinks, and alcoholic beverages during the study, and to use only very mild soaps or soapless cleansing lotion for facial cleansing.

The primary efficacy endpoints were both 1) change from baseline in inflammatory lesion counts and 2) success defined as a score of clear or minimal with at least a 2 step reduction from baseline on the investigator's Global Assessment (IGA):

CLEAR:
No papules and/or pustules; no or residual erythema; no or mild to moderate telangiectasia

MINIMAL:
Rare papules and/or pustules; residual to mild erythema; mild to moderate telangiectasia

MILD:
Few papules and/or pustules; mild erythema; mild to moderate telangiectasia

MILD TO MODERATE:
Distinct number of papules and/or pustules; mild to moderate erythema; mild to moderate telangiectasia

MODERATE:
Pronounced number of papules and/or pustules; moderate erythema; mild to moderate telangiectasia

MODERATE TO SEVERE:
Many papules and/or pustules, occasionally with large inflamed lesions; moderate erythema; moderate degree of telangiectasia

SEVERE:
Numerous papules and/or pustules, occasionally with confluent areas of inflamed lesions; moderate or severe erythema; moderate or severe telangiectasia

Primary efficacy assessment was based on the intent-to-treat (ITT) population with last observation carried forward (LOCF).

Both studies demonstrated a statistically significant difference in favor of FINACEA™ Gel, 15%, over its vehicle in reducing the number of inflammatory papules and pustules associated with rosacea and with success on the IGA in the ITT-LOCF population at the end of treatment.
[See table 1 at top of next page]

FINACEA™ Gel, 15%, was superior to the vehicle with regard to success based on the investigator's global assessment of rosacea on a 7-point static score at the end of treatment, (ITT population; Table 2).
[See table 2 at top of next page]

INDICATIONS AND USAGE

FINACEA™ Gel, 15%, is indicated for topical treatment of inflammatory papules and pustules of mild to moderate rosacea. Patients should be instructed to avoid spicy foods,

Continued on next page

Finacea—Cont.

thermally hot foods and drinks, alcoholic beverages and to use only very mild soaps or soapless cleansing lotion for facial cleansing.

CONTRAINDICATIONS

FINACEA™ Gel, 15%, is contraindicated in individuals with a history of hypersensitivity to propylene glycol or any other component of the formulation.

WARNINGS

FINACEA™ Gel, 15%, is for dermatologic use only, and not for ophthalmic, oral or intravaginal use.

There have been isolated reports of hypopigmentation after use of azelaic acid. Since azelaic acid has not been well studied in patients with dark complexion, these patients should be monitored for early signs of hypopigmentation.

PRECAUTIONS

General: Contact with the eyes should be avoided. If sensitivity or severe irritation develops with the use of FINACEA™ Gel, 15%, treatment should be discontinued and appropriate therapy instituted. The safety and efficacy of FINACEA™ Gel, 15%, has not been studied beyond 12 weeks.

Information for Patients: Patients using FINACEA™ Gel, 15%, should receive the following information and instructions:

- FINACEA™ Gel, 15%, is to be used only as directed by the physician.
- FINACEA™ Gel, 15%, is for external use only. It is not to be used orally, intravaginally, or for the eyes.
- Cleanse affected area(s) with a very mild soap or a soapless cleansing lotion and pat dry with a soft towel before applying FINACEA™ Gel, 15%. Avoid alcoholic cleansers, tinctures and astringents, abrasives and peeling agents.
- Avoid contact of FINACEA™ Gel, 15%, with the mouth, eyes and other mucous membranes. If it does come in contact with the eyes, wash the eyes with large amounts of water and consult a physician if eye irritation persists.
- The hands should be washed following application of FINACEA™ Gel, 15%.
- Cosmetics may be applied after FINACEA™ Gel, 15%, has dried.
- Skin irritation (e.g., pruritus, burning, or stinging) may occur during use of FINACEA™ Gel, 15%, usually during the first few weeks of treatment. If irritation is excessive or persists, use of FINACEA™ Gel, 15%, should be discontinued, and patients should consult their physician (see **ADVERSE REACTIONS**).
- Avoid any foods and beverages that might provoke erythema, flushing, and blushing (including spicy food, alcoholic beverages, and thermally hot drinks, including hot coffee and tea).
- Patients should report abnormal changes in skin color to their physician
- Avoid the use of occlusive dressings or wrappings.

Drug Interactions: There have been no formal studies of the interaction of FINACEA™ Gel, 15%, with other drugs.

Carcinogenesis, Mutagenesis, Impairment of Fertility: Long-term animal studies have not been performed to evaluate the carcinogenic potential of FINACEA™ Gel, 15%. Azelaic acid was not mutagenic or clastogenic in a battery of *in vitro* (Ames assay, HGPRT in V79 cells (Chinese hamster lung cells), and chromosomal aberration assay in human lymphocytes) and *in vivo* (dominant lethal assay in mice and mouse micronucleus assay) genotoxicity tests.

Oral administration of azelaic acid at dose levels up to 2500 mg/kg/day (162 times the maximum recommended human dose based on body surface area) did not affect fertility or reproductive performance in male or female rats.

Pregnancy: Teratogenic Effects: Pregnancy Category B

There are no adequate and well-controlled studies of topically administered azelaic acid in pregnant women. The experience with FINACEA™ Gel, 15%, when used by pregnant women is too limited to permit assessment of the safety of its use during pregnancy.

Dermal embryofetal developmental toxicology studies have not been performed with azelaic acid, 15%, gel. Oral embryofetal developmental studies were conducted with azelaic acid in rats, rabbits, and cynomolgus monkeys. Azelaic acid was administered during the period of organogeneisis in all three animal species. Embryotoxicity was observed in rats, rabbits, and monkeys at oral doses of azelaic acid that generated some maternal toxicity. Embryotoxicity was observed in rats given 2500 mg/kg/day (162 times the maximum recommended human dose based on body surface area), rabbits given 150 or 500 mg/kg/day (19 or 65 times the maximum recommended human dose based on body surface area) and cynomolgus monkeys given 500 mg/kg/day (65 times the maximum recommended human dose based on body surface area) azelaic acid. No teratogenic effects were observed in the oral embryofetal developmental studies conducted in rats, rabbits and cynomolgus monkeys.

An oral peri- and post-natal developmental study was conducted in rats. Azelaic acid was administered from gestational day 15 through day 21 postpartum up to a dose level of 2500 mg/kg/day. Embryotoxicity was observed in rats at an oral dose that generated some maternal toxicity (2500 mg/kg/day; 162 times the maximum recommended human dose based on body surface area). In addition, slight disturbances in the post-natal development of fetuses was noted in rats at oral doses that generated some maternal toxicity (500 and 2500 mg/kg/day; 32 and 162 times the maximum recommended human dose based on body surface area). No effects on sexual maturation of the fetuses were noted in this study.

Because animal reproduction studies are not always predictive of human response, this drug should be used only if clearly needed during pregnancy.

Nursing Mothers: Equilibrium dialysis was used to assess human milk partitioning *in vitro*. At an azelaic acid concentration of 25 µg/mL, the milk/plasma distribution coefficient was 0.7 and the milk/buffer distribution was 1.0, indicating that passage of drug into maternal milk may occur. Since less than 4% of a topically applied dose of AZELEX® Cream, 20%, is systemically absorbed, the uptake of azelaic acid into maternal milk is not expected to cause a significant change from baseline azelaic acid levels in the milk. However, caution should be exercised when FINACEA™ Gel, 15%, is administered to a nursing mother.

Pediatric Use: Safety and effectiveness of FINACEA™ Gel, 15%, in pediatric patients have not been established.

Geriatric: Clinical studies of FINACEA™ Gel, 15%, did not include sufficient numbers of subjects aged 65 and over to determine whether they respond differently from younger subjects.

ADVERSE REACTIONS

In the 2 vehicle controlled, identically designed U.S. clinical studies, treatment safety was monitored in 664 patients who used FINACEA™ Gel, 15%, (N=333), or the gel vehicle (N=331), twice daily for 12 weeks.
[See table 3 above]

FINACEA™ Gel, 15%, and its vehicle caused irritant reactions at the application site in human dermal safety studies. FINACEA™ Gel, 15%, caused significantly more irritation than its vehicle in a cumulative irritation study. Some improvement in irritation was demonstrated over the course of the clinical studies, but this improvement might be attributed to subject dropouts. No phototoxicity or photoallergenicity were reported in human dermal safety studies.

In patients using azelaic acid formulations, the following additional adverse experiences have been reported rarely: worsening of asthma, vitiligo depigmentation, small depigmented spots, hypertrichosis, reddening (signs of keratosis pilaris), and exacerbation of recurrent herpes labialis.

OVERDOSAGE

FINACEA™ Gel, 15%, is intended for cutaneous use only. If pronounced local irritation occurs, patients should be directed to discontinue use and appropriate therapy should be instituted (see **PRECAUTIONS**).

DOSAGE AND ADMINISTRATION

A thin layer of FINACEA™ Gel, 15%, should be gently massaged into the affected areas on the face twice daily, in the morning and evening. FINACEA™ Gel, 15%, has only been studied up to 12 weeks in patients with mild to moderate rosacea (See **CLINICAL STUDIES**).

HOW SUPPLIED

FINACEA™ Gel, 15%, is supplied in tubes in the following size: 30 g – NDC 50419-825-01

Storage

Store at 25°C (77°F); excursions permitted between 15°-30° C (59°-86°F) [See USP Controlled Room Temperature].

Distributed under license; *U.S. Patent No 4,713,394*

© 2003, Berlex Laboratories. All rights reserved.

January 2003

AZELEX® is a registered trademark of Allergan, Inc.
Manufactured by Schering S.p.A., Segrate, Milan, Italy
Distributed by:
BERLEX® Laboratories, Montville, NJ 07045
2189827   6058000

Table 1. Inflammatory Papules and Pustules (ITT population)[1]

	Study One FINACEA™ Gel, 15% N = 164	Study One VEHICLE N = 165	Study Two FINACEA™ Gel, 15% N = 169	Study Two VEHICLE N = 166
Mean Lesion Count Baseline	17.5	17.6	17.9	18.5
End of Treatment[1]	6.8	10.5	9.0	12.1
Mean Percent Reduction End of Treatment[1]	57.9%	39.9%	50.0%	38.2%

[1]ITT population with last observation carried forward (LOCF);

Table 2. Investigator's Global Assessment at the End of Treatment[1]

	Study One FINACEA™ Gel, 15% N = 164	Study One VEHICLE N = 165	Study Two FINACEA™ Gel, 15% N = 169	Study Two VEHICLE N = 166
Clear, Minimal or Mild at End of Treatment (% of Patients)	61%	40%	62%	48%

[1]ITT population with last observation carried forward (LOCF);

Table 3. Cutaneous Adverse Events Occurring in ≥1% of Subjects in the Rosacea Trials by Treatment Group and Maximum Intensity*

	FINACEA™ Gel, 15% N=333 (100%)			Vehicle N=331 (100%)		
	Mild n=86 (26%)	Moderate n=44 (13%)	Severe n=20 (6%)	Mild n=49 (15%)	Moderate n=27 (8%)	Severe n=5 (2%)
Burning/stinging/tingling	66 (20%)	30 (9%)	12 (4%)	8 (2%)	6 (2%)	2 (1%)
Pruritus	24 (7%)	14 (4%)	3 (1%)	9 (3%)	6 (2%)	0 (0%)
Scaling/dry skin/xerosis	21 (6%)	8 (2%)	4 (1%)	33 (10%)	12 (4%)	1 (0%)
Erythema/irritation	6 (2%)	6 (2%)	1 (0%)	8 (2%)	4 (1%)	2 (1%)
Edema	3 (1%)	2 (1%)	0 (0%)	3 (1%)	0 (0%)	0 (0%)
Contact dermatitis	2 (1%)	2 (1%)	0 (0%)	1 (0%)	0 (0%)	0 (0%)
Acne	2 (1%)	1 (0%)	0 (0%)	1 (0%)	0 (0%)	0 (0%)
Seborrhea	2 (1%)	0 (0%)	0 (0%)	0 (0%)	0 (0%)	0 (0%)
Photo-sensitivity	1 (0%)	0 (0%)	0 (0%)	3 (1%)	1 (0%)	1 (0%)
Skin disease	1 (0%)	0 (0%)	0 (0%)	1 (0%)	2 (1%)	0 (0%)

*Subjects may have >1 cutaneous adverse event; thus, the sum of the frequencies of preferred terms may exceed the number of subjects with at least 1 cutaneous adverse event

---

To keep your **PDR** up to date throughout the year, note these revisions on the corresponding pages of the annual volume. Simply write **"See Supplement A"** next to the product heading.

Biogen, Inc.
14 CAMBRIDGE CENTER
CAMBRIDGE, MA 02142

Direct Inquiries to:
Customer Service (800) 456-2255
Fax (617) 679-3100

AMEVIVE® ℞
[ă' mĕ-vēv]
(alefacept)
℞ only

DESCRIPTION
AMEVIVE® (alefacept) is an immunosuppressive dimeric fusion protein that consists of the extracellular CD2-binding portion of the human leukocyte function antigen-3 (LFA-3) linked to the Fc (hinge, C_H2 and C_H3 domains) portion of human IgG1. Alefacept is produced by recombinant DNA technology in a Chinese Hamster Ovary (CHO) mammalian cell expression system. The molecular weight of alefacept is 91.4 kilodaltons.
AMEVIVE® is supplied as a sterile, white-to-off-white, preservative-free, lyophilized powder for parenteral administration. After reconstitution with 0.6 mL of the supplied Sterile Water for Injection, USP, the solution of AMEVIVE® is clear, with a pH of approximately 6.9.
AMEVIVE® is available in two formulations. AMEVIVE® for intramuscular injection contains 15 mg alefacept per 0.5 mL of reconstituted solution. AMEVIVE® for intravenous injection contains 7.5 mg alefacept per 0.5 mL of reconstituted solution. Both formulations also contain 12.5 mg sucrose, 5.0 mg glycine, 3.6 mg sodium citrate dihydrate, and 0.06 mg citric acid monohydrate per 0.5 mL.

CLINICAL PHARMACOLOGY
AMEVIVE® interferes with lymphocyte activation by specifically binding to the lymphocyte antigen, CD2, and inhibiting LFA-3/CD2 interaction. Activation of T lymphocytes involving the interaction between LFA-3 on antigen-presenting cells and CD2 on T lymphocytes plays a role in the pathophysiology of chronic plaque psoriasis. The majority of T lymphocytes in psoriatic lesions are of the memory effector phenotype characterized by the presence of the CD45RO marker[1], express activation markers (e.g., CD25, CD69) and release inflammatory cytokines, such as interferon γ.
AMEVIVE® also causes a reduction in subsets of CD2+ T lymphocytes (primarily CD45RO+), presumably by bridging between CD2 on target lymphocytes and immunoglobulin Fc receptors on cytotoxic cells, such as natural killer cells. Treatment with AMEVIVE® results in a reduction in circulating total CD4+ and CD8+ T lymphocyte counts. CD2 is also expressed at low levels on the surface of natural killer cells and certain bone marrow B lymphocytes. Therefore, the potential exists for AMEVIVE® to affect the activation and numbers of cells other than T lymphocytes. In clinical studies of AMEVIVE®, minor changes in the numbers of circulating cells other than T lymphocytes have been observed.

Pharmacokinetics
In patients with moderate to severe plaque psoriasis, following a 7.5 mg intravenous (IV) administration, the mean volume of distribution of alefacept was 94 mL/kg, the mean clearance was 0.25 mL/h/kg, and the mean elimination half-life was approximately 270 hours. Following an intramuscular (IM) injection, bioavailability was 63%.
The pharmacokinetics of alefacept in pediatric patients have not been studied. The effects of renal or hepatic impairment on the pharmacokinetics of alefacept have not been studied.

Pharmacodynamics
At doses tested in clinical trials, AMEVIVE® therapy resulted in a dose-dependent decrease in circulating total lymphocytes[2]. This reduction predominantly affected the memory effector subset of the CD4+ and CD8+ T lymphocyte compartments (CD4+CD45RO+ and CD8+CD45RO+), the predominant phenotype in psoriatic lesions. Circulating naïve T lymphocyte and natural killer cell counts appeared to be only minimally susceptible to AMEVIVE® treatment, while circulating B lymphocyte counts appeared not to be affected by AMEVIVE® (see **ADVERSE REACTIONS, Effect on Lymphocyte Counts**).

CLINICAL STUDIES
AMEVIVE® was evaluated in two randomized, double-blind, placebo-controlled studies in adults with chronic (≥1 year) plaque psoriasis and a minimum body surface area involvement of 10% who were candidates for or had previously received systemic therapy or phototherapy. Each course consisted of once-weekly administration for 12 weeks (IV for Study 1, IM for Study 2) of placebo or AMEVIVE®. Patients could receive concomitant low potency topical steroids. Concomitant phototherapy or systemic therapy was not allowed.
In Study 1, patients were randomized to receive one or two courses of AMEVIVE® 7.5 mg administered by IV bolus. The first and second courses in the two-course cohort were separated by at least a 12-week post-dosing interval. A total of 553 patients were randomized into three cohorts (Table 1).

Table 2. Percentage of Patients Responding to the First Course of Treatment in Study 1 (the Intravenous Study) and Study 2 (the Intramuscular Study) Two Weeks Post Dosing

	Study 1			Study 2		
Treatment response: (reduction in disease activity from baseline)	Placebo (N=186)	AMEVIVE® 7.5 mg IV (N=367)[1]	Difference (95% CI)	Placebo (N=168)	AMEVIVE® 15 mg IM (N=166)	Difference (95% CI)
≥75% reduction PASI	4%	14%	10* (6, 15)	5%	21%	16* (9, 23)
≥50% reduction PASI	10%	38%	28* (22, 35)	18%	42%	24* (14, 33)
PGA "almost clear" or "clear"	4%	11%	7+(3, 12)	5%	14%	9$(3, 15)

[1]Cohorts 1 and 2 are combined.
*p values <0.001
+p value 0.004
$p value 0.006

Table 1. Treatment Group and Number of Patients Dosed in Study 1

	Course 1 (No. of patients)	Course 2 (No. of patients)
Cohort 1	AMEVIVE® (183)	AMEVIVE® (154)
Cohort 2	AMEVIVE® (184)	Placebo (142)
Cohort 3	Placebo (186)	AMEVIVE®(153)

Study 2 provided a basis for comparison of patients treated with either 10 mg or 15 mg AMEVIVE® IM. One hundred seventy-three patients were randomized to receive 10 mg of AMEVIVE® IM, 166 to receive 15 mg of AMEVIVE® IM, and 168 to receive placebo.
In Studies 1 and 2, 77% of patients had previously received systemic therapy and/or phototherapy for psoriasis. Of these, 23% and 19%, respectively, had failed to respond to at least one of these previous therapies.
Table 2 shows the treatment response in the first course of Study 1 and Study 2. Response to treatment in both studies was defined as the proportion of patients with a reduction in score on the Psoriasis Area and Severity Index (PASI)[3] of at least 75% from baseline at two weeks following the 12-week treatment period.
Other treatment responses included the proportion of patients who achieved a scoring of "almost clear" or "clear" by Physician Global Assessment (PGA) and the proportion of patients with a reduction in PASI of at least 50% from baseline two weeks after the 12-week treatment period.
[See table above]
In Study 2, the proportion of responders to the 10 mg IM dose was higher than placebo, but the difference was not statistically significant.
In both studies, onset of response to AMEVIVE® treatment (at least a 50% reduction of baseline PASI) began 60 days after the start of therapy.
With one course of therapy in Study 1 (IV route), the median duration of response (defined as maintenance of a 75% or greater reduction in PASI) was 3.5 months for AMEVIVE®-treated patients and 1 month for placebo-treated patients. In Study 2 (IM route), the median duration of response was approximately 2 months for both AMEVIVE®-treated patients and placebo-treated patients. Most patients who had responded to either AMEVIVE® or placebo maintained a 50% or greater reduction in PASI through the 3-month observation period.
The responders (n=52) in a subset of patients in Study 1 who crossed over to placebo for course 2 (Cohort 2) maintained a 50% or greater reduction in PASI for a median of 7 months.
Some patients achieved their maximal response beyond 2 weeks post-dosing. In Studies 1 and 2, an additional 11% (42/367) and 7% (12/166) of patients treated with AMEVIVE®, respectively, achieved a 75% reduction from baseline PASI score at one or more visits after the first 2 weeks of the follow-up period.

Retreatment
Patients in Study 1 who had completed the first IV treatment course were eligible to receive a second treatment course if their psoriasis was less than "clear" by PGA and their CD4+ T lymphocyte count was above the lower limit of normal. The level of response (decrease in median PASI score) over the two courses of IV treatment is shown in Figure 1. The median reduction in PASI score was greater in patients who received a second course of AMEVIVE® treatment (see Cohort 1) compared to patients who received placebo (see Cohort 2).
Data on the safety and efficacy of AMEVIVE® treatment beyond two courses are limited.
[See figure 1 at bottom of next page]

INDICATIONS AND USAGE
AMEVIVE® is indicated for the treatment of adult patients with moderate to severe chronic plaque psoriasis who are candidates for systemic therapy or phototherapy.

CONTRAINDICATIONS
AMEVIVE® should not be administered to patients with known hypersensitivity to AMEVIVE® or any of its components.

WARNINGS
LYMPHOPENIA
AMEVIVE® INDUCES DOSE-DEPENDENT REDUCTIONS IN CIRCULATING CD4+ AND CD8+ T LYMPHOCYTE COUNTS.
A COURSE OF AMEVIVE® THERAPY SHOULD NOT BE INITIATED IN PATIENTS WITH A CD4+ T LYMPHOCYTE COUNT BELOW NORMAL. THE CD4+ T LYMPHOCYTE COUNTS OF PATIENTS RECEIVING AMEVIVE® SHOULD BE MONITORED WEEKLY THROUGHOUT THE COURSE OF THE 12-WEEK DOSING REGIMEN. DOSING SHOULD BE WITHHELD IF CD4+ T LYMPHOCYTE COUNTS ARE BELOW 250 CELLS/µL. THE DRUG SHOULD BE DISCONTINUED IF THE COUNTS REMAIN BELOW 250 CELLS/µL FOR ONE MONTH (SEE DOSAGE AND ADMINISTRATION).

Malignancies
AMEVIVE® may increase the risk of malignancies. Some patients who received AMEVIVE® in clinical studies developed malignancies (**see ADVERSE REACTIONS, Malignancies**). In preclinical studies, animals developed B cell hyperplasia, and one animal developed a lymphoma (**see PRECAUTIONS, Carcinogenesis, Mutagenesis, and Fertility**). AMEVIVE® should not be administered to patients with a history of systemic malignancy. Caution should be exercised when considering the use of AMEVIVE® in patients at high risk for malignancy. If a patient develops a malignancy, AMEVIVE® should be discontinued.

Serious Infections
AMEVIVE® is an immunosuppressive agent and, therefore, has the potential to increase the risk of infection and reactivate latent, chronic infections. AMEVIVE® should not be administered to patients with a clinically important infection. Caution should be exercised when considering the use of AMEVIVE® in patients with chronic infections or a history of recurrent infection. Patients should be monitored for signs and symptoms of infection during or after a course of AMEVIVE®. New infections should be closely monitored. If a patient develops a serious infection, AMEVIVE® should be discontinued (see **ADVERSE REACTIONS, Infections**).

PRECAUTIONS
Effects on the Immune System
Patients receiving other immunosuppressive agents or phototherapy should not receive concurrent therapy with AMEVIVE® because of the possibility of excessive immunosuppression. The duration of the period following treatment with AMEVIVE® before one should consider starting other immunosuppressive therapy has not been evaluated.
The safety and efficacy of vaccines, specifically live or live-attenuated vaccines, administered to patients being treated with AMEVIVE® have not been studied. In a study of 46 patients with chronic plaque psoriasis, the ability to mount immunity to tetanus toxoid (recall antigen) and an experimental neo-antigen was preserved in those patients undergoing AMEVIVE® therapy.

Allergic Reactions
Hypersensitivity reactions (urticaria, angioedema) were associated with the administration of AMEVIVE®. If an anaphylactic reaction or other serious allergic reaction occurs, administration of AMEVIVE® should be discontinued immediately and appropriate therapy initiated.

Information for Patients
Patients should be informed of the need for regular monitoring of white blood cell (lymphocyte) counts during therapy and that AMEVIVE® must be administered under the supervision of a physician. Patients should also be informed that AMEVIVE® reduces lymphocyte counts, which could increase their chances of developing an infection or a malignancy. Patients should be advised to inform their physician promptly if they develop any signs of an infection or malignancy while undergoing a course of treatment with AMEVIVE®.

Continued on next page

Amevive—Cont.

Female patients should also be advised to notify their physicians if they become pregnant while taking AMEVIVE® (or within 8 weeks of discontinuing AMEVIVE®) and be advised of the existence of and encouraged to enroll in the Pregnancy Registry. Call 1-866-AMEVIVE (1-866-263-8483) to enroll into the Registry (see **PRECAUTIONS, Pregnancy**).

Laboratory Tests
CD4+ T lymphocyte counts should be monitored weekly during the 12-week dosing period and used to guide dosing. Patients should have normal CD4+ T lymphocyte counts prior to an initial or a subsequent course of treatment with AMEVIVE®. Dosing should be withheld if CD4+ T lymphocyte counts are below 250 cells/μL. AMEVIVE® should be discontinued if CD4+ T lymphocyte counts remain below 250 cells/μL for one month.

Drug Interactions
No formal interaction studies have been performed. The duration of the period following treatment with AMEVIVE® before one should consider starting other immunosuppressive therapy has not been evaluated.

Carcinogenesis, Mutagenesis, and Fertility
In a chronic toxicity study, cynomolgus monkeys were dosed weekly for 52 weeks with intravenous alefacept at 1 mg/kg/dose or 20 mg/kg/dose. One animal in the high dose group developed a B-cell lymphoma that was detected after 28 weeks of dosing. Additional animals in both dose groups developed B-cell hyperplasia of the spleen and lymph nodes. All animals in the study were positive for an endemic primate gammaherpes virus also known as lymphocryptovirus (LCV). Latent LCV infection is generally asymptomatic, but can lead to B-cell lymphomas when animals are immune suppressed.

In a separate study, baboons given 3 doses of alefacept at 1 mg/kg every 8 weeks were found to have centroblast proliferation in B-cell dependent areas in the germinal centers of the spleen following a 116-day washout period.

The role of AMEVIVE® in the development of the lymphoid malignancy and the hyperplasia observed in non-human primates and the relevance to humans is unknown. Immunodeficiency-associated lymphocyte disorders (plasmacytic hyperplasia, polymorphic proliferation, and B-cell lymphomas) occur in patients who have congenital or acquired immunodeficiencies including those resulting from immunosuppressive therapy.

No carcinogenicity or fertility studies were conducted. Mutagenicity studies were conducted *in vitro* and *in vivo*; no evidence of mutagenicity was observed.

Pregnancy (Category B)
Women of childbearing potential make up a considerable segment of the patient population affected by psoriasis. Since the effect of AMEVIVE® on pregnancy and fetal development, including immune system development, is not known, health care providers are encouraged to enroll patients currently taking AMEVIVE® who become pregnant into the Biogen Pregnancy Registry by calling 1-866-AMEVIVE (1-866-263-8483).

Reproductive toxicology studies have been performed in cynomolgus monkeys at doses up to 5 mg/kg/week (about 62 times the human dose based on body weight) and have revealed no evidence of impaired fertility or harm to the fetus due to AMEVIVE®. No abortifacient or teratogenic effects were observed in cynomolgus monkeys following intravenous bolus injections of AMEVIVE® administered weekly during the period of organogenesis to gestation. AMEVIVE® underwent trans-placental passage and produced *in utero* exposure in the developing monkeys. *In utero*, serum levels of exposure in these monkeys were 23% of maternal serum levels. No evidence of fetal toxicity including adverse effects on immune system development was observed in any of these animals.

Animal reproduction studies, however, are not always predictive of human response and there are no adequate and well-controlled studies in pregnant women. Because the risk to the development of the fetal immune system and postnatal immune function in humans is unknown, AMEVIVE® should be used during pregnancy only if clearly needed. If pregnancy occurs while taking AMEVIVE®, continued use of the drug should be assessed.

Nursing Mothers
It is not known whether AMEVIVE® is excreted in human milk. Because many drugs are excreted in human milk, and because there exists the potential for serious adverse reactions in nursing infants from AMEVIVE®, a decision should be made whether to discontinue nursing while taking the drug or to discontinue the use of the drug, taking into account the importance of the drug to the mother.

Geriatric Use
Of the 1357 patients who received AMEVIVE® in clinical trials, a total of 100 patients were ≥ 65 years of age and 13 patients were ≥ 75 years of age. No differences in safety or efficacy were observed between older and younger patients, but there were not sufficient data to exclude important differences. Because the incidence of infections and certain malignancies is higher in the elderly population, in general, caution should be used in treating the elderly.

Pediatric Use
The safety and efficacy of AMEVIVE® in pediatric patients have not been studied. AMEVIVE® is not indicated for pediatric patients.

ADVERSE REACTIONS

The most serious adverse reactions were:

- Lymphopenia (see **WARNINGS**)
- Malignancies (see **WARNINGS**)
- Serious Infections requiring hospitalization (see **WARNINGS**)
- Hypersensitivity Reactions (see **PRECAUTIONS, Allergic Reactions**)

Commonly observed adverse events seen in the first course of placebo-controlled clinical trials with at least a 2% higher incidence in the AMEVIVE®-treated patients compared to placebo-treated patients were: pharyngitis, dizziness, increased cough, nausea, pruritus, myalgia, chills, injection site pain, injection site inflammation, and accidental injury. The only adverse event that occurred at a 5% or higher incidence among AMEVIVE®-treated patients compared to placebo-treated patients was chills (1% placebo *vs.* 6% AMEVIVE®), which occurred predominantly with intravenous administration.

The adverse reactions which most commonly resulted in clinical intervention were cardiovascular events including coronary artery disorder in <1% of patients and myocardial infarct in <1% of patients. These events were not observed in any of the 413 placebo-treated patients. The total number of patients hospitalized for cardiovascular events in the AMEVIVE®-treated group was 1.2% (11/876).

The most common events resulting in discontinuation of treatment with AMEVIVE® were CD4+ T lymphocyte levels below 250 cells/μL (see **WARNINGS**, and **ADVERSE REACTIONS, Effect on Lymphocyte Counts**), headache (0.2%), and nausea (0.2%).

Because clinical trials are conducted under widely varying conditions, adverse event rates observed in the clinical trials of a drug cannot be directly compared to rates in the clinical trials of another drug and may not reflect the rates observed in practice. The adverse reaction information does, however, provide a basis for identifying the adverse events that appear to be related to drug use and a basis for approximating rates.

The data described below reflect exposure to AMEVIVE® in a total of 1357 psoriasis patients, 85% of whom received 1 to 2 courses of therapy and the rest received 3 to 6 courses and were followed for up to three years. Of the 1357 total patients, 876 received their first course in placebo-controlled studies. The population studied ranged in age from 16 to 84 years, and included 69% men and 31% women. The patients were mostly Caucasian (89%), reflecting the general psoriatic population. Disease severity at baseline was moderate to severe psoriasis.

Effect on Lymphocyte Counts
In the intramuscular study (Study 2), 4% of patients temporarily discontinued treatment and no patients permanently discontinued treatment due to CD4+ T lymphocyte counts below the specified threshold of 250 cells/μL. In Study 2, 10%, 28%, and 42% of patients had total lymphocyte, CD4+, and CD8+ T lymphocyte counts below normal, respectively. Twelve weeks after a course of therapy (12 weekly doses), 2%, 8%, and 21% of patients had total lymphocyte, CD4+, and CD8+ T cell counts below normal.

In the first course of the intravenous study (Study 1), 10% of patients temporarily discontinued treatment and 2% permanently discontinued treatment due to CD4+ T lymphocyte counts below the specified threshold of 250 cells/μL. During the first course of Study 1, 22% of patients had total lymphocyte counts below normal, 48% had CD4+ T lymphocyte counts below normal and 59% had CD8+ T lymphocyte counts below normal. The maximal effect on lymphocytes was observed within 6 to 8 weeks of initiation of treatment. Twelve weeks after a course of therapy (12 weekly doses), 4% of patients had total lymphocyte counts below normal, 19% had CD4+ T lymphocyte counts below normal, and 36% had CD8+ T lymphocyte counts below normal.

For patients receiving a second course of AMEVIVE® in Study 1, 17% of patients had total lymphocyte counts below normal, 44% had CD4+ T lymphocyte counts below normal, and 56% had CD8+ T lymphocyte counts below normal. Twelve weeks after completing dosing, 3% of patients had total lymphocyte counts below normal, 17% had CD4+ T lymphocyte counts below normal, and 35% had CD8+ T lymphocyte counts below normal (see **WARNINGS**, and **PRECAUTIONS, Laboratory Tests**).

Malignancies
In the 24-week period constituting the first course of placebo-controlled studies, 13 malignancies were diagnosed in 11 AMEVIVE®-treated patients. The incidence of malignancies was 1.3% (11/876) for AMEVIVE®-treated patients compared to 0.5% (2/413) in the placebo group.

Among 1357 patients who received AMEVIVE®, 25 patients were diagnosed with 35 treatment-emergent malignancies. The majority of these malignancies (23 cases) were basal (6) or squamous cell cancers (17) of the skin. Three cases of lymphoma were observed; one was classified as non-Hodgkin's follicle-center cell lymphoma and two were classified as Hodgkin's disease.

Infections
In the 24-week period constituting the first course of placebo-controlled studies, serious infections (infections requiring hospitalization) were seen at a rate of 0.9% (8/876) in AMEVIVE®-treated patients and 0.2% (1/413) in the placebo group. In patients receiving repeated courses of AMEVIVE® therapy, the rates of serious infections were 0.7% (5/756) and 1.5% (3/199) in the second and third course of therapy, respectively. Serious infections among 1357 AMEVIVE®-treated patients included necrotizing cellulitis, peritonsillar abscess, post-operative and burn wound infection, toxic shock, pneumonia, appendicitis, pre-septal cellulitis, cholecystitis, gastroenteritis and herpes simplex infection.

Hypersensitivity Reactions
In clinical studies two patients were reported to experience angioedema, one of whom was hospitalized. In the 24-week period constituting the first course of placebo-controlled studies, urticaria was reported in 6 (<1%) AMEVIVE®-treated patients *vs.* 1 patient in the control group. Urticaria resulted in discontinuation of therapy in one of the AMEVIVE®-treated patients.

Injection Site Reactions
In the intramuscular study (Study 2), 16% of AMEVIVE®-treated patients and 8% of placebo-treated patients reported injection site reactions. Reactions at the site of injection were generally mild, typically occurred on single occasions, and included either pain (7%), inflammation (4%), bleeding (4%), edema (2%), non-specific reaction (2%), mass (1%), or skin hypersensitivity (<1%). In the clinical trials, a single case of injection site reaction led to the discontinuation of AMEVIVE®.

Immunogenicity
Approximately 3% (35/1306) of patients receiving AMEVIVE® developed low-titer antibodies to alefacept. No

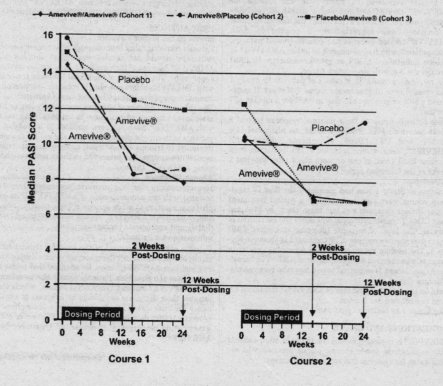

Figure 1. Median PASI Score Over Time

apparent correlation of antibody development and clinical response or adverse events was observed. The long-term immunogenicity of AMEVIVE® is unknown.

The data reflect the percentage of patients whose test results were considered positive for antibodies to alefacept in an ELISA assay, and are highly dependent on the sensitivity and specificity of the assay. Additionally, the observed incidence of antibody positivity in an assay may be influenced by several factors including sample handling, timing of sample collection, concomitant medications, and underlying disease. For these reasons, comparison of the incidence of antibodies to alefacept with the incidence of antibodies to other products may be misleading.

Other Observed Adverse Reactions from Clinical Trials

Less common events that were observed at a higher rate in AMEVIVE®-treated patients include rare cases (9) of transaminase elevations to 5 to 10 times the upper limit of normal.

OVERDOSAGE

The highest dose tested in humans (0.75 mg/kg IV) was associated with chills, headache, arthralgia, and sinusitis within one day of dosing. Patients who have been inadvertently administered an excess of the recommended dose should be closely monitored for effects on total lymphocyte count and CD4+ T lymphocyte count.

DOSAGE AND ADMINISTRATION

AMEVIVE® should only be used under the guidance and supervision of a physician.

The recommended dose of AMEVIVE® is 7.5 mg given once weekly as an IV bolus or 15 mg given once weekly as an IM injection. The recommended regimen is a course of 12 weekly injections. Retreatment with an additional 12-week course may be initiated provided that CD4+ T lymphocyte counts are within the normal range, and a minimum of a 12-week interval has passed since the previous course of treatment. Data on retreatment beyond two cycles are limited.

The CD4+ T lymphocyte counts of patients receiving AMEVIVE® should be monitored weekly before initiating dosing and throughout the course of the 12-week dosing regimen. Dosing should be withheld if CD4+ T lymphocyte counts are below 250 cells/µL. The drug should be discontinued if the counts remain below 250 cells/µL for one month (see **PRECAUTIONS, Laboratory Tests**).

Preparation Instructions

AMEVIVE® should be reconstituted by a health care professional using aseptic technique. Each vial is intended for single patient use only.

Do not use an AMEVIVE® dose tray beyond the date stamped on the carton, dose tray lid, AMEVIVE® vial label, or diluent container label.

AMEVIVE® 15 mg lyophilized powder for IM administration should be reconstituted with 0.6 mL of the supplied diluent (Sterile Water for Injection, USP). 0.5 mL of the reconstituted solution contains 15 mg of alefacept.

AMEVIVE® 7.5 mg lyophilized powder for IV administration should be reconstituted with 0.6 mL of the supplied diluent. 0.5 mL of the reconstituted solution contains 7.5 mg of alefacept.

Do not add other medications to solutions containing AMEVIVE®. Do not reconstitute AMEVIVE® with other diluents. Do not filter reconstituted solution during preparation or administration.

All procedures require the use of aseptic technique. Using the supplied syringe and one of the supplied needles, withdraw **only 0.6 mL** of the supplied diluent, (Sterile Water for Injection, USP). Keeping the needle pointed at the sidewall of the vial, slowly inject the diluent into the vial of AMEVIVE®. Some foaming will occur, which is normal. To avoid excessive foaming, do not shake or vigorously agitate. The contents should be swirled gently during dissolution. Generally, dissolution of AMEVIVE® takes less than two minutes. The solution should be used as soon as possible after reconstitution.

The reconstituted solution should be clear and colorless to slightly yellow. Visually inspect the solution for particulate matter and discoloration prior to administration. The solution should not be used if discolored or cloudy, or if undissolved material remains.

Following reconstitution, the product should be used immediately or within 4 hours if stored in the vial at 2-8°C (36-46°F). AMEVIVE® NOT USED WITHIN 4 HOURS OF RECONSTITUTION SHOULD BE DISCARDED.

Remove the needle used for reconstitution and attach the other supplied needle. Withdraw 0.5 mL of the AMEVIVE® solution into the syringe. Some foam or bubbles may remain in the vial.

Administration Instructions

For intramuscular use, inject the full 0.5 mL of solution. Rotate injection sites so that a different site is used for each new injection. New injections should be given at least 1 inch from an old site and never into areas where the skin is tender, bruised, red, or hard.

For intravenous use,

- Prepare 2 syringes with 3.0 mL Normal Saline, USP for pre- and post-administration flush.
- Prime the winged infusion set with 3.0 mL saline and insert the set into the vein.
- Attach the AMEVIVE®-filled syringe to the infusion set and administer the solution over no more than 5 seconds.
- Flush the infusion set with 3.0 mL saline, USP.

HOW SUPPLIED

AMEVIVE® for IV administration is supplied in either a carton containing four administration dose packs, or in a carton containing one administration dose pack. Each dose pack contains one 7.5-mg single-use vial of AMEVIVE®, one 10 mL single-use diluent vial (Sterile Water for Injection, USP), one syringe, one 23 gauge, ¾ inch winged infusion set, and two 23 gauge, 1 ¼ inch needles. The NDC number for the four administration dose pack carton is 59627-020-01. The NDC number for the one administration dose pack carton is 59627-020-02.

AMEVIVE® for IM administration is supplied in either a carton containing four administration dose packs, or in a carton containing one administration dose pack. Each dose pack contains one 15-mg single-use vial of AMEVIVE®, one 10 mL single-use diluent vial (Sterile Water for Injection, USP), one syringe, and two 23 gauge, 1 ¼ inch needles. The NDC number for the four administration dose pack carton is 59627-021-03. The NDC number for the one administration dose pack carton is 59627-021-04.

AMEVIVE® is reconstituted with 0.6 mL of the 10 mL single-use diluent.

Storage

The dose tray containing AMEVIVE® (lyophilized powder) should be stored at controlled room temperature (15-30°C; 59-86°F). PROTECT FROM LIGHT. Retain in carton until time of use.

Rx only

REFERENCES

1. Bos JD, Hagenaars C, Das PK, et al. Predominance of "memory" T cells (CD4+, CDw29+) over "naïve" T cells (CD4+, CD45R+) in both normal and diseased human skin. Arch Dermatol Res 1989; 281:24-30.
2. Ellis C, Krueger GG. Treatment of chronic plaque psoriasis by selective targeting of memory effector T lymphocytes. N Engl J Med 2001; 345:248-255.
3. Fredriksson T, Pettersson U. Severe psoriasis–oral therapy with a new retinoid. Dermatologica 1978; 157:238-244.

Issued: February/2003
AMEVIVE® (alefacept)
Manufactured by:
BIOGEN, INC.
14 Cambridge Center
Cambridge, MA 02142 USA
©2003 Biogen, Inc. All rights reserved.
1-866-263-8483
U.S. Patents:
4,956,281
5,547,853
5,728,677
5,914,111
5,928,643
6,162,432
Additional U.S. Patents Pending
I63007-1

Biovail Pharmaceuticals, Inc.

170 SOUTHPORT DRIVE
MORRISVILLE, NC 27560

For direct inquiries contact:
Phone: 1-866-Biovail
1-866-246-8245
For Medical Information & Adverse Drug Experiences Contact:
Biovail Medical Information Line
1-866-276-1030
Fax: 800-347-9315

ZOVIRAX® ℞

[zō'vī-rāks]
(acyclovir)
Cream 5%
USE ONLY FOR COLD SORES

DESCRIPTION

ZOVIRAX is the brand name for acyclovir, a synthetic nucleoside analogue active against herpesviruses. ZOVIRAX Cream 5% is a formulation for topical administration. Each gram of ZOVIRAX Cream 5% contains 50 mg of acyclovir and the following inactive ingredients: cetostearyl alcohol, mineral oil, poloxamer 407, propylene glycol, sodium lauryl sulfate, water, and white petrolatum.

Acyclovir is a white, crystalline powder with the molecular formula $C_8H_{11}N_5O_3$ and a molecular weight of 225. The maximum solubility in water at 37°C is 2.5 mg/mL. The pKa's of acyclovir are 2.27 and 9.25.

The chemical name of acyclovir is 2-amino-1,9-dihydro-9-[(2-hydroxyethoxy)methyl]-6*H*-purin-6-one; it has the following structural formula:

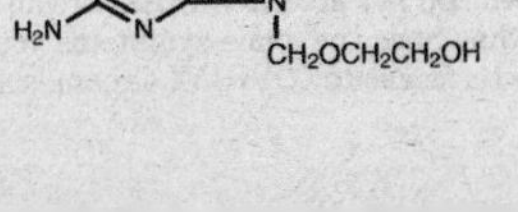

VIROLOGY

Mechanism of Antiviral Action: Acyclovir is a synthetic purine nucleoside analogue with in vitro and in vivo inhibitory activity against herpes simplex virus types 1 (HSV-1), 2 (HSV-2), and varicella-zoster virus (VZV).

The inhibitory activity of acyclovir is highly selective due to its affinity for the enzyme thymidine kinase (TK) encoded by HSV and VZV. This viral enzyme converts acyclovir into acyclovir monophosphate, a nucleotide analogue. The monophosphate is further converted into diphosphate by cellular guanylate kinase and into triphosphate by a number of cellular enzymes. In vitro, acyclovir triphosphate stops replication of herpes viral DNA. This is accomplished in 3 ways: 1) competitive inhibition of viral DNA polymerase, 2) incorporation into and termination of the growing viral DNA chain, and 3) inactivation of the viral DNA polymerase. The greater antiviral activity of acyclovir against HSV compared with VZV is due to its more efficient phosphorylation by the viral TK.

Antiviral Activities: The quantitative relationship between the in vitro susceptibility of herpes viruses to antivirals and the clinical response to therapy has not been established in humans, and virus sensitivity testing has not been standardized. Sensitivity testing results, expressed as the concentration of drug required to inhibit by 50% the growth of virus in cell culture (IC_{50}), vary greatly depending upon a number of factors. Using plaque-reduction assays, the IC_{50} against herpes simplex virus isolates ranges from 0.02 to 13.5 mcg/mL for HSV-1 and from 0.01 to 9.9 mcg/mL for HSV-2. The IC_{50} for acyclovir against most laboratory strains and clinical isolates of VZV ranges from 0.12 to 10.8 mcg/mL. Acyclovir also demonstrates activity against the Oka vaccine strain of VZV with a mean IC_{50} of 1.35 mcg/mL.

Drug Resistance: Resistance of HSV and VZV to acyclovir can result from qualitative and quantitative changes in the viral TK and/or DNA polymerase. Clinical isolates of HSV and VZV with reduced susceptibility to acyclovir have been recovered from immunocompromised patients, especially with advanced HIV infection. While most of the acyclovir-resistant mutants isolated thus far from immunocompromised patients have been found to be TK-deficient mutants, other mutants involving the viral TK gene (TK partial and TK altered) and DNA polymerase have been isolated. TK-negative mutants may cause severe disease in infants and immunocompromised adults. The possibility of viral resistance to acyclovir should be considered in patients who show poor clinical response during therapy.

CLINICAL PHARMACOLOGY

Pharmacokinetics: ***Adults:*** A clinical pharmacology study was performed with ZOVIRAX Cream in adult volunteers to evaluate the percutaneous absorption of acyclovir. In this study, which included 6 male volunteers, the cream was applied to an area of 710 cm² on the backs of the volunteers 5 times daily at intervals of 2 hours for a total of 4 days. The weight of cream applied and urinary excretion of acyclovir were measured daily. Plasma concentration of acyclovir was assayed 1 hour after the final application. The average daily urinary excretion of acyclovir was approximately 0.04% of the daily applied dose. Plasma acyclovir concentrations were below the limit of detection (0.01 µM) in 5 subjects and barely detectable (0.014 µM) in 1 subject. Systemic absorption of acyclovir from ZOVIRAX Cream is minimal in adults.

Pediatric Patients: The systemic absorption of acyclovir following topical application of cream has not been evaluated in patients <18 years of age.

CLINICAL TRIALS

Adults: ZOVIRAX Cream was evaluated in 2 double-blind, randomized, placebo (vehicle)-controlled trials for the treatment of recurrent herpes labialis. The average patient had 5 episodes of herpes labialis in the previous 12 months. In the first study, median age was 37 years (range 18 to 81 years), 74% were female, and 94% were Caucasian. In the second study, median age was 38 years (range 18 to 87 years), 73% were female, and 94% were Caucasian. Subjects were instructed to initiate treatment within 1 hour of noticing signs or symptoms and continue treatment for 4 days, with application of study medication 5 times per day. In both studies, the mean duration of the recurrent herpes labialis episode was approximately one-half day shorter in the subjects treated with ZOVIRAX Cream (n = 682) compared with subjects treated with placebo (n = 703) (approximately 4.5 days versus 5 days, respectively). No significant difference was observed between subjects receiving ZOVIRAX Cream or vehicle in the prevention of progression of cold sore lesions.

Pediatric Patients: An open-label, uncontrolled trial with ZOVIRAX Cream 5% was conducted in 113 patients aged 12 to 17 years with herpes labialis. In this study, therapy was applied using the same dosing regimen as in adults and subjects were followed for adverse events. The safety profile was similar to that observed in adults.

INDICATIONS AND USAGE

ZOVIRAX Cream is indicated for the treatment of recurrent herpes labialis (cold sores) in adults and adolescents (12 years of age and older).

CONTRAINDICATIONS

ZOVIRAX Cream is contraindicated in patients with known hypersensitivity to acyclovir, valacyclovir, or any component of the formulation.

Continued on next page

Zovirax—Cont.

PRECAUTIONS

General: ZOVIRAX Cream is intended for cutaneous use only and should not be used in the eye or inside the mouth or nose. ZOVIRAX Cream should only be used on herpes labialis on the affected external aspects of the lips and face. Because no data are available, application to human mucous membranes is not recommended. ZOVIRAX Cream has a potential for irritation and contact sensitization (see ADVERSE REACTIONS). The effect of ZOVIRAX Cream has not been established in immunocompromised patients.

Information for Patients: Please see **Patient Information About ZOVIRAX Cream.**

Drug Interactions: Clinical experience has identified no interactions resulting from topical or systemic administration of other drugs concomitantly with ZOVIRAX Cream.

Carcinogenesis, Mutagenesis, Impairment of Fertility: Systemic exposure following topical administration of acyclovir is minimal. Dermal carcinogenicity studies were not conducted. Results from the studies of carcinogenesis, mutagenesis and fertility are not included in the full prescribing information for ZOVIRAX Cream due to the minimal exposures of acyclovir that result from dermal application. Information on these studies is available in the full prescribing information for ZOVIRAX Capsules, Tablets, and Suspension and ZOVIRAX for Injection.

Pregnancy: *Teratogenic Effects:* Pregnancy Category B. Acyclovir was not teratogenic in the mouse, rabbit, or rat at exposures greatly in excess of human exposure. There are no adequate and well-controlled studies of systemic acyclovir in pregnant women. A prospective epidemiologic registry of acyclovir use during pregnancy was established in 1984 and completed in April 1999. There were 749 pregnancies followed in women exposed to systemic acyclovir during the first trimester of pregnancy resulting in 756 outcomes. The occurrence rate of birth defects approximates that found in the general population. However, the small size of the registry is insufficient to evaluate the risk for less common defects or to permit reliable or definitive conclusions regarding the safety of acyclovir in pregnant women and their developing fetuses. Systemic acyclovir should be used during pregnancy only if the potential benefit justifies the potential risk to the fetus.

Nursing Mothers: It is not known whether topically applied acyclovir is excreted in breast milk. Systemic exposure following topical administration is minimal.

After oral administration of ZOVIRAX, acyclovir concentrations have been documented in breast milk in 2 women an ranged from 0.6 to 4.1 times the corresponding plasma levels. These concentrations would potentially expose the nursing infant to a dose of acyclovir up to 0.3 mg/kg/day. Nursing mothers who have active herpetic lesions near or on the breast should avoid nursing.

Geriatric Use: Clinical studies of acyclovir cream did not include sufficient numbers of subjects aged 65 and over to determine whether they respond differently from younger subjects. Other reported clinical experience has not identified differences in responses between the elderly and younger patients. Systemic absorption of acyclovir after topical administration is minimal (see CLINICAL PHARMACOLOGY).

Pediatric Use: Safety and effectiveness in pediatric patients less than 12 years of age have not been established.

ADVERSE REACTIONS

In 5 double-blind, placebo-controlled trials, 1,124 patients were treated with ZOVIRAX Cream and 1,161 with placebo (vehicle) cream. ZOVIRAX Cream was well tolerated; 5% of patients on ZOVIRAX Cream and 4% of patients on placebo reported local application site reactions.

The most common adverse reactions at the site of topical application were dry lips, desquamation, dryness of skin, cracked lips, burning skin, pruritus, flakiness of skin, and stinging on skin; each event occurred in less than 1% of patients receiving ZOVIRAX Cream and vehicle. Three patients on ZOVIRAX Cream and 1 patient on placebo discontinued treatment due to an adverse event.

An additional study, enrolling 22 healthy adults, was conducted to evaluate the dermal tolerance of ZOVIRAX Cream compared with vehicle using single occluded and semi-occluded patch testing methodology. Both ZOVIRAX Cream and vehicle showed a high and cumulative irritation potential. Another study, enrolling 251 healthy adults, was conducted to evaluate the contact sensitization potential of ZOVIRAX Cream using repeat insult patch testing methodology. Of 202 evaluable subjects, possible cutaneous sensitization reactions were observed in the same 4 (2%) subjects with both ZOVIRAX Cream and vehicle, and these reactions to both ZOVIRAX Cream and vehicle were confirmed in 3 subjects upon rechallenge. The sensitizing ingredient(s) has not been identified.

The safety profile in patients 12 to 17 years of age was similar to that observed in adults.

Observed During Clinical Practice: In addition to adverse events reported from clinical trials, the following events have been identified during post-approval use of acyclovir cream. Because they are reported voluntarily from a population of unknown size, estimates of frequency cannot be made. These events have been chosen for inclusion due to a combination of their seriousness, frequency of reporting, or potential causal connection to acyclovir cream

General: Angioedema, anaphylaxis.

Skin: Contact dermatitis, eczema, application site reactions including signs and symptoms of inflammation.

OVERDOSAGE

Overdosage by topical application of ZOVIRAX Cream is unlikely because of minimal systemic exposure (see CLINICAL PHARMACOLOGY).

DOSAGE AND ADMINISTRATION

ZOVIRAX Cream should be applied 5 times per day for 4 days. Therapy should be initiated as early as possible following onset of signs and symptoms (i.e., during the prodrome or when lesions appear). For adolescents 12 years of age and older, the dosage is the same as in adults.

HOW SUPPLIED

Each gram of ZOVIRAX Cream 5% contains 50 mg acyclovir in an aqueous cream base. ZOVIRAX Cream is supplied as follows:

2-g tubes (NDC 64455-994-42).

Store at or below 25°C (77°F); excursions permitted to 15° to 30°C (59° to 86°F) (see USP Controlled Room Temperature).

Manufactured by
GlaxoSmithKline
Research Triangle Park, NC 27709
for
Biovail
Pharmaceuticals, Inc.
Morrisville, NC 27560
©Copyright 2002, GlaxoSmithKline. All rights reserved.
December 2002   RL-1167

PATIENT INFORMATION ABOUT ZOVIRAX® (ACYCLOVIR) CREAM 5%

USE ONLY FOR COLD SORES. FOR EXTERNAL USE ONLY.
Read this information before you start using ZOVIRAX (acyclovir) Cream and each time you refill your prescription. There may be new information. This summary is not meant to take the place of your doctor's advice.

What is ZOVIRAX Cream?
ZOVIRAX Cream is a prescription medicine that is applied to the skin to treat cold sores (herpes labialis) that occur on the face or lips. However, ZOVIRAX Cream is not a cure for cold sores.

Who should not use ZOVIRAX Cream?
Do not use ZOVIRAX Cream if you are allergic to ZOVIRAX (also known as acyclovir), VALTREX® (also known as valacyclovir), or any of the ingredients of ZOVIRAX Cream. Ask your doctor or pharmacist about the inactive ingredients.
Before you start using ZOVIRAX Cream, tell your doctor if you are pregnant, planning to become pregnant, or are breast feeding.
The safety and efficacy of ZOVIRAX Cream have not been studied in patients younger than 12 years of age or in patients whose immune system is not normal.

How do I use ZOVIRAX Cream?
ZOVIRAX Cream is most effective when used early, at the start of a cold sore. For best results, apply the cream at the first sign of a cold sore (such as tingle, redness, bump, or itch).
- Wash your hands before using ZOVIRAX Cream.
- Apply ZOVIRAX Cream to clean, dry skin.
- Apply a layer of ZOVIRAX Cream to cover only the cold sore or cover only the area of tingling (or other symptoms) before the cold sore appears. Rub the cream in until it disappears.
- Apply the cream 5 times a day for 4 days.
- Wash your hands with soap and water after applying ZOVIRAX Cream. This should remove any cream left on the hands.

What Should I Avoid While Using ZOVIRAX Cream?
- Use ZOVIRAX Cream only on your affected skin. Do not swallow ZOVIRAX Cream. Do not apply ZOVIRAX Cream to the eyes, inside the mouth or nose, or on unaffected skin. Do not use ZOVIRAX Cream for genital herpes.
- Do not cover the cold sore area with a bandage or dressing unless otherwise instructed by your doctor.
- Do not apply another type of skin product (for example, cosmetics, sun screens, or lip balms) or other skin medication to the cold sore area while using ZOVIRAX Cream unless otherwise instructed by your doctor.
- Avoid irritation of the cold sore area while using ZOVIRAX Cream.
- Do not bathe, shower, or swim right after applying ZOVIRAX Cream. This could wash off the medicine.

What Are the Possible Side Effects of ZOVIRAX Cream?
ZOVIRAX Cream was well tolerated in studies in patients with cold sores. The most common skin-related side effects of ZOVIRAX Cream are dry or cracked lips, flakiness or dryness of skin, a burning or stinging feeling, or itching of the skin. Each event occurred in fewer than 1 in 100 patients in clinical studies. Ask a doctor or pharmacist about any concerns about ZOVIRAX Cream.

How Should I Store ZOVIRAX Cream?
Store ZOVIRAX Cream at room temperature (59° to 86°F). Never leave ZOVIRAX Cream in your car in cold or hot weather. Make sure the cap on the tube is tightly closed. Keep ZOVIRAX Cream out of the reach of children.

General Advice about Prescription Medicines
Do not use ZOVIRAX Cream for a condition for which it was not prescribed. Do not give ZOVIRAX Cream to other people, even if they have the same symptoms you have. If you have any concerns about ZOVIRAX Cream, ask your doctor.

Your doctor or pharmacist can give you additional information about ZOVIRAX Cream that was written for healthcare professionals.
Manufactured by
GlaxoSmithKline
Research Triangle Park, NC 27709
for
Biovail Pharmaceuticals, Inc.
Morrisville, NC 27560
December 2002   RL-1167

Bristol-Myers Squibb Company
P.O. BOX 4500
PRINCETON, NJ 08543-4500

For Medical Information Contact:
Generally:
Bristol-Myers Squibb Drug Information Department
P.O. Box 4500
Princeton, NJ 08543-4500
(800) 321–1335

Adverse Drug Experiences
and Product Defects Reporting call
between 8:30 AM–4:30 PM EST:
(609) 818-3737

Sales and Ordering:
Orders may be placed by:
1. Calling your purchase orders toll-free between 8:30 AM–5:00 PM EST:
(800) 631-5244
2. Mailing your purchase orders to:
Bristol-Myers Squibb U.S. Pharmaceuticals
Attn: Customer Service
P.O. Box 5250
Princeton, NJ 08543-5250
3. Faxing your purchase orders to:
(800) 523-2965
4. Transmitting computer-to-computer on the NWDA and UCS formats through Ordernet Services use:
DEA#PE0048579

ABILIFY™
(aripiprazole) Tablets
Rx only   ℞

DESCRIPTION

ABILIFY™ (aripiprazole) is a psychotropic drug that is available as tablets for oral administration. Aripiprazole is 7-[4-[4-(2,3-dichlorophenyl)-1-piperazinyl]butoxy]-3,4-dihydrocarbostyril. The empirical formula is $C_{23}H_{27}C_{12}N_3O_2$ and its molecular weight is 448.38. The chemical structure is:

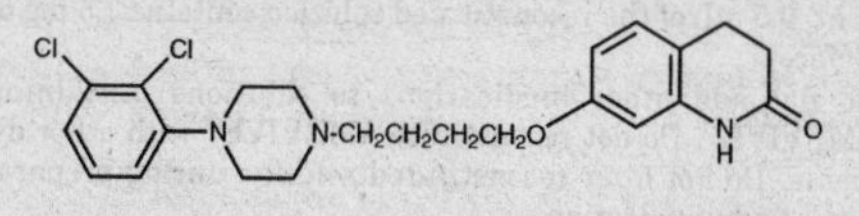

ABILIFY tablets are available in 10-mg, 15-mg, 20-mg, and 30-mg strengths. Inactive ingredients include lactose monohydrate, cornstarch, microcrystalline cellulose, hydroxypropyl cellulose, and magnesium stearate. Colorants include ferric oxide (yellow or red).

CLINICAL PHARMACOLOGY
Pharmacodynamics
Aripiprazole exhibits high affinity for dopamine D_2 and D_3, serotonin $5-HT_{1A}$ and $5-HT_{2A}$ receptors (K_i values of 0.34, 0.8, 1.7, and 3.4 nM, respectively), moderate affinity for dopamine D_4, serotonin $5-HT_{2C}$ and $5-HT_7$, alpha$_1$-adrenergic and histamine H_1 receptors (K_i values of 44, 15, 39, 57, and 61 nM, respectively), and moderate affinity for the serotonin reuptake site ($K_i = 98$ nM). Aripiprazole has no appreciable affinity for cholinergic muscarinic receptors (IC$_{50}$ > 1000 nM). Aripiprazole functions as a partial agonist at the dopamine D_2 and the serotonin $5-HT_{1A}$ receptors, and as an antagonist at serotonin $5-HT_{2A}$ receptor.

The mechanism of action of aripiprazole, as with other drugs having efficacy in schizophrenia, is unknown. However, it has been proposed that the efficacy of aripiprazole is mediated through a combination of partial agonist activity at D_2 and $5-HT_{1A}$ receptors and antagonist activity at $5-HT_{2A}$ receptors. Actions at receptors other than D_2, $5-HT_{1A}$, and $5-HT_{2A}$ may explain some of the other clinical effects of aripiprazole, e.g., the orthostatic hypotension observed with aripiprazole may be explained by its antagonist activity at adrenergic alpha$_1$ receptors.

Pharmacokinetics
ABILIFY activity is presumably primarily due to the parent drug, aripiprazole, and to a lesser extent, to its major metabolite, dehydro-aripiprazole, which has been shown to have affinities for D_2 receptors similar to the parent drug and represents 40% of the parent drug exposure in plasma. The mean elimination half-lives are about 75 hours and 94 hours for aripiprazole and dehydro-aripiprazole, respectively. Steady-state concentrations are attained within 14 days of dosing for both active moieties. Aripiprazole accumulation is predictable from single-dose pharmacokinetics. At steady state, the pharmacokinetics of aripiprazole are

dose-proportional. Elimination of aripiprazole is mainly through hepatic metabolism involving two P450 isozymes, CYP2D6 and CYP3A4.

Absorption

Aripiprazole is well absorbed, with peak plasma concentrations occurring within 3 to 5 hours; the absolute oral bioavailability of the tablet formulation is 87%. ABILIFY can be administered with or without food. Administration of a 15-mg ABILIFY tablet with a standard high-fat meal did not significantly affect the C_{max} or AUC of aripiprazole or its active metabolite, dehydro-aripiprazole, but delayed T_{max} by 3 hours for aripiprazole and 12 hours for dehydro-aripiprazole.

Distribution

The steady-state volume of distribution of aripiprazole following intravenous administration is high (404 L or 4.9 L/kg), indicating extensive extravascular distribution. At therapeutic concentrations, aripiprazole and its major metabolite are greater than 99% bound to serum proteins, primarily to albumin. In healthy human volunteers administered 0.5 to 30 mg/day aripiprazole for 14 days, there was dose-dependent D_2-receptor occupancy indicating brain penetration of aripiprazole in humans.

Metabolism and Elimination

Aripiprazole is metabolized primarily by three biotransformation pathways: dehydrogenation, hydroxylation, and N-dealkylation. Based on *in vitro* studies, CYP3A4 and CYP2D6 enzymes are responsible for dehydrogenation and hydroxylation of aripiprazole, and N-dealkylation is catalyzed by CYP3A4. Aripiprazole is the predominant drug moiety in the systemic circulation. At steady state, dehydro-aripiprazole, the active metabolite, represents about 40% of aripiprazole AUC in plasma.

Approximately 8% of Caucasians lack the capacity to metabolize CYP2D6 substrates and are classified as poor metabolizers (PM), whereas the rest are extensive metabolizers (EM). PMs have about an 80% increase in aripiprazole exposure and about a 30% decrease in exposure to the active metabolite compared to EMs, resulting in about a 60% higher exposure to the total active moieties from a given dose of aripiprazole compared to EMs. Coadministration of ABILIFY (aripiprazole) with known inhibitors of CYP2D6, like quinidine in EMs, results in a 112% increase in aripiprazole plasma exposure, and dosing adjustment is needed (see **PRECAUTIONS: Drug-Drug Interactions**). The mean elimination half-lives are about 75 hours and 146 hours for aripiprazole in EMs and PMs, respectively. Aripiprazole does not inhibit or induce the CYP2D6 pathway.

Following a single oral dose of [^{14}C]-labeled aripiprazole, approximately 25% and 55% of the administered radioactivity was recovered in the urine and feces, respectively. Less than 1% of unchanged aripiprazole was excreted in the urine and approximately 18% of the oral dose was recovered unchanged in the feces.

Special Populations

In general, no dosage adjustment for ABILIFY (aripiprazole) Tablets is required on the basis of a patient's age, gender, race, smoking status, hepatic function, or renal function (see **DOSAGE AND ADMINISTRATION: Dosage in Special Populations**). The pharmacokinetics of aripiprazole in special populations are described below.

Hepatic Impairment

In a single-dose study (15 mg of aripiprazole) in subjects with varying degrees of liver cirrhosis (Child-Pugh Classes A, B, and C) the AUC of aripiprazole, compared to healthy subjects, increased 31% in mild HI, increased 8% in moderate HI, and decreased 20% in severe HI. None of these differences would require dose adjustment.

Renal Impairment

In patients with severe renal impairment (creatinine clearance <30 mL/min), C_{max} of aripiprazole (given in a single dose of 15 mg) and dehydro-aripiprazole increased by 36% and 53%, respectively, but AUC was 15% lower for aripiprazole and 7% higher for dehydro-aripiprazole. Renal excretion of both unchanged aripiprazole and dehydro-aripiprazole is less than 1% of the dose. No dosage adjustment is required in subjects with renal impairment.

Elderly

In formal single-dose pharmacokinetic studies (with aripiprazole given in a single dose of 15 mg), aripiprazole clearance was 20% lower in elderly (≥65 years) subjects compared to younger adult subjects (18 to 64 years). There was no detectable age effect, however, in the population pharmacokinetic analysis in schizophrenia patients. Also, the pharmacokinetics of aripiprazole after multiple doses in elderly patients appeared similar to that observed in young, healthy subjects. No dosage adjustment is recommended for elderly patients (see **PRECAUTIONS: Geriatric Use**).

Gender

C_{max} and AUC of aripiprazole and its active metabolite, dehydro-aripiprazole, are 30 to 40% higher in women than in men, and correspondingly, the apparent oral clearance of aripiprazole is lower in women. These differences, however, are largely explained by differences in body weight (25%) between men and women. No dosage adjustment is recommended based on gender.

Race

Although no specific pharmacokinetic study was conducted to investigate the effects of race on the disposition of aripiprazole, population pharmacokinetic evaluation revealed no evidence of clinically significant race-related differences in the pharmacokinetics of aripiprazole. No dosage adjustment is recommended based on race.

Smoking

Based on studies utilizing human liver enzymes *in vitro*, aripiprazole is not a substrate for CYP1A2 and also does not undergo direct glucuronidation. Smoking should, therefore, not have an effect on the pharmacokinetics of aripiprazole. Consistent with these *in vitro* results, population pharmacokinetic evaluation did not reveal any significant pharmacokinetic differences between smokers and nonsmokers. No dosage adjustment is recommended based on smoking status.

Drug-Drug Interactions

Potential for Other Drugs to Affect ABILIFY (aripiprazole)

Aripiprazole is not a substrate of CYP1A1, CYP1A2, CYP2A6, CYP2B6, CYP2C8, CYP2C9, CYP2C19, or CYP2E1 enzymes. Aripiprazole also does not undergo direct glucuronidation. This suggests that an interaction of aripiprazole with inhibitors or inducers of these enzymes, or other factors, like smoking, is unlikely.

Both CYP3A4 and CYP2D6 are responsible for aripiprazole metabolism. Agents that induce CYP3A4 (e.g., carbamazepine) could cause an increase in aripiprazole clearance and lower blood levels. Inhibitors of CYP3A4 (e.g., ketoconazole) or CYP2D6 (e.g., quinidine, fluoxetine, or paroxetine) can inhibit aripiprazole elimination and cause increased blood levels.

Potential for ABILIFY (aripiprazole) to Affect Other Drugs

Aripiprazole is unlikely to cause clinically important pharmacokinetic interactions with drugs metabolized by cytochrome P450 enzymes. In *in vivo* studies, 10- to 30-mg/day doses of aripiprazole had no significant effect on metabolism by CYP2D6 (dextromethorphan), CYP2C9 (warfarin), CYP2C19 (omeprazole, warfarin), and CYP3A4 (dextromethorphan) substrates. Additionally, aripiprazole and dehydro-aripiprazole did not show potential for altering CYP1A2-mediated metabolism *in vitro* (see **PRECAUTIONS: Drug-Drug Interactions**).

Aripiprazole had no clinically important interactions with the following drugs:

Famotidine: Coadministration of aripiprazole (given in a single dose of 15 mg) with a 40-mg single dose of the H_2 antagonist famotidine, a potent gastric acid blocker, decreased the solubility of aripiprazole and, hence, its rate of absorption, reducing by 37% and 21% the C_{max} of aripiprazole and dehydro-aripiprazole, respectively, and by 13% and 15%, respectively, the extent of absorption (AUC). No dosage adjustment of aripiprazole is required when administered concomitantly with famotidine.

Valproate: When valproate (500–1500 mg/day) and aripiprazole (30 mg/day) were coadministered at steady state, the C_{max} and AUC of aripiprazole were decreased by 25%. No dosage adjustment of aripiprazole is required when administered concomitantly with valproate.

Lithium: A pharmacokinetic interaction of aripiprazole with lithium is unlikely because lithium is not bound to plasma proteins, is not metabolized, and is almost entirely excreted unchanged in urine. Coadministration of therapeutic doses of lithium (1200–1800 mg/day) for 21 days with aripiprazole (30 mg/day) did not result in clinically significant changes in the pharmacokinetics of aripiprazole or its active metabolite, dehydro-aripiprazole (C_{max} and AUC increased by less than 20%). No dosage adjustment of aripiprazole is required when administered concomitantly with lithium.

Dextromethorphan: Aripiprazole at doses of 10 to 30 mg per day for 14 days had no effect on dextromethorphan's O-dealkylation to its major metabolite, dextrorphan, a pathway known to be dependent on CYP2D6 activity. Aripiprazole also had no effect on dextromethorphan's N-demethylation to its metabolite 3-methyoxymorphan, a pathway known to be dependent on CYP3A4 activity. No dosage adjustment of dextromethorphan is required when administered concomitantly with aripiprazole.

Warfarin: Aripiprazole 10 mg per day for 14 days had no effect on the pharmacokinetics of R- and S-warfarin or on the pharmacodynamic end point of International Normalized Ratio, indicating the lack of a clinically relevant effect of aripiprazole on CYP2C9 and CYP2C19 metabolism or the binding of highly protein-bound warfarin. No dosage adjustment of warfarin is required when administered concomitantly with aripiprazole.

Omeprazole: Aripiprazole 10 mg per day for 15 days had no effect on the pharmacokinetics of a single 20-mg dose of omeprazole, a CYP2C19 substrate, in healthy subjects. No dosage adjustment of omeprazole is required when administered concomitantly with aripiprazole.

Clinical Studies

The efficacy of ABILIFY (aripiprazole) in the treatment of schizophrenia was evaluated in four short-term (4- and 6-week), placebo-controlled trials of acutely relapsed inpatients who predominantly met DSM-III/IV criteria for schizophrenia. Three of the four trials were able to distinguish aripiprazole from placebo, but one study, the smallest, did not. Three of these studies also included an active control group consisting of either risperidone (one trial) or haloperidol (two trials), but they were not designed to allow for a comparison of ABILIFY and the active comparators.

In the three positive trials for ABILIFY, four primary measures were used for assessing psychiatric signs and symptoms. The Positive and Negative Syndrome Scale (PANSS) is a multi-item inventory of general psychopathology used to evaluate the effects of drug treatment in schizophrenia. The PANSS positive subscale is a subset of items in the PANSS that rates seven positive symptoms of schizophrenia (delusions, conceptual disorganization, hallucinatory behavior, excitement, grandiosity, suspiciousness/persecution, and hostility). The PANSS negative subscale is a subset of items in the PANSS that rates seven negative symptoms of schizophrenia (blunted affect, emotional withdrawal, poor rapport, passive apathetic withdrawal, difficulty in abstract thinking, lack of spontaneity/flow of conversation, stereotyped thinking). The Clinical Global Impression (CGI) assessment reflects the impression of a skilled observer, fully familiar with the manifestations of schizophrenia, about the overall clinical state of the patient.

In a 4-week trial (n=414) comparing two fixed doses of ABILIFY (15 or 30 mg/day) and haloperidol (10 mg/day) to placebo, both doses of ABILIFY were superior to placebo in the PANSS total score, PANSS positive subscale, and CGI-severity score. In addition, the 15-mg dose was superior to placebo in the PANSS negative subscale.

In a 4-week trial (n=404) comparing two fixed doses of ABILIFY (20 or 30 mg/day) and risperidone (6 mg/day) to placebo, both doses of ABILIFY were superior to placebo in the PANSS total score, PANSS positive subscale, PANSS negative subscale, and CGI-severity score.

In a 6-week trial (n=420) comparing three fixed doses of ABILIFY (10, 15, or 20 mg/day) to placebo, all three doses of ABILIFY were superior to placebo in the PANSS total score, PANSS positive subscale, and the PANSS negative subscale.

In a fourth study, a 4-week trial (n=103) comparing ABILIFY in a range of 5 to 30 mg/day or haloperidol 5 to 20 mg/day to placebo, haloperidol was superior to placebo, in the Brief Psychiatric Rating Scale (BPRS), a multi-item inventory of general psychopathology traditionally used to evaluate the effects of drug treatment in psychosis, and in a responder analysis based on the CGI-severity score, the primary outcomes for that trial. ABILIFY was only significantly different compared to placebo in a responder analysis based on the CGI-severity score.

Thus, the efficacy of 15-mg, 20-mg, and 30-mg daily doses was established in two studies for each dose, whereas the efficacy of the 10-mg dose was established in one study. There was no evidence in any study that the higher dose groups offered any advantage over the lowest dose group.

An examination of population subgroups did not reveal any clear evidence of differential responsiveness on the basis of age, gender, or race.

INDICATIONS AND USAGE

ABILIFY (aripiprazole) is indicated for the treatment of schizophrenia. The efficacy of ABILIFY in the treatment of schizophrenia was established in short-term (4- and 6-week) controlled trials of schizophrenic inpatients (see **CLINICAL PHARMACOLOGY: Clinical Studies**).

The long-term efficacy of aripipazole in the treatment of schizophrenia has not been established. The physician who elects to use ABILIFY for extended periods should periodically re-evaluate the long-term usefulness of the drug for the individual patient.

CONTRAINDICATIONS

ABILIFY is contraindicated in patients with a known hypersensitivity to the product.

WARNINGS

Neuroleptic Malignant Syndrome (NMS)

A potentially fatal symptom complex sometimes referred to as Neuroleptic Malignant Syndrome (NMS) has been reported in association with administration of antipsychotic drugs, including aripiprazole. Two possible cases of NMS occurred during aripiprazole treatment in the premarketing worldwide clinical database. Clinical manifestations of NMS are hyperpyrexia, muscle rigidity, altered mental status, and evidence of autonomic instability (irregular pulse or blood pressure, tachycardia, diaphoresis, and cardiac dysrhythmia). Additional signs may include elevated creatine phosphokinase, myoglobinuria (rhabdomyolysis), and acute renal failure.

The diagnostic evaluation of patients with this syndrome is complicated. In arriving at a diagnosis, it is important to exclude cases where the clinical presentation includes both serious medical illness (e.g., pneumonia, systemic infection, etc) and untreated or inadequately treated extrapyramidal signs and symptoms (EPS). Other important considerations in the differential diagnosis include central anticholinergic toxicity, heat stroke, drug fever, and primary central nervous system pathology.

The management of NMS should include: 1) immediate discontinuation of antipsychotic drugs and other drugs not essential to concurrent therapy; 2) intensive symptomatic treatment and medical monitoring; and 3) treatment of any concomitant serious medical problems for which specific treatments are available. There is no general agreement about specific pharmacological treatment regimens for uncomplicated NMS.

If a patient requires antipsychotic drug treatment after recovery from NMS, the potential reintroduction of drug therapy should be carefully considered. The patient should be carefully monitored, since recurrences of NMS have been reported.

Tardive Dyskinesia

A syndrome of potentially irreversible, involuntary, dyskinetic movements may develop in patients treated with antipsychotic drugs. Although the prevalence of the syndrome appears to be highest among the elderly, especially elderly women, it is impossible to rely upon prevalence estimates to predict, at the inception of antipsychotic treatment, which

Continued on next page

Abilify—Cont.

patients are likely to develop the syndrome. Whether antipsychotic drug products differ in their potential to cause tardive dyskinesia is unknown.

The risk of developing tardive dyskinesia and the likelihood that it will become irreversible are believed to increase as the duration of treatment and the total cumulative dose of antipsychotic drugs administered to the patient increase. However, the syndrome can develop, although much less commonly, after relatively brief treatment periods at low doses.

There is no known treatment for established cases of tardive dyskinesia, although the syndrome may remit, partially or completely, if antipsychotic treatment is withdrawn. Antipsychotic treatment, itself, however, may suppress (or partially suppress) the signs and symptoms of the syndrome and, thereby, may possibly mask the underlying process. The effect that symptomatic suppression has upon the long-term course of the syndrome is unknown.

Given these considerations, ABILIFY should be prescribed in a manner that is most likely to minimize the occurrence of tardive dyskinesia. Chronic antipsychotic treatment should generally be reserved for patients who suffer from a chronic illness that (1) is known to respond to antipsychotic drugs, and (2) for whom alternative, equally effective, but potentially less harmful treatments are not available or appropriate. In patients who do require chronic treatment, the smallest dose and the shortest duration of treatment producing a satisfactory clinical response should be sought. The need for continued treatment should be reassessed periodically.

If signs and symptoms of tardive dyskinesia appear in a patient on ABILIFY, drug discontinuation should be considered. However, some patients may require treatment with ABILIFY despite the presence of the syndrome.

PRECAUTIONS
General
Orthostatic Hypotension
Aripiprazole may be associated with orthostatic hypotension, perhaps due to its α_1-adrenergic receptor antagonism. The incidence of orthostatic hypotension associated events from five short-term, placebo-controlled trials in schizophrenia (n=926) on ABILIFY (aripiprazole) included: orthostatic hypotension (placebo 1%, aripiprazole 1.9%); orthostatic lightheadedness (placebo 1%, aripiprazole 0.9%), and syncope (placebo 1%, aripiprazole 0.6%). The incidence of a significant orthostatic change in blood pressure (defined as a decrease of at least 30 mmHg in systolic blood pressure when changing from a supine to standing position) for aripiprazole was not statistically different from placebo (14% among aripiprazole-treated patients and 12% among placebo-treated patients).

Aripiprazole should be used with caution in patients with known cardiovascular disease (history of myocardial infarction or ischemic heart disease, heart failure or conduction abnormalities), cerebrovascular disease, or conditions which would predispose patients to hypotension (dehydration, hypovolemia, and treatment with antihypertensive medications).

Seizure
Seizures occurred in 0.1% (1/926) of aripiprazole-treated patients in short-term, placebo-controlled trials. As with other antipsychotic drugs, aripiprazole should be used cautiously in patients with a history of seizures or with conditions that lower the seizure threshold, e.g., Alzheimer's dementia. Conditions that lower the seizure threshold may be more prevalent in a population of 65 years or older.

Potential for Cognitive and Motor Impairment
In short-term, placebo-controlled trials, somnolence was reported in 11% of patients on ABILIFY (aripiprazole) compared to 8% of patients on placebo; somnolence led to discontinuation in 0.1% (1/926) of patients on ABILIFY in short-term, placebo-controlled trials. Despite the relatively modest increased incidence of somnolence compared to placebo, ABILIFY, like other antipsychotics, may have the potential to impair judgment, thinking, or motor skills. Patients should be cautioned about operating hazardous machinery, including automobiles, until they are reasonably certain that therapy with ABILIFY does not affect them adversely.

Body Temperature Regulation
Disruption of the body's ability to reduce core body temperature has been attributed to antipsychotic agents. Appropriate care is advised when prescribing aripiprazole for patients who will be experiencing conditions which may contribute to an elevation in core body temperature, e.g., exercising strenuously, exposure to extreme heat, receiving concomitant medication with anticholinergic activity, or being subject to dehydration.

Dysphagia
Esophageal dysmotility and aspiration have been associated with antipsychotic drug use. Aspiration pneumonia is a common cause of morbidity and mortality in elderly patients, in particular those with advanced Alzheimer's dementia. Aripiprazole and other antipsychotic drugs should be used cautiously in patients at risk for aspiration pneumonia (see **PRECAUTIONS**: Use in Patients with Concomitant Illness).

Suicide
The possibility of a suicide attempt is inherent in psychotic illnesses, and close supervision of high-risk patients should accompany drug therapy. Prescriptions for ABILIFY should be written for the smallest quantity of tablets consistent with good patient management in order to reduce the risk of overdose.

Use in Patients with Concomitant Illness
Safety Experience in Elderly Patients with Psychosis Associated with Alzheimer's Disease:
In a flexible dose (2 to 15 mg/day), 10-week, placebo-controlled study of aripiprazole in elderly patients (mean age: 81.5 years; range: 56 to 95 years) with psychosis associated with Alzheimer's dementia, 4 of 105 patients (3.8%) who received ABILIFY died compared to no deaths among 102 patients who received placebo during or within 30 days after termination of the double-blind portion of the study. Three of the patients (age 92, 91, and 87 years) died following the discontinuation of ABILIFY in the double-blind phase of the study (causes of death were pneumonia, heart failure, and shock). The fourth patient (age 78 years) died following hip surgery while in the double-blind portion of the study. The treatment-emergent adverse events that were reported at an incidence of ≥5% and having a greater incidence than placebo in this study were accidental injury, somnolence, and bronchitis. Eight percent of the ABILIFY-treated patients reported somnolence compared to one percent of placebo patients. In a small pilot, open-label, ascending-dose cohort study (n=30) in elderly patients with dementia, ABILIFY was associated in a dose-related fashion with somnolence.

The safety and efficacy of ABILIFY in the treatment of patients with psychosis associated with dementia have not been established. If the prescriber elects to treat such patients with ABILIFY, vigilance should be exercised, particularly for the emergence of difficulty swallowing or excessive somnolence, which could predispose to accidental injury or aspiration.

Clinical experience with ABILIFY in patients with certain concomitant systemic illnesses (see **CLINICAL PHARMACOLOGY: Special Populations:** *Renal Impairment* and *Hepatic Impairment*) is limited.

ABILIFY has not been evaluated or used to any appreciable extent in patients with a recent history of myocardial infarction or unstable heart disease. Patients with these diagnoses were excluded from premarketing clinical studies.

Information for Patients
Physicians are advised to discuss the following issues with patients for whom they prescribe ABILIFY (aripiprazole):
Interference with Cognitive and Motor Performance
Because aripiprazole may have the potential to impair judgment, thinking, or motor skills, patients should be cautioned about operating hazardous machinery, including automobiles, until they are reasonably certain that aripiprazole therapy does not affect them adversely.

Pregnancy
Patients should be advised to notify their physician if they become pregnant or intend to become pregnant during therapy with ABILIFY.

Nursing
Patients should be advised not to breast-feed an infant if they are taking ABILIFY.

Concomitant Medication
Patients should be advised to inform their physicians if they are taking, or plan to take, any prescription or over-the-counter drugs, since there is a potential for interactions.

Alcohol
Patients should be advised to avoid alcohol while taking ABILIFY.

Heat Exposure and Dehydration
Patients should be advised regarding appropriate care in avoiding overheating and dehydration.

Drug-Drug Interactions
Given the primary CNS effects of aripiprazole, caution should be used when ABILIFY (aripiprazole) is taken in combination with other centrally acting drugs and alcohol. Due to its α_1-adrenergic receptor antagonism, aripiprazole has the potential to enhance the effect of certain antihypertensive agents.

Potential for Other Drugs to Affect ABILIFY
Aripiprazole is not a substrate of CYP1A1, CYP1A2, CYP2A6, CYP2B6, CYP2C8, CYP2C9, CYP2C19, or CYP2E1 enzymes. Aripiprazole also does not undergo direct glucuronidation. This suggests that an interaction of aripiprazole with inhibitors or inducers of these enzymes, or other factors, like smoking, is unlikely.

Both CYP3A4 and CYP2D6 are responsible for aripiprazole metabolism. Agents that induce CYP3A4 (e.g., carbamazepine) could cause an increase in aripiprazole clearance and lower blood levels. Inhibitors of CYP3A4 (e.g., ketoconazole) or CYP2D6 (e.g., quinidine, fluoxetine, or paroxetine) can inhibit aripiprazole elimination and cause increased blood levels.

Ketoconazole: Coadministration of ketoconazole (200 mg/day for 14 days) with a 15-mg single dose of aripiprazole increased the AUC of aripiprazole and its active metabolite by 63% and 77%, respectively. The effect of a higher ketoconazole dose (400 mg/day) has not been studied. When concomitant administration of ketoconazole with aripiprazole occurs, aripiprazole dose should be reduced to one-half of its normal dose. Other strong inhibitors of CYP3A4 (itraconazole) would be expected to have similar effects and need similar dose reductions; weaker inhibitors (erythromycin, grapefruit juice) have not been studied. When the CYP3A4 inhibitor is withdrawn from the combination therapy, aripiprazole dose should then be increased.

Quinidine: Coadministration of a 10-mg single dose of aripiprazole with quinidine (166 mg/day for 13 days), a potent inhibitor of CYP2D6, increased the AUC of aripiprazole by 112% but decreased the AUC of its active metabolite, dehydro-aripiprazole, by 35%. Aripiprazole dose should be reduced to one-half of its normal dose when concomitant administration of quinidine with aripiprazole occurs. Other significant inhibitors of CYP2D6, such as fluoxetine or paroxetine, would be expected to have similar effects and, therefore, should be accompanied by similar dose reductions. When the CYP2D6 inhibitor is withdrawn from the combination therapy, aripiprazole dose should then be increased.

Carbamazepine: Coadministration of carbamazepine (200 mg BID), a potent CYP3A4 inducer, with aripiprazole (30 mg QD) resulted in an approximate 70% decrease in C_{max} and AUC values of both aripiprazole and its active metabolite, dehydro-aripiprazole. When carbamazepine is added to aripiprazole therapy, aripiprazole dose should be doubled. Additional dose increases should be based on clinical evaluation. When carbamazepine is withdrawn from the combination therapy, aripiprazole dose should then be reduced.

No clinically significant effect of famotidine, valproate, or lithium was seen on the pharmacokinetics of aripiprazole (see **CLINICAL PHARMACOLOGY: Drug-Drug Interactions**).

Potential for ABILIFY to Affect Other Drugs
Aripiprazole is unlikely to cause clinically important pharmacokinetic interactions with drugs metabolized by cytochrome P450 enzymes. In *in vivo* studies, 10- to 30-mg/day doses of aripiprazole had no significant effect on metabolism by CYP2D6 (dextromethorphan), CYP2C9 (warfarin), CYP2C19 (omeprazole, warfarin), and CYP3A4 (dextromethorphan) substrates. Additionally, aripiprazole and dehydro-aripiprazole did not show potential for altering CYP1A2-mediated metabolism *in vitro* (see **CLINICAL PHARMACOLOGY: Drug-Drug Interactions**).

Alcohol: There was no significant difference between aripiprazole coadministered with ethanol and placebo coadministered with ethanol on performance of gross motor skills or stimulus response in healthy subjects. As with most psychoactive medications, patients should be advised to avoid alcohol while taking ABILIFY (aripiprazole).

Carcinogenesis, Mutagenesis, Impairment of Fertility
Carcinogenesis
Lifetime carcinogenicity studies were conducted in ICR mice and in Sprague-Dawley (SD) and F344 rats. Aripiprazole was administered for 2 years in the diet at doses of 1, 3, 10, and 30 mg/kg/day to ICR mice and 1, 3, and 10 mg/kg/day to F344 rats (0.2 to 5 and 0.3 to 3 times the maximum recommended human dose [MRHD] based on mg/m^2, respectively). In addition, SD rats were dosed orally for 2 years at 10, 20, 40, and 60 mg/kg/day (3 to 19 times the MRHD based on mg/m^2). Aripiprazole did not induce tumors in male mice or rats. In female mice, the incidences of pituitary gland adenomas and mammary gland adenocarcinomas and adenoacanthomas were increased at dietary doses of 3 to 30 mg/kg/day (0.1 to 0.9 times human exposure at MRHD based on AUC and 0.5 to 5 times the MRHD based on mg/m^2). In female rats, the incidence of mammary gland fibroadenomas was increased at a dietary dose of 10 mg/kg/day (0.1 times human exposure at MRHD based on AUC and 3 times the MRHD based on mg/m^2); and the incidences of adrenocortical carcinomas and combined adrenocortical adenomas/carcinomas were increased at an oral dose of 60 mg/kg/day (14 times human exposure at MRHD based on AUC and 19 times the MRHD based on mg/m^2).

Proliferative changes in the pituitary and mammary gland of rodents have been observed following chronic administration of other antipsychotic agents and are considered prolactin-mediated. Serum prolactin was not measured in the aripiprazole carcinogenicity studies. However, increases in serum prolactin levels were observed in female mice in a 13-week dietary study at the doses associated with mammary gland and pituitary tumors. Serum prolactin was not increased in female rats in 4- and 13-week dietary studies at the dose associated with mammary gland tumors. The relevance for human risk of the findings of prolactin-mediated endocrine tumors in rodents is unknown.

Mutagenesis
The mutagenic potential of aripiprazole was tested in the *in vitro* bacterial reverse-mutation assay, the *in vitro* bacterial DNA repair assay, the *in vitro* forward gene mutation assay in mouse lymphoma cells, the *in vitro* chromosomal aberration assay in Chinese hamster lung (CHL) cells, the *in vivo* micronucleus assay in mice, and the unscheduled DNA synthesis assay in rats. Aripiprazole and a metabolite (2,3-DCPP) were clastogenic in the *in vitro* chromosomal aberration assay in CHL cells with and without metabolic activation. The metabolite, 2,3-DCPP, produced increases in numerical aberrations in the *in vitro* assay in CHL cells in the absence of metabolic activation. A positive response was obtained in the *in vivo* micronucleus assay in mice, however, the response was shown to be due to a mechanism not considered relevant to humans.

Impairment of Fertility
Female rats were treated with oral doses of 2, 6, and 20 mg/kg/day (0.6, 2, and 6 times the maximum recommended human dose [MRHD] on a mg/m^2 basis) of aripiprazole from 2 weeks prior to mating through day 7 of gestation. Estrus cycle irregularities and increased corpora lutea were seen at all doses, but no impairment of fertility was seen. Increased preimplantation loss was seen at 6 and 20 mg/kg, and decreased fetal weight was seen at 20 mg/kg.

Male rats were treated with oral doses of 20, 40, and 60 mg/kg/day (6, 13, and 19 times the MRHD on a mg/m^2 basis) of aripiprazole from 9 weeks prior to mating through mating.

Disturbances in spermatogenesis were seen at 60 mg/kg, and prostate atrophy was seen at 40 and 60 mg/kg, but no impairment of fertility was seen.

Pregnancy

Pregnancy Category C

In animal studies, aripiprazole demonstrated developmental toxicity, including possible teratogenic effects in rats and rabbits.

Pregnant rats were treated with oral doses of 3, 10, and 30 mg/kg/day (1, 3, and 10 times the maximum recommended human dose [MRHD] on a mg/m^2 basis) of aripiprazole during the period of organogenesis. Gestation was slightly prolonged at 30 mg/kg. Treatment caused a slight delay in fetal development, as evidenced by decreased fetal weight (30 mg/kg), undescended testes (30 mg/kg), and delayed skeletal ossification (10 and 30 mg/kg). There were no adverse effects on embryofetal or pup survival. Delivered offspring had decreased bodyweights (10 and 30 mg/kg), and increased incidences of hepatodiaphragmatic nodules and diaphragmatic hernia at 30 mg/kg (the other dose groups were not examined for these findings). (A low incidence of diaphragmatic hernia was also seen in the fetuses exposed to 30 mg/kg.) Postnatally, delayed vaginal opening was seen at 10 and 30 mg/kg and impaired reproductive performance (decreased fertility rate, corpora lutea, implants, and live fetuses, and increased post-implantation loss, likely mediated through effects on female offspring) was seen at 30 mg/kg. Some maternal toxicity was seen at 30 mg/kg, however, there was no evidence to suggest that these developmental effects were secondary to maternal toxicity.

Pregnant rabbits were treated with oral doses of 10, 30, and 100 mg/kg/day (2, 3, and 11 times human exposure at MRHD based on AUC and 6, 19, and 65 times the MRHD based on mg/m^2) of aripiprazole during the period of organogenesis. Decreased maternal food consumption and increased abortions were seen at 100 mg/kg. Treatment caused increased fetal mortality (100 mg/kg), decreased fetal weight (30 and 100 mg/kg), increased incidence of skeletal abnormality (fused sternebrae at 30 and 100 mg/kg) and minor skeletal variations (100 mg/kg).

In a study in which rats were treated with oral doses of 3, 10, and 30 mg/kg/day (1, 3, and 10 times the MRHD on a mg/m^2 basis) of aripiprazole perinatally and postnatally (from day 17 of gestation through day 21 postpartum), slight maternal toxicity and slightly prolonged gestation were seen at 30 mg/kg. An increase in stillbirths, and decreases in pup weight (persisting into adulthood) and survival, were seen at this dose.

There are no adequate and well-controlled studies in pregnant women. It is not known whether aripiprazole can cause fetal harm when administered to a pregnant woman or can affect reproductive capacity. Aripiprazole should be used during pregnancy only if the potential benefit outweighs the potential risk to the fetus.

Labor and Delivery

The effect of aripiprazole on labor and delivery in humans is unknown.

Nursing Mothers

Aripiprazole was excreted in milk of rats during lactation. It is not known whether aripiprazole or its metabolites are excreted in human milk. It is recommended that women receiving aripiprazole should not breast-feed.

Pediatric Use

Safety and effectiveness in pediatric and adolescent patients have not been established.

Geriatric Use

Of the 5592 patients treated with aripiprazole in premarketing clinical trials, 659 (12%) were ≥65 years old and 525 (9%) were ≥75 years old. The majority (91%) of the 659 patients were diagnosed with dementia of the Alzheimer's type.

Placebo-controlled studies of aripiprazole in schizophrenia did not include sufficient numbers of subjects aged 65 and over to determine whether they respond differently from younger subjects. There was no effect of age on the pharmacokinetics of a single 15-mg dose of aripiprazole. Aripiprazole clearance was decreased by 20% in elderly subjects (≥65 years) compared to younger adult subjects (18 to 64 years), but there was no detectable effect of age in the population pharmacokinetic analysis in schizophrenia patients.

Studies of elderly patients with psychosis associated with Alzheimer's disease, have suggested that there may be a different tolerability profile in this population compared to younger patients with schizophrenia (see **PRECAUTIONS:** *Use in Patients with Concomitant Illness*). The safety and efficacy of ABILIFY (aripiprazole) in the treatment of patients with psychosis associated with Alzheimer's disease has not been established. If the prescriber elects to treat such patients with ABILIFY, vigilance should be exercised.

ADVERSE REACTIONS

Aripiprazole has been evaluated for safety in 5592 patients who participated in multiple-dose, premarketing trials in schizophrenia, bipolar mania, and dementia of the Alzheimer's type, and who had approximately 3639 patient-years of exposure. A total of 1887 aripiprazole-treated patients were treated for at least 180 days and 1251 aripiprazole-treated patients had at least 1 year of exposure.

The conditions and duration of treatment with aripiprazole included (in overlapping categories) double-blind, comparative and noncomparative open-label studies, inpatient and outpatient studies, fixed- and flexible-dose studies, and short- and longer-term exposure.

Adverse events during exposure were obtained by collecting volunteered adverse events, as well as results of physical examinations, vital signs, weights, laboratory analyses, and ECG. Adverse experiences were recorded by clinical investigators using terminology of their own choosing. In the tables and tabulations that follow, modified COSTART dictionary terminology has been used initially to classify reported adverse events into a smaller number of standardized event categories, in order to provide a meaningful estimate of the proportion of individuals experiencing adverse events.

The stated frequencies of adverse events represent the proportion of individuals who experienced at least once, a treatment-emergent adverse event of the type listed. An event was considered treatment emergent if it occurred for the first time or worsened while receiving therapy following baseline evaluation. There was no attempt to use investigator causality assessments; ie, all reported events are included.

The prescriber should be aware that the figures in the tables and tabulations cannot be used to predict the incidence of side effects in the course of usual medical practice where patient characteristics and other factors differ from those that prevailed in the clinical trials. Similarly, the cited frequencies cannot be compared with figures obtained from other clinical investigations involving different treatment, uses, and investigators. The cited figures, however, do provide the prescribing physician with some basis for estimating the relative contribution of drug and nondrug factors to the adverse event incidence in the population studied.

Adverse Findings Observed in Short-Term, Placebo-Controlled Trials of Patients with Schizophrenia

The following findings are based on a pool of five placebo-controlled trials (four 4-week and one 6-week) in which aripiprazole was administered in doses ranging from 2 to 30 mg/day.

Adverse Events Associated with Discontinuation of Treatment in Short-Term, Placebo-Controlled Trials

Overall, there was no difference in the incidence of discontinuation due to adverse events between aripiprazole-treated (7%) and placebo-treated (9%) patients. The types of adverse events that led to discontinuation were similar between the aripiprazole and placebo-treated patients.

Adverse Events Occurring at an Incidence of 2% or More Among Aripiprazole-Treated Patients and Greater than Placebo in Short-Term Placebo-Controlled Trials

Table 1 enumerates the incidence, rounded to the nearest percent, of treatment-emergent adverse events that occurred during acute therapy (up to 6 weeks), including only those events that occurred in 2% or more of patients treated with aripiprazole (doses ≥2 mg/day) and for which the incidence in patients treated with aripiprazole was greater than the incidence in patients treated with placebo.

Table 1: Treatment-Emergent Adverse Events in Short-Term, Placebo-Controlled Trials

Body System Adverse Event	Percentage of Patients Reporting Event[a] Aripiprazole (n=926)	Placebo (n=413)
Body as a Whole		
Headache	32	25
Asthenia	7	5
Fever	2	1
Digestive System		
Nausea	14	10
Vomiting	12	7
Constipation	10	8
Nervous System		
Anxiety	25	24
Insomnia	24	19
Lightheadedness	11	7
Somnolence	11	8
Akathisia	10	7
Tremor	3	2
Respiratory System		
Rhinitis	4	3
Coughing	3	2
Skin and Appendages		
Rash	6	5
Special Senses		
Blurred vision	3	1

[a] Events reported by at least 2% of patients treated with aripiprazole, except the following events, which had an incidence equal to or less than placebo: abdominal pain, accidental injury, back pain, dental pain, dyspepsia, diarrhea, dry mouth, myalgia, agitation, psychosis, extrapyramidal syndrome, hypertonia, pharyngitis, upper respiratory tract infection, dysmenorrhea, vaginitis.

An examination of population subgroups did not reveal any clear evidence of differential adverse event incidence on the basis of age, gender, or race.

Dose-Related Adverse Events

Dose response relationships for the incidence of treatment-emergent adverse events were evaluated from four trials comparing various fixed doses (2, 10, 15, 20, and 30 mg/day) of aripiprazole to placebo. This analysis, stratified by study, indicated that the only adverse event to have a possible dose response relationship, and then most prominent only with 30 mg, was somnolence (placebo, 7.7%; 15 mg, 8.7%; 20 mg, 7.5%; 30 mg, 15.3%).

Extrapyramidal Symptoms

In the short-term, placebo-controlled trials the incidence of reported EPS for aripiprazole-treated patients was 6% vs. 6% for placebo. Objectively collected data from those trials on the Simpson Angus Rating Scale (for EPS), the Barnes Akathisia Scale (for akathisia), and the Assessments of Involuntary Movement Scales (for dyskinesias) also did not show a difference between aripiprazole and placebo, with the exception of the Barnes Akathisia Scale (aripiprazole, 0.08; placebo, -0.05).

Laboratory Test Abnormalities

A between group comparison for 4- to 6-week placebo-controlled trials revealed no medically important differences between the aripiprazole and placebo groups in the proportions of patients experiencing potentially clinically significant changes in routine serum chemistry, hematology, or urinalysis parameters. Similarly, there were no aripiprazole/placebo differences in the incidence of discontinuations for changes in serum chemistry, hematology, or urinalysis.

Weight Gain

In short-term trials, there was a slight difference in mean weight gain between aripiprazole and placebo patients (+0.7 kg vs. -0.05 kg, respectively), and also a difference in the proportion of patients meeting a weight gain criterion of ≥7% of body weight [aripiprazole (8%) compared to placebo (3%)]. The following table provides the weight change results from a long-term (52-week) study of aripiprazole, both mean change from baseline and proportions of patients meeting a weight gain criterion of ≥7% of body weight relative to baseline, categorized by BMI at baseline:

Table 2: Weight Change Results Categorized by BMI at Baseline

	BMI<23	BMI 23–27	BMI>27
Mean change from baseline (kg)	2.6	1.4	-1.2
% with ≥7% increase BW	30%	19%	8%

ECG Changes

Between group comparisons for pooled, placebo-controlled trials revealed no significant differences between aripiprazole and placebo in the proportion of patients experiencing potentially important changes in ECG parameters; in fact, within the dose range of 10 to 30 mg/day, aripiprazole tended to slightly shorten the QT_c interval. Aripiprazole was associated with a median increase in heart rate of 4 beats per minute compared to a 1 beat per minute increase among placebo patients.

Other Adverse Events Observed During the Premarketing Evaluation of Aripiprazole

Following is a list of modified COSTART terms that reflect treatment-emergent adverse events as defined in the introduction to the **ADVERSE REACTIONS** section reported by patients treated with aripiprazole at multiple doses ≥2 mg/day during any phase of a trial within the database of 5592 patients. All reported events are included except those already listed in Table 1, or other parts of the **ADVERSE REACTIONS** section, those considered in the **WARNINGS** or **PRECAUTIONS**, those event terms which were so general as to be uninformative, events reported with an incidence of <0.05% and which did not have a substantial probability of being acutely life-threatening, events that are otherwise common as background events, and events considered unlikely to be drug related. It is important to emphasize that, although the events reported occurred during treatment with aripiprazole, they were not necessarily caused by it.

Events are further categorized by body system and listed in order of decreasing frequency according to the following definitions: frequent adverse events are those occurring in at least 1/100 patients (only those not already listed in the tabulated results from placebo-controlled trials appear in this listing); infrequent adverse events are those occurring in 1/100 to 1/1000 patients; rare events are those occurring in fewer than 1/1000 patients.

Body as a Whole: Frequent—flu syndrome, peripheral edema, chest pain, neck pain, neck rigidity; *Infrequent*—pelvic pain, suicide attempt, face edema, malaise, photosensitivity, arm rigidity, jaw pain, chills, bloating, jaw tightness, enlarged abdomen, chest tightness; *Rare*—throat pain, back tightness, head heaviness, moniliasis, throat tightness, leg rigidity, neck tightness, Mendelson's syndrome, heat stroke.

Cardiovascular System: Frequent—hypertension, tachycardia, hypotension, bradycardia; *Infrequent*—palpitation, hemorrhage, myocardial infarction, prolonged QT interval, cardiac arrest, atrial fibrillation, heart failure, AV block, myocardial ischemia, phlebitis, deep vein thrombosis, angina pectoris, extrasystoles; *Rare*—vasovagal reaction, cardiomegaly, atrial flutter, thrombophlebitis.

Digestive System: Frequent—anorexia, nausea and vomiting; *Infrequent*—increased appetite, gastroenteritis, dysphagia, flatulence, gastritis, tooth caries, gingivitis, hemorrhoids, gastroesophageal reflux, gastrointestinal hemorrhage, periodontal abscess, tongue edema, fecal incontinence, colitis, rectal hemorrhage, stomatitis, mouth ulcer, cholecystitis, fecal impaction, oral moniliasis, cholelithiasis, eructation, intestinal obstruction, peptic ulcer;

Continued on next page

Abilify—Cont.

Rare—esophagitis, gum hemorrhage, glossitis, hematemesis, melena, duodenal ulcer, cheilitis, hepatitis, hepatomegaly, pancreatitis, intestinal perforation.
Endocrine System: Infrequent—hypothroidism; *Rare*—goiter, hyperthyroidism.
Hemic/Lymphatic System: Frequent—ecchymosis, anemia; *Infrequent*—hypochromic anemia, leukopenia, leukocytosis, lymphadenopathy, thrombocytopenia; *Rare*—eosinophilia, thrombocythemia, macrocytic anemia.
Metabolic and Nutritional Disorders: Frequent—weight loss, creatine phosphokinase increased; *Infrequent*—dehydration, edema, hypercholesteremia, hyperglycemia, hypokalemia, diabetes mellitus, SGPT increased, hyperlipemia, hypoglycemia, thirst, BUN increased, hyponatremia, SGOT increased, alkaline phosphatase increased, iron deficiency anemia, creatinine increased, bilirubinemia, lactic dehydrogenase increased, obesity; *Rare*—hyperkalemia, gout, hypernatremia, cyanosis, hyperuricemia, hypoglycemic reaction.
Musculoskeletal System: Frequent—muscle cramp; *Infrequent*—arthralgia, bone pain, myasthenia, arthritis, arthrosis, muscle weakness, spasm, bursitis; *Rare*—rhabdomyolysis, tendonitis, tenosynovitis, rheumatoid arthritis, myopathy.
Nervous System: Frequent—depression, nervousness, increased salivation, hostility, suicidal thought, manic reaction, abnormal gait, confusion, cogwheel rigidity; *Infrequent*—dystonia, twitch, impaired concentration, paresthesia, vasodilation, hyperesthesia, extremity tremor, impotence, bradykinesia, decreased libido, panic attack, apathy, dyskinesia, hypersomnia, vertigo, dysarthria, tardive dyskinesia, ataxia, impaired memory, stupor, increased libido, amnesia, cerebrovascular accident, hyperactivity, depersonalization, hypokinesia, restless leg, myoclonus, dysphoria, neuropathy, increased reflexes, slowed thinking, hyperkinesia, hyperesthesia, hypotonia, oculogyric crisis; *Rare*—delirium, euphoria, buccoglossal syndrome, akinesia, blunted affect, decreased consciousness, incoordination, cerebral ischemia, decreased reflexes, obsessive thought, intracranial hemmorage.
Respiratory System: Frequent—dyspnea, pneumonia; *Infrequent*—asthma, epistaxis, hiccup, laryngitis; *Rare*—hemoptysis, aspiration pneumonia, increased sputum, dry nasal passages, pulmonary edema, pulmonary embolism, hypoxia, respiratory failure, apnea.
Skin and Appendages: Frequent—dry skin, pruritis, sweating, skin ulcer; *Infrequent*—acne, vesiculobullous rash, eczema, alopecia, psoriasis, seborrhea; *Rare*—maculopapular rash, exfoliative dermatitis, urticaria.
Special Senses: Frequent—conjunctivitus, ear pain; *Infrequent*—dry eye, eye pain, tinnitus, otitis media, cataract, altered taste, blepharitis; *Rare*—increased lacrimation, frequent blinking, otitis externa, amblyopia, deafness, diplopia, eye hemorrhage, photophobia.
Urogenital System: Frequent—urinary incontinence; *Infrequent*—cystitis, urinary frequency, leukorrhea, urinary retention, hematuria, dysuria, amenorrhea, abnormal ejaculation, vaginal hemorrhage, vaginal moniliasis, kidney failure, uterus hemorrhage, menorrhagia, albuminuria, kidney calculus, nocturia, polyuria, urinary urgency; *Rare*—breast pain, cervicitis, female lactation, anorgasmy, urinary burning, glycosuria, gynecomastia, urolithiasis, priapism.

DRUG ABUSE AND DEPENDENCE

Controlled Substance

ABILIFY (aripiprazole) is not a controlled substance.

Abuse and Dependence

Aripiprazole has not been systematically studied in humans for its potential for abuse, tolerance, or physical dependence. In physical dependence studies in monkeys, withdrawal symptoms were observed upon abrupt cessation of dosing. While the clinical trials did not reveal any tendency for any drug-seeking behavior, these observations were not systematic and it is not possible to predict on the basis of this limited experience the extent to which a CNS-active drug will be misused, diverted, and/or abused once marketed. Consequently, patients should be evaluated carefully for a history of drug abuse, and such patients should be observed closely for signs of ABILIFY misuse or abuse (e.g., development of tolerance, increases in dose, drug-seeking behavior).

OVERDOSAGE

Human Experience

In premarketing clinical studies, involving more than 5500 patients, accidental or intentional acute overdosage of aripiprazole was identified in seven patients. In the two patients taking the largest identified amount, 180 mg, the only symptoms reported were somnolence and vomiting in one of the two patients. In the patients who were evaluated in hospital settings, including the two patients taking 180 mg, there were no observations indicating an adverse change in vital signs, laboratory assessments, or ECG. An uneventful, accidental overdose (15 mg) occurred in a non-patient, an 18-month-old child, with concomitant ingestion of ATIVAN® (2 mg).

ATIVAN® is a registered trademark of Wyeth Laboratories, a Wyeth-Ayerst Company.

Management of Overdosage

No specific information is available on the treatment of overdose with aripiprazole. An electrocardiogram should be obtained in case of overdosage and, if QT_c interval prolongation is present, cardiac monitoring should be instituted. Otherwise, management of overdose should concentrate on supportive therapy, maintaining an adequate airway, oxygenation and ventilation, and management of symptoms. Close medical supervision and monitoring should continue until the patient recovers.
Charcoal: In the event of an overdose of ABILIFY (aripiprazole), an early charcoal administration may be useful in partially preventing the absorption of aripiprazole. Administration of 50 g of activated charcoal, one hour after a single 15-mg oral dose of aripiprazole, decreased the mean AUC and C_{max} of aripiprazole by 50%.
Hemodialysis: Although there is no information on the effect of hemodialysis in treating an overdose with aripiprazole, hemodialysis is unlikely to be useful in overdose management since aripiprazole is highly bound to plasma proteins.

DOSAGE AND ADMINISTRATION

Usual Dose

The recommended starting and target dose for ABILIFY is 10 or 15 mg/day administered on a once-a-day schedule without regard to meals. ABILIFY has been systematically evaluated and shown to be effective in a dose range of 10 to 30 mg/day; however, doses higher than 10 or 15 mg/day, the lowest doses in these trials, were not more effective than 10 or 15 mg/day. Dosage increases should not be made before 2 weeks, the time needed to achieve steady state.

Dosage in Special Populations

Dosage adjustments are not routinely indicated on the basis of age, gender, race, or renal or hepatic impairment status (see **CLINICAL PHARMACOLOGY: Special Populations**).
Dosage adjustment for patients taking aripiprazole concomitantly with potential CYP3A4 inhibitors: When concomitant administration of ketoconazole with aripiprazole occurs, aripiprazole dose should be reduced to one-half of the usual dose. When the CYP3A4 inhibitor is withdrawn from the combination therapy, aripiprazole dose should then be increased.
Dosage adjustment for patients taking aripiprazole concomitantly with potential CYP2D6 inhibitors: When concomitant administration of potential CYP2D6 inhibitors such as quinidine, fluoxetine, or paroxetine with aripiprazole occurs, aripiprazole dose should be reduced at least to one-half of its normal dose. When the CYP2D6 inhibitor is withdrawn from the combination therapy, aripiprazole dose should then be increased.
Dosage adjustment for patients taking potential CYP3A4 inducers: When a potential CYP3A4 inducer such as carbamazepine is added to aripiprazole therapy, the aripiprazole dose should be doubled (to 20 to 30 mg). Additional dose increases should be based on clinical evaluation. When carbamazepine is withdrawn from the combination therapy, the aripiprazole dose should be reduced to 10 to 15 mg.

Maintenance Therapy

There is no body of evidence available from controlled trials to answer the question of how long a patient treated with aripiprazole should remain on it. It is generally agreed, however, that pharmacological treatment for episodes of acute schizophrenia should continue for up to 6 months or longer. Patients should be periodically reassessed to determine the need for maintenance treatment.

Switching from Other Antipsychotics

There are no systematically collected data to specifically address switching patients with schizophrenia from other antipsychotics to ABILIFY or concerning concomitant administration with other antipsychotics. While immediate discontinuation of the previous antipsychotic treatment may be acceptable for some patients with schizophrenia, more gradual discontinuation may be most appropriate for others. In all cases, the period of overlapping antipsychotic administration should be minimized.

ANIMAL TOXICOLOGY

Aripiprazole produced retinal degeneration in albino rats in a 26-week chronic toxicity study at a dose of 60 mg/kg and in a 2-year carcinogenicity study at doses of 40 and 60 mg/kg. The 40- and 60-mg/kg doses represent 13 and 19 times the maximum recommended human dose (MRHD) based on mg/m^2 and 7 to 14 times human exposure at MRHD based on AUC. Evaluation of the retinas of albino mice and monkeys did not reveal evidence of retinal degeneration. Additional studies to further evaluate the mechanism have not been performed. The relevance of this finding to human risk is unknown.

HOW SUPPLIED

ABILIFY™ (aripiprazole) Tablets are available in the following strengths and packages.

The 10-mg ABILIFY tablets are pink, modified rectangular tablets, debossed on one side with "A-008" and "10".

Bottles of 30	NDC 59148-008-13
Blister of 100	NDC 59148-008-35

The 15-mg ABILIFY tablets are yellow, round tablets, debossed on one side with "A-009" and "15".

Bottles of 30	NDC 59148-009-13
Blister of 100	NDC 59148-009-35

The 20-mg ABILIFY tablets are white, round tablets, debossed on one side with "A-010" and "20".

Bottles of 30	NDC 59148-010-13
Blister of 100	NDC 59148-010-35

The 30-mg ABILIFY tablets are pink, round tablets, debossed on one side with "A-011" and "30".

Bottles of 30	NDC 59148-011-13
Blister of 100	NDC 59148-011-35

Storage

Store at 25° C (77° F); excursions permitted to 15–30° C (59–86° F) [see USP Controlled Room Temperature].

Marketed by Otsuka America Pharmaceutical, Inc, Rockville, MD 20850 USA
and Bristol-Myers Squibb Co, Princeton, NJ 08543 USA
Manufactured by Otsuka Pharmaceutical Co, Ltd, Tokyo, 101-8535 Japan
Distributed by Bristol-Myers Squibb Co, Princeton, NJ 08543 USA
U.S. Patent Nos. 4,734,416 and 5,006,528
D6-B0001-11-02 Issued: November 2002
A4114/10-02

METAGLIP™ ℞

(glipizide and metformin HCl) Tablets
2.5 mg/250 mg
2.5 mg/500 mg
5 mg/500 mg

DESCRIPTION

METAGLIP™ (glipizide and metformin HCl) Tablets contains two oral antihyperglycemic drugs used in the management of type 2 diabetes, glipizide and metformin hydrochloride.

Glipizide is an oral antihyperglycemic drug of the sulfonylurea class. The chemical name for glipizide is 1-cyclohexyl-3-[[*p*-[2-(5-methylpyrazinecarboxamido)ethyl]phenyl]sulfonyl]urea. Glipizide is a whitish, odorless powder with a molecular formula of $C_{21}H_{27}N_5O_4S$, a molecular weight of 445.55 and a pK_a of 5.9. It is insoluble in water and alcohols, but soluble in 0.1 *N* NaOH; it is freely soluble in dimethylformamide. The structural formula is represented below.

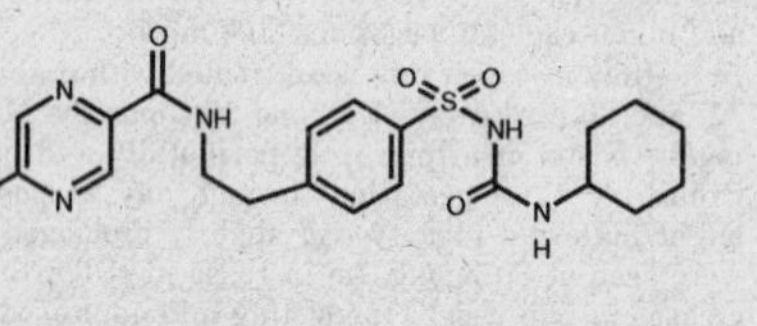

Glipizide

Metformin hydrochloride is an oral antihyperglycemic drug used in the management of type 2 diabetes. Metformin hydrochloride (*N,N*-dimethylimidodicarbonimidic diamide mono-hydrochloride) is not chemically or pharmacologically related to sulfonylureas, thiazolidinediones, or α-glucosidase inhibitors. It is a white to off-white crystalline compound with a molecular formula of $C_4H_{12}ClN_5$ (monohydrochloride) and a molecular weight of 165.63. Metformin hydrochloride is freely soluble in water and is practically insoluble in acetone, ether, and chloroform. The pK_a of metformin is 12.4. The pH of a 1% aqueous solution of metformin hydrochloride is 6.68. The structural formula is as shown:

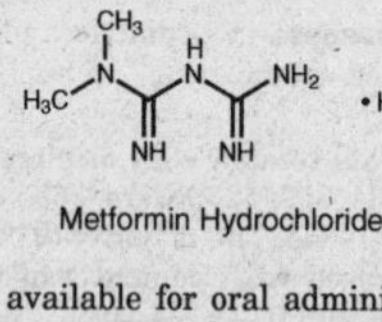

Metformin Hydrochloride

METAGLIP is available for oral administration in tablets containing 2.5 mg glipizide with 250 mg metformin hydrochloride, 2.5 mg glipizide with 500 mg metformin hydrochloride, and 5 mg glipizide with 500 mg metformin hydrochloride. In addition, each tablet contains the following inactive ingredients: microcrystalline cellulose, povidone, croscarmellose sodium, and magnesium stearate. The tablets are film coated, which provides color differentiation.

CLINICAL PHARMACOLOGY

Mechanism of Action

METAGLIP (glipizide and metformin HCl) combines glipizide and metformin hydrochloride, two antihyperglycemic agents with complementary mechanisms of action, to improve glycemic control in patients with type 2 diabetes.

Glipizide appears to lower blood glucose acutely by stimulating the release of insulin from the pancreas, an effect dependent upon functioning beta cells in the pancreatic islets. Extrapancreatic effects may play a part in the mechanism of action of oral sulfonylurea hypoglycemic drugs. The mechanism by which glipizide lowers blood glucose during long-term administration has not been clearly established. In man, stimulation of insulin secretion by glipizide in response to a meal is undoubtedly of major importance. Fasting insulin levels are not elevated even on long-term glipizide administration, but the postprandial insulin response continues to be enhanced after at least 6 months of treatment.

Metformin hydrochloride is an antihyperglycemic agent that improves glucose tolerance in patients with type 2 diabetes, lowering both basal and postprandial plasma glucose. Metformin hydrochloride decreases hepatic glucose production, decreases intestinal absorption of glucose, and improves insulin sensitivity by increasing peripheral glucose uptake and utilization.

Pharmacokinetics
Absorption and Bioavailability
METAGLIP
In a single dose study in healthy subjects, the glipizide and metformin components of METAGLIP 5 mg/500 mg were bioequivalent to coadministered GLUCOTROL® and GLUCOPHAGE®. Following administration of a single METAGLIP 5 mg/500 mg tablet in healthy subjects with either a 20% glucose solution or a 20% glucose solution with food, there was a small effect of food on peak plasma concentration (C_{max}) and no effect of food on area under the curve (AUC) of the glipizide component. Time to peak plasma concentration (T_{max}) for the glipizide component was delayed 1 hour with food relative to the same tablet strength administered fasting with a 20% glucose solution. C_{max} for the metformin component was reduced approximately 14% by food whereas AUC was not affected. T_{max} for the metformin component was delayed 1 hour after food.

Glipizide
Gastrointestinal absorption of glipizide is uniform, rapid, and essentially complete. Peak plasma concentrations occur 1–3 hours after a single oral dose. Glipizide does not accumulate in plasma on repeated oral administration. Total absorption and disposition of an oral dose was unaffected by food in normal volunteers, but absorption was delayed by about 40 minutes.

Metformin hydrochloride
The absolute bioavailability of a 500 mg metformin hydrochloride tablet given under fasting conditions is approximately 50–60%. Studies using single oral doses of metformin tablets of 500 mg and 1500 mg, and 850 mg to 2550 mg, indicate that there is a lack of dose proportionality with increasing doses, which is due to decreased absorption rather than an alteration in elimination. Food decreases the extent of and slightly delays the absorption of metformin, as shown by approximately a 40% lower peak concentration and a 25% lower AUC in plasma and a 35-minute prolongation of time to peak plasma concentration following administration of a single 850 mg tablet of metformin with food, compared to the same tablet strength administered fasting. The clinical relevance of these decreases is unknown.

Distribution
Glipizide
Protein binding was studied in serum from volunteers who received either oral or intravenous glipizide and found to be 98–99% one hour after either route of administration. The apparent volume of distribution of glipizide after intravenous was 11 liters, indicative of localization within the extracellular fluid compartment. In mice, no glipizide or metabolites were detectable autoradiographically in the brain or spinal cord of males or females, nor in the fetuses of pregnant females. In another study, however, very small amounts of radioactivity were detected in the fetuses of rats given labeled drug.

Metformin hydrochloride
The apparent volume of distribution (V/F) of metformin following single oral doses of 850 mg averaged 654 ± 358 L. Metformin is negligibly bound to plasma proteins. Metformin partitions into erythrocytes, most likely as a function of time. At usual clinical doses and dosing schedules of metformin, steady state plasma concentrations of metformin are reached within 24–48 hours and are generally <1 µg/mL. During controlled clinical trials, maximum metformin plasma levels did not exceed 5 µg/mL, even at maximum doses.

Metabolism and Elimination
Glipizide
The metabolism of glipizide is extensive and occurs mainly in the liver. The primary metabolites are inactive hydroxylation products and polar conjugates and are excreted mainly in the urine. Less than 10% unchanged glipizide is found in the urine. The half-life of elimination ranges from 2–4 hours in normal subjects, whether given intravenously or orally. The metabolic and excretory patterns are similar with the two routes of administration, indicating that first-pass metabolism is not significant.

Metformin hydrochloride
Intravenous single-dose studies in normal subjects demonstrate that metformin is excreted unchanged in the urine and does not undergo hepatic metabolism (no metabolites have been identified in humans) nor biliary excretion. Renal clearance (see **Table 1**) is approximately 3.5 times greater than creatinine clearance, which indicates that tubular secretion is the major route of metformin elimination. Following oral administration, approximately 90% of the absorbed drug is eliminated via the renal route within the first 24 hours, with a plasma elimination half-life of approximately 6.2 hours. In blood, the elimination half-life is approximately 17.6 hours, suggesting that the erythrocyte mass may be a compartment of distribution.

Special Populations
Patients With Type 2 Diabetes
In the presence of normal renal function, there are no differences between single- or multiple-dose pharmacokinetics of metformin between patients with type 2 diabetes and normal subjects (see **Table 1**), nor is there any accumulation of metformin in either group at usual clinical doses.

Hepatic Insufficiency
The metabolism and excretion of glipizide may be slowed in patients with impaired hepatic function (see **PRECAUTIONS**). No pharmacokinetic studies have been conducted in patients with hepatic insufficiency for metformin.

Renal Insufficiency
The metabolism and excretion of glipizide may be slowed in patients with impaired renal function (see **PRECAUTIONS**).

In patients with decreased renal function (based on creatinine clearance), the plasma and blood half-life of metformin is prolonged and the renal clearance is decreased in proportion to the decrease in creatinine clearance (see **Table 1**; also see **WARNINGS**).

Geriatrics
There is no information on the pharmacokinetics of glipizide in elderly patients.
Limited data from controlled pharmacokinetic studies of metformin in healthy elderly subjects suggest that total plasma clearance is decreased, the half-life is prolonged, and C_{max} is increased, compared to healthy young subjects. From these data, it appears that the change in metformin pharmacokinetics with aging is primarily accounted for by a change in renal function (see **Table 1**). Metformin treatment should not be initiated in patients ≥80 years of age unless measurement of creatinine clearance demonstrates that renal function is not reduced.
[See table 1 above]

Pediatrics
No data from pharmacokinetic studies in pediatric subjects are available for either glipizide or metformin.

Gender
There is no information on the effect of gender on the pharmacokinetics of glipizide.
Metformin pharmacokinetic parameters did not differ significantly in subjects with or without type 2 diabetes when analyzed according to gender (males = 19, females = 16). Similarly, in controlled clinical studies in patients with type 2 diabetes, the antihyperglycemic effect of metformin was comparable in males and females.

Race
No information is available on race differences in the pharmacokinetics of glipizide.
No studies of metformin pharmacokinetic parameters according to race have been performed. In controlled clinical studies of metformin in patients with type 2 diabetes, the antihyperglycemic effect was comparable in whites (n=249), blacks (n=51), and Hispanics (n=24).

CLINICAL STUDIES
Initial Therapy
In a 24-week, double-blind, active-controlled, multicenter international clinical trial, patients with type 2 diabetes, whose hyperglycemia was not adequately controlled with diet and exercise alone (hemoglobin A_{1c} [HbA_{1c}] >7.5% and ≤12% and fasting plasma glucose [FPG] <300 mg/dL) were randomized to receive initial therapy with glipizide 5 mg, metformin 500 mg, METAGLIP 2.5 mg/250 mg, or METAGLIP 2.5 mg/500 mg. After two weeks, the dose was progressively increased (up to the 12-week visit) to a maximum of four tablets daily in divided doses as needed to reach a target mean daily glucose (MDG) of ≤130 mg/dL. Trial data at 24 weeks are summarized in **Table 2**.
[See table 2 above]

After 24 weeks, treatment with METAGLIP (glipizide and metformin HCl) Tablets 2.5 mg/250 mg and 2.5 mg/500 mg resulted in significantly greater reduction in HbA_{1c} compared to glipizide and to metformin therapy. Also, METAGLIP 2.5 mg/250 mg therapy resulted in significant reductions in FPG versus metformin therapy.

Increases above fasting glucose and insulin levels were determined at baseline and final study visits by measurement of plasma glucose and insulin for three hours following a standard mixed liquid meal. Treatment with METAGLIP lowered the three-hour postprandial glucose AUC, compared to baseline, to a significantly greater extent than did the glipizide and the metformin therapies. Compared to baseline, METAGLIP enhanced the postprandial insulin response, but did not significantly affect fasting insulin levels.

Continued on next page

Table 1: Select Mean (±S.D.) Metformin Pharmacokinetic Parameters Following Single or Multiple Oral Doses of Metformin

Subject Groups: Metformin Dose[a] (Number of Subjects)	C_{max}[b] (µg/mL)	T_{max}[c] (hrs)	Renal Clearance (mL/min)
Healthy, Nondiabetic Adults:			
500 mg SD[d] (24)	1.03 (±0.33)	2.75 (±0.81)	600 (±132)
850 mg SD (74)[e]	1.60 (±0.38)	2.64 (±0.82)	552 (±139)
850 mg t.i.d. for 19 doses[f] (9)	2.01 (±0.42)	1.79 (±0.94)	642 (±173)
Adults and Type 2 Diabetes:			
850 mg SD (23)	1.48 (±0.5)	3.32 (±1.08)	491 (±138)
850 mg t.i.d. for 19 doses[f] (9)	1.90 (±0.62)	2.01 (±1.22)	550 (±160)
Elderly[g], Healthy Nondiabetic Adults:			
850 mg SD (12)	2.45 (±0.70)	2.71 (±1.05)	412 (±98)
Renal-impaired Adults:			
850 mg SD			
Mild (CL_{cr}[h] 61–90 mL/min (5)	1.86 (±0.52)	3.20 (±0.45)	384 (±122)
Moderate (CL_{cr} 31–60 mL/min (4)	4.12 (±1.83)	3.75 (±0.50)	108 (±57)
Severe (CL_{cr} 10–30 mL/min (6)	3.93 (±0.92)	4.01 (±1.10)	130 (±90)

[a] All doses given fasting except the first 18 doses of the multiple-dose studies
[b] Peak plasma concentration
[c] Time to peak plasma concentration
[d] SD = single dose
[e] Combined results (average means) of five studies: mean age 32 years (range 23–59 years)
[f] Kinetic study done following dose 19, given fasting
[g] Elderly subjects, mean age 71 years (range 65–81 years)
[h] CL_{cr} = creatinine clearance normalized to body surface area of 1.73 m²

Table 2: Active-Controlled Trial of METAGLIP as Initial Therapy: Summary of Trial Data at 24 Weeks

	Glipizide 5 mg tablets	Metformin 500 mg tablets	METAGLIP 2.5 mg/250 mg tablets	METAGLIP 2.5 mg/500 mg tablets
Mean Final Dose	16.7 mg	1749 mg	7.9 mg/791 mg	7.4 mg/1477 mg
Hemoglobin A_{1c} (%)	N=168	N=171	N=166	N=163
Baseline Mean	9.17	9.15	9.06	9.10
Final Mean	7.36	7.67	6.93	6.95
Adjusted Mean Change from Baseline	−1.77	−1.46	−2.15	−2.14
Difference from Glipizide			−0.38[a]	−0.37[a]
Difference from Metformin			−0.70[a]	−0.69[a]
% Patients with Final HbA_{1c} <7%	43.5%	35.1%	59.6%	57.1%
Fasting Plasma Glucose (mg/dL)	N=169	N=176	N=170	N=169
Baseline Mean	210.7	207.4	206.8	203.1
Final Mean	162.1	163.8	152.1	148.7
Adjusted Mean Change from Baseline	−46.2	−42.9	−54.2	−56.5
Difference from Glipizide			−8.0	−10.4
Difference from Metformin			−11.3	−13.6

[a] $p < 0.001$

Metaglip—Cont.

There were no clinically meaningful differences in changes from baseline for all lipid parameters between METAGLIP (glipizide and metformin HCl) therapy and either metformin therapy or glipizide therapy. The adjusted mean changes from baseline in body weight were: METAGLIP 2.5 mg/250 mg, −0.4 kg; METAGLIP 2.5 mg/500 mg, −0.5 kg; glipizide, −0.2 kg; and metformin, −1.9 kg. Weight loss was greater with metformin than with METAGLIP.

Second-Line Therapy

In an 18-week, double-blind, active-controlled U.S. clinical trial, a total of 247 patients with type 2 diabetes not adequately controlled (HbA_{1c} ≥7.5% and ≤12% and FPG <300 mg/dL) while being treated with at least one-half the maximum labeled dose of a sulfonylurea (e.g. glyburide 10 mg, glipizide 20 mg) were randomized to receive glipizide (fixed dose, 30 mg), metformin (500 mg), or METAGLIP 5 mg/500 mg. The doses of metformin and METAGLIP were titrated (up to the eight-week visit) to a maximum of four tablets daily as needed to achieve MDG ≤130 mg/dL. Trial data at 18 weeks are summarized in **Table 3**.

[See table 3 above]

Table 3: METAGLIP as Second-Line Therapy: Summary of Trial Data at 18 Weeks

	Glipizide 5 mg tablets	Metformin 500 mg tablets	METAGLIP 5 mg/500 mg tablets
Mean Final Dose	30.0 mg	1927 mg	17.5 mg/1747 mg
Hemoglobin A_{1c} (%)	N=79	N=71	N=80
Baseline Mean	8.87	8.61	8.66
Final Adjusted Mean	8.45	8.36	7.39
Difference from Glipizide			−1.06[a]
Difference from Metformin			−0.98[a]
% Patients with Final HbA_{1c} <7%	8.9%	9.9%	36.3%
Fasting Plasma Glucose (mg/dL)	N=82	N=75	N=81
Baseline Mean	203.6	191.3	194.3
Adjusted Mean Change from Baseline	7.0	6.7	−30.4
Difference from Glipizide			−37.4
Difference from Metformin			−37.2

[a] $p < 0.001$

After 18 weeks, treatment with METAGLIP at doses up to 20 mg/2000 mg per day resulted in significantly lower mean final HbA_{1c} and significantly greater mean reductions in FPG compared to glipizide and to metformin therapy. Treatment with METAGLIP lowered the three-hour postprandial glucose AUC, compared to baseline, to a significantly greater extent than did the glipizide and the metformin therapies. METAGLIP did not significantly affect fasting insulin levels.

There were no clinically meaningful differences in changes from baseline for all lipid parameters between METAGLIP therapy and either metformin therapy or glipizide therapy. The adjusted mean changes from baseline in body weight were: METAGLIP 5 mg/500 mg, −0.3 kg; glipizide, −0.4 kg; and metformin, −2.7 kg. Weight loss was greater with metformin than with METAGLIP.

INDICATIONS AND USAGE

METAGLIP (glipizide and metformin HCl) Tablets is indicated as initial therapy, as an adjunct to diet and exercise, to improve glycemic control in patients with type 2 diabetes whose hyperglycemia cannot be satisfactorily managed with diet and exercise alone.

METAGLIP is indicated as second-line therapy when diet, exercise, and initial treatment with sulfonylurea or metformin do not result in adequate glycemic control in patients with type 2 diabetes.

CONTRAINDICATIONS

METAGLIP is contraindicated in patients with:

1. Renal disease or renal dysfunction (e.g., as suggested by serum creatinine levels ≥1.5 mg/dL [males], ≥1.4 mg/dL [females], or abnormal creatinine clearance) which may also result from conditions such as cardiovascular collapse (shock), acute myocardial infarction, and septicemia (see **WARNINGS** and **PRECAUTIONS**).
2. Congestive heart failure requiring pharmacologic treatment.
3. Known hypersensitivity to glipizide or metformin hydrochloride.
4. Acute or chronic metabolic acidosis, including diabetic ketoacidosis, with or without coma. Diabetic ketoacidosis should be treated with insulin.

METAGLIP should be temporarily discontinued in patients undergoing radiologic studies involving intravascular administration of iodinated contrast materials, because use of such products may result in acute alteration of renal function. (See also **PRECAUTIONS**).

WARNINGS

Metformin Hydrochloride

Lactic acidosis:

Lactic acidosis is a rare, but serious, metabolic complication that can occur due to metformin accumulation during treatment with METAGLIP (glipizide and metformin HCl) Tablets; when it occurs, it is fatal in approximately 50% of cases. Lactic acidosis may also occur in association with a number of pathophysiologic conditions, including diabetes mellitus, and whenever there is significant tissue hypoperfusion and hypoxemia. Lactic acidosis is characterized by elevated blood lactate levels (>5 mmol/L), decreased blood pH, electrolyte disturbances with an increased anion gap, and an increased lactate/pyruvate ratio. When metformin is implicated as the cause of lactic acidosis, metformin plasma levels >5 µg/mL are generally found.

The reported incidence of lactic acidosis in patients receiving metformin hydrochloride is very low (approximately 0.03 cases/1000 patient-years, with approximately 0.015 fatal cases/1000 patient-years). Reported cases have occurred primarily in diabetic patients with significant renal insufficiency, including both intrinsic renal disease and renal hypoperfusion, often in the setting of multiple concomitant medical/surgical problems and multiple concomitant medications. Patients with congestive heart failure requiring pharmacologic management, in particular those with unstable or acute congestive heart failure who are at risk of hypoperfusion and hypoxemia, are at increased risk of lactic acidosis. The risk of lactic acidosis increases with the degree of renal dysfunction and the patient's age. The risk of lactic acidosis may, therefore, be significantly decreased by regular monitoring of renal function in patients taking metformin and by use of the minimum effective dose of metformin. In particular, treatment of the elderly should be accompanied by careful monitoring of renal function. METAGLIP treatment should not be initiated in patients ≥80 years of age unless measurement of creatinine clearance demonstrates that renal function is not reduced, as these patients are more susceptible to developing lactic acidosis. In addition, METAGLIP should be promptly withheld in the presence of any condition associated with hypoxemia, dehydration, or sepsis. Because impaired hepatic function may significantly limit the ability to clear lactate, METAGLIP (glipizide and metformin HCl) should generally be avoided in patients with clinical or laboratory evidence of hepatic disease. Patients should be cautioned against excessive alcohol intake, either acute or chronic, when taking METAGLIP, since alcohol potentiates the effects of metformin hydrochloride on lactate metabolism. In addition, METAGLIP should be temporarily discontinued prior to any intravascular radiocontrast study and for any surgical procedures (see also PRECAUTIONS).

The onset of lactic acidosis often is subtle, and accompanied only by nonspecific symptoms such as malaise, myalgias, respiratory distress, increasing somnolence, and nonspecific abdominal distress. There may be associated hypothermia, hypotension, and resistant bradyarrhythmias with more marked acidosis. The patient and the patient's physician must be aware of the possible importance of such symptoms and the patient should be instructed to notify the physician immediately if they occur (see also PRECAUTIONS). METAGLIP should be withdrawn until the situation is clarified. Serum electrolytes, ketones, blood glucose, and if indicated, blood pH, lactate levels, and even blood metformin levels may be useful. Once the patient is stabilized on any dose level of METAGLIP, gastrointestinal symptoms, which are common during initiation of therapy with metformin, are unlikely to be drug related. Later occurrence of gastrointestinal symptoms could be due to lactic acidosis or other serious disease.

Levels of fasting venous plasma lactate above the upper limit of normal but less than 5 mmol/L in patients taking METAGLIP do not necessarily indicate impending lactic acidosis and may be explainable by other mechanisms, such as poorly controlled diabetes or obesity, vigorous physical activity, or technical problems in sample handling. (See also PRECAUTIONS).

Lactic acidosis should be suspected in any diabetic patient with metabolic acidosis lacking evidence of ketoacidosis (ketonuria and ketonemia).

Lactic acidosis is a medical emergency that must be treated in a hospital setting. In a patient with lactic acidosis who is taking METAGLIP, the drug should be discontinued immediately and general supportive measures promptly instituted. Because metformin hydrochloride is dialyzable (with a clearance of up to 170 mL/min under good hemodynamic conditions), prompt hemodialysis is recommended to correct the acidosis and remove the accumulated metformin. Such management often results in prompt reversal of symptoms and recovery. (See also CONTRAINDICATIONS and PRECAUTIONS).

SPECIAL WARNING ON INCREASED RISK OF CARDIOVASCULAR MORTALITY

The administration of oral hypoglycemic drugs has been reported to be associated with increased cardiovascular mortality as compared to treatment with diet alone or diet plus insulin. This warning is based on the study conducted by the University Group Diabetes Program (UGDP), a long-term prospective clinical trial designed to evaluate the effectiveness of glucose-lowering drugs in preventing or delaying vascular complications in patients with non-insulin-dependent diabetes. The study involved 823 patients who were randomly assigned to one of four treatment groups (*Diabetes* 19 (Suppl. 2):747–830, 1970).

UGDP reported that patients treated for 5 to 8 years with diet plus a fixed dose of tolbutamide (1.5 grams per day) had a rate of cardiovascular mortality approximately 2½ times that of patients treated with diet alone. A significant increase in total mortality was not observed, but the use of tolbutamide was discontinued based on the increase in cardiovascular mortality, thus limiting the opportunity for the study to show an increase in overall mortality. Despite controversy regarding the interpretation of these results, the findings of the UGDP study provide an adequate basis for this warning. The patient should be informed of the potential risks and benefits of glipizide and of alternative modes of therapy.

Although only one drug in the sulfonylurea class (tolbutamide) was included in this study, it is prudent from a safety standpoint to consider that this warning may also apply to other hypoglycemic drugs in this class, in view of their close similarities in mode of action and chemical structure.

PRECAUTIONS

General

METAGLIP

Hypoglycemia

METAGLIP (glipizide and metformin HCl) Tablets is capable of producing hypoglycemia, therefore, proper patient selection, dosing, and instructions are important to avoid potential hypoglycemic episodes. The risk of hypoglycemia is increased when caloric intake is deficient, when strenuous exercise is not compensated by caloric supplementation, or during concomitant use with other glucose-lowering agents or ethanol. Renal insufficiency may cause elevated drug levels of both glipizide and metformin hydrochloride. Hepatic insufficiency may increase drug levels of glipizide and may also diminish gluconeogenic capacity, both of which increase the risk of hypoglycemic reactions. Elderly, debilitated, or malnourished patients and those with adrenal or pituitary insufficiency or alcohol intoxication are particularly susceptible to hypoglycemic effects. Hypoglycemia may be difficult to recognize in the elderly, and in people who are taking beta-adrenergic blocking drugs.

Glipizide

Renal and hepatic disease

The metabolism and excretion of glipizide may be slowed in patients with impaired renal and/or hepatic function. If hypoglycemia should occur in such patients, it may be prolonged and appropriate management should be instituted.

Metformin Hydrochloride

Monitoring of renal function

Metformin is known to be substantially excreted by the kidney, and the risk of metformin accumulation and lactic acidosis increases with the degree of impairment of renal function. Thus, patients with serum creatinine levels above the upper limit of normal for their age should not receive METAGLIP (glipizide and metformin HCl). In patients with advanced age, METAGLIP should be carefully titrated to establish the minimum dose for adequate glycemic effect, because aging is associated with reduced renal function. In elderly patients, particularly those ≥ 80 years of age, renal function should be monitored regularly and, generally, METAGLIP should not be titrated to the maximum dose (see **WARNINGS** and **DOSAGE AND ADMINISTRATION**). Before initiation of METAGLIP therapy and at least annually thereafter, renal function should be assessed and verified as normal. In patients in whom development of renal dysfunction is anticipated, renal function should be assessed more frequently and METAGLIP discontinued if evidence of renal impairment is present.

Use of concomitant medications that may affect renal function or metformin disposition

Concomitant medication(s) that may affect renal function or result in significant hemodynamic change or may interfere with the disposition of metformin, such as cationic drugs that are eliminated by renal tubular secretion (see **PRECAUTIONS: Drug Interactions**), should be used with caution.

Radiologic studies involving the use of intravascular iodinated contrast materials (for example, intravenous urogram, intravenous cholangiography, angiography, and computed tomography (CT) scans with intravascular contrast materials)

Intravascular contrast studies with iodinated materials can lead to acute alteration of renal function and have been associated with lactic acidosis in patients receiving metformin (see **CONTRAINDICATIONS**). Therefore, in patients in whom any such study is planned, METAGLIP should be temporarily discontinued at the time of or prior to the procedure, and withheld for 48 hours subsequent to the procedure and reinstituted only after renal function has been reevaluated and found to be normal.

Hypoxic states

Cardiovascular collapse (shock) from whatever cause, acute congestive heart failure, acute myocardial infarction, and other conditions characterized by hypoxemia have been associated with lactic acidosis and may also cause azotemia. When such events occur in patients on METAGLIP therapy, the drug should be promptly discontinued.

Surgical procedures

METAGLIP therapy should be temporarily suspended for any surgical procedure (except minor procedures not associated with restricted intake of food and fluids) and should not be restarted until the patient's oral intake has resumed and renal function has been evaluated as normal.

Alcohol intake

Alcohol is known to potentiate the effect of metformin on lactate metabolism. Patients, therefore, should be warned against excessive alcohol intake, acute or chronic, while receiving METAGLIP. Due to its effect on the gluconeogenic capacity of the liver, alcohol may also increase the risk of hypoglycemia.

Impaired hepatic function

Since impaired hepatic function has been associated with some cases of lactic acidosis, METAGLIP should generally be avoided in patients with clinical or laboratory evidence of hepatic disease.

Vitamin B_{12} levels

In controlled clinical trials with metformin of 29 weeks duration, a decrease to subnormal levels of previously normal serum Vitamin B_{12}, without clinical manifestations, was observed in approximately 7% of patients. Such decrease, possibly due to interference with B_{12} absorption from the B_{12}-intrinsic factor complex, is, however, very rarely associated with anemia and appears to be rapidly reversible with discontinuation of metformin or Vitamin B_{12} supplementation. Measurement of hematologic parameters on an annual basis is advised in patients on metformin and any apparent abnormalities should be appropriately investigated and managed (see **PRECAUTIONS: Laboratory Tests**).

Certain individuals (those with inadequate Vitamin B_{12} or calcium intake or absorption) appear to be predisposed to developing subnormal Vitamin B_{12} levels. In these patients, routine serum Vitamin B_{12} measurements at two- to three-year intervals may be useful.

Change in clinical status of patients with previously controlled type 2 diabetes

A patient with type 2 diabetes previously well-controlled on metformin who develops laboratory abnormalities or clinical illness (especially vague and poorly defined illness) should be evaluated promptly for evidence of ketoacidosis or lactic acidosis. Evaluation should include serum electrolytes and ketones, blood glucose and, if indicated, blood pH, lactate, pyruvate, and metformin levels. If acidosis of either form occurs, METAGLIP (glipizide and metformin HCl) Tablets must be stopped immediately and other appropriate corrective measures initiated (see also **WARNINGS**).

Information for Patients

METAGLIP

Patients should be informed of the potential risks and benefits of METAGLIP (glipizide and metformin HCl) and of alternative modes of therapy. They should also be informed about the importance of adherence to dietary instructions, or a regular exercise program, and of regular testing of blood glucose, glycosylated hemoglobin, renal function, and hematologic parameters.

The risks of lactic acidosis associated with metformin therapy, its symptoms, and conditions that predispose to its development, as noted in the **WARNINGS** and **PRECAUTIONS** sections, should be explained to patients. Patients should be advised to discontinue METAGLIP immediately and to promptly notify their health practitioner if unexplained hyperventilation, myalgia, malaise, unusual somnolence, or other nonspecific symptoms occur. Once a patient is stabilized on any dose level of METAGLIP, gastrointestinal symptoms, which are common during initiation of metformin therapy, are unlikely to be drug related. Later occurrence of gastrointestinal symptoms could be due to lactic acidosis or other serious disease.

The risks of hypoglycemia, its symptoms and treatment, and conditions that predispose to its development should be explained to patients and responsible family members.

Patients should be counseled against excessive alcohol intake, either acute or chronic, while receiving METAGLIP. (See **Patient Information** printed below.)

Laboratory Tests

Periodic fasting blood glucose and glycosylated hemoglobin (HbA_{1c}) measurements should be performed to monitor therapeutic response.

Initial and periodic monitoring of hematologic parameters (e.g., hemoglobin/hematocrit and red blood cell indices) and renal function (serum creatinine) should be performed, at least on an annual basis. While megaloblastic anemia has rarely been seen with metformin therapy, if this is suspected, Vitamin B_{12} deficiency should be excluded.

Drug Interactions

METAGLIP

Certain drugs tend to produce hyperglycemia and may lead to loss of blood glucose control. These drugs include the thiazides and other diuretics, corticosteroids, phenothiazines, thyroid products, estrogens, oral contraceptives, phenytoin, nicotinic acid, sympathomimetics, calcium channel blocking drugs, and isoniazid. When such drugs are administered to a patient receiving METAGLIP (glipizide and metformin HCl), the patient should be closely observed for loss of blood glucose control. When such drugs are withdrawn from a patient receiving METAGLIP, the patient should be observed closely for hypoglycemia. Metformin is negligibly bound to plasma proteins and is, therefore, less likely to interact with highly protein-bound drugs such as salicylates, sulfonamides, chloramphenicol, and probenecid as compared to sulfonylureas, which are extensively bound to serum proteins.

Glipizide

The hypoglycemic action of sulfonylureas may be potentiated by certain drugs including nonsteroidal anti-inflammatory agents, some azoles, and other drugs that are highly protein bound, salicylates, sulfonamides, chloramphenicol, probenecid, coumarins, monoamine oxidase inhibitors, and beta adrenergic blocking agents. When such drugs are administered to a patient receiving METAGLIP (glipizide and metformin HCl), the patient should be observed closely for hypoglycemia. When such drugs are withdrawn from a patient receiving METAGLIP, the patient should be observed closely for loss of blood glucose control. *In vitro* binding studies with human serum proteins indicate that glipizide binds differently than tolbutamide and does not interact with salicylate or dicumarol. However, caution must be exercised in extrapolating these findings to the clinical situation and in the use of METAGLIP with these drugs.

A potential interaction between oral miconazole and oral hypoglycemic agents leading to severe hypoglycemia has been reported. Whether this interaction also occurs with the intravenous, topical, or vaginal preparations of miconazole is not known. The effect of concomitant administration of fluconazole and glipizide has been demonstrated in a placebo-controlled crossover study in normal volunteers. All subjects received glipizide alone and following treatment with 100 mg of fluconazole as a single oral daily dose for 7 days, the mean percent increase in the glipizide AUC after fluconazole administration was 56.9% (range: 35 to 81%).

Metformin Hydrochloride

Furosemide

A single-dose, metformin-furosemide drug interaction study in healthy subjects demonstrated that pharmacokinetic parameters of both compounds were affected by co-administration. Furosemide increased the metformin plasma and blood C_{max} by 22% and blood AUC by 15%, without any significant change in metformin renal clearance. When administered with metformin, the C_{max} and AUC of furosemide were 31% and 12% smaller, respectively, than when administered alone, and the terminal half-life was decreased by 32%, without any significant change in furosemide renal clearance. No information is available about the interaction of metformin and furosemide when co-administered chronically.

Nifedipine

A single-dose, metformin-nifedipine drug interaction study in normal healthy volunteers demonstrated that co-administration of nifedipine increased plasma metformin C_{max} and AUC by 20% and 9%, respectively, and increased the amount excreted in the urine. T_{max} and half-life were unaffected. Nifedipine appears to enhance the absorption of metformin. Metformin had minimal effects on nifedipine.

Cationic drugs

Cationic drugs (e.g., amiloride, digoxin, morphine, procainamide, quinidine, quinine, ranitidine, triamterene, trimethoprim, or vancomycin) that are eliminated by renal tubular secretion theoretically have the potential for interaction with metformin by competing for common renal tubular transport systems. Such interaction between metformin and oral cimetidine has been observed in normal healthy volunteers in both single- and multiple-dose, metformin-cimetidine drug interaction studies, with a 60% increase in peak metformin plasma and whole blood concentrations and a 40% increase in plasma and whole blood metformin AUC. There was no change in elimination half-life in the single-dose study. Metformin had no effect on cimetidine pharmacokinetics. Although such interactions remain theoretical (except for cimetidine), careful patient monitoring and dose adjustment of METAGLIP (glipizide and metformin HCl) Tablets and/or the interfering drug is recommended in patients who are taking cationic medications that are excreted via the proximal renal tubular secretory system.

Other

In healthy volunteers, the pharmacokinetics of metformin and propranolol and metformin and ibuprofen were not affected when co-administered in single-dose interaction studies.

Carcinogenesis, Mutagenesis, Impairment of Fertility

No animal studies have been conducted with the combined products in METAGLIP. The following data are based on findings in studies performed with the individual products.

Glipizide

A 20-month study in rats and an 18-month study in mice at doses up to 75 times the maximum human dose revealed no evidence of drug-related carcinogenicity. Bacterial and *in vivo* mutagenicity tests were uniformly negative. Studies in rats of both sexes at doses up to 75 times the human dose showed no effects on fertility.

Metformin Hydrochloride

Long-term carcinogenicity studies were performed with metformin alone in rats (dosing duration of 104 weeks) and mice (dosing duration of 91 weeks) at doses up to and including 900 mg/kg/day and 1500 mg/kg/day, respectively. These doses are both approximately four times the maximum recommended human daily dose of 2000 mg of the metformin component of METAGLIP based on body surface area comparisons. No evidence of carcinogenicity with metformin alone was found in either male or female mice. Similarly, there was no tumorigenic potential observed with metformin alone in male rats. There was, however, an increased incidence of benign stromal uterine polyps in female rats treated with 900 mg/kg/day of metformin alone.

There was no evidence of a mutagenic potential of metformin alone in the following *in vitro* tests: Ames test (*S. typhimurium*), gene mutation test (mouse lymphoma cells), or chromosomal aberrations test (human lymphocytes). Results in the *in vivo* mouse micronucleus test were also negative.

Fertility of male or female rats was unaffected by metformin alone when administered at doses as high as 600 mg/kg/day, which is approximately three times the maximum recommended human daily dose of the metformin component of METAGLIP based on body surface area comparisons.

Pregnancy

Teratogenic Effects: Pregnancy Category C

Recent information strongly suggests that abnormal blood glucose levels during pregnancy are associated with a higher incidence of congenital abnormalities. Most experts recommend that insulin be used during pregnancy to maintain blood glucose as close to normal as possible. Because animal reproduction studies are not always predictive of human response, METAGLIP should not be used during pregnancy unless clearly needed. (See below.)

There are no adequate and well-controlled studies in pregnant women with METAGLIP or its individual components. No animal studies have been conducted with the combined products in METAGLIP. The following data are based on findings in studies performed with the individual products.

Glipizide

Glipizide was found to be mildly fetotoxic in rat reproductive studies at all dose levels (5–50 mg/kg). This fetotoxicity has been similarly noted with other sulfonylureas, such as tolbutamide and tolazamide. The effect is perinatal and believed to be directly related to the pharmacologic (hypoglycemic) action of glipizide. In studies in rats and rabbits, no teratogenic effects were found.

Metformin hydrochloride

Metformin alone was not teratogenic in rats or rabbits at doses up to 600 mg/kg/day. This represents an exposure of about two and six times the maximum recommended human daily dose of 2000 mg of the metformin component of METAGLIP (glipizide and metformin HCl) Tablets based on body surface area comparisons for rats and rabbits, respectively. Determination of fetal concentrations demonstrated a partial placental barrier to metformin.

Nonteratogenic Effects

Prolonged severe hypoglycemia (4 to 10 days) has been reported in neonates born to mothers who were receiving a sulfonylurea drug at the time of delivery. This has been reported more frequently with the use of agents with prolonged half-lives. It is not recommended that METAGLIP be used during pregnancy. However, if it is used, METAGLIP should be discontinued at least one month before the expected delivery date. (See **Pregnancy; Teratogenic Effects: Pregnancy Category C.**)

Nursing Mothers

Although it is not known whether glipizide is excreted in human milk, some sulfonylurea drugs are known to be excreted in human milk. Studies in lactating rats show that metformin is excreted into milk and reaches levels comparable to those in plasma. Similar studies have not been conducted in nursing mothers. Because the potential for hypoglycemia in nursing infants may exist, a decision should be made whether to discontinue nursing or to discontinue METAGLIP, taking into account the importance of the drug to the mother. If METAGLIP is discontinued, and if diet alone is inadequate for controlling blood glucose, insulin therapy should be considered.

Pediatric Use

Safety and effectiveness of METAGLIP in pediatric patients have not been established.

Geriatric Use

Of the 345 patients who received METAGLIP 2.5 mg/250 mg and 2.5 mg/500 mg in the initial therapy trial, 67 (19.4%) were aged 65 and older while 5 (1.4%) were aged 75 and older. Of the 87 patients who received METAGLIP in the second-line therapy trial, 17 (19.5%) were aged 65 and older while one (1.1%) was at least aged 75. No overall differences in effectiveness or safety were observed between these patients and younger patients in either the initial therapy trial or the second-line therapy trial, and other reported clinical experience has not identified differences in

Continued on next page

Metaglip—Cont.

response between the elderly and younger patients, but greater sensitivity of some older individuals cannot be ruled out.

Metformin hydrochloride is known to be substantially excreted by the kidney and because the risk of serious adverse reactions to the drug is greater in patients with impaired renal function, METAGLIP should only be used in patients with normal renal function (see **CONTRAINDICATIONS, WARNINGS,** and **CLINICAL PHARMACOLOGY: Pharmacokinetics**). Because aging is associated with reduced renal function, METAGLIP (glipizide and metformin HCl) should be used with caution as age increases. Care should be taken in dose selection and should be based on careful and regular monitoring of renal function. Generally, elderly patients should not be titrated to the maximum dose of METAGLIP (see also **WARNINGS** and **DOSAGE AND ADMINISTRATION**).

ADVERSE REACTIONS
METAGLIP
In a double-blind 24-week clinical trial involving METAGLIP (glipizide and metformin HCl) Tablets as initial therapy, a total of 172 patients received METAGLIP 2.5 mg/250 mg, 173 received METAGLIP 2.5 mg/500 mg, 170 received glipizide, and 177 received metformin. The most common clinical adverse events in these treatment groups are listed in **Table 4**.
[See table 4 above]
In a double-blind 18-week clinical trial involving METAGLIP as second-line therapy, a total of 87 patients received METAGLIP, 84 received glipizide, and 75 received metformin. The most common clinical adverse events in this clinical trial are listed in **Table 5**.
[See table 5 above]

Hypoglycemia
In a controlled initial therapy trial of METAGLIP (glipizide and metformin HCl) 2.5 mg/250 mg and 2.5 mg/500 mg the numbers of patients with hypoglycemia documented by symptoms (such as dizziness, shakiness, sweating, and hunger) and a fingerstick blood glucose measurement ≤50 mg/dL were 5 (2.9%) for glipizide, 0 (0%) for metformin, 13 (7.6%) for METAGLIP 2.5 mg/250 mg, and 16 (9.3%) for METAGLIP 2.5 mg/500 mg. Among patients taking either METAGLIP 2.5 mg/250 mg or METAGLIP 2.5 mg/500 mg, nine (2.6%) patients discontinued METAGLIP due to hypoglycemic symptoms and one required medical intervention due to hypoglycemia. In a controlled second-line therapy trial of METAGLIP 5 mg/500 mg, the numbers of patients with hypoglycemia documented by symptoms and a fingerstick blood glucose measurement of ≤50 mg/dL were 0 (0%) for glipizide, 1 (1.3%) for metformin, and 11 (12.6%) for METAGLIP. One (1.1%) patient discontinued METAGLIP therapy due to hypoglycemic symptoms and none required medical intervention due to hypoglycemia. (See **PRECAUTIONS** section.)

Gastrointestinal Reactions
Among the most common clinical adverse events in the initial trial were diarrhea and nausea/vomiting; the incidences of these events were lower with both METAGLIP dosage strengths than with metformin therapy. There were 4 (1.2%) patients in the initial therapy trial who discontinued METAGLIP therapy due to GI adverse events. Gastrointestinal symptoms of diarrhea, nausea/vomiting, and abdominal pain were comparable among METAGLIP, glipizide and metformin in the second-line therapy trial. There were 4 (4.6%) patients in the second-line therapy trial who discontinued METAGLIP therapy due to GI adverse events.

OVERDOSAGE
Glipizide
Overdosage of sulfonylureas, including glipizide, can produce hypoglycemia. Mild hypoglycemic symptoms, without loss of consciousness or neurological findings, should be treated aggressively with oral glucose and adjustments in drug dosage and/or meal patterns. Close monitoring should continue until the physician is assured that the patient is out of danger. Severe hypoglycemic reactions with coma, seizure, or other neurological impairment occur infrequently, but constitute medical emergencies requiring immediate hospitalization. If hypoglycemic coma is diagnosed or suspected, the patient should be given a rapid intravenous injection of concentrated (50%) glucose solution. This should be followed by a continuous infusion of a more dilute (10%) glucose solution at a rate that will maintain the blood glucose at a level above 100 mg/dL. Patients should be closely monitored for a minimum of 24 to 48 hours, since hypoglycemia may recur after apparent clinical recovery. Clearance of glipizide from plasma would be prolonged in persons with liver disease. Because of the extensive protein binding of glipizide, dialysis is unlikely to be of benefit.

Metformin Hydrochloride
Among cases of overdosage of metformin hydrochloride, including ingestion of amounts greater than 100 grams, hypoglycemia was reported in approximately 10%, but no causal association with metformin hydrochloride has been established, although lactic acidosis has occurred in such circumstances (see **WARNINGS**.) Metformin is dialyzable with a clearance of up to 170 mL/min under good hemodynamic conditions. Therefore, hemodialysis may be useful for removal of accumulated drug from patients in whom metformin overdosage is suspected.

Table 4: Clinical Adverse Events >5% in any Treatment Group, by Primary Term, in Initial Therapy Study

Adverse Event	Number (%) of Patients			
	Glipizide 5 mg tablets N=170	Metformin 500 mg tablets N=177	METAGLIP 2.5 mg/250 mg tablets N=172	METAGLIP 2.5 mg/500 mg tablets N=173
Upper respiratory infection	12 (7.1)	15 (8.5)	17 (9.9)	14 (8.1)
Diarrhea	8 (4.7)	15 (8.5)	4 (2.3)	9 (5.2)
Dizziness	9 (5.3)	2 (1.1)	3 (1.7)	9 (5.2)
Hypertension	17 (10.0)	10 (5.6)	5 (2.9)	6 (3.5)
Nausea/vomiting	6 (3.5)	9 (5.1)	1 (0.6)	3 (1.7)

Table 5: Clinical Adverse Events >5% in any Treatment Group, by Primary Term, in Second-line Therapy Study

Adverse Event	Number (%) of Patients		
	Glipizide 5 mg tablets[a] N=84	Metformin 500 mg tablets[a] N=75	METAGLIP 5 mg/500 mg tablets[a] N=87
Diarrhea	11 (13.1)	13 (17.3)	16 (18.4)
Headache	5 (6.0)	4 (5.3)	11 (12.6)
Upper respiratory infection	11 (13.1)	8 (10.7)	9 (10.3)
Musculoskeletal pain	6 (7.1)	5 (6.7)	7 (8.0)
Nausea/vomiting	5 (6.0)	6 (8.0)	7 (8.0)
Abdominal pain	7 (8.3)	5 (6.7)	5 (5.7)
UTI	4 (4.8)	6 (8.0)	1 (1.1)

[a] The dose of glipizde was fixed at 30 mg daily; doses of metformin and METAGLIP were titrated.

DOSAGE AND ADMINISTRATION
General Considerations
Dosage of METAGLIP (glipizide and metformin HCl) Tablets must be individualized on the basis of both effectiveness and tolerance while not exceeding the maximum recommended daily dose of 20 mg glipizide/2000 mg metformin. METAGLIP should be given with meals and should be initiated at a low dose, with gradual dose escalation as described below, in order to avoid hypoglycemia (largely due to glipizide), to reduce GI side effects (largely due to metformin), and to permit determination of the minimum effective dose for adequate control of blood glucose for the individual patient.

With initial treatment and during dose titration, appropriate blood glucose monitoring should be used to determine the therapeutic response to METAGLIP and to identify the minimum effective dose for the patient. Thereafter, HbA_{1c} should be measured at intervals of approximately 3 months to assess the effectiveness of therapy. The therapeutic goal in all patients with type 2 diabetes is to decrease FPG, PPG, and HbA_{1c} to normal or as near normal as possible. Ideally, the response to therapy should be evaluated using HbA_{1c} (glycosylated hemoglobin), which is a better indicator of long-term glycemic control than FPG alone.

No studies have been performed specifically examining the safety and efficacy of switching to METAGLIP therapy in patients taking concomitant glipizide (or other sulfonylurea) plus metformin. Changes in glycemic control may occur in such patients, with either hyperglycemia or hypoglycemia possible. Any change in therapy of type 2 diabetes should be undertaken with care and appropriate monitoring.

METAGLIP as Initial Therapy
For patients with type 2 diabetes whose hyperglycemia cannot be satisfactorily managed with diet and exercise alone, the recommended starting dose of METAGLIP is 2.5 mg/250 mg once a day with a meal. For patients whose FPG is 280 to 320 mg/dL a starting dose of METAGLIP 2.5 mg/500 mg twice daily should be considered. The efficacy of METAGLIP (glipizide and metformin HCl) Tablets in patients whose FPG exceeds 320 mg/dL has not been established. Dosage increases to achieve adequate glycemic control should be made in increments of one tablet per day every two weeks up to maximum of 10 mg/1000 mg or 10 mg/2000 mg METAGLIP per day given in divided doses. In clinical trials of METAGLIP as initial therapy, there was no experience with total daily doses greater than 10 mg/2000 mg per day.

METAGLIP as Second-Line Therapy
For patients not adequately controlled on either glipizide (or another sulfonylurea) or metformin alone, the recommended starting dose of METAGLIP is 2.5 mg/500 mg or 5mg/500mg twice daily with the morning and evening meals. In order to avoid hypoglycemia, the starting dose of METAGLIP should not exceed the daily doses of glipizide or metformin already being taken. The daily dose should be titrated in increments of no more than 5 mg/500 mg up to the minimum effective dose to achieve adequate control of blood glucose or to a maximum dose of 20 mg/2000 mg per day.

Patients previously treated with combination therapy of glipizide (or another sulfonylurea) plus metformin may be switched to METAGLIP 2.5 mg/500 mg or 5 mg/500 mg; the starting dose should not exceed the daily dose of glipizide (or equivalent dose of another sulfonylurea) and metformin already being taken. The decision to switch to the nearest equivalent dose or to titrate should be based on clinical judgment. Patients should be monitored closely for signs and symptoms of hypoglycemia following such a switch and the dose of METAGLIP should be titrated as described above to achieve adequate control of blood glucose.

Specific Patient Populations
METAGLIP is not recommended for use during pregnancy or for use in pediatric patients. The initial and maintenance dosing of METAGLIP should be conservative in patients with advanced age, due to the potential for decreased renal function in this population. Any dosage adjustment requires a careful assessment of renal function. Generally, elderly, debilitated, and malnourished patients should not be titrated to the maximum dose of METAGLIP to avoid the risk of hypoglycemia. Monitoring of renal function is necessary to aid in prevention of metformin-associated lactic acidosis, particularly in the elderly. (See **WARNINGS**.)

HOW SUPPLIED
METAGLIP™ (glipizide and metformin HCl) Tablets
METAGLIP **2.5 mg/250 mg** tablet is a pink oval-shaped, biconvex film-coated tablet with "BMS" debossed on one side and "6081" debossed on the opposite side.
METAGLIP **2.5 mg/500 mg** tablet is a white oval-shaped, biconvex film-coated tablet with "BMS" debossed on one side and "6077" debossed on the opposite side.
METAGLIP **5 mg/500 mg** tablet is a pink oval-shaped, biconvex film-coated tablet with "BMS" debossed on one side and "6078" debossed on the opposite side.

METAGLIP		NDC 0087-xxxx-xx for unit of use
Glipizide (mg)	Metformin HCl (mg)	Bottle of 100
2.5	250	6081-31
2.5	500	6077-31
5.0	500	6078-31

STORAGE
Store at 20° C–25° C (68° F–77° F); excursions permitted to 15° C–30° C (59° F–86°F). [See USP Controlled Room Temperature.]

METAGLIP™ is a trademark of Merck Santé S.A.S., an associate of Merck KGaA of Darmstadt, Germany. Licensed to Bristol-Myers Squibb Company.

GLUCOPHAGE® is a registered trademark of Merck Santé S.A.S., an associate of Merck KGaA of Darmstadt, Germany. Licensed to Bristol-Myers Squibb Company.
GLUCOTROL® is a registered trademark of Pfizer Inc.

PATIENT INFORMATION ABOUT
METAGLIP™ (glipizide and metformin HCl) Tablets

> WARNING: A small number of people who have taken metformin hydrochloride have developed a serious condition called lactic acidosis. Properly functioning kidneys are needed to help prevent lactic acidosis. Most people with kidney problems should not take METAGLIP. (See Question Nos. 9–13.)

Q1. WHY DO I NEED TO TAKE METAGLIP?
Your doctor has prescribed METAGLIP to treat your type 2 diabetes. This is also known as non-insulin-dependent diabetes mellitus.

Q2. WHAT IS TYPE 2 DIABETES?
People with diabetes are not able to make enough insulin and/or respond normally to the insulin their body does make. When this happens, sugar (glucose) builds up in the blood. This can lead to serious medical problems including kidney damage, amputations, and blindness. Diabetes is also closely linked to heart disease. The main goal of treating diabetes is to lower your blood sugar to a normal level.

Q3. WHY IS IT IMPORTANT TO CONTROL TYPE 2 DIABETES?
The main goal of treating diabetes is to lower your blood sugar to a normal level. Studies have shown that good control of blood sugar may prevent or delay complications such as heart disease, kidney disease, or blindness.

Q4. HOW IS TYPE 2 DIABETES USUALLY CONTROLLED?
High blood sugar can be lowered by diet and exercise, by a number of oral medications, and by insulin injections. Before taking METAGLIP (glipizide and metformin HCl) you should first try to control your diabetes by exercise and weight loss. Even if you are taking METAGLIP, you should still exercise and follow the diet recommended for your diabetes.

Q5. DOES METAGLIP WORK DIFFERENTLY FROM OTHER GLUCOSE-CONTROL MEDICATIONS?
Yes it does. METAGLIP combines two glucose lowering drugs, glipizide and metformin. These two drugs work together to improve the different metabolic defects found in type 2 diabetes. Glipizide lowers blood sugar primarily by causing more of the body's own insulin to be released, and metformin lowers blood sugar, in part, by helping your body use your own insulin more effectively. Together, they are efficient in helping you achieve better glucose control.

Q6. WHAT HAPPENS IF MY BLOOD SUGAR IS STILL TOO HIGH?
When blood sugar cannot be lowered enough by METAGLIP your doctor may prescribe injectable insulin or take other measures to control your diabetes.

Q7. CAN METAGLIP CAUSE SIDE EFFECTS?
METAGLIP, like all blood sugar-lowering medications, can cause side effects in some patients. Most of these side effects are minor. However, there are also serious, but rare, side effects related to METAGLIP (see Question Nos. 9–13).

Q8. WHAT ARE THE MOST COMMON SIDE EFFECTS OF METAGLIP?
The most common side effects of METAGLIP are normally minor ones such as diarrhea, nausea, and upset stomach. If these side effects occur, they usually occur during the first few weeks of therapy. Taking your METAGLIP with meals can help reduce these side effects.
Symptoms of hypoglycemia (low blood sugar), such as light-headedness, dizziness, shakiness, or hunger may occur. The risk of hypoglycemic symptoms increases when meals are skipped, too much alcohol is consumed, or heavy exercise occurs without enough food. Following the advice of your doctor can help you to avoid these symptoms.

Q9. ARE THERE ANY SERIOUS SIDE EFFECTS THAT METAGLIP CAN CAUSE?
METAGLIP rarely causes serious side effects. The most serious side effect that METAGLIP can cause is called lactic acidosis.

Q10. WHAT IS LACTIC ACIDOSIS AND CAN IT HAPPEN TO ME?
Lactic acidosis is caused by a buildup of lactic acid in the blood. Lactic acidosis associated with metformin is rare and has occurred mostly in people whose kidneys were not working normally. Lactic acidosis has been reported in about one in 33,000 patients taking metformin over the course of a year. Although rare, if lactic acidosis does occur, it can be fatal in up to half the cases.
It's also important for your liver to be working normally when you take METAGLIP. Your liver helps remove lactic acid from your bloodstream.
Your doctor will monitor your diabetes and may perform blood tests on you from time to time to make sure your kidneys and your liver are functioning normally.
There is no evidence that METAGLIP causes harm to the kidneys or liver.

Q11. ARE THERE OTHER RISK FACTORS FOR LACTIC ACIDOSIS?
Your risk of developing lactic acidosis from taking METAGLIP (glipizide and metformin HCl) Tablets is very low as long as your kidneys and liver are healthy. However, some factors can increase your risk because they can affect kidney and liver function. You should discuss your risk with your physician.

You should not take METAGLIP if:
- You have chronic kidney or liver problems
- You have congestive heart failure which is treated with medications, e.g., digoxin (Lanoxin®) or furosemide (Lasix®)
- You drink alcohol excessively (all the time or short-term "binge" drinking)
- You are seriously dehydrated (have lost a large amount of body fluids)
- You are going to have certain x-ray procedures with injectable contrast agents
- You are going to have surgery
- You develop a serious condition such as a heart attack, severe infection, or a stroke
- You are ≥80 years of age and have NOT had your kidney function tested

Q12. WHAT ARE THE SYMPTOMS OF LACTIC ACIDOSIS?
Some of the symptoms include: feeling very weak, tired or uncomfortable; unusual muscle pain, trouble breathing, unusual or unexpected stomach discomfort, feeling cold, feeling dizzy or lightheaded, or suddenly developing a slow or irregular heartbeat.
If you notice these symptoms, or if your medical condition has suddenly changed, stop taking METAGLIP tablets and call your doctor right away. Lactic acidosis is a medical emergency that must be treated in a hospital.

Q13. WHAT DOES MY DOCTOR NEED TO KNOW TO DECREASE MY RISK OF LACTIC ACIDOSIS?
Tell your doctor if you have an illness that results in severe vomiting, diarrhea, and/or fever, or if your intake of fluids is significantly reduced. These situations can lead to severe dehydration, and it may be necessary to stop taking METAGLIP temporarily.
You should let your doctor know if you are going to have any surgery or specialized x-ray procedures that require injection of contrast agents. METAGLIP therapy will need to be stopped temporarily in such instances.

Q14. CAN I TAKE METAGLIP WITH OTHER MEDICATIONS?
Remind your doctor that you are taking METAGLIP when any new drug is prescribed or a change is made in how you take a drug already prescribed.
METAGLIP may interfere with the way some drugs work and some drugs may interfere with the action of METAGLIP.

Q15. WHAT IF I BECOME PREGNANT WHILE TAKING METAGLIP?
Tell your doctor if you plan to become pregnant or have become pregnant. As with other oral glucose-control medications, you should not take METAGLIP (glipizide and metformin HCl) during pregnancy.
Usually your doctor will prescribe insulin while you are pregnant. As with all medications. you and your doctor should discuss the use of METAGLIP if you are nursing a child.

Q16. HOW DO I TAKE METAGLIP?
Your doctor will tell you how many METAGLIP tablets to take and how often.
This should also be printed on the label of your prescription. You will probably be started on a low dose of METAGLIP and your dosage will be increased gradually until your blood sugar is controlled.

Q17. WHERE CAN I GET MORE INFORMATION ABOUT METAGLIP?
This leaflet is a summary of the most important information about METAGLIP.
If you have any questions or problems, you should talk to your doctor or other healthcare provider about type 2 diabetes as well as METAGLIP and its side effects. There is also a leaflet (package insert) written for health professionals that your pharmacist can let you read.
METAGLIP™ is a trademark of Merck Santé S.A.S., an associate of Merck KGaA of Darmstadt, Germany. Licensed to Bristol-Myers Squibb Company.
Bristol-Myers Squibb Company
Distributed by
Bristol-Myers Squibb Company
Princeton, NJ 08543 USA
M1-B0001-10-02   Issued: October 2002

In the PDR annual,
the **Brand and Generic Name Index**
(PINK section)
alphabetizes drugs under both
brand and generic names.

Clay-Park Labs, Inc.
1700 BATHGATE AVENUE
BRONX, NY 10457

Direct Inquiries to:
1-800-933-5550

Products:
Name/Product Description
How Supplied

Ammonium Lactate Cream, 12%
385 g pump bottle and 280 g carton (2–140 g tubes)

Antipyrine/Benzocaine Otic Drops
15 ml

Betamethasone Dipropionate Lotion USP, 0.05%
20 ml and 60 ml bottles

Clindamycin Phosphate Pledgets, 1%
60's and 69's

Desonide Cream 0.05%
15 g and 60 g tubes

Desonide Ointment 0.05%
15 g and 60 g tubes

Erythromycin-Benzoyl Peroxide Topical Gel
23.3 g and 46.6 g jars

Erythromycin Topical Solution USP, 2%
60 ml bottle

Gentamicin Sulfate Cream, USP
15g and 30g tubes

Gentamicin Sulfate Ointment, USP
15g and 30g tubes

Hydrocortisone Acetate Suppositories, 25 mg
12's and 24's

Hydrocortisone Cream USP, 2.5%
20 g and 1 oz. tubes

Hydrocortisone Ointment USP, 2.5%
20 g tube and 1 lb. jar

Hydrocortisone Valerate Cream USP, 0.2%
15 g, 45 g and 60 g tubes

Mometasone Furoate Ointment USP, 0.1%
15 g and 45 g tubes

Nystatin Cream, USP
15 g and 30 g tubes

Nystatin Ointment, USP
15 g and 30 g tubes

Permethrin Cream, 5%
60 g tube

Selenium Sulfide Lotion USP, 2.5%
4 oz. bottle

Trimethobenzamide Suppositories, 100 mg
10's and 50's

Trimethobenzamide Suppositories, 200 mg
10's and 50's

Triamcinolone Acetonide Cream USP, 0.025%
15 g and 80 g tubes; 1 lb. jar

Triamcinolone Acetonide Cream USP, 0.1%
15 g and 80 g tubes; 1 lb. and 5 lb. jars

Triamcinolone Acetonide Cream USP, 0.5%
15 g tube

Triamcinolone Acetonide Ointment USP, 0.025%
15 g and 80 g tubes; 1 lb. jar

Triamcinolone Acetonide Ointment USP, 0.1%
15 g and 80 g tubes; 1 lb. jar

Triamcinolone Acetonide Ointment USP, 0.5%
15 g tube

Tridesilon® (desonide) Cream 0.05%
15 g and 60 g tubes

Tridesilon® (desonide) Ointment 0.05%
15 g and 60 g tubes

To keep your **PDR** up to date
throughout the year, note these revisions
on the corresponding pages of the annual
volume. Simply write **"See Supplement A"**
next to the product heading.

ESP Pharma
2035 LINCOLN HIGHWAY
SUITE 2150
EDISON, NJ 08817

Direct Inquiries to:
phone: (732) 650-1377

The following list of products is also available from ESP Pharma:

Ismo
Sectal
Tenex

For full prescribing information, please refer to the ESP Pharma website, www.esppharma.com

CARDENE® I.V. ℞
(nicardipine hydrochloride)

℞ only

DESCRIPTION

Cardene (nicardipine HCl) is a calcium ion influx inhibitor (slow channel blocker or calcium channel blocker). Cardene I.V. for intravenous administration contains 2.5 mg/mL of nicardipine hydrochloride. Nicardipine hydrochloride is a dihydropyridine derivative with IUPAC (International Union of Pure and Applied Chemistry) chemical name (±)-2-(benzyl-methyl amino) ethyl methyl 1,4-dihydro-2,6-dimethyl-4-(*m*-nitrophenyl)-3,5-pyridinedicarboxylate monohydrochloride and has the following structure:

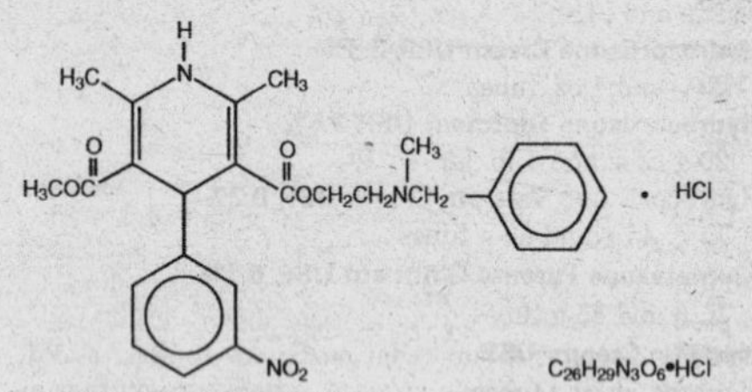

$C_{26}H_{29}N_3O_6 \cdot HCl$

Nicardipine hydrochloride is a greenish-yellow, odorless, crystalline powder that melts at about 169° C. It is freely soluble in chloroform, methanol, and glacial acetic acid, sparingly soluble in anhydrous ethanol, slightly soluble in n-butanol, water, 0.01 M potassium dihydrogen phosphate, acetone, and dioxane, very slightly soluble in ethyl acetate, and practically insoluble in benzene, ether, and hexane. It has a molecular weight of 515.99.

Cardene I.V. is available as a sterile, non-pyrogenic, clear, yellow solution in 10 mL ampuls for intravenous infusion after dilution. Each mL contains 2.5 mg nicardipine hydrochloride in Water for Injection, USP with 48.00 mg Sorbitol, NF, buffered to pH 3.5 with 0.525 mg citric acid monohydrate, USP and 0.09 mg sodium hydroxide, NF. Additional citric acid and/or sodium hydroxide may have been added to adjust pH.

CLINICAL PHARMACOLOGY

MECHANISM OF ACTION

Nicardipine inhibits the transmembrane influx of calcium ions into cardiac muscle and smooth muscle without changing serum calcium concentrations. The contractile processes of cardiac muscle and vascular smooth muscle are dependent upon the movement of extracellular calcium ions into these cells through specific ion channels. The effects of nicardipine are more selective to vascular smooth muscle than cardiac muscle. In animal models, nicardipine produced relaxation of coronary vascular smooth muscle at drug levels which cause little or no negative inotropic effect.

PHARMACOKINETICS AND METABOLISM

Following infusion, nicardipine plasma concentrations decline tri-exponentially, with a rapid early distribution phase (α-half-life of 2.7 minutes), an intermediate phase (β-half-life of 44.8 minutes), and a slow terminal phase (γ-half-life of 14.4 hours) that can only be detected after long-term infusions. Total plasma clearance (Cl) is 0.4 L/hr•kg, and the apparent volume of distribution (V_d) using a non-compartment model is 8.3 L/kg. The pharmacokinetics of Cardene I.V. are linear over the dosage range of 0.5 to 40.0 mg/hr.

Rapid dose-related increases in nicardipine plasma concentrations are seen during the first two hours after the start of an infusion of Cardene I.V. Plasma concentrations increase at a much slower rate after the first few hours, and approach steady state at 24 to 48 hours. On termination of the infusion, nicardipine concentrations decrease rapidly, with at least a 50% decrease during the first two hours post-infusion. The effects of nicardipine on blood pressure significantly correlate with plasma concentrations.

Nicardipine is highly protein bound (>95%) in human plasma over a wide concentration range.

Cardene I.V. has been shown to be rapidly and extensively metabolized by the liver. After coadministration of a radioactive intravenous dose of Cardene I.V. with an oral 30 mg dose given every 8 hours, 49% of the radioactivity was recovered in the urine and 43% in the feces within 96 hours. None of the dose was recovered as unchanged nicardipine. Nicardipine does not induce or inhibit its own metabolism and does not induce or inhibit hepatic microsomal enzymes. The steady-state pharmacokinetics of nicardipine are similar in elderly hypertensive patients (>65 years) and young healthy adults.

HEMODYNAMICS

Cardene I.V. produces significant decreases in systemic vascular resistance. In a study of intra-arterially administered Cardene I.V., the degree of vasodilation and the resultant decrease in blood pressure were more prominent in hypertensive patients than in normotensive volunteers. Administration of Cardene I.V. to normotensive volunteers at dosages of 0.25 to 3.0 mg/hr for eight hours produced changes of <5 mmHg in systolic blood pressure and <3 mmHg in diastolic blood pressure.

An increase in heart rate is a normal response to vasodilation and decrease in blood pressure; in some patients these increases in heart rate may be pronounced. In placebo-controlled trials, the mean increases in heart rate were 7 ± 1 bpm in postoperative patients and 8 ± 1 bpm in patients with severe hypertension at the end of the maintenance period.

Hemodynamic studies following intravenous dosing in patients with coronary artery disease and normal or moderately abnormal left ventricular function have shown significant increases in ejection fraction and cardiac output with no significant change, or a small decrease, in left ventricular end-diastolic pressure (LVEDP). There is evidence that Cardene increases blood flow. Coronary dilatation induced by Cardene I.V. improves perfusion and aerobic metabolism in areas with chronic ischemia, resulting in reduced lactate production and augmented oxygen consumption. In patients with coronary artery disease, Cardene I.V., administered after beta-blockade, significantly improved systolic and diastolic left ventricular function.

In congestive heart failure patients with impaired left ventricular function, Cardene I.V. increased cardiac output both at rest and during exercise. Decreases in left ventricular end-diastolic pressure were also observed. However, in some patients with severe left ventricular dysfunction, it may have a negative inotropic effect and could lead to worsened failure.

"Coronary steal" has not been observed during treatment with Cardene I.V. (Coronary steal is the detrimental redistribution of coronary blood flow in patients with coronary artery disease from underperfused areas toward better perfused areas.) Cardene I.V. has been shown to improve systolic shortening in both normal and hypokinetic segments of myocardial muscle. Radionuclide angiography has confirmed that wall motion remained improved during increased oxygen demand. (Occasional patients have developed increased angina upon receiving Cardene capsules. Whether this represents coronary steal in these patients, or is the result of increased heart rate and decreased diastolic pressure, is not clear.)

In patients with coronary artery disease, Cardene I.V. improves left ventricular diastolic distensibility during the early filling phase, probably due to a faster rate of myocardial relaxation in previously underperfused areas. There is little or no effect on normal myocardium, suggesting the improvement is mainly by indirect mechanisms such as afterload reduction and reduced ischemia. Cardene I.V. has no negative effect on myocardial relaxation at therapeutic doses. The clinical benefits of these properties have not yet been demonstrated.

ELECTROPHYSIOLOGIC EFFECTS

In general, no detrimental effects on the cardiac conduction system have been seen with Cardene I.V. During acute electrophysiologic studies, it increased heart rate and prolonged the corrected QT interval to a minor degree. It did not affect sinus node recovery or SA conduction times. The PA, AH, and HV intervals* or the function and effective refractory periods of the atrium were not prolonged. The relative and effective refractory periods of the His-Purkinje system were slightly shortened.

HEPATIC FUNCTION

Because nicardipine is extensively metabolized by the liver, plasma concentrations are influenced by changes in hepatic function. In a clinical study with Cardene capsules in patients with severe liver disease, plasma concentrations were elevated and the half-life was prolonged (see **"PRECAUTIONS"**). Similar results were obtained in patients with hepatic disease when Cardene I.V. (nicardipine hydrochloride) was adminstered for 24 hours at 0.6 mg/hr.

RENAL FUNCTION

When Cardene I.V. was given to mild to moderate hypertensive patients with moderate degrees of renal impairment, significant reduction in glomerular filtration rate (GFR) and effective renal plasma flow (RPF) was observed. No significant differences in liver blood flow were observed in these patients. A significantly lower systemic clearance and higher area under the curve (AUC) were observed.

When Cardene capsules (20 mg or 30 mg TID) were given to hypertensive patients with impaired renal function, mean plasma concentrations, AUC, and C_{max} were approximately two-fold higher than in healthy controls. There is a transient increase in electrolyte excretion, including sodium (see **"PRECAUTIONS"**).

Acute bolus administration of Cardene I.V. (2.5 mg) in healthy volunteers decreased mean arterial pressure and renal vascular resistance; glomerular filtration rate (GFR), renal plasma flow (RPF), and the filtration fraction were unchanged. In healthy patients undergoing abdominal surgery, Cardene I.V. (10 mg over 20 minutes) increased GFR with no change in RPF when compared with placebo. In hypertensive type II diabetic patients with nephropathy, Cardene capsules (20 mg TID) did not change RPF and GFR, but reduced renal vascular resistance.

PULMONARY FUNCTION

In two well-controlled studies of patients with obstructive airway disease treated with Cardene capsules, no evidence of increased bronchospasm was seen. In one of the studies, Cardene capsules improved forced expiratory volume 1 second (FEV_1) and forced vital capacity (FVC) in comparison with metoprolol. Adverse experiences reported in a limited number of patients with asthma, reactive airway disease, or obstructive airway disease are similar to all patients treated with Cardene capsules.

EFFECTS IN HYPERTENSION

In patients with mild to moderate chronic stable essential hypertension, Cardene I.V. (0.5 to 4.0 mg/hr) produced dose-dependent decreases in blood pressure, although only the decreases at 4.0 mg/hr were statistically different from placebo. At the end of a 48-hour infusion at 4.0 mg/hr, the decreases were 26.0 mmHg (17%) in systolic blood pressure at 20.7 mmHg (20%) in diastolic blood pressure. In other settings (e.g., patients with severe or postoperative hypertension), Cardene I.V. (5 to 15 mg/hr) produced dose-dependent decreases in blood pressure. Higher infusion rates produced therapeutic responses more rapidly. The mean time to therapeutic response for severe hypertension, defined as diastolic blood pressure ≤ 95 mmHg or ≥ 25 mmHg decrease and systolic blood pressure ≤160 mmHg, was 77 ± 5.2 minutes. The average maintenance dose was 8.0 mg/hr. The mean time to therapeutic response for postoperative hypertension, defined as ≥15% reduction in diastolic or systolic blood pressure, was 11.5 ± 0.8 minutes. The average maintenance dose was 3.0 mg/hr.

*PA = conduction time from high to low right atrium; AH = conduction time from low right atrium to His bundle deflection, or AV nodal conduction time; HV = conduction time through the His bundle branch-Purkinje system.

INDICATION AND USAGE

Cardene I.V. is indicated for the short-term treatment of hypertension when oral therapy is not feasible or not desirable.

For prolonged control of blood pressure, patients should be transferred to oral medication as soon as their clinical condition permits (see **"DOSAGE AND ADMINISTRATION"**).

CONTRAINDICATIONS

Cardene I.V. is contraindicated in patients with known hypersensitivity to the drug. Cardene I.V. is also contraindicated in patients with advanced aortic stenosis because part of the effect of Cardene I.V. is secondary to reduced afterload. Reduction of diastolic pressure in these patients may worsen rather than improve myocardial oxygen balance.

WARNINGS

BETA-BLOCKER WITHDRAWAL

Nicardipine is not a beta-blocker and therefore gives no protection against the dangers of abrupt beta-blocker withdrawal; any such withdrawal should be by gradual reduction dose of beta-blocker.

RAPID DECREASES IN BLOOD PRESSURE

No clinical events have been reported suggestive of a too rapid decreases in blood pressure with Cardene I.V. However, as with any antihypertensive agent, blood pressure lowering should be accomplished over as long a time as is compatible with the patient's clinical status.

USE IN PATIENTS WITH ANGINA

Increases in frequency, duration, or severity of angina have been seen in chronic oral therapy with Cardene capsules. Induction or exacerbation of angina has been seen in less than 1% of coronary artery disease patients treated with Cardene I.V. The mechanism of this effect has not been established.

USE IN PATIENTS WITH CONGESTIVE HEART FAILURE

Cardene I.V. reduced afterload without impairing myocardial contractility in preliminary hemodynamic studies of CHF patients. However, *in vitro* and in some patients, a negative inotropic effect has been observed. Therefore, caution should be exercised when using Cardene I.V., particularly in combination with a beta-blocker, in patients with CHF or significant left ventricular dysfunction.

USE IN PATIENTS WITH PHEOCHROMOCYTOMA

Only limited clinical experience exists in use of Cardene I.V. for patients with hypertension associated with pheochromocytoma. Caution should therefore be exercised when using the drug in these patients.

PERIPHERAL VEIN INFUSION SITE

To minimize the risk of peripheral venous irritation, it is recommended that the site of infusion of Cardene I.V., be changed every 12 hours.

PRECAUTIONS

GENERAL

Blood Pressure: Because Cardene I.V. decreases peripheral resistance, monitoring of blood pressure during administration is required. Cardene I.V., like other calcium channel blockers, may occasionally produce symptomatic hypotension. Caution is advised to avoid systemic hypotension when administering the drug to patients who have sustained an acute cerebral infarction or hemorrhage.

Use in Patients with Impaired Hepatic Function: Since nicardipine is metabolized in the liver, the drug should be used with caution in patients with impaired liver function or reduced hepatic blood flow. The use of lower dosages should be considered.

Nicardipine administered intravenously has been reported to increase hepatic venous pressure gradient by 4 mmHg in cirrhotic patients at high doses (5 mg/20 min). Cardene I.V. should therefore be used with caution in patients with portal hypertension.

Use in Patients with Impaired Renal Function: When Cardene I.V. was given to mild to moderate hypertensive patients with moderate renal impairment, a significantly lower systemic clearance and higher AUC was observed. These results are consistent with those seen after oral administration of nicardipine. Careful dose titration is advised when treating renal impaired patients.

DRUG INTERACTIONS

Since Cardene I.V. may be administered to patients already being treated with other medications, including other antihypertensive agents, careful monitoring of these patients is necessary to detect and promptly treat any undesired effects from concomitant administration.

BETA-BLOCKERS

In most patients, Cardene I.V. can safely be used concomitantly with beta-blockers. However, caution should be exercised when using Cardene I.V. in combination with a beta-blocker in congestive heart failure patients (see "WARNINGS").

CIMETIDINE

Cimetidine has been shown to increase nicardipine plasma concentrations with Cardene capsule administration. Patients receiving the two drugs concomitantly should be carefully monitored. Data with other histamine-2 antagonists are not available.

DIGOXIN

Studies have shown that Cardene capsules usually do not alter digoxin plasma concentrations. However, as a precaution, digoxin levels should be evaluated when concomitant therapy with Cardene I.V. is initiated.

FENTANYL ANESTHESIA

Hypotension has been reported during fentanyl anesthesia with concomitant use of a beta-blocker and a calcium channel blocker. Even though such interactions were not seen during clinical studies with Cardene I.V. (nicardipine hydrochloride), an increased volume of circulating fluids might be required if such an interaction were to occur.

CYCLOSPORINE

Concomitant administration of Cardene capsules and cyclosporine results in elevated plasma cyclosporine levels. Plasma concentrations of cyclosporine should therefore be closely monitored during Cardene I.V. administration, and the dose of cyclosporine reduced accordingly.

IN VITRO INTERACTION

The plasma protein binding of nicardipine was not altered when therapeutic concentrations of furosemide, propranolol, dipyridamole, warfarin, quinidine, or naproxen were added to human plasma *in vitro*.

CARCINOGENESIS, MUTAGENESIS, IMPAIRMENT OF FERTILITY

Rats treated with nicardipine in the diet (at concentrations calculated to provide daily dosage levels of 5, 15, or 45 mg/kg/day) for two years showed a dose-dependent increase in thyroid hyperplasia and neoplasia (follicular adenoma/carcinoma). One- and three-month studies in the rat have suggested that these results are linked to a nicardipine-induced reduction in plasma thyroxine (T4) levels with a consequent increase in plasma levels of thyroid stimulating hormone (TSH). Chronic elevation of TSH is known to cause hyperstimulation of the thyroid. In rats on an iodine deficient diet, nicardipine administration for one month was associated with thyroid hyperplasia that was prevented by T4 supplementation. Mice treated with nicardipine in the diet (at concentrations calculated to provide daily dosage levels of up to 100 mg/kg/day) for up to 18 months showed no evidence of neoplasia of any tissue and no evidence of thyroid changes. There was no evidence of thyroid pathology in dogs treated with up to 25 mg nicardipine/kg/day for one year and no evidence of effects of nicardipine on thyroid function (plasma T4 and TSH) in man. There was no evidence of a mutagenic potential of nicardipine in a battery of genotoxicity tests conducted on microbial indicator organisms, in micronucleus tests in mice and hamsters, or in a sister chromatid exchange study in hamsters. No impairment of fertility was seen in male or female rats administered nicardipine at oral doses as high as 100 mg/kg/day (50 times the 40 mg TID maximum recommended dose in man, assuming a patient weight of 60 kg).

Pregnancy Category C: Cardene® I.V. at doses up to 5 mg/kg/day to pregnant rats and up to 0.5 mg/kg/day to pregnant rabbits produced no embryotoxicity or teratogenicity. Embryotoxicity was seen at 10 mg/kg/day in rats and at 1 mg/kg/day in rabbits, but no teratogenicity was observed at these doses.

Nicardipine was embryocidal when administered orally to pregnant Japanese White rabbits, during organogenesis, at 150 mg/kg/day (a dose associated with marked body weight gain suppression in the treated doe), but not at 50 mg/kg/day (25 times the maximum recommended dose in man). No adverse effects on the fetus were observed when New Zealand albino rabbits were treated, during organogenesis, with up to 100 mg nicardipine/kg/day (a dose associated with significant mortality in the treated doe). In pregnant rats administered nicardipine orally at up to 100 mg/kg/day (50 times the maximum recommended human dose) there was no evidence of embryolethality or teratogenicity. However, dystocia, reduced birth weights, reduced neonatal survival, and reduced neonatal weight gain were noted. There are no adequate and well-controlled studies in pregnant women. Cardene should be used during pregnancy only if the potential benefit justifies the potential risk to the fetus.

NURSING MOTHERS

Studies in rats have shown significant concentrations of nicardipine in maternal milk. For this reason, it is recommended that women who wish to breastfeed should not be given this drug.

PEDIATRIC USE

Safety and efficacy in patients under the age of 18 have not been established.

USE IN THE ELDERLY

No significant difference has been observed in the antihypertensive effect of Cardene I.V. in elderly patients (≥ 65 years) compared with other adult patients in clinical studies.

Adverse Experiences

Two hundred forty-four patients participated in two multicenter, double-blind, placebo-controlled trials of Cardene I.V. Adverse experiences were generally not serious and most were expected consequences of vasodilation. Adverse experiences occasionally required dosage adjustment. Therapy was discontinued in approximately 12% of patients, mainly due to hypotension, headache, and tachycardia.

Percent of Patients with Adverse Experiences During the Double-Blind Portion of Controlled Trials

Adverse Experience	Cardene (n=144)	Placebo (n=100)
Body as a Whole		
Headache	14.6	2.0
Asthenia	0.7	0.0
Abdominal pain	0.7	0.0
Chest pain	0.7	0.0
Cardiovascular		
Hypotension	5.6	1.0
Tachycardia	3.5	0.0
ECG abnormality	1.4	0.0
Postural hypotension	1.4	0.0
Ventricular extrasystoles	1.4	0.0
Extrasystoles	0.7	0.0
Hemopericardium	0.7	0.0
Hypertension	0.7	0.0
Supraventricular tachycardia	0.7	0.0
Syncope	0.7	0.0
Vasodilation	0.7	0.0
Ventricular tachycardia	0.7	0.0
Digestive		
Nausea/vomiting	4.9	1.0
Injection Site		
Injection site reaction	1.4	0.0
Injection site pain	0.7	0.0
Metabolic and Nutritional		
Hypokalemia	0.7	0.0
Nervous		
Dizziness	1.4	0.0
Hypesthesia	0.7	0.0
Intracranial hemorrhage	0.7	0.0
Paresthesia	0.7	0.0
Respiratory		
Dyspnea	0.7	0.0
Skin and Appendages		
Sweating	1.4	0.0
Urogenital		
Polyuria	1.4	0.0
Hematuria	0.7	0.0

RARE EVENTS

The following rare events have been reported in clinical trials or in the literature in association with the use of intravenously administered nicardipine.

Body as a Whole: fever, neck pain
Cardiovascular: angina pectoris, atrioventricular block, ST segment depression, inverted T wave, deep-vein thrombophlebitis
Digestive: dyspepsia
Hemic and Lymphatic: thrombocytopenia
Metabolic and Nutritional: hypophosphatemia, peripheral edema
Nervous: confusion, hypertonia
Respiratory: respiratory disorder
Special Senses: conjunctivitis, ear disorder, tinnitus
Urogenital: urinary frequency

Sinus node dysfunction and myocardial infarction, which may be due to disease progression, have been seen in patients on chronic therapy with orally administered nicardipine.

OVERDOSAGE

Several overdosages with orally administered nicardipine have been reported. One adult patient allegedly ingested 600 mg of nicardipine [standard (immediate release) capsules], and another patient, 2160 mg of the sustained release formulation of nicardipine. Symptoms included marked hypotension, bradycardia, palpitations, flushing, drowsiness, confusion and slurred speech. All symptoms resolved without sequelae. An overdosage occurred in a one-year-old child who ingested half of the powder in a 30 mg nicardipine standard capsule. The child remained asymptomatic.

Based on results obtained in laboratory animals, lethal overdose may cause systemic hypotension, bradycardia (following initial tachycardia) and progressive atrioventricular conduction block. Reversible hepatic function abnormalities and sporadic focal hepatic necrosis were noted in some animal species receiving very large doses of nicardipine.

For treatment of overdosage, standard measures including monitoring of cardiac and respiratory functions should be implemented. The patient should be positioned so as to avoid cerebral anoxia.

Frequent blood pressure determinations are essential. Vasopressors are clinically indicated for patients exhibiting profound hypotension. Intravenous calcium gluconate may help reverse the effects of calcium entry blockade.

DOSAGE AND ADMINISTRATION

Cardene I.V. (nicardipine hydrochloride) is intended for intravenous use. DOSAGE MUST BE INDIVIDUALIZED depending upon the severity of hypertension and the response of the patient during dosing. Blood pressure should be monitored both during and after the infusion; too rapid or excessive reduction in either systolic or diastolic blood pressure during parenteral treatment should be avoided.

PREPARATION

WARNING: AMPULS MUST BE DILUTED BEFORE INFUSION

Dilution: Cardene I.V. is administered by slow continuous infusion at a CONCENTRATION OF 0.1 MG/ML. Each ampul (25 mg) should be diluted with 240 mL of compatible intravenous fluid (see below), resulting in 250 mL of solution at a concentration of 0.1 mg/mL.

Cardene I.V. has been found to be compatible and stable in glass or polyvinyl chloride containers for 24 hours at controlled room temperature with:

Dextrose (5%) Injection, USP
Dextrose (5%) and Sodium Chloride (0.45%) Injection, USP
Dextrose (5%) and Sodium Chloride (0.9%) Injection, USP
Dextrose (5%) and 40 mEq Potassium, USP
Sodium Chloride (0.45%) Injection, USP
Sodium Chloride (0.9%) Injection, USP

Cardene I.V. is NOT compatible with Sodium Bicarbonate (5%) Injection, USP or Lactated Ringer's Injection, USP.

THE DILUTED SOLUTION IS STABLE FOR 24 HOURS AT ROOM TEMPERATURE.

Inspection: As with all parenteral drugs, Cardene I.V. should be inspected visually for particulate matter and discoloration prior to administration, whenever solution and container permit. Cardene I.V. is normally light yellow in color.

DOSAGE

As a Substitute for Oral Nicardipine Therapy

The intravenous infusion rate required to produce an average plasma concentration equivalent to a given oral dose at steady state is shown in the following table:

Oral Cardene Dose	Equivalent I.V. Infusion Rate
20 mg q8h	0.5 mg/hr
30 mg q8h	1.2 mg/hr
40 mg q8h	2.2 mg/hr

For Initiation of Therapy in a Drug Free Patient

The time course of blood pressure decrease is dependent on the initial rate of infusion and the frequency of dosage adjustment.

Cardene I.V. is administered by slow continuous infusion at a CONCENTRATION OF 0.1 MG/ML. With constant infusion, blood pressure begins to fall within minutes. It reaches about 50% of its ultimate decrease in about 45 minutes and does not reach final steady state for about 50 hours.

When treating acute hypertensive episodes in patients with chronic hypertension, discontinuation of infusion is followed by a 50% offset of action in 30 ± 7 minutes but plasma levels of drug and gradually decreasing antihypertensive effects exist for about 50 hours.

Titration: For gradual reduction in blood pressure, initiate therapy at 50 mL/hr (5.0 mg/hr). If desired blood pressure reduction is not achieved at this dose, the infusion rate may be increased by 25 mL/hr (2.5 mg/hr) every 15 minutes up to a maximum of 150 mL/hr (15.0 mg/hr), until desired blood pressure reduction is achieved.

For more rapid blood pressure reduction, initiate therapy at 50 mL/hr (5.0 mg/hr). If desired blood pressure reduction is not achieved at this dose, the infusion rate may be increased by 25 mL/hr (2.5 mg/hr) every 5 minutes up to a maximum of 150 mL/hr (15.0 mg/hr), until desired blood pressure reduction is achieved. Following achievement of the blood pressure goal, the infusion rate should be decreased to 30 mL/hr (3 mg/hr).

Maintenance: The rate of infusion should be adjusted as needed to maintain desired response.

CONDITIONS REQUIRING INFUSION ADJUSTMENT

Hypotension or Tachycardia: If there is concern of impending hypotension or tachycardia, the infusion should be discontinued. When blood pressure has stabilized, infusion of Cardene I.V. may be restarted at low doses such as 30 - 50 mL/hr (3.0 - 5.0 mg/hr) and adjusted to maintain desired blood pressure.

Infusion Site Changes: Cardene I.V. should be continued as long as blood pressure control is needed. The infusion site should be changed every 12 hours if administered via peripheral vein.

Continued on next page

Cardene—Cont.

Impaired Cardiac, Hepatic, or Renal Function: Caution is advised when titrating Cardene I.V. in patients with congestive heart failure or impaired hepatic or renal function (see "**PRECAUTIONS**").

TRANSFER TO ORAL ANTIHYPERTENSIVE AGENTS

If treatment includes transfer to an oral antihypertensive agent other than CARDENE capsules, therapy should generally be initiated upon discontinuation of Cardene I.V.

If Cardene capsules are to be used, the first dose of a TID regimen should be administered 1 hour prior to discontinuation of the infusion.

HOW SUPPLIED

Cardene® I.V. (nicardipine hydrochloride) is available in packages of 10 ampuls of 10 mL as follows:
25 mg (2.5 mg/mL), NDC 67286-0812-3.

Store at controlled room temperature 20° to 25°C (68° to 77°F).

Freezing does not adversely affect the product, but exposure to elevated temperatures should be avoided.

Protect from light. Store ampuls in carton until used.

U S Patent Nos.: 3,985,758; 4,880,823; and 5,164,405
Cardene® is a registered trademark of Roche Palo Alto LLC
Manufactured under license
from Roche Palo Alto LLC
Baxter Healthcare Corporation
Deerfield, IL 60015 USA
CI 4806-2
Marketed by:
ESP Pharma, Inc.
Edison, NJ 08817

CIV0021 Revised March 20, 2002

GATE Pharmaceuticals

Div. of TEVA Pharmaceuticals USA
650 CATHILL ROAD
SELLERSVILLE, PA 18960

Direct Inquiries to:
1090 Horsham Road
P. O. Box 1090
North Wales, PA 19454
(800) 292-4283

LOFIBRA™ ℞

[lō'fĭ-bră]
[Fenofibrate capsules (micronized)]
℞ Only

DESCRIPTION

LOFIBRA™ [Fenofibrate capsules (micronized)] is a lipid regulating agent available as capsules for oral administration. The chemical name for fenofibrate is 2-[4-(4-chlorobenzoyl) phenoxy]-2-methyl-propanoic acid, 1-methylethyl ester with the following structural formula:

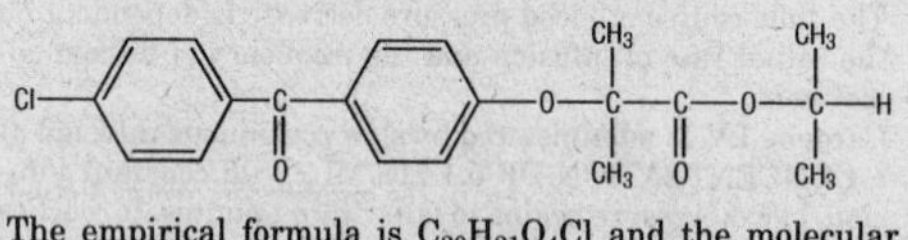

The empirical formula is $C_{20}H_{21}O_4Cl$ and the molecular weight is 360.83; fenofibrate is insoluble in water. The melting point is 79 to 82°C. Fenofibrate is a white solid which is stable under ordinary conditions.

Each 67 mg LOFIBRA™ contains the following inactive ingredients: croscarmellose sodium, crospovidone, lactose monohydrate, magnesium stearate, povidone, pregelatinized starch, sodium lauryl sulfate, talc, D&C Red #28, FD&C Blue #1, FD&C Red #40, titanium dioxide and gelatin.

Each 134 mg LOFIBRA™ contains the following inactive ingredients: croscarmellose sodium, crospovidone, lactose monohydrate, magnesium stearate, povidone, pregelatinized starch, sodium lauryl sulfate, talc, D&C Red #28, FD&C Blue #1, titanium dioxide and gelatin.

Each 200 mg LOFIBRA™ contains the following inactive ingredients: croscarmellose sodium, crospovidone, lactose monohydrate, magnesium stearate, povidone, pregelatinized starch, sodium lauryl sulfate, talc, FD&C Red #40, D&C Red #28, FDA/E172 yellow iron oxide, titanium dioxide and gelatin.

CLINICAL PHARMACOLOGY

A variety of clinical studies have demonstrated that elevated levels of total cholesterol (total-C), low density lipoprotein cholesterol (LDL-C), and apolipoprotein B (apo B), an LDL membrane complex, are associated with human atherosclerosis. Similarly, decreased levels of high density lipoprotein cholesterol (HDL-C) and its transport complex, apolipoprotein A (apo AI and apo AII) are associated with the development of atherosclerosis. Epidemiologic investigations have established that cardiovascular morbidity and mortality vary directly with the level of total-C, LDL-C, and triglycerides, and inversely with the level of HDL-C. The independent effect of raising HDL-C or lowering triglycerides (TG) on the risk of cardiovascular morbidity and mortality has not been determined.

Table 1

Mean Percent Change in lipid Parameters at End of Treatment†

Treatment Group	Total-C	LDL-C	HDL-C	TG
Pooled Cohort				
Mean baseline lipid values (n=646)	306.9 mg/dL	213.8 mg/dL	52.3 mg/dL	191.0 mg/dL
All FEN (n=361)	-18.7%*	-20.6%*	+11.0%*	-28.9%*
Placebo (n=285)	-0.4%	-2.2%	+0.7%	+7.7%
Baseline LDL-C > 160 mg/dL and TG < 150 mg/dL (Type IIa)				
Mean baseline lipid values (n=334)	307.7 mg/dL	227.7 mg/dL	58.1 mg/dL	101.7 mg/dL
All FEN (n=193)	-22.4%*	-31.4%*	+9.8%	-23.5%*
Placebo (n=141)	+0.2%	-2.2%	+2.6%	+11.7%
Baseline LDL-C > 160 mg/dL and TG < 150 mg/dL (Type IIb)				
Mean baseline lipid values (n=242)	312.8 mg/dL	219.8 mg/dL	46.7 mg/dL	231.9 mg/dL
All FEN (n=126)	-16.8%*	-20.1%*	+14.6%*	-35.9%*
Placebo (n=116)	-3.0%	-6.6%	+2.3%	+0.9%

†Duration of study treatment was 3 to 6 months
*p = <0.05 vs. Placebo

Fenofibric acid, the active metabolite of fenofibrate, produces reductions in total cholesterol, LDL cholesterol, apolipoprotein B, total triglycerides and triglyceride rich lipoprotein (VLDL) in treated patients. In addition, treatment with fenofibrate results in increases in high density lipoprotein (HDL) and apoproteins apo AI and apo AII.

The effects of fenofibric acid seen in clinical practice have been explained *in vivo* in transgenic mice and *in vitro* in human hepatocyte cultures by the activation of peroxisome proliferator activated receptor α (PPARα). Through this mechanism, fenofibrate increases lipolysis and elimination of triglyceride-rich particles from plasma by activating lipoprotein lipase and reducing production of apoproteins C-III (an inhibitor of lipoprotein lipase activity). The resulting fall in triglycerides produces an alteration in the size and composition of LDL from small, dense particles (which are thought to be atherogenic due to their susceptibility to oxidation), to large buoyant particles. These larger particles have a greater affinity for cholesterol receptors and are catabolized rapidly. Activation of PPARα also induces an increase in the synthesis of apoproteins A-I, A-II and HDL-cholesterol.

Fenofibrate also reduces serum uric acid levels in hyperuricemic and normal individuals by increasing the urinary excretion of uric acid.

Pharmacokinetics/Metabolism

Clinical experience has been obtained with two different formulations of fenofibrate: a "micronized" and "non-micronized" formulation, which have been demonstrated to be bioequivalent. Comparisons of blood levels following oral administration of both formulations in healthy volunteers demonstrate that a single capsule containing 67 mg of the "micronized" formulation is bioequivalent to 100 mg of the "non-micronized" formulation. Three capsules containing 67 mg LOFIBRA™ are bioequivalent to a single 200 mg LOFIBRA™ capsule.

Absorption

The absolute bioavailability of fenofibrate cannot be determined as the compound is virtually insoluble in aqueous media suitable for injection. However, fenofibrate is well absorbed from the gastrointestinal tract. Following oral administration in healthy volunteers, approximately 60% of a single dose of radiolabelled fenofibrate appeared in urine, primarily as fenofibric acid and its glucuronate conjugate, and 25% was excreted in the feces. Peak plasma levels of fenofibric acid occur within 6 to 8 hours after administration.

The absorption of fenofibrate is increased when administered with food. With micronized fenofibrate, the absorption is increased by approximately 35% under fed as compared to fasting conditions.

Distribution

In healthy volunteers, steady-state plasma levels of fenofibric acid were shown to be achieved within 5 days of dosing with single oral doses equivalent to 67 mg fenofibrate and did not demonstrate accumulation across time following multiple dose administration. Serum protein binding was approximately 99% in normal and hyperlipidemic subjects.

Metabolism

Following oral administration, fenofibrate is rapidly hydrolyzed by esterases to the active metabolite, fenofibric acid; no unchanged fenofibrate is detected in plasma.

Fenofibric acid is primarily conjugated with glucuronic acid and then excreted in urine. A small amount of fenofibric acid is reduced at the carbonyl moiety to a benzhydrol metabolite which is, in turn, conjugated with glucuronic acid and excreted in urine.

In vivo metabolism data indicate that neither fenofibrate nor fenofibric acid undergo oxidative metabolism (e.g., cytochrome P450) to a significant extent.

Excretion

After absorption, fenofibrate is mainly excreted in the urine in the form of metabolites, primarily fenofibric acid and fenofibric acid glucuronide. After administration of radiolabelled fenofibrate, approximately 60% of the dose appeared in the urine and 25% was excreted in the feces.

Fenofibric acid is eliminated with a half-life of 20 hours, allowing once daily administration in a clinical setting.

Special populations

Geriatrics

In elderly volunteers 77 to 87 years of age, the oral clearance of fenofibric acid following a single oral dose of fenofibrate was 1.2 L/h, which compares to 1.1 L/h in young adults. This indicates that a similar dosage regimen can be used in the elderly, without increasing accumulation of the drug or metabolites.

Pediatrics

Fenofibrate has not been investigated in adequate and well-controlled trials in pediatric patients.

Gender

No pharmacokinetic difference between males and females has been observed for fenofibrate.

Race

The influence of race on the pharmacokinetics of fenofibrate has not been studied, however fenofibrate is not metabolized by enzymes known for exhibiting inter-ethnic variability. Therefore, inter-ethnic pharmacokinetic differences are very unlikely.

Renal insufficiency

In a study in patients with severe renal impairment (creatinine clearance < 50 mL/min), the rate of clearance of fenofibric acid was greatly reduced, and the compound accumulated during chronic dosage. However, in patients having moderate renal impairment (creatinine clearance of 50 to 90 mL/min), the oral clearance and the oral volume of distribution of fenofibric acid are increased compared to healthy adults (2.1 L/h and 95 L versus 1.1 L/h and 30 L, respectively). Therefore, the dosage of fenofibrate should be minimized in patients who have severe renal impairment, while no modification of dosage is required in patients having moderate renal impairment.

Hepatic insufficiency

No pharmacokinetic studies have been conducted in patients having hepatic insufficiency.

Drug-drug interactions

In vitro studies using human liver microsomes indicate that fenofibrate and fenofibric acid are not inhibitors of cytochrome (CYP) P450 isoforms CYP3A4, CYP2D6, CYP2E1, or CYP1A2. They are weak inhibitors of CYP2C19 and CYP2A6, and mild-to-moderate inhibitors of CYP2C9 at therapeutic concentrations.

Potentiation of coumarin-type anti-coagulants has been observed with prolongation of the prothrombin time/INR.

Bile acid sequestrants have been shown to bind other drugs given concurrently. Therefore, fenofibrate should be taken at least 1 hour before or 4 to 6 hours after a bile acid binding resin to avoid impeding its absorption. (See **WARNINGS** and **PRECAUTIONS**).

Clinical Trials

Hypercholesterolemia (Heterozygous Familial and Nonfamilial) and Mixed Dyslipidemia (Freckson Types IIa and IIb)

The effects of fenofibrate at a dose equivalent to 200 mg fenofibrate per day were assessed from four randomized, placebo-controlled, double-blind, parallel-group studies including patients with the following mean baseline lipid values: total-C 306.9 mg/dL; LDL-C 213.8 mg/dL; HDL-C 52.3 mg/dL; and triglycerides 191.0 mg/dL. Fenofibrate therapy lowered LDL-C, Total-C, and the LDL-C/HDL-C ratio. Fenofibrate therapy also lowered triglycerides and raised HDL-C (see Table 1).

[See table 1 above]

In a subset of the subjects, measurements of apo B were conducted. Fenofibrate treatment significantly reduced apo B from baseline to endpoint as compared with placebo (-25.1% vs. 2.4%, p<0.0001, n=213 and 143 respectively).

Hypertriglyceridemia (Fredrickson Type IV and V)

The effects of fenofibrate on serum triglycerides were studied in two randomized, double-blind, placebo-controlled clinical trials 1 of 147 hypertriglyceridemia patients (Fredrickson Type IV and V). Patients were treated for eight weeks under protocols that differed only in that one entered patients with baseline triglyceride (TG) levels of 500 to 1500 mg/dL, and the other TG levels of 350 to 500 mg/dL. In patients with hypertriglyceridemia and normal cholesterolemia with or without hyperchylomicronemia (Type IV/V hyperlipidemia), treatment with fenofibrate at dosages equivalent to 200 mg fenofibrate per day decreased primarily very low density lipoprotine (VLDL) triglycerides and VLDL cholesterol. Treatment of patients with type IV hyperlipoproteinemia and elevated triglycerides often results in an increase of low density lipoprotein (LDL) cholesterol (see Table 2).

[See table 2 above]

The effect of fenofibrate on cardiovascular morbidity and mortality has not been determined.

INDICATIONS AND USAGE

Treatment of Hypercholesterolemia

Fenofibrate capsules (micronized) is indicated as adjunctive therapy to diet for the reduction of LDL-C, Total-C, Triglycerides and Apo B in adult patients with primary hypercholesterolemia or mixed dyslipidemia (Fredrickson Types IIa and IIb. Lipid-altering agents should be used in addition to a diet restricted in saturated fat and cholesterol when response to diet and non-pharmacological interventions alone has been inadequate (see National Cholesterol Education Program [NCEP] Treatment Guidelines, below).

Treatment of Hypertriglyceridemia

Fenofibrate capsules (micronized) is also indicated as adjunctive therapy to diet for treatment of adult patients with hypertriglyceridemia (Fredrickson Types IV and V hyperlipidemia). Improving glycemic control in diabetic patients showing fasting chylomicronemia will usually reduce fasting triglycerides and eliminate chylomicronemia thereby obviating the need for pharmacologic intervention.

Markedly elevated levels of serum triglycerides (e.g. > 2,000 mg/dL) may increase the risk of developing pancreatitis. The effect of fenofibrate therapy on reducing this risk has not been adequately studied.

Drug therapy is not indicated for patients with Type I hyperlipoproteinemia, who have elevations of chylomicrons and plasma triglycerides, but who have normal levels of very low density lipoprotein (VLDL). Inspection of plasma refrigerated for 14 hours is helpful in distinguishing Types I, IV and V hyperlipoproteinemia[2].

The initial treatment for dyslipidemia is dietary therapy specific for the type of lipoprotein abnormality. Excess body weight and excess alcoholic intake may be important factors in hypertriglyceridemia and should be addressed prior to any drug therapy. Physical exercise can be an important ancillary measure. Diseases contributory to hyperlipidemia, such as hypothyroidism or diabetes mellitus should be looked for and adequately treated. Estrogen therapy, like thiazide diuretics and beta-blockers, is sometimes associated with massive rises in plasma triglycerides, especially in subjects with familial hypertriglyceridemia. In such cases, discontinuation of the specific etiologic agent may obviate the need for specific drug therapy of hypertriglyceridemia.

The use of drugs should be considered only when reasonable attempts have been made to obtain satisfactory results with non-drug methods. If the decision is made to use drugs, the patient should be instructed that this does not reduce the importance of adhering to diet (See **WARNINGS** and **PRECAUTIONS**).

Fredrickson Classification of Hyperlipoproteinemias

Type	Lipoprotein Elevated	Lipid Elevation Major	Lipid Elevation Minor
I(rare)	Chylomicrons	TG	↑↔C
IIa	LDL	C	-
IIb	LDL, VLDL	C	TG
III (rare)	IDL	C, TG	-
IV	VLDL	TG	↑↔C
V(rare)	chylomicrons, VLDL	TG	↑↔

C = cholesterol
TG = triglycerides
LDL = low density lipoprotein
VLDL = very low density lipoprotein
IDL = intermediate density lipoprotein

The NCEP Treatment Guidelines

Definite Athero-sclerotic Disease[a]	Two or More Other Risk Factors[b]	LDL-Cholesterol mg/dL (mmol/L) Initiation Level	LDL-Cholesterol mg/dL (mmol/L) Goal
No	No	≥190 (≥4.9)	<160 (<4.1)
No	Yes	≥160 (≥4.1)	<130 (<3.4)
Yes	Yes or No	≥130[c] (≥3.4)	<100 (<2.6)

(a) Coronary heart disease or peripheral vascular disease (including symptomatic carotid artery disease).

(b) Other risk factors for coronary heart disease (CHD) include: age (males: ≥45 years; females: ≥55 years or premature menopause without estrogen replacement therapy); family history of premature CHD; current cigarette smoking; hypertension; confirmed HDL-C <35 mg/dL (<0.91 mmol/L); and diabetes mellitus. Subtract 1 risk factor if HDL-C is ≥60 mg/dL (≥1.6 mmol/L).

(c) In CHD patients with LDL-C levels 100 to 129 mg/dL, the physician should exercise clinical judgment in deciding whether to initiate drug treatment.

CONTRAINDICATIONS

LOFIBRA™ is contraindicated in patients who exhibit hypersensitivity to fenofibrate.

Table 2
Effects of Fenofibrate Capsules (micronized) in Patients With Fredrickson Type IV/V Hyperlipidemia

Study 1	Placebo				Fenofibrate Capsules (micronized)			
Baseline TG Levels 350 to 499 mg/dL	**N**	**Baseline (Mean)**	**Endpoint (Mean)**	**% Change (Mean)**	**N**	**Baseline (Mean)**	**Endpoint (Mean)**	**% Change (Mean)**
Triglycerides	28	449	450	-0.5	27	432	223	-46.2*
VLDL Triglycerides	19	367	350	2.7	19	350	178	-44.1*
Total Cholesterol	28	255	261	2.8	27	252	227	-9.1*
HDL Cholesterol	28	35	36	4	27	34	40	19.6*
LDL Cholesterol	28	120	129	12	27	128	137	14.5
VLDL Cholesterol	27	99	99	5.8	27	92	46	-44.7*
Study 2	**Placebo**				**Fenofibrate Capsules (micronized)**			
Baseline TG Levels 500 to 1500 mg/dL	**N**	**Baseline (Mean)**	**Endpoint (Mean)**	**% Change (Mean)**	**N**	**Baseline (Mean)**	**Endpoint (Mean)**	**% Change (Mean)**
Triglycerides	44	710	750	7.2	48	726	308	-54.5*
VLDL Triglycerides	29	537	571	18.7	33	543	205	-50.6*
Total Cholesterol	44	272	271	0.4	48	261	223	-13.8*
HDL Cholesterol	44	27	28	5.0	48	30	36	22.9*
LDL Cholesterol	42	100	90	-4.2	45	103	131	45.0*
VLDL Cholesterol	42	137	142	11.0	45	126	54	-49.4*

* = p<0.05 vs. Placebo

LOFIBRA™ is contraindicated in patients with hepatic or severe renal dysfunction, including primary biliary cirrhosis, and patients with unexplained persistent liver function abnormality.

LOFIBRA™ is contraindicated in patients with preexisting gallbladder disease (see **WARNINGS**).

WARNINGS

Liver Function: LOFIBRA™ at doses equivalent to 134 mg to 200 mg fenofibrate per day has been associated with increases in serum transaminases [AST (SGOT) or ALT (SGPT)]. In a pooled analysis of 10 placebo-controlled trials, increases to > 3 times the upper limit of normal occurred in 5.3% of patients taking fenofibrate versus 1.1% of patients treated with placebo.

When transaminase determinations were followed either after discontinuation of treatment or during continued treatment, a return to normal limits was usually observed. The incidence of increases in transaminase related to fenofibrate therapy appear to be dose related. In an 8-week dose-ranging study, the incidence of ALT or AST elevations to at least three times the upper limit of normal was 13% in patients receiving dosages equivalent to 134 mg to 200 mg fenofibrate per day and was 0% in those receiving dosages equivalent to 34 mg or 67 mg of fenofibrate per day or placebo. Hepatocellular, chronic active and cholestatic hepatitis associated with fenofibrate therapy have been reported after exposures of weeks to several years. In extremely rare cases, cirrhosis has been reported in association with chronic active hepatitis.

Regular periodic monitoring of liver function, including serum ALT (SGPT) should be performed for the duration of therapy with fenofibrate, and therapy discontinued if enzyme levels persist above three times the normal limit.

Cholelithiasis: Fenofibrate, like clofibrate and gemfibrozil, may increase cholesterol excretion into the bile, leading to cholelithiasis. If cholelithiasis is suspected, gallbladder studies are indicated. Fenofibrate therapy should be discontinued if gallstones are found.

Concomitant Oral Anticoagulants: Caution should be exercised when anticoagulants are given in conjunction with fenofibrate because of the potentiation of coumarin-type anticoagulants in prolonging the prothrombin time/INR. The dosage of the anticoagulant should be reduced to maintain the prothrombin time/INR at the desired level to prevent bleeding complications. Frequent prothrombin time/INR determinations are advisable until it has been definitely determined that the prothrombin time/INR has stabilized.

Concomitant HMG-CoA reductase inhibitors: The combined use of fenofibrate and HMG-CoA reductase inhibitors should be avoided unless the benefit of further alterations in lipid levels is likely to outweigh the increased risk of this drug combination.

In a single-dose drug interaction study in 23 healthy adults the concomitant administration of fenofibrate and pravastatin resulted in no clinically important difference in the pharmacokinetics of fenofibric acid, pravastatin or its active metabolite 3α-hydroxy isopravastatin when compared to either drug given alone.

The combined use of fibric acid derivatives and HMG-CoA reductase inhibitors has been associated, in the absences of a marked pharmacokinetic interaction, in numerous case reports, with rhabdomyolysis, markedly elevated creatine kinase (CK) levels and myoglobinuria, leading in a high proportion of cases to acute renal failure.

The use of fibrates alone, including fenofibrate capsules (micronized) may occasionally be associated with myositis, myopathy, or rhabdomyolysis. Patients receiving fenofibrate and complaining of muscle pain, tenderness, or weakness should have prompt medical evaluation for myopathy, including serum creatine kinase level determination. If myopathy/myositis is suspected or diagnosed, fenofibrate therapy should be stopped.

Mortality: The effect of fenofibrate on coronary heart disease morbidity and mortality and non-cardiovascular mortality has not been established.

Other Considerations: In the Coronary Drug Project, a large study of post myocardial infarction of patients treated for 5 years with clofibrate, there was no difference in mortality seen between the clofibrate group and the placebo group. There was however, a difference in the rate of cholelithiasis and cholecystitis requiring surgery between the two groups (3.0% vs. 1.8%).

Because of chemical, pharmacological, and clinical similarities between fenofibrate, clofibrate, and gemfibrozil, the adverse findings in 4 large randomized, placebo-controlled clinical studies with these other fibrate drugs may also apply to fenofibrate.

In a study conducted by the World Health Organization (WHO), 5000 subjects without known coronary artery disease were treated with placebo or clofibrate for 5 years and followed for an additional one year. There was a statistically significant, higher age-adjusted all-cause mortality in the clofibrate group compared with the placebo group (5.70% vs. 3.96%, p=<0.01). Excess mortality was due to a 33% increase in non-cardiovascular causes, including malignancy, post-cholecystectomy complications, and pancreatitis. This appeared to confirm the higher risk of gallbladder disease seen in clofibrate-treated patients studied in the Coronary Drug Project.

The Helsinki Heart Study was a large (n=4081) study of middle-aged men without a history of coronary artery disease. Subjects received either placebo or gemfibrozil for 5 years, with a 3.5 year open extension afterward. Total mortality was numerically higher in the gemfibrozil randomization group but did not achieve statistical significance (p=0.19, 95% confidence interval for relative risk G:P=.91-1.64). Although cancer deaths trended higher in the gemfibrozil group (p=0.11), cancers (excluding basal cell carcinoma) were diagnosed with equal frequency in both study groups. Due to the limited size of the study, the relative risk of death from any cause was not shown to be different than that seen in the 9 year follow-up data from World Health Organization study (RR=1.29). Similarly, the numerical excess of gallbladder surgeries in the gemfibrozil group did not differ statistically from that observed in the WHO study.

A secondary prevention component of the Helsinki Heart Study enrolled middle-aged men excluded from the primary prevention study because of known or suspected coronary heart disease. Subjects received gemfibrozil or placebo for 5 years. Although cardiac deaths trended higher in the gemfibrozil group, this was not statistically significant (hazard ratio 2.2, 95% confidence interval: 0.94-5.05). The rate of gallbladder surgery was not statistically significant between study groups, but did trend higher in the gemfibrozil group, (1.9% vs. 0.3%, p=0.07). There was a statistically significant difference in the number of appendectomies in the gemfibrozil group (6/311 vs. 0/317, p=0.029).

PRECAUTIONS

Initial therapy: Laboratory studies should be done to ascertain that the lipid levels are consistently abnormal before instituting fenofibrate therapy. Every attempt should be made to control serum lipids with appropriate diet, exercise, weight loss in obese patients, and control of any medical problems such as diabetes mellitus and hypothyroidism that are contributing to the lipid abnormalities. Medications known to exacerbate hypertriglyceridemia (beta-blockers, thiazides, estrogens) should be discontinued or changed if possible prior to consideration of triglyceride-lowering drug therapy.

Continued therapy: Periodic determination of serum lipids should be obtained during initial therapy in order to establish the lowest effective dose of LOFIBRA™ [Fenofibrate capsules (micronized)]. Therapy should be withdrawn in patients who do not have an adequate response after two months of treatment with the maximum recommended dose of 200 mg per day.

Pancreatitis: Pancreatitis has been reported in patients taking fenofibrate, gemfibrozil, and clofibrate. This occur-

Continued on next page

Lofibra—Cont.

rence may represent a failure of efficacy in patients with severe hypertriglyceridemia, a direct drug effect, or a secondary phenomenon mediated through biliary tract stone or sludge formation with obstruction of the common bile duct.

Hypersensitivity Reactions: Acute hypersensitivity reactions including severe skin rashes requiring patient hospitalization and treatment with steroids have occurred very rarely during treatment with fenofibrate, including rare spontaneous reports of Stevens-Johnson syndrome, and toxic epidermal necrolysis. Urticaria was seen in 1.1 vs. 0%, and rash in 1.4 vs. 0.8% of fenofibrate and placebo patients respectively in controlled trials.

Hematologic Changes: Mild to moderate hemoglobin, hematocrit, and white blood cell decreases have been observed in patients following initiation of fenofibrate therapy. However, these levels stabilize during long-term administration. Extremely rare spontaneous reports of thrombocytopenia and agranulocytosis have been received during post-marketing surveillance outside of the U.S. Periodic blood counts are recommended during the first 12 months of fenofibrate administration.

Skeletal muscle: The use of fibrates alone, including fenofibrate, may occasionally be associated with myopathy. Treatment with drugs of the fibrate class has been associated on rare occasions with rhabdomyolysis, usually in patients with impaired renal function. Myopathy should be considered in any patient with diffuse myalgias, muscle tenderness or weakness, and/or marked elevations of creatine phosphokinase levels.

Patients should be advised to report promptly unexplained muscle pain, tenderness or weakness, particularly if accompanied by malaise or fever. CPK levels should be assessed in patients reporting these symptoms, and fenofibrate therapy should be discontinued if markedly elevated CPK levels occur or myopathy is diagnosed.

Drug Interactions

Oral Anticoagulants: CAUTION SHOULD BE EXERCISED WHEN COUMARIN ANTICOAGULANTS ARE GIVEN IN CONJUNCTION WITH LOFIBRA™. THE DOSAGE OF THE ANTICOAGULANTS SHOULD BE REDUCED TO MAINTAIN THE PROTHROMBIN TIME/INR AT THE DESIRED LEVEL TO PREVENT BLEEDING COMPLICATIONS. FREQUENT PROTHROMBIN TIME/INR DETERMINATIONS ARE ADVISABLE UNTIL IT HAS BEEN DEFINITELY DETERMINED THAT THE PROTHROMBIN TIME/INR HAS STABILIZED.

HMG-CoA reductase inhibitors: The combined use of fenofibrate and HMG-CoA reductase inhibitors should be avoided unless the benefit of further alterations in lipid levels is likely to outweigh the increased risk of this drug combination (see WARNINGS).

Resins: Since bile acid sequestrants may bind other drugs given concurrently, patients should take LOFIBRA™ at least 1 hour before or 4 to 6 hours after a bile acid binding resin to avoid impeding its absorption.

Cyclosporine: Because cyclosporine can produce nephrotoxicity with decreases in creatinine clearance and rises in serum creatinine, and because renal excretion is the primary elimination route of fibrate drugs including fenofibrate, there is a risk that an interaction will lead to deterioration. The benefits and risks of using fenofibrate with immunosuppressants and other potentially nephrotoxic agents should be carefully considered, and the lowest effective dose employed.

Carcinogenesis, Mutagenesis, Impairment of Fertility: In a 24-month study in rats (10, 45, and 200 mg/kg; 0.3, 1, and 6 times the maximum recommended human dose on the basis of mg/meter^2 of surface area), the incidence of liver carcinoma was significantly increased at 6 times the maximum recommended human dose in males and females. A statistically significant increase in pancreatic carcinomas occurred in males at 1 and 6 times the maximum recommended human dose; there were also increases in pancreatic adenomas and benign testicular interstitial cell tumors at 6 times the maximum recommended human dose in males. In a second 24-month study in a different strain of rats (doses of 10 and 60 mg/kg; 0.3 and 2 times the maximum recommended human dose based on mg/meter^2 surface area), there were significant increases in the incidence of pancreatic acinar adenomas in both sexes and increases in interstitial cell tumors of the testes at 2 times the maximum recommended human dose.

A comparative carcinogenicity study was done in rats comparing three drugs: fenofibrate (10 and 70 mg/kg; 0.3 and 1.6 times the maximum recommended human dose), clofibrate (400 mg/kg; 1.6 times the human dose), and gemfibrozil (250 mg/kg; 1.7 times the human dose) (multiples based on mg/meter^2 surface area). Pancreatic acinar adenomas were increased in males and females on fenofibrate; hepatocellular carcinoma and pancreatic acinar adenomas were increased in males and hepatic neoplastic nodules in females treated with clofibrate; hepatic neoplastic nodules were increased in males and females treated with gemfibrozil while testicular interstitial cell tumors were increased in males on all three drugs.

In a 21-month study in mice at doses of 10, 45, and 200 mg/kg (approximately 0.2, 0.7 and 3 times the maximum recommended human dose on the basis of mg/meter^2 surface area), there were statistically significant increases in liver carcinoma at 3 times the maximum recommended human dose in both males and females. In a second 18-month study at the same doses, there was a significant increase in liver carcinoma in male mice and liver adenoma in female mice at 3 times the maximum recommended human dose. Electron microscopy studies have demonstrated peroxisomal proliferation following fenofibrate administration to the rat. An adequate study to test for peroxisome proliferation in humans has not been done, but changes in peroxisome morphology and numbers have been observed in humans after treatment with other members of the fibrate class when liver biopsies were compared before and after treatment in the same individual.

Fenofibrate has been demonstrated to be devoid of mutagenic potential in the following tests: Ames, mouse lymphoma, chromosomal aberration and unscheduled DNA synthesis.

Pregnancy Category C: Fenofibrate has been shown to be embryocidal and teratogenic in rats when given in doses 7 to 10 times the maximum recommended human dose and embryocidal in rabbits when given at 9 times the maximum recommended human dose (on the basis of mg/meter^2 surface area). There are no adequate and well-controlled studies in pregnant women. Fenofibrate should be used during pregnancy only if the potential benefit justifies the potential risk to the fetus.

Administration of 9 times the maximum recommended human dose of fenofibrate to female rats before and throughout gestation caused 100% of dams to delay delivery and resulted in a 60% increase in post-implantation loss, a decrease in litter size, a decrease in birth weight, a 40% survival of pups at birth, a 4% survival of pups as neonates, and a 0% survival of pups to weaning, and an increase in spina bifida.

Administration of 10 times the maximum recommended human dose to female rats on days 6 to 15 of gestation caused an increase in gross, visceral and skeletal findings in fetuses (domed head/hunched shoulders/rounded body/abnormal chest, kyphosis, stunted fetuses, elongated sternal ribs, malformed sternebrae, extra foramen in palatine, misshapen vertebrae, supernumerary ribs).

Administration of 7 times the maximum recommended human dose to female rats from day 15 of gestation through weaning caused a delay in delivery, a 40% decrease in live births, a 75% decrease in neonatal survival, and decreases in pup weight, at birth as well as on days 4 and 21 postpartum.

Administration of 9 and 18 times the maximum recommended human dose to female rabbits caused abortions in 10% of dams at 9 times and 25% of dams at 18 times the maximum recommended human dose and death of 7% of fetuses at 18 times the maximum recommended human dose.

Nursing mothers: Fenofibrate should not be used in nursing mothers. Because of the potential for tumorigenicity seen in animal studies, a decision should be made whether to discontinue nursing or to discontinue the drug.

Pediatric Use: Safety and efficacy in pediatric patients have not been established.

Geriatric Use: Fenofibric acid is known to be substantially excreted by the kidney, and the risk of adverse reactions to this drug may be greater in patients with impaired renal function. Because elderly patients are more likely to have decreased renal function, care should be taken in dose selection.

ADVERSE REACTIONS

CLINICAL: Adverse events reported by 2% or more of patients treated with fenofibrate during the double-blind, placebo-controlled trials, regardless of causality, are listed in the table below. Adverse events led to discontinuation of treatment in 5.0% of patients treated with fenofibrate and in 3.0% treated with placebo. Increases in liver function tests were the most frequent events, causing discontinuation of fenofibrate treatment in 1.6% of patients in double-blind trials.

BODY SYSTEM Adverse Event	Fenofibrate* (N=439)	PLACEBO (N=365)
BODY AS A WHOLE		
Abdominal Pain	4.6%	4.4%
Back pain	3.4%	2.5%
Headache	3.2%	2.7%
Asthenia	2.1%	3.0%
Flu Syndrome	2.1%	2.7%
DIGESTIVE		
Liver Function Tests		
Abnormal	7.5%**	1.4%
Diarrhea	2.3%	4.1%
Nausea	2.3%	1.9%
Constipation	2.1%	1.4%
METABOLIC AND NUTRITIONAL DISORDERS		
SPGT Increased	3.0%	1.6%
Creatine Phosphokinase		
Increased	3.0%	1.4%
SGOT Increased	3.4%**	0.5%
RESPIRATORY		
Respiratory Disorder	6.2%	5.5%
Rhinitis	2.3%	1.1%

*Dosage equivalent to 200 mg LOFIBRA™ [Fenofibrate capsules (micronized)]
**Significantly different from Placebo

Additional adverse events reported by three or more patients in placebo-controlled trials or reported in other controlled or open trials, regardless of causality are listed below.

BODY AS A WHOLE: Chest pain, pain (unspecified), infection, malaise, allergic reaction, cyst, hernia, fever, photosensitivity reaction, and accidental injury.

CARDIOVASCULAR SYSTEM: Angina pectoris, hypertension, vasodilatation, coronary artery disorder, electrocardiogram abnormal, ventricular extrasystoles, myocardial infarct, peripheral vascular disorder, migraine, varicose vein, cardiovascular disorder, hypotension, palpitation, vascular disorder, arrhythmia, phlebitis, tachycardia, extrasystoles, and atrial fibrillation.

DIGESTIVE SYSTEM: Dyspepsia, flatulence, nausea, increased appetite, gastroenteritis, cholelithiasis, rectal disorder, esophagitis, gastritis, colitis, tooth disorder, vomiting, anorexia, gastrointestinal disorder, duodenal ulcer, nausea and vomiting, peptic ulcer, rectal hemorrhage, liver fatty deposit, cholecystitis, eructation, gamma glutamyl transpeptidase, and diarrhea.

ENDOCRINE SYSTEM: Diabetes mellitus

HEMIC AND LYMPHATIC SYSTEM: Anemia, leukopenia, ecchymosis, eosinophilia, lymphadenopathy, and thrombocytopenia.

METABOLIC AND NUTRITIONAL DISORDERS: Creatinine increased, weight gain, hypoglycemia, gout, weight loss, edema, hyperuricemia, and peripheral edema.

MUSCULOSKELETAL SYSTEM: Myositis, myalgia, arthralgia, arthritis, tenosynovitis, joint disorder, arthrosis, leg cramps, bursitis, and myasthenia.

NERVOUS SYSTEM: Dizziness, insomnia, depression, vertigo, libido decreased, anxiety, paresthesia, dry mouth, hypertonia, nervousness, neuralgia, and somnolence.

RESPIRATORY SYSTEM: Pharyngitis, bronchitis, cough increased, dyspnea, asthma, pneumonia, laryngitis, and sinusitis.

SKIN AND APPENDAGES: Rash, pruritus, eczema, herpes zoster, urticaria, acne, sweating, fungal dermatitis, skin disorder, alopecia, contact dermatitis, herpes simplex, maculopapular rash, nail disorder, and skin ulcer.

SPECIAL SENSES: Conjunctivitis, eye disorder, amblyopia, ear pain, otitis media, abnormal vision, cataract specified, and refraction disorder.

UROGENITAL SYSTEM: Urinary frequency, prostatic disorder, dysuria, kidney function abnormal, urolithiasis, gynecomastia, unintended pregnancy, vaginal moniliasis, and cystitis.

OVERDOSAGE

There is no specific treatment for overdose with fenofibrate. General supportive care of the patient is indicated, including monitoring of vital signs and observation of clinical status, should an overdose occur. If indicated, elimination of unabsorbed drug should be achieved by emesis or gastric lavage; usual precautions should be observed to maintain the airway. Because fenofibrate is highly bound to plasma proteins, hemodialysis should not be considered.

DOSAGE AND ADMINISTRATION

Patients should be placed on an appropriate lipid-lowering diet before receiving LOFIBRA™ [Fenofibrate capsules (micronized)], and should continue this diet during treatment with LOFIBRA™. LOFIBRA™ should be given with meals, thereby optimizing the bioavailability of the medication.

For the treatment of adult patients with primary hypercholesterolemia or mixed hyperlipidemia, the initial dose of LOFIBRA™ is 200 mg per day.

For adult patients with hypertriglyceridemia, the initial dose is 67 to 200 mg per day. Dosage should be individualized according to patient response, and should be adjusted if necessary following repeat lipid determinations at 4 to 8 week intervals. The maximum dose is 200 mg per day. Treatment with LOFIBRA™ should be initiated at a dose of 67 mg/day in patients having impaired renal function, and increased only after evaluation of the effects on renal function and lipid levels at this dose. In the elderly, the initial dose should likewise be limited to 67 mg/day.

Lipid levels should be monitored periodically and consideration should be given to reducing the dosage of LOFIBRA™ if lipid levels fall significantly below the targeted range.

HOW SUPPLIED

LOFIBRA™, 67 mg are opaque pink cap and body, hard gelatin capsules, printed in black ink **N** over **240** and **67** on opposing cap and body portions of the capsule. They are supplied as follows:
  NDC 57844-322-01 Bottles of 100 capsules
LOFIBRA™, 134 mg are opaque light blue cap and body, hard gelatin capsules, printed in black ink **N** over **411** and **134** on opposing cap and body portions of the capsule. They are supplied as follows:
  NDC 57844-323-01 Bottles of 100 capsules
LOFIBRA™, 200 mg are opaque orange cap and body, hard gelatin capsules, printed in black ink **N** over **412** and **200** on opposing cap and body portions of the capsule. They are supplied as follows:
  NDC 57844-324-01 Bottles of 100 capsules

STORAGE

Store at controlled room temperature, between 20° and 25°C (68° and 77°F) (see USP). Keep out of the reach of children. Protect from moisture.

Manufactured by:
NOVOPHARM LIMITED
Toronto, Canada
M1B 2K9
Manufactured for:
GATE PHARMACEUTICALS
Div. of TEVA PHARMACEUTICALS USA
Sellersville, PA 18960

REFERENCES

1. GOLDBERG AC, *et al.* Fenofibrate for the Treatment of Type IV and V Hyperlipoproteinemias: A Double-Blind, Placebo-Controlled Multicenter US Study. *Clinical Therapeutics*, 11, pp. 69-83, 1989.
2. NIKKILA EA. Familial Lipoprotein Lipase Deficiency and Related Disorders of Chylomicron Metabolism. In Stanbury J.B., *et al.* (eds.): *The Metabolic Basis of Inherited Disease*, 5th edition, McGraw-Hill, 1983, Chap. 30, pp. 622-642.
3. BROWN WV, *et al.* Effects of Fenofibrate on Plasma Lipids: Double-Blind, Multicenter Study In Patients with Type IIA or IIB Hyperlipidemia. *Arteriosclerosis*. 6, pp. 670-678, 1986.

72204IN-2600 Rev. 00
Rev. C 4/2003

Gilead Sciences, Inc.

333 LAKESIDE DRIVE
FOSTER CITY, CA 94404

Direct Inquiries To:
Customer Service
(800) GILEAD5

Medical Emergency Contact:
Director, Medical Information
(800) GILEAD5
FAX: (650) 522-5477

HEPSERA™ ℞

[hĕp' sĕră]
adefovir dipivoxil Tablets
℞ Only

WARNINGS

1. SEVERE ACUTE EXACERBATIONS OF HEPATITIS HAVE BEEN REPORTED IN PATIENTS WHO HAVE DISCONTINUED ANTI-HEPATITIS B THERAPY, INCLUDING THERAPY WITH HEPSERA. HEPATIC FUNCTION SHOULD BE MONITORED CLOSELY IN PATIENTS WHO DISCONTINUE ANTI-HEPATITIS B THERAPY. IF APPROPRIATE, RESUMPTION OF ANTI-HEPATITIS B THERAPY MAY BE WARRANTED (SEE WARNINGS).

2. IN PATIENTS AT RISK OF OR HAVING UNDERLYING RENAL DYSFUNCTION, CHRONIC ADMINISTRATION OF HEPSERA MAY RESULT IN NEPHROTOXICITY. THESE PATIENTS SHOULD BE MONITORED CLOSELY FOR RENAL FUNCTION AND MAY REQUIRE DOSE ADJUSTMENT (SEE WARNINGS AND DOSAGE AND ADMINISTRATION).

3. HIV RESISTANCE MAY EMERGE IN CHRONIC HEPATITIS B PATIENTS WITH UNRECOGNIZED OR UNTREATED HUMAN IMMUNODEFICIENCY VIRUS (HIV) INFECTION TREATED WITH ANTI-HEPATITIS B THERAPIES, SUCH AS THERAPY WITH HEPSERA, THAT MAY HAVE ACTIVITY AGAINST HIV (SEE WARNINGS).

4. LACTIC ACIDOSIS AND SEVERE HEPATOMEGALY WITH STEATOSIS, INCLUDING FATAL CASES, HAVE BEEN REPORTED WITH THE USE OF NUCLEOSIDE ANALOGS ALONE OR IN COMBINATION WITH OTHER ANTIRETROVIRALS (SEE WARNINGS).

DESCRIPTION

HEPSERA is the tradename for adefovir dipivoxil, a diester prodrug of adefovir. Adefovir is an acyclic nucleotide analog with activity against human hepatitis B virus (HBV).

The chemical name of adefovir dipivoxil is 9-[2-[bis[(pivaloyloxy)methoxy]phosphinyl]methoxy]ethyl]adenine. It has a molecular formula of $C_{20}H_{32}N_5O_8P$, a molecular weight of 501.48 and the following structural formula:

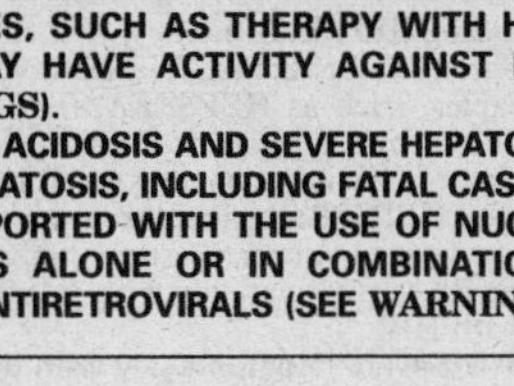

Adefovir dipivoxil is a white to off-white crystalline powder with an aqueous solubility of 19 mg/mL at pH 2.0 and 0.4 mg/mL at pH 7.2. It has an octanol/aqueous phosphate buffer (pH 7) partition coefficient (log p) of 1.91.

HEPSERA tablets are for oral administration. Each tablet contains 10 mg of adefovir dipivoxil and the following inactive ingredients: croscarmellose sodium, lactose monohydrate, magnesium stearate, pregelatinized starch, and talc.

Microbiology

Mechanism of Action:

Adefovir is an acyclic nucleotide analog of adenosine monophosphate. Adefovir is phosphorylated to the active metabolite, adefovir diphosphate, by cellular kinases. Adefovir diphosphate inhibits HBV DNA polymerase (reverse transciptase) by competing with the natural substrate deoxyadenosine triphosphate and by causing DNA chain termination after its incorporation into viral DNA. The inhibition constant (K_i) for adefovir diphosphate for HBV DAN polymerase was 0.1 μM. Adefovir diphosphate is a weak inhibitor of human DNA polymerases α and γ with K_i values of 1.18 μM and 0.97 μM, respectively.

Table 1. Pharmacokinetic Parameters (Mean ± SD) of Adefovir in Patients with Varying Degrees of Renal Function

Renal Function Group	Unimpaired	Mild	Moderate	Severe
Baseline Creatinine Clearance (mL/min)	> 80 (n = 7)	50 – 80 (n = 8)	30 – 49 (n = 7)	10 – 29 (n = 10)
C_{max} (ng/mL)	17.8 ± 3.22	22.4 ± 4.04	28.5 ± 8.57	51.6 ± 10.3
$AUC_{0-\infty}$ (ng•h/mL)	201 ± 40.8	266 ± 55.7	455 ± 176	1240 ± 629
CL/F (mL/min)	469 ± 99.0	356 ± 85.6	237 ± 118	91.7 ± 51.3
CL_{renal} (mL/min)	231 ± 48.9	148 ± 39.3	83.9 ± 27.5	37.0 ± 18.4

Antiviral Activity:

The *in vitro* antiviral activity of adefovir was determined in HBV transfected human hepatoma cell lines. The concentration of adefovir that inhibited 50% of viral DNA synthesis (IC_{50}) varied from 0.2 to 2.5 μM.

Drug Resistance:

Clinical Studies 437 & 438

Genotypic and phenotypic analyses of serum HBV DNA from adefovir dipivoxil (10 mg or 30 mg) treated HBeAg-positive patients (n = 215; study 437) and HBeAg-negative patients (n = 56; study 438) at baseline and week 48 did not identify mutations in the HBV DNA polymerase gene that may confer reduced susceptibility to adefovir. An unconfirmed increase of ≥ 1 $\log_{10}$ copies/mL in serum HBV DNA was observed in some patients. The molecular basis and/or the clinical significance for the observed unconfirmed increases are not known.

Cross-resistance:

Recombinant HBV variants containing lamivudine-resistance-associated mutations (L528M, M552I, M552V, L528M + M552V) in the HBV DNA polymerase gene were susceptible to adefovir *in vitro*. Adefovir has also demonstrated anti-HBV activity (median reduction in serum HBV DNA of 4.3 $\log_{10}$ copies/mL) against clinical isolates of HBV containing lamivudine-resistance-associated mutations (study 435). HBV variants with DNA polymerase mutations T476N and R or W501Q associated with resistance to hepatitis B immunoglobulin were susceptible to adefovir *in vitro*.

CLINICAL PHARMACOLOGY

Pharmacokinetics

The pharmacokinetics of adefovir have been evaluated in healthy volunteers and patients with chronic hepatitis B. Adefovir pharmacokinetics are similar between these populations.

Absorption:

Adefovir dipivoxil is a diester prodrug of the active moiety adefovir. Based on a cross study comparison, the approximate oral bioavailability of adefovir from a 10 mg single dose of HEPSERA is 59%.

Following oral administration of a 10 mg single dose of HEPSERA to chronic hepatitis B patients (n = 14), the peak adefovir plasma concentration (C_{max}) was 18.4 ± 6.26 ng/mL (mean ± SD) and occurred between 0.58 and 4.00 hours (median = 1.75 hours) post dose. The adefovir area under the plasma concentration-time curve ($AUC_{0-\infty}$) was 220 ± 70.0 ng•h/mL. Plasma adefovir concentrations declined in a biexponential manner with a terminal elimination half-life of 7.48 ± 1.65 hours.

The pharmacokinetics of adefovir in subjects with adequate renal function were not affected by once daily dosing of 10 mg HEPSERA over seven days. The impact of long-term once daily administration of 10 mg HEPSERA on adefovir pharmacokinetics has not been evaluated.

Effects of Food on Oral Absorption:

Adefovir exposure was unaffected when a 10 mg single dose of HEPSERA was administered with food (an approximately 1000 kcal high-fat meal). HEPSERA may be taken without regard to food.

Distribution:

In vitro binding of adefovir to human plasma or human serum proteins is ≤ 4% over the adefovir concentration range of 0.1 to 25 μg/mL. The volume of distribution at steady-state following intravenous administration of 1.0 or 3.0 mg/kg/day is 392 ± 75 and 352 ± 9 mL/kg, respectively.

Metabolism and Elimination:

Following oral administration, adefovir dipivoxil is rapidly converted to adefovir. Forty-five percent of the dose is recovered as adefovir in the urine over 24 hours at steady-state following 10 mg oral doses of HEPSERA. Adefovir is renally excreted by a combination of glomerular filtration and active tubular secretion (**See Drug Interactions**).

Special Populations:

Gender

The pharmacokinetics of adefovir were similar in male and female patients.

Race

Insufficient data are available to determine the effect of race on the pharmacokinetics of adefovir.

Pediatric and Geriatric Patients

Pharmacokinetic studies have not been conducted in children or in the elderly.

Renal Impairment

In subjects with moderately or severely impaired renal function or with end-stage renal disease (ESRD) requiring hemodialysis, C_{max}, AUC, and half-life ($T_{1/2}$) were increased compared to subjects with normal renal function. It is recommended that the dosing interval of HEPSERA be modified in these patients (**See DOSAGE AND ADMINISTRATION**).

The pharmacokinetics of adefovir in non-chronic hepatitis B patients with varying degrees of renal impairment are described in Table 1. In this study, subjects received a 10 mg single dose of HEPSERA.

[See table 1 above]

A four-hour period of hemodialysis removed approximately 35% of the adefovir dose. The effect of peritoneal dialysis on adefovir removal has not been evaluated.

Hepatic Impairment

The pharmacokinetics of adefovir following a 10 mg single dose of HEPSERA have been studied in non-chronic hepatitis B patients with hepatic impairment. There were no substantial alterations in adefovir pharmacokinetics in patients with moderate and severe hepatic impairment compared to unimpaired patients. No change in HEPSERA dosing is required in patients with hepatic impairment.

Drug Interactions:

Adefovir dipivoxil is rapidly converted to adefovir *in vivo*. At concentrations substantially higher (> 4000 fold) than those observed *in vivo*, adefovir did not inhibit any of the common human CYP450 enzymes, CYP1A2, CYP2C9, CYP2C19, CYP2D6, and CYP3A4. Adefovir is not a substrate for these enzymes. However, the potential for adefovir to induce CYP450 enzymes is unknown. Based on the results of these *in vitro* experiments and the renal elimination pathway of adefovir, the potential for CYP450 mediated interactions involving adefovir as an inhibitor or substrate with other medicinal products is low.

The pharmacokinetics of adefovir have been evaluated following multiple dose administration of HEPSERA (10 mg once daily) in combination with lamivudine (100 mg once daily), trimethoprim/sulfamethoxazole (160/800 mg twice daily), acetaminophen (1000 mg four times daily) and ibuprofen (800 mg three times daily) in healthy volunteers (n = 18 per study).

Adefovir did not alter the pharmacokinetics of lamivudine, trimethoprim/sulfamethoxazole, acetaminophen and ibuprofen.

The pharmacokinetics of adefovir were unchanged when HEPSERA was co-administered with lamivudine, trimethoprim/sulfamethoxazole and acetaminophen. When HEPSERA was co-administered with ibuprofen (800 mg three times daily) increases in adefovir C_{max} (33%), AUC (23%) and urinary recovery were observed. This increase appears to be due to higher oral bioavailability, not a reduction in renal clearance of adefovir.

INDICATIONS AND USAGE

HEPSERA is indicated for the treatment of chronic hepatitis B in adults with evidence of active viral replication and either evidence of persistent elevations in serum aminotransferases (ALT or AST) or histologically active disease. This indication is based on histological, virological, biochemical, and serological responses in adult patients with HBeAg+ and HBeAg- chronic hepatitis B with compensated liver function, and in adult patients with clinical evidence of lamivudine-resistant hepatitis B virus with either compensated or decompensated liver function.

Description of Clinical Studies

HBeAg-positive Chronic Hepatitis B:

Study 437 was a randomized, double-blind, placebo-controlled, three-arm study in patients with HBeAg-positive chronic hepatitis B that allowed for a comparison between placebo and HEPSERA. The median age of patients was 33 years. Seventy-four percent were male, 59% were Asian, 36% were Caucasian and 24% has prior interferon-α treatment. At baseline, patients had a median total Knodell Histology Activity Index (HAI) score of 10, a median serum HBV DNA level as measured by an experimental polymerase chain reaction assay of 8.36 $\log_{10}$ copies/mL and a median ALT level of 2.3 times the upper limit of normal.

HBeAg-negative (anti-HBe positive/HBV DNA positive) Chronic Hepatitis B:

Study 438 was a randomized, double-blind, placebo-controlled study in patients who were HBeAg-negative at screening, and anti-HBe positive. The median age of patients was 46 years. Eight-three percent were male, 66%

Continued on next page

Hepsera—Cont.

were Caucasian, 30% were Asian and 41% had prior interferon-α treatment. At baseline, the median total Knodell HAI score was 10, the median serum HBV DNA level as measured by an experimental polymerase chain reaction assay was 7.08 $\log_{10}$ copies/mL, and the median ALT was 2.3 times the upper limit of normal.

The primary efficacy endpoint in both studies was histological improvement at week 48; results of which are shown in Table 2.
[See table 2 at right]
Table 3 illustrates the changes in Ishak Fibrosis Score by treatment group.
[See table 3 at right]
At week 48, improvement was seen in respect to mean change in serum HBV DNA ($\log_{10}$ copies/mL), normalization of ALT, and HBeAg seroconversion as compared to placebo in patients receiving HEPSERA (Table 4).
[See table 4 at right]
In studies 437 and 438, continued treatment with HEPSERA to 72 weeks resulted in continued maintenance of mean reductions in serum HBV DNA observed at week 48. An increase in the proportion of patients with ALT normalization was also observed in study 437. The effect of continued treatment with HEPSERA on seroconversion is unknown.

Pre- and Post-Liver Transplantation Patients:
HEPSERA was also evaluated in an open-label, uncontrolled study of 324 chronic hepatitis B patients pre- (n = 128) and post- (n = 196) liver transplantation with clinical evidence of lamivudine-resistant hepatitis B virus (study 435). The median baseline HBV DNA as measured by an experimental polymerase chain reaction assay was 7.4 and 8.2 $\log_{10}$ copies/mL, and the median baseline ALT was 1.8 and 2.1 times the upper limit of normal in pre- and post-liver transplantation patients, respectively. Results of this study are displayed in Table 5. Treatment with HEPSERA resulted in a similar reduction in serum HBV DNA regardless of the patterns of lamivudine-resistant HBV DNA polymerase mutations at baseline. The clinical significance of these findings as they relate to histological improvement is not known.

Table 5. Efficacy in Pre- and Post-Liver Transplantation Patients at Week 48

Efficacy Parameter	Pre-Liver Transplantation	Post-Liver Transplantation
	(n = 128)	(n = 196)
Mean change ± SD in serum HBV DNA from baseline ($\log_{10}$ copies/mL)	-3.8 ± 1.4	-4.1 ± 1.6
Stable or improved Child-Pugh-Turcotte score	92%*	96%
Normalization of:**		
ALT	76%	49%
Albumin	81%	76%
Bilirubin	50%	75%
Prothrombin time	83%	20%

* 24 week data
** Denominator in patients with abnormal values at baseline

Clinical Evidence of Lamivudine Resistance:
In study 461, an ongoing double-blind, active-controlled study in 59 chronic hepatitis B patients with clinical evidence of lamivudine-resistant hepatitis B virus, patients were randomized to receive either HEPSERA monotherapy or HEPSERA in combination with lamivudine 100 mg or lamivudine 100 mg alone. At week 16, the mean ± SD decrease in serum HBV DNA as measured by an experimental polymerase chain reaction assay was 3.11 ± 0.94 $\log_{10}$ copies/mL for patients treated with HEPSERA and 2.95 ± 0.64 $\log_{10}$ copies/mL for patients treated with HEPSERA in combination with lamivudine. There was a mean decrease in serum HBV DNA of 0.00 ± 0.28 $\log_{10}$ copies/mL in patients receiving lamivudine alone. The clinical significance of these observed changes in serum HBV DNA has not yet been established.

CONTRAINDICATIONS
HEPSERA is contraindicated in patients with previously demonstrated hypersensitivity to any of the components of the product.

WARNINGS
Exacerbations of Hepatitis after Discontinuation of Treatment
Severe acute exacerbation of hepatitis has been reported in patients who have discontinued anti-hepatitis B therapy, including therapy with HEPSERA. Patients who discontinue HEPSERA should be monitored at repeated intervals over a period of time for hepatic function. If appropriate, resumption of anti-hepatitis B therapy may be warranted.

Table 2. Histological Response at Week 48*

	Study 437		Study 438	
	HEPSERA 10 mg	Placebo	HEPSERA 10 mg	Placebo
	(n = 168)	(n = 161)	(n = 121)	(n = 57)
Improvement**	53%	25%	64%	35%
No Improvement	37%	67%	29%	63%
Missing/Unassessable Data	10%	7%	7%	2%

* Intent-to-Treat population (patients with ≥ 1 dose of study drug) with assessable baseline biopsies
** Histological improvement defined as ≥ 2 point decrease in the Knodell necro-inflammatory score with no worsening of the Knodell fibrosis score

Table 3. Changes in Ishak Fibrosis Score at Week 48

	Study 437		Study 438	
	HEPSERA 10 mg	Placebo	HEPSERA 10 mg	Placebo
Number of adequate biopsy pairs	(n = 150)	(n = 146)	(n = 112)	(n = 55)
Ishak Fibrosis Score Improved*	34%	19%	34%	14%
Unchanged	55%	60%	62%	50%
Worsened	11%	21%	4%	36%

* Change of 1 point or more in Ishak Fibrosis Score

Table 4. Change in Serum HBV DNA, ALT Normalization, and HBeAg Seroconversion at Week 48

	Study 437		Study 438	
	HEPSERA 10 mg	Placebo	HEPSERA 10 mg	Placebo
	(n = 167)	(n = 171)	(n = 123)	(n = 61)
Mean change ± SD in serum HBV DNA from baseline ($\log_{10}$ copies/mL)	-3.57 ± 1.64	-0.98 ± 1.32	-3.65 ± 1.14	-1.32 ± 1.25
ALT Normalization	48%	16%	72%	29%
HBeAg Seroconversion	12%	6%	NA*	NA*

* Patients with HBeAg-negative disease cannot undergo HBeAg seroconversion

In clinical trials of HEPSERA, exacerbations of hepatitis (ALT elevations 10 times the upper limit of normal or greater) occurred in up to 25% of patients after discontinuation of HEPSERA. Most of these events occurred within 12 weeks of drug discontinuation. These exacerbations generally occurred in the absence of HBeAg seroconversion, and presented as serum ALT elevations in addition to re-emergence of viral replication. In the HBeAg-positive and HBeAg-negative studies in patients with compensated liver function, the exacerbations were not generally accompanied by hepatic decompensation. However, patients with advanced liver disease or cirrhosis may be at higher risk for hepatic decompensation. Although most events appear to have been self-limited or resolved with re-initiation of treatment, severe hepatitis exacerbations, including fatalities, have been reported. Therefore, patients should be closely monitored after stopping treatment.

Nephrotoxicity
Nephrotoxicity characterized by a delayed onset of gradual increases in serum creatinine and decreases in serum phosphorus was historically shown to be the treatment-limiting toxicity of adefovir dipivoxil therapy at substantially higher doses in HIV-infected patients (60 and 120 mg daily) and in chronic hepatitis B patients (30 mg daily). Chronic administration of HEPSERA (10 mg once daily) may result in nephrotoxicity. The overall risk of nephrotoxicity in patients with adequate renal function is low. However, this is of special importance in patients at risk of or having underlying renal dysfunction and patients taking concomitant nephrotoxic agents such as cyclosporine, tacrolimus, aminoglycosides, vancomycin and non-steroidal anti-inflammatory drugs **(See ADVERSE REACTIONS).**

It is important to monitor renal function for all patients during treatment with HEPSERA, particularly for those with pre-existing or other risks for renal impairment. Patients with renal insufficiency at baseline or during treatment may require dose adjustment **(See DOSAGE AND ADMINISTRATION).** The risks and benefits of HEPSERA treatment should be carefully evaluated prior to discontinuing HEPSERA in a patient with treatment-emergent nephrotoxicity.

HIV Resistance
Prior to initiating HEPSERA therapy, HIV antibody testing should be offered to all patients. Treatment with anti-hepatitis B therapies, such as HEPSERA, that have activity against HIV in a chronic hepatitis B patient with unrecognized or untreated HIV infection may result in emergence of HIV resistance. HEPSERA has not been shown to suppress HIV RNA in patients; however, there are limited data on the use of HEPSERA to treat patients with chronic hepatitis B co-infected with HIV.

Lactic Acidosis/Severe Hepatomegaly with Steatosis
Lactic acidosis and severe hepatomegaly with steatosis, including fatal cases, have been reported with the use of nucleoside analogs alone or in combination with antiretrovirals.

A majority of these cases have been in women. Obesity and prolonged nucleoside exposure may be risk factors. Particular caution should be exercised when administering nucleoside analogs to any patient with known risk factors for liver disease; however, cases have also been reported in patients with no known risk factors. Treatment with HEPSERA should be suspended in any patient who develops clinical or laboratory findings suggestive of lactic acidosis or pronounced hepatotoxicity (which may include hepatomegaly and steatosis even in the absence of marked transaminase elevations).

PRECAUTIONS
Drug Interactions
Since adefovir is eliminated by the kidney, co-administration of HEPSERA with drugs that reduce renal function or compete for active tubular secretion may increase serum concentrations of either adefovir and/or these co-administered drugs.

Apart from lamivudine, trimethoprim/sulfamethoxazole and acetaminophen, the effects of co-administration of HEPSERA with drugs that are excreted renally, or other drugs known to affect renal function have not been evaluated **(See CLINICAL PHARMACOLOGY).**

Patients should be monitored closely for adverse events when HEPSERA is co-administered with drugs that are excreted renally or with other drugs known to affect renal function.

Ibuprofen 800 mg three times daily increased adefovir exposure by approximately 23%. The clinical significance of this increase in adefovir exposure is unknown **(See CLINICAL PHARMACOLOGY).**

While adefovir does not inhibit common CYP450 enzymes, the potential for adefovir to induce CYP450 enzymes is not known.

The effect of adefovir on cyclosporine and tacrolimus concentrations is not known.

Duration of Treatment
The optimal duration of HEPSERA treatment and the relationship between treatment response and long-term outcomes such as hepatocellular carcinoma or decompensated cirrhosis are not known.

Animal Toxicology
Renal tubular nephropathy characterized by histological alterations and/or increases in BUN and serum creatinine was the primary dose-limiting toxicity associated with administration of adefovir dipivoxil in animals. Nephrotoxicity was observed in animals at systemic exposures approximately 3–10 times higher than those in humans at the recommended therapeutic dose of 10 mg/day.

Carcinogenesis, Mutagenesis, Impairment of Fertility
Carcinogenicity studies in mice and rats receiving adefovir have been conducted. In mice, at dose levels of 1, 3, or 10 mg/kg/day, no treatment-related increases in tumor incidence were found at 10 mg/kg/day (systemic exposure was 10 times that achieved in humans at a therapeutic dose of 10 mg/day). In rats dosed at levels of 0.5, 1.5, or 5 mg/kg/day, no drug-related increase in tumor incidence was observed. The exposure at the high dose was four times that at the human therapeutic dose. Adefovir dipivoxil was mutagenic in the in vitro mouse lymphoma cell assay (with or without metabolic activation). Adefovir induced chromosomal aberrations in the in vitro human peripheral blood lymphocyte assay without metabolic activation. Adefovir was not clastogenic in the in vivo mouse micronucleus assay at doses up to 2,000 mg/kg and it was not mutagenic in the Ames bacterial reverse mutation assay using S. typhimurium and E. coli strains in the presence and absence of metabolic activation. In reproductive toxicology studies, no evidence of impaired fertility was seen in male or female rats at doses up to 30 mg/kg/day (systemic exposure 19 times that achieved in humans at the therapeutic dose).

Pregnancy
Pregnancy Category C:
Reproduction studies conducted with adefovir dipivoxil administered orally have shown no embryotoxicity or teratogenicity in rats at doses up to 35 mg/kg/day (systemic exposure approximately 23 times that achieved in humans at the therapeutic dose of 10 mg/day), or in rabbits at 20 mg/kg/day (systemic exposure 40 times human).

When adefovir was administered intravenously to pregnant rats at doses associated with notable maternal toxicity (20 mg/kg/day, systemic exposure 38 times human), embryotoxicity and an increased incidence of fetal malformations (anasarca, depressed eye bulge, umbilical hernia and kinked tail) were observed. No adverse effects on development were seen with adefovir administered intravenously to pregnant rats at 2.5 mg/kg/day (systemic exposure 12 times human).

There are no adequate and well-controlled studies in pregnant women. Because animal reproduction studies are not always predictive of human response, HEPSERA should be used during pregnancy only if clearly needed and after careful consideration of the risks and benefits.

Pregnancy Registry
To monitor fetal outcomes of pregnant women exposed to HEPSERA, a pregnancy registry has been established. Healthcare providers are encouraged to register patients by calling 1-800-258-4263.

Labor and Delivery
There are no studies in pregnant women and no data on the effect of HEPSERA on transmission of HBV from mother to infant. Therefore, appropriate infant immunizations should be used to prevent neonatal acquisition of hepatitis B virus.

Lactating Women
It is not known whether adefovir is excreted in human milk. Mothers should be instructed not to breast-feed if they are taking HEPSERA.

Pediatric Use
Safety and effectiveness in pediatric patients have not been established.

Geriatric Use
Clinical studies of HEPSERA did not include sufficient numbers of patients aged 65 and over to determine whether they respond differently from younger patients. In general, caution should be exercised when prescribing to elderly patients since they have greater frequency of decreased renal or cardiac function due to concomitant disease or other drug therapy.

ADVERSE REACTIONS
Assessment of adverse reactions is based on two studies (437 and 438) in which 522 patients with chronic hepatitis B received double-blind treatment with HEPSERA (n = 294) or placebo (n = 228) for 48 weeks. With extended therapy in the second 48 week treatment period, 492 patients were treated for up to 109 weeks, with a median time on treatment of 49 weeks.

In addition to specific adverse events described under the WARNINGS section, all treatment-related clinical adverse events that occurred in 3% or greater of HEPSERA-treated patients compared with placebo are listed in Table 6. A summary of grade 3 and 4 laboratory abnormalities during therapy with HEPSERA compared with placebo is listed in Table 7.

Table 8. Dosing Interval Adjustment of HEPSERA in Patients with Renal Impairment

	Creatinine Clearance (mL/min)*			
	≥ 50	20–49	10–19	Hemodialysis Patients
Recommended Dose and Dosing Interval	10 mg every 24 hours	10 mg every 48 hours	10 mg every 72 hours	10 mg every 7 days following dialysis

* Creatinine clearance calculated by Cockcroft-Gault method using lean or ideal body weight

Table 6. Treatment-Related Adverse Events (Grades 1–4) Reported in ≥ 3% of All HEPSERA-Treated Patients in the Pooled 437 – 438 Studies (0–48 Weeks)

	HEPSERA 10 mg	Placebo
	(n = 294)	(n = 228)
Asthenia	13%	14%
Headache	9%	10%
Abdominal pain	9%	11%
Nausea	5%	8%
Flatulence	4%	4%
Diarrhea	3%	4%
Dyspepsia	3%	2%

Laboratory Abnormalities

Table 7. Grade 3–4 Laboratory Abnormalities Reported in ≥ 1% of All HEPSERA-Treated Patients in the Pooled 437 – 438 Studies (0–48 Weeks)

	HEPSERA 10 mg	Placebo
	(n = 294)	(n = 228)
ALT (> 5 × ULN)	20%	41%
Hematuria (≥ 3+)	11%	10%
AST (> 5 × ULN)	8%	23%
Creatine Kinase (> 4 × ULN)	7%	7%
Amylase (> 2 × ULN)	4%	4%
Glycosuria (≥ 3+)	1%	3%

In patients with adequate renal function, increases in serum creatinine ≥ 0.3 mg/dL from baseline were observed in 4% of patients treated with HEPSERA 10 mg daily compared with 2% of patients in the placebo group by week 48. No patients developed a serum creatinine increase ≥ 0.5 mg/dL from baseline by week 48. By week 96, 10% and 2% of HEPSERA-treated patients, by Kaplan-Meier estimate, had increases in serum creatinine ≥ 0.3 mg/dL and ≥ 0.5 mg/dL from baseline, respectively (no placebo-controlled results were available for comparison beyond week 48). Of the 29 of 492 patients with elevations in serum creatinine ≥ 0.3 mg/dL from baseline, 20 out of 29 resolved on continued treatment (≤ 0.2 mg/dL from baseline), 8 of 29 remained unchanged and 1 of 29 resolved on discontinuing treatment **(See Special Risk Patients section below for changes in serum creatinine in patients with underlying renal insufficiency at baseline).**

Special Risk Patients
Pre- (n = 128) and post-liver transplantation patients (n = 196) with chronic hepatitis B and clinical evidence of lamivudine-resistant hepatitis B virus were treated in an open-label study with HEPSERA for up to 129 weeks, with a median time on treatment of 19 and 56 weeks, respectively. The majority of these patients had some degree of underlying renal insufficiency at baseline or other risk factors for renal dysfunction during treatment. Increases in serum creatinine ≥ 0.3 mg/dL from baseline were observed in 26% of these patients by week 48 and 37% by week 96 by Kaplan-Meier estimates. Increases in serum creatinine ≥ 0.5 mg/dL from baseline were observed in 16% of these patients by week 48 and 31% by week 96. Of the 41 of 324 patients with elevations in serum creatinine ≥ 0.5 mg/dL from baseline, 7 of 41 resolved on continued treatment (≤ 0.3 mg/dL from baseline), 18 of 41 remained unchanged and 16 of 41 had not resolved. Additionally, decreases in serum phosphorus were observed in 4% of these patients by week 48, and 6% by week 96 by Kaplan-Meier estimates. One percent (3 of 324) of pre- and post-liver transplantation patients discontinued HEPSERA due to renal events.

Due to the presence of multiple concomitant risk factors for renal dysfunction in these patients, the contributory role of HEPSERA to these changes in serum creatinine and serum phosphorus is difficult to assess.

The most common treatment-related adverse events reported in pre- and post-liver transplantation patients treated with HEPSERA with a 2% frequency or higher include:

Body as a whole: asthenia, abdominal pain, headache, fever
Gastrointestinal: nausea, vomiting, diarrhea, flatulence, hepatic failure
Metabolic and Nutritional: increases in ALT and AST, abnormal liver function
Respiratory: increased cough, pharyngitis, sinusitis
Skin and Appendages: pruritus, rash
Urogenital: increases in creatinine, renal failure, renal insufficiency

OVERDOSAGE
Doses of adefovir dipivoxil 500 mg daily for 2 weeks and 250 mg daily for 12 weeks have been associated with gastrointestinal side effects. If overdose occurs the patient must be monitored for evidence of toxicity, and standard supportive treatment applied as necessary.

Following a 10 mg single dose of HEPSERA, a four-hour hemodialysis session removed approximately 35% of the adefovir dose.

DOSAGE AND ADMINISTRATION
The recommended dose of HEPSERA in chronic hepatitis B patients with adequate renal function is 10 mg, once daily, taken orally, without regard to food. The optimal duration of treatment is unknown.

Dose Adjustment in Renal Impairment
Significantly increased drug exposures were seen when HEPSERA was administered to patients with renal impairment **(See Pharmacokinetics).** Therefore, the dosing interval of HEPSERA should be adjusted in patients with baseline creatinine clearance < 50 mL/min using the following suggested guidelines (See Table 8). The safety and effectiveness of these dosing interval adjustment guidelines have not been clinically evaluated. Additionally, it is important to note that these guidelines were derived from data in patients with pre-existing renal impairment at baseline. They may not be appropriate for patients in whom renal insufficiency evolves during treatment with HEPSERA. Therefore, clinical response to treatment and renal function should be closely monitored in these patients.

[See table 8 above]

The pharmacokinetics of adefovir have not been evaluated in non-hemodialysis patients with creatinine clearance < 10 mL/min; therefore, no dosing recommendation is available for these patients.

HOW SUPPLIED
HEPSERA is available as tablets. Each tablet contains 10 mg of adefovir dipivoxil. The tablets are white and debossed with "10" and "GILEAD" on one side and the stylized figure of a liver on the other side. They are packaged as follows: Bottles of 30 tablets (NDC 61958-0501-1) containing desiccant (silica gel) and closed with a child-resistant closure.

Store in original container at 25 °C (77 °F), excursions permitted to 15–30 °C (59–86 °F) (See USP Controlled Room Temperature).

Gilead Sciences, Inc.
Foster City, CA 94404
September 2002
HEPSERA™ is a trademark of Gilead Sciences
©2002 Gilead Sciences, Inc.
GILEAD

In the PDR annual,
the **Brand and Generic Name Index**
(PINK section)
alphabetizes drugs under both
brand and generic names.

GlaxoSmithKline
FIVE MOORE DRIVE
RESEARCH TRIANGLE PARK, NC 27709

For Medical Emergencies, Medical Information for Healthcare Professionals, and Consumer Inquiries, Contact:
1-888-825-5249
www.druginfo.gsk.com

AUGMENTIN XR™ ℞

[ăg-mint'in]
amoxicillin/clavulanate potassium
Extended Release Tablets

DESCRIPTION

Augmentin XR is an oral antibacterial combination consisting of the semisynthetic antibiotic amoxicillin (present as amoxicillin trihydrate and amoxicillin sodium) and the β-lactamase inhibitor, clavulanate potassium (the potassium salt of clavulanic acid). Amoxicillin is an analog of ampicillin, derived from the basic penicillin nucleus, 6-aminopenicillanic acid. The amoxicillin trihydrate molecular formula is $C_{16}H_{19}N_3O_5S \bullet 3H_2O$ and the molecular weight is 419.45. Chemically, amoxicillin trihydrate is (2*S*,5*R*,6*R*)-6-[(*R*)-(-)-2-Amino-2-(*p*-hydroxyphenyl)acetamido]-3,3-dimethyl-7-oxo-4-thia-1-azabicyclo[3.2.0]heptane-2-carboxylic acid trihydrate and may be represented structurally as:

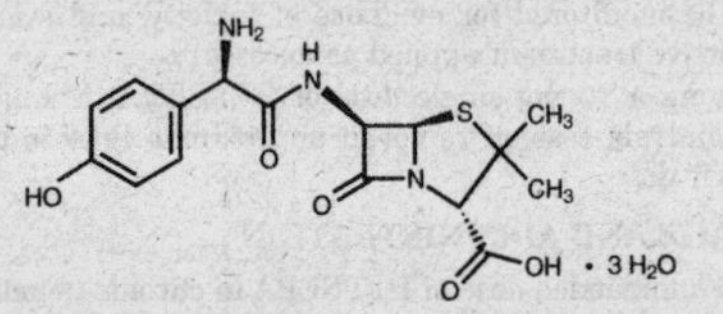

The amoxicillin sodium molecular formula is $C_{16}H_{18}N_3NaO_5S$ and the molecular weight is 387.39. Chemically, amoxicillin sodium is [2*S*-[2α,5α,6β(*S**)]]-6-[[Amino(4-hydroxyphenyl)acetyl]amino]-3,3-dimethyl-7-oxo-4-thia-1-azabicyclo[3.2.0]heptane-2-carboxylic acid monosodium salt and may be represented structurally as:

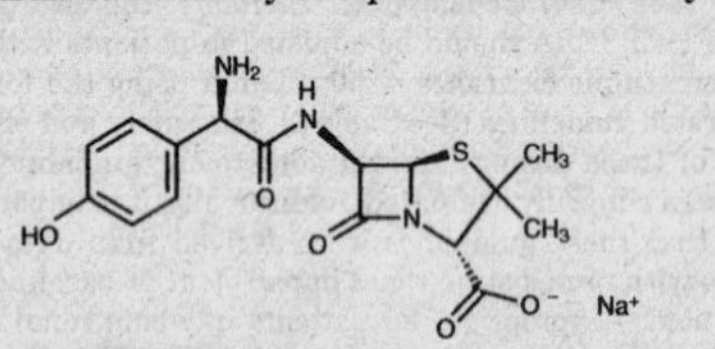

Clavulanic acid is produced by the fermentation of *Streptomyces clavuligerus*. It is a β-lactam structurally related to the penicillins and possesses the ability to inactivate a wide variety of β-lactamases by blocking the active sites of these enzymes. Clavulanic acid is particularly active against the clinically important plasmid mediated β-lactamases frequently responsible for transferred drug resistance to penicillins and cephalosporins. The clavulanate potassium molecular formula is $C_8H_8KNO_5$ and the molecular weight is 237.25. Chemically, clavulanate potassium is potassium (*Z*)-(2*R*, 5*R*)-3-(2-hydroxyethylidene)-7-oxo-4-oxa-1-azabicyclo[3.2.0]-heptane-2-carboxylate, and may be represented structurally as:

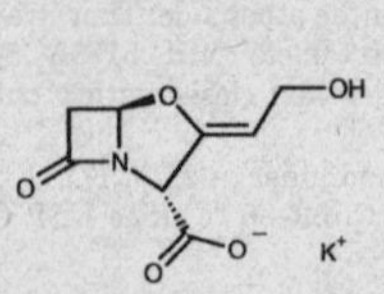

Inactive Ingredients: Citric acid, colloidal silicon dioxide, hypromellose, magnesium stearate, microcrystalline cellulose, polyethylene glycol, sodium starch glycolate, titanium dioxide, xanthan gum.

Each Augmentin XR (amoxicillin/clavulanate potassium) tablet contains 12.6 mg (0.32 mEq) of potassium and 29.3 mg (1.27 mEq) of sodium.

CLINICAL PHARMACOLOGY

Amoxicillin and clavulanate potassium are well absorbed from the gastrointestinal tract after oral administration of *Augmentin XR*.

Augmentin XR is an extended-release formulation which provides sustained plasma concentrations of amoxicillin. Amoxicillin systemic exposure achieved with *Augmentin XR* is similar to that produced by the oral administration of equivalent doses of amoxicillin alone. In a study of healthy adult volunteers, the pharmacokinetics of *Augmentin XR* were compared when administered in a fasted state, at the start of a standardized meal (612 kcal, 89.3 g carb, 24.9 g fat, 14.0 g protein), or 30 minutes after a high-fat meal. When the systemic exposure to both amoxicillin and clavulanate is taken into consideration, *Augmentin XR* is optimally administered at the start of a standardized meal. Absorption of amoxicillin is decreased in the fasted state. *Augmentin XR* is not recommended to be taken with a high-fat meal, because clavulanate absorption is decreased. The pharmacokinetics of the components of *Augmentin XR* following administration of two *Augmentin XR* tablets at the start of a standardized meal are presented below.

Mean (SD) Pharmacokinetic Parameters for Amoxicillin and Clavulanate Following Oral Administration of Two *Augmentin XR* Tablets (2000/125 mg) to Healthy Adult Volunteers [n = 55] Fed a Standardized Meal

Parameter (units)	Amoxicillin	Clavulanate
AUC (0-inf) (µg.h/mL)	71.6 (16.5)	5.29 (1.55)
C_{max} (µg/mL)	17.0 (4.0)	2.05 (0.80)
T_{max} (hours)†	1.50 (1.00–6.00)	1.03 (0.75–3.00)
$T_{1/2}$ (hours)	1.27 (0.20)	1.03 (0.17)

† median (range).

The half-life of amoxicillin after the oral administration of *Augmentin XR* is approximately 1.3 hours, and that of clavulanate is approximately 1.0 hour.

Clearance of amoxicillin is predominantly renal, with approximately 60% to 80% of the dose being excreted unchanged in urine, whereas clearance of clavulanate has both a renal (30% to 50%) and a non-renal component.

Concurrent administration of probenecid delays amoxicillin excretion but does not delay renal excretion of clavulanate.

In a study of adults, the pharmacokinetics of amoxicillin and clavulanate were not affected by administration of an antacid (Maalox®), either simultaneously with or two hours after Augmentin XR (amoxicillin/clavulanate potassium).

Neither component in *Augmentin XR* is highly protein-bound; clavulanate has been found to be approximately 25% bound to human serum and amoxicillin approximately 18% bound.

Amoxicillin diffuses readily into most body tissues and fluids with the exception of the brain and spinal fluid. The results of experiments involving the administration of clavulanic acid to animals suggest that this compound, like amoxicillin, is well distributed in body tissues.

Microbiology

Amoxicillin is a semisynthetic antibiotic with a broad spectrum of bactericidal activity against many gram-positive and gram-negative microorganisms. Amoxicillin is, however, susceptible to degradation by β-lactamases, and therefore, the spectrum of activity does not include organisms which produce these enzymes. Clavulanic acid is a β-lactam, structurally related to the penicillins, which possesses the ability to inactivate a wide range of β-lactamase enzymes commonly found in microorganisms resistant to penicillins and cephalosporins. In particular, it has good activity against the clinically important plasmid mediated β-lactamases frequently responsible for transferred drug resistance.

The clavulanic acid component in *Augmentin XR* protects amoxicillin from degradation by β-lactamase enzymes and effectively extends the antibiotic spectrum of amoxicillin to include many bacteria normally resistant to amoxicillin and other β-lactam antibiotics.

Amoxicillin/clavulanic acid has been shown to be active against most strains of the following microorganisms, both *in vitro* and in clinical infections as described in the INDICATIONS AND USAGE section.

Aerobic Gram-positive Microorganisms

Streptococcus pneumoniae (including isolates with penicillin MICs ≤2 µg/mL)

Staphylococcus aureus (including β-lactamase producing strains)

NOTE: Staphylococci which are resistant to methicillin/oxacillin must be considered resistant to amoxicillin/clavulanic acid.

Aerobic Gram-negative Microorganisms

Haemophilus influenzae (including β-lactamase producing strains)

Moraxella catarrhalis (including β-lactamase producing strains)

Haemophilus parainfluenzae (including β-lactamase producing strains)

Klebsiella pneumoniae (all known strains are β-lactamase producing)

The following *in vitro* data are available, **but their clinical significance is unknown.**

Amoxicillin/clavulanic acid exhibits *in vitro* minimal inhibitory concentrations (MICs) of 2.0 µg/mL or less against most (≥90%) strains of *Streptococcus pyogenes* and MICs of 4.0 µg/mL or less against most (≥90%) strains of the anaerobic bacteria listed below.

Aerobic Gram-positive Microorganisms

Streptococcus pyogenes

Anaerobic Microorganisms

Bacteroides fragilis (including β-lactamase producing strains)

Fusobacterium nucleatum (including β-lactamase producing strains)

Peptostreptococcus magnus

Peptostreptococcus micros

NOTE: *S. pyogenes*, *P. magnus* and *P. micros* do not produce β-lactamase, and therefore, are susceptible to amoxicillin alone. Adequate and well-controlled clinical trials have established the effectiveness of amoxicillin alone in treating certain clinical infections due to *S. pyogenes*.

Susceptibility Testing

Dilution Techniques: Quantitative methods are used to determine antimicrobial minimum inhibitory concentrations (MICs). These MICs provide estimates of the susceptibility of bacteria to antimicrobial compounds. The MICs should be determined using a standardized procedure.[1,2] Standardized procedures are based on a dilution method (broth or agar; broth for *S. pneumoniae* and *Haemophilus* species) or equivalent with standardized inoculum concentrations and standardized concentrations of amoxicillin/clavulanate potassium powder.

The recommended dilution pattern utilizes a constant amoxicillin/clavulanate potassium ratio of 2 to 1 in all tubes with varying amounts of amoxicillin. MICs are expressed in terms of the amoxicillin concentration in the presence of clavulanic acid at a constant 2 parts amoxicillin to 1 part clavulanic acid.

The MIC values should be interpreted according to the following criteria:

For testing *Klebsiella pneumoniae*:

MIC (µg/mL)	Interpretation
≤8/4	Susceptible (S)
16/8	Intermediate (I)
≥32/16	Resistant (R)

For testing *Streptococcus pneumoniae*[a]:

MIC (µg/mL)	Interpretation
≤2/1	Susceptible (S)
4/2	Intermediate (I)
≥8/4	Resistant (R)

[a] These interpretive standards are applicable only to broth microdilution susceptibility tests using cation-adjusted Mueller-Hinton broth with 2–5% lysed horse blood.[2]

For testing *Staphylococcus* species and *Haemophilus* species[b]:

MIC (µg/mL)	Interpretation
≤4/2	Susceptible (S)
≥8/4	Resistant (R)

[b] These interpretive standards are applicable only to broth microdilution susceptibility tests with *Haemophilus* spp. using *Haemophilus* Test Medium (HTM).[2]

NOTE: Staphylococci which are resistant to methicillin/oxacillin must be considered resistant to amoxicillin/clavulanic acid.

A report of "Susceptible" indicates that the pathogen is likely to be inhibited if the antimicrobial compound in the blood reaches the concentration usually achievable. A report of "Intermediate" indicates that the result should be considered equivocal, and if the microorganism is not fully susceptible to alternative, clinically feasible drugs, the test should be repeated. This category implies possible clinical applicability in body sites where the drug is physiologically concentrated or in situations where high dosage of drug can be used. This category also provides a buffer zone which prevents small uncontrolled technical factors from causing major discrepancies in interpretation. A report of "Resistant" indicates that the pathogen is not likely to be inhibited if the antimicrobial compound in the blood reaches the concentrations usually achievable; other therapy should be selected.

Standardized susceptibility test procedures require the use of laboratory control microorganisms to control the technical aspects of the laboratory procedures. Standard amoxicillin/clavulanate potassium powder should provide the following MIC values:

Microorganism	MIC Range (µg/mL)[c]
Escherichia coli ATCC 35218	4 to 16
Escherichia coli ATCC 25922	2 to 8
Haemophilus influenzae[d] ATCC 49247	2 to 16
Staphylococcus aureus ATCC 29213	0.12 to 0.5
Streptococcus pneumoniae[e] ATCC 49619	0.03 to 0.12

[c] Expressed as concentration of amoxicillin in the presence of clavulanic acid at a constant 2 parts amoxicillin to 1 part clavulanic acid.

[d] This quality control range is applicable to *H. influenzae* ATCC 49247 tested by a broth microdilution procedure using HTM.[2]

[e] This quality control range is applicable to *S. pneumoniae* ATCC 49619 tested by a broth microdilution procedure using cation-adjusted Mueller-Hinton broth with 2–5% lysed horse blood.[2]

Diffusion Techniques: Quantitative methods that require measurement of zone diameters also provide reproducible estimates of the susceptibility of bacteria to antimicrobial compounds. One such standardized procedure[3] requires the use of standardized inoculum concentrations. This procedure uses paper disks impregnated with 30 µg of amoxicillin/clavulanate potassium (20 µg amoxicillin plus 10 µg clavulanate potassium) to test the susceptibility of microorganisms to amoxicillin/clavulanic acid.

Reports from the laboratory providing results of the standard single-disk susceptibility test with a 30 µg amoxicillin/clavulanate potassium (20 µg amoxicillin plus 10 µg clavulanate potassium) disk should be interpreted according to the following criteria:

For testing *Klebsiella pneumoniae*:

Zone Diameter (mm)	Interpretation
≥18	Susceptible (S)
14–17	Intermediate (I)
≤13	Resistant (R)

For testing *Staphylococcus* and *Haemophilus*[f] species:

Zone Diameter (mm)	Interpretation
≥20	Susceptible (S)
≤19	Resistant (R)

[f] These zone diameter standards are applicable only to tests conducted with *Haemophilus* spp. using HTM.[2]

NOTE: Staphylococci which are resistant to methicillin/oxacillin must be considered resistant to amoxicillin/clavulanic acid.

NOTE: Beta-lactamase negative, ampicillin-resistant *H. influenzae* strains must be considered resistant to amoxicillin/clavulanic acid.

For testing *Streptococcus pneumoniae:*

Susceptibility of *S. pneumoniae* should be determined using a 1 µg oxacillin disk. Isolates with oxacillin zone sizes of ≥20 mm are susceptible to amoxicillin/clavulanic acid.[g] An amoxicillin/clavulanic acid MIC should be determined on isolates of *S. pneumoniae* with oxacillin zone sizes of ≤19 mm.

[g] These zone diameter standards for *S. pneumoniae* apply only to tests performed using Mueller-Hinton agar supplemented with 5% sheep blood incubated in 5% CO_2.[2]

Interpretation should be as stated above for results using dilution techniques. Interpretation involves correlation of the diameter obtained in the disk test with the MIC for amoxicillin/clavulanic acid.

As with standardized dilution techniques, diffusion methods require the use of laboratory control microorganisms that are used to control the technical aspects of the laboratory procedures. For the diffusion technique, the 30 µg amoxicillin/clavulanate potassium (20 µg amoxicillin plus 10 µg clavulanate potassium) disk should provide the following zone diameters in these laboratory quality control strains:

Microorganism	Zone Diameter (mm)
Escherichia coli ATCC 35218	17 to 22
Escherichia coli ATCC 25922	18 to 24
Staphylococcus aureus ATCC 25923	28 to 36
Haemophilus influenzae[h] ATCC 49247	15 to 23

[h] This quality control limit applies only to tests conducted with *H. influenzae* ATCC 49247 using HTM.[2]

INDICATIONS AND USAGE

Augmentin XR Extended Release Tablets are indicated for the treatment of patients with community-acquired pneumonia or acute bacterial sinusitis due to confirmed, or suspected β-lactamase producing pathogens (i.e., *H. influenzae, M. catarrhalis, H. parainfluenzae, K. pneumoniae*, or methicillin-susceptible *S. aureus*) and *S. pneumoniae* with reduced susceptibility to penicillin (i.e., penicillin MICs = 2 µg/mL). *Augmentin XR* is not indicated for the treatment of infections due to *S. pneumoniae* with penicillin MICs ≥4 µg/mL. Data are limited with regard to infections due to *S. pneumoniae* with penicillin MICs ≥4 µg/mL (see CLINICAL STUDIES section).

Of the common epidemiological risk factors for patients with resistant pneumococcal infections, only age >65 years was studied. Patients with other common risk factors for resistant pneumococcal infections (e.g., alcoholism, immune-suppressive illness, and presence of multiple co-morbid conditions) were not studied.

In patients with community-acquired pneumonia in whom penicillin-resistant *S. pneumoniae* is suspected, bacteriological studies should be performed to determine the causative organisms and their susceptibility when *Augmentin XR* is prescribed. Once the results are known, therapy should be adjusted appropriately.

Acute bacterial sinusitis or community-acquired pneumonia due to a penicillin-susceptible strain of *S. pneumoniae* plus a β-lactamase producing pathogen can be treated with another *Augmentin* product containing lower daily doses of amoxicillin (i.e., 500 mg q8h or 875 mg q12h). Acute bacterial sinusitis or community-acquired pneumonia due to *S. pneumoniae* alone can be treated with amoxicillin.

CONTRAINDICATIONS

Augmentin XR is contraindicated in patients with a history of allergic reactions to any penicillin. It is also contraindicated in patients with a previous history of cholestatic jaundice/hepatic dysfunction associated with treatment with amoxicillin/clavulanate.

Augmentin XR (amoxicillin/clavulanate potassium) is contraindicated in patients with severe renal impairment (creatinine clearance <30 mL/minute) and in hemodialysis patients.

WARNINGS

SERIOUS AND OCCASIONALLY FATAL HYPERSENSITIVITY (ANAPHYLACTIC) REACTIONS HAVE BEEN REPORTED IN PATIENTS ON PENICILLIN THERAPY. THESE REACTIONS ARE MORE LIKELY TO OCCUR IN INDIVIDUALS WITH A HISTORY OF PENICILLIN HYPERSENSITIVITY AND/OR A HISTORY OF SENSITIVITY TO MULTIPLE ALLERGENS. THERE HAVE BEEN REPORTS OF INDIVIDUALS WITH A HISTORY OF PENICILLIN HYPERSENSITIVITY WHO HAVE EXPERIENCED SEVERE REACTIONS WHEN TREATED WITH CEPHALOSPORINS. BEFORE INITIATING THERAPY WITH *AUGMENTIN XR*, CAREFUL INQUIRY SHOULD BE MADE CONCERNING PREVIOUS HYPERSENSITIVITY REACTIONS TO PENICILLINS, CEPHALOSPORINS OR OTHER ALLERGENS. IF AN ALLERGIC REACTION OCCURS, *AUGMENTIN XR* SHOULD BE DISCONTINUED AND THE APPROPRIATE THERAPY INSTITUTED. **SERIOUS ANAPHYLACTIC REACTIONS REQUIRE IMMEDIATE EMERGENCY TREATMENT WITH EPINEPHRINE. OXYGEN, INTRAVENOUS STEROIDS AND AIRWAY MANAGEMENT, INCLUDING INTUBATION, SHOULD ALSO BE ADMINISTERED AS INDICATED.**

Pseudomembranous colitis has been reported with nearly all antibacterial agents, including amoxicillin/clavulanate potassium, and has ranged in severity from mild to life-threatening. Therefore, it is important to consider this diagnosis in patients who present with diarrhea subsequent to the administration of antibacterial agents.

Treatment with antibacterial agents alters the normal flora of the colon and may permit overgrowth of clostridia. Studies indicate that a toxin produced by *Clostridium difficile* is one primary cause of "antibiotic associated colitis."

After the diagnosis of pseudomembranous colitis has been established, appropriate therapeutic measures should be initiated. Mild cases of pseudomembranous colitis usually respond to drug discontinuation alone. In moderate to severe cases, consideration should be given to management with fluids and electrolytes, protein supplementation and treatment with an antibacterial drug clinically effective against *Clostridium difficile* colitis.

Augmentin XR should be used with caution in patients with evidence of hepatic dysfunction. Hepatic toxicity associated with the use of amoxicillin/clavulanate potassium is usually reversible. On rare occasions, deaths have been reported (less than 1 death reported per estimated 4 million prescriptions worldwide). These have generally been cases associated with serious underlying diseases or concomitant medications (see CONTRAINDICATIONS and ADVERSE REACTIONS–Liver).

PRECAUTIONS

General: While amoxicillin/clavulanate possesses the characteristic low toxicity of the penicillin group of antibiotics, periodic assessment of organ system functions, including renal, hepatic and hematopoietic function, is advisable if therapy is for longer than the drug is approved for administration.

A high percentage of patients with mononucleosis who receive ampicillin develop an erythematous skin rash. Thus, ampicillin class antibiotics should not be administered to patients with mononucleosis.

The possibility of superinfections with mycotic or bacterial pathogens should be kept in mind during therapy. If superinfections occur (usually involving *Pseudomonas* or *Candida*), the drug should be discontinued and/or appropriate therapy instituted.

Information for Patients: *Augmentin XR* should be taken every 12 hours with a meal or snack to reduce the possibility of gastrointestinal upset. If diarrhea develops and is severe or lasts more than 2 or 3 days, call your doctor. The entire prescribed course of treatment should be completed, even if you begin to feel better after a few days. Discard any unused medicine.

Drug Interactions: Probenecid decreases the renal tubular secretion of amoxicillin. Concurrent use with *Augmentin XR* may result in increased and prolonged blood levels of amoxicillin. Co-administration of probenecid cannot be recommended.

The concurrent administration of allopurinol and ampicillin increases substantially the incidence of rashes in patients receiving both drugs as compared to patients receiving ampicillin alone. It is not known whether this potentiation of ampicillin rashes is due to allopurinol or the hyperuricemia present in these patients. In *Augmentin XR* controlled clinical trials, 22 patients received concomitant allopurinol and *Augmentin XR*. No rashes were reported in these patients. However, this sample size is too small to allow for any conclusions to be drawn regarding the risk of rashes with concomitant *Augmentin XR* and allupurinol use.

In common with other broad-spectrum antibiotics, Augmentin XR (amoxicillin/clavulanate potassium) may reduce the efficacy of oral contraceptives.

Drug/Laboratory Test Interactions: Oral administration of *Augmentin XR* will result in high urine concentrations of amoxicillin. High urine concentrations of ampicillin may result in false-positive reactions when testing for the presence of glucose in urine using Clinitest®, Benedict's Solution or Fehling's Solution. Since this effect may also occur with amoxicillin and therefore *Augmentin XR*, it is recommended that glucose tests based on enzymatic glucose oxidase reactions (such as Clinistix®) be used.

Following administration of ampicillin to pregnant women, a transient decrease in plasma concentration of total conjugated estriol, estriol-glucuronide, conjugated estrone and estradiol has been noted. This effect may also occur with amoxicillin and therefore *Augmentin XR*.

Carcinogenesis, Mutagenesis, Impairment of Fertility: Long-term studies in animals have not been performed to evaluate carcinogenic potential. The mutagenic potential of *Augmentin* was investigated *in vitro* with an Ames test, a human lymphocyte cytogenetic assay, a yeast test and a mouse lymphoma forward mutation assay, and *in vivo* with mouse micronucleus tests and a dominant lethal test. All were negative apart from the *in vitro* mouse lymphoma assay where weak activity was found at very high, cytotoxic concentrations. *Augmentin* at oral doses of up to 1200 mg/kg/day (1.9 times the maximum human dose of amoxicillin and 15 times the maximum human dose of clavulanate based on body surface area) was found to have no effect on fertility and reproductive performance in rats dosed with a 2:1 ratio formulation of amoxicillin:clavulanate.

Teratogenic effects. Pregnancy (Category B): Reproduction studies performed in pregnant rats and mice given *Augmentin* at oral doses up to 1200 mg/kg/day revealed no evidence of harm to the fetus due to *Augmentin*. In terms of body surface area, the doses in rats were 1.6 times the maximum human oral dose of amoxicillin and 13 times the maximum human dose for clavulanate. For mice, these doses were 0.9 and 7.4 times the maximum human oral dose of amoxicillin and clavulanate, respectively. There are, however, no adequate and well-controlled studies in pregnant women. Because animal reproduction studies are not always predictive of human response, this drug should be used during pregnancy only if clearly needed.

Labor and Delivery: Oral ampicillin class antibiotics are generally poorly absorbed during labor. Studies in guinea pigs have shown that intravenous administration of ampicillin decreased the uterine tone, frequency of contractions, height of contractions and duration of contractions. However, it is not known whether the use of *Augmentin XR* in humans during labor or delivery has immediate or delayed adverse effects on the fetus, prolongs the duration of labor, or increases the likelihood that forceps delivery or other obstetrical intervention or resuscitation of the newborn will be necessary. In a single study in women with premature rupture of fetal membranes, it was reported that prophylactic treatment with *Augmentin* may be associated with an increased risk of necrotizing enterocolitis in neonates.

Nursing Mothers: Ampicillin class antibiotics are excreted in the milk; therefore, caution should be exercised when Augmentin XR (amoxicillin/clavulanate potassium) is administered to a nursing woman.

Pediatric Use: Safety and effectiveness in pediatric patients below the age of 16 years have not been established.

Geriatric Use: Of the total number of subjects in clinical studies of *Augmentin XR*, 19.2% were 65 and over and 7.9% were 75 and older. No overall differences in safety and effectiveness were observed between these subjects and younger subjects, and other clinical experience has not reported differences in responses between the elderly and younger patients, but a greater sensitivity of some older individuals cannot be ruled out.

This drug is known to be substantially excreted by the kidney, and the risk of dose-dependent toxic reactions to this drug may be greater in patients with impaired renal function. Because elderly patients are more likely to have decreased renal function, it may be useful to monitor renal function.

Each *Augmentin XR* tablet contains 29.3 mg (1.27 mEq) of sodium.

ADVERSE REACTIONS

In clinical trials, 4,144 patients have been treated with *Augmentin XR*. The majority of side effects observed in clinical trials were of a mild and transient nature; 2% of patients discontinued therapy because of drug-related side effects. The most frequently reported adverse effects which were suspected or probably drug-related were diarrhea (15.6%), nausea (2.2%), genital moniliasis (2.1%) and abdominal pain (1.6%). *Augmentin XR* had a higher rate of diarrhea which required corrective therapy (4.0% vs. 2.4% for *Augmentin XR* and all comparators, respectively).

The following adverse reactions have been reported for ampicillin class antibiotics:

Gastrointestinal: Diarrhea, nausea, vomiting, indigestion, gastritis, stomatitis, glossitis, black "hairy" tongue, mucocutaneous candidiasis, enterocolitis, and hemorrhagic/pseudomembranous colitis. Onset of pseudomembranous colitis symptoms may occur during or after antibiotic treatment (see WARNINGS).

Hypersensitivity Reactions: Skin rashes, pruritus, urticaria, angioedema, serum sickness-like reactions (urticaria or skin rash accompanied by arthritis, arthralgia, myalgia and frequently fever), erythema multiforme (rarely Stevens-Johnson syndrome), acute generalized exanthematous pustulosis, and an occasional case of exfoliative dermatitis (including toxic epidermal necrolysis) have been reported. Whenever such reactions occur, the drug should be discontinued, unless the opinion of the physician dictates otherwise. Serious and occasional fatal hypersensitivity (anaphylactic) reactions can occur with oral penicillin (see WARNINGS).

Liver: A moderate rise in AST (SGOT) and/or ALT (SGPT) has been noted in patients treated with ampicillin class antibiotics but the significance of these findings is unknown. Hepatic dysfunction, including increases in serum transaminases (AST and/or ALT), serum bilirubin and/or alkaline phosphatase, has been infrequently reported with *Augmentin* or *Augmentin XR*. It has been reported more commonly in the elderly, in males, or in patients on prolonged treatment. The histologic findings on liver biopsy have consisted of predominantly cholestatic, hepatocellular, or mixed cholestatic-hepatocellular changes. The onset of signs/symptoms of hepatic dysfunction may occur during or several weeks after therapy has been discontinued. The hepatic dysfunction, which may be severe, is usually reversible. On rare occasions, deaths have been reported (less than 1 death reported per estimated 4 million prescriptions worldwide). These have generally been cases associated with serious underlying diseases or concomitant medications.

Renal: Interstitial nephritis and hematuria have been reported rarely.

Hemic and Lymphatic Systems: Anemia, including hemolytic anemia, thrombocytopenia, thrombocytopenic purpura, eosinophilia, leukopenia and agranulocytosis have been reported during therapy with penicillins. These reactions are

Continued on next page

Augmentin XR—Cont.

usually reversible on discontinuation of therapy and are believed to be hypersensitivity phenomena. Mild to moderate thrombocytosis was noted in <1% of patients treated with *Augmentin* and 3.6% of patients treated with *Augmentin XR*. There have been reports of increased prothrombin time in patients receiving *Augmentin* and anticoagulant therapy concomitantly.

Central Nervous System: Agitation, anxiety, behavioral changes, confusion, convulsions, dizziness, headache, insomnia, and reversible hyperactivity have been reported rarely.

OVERDOSAGE

Following overdosage, patients have experienced primarily gastrointestinal symptoms including stomach and abdominal pain, vomiting, and diarrhea. Rash, hyperactivity, or drowsiness have also been observed in a small number of patients.

In the case of overdosage, discontinue *Augmentin XR*, treat symptomatically, and institute supportive measures as required. If the overdosage is very recent and there is no contraindication, an attempt at emesis or other means of removal of drug from the stomach may be performed. A prospective study of 51 pediatric patients at a poison control center suggested that overdosages of less than 250 mg/kg of amoxicillin are not associated with significant clinical symptoms and do not require gastric emptying.[4]

Interstitial nephritis resulting in oliguric renal failure has been reported in a small number of patients after overdosage with amoxicillin. Renal impairment appears to be reversible with cessation of drug administration. High blood levels may occur more readily in patients with impaired renal function because of decreased renal clearance of both amoxicillin and clavulanate. Both amoxicillin and clavulanate are removed from the circulation by hemodialysis (see DOSAGE AND ADMINISTRATION).

DOSAGE AND ADMINISTRATION

Augmentin XR should be taken at the start of a meal to enhance the absorption of amoxicillin and to minimize the potential for gastrointestinal intolerance. Absorption of the amoxicillin component is decreased when *Augmentin XR* is taken on an empty stomach (see CLINICAL PHARMACOLOGY).

The recommended dose of Augmentin XR (amoxicillin/clavulanate potassium) is 4000 mg/250 mg daily according to the following table:

Indication	Dose	Duration
Acute Bacterial Sinusitis	2 tablets q12h	10 days
Community-Acquired Pneumonia	2 tablets q12h	7–10 days

***Augmentin* Tablets (250 mg or 500 mg) CANNOT be used to provide the same dosages as *Augmentin XR* Extended Release Tablets. This is because *Augmentin XR* contains 62.5 mg of clavulanic acid, while the *Augmentin* 250 mg and 500 mg tablets each contain 125 mg of clavulanic acid. In addition, the Extended Release Tablet provides an extended time course of plasma amoxicillin concentrations compared to immediate-release Tablets. Thus, two *Augmentin* 500 mg tablets are not equivalent to one *Augmentin XR* tablet.**

Renally impaired patients: The pharmacokinetics of *Augmentin XR* have not been studied in patients with renal impairment. *Augmentin XR* is contraindicated in severely impaired patients with a creatinine clearance of <30 mL/minute and in hemodialysis patients (see CONTRAINDICATIONS).

Hepatically impaired patients: Hepatically impaired patients should be dosed with caution and hepatic function monitored at regular intervals (see WARNINGS).

Pediatric Use: Safety and effectiveness in pediatric patients below the age of 16 years have not been established.

Geriatric Use: No dosage adjustment is required for the elderly (see PRECAUTIONS).

HOW SUPPLIED

AUGMENTIN XR (amoxicillin/clavulanate potassium) EXTENDED RELEASE TABLETS: Each white, oval filmcoated bilayer tablet, debossed with AC 1000/62.5, contains amoxicillin trihydrate and amoxicillin sodium equivalent to a total of 1000 mg of amoxicillin and clavulanate potassium equivalent to 62.5 mg of clavulanic acid.

NDC 0029-6096-28 Bottles of 28 (7 day XR pack)
NDC 0029-6096-40 Bottles of 40 (10 day XR pack)

STORAGE

Store tablets at or below 25°C (77°F). Dispense in original container.

CLINICAL STUDIES

Community-Acquired Pneumonia

Three randomized, controlled, double-blind clinical studies and one non-comparative study were conducted in adults with community-acquired pneumonia (CAP). In comparative studies, 582 patients received *Augmentin XR* at a dose of 2000/125 mg orally every 12 hours for 7 or 10 days. In the non-comparative study to assess both clinical and bacteriological efficacy, 1,122 patients received *Augmentin XR* 2000/125 mg orally every 12 hours for 7 days. In the three comparative studies, the combined clinical success rate at test of cure ranged from 86.3% to 94.7% in clinically evaluable patients in the *Augmentin XR* group; in the non-comparative study, the clinical success rate was 85.6%.

Clinical Outcome for CAP due to *S. pneumoniae*

Penicillin MICs of *S. pneumoniae* Isolates	Intent-To-Treat			Clinically Evaluable		
	n/N*	%	95% CI†	n/N*	%	95% CI†
All *S. pneumoniae*	184/214	86.0	—	157/172	91.3	—
MIC ≥2.0 µg/mL‡	17/20	85.0	62.1, 96.8	14/15	93.3	68.1, 99.8
MIC = 2.0 µg/mL	13/14	92.9	66.1, 99.8	10/10	100	69.2, 100
MIC = 4.0 µg/mL	4/6	66.7	22.3, 95.7	4/5	80.0	28.4, 99.5

* n/N = patients with pathogen eradicated or presumed eradicated/total number of patients.
† Confidence limits calculated using exact probabilities.
‡ *S. pneumoniae* strains with penicillin MICs of ≥2 µg/mL are considered resistant to penicillin.

Clinical Outcome for ABS

Penicillin MICs of *S. pneumoniae* Isolates	Intent-To-Treat			Clinically Evaluable		
	n/N*	%	95% CI†	n/N*	%	95% CI†
All *S. pneumoniae*	222/240	92.5	—	210/215	97.7	—
MIC ≥2.0 µg/mL‡	25/26	96.2	80.4, 99.9	22/23	95.7	78.1, 99.9
MIC = 2.0 µg/mL	16/17	94.1	71.3, 99.9	13/14	92.9	66.1, 99.8
MIC ≥4.0 µg/mL§	9/9	100	66.4, 100	9/9	100	66.4, 100
H. influenzae	177/203	87.2	—	160/170	94.1	—
M. catarrhalis	67/74	90.5	—	61/62	98.4	—

* n/N = patients with pathogen eradicated or presumed eradicated/total number of patients.
† Confidence limits calculated using exact probabilities.
‡ *S. pneumoniae* strains with penicillin MICs of ≥2 µg/mL are considered resistant to penicillin.
§ Includes one patient each with *S. pneumoniae* penicillin MICs of 8 and 16 µg/mL.

Data on the efficacy of *Augmentin XR* in the treatment of community-acquired pneumonia due to *Streptococcus pneumoniae* with reduced susceptibility to penicillin were accrued from the three controlled clinical studies and the one non-comparative study. The majority of these cases were accrued from the non-comparative study.

[See first table above]

Acute Bacterial Sinusitis

Adults with a diagnosis of Acute Bacterial Sinusitis (ABS) were evaluated in three clinical studies. In one study, 363 patients were randomized to receive either *Augmentin XR* 2000/125 mg orally q12h or levofloxacin 500 mg orally daily for 10 days in a double-blind, multicenter prospective trial. These patients were clinically and radiologically evaluated at the test of cure (day 17-28) visit. The combined clinical and radiological responses were 83.7% for *Augmentin XR* and 84.3% for levofloxacin at the test of cure visit in clinically evaluable patients (95% CI for the treatment difference = -9.4, 8.3). The clinical response rates at the test of cure were 87.0% and 88.6%, respectively.

The other two trials were non-comparative, multicenter studies designed to assess the bacteriological and clinical efficacy of *Augmentin XR* (2000/125 mg orally q12h for 10 days) in the treatment of 1,554 patients with ABS. Evaluation timepoints were the same as in the prior study. Patients underwent maxillary sinus puncture for culture prior to receiving study medication. At test of cure, the clinical success rates were 87.5% and 87.1% (intention-to-treat) and 92.5% and 94.0% (per protocol populations).

Patients with acute bacterial sinusitis due to *S. pneumoniae* with reduced susceptibility to penicillin were accrued through enrollment in these two open-label non-comparative clinical trials. Microbiologic eradication rates for key pathogens in these studies are shown in the following table:

[See second table above]

Safety

In a randomized, double-blind, multicenter study, *Augmentin XR* (2000/125 mg orally q12h, n = 255) was compared to *Augmentin* (875/125 mg orally q12h, n = 259), administered for 7 days for the treatment of community-acquired pneumonia. Adverse events, regardless of relationship to test drug, were reported by 49.4% of patients in the *Augmentin XR* group (vs. 51.4% in comparator group). Treatment-related adverse events were reported in 25.1% of patients in the *Augmentin XR* group (vs. 24.7% in comparator group); most were mild and transient in nature. Adverse events which led to withdrawal were reported by 2.4% of patients in the *Augmentin XR* group (vs. 5.4% in comparator group). In each group, the most frequently reported adverse events were diarrhea (18.0% vs. 14.3%, p = 0.28), nausea (4.3% vs. 5.4%), and headache (4.3% vs. 5.0%). Only one patient (0.4%) in the Augmentin XR (amoxicillin/clavulanate potassium) group and two patients (0.8%) in the comparator group withdrew due to diarrhea. Serious adverse events considered suspected or probably related to test drug were reported in 0.8% of patients (vs. 0.4% in comparator).

REFERENCES

1. National Committee for Clinical Laboratory Standards. Methods for Dilution Antimicrobial Susceptibility Tests for Bacteria that Grow Aerobically—Fifth Edition. Approved Standard NCCLS Document M7-A5, Vol. 20, No. 2. NCCLS, Wayne, PA, Jan. 2000.
2. National Committee for Clinical Laboratory Standards. Performance Standards for Antimicrobial Susceptibility Testing – Twelfth Informational Standard. M100-S12, Vol. 22, No. 1. NCCLS, Wayne, PA, Jan. 2002.
3. National Committee for Clinical Laboratory Standards. Performance Standards for Antimicrobial Disk Susceptibility Tests—Seventh Edition. Approved Standard NCCLS Document M2-A7, Vol. 20, No. 1. NCCLS, Wayne, PA, Jan. 2000.
4. Swanson-Biearman B, Dean BS, Lopez G, Krenzelok EP. The effects of penicillin and cephalosporin ingestions in children less than six years of age. *Vet Hum Toxicol* 1988;30:66-67.

Maalox is a registered trademark of Novartis Consumer Health, Inc.

GlaxoSmithKline, Research Triangle Park, NC 27709

©2002, GlaxoSmithKline. All rights reserved.

November 2002/AX:L2

AVANDAMET™ ℞

[*ə văn' də mət*]

brand of
rosiglitazone maleate and metformin hydrochloride tablets

DESCRIPTION

AVANDAMET™ (rosiglitazone maleate and metformin HCl) tablets contain two oral antihyperglycemic drugs used in the management of type 2 diabetes: Rosiglitazone maleate and metformin hydrochloride. The combination of rosiglitazone maleate and metformin hydrochloride has been previously approved based on clinical trials in people with type 2 diabetes mellitus inadequately controlled on metformin alone. Additional efficacy and safety information about rosiglitazone and metformin monotherapies may be found in the prescribing information for each individual drug.

Rosiglitazone maleate is an oral antidiabetic agent, which acts primarily by increasing insulin sensitivity. Rosiglitazone improves glycemic control while reducing circulating insulin levels. Pharmacologic studies in animal models indicate that rosiglitazone improves sensitivity to insulin in muscle and adipose tissue and inhibits hepatic gluconeogenesis. Rosiglitazone maleate is not chemically or functionally related to the sulfonylureas, the biguanides, or the α-glucosidase inhibitors.

Chemically, rosiglitazone maleate is (±)-5-[[4-[2-(methyl-2-pyridinylamino)ethoxy]phenyl]methyl]-2,4-thiazolidinedione, (*Z*)-2-butenedioate (1:1) with a molecular weight of 473.52 (357.44 free base). The molecule has a single chiral center and is present as a racemate. Due to rapid interconversion, the enantiomers are functionally indistinguishable. The molecular formula is $C_{18}H_{19}N_3O_3S{\bullet}C_4H_4O_4$. Rosiglitazone maleate is a white to off-white solid with a melting point range of 122° to 123°C. The pK_a values of rosiglitazone maleate are 6.8 and 6.1. It is readily soluble in ethanol and a buffered aqueous solution with pH of 2.3; solubility decreases with increasing pH in the physiological range. The structural formula is:

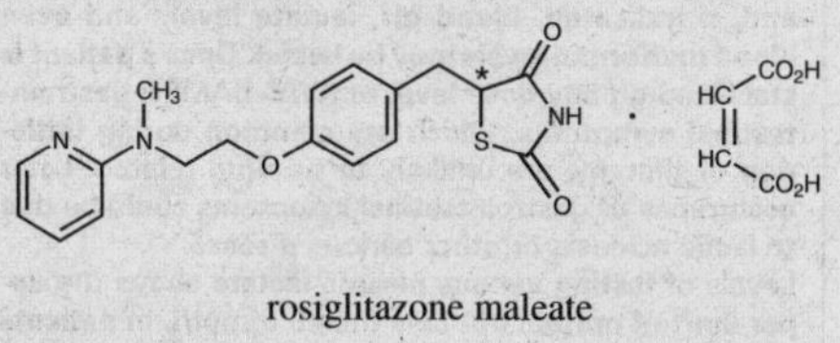

rosiglitazone maleate

Metformin hydrochloride (N,N-dimethylimidodicarbonimidic diamide hydrochloride) is not chemically or pharmacologically related to any other classes of oral antihyperglycemic agents. Metformin hydrochloride is a white to off-white crystalline compound with a molecular formula of $C_4H_{11}N_5$•HCl and a molecular weight of 165.63. Metformin hydrochloride is freely soluble in water and is practically insoluble in acetone, ether and chloroform. The pK_a of metformin is 12.4. The pH of a 1% aqueous solution of metformin hydrochloride is 6.68. The structural formula is:

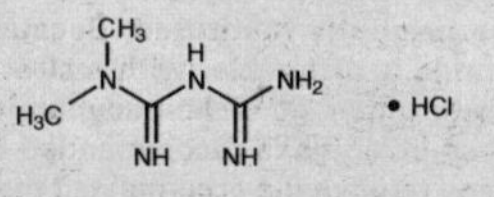

metformin hydrochloride

AVANDAMET is available for oral administration as tablets containing rosiglitazone maleate and metformin hydrochloride equivalent to: 1 mg rosiglitazone with 500 mg metformin hydrochloride (1 mg/500 mg), 2 mg rosiglitazone with 500 mg metformin hydrochloride (2 mg/500 mg), and 4 mg rosiglitazone with 500 mg metformin hydrochloride (4 mg/500 mg). In addition, each tablet contains the following inactive ingredients: Hypromellose, lactose monohydrate, magnesium stearate, microcrystalline cellulose, polyethylene glycol 400, povidone 29-32, sodium starch glycolate, titanium dioxide and one or more of the following: Red and yellow iron oxides.

CLINICAL PHARMACOLOGY

Mechanism of Action: AVANDAMET combines two antidiabetic agents with different mechanisms of action to improve glycemic control in patients with type 2 diabetes: Rosiglitazone maleate, a member of the thiazolidinedione class and metformin hydrochloride, a member of the biguanide class. Thiazolidinediones are insulin sensitizing agents that act primarily by enhancing peripheral glucose utilization, whereas biguanides act primarily by decreasing endogenous hepatic glucose production.

Rosiglitazone, a member of the thiazolidinedione class of antidiabetic agents, improves glycemic control by improving insulin sensitivity while reducing circulating insulin levels. Rosiglitazone is a highly selective and potent agonist for the peroxisome proliferator-activated receptor-gamma (PPARγ). In humans, PPAR receptors are found in key target tissues for insulin action such as adipose tissue, skeletal muscle and liver. Activation of PPARγ nuclear receptors regulates the transcription of insulin-responsive genes involved in the control of glucose production, transport, and utilization. In addition, PPARγ-responsive genes also participate in the regulation of fatty acid metabolism.

Insulin resistance is a common feature characterizing the pathogenesis of type 2 diabetes. The antidiabetic activity of rosiglitazone has been demonstrated in animal models of type 2 diabetes in which hyperglycemia and/or impaired glucose tolerance is a consequence of insulin resistance in target tissues. Rosiglitazone reduces blood glucose concentrations and reduces hyperinsulinemia in the ob/ob obese mouse, db/db diabetic mouse, and fa/fa fatty Zucker rat.

In animal models, rosiglitazone's antidiabetic activity was shown to be mediated by increased sensitivity to insulin's action in the liver, muscle and adipose tissue. The expression of the insulin-regulated glucose transporter GLUT-4 was increased in adipose tissue. Rosiglitazone did not induce hypoglycemia in animal models of type 2 diabetes and/or impaired glucose tolerance.

Metformin hydrochloride is an antihyperglycemic agent, which improves glucose tolerance in patients with type 2 diabetes, lowering both basal and postprandial plasma glucose. Its pharmacologic mechanisms of action are different from other classes of oral antihyperglycemic agents. Metformin decreases hepatic glucose production, decreases intestinal absorption of glucose and increases peripheral glucose uptake and utilization. Unlike sulfonylureas, metformin does not produce hypoglycemia in either patients with type 2 diabetes or normal subjects (except in special circumstances, see PRECAUTIONS) and does not cause hyperinsulinemia. With metformin therapy, insulin secretion remains unchanged while fasting insulin levels and daylong plasma insulin response may actually decrease.

Pharmacokinetics

Absorption and Bioavailability: ***AVANDAMET:*** In a bioequivalence and dose proportionality study of AVANDAMET 4 mg/500 mg, both the rosiglitazone component and the metformin component were bioequivalent to coadministered 4 mg rosiglitazone maleate tablet and 500 mg metformin hydrochloride tablet under fasted conditions (see Table 1). In this study, dose proportionality of rosiglitazone in the combination formulations of 1 mg/500 mg and 4 mg/500 mg was demonstrated.

[See table 1 above]

Table 1. Mean (SD) Pharmacokinetic Parameters for Rosiglitazone and Metformin

		Pharmacokinetic Parameter			
Regimen	**N**	**AUC (0-inf) (ng.h/mL)**	**C_{max} (ng/mL)**	**T_{max}* (h)**	**T1/2 (h)**
Rosiglitazone					
A	25	1442 (324)	242 (70)	0.95 (0.48-2.47)	4.26 (1.18)
B	25	1398 (340)	254 (69)	0.57 (0.43-2.58)	3.95 (0.81)
C	24	349 (91)	63.0 (15.0)	0.57 (0.47-1.45)	3.87 (0.88)
Metformin					
A	25	7116 (2096)	1106 (329)	2.97 (1.02-4.02)	3.46 (0.96)
B	25	7413 (1838)	1135 (253)	2.50 (1.03-3.98)	3.36 (0.54)
C	24	6945 (2045)	1080 (327)	2.97 (1.00-5.98)	3.35 (0.59)

* = Median and range presented for T_{max}

Regimen Key: Regimen A = 4 mg/500 mg AVANDAMET
Regimen B = 4 mg rosiglitazone maleate tablet + 500 mg metformin hydrochloride tablet
Regimen C = 1 mg/500 mg AVANDAMET

Administration of AVANDAMET 4 mg/500 mg with food resulted in no change in overall exposure (AUC) for either rosiglitazone or metformin. However, there were decreases in C_{max} of both components (22% for rosiglitazone and 15% for metformin, respectively) and a delay in T_{max} of both components (1.5 hrs for rosiglitazone and 0.5 hrs for metformin, respectively). These changes are not likely to be clinically significant. The pharmacokinetics of both the rosiglitazone component and the metformin component of AVANDAMET when taken with food were similar to the pharmacokinetics of rosiglitazone and metformin when administered concomitantly as separate tablets with food.

Rosiglitazone maleate: The absolute bioavailability of rosiglitazone is 99%. Peak plasma concentrations are observed about 1 hour after dosing. Maximum plasma concentration (C_{max}) and the area under the curve (AUC) of rosiglitazone increase in a dose-proportional manner over the therapeutic dose range. The elimination half-life is 3 to 4 hours and is independent of dose.

Metformin hydrochloride: The absolute bioavailability of a 500 mg metformin hydrochloride tablet given under fasting conditions is approximately 50-60%. Studies using single oral doses of metformin hydrochloride tablets of 500 mg and 1500 mg, and 850 mg to 2550 mg, indicate that there is a lack of dose proportionality with increasing doses, which is due to decreased absorption rather than an alteration in elimination.

Distribution: ***Rosiglitazone maleate:*** The mean (CV%) oral volume of distribution (Vss/F) of rosiglitazone is approximately 17.6 (30%) liters, based on a population pharmacokinetic analysis. Rosiglitazone is approximately 99.8% bound to plasma proteins, primarily albumin.

Metformin hydrochloride: The apparent volume of distribution (V/F) of metformin following single oral doses of 850 mg metformin hydrochloride averaged 654 ± 358 L. Metformin is negligibly bound to plasma proteins. Metformin partitions into erythrocytes, most likely as a function of time. At usual clinical doses and dosing schedules of metformin, steady state plasma concentrations of metformin are reached within 24-48 hours and are generally <1 µg/mL. During controlled clinical trials, maximum metformin plasma levels did not exceed 5 µg/mL, even at maximum doses.

Metabolism and Excretion: ***Rosiglitazone maleate:*** Rosiglitazone is extensively metabolized with no unchanged drug excreted in the urine. The major routes of metabolism were N-demethylation and hydroxylation, followed by conjugation with sulfate and glucuronic acid. All the circulating metabolites are considerably less potent than parent and, therefore, are not expected to contribute to the insulin-sensitizing activity of rosiglitazone. *In vitro* data demonstrate that rosiglitazone is predominantly metabolized by Cytochrome P_{450} (CYP) isoenzyme 2C8, with CYP2C9 contributing as a minor pathway. Following oral or intravenous administration of [^{14}C]rosiglitazone maleate, approximately 64% and 23% of the dose was eliminated in the urine and in the feces, respectively. The plasma half-life of [^{14}C]related material ranged from 103 to 158 hours.

Metformin hydrochloride: Intravenous single-dose studies in normal subjects demonstrate that metformin is excreted unchanged in the urine and does not undergo hepatic metabolism (no metabolites have been identified in humans) nor biliary excretion. Renal clearance is approximately 3.5 times greater than creatinine clearance which indicates that tubular secretion is the major route of metformin elimination. Following oral administration, approximately 90% of the absorbed drug is eliminated via the renal route within the first 24 hours, with a plasma elimination half-life of approximately 6.2 hours. In blood, the elimination half-life is approximately 17.6 hours, suggesting that the erythrocyte mass may be a compartment of distribution.

Special Populations: **Renal Impairment:** In subjects with decreased renal function (based on measured creatinine clearance), the plasma and blood half-life of metformin is prolonged and the renal clearance is decreased in proportion to the decrease in creatinine clearance (see WARNINGS, also see GLUCOPHAGE[1] prescribing information, CLINICAL PHARMACOLOGY, Pharmacokinetics). Since metformin is contraindicated in patients with renal impairment, administration of AVANDAMET is contraindicated in these patients.

Hepatic Impairment: Unbound oral clearance of rosiglitazone was significantly lower in patients with moderate to severe liver disease (Child-Pugh Class B/C) compared to healthy subjects. As a result, unbound C_{max} and AUC_{0-inf} were increased 2- and 3-fold, respectively. Elimination half-life for rosiglitazone was about 2 hours longer in patients with liver disease, compared to healthy subjects.

Therapy with AVANDAMET should not be initiated if the patient exhibits clinical evidence of active liver disease or increased serum transaminase levels (ALT >2.5X upper limit of normal) at baseline (see PRECAUTIONS, Hepatic effects).

No pharmacokinetic studies of metformin have been conducted in subjects with hepatic insufficiency.

Geriatrics: Results of the population pharmacokinetics analysis (n = 716 <65 years; n = 331 ≥65 years) showed that age does not significantly affect the pharmacokinetics of rosiglitazone. However, limited data from controlled pharmacokinetic studies of metformin hydrochloride in healthy elderly subjects suggest that total plasma clearance of metformin is decreased, the half-life is prolonged and C_{max} is increased, compared to healthy young subjects. From these data, it appears that the change in metformin pharmacokinetics with aging is primarily accounted for by a change in renal function (see GLUCOPHAGE[1] prescribing information, CLINICAL PHARMACOLOGY, Pharmacokinetics). Metformin treatment and therefore treatment with AVANDAMET should not be initiated in patients ≥80 years of age unless measurement of creatinine clearance demonstrates that renal function is not reduced (see WARNINGS and DOSAGE AND ADMINISTRATION).

Gender: Results of the population pharmacokinetics analysis showed that the mean oral clearance of rosiglitazone in female patients (n = 405) was approximately 6% lower compared to male patients of the same body weight (n = 642). In rosiglitazone and metformin combination studies, efficacy was demonstrated with no gender differences in glycemic response.

Metformin pharmacokinetic parameters did not differ significantly between normal subjects and patients with type 2 diabetes when analyzed according to gender (males = 19, females = 16). Similarly, in controlled clinical studies in patients with type 2 diabetes, the antihyperglycemic effect of metformin hydrochloride tablets was comparable in males and females.

Race: Results of a population pharmacokinetic analysis including subjects of white, black, and other ethnic origins indicate that race has no influence on the pharmacokinetics of rosiglitazone.

No studies of metformin pharmacokinetic parameters according to race have been performed. In controlled clinical studies of metformin hydrochloride in patients with type 2 diabetes, the antihyperglycemic effect was comparable in whites (n = 249), blacks (n = 51) and Hispanics (n = 24).

Pediatrics: No pharmacokinetic data from studies in pediatric subjects are available for either rosiglitazone or metformin.

CLINICAL STUDIES

There have been no clinical efficacy trials conducted with AVANDAMET tablets. However, studies utilizing the sepa-

Continued on next page

Avandamet—Cont.

rate components have established the effective and safe use, and the additive benefit of the combination has been shown in patients with diabetes mellitus inadequately controlled with fasting plasma glucose between 140 and 300 mg/dL despite maximal metformin therapy alone (2500 mg/day). Bioequivalence of AVANDAMET with coadministered rosiglitazone maleate tablets and metformin hydrochloride tablets was demonstrated (see CLINICAL PHARMACOLOGY, Pharmacokinetics).

The addition of rosiglitazone to metformin resulted in significant improvements in glucose concentrations compared to either of these agents alone. These results are consistent with an additive effect on glycemic control when rosiglitazone is used in combination with metformin. No clinical trials have been conducted with combination rosiglitazone and metformin therapy as initial therapy in patients with type 2 diabetes mellitus. No controlled clinical trials have been conducted in which metformin was added to patients inadequately controlled with rosiglitazone alone. The pattern of LDL and HDL changes following therapy with rosiglitazone in combination with metformin was generally similar to those seen with rosiglitazone in monotherapy.

Clinical Trials of Rosiglitazone Add-on Therapy in Patients Not Adequately Controlled on Metformin Alone: A total of 670 patients with type 2 diabetes participated in two 26-week, randomized, double-blind, placebo/active-controlled studies designed to assess the efficacy of rosiglitazone in combination with metformin. Rosiglitazone maleate, administered in either once-daily or twice-daily dosing regimens, was added to the therapy of patients who were inadequately controlled on 2.5 grams/day of metformin hydrochloride.

In one study, patients inadequately controlled on 2.5 grams/day of metformin hydrochloride (mean baseline FPG 216 mg/dL and mean baseline HbA1c 8.8%) were randomized to receive rosiglitazone 4 mg once daily, rosiglitazone 8 mg once daily, or placebo in addition to metformin. A statistically significant improvement in FPG and HbA1c was observed in patients treated with the combinations of metformin and rosiglitazone 4 mg once daily and rosiglitazone 8 mg once daily, versus patients continued on metformin alone (Table 2).

[See table 2 below]

In a second 26-week study, patients with type 2 diabetes inadequately controlled on 2.5 grams/day of metformin hydrochloride who were randomized to receive the combination of rosiglitazone 4 mg twice daily and metformin (N = 105) showed a statistically significant improvement in glycemic control with a mean treatment effect for FPG of -56 mg/dL and a mean treatment effect for HbA1c of -0.8% over metformin alone. The combination of metformin and rosiglitazone resulted in lower levels of FPG and HbA1c than either agent alone.

INDICATIONS AND USAGE

AVANDAMET is indicated as an adjunct to diet and exercise to improve glycemic control in patients with type 2 diabetes mellitus who are already treated with combination rosiglitazone and metformin or who are not adequately controlled on metformin alone.

Management of type 2 diabetes mellitus should include diet control. Caloric restriction, weight loss, and exercise are essential for the proper treatment of the diabetic patient because they help improve insulin sensitivity. This is important not only in the primary treatment of type 2 diabetes, but also in maintaining the efficacy of drug therapy. Prior to initiation or escalation of oral antidiabetic therapy in patients with type 2 diabetes mellitus, secondary causes of poor glycemic control, e.g., infection, should be investigated and treated.

The safety and efficacy of AVANDAMET as initial pharmacologic therapy for patients with type 2 diabetes mellitus after a trial of caloric restriction, weight loss, and exercise has not been established.

CONTRAINDICATIONS

AVANDAMET (rosiglitazone maleate and metformin hydrochloride) tablets are contraindicated in patients with:

1. Renal disease or renal dysfunction (e.g., as suggested by serum creatinine levels ≥1.5 mg/dL [males], ≥1.4 mg/dL [females] or abnormal creatinine clearance) which may also result from conditions such as cardiovascular collapse (shock), acute myocardial infarction, and septicemia (see WARNINGS and PRECAUTIONS).
2. Congestive heart failure requiring pharmacologic treatment.
3. Known hypersensitivity to rosiglitazone maleate or metformin hydrochloride.
4. Acute or chronic metabolic acidosis, including diabetic ketoacidosis, with or without coma. Diabetic ketoacidosis should be treated with insulin.

AVANDAMET should be temporarily discontinued in patients undergoing radiologic studies involving intravascular administration of iodinated contrast materials, because use of such products may result in acute alteration of renal function (see also PRECAUTIONS).

WARNINGS

Metformin hydrochloride

Lactic Acidosis

Lactic acidosis is a rare, but serious, metabolic complication that can occur due to metformin accumulation during treatment with AVANDAMET; when it occurs, it is fatal in approximately 50% of cases. Lactic acidosis may also occur in association with a number of pathophysiologic conditions, including diabetes mellitus, and whenever there is significant tissue hypoperfusion and hypoxemia. Lactic acidosis is characterized by elevated blood lactate levels (>5 mmol/L), decreased blood pH, electrolyte disturbances with an increased anion gap, and an increased lactate/pyruvate ratio. When metformin is implicated as the cause of lactic acidosis, metformin plasma levels >5 µg/mL are generally found.

The reported incidence of lactic acidosis in patients receiving metformin hydrochloride is very low (approximately 0.03 cases/1000 patient-years, with approximately 0.015 fatal cases/1000 patient-years). Reported cases have occurred primarily in diabetic patients with significant renal insufficiency, including both intrinsic renal disease and renal hypoperfusion, often in the setting of multiple concomitant medical/surgical problems and multiple concomitant medications. Patients with congestive heart failure requiring pharmacologic management, in particular those with unstable or acute congestive heart failure who are at risk of hypoperfusion and hypoxemia, are at increased risk of lactic acidosis. The risk of lactic acidosis increases with the degree of renal dysfunction and the patient's age. The risk of lactic acidosis may, therefore, be significantly decreased by regular monitoring of renal function in patients taking AVANDAMET and by use of the minimum effective dose of AVANDAMET. In particular, treatment of the elderly should be accompanied by careful monitoring of renal function. Treatment with AVANDAMET should not be initiated in patients ≥80 years of age unless measurement of creatinine clearance demonstrates that renal function is not reduced, as these patients are more susceptible to developing lactic acidosis. In addition, AVANDAMET should be promptly withheld in the presence of any condition associated with hypoxemia, dehydration or sepsis. Because impaired hepatic function may significantly limit the ability to clear lactate, AVANDAMET should generally be avoided in patients with clinical or laboratory evidence of hepatic disease. Patients should be cautioned against excessive alcohol intake, either acute or chronic, when taking AVANDAMET, since alcohol potentiates the effects of metformin hydrochloride on lactate metabolism. In addition, AVANDAMET should be temporarily discontinued prior to any intravascular radiocontrast study and for any surgical procedure (see also PRECAUTIONS).

The onset of lactic acidosis often is subtle, and accompanied only by nonspecific symptoms such as malaise, myalgias, respiratory distress, increasing somnolence and nonspecific abdominal distress. There may be associated hypothermia, hypotension and resistant bradyarrhythmias with more marked acidosis. The patient and the patient's physician must be aware of the possible importance of such symptoms and the patient should be instructed to notify the physician immediately if they occur (see also PRECAUTIONS). AVANDAMET should be withdrawn until the situation is clarified. Serum electrolytes, ketones, blood glucose and, if indicated, blood pH, lactate levels and even blood metformin levels may be useful. Once a patient is stabilized on any dose level of AVANDAMET, gastrointestinal symptoms, which are common during initiation of therapy, are unlikely to be drug related. Later occurrence of gastrointestinal symptoms could be due to lactic acidosis or other serious disease.

Levels of fasting venous plasma lactate above the upper limit of normal but less than 5 mmol/L in patients taking AVANDAMET do not necessarily indicate impending lactic acidosis and may be explainable by other mechanisms, such as poorly controlled diabetes or obesity, vigorous physical activity or technical problems in sample handling (see also PRECAUTIONS).

Lactic acidosis should be suspected in any diabetic patient with metabolic acidosis lacking evidence of ketoacidosis (ketonuria and ketonemia).

Lactic acidosis is a medical emergency that must be treated in a hospital setting. In a patient with lactic acidosis who is taking AVANDAMET, the drug should be discontinued immediately and general supportive measures promptly instituted. Because metformin hydrochloride is dialyzable (with a clearance of up to 170 mL/min under good hemodynamic conditions), prompt hemodialysis is recommended to correct the acidosis and remove the accumulated metformin. Such management often results in prompt reversal of symptoms and recovery (see also CONTRAINDICATIONS and PRECAUTIONS).

Rosiglitazone maleate

Cardiac Failure and Other Cardiac Effects: Rosiglitazone, like other thiazolidinediones, can cause fluid retention, which may exacerbate or lead to heart failure. Patients should be observed for signs and symptoms of heart failure. AVANDAMET should be discontinued if any deterioration in cardiac status occurs.

Patients with New York Heart Association (NYHA) Class 3 and 4 cardiac status were not studied during the clinical trials with rosiglitazone maleate. In patients requiring pharmacologic treatment for congestive heart failure, AVANDAMET should not be used (see CONTRAINDICATIONS).

In two 26-week U.S. trials involving 611 patients with type 2 diabetes, rosiglitazone maleate plus insulin therapy was compared with insulin therapy alone. These trials included patients with long-standing diabetes and a high prevalence of pre-existing medical conditions, including peripheral neuropathy (34%), retinopathy (19%), ischemic heart disease (14%), vascular disease (9%), and congestive heart failure (2.5%). In these clinical studies, an increased incidence of cardiac failure and other cardiovascular adverse events were seen in patients on rosiglitazone and insulin combination therapy compared to insulin and placebo. Patients who experienced heart failure were on average older, had a longer duration of diabetes, and were mostly on the higher 8 mg daily dose of rosiglitazone. In this population, however, it was not possible to determine specific risk factors that could be used to identify all patients at risk of heart failure on combination therapy. Three of 10 patients who developed cardiac failure on combination therapy during the double-blind part of the studies had no known prior evidence of congestive heart failure, or pre-existing cardiac condition. **The use of rosiglitazone maleate in combination therapy with insulin is not indicated (see ADVERSE REACTIONS), therefore, AVANDAMET is not indicated for use in combination with insulin.**

PRECAUTIONS

General: ***Metformin hydrochloride***

Monitoring of renal function: Metformin is known to be substantially excreted by the kidney, and the risk of metformin accumulation and lactic acidosis increases with the degree of impairment of renal function. Thus, patients with serum creatinine levels above the upper limit of normal for their age should not receive AVANDAMET. In patients with advanced age, AVANDAMET should be carefully titrated to establish the minimum dose for adequate glycemic effect, because aging is associated with reduced renal function. In elderly patients, particularly those ≥80 years of age, renal function should be monitored regularly and, generally, AVANDAMET should not be titrated to the maximum dose of the metformin component, i.e., 2000 mg (see WARNINGS and DOSAGE AND ADMINISTRATION).

Before initiation of therapy with AVANDAMET and at least annually thereafter, renal function should be assessed and verified as normal. In patients in whom development of renal dysfunction is anticipated, renal function should be assessed more frequently and AVANDAMET discontinued if evidence of renal impairment is present.

Use of concomitant medications that may affect renal function or metformin disposition: Concomitant medication(s) that may affect renal function or result in significant hemodynamic change or may interfere with the disposition of metformin, such as cationic drugs that are eliminated by renal tubular secretion (see PRECAUTIONS, Drug Interactions), should be used with caution.

Radiologic studies involving the use of intravascular iodinated contrast materials (for example, intravenous urogram, intravenous cholangiography, angiography, and computed tomography (CT) scans with contrast materials): Intravascular contrast studies with iodinated materials can lead to acute alteration of renal function and have been as-

Table 2. Glycemic Parameters in a 26-Week Rosiglitazone maleate + Metformin hydrochloride Combination Study

	Metformin	Rosiglitazone 4 mg once daily +metformin	Rosiglitazone 8 mg once daily +metformin
N	113	116	110
FPG (mg/dL)			
Baseline (mean)	214	215	220
Change from baseline (mean)	6	-33	-48
Difference from metformin alone (adjusted mean)		-40*	-53*
Responders (≥30 mg/dL decrease from baseline)	20%	45%	61%
HbA1c (%)			
Baseline (mean)	8.6	8.9	8.9
Change from baseline (mean)	0.5	-0.6	-0.8
Difference from metformin alone (adjusted mean)		-1.0*	-1.2*
Responders (≥0.7% decrease from baseline)	11%	45%	52%

*p<0.0001 compared to metformin.

sociated with lactic acidosis in patients receiving metformin (see CONTRAINDICATIONS). Therefore, in patients in whom any such study is planned, AVANDAMET should be temporarily discontinued at the time of or prior to the procedure, and withheld for 48 hours subsequent to the procedure and reinstituted only after renal function has been re-evaluated and found to be normal.

Hypoxic states: Cardiovascular collapse (shock) from whatever cause, acute congestive heart failure, acute myocardial infarction and other conditions characterized by hypoxemia have been associated with lactic acidosis and may also cause prerenal azotemia. When such events occur in patients receiving AVANDAMET, the drug should be promptly discontinued.

Surgical procedures: Use of AVANDAMET should be temporarily suspended for any surgical procedure (except minor procedures not associated with restricted intake of food and fluids) and should not be restarted until the patient's oral intake has resumed and renal function has been evaluated as normal.

Alcohol intake: Alcohol is known to potentiate the effect of metformin on lactate metabolism. Patients, therefore, should be warned against excessive alcohol intake, acute or chronic, while receiving AVANDAMET.

Impaired hepatic function: Since impaired hepatic function has been associated with some cases of lactic acidosis, AVANDAMET should generally be avoided in patients with clinical or laboratory evidence of hepatic disease.

Vitamin B_{12} levels: In controlled clinical trials of metformin hydrochloride of 29 weeks' duration, a decrease to subnormal levels of previously normal serum vitamin B_{12} levels, without clinical manifestations, was observed in approximately 7% of patients. Such decrease, possibly due to interference with B_{12} absorption from the B_{12}-intrinsic factor complex, is, however, very rarely associated with anemia and appears to be rapidly reversible with discontinuation of metformin or vitamin B_{12} supplementation. Measurement of hematologic parameters on an annual basis is advised in patients on AVANDAMET and any apparent abnormalities should be appropriately investigated and managed (see PRECAUTIONS, Laboratory Tests). Certain individuals (those with inadequate vitamin B_{12} or calcium intake or absorption) appear to be predisposed to developing subnormal vitamin B_{12} levels. In these patients, routine serum vitamin B_{12} measurements at two- to three-year intervals may be useful.

Change in clinical status of previously controlled diabetic: A patient with type 2 diabetes previously well-controlled on AVANDAMET who develops laboratory abnormalities or clinical illness (especially vague and poorly defined illness) should be evaluated promptly for evidence of ketoacidosis or lactic acidosis. Evaluation should include serum electrolytes and ketones, blood glucose and, if indicated, blood pH, lactate, pyruvate and metformin levels. If acidosis of either form occurs, AVANDAMET must be stopped immediately and other appropriate corrective measures initiated (see also WARNINGS).

Hypoglycemia: Hypoglycemia does not occur in patients receiving metformin hydrochloride alone under usual circumstances of use, but could occur when caloric intake is deficient, when strenuous exercise is not compensated by caloric supplementation, or during concomitant use with hypoglycemic agents (such as sulfonylureas or insulin) or ethanol. Elderly, debilitated or malnourished patients, and those with adrenal or pituitary insufficiency or alcohol intoxication are particularly susceptible to hypoglycemic effects. Hypoglycemia may be difficult to recognize in the elderly, and in people who are taking beta-adrenergic blocking drugs.

Loss of control of blood glucose: When a patient stabilized on any diabetic regimen is exposed to stress such as fever, trauma, infection, or surgery, a temporary loss of glycemic control may occur. At such times, it may be necessary to withhold AVANDAMET and temporarily administer insulin. AVANDAMET may be reinstituted after the acute episode is resolved.

Rosiglitazone maleate: General: Due to its mechanism of action, rosiglitazone is active only in the presence of endogenous insulin. Therefore, AVANDAMET should not be used in patients with type 1 diabetes.

Edema: AVANDAMET should be used with caution in patients with edema. In a clinical study in healthy volunteers who received rosiglitazone 8 mg once daily for 8 weeks, there was a statistically significant increase in median plasma volume compared to placebo. Since thiazolidinediones, including rosiglitazone, can cause fluid retention, which can exacerbate or lead to congestive heart failure, AVANDAMET should be used with caution in patients at risk for heart failure. Patients should be monitored for signs and symptoms of heart failure (see WARNINGS, Cardiac Failure and Other Cardiac Effects and PRECAUTIONS, Information for Patients).

In controlled clinical trials of patients with type 2 diabetes, mild to moderate edema was reported in patients treated with rosiglitazone maleate, and may be dose related. Patients with ongoing edema are more likely to have adverse events associated with edema if started on combination therapy with insulin and rosiglitazone (see ADVERSE REACTIONS).

Weight gain: Dose-related weight gain was seen with rosiglitazone alone or in combination with other hypoglycemic agents (Table 3). The mechanism of weight gain is unclear but probably involves a combination of fluid retention and fat accumulation.

Table 3. Weight Changes (kg) from Baseline During Clinical Trials with Rosiglitazone maleate

		Control Group		Rosiglitazone 4 mg	Rosiglitazone 8 mg
Monotherapy	Duration		Median (25th, 75th percentile)	Median (25th, 75th percentile)	Median (25th, 75th percentile)
	26 weeks	placebo	-0.9 (-2.8, 0.9)	1.0 (-0.9, 3.6)	3.1 (1.1, 5.8)
	52 weeks	sulfonylurea	2.0 (0, 4.0)	2.0 (-0.6, 4.0)	2.6 (0, 5.3)
Combination therapy					
sulfonylurea	26 weeks	sulfonylurea	0 (-1.3, 1.2)	1.8 (0, 3.1)	–
metformin	26 weeks	metformin	-1.4 (-3.2, 0.2)	0.8 (-1.0, 2.6)	2.1 (0, 4.3)
insulin	26 weeks	insulin	0.9 (-0.5, 2.7)	4.1 (1.4, 6.3)	5.4 (3.4, 7.3)

In postmarketing experience with rosiglitazone alone or in combination with other hypoglycemic agents, there have been rare reports of unusually rapid increases in weight and increases in excess of that generally observed in clinical trials. Patients who experience such increases should be assessed for fluid accumulation and volume-related events such as excessive edema and congestive heart failure.
[See table 3 above]

Hematologic: Across all controlled clinical studies, decreases in hemoglobin and hematocrit (mean decreases in individual studies ≤ 1.0 gram/dL and $\leq 3.3\%$, respectively) were observed for rosiglitazone maleate alone and in combination with other hypoglycemic agents. The changes occurred primarily during the first 3 months following initiation of rosiglitazone therapy or following an increase in rosiglitazone dose. White blood cell counts also decreased slightly in patients treated with rosiglitazone. The observed changes may be related to the increased plasma volume observed with treatment with rosiglitazone and may be dose related (see ADVERSE REACTIONS, Laboratory Abnormalities).

Ovulation: Therapy with rosiglitazone, like other thiazolidinediones, may result in ovulation in some premenopausal anovulatory women. As a result, these patients may be at an increased risk for pregnancy while taking AVANDAMET (see PRECAUTIONS, Pregnancy, Pregnancy Category C). Thus, adequate contraception in premenopausal women should be recommended. This possible effect has not been specifically investigated in clinical studies so the frequency of this occurrence is not known.

Although hormonal imbalance has been seen in preclinical studies (see PRECAUTIONS, Carcinogenesis, Mutagenesis, Impairment of Fertility), the clinical significance of this finding is not known. If unexpected menstrual dysfunction occurs, the benefits of continued therapy with AVANDAMET should be reviewed.

Hepatic effects: Another drug of the thiazolidinedione class, troglitazone, was associated with idiosyncratic hepatotoxicity, and very rare cases of liver failure, liver transplants, and death were reported during clinical use. In pre-approval controlled clinical trials in patients with type 2 diabetes, troglitazone was more frequently associated with clinically significant elevations in liver enzymes (ALT >3X upper limit of normal) compared to placebo. Very rare cases of reversible jaundice were also reported.

In pre-approval clinical studies in 4598 patients treated with rosiglitazone maleate, encompassing approximately 3600 patient years of exposure, there was no signal of drug-induced hepatotoxicity or elevation of ALT levels. In the pre-approval controlled trials, 0.2% of patients treated with rosiglitazone had elevations in ALT >3X the upper limit of normal compared to 0.2% on placebo and 0.5% on active comparators. The ALT elevations in patients treated with rosiglitazone were reversible and were not clearly causally related to therapy with rosiglitazone.

In postmarketing experience with rosiglitazone maleate, reports of hepatitis and of hepatic enzyme elevations to three or more times the upper limit of normal have been received. Very rarely, these reports have involved hepatic failure with and without fatal outcome, although causality has not been established. Rosiglitazone is structurally related to troglitazone, a thiazolidinedione no longer marketed in the United States, which was associated with idiosyncratic hepatotoxicity and rare cases of liver failure, liver transplants, and death during clinical use. Pending the availability of the results of additional large, long-term controlled clinical trials and additional postmarketing safety data, it is recommended that patients treated with AVANDAMET undergo periodic monitoring of liver enzymes.

Liver enzymes should be checked prior to the initiation of therapy with AVANDAMET in all patients. Therapy with AVANDAMET should not be initiated in patients with increased baseline liver enzyme levels (ALT >2.5X upper limit of normal). In patients with normal baseline liver enzymes, following initiation of therapy with AVANDAMET, it is recommended that liver enzymes be monitored every 2 months for the first 12 months, and periodically thereafter. Patients with mildly elevated liver enzymes (ALT levels ≤ 2.5X upper limit of normal) at baseline or during therapy with AVANDAMET should be evaluated to determine the cause of the liver enzyme elevation. Initiation of, or continuation of, therapy with AVANDAMET in patients with mild liver enzyme elevations should proceed with caution and include close clinical follow-up, including more frequent liver enzyme monitoring, to determine if the liver enzyme elevations resolve or worsen. If at any time ALT levels increase to >3X the upper limit of normal in patients on therapy with AVANDAMET, liver enzyme levels should be rechecked as soon as possible. If ALT levels remain >3X the upper limit of normal, therapy with AVANDAMET should be discontinued. There are no data available from clinical trials to evaluate the safety of AVANDAMET in patients who experienced liver abnormalities, hepatic dysfunction, or jaundice while on troglitazone. AVANDAMET should not be used in patients who experienced jaundice while taking troglitazone. If any patient develops symptoms suggesting hepatic dysfunction, which may include unexplained nausea, vomiting, abdominal pain, fatigue, anorexia and/or dark urine, liver enzymes should be checked. If jaundice is observed, drug therapy should be discontinued.

In addition, if the presence of hepatic disease or hepatic dysfunction of sufficient magnitude to predispose to lactic acidosis is confirmed, therapy with AVANDAMET should be discontinued.

Laboratory Tests: Periodic fasting blood glucose and HbA1c measurements should be performed to monitor therapeutic response.

Liver enzyme monitoring is recommended prior to initiation of therapy with AVANDAMET in all patients and periodically thereafter (see PRECAUTIONS, Hepatic effects and ADVERSE REACTIONS, Serum Transaminase Levels).

Initial and periodic monitoring of hematologic parameters (e.g., hemoglobin/hematocrit and red blood cell indices) and renal function (serum creatinine) should be performed, at least on an annual basis. While megaloblastic anemia has rarely been seen with metformin therapy, if this is suspected, vitamin B_{12} deficiency should be excluded.

Information for Patients: Patients should be informed of the potential risks and advantages of AVANDAMET and of alternative modes of therapy. They should also be informed about the importance of adherence to dietary instructions, weight loss, and a regular exercise program because they help improve insulin sensitivity. The importance of regular testing of blood glucose, glycosylated hemoglobin (HbA1c), renal function and hematologic parameters should be emphasized. Patients should be advised that AVANDAMET can begin to take effect 1-2 weeks after initiation, however it can take 2-3 months to see the full effect of glycemic improvement.

The risks of lactic acidosis, its symptoms, and conditions that predispose to its development, as noted in the WARNINGS and PRECAUTIONS sections, should be explained to patients. Patients should be advised to discontinue AVANDAMET immediately and to promptly notify their health practitioner if unexplained hyperventilation, myalgia, malaise, unusual somnolence or other nonspecific symptoms occur. Once a patient is stabilized on any dose level of AVANDAMET, gastrointestinal symptoms, which are common during initiation of metformin therapy, are unlikely to be drug related. Later occurrence of gastrointestinal symptoms could be due to lactic acidosis or other serious disease.

Patients should be counselled against excessive alcohol intake, either acute or chronic, while receiving AVANDAMET. Patients should be informed that blood will be drawn to check their liver function prior to the start of therapy and every 2 months for the first 12 months, and periodically thereafter. Patients with unexplained symptoms of nausea, vomiting, abdominal pain, fatigue, anorexia, or dark urine should immediately report these symptoms to their physician.

Patients who experience an unusually rapid increase in weight or edema or who develop shortness of breath or other symptoms of heart failure while on AVANDAMET should immediately report these symptoms to their physician.

Therapy with AVANDAMET, like other thiazolidinediones, may result in ovulation in some premenopausal anovulatory women. As a result, these patients may be at an increased risk for pregnancy while taking AVANDAMET (see PRECAUTIONS, Pregnancy, Pregnancy Category C). Thus, adequate contraception in premenopausal women should be recommended. This possible effect has not been specifically investigated in clinical studies so the frequency of this occurrence is not known.

Continued on next page

Avandamet—Cont.

Drug Interactions: ***Rosiglitazone maleate:*** Drugs Metabolized by Cytochrome P_{450}: *In vitro* drug metabolism studies suggest that rosiglitazone does not inhibit any of the major P_{450} enzymes at clinically relevant concentrations. *In vitro* data demonstrate that rosiglitazone is predominantly metabolized by CYP2C8, and to a lesser extent, 2C9.

Rosiglitazone (4 mg twice daily) was shown to have no clinically relevant effect on the pharmacokinetics of nifedipine and oral contraceptives (ethinylestradiol and norethindrone), which are predominantly metabolized by CYP3A4.

Metformin hydrochloride: Furosemide: A single-dose, metformin-furosemide drug interaction study in healthy subjects demonstrated that pharmacokinetic parameters of both compounds were affected by coadministration. Furosemide increased the metformin plasma and blood C_{max} by 22% and blood AUC by 15%, without any significant change in metformin renal clearance. When administered with metformin, the C_{max} and AUC of furosemide were 31% and 12% smaller, respectively, than when administered alone, and the terminal half-life was decreased by 32%, without any significant change in furosemide renal clearance. No information is available about the interaction of metformin and furosemide when coadministered chronically.

Nifedipine: A single-dose, metformin-nifedipine drug interaction study in normal healthy volunteers demonstrated that coadministration of nifedipine increased plasma metformin C_{max} and AUC by 20% and 9%, respectively, and increased the amount excreted in the urine. T_{max} and half-life were unaffected. Nifedipine appears to enhance the absorption of metformin. Metformin had minimal effects on nifedipine.

Cationic Drugs: Cationic drugs (e.g., amiloride, digoxin, morphine, procainamide, quinidine, quinine, ranitidine, triamterene, trimethoprim, and vancomycin) that are eliminated by renal tubular secretion theoretically have the potential for interaction with metformin by competing for common renal tubular transport systems. Such interaction between metformin and oral cimetidine has been observed in normal healthy volunteers in both single- and multiple-dose, metformin-cimetidine drug interaction studies, with a 60% increase in peak metformin plasma and whole blood concentrations and a 40% increase in plasma and whole blood metformin AUC. There was no change in elimination half-life in the single-dose study. Metformin had no effect on cimetidine pharmacokinetics. Although such interactions remain theoretical (except for cimetidine), careful patient monitoring and dose adjustment of AVANDAMET and/or the interfering drug is recommended in patients who are taking cationic medications that are excreted via the proximal renal tubular secretory system.

Other: Certain drugs tend to produce hyperglycemia and may lead to loss of glycemic control. These drugs include thiazides and other diuretics, corticosteroids, phenothiazines, thyroid products, estrogens, oral contraceptives, phenytoin, nicotinic acid, sympathomimetics, calcium channel blocking drugs, and isoniazid. When such drugs are administered to a patient receiving AVANDAMET, the patient should be closely observed to maintain adequate glycemic control.

In healthy volunteers, the pharmacokinetics of metformin and propranolol and metformin and ibuprofen were not affected when coadministered in single-dose interaction studies.

Metformin is negligibly bound to plasma proteins and is therefore, less likely to interact with highly protein-bound drugs such as salicylates, sulfonamides, chloramphenicol and probenecid.

Carcinogenesis, Mutagenesis, Impairment of Fertility: No animal studies have been conducted with the combined products in AVANDAMET. The following data are based on findings in studies performed with rosiglitazone or metformin individually.

Rosiglitazone maleate: A 2-year carcinogenicity study was conducted in Charles River CD-1 mice at doses of 0.4, 1.5, and 6 mg/kg/day in the diet (highest dose equivalent to approximately 12 times human AUC at the maximum recommended human daily dose of the rosiglitazone component of AVANDAMET). Sprague-Dawley rats were dosed for 2 years by oral gavage at doses of 0.05, 0.3, and 2 mg/kg/day (highest dose equivalent to approximately 10 and 20 times human AUC at the maximum recommended human daily dose of the rosiglitazone component of AVANDAMET for male and female rats, respectively).

Rosiglitazone was not carcinogenic in the mouse. There was an increase in incidence of adipose hyperplasia in the mouse at doses ≥1.5 mg/kg/day (approximately 2 times human AUC at the maximum recommended human daily dose of the rosiglitazone component of AVANDAMET). In rats, there was a significant increase in the incidence of benign adipose tissue tumors (lipomas) at doses ≥0.3 mg/kg/day (approximately 2 times human AUC at the maximum recommended human daily dose of the rosiglitazone component of AVANDAMET). These proliferative changes in both species are considered due to the persistent pharmacological overstimulation of adipose tissue.

Rosiglitazone was not mutagenic or clastogenic in the *in vitro* bacterial assays for gene mutation, the *in vitro* chromosome aberration test in human lymphocytes, the *in vivo* mouse micronucleus test, and the *in vivo*/*in vitro* rat UDS assay. There was a small (about 2-fold) increase in mutation in the *in vitro* mouse lymphoma assay in the presence of metabolic activation.

Rosiglitazone had no effects on mating or fertility of male rats given up to 40 mg/kg/day (approximately 116 times human AUC at the maximum recommended human daily dose of the rosiglitazone component of AVANDAMET). Rosiglitazone altered estrous cyclicity (2 mg/kg/day) and reduced fertility (40 mg/kg/day) of female rats in association with lower plasma levels of progesterone and estradiol (approximately 20 and 200 times human AUC at the maximum recommended human daily dose of the rosiglitazone component of AVANDAMET, respectively). No such effects were noted at 0.2 mg/kg/day (approximately 3 times human AUC at the maximum recommended human daily dose of the rosiglitazone component of AVANDAMET). In monkeys, rosiglitazone (0.6 and 4.6 mg/kg/day; approximately 3 and 15 times human AUC at the maximum recommended human daily dose of the rosiglitazone component of AVANDAMET, respectively) diminished the follicular phase rise in serum estradiol with consequential reduction in the luteinizing hormone surge, lower luteal phase progesterone levels, and amenorrhea. The mechanism for these effects appears to be direct inhibition of ovarian steroidogenesis.

Metformin hydrochloride: Long-term carcinogenicity studies have been performed in rats (dosing duration of 104 weeks) and mice (dosing duration of 91 weeks) at doses up to and including 900 mg/kg/day and 1500 mg/kg/day, respectively. These doses are both approximately four times the maximum recommended human daily dose of 2000 mg of the metformin component of AVANDAMET based on body surface area comparisons. No evidence of carcinogenicity with metformin was found in either male or female mice. Similarly, there was no tumorigenic potential observed with metformin in male rats. There was, however, an increased incidence of benign stromal uterine polyps in female rats treated with 900 mg/kg/day.

There was no evidence of mutagenic potential of metformin in the following *in vitro* tests: Ames test (*S. typhimurium*), gene mutation test (mouse lymphoma cells), or chromosomal aberrations test (human lymphocytes). Results in the *in vivo* mouse micronucleus test were also negative.

Fertility of male or female rats was unaffected by metformin when administrated at doses as high as 600 mg/kg/day, which is approximately three times the maximum recommended human daily dose of the metformin component of AVANDAMET based on body surface area comparisons.

Animal Toxicology: Heart weights were increased in mice (3 mg/kg/day), rats (5 mg/kg/day), and dogs (2 mg/kg/day) with rosiglitazone treatments (approximately 5, 22, and 2 times human AUC at the maximum recommended human daily dose of the rosiglitazone component of AVANDAMET, respectively). Morphometric measurement indicated that there was hypertrophy in cardiac ventricular tissues, which may be due to increased heart work as a result of plasma volume expansion.

Pregnancy: Pregnancy Category C: Because current information strongly suggests that abnormal blood glucose levels during pregnancy are associated with a higher incidence of congenital anomalies as well as increased neonatal morbidity and mortality, most experts recommend that insulin monotherapy be used during pregnancy to maintain blood glucose levels as close to normal as possible. AVANDAMET should not be used during pregnancy unless the potential benefit justifies the potential risk to the fetus.

There are no adequate and well-controlled studies in pregnant women with AVANDAMET or its individual components. No animal studies have been conducted with the combined products in AVANDAMET. The following data are based on findings in studies performed with rosiglitazone or metformin individually.

Rosiglitazone maleate: There was no effect on implantation or the embryo with rosiglitazone treatment during early pregnancy in rats, but treatment during mid-late gestation was associated with fetal death and growth retardation in both rats and rabbits. Teratogenicity was not observed at doses up to 3 mg/kg in rats and 100 mg/kg in rabbits (approximately 20 and 75 times human AUC at the maximum recommended human daily dose of the rosiglitazone component of AVANDAMET, respectively). Rosiglitazone caused placental pathology in rats (3 mg/kg/day). Treatment of rats during gestation through lactation reduced litter size, neonatal viability, and postnatal growth, with growth retardation reversible after puberty. For effects on the placenta, embryo/fetus, and offspring, the no-effect dose was 0.2 mg/kg/day in rats and 15 mg/kg/day in rabbits. These no-effect levels are approximately 4 times human AUC at the maximum recommended human daily dose of the rosiglitazone component of AVANDAMET.

Metformin hydrochloride: Metformin was not teratogenic in rats and rabbits at doses up to 600 mg/kg/day. This represents an exposure of about two and six times the maximum recommended human daily dose of 2000 mg based on body surface area comparisons for rats and rabbits, respectively. Determination of fetal concentrations demonstrated a partial placental barrier to metformin.

Labor and Delivery: The effect of AVANDAMET or its components on labor and delivery in humans is unknown.

Nursing Mothers: No studies have been conducted with the combined components of AVANDAMET. In studies performed with the individual components, both rosiglitazone-related material and metformin were detectable in milk from lactating rats. It is not known whether rosiglitazone and/or metformin is excreted in human milk. Because many drugs are excreted in human milk, AVANDAMET should not be administered to a nursing woman. If AVANDAMET is discontinued, and if diet alone is inadequate for controlling blood glucose, insulin therapy should be considered.

Pediatric Use: Safety and effectiveness of AVANDAMET in pediatric patients have not been established.

Geriatric Use: Metformin is known to be substantially excreted by the kidney and because the risk of serious adverse reactions to the drug is greater in patients with impaired renal function, AVANDAMET should only be used in patients with normal renal function (see CONTRAINDICATIONS, WARNINGS, and CLINICAL PHARMACOLOGY, Pharmacokinetics). Because aging is associated with reduced renal function, AVANDAMET should be used with caution as age increases. Care should be taken in dose selection and should be based on careful and regular monitoring of renal function. Generally, elderly patients should not be titrated to the maximum dose of AVANDAMET (see also WARNINGS, DOSAGE AND ADMINISTRATION).

ADVERSE REACTIONS

The incidence and types of adverse events reported in controlled, 26-week clinical trials in association with rosiglitazone maleate in combination with doses of metformin hydrochloride of 2500 mg/day are shown in Table 4, in comparison to adverse reactions reported in association with rosiglitazone and metformin monotherapies.

[See table 4 below]

Reports of hypoglycemia in patients treated with rosiglitazone and maximum metformin combination therapy were more frequent than in patients treated with rosiglitazone or metformin monotherapies. In double-blind studies, hypoglycemia was reported by 3.0% of patients receiving rosiglitazone in combination with maximum doses of metformin, by 1.3% of patients receiving metformin monotherapy, by 0.6% of patients receiving rosiglitazone as monotherapy, and by 0.2% of patients receiving placebo.

There were a small number of patients treated with rosiglitazone who had adverse events of anemia and edema. Overall, these events were generally mild to moderate in severity and usually did not require discontinuation of treatment with rosiglitazone.

Edema was reported in 4.8% of patients receiving rosiglitazone compared to 1.3% on placebo, and 2.2% on metformin monotherapy and 4.4% on rosiglitazone in combination with maximum doses of metformin. Overall, the types of adverse experiences reported when rosiglitazone was used in combination with metformin were similar to those during monotherapy with rosiglitazone. Reports of anemia (7.1%) were greater in patients treated with a combination of rosiglitazone and metformin compared to monotherapy with rosiglitazone.

Lower pre-treatment hemoglobin/hematocrit levels in patients enrolled in the metformin combination clinical trials may have contributed to the higher reporting rate of anemia in these studies (see ADVERSE REACTIONS, Laboratory Abnormalities, Hematologic).

In 26-week double-blind studies, edema was reported with higher frequency in the rosiglitazone plus insulin combination trials (insulin, 5.4%; and rosiglitazone in combination with insulin, 14.7%). Reports of new onset or exacerbation of congestive heart failure occurred at rates of 1% for insulin alone, and 2% (4 mg) and 3% (8 mg) for insulin in combination with rosiglitazone (see WARNINGS, Cardiac Failure and Other Cardiac Effects).

Table 4. Adverse Events (≥5% in Any Treatment Group) Reported by Patients in 26-week Double-blind Clinical Trials

	Rosiglitazone monotherapy N = 2526	Placebo N = 601	Metformin monotherapy N = 225	Rosiglitazone plus metformin N = 338
Preferred term	%	%	%	%
Upper respiratory tract infection	9.9	8.7	8.9	16.0
Injury	7.6	4.3	7.6	8.0
Headache	5.9	5.0	8.9	6.5
Back pain	4.0	3.8	4.0	5.0
Hyperglycemia	3.9	5.7	4.4	2.1
Fatigue	3.6	5.0	4.0	5.9
Sinusitis	3.2	4.5	5.3	6.2
Diarrhea	2.3	3.3	15.6	12.7
Viral infection	3.2	4.0	3.6	5.0
Arthralgia	3.0	4.0	2.2	5.0
Anemia	1.9	0.7	2.2	7.1

In postmarketing experience with rosiglitazone maleate, adverse events potentially related to volume expansion (e.g., congestive heart failure, pulmonary edema, and pleural effusions) have been reported.

(See also GLUCOPHAGE[1] prescribing information, ADVERSE REACTIONS).

Laboratory Abnormalities: Hematologic: Decreases in mean hemoglobin and hematocrit occurred in a dose-related fashion in patients treated with rosiglitazone maleate (mean decreases in individual studies up to 1.0 gram/dL hemoglobin and up to 3.3% hematocrit). The time course and magnitude of decreases were similar in patients treated with a combination of rosiglitazone and other hypoglycemic agents or rosiglitazone monotherapy. Pre-treatment levels of hemoglobin and hematocrit were lower in patients in metformin combination studies and may have contributed to the higher reporting rate of anemia. White blood cell counts also decreased slightly in patients treated with rosiglitazone. Decreases in hematologic parameters may be related to increased plasma volume observed with rosiglitazone treatment.

In controlled clinical trials of metformin hydrochloride of 29 weeks' duration, a decrease to subnormal levels of previously normal serum vitamin B_{12} levels, without clinical manifestations, was observed in approximately 7% of patients. Such decrease, possibly due to interference with B_{12} absorption from the B_{12}-intrinsic factor complex, is, however, very rarely associated with anemia and appears to be rapidly reversible with discontinuation of metformin or vitamin B_{12} supplementation.

Lipids: Changes in serum lipids have been observed following treatment with rosiglitazone maleate (see CLINICAL STUDIES).

Serum Transaminase Levels: In clinical studies in 4598 patients treated with rosiglitazone maleate encompassing approximately 3600 patient years of exposure, there was no evidence of drug-induced hepatotoxicity or elevated ALT levels.

In controlled trials, 0.2% of patients treated with rosiglitazone maleate had reversible elevations in ALT >3X the upper limit of normal compared to 0.2% on placebo and 0.5% on active comparators. Hyperbilirubinemia was found in 0.3% of patients treated with rosiglitazone compared with 0.9% treated with placebo and 1% in patients treated with active comparators.

In the clinical program including long-term, open-label experience, the rate per 100 patient years' exposure of ALT increase to >3X the upper limit of normal was 0.35 for patients treated with rosiglitazone maleate, 0.59 for placebo-treated patients, and 0.78 for patients treated with active comparator agents.

In pre-approval clinical trials, there were no cases of idiosyncratic drug reactions leading to hepatic failure. In postmarketing experience with rosiglitazone maleate, reports of hepatic enzyme elevations three or more times the upper limit of normal and hepatitis have been received (see PRECAUTIONS, Hepatic effects).

OVERDOSAGE

Rosiglitazone maleate: Limited data are available with regard to overdosage in humans. In clinical studies in volunteers, rosiglitazone has been administered at single oral doses of up to 20 mg and was well-tolerated. In the event of an overdose, appropriate supportive treatment should be initiated as dictated by the patients clinical status.

Metformin hydrochloride: Hypoglycemia has not been seen with ingestion of up to 85 grams of metformin hydrochloride, although lactic acidosis has occurred in such circumstances (see WARNINGS). Metformin is dialyzable with a clearance of up to 170 mL/min under good hemodynamic conditions. Therefore, hemodialysis may be useful for removal of accumulated metformin from patients in whom metformin overdosage is suspected.

DOSAGE AND ADMINISTRATION

General

The selection of the dose of AVANDAMET should be based on the patient's current doses of rosiglitazone and/or metformin.

The safety and efficacy of AVANDAMET as initial therapy for patients with type 2 diabetes melllitus have not been established.

The following recommendations regarding the use of AVANDAMET in patients inadequately controlled on rosiglitazone and metformin monotherapies are based on clinical practice experience with rosiglitazone and metformin combination therapy.

- The dosage of antidiabetic therapy with AVANDAMET should be individualized on the basis of effectiveness and tolerability while not exceeding the maximum recommended daily dose of 8 mg/2000 mg.
- AVANDAMET should be given in divided doses with meals, with gradual dose escalation. This reduces GI side effects (largely due to metformin) and permits determination of the minimum effective dose for the individual patient.
- Sufficient time should be given to assess adequacy of therapeutic response. Fasting plasma glucose (FPG) should be used to determine the therapeutic response to AVANDAMET. After an increase in metformin dosage, dose titration is recommended if patients are not adequately controlled after 1-2 weeks. After an increase in rosiglitazone dosage, dose titration is recommended if patients are not adequately controlled after 8-12 weeks.

Dosage Recommendations

For patients inadequately controlled on metformin monotherapy: the usual starting dose of AVANDAMET is 4 mg rosiglitazone (total daily dose) plus the dose of metformin already being taken (see Table 5).

For patients inadequately controlled on rosiglitazone monotherapy: the usual starting dose of AVANDAMET is 1000 mg metformin (total daily dose) plus the dose of rosiglitazone already being taken (see Table 5).

Table 5. AVANDAMET Starting Dose

PRIOR THERAPY	Usual AVANDAMET Starting Dose	
Total daily dose	Tablet strength	Number of tablets
Metformin HCl*		
1000 mg/day	2 mg/500 mg	1 tablet b.i.d.
2000 mg/day	1 mg/500 mg	2 tablets b.i.d.
Rosiglitazone		
4 mg/day	2 mg/500 mg	1 tablet b.i.d.
8 mg/day	4 mg/500 mg	1 tablet b.i.d.

*For patients on doses of metformin HCl between 1000 and 2000 mg/day, initiation of AVANDAMET requires individualization of therapy.

When switching from combination therapy of rosiglitazone plus metformin as separate tablets: the usual starting dose of AVANDAMET is the dose of rosiglitazone and metformin already being taken.

If additional glycemic control is needed: the daily dose of AVANDAMET may be increased by increments of 4 mg rosiglitazone and/or 500 mg metformin, up to the maximum recommended total daily dose of 8 mg/2000 mg.

No studies have been performed specifically examining the safety and efficacy of AVANDAMET in patients previously treated with other oral hypoglycemic agents and switched to AVANDAMET. Any change in therapy of type 2 diabetes should be undertaken with care and appropriate monitoring as changes in glycemic control can occur.

Specific Patient Populations

AVANDAMET is not recommended for use in pregnancy or for use in pediatric patients.

The initial and maintenance dosing of AVANDAMET should be conservative in patients with advanced age, due to the potential for decreased renal function in this population. Any dosage adjustment should be based on a careful assessment of renal function. Generally, elderly, debilitated, and malnourished patients should not be titrated to the maximum dose of AVANDAMET. Monitoring of renal function is necessary to aid in prevention of metformin-associated lactic acidosis, particularly in the elderly (see WARNINGS).

Therapy with AVANDAMET should not be initiated if the patient exhibits clinical evidence of active liver disease or increased serum transaminase levels (ALT >2.5X upper limit of normal at start of therapy) (see PRECAUTIONS, Hepatic effects and CLINICAL PHARMACOLOGY, Hepatic Impairment). Liver enzyme monitoring is recommended in all patients prior to initiation of therapy with AVANDAMET and periodically thereafter (see PRECAUTIONS, Hepatic effects).

HOW SUPPLIED

Tablets: Each tablet contains rosiglitazone as the maleate and metformin hydrochloride as follows:

1 mg/500 mg — yellow, film coated oval tablet, debossed with gsk on one side and 1/500 on the other.

2 mg/500 mg — pale pink, film coated oval tablet, debossed with gsk on one side and 2/500 on the other.

4 mg/500 mg — orange, film coated oval tablet, debossed with gsk on one side and 4/500 on the other.

1 mg/500 mg bottles of 60: NDC 0007-3166-18
1 mg/500 mg bottles of 100: NDC 0007-3166-20
1 mg/500 mg SUP 100s: NDC 0007-3166-21

2 mg/500 mg bottles of 60: NDC 0007-3167-18
2 mg/500 mg bottles of 100: NDC 0007-3167-20
2 mg/500 mg SUP 100s: NDC 0007-3167-21

4 mg/500 mg bottles of 60: NDC 0007-3168-18
4 mg/500 mg bottles of 100: NDC 0007-3168-20
4 mg/500 mg SUP 100s: NDC 0007-3168-21

STORAGE

Store at 25°C (77°F); excursions permitted to 15-30°C (59-86°F).

Dispense in a tight, light-resistant container.

[1]GLUCOPHAGE® is a registered trademark of Merck Santé S.A.S., an associate of Merck KGaA of Darmstadt, Germany. Licensed to Bristol-Myers Squibb Company.

GlaxoSmithKline, Research Triangle Park, NC 27709
©2002, GlaxoSmithKline. All rights reserved.
October 2002/AT:L1

AVODART™ ℞

[*av' ō dart*]
(dutasteride)
Soft Gelatin Capsules

DESCRIPTION

AVODART (dutasteride) is a synthetic 4-azasteroid compound that is a selective inhibitor of both the type 1 and type 2 isoforms of steroid 5α-reductase (5AR), an intracellular enzyme that converts testosterone to 5α-dihydrotestosterone (DHT).

Dutasteride is chemically designated as (5α,17β)-N-{2,5 bis(trifluoromethyl)phenyl}-3-oxo-4-azaandrost-1-ene-17-carboxamide. The empirical formula of dutasteride is $C_{27}H_{30}F_6N_2O_2$, representing a molecular weight of 528.5 with the following structural formula:

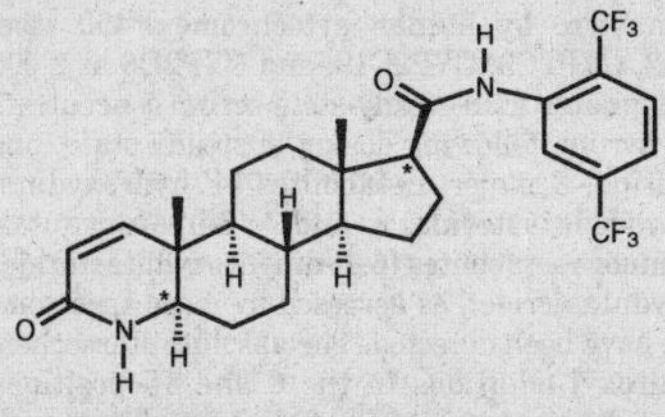

Dutasteride is a white to pale yellow powder with a melting point of 242° to 250°C. It is soluble in ethanol (44 mg/mL), methanol (64 mg/mL) and polyethylene glycol 400 (3 mg/mL), but it is insoluble in water.

AVODART Soft Gelatin Capsules for oral administration contain 0.5 mg of the active ingredient dutasteride in yellow capsules with red print. Each capsule contains 0.5 mg dutasteride dissolved in a mixture of mono-di-glycerides of caprylic/capric acid and butylated hydroxytoluene. The inactive excipients in the capsule shell are gelatin (from certified BSE-free bovine sources), glycerin, and ferric oxide (yellow). The soft gelatin capsules are printed with edible red ink.

CLINICAL PHARMACOLOGY

Pharmacodynamics: ***Mechanism of Action:*** Dutasteride inhibits the conversion of testosterone to 5α-dihydrotestosterone (DHT). DHT is the androgen primarily responsible for the initial development and subsequent enlargement of the prostate gland. Testosterone is converted to DHT by the enzyme 5α-reductase, which exists as 2 isoforms, type 1 and type 2. The type 2 isoenzyme is primarily active in the reproductive tissues while the type 1 isoenzyme is also responsible for testosterone conversion in the skin and liver. Dutasteride is a competitive and specific inhibitor of both type 1 and type 2 5α-reductase isoenzymes, with which it forms a stable enzyme complex. Dissociation from this complex has been evaluated under in vitro and in vivo conditions and is extremely slow. Dutasteride does not bind to the human androgen receptor.

Effect on DHT and Testosterone: The maximum effect of daily doses of dutasteride on the reduction of DHT is dose dependent and is observed within 1 to 2 weeks. After 1 and 2 weeks of daily dosing with dutasteride 0.5 mg, median serum DHT concentrations were reduced by 85% and 90%, respectively. In patients with BPH treated with dutasteride 0.5 mg/day for 2 years, the median decrease in serum DHT was 94% at 1 year and 93% at 2 years. The median increase in serum testosterone was 19% at both 1 and 2 years but remained within the physiologic range.

In BPH patients treated with 5 mg/day of dutasteride or placebo for up to 12 weeks prior to transurethral resection of the prostate, mean DHT concentrations in prostatic tissue were significantly lower in the dutasteride group compared with placebo (784 and 5,793 pg/g, respectively, $p<0.001$). Mean prostatic tissue concentrations of testosterone were significantly higher in the dutasteride group compared with placebo (2,073 and 93 pg/g, respectively, $p<0.001$).

Adult males with genetically inherited type 2 5α-reductase deficiency also have decreased DHT levels. These 5α-reductase deficient males have a small prostate gland throughout life and do not develop BPH. Except for the associated urogenital defects present at birth, no other clinical abnormalities related to 5α-reductase deficiency have been observed in these individuals.

Other Effects: Plasma lipid panel and bone mineral density were evaluated following 52 weeks of dutasteride 0.5 mg once daily in healthy volunteers. There was no change in bone mineral density as measured by dual energy x-ray absorptiometry (DEXA) compared with either placebo or baseline. In addition, the plasma lipid profile (i.e., total cholesterol, low density lipoproteins, high density lipoproteins, and triglycerides) was unaffected by dutasteride. No clinically significant changes in adrenal hormone responses to ACTH stimulation were observed in a subset population (n = 13) of the one-year healthy volunteer study.

Pharmacokinetics: ***Absorption:*** Following administration of a single 0.5-mg dose of a soft gelatin capsule, time to peak serum concentrations (T_{max}) of dutasteride occurs within 2 to 3 hours. Absolute bioavailability in 5 healthy subjects is approximately 60% (range 40% to 94%). When the drug is administered with food, the maximum serum concentrations were reduced by 10% to 15%. This reduction is of no clinical significance.

Distribution: Pharmacokinetic data following single and repeat oral doses show that dutasteride has a large volume of distribution (300 to 500 L). Dutasteride is highly bound to plasma albumin (99.0%) and alpha-1 acid glycoprotein (96.6%).

In a study of healthy subjects (n = 26) receiving dutasteride 0.5 mg/day for 12 months, semen dutasteride concentrations averaged 3.4 ng/mL (range 0.4 to 14 ng/mL) at 12 months and, similar to serum, achieved steady-state con-

Continued on next page

Avodart—Cont.

centrations at 6 months. On average, at 12 months, 11.5% of serum dutasteride concentrations partitioned into semen.

Metabolism and Elimination: Dutasteride is extensively metabolized in humans. While not all metabolic pathways have been identified, in vitro studies showed that dutasteride is metabolized by the CYP3A4 isoenzyme to 2 minor mono-hydroxylated metabolites. Dutasteride is not metabolized in vitro by human cytochrome P450 isoenzymes CYP1A2, CYP2C9, CYP2C19, and CYP2D6 at 2,000 ng/mL (50-fold greater than steady-state serum concentrations). In human serum, following dosing to steady state, unchanged dutasteride, 3 major metabolites (4′-hydroxydutasteride, 1,2-dihydrodutasteride, and 6-hydroxydutasteride), and 2 minor metabolites (6,4′-dihydroxydutasteride and 15-hydroxydutasteride), as assessed by mass spectrometric response, have been detected. The absolute stereochemistry of the hydroxyl additions in the 6 and 15 positions is not known. In vitro, the 4′-hydroxydutasteride and 1, 2-dihydrodutasteride metabolites are much less potent than dutasteride against both isoforms of human 5AR. The activity of 6β-hydroxydutasteride is comparable to that of dutasteride.

Dutasteride and its metabolites were excreted mainly in feces. As a percent of dose, there was approximately 5% unchanged dutasteride (~1% to ~15%) and 40% as dutasteride-related metabolites (~2% to ~90%). Only trace amounts of unchanged dutasteride were found in urine (<1%). Therefore, on average, the dose unaccounted for approximated 55% (range 5% to 97%).

The terminal elimination half-life of dutasteride is approximately 5 weeks at steady state. The average steady-state serum dutasteride concentration was 40 ng/mL following 0.5 mg/day for 1 year. Following daily dosing, dutasteride serum concentrations achieve 65% of steady-state concentration after 1 month and approximately 90% after 3 months. Due to the long half-life of dutasteride, serum concentrations remain detectable (greater than 0.1 ng/mL) for up to 4 to 6 months after discontinuation of treatment.

Special Populations: ***Pediatric:*** Dutasteride pharmacokinetics have not been investigated in subjects less than 18 years of age.

Geriatric: No dose adjustment is necessary in the elderly. The pharmacokinetics and pharmacodynamics of dutasteride were evaluated in 36 healthy male subjects between the ages of 24 and 87 years following administration of a single 5-mg dose of dutasteride. In this single-dose study, dutasteride half-life increased with age (approximately 170 hours in men 20 to 49 years of age, approximately 260 hours in men 50 to 69 years of age, and approximately 300 hours in men over 70 years of age). Of 2,167 men treated with dutasteride in the 3 pivotal studies, 60% were age 65 and over and 15% were age 75 and over. No overall differences in safety or efficacy were observed between these patients and younger patients.

Gender: AVODART is not indicated for use in women (see WARNINGS and PRECAUTIONS). The pharmacokinetics of dutasteride in women have not been studied.

Race: The effect of race on dutasteride pharmacokinetics has not been studied.

Renal Impairment: The effect of renal impairment on dutasteride pharmacokinetics has not been studied. However, less than 0.1% of a steady-state 0.5-mg dose of dutasteride is recovered in human urine, so no adjustment in dosage is anticipated for patients with renal impairment.

Hepatic Impairment: The effect of hepatic impairment on dutasteride pharmacokinetics has not been studied. Because dutasteride is extensively metabolized, exposure could be higher in hepatically impaired patients (see PRECAUTIONS: Use in Hepatic Impairment).

Drug Interactions: In vitro drug metabolism studies reveal that dutasteride is metabolized by human cytochrome P450 isoenzyme CYP3A4. In a human mass balance analysis (n = 8), dutasteride was extensively metabolized. Less than 20% of the dose was excreted unchanged in the feces. No clinical drug interaction studies have been performed to evaluate the impact of CYP3A4 enzyme inhibitors on dutasteride pharmacokinetics. However, based on the in vitro data, blood concentrations of dutasteride may increase in the presence of inhibitors of CYP3A4 such as ritonavir, ketoconazole, verapamil, diltiazem, cimetidine, and ciprofloxacin. Dutasteride is not metabolized in vitro by human cytochrome P450 isoenzymes CYP1A2, CYP2C9, CYP2C19, and CYP2D6 at 2,000 ng/mL (50-fold greater than steady-state serum concentrations).

Clinical drug interaction studies have shown no pharmacokinetic or pharmacodynamic interactions between dutasteride and tamsulosin, terazosin, warfarin, digoxin, and cholestyramine (see PRECAUTIONS: Drug Interactions).

Dutasteride does not inhibit the in vitro metabolism of model substrates for the major human cytochrome P450 isoenzymes (CYP1A2, CYP2C9, CYP2C19, CYP2D6, and CYP3A4) at a concentration of 1,000 ng/mL, 25 times greater than steady-state serum concentrations in humans.

CLINICAL STUDIES

Dutasteride 0.5 mg/day (n = 2,167) or placebo (n = 2,158) was evaluated in male subjects with BPH in three 2-year multicenter, placebo-controlled, double-blind studies, each with 2-year open-label extensions. Data from the first 24 months of the trials are presented. More than 90% of the study population was Caucasian. Subjects were at least 50 years of age with a serum PSA ≥1.5 ng/mL and <10 ng/mL, and BPH diagnosed by medical history and physical examination, including enlarged prostate (≥30 cc) and BPH symptoms that were moderate to severe according to the American Urological Association Symptom Index (AUA-SI). Most of the 4,325 subjects randomly assigned to receive either dutasteride or placebo completed 2 years of treatment (70% and 67%, respectively).

Effect on Symptom Scores: Symptoms were quantified using the AUA-SI, a questionnaire that evaluates urinary symptoms (incomplete emptying, frequency, intermittency, urgency, weak stream, straining, and nocturia) by rating on a 0 to 5 scale for a total possible score of 35. The baseline AUA-SI score across the 3 studies was approximately 17 units in both treatment groups.

Subjects receiving dutasteride achieved statistically significant improvement in symptoms versus placebo by Month 3 in one study, and by Month 12 in the other 2 pivotal studies. At Month 12, the mean decrease from baseline in AUA-SI symptom scores across the 3 studies pooled was -3.3 units for dutasteride and -2.0 units for placebo with a mean difference between the 2 treatment groups of -1.3 (range, -1.1 to -1.5 units in each of the 3 studies, p<0.001) and was consistent across the 3 studies. At Month 24, the mean decrease from baseline was -3.8 units for dutasteride and -1.7 units for placebo with a mean difference of -2.1 (range, -1.9 to -2.2 units in each of the 3 studies, p<0.001). See Figure 1.

These studies were prospectively designed to evaluate effects on symptoms based on prostate size at baseline. In men with prostate volumes ≥40 cc, the mean decrease was -3.8 units for dutasteride and -1.6 units for placebo with a mean difference between the 2 treatment groups of -2.2 at Month 24. In men with prostate volumes <40 cc, the mean decrease was -3.7 units for dutasteride and -2.2 units for placebo with a mean difference between the 2 treatment groups of -1.5 at Month 24.

Figure 1. AUA Symptom Score* Change from Baseline (Pivotal Studies Pooled)

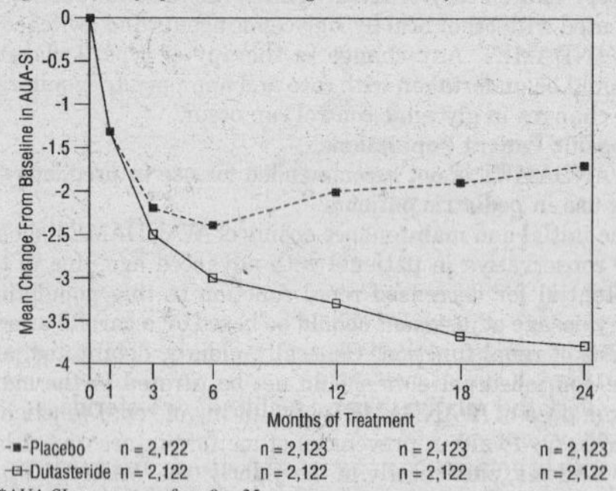

*AUA-SI score ranges from 0 to 35.

Effect on Acute Urinary Retention and the Need for Surgery: Efficacy was also assessed after 2 years of treatment by the incidence of acute urinary retention requiring catheterization and BPH-related urological surgical intervention. Compared with placebo, AVODART was associated with a statistically significantly lower incidence of acute urinary retention (1.8% for AVODART vs. 4.2% for placebo, p<0.001; 57% reduction in risk, 95% CI: [38-71%]) and with a statistically significantly lower incidence of surgery (2.2% for AVODART vs. 4.1% for placebo, p<0.001; 48% reduction in risk, 95% CI: [26-63%]). See Figures 2 and 3.

Figure 2. Percent of Subjects Developing Acute Urinary Retention Over a 24-Month Period (Pivotal Studies Pooled)

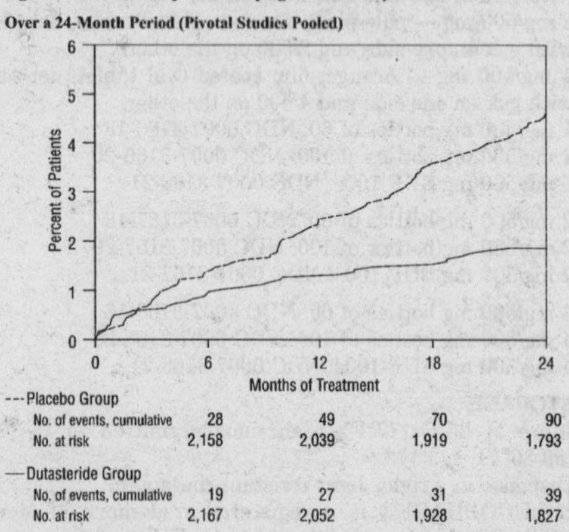

[See figure 3 at top of next column]

Effect on Prostate Volume: A prostate volume of at least 30 cc measured by transrectal ultrasound was required for study entry. The mean prostate volume at study entry was approximately 54 cc.

Statistically significant differences (dutasteride versus placebo) were noted at the earliest post-treatment prostate volume measurement in each study (Month 1, Month 3, or Month 6) and continued through Month 24. At Month 12, the mean percent change in prostate volume across the 3 studies pooled was -24.7% for dutasteride and -3.4% for placebo; the mean difference (dutasteride minus placebo) was -21.3% (range, -21.0% to -21.6% in each of the 3 studies, p<0.001). At Month 24, the mean percent change in prostate volume across the 3 studies pooled was -26.7% for

Figure 3. Percent of Subjects Having Surgery for BPH Over a 24-Month Period (Pivotal Studies Pooled)

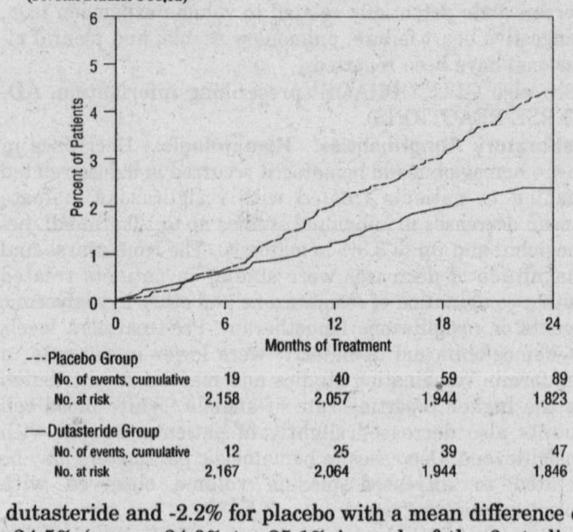

dutasteride and -2.2% for placebo with a mean difference of -24.5% (range -24.0% to -25.1% in each of the 3 studies, p<0.001). See Figure 4.

Figure 4. Prostate Volume Percent Change from Baseline (Pivotal Studies Pooled)

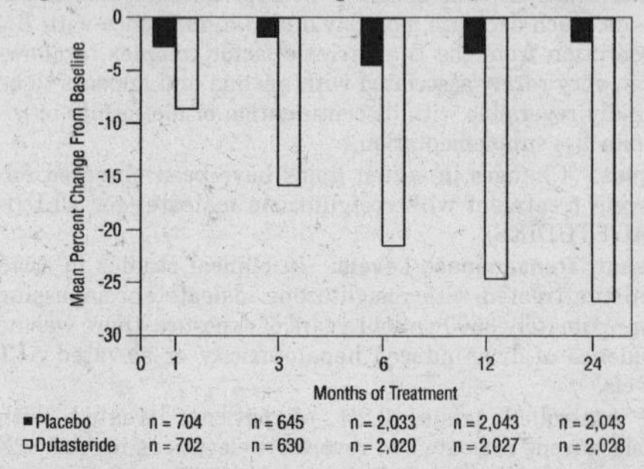

Effect on Maximum Urine Flow Rate: A mean peak urine flow rate (Q_{max}) of ≤15 mL/sec was required for study entry. Q_{max} was approximately 10 mL/sec at baseline across the 3 pivotal studies.

Differences between the 2 groups were statistically significant from baseline at Month 3 in all 3 studies and were maintained through Month 12. At Month 12, the mean increase in Q_{max} across the 3 studies pooled was 1.6 mL/sec for dutasteride and 0.7 mL/sec for placebo; the mean difference (dutasteride minus placebo) was 0.8 mL/sec (range, 0.7 to 1.0 mL/sec in each of the 3 studies, p<0.001). At Month 24, the mean increase in Q_{max} was 1.8 mL/sec for dutasteride and 0.7 mL/sec for placebo, with a mean difference of 1.1 mL/sec (range, 1.0 to 1.2 mL/sec in each of the 3 studies, p<0.001). See Figure 5.

Figure 5. Q_{max} Change from Baseline (Pivotal Studies Pooled)

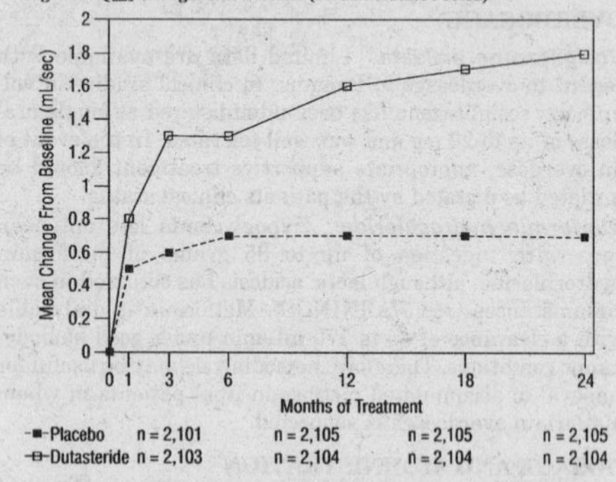

Summary of Clinical Studies: Data from 3 large, well-controlled efficacy studies demonstrate that treatment with AVODART (0.5 mg once daily) reduces the risk of both AUR and BPH-related surgical intervention relative to placebo, improves BPH-related symptoms, decreases prostate volume, and increases maximum urinary flow rates. These data suggest that AVODART arrests the disease process of BPH in men with an enlarged prostate.

INDICATIONS AND USAGE

AVODART is indicated for the treatment of symptomatic benign prostatic hyperplasia (BPH) in men with an enlarged prostate to:

- Improve symptoms
- Reduce the risk of acute urinary retention
- Reduce the risk of the need for BPH-related surgery

CONTRAINDICATIONS

AVODART is contraindicated for use in women and children.

AVODART is contraindicated for patients with known hypersensitivity to dutasteride, other 5α-reductase inhibitors, or any component of the preparation.

WARNINGS

Exposure of Women-Risk to Male Fetus: Dutasteride is absorbed through the skin. Therefore, women who are pregnant or may be pregnant should not handle AVODART Soft Gelatin Capsules because of the possibility of absorption of dutasteride and the potential risk of a fetal anomaly to a male fetus (see CONTRAINDICATIONS). In addition, women should use caution whenever handling AVODART Soft Gelatin Capsules. If contact is made with leaking capsules, the contact area should be washed immediately with soap and water.

PRECAUTIONS

General: Lower urinary tract symptoms of BPH can be indicative of other urological diseases, including prostate cancer. Patients should be assessed to rule out other urological diseases prior to treatment with AVODART. Patients with a large residual urinary volume and/or severely diminished urinary flow may not be good candidates for 5α-reductase inhibitor therapy and should be carefully monitored for obstructive uropathy.

Blood Donation: Men being treated with dutasteride should not donate blood until at least 6 months have passed following their last dose. The purpose of this deferred period is to prevent administration of dutasteride to a pregnant female transfusion recipient.

Use in Hepatic Impairment: The effect of hepatic impairment on dutasteride pharmacokinetics has not been studied. Because dutasteride is extensively metabolized and has a half-life of approximately 5 weeks at steady state, caution should be used in the administration of dutasteride to patients with liver disease.

Use with Potent CYP3A4 Inhibitors: Although dutasteride is extensively metabolized, no metabolically-based drug interaction studies have been conducted. The effect of potent CYP3A4 inhibitors has not been studied. Because of the potential for drug-drug interactions, care should be taken when administering dutasteride to patients taking potent, chronic CYP3A4 enzyme inhibitors (e.g., ritonavir).

Effects on PSA and Prostate Cancer Detection: Digital rectal examinations, as well as other evaluations for prostate cancer, should be performed on patients with BPH prior to initiating therapy with AVODART and periodically thereafter.

Dutasteride reduces total serum PSA concentration by approximately 40% following 3 months of treatment and approximately 50% following 6, 12, and 24 months of treatment. This decrease is predictable over the entire range of PSA values, although it may vary in individual patients. Therefore, for interpretation of serial PSAs in a man taking AVODART, a new baseline PSA concentration should be established after 3 to 6 months of treatment, and this new value should be used to assess potentially cancer-related changes in PSA. To interpret an isolated PSA value in a man treated with AVODART for 6 months or more, the PSA value should be doubled for comparison with normal values in untreated men.

Information for Patients: Physicians should instruct their patients to read the Patient Information leaflet before starting therapy with AVODART and to reread it upon prescription renewal for new information regarding the use of AVODART.

AVODART Soft Gelatin Capsules should not be handled by a woman who is pregnant or who may become pregnant because of the potential for absorption of dutasteride and the subsequent potential risk to a developing male fetus (see CONTRAINDICATIONS and WARNINGS: Exposure Of Women—Risk To Male Fetus).

Physicians should inform patients that ejaculate volume might be decreased in some patients during treatment with AVODART. This decrease does not appear to interfere with normal sexual function. In clinical trials, impotence and decreased libido, considered by the investigator to be drug-related, occurred in a small number of patients treated with AVODART or placebo (see ADVERSE REACTIONS, Table 1).

Men treated with dutasteride should not donate blood until at least 6 months have passed following their last dose to prevent pregnant women from receiving dutasteride through blood transfusion (see PRECAUTIONS: Blood Donation).

Drug Interactions: Care should be taken when administering dutasteride to patients taking potent, chronic CYP3A4 inhibitors (see PRECAUTIONS: Use with Potent CYP3A4 Inhibitors).

Dutasteride does not inhibit the in vitro metabolism of model substrates for the major human cytochrome P450 isoenzymes (CYP1A2, CYP2C9, CYP2C19, CYP2D6, and CYP3A4) at a concentration of 1,000 ng/mL, 25 times greater than steady-state serum concentrations in humans. In vitro studies demonstrate that dutasteride does not displace warfarin, diazepam, or phenytoin from plasma protein binding sites, nor do these model compounds displace dutasteride.

Digoxin: In a study of 20 healthy volunteers, AVODART did not alter the steady-state pharmacokinetics of digoxin when administered concomitantly at a dose of 0.5 mg/day for 3 weeks.

Warfarin: In a study of 23 healthy volunteers, 3 weeks of treatment with AVODART 0.5 mg/day did not alter the steady-state pharmacokinetics of the S- or R-warfarin isomers or alter the effect of warfarin on prothrombin time when administered with warfarin.

Alpha Adrenergic Blocking Agents: In a single sequence, cross-over study in healthy volunteers, the administration of tamsulosin or terazosin in combination with AVODART had no effect on the steady-state pharmacokinetics of either alpha adrenergic blocker. The percent change in DHT concentrations was similar for AVODART alone compared with the combination treatment.

Table 1. Drug-related Adverse Events* Reported in ≥1% Subjects Over a 24-Month Period and More Frequently in the Dutasteride Group than the Placebo Group (Pivotal Studies Pooled)

	Adverse Event Onset			
Adverse Events Dutasteride (n) Placebo (n)	Month 0-6 (n = 2,167) (n = 2,158)	Month 7-12 (n = 1,901) (n = 1,922)	Month 13-18 (n = 1,725) (n = 1,714)	Month 19-24 (n = 1,605) (n = 1,555)
Impotence				
Dutasteride	4.7%	1.4%	1.0%	0.8%
Placebo	1.7%	1.5%	0.5%	0.9%
Decreased libido				
Dutasteride	3.0%	0.7%	0.3%	0.3%
Placebo	1.4%	0.6%	0.2%	0.1%
Ejaculation disorder				
Dutasteride	1.4%	0.5%	0.5%	0.1%
Placebo	0.5%	0.3%	0.1%	0.0%
Gynecomastia[†]				
Dutasteride	0.5%	0.8%	1.1%	0.6%
Placebo	0.2%	0.3%	0.3%	0.1%

* **A drug-related adverse event is one considered by the investigator to have a reasonable possibility of being caused by the study medication. In assessing causality, investigators were asked to select from one of two options: reasonably related to study medication or unrelated to study medication.**

[†] Includes breast tenderness and breast enlargement.

A clinical trial was conducted in which dutasteride and tamsulosin were administered concomitantly for 24 weeks followed by 12 weeks of treatment with either the dutasteride and tamsulosin combination or dutasteride monotherapy. Results from the second phase of the trial revealed no excess of serious adverse events or discontinuations due to adverse events in the combination group compared to the dutasteride monotherapy group.

Calcium Channel Antagonists: In a population PK analysis, a decrease in clearance of dutasteride was noted when co-administered with the CYP3A4 inhibitors verapamil (-37%, n = 6) and diltiazem (-44%, n = 5). In contrast, no decrease in clearance was seen when amlodipine, another calcium channel antagonist that is not a CYP3A4 inhibitor, was co-administered with dutasteride (+7%, n = 4).

The decrease in clearance and subsequent increase in exposure to dutasteride in the presence of verapamil and diltiazem is not considered to be clinically significant. No dose adjustment is recommended.

Cholestyramine: Administration of a single 5-mg dose of AVODART followed 1 hour later by 12 g cholestyramine did not affect the relative bioavailability of dutasteride in 12 normal volunteers.

Other Concomitant Therapy: Although specific interaction studies were not performed with other compounds, approximately 90% of the subjects in the 3 Phase III pivotal efficacy studies receiving AVODART were taking other medications concomitantly. No clinically significant adverse interactions could be attributed to the combination of AVODART and concurrent therapy when AVODART was co-administered with anti-hyperlipidemics, angiotensin-converting enzyme (ACE) inhibitors, beta-adrenergic blocking agents, calcium channel blockers, corticosteroids, diuretics, nonsteroidal anti-inflammatory drugs (NSAIDs), phosphodiesterase Type V inhibitors, and quinolone antibiotics.

Drug/Laboratory Test Interactions: *Effects on PSA:* PSA levels generally decrease in patients treated with AVODART as the prostate volume decreases. In approximately one-half of the subjects, a 20% decrease in PSA is seen within the first month of therapy. After 6 months of therapy, PSA levels stabilize to a new baseline that is approximately 50% of the pre-treatment value. Results of subjects treated with AVODART for up to 2 years indicate this 50% reduction in PSA is maintained. Therefore, a new baseline PSA concentration should be established after 3 to 6 months of treatment with AVODART (see PRECAUTIONS: Effects on PSA and Prostate Cancer Detection).

Hormone Levels: In healthy volunteers, 52 weeks of treatment with dutasteride 0.5 mg/day (n = 26) resulted in no clinically significant change compared with placebo (n = 23) in sex hormone binding globulin, estradiol, luteinizing hormone, follicle-stimulating hormone, thyroxine (free T4), and dehydroepiandrosterone. Statistically significant, baseline-adjusted mean increases compared with placebo were observed for total testosterone at 8 weeks (97.1 ng/dL, $p<0.003$) and thyroid-stimulating hormone (TSH) at 52 weeks (0.4 mcIU/mL, $p<0.05$). The median percentage changes from baseline within the dutasteride group were 17.9% for testosterone at 8 weeks and 12.4% for TSH at 52 weeks. The mean levels of testosterone and TSH had returned to baseline at the 24-week post-treatment follow-up period in the group of subjects with available data at the visit. In BPH patients treated with dutasteride in a large Phase III trial, there was a median percent increase in luteinizing hormone of 12% at 6 months and 19% at both 12 and 24 months.

Reproductive Function: The effects of dutasteride 0.5 mg/day on reproductive function were evaluated in normal volunteers aged 18 to 52 (n = 26) throughout 52 weeks of treatment. Semen characteristics were evaluated at 3 timepoints and indicated no clinically meaningful changes in sperm concentration, sperm motility, or sperm morphology. A 0.8 mL (25%) mean decrease in ejaculate volume with a concomitant reduction in total sperm per ejaculate was observed at 52 weeks, but remained within the normal range. At the 24-week post-treatment follow-up visit, mean values for both parameters had returned to baseline in the group of subjects with available data at that visit.

CNS Toxicity: In rats and dogs, repeated oral administration of dutasteride resulted in some animals showing signs of non-specific, reversible, centrally-mediated toxicity, without associated histopathological changes at exposure 425- and 315-fold the expected clinical exposure (of parent drug), respectively.

Carcinogenesis, Mutagenesis, Impairment of Fertility: ***Carcinogenesis:*** In a 2-year carcinogenicity study in B6C3F1 mice, at doses of 3, 35, 250, and 500 mg/kg/day for males and 3, 35, and 250 mg/kg/day for females. An increased incidence of benign hepatocellular adenomas was noted at 250 mg/kg/day (290-fold the expected clinical exposure to a 0.5 mg daily dose) in females only. Two of the 3 major human metabolites have been detected in mice. The exposure to these metabolites in mice is either lower than in humans or is not known.

In a 2-year carcinogenicity study in Han Wistar rats, at doses of 1.5, 7.5, and 53 mg/kg/day for males and 0.8, 6.3, and 15 mg/kg/day for females there was an increase in Leydig cell adenomas in the testes at 53 mg/kg/day (135-fold the expected clinical exposure). An increased incidence of Leydig cell hyperplasia was present at 7.5 mg/kg/day (52-fold the expected clinical exposure) and 53 mg/kg/day in male rats. A positive correlation between proliferative changes in the Leydig cells and an increase in circulating luteinizing hormone levels has been demonstrated with 5α-reductase inhibitors and is consistent with an effect on the hypothalamic-pituitary-testicular axis following 5α-reductase inhibition. At tumorigenic doses in rats, luteinizing hormone levels in rats were increased by 167%. In this study, the major human metabolites were tested for carcinogenicity at approximately 1 to 3 times the expected clinical exposure.

Mutagenesis: Dutasteride was tested for genotoxicity in a bacterial mutagenesis assay (Ames test), a chromosomal aberration assay in CHO cells, and a micronucleus assay in rats. The results did not indicate any genotoxic potential of the parent drug. Two major human metabolites were also negative in either the Ames test or an abbreviated Ames test.

Impairment of Fertility: Treatment of sexually mature male rats with dutasteride at doses of 0.05, 10, 50, and 500 mg/kg/day (0.1 to 110-fold the expected clinical exposure of parent drug) for up to 31 weeks resulted in dose- and time-dependent decreases in fertility, reduced cauda epididymal (absolute) sperm counts but not sperm concentration (at 50 and 500 mg/kg/day), reduced weights of the epididymis, prostate and seminal vesicles, and microscopic changes in the male reproductive organs. The fertility effects were reversed by recovery week 6 at all doses, and sperm counts were normal at the end of a 14-week recovery period. The 5α-reductase-related changes consisted of cytoplasmic vacuolation of tubular epithelium in the epididymides and decreased cytoplasmic content of epithelium, consistent with decreased secretory activity in the prostate and seminal vesicles. The microscopic changes were no longer present at recovery week 14 in the low-dose group and were partly recovered in the remaining treatment groups. Low levels of dutasteride (0.6 to 17 ng/mL) were detected in the serum of untreated female rats mated to males dosed at 10, 50, or 500 mg/kg/ day for 29 to 30 weeks.

In a fertility study in female rats, oral administration of dutasteride at doses of 0.05, 2.5, 12.5, and 30 mg/kg/day resulted in reduced litter size, increased embryo resorption and feminization of male fetuses (decreased anogenital distance) at doses of ≥2.5 mg/kg/day (2- to 10-fold the clinical exposure of parent drug in men). Fetal body weights were also reduced at ≥0.05 mg/kg/day in rats (<0.02-fold the human exposure).

Pregnancy: Pregnancy Category **X** (see CONTRAINDICATIONS). AVODART is contraindicated for use in women.

Continued on next page

Avodart—Cont.

AVODART has not been studied in women because preclinical data suggest that the suppression of circulating levels of dihydrotestosterone may inhibit the development of the external genital organs in a male fetus carried by a woman exposed to dutasteride.

In an intravenous embryo-fetal development study in the rhesus monkey (12/group), administration of dutasteride at 400, 780, 1,325, or 2,010 ng/day on gestation days 20 to 100 did not adversely affect development of male external genitalia. Reduction of fetal adrenal weights, reduction in fetal prostate weights, and increases in fetal ovarian and testis weights were observed in monkeys treated with the highest dose. Based on the highest measured semen concentration of dutasteride in treated men (14 ng/mL) these doses represent 0.8 to 16 times based on blood levels of parent drug (32 to 186 times based on a ng/kg daily dose) the potential maximum exposure of a 50-kg human female to 5 mL semen daily from a dutasteride-treated man, assuming 100% absorption. Dutasteride is highly bound to proteins in human semen (>96%), potentially reducing the amount of dutasteride available for vaginal absorption.

In an embryo-fetal development study in female rats, oral administration of dutasteride at doses of 0.05, 2.5, 12.5, and 30 mg/kg/day resulted in feminization of male fetuses (decreased anogenital distance) and male offspring (nipple development, hypospadias, and distended preputial glands) at all doses (0.07- to 111-fold the expected male clinical exposure). An increase in stillborn pups was observed at 30 mg/kg/day, and reduced fetal body weight was observed at doses $\geq$2.5 mg/kg/day (15- to 111-fold the expected clinical exposure). Increased incidences of skeletal variations considered to be delays in ossification associated with reduced body weight were observed at doses of 12.5 and 30 mg/kg/day (56- to 111-fold the expected clinical exposure).

In an oral pre- and post-natal development study in rats, dutasteride doses of 0.05, 2.5, 12.5, or 30 mg/kg/day were administered. Unequivocal evidence of feminization of the genitalia (i.e., decreased anogenital distance, increased incidence of hypospadias, nipple development) of F1 generation male offspring occurred at doses $\geq$2.5 mg/kg/day (14- to 90-fold the expected clinical exposure in men). At a daily dose of 0.05 mg/kg/day (0.05-fold the expected clinical exposure), evidence of feminization was limited to a small, but statistically significant, decrease in anogenital distance. Doses of 2.5 to 30 mg/kg/day resulted in prolonged gestation in the parental females and a decrease in time to vaginal patency for female offspring and decrease prostate and seminal vesicle weights in male offspring. Effects on newborn startle response were noted at doses greater than or equal to 12.5 mg/kg/day. Increased stillbirths were noted at 30 mg/kg/day.

Feminization of male fetuses is an expected physiological consequence of inhibition of the conversion of testosterone to DHT by 5α-reductase inhibitors. These results are similar to observations in male infants with genetic 5α-reductase deficiency.

In the rabbit, embryo-fetal study doses of 30, 100, and 200 mg/kg (28- to 93-fold the expected clinical exposure in men) were administered orally on days 7 to 29 of pregnancy to encompass the late period of external genitalia development. Histological evaluation of the genital papilla of fetuses revealed evidence of feminization of the male fetus at all doses. A second embryo-fetal study in rabbits at doses of 0.05, 0.4, 3.0, and 30 mg/kg/day (0.3- to 53-fold the expected clinical exposure) also produced evidence of feminization of the genitalia in male fetuses at all doses. It is not known whether rabbits or rhesus monkeys produce any of the major human metabolites.

Nursing Mothers: AVODART is not indicated for use in women. It is not known whether dutasteride is excreted in human breast milk.

Pediatric Use: AVODART is not indicated for use in the pediatric population. Safety and effectiveness in the pediatric population have not been established.

Geriatric Use: Of 2,167 male subjects treated with AVODART in 3 clinical studies, 60% were 65 and over and 15% were 75 and over. No overall differences in safety or efficacy were observed between these subjects and younger subjects. Other reported clinical experience has not identified differences in responses between the elderly and younger patients.

ADVERSE REACTIONS

Most adverse reactions were mild or moderate and generally resolved while on treatment in both the AVODART and placebo groups. The most common adverse events leading to withdrawal in both treatment groups were associated with the reproductive system.

Over 4,300 male subjects with BPH were randomly assigned to receive placebo or 0.5-mg daily doses of AVODART in 3 identical, placebo-controlled Phase III treatment studies. Of this group, 2,167 male subjects were exposed to AVODART, including 1,772 exposed for 1 year and 1,510 exposed for 2 years. The population was aged 47 to 94 years (mean age 66 years) and greater than 90% Caucasian. Over the 2-year treatment period, 376 subjects (9% of each treatment group) were withdrawn from the studies due to adverse experiences, most commonly associated with the reproductive system. Withdrawals due to adverse events considered by the investigator to have a reasonable possibility of being caused by the study medication occurred in 4% of the subjects receiving AVODART and in 3% of the subjects receiving placebo. Table 1 summarizes clinical adverse reactions that were reported by the investigator as drug-related in at least 1% of subjects receiving AVODART and at a higher incidence than subjects receiving placebo.

[See table 1 at top of previous page]

Long-Term Treatment: The incidence of most drug-related sexual adverse events (impotence, decreased libido and ejaculation disorder) decreased with duration of treatment. The incidence of drug-related gynecomastia remained constant over the treatment period (see Table 1). The relationship between long-term use of dutasteride and male breast neoplasia is currently unknown.

OVERDOSAGE

In volunteer studies, single doses of dutasteride up to 40 mg (80 times the therapeutic dose) for 7 days have been administered without significant safety concerns. In a clinical study, daily doses of 5 mg (10 times the therapeutic dose) were administered to 60 subjects for 6 months with no additional adverse effects to those seen at therapeutic doses of 0.5 mg.

There is no specific antidote for dutasteride. Therefore, in cases of suspected overdosage symptomatic and supportive treatment should be given as appropriate, taking the long half-life of dutasteride into consideration.

DOSAGE AND ADMINISTRATION

The recommended dose of AVODART is 1 capsule (0.5 mg) taken orally once a day. The capsules should be swallowed whole. AVODART may be administered with or without food.

No dosage adjustment is necessary for subjects with renal impairment or for the elderly (see CLINICAL PHARMACOLOGY: Pharmacokinetics: Geriatric and Renal Impairment). Due to the absence of data in patients with hepatic impairment, no dosage recommendation can be made (see PRECAUTIONS: General).

HOW SUPPLIED

AVODART Soft Gelatin Capsules 0.5 mg are oblong, opaque, dull yellow, gelatin capsules imprinted with "GX CE2" in red ink on one side packaged in bottles of 100 (NDC 0173-0712-00) with child-resistant closures and unit dose blister packs of 70 capsules (NDC 0173-0712-01).

Storage and Handling: Store at 25°C (77°F); excursions permitted to 15-30°C (59-86°F) [see USP Controlled Room Temperature].

Dutasteride is absorbed through the skin. AVODART Soft Gelatin capsules should not be handled by women who are pregnant or who may become pregnant because of the potential for absorption of dutasteride and the subsequent potential risk to a developing male fetus (see CLINICAL PHARMACOLOGY: Pharmacokinetics, WARNINGS: Exposure of Women—Risk to Male Fetus, and PRECAUTIONS: Information for Patients and Pregnancy).

Manufactured by: RP Scherer, Beinheim, France for GlaxoSmithKline, Research Triangle Park, NC 27709
©2002, GlaxoSmithKline. All rights reserved.
October 2002/RL-1146

PEDIARIX™ ℞
[pĕd'ē ə rix]
[Diphtheria and Tetanus Toxoids and Acellular Pertussis Adsorbed, Hepatitis B (Recombinant) and Inactivated Poliovirus Vaccine Combined]

DESCRIPTION

PEDIARIX™ [Diphtheria and Tetanus Toxoids and Acellular Pertussis Adsorbed, Hepatitis B (Recombinant) and Inactivated Poliovirus Vaccine Combined] is a noninfectious, sterile, multivalent vaccine for intramuscular administration manufactured by SmithKline Beecham Biologicals. It contains diphtheria and tetanus toxoids, 3 pertussis antigens (inactivated pertussis toxin [PT], filamentous hemagglutinin [FHA], and pertactin [69 kiloDalton outer membrane protein]), hepatitis B surface antigen, plus poliovirus Type 1 (Mahoney), Type 2 (MEF-1), and Type 3 (Saukett). The diphtheria toxoid, tetanus toxoid, and pertussis antigens are the same as those in INFANRIX® (Diphtheria and Tetanus Toxoids and Acellular Pertussis Vaccine Adsorbed). The hepatitis B surface antigen is the same as that in ENGERIX-B® [Hepatitis B Vaccine (Recombinant)].

The diphtheria toxin is produced by growing Corynebacterium diphtheriae in Fenton medium containing a bovine extract. Tetanus toxin is produced by growing Clostridium tetani in a modified Latham medium derived from bovine casein. The bovine materials used in these extracts are sourced from countries which the United States Department of Agriculture (USDA) has determined neither have nor are at risk of bovine spongiform encephalopathy (BSE). Both toxins are detoxified with formaldehyde, concentrated by ultrafiltration, and purified by precipitation, dialysis, and sterile filtration.

The 3 acellular pertussis antigens (PT, FHA, and pertactin) are isolated from Bordetella pertussis culture grown in modified Stainer-Scholte liquid medium. PT and FHA are isolated from the fermentation broth; pertactin is extracted from the cells by heat treatment and flocculation. The antigens are purified in successive chromatographic and precipitation steps. PT is detoxified using glutaraldehyde and formaldehyde. FHA and pertactin are treated with formaldehyde.

The hepatitis B surface antigen (HBsAg) is obtained by culturing genetically engineered Saccharomyces cerevisiae cells, which carry the surface antigen gene of the hepatitis B virus, in synthetic medium. The surface antigen expressed in the S. cerevisiae cells is purified by several physiochemical steps, which include precipitation, ion exchange chromatography, and ultrafiltration. The purified HBsAg undergoes dialysis with cysteine to remove residual thimerosal.

The inactivated poliovirus component of PEDIARIX is an enhanced potency component. Each of the 3 strains of poliovirus is individually grown in VERO cells, a continuous line of monkey kidney cells, cultivated on microcarriers. Calf serum and lactalbumin hydrolysate are used during VERO cell culture and/or virus culture. Calf serum is sourced from countries the USDA has determined neither have nor are at risk of BSE. After clarification, each viral suspension is purified by ultrafiltration, diafiltration, and successive chromatographic steps, and inactivated with formaldehyde. The 3 purified viral strains are then pooled to form a trivalent concentrate.

The diphtheria, tetanus, and pertussis antigens are individually adsorbed onto aluminum hydroxide; hepatitis B component is adsorbed onto aluminum phosphate. All antigens are then diluted and combined to produce the final formulated vaccine. Each 0.5-mL dose is formulated to contain 25 Lf of diphtheria toxoid, 10 Lf of tetanus toxoid, 25 mcg of inactivated PT, 25 mcg of FHA, 8 mcg of pertactin, 10 mcg of HBsAg, 40 D-antigen Units (DU) of Type 1 poliovirus, 8 DU of Type 2 poliovirus, and 32 DU of Type 3 poliovirus.

Diphtheria and tetanus toxoid potency is determined by measuring the amount of neutralizing antitoxin in previously immunized guinea pigs. The potency of the acellular pertussis components (PT, FHA, and pertactin) is determined by enzyme-linked immunosorbent assay (ELISA) on sera from previously immunized mice. Potency of the hepatitis B component is established by HBsAg ELISA. The potency of the inactivated poliovirus component is determined by using the D-antigen ELISA and by a poliovirus neutralizing cell culture assay on sera from previously immunized rats.

Each 0.5-mL dose also contains 2.5 mg of 2-phenoxyethanol as a preservative, 4.5 mg of NaCl, and aluminum adjuvant (not more than 0.85 mg aluminum by assay). Each dose also contains $\leq$100 mcg of residual formaldehyde and $\leq$100 mcg of polysorbate 80 (Tween 80). Thimerosal is used at the early stages of manufacture and is removed by subsequent purification steps to below the analytical limit of detection (<25 ng of mercury/20 mcg HBsAg) which upon calculation is <12.5 ng mercury per dose. Neomycin sulfate and polymyxin B are used in the polio vaccine manufacturing process and may be present in the final vaccine at $\leq$0.05 ng neomycin and $\leq$0.01 ng polymyxin B per dose. The procedures used to manufacture the HBsAg antigen result in a product that contains $\leq$5% yeast protein.

The vaccine must be well shaken before administration and is a turbid white suspension after shaking.

Diphtheria and Tetanus Toxoids Adsorbed Bulk Concentrate (For Further Manufacturing) is manufactured by Chiron Behring GmbH & Co, Marburg, Germany. The acellular pertussis antigens, the hepatitis B surface antigen, and the inactivated poliovirus antigens are manufactured by SmithKline Beecham Biologicals, Rixensart, Belgium. Formulation, filling, testing, packaging, and release of the vaccine are performed by SmithKline Beecham Biologicals Manufacturing (wholly-owned subsidiary of SmithKline Beecham Biologicals).

CLINICAL PHARMACOLOGY

The efficacy of PEDIARIX is based on the immunogenicity of the individual antigens compared to licensed vaccines. The efficacy of the pertussis component, which does not have a well established correlate of protection, was determined in clinical trials of INFANRIX. The efficacy of the HBsAg was determined in clinical studies of ENGERIX-B. Serological correlates of protection exist for the diphtheria, tetanus, hepatitis B, and poliovirus components.

Diphtheria: Diphtheria is an acute toxin-mediated infectious disease caused by toxigenic strains of C. diphtheriae. Although the incidence of diphtheria in the United States has decreased from more than 200,000 cases reported in 1921,[1] before the general use of diphtheria toxoid, to only 51 cases of respiratory diphtheria reported from 1980 through 2000,[2] the case-fatality rate has remained constant at about 10%. Of 41 cases reported between 1980 and 1994, 15 (37%) patients had never been immunized, 21 (51%) had been inadequately immunized, and immunization history was unknown for 5 (12%). All 4 (10%) fatalities in this time period occurred in unvaccinated children 9 years and younger.[3] Although diphtheria is rare in the United States, toxigenic C. diphtheriae strains continue to circulate in previously endemic areas.[4] Protection against disease is due to the development of neutralizing antibodies to the diphtheria toxin. Following adequate immunization with diphtheria toxoid, it is thought that protection persists for at least 10 years. A serum diphtheria antitoxin level of 0.01 IU/mL is the lowest level giving some degree of protection.[5] Antitoxin levels of at least 0.1 IU/mL are generally regarded as protective.[5] Immunization with diphtheria toxoid does not, however, eliminate carriage of C. diphtheriae in the pharynx or nares or on the skin.[1]

Efficacy of diphtheria toxoid used in INFANRIX was determined on the basis of immunogenicity studies. A VERO cell toxin neutralizing test confirmed the ability of infant sera (N = 45), obtained 1 month after a 3-dose primary series, to neutralize diphtheria toxin. Levels of diphtheria antitoxin $\geq$0.01 IU/mL were achieved in 100% of the sera tested.

Tetanus: Tetanus is a condition manifested primarily by neuromuscular dysfunction caused by a potent exotoxin released by *C. tetani*. Following the introduction of vaccination with tetanus toxoid in the 1940s, the overall incidence of tetanus declined from 0.4 per 100,000 population in 1947 to 0.02 during the latter half of the 1990s.[6] Adults 60 years of age and older are at greatest risk for tetanus and tetanus-related mortality.[6] Of 124 cases of tetanus reported from 1995 through 1997, 12 (9.7%) occurred among persons younger than 25 years, one of which was a case of neonatal tetanus.[7] Overall, the case-fatality rate was 11%. The disease continues to occur almost exclusively among persons who are unvaccinated, inadequately vaccinated, or whose vaccination histories are unknown or uncertain.[7]

Spores of *C. tetani* are ubiquitous. Naturally acquired immunity to tetanus toxin does not occur. Thus, universal primary immunization and timed booster doses to maintain adequate tetanus antitoxin levels are necessary to protect all age groups.[1] Protection against disease is due to the development of neutralizing antibodies to the tetanus toxin. A serum tetanus antitoxin level of at least 0.01 IU/mL, measured by neutralization assays, is considered the minimum protective level.[8,9] More recently a level ≥0.1 to 0.2 IU/mL has been considered as protective.[10] It is thought that protection persists for at least 10 years.[1]

Efficacy of tetanus toxoid used in INFANRIX was determined on the basis of immunogenicity studies. An in vivo mouse neutralization assay confirmed the ability of infant sera (N = 45), obtained 1 month after a 3-dose primary series, to neutralize tetanus toxin. Levels of tetanus antitoxin ≥0.01 IU/mL were achieved in 100% of the sera tested.

Pertussis: Pertussis (whooping cough) is a disease of the respiratory tract caused by *B. pertussis*. Pertussis is highly communicable (attack rates in unimmunized household contacts of up to 100% have been reported[1,11]) and can cause severe disease, particularly in young infants.[1] Since immunization against pertussis became widespread, the number of reported cases and associated mortality in the United States has declined from an average annual incidence and mortality of 150 cases and 6 deaths per 100,000 population, respectively, in the early 1940s to an annual reported incidence of 2.7 cases per 100,000 population in 2000.[12] Of 28,187 cases of pertussis reported among all ages from 1997 to 2000, 62 (0.2%) resulted in death.[12] The highest number of pertussis cases (7,867) since 1967 was reported in 2000. From 1997 to 2000, infants younger than 1 year had the highest average annual incidence rate (55.5 cases per 100,000 population). During this period, of the 8,276 pertussis cases reported nationally in infants younger than 1 year, 59% were hospitalized, 11% had pneumonia, 1.3% had seizures, 0.2% had encephalopathy, and 0.7% died. Older children, adolescents, and adults, in whom classic signs are often absent, may go undiagnosed and may serve as reservoirs of disease.[1,13] The incidence of reported pertussis among adolescents and adults increased during the 1980s and 1990s.[12,14]

The role of the different components produced by *B. pertussis* in either the pathogenesis of, or the immunity to, pertussis is not well understood.

Efficacy of a 3-dose primary series of INFANRIX has been assessed in 2 clinical studies.[15,16]

A double-blind, randomized, active Diphtheria and Tetanus Toxoids (DT)-controlled trial conducted in Italy, sponsored by the National Institutes of Health (NIH), assessed the absolute protective efficacy of INFANRIX when administered at 2, 4, and 6 months of age.[15] A total of 15,601 infants were immunized with 1 of 2 acellular DTP (DTaP) vaccines, a US-licensed whole-cell DTP vaccine, or with DT vaccine alone. The mean length of follow-up was 17 months (mean age 24 months), beginning 30 days after the third dose of vaccine. The population used in the primary analysis of the efficacy of INFANRIX included 4,481 infants vaccinated with INFANRIX and 1,470 DT vaccinees. After 3 doses, the absolute protective efficacy of INFANRIX against WHO-defined typical pertussis (21 days or more of paroxysmal cough with infection confirmed by culture and/or serologic testing) was 84% (95% CI: 76% to 89%). When the definition of pertussis was expanded to include clinically milder disease with respect to type and duration of cough, with infection confirmed by culture and/or serologic testing, the efficacy of INFANRIX was calculated to be 71% (95% CI: 60% to 78%) against >7 days of any cough and 73% (95% CI: 63% to 80%) against ≥14 days of any cough. A second follow-up period to a mean age of 33 months was conducted in a partially unblinded cohort (children who received DT were offered pertussis vaccine and those who declined were retained in the study cohort). A longer unblinded follow-up period showed that after 3 doses and with no booster dose in the second year of life, the efficacy of INFANRIX against WHO-defined pertussis was 86% (95% CI: 79% to 91%) among children followed to 6 years of age.[17]

A prospective efficacy trial was also conducted in Germany employing a household contact study design.[16] In preparation for this study, 3 doses of INFANRIX were administered at 3, 4, and 5 months of age to more than 22,000 children living in 6 areas of Germany in a safety and immunogenicity study. Infants who did not participate in the safety and immunogenicity study could have received a whole-cell DTP vaccine or DT vaccine. Index cases were identified by spontaneous presentation to a physician. Households with at least one other member (i.e., besides index case) aged 6 through 47 months were enrolled. Household contacts of index cases were monitored for incidence of pertussis by a physician who was blinded to the vaccination status of the household. Calculation of vaccine efficacy was based on attack rates of pertussis in household contacts classified by vaccination status. Of the 173 household contacts who had not received a pertussis vaccine, 96 developed WHO-defined pertussis, as compared to 7 of 112 contacts vaccinated with INFANRIX. The protective efficacy of INFANRIX was calculated to be 89% (95% CI: 77% to 95%), with no indication of waning of protection up until the time of the booster vaccination. The average age of infants vaccinated with INFANRIX at the end of follow-up in this trial was 13 months (range 6 to 25 months). When the definition of pertussis was expanded to include clinically milder disease, with infection confirmed by culture and/or serologic testing, the efficacy of INFANRIX against ≥7 days of any cough was 67% (95% CI: 52% to 78%) and against ≥7 days of paroxysmal cough was 81% (95% CI: 68% to 89%). The corresponding efficacy rates of INFANRIX against ≥14 days of any cough or paroxysmal cough were 73% (95% CI: 59% to 82%) and 84% (95% CI: 71% to 91%), respectively.

Hepatitis B: Several hepatitis viruses are known to cause a systemic infection resulting in major pathologic changes in the liver (e.g., A, B, C, D, and E). The estimated lifetime risk of hepatitis B infection in the United States varies from almost 100% for the highest-risk groups to approximately 5% for the population as a whole.[18] The modes of transmission of hepatitis B include sexual contact (contaminated body secretions including semen, vaginal secretions, blood, and saliva); parenteral exposure (e.g., blood transfusions, accidental needlesticks or sharing needles from infected individuals); or maternal-neonatal transmission.[19] Hepatitis B infection can have serious consequences including acute massive hepatic necrosis, chronic active hepatitis, and cirrhosis of the liver. Up to 90% of neonates, 30% to 50% of children aged 1 to 5 years, and 6% to 10% of older children and adults who are infected in the United States will become hepatitis B virus carriers.[19] It has been estimated that 200 to 300 million people in the world are chronically infected with hepatitis B virus,[19] and that there are approximately 1.25 million chronic carriers of hepatitis B virus in the United States.[20] Those patients who become chronic carriers can infect others and are at increased risk of developing primary hepatocellular carcinoma. Among other factors, infection with hepatitis B may be the single most important factor for development of this carcinoma.[20,21]

Mothers infected with hepatitis B virus can infect their infants at, or shortly after, birth if they are carriers of the HBsAg or develop an active infection during the third trimester of pregnancy. Infected infants usually become chronic carriers. Therefore, screening of pregnant women for hepatitis B is recommended.[10] There is no specific treatment for acute hepatitis B infection. Persons who develop anti-HBs antibodies after active infection are usually protected against subsequent infection. Antibody concentrations ≥10 mIU/mL against HBsAg are recognized as conferring protection against hepatitis B.[22]

Protective efficacy with ENGERIX-B has been demonstrated in a clinical trial in neonates at high risk of hepatitis B infection.[23,24] Fifty-eight neonates born of mothers who were both HBsAg- and HBeAg-positive were given ENGERIX-B (10 mcg at 0, 1, and 2 months) without concomitant hepatitis B immune globulin. Two infants became chronic carriers in the 12-month follow-up period after initial inoculation. Assuming an expected carrier rate of 70%, the protective efficacy rate against the chronic carrier state during the first 12 months of life was 95%.

Reduced Risk of Hepatocellular Carcinoma: According to the Centers for Disease Control and Prevention (CDC), hepatitis B vaccine is recognized as the first anti-cancer vaccine because it can prevent primary liver cancer.[25] A clear link has been demonstrated between chronic hepatitis B infection and the occurrence of hepatocellular carcinoma. In a Taiwanese study, the institution of universal childhood immunization against hepatitis B virus has been shown to decrease the incidence of hepatocellular carcinoma among children.[26] In a Korean study in adult males, vaccination against the hepatitis B virus has been shown to decrease the incidence and risk of developing hepatocellular carcinoma in adults.[27]

Poliomyelitis: Poliovirus is an enterovirus that belongs to the picornavirus family.[28] Three serotypes of poliovirus have been identified (Types 1, 2, and 3). Poliovirus is highly contagious with the predominant mode of transmission being person-to-person via the fecal-oral route. The virus may also be spread indirectly through contact with infectious saliva or feces or by contaminated water or sewage.[29]

Replication of poliovirus in the pharynx and intestine is followed by a viremic phase in which involvement of the central nervous system (CNS) can occur. Whereas poliovirus infections are asymptomatic or cause nonspecific symptoms (low-grade fever, malaise, anorexia, and sore throat) in 90% to 95% of individuals, up to 2% of infected persons develop paralytic disease.[28]

As a result of the introduction of poliovirus vaccines in the 1950s and 1960s, and their subsequent widespread use, poliomyelitis control has been achieved in the United States.[30,31] After introduction of conventional (non-enhanced) inactivated poliovirus vaccine (IPV) in 1955, the annual incidence of paralytic disease of 11.4 cases per 100,000 population declined to 0.5 cases per 100,000 population in 1961, when oral poliovirus vaccine (OPV) was introduced. Incidence continued to decline thereafter, with rates of 0.00–0.01 cases per 100,000 population during the years 1990–2000.[32] Evidence suggests that endemic circulation of wild polioviruses ceased in the United States in the 1960s. The last indigenously acquired cases of poliomyelitis caused by wild poliovirus were detected in 1979 and were due to imported viruses. Since then, vaccine-associated paralytic poliomyelitis (VAPP) attributable to live OPV has been the only indigenous form of the disease in the United States.[33] To eliminate the risk for VAPP, since 2000, an all IPV schedule has been recommended for routine childhood polio vaccination in the United States. Although the likelihood of poliovirus importation has decreased substantially since 1997 as a result of decreases in the number of polio cases worldwide, the potential for importation will remain until global eradication is achieved.

IPV induces the production of neutralizing antibodies against each poliovirus serotype; these neutralizing antibodies are recognized as conferring protection against poliomyelitis disease.[34]

Immune Response to PEDIARIX Administered as a 3-Dose Primary Series: In a study conducted in the United States, the immune responses to each of the antigens contained in PEDIARIX were evaluated in sera obtained 1 month after the third dose of vaccine and were compared to those following administration of US-licensed vaccines (INFANRIX and ENGERIX-B concomitantly at separate sites, and OPV [Poliovirus Vaccine Live Oral Trivalent, Lederle Laboratories]).[35] Both groups received a US-licensed *Haemophilus influenzae* type b (Hib) vaccine (Aventis Pasteur) concomitantly at separate sites. The schedule of administration was 2, 4, and 6 months of age. One month after the third dose of PEDIARIX, vaccine response rates for each of the pertussis antigens (with the exception of FHA), geometric mean antibody concentrations for each of the pertussis antigens, and seroprotection rates for diphtheria, tetanus, hepatitis B, and the polioviruses, were shown to be non-inferior to those achieved following separately administered vaccines (see Table 1). The vaccine response to FHA marginally exceeded the 10% limit for non-inferiority.[35]

Table 1. Antibody Responses to Each Antigen Following PEDIARIX as Compared to INFANRIX, ENGERIX-B, and OPV (One Month After Administration of Dose 3) in US Infants Vaccinated at 2, 4, and 6 Months of Age

	PEDIARIX (N = 86–91)	INFANRIX, ENGERIX-B, OPV (N = 73–78)
Anti-Diphtheria % ≥0.1 IU/mL*	98.9	100
Anti-Tetanus % ≥0.1 IU/mL*	100	100
Anti-PT % VR*	98.9	98.7
GMC†	97.1	47.5
Anti-FHA % VR	95.6	100
GMC†	119.1	153.2
Anti-Pertactin % VR*	95.6	91.0
GMC†	150.4	108.6
Anti-HBsAg % ≥10 mIU/mL*	100	100
GMC†	1661.2	804.9
Anti-Polio 1 % ≥1:8*‡	100	98.6
Anti-Polio 2 % ≥1:8*‡	98.8	100
Anti-Polio 3 % ≥1:8*‡	100	100

Both groups received Hib vaccine (Aventis Pasteur) concomitantly at a separate site.
OPV manufactured by Lederle Laboratories.
VR = Vaccine response: In initially seronegative infants, appearance of antibodies (concentration ≥5 EL.U./mL); in initially seropositive infants, at least maintenance of pre-vaccination concentration.
GMC = Geometric mean antibody concentration.
* Seroprotection rate or vaccine response rate to PEDIARIX not inferior to separately administered vaccines (upper limit of 90% CI on the difference for separate administration minus PEDIARIX <10%).
† GMC in the group that received PEDIARIX not inferior to separately administered vaccines (upper limit of 90% CI on the ratio of GMC for separate administration/PEDIARIX <1.5 for anti-PT, anti-FHA, and anti-pertactin, and <2.0 for anti-HBsAg).
‡ Poliovirus neutralizing antibody titer.

Immune Response to Concomitantly Administered Vaccines: In a clinical trial in the United States, PEDIARIX was given concomitantly, at separate sites, with Hib vaccine (Aventis Pasteur) to infants at 2, 4, and 6 months of age.[35] Immunogenicity data are available in 90 infants one month after the third dose of the vaccines; 98.9% (95% CI: 94% to 100%) of infants demonstrated anti-PRP antibodies ≥0.15 mcg/mL and 94.4% (95% CI: 87.5% to 98.2%) demonstrated anti-PRP antibodies ≥1.0 mcg/mL.

Continued on next page

Pediarix—Cont.

Immunogenicity data are not available on the concurrent administration of PEDIARIX with pneumococcal conjugate vaccine.

INDICATIONS AND USAGE
PEDIARIX is indicated for active immunization against diphtheria, tetanus, pertussis (whooping cough), all known subtypes of hepatitis B virus, and poliomyelitis caused by poliovirus Types 1, 2, and 3 as a three-dose primary series in infants born of HBsAg-negative mothers, beginning as early as 6 weeks of age. PEDIARIX should not be administered to any infant before the age of 6 weeks, or to individuals 7 years of age or older.

Infants born of HBsAg-positive mothers should receive Hepatitis B Immune Globulin (Human) (HBIG) and monovalent Hepatitis B Vaccine (Recombinant) within 12 hours of birth and should complete the hepatitis B vaccination series according to a particular schedule.[36] (See manufacturer's prescribing information for Hepatitis B Vaccine [Recombinant]) (see DOSAGE AND ADMINISTRATION).

Infants born of mothers of unknown HBsAg status should receive monovalent Hepatitis B Vaccine (Recombinant) within 12 hours of birth and should complete the hepatitis B vaccination series according to a particular schedule.[36] (See manufacturer's prescribing information for Hepatitis B Vaccine [Recombinant]) (see DOSAGE AND ADMINISTRATION).

PEDIARIX will not prevent hepatitis caused by other agents, such as hepatitis A, C, and E viruses, or other pathogens known to infect the liver. As hepatitis D (caused by the delta virus) does not occur in the absence of hepatitis B infection, hepatitis D will also be prevented by vaccination with PEDIARIX.

Hepatitis B has a long incubation period. Vaccination with PEDIARIX may not prevent hepatitis B infection in individuals who had an unrecognized hepatitis B infection at the time of vaccine administration.

When passive protection against tetanus or diphtheria is required, Tetanus Immune Globulin or Diphtheria Antitoxin, respectively, should be administered at separate sites.[1]

As with any vaccine, PEDIARIX may not protect 100% of individuals receiving the vaccine, and is not recommended for treatment of actual infections.

CONTRAINDICATIONS
Hypersensitivity to any component of the vaccine, including yeast, neomycin, and polymyxin B, is a contraindication (see DESCRIPTION).

It is a contraindication to use this vaccine after a serious allergic reaction (e.g., anaphylaxis) temporally associated with a previous dose of this vaccine or with any components of this vaccine. Because of the uncertainty as to which component of the vaccine might be responsible, no further vaccination with any of these components should be given. Alternatively, such individuals may be referred to an allergist for evaluation if further immunizations are to be considered.[1]

In addition, the following events are contraindications to administration of any pertussis-containing vaccine, including PEDIARIX:[10]
- Encephalopathy (e.g., coma, decreased level of consciousness, prolonged seizures) within 7 days of administration of a previous dose of a pertussis-containing vaccine that is not attributable to another identifiable cause;
- Progressive neurologic disorder, including infantile spasms, uncontrolled epilepsy, or progressive encephalopathy. Pertussis vaccine should not be administered to individuals with such conditions until a treatment regimen has been established and the condition has stabilized.

PEDIARIX is not contraindicated for use in individuals with HIV infection.[10,37]

WARNINGS
Administration of PEDIARIX is associated with higher rates of fever relative to separately administered vaccines. In one study that evaluated medically attended fever after the first dose of PEDIARIX or separately administered vaccines, infants who received PEDIARIX had a higher rate of medical encounters for fever within the first 4 days following vaccination. In some infants, these encounters included the performance of diagnostic studies to evaluate other causes of fever (see ADVERSE REACTIONS).

The vial stopper is latex-free. The tip cap and the rubber plunger of the needleless prefilled syringes contain dry natural latex rubber that may cause allergic reactions in latex sensitive individuals.

If any of the following events occur in temporal relation to receipt of whole-cell DTP or a vaccine containing an acellular pertussis component, the decision to give subsequent doses of PEDIARIX or any vaccine containing a pertussis component should be based on careful consideration of the potential benefits and possible risks:[38,39]
- Temperature of ≥40.5°C (105°F) within 48 hours not due to another identifiable cause;
- Collapse or shock-like state (hypotonic-hyporesponsive episode) within 48 hours;
- Persistent, inconsolable crying lasting ≥3 hours, occurring within 48 hours;
- Seizures with or without fever occurring within 3 days.

When a decision is made to withhold pertussis vaccine, immunization with DT vaccine, hepatitis B vaccine, and IPV should be continued.

Table 2. Percentage of Infants in a German Safety Study With Solicited Local Reactions or Selected Systemic Adverse Events Within 4 Days of Vaccination* at 3, 4, and 5 Months of Age With PEDIARIX Administered Concomitantly With Hib Vaccine or With Separate Concomitant Administration of INFANRIX, Hib Vaccine, and OPV (ITT Cohort)

	PEDIARIX & Hib			INFANRIX, Hib, & OPV		
	Dose 1	Dose 2	Dose 3	Dose 1	Dose 2	Dose 3
N	4,666	4,619	4,574	768	757	750
Local†						
Pain, any	14.0	10.2	9.9	14.2	9.8	8.1
Pain, grade 2 or 3	2.9	1.2	1.5	3.6	1.7	1.1
Pain, grade 3	0.7	0.3	0.3	1.3	0.4	0.1
Redness, any	18.6	26.6	25.6	16.1	21.4	20.8
Redness, >5 mm	6.7	9.9	9.0	5.9	8.2	7.7
Redness, >20 mm	1.2	1.0	1.1	1.8	0.7	1.1
Swelling, any	12.7	18.5	18.4	9.6	12.9	13.6
Swelling, >5 mm	5.6	7.7	7.8	3.6	5.2	4.8
Swelling, >20 mm	1.2	1.6	1.5	1.3	1.1	1.2
Systemic						
Restlessness, any	41.4	32.0	26.7	46.4	35.0	27.6
Restlessness, grade 2 or 3	14.4	10.0	8.9	20.2	11.5	8.4
Restlessness, grade 3	3.0	1.5	1.6	5.7	3.0	1.7
Fever‡, ≥100.4°F	25.1	19.3	19.7	13.2	13.1	11.2
Fever‡, >101.3°F	5.8	4.1	4.6	2.2	2.8	2.1
Fever‡, >103.1°F	0.3	0.5	0.7	0.3	0.3	0.5
Unusual cry§, any	24.9	16.5	13.1	36.5	19.7	14.3
Unusual cry§, grade 2 or 3	12.7	7.1	5.7	20.8	10.0	5.7
Unusual cry§, grade 3	3.9	1.7	1.4	6.8	2.1	1.1
Loss of appetite, any	17.9	13.3	12.5	19.1	16.2	11.3
Loss of appetite, grade 2 or 3	4.0	2.9	2.7	4.4	2.9	2.3
Loss of appetite, grade 3	0.6	0.5	0.4	0.5	0.7	0.0

N = number of infants in the intent-to-treat (ITT) cohort (infants who received the indicated vaccine and for whom at least one symptom sheet was completed).
Grade 2 defined as sufficiently discomforting to interfere with daily activities.
Grade 3 defined as preventing normal daily activities.
* Within 4 days of vaccination defined as day of vaccination and the next 3 days.
† Local reactions at the injection site for PEDIARIX or INFANRIX.
‡ Rectal temperatures.
§ Unusual cry lasting >1 hour.

If Guillain-Barré syndrome occurs within 6 weeks of receipt of prior vaccine containing tetanus toxoid, the decision to give subsequent doses of PEDIARIX or any vaccine containing tetanus toxoid should be based on careful consideration of the potential benefits and possible risks.[10]

A committee of the Institute of Medicine (IOM) has concluded that evidence is consistent with a causal relationship between whole-cell DTP vaccine and acute neurologic illness, and under special circumstances, between whole-cell DTP vaccine and chronic neurologic disease in the context of the National Childhood Encephalopathy Study (NCES) report.[40,41] However, the IOM committee concluded that the evidence was insufficient to indicate whether or not whole-cell DTP vaccine increased the overall risk of chronic neurologic disease.[41] Acute encephalopathy and permanent neurologic damage have not been reported causally linked or in temporal association with administration of PEDIARIX, but the experience with PEDIARIX is insufficient to rule this out. Encephalopathy has been reported following INFANRIX (see ADVERSE REACTIONS, Postmarketing Reports), but data are not sufficient to evaluate a causal relationship.

The decision to administer a pertussis-containing vaccine to children with stable CNS disorders must be made by the physician on an individual basis, with consideration of all relevant factors, and assessment of potential risks and benefits for that individual. The Advisory Committee on Immunization Practices (ACIP) and the Committee on Infectious Diseases of the American Academy of Pediatrics (AAP) have issued guidelines for such children.[38,42] The parent or guardian should be advised of the potential increased risk involved (see PRECAUTIONS, Information for Vaccine Recipients and Parents or Guardians).

A family history of seizures or other CNS disorders is not a contraindication to pertussis vaccine.[38]

For children at higher risk for seizures than the general population, an appropriate antipyretic may be administered at the time of vaccination with a vaccine containing an acellular pertussis component (including PEDIARIX) and for the ensuing 24 hours according to the respective prescribing information recommended dosage to reduce the possibility of post-vaccination fever.[10,38]

Vaccination should be deferred during the course of a moderate or severe illness with or without fever. Such children should be vaccinated as soon as they have recovered from the acute phase of the illness.[10]

As with other intramuscular injections, PEDIARIX should not be given to children on anticoagulant therapy unless the potential benefit clearly outweighs the risk of administration (see PRECAUTIONS).

PRECAUTIONS
PEDIARIX should be given with caution in children with bleeding disorders such as hemophilia or thrombocytopenia, with steps taken to avoid the risk of hematoma following the injection.

Before the injection of any biological, the physician should take all reasonable precautions to prevent allergic or other adverse reactions, including understanding the use of the biological concerned, and the nature of the side effects and adverse reactions that may follow its use.

Prior to immunization, the patient's current health status and medical history should be reviewed. The physician should review the patient's immunization history for possible vaccine sensitivity, previous vaccination-related adverse reactions and occurrence of any adverse–event-related symptoms and/or signs, in order to determine the existence of any contraindication to immunization with PEDIARIX and to allow an assessment of benefits and risks. Epinephrine injection (1:1000) and other appropriate agents used for the control of immediate allergic reactions must be immediately available should an acute anaphylactic reaction occur.

A separate sterile syringe and sterile disposable needle or a sterile disposable unit should be used for each individual patient to prevent transmission of hepatitis or other infectious agents from one person to another. Needles should be disposed of properly and should not be recapped.

Special care should be taken to prevent injection into a blood vessel.

As with any vaccine, if administered to immunosuppressed persons, including individuals receiving immunosuppressive therapy, the expected immune response may not be obtained.[37]

Information for Vaccine Recipients and Parents or Guardians: Parents or guardians should be informed by the healthcare provider of the potential benefits and risks of the vaccine, and of the importance of completing the immunization series. When a child returns for the next dose in a series, it is important that the parent or guardian be questioned concerning occurrence of any symptoms and/or signs of an adverse reaction after a previous dose of the same vaccine. The physician should inform the parents or guardians about the potential for adverse events that have been temporally associated with administration of PEDIARIX or other vaccines containing similar components. The parent or guardian accompanying the recipient should be told to report severe or unusual adverse events to the physician or clinic where the vaccine was administered.

The parent or guardian should be given the Vaccine Information Statements, which are required by the National Childhood Vaccine Injury Act of 1986 to be given prior to immunization. These materials are available free of charge at the CDC website (www.cdc.gov/nip).

The US Department of Health and Human Services has established a Vaccine Adverse Event Reporting System (VAERS) to accept all reports of suspected adverse events after the administration of any vaccine, including but not limited to the reporting of events required by the National Childhood Vaccine Injury Act of 1986.[10] The VAERS toll-free number is 1-800-822-7967.

Drug Interactions: For information regarding concomitant administration with other vaccines, refer to DOSAGE AND ADMINISTRATION.

PEDIARIX should not be mixed with any other vaccine in the same syringe or vial.

Immunosuppressive therapies, including irradiation, antimetabolites, alkylating agents, cytotoxic drugs, and corticosteroids (used in greater than physiologic doses), may reduce the immune response to vaccines. Although no specific data from studies with PEDIARIX under these conditions are available, if immunosuppressive therapy will be discontinued shortly, it would be reasonable to defer immunization until the patient has been off therapy for 3 months; otherwise, the patient should be vaccinated while still on therapy.[37] If PEDIARIX is administered to a person receiving immunosuppressive therapy, or who received a recent injection of immune globulin, or who has an immunodeficiency disorder, an adequate immunologic response may not be obtained.

Tetanus Immune Globulin or Diphtheria Antitoxin, if needed, should be given at a separate site, with a separate needle and syringe.

Carcinogenesis, Mutagenesis, Impairment of Fertility: PEDIARIX has not been evaluated for carcinogenic or mutagenic potential, or for impairment of fertility.

Pregnancy: Pregnancy Category C: PEDIARIX is not indicated for women of child-bearing age. Animal reproduction studies have not been conducted with PEDIARIX. It is not known whether PEDIARIX can cause fetal harm when administered to a pregnant woman or if PEDIARIX can affect reproductive capacity.

Geriatric Use: PEDIARIX is not indicated for use in adult populations.

Pediatric Use: Safety and effectiveness of PEDIARIX in infants younger than 6 weeks of age have not been evaluated (see DOSAGE AND ADMINISTRATION). PEDIARIX is not recommended for persons 7 years of age or older. Tetanus and Diphtheria Toxoids Adsorbed (Td) For Adult Use, IPV, and Hepatitis B Vaccine (Recombinant) should be used in individuals 7 years of age or older.

ADVERSE REACTIONS

A total of 20,739 doses of PEDIARIX have been administered to 7,028 infants as a 3-dose primary series. The most common adverse reactions observed in clinical trials were local injection site reactions (pain, redness, or swelling), fever, and fussiness. In comparative studies, administration of PEDIARIX was associated with higher rates of fever relative to separately administered vaccines (see WARNINGS; see ADVERSE REACTIONS Tables 2 and 4). The prevalence of fever was highest on the day of vaccination and the day following vaccination. More than 98% of episodes of fever resolved within the 4-day period following vaccination (i.e., the period including the day of vaccination and the next 3 days). Rates of most other solicited adverse events following PEDIARIX were comparable to rates observed following separately administered US-licensed vaccines (see ADVERSE REACTIONS Table 2).

The adverse event information from clinical trials provides a basis for identifying adverse events that appear to be related to vaccine use and for approximating rates. However, because clinical trials are conducted under widely varying conditions, adverse event rates observed in the clinical trials of a vaccine cannot be directly compared to rates in the clinical trials of another vaccine, and may not reflect the rates observed in practice.

A total of 5,472 infants were enrolled in a German safety study that was originally designed to compare the safety and reactogenicity of PEDIARIX administered concomitantly at separate sites with 1 of 4 Hib vaccines (SmithKline Beecham Biologicals [not US-licensed]; Lederle Laboratories, Aventis Pasteur, or Merck & Co [all US-licensed]) at 3, 4, and 5 months of age.[43] After enrollment of 1,569 infants, the study was amended to include a control group that received separate US-licensed vaccines (INFANRIX, Hib vaccine [Aventis Pasteur], and OPV [Lederle Laboratories]). Infants in the separate administration group received one less antigen (hepatitis B) than the infants who received PEDIARIX. Safety data were available for 4,666 infants who received PEDIARIX administered concomitantly at separate sites with 1 of 4 Hib vaccines and for 768 infants in the control group that received separate vaccines. Data on adverse events were collected by parents using standardized diary cards for 4 consecutive days following each vaccine dose (i.e., day of vaccination and the next 3 days).

The primary end-point of the study was the percentage of infants with any grade 3 solicited symptom (redness or swelling >20 mm, fever >103.1°F, or crying, pain, vomiting, diarrhea, loss of appetite, or restlessness that prevented normal daily activities) over the 3-dose primary series in infants who received PEDIARIX (4 groups that received PEDIARIX and Hib vaccines pooled) compared to the group that received INFANRIX and Hib vaccine separately with OPV. Analysis for the primary end-point was performed on the according-to-protocol (ATP) cohort that included only those infants who were enrolled after the protocol amendment to include a control group. Of 3,773 infants in the ATP cohort for whom safety data were available, 16.2% (95% CI: 14.9% to 17.5%) of 3,029 infants who received PEDIARIX and Hib vaccine compared to 20.3% (95% CI: 17.5% to 23.4%) of 744 infants who received separate vaccines were reported to have had at least one grade 3 solicited symptom within 4 days of vaccination (i.e., day of vaccination and the next 3 days). The difference between groups in the rate of grade 3 symptoms was 4.1% (90% CI: 1.4% to 7.1%).

Table 3. Percentage of Infants in a US Lot Consistency Study With Solicited Local Reactions or Selected Systemic Adverse Events Within 4 Days of Vaccination* at 2, 4, and 6 Months of Age With PEDIARIX Administered Concomitantly With Hib Vaccine (ITT Cohort)

	PEDIARIX & Hib		
	Dose 1	Dose 2	Dose 3
Local[†]	N = 482	N = 469	N = 466
Pain, any	30.5	25.4	23.0
Pain, grade 2 or 3	6.2	5.5	3.6
Pain, grade 3	1.2	0.6	0.6
Redness, any	25.3	32.6	35.6
Redness, >5 mm	9.3	10.4	8.6
Redness, >20 mm	0.6	1.5	1.3
Swelling, any	15.1	16.6	22.3
Swelling, >5 mm	6.8	6.2	6.4
Swelling, >20 mm	1.0	1.3	1.3
Systemic	N = 482	N = 469	N = 467
Restlessness, any	28.8	30.3	28.5
Restlessness, grade 2 or 3	7.1	9.0	9.4
Restlessness, grade 3	1.0	1.1	0.6
Fever[‡], ≥100.4°F	26.6	31.3	25.9
Fever[‡], >101.3°F	2.9	6.2	4.7
Fever[‡], >103.1°F	0.0	0.2	0.6
Fussiness, any	61.8	63.8	57.0
Fussiness, grade 2 or 3	14.9	21.5	17.1
Fussiness, grade 3	2.7	3.4	1.7
Loss of appetite, any	21.6	19.8	18.8
Loss of appetite, grade 2 or 3	3.1	3.2	2.4
Loss of appetite, grade 3	0.2	0.4	0.0
Sleeping more than usual, any	46.7	31.8	28.1
Sleeping more than usual, grade 2 or 3	10.2	6.0	4.7
Sleeping more than usual, grade 3	1.7	0.4	0.6

N = number of infants in the intent-to-treat (ITT) cohort (infants who received the indicated vaccine and for whom at least one symptom sheet was completed).
Grade 2 defined as sufficiently discomforting to interfere with daily activities.
Grade 3 defined as preventing normal daily activities.
* Within 4 days of vaccination defined as day of vaccination and the next 3 days.
† Local reactions at the injection site for PEDIARIX.
‡ Rectal temperatures.

Data for selected solicited symptoms following each dose in a 3-dose primary series are presented in Table 2 for the intent-to-treat (ITT) cohort (includes all infants enrolled before and after the amendment who received the indicated vaccine and for whom at least one symptom sheet was completed).
[See table 2 at top of previous page]

In this study, infants were also monitored for unsolicited adverse events that occurred within 30 days following vaccination using diaries which were returned at subsequent visits and were supplemented by spontaneous reports and a medical history as reported by parents. Over the entire study period, 6 subjects in the group that received PEDIARIX reported seizures. Two of these subjects had a febrile seizure, 1 of whom also developed afebrile seizures. The remaining 4 subjects had afebrile seizures, including 2 with infantile spasms. Two subjects reported seizures within 7 days following vaccination (1 subject had both febrile and afebrile seizures, and 1 subject had afebrile seizures), corresponding to a rate of 0.22 seizures per 1,000 doses (febrile seizures 0.07 per 1,000 doses, afebrile seizures 0.14 per 1,000 doses). No subject who received concomitant INFANRIX, Hib vaccine, and OPV reported seizures. In a separate German study that evaluated the safety of INFANRIX in 22,505 infants who received 66,867 doses of INFANRIX administered as a 3-dose primary series, the rate of seizures within 7 days of vaccination with INFANRIX was 0.13 per 1,000 doses (febrile seizures 0.0 per 1,000 doses, afebrile seizures 0.13 per 1,000 doses).

No cases of hypotonic-hyporesponsiveness, encephalopathy, or anaphylaxis were reported in the German study that evaluated the safety of PEDIARIX.

Rates of serious adverse events that are less common than those reported in this safety study are not known at this time.

Additional safety data for PEDIARIX are available for 482 infants enrolled in a US study designed to evaluate lot-to-lot consistency and a bridge for a new manufacturing step. Table 3 presents the local reactions and selected adverse events within 4 days of vaccination with PEDIARIX administered concomitantly with a US-licensed Hib vaccine (Aventis Pasteur) at 2, 4, and 6 months of age. Data on adverse events were collected by parents using standardized diaries for 4 consecutive days after each vaccine dose (i.e., day of vaccination and the next 3 days) with follow-up telephone calls made by study personnel between days 1 and 3.
[See table 3 above]

Post-dose 1 safety data are available from a US study initiated in December 2001, which was designed to assess the safety of PEDIARIX administered concomitantly at separate sites with Hib and pneumococcal conjugate vaccines (Lederle Laboratories), relative to separately administered INFANRIX, ENGERIX-B, IPV (Aventis Pasteur), Hib vaccine (Lederle Laboratories), and pneumococcal conjugate vaccine (Lederle Laboratories) at 2, 4, and 6 months of age. The study was powered to evaluate fever >101.3°F. Enrollment for this study is complete, with 673 infants in the group that received PEDIARIX and 335 infants in the separate vaccines group. Safety data following the second and third doses are expected in 2003. Data for fever within 4 days following dose 1 (i.e., day of vaccination and the next 3 days) are presented in Table 4.
[See table 4 at top of next page]

In this study, medical attention (a visit to or from medical personnel) for fever within 4 days following vaccination was sought for 8 infants who received PEDIARIX (1.2%) and no infants who received separately administered vaccines. Four infants were seen by medical personnel in an office setting; no diagnostic tests were performed in 2 of the infants and a complete blood count (CBC) was done in the other 2 infants. Of 3 infants who were seen in an emergency room, all had a CBC and a blood and urine culture performed; chest X-rays were done in 2 of the infants and a nasopharyngeal specimen was tested for Respiratory Syncytial Virus in one of the infants. One infant was hospitalized for a work-up that included a CBC, blood and urine cultures, a lumbar puncture, and a chest X-ray. All episodes of medically attended fever resolved within 4 days post-vaccination.

In 12 clinical trials, 5 deaths were reported in 7,028 (0.07%) recipients of PEDIARIX and 1 death was reported in 1,764 (0.06%) recipients of comparator vaccines. Causes of death in the group that received PEDIARIX included 2 cases of Sudden Infant Death Syndrome (SIDS) and one case of each of the following: Convulsive disorder, congenital immunodeficiency with sepsis, and neuroblastoma. One case of SIDS was reported in the comparator group. The rate of SIDS among all recipients of PEDIARIX across the 12 trials was 0.3/1,000. The rate of SIDS observed for recipients of PEDIARIX in the German safety study was 0.2/1,000 infants (reported rate of SIDS in Germany in the latter part of the 1990s was 0.7/1,000 newborns).[44] The reported rate of SIDS in the United States from 1990 to 1994 was 1.2/1,000 live births.[45] By chance alone, some cases of SIDS can be expected to follow receipt of pertussis-containing vaccines.[39] Limited data are available on the safety of administering PEDIARIX after a birth dose of hepatitis B vaccine (see Table 5). In a study conducted in Moldova, 160 infants received a dose of hepatitis B vaccine within 48 hours of birth followed by 3 doses of PEDIARIX at 6, 10, and 14 weeks of age. No information was collected on the HBsAg status of mothers of enrolled infants.
[See table 5 at top of next page]

Although there was no comparator group who received PEDIARIX without a birth dose of hepatitis B vaccine, available data suggest that some local adverse events may occur at a higher rate when PEDIARIX is administered after a birth dose of hepatitis B vaccine.

Continued on next page

Pediarix—Cont.

As with any vaccine, there is the possibility that broad use of PEDIARIX could reveal adverse events not observed in clinical trials.

Additional Adverse Events: Rarely, an anaphylactic reaction (i.e., hives, swelling of the mouth, difficulty breathing, hypotension, or shock) has been reported after receiving preparations containing diphtheria, tetanus, and/or pertussis antigens.[39] Arthus-type hypersensitivity reactions, characterized by severe local reactions, may follow receipt of tetanus toxoid. A review by the IOM found evidence for a causal relationship between receipt of tetanus toxoid and both brachial neuritis and Guillain-Barré syndrome.[46] A few cases of demyelinating diseases of the CNS have been reported following some tetanus toxoid-containing vaccines or tetanus and diphtheria toxoid-containing vaccines, although the IOM concluded that the evidence was inadequate to accept or reject a causal relationship.[46] A few cases of peripheral mononeuropathy and of cranial mononeuropathy have been reported following tetanus toxoid administration, although the IOM concluded that the evidence was inadequate to accept or reject a causal relationship.

Postmarketing Reports: Worldwide voluntary reports of adverse events received for INFANRIX and ENGERIX-B in children younger than 7 years of age since market introduction of these US-licensed vaccines are listed below. This list includes adverse events for which 20 or more reports were received with the exception of intussusception, idiopathic thrombocytopenic purpura, thrombocytopenia, anaphylactic reaction, angioedema, encephalopathy, hypotonic-hyporesponsive episode, and alopecia for which fewer than 20 reports were received. These latter events are included either because of the seriousness of the event or the strength of causal connection to components of this or other vaccines or drugs.

Body as a whole: Asthenia[b], fever[a+b], lethargy[b], malaise[b], Sudden Infant Death Syndrome[a+b].
Cardiovascular system: Cyanosis[a+b], edema[b], pallor[b].
Gastrointestinal system: Abdominal pain[b], anorexia[b], diarrhea[a+b], intussusception[a+b], nausea[b], vomiting[a+b].
Hematologic/lymphatic: Idiopathic thrombocytopenic purpura[a+b], lymphadenopathy[a], thrombocytopenia[a+b].
Hepatic: Jaundice[b], liver function tests abnormal[b].
Hypersensitivity: Anaphylactic reaction[a+b], angioedema[b], hypersensitivity[a].
Infections: Cellulitis[a].
Injection site reactions: Injection site reactions[a+b].
Musculoskeletal: Arthralgia[b], limb swelling[a+b].
Nervous system: Convulsions[a+b], encephalopathy[a], headache[b], hypotonia[a+b], hypotonic hyporesponsive episode[a], somnolence[a+b].
Psychiatric: Crying[a+b], irritability[a+b].
Respiratory system: Respiratory tract infection[a].
Skin and appendages: Alopecia[b], erythema[a+b], erythema multiforme[b], petechiae[b], pruritis[a+b], rash[a+b], urticaria[a+b].
Special senses: Ear pain[a].

[a] Following INFANRIX.
[b] Following ENGERIX-B.
[a+b] Following either INFANRIX or ENGERIX-B.

These reactions were reported voluntarily from a population of uncertain size; therefore, it is not always possible to reliably estimate their frequency or establish a causal relationship to vaccination.

Reporting Adverse Events: The National Childhood Vaccine Injury Act requires that the manufacturer and lot number of the vaccine administered be recorded by the healthcare provider in the vaccine recipient's permanent medical record, along with the date of administration of the vaccine and the name, address, and title of the person administering the vaccine.[47] The Act further requires the healthcare provider to report to the US Department of Health and Human Services via VAERS the occurrence following immunization of any event set forth in the Vaccine Injury Table including: Anaphylaxis or anaphylactic shock within 7 days, encephalopathy or encephalitis within 7 days, brachial neuritis within 28 days, or an acute complication or sequelae (including death) of an illness, disability, injury, or condition referred to above, or any events that would contraindicate further doses of vaccine, according to this prescribing information.[47,48] The VAERS toll-free number is 1-800-822-7967.

Table 4. Percentage of Infants in a US Coadministration Safety Study With Fever Within 4 Days of Dose 1* at 2 Months of Age With PEDIARIX Administered Concomitantly With Hib Vaccine and Pneumococcal Conjugate Vaccine or With Separate Concomitant Administration of INFANRIX, ENGERIX-B, IPV, Hib Vaccine, and Pneumococcal Conjugate Vaccine

	PEDIARIX, Hib, & Pneumococcal Conjugate (N = 667)	INFANRIX, ENGERIX-B, IPV, Hib, & Pneumococcal Conjugate (N = 333)	Separate Vaccine Group Minus Combination Vaccine Group
Fever†	%	%	Difference (95% CI)
≥100.4°F‡	27.9	19.8	−8.07 (−13.54, −2.60)
>101.3°F	7.0	4.5	−2.54 (−5.50, 0.41)
>102.2°F‡	2.2	0.3	−1.95 (−3.22, −0.68)
>103.1°F	0.4	0.0	−0.45 (−0.96, 0.06)
M.A.‡	1.2	0.0	−1.20 (−2.03, −0.37)

N = number of infants for whom at least one symptom sheet was completed, excluding 3 infants for whom temperature was not measured and 3 infants whose temperature was measured by the tympanic method.
* Within 4 days of dose 1 defined as day of vaccination and the next 3 days.
† Rectal temperatures.
‡ The group that received PEDIARIX compared to separate vaccine group p value <0.05 (2-sided Fisher Exact test) or the 95% confidence interval on the difference between groups does not include 0.
M.A. = Medically attended (a visit to or from medical personnel).

Table 5. Percentage of Infants in a Moldovan Study With Solicited Local Reactions or Selected Systemic Adverse Events Within 4 Days of Vaccination* at 6, 10, and 14 Weeks of Age With PEDIARIX Administered Concomitantly With Hib Vaccine Following a Birth Dose of Hepatitis B Vaccine (ITT Cohort)

	PEDIARIX & Hib		
	Dose 1	Dose 2	Dose 3
N	160	158	157
Local†			
Pain, any	25.6	18.4	14.0
Pain, grade 3	3.1	0.6	1.9
Redness, any	41.9	41.8	47.1
Redness, >20 mm	1.9	2.5	4.5
Swelling, any	20.6	18.4	28.0
Swelling, >20 mm	4.4	2.5	7.0
Systemic			
Restlessness, any	13.1	10.8	8.9
Restlessness, grade 3	1.3	0.6	0.6
Fever‡, ≥100.4°F	14.4	11.4	5.1
Fever‡, >103.1°F	0.0	0.6	0.0
Fussiness, any	25.0	21.5	17.8
Fussiness, grade 3	2.5	0.6	0.6

N = number of infants in the intent-to-treat (ITT) cohort (infants who received the indicated vaccine and for whom at least one symptom sheet was completed).
Grade 3 defined as preventing normal daily activities.
* Within 4 days of vaccination defined as day of vaccination and the next 3 days.
† Local reactions at the injection site for PEDIARIX.
‡ Rectal temperatures.

DOSAGE AND ADMINISTRATION

Preparation for Administration: PEDIARIX contains an adjuvant; therefore shake vigorously to obtain a homogeneous, turbid, white suspension. DO NOT USE IF RESUSPENSION DOES NOT OCCUR WITH VIGOROUS SHAKING. Inspect visually for particulate matter or discoloration prior to administration. After removal of the dose, any vaccine remaining in the vial should be discarded.

PEDIARIX should be administered by intramuscular injection. The preferred sites are the anterolateral aspects of the thigh or the deltoid muscle of the upper arm. The vaccine should not be injected in the gluteal area or areas where there may be a major nerve trunk. Gluteal injections may result in suboptimal hepatitis B immune response. Before injection, the skin at the injection site should be cleaned and prepared with a suitable germicide. After insertion of the needle, aspirate to ensure that the needle has not entered a blood vessel.

Do not administer this product subcutaneously or intravenously.

Recommended Schedule: The primary immunization series for PEDIARIX is 3 doses of 0.5 mL, given intramuscularly, at 6- to 8-week intervals (preferably 8 weeks). The customary age for the first dose is 2 months of age, but it may be given starting at 6 weeks of age.

PEDIARIX should not be administered to any infant before the age of 6 weeks. Only monovalent hepatitis B vaccine can be used for the birth dose.

Infants born of HBsAg-positive mothers should receive HBIG and Hepatitis B Vaccine (Recombinant) within 12 hours of birth at separate sites and should complete the hepatitis B vaccination series according to a particular schedule.[36] (See manufacturer's prescribing information for Hepatitis B Vaccine [Recombinant]).

Infants born of mothers of unknown HBsAg status should receive Hepatitis B Vaccine (Recombinant) within 12 hours of birth and should complete the hepatitis B vaccination series according to a particular schedule.[36] (See manufacturer's prescribing information for Hepatitis B Vaccine [Recombinant]).

The administration of PEDIARIX for completion of the hepatitis B vaccination series in infants who were born of HBsAg-positive mothers and who received monovalent Hepatitis B Vaccine (Recombinant) and HBIG has not been studied.

Modified Schedules: ***Children Previously Vaccinated With One or More Doses of Hepatitis B Vaccine:*** Infants born of HBsAg-negative mothers and who received a dose of hepatitis B vaccine at or shortly after birth may be administered 3 doses of PEDIARIX according to the recommended schedule. However, data are limited regarding the safety of PEDIARIX in such infants (see ADVERSE REACTIONS). There are no data to support the use of a 3-dose series of PEDIARIX in infants who have previously received more than one dose of hepatitis B vaccine. PEDIARIX may be used to complete a hepatitis B vaccination series in infants who have received 1 or more doses of Hepatitis B Vaccine (Recombinant) and who are also scheduled to receive the other vaccine components of PEDIARIX. However, the safety and efficacy of PEDIARIX in such infants have not been studied.

Children Previously Vaccinated With One or More Doses of INFANRIX: PEDIARIX may be used to complete the first 3 doses of the DTaP series in infants who have received 1 or 2 doses of INFANRIX and are also scheduled to receive the other vaccine components of PEDIARIX. However, the safety and efficacy of PEDIARIX in such infants have not been evaluated.

Children Previously Vaccinated With One or More Doses of IPV: PEDIARIX may be used to complete the first 3 doses of the IPV series in infants who have received 1 or 2 doses of IPV and are also scheduled to receive the other vaccine components of PEDIARIX. However, the safety and efficacy of PEDIARIX in such infants have not been studied.

Interchangeability of PEDIARIX and Licensed DTaP, IPV, or Recombinant Hepatitis B Vaccines: It is recommended that PEDIARIX be given for all 3 doses because data are limited regarding the safety and efficacy of using acellular pertussis vaccines from different manufacturers for successive doses of the pertussis vaccination series. PEDIARIX is not recommended for completion of the first 3 doses of the DTaP vaccination series initiated with a DTaP vaccine from a different manufacturer because no data are available regarding the safety or efficacy of using such a regimen.

PEDIARIX may be used to complete a hepatitis B vaccination series initiated with a licensed Hepatitis B Vaccine (Recombinant) vaccine from a different manufacturer.

PEDIARIX may be used to complete the first 3 doses of the IPV vaccination series initiated with IPV from a different manufacturer.

Additional Dosing Information: If any recommended dose of pertussis vaccine cannot be given, DT (For Pediatric Use), Hepatitis B (Recombinant), and inactivated poliovirus vaccines should be given as needed to complete the series.

Interruption of the recommended schedule with a delay between doses should not interfere with the final immunity

achieved with PEDIARIX. There is no need to start the series over again, regardless of the time elapsed between doses.
The use of reduced volume (fractional doses) is not recommended. The effect of such practices on the frequency of serious adverse events and on protection against disease has not been determined.[10]
Preterm infants should be vaccinated according to their chronological age from birth.[10]
PEDIARIX is not indicated for use as a booster dose following a 3-dose primary series of PEDIARIX. Children who have received a 3-dose primary series of PEDIARIX should receive a fourth dose of IPV at 4 to 6 years of age and a fourth dose of DTaP vaccine at 15 to 18 months of age. Because the pertussis antigen components of INFANRIX are the same as those components in PEDIARIX, these children should receive INFANRIX as their fourth dose of DTaP. However, data are insufficient to evaluate the safety of INFANRIX following 3 doses of PEDIARIX.
Concomitant Vaccine Administration: In clinical trials, PEDIARIX was routinely administered, at separate sites, concomitantly with Hib vaccine (see CLINICAL PHARMACOLOGY). Safety data are available following the first dose of PEDIARIX administered concomitantly, at separate sites, with Hib and pneumococcal conjugate vaccines (see ADVERSE REACTIONS).
When concomitant administration of other vaccines is required, they should be given with separate syringes and at different injection sites.

STORAGE

Store PEDIARIX refrigerated between 2° and 8°C (36° and 46°F). **Do not freeze.** Discard if the vaccine has been frozen. Do not use after expiration date shown on the label.

HOW SUPPLIED

PEDIARIX is supplied as a turbid white suspension in single-dose (0.5 mL) vials and disposable prefilled Tip-Lok® syringes.
Single-Dose Vials
NDC 58160-841-11 (package of 10)
Single-Dose Prefilled Disposable Tip-Lok® Syringes (packaged without needles)
NDC 58160-841-46 (package of 5)
NDC 58160-841-50 (package of 25)
Single-Dose Prefilled Disposable Tip-Lok® Syringes with 1-inch 25-gauge BD SafetyGlide™ Needles
NDC 58160-841-56 (package of 25)
Single-Dose Prefilled Disposable Tip-Lok® Syringes with 5/8-inch 25-gauge BD SafetyGlide™ Needles
NDC 58160-841-57 (package of 25)

REFERENCES

1. Centers for Disease Control. Diphtheria, tetanus, and pertussis: Recommendations for vaccine use and other preventive measures — Recommendations of the Immunization Practices Advisory Committee (ACIP). *MMWR* 1991;40(RR-10):1-28. **2.** Centers for Disease Control and Prevention. Diphtheria. In: Atkinson W and Wolfe C, eds. *Epidemiology and prevention of vaccine-preventable diseases*. 7th ed. Atlanta, GA: Public Health Foundation; 2002:39-48. **3.** Bisgard KM, Hardy I, Popovic T, et al. Respiratory diphtheria in the United States, 1980 through 1995. *Am J Public Health* 1998;88(5):787-791. **4.** Centers for Disease Control and Prevention. Toxigenic *Corynebacterium diphtheriae* — Northern Plains Indian community, August-October 1996. *MMWR* 1997;46(22):506-510. **5.** Mortimer EA and Wharton M. Diphtheria Toxoid. In: Plotkin SA and Orenstein WA, eds. *Vaccines*. 3rd ed. Philadelphia, PA: W.B. Saunders Company; 1999:140-157. **6.** Centers for Disease Control and Prevention. Tetanus — Puerto Rico, 2002. *MMWR* 2002;51(28):613-615. **7.** Centers for Disease Control and Prevention. Tetanus surveillance — United States, 1995-1997. *MMWR* 1998;47(SS-2):1-13. **8.** Wassilak SGF, Orenstein WA, and Sutter RW. Tetanus Toxoid. In: Plotkin SA and Orenstein WA, eds. *Vaccines*. 3rd ed. Philadelphia, PA: W.B. Saunders Company; 1999:441-474. **9.** Department of Health and Human Services, Food and Drug Administration. Biological products; Bacterial vaccines and toxoids; Implementation of efficacy review; Proposed rule. *Federal Register* December 13, 1985;50(240):51002-51117. **10.** Centers for Disease Control and Prevention. General recommendations on immunization: Recommendations of the Advisory Committee on Immunization Practices (ACIP) and the American Academy of Family Physicians (AAFP). *MMWR* 2002;51(RR-2):1-35. **11.** Long SS. Pertussis (*Bordetella pertussis* and *B. parapertussis*). In: Behrman RE, Kliegman RM, Jenson HB, eds. *Nelson Textbook of Pediatrics*. 16th ed. Philadelphia, PA: W.B. Saunders; 2000:838-842. **12.** Centers for Disease Control and Prevention. Pertussis — United States, 1997-2000. *MMWR* 2002;51(4):73-76. **13.** Nennig ME, Shinefield HR, Edwards KM, et al. Prevalence and incidence of adult pertussis in an urban population. *JAMA* 1996;275(21):1672-1674. **14.** Güris D, Strebel PM, Bardenheier B, et al. Changing epidemiology of pertussis in the United States: Increasing reported incidence among adolescents and adults, 1990-1996. *Clin Infect Dis* 1999;28:1230-1237. **15.** Greco D, Salmaso S, Mastrantonio P, et al. A controlled trial of two acellular vaccines and one whole-cell vaccine against pertussis. *N Engl J Med* 1996;334(6):341-348. **16.** Schmitt H-J, von König CHW, Neiss A, et al. Efficacy of acellular pertussis vaccine in early childhood after household exposure. *JAMA* 1996;275(1):37-41. **17.** Salmaso S, Mastrantonio P, Tozzi AE, et al. Sustained efficacy during the first 6 years of life of 3-component acellular pertussis vaccines administered in infancy: The Italian experience. *Pediatrics* 2001;108(5):E81.**18.** Centers for Disease Control. Recommendations for protection against viral hepatitis: Recommendation of the Immunization Practices Advisory Committee (ACIP). *MMWR* 1985;34(22):313-324. **19.** Centers for Disease Control and Prevention. Hepatitis B. In: Atkinson W and Wolfe C, eds. *Epidemiology and prevention of vaccine-preventable diseases*. 7th ed. Atlanta, GA: Public Health Foundation; 2002:169-189. **20.** Lee WM. Hepatitis B virus infection. *N Engl J Med* 1997;337(24):1733-1745. **21.** Centers for Disease Control. Protection against viral hepatitis: Recommendations of the Immunization Practices Advisory Committee (ACIP). *MMWR* 1990;39(RR-2):1-26. **22.** Ambrosch F, Frisch-Niggemeyer W, Kremsner P, et al. Persistence of vaccine-induced antibodies to hepatitis B surface antigen and the need for booster vaccination in adult subjects. *Postgrad Med J* 1987;63(Suppl. 2):129-135. **23.** Andre FE and Safary A. Clinical experience with a yeast-derived hepatitis B vaccine. In: Zuckerman AJ, ed. *Viral hepatitis and liver disease*. New York, NY: Alan R Liss, Inc.; 1988:1025-1030. **24.** Poovorawan Y, Sanpavat S, Pongpunlert W, et al. Protective efficacy of a recombinant DNA hepatitis B vaccine in neonates of HBe antigen-positive mothers. *JAMA* 1989;261(22):3278-3281. **25.** Centers for Disease Control and Prevention. Proposed vaccine information materials for hepatitis B, Haemophilus influenza type B (Hib), varicella (chickenpox), and measles, mumps, rubella (MMR) vaccines. *Federal Register* September 3, 1998;63(171):47026-47031. **26.** Chang MH, Chen CJ, Lai MS. Universal hepatitis B vaccination in Taiwan and the incidence of hepatocellular carcinoma in children. *N Engl J Med* 1997;336:1855-1859. **27.** Lee MS, Kim DH, Kim H, et al. Hepatitis B vaccination and reduced risk of primary liver cancer among male adults: A cohort study in Korea. *Int J Epidemiol* 1998;27(2):316-319. **28.** Centers for Disease Control and Prevention. Poliomyelitis. In: Atkinson W and Wolfe C, eds. *Epidemiology and prevention of vaccine-preventable diseases*. 7th ed. Atlanta, GA: Public Health Foundation; 2002:71-82. **29.** Centers for Disease Control and Prevention. Poliomyelitis prevention in the United States: Introduction of a sequential vaccination schedule of inactivated poliovirus vaccine followed by oral poliovirus vaccine — Recommendations of the Advisory Committee on Immunization Practices (ACIP). *MMWR* 1997;46(RR-3):1-25. **30.** Kim-Farley RJ, Bart KJ, Schonberger LP, et al. Poliomyelitis in the USA: Virtual elimination of disease caused by wild virus. *Lancet* 1984;2:1315-1317. **31.** Nathanson N, Martin JR. The epidemiology of poliomyelitis: Enigmas surrounding its appearance, epidemiology, and disappearance. *Am J Epidemiol* 1979;110(6):672-692. **32.** Centers for Disease Control and Prevention. Summary of notifiable diseases, United States, 2000. *MMWR* 2000;49(53):83. **33.** Centers for Disease Control and Prevention. Poliomyelitis prevention in the United States: Updated recommendations of the Advisory Committee on Immunization Practices (ACIP). *MMWR* 2000;49(RR-5):1-22. **34.** Sutter RW, Pallansch MA, Sawyer LA, et al. Defining surrogate serologic tests with respect to predicting protective vaccine efficacy: Poliovirus vaccination. In: Williams JC, Goldenthal KL, Burns DL, Lewis Jr BP, eds. Combined vaccines and simultaneous administration. Current issues and perspectives. New York, NY: The New York Academy of Sciences; 1995:289-299. **35.** Yeh SH, Ward JI, Partridge S, et al. Safety and immunogenicity of a pentavalent diphtheria, tetanus, pertussis, hepatitis B and polio combination vaccine in infants. *Pediatr Infect Dis J* 2001;20:973-980. **36.** Centers for Disease Control and Prevention. Recommended childhood immunization schedule — United States, 2002. *MMWR* 2002;51(2):31-33. **37.** Centers for Disease Control and Prevention. Use of vaccines and immune globulins in persons with altered immunocompetence: Recommendations of the Advisory Committee on Immunization Practices (ACIP). *MMWR* 1993;42(RR-4):1-18. **38.** Centers for Disease Control and Prevention. Pertussis vaccination: Use of acellular pertussis vaccines among infants and young children — Recommendations of the Advisory Committee on Immunization Practices (ACIP). *MMWR* 1997;46(RR-7):1-25. **39.** Centers for Disease Control and Prevention. Update: Vaccine side effects, adverse reactions, contraindications, and precautions — Recommendations of the Advisory Committee on Immunization Practices (ACIP). *MMWR* 1996;45(RR-12):1-35. **40.** Institute of Medicine (IOM). Howson CP, Howe CJ, Fineberg HV, eds. *Adverse effects of pertussis and rubella vaccines*. Washington, DC: National Academy Press; 1991. **41.** Institute of Medicine (IOM). Stratton KR, Howe CJ, Johnston RB, eds. *DPT vaccine and chronic nervous dysfunction: A new analysis*. Washington, DC: National Academy Press; 1994. **42.** American Academy of Pediatrics. Pertussis. In: Pickering LK, ed. *2000 Red Book: Report of the Committee on Infectious Diseases*. 25th ed. Elk Grove Village, IL: American Academy of Pediatrics; 2000:442-448. **43.** Zepp F, Schuind A, Meyer C, et al. Safety and reactogenicity of a novel DTPa-HBV-IPV combined vaccine given along with commercial Hib vaccines in comparison with separate concomitant administration of DTPa, Hib, and OPV vaccines in infants. *Pediatrics* 2002;109(4):E58. **44.** Poets CF. Plötzlicher Säuglingstod. Neue Erkenntnisse. *Pädiat prax* 2001;60:285-292. **45.** Centers for Disease Control and Prevention. Sudden Infant Death Syndrome — United States, 1983-94. *MMWR* 1996;45(40):859-863. **46.** Institute of Medicine (IOM). Stratton KR, Howe CJ, Johnston RB, eds. *Adverse events associated with childhood vaccines. Evidence bearing on causality*. Washington, DC: National Academy Press; 1994. **47.** Centers for Disease Control. National Childhood Vaccine Injury Act: Requirements for permanent vaccination records and for reporting of selected events after vaccination. *MMWR* 1988;37(13):197-200. **48.** National Vaccine Injury Compensation Program: Vaccine injury table. www.hrsa.gov/osp/vicp/table.htm. Accessed April 29, 2002.

Manufactured by **SmithKline Beecham Biologicals**
Rixensart, Belgium, US License 1090, and
Chiron Behring GmbH & Co
Marburg, Germany, US License 0097
Distributed by **SmithKline Beecham Pharmaceuticals**, Philadelphia, PA 19101
PEDIARIX is a trademark and TIP-LOK, INFANRIX, and ENGERIX-B are registered trademarks of SmithKline Beecham.
SAFETYGLIDE is a trademark of Becton, Dickinson and Company.

December 2002/PE:L1

Eli Lilly and Company

LILLY CORPORATE CENTER
INDIANAPOLIS, IN 46285

Direct Inquiries to:
Lilly Corporate Center
Indianapolis, IN 46285
(317) 276-2000
www.lilly.com
For Medical Information Contact:
Lilly Research Laboratories
Lilly Corporate Center
Indianapolis, IN 46285
(800) 545-5979

FORTEO™ ℞

[for-tay-o]
teriparatide (rDNA origin)
injection 750 mcg/3 mL

WARNING
In male and female rats, teriparatide caused an increase in the incidence of osteosarcoma (a malignant bone tumor) that was dependent on dose and treatment duration. The effect was observed at systemic exposures to teriparatide ranging from 3 to 60 times the exposure in humans given a 20-mcg dose. Because of the uncertain relevance of the rat osteosarcoma finding to humans, teriparatide should be prescribed only to patients for whom the potential benefits are considered to outweigh the potential risk. Teriparatide should not be prescribed for patients who are at increased baseline risk for osteosarcoma (including those with Paget's disease of bone or unexplained elevations of alkaline phosphatase, open epiphyses, or prior radiation therapy involving the skeleton) (*see* WARNINGS *and* PRECAUTIONS, Carcinogenesis).

DESCRIPTION

FORTEO™ [teriparatide (rDNA origin) injection] contains recombinant human parathyroid hormone (1-34), [rhPTH (1-34)], which has an identical sequence to the 34 N-terminal amino acids (the biologically active region) of the 84-amino acid human parathyroid hormone.
Teriparatide has a molecular weight of 4117.8 daltons and its amino acid sequence is shown below:

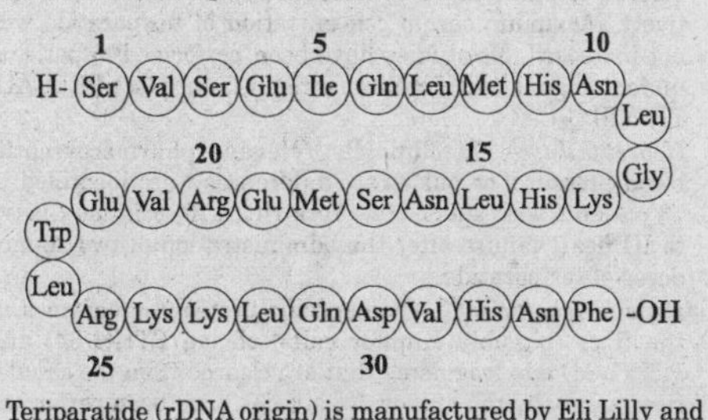
1 5 10
H- Ser Val Ser Glu Ile Gln Leu Met His Asn
Leu
20 15
Gly
Glu Val Arg Glu Met Ser Asn Leu His Lys
Trp
Leu
Arg Lys Lys Leu Gln Asp Val His Asn Phe -OH
25 30

Teriparatide (rDNA origin) is manufactured by Eli Lilly and Company using a strain of *Escherichia coli* modified by recombinant DNA technology. FORTEO is supplied as a sterile, colorless, clear, isotonic solution in a glass cartridge which is pre-assembled into a disposable pen device for subcutaneous injection. Each prefilled delivery device is filled with 3.3 mL to deliver 3 mL. Each mL contains 250 mcg teriparatide (corrected for acetate, chloride, and water content), 0.41 mg glacial acetic acid, 0.10 mg sodium acetate (anhydrous), 45.4 mg mannitol, 3.0 mg Metacresol, and Water for Injection. In addition, hydrochloric acid solution 10% and/or sodium hydroxide solution 10% may have been added to adjust the product to pH 4.
Each cartridge pre-assembled into a pen device delivers 20 mcg of teriparatide per dose each day for up to 28 days.
See accompanying User Manual: Instructions for Use.

CLINICAL PHARMACOLOGY

Mechanism of Action—Endogenous 84-amino-acid parathyroid hormone (PTH) is the primary regulator of calcium and

Continued on next page

Forteo—Cont.

phosphate metabolism in bone and kidney. Physiological actions of PTH include regulation of bone metabolism, renal tubular reabsorption of calcium and phosphate, and intestinal calcium absorption. The biological actions of PTH and teriparatide are mediated through binding to specific high-affinity cell-surface receptors. Teriparatide and the 34 N-terminal amino acids of PTH bind to these receptors with the same affinity and have the same physiological actions on bone and kidney. Teriparatide is not expected to accumulate in bone or other tissues.

The skeletal effects of teriparatide depend upon the pattern of systemic exposure. Once-daily administration of teriparatide stimulates new bone formation on trabecular and cortical (periosteal and/or endosteal) bone surfaces by preferential stimulation of osteoblastic activity over osteoclastic activity. In monkey studies, teriparatide improved trabecular microarchitecture and increased bone mass and strength by stimulating new bone formation in both cancellous and cortical bone. In humans, the anabolic effects of teriparatide are manifest as an increase in skeletal mass, an increase in markers of bone formation and resorption, and an increase in bone strength. By contrast, continuous excess of endogenous PTH, as occurs in hyperparathyroidism, may be detrimental to the skeleton because bone resorption may be stimulated more than bone formation.

Human Pharmacokinetics—Teriparatide is extensively absorbed after subcutaneous injection; the absolute bioavailability is approximately 95% based on pooled data from 20-, 40-, and 80-mcg doses. The rates of absorption and elimination are rapid. The peptide reaches peak serum concentrations about 30 minutes after subcutaneous injection of a 20-mcg dose and declines to non-quantifiable concentrations within 3 hours.

Systemic clearance of teriparatide (approximately 62 L/hr in women and 94 L/hr in men) exceeds the rate of normal liver plasma flow, consistent with both hepatic and extrahepatic clearance. Volume of distribution, following intravenous injection, is approximately 0.12 L/kg. Intersubject variability in systemic clearance and volume of distribution is 25% to 50%. The half-life of teriparatide in serum is 5 minutes when administered by intravenous injection and approximately 1 hour when administered by subcutaneous injection. The longer half-life following subcutaneous administration reflects the time required for absorption from the injection site.

No metabolism or excretion studies have been performed with teriparatide. However, the mechanisms of metabolism and elimination of PTH(1-34) and intact PTH have been extensively described in published literature. Peripheral metabolism of PTH is believed to occur by non-specific enzymatic mechanisms in the liver followed by excretion via the kidneys.

Special Populations—*Pediatric*—Pharmacokinetic data in pediatric patients are not available (*see* WARNINGS).

Geriatric—No age-related differences in teriparatide pharmacokinetics were detected (range 31 to 85 years).

Gender—Although systemic exposure to teriparatide was approximately 20% to 30% lower in men than women, the recommended dose for both genders is 20 mcg/day.

Race—The populations included in the pharmacokinetic analyses were 98.5% Caucasian. The influence of race has not been determined.

Renal insufficiency—No pharmacokinetic differences were identified in 11 patients with mild or moderate renal insufficiency [creatinine clearance (CrCl) 30 to 72 mL/min] administered a single dose of teriparatide, in 5 patients with severe renal insufficiency (CrCl < 30 mL/min), the AUC and T1/2 of teriparatide were increased by 73% and 77%, respectively. Maximum serum concentration of teriparatide was not increased. No studies have been performed in patients undergoing dialysis for chronic renal failure (*see* PRECAUTIONS).

Heart failure—No clinically relevant pharmacokinetic, blood pressure, or pulse rate differences were identified in 13 patients with stable New York Heart Association Class I to III heart failure after the administration of two 20-mcg doses of teriparatide.

Hepatic insufficiency—Non-specific proteolytic enzymes in the liver (possibly Kupffer cells) cleave PTH(1-34) and PTH(1-84) into fragments that are cleared from the circulation mainly by the kidney. No studies have been performed in patients with hepatic impairment.

Drug Interactions—*Hydrochlorothiazide*—In a study of 20 healthy people, the coadministration of hydrochlorothiazide 25 mg with teriparatide did not affect the serum calcium response to teriparatide 40 mcg. The 24-hour urine excretion of calcium was reduced by a clinically unimportant amount (15%). The effect of coadministration of a higher dose of hydrochlorothiazide with teriparatide on serum calcium levels has not been studied.

Furosemide—In a study of 9 healthy people and 17 patients with mild, moderate, or severe renal insufficiency (CrCl 13 to 72 mL/min), coadministration of intravenous furosemide (20 to 100 mg) with teriparatide 40 mcg resulted in small increases in the serum calcium (2%) and 24-hour urine calcium (37%) responses to teriparatide that did not appear to be clinically important.

Human Pharmacodynamics—*Effects on mineral metabolism*—Teriparatide affects calcium and phosphorus metabolism in a pattern consistent with the known actions of endogenous PTH (eg, increases serum calcium and decreases serum phosphorus).

Table 1. Effect of FORTEO on Risk of Vertebral Fractures in Postmenopausal Women with Osteoporosis

	Percent of Women With Fracture			
	FORTEO (N=444)	Placebo (N=448)	Absolute Risk Reduction (%, 95% CI)	Relative Risk Reduction (%, 95% CI)
New fracture (≥1)	5.0[a]	14.3	9.3 (5.5-13.1)	65 (45-78)
1 fracture	3.8	9.4		
2 fractures	0.9	2.9		
≥3 fractures	0.2	2.0		

[a]p≤0.001 compared with placebo

Serum calcium concentrations—When teriparatide 20 mcg is administered once daily, the serum calcium concentration increases transiently, beginning approximately 2 hours after dosing and reaching a maximum concentration between 4 and 6 hours (median increase, 0.4 mg/dL). The serum calcium concentration begins to decline approximately 6 hours after dosing and returns to baseline by 16 to 24 hours after each dose.

In a clinical study of postmenopausal women with osteoporosis, the median peak serum calcium concentration measured 4 to 6 hours after dosing with FORTEO (teriparatide 20 mcg) was 2.42 mmol/L (9.68 mg/dL) at 12 months. The peak serum calcium remained below 2.76 mmol/L (11.0 mg/dL) in >99% of women at each visit. Sustained hypercalcemia was not observed.

In this study, 11.1% of women treated with FORTEO had at least 1 serum calcium value above the upper limit of normal [2.64 mmol/L (10.6 mg/dL)] compared with 1.5% of women treated with placebo. The percentage of women treated with FORTEO whose serum calcium was above the upper limit of normal on consecutive 4- to 6-hour post-dose measurements was 3.0% compared with 0.2% of women treated with placebo. In these women, calcium supplements and/or FORTEO doses were reduced. The timing of these dose reductions was at the discretion of the investigator. FORTEO dose adjustments were made at varying intervals after the first observation of increased serum calcium (median 21 weeks). During these intervals, there was no evidence of progressive increases in serum calcium.

In a clinical study of men with either primary or hypogonadal osteoporosis, the effects on serum calcium were similar to those observed in postmenopausal women. The median peak serum calcium concentration measured 4 to 6 hours after dosing with FORTEO was 2.35 mmol/L (9.44 mg/dL) at 12 months. The peak serum calcium remained below 2.76 mmol/L (11.0 mg/dL) in 98% of men at each visit. Sustained hypercalcemia was not observed.

In this study, 6.0% of men treated with FORTEO daily had at least 1 serum calcium value above the upper limit of normal [2.64 mmol/L (10.6 mg/dL)] compared with none of the men treated with placebo. The percentage of men treated with FORTEO whose serum calcium was above the upper limit of normal on consecutive measurements was 1.3% (2 men) compared with none of the men treated with placebo. Although calcium supplements and/or FORTEO doses could have been reduced in these men, only calcium supplementation was reduced (*see* PRECAUTIONS *and* ADVERSE EVENTS).

In a clinical study of women previously treated for 18 to 39 months with raloxifene (n=26) or alendronate (n=33), mean serum calcium >12 hours after FORTEO injection was increased by 0.09 to 0.14 mmol/L (0.36 to 0.56 mg/dL), after 1 to 6 months of FORTEO treatment compared with baseline. Of the women pretreated with raloxifene, 3 (11.5%) had a serum calcium >2.76 mmol/L (11.0 mg/dL), and of those pretreated with alendronate, 3 (9.1%) had a serum calcium >2.76 mmol/L (11.0 mg/dL). The highest serum calcium reported was 3.12 mmol/L (12.5 mg/dL). None of the women had symptoms of hypercalcemia. There were no placebo controls in this study.

Urinary calcium excretion—In a clinical study of postmenopausal women with osteoporosis who received 1000 mg of supplemental calcium and at least 400 IU of vitamin D, daily FORTEO increased urinary calcium excretion. The median urinary excretion of calcium was 4.8 mmol/day (190 mg/day) at 6 months and 4.2 mmol/day (170 mg/day) at 12 months. These levels were 0.76 mmol/day (30 mg/day) and 0.30 mmol/day (12 mg/day) higher, respectively, than in women treated with placebo. The incidence of hypercalciuria (>7.5 mmol Ca/day or 300 mg/day) was similar in the women treated with FORTEO or placebo.

In a clinical study of men with either primary or hypogonadal osteoporosis who received 1000 mg of supplemental calcium and at least 400 IU of vitamin D, daily FORTEO had inconsistent effects on urinary calcium excretion. The median urinary excretion of calcium was 5.6 mmol/day (220 mg/day) at 1 month and 5.3 mmol/day (210 mg/day) at 6 months. These levels were 0.50 mmol/day (20 mg/day) higher and 0.20 mmol/day (8.0 mg/day) lower, respectively, than in men treated with placebo. The incidence of hypercalciuria (>7.5 mmol Ca/day or 300 mg/day) was similar in the men treated with FORTEO or placebo.

Phosphorus and vitamin D—In single-dose studies, teriparatide produced transient phosphaturia and mild transient reductions in serum phosphorus concentration. However, hypophosphatemia (<0.74 mmol/L or 2.4 mg/dL) was not observed in clinical trials with FORTEO.

In clinical trials of daily FORTEO, the median serum concentration of 1,25-dihydroxyvitamin D was increased at 12 months by 19% in women and 14% in men, compared with baseline. In the placebo group, this concentration decreased by 2% in women and increased by 5% in men. The median serum 25-hydroxyvitamin D concentration at 12 months was decreased by 19% in women and 10% in men compared with baseline. In the placebo group, this concentration was unchanged in women and increased by 1% in men.

Effects on markers of bone turnover—Daily administration of FORTEO to men and postmenopausal women with osteoporosis in clinical studies stimulated bone formation, as shown by increases in the formation markers serum bone-specific alkaline phosphatase (BSAP) and procollagen I carboxy-terminal propeptide (PICP). Data on biochemical markers of bone turnover were available for the first 12 months of treatment. Peak concentrations of PICP at 1 month of treatment were approximately 41% above baseline, followed by a decline to near-baseline values by 12 months. BSAP concentrations increased by 1 month of treatment and continued to rise more slowly from 6 through 12 months. The maximum increases of BSAP were 45% above baseline in women and 23% in men. After discontinuation of therapy, BSAP concentrations returned toward baseline. The increases in formation markers were accompanied by secondary increases in the markers of bone resorption: urinary N-telopeptide (NTX) and urinary deoxypyridinoline (DPD), consistent with the physiological coupling of bone formation and resorption in skeletal remodeling. Changes in BSAP, NTX, and DPD were lower in men than in women, possibly because of lower systemic exposure to teriparatide in men.

CLINICAL STUDIES

Treatment of Osteoporosis in Postmenopausal Women—The safety and efficacy of once-daily FORTEO, median exposure of 19 months, were examined in a double-blind, placebo-controlled clinical study of 1637 postmenopausal women with osteoporosis [FORTEO 20 mcg, n = 541].

This multicenter study was performed in the US and 16 other countries. All women received 1000 mg of calcium per day and at least 400 IU of vitamin D per day. Baseline and endpoint spinal radiographs were evaluated using the semiquantitative scoring method of Genant et al [*J Bone Miner Res* 1993:8(9):1137–48]. Ninety percent of the women in the study had one or more radiographically diagnosed vertebral fractures at baseline. The primary efficacy endpoint was the occurrence of new radiographically diagnosed vertebral fractures defined as changes in the height of previously undeformed vertebrae. Such fractures are not necessarily symptomatic.

Effect on fracture incidence—*New vertebral fractures*—FORTEO, when taken with calcium and vitamin D and compared with calcium and vitamin D alone, reduced the risk of 1 or more new vertebral fractures from 14.3% of women in the placebo group to 5.0% in the FORTEO group. This difference was statistically significant (p<0.001); the absolute reduction in risk was 9.3% and the relative reduction was 65%. FORTEO was effective in reducing the risk for vertebral fractures regardless of age, baseline rate of bone turnover, or baseline BMD.

[See table 1 above]

New nonvertebral osteoporotic fractures—Table 2 shows the effect of FORTEO on the risk of nonvertebral fractures. FORTEO significantly reduced the risk of any nonvertebral fracture from 5.5% in the placebo group to 2.6% in the FORTEO group (p<0.05). The absolute reduction in risk was 2.9% and the relative reduction was 53%.

Table 2. Effects of FORTEO on Risk of New Nonvertebral Fractures in Postmenopausal Women with Osteoporosis

Skeletal site	FORTEO[a] N=541	Placebo[a] N=544
Wrist	2 (0.4%)	7 (1.3%)
Ribs	3 (0.6%)	5 (0.9%)
Hip	1 (0.2%)	4 (0.7%)
Ankle/Foot	1 (0.2%)	4 (0.7%)
Humerus	2 (0.4%)	2 (0.4%)
Pelvis	0	3 (0.6%)

Other	6 (1.1%)	8 (1.5%)
Total	14 (2.6%)[b]	30 (5.5%)

[a]Data shown as number (%) of women with fractures.
[b]$p<0.05$ compared with placebo.

The cumulative percentage of postmenopausal women with osteoporosis who sustained new nonvertebral fractures was lower in women treated with FORTEO than in women treated with placebo (see Figure 1).

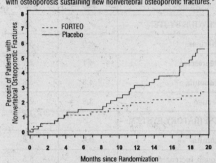

Figure 1. Cumulative percentage of postmenopausal women with osteoporosis sustaining new nonvertebral osteoporotic fractures.*

*This graph includes all fractures listed above in Table 2.

Effect on bone mineral density (BMD)—FORTEO increased lumbar spine BMD in postmenopausal women with osteoporosis. Statistically significant increases were seen at 3 months and continued throughout the treatment period, as shown in Figure 2.

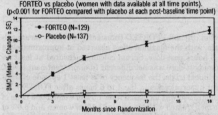

Postmenopausal women with osteoporosis who were treated with FORTEO also had statistically significant increases in BMD at the femoral neck, total hip, and total body (see Table 3).

Table 3. Mean Percent Change in BMD from Baseline to Endpoint* in Postmenopausal Women with Osteoporosis, Treated with FORTEO or Placebo

	FORTEO N=541	Placebo N=544
Lumber spine BMD	9.7[a]	1.1
Femoral neck BMD	2.8[b]	-0.7
Total hip BMD	2.6[b]	-1.0
Trochanter BMD	3.5[b]	-0.2
Intertrochanter BMD	2.6[b]	-1.3
Ward's triangle BMD	4.2[b]	-0.8
Total body BMD	0.6[b]	-0.5
Distal 1/3 radius BMD	-2.1	-1.3
Ultradistal radius BMD	-0.1	-1.6

*Intent-to-treat analysis, last observation carried forward.
[a]$p<0.001$ compared with placebo.
[b]$p<0.05$ compared with placebo.

Figure 3 shows the cumulative distribution of the percentage change from baseline of lumbar spine BMD for the FORTEO and placebo groups. FORTEO treatment increased lumbar spine BMD from baseline in 96% of postmenopausal women treated (see Figure 3). Seventy-two percent of patients treated with FORTEO achieved at least a 5% increase in spine BMD, and 44% gained 10% or more. [See figure 3 at top of next column]

Both treatment groups lost height during the trial. The mean decreases were 3.61 and 2.81 mm in the placebo and FORTEO groups, respectively.

Bone histology—The effects of teriparatide on bone histology were evaluated in iliac crest biopsies of 35 postmenopausal women treated for 12 to 24 months with calcium and vitamin D and teriparatide 20 or 40 mcg/day. Normal mineralization was observed with no evidence of cellular toxicity. The new bone formed with teriparatide was of normal quality (as evidenced by the absence of woven bone and marrow fibrosis).

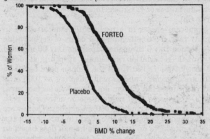

Figure 3. Percent of postmenopausal women with osteoporosis attaining a lumbar spine BMD percent change from baseline at least as great as the value on the x-axis (median duration of treatment 19 months).

Treatment to increase bone mass in men with primary or hypogonadal osteoporosis—The safety and efficacy of once-daily FORTEO, median exposure of 10 months, were examined in a double-blind, placebo-controlled clinical study of 437 men with either primary (idiopathic) or hypogonadal osteoporosis (FORTEO 20 mcg, n = 151). This multicenter efficacy study was performed in the US and 10 other countries. All men received 1000 mg of calcium per day and at least 400 IU of vitamin D per day. The primary efficacy endpoint was change in lumbar spine BMD.

FORTEO increased lumbar spine BMD in men with primary or hypogonadal osteoporosis. Statistically significant increases were seen at 3 months and continued throughout the treatment period. FORTEO was effective in increasing lumbar spine BMD regardless of age, baseline rate of bone turnover, and baseline BMD. The effects of FORTEO at additional skeletal sites are shown in table 4.

Table 4. Mean Percent Change in BMD from Baseline to Endpoint* in Men with Primary or Hypogonadal Osteoporosis, Treated with FORTEO or Placebo for a Median of 10 Months

	FORTEO N=151	Placebo N=147
Lumber spine BMD	5.9[a]	0.5
Femoral neck BMD	1.5[b]	0.3
Total hip BMD	1.2	0.5
Trochanter BMD	1.3	1.1
Intertrochanter BMD	1.2	0.6
Ward's triangle BMD	2.8	1.1
Total body BMD	0.4	-0.4
Distal 1/3 radius BMD	-0.5	-0.2
Ultradistal radius BMD	-0.5	-0.3

*Intent-to-treat analysis, last observation carried forward.
[a]$p<0.001$ compared with placebo.
[b]$p<0.05$ compared with placebo.

Figure 4 shows the cumulative distribution of the percentage change from baseline of lumbar spine BMD for the FORTEO and placebo groups. FORTEO treatment for a median of 10 months increased lumbar spine BMD from baseline in 94% of men treated. Fifty-three percent of patients treated with FORTEO achieved at least a 5% increase in spine BMD, and 14% gained 10% or more.

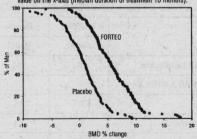

Figure 4. Percent of men with primary or hypogonadal osteoporosis attaining a lumbar spine BMD percent change from baseline at least as great as the value on the x-axis (median duration of treatment 10 months).

INDICATIONS AND USAGE

FORTEO is indicated for the treatment of postmenopausal women with osteoporosis who are at high risk for fracture. These include women with a history of osteoporotic fracture, or who have multiple risk factors for fracture, or who have failed or are intolerant of previous osteoporosis therapy, based upon physician assessment (see BLACK BOX WARNING). In postmenopausal women with osteoporosis, FORTEO increases BMD and reduces the risk of vertebral and nonvertebral fractures.

FORTEO is indicated to increase bone mass in men with primary or hypogonadal osteoporosis who are at high risk for fracture. These include men with a history of osteoporotic fracture, or who have multiple risk factors for fracture, or who have failed or are intolerant to previous osteoporosis therapy, based upon physician assessment (see BLACK BOX WARNING). In men with primary or hypogonadal osteoporosis, FORTEO increases BMD. The effects of FORTEO on risk for fracture in men have not been studied.

- FORTEO reduces the risk of vertebral fractures in postmenopausal women with osteoporosis.
- FORTEO reduces the risk of nonvertebral fractures in postmenopausal women with osteoporosis.
- FORTEO increases vertebral and femoral neck BMD in postmenopausal women with osteoporosis and in men with primary or hypogonadal osteoporosis.
- The effects of FORTEO on fracture risk have not been studied in men.

CONTRAINDICATIONS

FORTEO should not be given to patients with hypersensitivity to teriparatide or to any of its excipients.

WARNINGS

In male and female rats, teriparatide caused an increase in the incidence of osteosarcoma (a malignant bone tumor) that was dependent on dose and treatment duration. (see BLACK BOX WARNING and PRECAUTIONS; Carcinogenesis).

The following categories of patients have increased baseline risk of osteosarcoma and therefore should not be treated with FORTEO:

- Paget's disease of bone. FORTEO should not be given to patients with Paget's disease of bone. Unexplained elevations of alkaline phosphatase may indicate Paget's disease of bone.
- Pediatric populations. FORTEO has not been studied in pediatric populations. FORTEO should not be used in pediatric patients or young adults with open epiphyses.
- Prior radiation therapy. Patients with a prior history of radiation therapy involving the skeleton should be excluded from treatment with FORTEO.

Patients with bone metastases or a history of skeletal malignancies should be excluded from treatment with FORTEO.

Patients with metabolic bone diseases other than osteoporosis should be excluded from treatment with FORTEO.

FORTEO has not been studied in patients with pre-existing hypercalcemia. These patients should be excluded from treatment with FORTEO because of the possibility of exacerbating hypercalcemia.

PRECAUTIONS

General—The safety and efficacy of FORTEO have not been evaluated beyond 2 years of treatment. Consequently, use of the drug for more than 2 years is not recommended.

In clinical trials, the frequency of urolithiasis was similar in patients treated with FORTEO and placebo. However, FORTEO has not been studied in patients with active urolithiasis. If active urolithiasis or pre-existing hypercalciuria are suspected, measurement of urinary calcium excretion should be considered. FORTEO should be used with caution in patients with active or recent urolithiasis because of the potential to exacerbate this condition.

Hypotension—In short-term clinical pharmacology studies with teriparatide, transient episodes of symptomatic orthostatic hypotension were observed infrequently. Typically, an event began within 4 hours of dosing and spontaneously resolved within a few minutes to a few hours. When transient orthostatic hypotension occurred, it happened within the first several doses, it was relieved by placing the person in a reclining position, and it did not preclude continued treatment.

Concomitant treatment with digitalis—In a study of 15 healthy people administered digoxin daily to steady state, a single FORTEO dose did not alter the effect of digoxin on the systolic time interval (from electrocardiographic Q-wave onset to aortic valve closure, a measure of digoxin's calcium-mediated cardiac effect). However, sporadic case reports have suggested that hypercalcemia may predispose patients to digitalis toxicity. Because FORTEO transiently increases serum calcium, FORTEO should be used with caution in patients taking digitalis.

Hepatic, renal, and cardiac—Limited information is available to evaluate safety in patients with hepatic, renal, and cardiac disease.

Information for Patients—For safe and effective use of FORTEO, the physician should inform patients about the following:

General—Patients should read the Medication Guide and pen User Manual before starting therapy with FORTEO and re-read them each time the prescription is renewed.

Osteosarcomas in rats—Patients should be made aware that FORTEO caused osteosarcomas in rats and that the clinical relevance of these findings is unknown.

Orthostatic hypotension—FORTEO should be administered initially under circumstances where the patient can immediately sit or lie down if symptoms occur. Patients should be instructed that if they feel lightheaded or have palpitations after the injection, they should sit or lie down until the symptoms resolve. If symptoms persist or worsen, patients should be instructed to consult a physician before continuing treatment (see PRECAUTIONS, General).

Continued on next page

Forteo—Cont.

Hypercalcemia—Although symptomatic hypercalcemia was not observed in clinical trials, physicians should instruct patients to contact a health care provider if they develop persistent symptoms of hypercalcemia (ie, nausea, vomiting, constipation, lethargy, muscle weakness).

Use of the pen—Patients should be instructed on how to properly use the delivery device (refer to User Manual), properly dispose of needles, and be advised not to share their pens with other patients.

Other osteoporosis treatments—Patients should be informed regarding the roles of supplemental calcium and/or vitamin D, weight-bearing exercise, and modification of certain behavioral factors such as cigarette smoking and/or alcohol consumption.

Laboratory Tests—*Serum calcium*—FORTEO transiently increases serum calcium, with the maximal effect observed at approximately 4 to 6 hours post-dose. By 16 hours post-dose, serum calcium generally has returned to or near baseline. These effects should be kept in mind because serum calcium concentrations observed within 16 hours after a dose may reflect the pharmacologic effect of teriparatide. Persistent hypercalcemia was not observed in clinical trials with FORTEO. If persistent hypercalcemia is detected, treatment with FORTEO should be discontinued pending further evaluation of the cause of hypercalcemia.

Patients known to have an underlying hypercalcemic disorder, such as primary hyperparathyroidism, should not be treated with FORTEO (see WARNINGS).

Urinary calcium—FORTEO increases urinary calcium excretion, but the frequency of hypercalciuria in clinical trials was similar for patients treated with FORTEO and placebo (see CLINICAL PHARMACOLOGY, Human Pharmacodynamics).

Renal function—No clinically important adverse renal effects were observed in clinical studies. Assessments included creatinine clearance; measurements of blood urea nitrogen (BUN), creatinine, and electrolytes in serum; urine specific gravity and pH; and examination of urine sediment. Long-term evaluation of patients with severe renal insufficiency, patients undergoing acute or chronic dialysis, or patients who have functioning renal transplants has not been performed.

Serum uric acid—FORTEO increases serum uric acid concentrations. In clinical trials, 2.8% of FORTEO patients had serum uric acid concentrations above the upper limit of normal compared with 0.7% of placebo patients. However, the hyperuricemia did not result in an increase in gout, arthralgia, or urolithiasis.

Carcinogenesis, Mutagenesis, Impairment of Fertility:
Carcinogenesis—Two carcinogenicity bioassays were conducted in Fischer 344. In the first study, male and female rats were given daily subcutaneous teriparatide injections of 5, 30, or 75 mcg/kg/day for 24 months from 2 months of age. These doses resulted in systemic exposures that were, respectively, 3, 20, and 60 times higher than the systemic exposure observed in humans following a subcutaneous dose of 20 mcg (based on AUC comparison). Teriparatide treatment resulted in a marked dose-related increase in the incidence of osteosarcoma, a rare malignant bone tumor, in both male and female rats. Osteosarcomas were observed at all doses and the incidence reached 40% to 50% in the high-dose groups. Teriparatide also caused a dose-related increase in osteoblastoma and osteoma in both sexes. No osteosarcomas, osteoblastomas or osteomas were observed in untreated control rats. The bone tumors in rats occurred in association with a large increase in bone mass and focal osteoblast hyperplasia.

The second 2-year study was carried out in order to determine the effect of treatment duration and animal age on the development of bone tumors. Female rats were treated for different periods between 2 and 26 months of age with subcutaneous doses and 5 and 30 mcg/kg (equivalent to 3 and 20 times the human exposure at the 20-mcg dose, based on AUC comparison). The study showed that the occurrence of osteosarcoma, osteoblastoma and osteoma was dependent upon dose and duration of exposure. Bone tumors were observed when immature 2-month old rats were treated with 30 mcg/kg/day for 24 months or with 5 or 30 mcg/kg/day for 6 months. Bone tumors were also observed when mature 6-month old rats were treated with 30 mcg/kg/day for 6 or 20 months. Tumors were not detected when mature 6-month old rats were treated with 5 mcg/kg/day for 6 or 20 months. The results did not demonstrate a difference in susceptibility to bone tumor formation, associated with teriparatide treatment, between mature and immature rats.

The relevance of these rat findings to humans is uncertain.

Mutagenesis—Teriparatide was not genotoxic in any of the following test systems: the Ames test for bacterial mutagenesis; the mouse lymphoma assay for mammalian cell mutation, the chromosomal aberration assay in Chinese hamster ovary cells, with and without metabolic activation, and the in vivo micronucleus test in mice.

Impairment of fertility—No effects on fertility were observed in male and female rats given subcutaneous teriparatide doses of 30, 100, or 300 mcg/kg/day prior to mating and in females continuing through gestation Day 6 (16 to 160 times the human dose of 20 mcg based on surface area, mcg/m^2).

Pregnancy: *Pregnancy Category C*—In pregnant rats given subcutaneous teriparatide doses up to 1000 mcg/kg/day, there were no findings. In pregnant mice given subcutaneous doses of 225 or 1000 mcg/kg/day (≥60 times the human dose based on surface area, mcg/m^2) from gestation Day 6 through 15, the fetuses showed an increased incidence of skeletal deviations or variations (interrupted rib, extra vertebra or rib).

Developmental effects in a perinatal/postnatal study in pregnant rats given subcutaneous doses of teriparatide from gestation Day 6 through postpartum Day 20 included mild growth retardation in female offspring at doses ≥225 mcg/kg/day (≥120 times the human dose based on surface area, mcg/m^2), and in male offspring at 1000 mcg/kg/day (540 times the human dose based on surface area, mcg/m^2). There was also reduced motor activity in both male and female offspring at 1000 mcg/kg/day. There were no developmental or reproductive effects in mice or rats at a dose of 30 mcg/kg (8 or 16 times the human dose based on surface area, mcg/m^2). The effect of teriparatide treatment on human fetal development has not been studied. FORTEO is not indicated for use in pregnancy.

Nursing Mothers: Because FORTEO is indicated for the treatment of osteoporosis in postmenopausal women, it should not be administered to women who are nursing their children. There have been no clinical studies to determine if teriparatide is secreted into breast milk.

Pediatric Use: The safety and efficacy of FORTEO have not been established in pediatric populations. FORTEO is not indicated for use in pediatric patients (see WARNINGS).

Geriatric Use: Of the patients receiving FORTEO in the osteoporosis trial of 1637 postmenopausal women, 75% were 65 years of age and over and 23% were 75 years of age and over. Of the patients receiving FORTEO in the osteoporosis trial of 437 men, 39% were 65 years of age and over and 13% were 75 years of age and over. No significant differences in bone response or adverse reactions were seen in geriatric patients receiving FORTEO as compared with younger patients. Nonetheless, as with many medications, elderly patients may have greater sensitivity to the adverse effects of FORTEO.

ADVERSE EVENTS

The safety of teriparatide has been evaluated in 24 clinical trials that enrolled over 2800 women and men. Four long-term Phase 3 clinical trials included 1 large placebo-controlled, double-blind, multinational trial with 1637 postmenopausal women; 1 placebo-controlled, double-blind, multinational trial with 437 men; and 2 active-controlled trials including 393 postmenopausal women. Teriparatide doses ranged from 5 to 100 mcg/day in short-term trials and 20 to 40 mcg/day in the other trials. A total of 1943 of the patients studied received teriparatide, including 815 patients at 20 mcg/day and 1107 patients at 40 mcg/day. In the clinical trials, a total of 1432 patients were treated with teriparatide for 3 months to 2 years, of whom 1137 were treated for greater than 1 year (500 at 20 mcg/day and 637 at 40 mcg/day). The maximum duration of treatment was 2 years. Adverse events associated with FORTEO usually were mild and generally did not require discontinuation of therapy.

In the two Phase 3, placebo-controlled clinical trials in men and postmenopausal women, early discontinuation due to adverse events occurred in 5.6% of patients assigned to placebo and 7.1% of patients assigned to FORTEO. Reported adverse events that appeared to be increased by FORTEO treatment were dizziness and leg cramps.

Table 5 lists adverse events that occurred in the two Phase 3, placebo-controlled clinical trials in men and postmenopausal women at a frequency ≥2.0% in the FORTEO groups and in more FORTEO-treated patients than in placebo-treated patients, without attribution of causality.

Table 5. Percentage of Patients with Adverse Events Reported by at Least 2% of FORTEO-Treated Patients and in More FORTEO-Treated Patients than Placebo-Treated Patients from the Two Principal Osteoporosis Trials in Women and Men
Adverse events are shown without attribution of causality

	FORTEO	Placebo
	N=691	N=691
Event Classification	(%)	(%)
BODY AS A WHOLE		
Pain	21.3	20.5
Headache	7.5	7.4
Asthenia	8.7	6.8
Neck Pain	3.0	2.7
CARDIOVASCULAR		
Hypertension	7.1	6.8
Angina Pectoris	2.5	1.6
Syncope	2.6	1.4
DIGESTIVE SYSTEM		
Nausea	8.5	6.7
Constipation	5.4	4.5
Diarrhea	5.1	4.6
Dyspepsia	5.2	4.1
Vomiting	3.0	2.3
Gastrointestinal Disorder	2.3	2.0
Tooth Disorder	2.0	1.3
MUSCULOSKELETAL		
Arthralgia	10.1	8.4
Leg Cramps	2.6	1.3
NERVOUS SYSTEM		
Dizziness	8.0	5.4
Depression	4.1	2.7
Insomnia	4.3	3.6
Vertigo	3.8	2.7
RESPIRATORY SYSTEM		
Rhinitis	9.6	8.8
Cough Increased	6.4	5.5
Pharyngitis	5.5	4.8
Dyspnea	3.6	2.6
Pneumonia	3.9	3.3
SKIN AND APPENDAGES		
Rash	4.9	4.5
Sweating	2.2	1.7

Serum calcium—FORTEO transiently increases serum calcium, with the maximal effect observed at approximately 4 to 6 hours post-dose. Serum calcium measured at least 16 hours post-dose was not different from pretreatment levels. In clinical trials, the frequency of at least 1 episode of transient hypercalcemia in the 4 to 6 hours after FORTEO administration was increased from 1.5% of women and none of the men treated with placebo to 11.1% of women and 6.0% of men treated with FORTEO. The number of patients treated with FORTEO whose transient hypercalcemia was verified on consecutive measurements was 3.0% of women and 1.3% of men.

Immunogenicity—In a large clinical trial, antibodies that cross-reacted with teriparatide were detected in 2.8% of women receiving FORTEO. Generally, antibodies were first detected following 12 months of treatment and diminished after withdrawal of therapy. There was no evidence of hypersensitivity reactions, allergic reactions, effects on serum calcium, or effects on BMD response.

OVERDOSAGE

Incidents of overdose in humans have not been reported in clinical trials. Teriparatide has been administered in single doses of up to 100 mcg and in repeated doses of up to 60 mcg/day for 6 weeks. The effects of overdose that might be expected include a delayed hypercalcemic effect and risk of orthostatic hypotension. Nausea, vomiting, dizziness, and headache might also occur.

In single-dose rodent studies using subcutaneous injection of teriparatide, no mortality was seen in rats given doses of 1000 mcg/kg (540 times the human dose based on surface area, mcg/m^2) or in mice given 10,000 mcg/kg (2700 times the human dose based on surface area, mcg/m^2).

Overdose management—There is no specific antidote for teriparatide. Treatment of suspected overdose should include discontinuation of FORTEO, monitoring of serum calcium and phosphorus, and implementation of appropriate supportive measures, such as hydration.

DOSAGE AND ADMINISTRATION

FORTEO should be administered as a subcutaneous injection into the thigh or abdominal wall. The recommended dosage is 20 mcg once a day.

FORTEO should be administered initially under circumstances in which the patient can sit or lie down if symptoms of orthostatic hypotension occur (see PRECAUTIONS, Information for the Patient).

FORTEO is a clear and colorless liquid. Do not use if solid particles appear or if the solution is cloudy or colored. The FORTEO pen should not be used past the stated expiration date.

No data are available on the safety or efficacy of intravenous or intramuscular injection of FORTEO.

The safety and efficacy of FORTEO have not been evaluated beyond 2 years of treatment. Consequently, use of the drug for more than 2 years is not recommended.

INSTRUCTIONS FOR PEN USE

Patients and caregivers who administer FORTEO should receive appropriate training and instruction on the proper use of the FORTEO pen from a qualified health professional. It is important to read, understand, and follow the instructions in the FORTEO pen User Manual for priming the pen and dosing. Failure to do so may result in inaccurate dosing. Each FORTEO pen can be used for up to 28 days after the first injection. After the 28-day use period, discard the FORTEO pen, even if it still contains some unused solution. Never share a FORTEO pen.

STORAGE: The FORTEO pen should be stored under refrigeration at 2° to 8°C (36° to 46°F) at all times. Recap the pen when not in use to protect the cartridge from physical damage and light. During the use period, time out of the refrigerator should be minimized; the dose may be delivered immediately following removal from the refrigerator.

Do not freeze. Do not use FORTEO if it has been frozen.

HOW SUPPLIED
The FORTEO pen is available in the following package size:
One 3 mL prefilled pen
delivery device   NDC 0002-8971-01 (MS8971)

Literature issued November 2002
Manufactured by Lilly France S.A.S.
F-67640 Fegersheim, France
for Eli Lilly and Company
Indianapolis, IN 46285, USA
www.lilly.com
PA 9241 FSAMP

Medication Guide
FORTEO™
Generic name: teriparatide (rDNA origin) injection

Read this information carefully before you start taking FORTEO (for-TAY-o) to learn about the benefits and risks of FORTEO. Before beginning therapy, read the FORTEO pen User Manual for information on how to use the pen to inject your medicine. Read the information you get with FORTEO each time you get a refill, in case something has changed. Talk with your health care provider if there is something you do not understand or if you want to learn more about FORTEO.

What is the most important information I should know about FORTEO?
As part of drug testing, teriparatide, the active ingredient in FORTEO, was given to rats for a significant part of their lifetime. **In these studies, teriparatide caused some rats to develop osteosarcoma, a bone cancer.** Osteosarcoma in humans is a serious but very rare cancer. Osteosarcoma occurs in about 4 out of every million older adults each year. **It is not known if humans treated with FORTEO also have a higher chance of getting osteosarcoma.**

FORTEO is approved for use in both men and postmenopausal (after the "change of life") women with osteoporosis who are at high risk for having broken bones (fractures) from osteoporosis.

Before starting treatment, talk with your doctor about the possible benefits and risks of FORTEO so you can decide if it is right for you.

What is Osteoporosis?
Osteoporosis is a disease in which the bones become thin and weak, increasing the chance of having a broken bone. Osteoporosis usually causes no symptoms until a fracture happens. The most common fractures are in the spine (backbone). They can shorten height, even without causing pain. Over time, the spine can become curved or deformed and the body bent over. Fractures from osteoporosis can also happen in almost any bone in the body, for example, the wrist, rib, or hip. Once you have had a fracture, the chance for more fractures greatly increases.

The following risk factors increase your chance of getting fractures from osteoporosis:
- past broken bones from osteoporosis
- very low bone mineral density (BMD)
- frequent falls
- limited movement, such as using a wheelchair
- medical conditions likely to cause bone loss, such as some kinds of arthritis
- medicines that may cause bone loss, for example: seizure medicines (such as phenytoin), blood thinners (such as heparin), steroids (such as prednisone), or high doses of vitamins A or D.

What is FORTEO?
FORTEO is a prescription medicine used to treat osteoporosis by forming new bone. FORTEO is the brand name for teriparatide, which is the same as the active part of a natural hormone called parathyroid hormone or "PTH." FORTEO forms new bone, increases bone mineral density and bone strength, and as a result, reduces the chance of getting a fracture. In a study of postmenopausal (after the "change of life") women with osteoporosis, FORTEO reduced the number of fractures of the spine and other bones. The effect on fractures has not been studied in men.

FORTEO is approved for use in both men and postmenopausal women with osteoporosis who are at high risk for having fractures. FORTEO can be used by people who have had a fracture related to osteoporosis, or who have multiple risk factors for fracture (See "What is osteoporosis?"), or who cannot use other osteoporosis treatments.

Who should not use FORTEO?
Do not use FORTEO if you:
- have Paget's disease of the bone
- have unexplained high levels of alkaline phosphatase in your blood, which means you might have Paget's disease. If you are not sure, ask your doctor.
- are a child or growing adult
- have ever been diagnosed with bone cancer or other cancers that have spread (metastasized) to your bones
- have had radiation therapy involving your bones
- have certain bone diseases. If you have a bone disease, tell your doctor.
- have too much calcium in your blood (hypercalcemia)
- are pregnant or nursing
- have had an allergic reaction to FORTEO or one of its ingredients (See the ingredients section at the end of this Medication Guide)
- have trouble injecting yourself and do not have someone who can help you.

FORTEO should not be used to prevent osteoporosis or to treat patients who are not considered to be at high risk for fracture.

Tell your health care provider and pharmacist about all the medicines you are taking when you start taking FORTEO, and if you start taking a new medicine after you start FORTEO treatment. Tell them about all medicines you get with prescriptions and without prescriptions, as well as herbal or natural remedies. Your doctor and pharmacist need this information to help keep you from taking a combination of products that may harm you.

How should I take FORTEO?
- Take FORTEO once a day for as long as your doctor prescribes it for you. Use of FORTEO for more than 2 years is not recommended. Your health care professional (doctor, nurse, or pharmacist) should teach you how to use the FORTEO pen (prefilled delivery device). (See the User Manual for written instructions on how to use the FORTEO pen.)
- Some patients get dizzy or get a fast heartbeat after the first few doses. For the first few doses, inject FORTEO where you can sit or lie down right away if you get dizzy.
- Inject FORTEO once each day in your thigh or abdomen (lower stomach area).
- You can take FORTEO with or without food or drink.
- You can take FORTEO at any time of the day. To help you remember to take FORTEO, take it at about the same time each day.
- Do not use FORTEO if it has solid particles in it, or if it is cloudy or colored. It should be clear and colorless.
- Do not use FORTEO after the expiration date printed on the pen and pen packaging.
- Throw away any FORTEO pen that you started using more than 28 days earlier, even if it still has medicine in it (See the User Manual).
- Inject FORTEO shortly after you take the pen out of the refrigerator. Recap the pen and put it back into the refrigerator right after use (See the User Manual).
- If you forget or are unable to take FORTEO at your usual time, take it as soon as possible on that day. Do not take more than one injection in the same day.
- Talk with your health care provider about other ways you can help your osteoporosis, such as exercise, diet, supplements, and reducing or stopping your use of tobacco and alcohol. If your health care provider recommends calcium and vitamin D supplements, you can take them at the same time as FORTEO.

What are the possible side effects of FORTEO?
Most side effects are mild and include dizziness and leg cramps. If you become lightheaded or have fast heartbeats after your injection, sit or lie down until you feel better. If you do not feel better, call your health care provider before continuing treatment.

Contact your health care provider if you have continuing nausea, vomiting, constipation, low energy, or muscle weakness. These may be signs there is too much calcium in your blood.

These are not all the possible side effects of FORTEO. For more information, ask your health care provider or pharmacist.

Your health care provider may take samples of blood and urine during treatment to check your response to FORTEO. Also, your health care provider may ask you to have follow-up tests of bone mineral density.

How should I store FORTEO?
- Keep your FORTEO pen in the refrigerator at 36° to 46°F (2° to 8°C).
- Do not freeze the pen. Do not use FORTEO if it has been frozen.
- You can use your FORTEO pen for up to 28 days after the first injection from the pen.
- Throw away the pen properly (See the User Manual) after 28 days of use, even if it is not completely empty.
- Recap the pen after each use (See the User Manual) to protect from physical damage.

General information about using FORTEO safely and effectively
Medicines are sometimes prescribed for conditions that are not mentioned in Medication Guides. Do not use FORTEO for a condition for which it was not prescribed. Do not give FORTEO to other people, even if they have the same condition you have.

This Medication Guide summarizes the most important information about FORTEO. If you would like more information, talk with your doctor, nurse, or pharmacist. You can ask your pharmacist or health care provider for information about FORTEO that is written for health care professionals. You can also call Lilly toll free at 1-866-4FORTEO (1-866-436-7836).

Ingredients
In addition to the active ingredient teriparatide, inactive ingredients are glacial acetic acid, sodium acetate (anhydrous), mannitol, Metacresol, and Water for Injection. In addition, hydrochloric acid solution 10% and/or sodium hydroxide solution 10% may have been added to adjust product pH.

This Medication Guide has been approved by the US Food and Drug Administration.

Literature issued November 2002
Manufactured by Lilly France S.A.S.
F-67640 Fegersheim, France
for Eli Lilly and Company
Indianapolis, IN 46285, USA
www.lilly.com
PA 9241 FSAMP

Copyright © 2002, Eli Lilly and Company. All rights reserved.

Prescriptions for the FORTEO Pen and pen needles should be written as shown in the samples below. Needle prescriptions should be written separately from FORTEO prescriptions.

SAMPLE FORTEO PEN PRESCRIPTION

℞ Pat Smith, MD
123 Maple St.
Anytown, USA

(321) 555-1234

DISP: FORTEO 3mL Pen

#: 1

DOSE: 20-mcg SQ Daily

REFILL 11 TIMES

SAMPLE NEEDLE PRESCRIPTION

℞ Pat Smith, MD
123 Maple St.
Anytown, USA

(321) 555-1234

DISP: <Brand Name> Pen Needles
31 Gauge 5mm

#: 1 Box of 100 Needles

DOSE: Use 1 needle daily with FORTEO Pen as directed

REFILL 3 TIMES

STRATTERA™   ℞
[strǎ-těr-ǎ]
(atomoxetine HCl)

DESCRIPTION
STRATTERA™ (atomoxetine HCl) is a selective norepinephrine reuptake inhibitor. Atomoxetine HCl is the $R(-)$ isomer as determined by x-ray diffraction. The chemical designation is $(-)$-N-methyl-3-phenyl-3-(o-tolyloxy)-propylamine hydrochloride. The molecular formula is $C_{17}H_{21}NO \cdot HCl$, which corresponds to a molecular weight of 291.82. The chemical structure is:

Continued on next page

Strattera—Cont.

Atomoxetine HCl is a white to practically white solid, which has a solubility of 27.8 mg/mL in water.

STRATTERA capsules are intended for oral administration only.

Each capsule contains atomoxetine HCl equivalent to 10, 18, 25, 40, or 60 mg of atomoxetine. The capsules also contain pregelatinized starch and dimethicone. The capsule shells contain gelatin, sodium lauryl sulfate, and other inactive ingredients. The capsule shells also contain one or more of the following: FD&C Blue No. 2, synthetic yellow iron oxide, titanium dioxide. The capsules are imprinted with edible black ink.

CLINICAL PHARMACOLOGY

Pharmacodynamics and Mechanism of Action—The precise mechanism by which atomoxetine produces its therapeutic effects in Attention-Deficit/Hyperactivity Disorder (ADHD) is unknown, but is thought to be related to selective inhibition of the pre-synaptic norepinephrine transporter, as determined in ex vivo uptake and neurotransmitter depletion studies.

Human Pharmacokinetics—Atomoxetine is well-absorbed after oral administration and is minimally affected by food. It is eliminated primarily by oxidative metabolism through the cytochrome P450 2D6 (CYP2D6) enzymatic pathway and subsequent glucuronidation. Atomoxetine has a half-life of about 5 hours. A fraction of the population (about 7% of Caucasians and 2% of African Americans) are poor metabolizers (PMs) of CYP2D6 metabolized drugs. These individuals have reduced activity in this pathway resulting in 10-fold higher AUCs, 5-fold higher peak plasma concentrations, and slower elimination (plasma half-life of about 24 hours) of atomoxetine compared with people with normal activity [extensive metabolizers (EMs)]. Drugs that inhibit CYP2D6, such as fluoxetine, paroxetine, and quinidine, cause similar increases in exposure.

The pharmacokinetics of atomoxetine have been evaluated in more than 400 children and adolescents in selected clinical trials, primarily using population pharmacokinetic studies. Single-dose and steady-state individual pharmacokinetic data were also obtained in children, adolescents, and adults. When doses were normalized to a mg/kg basis, similar half-life, C_{max}, and AUC values were observed in children, adolescents, and adults. Clearance and volume of distribution after adjustment for body weight were also similar.

Absorption and Distribution—Atomoxetine is rapidly absorbed after oral administration, with absolute bioavailability of about 63% in EMs and 94% in PMs. Maximal plasma concentrations (C_{max}) are reached approximately 1 to 2 hours after dosing.

STRATTERA can be administered with or without food. Administration of STRATTERA with a standard high-fat meal in adults did not affect the extent of oral absorption of atomoxetine (AUC), but did decrease the rate of absorption, resulting in a 37% lower C_{max}, and delayed T_{max} by 3 hours. In clinical trials with children and adolescents, administration of STRATTERA with food resulted in a 9% lower C_{max}. The steady-state volume of distribution after intravenous administration is 0.85 L/kg indicating that atomoxetine distributes primarily into total body water. Volume of distribution is similar across the patient weight range after normalizing for body weight.

At therapeutic concentrations, 98% of atomoxetine in plasma is bound to protein, primarily albumin.

Metabolism and Elimination—Atomoxetine is metabolized primarily through the CYP2D6 enzymatic pathway. People with reduced activity in this pathway (PMs) have higher plasma concentrations of atomoxetine compared with people with normal activity (EMs). For PMs, AUC of atomoxetine is approximately 10-fold and $C_{ss,max}$ is about 5-fold greater than EMs. Laboratory tests are available to identify CYP2D6 PMs. Coadministration of STRATTERA with potent inhibitors of CYP2D6, such as fluoxetine, paroxetine, or quinidine, results in a substantial increase in atomoxetine plasma exposure, and dosing adjustment may be necessary (see Drug-Drug Interactions). Atomoxetine did not inhibit or induce the CYP2D6 pathway.

The major oxidative metabolite formed, regardless of CYP2D6 status, is 4-hydroxyatomoxetine, which is glucuronidated. 4-Hydroxyatomoxetine is equipotent to atomoxetine as an inhibitor of the norepinephrine transporter but circulates in plasma at much lower concentrations (1% of atomoxetine concentration in EMs and 0.1% of atomoxetine concentration in PMs). 4-Hydroxyatomoxetine is primarily formed by CYP2D6, but in PMs, 4-hydroxyatomoxetine is formed at a slower rate by several other cytochrome P450 enzymes. N-desmethylatomoxetine is formed by CYP2C19 and other cytochrome P450 enzymes, but has substantially less pharmacological activity compared with atomoxetine and circulates in plasma at lower concentrations (5% of atomoxetine concentration in EMs and 45% of atomoxetine concentration in PMs).

Mean apparent plasma clearance of atomoxetine after oral administration in adult EMs is 0.35 L/hr/kg and the mean half-life is 5.2 hours. Following oral administration of atomoxetine to PMs, mean apparent plasma clearance is 0.03 L/hr/kg and mean half-life is 21.6 hours. For PMs, AUC of atomoxetine is approximately 10-fold and $C_{ss,max}$ is about 5-fold greater than EMs. The elimination half-life of 4-hydroxyatomoxetine is similar to that of N-desmethylatomoxetine (6 to 8 hours) in EM subjects, while the half-life of N-desmethylatomoxetine is much longer in PM subjects (34 to 40 hours).

Atomoxetine is excreted primarily as 4-hydroxyatomoxetine-O-glucuronide, mainly in the urine (greater than 80% of the dose) and to a lesser extent in the feces (less than 17% of the dose). Only a small fraction of the STRATTERA dose is excreted as unchanged atomoxetine (less than 3% of the dose), indicating extensive biotransformation.

Special Populations—Hepatic Insufficiency—Atomoxetine exposure (AUC) is increased, compared with normal subjects, in EM subjects with moderate (Child-Pugh Class B) (2-fold increase) and severe (Child-Pugh Class C) (4-fold increase) hepatic insufficiency. Dosage adjustment is recommended for patients with moderate or severe hepatic insufficiency (see DOSAGE AND ADMINISTRATION).

Renal Insufficiency—EM subjects with end stage renal disease had higher systemic exposure to atomoxetine than healthy subjects (about a 65% increase), but there was no difference when exposure was corrected for mg/kg dose. STRATTERA can therefore be administered to ADHD patients with end stage renal disease or lesser degrees of renal insufficiency using the normal dosing regimen.

Geriatric—The pharmacokinetics of atomoxetine have not been evaluated in the geriatric population.

Pediatric—The pharmacokinetics of atomoxetine in children and adolescents are similar to those in adults. The pharmacokinetics of atomoxetine have not been evaluated in children under 6 years of age.

Gender—Gender did not influence atomoxetine disposition.

Ethnic Origin—Ethnic origin did not influence atomoxetine disposition (except that PMs are more common in Caucasians).

Drug-Drug Interactions—CYP2D6 Activity and Atomoxetine Plasma Concentration—Atomoxetine is primarily metabolized by the CYP2D6 pathway to 4-hydroxyatomoxetine. In EMs, inhibitors of CYP2D6 increase atomoxetine steady-state plasma concentrations to exposures similar to those observed in PMs. Dosage adjustment of STRATTERA in EMs may be necessary when coadministered with CYP2D6 inhibitors, e.g., paroxetine, fluoxetine, and quinidine (see Drug Interactions under PRECAUTIONS). In vitro studies suggest that coadministration of cytochrome P450 inhibitors to PMs will not increase the plasma concentrations of atomoxetine.

Effect of Atomoxetine on P450 enzymes—Atomoxetine did not cause clinically important inhibition or induction of cytochrome P450 enzymes, including CYP1A2, CYP3A, CYP2D6, and CYP2C9.

Albuterol—Albuterol (600 mcg iv over 2 hours) induced increases in heart rate and blood pressure. These effects were potentiated by atomoxetine (60 mg BID for 5 days) and were most marked after the initial coadministration of albuterol and atomoxetine (see Drug-Drug Interactions under PRECAUTIONS).

Alcohol—Consumption of ethanol with STRATTERA did not change the intoxicating effects of ethanol.

Desipramine—Coadministration of STRATTERA (40 or 60 mg BID for 13 days) with desipramine, a model compound for CYP2D6 metabolized drugs (single dose of 50 mg), did not alter the pharmacokinetics of desipramine. No dose adjustment is recommended for drugs metabolized by CYP2D6.

Methylphenidate—Coadministration of methylphenidate with STRATTERA did not increase cardiovascular effects beyond those seen with methylphenidate alone.

Midazolam—Coadministration of STRATTERA (60 mg BID for 12 days) with midazolam, a model compound for CYP3A4 metabolized drugs, (single dose of 5 mg) resulted in 15% increase in AUC of midazolam. No dose adjustment is recommended for drugs metabolized by CYP3A.

Drugs Highly Bound to Plasma Protein—In vitro drug-displacement studies were conducted with atomoxetine and other highly-bound drugs at therapeutic concentrations. Atomoxetine did not affect the binding of warfarin, acetylsalicylic acid, phenytoin, or diazepam to human albumin. Similarly, these compounds did not affect the binding of atomoxetine to human albumin.

Drugs that Affect Gastric pH—Drugs that elevate gastric pH (magnesium hydroxide/aluminum hydroxide, omeprazole) had no effect on STRATTERA bioavailability.

CLINICAL STUDIES

The effectiveness of STRATTERA in the treatment of ADHD was established in 6 randomized, double-blind, placebo-controlled studies in children, adolescents, and adults who met Diagnostic and Statistical Manual 4th edition (DSM-IV) criteria for ADHD. (See INDICATIONS AND USAGE)

Children and Adolescents—The effectiveness of STRATTERA in the treatment of ADHD was established in 4 randomized, double-blind, placebo-controlled studies of pediatric patients (ages 6 to 18). Approximately one-third of the patients met DSM-IV criteria for inattentive subtype and two-thirds met criteria for both inattentive and hyperactive/impulsive subtypes. (See INDICATIONS AND USAGE)

Signs and symptoms of ADHD were evaluated by a comparison of mean change from baseline to endpoint for STRATTERA and placebo-treated patients using an intent-to-treat analysis of the primary outcome measure, the investigator administered and scored ADHD Rating Scale-IV-Parent Version (ADHDRS) total score including hyperactive/impulsive and inattentive sub-scales. Each item on the ADHDRS maps directly to one symptom criterion for ADHD in the DSM-IV.

In Study 1, an 8-week randomized, double-blind, placebo-controlled, dose-response, acute treatment study of children and adolescents aged 8 to 18 (N=297), patients received either a fixed dose of STRATTERA (0.5, 1.2, or 1.8 mg/kg/day) or placebo. STRATTERA was administered as a divided dose in the early morning and late afternoon/early evening. At the 2 higher doses, improvements in ADHD symptoms were statistically significantly superior in STRATTERA-treated patients compared with placebo-treated patients as measured on the ADHDRS scale. The 1.8-mg/kg/day STRATTERA dose did not provide any additional benefit over that observed with the 1.2-mg/kg/day dose. The 0.5-mg/kg/day STRATTERA dose was not superior to placebo.

In Study 2, a 6-week randomized, double-blind, placebo-controlled, acute treatment study of children and adolescents aged 6 to 16 (N=171), patients received either STRATTERA or placebo. STRATTERA was administered as a single dose in the early morning and titrated on a weight-adjusted basis according to clinical response, up to a maximum dose of 1.5 mg/kg/day. The mean final dose of STRATTERA was approximately 1.3 mg/kg/day. ADHD symptoms were statistically significantly improved on STRATTERA compared with placebo, as measured on the ADHDRS scale. This study shows that STRATTERA is effective when administered once daily in the morning.

In 2 identical, 9-week, acute, randomized, double-blind, placebo-controlled studies of children aged 7 to 13 (Study 3, N=147; Study 4, N=144), STRATTERA and methylphenidate were compared with placebo. STRATTERA was administered as a divided dose in the early morning and late afternoon (after school) and titrated on a weight adjusted basis according to clinical response. The maximum recommended STRATTERA dose was 2.0 mg/kg/day. The mean final dose of STRATTERA for both studies was approximately 1.6 mg/kg/day. In both studies, ADHD symptoms statistically significantly improved more on STRATTERA than on placebo, as measured on the ADHDRS scale.

Examination of population subsets based on gender and age (<12 and 12 to 17) did not reveal any differential responsiveness on the basis of these subgroupings. There was not sufficient exposure of ethnic groups other than Caucasian to allow exploration of differences in these subgroups.

Adults—The effectiveness of STRATTERA in the treatment of ADHD was established in 2 randomized, double-blind, placebo-controlled clinical studies of adult patients, age 18 and older, who met DSM-IV criteria for ADHD.

Signs and symptoms of ADHD were evaluated using the investigator-administered Conners Adult ADHD Rating Scale Screening Version (CAARS), a 30-item scale. The primary effectiveness measure was the 18-item Total ADHD Symptom score (the sum of the inattentive and hyperactivity/impulsivity subscales from the CAARS) evaluated by a comparison of mean change from baseline to endpoint using an intent-to-treat analysis.

In 2 identical, 10-week, randomized, double-blind, placebo-controlled acute treatment studies (Study 5, N=280; Study 6, N=256), patients received either STRATTERA or placebo. STRATTERA was administered as a divided dose in the early morning and late afternoon/early evening and titrated according to clinical response in a range of 60 to 120 mg/day. The mean final dose of STRATTERA for both studies was approximately 95 mg/day. In both studies, ADHD symptoms were statistically significantly improved on STRATTERA, as measured on the ADHD Symptom score from the CAARS scale.

Examination of population subsets based on gender and age (<42 and ≥42) did not reveal any differential responsiveness on the basis of these subgroupings. There was not sufficient exposure of ethnic groups other than Caucasian to allow exploration of differences in these subgroups.

INDICATIONS AND USAGE

STRATTERA is indicated for the treatment of Attention-Deficit/Hyperactivity Disorder (ADHD).

The effectiveness of STRATTERA in the treatment of ADHD was established in 2 placebo-controlled trials in children, 2 placebo-controlled trials in children and adolescents, and 2 placebo-controlled trials in adults who met DSM-IV criteria for ADHD (see CLINICAL STUDIES).

A diagnosis of ADHD (DSM-IV) implies the presence of hyperactive-impulsive or inattentive symptoms that cause impairment and that were present before age 7 years. The symptoms must be persistent, must be more severe than is typically observed in individuals at a comparable level of development, must cause clinically significant impairment, e.g., in social, academic, or occupational functioning, and must be present in 2 or more settings, e.g., school (or work) and at home. The symptoms must not be better accounted for by another mental disorder. For the Inattentive Type, at least 6 of the following symptoms must have persisted for at least 6 months: lack of attention to details/careless mistakes, lack of sustained attention, poor listener, failure to follow through on tasks, poor organization, avoids tasks requiring sustained mental effort, loses things, easily distracted, forgetful. For the Hyperactive-Impulsive Type, at least 6 of the following symptoms must have persisted for at least 6 months: fidgeting/squirming, leaving seat, inappropriate running/climbing, difficulty with quiet activities, "on the go," excessive talking, blurting answers, can't wait turn, intrusive. For a Combined Type diagnosis, both inattentive and hyperactive-impulsive criteria must be met.

Special Diagnostic Considerations—The specific etiology of ADHD is unknown, and there is no single diagnostic test. Adequate diagnosis requires the use not only of medical but also of special psychological, educational, and social resources. Learning may or may not be impaired. The diagnosis must be based upon a complete history and evaluation of the patient and not solely on the presence of the required number of DSM-IV characteristics.

Need for Comprehensive Treatment Program—STRATTERA is indicated as an integral part of a total treatment program for ADHD that may include other measures (psychological, educational, social) for patients with this syndrome. Drug treatment may not be indicated for all patients with this syndrome. Drug treatment is not intended for use in the patient who exhibits symptoms secondary to environmental factors and/or other primary psychiatric disorders, including psychosis. Appropriate educational placement is essential in children and adolescents with this diagnosis and psychosocial intervention is often helpful. When remedial measures alone are insufficient, the decision to prescribe drug treatment medication will depend upon the physician's assessment for the chronicity and severity of the patient's symptoms.

Long-term Use—The effectiveness of STRATTERA for long-term use, ie, for more than 9 weeks in child and adolescent patients and 10 weeks in adult patients, has not been systematically evaluated in controlled trials. Therefore, the physician who elects to use STRATTERA for extended periods should periodically reevaluate the long-term usefulness of the drug for the individual patient (see DOSAGE AND ADMINISTRATION).

CONTRAINDICATIONS

Hypersensitivity—STRATTERA is contraindicated in patients known to be hypersensitive to atomoxetine or other constituents of the product (see WARNINGS).

Monoamine Oxidase Inhibitors (MAOI)—STRATTERA should not be taken with an MAOI, or within 2 weeks after discontinuing an MAOI. Treatment with an MAOI should not be initiated within 2 weeks after discontinuing STRATTERA. With other drugs that affect brain monoamine concentrations, there have been reports of serious, sometimes fatal, reactions (including hyperthermia, rigidity, myoclonus, autonomic instability with possible rapid fluctuations of vital signs, and mental status changes that include extreme agitation progressing to delirium and coma) when taken in combination with an MAOI. Some cases presented with features resembling neuroleptic malignant syndrome. Such reactions may occur when these drugs are given concurrently or in close proximity.

Narrow Angle Glaucoma—In clinical trials, STRATTERA use was associated with an increased risk of mydriasis and therefore its use is not recommended in patients with narrow angle glaucoma.

WARNINGS

Allergic Events—Although uncommon, allergic reactions, including angioneurotic edema, urticaria, and rash, have been reported in patients taking STRATTERA.

Growth—Growth should be monitored during treatment with STRATTERA. During acute treatment studies (up to 9 weeks), STRATTERA-treated patients lost an average of 0.4 kg, while placebo patients gained an average of 1.5 kg. In a controlled trial that randomized patients to placebo or 1 of 3 atomoxetine doses, 1.3%, 7.1%, 19.3%, and 29.1% of patients lost at least 3.5% of their body weight in the placebo, 0.5, 1.2, and 1.8 mg/kg/day STRATTERA dose groups, respectively. During acute treatment studies, STRATTERA-treated patients grew an average of 0.9 cm, while placebo-treated patients grew an average of 1.1 cm. There are no long-term, placebo-controlled data to evaluate the effect of STRATTERA on growth. Weight and height were assessed during open-label studies of 12 and 18 months, and mean rates of growth were compared to normal growth curves. Patients treated with STRATTERA for at least 18 months gained an average of 6.5 kg while mean weight percentile decreased slightly from 68 to 60. For this same group of patients, the average gain in height was 9.3 cm with a slight decrease in mean height percentile from 54 to 50. Among patients treated for at least 6 months, mean weight gain was lower for poor metabolizer (PM) patients compared with extensive metabolizer (EM) patients (+0.7 kg compared with +3.0 kg), while mean growth for PM patients was 4.3 cm and mean growth for EM patients was 4.4 cm. Whether final adult height or weight is affected by treatment with STRATTERA is unknown. Patients requiring long-term therapy should be monitored, and consideration should be given to interrupting therapy in patients who are not growing or gaining weight satisfactorily.

PRECAUTIONS

General—Effects on Blood Pressure and Heart Rate—STRATTERA should be used with caution in patients with hypertension, tachycardia, or cardiovascular or cerebrovascular disease because it can increase blood pressure and heart rate. Pulse and blood pressure should be measured at baseline, following STRATTERA dose increases, and periodically while on therapy.

In pediatric placebo-controlled trials, STRATTERA-treated subjects experienced a mean increase in heart rate of about 6 beats/minute compared with placebo subjects. At the final study visit before drug discontinuation, 3.6% (12/335) of STRATTERA-treated subjects had heart rate increases of at least 25 beats/minute and a heart rate of at least 110 beats/minute, compared with 0.5% (1/204) of placebo subjects. No pediatric subject had a heart rate increase of at least 25 beats/minute and a heart rate of at least 110 beats/minute on more than one occasion. Tachycardia was identified as an adverse event for 1.5% (5/340) of these pediatric subjects compared with 0.5% (1/207) of placebo subjects. The mean heart rate increase in extensive metabolizer (EM) patients was 6.7 beats/minute, and in poor metabolizer (PM) patients 10.4 beats/minute.

STRATTERA-treated pediatric subjects experienced mean increases of about 1.5 mm Hg in systolic and diastolic blood pressures compared with placebo. At the final study visit before drug discontinuation, 6.8% (22/324) of STRATTERA-treated pediatric subjects had high systolic blood pressure measurements compared with 3.0% (6/197) of placebo subjects. High systolic blood pressures were measured on 2 or more occasions in 8.6% (28/324) of Strattera-treated subjects and 3.6% (7/197) of placebo subjects. At the final study visit before drug discontinuation, 2.8% (9/326) of STRATTERA-treated pediatric subjects had high diastolic blood pressure measurements compared with 0.5% (1/200) of placebo subjects. High diastolic blood pressures were measured on 2 or more occasions in 5.2% (17/326) of Strattera-treated subjects and 1.5% (3/200) placebo subjects. [High systolic and diastolic blood pressure measurements were defined as those exceeding the 95th percentile, stratified by age, gender, and height percentile - National High Blood Pressure Education Working Group on Hypertension Control in Children and Adolescents.]

In adult placebo-controlled trials, STRATTERA-treated subjects experienced a mean increase in heart rate of 5 beats/minute compared with placebo subjects. Tachycardia was identified as an adverse event for 3% (8/269) of these adult atomoxetine subjects compared with 0.8% (2/263) of placebo subjects.

STRATTERA-treated adult subjects experienced mean increases in systolic (about 3 mm Hg) and diastolic (about 1 mm Hg) blood pressures compared with placebo. At the final study visit before drug discontinuation, 1.9% (5/258) of STRATTERA-treated adult subjects had systolic blood pressure measurements ≥150 mm Hg compared with 1.2% (3/256) of placebo subjects. At the final study visit before drug discontinuation, 0.8% (2/257) of STRATTERA-treated adult subjects had diastolic blood pressure measurements ≥100 mm Hg compared with 0.4% (1/257) of placebo subjects. No adult subject had a high systolic or diastolic blood pressure detected on more than one occasion.

Orthostatic hypotension has been reported in subjects taking STRATTERA. In short-term child- and adolescent-controlled trials, 1.8% (6/340) of STRATTERA-treated subjects experienced symptoms of postural hypotension compared with 0.5% (1/207) of placebo-treated subjects. STRATTERA should be used with caution in any condition that may predispose patients to hypotension.

Effects on Urine Outflow from the Bladder—In adult ADHD controlled trials, the rates of urinary retention (3%, 7/269) and urinary hesitation (3%, 7/269) were increased among atomoxetine subjects compared with placebo subjects (0%, 0/263). Two adult atomoxetine subjects and no placebo subjects discontinued from controlled clinical trials because of urinary retention. A complaint of urinary retention or urinary hesitancy should be considered potentially related to atomoxetine.

Information for Patients—Patients should read *information for Patients* before starting therapy with STRATTERA and when the prescription is renewed.

Patients should consult a physician if they are taking or plan to take any prescription or over-the-counter medicines, dietary supplements, or herbal remedies.

Patients should consult a physician if they are nursing, pregnant, or thinking of becoming pregnant while taking STRATTERA.

Patients may take STRATTERA with or without food.

If patients miss a dose, they should take it as soon as possible, but should not take more than the prescribed total daily amount of STRATTERA in any 24-hour period.

Patients should use caution when driving a car or operating hazardous machinery until they are reasonably certain that their performance is not affected by atomoxetine.

Laboratory Tests—Routine laboratory tests are not required.

CYP2D6 Metabolism—Poor metabolizers (PMs) of CYP2D6 have a 10-fold higher AUC and a 5-fold higher peak concentration to a given dose of STRATTERA compared with extensive metabolizers (EMs). Approximately 7% of a Caucasian population are PMs. Laboratory tests are available to identify CYP2D6 PMs. The blood levels in PMs are similar to those attained by taking strong inhibitors of CYP2D6. The higher blood levels in PMs lead to a higher rate of some adverse effects of STRATTERA (see ADVERSE REACTIONS).

Drug-Drug Interactions: *Albuterol*—STRATTERA should be administered with caution to patients being treated with systemically-administered (oral or intravenous) albuterol (or other beta$_2$ agonists) because the action of albuterol on the cardiovascular system can be potentiated.

CYP2D6 Inhibitors—Atomoxetine is primarily metabolized by the CYP2D6 pathway to 4-hydroxyatomoxetine. In EMs, selective inhibitors of CYP2D6 increase atomoxetine steady-state plasma concentrations to exposures similar to those observed in PMs. Dosage adjustment of STRATTERA may be necessary when coadministered with CYP2D6 inhibitors, e.g., paroxetine, fluoxetine, and quinidine. (See DOSAGE AND ADMINISTRATION) In EM individuals treated with paroxetine or fluoxetine, the AUC of atomoxetine is approximately 6- to 8-fold and $C_{ss,max}$ is about 3- to 4-fold greater than atomoxetine alone.

In vitro studies suggest that coadministration of cytochrome P450 inhibitors to PMs will not increase the plasma concentrations of atomoxetine.

Monoamine oxidase inhibitors—See CONTRAINDICATIONS.

Pressor agents—Because of possible effects on blood pressure, STRATTERA should be used cautiously with pressor agents.

Carcinogenesis, Mutagenesis, Impairment of Fertility:
Carcinogenesis—Atomoxetine HCl was not carcinogenic in rats and mice when given in the diet for 2 years at time-weighted average doses up to 47 and 458 mg/kg/day, respectively. The highest dose used in rats is approximately 8 and 5 times the maximum human dose in children and adults, respectively, on a mg/m^2 basis. Plasma levels (AUC) of atomoxetine at this dose in rats are estimated to be 1.8 times (extensive metabolizers) or 0.2 times (poor metabolizers) those in humans receiving the maximum human dose. The highest dose used in mice is approximately 39 and 26 times the maximum human dose in children and adults, respectively, on a mg/m^2 basis.

Mutagenesis—Atomoxetine HCl was negative in a battery of genotoxicity studies that included a reverse point mutation assay (Ames Test), an in vitro mouse lymphoma assay, a chromosomal aberration test in Chinese hamster ovary cells, an unscheduled DNA synthesis test in rat hepatocytes, and an in vivo micronucleus test in mice. However, there was a slight increase in the percentage of Chinese hamster ovary cells with diplochromosomes, suggesting endoreduplication (numerical aberration).

The metabolite N-desmethylatomoxetine HCl was negative in the Ames Test, mouse lymphoma assay, and unscheduled DNA synthesis test.

Impairment of Fertility—Atomoxetine HCl did not impair fertility in rats when given in the diet at doses of up to 57 mg/kg/day, which is approximately 6 times the maximum human dose on a mg/m^2 basis.

Pregnancy: *Pregnancy Category C*—Pregnant rabbits were treated with up to 100 mg/kg/day of atomoxetine by gavage throughout the period of organogenesis. At this dose, in 1 of 3 studies, a decrease in live fetuses and an increase in early resorption was observed. Slight increases in the incidences of atypical origin of carotid artery and absent subclavian artery were observed. These findings were observed at doses that caused slight maternal toxicity. The no-effect dose for these findings was 30 mg/kg/day. The 100 mg/kg dose is approximately 23 times the maximum human dose on a mg/m^2 basis; plasma levels (AUC) of atomoxetine at this dose in rabbits are estimated to be 3.3 times (extensive metabolizers) or 0.4 times (poor metabolizers) those in humans receiving the maximum human dose.

Rats were treated with up to approximately 50 mg/kg/day of atomoxetine (approximately 6 times the maximum human dose on a mg/m^2 basis) in the diet from 2 weeks (females) or 10 weeks (males) prior to mating through the periods of organogenesis and lactation. In 1 of 2 studies, decreases in pup weight and pup survival were observed. The decreased pup survival was also seen at 25 mg/kg (but not at 13 mg/kg). In a study in which rats were treated with atomoxetine in the diet from 2 weeks (females) or 10 weeks (males) prior to mating throughout the period of organogenesis, a decrease in fetal weight (female only) and an increase in the incidence of incomplete ossification of the vertebral arch in fetuses were observed at 40 mg/kg/day (approximately 5 times the maximum human dose on a mg/m^2 basis) but not at 20 mg/kg/day.

No adverse fetal effects were seen when pregnant rats were treated with up to 150 mg/kg/day (approximately 17 times the maximum human dose on a mg/m^2 basis) by gavage throughout the period of organogenesis.

No adequate and well-controlled studies have been conducted in pregnant women. STRATTERA should not be used during pregnancy unless the potential benefit justifies the potential risk to the fetus.

Labor and Delivery—Parturition in rats was not affected by atomoxetine. The effect of STRATTERA on labor and delivery in humans is unknown.

Nursing Mothers—Atomoxetine and/or its metabolites were excreted in the milk of rats. It is not known if atomoxetine is excreted in human milk. Caution should be exercised if STRATTERA is administered to a nursing woman.

Pediatric Use—The safety and efficacy of STRATTERA in pediatric patients less than 6 years of age have not been established. The efficacy of STRATTERA beyond 9 weeks and safety of STRATTERA beyond 1 year of treatment have not been systematically evaluated.

A study was conducted in young rats to evaluate the effects of atomoxetine on growth and neurobehavioral and sexual development. Rats were treated with 1, 10, or 50 mg/kg/day (approximately 0.2, 2, an 8 times, respectively, the maximum human dose on a mg/m^2 basis) of atomoxetine given by gavage from the early postnatal period (Day 10 of age) through adulthood. Slight delays in onset of vaginal patency (all doses) and preputial separation (10 and 50 mg/kg), slight decreases in epididymal weight and sperm number (10 and 50 mg/kg), and a slight decrease in corpora lutea (50 mg/kg) were seen, but there were no effects on fertility or reproductive performance. A slight delay in onset of incisor eruption was seen at 50 mg/kg. A slight increase in motor activity was seen on day 15 (males at 10 and 50 mg/kg and females at 50 mg/kg) and on day 30 (females at 50 mg/kg) but not on day 60 of age. There were no effects on learning and memory tests. The significance of these findings to humans is unknown.

Geriatric Use—The safety and efficacy of STRATTERA in geriatric patients have not been established.

ADVERSE REACTIONS

STRATTERA was administered to 2067 children or adolescent patients with ADHD and 270 adults with ADHD in clinical studies. During the ADHD clinical trials, 169 patients were treated for longer than 1 year and 526 patients were treated for over 6 months.

The data in the following tables and text cannot be used to predict the incidence of side effects in the course of usual medical practice where patient characteristics and other factors differ from those that prevailed in the clinical trials.

Continued on next page

Strattera—Cont.

Similarly, the cited frequencies cannot be compared with data obtained from other clinical investigations involving different treatments, uses, or investigators. The cited data provide the prescribing physician with some basis for estimating the relative contribution of drug and non-drug factors to the adverse event incidence in the population studied.

Child and Adolescent Clinical Trials—Reasons for discontinuation of treatment due to adverse events in child and adolescent clinical trials—In acute child and adolescent placebo-controlled trials, 3.5% (15/427) of atomoxetine subjects and 1.4% (4/294) placebo subjects discontinued for adverse events. For all studies, (including open-label and long-term studies), 5% of extensive metabolizer (EM) patients and 7% of poor metabolizer (PM) patients discontinued because of an adverse event. Among STRATTERA-treated patients, aggression (0.5%, N=2); irritability (0.5%, N=2); somnolence (0.5%, N=2); and vomiting (0.5%, N=2) were the reasons for discontinuation reported by more than 1 patient.

Commonly observed adverse events in acute child and adolescent, placebo-controlled trials—Commonly observed adverse events associated with the use of STRATTERA (incidence of 2% or greater) and not observed at an equivalent incidence among placebo-treated patients (STRATTERA incidence greater than placebo) are listed in Table 1 for BID trials. Results were similar in the QD trial except as shown in Table 2, which shows both BID and QD results for selected adverse events. The most commonly observed adverse events in patients treated with STRATTERA (incidence of 5% or greater and at least twice the incidence in placebo patients, for either BID or QD dosing) were: dyspepsia, nausea, vomiting, fatigue, appetite decreased, dizziness, and mood swings (see Tables 1 and 2).

TABLE 1 Common Treatment-Emergent Adverse Events Associated with the Use of STRATTERA in Acute (up to 9 weeks) Child and Adolescent Trials

Adverse Event[1]	Percentage of Patients Reporting Events from BID Trials	
	STRATTERA (N=340)	Placebo (N=207)
Gastrointestinal Disorders		
Abdominal pain upper	20	16
Constipation	3	1
Dyspepsia	4	2
Vomiting	11	9
Infections		
Ear infection	3	1
Influenza	3	1
Investigations		
Weight decreased	2	0
Metabolism and Nutritional Disorders		
Appetite decreased	14	6
Nervous System Disorders		
Dizziness (exc vertigo)	6	3
Headache	27	25
Somnolence	7	5
Psychiatric Disorders		
Crying	2	1
Irritability	8	5
Mood swings	2	0
Respiratory, Thoracic, and Mediastinal Disorders		
Cough	11	7
Rhinorrhea	4	3
Skin and Subcutaneous Tissue Disorders		
Dermatitis	4	1

[1] Events reported by at least 2% of patients treated with atomoxetine, and greater than placebo. The following events did not meet this criterion but were reported by more atomoxetine-treated patients than placebo-treated patients and are possibly related to atomoxetine treatment: anorexia, blood pressure increased, early morning awakening, flushing, mydriasis, sinus tachycardia, tearfulness. The following events were reported by at least 2% of patients treated with atomoxetine, and equal to or less than placebo: arthralgia, gastroenteritis viral, insomnia, sore throat, nasal congestion, nasopharyngitis, pruritus, sinus congestion, upper respiratory tract infection.

[See table 2 above]

The following adverse events occurred in at least 2% of PM patients and were either twice as frequent or statistically significantly more frequent in PM patients compared with EM patients: decreased appetite (23% of PMs, 16% of EMs); insomnia (13% of PMs, 7% of EMs); sedation (4% of PMs, 2% of EMs); depression (6% of PMs, 2% of EMs); tremor (4% of PMs, 1% of EMs); early morning awakening (3% of PMs, 1% of EMs); pruritus (2% of PMs, 1% of EMs); mydriasis (2% of PMs, 1% of EMs).

Adult Clinical Trials—Reasons for discontinuation of treatment due to adverse events in acute adult placebo-controlled trials—In the acute adult placebo-controlled trials, 8.5% (23/270) atomoxetine subjects and 3.4% (9/266) placebo subjects discontinued for adverse events. Among STRATTERA-treated patients, insomnia (1.1%, N=3); chest pain (0.7%, N=2); palpitations (0.7%, N=2); and urinary retention (0.7%, N=2) were the reasons for discontinuation reported by more than 1 patient.

Commonly observed adverse events in acute adult placebo-controlled trials—Commonly observed adverse events associated with the use of STRATTERA (incidence of 2% or greater) and not observed at an equivalent incidence among placebo-treated patients (STRATTERA incidence greater than placebo) are listed in Table 3. The most commonly observed adverse events in patients treated with STRATTERA (incidence of 5% or greater and at least twice the incidence in placebo patients) were: constipation, dry mouth, nausea, appetite decreased, dizziness, insomnia, decreased libido, ejaculatory problems, impotence, urinary hesitation and/or urinary retention and/or difficulty in micturition, and dysmenorrhea (see Table 3).

TABLE 2 Common Treatment-Emergent Adverse Events Associated with the Use of STRATTERA in Acute (up to 9 weeks) Child and Adolescent Trials

Adverse Event	Percentage of Patients Reporting Events from BID Trials		Percentage of Patients Reporting Events from QD Trials	
	STRATTERA (N=340)	Placebo (N=207)	STRATTERA (N=85)	Placebo (N=85)
Gastrointestinal Disorders				
Abdominal pain upper	20	16	16	9
Constipation	3	1	0	0
Diarrhea	3	6	4	1
Dry mouth	1	2	4	1
Dyspepsia	4	2	8	0
Nausea	7	8	12	2
Vomiting	11	9	15	1
General Disorders				
Fatigue	4	5	9	1
Psychiatric Disorders				
Mood swings	2	0	5	2

	STRATTERA™ Capsules				
	10 mg*	18 mg*	25 mg*	40 mg*	60 mg*
Color	Opaque White Opaque White	Gold Opaque White	Opaque Blue Opaque White	Opaque Blue Opaque Blue	Opaque Blue, Gold
Identification	LILLY 3227	LILLY 3238	LILLY 3228	LILLY 3229	LILLY 3239
NDC Codes: Bottles of 30	NDC-0002-3227-30	NDC-0002-3238-30	NDC-0002-3228-30	NDC-0002-3229-30	NDC-0002-3239-30

*Atomoxetine base equivalent.

TABLE 3 Common Treatment-Emergent Adverse Events Associated with the Use of STRATTERA in Acute (up to 10 weeks) Adult Trials

Adverse Event[1]	Percentage of Patients Reporting Events	
System Organ Class/ Adverse Event	STRATTERA (N=269)	Placebo (N=263)
Cardiac Disorders		
Palpitations	4	1
Gastrointestinal Disorders		
Constipation	10	4
Dry mouth	21	6
Dyspepsia	6	4
Flatulence	2	1
Nausea	12	5
General Disorders and Administration Site Conditions		
Fatigue and/or lethargy	7	4
Pyrexia	3	2
Rigors	3	1
Infections		
Sinusitis	6	4
Investigations		
Weight decreased	2	1
Metabolism and Nutritional Disorders		
Appetite decreased	10	3
Musculoskeletal, Connective Tissue, and Bone Disorders		
Myalgia	3	2
Nervous System Disorders		
Dizziness	6	2
Headache	17	17
Insomnia and/or middle insomnia	16	8
Paraesthesia	4	2
Sinus headache	3	1
Psychiatric Disorders		
Abnormal dreams	4	3
Libido decreased	6	2
Sleep disorder	4	2
Renal and Urinary Disorders		
Urinary hesitation and/or urinary retention and/or difficulty in micturition	8	0

	STRATTERA	Placebo
Reproductive System and Breast Disorders		
Dysmenorrhea[3]	7	3
Ejaculation failure[2] and/or ejaculation disorder[2]	5	2
Erectile disturbance[2]	7	1
Impotence[2]	3	0
Menses delayed[3]	2	1
Menstrual disorder[3]	3	2
Menstruation irregular[3]	2	0
Orgasm abnormal	2	1
Prostatitis[2]	3	0
Skin and Subcutaneous Tissue Disorders		
Dermatitis	2	1
Sweating increased	4	1
Vascular Disorders		
Hot flushes	3	1

[1] Events reported by at least 2% of patients treated with atomoxetine, and greater than placebo. The following events did not meet this criterion but were reported by more atomoxetine-treated patients than placebo-treated patients and are possibly related to atomoxetine treatment: early morning awakening, peripheral coldness, tachycardia. The following events were reported by at least 2% of patients treated with atomoxetine, and equal to or less than placebo: abdominal pain upper, arthralgia, back pain, cough, diarrhea, influenza, irritability, nasopharyngitis, sore throat, upper respiratory tract infection, vomiting.
[2] Based on total number of males (STRATTERA, N=174; placebo, N=172).
[3] Based on total number of females (STRATTERA, N=95; placebo, N=91).

Male and Female Sexual Dysfunction—Atomoxetine appears to impair sexual function in some patients. Changes in sexual desire, sexual performance, and sexual satisfaction are not well assessed in most clinical trials because they need special attention and because patients and physicians may be reluctant to discuss them. Accordingly, estimates of the incidence of untoward sexual experience and performance cited in product labeling are likely to underestimate the actual incidence. The table below displays the incidence of sexual side effects reported by at least 2% of adult patients taking STRATTERA in placebo-controlled trials.

TABLE 4

	STRATTERA	Placebo
Erectile disturbance[1]	7%	1%
Impotence[1]	3%	0%
Orgasm abnormal	2%	1%

[1] Males only.

There are no adequate and well-controlled studies examining sexual dysfunction with STRATTERA treatment. While it is difficult to know the precise risk of sexual dysfunction associated with the use of STRATTERA, physicians should routinely inquire about such possible side effects.

DRUG ABUSE AND DEPENDENCE
Controlled Substance Class—STRATTERA is not a controlled substance.
Physical and Psychological Dependence—In a randomized, double-blind, placebo-controlled, abuse-potential study in adults comparing effects of STRATTERA and placebo, STRATTERA was not associated with a pattern of response that suggested stimulant or euphoriant properties.
Clinical study data in over 2000 children, adolescents, and adults with ADHD and over 1200 adults with depression showed only isolated incidents of drug diversion or inappropriate self-administration associated with STRATTERA. There was no evidence of symptom rebound or adverse events suggesting a drug-discontinuation or withdrawal syndrome.
Animal Experience—Drug discrimination studies in rats and monkeys showed inconsistent stimulus generalization between atomoxetine and cocaine.

OVERDOSAGE
The effects of overdose greater than twice the maximum recommended daily dose in humans are unknown.
No specific information is available on the treatment of overdose with atomoxetine. Patients who overdose with atomoxetine should be monitored carefully and receive supportive care. Gastric emptying and repeated activated charcoal (with/without cathartics) may prevent systemic absorption.

DOSAGE AND ADMINISTRATION
Initial Treatment—Dosing of Children and Adolescents up to 70 kg Body Weight—STRATTERA should be initiated at a total daily dose of approximately 0.5 mg/kg and increased after a minimum of 3 days to a target total daily dose of approximately 1.2 mg/kg administered either as a single daily dose in the morning or as evenly divided doses in the morning and late afternoon/early evening. No additional benefit has been demonstrated for doses higher than 1.2 mg/kg/day (see CLINICAL STUDIES).
The total daily dose in children and adolescents should not exceed 1.4 mg/kg/day or 100 mg, whichever is less.
Dosing of Children and Adolescents Over 70 kg Body Weight and Adults—STRATTERA should be initiated at a total daily dose of 40 mg and increased after a minimum of 3 days to a target total daily dose of approximately 80 mg administered either as a single daily dose in the morning or as evenly divided doses in the morning and late afternoon/early evening. After 2 to 4 additional weeks, the dose may be increased to a maximum of 100 mg in patients who have not achieved an optimal response. There are no data that support increased effectiveness at higher doses (see CLINICAL STUDIES).
The maximum recommended total daily dose in children and adolescents over 70 kg and adults is 100 mg.
Maintenance/Extended Treatment—There is no evidence available from controlled trials to indicate how long the patient with ADHD should be treated with STRATTERA. It is generally agreed, however, that pharmacological treatment of ADHD may be needed for extended periods. Nevertheless, the physician who elects to use STRATTERA for extended periods should periodically reevaluate the long-term usefulness of the drug for the individual patient.
General Dosing Information—STRATTERA may be taken with or without food.
The safety of single doses over 120 mg and total daily doses above 150 mg have not been systematically evaluated.
Dosing Adjustment for the Hepatically Impaired Patients—For those ADHD patients who have hepatic insufficiency (HI), dosage adjustment is recommended as follows—For patients with moderate HI (Child-Pugh Class B), initial and target doses should be reduced to 50% of the normal dose (for patients without HI). For patients with severe HI (Child-Pugh Class C), initial dose and target doses should be reduced to 25% of normal (see Special Populations under CLINICAL PHARMACOLOGY).
Dosing Adjustment for Use with a Strong CYP2D6 Inhibitor—In children and adolescents up to 70 kg body weight administered strong CYP2D6 inhibitors, e.g., paroxetine, fluoxetine, and quinidine, STRATTERA should be initiated at 0.5 mg/kg/day and only increased to the usual target dose of 1.2 mg/kg/day if symptoms fail to improve after 4 weeks and the initial dose is well tolerated. In children and adolescents over 70 kg body weight and adults administered strong CYP2D6 inhibitors, e.g., paroxetine, fluoxetine, and quinidine, STRATTERA should be initiated at 40 mg/day and only increased to the usual target dose of 80 mg/day if symptoms fail to improve after 4 weeks and the initial dose is well tolerated.
Atomoxetine can be discontinued without being tapered.

HOW SUPPLIED
STRATTERA capsules are supplied in 10-, 18-, 25-, 40-, and 60-mg strengths.
Store at 25°C (77°F); excursions permitted to 15° to 30°C (59° to 86°F)
[see USP Controlled Room Temperature].
[See second table at top of previous page]
Literature Revised March 5, 2003
Eli Lilly and Company
Indianapolis, IN 46285
www.strattera.com
PV 3752 AMP
Copyright © 2003, Eli Lilly and Company.
All rights reserved.

To keep your **PDR** up to date throughout the year, note these revisions on the corresponding pages of the annual volume. Simply write **"See Supplement A"** next to the product heading.

Merck/Schering-Plough Pharmaceuticals
PO BOX 1000
UG4B–75A
351 N. SUMNEYTOWN PIKE
NORTH WALES, PA 19454

For Product and Service Information, Medical Information, and Adverse Drug Experience Reporting:
Call: Merck/Schering-Plough National Service Center
Monday through Friday, 8:00 AM to 7:00 PM (ET)
866-637-2501
Fax: 800-637-2568
For 24-hour emergency information, healthcare professionals should call:
Merck/Schering-Plough National Service Center at 866-637-2501
For Product Ordering,
Call: Merck Order Management Center
Monday through Friday, 8:00 AM to 7:00 PM (ET)
800-637-2579

ZETIA™ ℞
[zĕt' ē ă]
(EZETIMIBE)
TABLETS

DESCRIPTION
ZETIA (ezetimibe) is in a class of lipid-lowering compounds that selectively inhibits the intestinal absorption of cholesterol and related phytosterols. The chemical name of ezetimibe is 1-(4-fluorophenyl)-3(R)-[3-(4-fluorophenyl)-3(S)-hydroxypropyl]-4(S)-(4-hydroxyphenyl)-2-azetidinone. The empirical formula is $C_{24}H_{21}F_2NO_3$. Its molecular weight is 409.4 and its structural formula is:

Ezetimibe is a white, crystalline powder that is freely to very soluble in ethanol, methanol, and acetone and practically insoluble in water. Ezetimibe has a melting point of about 163°C and is stable at ambient temperature. ZETIA is available as a tablet for oral administration containing 10 mg of ezetimibe and the following inactive ingredients: croscarmellose sodium NF, lactose monohydrate NF, magnesium stearate NF, microcrystalline cellulose NF, povidone USP, and sodium lauryl sulfate NF.

CLINICAL PHARMACOLOGY
Background
Clinical studies have demonstrated that elevated levels of total cholesterol (total-C), low density lipoprotein cholesterol (LDL-C) and apolipoprotein B (Apo B), the major protein constituent of LDL, promote human atherosclerosis. In addition, decreased levels of high density lipoprotein cholesterol (HDL-C) are associated with the development of atherosclerosis. Epidemiologic studies have established that cardiovascular morbidity and mortality vary directly with the level of total-C and LDL-C and inversely with the level of HDL-C. Like LDL, cholesterol-enriched triglyceride-rich lipoproteins, including very-low-density lipoproteins (VLDL), intermediate-density lipoproteins (IDL), and remnants, can also promote atherosclerosis. The independent effect of raising HDL-C or lowering triglycerides (TG) on the risk of coronary and cardiovascular morbidity and mortality has not been determined.
ZETIA reduces total-C, LDL-C, Apo B, and TG, and increases HDL-C in patients with hypercholesterolemia. Administration of ZETIA with an HMG-CoA reductase inhibitor is effective in improving serum total-C, LDL-C, Apo B, TG, and HDL-C beyond treatment alone. The effects of ezetimibe given either alone or in addition to an HMG-CoA reductase inhibitor on cardiovascular morbidity and mortality have not been established.
Mode of Action
Ezetimibe reduces blood cholesterol by inhibiting the absorption of cholesterol by the small intestine. In a 2-week clinical study in 18 hypercholesterolemic patients, ZETIA inhibited intestinal cholesterol absorption by 54%, compared with placebo. ZETIA had no clinically meaningful effect on the plasma concentrations of the fat-soluble vitamins A, D, and E (in a study of 113 patients), and did not impair adrenocortical steroid hormone production (in a study of 118 patients).
The cholesterol content of the liver is derived predominantly from three sources. The liver can synthesize cholesterol, take up cholesterol from the blood from circulating lipoproteins, or take up cholesterol absorbed by the small intestine. Intestinal cholesterol is derived primarily from cholesterol secreted in the bile and from dietary cholesterol. Ezetimibe has a mechanism of action that differs from those of other classes of cholesterol-reducing compounds (HMG-CoA reductase inhibitors, bile acid sequestrants [resins], fibric acid derivatives, and plant stanols).

Continued on next page

Zetia—Cont.

Ezetimibe does not inhibit cholesterol synthesis in the liver, or increase bile acid excretion. Instead, ezetimibe localizes and appears to act at the brush border of the small intestine and inhibits the absorption of cholesterol, leading to a decrease in the delivery of intestinal cholesterol to the liver. This causes a reduction of hepatic cholesterol stores and an increase in clearance of cholesterol from the blood; this distinct mechanism is complementary to that of HMG-CoA reductase inhibitors (see CLINICAL STUDIES).

Pharmacokinetics

Absorption

After oral administration, ezetimibe is absorbed and extensively conjugated to a pharmacologically active phenolic glucuronide (ezetimibe-glucuronide). After a single 10-mg dose of ZETIA to fasted adults, mean ezetimibe peak plasma concentrations (C_{max}) of 3.4 to 5.5 ng/mL were attained within 4 to 12 hours (T_{max}). Ezetimibe-glucuronide mean C_{max} values of 45 to 71 ng/mL were achieved between 1 and 2 hours (T_{max}). There was no substantial deviation from dose proportionality between 5 and 20 mg. The absolute bioavailability of ezetimibe cannot be determined, as the compound is virtually insoluble in aqueous media suitable for injection. Ezetimibe has variable bioavailability; the coefficient of variation, based on inter-subject variability, was 35 to 60% for AUC values.

Effect of Food on Oral Absorption

Concomitant food administration (high fat or non-fat meals) had no effect on the extent of absorption of ezetimibe when administered as ZETIA 10-mg tablets. The C_{max} value of ezetimibe was increased by 38% with consumption of high fat meals. ZETIA can be administered with or without food.

Distribution

Ezetimibe and ezetimibe-glucuronide are highly bound (>90%) to human plasma proteins.

Metabolism and Excretion

Ezetimibe is primarily metabolized in the small intestine and liver via glucuronide conjugation (a phase II reaction) with subsequent biliary and renal excretion. Minimal oxidative metabolism (a phase I reaction) has been observed in all species evaluated.

In humans, ezetimibe is rapidly metabolized to ezetimibe-glucuronide. Ezetimibe and ezetimibe-glucuronide are the major drug-derived compounds detected in plasma, constituting approximately 10 to 20% and 80 to 90% of the total drug in plasma, respectively. Both ezetimibe and ezetimibe-glucuronide are slowly eliminated from plasma with a half-life of approximately 22 hours for both ezetimibe and ezetimibe-glucuronide. Plasma concentration-time profiles exhibit multiple peaks, suggesting enterohepatic recycling.

Following oral administration of ^{14}C-ezetimibe (20 mg) to human subjects, total ezetimibe (ezetimibe + ezetimibe-glucuronide) accounted for approximately 93% of the total radioactivity in plasma. After 48 hours, there were no detectable levels of radioactivity in the plasma.

Approximately 78% and 11% of the administered radioactivity were recovered in the feces and urine, respectively, over a 10-day collection period. Ezetimibe was the major component in feces and accounted for 69% of the administered dose, while ezetimibe-glucuronide was the major component in urine and accounted for 9% of the administered dose.

Special Populations

Geriatric Patients

In a multiple dose study with ezetimibe given 10 mg once daily for 10 days, plasma concentrations for total ezetimibe were about 2-fold higher in older (≥65 years) healthy subjects compared to younger subjects.

Pediatric Patients

In a multiple dose study with ezetimibe given 10 mg once daily for 7 days, the absorption and metabolism of ezetimibe were similar in adolescents (10 to 18 years) and adults. Based on total ezetimibe, there are no pharmacokinetic differences between adolescents and adults. Pharmacokinetic data in the pediatric population <10 years of age are not available.

Gender

In a multiple dose study with ezetimibe given 10 mg once daily for 10 days, plasma concentrations for total ezetimibe were slightly higher (<20%) in women than in men.

Race

Based on a meta-analysis of multiple-dose pharmacokinetic studies, there were no pharmacokinetic differences between Blacks and Caucasians. There were too few patients in other racial or ethnic groups to permit further pharmacokinetic comparisons.

Hepatic Insufficiency

After a single 10-mg dose of ezetimibe, the mean area under the curve (AUC) for total ezetimibe was increased approximately 1.7-fold in patients with mild hepatic insufficiency (Child-Pugh score 5 to 6), compared to healthy subjects. The mean AUC values for total ezetimibe and ezetimibe were increased approximately 3-4 fold and 5-6 fold, respectively, in patients with moderate (Child-Pugh score 7 to 9) or severe hepatic impairment (Child-Pugh score 10 to 15). In a 14-day, multiple-dose study (10 mg daily) in patients with moderate hepatic insufficiency, the mean AUC values for total ezetimibe and ezetimibe were increased approximately 4-fold on Day 1 and Day 14 compared to healthy subjects. Due to the unknown effects of the increased exposure to ezetimibe in patients with moderate or severe hepatic insufficiency, ZETIA is not recommended in these patients (see CONTRAINDICATIONS and PRECAUTIONS, *Hepatic Insufficiency*).

Table 1
Response to ZETIA in Patients with Primary Hypercholesterolemia
(Mean[a] % Change from Untreated Baseline[b])

	Treatment group	N	Total-C	LDL-C	Apo B	TG[a]	HDL-C
Study 1[c]	Placebo	205	+1	+1	−1	−1	−1
	Ezetimibe	622	−12	−18	−15	−7	+1
Study 2[c]	Placebo	226	+1	+1	−1	+2	−2
	Ezetimibe	666	−12	−18	−16	−9	+1
Pooled Data[c] (Studies 1 & 2)	Placebo	431	0	+1	−2	0	−2
	Ezetimibe	1288	−13	−18	−16	−8	+1

[a] For triglycerides, median % change from baseline
[b] Baseline - on no lipid-lowering drug
[c] ZETIA significantly reduced total-C, LDL-C, Apo B, and TG, and increased HDL-C compared to placebo.

Table 2
Response to Addition of ZETIA to On-going HMG-CoA Reductase Inhibitor Therapy[a] in Patients with Hypercholesterolemia
(Mean[b] % Change from Treated Baseline[c])

Treatment (Daily Dose)	N	Total-C	LDL-C	Apo B	TG[b]	HDL-C
On-going HMG-CoA reductase inhibitor +Placebo[d]	390	−2	−4	−3	−3	+1
On-going HMG-CoA reductase inhibitor +ZETIA[d]	379	−17	−25	−19	−14	+3

[a] Patients receiving each HMG-CoA reductase inhibitor: 40% atorvastatin, 31% simvastatin, 29% others (pravastatin, fluvastatin, cerivastatin, lovastatin)
[b] For triglycerides, median % change from baseline
[c] Baseline - on an HMG-CoA reductase inhibitor alone.
[d] ZETIA + HMG-CoA reductase inhibitor significantly reduced total-C, LDL-C, Apo B, and TG, and increased HDL-C compared to HMG-CoA reductase inhibitor alone.

Renal Insufficiency

After a single 10-mg dose of ezetimibe in patients with severe renal disease (n=8; mean CrCl ≤30 mL/min/1.73 m^2), the mean AUC values for total ezetimibe, ezetimibe-glucuronide, and ezetimibe were increased approximately 1.5-fold, compared to healthy subjects (n=9).

Drug Interactions (See also PRECAUTIONS, *Drug Interactions*)

ZETIA had no significant effect on a series of probe drugs (caffeine, dextromethorphan, tolbutamide, and IV midazolam) known to be metabolized by cytochrome P450 (1A2, 2D6, 2C8/9 and 3A4) in a "cocktail" study of twelve healthy adult males. This indicates that ezetimibe is neither an inhibitor nor an inducer of these cytochrome P450 isozymes, and it is unlikely that ezetimibe will affect the metabolism of drugs that are metabolized by these enzymes.

Warfarin: Concomitant administration of ezetimibe (10 mg once daily) had no significant effect on bioavailability of warfarin and prothrombin time in a study of twelve healthy adult males.

Digoxin: Concomitant administration of ezetimibe (10 mg once daily) had no significant effect on the bioavailability of digoxin and the ECG parameters (HR, PR, QT, and QTc intervals) in a study of twelve healthy adult males.

Gemfibrozil: In a study of twelve healthy adult males, concomitant administration of gemfibrozil (600 mg twice daily) significantly increased the oral bioavailability of total ezetimibe by a factor of 1.7. Ezetimibe (10 mg once daily) did not significantly affect the bioavailability of gemfibrozil.

Oral Contraceptives: Co-administration of ezetimibe (10 mg once daily) with oral contraceptives had no significant effect on the bioavailability of ethinyl estradiol or levonorgestrel in a study of eighteen healthy adult females.

Cimetidine: Multiple doses of cimetidine (400 mg twice daily) had no significant effect on the oral bioavailability of ezetimibe and total ezetimibe in a study of twelve healthy adults.

Antacids: In a study of twelve healthy adults, a single dose of antacid (Supralox™ 20 mL) administration had no significant effect on the oral bioavailability of total ezetimibe, ezetimibe-glucuronide, or ezetimibe based on AUC values. The C_{max} value of total ezetimibe was decreased by 30%.

Glipizide: In a study of twelve healthy adult males, steady-state levels of ezetimibe (10 mg once daily) had no significant effect on the pharmacokinetics and pharmacodynamics of glipizide. A single dose of glipizide (10 mg) had no significant effect on the exposure to total ezetimibe or ezetimibe.

HMG-CoA reductase inhibitors: In studies of healthy hypercholesterolemic (LDL-C ≥130 mg/dl) adult subjects, concomitant administration of ezetimibe (10 mg once daily) had no significant effect on the bioavailability of either lovastatin, simvastatin, pravastatin, atorvastatin, or fluvastatin. No significant effect on the bioavailability of total ezetimibe and ezetimibe was demonstrated by either lovastatin (20 mg once daily), pravastatin (20 mg once daily), atorvastatin (10 mg once daily), or fluvastatin (20 mg once daily).

Fenofibrate: In a study of thirty-two healthy hypercholesterolemic (LDL-C ≥130 mg/dl) adult subjects, concomitant fenofibrate (200 mg once daily) administration increased the mean C_{max} and AUC values of total ezetimibe approximately 64% and 48%, respectively. Pharmacokinetics of fenofibrate were not significantly affected by ezetimibe (10 mg once daily).

Cholestyramine: In a study of forty healthy hypercholesterolemic (LDL-C ≥130 mg/dl) adult subjects, concomitant cholestyramine (4 g twice daily) administration decreased the mean AUC values of total ezetimibe and ezetimibe approximately 55% and 80%, respectively.

ANIMAL PHARMACOLOGY

The hypocholesterolemic effect of ezetimibe was evaluated in cholesterol-fed Rhesus monkeys, dogs, rats, and mouse models of human cholesterol metabolism. Ezetimibe was found to have an ED_{50} value of 0.5 μg/kg/day for inhibiting the rise in plasma cholesterol levels in monkeys. The ED_{50} values in dogs, rats, and mice were 7, 30, and 700 μg/kg/day, respectively. These results are consistent with ZETIA being a potent cholesterol absorption inhibitor.

In a rat model, where the glucuronide metabolite of ezetimibe (SCH 60663) was administered intraduodenally, the metabolite was as potent as the parent compound (SCH 58235) in inhibiting the absorption of cholesterol, suggesting that the glucuronide metabolite had activity similar to the parent drug.

In 1-month studies in dogs given ezetimibe (0.03–300 mg/kg/day), the concentration of cholesterol in gallbladder bile increased ~2- to 4-fold. However, a dose of 300 mg/kg/day administered to dogs for one year did not result in gallstone formation or any other adverse hepatobiliary effects. In a 14-day study in mice given ezetimibe (0.3–5 mg/kg/day) and fed a low-fat or cholesterol-rich diet, the concentration of cholesterol in gallbladder bile was either unaffected or reduced to normal levels, respectively.

A series of acute preclinical studies was performed to determine the selectivity of ZETIA for inhibiting cholesterol absorption. Ezetimibe inhibited the absorption of C14 cholesterol with no effect on the absorption of triglycerides, fatty acids, bile acids, progesterone, ethyl estradiol, or the fat-soluble vitamins A and D.

In 4- to 12-week toxicity studies in mice, ezetimibe did not induce cytochrome P450 drug metabolizing enzymes. In toxicity studies, a pharmacokinetic interaction of ezetimibe with HMG-CoA reductase inhibitors (parents or their active hydroxy acid metabolites) was seen in rats, dogs, and rabbits.

CLINICAL STUDIES

Primary Hypercholesterolemia

ZETIA reduces total-C, LDL-C, Apo B, and TG, and increases HDL-C in patients with hypercholesterolemia. Maximal to near maximal response is generally achieved within 2 weeks and maintained during chronic therapy.

ZETIA is effective in patients with hypercholesterolemia, in men and women, in younger and older patients, alone or administered with an HMG-CoA reductase inhibitor. Experience in pediatric and adolescent patients (ages 9 to 17) has been limited to patients with homozygous familial hypercholesterolemia (HoFH) or sitosterolemia.

Experience in non-Caucasians is limited and does not permit a precise estimate of the magnitude of the effects of ZETIA.

Monotherapy
In two, multicenter, double-blind, placebo-controlled, 12-week studies in 1719 patients with primary hypercholesterolemia, ZETIA significantly lowered total-C, LDL-C, Apo B, and TG, and increased HDL-C compared to placebo (see Table 1). Reduction in LDL-C was consistent across age, sex, and baseline LDL-C.
[See table 1 at top of previous page]
Combination with HMG-CoA Reductase Inhibitors
ZETIA Added to On-going HMG-CoA Reductase Inhibitor Therapy
In a multicenter, double-blind, placebo-controlled, 8-week study, 769 patients with primary hypercholesterolemia, known coronary heart disease or multiple cardiovascular risk factors who were already receiving HMG-CoA reductase inhibitor monotherapy, but who had not met their NCEP ATP II target LDL-C goal were randomized to receive either ZETIA or placebo in addition to their on-going HMG-CoA reductase inhibitor therapy.
ZETIA, added to on-going HMG-CoA reductase inhibitor therapy, significantly lowered total-C, LDL-C, Apo B, and TG, and increased HDL-C compared with an HMG-CoA reductase inhibitor administered alone (see Table 2). LDL-C reductions induced by ZETIA were generally consistent across all HMG-CoA reductase inhibitors.
[See table 2 at top of previous page]
ZETIA Initiated Concurrently with an HMG-CoA Reductase Inhibitor
In four, multicenter, double-blind, placebo-controlled, 12-week trials, in 2382 hypercholesterolemic patients, ZETIA or placebo was administered alone or with various doses of atorvastatin, simvastatin, pravastatin, or lovastatin.
When all patients receiving ZETIA with an HMG-CoA reductase inhibitor were compared to all those receiving the corresponding HMG-CoA reductase inhibitor alone, ZETIA significantly lowered total-C, LDL-C, Apo B, and TG, and, with the exception of pravastatin, increased HDL-C compared to the HMG-CoA reductase inhibitor administered alone. LDL-C reductions induced by ZETIA were generally consistent across all HMG-CoA reductase inhibitors. (See footnote c, Tables 3 to 6.)
[See table 3 above]
[See table 4 above]
[See table 5 at top of next page]
[See table 6 at top of next page]
Homozygous Familial Hypercholesterolemia (HoFH)
A study was conducted to assess the efficacy of ZETIA in the treatment of HoFH. This double-blind, randomized, 12-week study enrolled 50 patients with a clinical and/or genotypic diagnosis of HoFH, with or without concomitant LDL apheresis, already receiving atorvastatin or simvastatin (40 mg). Patients were randomized to one of three treatment groups, atorvastatin or simvastatin (80 mg), ZETIA administered with atorvastatin or simvastatin (40 mg), or ZETIA administered with atorvastatin or simvastatin (80 mg). Due to decreased bioavailability of ezetimibe in patients concomitantly receiving cholestyramine (see PRECAUTIONS), ezetimibe was dosed at least 4 hours before or after administration of resins. Mean baseline LDL-C was 341 mg/dL in those patients randomized to atorvastatin 80 mg or simvastatin 80 mg alone and 316 mg/dL in the group randomized to ZETIA plus atorvastatin 40 or 80 mg or simvastatin 40 or 80 mg. ZETIA, administered with atorvastatin or simvastatin (40 and 80 mg statin groups, pooled), significantly reduced LDL-C (21%) compared with increasing the dose of simvastatin or atorvastatin monotherapy from 40 to 80 mg (7%). In those treated with ZETIA plus 80 mg atorvastatin or with ZETIA plus 80 mg simvastatin, LDL-C was reduced by 27%.
Homozygous Sitosterolemia (Phytosterolemia)
A study was conducted to assess the efficacy of ZETIA in the treatment of homozygous sitosterolemia. In this multicenter, double-blind, placebo-controlled, 8-week trial, 37 patients with homozygous sitosterolemia with elevated plasma sitosterol levels (>5 mg/dL) on their current therapeutic regimen (diet, bile-acid-binding resins, HMG-CoA reductase inhibitors, ileal bypass surgery and/or LDL apheresis), were randomized to receive ZETIA (n=30) or placebo (n=7). Due to decreased bioavailability of ezetimibe in patients concomitantly receiving cholestyramine (see PRECAUTIONS), ezetimibe was dosed at least 2 hours before or 4 hours after resins were administered. Excluding the one subject receiving LDL-apheresis, ZETIA significantly lowered plasma sitosterol and campesterol, by 21% and 24% from baseline, respectively. In contrast, patients who received placebo had increases in sitosterol and campesterol of 4% and 3% from baseline, respectively. For patients treated with ZETIA, mean plasma levels of plant sterols were reduced progressively over the course of the study. The effects of reducing plasma sitosterol and campesterol on reducing the risks of cardiovascular morbidity and mortality have not been established.
Reductions in sitosterol and campesterol were consistent between patients taking ZETIA concomitantly with bile acid sequestrants (n=8) and patients not on concomitant bile acid sequestrant therapy (n=21).

INDICATIONS AND USAGE
Primary Hypercholesterolemia
Monotherapy
ZETIA, administered alone is indicated as adjunctive therapy to diet for the reduction of elevated total-C, LDL-C, and Apo B in patients with primary (heterozygous familial and non-familial) hypercholesterolemia.

Table 3
Response to ZETIA and Atorvastatin Initiated Concurrently in Patients with Primary Hypercholesterolemia (Mean[a] % Change from Untreated Baseline[b])

Treatment (Daily Dose)	N	Total-C	LDL-C	Apo B	TG[a]	HDL-C
Placebo	60	+4	+4	+3	−6	+4
ZETIA	65	−14	−20	−15	−5	+4
Atorvastatin 10 mg	60	−26	−37	−28	−21	+6
ZETIA + Atorvastatin 10 mg	65	−38	−53	−43	−31	+9
Atorvastatin 20 mg	60	−30	−42	−34	−23	+4
ZETIA + Atorvastatin 20 mg	62	−39	−54	−44	−30	+9
Atorvastatin 40 mg	66	−32	−45	−37	−24	+4
ZETIA + Atorvastatin 40 mg	65	−42	−56	−45	−34	+5
Atorvastatin 80 mg	62	−40	−54	−46	−31	+3
ZETIA + Atorvastatin 80 mg	63	−46	−61	−50	−40	+7
Pooled data (All Atorvastatin Doses)[c]	248	−32	−44	−36	−24	+4
Pooled data (All ZETIA + Atorvastatin Doses)[c]	255	−41	−56	−45	−33	+7

[a] For triglycerides, median % change from baseline
[b] Baseline - on no lipid-lowering drug
[c] ZETIA + all doses of atorvastatin pooled (10–80 mg) significantly reduced total-C, LDL-C, Apo B, and TG, and increased HDL-C compared to all doses of atorvastatin pooled (10–80 mg).

Table 4
Response to ZETIA and Simvastatin Initiated Concurrently in Patients with Primary Hypercholesterolemia (Mean[a] % Change from Untreated Baseline[b])

Treatment (Daily Dose)	N	Total-C	LDL-C	Apo B	TG[a]	HDL-C
Placebo	70	−1	−1	0	+2	+1
ZETIA	61	−13	−19	−14	−11	+5
Simvastatin 10 mg	70	−18	−27	−21	−14	+8
ZETIA + Simvastatin 10 mg	67	−32	−46	−35	−26	+9
Simvastatin 20 mg	61	−26	−36	−29	−18	+6
ZETIA + Simvastatin 20 mg	69	−33	−46	−36	−25	+9
Simvastatin 40 mg	65	−27	−38	−32	−24	+6
ZETIA + Simvastatin 40 mg	73	−40	−56	−45	−32	+11
Simvastatin 80 mg	67	−32	−45	−37	−23	+8
ZETIA + Simvastatin 80 mg	65	−41	−58	−47	−31	+8
Pooled data (All Simvastatin Doses)[c]	263	−26	−36	−30	−20	+7
Pooled data (All ZETIA + Simvastatin Doses)[c]	274	−37	−51	−41	−29	+9

[a] For triglycerides, median % change from baseline
[b] Baseline - on no lipid-lowering drug
[c] ZETIA + all doses of simvastatin pooled (10–80 mg) significantly reduced total-C, LDL-C, Apo B, and TG, and increased HDL-C compared to all doses of simvastatin pooled (10–80 mg).

Combination therapy with HMG-CoA reductase inhibitors
ZETIA, administered in combination with an HMG-CoA reductase inhibitor, is indicated as adjunctive therapy to diet for the reduction of elevated total-C, LDL-C, and Apo B in patients with primary (heterozygous familial and non-familial) hypercholesterolemia.
Homozygous Familial Hypercholesterolemia (HoFH)
The combination of ZETIA and atorvastatin or simvastatin, is indicated for the reduction of elevated total-C and LDL-C levels in patients with HoFH, as an adjunct to other lipid-lowering treatments (e.g., LDL apheresis) or if such treatments are unavailable.
Homozygous Sitosterolemia
ZETIA is indicated as adjunctive therapy to diet for the reduction of elevated sitosterol and campesterol levels in patients with homozygous familial sitosterolemia.

Therapy with lipid-altering agents should be a component of multiple risk-factor intervention in individuals at increased risk for atherosclerotic vascular disease due to hypercholesterolemia. Lipid-altering agents should be used in addition to an appropriate diet (including restriction of saturated fat and cholesterol) and when the response to diet and other non-pharmacological measures has been inadequate. (See NCEP Adult Treatment Panel (ATP) III Guidelines, summarized in Table 7.)
[See table 7 at top of page 61]
Prior to initiating therapy with ZETIA, secondary causes for dyslipidemia (i.e., diabetes, hypothyroidism, obstructive liver disease, chronic renal failure, and drugs that increase LDL-C and decrease HDL-C [progestins, anabolic steroids,

Continued on next page

Zetia—Cont.

and corticosteroids]), should be excluded or, if appropriate, treated. A lipid profile should be performed to measure total-C, LDL-C, HDL-C and TG. For TG levels >400 mg/dL (>4.5 mmol/L), LDL-C concentrations should be determined by ultracentrifugation.

At the time of hospitalization for an acute coronary event, lipid measures should be taken on admission or within 24 hours. These values can guide the physician on initiation of LDL-lowering therapy before or at discharge.

CONTRAINDICATIONS
Hypersensitivity to any component of this medication.

The combination of ZETIA with an HMG-CoA reductase inhibitor is contraindicated in patients with active liver disease or unexplained persistent elevations in serum transaminases.

All HMG-CoA reductase inhibitors are contraindicated in pregnant and nursing women. When ZETIA is administered with an HMG-CoA reductase inhibitor in a woman of childbearing potential, refer to the pregnancy category and product labeling for the HMG-CoA reductase inhibitor. (See PRECAUTIONS, *Pregnancy*.)

PRECAUTIONS
Concurrent administration of ZETIA with a specific HMG-CoA reductase inhibitor should be in accordance with the product labeling for that HMG-CoA reductase inhibitor.

Liver Enzymes
In controlled clinical monotherapy studies, the incidence of consecutive elevations (≥3 × the upper limit of normal [ULN]) in serum transaminases was similar between ZETIA (0.5%) and placebo (0.3%).

In controlled clinical combination studies of ZETIA initiated concurrently with an HMG-CoA reductase inhibitor, the incidence of consecutive elevations (≥3 × ULN) in serum transaminases was 1.3% for patients treated with ZETIA administered with HMG-CoA reductase inhibitors and 0.4% for patients treated with HMG-CoA reductase inhibitors alone. These elevations in transaminases were generally asymptomatic, not associated with cholestasis, and returned to baseline after discontinuation of therapy or with continued treatment. When ZETIA is co-administered with an HMG-CoA reductase inhibitor, liver function tests should be performed at initiation of therapy and according to the recommendations of the HMG-CoA reductase inhibitor.

Skeletal Muscle
In clinical trials, there was no excess of myopathy or rhabdomyolysis associated with ZETIA compared with the relevant control arm (placebo or HMG-CoA reductase inhibitor alone). However, myopathy and rhabdomyolysis are known adverse reactions to HMG-CoA reductase inhibitors and other lipid-lowering drugs. In clinical trials, the incidence of CPK >10 × ULN was 0.2% for ZETIA vs 0.1% for placebo, and 0.1% for ZETIA co-administered with an HMG-CoA reductase inhibitor vs 0.4% for HMG-CoA reductase inhibitors alone.

Hepatic Insufficiency
Due to the unknown effects of the increased exposure to ezetimibe in patients with moderate or severe hepatic insufficiency, ZETIA is not recommended in these patients. (See CLINICAL PHARMACOLOGY, *Special Populations*.)

Drug Interactions (See also CLINICAL PHARMACOLOGY, *Drug Interactions*.)

Cholestyramine: Concomitant cholestyramine administration decreased the mean AUC of total ezetimibe approximately 55%. The incremental LDL-C reduction due to adding ezetimibe to cholestyramine may be reduced by this interaction.

Fibrates: The safety and effectiveness of ezetimibe administered with fibrates have not been established.

Fibrates may increase cholesterol excretion into the bile, leading to cholelithiasis. In a preclinical study in dogs, ezetimibe increased cholesterol in the gallbladder bile (see ANIMAL PHARMACOLOGY). Co-administration of ZETIA with fibrates is not recommended until use in patients is studied.

Fenofibrate: In a pharmacokinetic study, concomitant fenofibrate administration increased total ezetimibe concentrations approximately 1.5-fold.

Gemfibrozil: In a pharmacokinetic study, concomitant gemfibrozil administration increased total ezetimibe concentrations approximately 1.7-fold.

HMG-CoA reductase inhibitors: No clinically significant pharmacokinetic interactions were seen when ezetimibe was co-administered with atorvastatin, simvastatin, pravastatin, lovastatin, or fluvastatin.

Cyclosporine: The total ezetimibe level increased 12-fold in one renal transplant patient receiving multiple medications, including cyclosporine. Patients who take both ezetimibe and cyclosporine should be carefully monitored.

Carcinogenesis, Mutagenesis, Impairment of Fertility
A 104-week dietary carcinogenicity study with ezetimibe was conducted in rats at doses up to 1500 mg/kg/day (males) and 500 mg/kg/day (females) (~20 times the human exposure at 10 mg daily based on AUC_{0-24hr} for total ezetimibe). A 104-week dietary carcinogenicity study with ezetimibe was also conducted in mice at doses up to 500 mg/kg/day (>150 times the human exposure at 10 mg daily based on AUC_{0-24hr} for total ezetimibe). There were no statistically significant increases in tumor incidences in drug-treated rats or mice.

No evidence of mutagenicity was observed *in vitro* in a microbial mutagenicity (Ames) test with *Salmonella typhimurium* and *Escherichia coli* with or without metabolic activation. No evidence of clastogenicity was observed *in vitro* in a chromosomal aberration assay in human peripheral blood lymphocytes with or without metabolic activation. In addition, there was no evidence of genotoxicity in the *in vivo* mouse micronucleus test.

In oral (gavage) fertility studies of ezetimibe conducted in rats, there was no evidence of reproductive toxicity at doses up to 1000 mg/kg/day in male or female rats (~7 times the human exposure at 10 mg daily based on AUC_{0-24hr} for total ezetimibe).

Pregnancy
Pregnancy Category: C
There are no adequate and well-controlled studies of ezetimibe in pregnant women. Ezetimibe should be used during pregnancy only if the potential benefit justifies the risk to the fetus.

In oral (gavage) embryo-fetal development studies of ezetimibe conducted in rats and rabbits during organogenesis, there was no evidence of embryolethal effects at the doses tested (250, 500, 1000 mg/kg/day). In rats, increased incidences of common fetal skeletal findings (extra pair of thoracic ribs, unossified cervical vertebral centra, shortened ribs) were observed at 1000 mg/kg/day (~10 times the human exposure at 10 mg daily based on AUC_{0-24hr} for total ezetimibe). In rabbits treated with ezetimibe, an increased incidence of extra thoracic ribs was observed at 1000 mg/kg/day (150 times the human exposure at 10 mg daily based on AUC_{0-24hr} for total ezetimibe). Ezetimibe crossed the placenta when pregnant rats and rabbits were given multiple oral doses.

Multiple dose studies of ezetimibe given in combination with HMG-CoA reductase inhibitors (statins) in rats and rabbits during organogenesis result in higher ezetimibe and statin exposures. Reproductive findings occur at lower doses in combination therapy compared to monotherapy.

All HMG-CoA reductase inhibitors are contraindicated in pregnant and nursing women. When ZETIA is administered with an HMG-CoA reductase inhibitor in a woman of childbearing potential, refer to the pregnancy category and package labeling for the HMG-CoA reductase inhibitor. (See CONTRAINDICATIONS.)

Labor and Delivery
The effects of ZETIA on labor and delivery in pregnant women are unknown.

Nursing Mothers
In rat studies, exposure to total ezetimibe in nursing pups was up to half of that observed in maternal plasma. It is not known whether ezetimibe is excreted into human breast milk; therefore, ZETIA should not be used in nursing mothers unless the potential benefit justifies the potential risk to the infant.

Pediatric Use
The pharmacokinetics of ZETIA in adolescents (10 to 18 years) have been shown to be similar to that in adults.

Table 5
Response to ZETIA and Pravastatin Initiated Concurrently in Patients with Primary Hypercholesterolemia (Mean[a] % Change from Untreated Baseline[b])

Treatment (Daily Dose)	N	Total-C	LDL-C	Apo B	TG[a]	HDL-C
Placebo	65	0	−1	−2	−1	+2
ZETIA	64	−13	−20	−15	−5	+4
Pravastatin 10 mg	66	−15	−21	−16	−14	+6
ZETIA + Pravastatin 10 mg	71	−24	−34	−27	−23	+8
Pravastatin 20 mg	69	−15	−23	−18	−8	+8
ZETIA + Pravastatin 20 mg	66	−27	−40	−31	−21	+8
Pravastatin 40 mg	70	−22	−31	−26	−19	+6
ZETIA + Pravastatin 40 mg	67	−30	−42	−32	−21	+8
Pooled data (All Pravastatin Doses)[c]	205	−17	−25	−20	−14	+7
Pooled data (All ZETIA + Pravastatin Doses)[c]	204	−27	−39	−30	−21	+8

[a] For triglycerides, median % change from baseline
[b] Baseline - on no lipid-lowering drug
[c] ZETIA + all doses of pravastatin pooled (10–40 mg) significantly reduced total-C, LDL-C, Apo B, and TG compared to all doses of pravastatin pooled (10–40 mg).

Table 6
Response to ZETIA and Lovastatin Initiated Concurrently in Patients with Primary Hypercholesterolemia (Mean[a] % Change from Untreated Baseline[b])

Treatment (Daily Dose)	N	Total-C	LDL-C	Apo B	TG[a]	HDL-C
Placebo	64	+1	0	+1	+6	0
ZETIA	72	−13	−19	−14	−5	+3
Lovastatin 10 mg	73	−15	−20	−17	−11	+5
ZETIA + Lovastatin 10 mg	65	−24	−34	−27	−19	+8
Lovastatin 20 mg	74	−19	−26	−21	−12	+3
ZETIA + Lovastatin 20 mg	62	−29	−41	−34	−27	+9
Lovastatin 40 mg	73	−21	−30	−25	−15	+5
ZETIA + Lovastatin 40 mg	65	−33	−46	−38	−27	+9
Pooled data (All Lovastatin Doses)[c]	220	−18	−25	−21	−12	+4
Pooled data (All ZETIA + Lovastatin Doses)[c]	192	−29	−40	−33	−25	+9

[a] For triglycerides, median % change from baseline
[b] Baseline - on no lipid-lowering drug
[c] ZETIA + all doses of lovastatin pooled (10–40 mg) significantly reduced total-C, LDL-C, Apo B, and TG, and increased HDL-C compared to all doses of lovastatin pooled (10–40 mg).

Treatment experience with ZETIA in the pediatric population is limited to 4 patients (9 to 17 years) in the sitosterolemia study and 5 patients (11 to 17 years) in the HoFH study. Treatment with ZETIA in children (<10 years) is not recommended. (See CLINICAL PHARMACOLOGY, *Special Populations*.)
Geriatric Use
Of the patients who received ZETIA in clinical studies, 948 were 65 and older (this included 206 who were 75 and older). The effectiveness and safety of ZETIA were similar between these patients and younger subjects. Greater sensitivity of some older individuals cannot be ruled out. (See CLINICAL PHARMACOLOGY, *Special Populations*, and ADVERSE REACTIONS.)

ADVERSE REACTIONS
ZETIA has been evaluated for safety in more than 4700 patients in clinical trials. Clinical studies of ZETIA (administered alone or with an HMG-CoA reductase inhibitor) demonstrated that ZETIA was generally well tolerated. The overall incidence of adverse events reported with ZETIA was similar to that reported with placebo, and the discontinuation rate due to adverse events was also similar for ZETIA and placebo.
Monotherapy
Adverse experiences reported in ≥2% of patients treated with ZETIA and at an incidence greater than placebo in placebo-controlled studies of ZETIA, regardless of causality assessment, are shown in Table 8.

Table 8*
Clinical Adverse Events Occurring in ≥2% of Patients Treated with ZETIA and at an Incidence Greater than Placebo, Regardless of Causality

Body System/Organ Class Adverse Event	Placebo (%) n = 795	ZETIA 10 mg (%) n = 1691
Body as a whole – general disorders		
Fatigue	1.8	2.2
Gastro-intestinal system disorders		
Abdominal pain	2.8	3.0
Diarrhea	3.0	3.7
Infection and infestations		
Infection viral	1.8	2.2
Pharyngitis	2.1	2.3
Sinusitis	2.8	3.6
Musculo-skeletal system disorders		
Arthralgia	3.4	3.8
Back pain	3.9	4.1
Respiratory system disorders		
Coughing	2.1	2.3

*Includes patients who received placebo or ZETIA alone reported in Table 9.

The frequency of less common adverse events was comparable between ZETIA and placebo.
Combination with an HMG-CoA reductase Inhibitor
ZETIA has been evaluated for safety in combination studies in more than 2000 patients.
In general, adverse experiences were similar between ZETIA administered with HMG-CoA reductase inhibitors and HMG-CoA reductase inhibitors alone. However, the frequency of increased transaminases was slightly higher in patients receiving ZETIA administered with HMG-CoA reductase inhibitors than in patients treated with HMG-CoA reductase inhibitors alone. (See PRECAUTIONS, *Liver Enzymes*.)
Clinical adverse experiences reported in ≥2% of patients and at an incidence greater than placebo in four placebo-controlled trials where ZETIA was administered alone or initiated concurrently with various HMG-CoA reductase inhibitors, regardless of causality assessment, are shown in Table 9.
[See table 9 above]

OVERDOSAGE
No cases of overdosage with ZETIA have been reported. Administration of ezetimibe, 50 mg/day, to 15 subjects for up to 14 days was generally well tolerated. In the event of an overdose, symptomatic and supportive measures should be employed.

DOSAGE AND ADMINISTRATION
The patient should be placed on a standard cholesterol-lowering diet before receiving ZETIA and should continue on this diet during treatment with ZETIA.
The recommended dose of ZETIA is 10 mg once daily. ZETIA can be administered with or without food.
ZETIA may be administered with an HMG-CoA reductase inhibitor for incremental effect. For convenience, the daily dose of ZETIA may be taken at the same time as the HMG-CoA reductase inhibitor, according to the dosing recommendations for the HMG-CoA reductase inhibitor.
Patients with Hepatic Insufficiency
No dosage adjustment is necessary in patients with mild hepatic insufficiency (see PRECAUTIONS, *Hepatic Insufficiency*).
Patients with Renal Insufficiency
No dosage adjustment is necessary in patients with renal insufficiency (see CLINICAL PHARMACOLOGY, *Special Populations*).

Geriatric Patients
No dosage adjustment is necessary in geriatric patients (see CLINICAL PHARMACOLOGY, *Special Populations*).
Co-administration with Bile Acid Sequestrants
Dosing of ZETIA should occur either ≥2 hours before or ≥4 hours after administration of a bile acid sequestrant (see PRECAUTIONS, *Drug Interactions*).

HOW SUPPLIED
No. 3861 - Tablets ZETIA, 10 mg, are white to off-white, capsule-shaped tablets debossed with "414" on one side. They are supplied as follows:
NDC 66582-414-31 bottles of 30
NDC 66582-414-54 bottles of 90
NDC 66582-414-74 bottles of 500
NDC 66582-414-28 unit dose packages of 100.
Storage
Store at 25°C (77°F); excursions permitted to 15–30°C (59–86°F). [See USP Controlled Room Temperature.] Protect from moisture.
Issued October 2002   REV 00   25751809T
Manufactured for:
Merck/Schering-Plough Pharmaceuticals
North Wales, PA 19454, USA
By:
Schering Corporation
Kenilworth, NJ 07033, USA
Copyright © Merck/Schering-Plough Pharmaceuticals, 2001, 2002. All rights reserved.

ZETIA™ (ezetimibe) Tablets
Patient Information about ZETIA (zĕt´-ē-ă)
Generic name: ezetimibe (ĕ-zĕt´-ĕ-mīb)
Read this information carefully before you start taking ZETIA and each time you get more ZETIA. There may be new information. This information does not take the place of talking with your doctor about your medical condition or your treatment. If you have any questions about ZETIA, ask your doctor. Only your doctor can determine if ZETIA is right for you.

What is ZETIA?
ZETIA is a medicine used to lower levels of total cholesterol and LDL (bad) cholesterol in the blood. It is used for patients who cannot control their cholesterol levels by diet alone. It can be used by itself or with other medicines to treat high cholesterol. You should stay on a cholesterol-lowering diet while taking this medicine.
ZETIA works to reduce the amount of cholesterol your body absorbs. ZETIA does not help you lose weight.
For more information about cholesterol, see the "What should I know about high cholesterol?" section that follows.

Who should not take ZETIA?
- Do not take ZETIA if you are allergic to ezetimibe, the active ingredient in ZETIA, or to the inactive ingredients. For a list of inactive ingredients, see the "Inactive ingredients" section that follows.
- If you have active liver disease, do not take ZETIA while taking cholesterol-lowering medicines called statins.
- If you are pregnant or breast-feeding, do not take ZETIA while taking a statin.

What should I tell my doctor before and while taking ZETIA?
Tell your doctor about any prescription and non-prescription medicines you are taking or plan to take, including natural or herbal remedies.
Tell your doctor about all your medical conditions including allergies.
Tell your doctor if you:
- ever had liver problems. ZETIA may not be right for you.
- are pregnant or plan to become pregnant. Your doctor will decide if ZETIA is right for you.

Continued on next page

Table 7
Summary of NCEP ATP III Guidelines

Risk Category	LDL Goal (mg/dL)	LDL Level at Which to Initiate Therapeutic Lifestyle Changes[a] (mg/dL)	LDL level at Which to Consider Drug Therapy (mg/dL)
CHD or CHD risk equivalents[b] (10-year risk >20%)[c]	<100	≥100	≥130 (100–129: drug optional)[d]
2+ Risk factors[e] (10-year risk ≤20%)[c]	<130	≥130	10-year risk 10–20%: ≥130[c] 10-year risk <10%: ≥160[c]
0–1 Risk factor[f]	<160	≥160	≥190 (160–189: LDL-lowering drug optional)

[a] Therapeutic lifestyle changes include: 1) dietary changes: reduced intake of saturated fats (<7% of total calories) and cholesterol (<200 mg per day), and enhancing LDL lowering with plant stanols/sterols (2 g/d) and increased viscous (soluble) fiber (10–25 g/d), 2) weight reduction, and 3) increased physical activity.
[b] CHD risk equivalents comprise: diabetes, multiple risk factors that confer a 10-year risk for CHD >20%, and other clinical forms of atherosclerotic disease (peripheral arterial disease, abdominal aortic aneurysm and symptomatic carotid artery disease).
[c] Risk assessment for determining the 10-year risk for developing CHD is carried out using the Framingham risk scoring. Refer to JAMA, May 16, 2001; 285 (19): 2486–2497, or the NCEP website (http://www.nhlbi.nih.gov) for more details.
[d] Some authorities recommend use of LDL-lowering drugs in this category if an LDL cholesterol <100 mg/dL cannot be achieved by therapeutic lifestyle changes. Others prefer use of drugs that primarily modify triglycerides and HDL, e.g., nicotinic acid or fibrate. Clinical judgment also may call for deferring drug therapy in this subcategory.
[e] Major risk factors (exclusive of LDL cholesterol) that modify LDL goals include cigarette smoking, hypertension (BP ≥140/90 mm Hg or on anti-hypertensive medication), low HDL cholesterol (<40 mg/dL), family history of premature CHD (CHD in male first-degree relative <55 years; CHD in female first-degree relative <65 years), age (men ≥45 years; women ≥55 years). HDL cholesterol ≥60 mg/dL counts as a "negative" risk factor; its presence removes one risk factor from the total count.
[f] Almost all people with 0–1 risk factor have a 10-year risk <10%; thus, 10-year risk assessment in people with 0–1 risk factor is not necessary.

Table 9*
Clinical Adverse Events occurring in ≥2% of Patients and at an Incidence Greater than Placebo, Regardless of Causality, in ZETIA/Statin Combination Studies

Body System/Organ Class Adverse Event	Placebo (%) n=259	ZETIA 10 mg (%) n=262	All Statins** (%) n=936	ZETIA + All Statins** (%) n=925
Body as a whole – general disorders				
Chest pain	1.2	3.4	2.0	1.8
Dizziness	1.2	2.7	1.4	1.8
Fatigue	1.9	1.9	1.4	2.8
Headache	5.4	8.0	7.3	6.3
Gastro-intestinal system disorders				
Abdominal pain	2.3	2.7	3.1	3.5
Diarrhea	1.5	3.4	2.9	2.8
Infection and infestations				
Pharyngitis	1.9	3.1	2.5	2.3
Sinusitis	1.9	4.6	3.6	3.5
Upper respiratory tract infection	10.8	13.0	13.6	11.8
Musculo-skeletal system disorders				
Arthralgia	2.3	3.8	4.3	3.4
Back pain	3.5	3.4	3.7	4.3
Myalgia	4.6	5.0	4.1	4.5

*Includes four placebo-controlled combination studies in which ZETIA was initiated concurrently with an HMG-CoA reductase inhibitor.
**All Statins = all doses of all HMG-CoA reductase inhibitors.

Zetia—Cont.

- are breast-feeding. We do not know if ZETIA can pass to your baby through your milk. Your doctor will decide if ZETIA is right for you.
- experience unexplained muscle pain, tenderness, or weakness.

How should I take ZETIA?
- Take ZETIA once a day, with or without food. It may be easier to remember to take your dose if you do it at the same time every day, such as with breakfast, dinner, or at bedtime. If you also take another medicine to reduce your cholesterol, ask your doctor if you can take them at the same time.
- If you forget to take ZETIA, take it as soon as you remember. However, do not take more than one dose of ZETIA a day.
- Continue to follow a cholesterol-lowering diet while taking ZETIA. Ask your doctor if you need diet information.
- Keep taking ZETIA unless your doctor tells you to stop. It is important that you keep taking ZETIA even if you do not feel sick.

See your doctor regularly to check your cholesterol level and to check for side effects. Your doctor may do blood tests to check your liver before you start taking ZETIA with a statin and during treatment.

What are the possible side effects of ZETIA?
Patients reported few side effects while taking ZETIA. Tell your doctor if you are having stomach pain, are feeling tired, or have any other medical problems while on ZETIA. For a complete list of side effects, ask your doctor or pharmacist.

What should I know about high cholesterol?
Cholesterol is a type of fat found in your blood. Your total cholesterol is made up of LDL and HDL cholesterol.
LDL cholesterol is called "bad" cholesterol because it can build up in the wall of your arteries and form plaque. Over time, plaque build-up can cause a narrowing of the arteries. This narrowing can slow or block blood flow to your heart, brain, and other organs. High LDL cholesterol is a major cause of heart disease and stroke.
HDL cholesterol is called "good" cholesterol because it keeps the bad cholesterol from building up in the arteries.
Triglycerides also are fats found in your blood.

General Information about ZETIA
Medicines are sometimes prescribed for conditions that are not mentioned in patient information leaflets. Do not use ZETIA for a condition for which it was not prescribed. Do not give ZETIA to other people, even if they have the same condition you have. It may harm them.
This summarizes the most important information about ZETIA. If you would like more information, talk with your doctor. You can ask your pharmacist or doctor for information about ZETIA that is written for health professionals.

Inactive ingredients:
Croscarmellose sodium, lactose monohydrate, magnesium stearate, microcrystalline cellulose, povidone, and sodium lauryl sulfate.

Issued October 2002　　REV 00　　2575701T
Manufactured for:
Merck/Schering-Plough Pharmaceuticals
North Wales, PA 19454, USA
By:
Schering Corporation
Kenilworth, NJ 07033, USA
Copyright © Merck/Schering-Plough Pharmaceuticals, 2001, 2002. All rights reserved.

Odyssey Pharmaceuticals, Inc.
72 EAGLE ROCK AVE,
P.O. BOX 522
EAST HANOVER, NJ 07936

Direct Inquiries to:
(877) 427-9068

VOSPIRE ER™　℞
[vō'spēr]
(Albuterol Sulfate)
Extended-Release Tablets

DESCRIPTION
Albuterol extended-release tablets contain albuterol sulfate, the racemic form of albuterol and a relatively selective beta$_2$-adrenergic bronchodilator, in an extended-release formulation. Albuterol sulfate has the chemical name (±) α_1-[(*tert*-butylamino)methyl]-4-hydroxy-*m*-xylene-α, α'-diol sulfate (2:1) (salt), and the following structural formula:

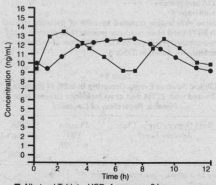

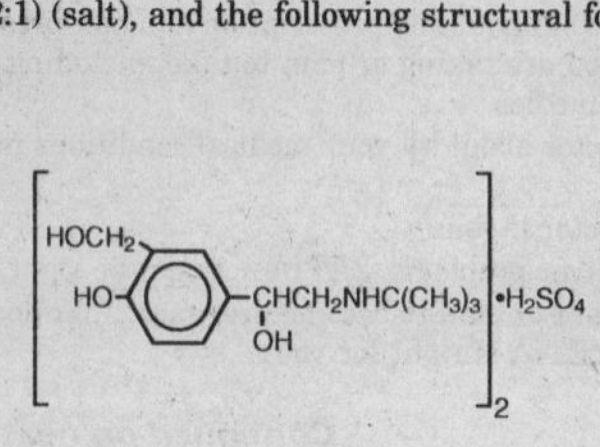

Albuterol sulfate has a molecular weight of 576.7, and the molecular formula is $(C_{13}H_{21}NO_3)_2 \cdot H_2SO_4$. Albuterol sulfate is a white crystalline powder, soluble in water and slightly soluble in ethanol.
The World Health Organization recommended name for albuterol base is salbutamol.
Each tablet for oral administration contains 4 mg or 8 mg of albuterol as 4.8 mg or 9.6 mg, respectively, of albuterol sulfate in a cellulosic material that serves as a diffusion-release membrane. In addition each tablet contains the following inactive ingredients: Calcium sulfate, carnauba wax, ethylcellulose, ferric oxide black, hydroxypropyl methylcellulose, ink-thinner XI, lactose monohydrate, magnesium stearate, polyethylene glycol, propylene glycol, shellac, stearic acid, titanium dioxide, triacetin, D&C Yellow #10, (4 mg only) and FD&C Blue #1 (4 mg only).

CLINICAL PHARMACOLOGY
In vitro studies and *in vivo* pharmacologic studies have demonstrated that albuterol has a preferential effect on beta$_2$-adrenergic receptors compared with isoproterenol. While it is recognized that beta$_2$-adrenergic receptors are the predominant receptors in bronchial smooth muscle, data indicates that there is a population of beta$_2$-receptors in the human heart existing in a concentration between 10% and 50%. The precise function of these receptors has not been established. (See Warnings).
The pharmacologic effects of beta-adrenergic agonist drugs, including albuterol, are at least in part attributable to stimulation through beta-adrenergic receptors on intracellular adenyl cyclase, the enzyme that catalyzes the conversion of adenosine triphosphate (ATP) to cyclic-3', 5'-adenosine monophosphate (cyclic AMP). Increased cyclic AMP levels are associated with relaxation of bronchial smooth muscle and inhibition of release of mediators of immediate hypersensitivity from cells, especially from mast cells.
Albuterol has been shown in most controlled clinical trials to have more effect on the respiratory tract, in the form of bronchial smooth muscle relaxation, than isoproterenol at comparable doses while producing fewer cardiovascular effects.
Albuterol is longer acting than isoproterenol in most patients by any route of administration because it is not a substrate for the cellular uptake processes for catecholamines nor for catechol-O-methyl transferase.
Preclinical: Intravenous studies in rats with albuterol sulfate have demonstrated that albuterol crosses the blood-brain barrier and reaches brain concentrations amounting to approximately 5.0% of the plasma concentrations. In structures outside the blood-brain barrier (pineal and pituitary glands), albuterol concentrations were found to be 100 times those in the whole brain.
Studies in laboratory animals (minipigs, rodents, and dogs) have demonstrated the occurrence of cardiac arrhythmias and sudden death (with histologic evidence of myocardial necrosis) when beta-agonists and methylxanthines were administered concurrently. The clinical significance of these findings is unknown.
Pharmacokinetics and Disposition: In a single-dose study comparing one 8 mg albuterol extended-release tablet with two 4 mg immediate-release albuterol tablets, USP in 17 normal adult volunteers, the extent of availability of albuterol extended-release tablets was shown to be about 80% of albuterol tablets, USP with or without food. In addition, lower mean peak plasma concentration and longer time to reach the peak level were observed with albuterol extended-release tablets as compared with albuterol tablets, USP. The single-dose study results also showed that food decreases the rate of absorption of albuterol from albuterol extended-release tablets without altering the extent of bioavailability. In addition, the study indicated that food causes a more gradual increase in the fraction of the available dose absorbed from the extended-release formulation as compared with the fasting condition.
In another single-dose study in adults, 8 mg and 4 mg albuterol extended-release tablets were shown to deliver dose-proportional plasma concentrations in the fasting state. Definitive studies for the effect of food on 4 mg albuterol extended-release tablets have not been conducted. However, since food lowers the rate of absorption of 8 mg albuterol extended-release tablets, it is expected that food reduces the rate of absorption of 4 mg albuterol extended-release tablets also.
Albuterol extended-release tablets have been formulated to provide duration of action of up to 12 hours. In an 8-day, multiple-dose, crossover study, 15 normal adult male volunteers were given 8 mg albuterol extended-release tablets every 12 hours or 4 mg albuterol tablets, USP every 6 hours. Each dose of albuterol extended-release tablets and the corresponding doses of albuterol tablets, USP were administered in the postprandial state. Steady-state plasma concentrations were reached within 2 days for both formulations. Fluctuations (C_{max}-C_{min}/$C_{average}$) in plasma concentrations were similar for albuterol extended-release tablets administered at 12-hour intervals and albuterol tablets, USP administered every 6 hours. In addition, the relative bioavailability of albuterol extended-release tablets was approximately 100% of the immediate-release tablet at steady state. A summary of these results is shown in the following table:
[See table above]
The mean plasma albuterol concentration versus time data at steady state after the administration of albuterol extended-release tablets 8 mg every 12 hours are displayed in the following graph:

	Mean Values at Steady State				
	C_{max} (ng/mL)	C_{min} (ng/mL)	T_{max} (h)	$T_{1/2}$ (h)	AUC (ng-h/mL)
Albuterol Extended-Release Tablets	13.7	8.1	6.0	9.3	134
Albuterol Tablets, USP	13.9	8.1	2.6	7.2	132

Mean Plasma Albuterol Concentration at Day 8

■ Albuterol Tablets, USP 4 mg every 6 hours
● Albuterol Extended-Release Tablets 8 mg every 12 hours

Pharmacokinetic studies of 4- and 8-mg albuterol extended-release tablets have not been conducted in pediatric patients. Bioavailability of 4- and 8-mg albuterol extended-release tablets in pediatric patients relative to 2- and 4-mg immediate release albuterol has been extrapolated from adult studies showing comparability at steady-state dosing and reduced bioavailability after single dose administration.

INDICATIONS AND USAGE
Albuterol extended-release tablets are indicated for the relief of bronchospasm in adults and children 6 years of age and older with reversible obstructive airway disease.

CONTRAINDICATIONS
Albuterol extended-release tablets are contraindicated in patients with a history of hypersensitivity to albuterol or any of its components.

WARNINGS
Immediate hypersensitivity reactions may occur after administration of albuterol, as demonstrated by rare cases of urticaria, angioedema, rash, bronchospasm, and oropharyngeal edema.
Cardiovascular Effects: Albuterol extended-release tablets, like all other beta-adrenergic agonists, can produce a clinically significant cardiovascular effect in some patients, as measured by pulse rate, blood pressure, and/or symptoms. Although such effects are uncommon after administration of albuterol extended-release tablets at recommended doses, if they occur, the drug may need to be discontinued. In addition, beta-agonists have been reported to produce electrocardiogram (ECG) changes, such as flattening of the T wave, prolongation of the QTc interval, and ST segment depression. The clinical significance of these findings is unknown. Therefore, albuterol extended-release tablets, like all sympathomimetic amines, should be used with caution in patients with cardiovascular disorders, especially coronary insufficiency, cardiac arrhythmias, and hypertension.
Deterioration of Asthma: Asthma may deteriorate acutely over a period of hours or chronically over several days or longer. If the patient needs more doses of albuterol extended-release tablets than usual, this may be a marker of destabilization of asthma and requires reevaluation of the patient and the treatment regimen, giving special consideration to the possible need for anti-inflammatory treatment; e.g., corticosteroids.
Use of Anti-Inflammatory Agents: The use of beta adrenergic agonist bronchodilators alone may not be adequate to control asthma in many patients. Early consideration should be given to adding anti-inflammatory agents; e.g., corticosteroids.
Paradoxical Bronchospasm: Albuterol extended-release tablets can produce paradoxical bronchospasm, which may be life threatening. If paradoxical bronchospasm occurs, albuterol extended-release tablets should be discontinued immediately and alternative therapy instituted.
Rarely, erythema multiforme and Stevens-Johnson syndrome have been associated with the administration of oral albuterol in children.

PRECAUTIONS

General: Albuterol, as with all sympathomimetic amines, should be used with caution in patients with cardiovascular disorders, especially coronary insufficiency, cardiac arrhythmias, and hypertension; in patients with convulsive disorders, hyperthyroidism, or diabetes mellitus; and in patients who are unusually responsive to sympathomimetic amines. Clinically significant changes in systolic and diastolic blood pressure have been seen and could be expected to occur in some patients after use of any beta-adrenergic bronchodilator.

In controlled clinical trials in adults, patients treated with albuterol extended-release tablets had increases in selected serum chemistry values and decreases in selected hematologic values. Increases in SGPT were more frequent among patients treated with albuterol extended-release tablets (12 of 247 patients, 4.9%) than among the theophylline (6 of 188 patients, 3.2%) and placebo (1 of 138 patients, 0.7%) groups. Increases in serum glucose concentration were also more frequent among patients treated with albuterol extended-release tablets (23 of 234 patients, 9.8%) than among theophylline (11 of 173 patients, 6.45%) and placebo (3 of 129 patients, 2.3%) groups. Increases in SGOT were also more frequent among patients treated with albuterol extended-release tablets (10 of 248 patients, 4%) and theophylline (5 of 193, 2.6%) than among patients treated with placebo. Decreases in white blood cell counts were more frequent in patients treated with albuterol extended-release tablets (10 of 247 patients, 4%) compared with patients receiving theophylline (2 of 185 patients, 1.1%) and patients receiving placebo (1 of 141 patients, 0.7%). Decreases in hemoglobin and hematocrit were more frequent in patients receiving albuterol extended-release tablets (16 of 228 patients, 7.0%, and 17 of 230 patients, 7.4%, respectively) than in patients receiving theophylline (5 of 171 patients, 2.9%, and 9 of 173 patients, 5.2%, respectively) and patients receiving placebo (5 of 129 patients, 3.9%, and 3 of 132 patients, 2.3%, respectively). The clinical significance of these results is unknown.

Large doses of intravenous albuterol have been reported to aggravate pre-existing diabetes mellitus and ketoacidosis. As with other beta-agonists, albuterol may produce significant hypokalemia in some patients, possibly through intracellular shunting, which has the potential to produce adverse cardiovascular effects. The decrease is usually transient, not requiring supplementation.

Information for Patients:

Albuterol extended-release tablets must be swallowed whole with the aid of liquids. DO NOT CHEW OR CRUSH THESE TABLETS.

The action of albuterol extended-release tablets should last up to 12 hours or longer. Albuterol extended-release tablets should not be used more frequently than recommended. Do not increase the dose or frequency of albuterol extended-release tablets without consulting your physician. If you find that treatment with albuterol extended-release tablets becomes less effective for symptomatic relief, your symptoms become worse, and/or you need to use the product more frequently than usual, you should seek medical attention immediately. While you are using albuterol extended-release tablets, other inhaled drugs and asthma medications should be taken only as directed by your physician. Common adverse effects include palpitations, chest pain, rapid heart rate, tremor or nervousness. If you are pregnant or nursing, contact your physician about use of albuterol extended-release tablets. Effective and safe use of albuterol extended-release tablets includes an understanding of the way that it should be administered.

Drug Interactions: The concomitant use of albuterol extended-release tablets and other oral sympathomimetic agents is not recommended since such combined use may lead to deleterious cardiovascular effects. This recommendation does not preclude the judicious use of an aerosol bronchodilator of the adrenergic stimulant type in patients receiving albuterol extended-release tablets. Such concomitant use, however, should be individualized and not given on a routine basis. If regular coadministration is required, then alternative therapy should be considered.

Monoamine Oxidase Inhibitors or Tricyclic Antidepressants: Albuterol should be administered with extreme caution to patients being treated with monoamine oxidase inhibitors or tricyclic antidepressants, or within 2 weeks of discontinuation of such agents, because the action of albuterol on the vascular system may be potentiated.

Beta Blockers: Beta-adrenergic receptor blocking agents not only block the pulmonary effect of beta-agonists, such as albuterol extended-release tablets, but may produce severe bronchospasm in asthmatic patients. Therefore, patients with asthma should not normally be treated with beta-blockers. However, under certain circumstances, e.g., as prophylaxis after myocardial infarction, there may be no acceptable alternatives to the use of beta-adrenergic blocking agents in patients with asthma. In this setting, cardioselective beta-blockers could be considered, although they should be administered with caution.

Diuretics: The ECG changes and/or hypokalemia that may result from the administration of non potassium-sparing diuretics (such as loop or thiazide diuretics) can be acutely worsened by beta-agonists, especially when the recommended dose of the beta-agonist is exceeded. Although the clinical significance of these effects is not known, caution is advised in the coadministration of beta-agonists with non potassium-sparing diuretics.

Digoxin: Mean decreases of 16% to 22% in serum digoxin levels were demonstrated after single dose intravenous and oral administration of albuterol, respectively, to normal volunteers who had received digoxin for 10 days. The clinical significance of these findings for patients with obstructive airway disease who are receiving albuterol and digoxin on a chronic basis is unclear. Nevertheless, it would be prudent to carefully evaluate the serum digoxin levels in patients who are currently receiving digoxin and albuterol.

Carcinogenesis, Mutagenesis, Impairment of Fertility: In a 2-year study in Sprague-Dawley rats, albuterol sulfate caused a significant dose-related increase in the incidence of benign leiomyomas of the mesovarium at dietary doses of 2.0, 10, and 50 mg/kg, (approximately 1/2, 3, and 15 times, respectively, the maximum recommended daily oral dose for adults on a mg/m^2 basis, or, approximately 2/5, 2, and 10 times, respectively, the maximum recommended daily oral dose for children on a mg/m^2 basis). In another study this effect was blocked by the coadministration of propranolol, a non-selective beta-adrenergic antagonist. In an 18 month study in CD-1 mice, albuterol sulfate showed no evidence of tumorigenicity at dietary doses of up to 500 mg/kg (approximately 65 times the maximum recommended daily oral dose for adults on a mg/m^2 basis, or, approximately 50 times the maximum recommended daily oral dose for children on a mg/m^2 basis). In a 22 month study in the Golden hamster, albuterol sulfate showed no evidence of tumorigenicity at dietary doses of 50 mg/kg, (approximately 7 times the maximum recommended daily oral dose for adults and children on a mg/m^2 basis).

Albuterol sulfate was not mutagenic in the Ames test with or without metabolic activation using tester strains *S. typhimurium* TA 1537, TA 1538, and TA98 or *E. coli* WP2, WP2uvrA, and WP67. No forward mutation was seen in yeast strain *S. cerevisiae* S9 nor any mitotic gene conversion in yeast strain *S. cerevisiae* JD1 with or without metabolic activation. Fluctuation assays in *S. typhimurium* TA98 and *E. coli* WP2, both with metabolic activation, were negative. Albuterol sulfate was not clastogenic in a human peripheral lymphocyte assay or in an AH1 strain mouse micronucleus assay at intraperitoneal doses of up to 200 mg/kg.

Reproduction studies in rats demonstrated no evidence of impaired fertility at oral doses up to 50 mg/kg, (approximately 15 times the maximum recommended daily oral dose for adults on a mg/m^2 basis).

Pregnancy: Teratogenic Effects: Pregnancy Category C: Albuterol Sulfate has been shown to be teratogenic in mice. A study in CD-1 mice at subcutaneous (SC) doses of 0.025, 0.25, and 2.5 mg/kg, (approximately 3/1000, 3/100, and 3/10 times the maximum recommended daily oral dose for adults on a mg/m^2 basis), showed cleft palate formation in 5 of 111 (4.5%) fetuses at 0.25 mg/kg and in 10 of 108 (9.3%) fetuses at 2.5 mg/kg. The drug did not induce cleft palate formation at the lowest dose, 0.025 mg/kg. Cleft palate also occurred in 22 of 72 (30.5%) fetuses of females treated with 2.5 mg/kg, of isoproterenol (positive control) subcutaneously (approximately 3/10 times the maximum recommended daily oral dose for adults on a mg/m^2 basis). A reproduction study in Stride Dutch rabbits revealed cranioschisis in 7/19 fetuses (37%) when albuterol sulfate was administered orally at a 50 mg/kg dose, (approximately 25 times the maximum recommended daily oral dose for adults on a mg/m^2 basis).

There are no adequate and well-controlled studies in pregnant women. Albuterol should be used during pregnancy only if the potential benefit justifies the potential risk to the fetus.

During worldwide marketing experience, various congenital anomalies, including cleft palate and limb defects, have been rarely reported in the offspring of patients being treated with albuterol. Some of the mothers were taking multiple medications during their pregnancies. No consistent pattern of defects can be discerned, and a relationship between albuterol use and congenital anomalies has not been established.

Labor and Delivery: Because of the potential for beta-agonist interference with uterine contractility, use of albuterol extended-release tablets for relief of bronchospasm during labor should be restricted to those patients in whom the benefits clearly outweigh the risks.

Tocolysis: Albuterol has not been approved for the management of pre-term labor. The benefit:risk ratio when albuterol is administered for tocolysis has not been established. Serious adverse reactions, including pulmonary edema, have been reported during or following treatment of premature labor with beta$_2$-agonists, including albuterol.

Nursing Mothers: It is not known whether albuterol is excreted in human milk. Because of the potential for tumorigenicity shown for albuterol in animal studies, a decision should be made whether to discontinue nursing or to discontinue the drug, taking into account the importance of the drug to the mother.

Pediatric Use: The safety and effectiveness of albuterol extended-release tablets have been established in pediatric patients 6 years of age or older. Use of albuterol extended-release tablets in these age groups is supported by evidence from adequate and well-controlled studies of albuterol extended-release tablets in adults; the likelihood that the disease course, pathophysiology, and the drug's effect in pediatric and adult patients are substantially similar; the established safety and effectiveness of immediate release albuterol tablets in pediatric patients 6 years of age and older; and clinical trials that support the safety of albuterol extended-release tablets in pediatric patients over 6 years of age. The recommended dose of albuterol extended-release tablets for the pediatric population is based upon the recommended pediatric dosing of immediate-release albuterol tablets and pharmacokinetic studies in adults showing comparable bioavailability at steadystate dosing and reduced bioavailability after single dose administration. Safety and effectiveness in pediatric patients below 6 years of age have not been established.

ADVERSE REACTIONS

The adverse reactions to albuterol are similar in nature to reactions to other sympathomimetic agents. The most frequent adverse reactions to albuterol are nervousness, tremor, headache, tachycardia, and palpitations. Less frequent adverse reactions are muscle cramps, insomnia, nausea, weakness, dizziness, drowsiness, flushing, restlessness, irritability, chest discomfort, and difficulty in micturition.

Rare cases of urticaria, angioedema, rash, bronchospasm, and oropharyngeal edema have been reported after the use of albuterol.

In addition, albuterol, like other sympathomimetic agents, can cause adverse reactions such as hypertension, angina, vomiting, vertigo, central nervous system stimulation, unusual taste, and drying or irritation of the oropharynx.

In controlled clinical trials of adult patients conducted in the United States, the following incidence of adverse events was reported:

[See table above]

Event (n=330)	Albuterol Extended-Release Tablets (n=197)	Theophylline (n=20)	Other Beta-agonists (n=178)	Placebo
Tremor	24.2%	6.1%	35.0%	1.1%
Headache	18.8%	26.9%	35.0%	20.8%
Nervousness	8.5%	5.1%	10.0%	2.8%
Nausea/Vomiting	4.2%	19.8%	5.0%	3.9%
Tachycardia	2.7%	0.5%	5.0%	0%
Muscle Cramps	2.7%	0.5%	5.0%	0.6%
Palpitations	2.4%	0.5%	0%	1.1%
Insomnia	2.4%	6.1%	0%	1.7%
Dizziness	1.5%	2.0%	0%	5.1%
Somnolence	0.3%	1.0%	0%	0.6%

A trend was observed among patients treated with albuterol extended-release tablets toward increasing frequency of muscle cramps with increasing patient age (12-20 years, 1.2%; 21-30 years, 2.6%; 31-40 years, 6.9%; 41-50 years, 6.9%), compared with no such events in the placebo group. Also observed was an increasing frequency of tremor with increasing patient age (12-20 years, 29.4%; 21-30 years, 29.9%; 31-40 years, 27.6%; 41-50 years, 37.9%), compared to 2.9% or less in the placebo group.

The reactions are generally transient in nature, and it is usually not necessary to discontinue treatment with albuterol extended-release tablets.

OVERDOSAGE

The expected symptoms with overdosage are those of excessive beta-adrenergic stimulation and/or occurrence or exaggeration of any of the symptoms listed under ADVERSE REACTIONS; e.g., seizures, angina, hypertension or hypotension, tachycardia with rates up to 200 beats per minute, arrhythmias, nervousness, headache, tremor, dry mouth, palpitation, nausea, dizziness, fatigue, malaise, and insomnia. Hypokalemia may also occur. As with all sympathomimetic aerosol medications, cardiac arrest and even death may be associated with abuse of albuterol extended-release tablets.

Treatment consists of discontinuation of albuterol extended-release tablets together with appropriate symptomatic therapy. The judicious use of a cardioselective beta-receptor blocker may be considered, bearing in mind that such medication can produce bronchospasm. There is insufficient evidence to determine if dialysis is beneficial for overdosage of albuterol extended-release tablets.

The oral median lethal dose of albuterol sulfate in mice is greater than 2000 mg/kg, (approximately 250 times the maximum recommended daily oral dose for adults on a mg/m^2 basis, or, approximately 200 times the maximum recommended daily oral dose for children on a mg/m^2 basis). In mature rats, the subcutaneous median lethal dose of albuterol sulfate is approximately 450 mg/kg (approximately 110 times the maximum recommended daily oral dose for adults on a mg/m^2 basis, or, approximately 90 times the maximum recommended daily oral dose for children on a mg/m^2 basis). In small young rats, the subcutaneous median lethal dose is approximately 2000 mg/kg, (approxi-

Continued on next page

Vospire ER—Cont.

mately 500 times the maximum recommended daily oral dose for adults on a mg/m^2 basis, or, approximately 400 times the maximum recommended daily oral dose for children on a mg/m^2 basis).

DOSAGE AND ADMINISTRATION

The following dosages of albuterol extended-release tablets are expressed in terms of albuterol base:

Usual Dosage:

Adults and Children over 12 years of age: The usual recommended dosage for adults and pediatric patients over 12 years of age is 8 mg every 12 hours. In some patients, 4 mg every 12 hours may be sufficient.

Children 6 to 12 years of age: The usual recommended dosage for children 6 through 12 years of age is 4 mg every 12 hours.

Dosage adjustment in Adults and Children over 12 years of age: In unusual circumstances, such as adults of low body weight, it may be desirable to use a starting dosage of 4 mg every 12 hours and progress to 8 mg every 12 hours according to response.

If control of reversible airway obstruction is not achieved with the recommended doses in patients on otherwise optimized asthma therapy, the doses may be cautiously increased stepwise under the control of the supervising physician to a maximum dose of 32 mg per day in divided doses (i.e., every 12 hours).

Dosage adjustment in Children 6 to 12 years of age: If control of reversible airway obstruction is not achieved with the recommended doses in patients on otherwise optimized asthma therapy, the doses may be cautiously increased stepwise under the control of the supervising physician to a maximum dose of 24 mg per day in divided doses (i.e., every 12 hours).

Switching from oral albuterol, USP products: Patients currently maintained on albuterol tablets, USP or albuterol sulfate syrup can be switched to albuterol extended-release tablets. For example, the administration of one 4 mg albuterol extended-release tablet every 12 hours is comparable to one 2 mg albuterol tablet, USP every 6 hours. Multiples of this regimen up to the maximum recommended daily dose also apply.

Albuterol extended-release tablets must be swallowed whole with the aid of liquids. **DO NOT CHEW OR CRUSH THESE TABLETS.**

HOW SUPPLIED

Albuterol Extended-Release Tablets, equivalent to 4 mg and 8 mg of Albuterol:

4 mg – Green, round, coated tablets in bottles of 100. Printed V on one side and 4 on the other side in black ink.

8 mg – White, round, coated tablets in bottles of 100. Printed V on one side and 8 on the other side in black ink.

Dispense in a well-closed, light-resistant container as defined in the USP. Replace cap securely after each opening. Store at controlled room temperature 15°-30°C (59°-86°F). Distributed by Odyssey Pharmaceuticals, Inc.
East Hanover, New Jersey 07936
Manufactured by:
PLIVA, Inc.
East Hanover, NJ 07936
Rev. 8/02

REFERENCES

1. Data on file, Odyssey Pharmaceuticals, Inc.
2. Volmax Prescribing Information. Available at: http://www.muropharm.com/pivol.pdf. Accessed August 7, 2002.
3. VoSpire ER [package insert]. East Hanover, NJ: Odyssey Pharmaceuticals, Inc; 2002.

Odyssey Pharmaceuticals is a wholly owned subsidiary of PLIVA, Inc.
72 Eagle Rock Avenue
East Hanover, NJ 07936
Tel: 1-877-427-9068
Fax: 1-877-427-9069

In the PDR annual,
the **Brand and Generic Name Index**
(PINK section)
alphabetizes drugs under both
brand and generic names.

Pfizer Inc.
235 EAST 42ND STREET
NEW YORK, NY 10017-5755

For Medical Information Contact:
(800) 438-1985
24 hours a day, seven days a week.

REBIF®
[rē-bĭf]
(interferon beta-1a)   ℞

DESCRIPTION

Rebif® (interferon beta-1a) is a purified 166 amino acid glycoprotein with a molecular weight of approximately 22,500 daltons. It is produced by recombinant DNA technology using genetically engineered Chinese Hamster Ovary cells into which the human interferon beta gene has been introduced. The amino acid sequence of Rebif® is identical to that of natural fibroblast derived human interferon beta. Natural interferon beta and interferon beta-1a (Rebif®) are glycosylated with each containing a single N-linked complex carbohydrate moiety.

Using a reference standard calibrated against the World Health Organization natural interferon beta standard (Second International Standard for Interferon, Human Fibroblast GB 23 902 531), Rebif® has a specific activity of approximately 270 million international units (MIU) of antiviral activity per mg of interferon beta-1a determined specifically by an in vitro cytopathic effect bioassay using WISH cells and Vesicular Stomatitis virus. Rebif® 44 mcg contains approximately 12 MIU of antiviral activity using this method.

Rebif® (interferon beta-1a) is formulated as a sterile solution in a prefilled syringe intended for subcutaneous (sc) injection. Each 0.5 ml (0.5 cc) of Rebif® contains either 44 mcg or 22 mcg of interferon beta-1a, 4 or 2 mg albumin (human) USP, 27.3 mg mannitol USP, 0.4 mg sodium acetate, Water for Injection USP.

CLINICAL PHARMACOLOGY

General

Interferons are a family of naturally occurring proteins that are produced by eukaryotic cells in response to viral infection and other biological inducers. Interferons possess immunomodulatory, antiviral and antiproliferative biological activities. They exert their biological effects by binding to specific receptors on the surface of cells. Three major groups of interferons have been distinguished: alpha, beta, and gamma. Interferons alpha and beta form the Type I interferons and interferon gamma is a Type II interferon. Type I interferons have considerably overlapping but also distinct biological activities. Interferon beta is produced naturally by various cell types including fibroblasts and macrophages. Binding of interferon beta to its receptors initiates a complex cascade of intracellular events that leads to the expression of numerous interferon-induced gene products and markers, including 2', 5'-oligoadenylate synthetase, beta 2-microglobulin and neopterin, which may mediate some of the biological activities. The specific interferon-induced proteins and mechanisms by which interferon beta-1a exerts its effects in multiple sclerosis have not been fully defined.

Pharmacokinetics

The pharmacokinetics of Rebif® (interferon beta-1a) in people with multiple sclerosis have not been evaluated. In healthy volunteer subjects, a single subcutaneous (sc) injection of 60 mcg of Rebif® (liquid formulation), resulted in a peak serum concentration (C_{max}) of 5.1 ± 1.7 IU/mL (mean ± SD), with a median time of peak serum concentration (T_{max}) of 16 hours. The serum elimination half-life ($t_{1/2}$) was 69 ± 37 hours, and the area under the serum concentration versus time curve (AUC) from zero to 96 hours was 294 ± 81 IU·h/mL. Following every other day sc injections in healthy volunteer subjects, an increase in AUC of approximately 240% was observed, suggesting that accumulation of interferon beta-1a occurs after repeat administration. Total clearance is approximately 33–55 L/hours. There have been no observed gender-related effects on pharmacokinetic parameters. Pharmacokinetics of Rebif® in pediatric and geriatric patients or patients with renal or hepatic insufficiency have not been established.

Pharmacodynamics

Biological response markers (e.g., 2', 5'-OAS activity, neopterin and beta 2-microglobulin) are induced by interferon beta-1a following parenteral doses administered to healthy volunteer subjects and to patients with multiple sclerosis. Following a single sc administration of 60 mcg of Rebif® intracellular 2', 5'-OAS activity peaked between 12 to 24 hours and beta-2-microglobulin and neopterin serum concentrations showed a maximum at approximately 24 to 48 hours. All three markers remained elevated for up to four days. Administration of Rebif® 22 mcg three times per week (tiw) inhibited mitogen-induced release of pro-inflammatory cytokines (IFN-γ, IL-1, IL-6, TNF-α and TNF-β) by peripheral blood mononuclear cells that, on average, was near double that observed with Rebif® administered once per week (qw) at either 22 or 66 mcg.

The relationships between serum interferon beta-1a levels and measurable pharmacodynamic activities to the mechanism(s) by which Rebif® exerts its effects in multiple sclerosis are unknown. No gender-related effects on pharmacodynamic parameters have been observed.

CLINICAL STUDIES

Two multicenter studies evaluated the safety and efficacy of Rebif® in patients with relapsing-remitting multiple sclerosis.

Study 1 was a randomized, double-blind, placebo controlled study in patients with multiple sclerosis for at least one year, Kurtzke Expanded Disability Status Scale (EDSS) scores ranging from 0 to 5, and at least 2 acute exacerbations in the previous 2 years.[1] Patients with secondary progressive multiple sclerosis were excluded from the study. Patients received sc injections of either placebo (n = 187), Rebif® 22 mcg (n = 189), or Rebif® 44 mcg (n = 184) administered tiw for two years. Doses of study agents were progressively increased to their target doses during the first 4 to 8 weeks for each patient in the study (see DOSAGE AND ADMINISTRATION).

The primary efficacy endpoint was the number of clinical exacerbations. Numerous secondary efficacy endpoints were also evaluated and included exacerbation-related parameters, effects of treatment on progression of disability and magnetic resonance imaging (MRI)-related parameters. Progression of disability was defined as an increase in the EDSS score of at least 1 point sustained for at least 3 months. Neurological examinations were completed every 3 months, during suspected exacerbations, and coincident with MRI scans. All patients underwent proton density T2-weighted (PD/T2) MRI scans at baseline and every 6 months. A subset of 198 patients underwent PD/T2 and T1 weighted gadolinium-enhanced (Gd)-MRI scans monthly for the first 9 months. Of the 560 patients enrolled, 533 (95%) provided 2 years of data and 502 (90%) received 2 years of study agent.

Study results are shown in Table 1 and Figure 1. Rebif® at doses of 22 mcg and 44 mcg administered sc tiw significantly reduced the number of exacerbations per patient as compared to placebo. Differences between the 22 mcg and 44 mcg groups were not significant (p >0.05).

The exact relationship between MRI findings and the clinical status of patients is unknown. Changes in lesion area often do not correlate with changes in disability progression. The prognostic significance of the MRI findings in these studies has not been evaluated.

[See table 1 below]

The time to onset of progression in disability sustained for three months was significantly longer in patients treated

Table 1: Clinical and MRI Endpoints from Study 1

	Placebo	22 mcg tiw	44 mcg tiw
	n = 187	n = 189	n = 184
Exacerbation-related			
Mean number of exacerbations per patient over 2 years[1,2]	2.56	1.82**	1.73***
(Percent reduction)		(29%)	(32%)
Percent (%) of patients exacerbation-free at 2 years[3]	15%	25%*	32%***
Median time to first exacerbation (months)[1,4]	4.5	7.6**	9.6***
MRI	n = 172	n = 171	n = 171
Median percent (%) change of MRI: PD-T2 lesion area at 2 years[5]	11.0	-1.2***	-3.8***

* p<0.05 compared to placebo
** p<0.001 compared to placebo
*** p<0.0001 compared to placebo
(1) Intent-to-treat analysis.
(2) Poisson regression model adjusted for center and time on study
(3) Logistic regression adjusted for center. Patients lost to follow-up prior to an exacerbation were excluded from this analysis (n = 185, 183, and 184 for the placebo, 22 mcg tiw, and 44 mcg tiw groups, respectively).
(4) Cox proportional hazard model adjusted for center
(5) ANOVA on ranks adjusted for center. Patients with missing scans were excluded from this analysis

with Rebif® than in placebo-treated patients. The Kaplan-Meier estimates of the proportions of patients with sustained disability are depicted in Figure 1.

Figure 1: Proportions of Patients with Sustained Disability Progression

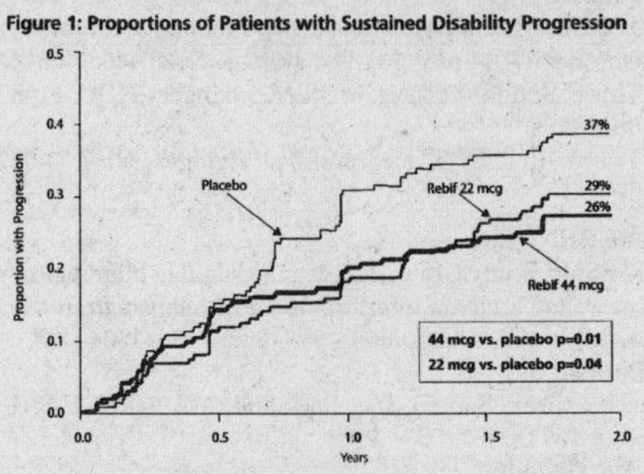

The safety and efficacy of treatment with Rebif® beyond 2 years have not been established.

Study 2 was a randomized, open-label, evaluator-blinded, active comparator study(2). Patients with relapsing-remitting multiple sclerosis with EDSS scores ranging from 0 to 5.5, and at least 2 exacerbations in the previous 2 years were eligible for inclusion. Patients with secondary progressive multiple sclerosis were excluded from the study. Patients were randomized to treatment with Rebif® 44 mcg tiw by sc injection (n=339) or Avonex® 30 mcg qw by intramuscular (im) injection (n=338). Study duration was 48 weeks.

The primary efficacy endpoint was the proportion of patients who remained exacerbation-free at 24 weeks. The principal secondary endpoint was the mean number per patient per scan of combined unique active MRI lesions through 24 weeks, defined as any lesion that was T1 active or T2 active. Neurological examinations were performed every three months by a neurologist blinded to treatment assignment. Patient visits were conducted monthly, and mid-month telephone contacts were made to inquire about potential exacerbations. If an exacerbation was suspected, the patient was evaluated with a neurological examination. MRI scans were performed monthly and analyzed in a treatment–blinded manner.

Patients treated with Rebif® 44 mcg sc tiw were more likely to remain relapse-free during the 24-week treatment period than were patients treated with Avonex® 30 mcg im qw (Table 2). The design of this study does not support any conclusion regarding effects on the accumulation of physical disability.

[See table 2 above]

The adverse reactions were generally similar between the two treatment groups. Exceptions included injection site disorders (80% of patients on Rebif® vs. 24% of patients on Avonex®), hepatic function disorders (14% on Rebif® vs. 7% on Avonex®), and leukopenia (3% on Rebif® vs. <1% on Avonex®), which were observed with greater frequency in the Rebif® group compared to the Avonex® group.

Table 2: Clinical and MRI Results from Study 2

	Rebif®	Avonex®	Absolute Difference	Risk of relapse on Rebif® relative to Avonex®
Relapses Proportion of patients relapse-free at 24 weeks[1]	N=339 75%	N=338 63%	12% (95% CI: 5%, 19%)	0.68 (95% CI: 0.54, 0.86)
MRI Median of the mean number of combined unique MRI lesions per patient per scan[2] (25th, 75th percentiles)	N=325 0.17* (0.00, 0.67)	N=325 0.33 (0.00, 1.29)		

* $p < 0.001$ Rebif® compared to Avonex®

(1) Logistic regression model adjusted for treatment and center, intent to treat analysis

(2) Nonparametric ANCOVA model adjusted for treatment, center, with baseline combined unique lesions as the single covariate.

INDICATIONS AND USAGE

Rebif® (interferon beta-1a) is indicated for the treatment of patients with relapsing forms of multiple sclerosis to decrease the frequency of clinical exacerbations and delay the accumulation of physical disability. Efficacy of Rebif® in chronic progressive multiple sclerosis has not been established.

CONTRAINDICATIONS

Rebif® (interferon beta-1a) is contraindicated in patients with a history of hypersensitivity to natural or recombinant interferon, human albumin, or any other component of the formulation.

WARNINGS

Depression

Rebif® (interferon beta-1a) should be used with caution in patients with depression, a condition that is common in people with multiple sclerosis. Depression, suicidal ideation, and suicide attempts have been reported to occur with increased frequency in patients receiving interferon compounds, including Rebif®. Patients should be advised to report immediately any symptoms of depression and/or suicidal ideation to the prescribing physician. If a patient develops depression, cessation of treatment with Rebif® should be considered.

Hepatic Injury

A case of fulminant hepatic failure requiring liver transplantation in a patient who initiated Rebif® therapy while taking another potentially hepato-toxic medication has been reported from a non-U.S. postmarketing source. Symptomatic hepatic dysfunction, primarily presenting as jaundice, has been reported as a rare complication of Rebif® use. Asymptomatic elevation of hepatic transaminases (particularly SGPT) is common with interferon therapy (see ADVERSE REACTIONS). Rebif® should be initiated with caution in patients with active liver disease, alcohol abuse, increased serum SGPT (> 2.5 times ULN), or a history of significant liver disease. Dose reduction should be considered if SGPT rises above 5 times the upper limit of normal. The dose may be gradually re-escalated when enzyme levels have normalized. Treatment with Rebif® should be stopped if jaundice or other clinical symptoms of liver dysfunction appear.

Anaphylaxis

Anaphylaxis has been reported as a rare complication of Rebif® use. Other allergic reactions have included skin rash and urticaria, and have ranged from mild to severe without a clear relationship to dose or duration of exposure. Several allergic reactions, some severe, have occurred after prolonged use.

Albumin (Human)

This product contains albumin, a derivative of human blood. Based on effective donor screening and product manufacturing processes, it carries an extremely remote risk for transmission of viral diseases. A theoretical risk for transmission of Creutzfeldt-Jakob disease (CJD) also is considered extremely remote. No cases of transmission of viral diseases or CJD have ever been identified for albumin.

PRECAUTIONS

General

Caution should be exercised when administering Rebif® to patients with pre-existing seizure disorders. Seizures have been associated with the use of beta interferons. A relationship between occurrence of seizures and the use of Rebif® has not been established. Leukopenia and new or worsening thyroid abnormalities have developed in some patients treated with Rebif® (see ADVERSE REACTIONS). Regular monitoring for these conditions is recommended (see PRECAUTIONS: Laboratory Tests).

Information for Patients

All patients should be instructed to read the Rebif® Medication Guide supplied to them. Patients should be cautioned not to change the dosage or the schedule of administration without medical consultation.

Patients should be informed of the most common and the most severe adverse reactions associated with the use of Rebif® (see WARNINGS and ADVERSE REACTIONS). Patients should be advised of the symptoms associated with these conditions, and to report them to their physician.

Female patients should be cautioned about the abortifacient potential of Rebif® (see PRECAUTIONS: Pregnancy).

Patients should be instructed in the use of aseptic technique when administering Rebif®. Appropriate instruction for self-injection or injection by another person should be provided, including careful review of the Rebif® Medication Guide. If a patient is to self-administer Rebif®, the physical and cognitive ability of that patient to self-administer and properly dispose of syringes should be assessed. The initial injection should be performed under the supervision of an appropriately qualified health care professional. Patients should be advised of the importance of rotating sites of injection with each dose, to minimize the likelihood of severe injection site reactions or necrosis. A puncture-resistant container for disposal of used needles and syringes should be supplied to the patient along with instructions for safe disposal of full containers. Patients should be instructed in the technique and importance of proper syringe disposal and be cautioned against reuse of these items.

Laboratory Tests

In addition to those laboratory tests normally required for monitoring patients with multiple sclerosis, blood cell counts and liver function tests are recommended at regular intervals (1, 3, and 6 months) following introduction of Rebif® therapy and then periodically thereafter in the absence of clinical symptoms. Thyroid function tests are recommended every 6 months in patients with a history of thyroid dysfunction or as clinically indicated. Patients with myelosuppression may require more intensive monitoring of complete blood cell counts, with differential and platelet counts.

Drug Interactions

No formal drug interaction studies have been conducted with Rebif®. Due to its potential to cause neutropenia and lymphopenia, proper monitoring of patients is required if Rebif® is given in combination with myelosuppressive agents.

Carcinogenesis, Mutagenesis, Impairment of Fertility

Carcinogenesis: No carcinogenicity data for Rebif® are available in animals or humans.

Mutagenesis: Rebif® was not mutagenic when tested in the Ames bacterial test and in an *in vitro* cytogenetic assay in human lymphocytes in the presence and absence of metabolic activation.

Impairment of Fertility: No studies have been conducted to evaluate the effects of Rebif® on fertility in humans. In studies in normally cycling female cynomolgus monkeys given daily sc injections of Rebif® for six months at doses of up to 9 times the recommended weekly human dose (based on body surface area), no effects were observed on either menstrual cycling or serum estradiol levels. The validity of extrapolating doses used in animal studies to human doses is not established. In male monkeys, the same doses of Rebif® had no demonstrable adverse effects on sperm count, motility, morphology, or function.

Pregnancy Category C

Rebif® treatment has been associated with significant increases in embryolethal or abortifacient effects in cynomolgus monkeys administered doses approximately 2 times the cumulative weekly human dose (based on either body weight or surface area) either during the period of organogenesis (gestation day 21–89) or later in pregnancy. There were no fetal malformations or other evidence of teratogenesis noted in these studies. These effects are consistent with the abortifacient effects of other type I interferons. There are no adequate and well-controlled studies of Rebif® in pregnant women. However, in Studies 1 and 2, there were 2 spontaneous abortions observed and 5 fetuses carried to term among 7 women in the Rebif® groups. If a woman becomes pregnant or plans to become pregnant while taking Rebif®, she should be informed about the potential hazards to the fetus and discontinuation of Rebif® should be considered.

Nursing Mothers

It is not known whether Rebif® is excreted in human milk. Because many drugs are excreted in human milk, caution should be exercised when Rebif® is administered to a nursing woman.

Pediatric Use: The safety and effectiveness of Rebif® in pediatric patients have not been studied.

Geriatric Use: Clinical studies of Rebif® did not include sufficient numbers of subjects aged 65 and over to determine whether they respond differently than younger subjects. In general, dose selection for an elderly patient should be cautious, usually starting at the low end of the dosing range, reflecting the greater frequency of decreased hepatic, renal or cardiac function, and of concomitant disease or other drug therapy.

ADVERSE REACTIONS

The most frequently reported serious adverse reactions with Rebif® were psychiatric disorders including depression and suicidal ideation or attempt (see WARNINGS). The incidence of depression of any severity in the Rebif®-treated groups and placebo-treated group was approximately 25%. The most commonly reported adverse reactions were injection site disorders, influenza-like symptoms (headache, fatigue, fever, rigors, chest pain, back pain, myalgia), abdominal pain, depression, elevation of liver enzymes and hematologic abnormalities. The most frequently reported adverse reactions resulting in clinical intervention (e.g., discontinuation of Rebif®, adjustment in dosage, or the need for concomitant medication to treat an adverse reaction symptom) were injection site disorders, influenza-like symptoms, depression and elevation of liver enzymes (see WARNINGS).

In Study 1, 6 patients randomized to Rebif® 44 mcg tiw (3%), and 2 patients who received Rebif® 22 mcg tiw (1%) developed injection site necrosis during two years of therapy. All events resolved with conservative management; none required skin debridement or grafting. Rebif® was continued in 7 patients and interrupted briefly in one patient. There were no reports of injection site necrosis in Study 2 during 24 weeks of Rebif® treatment.

The rates of adverse reactions and association with Rebif® in patients with relapsing-remitting multiple sclerosis are drawn from the placebo-controlled study (n = 560) and the active comparator-controlled study (n = 339).

The population encompassed an age range from 18 to 55 years. Nearly three-fourths of the patients were female, and more than 90% were Caucasian, largely reflecting the general demographics of the population of patients with multiple sclerosis.

Because clinical trials are conducted under widely varying conditions, adverse reaction rates observed in the clinical trials of Rebif® cannot be directly compared to rates in the clinical trials of other drugs and may not reflect the rates observed in practice.

Continued on next page

Rebif—Cont.

Table 3 enumerates adverse events and laboratory abnormalities that occurred at an incidence that was at least 2% more in either Rebif®-treated group than was observed in the placebo group.
[See table 3 below]
The adverse reactions were generally similar in Studies 1 and 2, taking into account the disparity in study durations.

Immunogenicity
As with all therapeutic proteins, there is a potential for immunogenicity. In study 1, the presence of neutralizing antibodies (NAb) to Rebif® was determined by collecting and analyzing serum pre-study and at 6 month time intervals during the 2 years of the clinical trial. Serum NAb were detected in 45/184 (24%) of Rebif®-treated patients at the 44 mcg tiw dose at one or more times during the study. The clinical significance of the presence of NAb to Rebif® is unknown.

The data reflect the percentage of patients whose test results were considered positive for antibodies to Rebif® using an antiviral cytopathic effect assay, and are highly dependent on the sensitivity and specificity of the assay. Additionally, the observed incidence of NAb positivity in an assay may be influenced by several factors including sample handling, timing of sample collection, concomitant medications and underlying disease. For these reasons, comparison of the incidence of antibodies to Rebif® with the incidence of antibodies to other products may be misleading.

Anaphylaxis and other allergic reactions have been observed with the use of Rebif® (see WARNINGS: Anaphylaxis).

DRUG ABUSE AND DEPENDENCE
There is no evidence that abuse or dependence occurs with Rebif® therapy. However, the risk of dependence has not been systematically evaluated.

OVERDOSAGE
Safety of doses higher than 44 mcg sc tiw have not been adequately evaluated. The maximum amount of Rebif® that can be safely administered has not been determined.

DOSAGE AND ADMINISTRATION
The recommended dosage of Rebif® is 44 mcg injected subcutaneously three times per week. Rebif® should be administered, if possible, at the same time (preferably in the late afternoon or evening) on the same three days (e.g. Monday, Wednesday, and Friday) at least 48 hours apart each week (see CLINICAL STUDIES). Generally, patients should be started at 8.8 mcg sc tiw and increased over a 4-week period to 44 mcg tiw (see Table 4). A Rebif® "Starter Pack" containing 22 mcg syringes, is available for use in titrating the dose during the first four weeks of treatment. Following the administration of each dose, any residual product remaining in the syringe should be discarded in a safe and proper manner.

Table 4: Schedule for Patient Titration

	Recommended Titration	Rebif® Dose	Volume	Syringe Strength (per 0.5 mL)
Weeks 1–2	20 %	8.8 mcg	0.2 mL	22 mcg
Weeks 3–4	50 %	22 mcg	0.5 mL	22 mcg
Weeks 5+	100 %	44 mcg	0.5 mL	44 mcg

Leukopenia or elevated liver function tests may necessitate dose reductions of 20–50% until toxicity is resolved (see WARNINGS: Hepatic Injury and PRECAUTIONS: General).

Rebif® is intended for use under the guidance and supervision of a physician. It is recommended that physicians or qualified medical personnel train patients in the proper technique for self-administering subcutaneous injections using the prefilled syringe. Patients should be advised to rotate sites for sc injections (see PRECAUTIONS: Information for Patients). Concurrent use of analgesics and/or antipyretics may help ameliorate flu-like symptoms on treatment days. Rebif® should be inspected visually for particulate matter and discoloration prior to administration.

Stability and Storage
Rebif® should be stored refrigerated between 2–8°C (36–46°F). DO NOT FREEZE. If a refrigerator is temporarily not available, such as while you are traveling, Rebif® should be kept cool (i.e., below 25°C/77°F) and away from heat and light.
Do not use beyond the expiration date printed on packages. Rebif® contains no preservatives. Each syringe is intended for single use. Unused portions should be discarded.

HOW SUPPLIED
Rebif® is supplied as a sterile, preservative-free solution packaged in graduated, ready to use 0.5 mL prefilled syringes with 27-gauge, 0.5 inch needle for subcutaneous injection. The following package presentations are available.

Rebif® (interferon beta -1a) Starter Pack (for initial dose escalation)
— Twelve Rebif® 22 mcg prefilled syringes, NDC 44087-0022-3

Rebif® (interferon beta -1a) 44 mcg Prefilled syringe
— One Rebif® 44 mcg prefilled syringe, NDC 44087-0044-1
— Three Rebif® 44 mcg prefilled syringes, NDC 44087-0044-2
— Twelve Rebif® 44 mcg prefilled syringes, NDC 44087-0044-3

REFERENCES
1. PRISMS Study Group. Randomized double-blind placebo-controlled study of interferon β-1a in relapsing/remitting multiple sclerosis. Lancet 1998; 352: 1498–1504.
2. Data on file.

Manufacturer: Serono, Inc. Rockland, MA 02370 U.S. Licence # 1574
Co-Marketed by:
Serono, Inc.
Rockland, MA 02370
Pfizer, Inc.
New York, NY 10017
Issued: August, 2002
*Avonex® is a registered trademark of Biogen, Inc.
SE0472-06

Medication Guide
Rebif®
Please read this leaflet carefully before you start to use Rebif® and each time your prescription is refilled since there may be new information. The information in this medication guide does not take the place of regularly talking with your doctor or healthcare professional.

What is the most important information I should know about Rebif®?
Rebif® will not cure multiple sclerosis (MS) but it has been shown to decrease the number of flare-ups and slow the occurrence of some of the physical disability that is common in people with MS. Rebif® can cause serious side effects, so before you start taking Rebif®, you should talk with your doctor about the possible benefits of Rebif® and its possible side effects to decide if Rebif® is right for you. Potential serious side effects include:

- **Depression.** Some patients treated with interferons, including Rebif®, have become seriously depressed (feeling sad). Some patients have had thoughts about or have attempted to kill themselves. Depression (a sinking of spirits or sadness) is not uncommon in people with multiple sclerosis. However, if you are feeling noticeably sadder or helpless, or feel like hurting yourself or others you should tell a family member or friend right away and call your doctor as soon as possible. Your doctor may ask that you stop using Rebif®. You should also tell your doctor if you have ever had any mental illness, including depression, and if you take any medications for depression.
- **Liver problems.** Your liver may be affected by taking Rebif®, so you may be asked to have regular blood tests to make sure that your liver is working properly. If your skin or the whites of your eyes become yellow or if you are bruising easily you should call your doctor right away.
- **Risk to pregnancy.** If you become pregnant while taking Rebif® you should stop using Rebif® immediately and call your doctor. Rebif® may cause you to lose your baby (miscarry) or may cause harm to your unborn child. You and your doctor will need to decide whether the potential benefit of taking Rebif® is greater than the risks to your unborn child.
- **Allergic reactions.** Some patients taking Rebif® have had severe allergic reactions leading to difficulty breathing, and loss of consciousness. Allergic reactions can happen after your first dose or may not happen until after you have taken Rebif® many times. Less severe allergic reactions such as itching, flushing or skin bumps can also happen at any time. If you think you are having an allergic reaction, stop using Rebif® immediately and call your doctor.
- **Injection site problems.** Rebif® may cause redness, pain or swelling at the place where an injection was given. A few patients have developed skin infections or areas of severe skin damage (necrosis). If one of your injection sites becomes swollen and painful or the area looks infected and it doesn't heal within a few days, you should call your doctor.

What is Rebif®?
Rebif® is a type of protein called beta interferon that occurs naturally in the body. It is used to treat relapsing forms of multiple sclerosis. It will not cure your MS but may decrease the number of flare-ups of the disease and slow the occurrence of some of the physical disability that is common in people with MS. MS is a life-long disease that affects your nervous system by destroying the protective covering (myelin) that surrounds your nerve fibers. The way Rebif® works in MS is not known.

Who should not take Rebif®?
Do not take Rebif® if you:
- have had an allergic reaction such as difficulty breathing, flushing or hives to another interferon beta or to human albumin.

Table 3. Adverse Reactions and Laboratory Abnormalities in Study 1

Body System Preferred Term	Placebo tiw (n=187)	Rebif® 22 mcg tiw (n=189)	Rebif® 44 mcg tiw (n=184)
BODY AS A WHOLE			
Influenza-like symptoms	51%	56%	59%
Headache	63%	65%	70%
Fatigue	36%	33%	41%
Fever	16%	25%	28%
Rigors	5%	6%	13%
Chest Pain	5%	6%	8%
Malaise	1%	4%	5%
INJECTION SITE DISORDERS			
Injection Site Reaction	39%	89%	92%
Injection Site Necrosis	0%	1%	3%
CENTRAL & PERIPH NERVOUS SYSTEM DISORDERS			
Hypertonia	5%	7%	6%
Coordination Abnormal	2%	5%	4%
Convulsions	2%	5%	4%
ENDOCRINE DISORDERS			
Thyroid Disorder	3%	4%	6%
GASTROINTESTINAL SYSTEM DISORDERS			
Abdominal Pain	17%	22%	20%
Dry Mouth	1%	1%	5%
LIVER AND BILIARY SYSTEM DISORDERS			
SGPT Increased	4%	20%	27%
SGOT Increased	4%	10%	17%
Hepatic Function Abnormal	2%	4%	9%
Bilirubinaemia	1%	3%	2%
MUSCULO-SKELETAL SYSTEM DISORDERS			
Myalgia	20%	25%	25%
Back Pain	20%	23%	25%
Skeletal Pain	10%	15%	10%
HEMATOLOGIC DISORDERS			
Leukopenia	14%	28%	36%
Lymphadenopathy	8%	11%	12%
Thrombocytopenia	2%	2%	8%
Anemia	3%	3%	5%
PSYCHIATRIC DISORDERS			
Somnolence	1%	4%	5%
SKIN DISORDERS			
Rash Erythematous	3%	7%	5%
Rash Maculo-Papular	2%	5%	4%
URINARY SYSTEM DISORDERS			
Micturition Frequency	4%	2%	7%
Urinary Incontinence	2%	4%	2%
VISION DISORDERS			
Vision Abnormal	7%	7%	13%
Xerophthalmia	0%	3%	1%

If you have any of the following conditions or serious medical problems, you should tell your doctor *before* taking Rebif®:

- Depression (a sinking feeling or sadness), anxiety (feeling uneasy or fearful for no reason), or trouble sleeping
- Liver diseases
- Problems with your thyroid gland
- Blood problems such as bleeding or bruising easily and anemia (low red blood cells) or low white blood cells
- Epilepsy
- Are planning to become pregnant

You should tell your doctor if you are taking any other prescription or non-prescription medicines. This includes any vitamin or mineral supplements, or herbal products.

How should I take Rebif®?

Rebif® is given by injection under the skin (subcutaneous injection) on the same three days a week (for example, Monday, Wednesday and Friday). Your injections should be at least 48 hours apart so it is best to take them the same time each day. Your doctor will tell you what dose of Rebif® to use, and may change the dose based on how your body responds. You should not change the dose without talking with your doctor.

If you miss a dose, you should take your next dose as soon as you remember or are able to take it, then skip the following day. **Do not take Rebif® on two consecutive days.** You should return to your regular schedule the following week.

If you accidentally take more than your prescribed dose, or take it on two consecutive days, call your doctor right away.

You should always follow your doctor's instructions and advice about how to take this medication. If your doctor feels that you, or a family member or friend may give you the injections then you and/or the other person should be trained by your doctor or healthcare provider in how to give an injection. Do not try to give yourself (or have another person give you) injections at home until you (or both of you) understand and are comfortable with how to prepare your dose and give the injections.

Always use a new, unopened, prefilled syringe of Rebif® for each injection. Never reuse syringes.

It is important that you change your injection site each time Rebif® is injected. This will lessen the chance of your having a serious skin reaction at the spot where you inject Rebif®. You should always avoid injecting Rebif® into an area of skin that is sore, reddened, infected or otherwise damaged.

At the end of this leaflet there are detailed instructions on how to prepare and give an injection of Rebif®. You should become familiar with these instructions and follow your doctor's orders before injecting Rebif®.

What should I avoid while taking Rebif®?

Pregnancy. You should avoid becoming pregnant while taking Rebif® until you have talked with your doctor. Rebif® can cause you to lose your baby (miscarry).

Breast feeding. You should talk to your doctor if you are breast feeding an infant. It is not known if the interferon in Rebif® can be passed to an infant in mother's milk, and it is not known whether the drug could harm the infant if it is passed to an infant.

What are the possible side effects of Rebif®?

- **Flu-like symptoms.** Most patients have flu-like symptoms (fever, chills, sweating, muscle aches and tiredness). For many patients, these symptoms will lessen or go away over time. You should talk to your doctor about whether you should take an over the counter medication for pain or fever reduction before or after taking your dose of Rebif®.
- **Skin reactions.** Soreness, redness, pain, bruising or swelling may occur at the place of injection. (see: *"What is the most important information I should know about Rebif®?"*)
- **Depression and anxiety.** Some patients taking interferons have become very depressed and or anxious. There have been patients taking interferons who have had thoughts about killing themselves. If you feel sad or hopeless you should tell a friend or family member right away and call your doctor immediately. (see: *"What is the most important information I should know about Rebif®?"*)
- **Liver problems.** Your liver function may be affected. Symptoms of changes in your liver include yellowing of the skin and whites of the eyes and easy bruising. (see: *"What is the most important information I should know about Rebif®?"*)
- **Blood problems.** You may have a drop in the levels of infection-fighting blood cells, red blood cells or cells that help to form blood clots. If the drop in levels are severe, they can lessen your ability to fight infections, make you feel tired or sluggish or cause you to bruise or bleed easily.
- **Thyroid problems.** Your thyroid function may change. Symptoms of changes in the function of your thyroid include feeling cold or hot all the time, change in your weight (gain or loss) without a change in your diet or amount of exercise you are getting.
- **Allergic reactions.** Some patients have had hives, rash, skin bumps or itching while they were taking Rebif®. Other patients have had more serious allergic reactions such as difficulty breathing, or feeling light-headed. You should tell your doctor if you think you are having an allergic reaction. (see: *"What is the most important information I should know about Rebif®?"*)

Whether you experience any of these side effects or not, you and your doctor should periodically talk about your general health. Your doctor may want to monitor you more closely and ask you to have blood tests done more frequently.

Storage Conditions

Rebif® is packaged in prefilled syringes with needles already attached to the syringe.

Rebif® should be stored refrigerated between 2–8°C (36–46°F). DO NOT FREEZE.

If a refrigerator is temporarily not available, such as while you are traveling, Rebif® should be kept cool (i.e., below 25°C/77°F) and away from heat and light.

General Information About Prescription Medicines

Medicines are sometimes prescribed for purposes other than those listed in a Medication Guide. This medication has been prescribed for your particular medical condition. Do not use it for another condition or give this drug to anyone else. If you have any questions you should speak with your doctor or health care professional. You may also ask your doctor or pharmacist for a copy of the information provided to them with the product.

Keep this and all drugs out of the reach of children.

Instructions for Preparing and Giving Yourself an Injection of Rebif®

Before you begin, gather all of the supplies listed below:

- Rebif® prefilled syringe with 27 gauge needle. You may wish to remove your syringe from the refrigerator 30 minutes prior to use and let it adjust to room temperature so the liquid is not cold. Do not heat or microwave a syringe.
- Alcohol swabs (wipes) or cotton balls and rubbing alcohol
- Small adhesive bandage strip (if desired)
- Puncture resistant safety container for disposal of used syringes
- Antibacterial soap
- An over-the-counter pain or fever reducing medication, if your doctor has recommended that you take this prior to, at the same time, or after you give yourself Rebif® to help minimize the fever, chills, sweating and muscle aches (flu-like symptoms) that may occur.

When first starting treatment with Rebif®, your doctor may prescribe a "Starter Pack" containing a lower strength version (22 mcg) of Rebif®. After that, you will be using syringes containing 44 mcg.

Preparing for an injection:

- Check the expiration date; **do not use if the medication is expired.** The expiration date is printed on the syringe, plastic syringe packaging and carton.
- Remove the Rebif® syringe from the plastic packaging. Keep the needle capped.
- Examine the contents of the syringe carefully. The liquid should be clear to slightly yellow. **Do not use if the liquid is cloudy, discolored or contains particles.**
- Choose the injection site. The best sites for giving yourself an injection are those areas with a layer of fat between the skin and muscle, like your thigh, the outer surface of your upper arm, your stomach or buttocks. Do not use the area near your navel or waistline. If you are very thin, use only the thigh or outer surface of the arm for injection. Use a different site each time you inject (thigh, hip, stomach or upper arm, see Figure below). Do not inject Rebif® into an area of your body where the skin is irritated, reddened, bruised, infected or abnormal in any way.
- Wash your hands thoroughly with antibacterial soap before preparing to inject the medication.
- Clean the injection site with an alcohol swab (wipe) or cotton ball with rubbing alcohol using a circular motion. To avoid stinging, you should let your skin dry before you inject Rebif®.

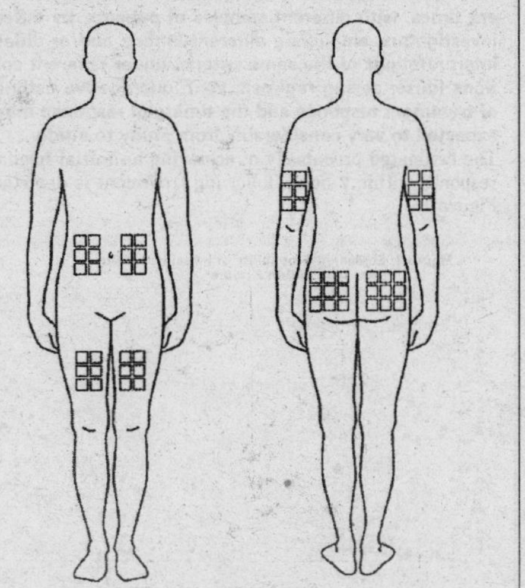

Giving yourself an injection of Rebif®

- Remove the needle cap from the syringe needle.
- If your doctor has told you to use less than the full 0.5ml dose, slowly push the plunger in until the amount of medication left in the syringe is the amount your doctor told you to use.

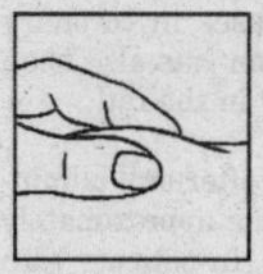

- Use your thumb and forefinger to pinch a pad of skin surrounding the cleaned injection site (see figure). Hold the syringe like a pencil with your other hand.

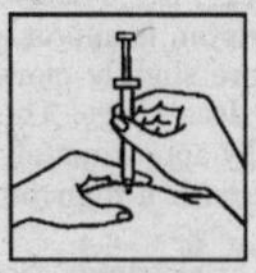

- While still pinching the skin, swiftly insert the needle like a dart at about a 90 degree angle (just under the skin) into the pad of tissue as shown.

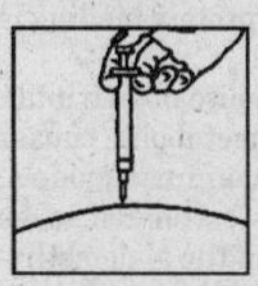

- After the needle is in, remove the hand that you used to pinch your skin and inject the drug using a slow, steady push on the plunger until all the medication is injected and the syringe is empty.

- Withdraw the needle and apply gentle pressure to the injection site with a dry cotton ball or sterile gauze. Applying a cold compress or ice pack to the injection site after injection may help reduce local skin reactions.
- Put a small adhesive bandage strip over the injection site, if desired.
- Discard the syringe and needle as you were instructed by your doctor or health care professional into a puncture resistant syringe disposal container.
- Keep a record of the date and location of each injection.
- After 2 hours, check the injection site for redness, swelling, or tenderness. If you have a skin reaction and it doesn't clear up in a few days, contact your doctor or nurse.

This Medication Guide has been approved by the U.S. Food and Drug Administration.

Co-Marketed by:
Serono, Inc.
Rockland, MA 02370
Pfizer, Inc.
New York, NY 10017
Rev (1), August 2002

RELPAX® ℞

[*rĕl-păks*]
(eletriptan hydrobromide)
Tablets

DESCRIPTION

RELPAX® (eletriptan) Tablets contain eletriptan hydrobromide, which is a selective 5-hydroxytryptamine 1B/1D (5-HT1B/1D) receptor agonist. Eletriptan is chemically designated as 3-[[(R)-1-Methyl-2-pyrrolidinyl]methyl]-5-[2-(phenylsulfonyl)ethyl]indole, monohydrobromide, and it has the following chemical structure:

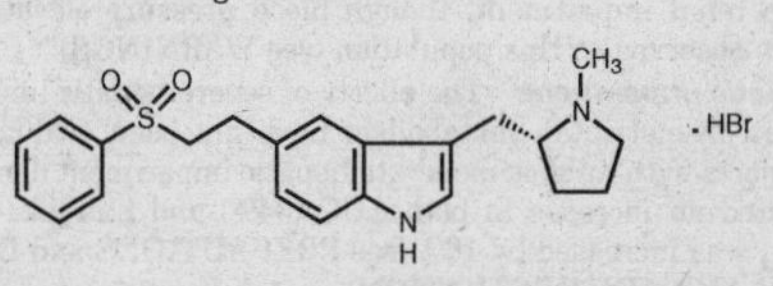

The empirical formula is $C_{22}H_{26}N_2O_2S$. HBr, representing a molecular weight of 463.40. Eletriptan hydrobromide is a white to light pale colored powder that is readily soluble in water.

Each RELPAX Tablet for oral administration contains 24.2 or 48.5 mg of eletriptan hydrobromide equivalent to 20 mg or 40 mg of eletriptan, respectively. Each tablet also contains the inactive ingredients microcrystalline cellulose NF, lactose NF, croscarmellose sodium NF, magnesium stearate NF, titanium dioxide USP, hydroxypropyl methylcellulose NF, triacetin USP and FD&C Yellow No. 6 aluminum lake.

CLINICAL PHARMACOLOGY

Mechanism of Action: Eletriptan binds with high affinity to $5\text{-}HT_{1B}$, $5\text{-}HT_{1D}$ and $5\text{-}HT_{1F}$ receptors, has modest affinity for $5\text{-}HT_{1A}$, $5\text{-}HT_{1E}$, $5\text{-}HT_{2B}$ and $5\text{-}HT_7$ receptors, and little or no affinity for $5\text{-}HT_{2A}$, $5\text{-}HT_{2C}$, $5\text{-}HT_3$, $5\text{-}HT_4$, $5\text{-}HT_{5A}$ and $5\text{-}HT_6$ receptors. Eletriptan has no significant affinity or pharmacological activity at adrenergic $alpha_1$, $alpha_2$, or beta; dopaminergic D_1 or D_2; muscarinic; or opioid receptors.

Two theories have been proposed to explain the efficacy of 5-HT receptor agonists in migraine. One theory suggests that activation of $5\text{-}HT_1$ receptors located on intracranial blood vessels, including those on the arteriovenous anastomoses, leads to vasoconstriction, which is correlated with the relief of migraine headache. The other hypothesis suggests that activation of $5\text{-}HT_1$ receptors on sensory nerve endings in the trigeminal system results in the inhibition of pro-inflammatory neuropeptide release. In the anesthetized dog, eletriptan has been shown to reduce carotid arterial blood flow, with only a small increase in arterial blood pressure at high doses. While the effect on blood flow was selec-

Continued on next page

Relpax—Cont.

tive for the carotid arterial bed, decreases in coronary artery diameter were observed. Eletriptan has also been shown to inhibit trigeminal nerve activity in the rat.

Pharmacokinetics:

Absorption: Eletriptan is well absorbed after oral administration with peak plasma levels occurring approximately 1.5 hours after dosing to healthy subjects. In patients with moderate to severe migraine the median T_{max} is 2.0 hours. The mean absolute bioavailability of eletriptan is approximately 50%. The oral pharmacokinetics are slightly more than dose proportional over the clinical dose range. The AUC and C_{max} of eletriptan are increased by approximately 20 to 30% following oral administration with a high fat meal.

Distribution: The volume of distribution of eletriptan following IV administration is 138L. Plasma protein binding is moderate and approximately 85%.

Metabolism: The N-demethylated metabolite of eletriptan is the only known active metabolite. This metabolite causes vasoconstriction similar to eletriptan in animal models. Though the half-life of the metabolite is estimated to be about 13 hours, the plasma concentration of the N-demethylated metabolite is 10-20% of parent drug and is unlikely to contribute significantly to the overall effect of the parent compound.

In vitro studies indicate that eletriptan is primarily metabolized by cytochrome P-450 enzyme CYP3A4 (see WARNINGS, DOSAGE AND ADMINISTRATION and CLINICAL PHARMACOLOGY: Drug Interactions).

Elimination: The terminal elimination half-life of eletriptan is approximately 4 hours. Mean renal clearance (CL_R) following oral administration is approximately 3.9 L/h. Non-renal clearance accounts for about 90% of the total clearance.

Special Populations:

Age: The pharmacokinetics of eletriptan are generally unaffected by age.

Eletriptan has been given to only 50 patients over the age of 65. Blood pressure was increased to a greater extent in elderly subjects than in young subjects. The pharmacokinetic disposition of eletriptan in the elderly is similar to that seen in younger adults (see PRECAUTIONS).

There is a statistically significant increased half-life (from about 4.4 hours to 5.7 hours) between elderly (65 to 93 years of age) and younger adult subjects (18 to 45 years of age) (see PRECAUTIONS).

Gender: The pharmacokinetics of eletriptan are unaffected by gender.

Race: A comparison of pharmacokinetic studies run in western countries with those run in Japan have indicated an approximate 35% reduction in the exposure of eletriptan in Japanese male volunteers compared to western males. Population pharmacokinetic analysis of two clinical studies indicates no evidence of pharmacokinetic differences between Caucasians and non Caucasian patients.

Menstrual Cycle: In a study of 16 healthy females, the pharmacokinetics of eletriptan remained consistent throughout the phases of the menstrual cycle.

Renal Impairment: There was no significant change in clearance observed in subjects with mild, moderate or severe renal impairment, though blood pressure elevations were observed in this population (see WARNINGS).

Hepatic Impairment: The effects of severe hepatic impairment on eletriptan metabolism have not been evaluated. Subjects with mild or moderate hepatic impairment demonstrated an increase in both AUC (34%) and half-life. The C_{max} was increased by 18% (see PRECAUTIONS and DOSAGE AND ADMINISTRATION).

Drug Interactions:

CYP3A4 inhibitors: *In vitro* studies have shown that eletriptan is metabolized by the CYP3A4 enzyme. A clinical study demonstrated about a 3-fold increase in C_{max} and about a 6-fold increase in the AUC of eletriptan when combined with ketoconazole. The half-life increased from 5 hours to 8 hours and the T_{max} increased from 2.8 hours to 5.4 hours. Another clinical study demonstrated about a 2-fold increase in C_{max} and about a 4-fold increase in AUC when erythromycin was co-administered with eletriptan. It has also been shown that co-administration of verapamil and eletriptan yields about a 2-fold increase in C_{max} and about a 3-fold increase in AUC of eletriptan, and that co-administration of fluconazole and eletriptan yields about a 1.4-fold increase in C_{max} and about a 2-fold increase in AUC of eletriptan.

Eletriptan should not be used within at least 72 hours of treatment with the following potent CYP3A4 inhibitors: ketoconazole, itraconazole, nefazodone, troleandomycin, clarithromycin, ritonavir and nelfinavir. Eletriptan should not be used within 72 hours with drugs that have demonstrated potent CYP3A4 inhibition and have this potent effect described in the CONTRAINDICATIONS, WARNINGS or PRECAUTIONS sections of their labeling (see WARNINGS and DOSAGE AND ADMINISTRATION).

Propranolol: The C_{max} and AUC of eletriptan were increased by 10 and 33% respectively in the presence of propranolol. No interactive increases in blood pressure were observed. No dosage adjustment appears to be needed for patients taking propranolol (see PRECAUTIONS).

The effect of eletriptan on other drugs: The effect of eletriptan on enzymes other than cytochrome P-450 has not been investigated. *In vitro* human liver microsome studies suggest that eletriptan has little potential to inhibit CYP1A2, 2C9, 2E1 and 3A4 at concentrations up to 100μM. While eletriptan has an effect on CYP2D6 at high concentration, this effect should not interfere with metabolism of other drugs when eletriptan is used at recommended doses. There is no *in vitro* or *in vivo* evidence that clinical doses of eletriptan will induce drug metabolizing enzymes. Therefore, eletriptan is unlikely to cause clinically important drug interactions mediated by these enzymes.

CLINICAL STUDIES

The efficacy of RELPAX in the acute treatment of migraines was evaluated in eight randomized, double-blind placebo-controlled studies. All eight studies used 40 mg. Seven studies evaluated an 80 mg dose and two studies included a 20 mg dose.

In all eight studies, randomized patients treated their headaches as outpatients. Seven studies enrolled adults and one study enrolled adolescents (age 11 to 17). Patients treated in the seven adult studies were predominantly female (85%) and Caucasian (94%) with a mean age of 40 years (range 18 to 78). In all studies, patients were instructed to treat a moderate to severe headache. Headache response, defined as a reduction in headache severity from moderate or severe pain to mild or no pain, was assessed up to 2 hours after dosing. Associated symptoms such as nausea, vomiting, photophobia and phonophobia were also assessed.

Maintenance of response was assessed for up to 24 hours post dose. In the adult studies, a second dose of RELPAX Tablets or other medication was allowed 2 to 24 hours after the initial treatment for both persistent and recurrent headaches. The incidence and time to use of these additional treatments were also recorded.

In the seven adult studies, the percentage of patients achieving headache response 2 hours after treatment was significantly greater among patients receiving RELPAX Tablets at all doses compared to those who received placebo. The two hour response rates from these controlled clinical studies are summarized in Table 1.

Table 1: Percentage of Patients with Headache Response (Mild or No Headache) 2 Hours Following Treatment

	Placebo	RELPAX 20 mg	RELPAX 40 mg	RELPAX 80 mg
Study 1	23.8% (n=126)	54.3%* (n=129)	65.0%* (n=117)	77.1%* (n=118)
Study 2	19.0% (n=232)	NA	61.6%* (n=430)	64.6%* (n=446)
Study 3	21.7% (n=276)	47.3%* (n=273)	61.9%* (n=281)	58.6%* (n=290)
Study 4	39.5% (n=86)	NA	62.3%* (n=175)	70.0%* (n=170)
Study 5	20.6% (n=102)	NA	53.9%* (n=206)	67.9%* (n=209)
Study 6	31.3% (n=80)	NA	63.9%* (n=169)	66.9%* (n=160)
Study 7	29.5% (n=122)	NA	57.5%* (n=492)	NA

* p value < 0.05 vs placebo
NA - Not Applicable

Comparisons of the performance of different drugs based upon results obtained in different clinical trials are never reliable. Because studies are generally conducted at different times, with different samples of patients, by different investigators, employing different criteria and/or different interpretations of the same criteria, under different conditions (dose, dosing regimen, etc.), quantitative estimates of treatment response and the timing of response may be expected to vary considerably from study to study.

The estimated probability of achieving an initial headache response within 2 hours following treatment is depicted in Figure 1.

Figure 1: Estimated Probability of Initial Headache Response Within 2 Hours*

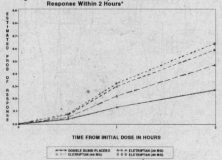

*Figure 1 shows the Kaplan-Meier plot of probability over time of obtaining headache response (no or mild pain) following treatment with eletriptan. The plot is based on 7 placebo-controlled, outpatient trials in adults providing evidence of efficacy (Studies 1 through 7). Patients not achieving headache response or taking additional treatment prior to 2 hours were censored at 2 hours.

For patients with migraine-associated photophobia, phonophobia, and nausea at baseline, there was a decreased incidence of these symptoms following administration of RELPAX as compared to placebo.

Two to 24 hours following the initial dose of study treatment, patients were allowed to use additional treatment for pain relief in the form of a second dose of study treatment or other medication. The estimated probability of taking a second dose or other medications for migraine over the 24 hours following the initial dose of study treatment is summarized in Figure 2.

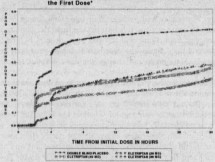

Figure 2: Estimated Probability of Taking a Second Dose/Other Medication Over the 24 Hours following the First Dose*

*This Kaplan-Meier plot is based on data obtained in 7 placebo-controlled trials in adults (Studies 1 through 7). Patients were instructed to take a second dose of study medication as follows: a) in the event of no response at 2 hours (studies 2 and 4-7) or at 4 hours (study 3); b) in the event of headache recurrence within 24 hours (studies 2-7). Patients not using additional treatments were censored at 24 hours. The plot includes both patients who had headache response at 2 hours and those who had no response to the initial dose. It should be noted that the protocols did not allow remedication within 2 hours post dose.

The efficacy of RELPAX was unaffected by the duration of attack; gender or age of the patient; relationship to menses; or concomitant use of estrogen replacement therapy/oral contraceptives or frequently used migraine prophylactic drugs.

In a single study in adolescents (n=274), there were no statistically significant differences between treatment groups. The headache response rate at 2 hours was 57% for both RELPAX 40 mg Tablets and placebo.

INDICATIONS AND USAGE

RELPAX is indicated for the acute treatment of migraine with or without aura in adults.

RELPAX is not intended for the prophylactic therapy of migraine or for use in the management of hemiplegic or basilar migraine (see CONTRAINDICATIONS). Safety and effectiveness of RELPAX Tablets have not been established for cluster headache, which is present in an older, predominantly male population.

CONTRAINDICATIONS

RELPAX Tablets should not be given to patients with ischemic heart disease (e.g., angina pectoris, history of myocardial infarction, or documented silent ischemia) or to patients who have symptoms, or findings consistent with ischemic heart disease, coronary artery vasospasm, including Prinzmetal's variant angina, or other significant underlying cardiovascular disease (see WARNINGS).

RELPAX Tablets should not be given to patients with cerebrovascular syndromes including (but not limited to) strokes of any type as well as transient ischemic attacks (see WARNINGS).

RELPAX Tablets should not be given to patients with peripheral vascular disease including (but not limited to) ischemic bowel disease (see WARNINGS).

Because RELPAX Tablets may increase blood pressure, it should not be given to patients with uncontrolled hypertension (see WARNINGS).

RELPAX Tablets should not be administered to patients with hemiplegic or basilar migraine.

RELPAX Tablets should not be used within 24 hours of treatment with another 5-HT$_1$ agonist, an ergotamine-containing or ergot-type medication such as dihydroergotamine (DHE) or methysergide.

RELPAX Tablets should not be used in patients with known hypersensitivity to eletriptan or any of its inactive ingredients.

RELPAX Tablets should not be given to patients with severe hepatic impairment.

WARNINGS

RELPAX Tablets should only be used where a clear diagnosis of migraine has been established.

CYP3A4 Inhibitors:

Eletriptan should not be used within at least 72 hours of treatment with the following potent CYP3A4 inhibitors: ketoconazole, itraconazole, nefazodone, troleandomycin, clarithromycin, ritonavir, and nelfinavir. Eletriptan should not be used within 72 hours with drugs that have demonstrated potent CYP3A4 inhibition and have this potent effect described in the CONTRAINDICATIONS, WARN-

INGS or PRECAUTIONS sections of their labeling (see CLINICAL PHARMACOLOGY: Drug Interactions and DOSAGE AND ADMINISTRATION).

In a coronary angiographic study of rapidly infused intravenous eletriptan to concentrations exceeding those achieved with 80 mg oral eletriptan in the presence of potent CYP3A4 inhibitors, a small dose-related decrease in coronary artery diameter similar to that seen with a 6 mg subcutaneous dose of sumatriptan was observed.

Risk of Myocardial Ischemia and/or Infarction and Other Cardiac Events: Because of the potential of 5-HT$_1$ agonists to cause coronary vasospasm, eletriptan should not be given to patients with documented ischemic or vasospastic coronary artery disease (CAD) (see CONTRAINDICATIONS). It is strongly recommended that eletriptan not be given to patients in whom unrecognized CAD is predicted by the presence of risk factors (e.g., hypertension, hypercholesterolemia, smoker, obesity, diabetes, strong family history of CAD, female with surgical or physiological menopause, or male over 40 years of age) unless a cardiovascular evaluation provides satisfactory clinical evidence that the patient is reasonably free of coronary artery and ischemic myocardial disease or other significant underlying cardiovascular disease. The sensitivity of cardiac diagnostic procedures to detect cardiovascular disease or predisposition to coronary artery vasospasm is modest, at best. If, during the cardiovascular evaluation, the patient's medical history, electrocardiographic, or other investigations reveal findings indicative of, or consistent with coronary artery vasospasm or myocardial ischemia, eletriptan should not be administered (see CONTRAINDICATIONS).

For patients with risk factors predictive of CAD, who are determined to have a satisfactory cardiovascular evaluation, it is strongly recommended that administration of the first dose of eletriptan take place in the setting of a physician's office or similar medically staffed and equipped facility unless the patient has previously received eletriptan. Because cardiac ischemia can occur in the absence of clinical symptoms, consideration should be given to obtaining on the first occasion of use an electrocardiogram (ECG) during the interval immediately following administration of RELPAX Tablets, in these patients with risk factors.

It is recommended that patients who are intermittent long-term users of 5-HT$_1$ agonists including RELPAX Tablets, and who have or acquire risk factors predictive of CAD, as described above, undergo periodic cardiovascular evaluation as they continue to use RELPAX Tablets.

The systematic approach described above is intended to reduce the likelihood that patients with unrecognized cardiovascular disease will be inadvertently exposed to eletriptan.

Cardiac Events and Fatalities Associated With 5-HT$_1$ Agonists: Serious adverse cardiac events, including acute myocardial infarction, life-threatening disturbances of cardiac rhythm, and death have been reported within a few hours following the administration of other 5-HT$_1$ agonists. Considering the extent of use of 5-HT$_1$ agonists in patients with migraine, the incidence of these events is extremely low. Premarketing experience with eletriptan among the 7,143 unique individuals who received eletriptan during premarketing clinical trials: In a clinical pharmacology study, in subjects undergoing diagnostic coronary angiography, a subject with a history of angina, hypertension and hypercholesterolemia, receiving intravenous eletriptan (Cmax of 127 ng/mL equivalent to 60 mg oral eletriptan), reported chest tightness and experienced angiographically documented coronary vasospasm with no ECG changes of ischemia. There was also one report of atrial fibrillation in a patient with a past history of atrial fibrillation.

Postmarketing experience with eletriptan: There was one report of myocardial infarction and death in a patient with cardiovascular risk factors (hypertension, hyperlipidemia, strong family history of CAD) in association with inappropriate concomitant use of eletriptan and sumatriptan. The uncontrolled nature of postmarketing surveillance, however, makes it impossible to determine definitively if the case was actually caused by eletriptan or to reliably assess causation in individual cases.

Cerebrovascular Events and Fatalities Associated With 5-HT$_1$ Agonists: Cerebral hemorrhage, subarachnoid hemorrhage, stroke, and other cerebrovascular events have been reported in patients treated with 5-HT$_1$ agonists, and some have resulted in fatalities. In a number of cases, it appears possible that the cerebrovascular events were primary, the agonist having been administered in the incorrect belief that the symptoms experienced were a consequence of migraine, when they were not. It should be noted that patients with migraine may be at increased risk of certain cerebrovascular events (e.g., stroke, hemorrhage, and transient ischemic attack).

Other Vasospasm-Related Events: 5-HT$_1$ agonists may cause vasospastic reactions other than coronary artery vasospasm. Both peripheral vascular ischemia and colonic ischemia with abdominal pain and bloody diarrhea have been reported with 5-HT$_1$ agonists.

Increase in Blood Pressure: Significant elevation in blood pressure, including hypertensive crisis, has been reported on rare occasion in patients receiving 5-HT$_1$ agonists with and without a history of hypertension. In clinical pharmacology studies, oral eletriptan (at doses of 60 mg or more) was shown to cause small, transient dose-related increases in blood pressure, predominantly diastolic, consistent with its mechanism of action and with other 5-HT$_{1B/1D}$ agonists. The effect was more pronounced in renally impaired and elderly subjects. A single patient with hepatic cirrhosis received eletriptan 80 mg and experienced a blood pressure of 220/96 mm Hg five hours after dosing. The treatment related event persisted for seven hours.

Eletriptan is contraindicated in patients with uncontrolled hypertension (see CONTRAINDICATIONS).

An 18% increase in mean pulmonary artery pressure was seen following dosing with another 5-HT$_1$ agonist in a study evaluating subjects undergoing cardiac catheterization.

PRECAUTIONS

General: As with other 5-HT$_1$ agonists, sensations of tightness, pain, pressure and heaviness have been reported after treatment with eletriptan in the precordium, throat, and jaw. Events that are localized to the chest, throat, neck and jaw have not been associated with arrhythmias or ischemic ECG changes in clinical trials; in a clinical pharmacology study of subjects undergoing diagnostic coronary angiography, one subject with a history of angina, hypertension and hypercholesterolemia, receiving intravenous eletriptan, reported chest tightness and experienced angiographically documented coronary vasospasm with no ECG changes of ischemia. Because 5-HT$_1$ agonists may cause coronary artery vasospasm, patients who experience signs or symptoms suggestive of angina following dosing should be evaluated for the presence of CAD or a predisposition to Prinzmetal's variant angina before receiving additional doses of medication, and should be monitored electrocardiographically if dosing is resumed and similar symptoms recur. Similarly, patients who experience other symptoms or signs suggestive of decreased arterial flow, such as ischemic bowel syndrome or Raynaud's syndrome following the use of any 5-HT$_1$ agonist are candidates for further evaluation (see CONTRAINDICATIONS and WARNINGS).

Hepatically Impaired Patients: The effects of severe hepatic impairment on eletriptan metabolism was not evaluated. Subjects with mild or moderate hepatic impairment demonstrated an increase in both AUC (34%) and half-life. The C$_{max}$ was increased by 18%. Eletriptan should not be used in patients with severe hepatic impairment. No dose adjustment is necessary in mild to moderate impairment (see DOSAGE AND ADMINISTRATION).

Binding to Melanin-Containing Tissues: In rats treated with a single intravenous (3 mg/kg) dose of radiolabeled eletriptan, elimination of radioactivity from the retina was prolonged, suggesting that eletriptan and/or its metabolites may bind to the melanin of the eye. Because there could be accumulation in melanin-rich tissues over time, this raises the possibility that eletriptan could cause toxicity in these tissues after extended use. Although no systematic monitoring of ophthalmologic function was undertaken in clinical trials, and no specific recommendations for ophthalmologic monitoring are offered, prescribers should be aware of the possibility of long-term ophthalmologic effects.

Corneal Opacities: Transient corneal opacities were seen in dogs receiving oral eletriptan at 5 mg/kg and above. They were observed during the first week of treatment, but were not present thereafter despite continued treatment. Exposure at the no-effect dose level of 2.5 mg/kg was approximately equal to that achieved in humans at the maximum recommended daily dose.

Information for Patients: See PATIENT INFORMATION at the end of this labeling for the text of the separate leaflet provided for patients.

Laboratory Tests: No specific laboratory tests are recommended.

Drug Interactions:

Ergot-containing drugs: Ergot-containing drugs have been reported to cause prolonged vasospastic reactions. Because these effects may be additive, use of ergotamine-containing or ergot-type medications (like dihydroergotamine [DHE] or methysergide) and eletriptan within 24 hours of each other is not recommended (see CONTRAINDICATIONS).

CYP3A4 Inhibitors: Eletriptan is metabolized primarily by CYP3A4 (see WARNINGS regarding use with potent CYP3A4 inhibitors).

Monoamine Oxidase Inhibitors: Eletriptan is not a substrate for monoamine oxidase (MAO) enzymes, therefore there is no expectation of an interaction between eletriptan and MAO inhibitors.

Propranolol: The C$_{max}$ and AUC of eletriptan were increased by 10 and 33% respectively in the presence of propranolol. No interactive increases in blood pressure were observed. No dosage adjustment appears to be needed for patients taking propranolol (see CLINICAL PHARMACOLOGY).

Other 5-HT$_1$ agonists: Concomitant use of other 5-HT$_1$ agonists within 24 hours of RELPAX treatment is not recommended (see CONTRAINDICATIONS).

Drug/Laboratory Test Interactions: RELPAX Tablets are not known to interfere with commonly employed clinical laboratory tests.

Carcinogenesis: Lifetime carcinogenicity studies, 104 weeks in duration, were carried out in mice and rats by administering eletriptan in the diet. In rats, the incidence of testicular interstitial cell adenomas was increased at the high dose of 75 mg/kg/day. The estimated exposure (AUC) to parent drug at that dose was approximately 6 times that achieved in humans receiving the maximum recommended daily dose (MRDD) of 80 mg, and at the no-effect dose of 15 mg/kg/day it was approximately 2 times the human exposure at the MRDD. In mice, the incidence of hepatocellular adenomas was increased at the high dose of 400 mg/kg/day. The exposure to parent drug (AUC) at that dose was approximately 18 times that achieved in humans receiving the MRDD, and the AUC at the no-effect dose of 90 mg/kg/day was approximately 7 times the human exposure at the MRDD.

Mutagenesis: Eletriptan was not mutagenic in bacterial or mammalian cell assays *in vitro*, testing negative in the Ames reverse mutation test and the hypoxanthine-guanine phosphoribosyl transferase (HGPRT) mutation test in Chinese hamster ovary cells. It was not clastogenic in two *in vivo* mouse micronucleus assays. Results were equivocal in *in vitro* human lymphocyte clastogenicity tests, in which the incidence of polyploidy was increased in the absence of metabolic activation (-S9 conditions), but not in the presence of metabolic activation.

Impairment of Fertility: In a rat fertility and early embryonic development study, doses tested were 50, 100 and 200 mg/kg/day, resulting in systemic exposures to parent drug in rats, based on AUC, that were 4, 8 and 16 times MRDD, respectively, in males and 7, 14 and 28 times MRDD, respectively, in females. There was a prolongation of the estrous cycle at the 200 mg/kg/day dose due to an increase in duration of estrus, based on vaginal smears. There were also dose-related, statistically significant decreases in mean numbers of corpora lutea per dam at all 3 doses, resulting in decreases in mean numbers of implants and viable fetuses per dam. This suggests a partial inhibition of ovulation by eletriptan. There was no effect on fertility of males and no other effect on fertility of females.

Pregnancy: *Pregnancy Category C:* In reproductive toxicity studies in rats and rabbits, oral administration of eletriptan was associated with developmental toxicity (decreased fetal and pup weights and an increased incidence of fetal structural abnormalities). Effects on fetal and pup weights were observed at doses that were, on a mg/m^2 basis, 6 to 12 times greater than the clinical maximum recommended daily dose (MRDD) of 80 mg. The increase in structural alterations occurred in the rat and rabbit at doses that, on a mg/m^2 basis, were 12 times greater than (rat) and approximately equal to (rabbit) the MRDD.

When pregnant rats were administered eletriptan during the period of organogenesis at doses of 10, 30 or 100 mg/kg/day, fetal weights were decreased and the incidences of vertebral and sternebral variations were increased at 100 mg/kg/day (approximately 12 times the MRDD on a mg/m^2 basis). The 100 mg/kg dose was also maternally toxic, as evidenced by decreased maternal body weight gain during gestation. The no-effect dose for developmental toxicity in rats exposed during organogenesis was 30 mg/kg, which is approximately 4 times the MRDD on a mg/m^2 basis.

When doses of 5, 10 or 50 mg/kg/day were given to New Zealand White rabbits throughout organogenesis, fetal weights were decreased at 50 mg/kg, which is approximately 12 times the MRDD on a mg/m^2 basis. The incidences of fused sternebrae and vena cava deviations were increased in all treated groups. Maternal toxicity was not produced at any dose. A no-effect dose for developmental toxicity in rabbits exposed during organogenesis was not established, and the 5 mg/kg dose is approximately equal to the MRDD on a mg/m^2 basis.

There are no adequate and well-controlled studies in pregnant women; therefore, eletriptan should be used during pregnancy only if the potential benefit justifies the potential risk to the fetus.

Nursing Mothers: Eletriptan is excreted in human breast milk. In one study of 8 women given a single dose of 80 mg, the mean total amount of eletriptan in breast milk over 24 hours in this group was approximately 0.02% of the administered dose. The ratio of eletriptan mean concentration in breast milk to plasma was 1:4, but there was great variability. The resulting eletriptan concentration-time profile was similar to that seen in the plasma over 24 hours, with very low concentrations of drug (mean 1.7 ng/mL) still present in the milk 18-24 hours post dose. The N-desmethyl active metabolite was not measured in the breast milk. Caution should be exercised when RELPAX is administered to nursing women.

Pediatric Use: Safety and effectiveness of RELPAX Tablets in pediatric patients have not been established; therefore, RELPAX is not recommended for use in patients under 18 years of age.

The efficacy of RELPAX Tablets (40 mg) in patients 11-17 was not established in a randomized, placebo-controlled trial of 274 adolescent migraineurs (see CLINICAL STUDIES). Adverse events observed were similar in nature to those reported in clinical trials in adults. Postmarketing experience with other triptans includes a limited number of reports that describe pediatric patients who have experienced clinically serious adverse events that are similar in nature to those reported rarely in adults. Long-term safety of eletriptan was studied in 76 adolescent patients who received treatment for up to one year. A similar profile of adverse events to that of adults was observed. The long-term safety of eletriptan in pediatric patients has not been established.

Geriatric Use: Eletriptan has been given to only 50 patients over the age of 65. Blood pressure was increased to a greater extent in elderly subjects than in young subjects. The pharmacokinetic disposition of eletriptan in the elderly is similar to that seen in younger adults (see CLINICAL PHARMACOLOGY). In clinical trials, there were no apparent differences in efficacy or the incidence of adverse events between patients under 65 years of age and those 65 and above (n=50).

There is a statistically significantly increased half-life (from about 4.4 hours to 5.7 hours) between elderly (65 to 93 years of age) and younger adult subjects (18 to 45 years of age) (see CLINICAL PHARMACOLOGY).

Continued on next page

Relpax—Cont.

ADVERSE REACTIONS

Serious cardiac events, including some that have been fatal, have occurred following the use of 5-HT₁ agonists. These events are extremely rare and most have been reported in patients with risk factors predictive of CAD. Events reported have included coronary artery vasospasm, transient myocardial ischemia, myocardial infarction, ventricular tachycardia, and ventricular fibrillation (see CONTRAINDICATIONS, WARNINGS and PRECAUTIONS).

Incidence in Controlled Clinical Trials:
Among 4,597 patients who treated the first migraine headache with RELPAX in short-term placebo-controlled trials, the most common adverse events reported with treatment with RELPAX were asthenia, nausea, dizziness, and somnolence. These events appear to be dose related.

In long-term open-label studies where patients were allowed to treat multiple migraine attacks for up to 1 year, 128 (8.3%) out of 1,544 patients discontinued treatment due to adverse events.

Table 2 lists adverse events that occurred in the subset of 5,125 migraineurs who received eletriptan doses of 20 mg, 40 mg and 80 mg or placebo in worldwide placebo-controlled clinical trials. The events cited reflect experience gained under closely monitored conditions of clinical trials in a highly selected patient population. In actual clinical practice or in other clinical trials, those frequency estimates may not apply, as the conditions of use, reporting behavior, and the kinds of patients treated may differ.

Only adverse events that were more frequent in a RELPAX treatment group compared to the placebo group with an incidence greater than or equal to 2% are included in Table 2.

Table 2: Adverse Experience Incidence in Placebo-Controlled Migraine Clinical Trials: Events Reported by ≥ 2% Patients Treated with RELPAX and More Than Placebo

Adverse Event Type	Placebo (n=988)	RELPAX 20 mg (n=431)	RELPAX 40 mg (n=1774)	RELPAX 80 mg (n=1932)
ATYPICAL SENSATIONS				
Paresthesia	2%	3%	3%	4%
Flushing/feeling of warmth	2%	2%	2%	2%
PAIN AND PRESSURE SENSATIONS				
Chest – tightness/pain/pressure	1%	1%	2%	4%
Abdominal – pain/discomfort/stomach pain/cramps/pressure	1%	1%	2%	2%
DIGESTIVE				
Dry mouth	2%	2%	3%	4%
Dyspepsia	1%	1%	2%	2%
Dysphagia – throat tightness/difficulty swallowing	0.2%	1%	2%	2%
Nausea	5%	4%	5%	8%
NEUROLOGICAL				
Dizziness	3%	3%	6%	7%
Somnolence	4%	3%	6%	7%
Headache	3%	4%	3%	4%
OTHER				
Asthenia	3%	4%	5%	10%

RELPAX is generally well-tolerated. Across all doses, most adverse reactions were mild and transient. The frequency of adverse events in clinical trials did not increase when up to 2 doses of RELPAX were taken within 24 hours. The incidence of adverse events in controlled clinical trials was not affected by gender, age, or race of the patients. Adverse event frequencies were also unchanged by concomitant use of drugs commonly taken for migraine prophylaxis (e.g., SSRIs, beta blockers, calcium channel blockers, tricyclic antidepressants), estrogen replacement therapy and oral contraceptives.

Other Events Observed in Association With the Administration of RELPAX Tablets:
In the paragraphs that follow, the frequencies of less commonly reported adverse clinical events are presented. Because the reports include events observed in open studies, the role of RELPAX Tablets in their causation cannot be reliably determined. Furthermore, variability associated with adverse event reporting, the terminology used to describe adverse events, etc., limit the value of the quantitative frequency estimates provided. Event frequencies are calculated as the number of patients reporting an event divided by the total number of patients (N=4,719) exposed to RELPAX. All reported events are included except those already listed in Table 2, those too general to be informative, and those not reasonably associated with the use of the drug. Events are further classified within body system categories and enumerated in order of decreasing frequency using the following definitions: frequent adverse events are those occurring in at least 1/100 patients, infrequent adverse events are those occurring in 1/100 to 1/1000 patients and rare adverse events are those occurring in fewer than 1/1000 patients.

General: Frequent were back pain, chills and pain. Infrequent were face edema and malaise. Rare were abdomen enlarged, abscess, accidental injury, allergic reaction, fever, flu syndrome, halitosis, hernia, hypothermia, lab test abnormal, moniliasis, rheumatoid arthritis and shock.

Cardiovascular: Frequent was palpitation. Infrequent were hypertension, migraine, peripheral vascular disorder and tachycardia. Rare were angina pectoris, arrhythmia, atrial fibrillation, AV block, bradycardia, hypotension, syncope, thrombophlebitis, cerebrovascular disorder, vasospasm and ventricular arrhythmia.

Digestive: Infrequent were anorexia, constipation, diarrhea, eructation, esophagitis, flatulence, gastritis, gastrointestinal disorder, glossitis, increased salivation and liver function tests abnormal. Rare were gingivitis, hematemesis, increased appetite, rectal disorder, stomatitis, tongue disorder, tongue edema and tooth disorder.

Endocrine: Rare were goiter, thyroid adenoma and thyroiditis.

Hemic and Lymphatic: Rare were anemia, cyanosis, leukopenia, lymphadenopathy, monocytosis and purpura.

Metabolic: Infrequent were creatine phosphokinase increased, edema, peripheral edema and thirst. Rare were alkaline phosphatase increased, bilirubinemia, hyperglycemia, weight gain and weight loss.

Musculoskeletal: Infrequent were arthralgia, arthritis, arthrosis, bone pain, myalgia and myasthenia. Rare were bone neoplasm, joint disorder, myopathy and tenosynovitis.

Neurological: Frequent were hypertonia, hypesthesia and vertigo. Infrequent were abnormal dreams, agitation, anxiety, apathy, ataxia, confusion, depersonalization, depression, emotional lability, euphoria, hyperesthesia, hyperkinesia, incoordination, insomnia, nervousness, speech disorder, stupor, thinking abnormal and tremor. Rare were abnormal gait, amnesia, aphasia, catatonic reaction, dementia, diplopia, dystonia, hallucinations, hemiplegia, hyperalgesia, hypokinesia, hysteria, manic reaction, neuropathy, neurosis, oculogyric crisis, paralysis, psychotic depression, sleep disorder and twitching.

Respiratory: Frequent was pharyngitis. Infrequent were asthma, dyspnea, respiratory disorder, respiratory tract infection, rhinitis, voice alteration and yawn. Rare were bronchitis, choking sensation, cough increased, epistaxis, hiccup, hyperventilation, laryngitis, sinusitis and sputum increased.

Skin and Appendages: Frequent was sweating. Infrequent were pruritus, rash and skin disorder. Rare were alopecia, dry skin, eczema, exfoliative dermatitis, maculopapular rash, psoriasis, skin discoloration, skin hypertrophy and urticaria.

Special Senses: Infrequent was abnormal vision, conjunctivitis, ear pain, eye pain, lacrimation disorder, photophobia, taste perversion and tinnitus. Rare were abnormality of accommodation, dry eyes, ear disorder, eye hemorrhage, otitis media, parosmia and ptosis.

Urogenital: Infrequent were impotence, polyuria, urinary frequency and urinary tract disorder. Rare were breast pain, kidney pain, leukorrhea, menorrhagia, menstrual disorder and vaginitis.

DRUG ABUSE AND DEPENDENCE

Although the abuse potential of RELPAX has not been assessed, no abuse of, tolerance to, withdrawal from, or drug-seeking behavior was observed in patients who received RELPAX in clinical trials or their extensions. The 5-HT$_{1B/1D}$ agonists, as a class, have not been associated with drug abuse.

OVERDOSAGE

No significant overdoses in premarketing clinical trials have been reported. Volunteers (N=21) have received single doses of 120 mg without significant adverse effects. Daily doses of 160 mg were commonly employed in Phase III trials. Based on the pharmacology of the 5-HT$_{1B/1D}$ agonists, hypertension or other more serious cardiovascular symptoms could occur on overdose.

The elimination half-life of eletriptan is about 4 hours (see CLINICAL PHARMACOLOGY) and therefore monitoring of patients after overdose with eletriptan should continue for at least 20 hours, or longer should symptoms or signs persist.

There is no specific antidote to eletriptan. In cases of severe intoxication, intensive care procedures are recommended, including establishing and maintaining a patent airway, ensuring adequate oxygenation and ventilation, and monitoring and support of the cardiovascular system.

It is unknown what effect hemodialysis or peritoneal dialysis has on the serum concentration of eletriptan.

DOSAGE AND ADMINISTRATION

In controlled clinical trials, single doses of 20 mg and 40 mg were effective for the acute treatment of migraine in adults. A greater proportion of patients had a response following a 40 mg dose than following a 20 mg dose (see CLINICAL STUDIES). Individuals may vary in response to doses of RELPAX Tablets. The choice of dose should therefore be made on an individual basis. An 80 mg dose, although also effective, was associated with an increased incidence of adverse events. Therefore, the maximum recommended single dose is 40 mg.

If after the initial dose, headache improves but then returns, a repeat dose may be beneficial. If a second dose is required, it should be taken at least 2 hours after the initial dose. If the initial dose is ineffective, controlled clinical trials have not shown a benefit of a second dose to treat the same attack. The maximum daily dose should not exceed 80 mg.

The safety of treating an average of more than 3 headaches in a 30-day period has not been established.

CYP3A4 Inhibitors: Eletriptan is metabolized by the CYP3A4 enzyme. Eletriptan should not be used within at least 72 hours of treatment with the following potent CYP3A4 inhibitors: ketoconazole, itraconazole, nefazodone, troleandomycin, clarithromycin, ritonavir and nelfinavir. Eletriptan should not be used within 72 hours with drugs that have demonstrated potent CYP3A4 inhibition and have this potent effect described in the CONTRAINDICATIONS, WARNINGS or PRECAUTIONS sections of their labeling (see WARNINGS and CLINICAL PHARMACOLOGY: Drug Interactions).

Hepatic Impairment: The drug should not be given to patients with severe hepatic impairment since the effect of severe hepatic impairment on eletriptan metabolism was not evaluated. No dose adjustment is necessary in mild to moderate impairment (see CLINICAL PHARMACOLOGY, CONTRAINDICATIONS and PRECAUTIONS).

HOW SUPPLIED

RELPAX® Tablets of 20 mg and 40 mg eletriptan (base) as the hydrobromide. RELPAX Tablets are orange, round, convex shaped, film-coated tablets with appropriate debossing. 20 mg Tablets are identified with "REP20" on one side and "Pfizer" on the reverse. They are supplied in displays containing 2 folded blister cards with 6 tablets on each card (NDC 0049-2330-34).

40 mg Tablets are identified with "REP40" on one side and "Pfizer" on the reverse. They are supplied in displays containing 2 folded blister cards with 6 tablets on each card (NDC 0049-2340-34).

Store at 25°C (77°F); excursions permitted to 15-30°C (59-86°F) [see USP Controlled Room Temperature].

PATIENT SUMMARY OF INFORMATION

RELPAX®
(eletriptan hydrobromide)

Please read this information before you start taking RELPAX and each time you renew your prescription. Remember, this summary does not take the place of discussions with your doctor. You and your doctor should discuss RELPAX when you start taking your medication and at regular checkups.

What is RELPAX?
RELPAX is a prescription medicine used to treat migraine headaches in adults. RELPAX is not for other types of headaches.

What is a Migraine Headache?
Migraine is an intense, throbbing headache. You may have pain on one or both sides of your head. You may have nausea and vomiting, and be sensitive to light and noise. The pain and symptoms of a migraine headache can be worse than a common headache. Some women get migraines around the time of their menstrual period. Some people have visual symptoms before the headache, such as flashing lights or wavy lines, called an aura.

How Does RELPAX Work?
Treatment with RELPAX reduces swelling of blood vessels surrounding the brain. This swelling is associated with the headache pain of a migraine attack. RELPAX blocks the release of substances from nerve endings that cause more pain and other symptoms like nausea, and sensitivity to light and sound.
It is thought that these actions contribute to relief of your symptoms by RELPAX.

Who should not take RELPAX?
Do not take RELPAX if you:
- have uncontrolled high blood pressure.
- have heart disease or a history of heart disease.
- have hemiplegic or basilar migraine (if you are not sure about this, ask your doctor).
- have or had a stroke or problems with your blood circulation.
- have serious liver problems.
- have taken any of the following medicines in the last 24 hours: other "triptans" like almotriptan (Axert®), frovatriptan (Frova™), naratriptan (Amerge®), rizatriptan (Maxalt®), sumatriptan (Imitrex®), zolmitriptan (Zomig®); ergotamines like Bellegral-S®, Cafergot®, Ergoma®, Wigraine®; dihydroergotamine like D.H.E. 45® or Migranal®; or methysergide (Sansert®). These medicines have side effects similar to RELPAX.*
- have taken the following medicines within at least 72 hours: ketoconazole (Nizoral®), itraconazole (Sporonox®), nefazodone (Serzone®), troleandomycin (TAO®), clarithromycin (Biaxin®), ritonavir (Norvir®),

and nelfinavir (Viracept®). These medicines may cause an increase in the amount of RELPAX in the blood.*
- are allergic to RELPAX or any of its ingredients. The active ingredient is eletriptan. The inactive ingredients are listed at the end of this leaflet.

Tell your doctor about all the medicines you take or plan to take, including prescription and non-prescription medicines, supplements, and herbal remedies. Your doctor will decide if you can take RELPAX with your other medicines. Tell your doctor if you know that you have any of the following: risk factors for heart disease like high cholesterol, diabetes, smoking, obesity, menopause, or a family history of heart disease or stroke.

How should I take RELPAX?
RELPAX comes in 20 mg and 40 mg tablets. When you have a migraine headache, take your medicine as directed by your doctor.
- Take one RELPAX tablet as soon as you feel a migraine coming on.
- If your headache improves and then comes back after 2 hours, you can take a second tablet.
- If the first tablet did not help your headache at all, do not take a second tablet without talking with your doctor.
- Do not take more than two RELPAX tablets in any 24-hour period.

What are the possible side effects of RELPAX?
RELPAX is generally well tolerated. As with any medicine, people taking RELPAX may have side effects. The side effects are usually mild and do not last long.

The most common side effects of RELPAX are:
- dizziness
- nausea
- weakness
- tiredness
- pain or pressure sensation (e.g., in the chest or throat)

In very rare cases, patients taking triptans may experience serious side effects, including heart attacks. **Call your doctor right away** if you have:
- severe chest pains
- shortness of breath

This is not a complete list of side effects. Talk to your doctor if you develop any symptoms that concern you.

What to do in case of an overdose?
Call your doctor or poison control center or go to the ER.

General advice about RELPAX
Medicines are sometimes prescribed for conditions that are not mentioned in patient information leaflets. Do not use RELPAX for a condition for which it was not prescribed. Do not give RELPAX to other people, even if they have the same symptoms you have.

This leaflet summarizes the most important information about RELPAX. If you would like more information about RELPAX, talk with your doctor. You can ask your doctor or pharmacist for information on RELPAX that is written for health professionals. You can also call 1-866-4RELPAX (1-866-473-5729) or visit our web site at www.RELPAX.com.

What are the ingredients in RELPAX?
Active ingredient: eletriptan hydrobromide
Inactive ingredients: microcrystalline cellulose, lactose, croscarmellose sodium, magnesium stearate, titanium oxide, hydroxypropyl methylcellulose, triacetin, and FD&C Yellow No. 6 aluminum lake.

Store RELPAX Tablets at room temperature 15-30°C (59-86°F).

*The brands listed are the trademarks of their respective owners and are not trademarks of Pfizer Inc.

© 2002 PFIZER INC
℞ Only
Distributed by
Pfizer Roerig
Division of Pfizer Inc, NY, NY 10017
70-5586-00-0   Issued December 2002

To keep your **PDR** up to date throughout the year, note these revisions on the corresponding pages of the annual volume. Simply write **"See Supplement A"** next to the product heading.

Pharmacia & Upjohn
100 ROUTE 206 NORTH
PEAPACK, NEW JERSEY 07977

Direct Inquiries to:
1-888-768-5501

For Medical and Pharmaceutical Information, Including Emergencies, Contact:
800-323-4204 or www.MEDINFO@pharmacia.com

SOMAVERT® ℞
[sō'mă-v'-ərt]
pegvisomant for injection
℞ only

DESCRIPTION
SOMAVERT contains pegvisomant for injection, an analog of human growth hormone (GH) that has been structurally altered to act as a GH receptor antagonist.

Pegvisomant is a protein of recombinant DNA origin containing 191 amino acid residues to which several polyethylene glycol (PEG) polymers are covalently bound (predominantly 4 to 6 PEG/protein molecule). The molecular weight of the protein of pegvisomant is 21,998 Daltons. The molecular weight of the PEG portion of pegvisomant is approximately 5000 Daltons. The predominant molecular weights of pegvisomant are thus approximately 42,000, 47,000, and 52,000 Daltons. The schematic shows the amino acid sequence of the pegvisomant protein (PEG polymers are shown attached to the 5 most probable attachment sites). Pegvisomant is synthesized by a specific strain of *Escherichia coli* bacteria that has been genetically modified by the addition of a plasmid that carries a gene for GH receptor antagonist. Biological potency is determined using a cell proliferation bioassay.
[See figure below]

SOMAVERT is supplied as a sterile, white lyophilized powder intended for subcutaneous injection after reconstitution with 1 mL of Sterile Water for Injection, USP. SOMAVERT is available in single-dose sterile vials containing 10, 15, or 20 mg of pegvisomant protein (approximately 10, 15, and 20 U activity, respectively). Vials containing 10, 15, and 20 mg of pegvisomant protein correspond to approximately 21, 32, and 43 mg pegvisomant, respectively. Each vial also contains 1.36 mg of glycine, 36.0 mg of mannitol, 1.04 mg of sodium phosphate dibasic anhydrous, and 0.36 mg of sodium phosphate monobasic monohydrate.

SOMAVERT is supplied in packages that include a plastic vial containing diluent. Sterile Water for Injection, USP, is a sterile, nonpyrogenic preparation of water for injection that contains no bacteriostat, antimicrobial agent, or added buffer, and is supplied in single-dose containers to be used as a diluent.

CLINICAL PHARMACOLOGY
Mechanism of Action
Pegvisomant selectively binds to growth hormone (GH) receptors on cell surfaces, where it blocks the binding of endogenous GH, and thus interferes with GH signal transduction. Inhibition of GH action results in decreased serum concentrations of insulin-like growth factor-I (IGF-I), as well as other GH-responsive serum proteins, including IGF binding protein-3 (IGFBP-3), and the acid-labile subunit (ALS).

Pharmacokinetics
Absorption: Following subcutaneous administration, peak serum pegvisomant concentrations are not generally attained until 33 to 77 hours after administration. The mean extent of absorption of a 20-mg subcutaneous dose was 57%, relative to a 10-mg intravenous dose.

Distribution: The mean apparent volume of distribution of pegvisomant is 7 L (12% coefficient of variation), suggesting that pegvisomant does not distribute extensively into tissues. After a single subcutaneous administration, exposure (C_{max}, AUC) to pegvisomant increases disproportionately with increasing dose. Mean ± SEM serum pegvisomant concentrations after 12 weeks of therapy with daily doses of 10, 15, and 20 mg were 6600 ± 1330; 16,000 ± 2200; and 27,000 ± 3100 ng/mL, respectively.

Metabolism and Elimination: The pegvisomant molecule contains covalently bound polyethylene glycol polymers in order to reduce the clearance rate. Clearance of pegvisomant following multiple doses is lower than seen following a single dose. The mean total body systemic clearance of pegvisomant following multiple doses is estimated to range between 36 to 28 mL/h for subcutaneous doses ranging from 10 to 20 mg/day, respectively. Clearance of pegvisomant was found to increase with body weight. Pegvisomant is eliminated from serum with a mean half-life of approximately 6 days following either single or multiple doses. Less than 1% of administered drug is recovered in the urine over 96 hours. The elimination route of pegvisomant has not been studied in humans.

Drug-Drug Interactions
In clinical studies, patients on opioids often needed higher serum pegvisomant concentrations to achieve appropriate IGF-I suppression compared with patients not receiving opioids. The mechanism of this interaction is not known (see **PRECAUTIONS, Drug Interactions**).

Special Populations
Renal: No pharmacokinetic studies have been conducted in patients with renal insufficiency.
Hepatic: No pharmacokinetic studies have been conducted in patients with hepatic insufficiency.
Geriatric: No pharmacokinetic studies have been conducted in elderly subjects.
Pediatric: No pharmacokinetic studies have been conducted in pediatric subjects.
Gender: No gender effect on the pharmacokinetics of pegvisomant was found in a population pharmacokinetic analysis.
Race: The effect of race on the pharmacokinetics of pegvisomant has not been studied.

CLINICAL STUDIES
One hundred twelve patients with acromegaly previously treated with surgery, radiation therapy, and/or medical therapies participated in a 12-week, randomized, double-blind, multi-center study comparing placebo and SOMAVERT. Following withdrawal from previous medical therapy, the 80 patients randomized to treatment with SOMAVERT received a subcutaneous (SC) loading dose, followed by 10, 15, or 20 mg/day SC. The three groups that received SOMAVERT showed dose-dependent reductions in serum levels of IGF-I, free IGF-I, IGFBP-3, and ALS compared with placebo at all post-baseline visits (Figure 1 and Table 1).

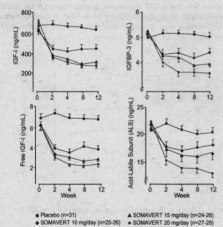

■ Placebo (n=31)   ▲ SOMAVERT 15 mg/day (n=24-26)
♦ SOMAVERT 10 mg/day (n=25-26)   ● SOMAVERT 20 mg/day (n=27-28)

Figure 1. Effects of SOMAVERT on Serum Markers (Mean ± Standard Error)

Continued on next page

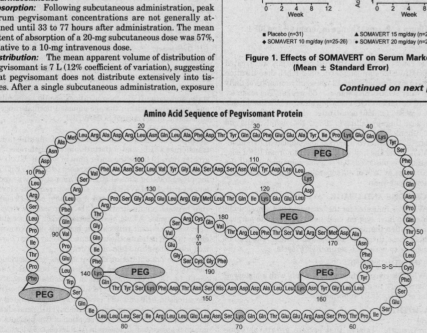

Amino Acid Sequence of Pegvisomant Protein

Stippled residues indicate PEG attachment sites (Phe_1, Lys_{38}, Lys_{41}, Lys_{70}, Lys_{115}, Lys_{120}, Lys_{140}, Lys_{145}, Lys_{158})

Somavert—Cont.

After 12 weeks of treatment, serum IGF-I levels were normalized in 10%, 39%, 75%, and 82% of subjects treated with placebo, 10, 15, or 20 mg/day of SOMAVERT, respectively (Figure 2).

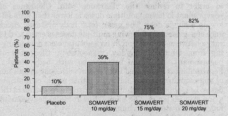

Figure 2. Percent of Patients Whose IGF-I Levels Normalized at Week 12

Table 2 shows the effect of treatment with SOMAVERT on ring size (standard jeweler's sizes converted to a numeric score ranging from 1 to 63), and on both the total and individual scores for signs and symptoms of acromegaly. Each individual score (for soft-tissue swelling, arthralgia, headache, perspiration and fatigue) was based on a nine-point ordinal rating scale (0 = absent and 8 = severe and incapacitating), and the total score was derived from the sum of the individual scores. Mean baseline scores were as follows: ring size = 47.1; total signs and symptoms = 15.2; soft tissue swelling = 2.5; arthralgia = 3.2; headache = 2.4; perspiration = 3.3; and fatigue = 3.7.
[See table 1 above]
[See table 2 above]
Ring size at week 12 was smaller (improved) in the groups treated with 15 or 20 mg of SOMAVERT, compared with placebo. The mean total score for signs and symptoms at week 12 was lower (improved) in each of the groups treated with SOMAVERT, compared with the group treated with placebo.

Serum growth hormone (GH) concentrations, as measured by research assays using antibodies that do not cross-react with pegvisomant (see **PRECAUTIONS, Drug/Laboratory Test Interactions**), rise within two weeks of beginning treatment with SOMAVERT. The largest GH response was seen in patients treated with doses of SOMAVERT greater than 20 mg/day. This effect is presumably the result of diminished inhibition of GH secretion as IGF-I levels fall. As shown in Figure 3, when patients with acromegaly were given a loading dose of SOMAVERT followed by a fixed daily dose, this rise in GH was inversely proportional to the fall in IGF-I and generally stabilized by week 2. Serum GH concentrations also remained stable in patients treated with SOMAVERT for up to 18 months.

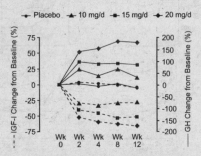

Figure 3. Percent Change in Serum GH and IGF-I Concentrations

Another cohort of 38 patients with acromegaly was treated with SOMAVERT in a long-term, open-label, dose-titration study and received at least 12 consecutive months of daily dosing with SOMAVERT (mean = 55 weeks). The mean (± standard deviation) IGF-I concentration at baseline in this cohort was 917 (± 356) ng/mL after withdrawal from previous medical therapy, falling to 268 (± 134) ng/mL at the end of treatment with SOMAVERT. Thirty-five of the 38 patients (92%) achieved a normal (age-adjusted) IGF-I concentration. After the first visit at which a normal IGF-I concentration was observed, IGF-I levels remained within the normal range at 92% of all subsequent visits over a mean duration of one year.

INDICATIONS AND USAGE
SOMAVERT is indicated for the treatment of acromegaly in patients who have had an inadequate response to surgery and/or radiation therapy and/or other medical therapies, or for whom these therapies are not appropriate. The goal of treatment is to normalize serum IGF-I levels.

CONTRAINDICATIONS
SOMAVERT is contraindicated in patients with a history of hypersensitivity to any of its components. The stopper on the vial of SOMAVERT contains latex.

PRECAUTIONS
General
Tumor Growth: Tumors that secrete growth hormone (GH) may expand and cause serious complications. Therefore, all patients with these tumors, including those who are receiving SOMAVERT, should be carefully monitored with periodic imaging scans of the sella turcica. During clinical studies of SOMAVERT, two patients manifested progressive tumor growth. Both patients had, at baseline, large globular tumors impinging on the optic chiasm, which had been relatively resistant to previous anti-acromegalic therapies. Overall, mean tumor size was unchanged during the course of treatment with SOMAVERT in the clinical studies.

Glucose Metabolism: GH opposes the effects of insulin on carbohydrate metabolism by decreasing insulin sensitivity; thus, glucose tolerance may increase in some patients treated with SOMAVERT. Although none of the acromegalic patients with diabetes mellitus who were treated with SOMAVERT during the clinical studies had clinically relevant hypoglycemia, these patients should be carefully monitored and doses of anti-diabetic drugs reduced as necessary.

GH Deficiency: A state of functional GH deficiency may result from administration of SOMAVERT, despite the presence of elevated serum GH levels. Therefore, during treatment with SOMAVERT, patients should be carefully observed for the clinical signs and symptoms of a GH-deficient state, and serum IGF-I concentrations should be monitored and maintained within the age-adjusted normal range (by adjustment of the dose of SOMAVERT).

Liver Tests (LTs)
Elevations of serum concentrations of alanine aminotransferase (ALT) and aspartate aminotransferase (AST) greater than 10 times the upper limit of normal (ULN) were reported in two patients (0.8%) exposed to SOMAVERT during pre-marketing clinical studies. One patient was rechallenged with SOMAVERT, and the recurrence of elevated transaminase levels suggested a probable causal relationship between administration of the drug and the elevation in liver enzymes. A liver biopsy performed on the second patient was consistent with chronic hepatitis of unknown etiology. In both patients, the transaminase elevations normalized after discontinuation of the drug.
During the pre-marketing clinical studies, the incidence of elevations in ALT greater than 3 times but less than or equal to 10 times the ULN in patients treated with SOMAVERT and placebo were 1.2% and 2.1%, respectively. Elevations in ALT and AST levels were not associated with increased levels of serum total bilirubin (TBIL) and alkaline phosphatase (ALP), with the exception of two patients with minimal associated increases in ALP levels (i.e., less than 3 times ULN). The transaminase elevations did not appear to be related to the dose of SOMAVERT administered, generally occurred within 4 to 12 weeks of initiation of therapy, and were not associated with any identifiable biochemical, phenotypic, or genetic predictors.
Baseline serum ALT, AST, TBIL, and ALP levels should be obtained prior to initiating therapy with SOMAVERT. Table 3 lists recommendations regarding initiation of treatment with SOMAVERT, based on the results of these liver tests (LTs).
If a patient develops LT elevations, or any other signs or symptoms of liver dysfunction while receiving SOMAVERT, the following patient management is recommended (Table 4).
[See table 3 above]
[See table 4 at top of next page]

Information for Patients
Patients and any other persons who may administer SOMAVERT should be carefully instructed by a health care professional on how to properly reconstitute and inject the product (see enclosed instructions).
Patients should be informed about the need for serial monitoring of LTs, and told to immediately discontinue therapy and contact their physician if they become jaundiced. In addition, patients should be made aware that serial IGF-I levels will need to be obtained to allow their physician to properly adjust the dose of SOMAVERT.

Laboratory Tests
Liver Tests: Recommendations for monitoring LTs are stated above (see **PRECAUTIONS, Liver Tests [LTs]**).
IGF-I Levels: Treatment with SOMAVERT should be evaluated by monitoring serum IGF-I concentrations four to six weeks after therapy is initiated or any dose adjustments are made and at least every six months after IGF-I levels have normalized. The goals of treatment should be to maintain a patient's serum IGF-I concentration within the age-adjusted normal range and to control the signs and symptoms of acromegaly.
GH Levels: Pegvisomant interferes with the measurement of serum GH concentrations by commercially available GH assays (see **Drug/Laboratory Test Interactions**). Furthermore, even when accurately determined, GH levels usually increase during therapy with SOMAVERT. Therefore, treatment with SOMAVERT should not be adjusted based on serum GH concentrations.

Drug Interactions
Acromegalic patients with diabetes mellitus being treated with insulin and/or oral hypoglycemic agents may require dose reductions of these therapeutic agents after the initiation of therapy with SOMAVERT.

Table 1. Mean Percent Change from Baseline in IGF-I at Week 12 for Intent-to-Treat Population

	SOMAVERT			Placebo n=31
	10 mg/day n=26	15 mg/day n=26	20 mg/day n=28	
Mean percent change from baseline in IGF-1 (SD)	-27 (28)	-48 (26)	-63 (21)	-4.0 (17)
SOMAVERT minus Placebo (95% CI for treatment difference)	-23* (-35, -11)	-44* (-56, -33)	-59** (-68, -49)	

* $P<0.01$

Table 2. Mean Change from Baseline (SD) at Week 12 for Ring Size and Signs and Symptoms of Acromegaly

	SOMAVERT			Placebo n=30
	10 mg/day n=26	15 mg/day n=25–25	20 mg/day n=26–27	
Ring size	-0.8 (1.6)	-1.9 (2.0)	-2.5 (3.3)	-0.1 (2.3)
Total score for signs and symptoms of acromegaly	-2.5 (4.3)	-4.4 (5.9)	-4.7 (4.7)	1.3 (6.0)
Soft-tissue swelling	-0.7 (1.6)	-1.2 (2.3)	-1.3 (1.3)	0.3 (2.3)
Arthralgia	-0.3 (1.8)	-0.5 (2.5)	-0.4 (2.1)	0.1 (1.8)
Headache	-0.4 (1.6)	-0.3 (1.4)	-0.3 (2.0)	0.1 (1.7)
Perspiration	-0.6 (1.6)	-1.1 (1.3)	-1.7 (1.6)	0.1 (1.7)
Fatigue	-0.5 (1.4)	-1.3 (1.7)	-1.0 (1.6)	0.7 (0.5)

Table 3. Initiation of Treatment with SOMAVERT Based on Results of Liver Tests

Baseline LT Levels	Recommendations
Normal	May treat with SOMAVERT. Monitor LTs at monthly intervals during the first 6 months of treatment, quarterly for the next 6 months, and then biannually for the next year.
Elevated, but less than or equal to 3 times ULN	May treat with SOMAVERT; however, monitor LTs monthly for at least one year after initiation of therapy and then biannually for the next year.
Greater than 3 times ULN	Do not treat with SOMAVERT until a comprehensive workup establishes the cause of the patient's liver dysfunction. Determine if the cholelithiasis or choledocholithiasis is present, particularly in patients with a history of prior therapy with somatostatin analogs. Based on the workup, consider initiation of therapy with SOMAVERT. If the decision is to treat, LTs and clinical symptoms should be monitored very closely.

In clinical studies, patients on opioids often needed higher serum pegvisomant concentrations to achieve appropriate IGF-I suppression compared with patients not receiving opioids. The mechanism of this interaction is not known.

Drug/Laboratory Test Interactions
Pegvisomant has significant structural similarity to GH, which causes it to cross-react in commercially available GH assays. Because serum concentrations of pegvisomant at therapeutically effective doses are generally 100 to 1000 times higher than endogenous serum GH levels seen in patients with acromegaly, commercially available GH assays will overestimate true GH levels. Treatment with SOMAVERT should therefore not be monitored or adjusted based on serum GH concentrations reported from these assays. Instead, monitoring and dose adjustments should only be based on serum IGF-I levels.

Carcinogenesis, Mutagenesis, Impairment of Fertility
Standard two-year rodent bioassays have not been performed with pegvisomant. Pegvisomant was not mutagenic in the Ames assay or clastogenic in the *in vitro* chromosomal aberration test in human lymphocytes. Pegvisomant was found to have no effect on fertility and reproductive performance of female rabbits at subcutaneous doses up to 10 mg/kg/day (10 times the maximum human therapeutic exposure based on body surface area, mg/m^2).

Pregnancy: Pregnancy Category B
Early embryonic development and teratology studies were conducted in pregnant rabbits with pegvisomant at subcutaneous doses of 1, 3, and 10 mg/kg/day. There was no evidence of teratogenic effects associated with pegvisomant treatment during organogenesis. At the 10-mg/kg/day dose (10 times the maximum human therapeutic dose based on body surface area), a reproducible, slight increase in postimplantation loss was observed in both studies. There are no adequate and well-controlled studies in pregnant women. Because animal reproduction studies are not always predictive of human responses, SOMAVERT should be used during pregnancy only if clearly needed.

Nursing Mothers
It is not known whether pegvisomant is excreted in human milk. Because many drugs are excreted in milk, caution should be exercised when SOMAVERT is administered to a nursing woman.

Pediatric Use
The safety and effectiveness of SOMAVERT in pediatric patients have not been established.

Geriatric Use
Clinical studies of SOMAVERT did not include sufficient numbers of subjects aged 65 and over to determine whether they respond differently from younger subjects. In general, dose selection for an elderly patient should be cautious, usually starting at the low end of the dosing range, reflecting the greater frequency of decreased hepatic, renal, or cardiac function, and of concomitant disease or other drug therapy.

ADVERSE REACTIONS
Laboratory Changes
Elevations of serum concentrations of ALT and AST greater than ten times the ULN were reported in two subjects (0.8%) exposed to SOMAVERT in pre-approval clinical studies (see **PRECAUTIONS, Liver Tests [LTs]**).

General
Nine acromegalic patients (9.6%) withdrew from pre-marketing clinical studies because of adverse events, including two patients with marked transaminase elevations (see **PRECAUTIONS, Liver Tests [LTs]**), one patient with lipohypertrophy at the injection sites, and one patient with substantial weight gain. The majority of reported adverse events were of mild to moderate intensity and limited duration. Most adverse events did not appear to be dose dependent. Table 5 shows the incidence of treatment-emergent adverse events that were reported in at least two patients treated with SOMAVERT and at frequencies greater than placebo during the 12-week, placebo-controlled study.
[See table 5 above]

Immunogenicity
In pre-marketing clinical studies, approximately 17% of the patients developed low titer, non-neutralizing anti-GH antibodies. Although the presence of these antibodies did not appear to impact the efficacy of SOMAVERT, the long-term clinical significance of these antibodies is not known. No assay for anti-pegvisomant antibodies is commercially available for patients receiving SOMAVERT.

OVERDOSAGE
In one reported incident of acute overdose with SOMAVERT during pre-marketing clinical studies, a patient self-administered 80 mg/day for seven days. The patient experienced a slight increase in fatigue, had no other complaints, and demonstrated no significant clinical laboratory abnormalities.
In cases of overdose, administration of SOMAVERT should be discontinued and not resumed until IGF-I levels return to within or above the normal range.

DRUG ABUSE AND DEPENDENCE
Available data do not demonstrate drug-abuse potential or psychological dependence with SOMAVERT. Radiolabeled pegvisomant does not cross the blood-brain barrier in rats.

DOSAGE AND ADMINISTRATION
A loading dose of 40 mg of SOMAVERT should be administered subcutaneously under physician supervision. The patient should then be instructed to begin daily subcutaneous injections of 10 mg of SOMAVERT. Serum IGF-I concentrations should be measured every four to six weeks, at which time the dosage of SOMAVERT should be adjusted in 5-mg increments if IGF-I levels are still elevated (or 5-mg decrements if IGF-I levels have decreased below the normal range). While the goals of therapy are to achieve (and then maintain) serum IGF-I concentrations within the age-adjusted normal range and to alleviate the signs and symptoms of acromegaly, titration of dosing should be based on IGF-I levels. It is unknown whether patients who remain symptomatic while achieving normalized IGF-I levels would benefit from increased dosing with SOMAVERT.
The maximum daily maintenance dose should not exceed 30 mg.
SOMAVERT is supplied as a lyophilized powder. Each vial of SOMAVERT should be reconstituted with 1 mL of the diluent provided in the package (Sterile Water for Injection, USP). Instructions regarding reconstitution and administration are included in the package of SOMAVERT and should be closely followed. To prepare the solution, withdraw 1 mL of Sterile Water for Injection, USP and inject it into the vial of SOMAVERT, aiming the stream of liquid against the glass wall. Hold the vial between the palms of both hands and gently roll it to dissolve the powder. **DO NOT SHAKE THE VIAL**, as this may cause denaturation of pegvisomant. Discard the diluent vial containing the remaining water for injection. After reconstitution, each vial of SOMAVERT contains 10, 15, or 20 mg of pegvisomant protein in one mL of solution. Parenteral drug products should be inspected visually for particulate matter and discoloration prior to administration. The solution should be clear after reconstitution. If the solution is cloudy, do not inject it. Only one dose should be administered from each vial. SOMAVERT should be administered within six hours after reconstitution.

HOW SUPPLIED
SOMAVERT is available in single-dose, sterile glass vials in the following strengths:
10 mg (as protein) vial   NDC 0009-5176-01
15 mg (as protein) vial   NDC 0009-5178-01
20 mg (as protein) vial   NDC 0009-5180-01
Each package of SOMAVERT also includes a single-dose LifeShield® plastic fliptop vial containing 10 mL of Sterile Water for Injection, USP.
The stopper on the vial of SOMAVERT contains latex.
Storage
Prior to reconstitution, SOMAVERT should be stored in a refrigerator at 2 to 8°C (36 to 46°F). Protect from freezing. After reconstitution, SOMAVERT should be administered within six hours. Only one dose should be administered from each vial.
Manufactured for:
Pharmacia & Upjohn Company
A subsidiary of Pharmacia Corporation
Kalamazoo, MI 49001, USA

Continued on next page

Table 4. Continuation of Treatment with SOMAVERT Based on Results of Liver Tests

LT Levels and Clinical Signs/Symptoms	Recommendations
Greater than or equal to 3 but less than 5 times ULN (without signs/symptoms of hepatitis or other liver injury, or increase in serum TBIL)	May continue therapy with SOMAVERT. However, monitor LTs weekly to determine if further increases occur (see below). In addition, perform a comprehensive hepatic workup to discern if an alternative cause of liver dysfunction is present.
At least 5 times ULN, or transaminase elevations at least 3 times ULN associated with any increase in serum TBIL (with or without signs/symptoms of hepatitis or other livery injury)	Discontinue SOMAVERT immediately. Perform a comprehensive hepatic workup, including serial LTs, to determine if and when serum levels return to normal. If LTs normalize (regardless of whether an alternative cause of the liver dysfunction is discovered), consider cautious reinitiation of therapy with SOMAVERT, with frequent LT monitoring.
Signs or symptoms suggestive of hepatitis or other liver injury (e.g., jaundice, bilirubinuria, fatigue, nausea, vomiting, right upper quadrant pain, ascites, unexplained edema, easy bruisability)	Immediately perform a comprehensive hepatic workup. If liver injury is confirmed, the drug should be discontinued.

Table 5. Number of Patients (%) with Acromegaly Reporting Adverse Events in a 12-week Placebo-controlled Study with SOMAVERT*

Event	SOMAVERT			Placebo n=32
	10 mg/day n=26	15 mg/day n=26	20 mg/day n=28	
Body as a whole				
Infection†	6 (23%)	0	0	2 (6%)
Pain	2 (8%)	1 (4%)	4 (14%)	2 (6%)
Injection site reaction	2 (8%)	1 (4%)	3 (11%)	0
Accidental injury	2 (8%)	1 (4%)	0	1 (3%)
Back pain	2 (8%)	0	1 (4%)	1 (3%)
Flu syndrome	1 (4%)	3 (12%)	2 (7%)	0
Chest pain	1 (4%)	2 (8%)	0	0
Digestive				
Abnormal liver function tests	3 (12%)	1 (4%)	1 (4%)	1 (3%)
Diarrhea	1 (4%)	0	4 (14%)	1 (3%)
Nausea	0	2 (8%)	4 (14%)	1 (3%)
Nervous				
Dizziness	2 (8%)	1 (4%)	1 (4%)	2 (6%)
Paresthesia	0	0	2 (7%)	2 (6%)
Metabolic and nutritional disorders				
Peripheral edema	2 (8%)	0	1 (4%)	0
Cardiovascular				
Hypertension	0	2 (8%)	0	0
Respiratory				
Sinusitis	2 (8%)	0	1 (4%)	1 (3%)

* Table includes only those events that were reported in at least 2 patients and at a higher incidence in patients treated with SOMAVERT than in patients treated with placebo.
† The 6 events coded as "infection" in the group treated with SOMAVERT 10 mg were reported as cold symptoms (3), upper respiratory infection (1), blister (1), and ear infection (1). The 2 events in the placebo group were reported as cold symptoms (1) and chest infection (1).

Somavert—Cont.

by:
Abbott Laboratories
North Chicago, IL 60064, USA
US Patent No. 5,849,535
March 2003
818 727 000
692842

XANAX XR® ℂⅣ ℞

[ză-nĕks]

alprazolam extended-release tablets

DESCRIPTION

XANAX XR Tablets contain alprazolam which is a triazolo analog of the 1,4 benzodiazepine class of central nervous system-active compounds.

The chemical name of alprazolam is 8-chloro-1-methyl-6-phenyl-4*H*-*s*-triazolo [4,3-α] [1,4] benzodiazepine. The molecular formula is $C_{17}H_{13}ClN_4$ which corresponds to a molecular weight of 308.76.

The structural formula is represented to the right:

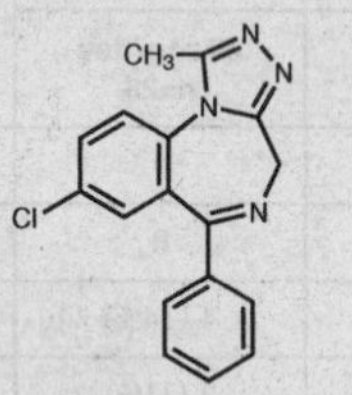

Alprazolam is a white crystalline powder, which is soluble in methanol or ethanol but which has no appreciable solubility in water at physiological pH.

Each XANAX XR extended-release tablet, for oral administration, contains 0.5 mg, 1 mg, 2 mg, or 3 mg of alprazolam. The inactive ingredients are lactose, magnesium stearate, colloidal silicon dioxide, and hypromellose. In addition, the 1 mg and 3 mg tablets contain D & C yellow No. 10 and the 2 mg and 3 mg tablets contain FD&C blue No. 2.

CLINICAL PHARMACOLOGY

Pharmacodynamics

CNS agents of the 1,4 benzodiazepine class presumably exert their effects by binding at stereospecific receptors at several sites within the central nervous system. Their exact mechanism of action is unknown. Clinically, all benzodiazepines cause a dose-related central nervous system depressant activity varying from mild impairment of task performance to hypnosis.

Pharmacokinetics

Absorption

Following oral administration of XANAX (immediate-release) Tablets, alprazolam is readily absorbed. Peak concentrations in the plasma occur in one to two hours following administration. Plasma levels are proportional to the dose given; over the dose range of 0.5 to 3.0 mg, peak levels of 8.0 to 37 ng/mL were observed. Using a specific assay methodology, the mean plasma elimination half-life of alprazolam has been found to be about 11.2 hours (range: 6.3–26.9 hours) in healthy adults.

The mean absolute bioavailability of alprazolam from XANAX XR Tablets is approximately 90%, and the relative bioavailability compared to XANAX Tablets is 100%. The bioavailability and pharmacokinetics of alprazolam following administration of XANAX XR Tablets are similar to that for XANAX Tablets, with the exception of a slower rate of absorption. The slower absorption rate results in a relatively constant concentration that is maintained between 5 and 11 hours after the dosing. The pharmacokinetics of alprazolam and two of its major active metabolites (4-hydroxyalprazolam and α-hydroxyalprazolam) are linear, and concentrations are proportional up to the recommended maximum daily dose of 10 mg given once daily. Multiple dose studies indicate that the metabolism and elimination of alprazolam are similar for the immediate-release and the extended-release products.

Food has a significant influence on the bioavailability of XANAX XR Tablets. A high-fat meal given up to 2 hours before dosing with XANAX XR Tablets increased the mean C_{max} by about 25%. The effect of this meal on T_{max} depended on the timing of the meal, with a reduction in T_{max} by about 1/3 for subjects eating immediately before dosing and an increase in T_{max} by about 1/3 for subjects eating 1 hour or more after dosing. The extent of exposure (AUC) and elimination half-life ($t_{1/2}$) were not affected by eating.

There were significant differences in absorption rate for the XANAX XR Tablet, depending on the time of day administered, with the C_{max} increased by 30% and the T_{max} decreased by an hour following dosing at night, compared to morning dosing.

Distribution

The apparent volume of distribution of alprazolam is similar for XANAX XR and XANAX Tablets. In vitro, alprazolam is bound (80%) to human serum protein. Serum albumin accounts for the majority of the binding.

Metabolism

Alprazolam is extensively metabolized in humans, primarily by cytochrome P450 3A4 (CYP3A4), to two major metabolites in the plasma: 4-hydroxyalprazolam and α-hydroxyalprazolam. A benzophenone derived from alprazolam is also found in humans.Their half-lives appear to be similar to that of alprazolam. The pharmacokinetic parameters at steady-state for the two hydroxylated metabolites of alprazolam (4-hydroxyalprazolam and α-hydroxy-alprazolam) were similar for XANAX and XANAX XR Tablets, indicating that the metabolism of alprazolam is not affected by absorption rate. The plasma concentrations of 4-hydroxyalprazolam and α-hydroxyalprazolam relative to unchanged alprazolam concentration after both XANAX XR and XANAX Tablets were always less than 10% and 4%, respectively. The reported relative potencies in benzodiazepine receptor binding experiments and in animal models of induced seizure inhibition are 0.20 and 0.66, respectively, for 4-hydroxyalprazolam and α-hydroxyalprazolam. Such low concentrations and the lesser potencies of 4-hydroxyalprazolam and α-hydroxyalprazolam suggest that they are unlikely to contribute much to the pharmacological effects of alprazolam. The benzophenone metabolite is essentially inactive.

Elimination

Alprazolam and its metabolites are excreted primarily in the urine. The mean plasma elimination half-life of alprazolam following administration of XANAX XR Tablet ranges from 10.7–15.8 hours in healthy adults.

Special Populations

While pharmacokinetic studies have not been performed in special populations with XANAX XR Tablets, the factors (such as age, gender, hepatic or renal impairment) that would affect the pharmacokinetics of alprazolam after the administration of XANAX Tablets would not be expected to be different with the administration of XANAX XR Tablets. Changes in the absorption, distribution, metabolism, and excretion of benzodiazepines have been reported in a variety of disease states including alcoholism, impaired hepatic function, and impaired renal function. Changes have also been demonstrated in geriatric patients. A mean half-life of alprazolam of 16.3 hours has been observed in healthy elderly subjects (range: 9.0–26.9 hours, n=16) compared to 11.0 hours (range: 6.3–15.8 hours, n=16) in healthy adult subjects. In patients with alcoholic liver disease the half-life of alprazolam ranged between 5.8 and 65.3 hours (mean: 19.7 hours, n=17) as compared to between 6.3 and 26.9 hours (mean=11.4 hours, n=17) in healthy subjects. In an obese group of subjects the half-life of alprazolam ranged between 9.9 and 40.4 hours (mean=21.8 hours, n=12) as compared to between 6.3 and 15.8 hours (mean=10.6 hours, n=12) in healthy subjects.

Because of its similarity to other benzodiazepines, it is assumed that alprazolam undergoes transplacental passage and that it is excreted in human milk.

Race—Maximal concentrations and half-life of alprazolam are approximately 15% and 25% higher in Asians compared to Caucasians.

Pediatrics—The pharmacokinetics of alprazolam after administration of the XANAX XR Tablet in pediatric patients have not been studied.

Gender—Gender has no effect on the pharmacokinetics of alprazolam.

Cigarette Smoking—Alprazolam concentrations may be reduced by up to 50% in smokers compared to non-smokers.

Drug-Drug Interactions

Alprazolam is primarily eliminated by metabolism via cytochrome P450 3A (CYP3A). Most of the interactions that have been documented with alprazolam are with drugs that inhibit or induce CYP3A4.

Compounds that are potent inhibitors of CYP3A would be expected to increase plasma alprazolam concentrations. Drug products that have been studied in vivo, along with their effect on increasing alprazolam AUC, are as follows: ketoconazole, 3.98 fold; itraconazole, 2.70 fold; nefazodone, 1.98 fold; fluvoxamine, 1.96 fold; and erythromycin, 1.61 fold (see CONTRAINDICATIONS, WARNINGS, and PRECAUTIONS–Drug Interactions).

CYP3A inducers would be expected to decrease alprazolam concentrations and this has been observed in vivo. The oral clearance of alprazolam (given in a 0.8 mg single dose) was increased from 0.90±0.21 mL/min/kg to 2.13±0.54 mL/min/kg and the elimination $t_{1/2}$ was shortened (from 17.1±4.9 to 7.7±1.7 h) following administration of 300 mg/day carbamazepine for 10 days (see PRECAUTIONS–Drug Interactions). However, the carbamazepine dose used in this study was fairly low compared to the recommended doses (1000–1200 mg/day); the effect at usual carbamazepine doses is unknown.

The ability of alprazolam to induce or inhibit human hepatic enzyme systems has not been determined. However, this is not a property of benzodiazepines in general. Further, alprazolam did not affect the prothrombin or plasma warfarin levels in male volunteers administered sodium warfarin orally.

CLINICAL EFFICACY TRIALS

The efficacy of XANAX XR Tablets in the treatment of panic disorder was established in two 6-week, placebo-controlled studies of XANAX XR in patients with panic disorder.

In two 6-week, flexible-dose, placebo-controlled studies in patients meeting DSM-III criteria for panic disorder, patients were treated with XANAX XR in a dose range of 1 to 10 mg/day, on a once-a-day basis. The effectiveness of XANAX XR was assessed on the basis of changes in various measures of panic attack frequency, on various measures of the Clinical Global Impression, and on the Overall Phobia Scale. In all, there were seven primary efficacy measures in these studies, and XANAX XR was superior to placebo on all seven outcomes in both studies. The mean dose of XANAX XR at the last treatment visit was 4.2 mg/day in the first study and 4.6 mg/day in the second.

In addition, there were two 8-week, fixed-dose, placebo-controlled studies of XANAX XR in patients with panic disorder, involving fixed XANAX XR doses of 4 and 6 mg/day, on a once-a-day basis, that did not show a benefit for either dose of XANAX XR.

The longer-term efficacy of XANAX XR in panic disorder has not been systematically evaluated.

Analyses of the relationship between treatment outcome and gender did not suggest any differential responsiveness on the basis of gender.

INDICATIONS AND USAGE

XANAX XR Tablets are indicated for the treatment of panic disorder, with or without agoraphobia.

This claim is supported on the basis of two positive studies with XANAX XR conducted in patients whose diagnoses corresponded closely to the DSM-III-R/IV criteria for panic disorder (see CLINICAL STUDIES).

Panic disorder (DSM-IV) is characterized by recurrent unexpected panic attacks, ie, a discrete period of intense fear or discomfort in which four (or more) of the following symptoms develop abruptly and reach a peak within 10 minutes: (1) palpitations, pounding heart, or accelerated heart rate; (2) sweating; (3) trembling or shaking; (4) sensations of shortness of breath or smothering; (5) feeling of choking; (6) chest pain or discomfort; (7) nausea or abdominal distress; (8) feeling dizzy, unsteady, lightheaded, or faint; (9) derealization (feelings of unreality) or depersonalization (being detached from oneself); (10) fear of losing control; (11) fear of dying; (12) paresthesias (numbness or tingling sensations); (13) chills or hot flushes.

The longer-term efficacy of XANAX XR has not been systematically evaluated. Thus, the physician who elects to use this drug for periods longer than 8 weeks should periodically reassess the usefulness of the drug for the individual patient.

CONTRAINDICATIONS

XANAX XR Tablets are contraindicated in patients with known sensitivity to this drug or other benzodiazepines. XANAX XR may be used in patients with open angle glaucoma who are receiving appropriate therapy, but is contraindicated in patients with acute narrow angle glaucoma.

XANAX XR is contraindicated with ketoconazole and itraconazole, since these medications significantly impair the oxidative metabolism mediated by cytochrome P450 3A (CYP3A) (see CLINICAL PHARMACOLOGY, WARNINGS and PRECAUTIONS–Drug Interactions).

WARNINGS

Dependence and Withdrawal Reactions, Including Seizures

Certain adverse clinical events, some life-threatening, are a direct consequence of physical dependence to alprazolam. These include a spectrum of withdrawal symptoms; the most important is seizure (see DRUG ABUSE AND DEPENDENCE). Even after relatively short-term use at doses of ≤4 mg/day, there is some risk of dependence. Spontaneous reporting system data suggest that the risk of dependence and its severity appear to be greater in patients treated with doses greater than 4 mg/day and for long periods (more than 12 weeks). However, in a controlled postmarketing discontinuation study of panic disorder patients who received XANAX Tablets, the duration of treatment (3 months compared to 6 months) had no effect on the ability of patients to taper to zero dose. In contrast, patients treated with doses of XANAX Tablets greater than 4 mg/day had more difficulty tapering to zero dose than those treated with less than 4 mg/day.

Relapse or return of illness was defined as a return of symptoms characteristic of panic disorder (primarily panic attacks) to levels approximately equal to those seen at baseline before active treatment was initiated. Rebound refers to a return of symptoms of panic disorder to a level substantially greater in frequency, or more severe in intensity than seen at baseline. Withdrawal symptoms were identified as those which were generally not characteristic of panic disorder and which occurred for the first time more frequently during discontinuation than at baseline.

The rate of relapse, rebound, and withdrawal in patients with panic disorder who received XANAX XR Tablets has not been systematically studied. Experience in randomized placebo-controlled discontinuation studies of patients with panic disorder who received XANAX Tablets showed a high rate of rebound and withdrawal symptoms compared to placebo treated patients.

In a controlled clinical trial in which 63 patients were randomized to XANAX Tablets and where withdrawal symptoms were specifically sought, the following were identified as symptoms of withdrawal: heightened sensory perception, impaired concentration, dysosmia, clouded sensorium, paresthesias, muscle cramps, muscle twitch, diarrhea, blurred vision, appetite decrease, and weight loss. Other symptoms, such as anxiety and insomnia, were frequently seen during discontinuation, but it could not be determined if they were due to return of illness, rebound, or withdrawal.

In two controlled trials of 6 to 8 weeks duration where the ability of patients to discontinue medication was measured, 71%–93% of patients treated with XANAX Tablets tapered completely off therapy compared to 89%–96% of placebo treated patients. In a controlled postmarketing discontinuation study of panic disorder patients treated with XANAX

Tablets, the duration of treatment (3 months compared to 6 months) had no effect on the ability of patients to taper to zero dose.

Seizures were reported for three patients in panic disorder clinical trials with XANAX XR. In two cases, the patients had completed 6 weeks of treatment with XANAX XR 6 mg/day before experiencing a single seizure. In one case, the patient abruptly discontinued XANAX XR, and in both cases, alcohol intake was implicated. The third case involved multiple seizures after the patient completed treatment with XANAX XR 4 mg/day and missed taking the medication on the first day of taper. All three patients recovered without sequelae.

Seizures have also been observed in association with dose reduction or discontinuation of XANAX Tablets, the immediate release form of alprazolam. Seizures attributable to XANAX were seen after drug discontinuance or dose reduction in 8 of 1980 patients with panic disorder or in patients participating in clinical trials where doses of XANAX greater than 4 mg/day for over 3 months were permitted. Five of these cases clearly occurred during abrupt dose reduction, or discontinuation from daily doses of 2 to 10 mg. Three cases occurred in situations where there was not a clear relationship to abrupt dose reduction or discontinuation. In one instance, seizure occurred after discontinuation from a single dose of 1 mg after tapering at a rate of 1 mg every three days from 6 mg daily. In two other instances, the relationship to taper is indeterminate; in both of these cases the patients had been receiving doses of 3 mg daily prior to seizure. The duration of use in the above 8 cases ranged from 4 to 22 weeks. There have been occasional voluntary reports of patients developing seizures while apparently tapering gradually from XANAX. The risk of seizure seems to be greatest 24–72 hours after discontinuation (see DOSAGE AND ADMINISTRATION for recommended tapering and discontinuation schedule).

Status Epilepticus
The medical event voluntary reporting system shows that withdrawal seizures have been reported in association with the discontinuation of XANAX Tablets. In most cases, only a single seizure was reported; however, multiple seizures and status epilepticus were reported as well.

Interdose Symptoms
Early morning anxiety and emergence of anxiety symptoms between doses of XANAX Tablets have been reported in patients with panic disorder taking prescribed maintenance doses. These symptoms may reflect the development of tolerance or a time interval between doses which is longer than the duration of clinical action of the administered dose. In either case, it is presumed that the prescribed dose is not sufficient to maintain plasma levels above those needed to prevent relapse, rebound, or withdrawal symptoms over the entire course of the interdosing interval.

Risk of Dose Reduction
Withdrawal reactions may occur when dosage reduction occurs for any reason. This includes purposeful tapering, but also inadvertent reduction of dose (eg, the patient forgets, the patient is admitted to a hospital). Therefore, the dosage of XANAX XR should be reduced or discontinued gradually (see DOSAGE AND ADMINISTRATION).

CNS Depression and Impaired Performance
Because of its CNS depressant effects, patients receiving XANAX XR should be cautioned against engaging in hazardous occupations or activities requiring complete mental alertness such as operating machinery or driving a motor vehicle. For the same reason, patients should be cautioned about the simultaneous ingestion of alcohol and other CNS depressant drugs during treatment with XANAX XR.

Risk of Fetal Harm
Benzodiazepines can potentially cause fetal harm when administered to pregnant women. If alprazolam is used during pregnancy, or if the patient becomes pregnant while taking this drug, the patient should be apprised of the potential hazard to the fetus. Because of experience with other members of the benzodiazepine class, alprazolam is assumed to be capable of causing an increased risk of congenital abnormalities when administered to a pregnant woman during the first trimester. Because use of these drugs is rarely a matter of urgency, their use during the first trimester should almost always be avoided. The possibility that a woman of childbearing potential may be pregnant at the time of institution of therapy should be considered. Patients should be advised that if they become pregnant during therapy or intend to become pregnant they should communicate with their physicians about the desirability of discontinuing the drug.

Alprazolam Interaction With Drugs That Inhibit Metabolism Via Cytochrome P450 3A
The initial step in alprazolam metabolism is hydroxylation catalyzed by cytochrome P450 3A (CYP3A). Drugs that inhibit this metabolic pathway may have a profound effect on the clearance of alprazolam. Consequently, alprazolam should be avoided in patients receiving very potent inhibitors of CYP3A. With drugs inhibiting CYP3A to a lesser but still significant degree, alprazolam should be used only with caution and consideration of appropriate dosage reduction. For some drugs, an interaction with alprazolam has been quantified with clinical data; for other drugs, interactions are predicted from in vitro data and/or experience with similar drugs in the same pharmacologic class.

The following are examples of drugs known to inhibit the metabolism of alprazolam and/or related benzodiazepines, presumably through inhibition of CYP3A.

Potent CYP3A Inhibitors
Azole antifungal agents—Ketoconazole and itraconazole are potent CYP3A inhibitors and have been shown in vivo to increase plasma alprazolam concentrations 3.98 fold and 2.70 fold, respectively. The coadministration of alprazolam with these agents is not recommended. Other azole-type antifungal agents should also be considered potent CYP3A inhibitors and the coadministration of alprazolam with them is not recommended (see CONTRAINDICATIONS).

Drugs demonstrated to be CYP3A inhibitors on the basis of clinical studies involving alprazolam (caution and consideration of appropriate alprazolam dose reduction are recommended during coadministration with the following drugs)

Nefazodone—Coadministration of nefazodone increased alprazolam concentration two-fold.

Fluvoxamine—Coadministration of fluvoxamine approximately doubled the maximum plasma concentration of alprazolam, decreased clearance by 49%, increased half-life by 71%, and decreased measured psychomotor performance.

Cimetidine—Coadministration of cimetidine increased the maximum plasma concentration of alprazolam by 86%, decreased clearance by 42%, and increased half-life by 16%.

Other Drugs Possibly Affecting Alprazolam Metabolism
Other drugs possibly affecting alprazolam metabolism by inhibition of CYP3A are discussed in the PRECAUTIONS section (see PRECAUTIONS–Drug Interactions).

PRECAUTIONS
General
Suicide
As with other psychotropic medications, the usual precautions with respect to administration of the drug and size of the prescription are indicated for severely depressed patients or those in whom there is reason to expect concealed suicidal ideation or plans. Panic disorder has been associated with primary and secondary major depressive disorders and increased reports of suicide among untreated patients.

Mania
Episodes of hypomania and mania have been reported in association with the use of XANAX Tablets in patients with depression.

Uricosuric Effect
Alprazolam has a weak uricosuric effect. Although other medications with weak uricosuric effect have been reported to cause acute renal failure, there have been no reported instances of acute renal failure attributable to therapy with alprazolam.

Use in Patients with Concomitant Illness
It is recommended that the dosage be limited to the smallest effective dose to preclude the development of ataxia or oversedation which may be a particular problem in elderly or debilitated patients (see DOSAGE AND ADMINISTRATION). The usual precautions in treating patients with impaired renal, hepatic, or pulmonary function should be observed. There have been rare reports of death in patients with severe pulmonary disease shortly after the initiation of treatment with XANAX Tablets. A decreased systemic alprazolam elimination rate (eg, increased plasma half-life) has been observed in both alcoholic liver disease patients and obese patients receiving XANAX Tablets (see CLINICAL PHARMACOLOGY).

Information for Patients
To assure safe and effective use of XANAX XR, the physician should provide the patient with the following guidance.
1. Inform your physician about any alcohol consumption and medicine you are taking now, including medication you may buy without a prescription. Alcohol should generally not be used during treatment with benzodiazepines.
2. Not recommended for use in pregnancy. Therefore, inform your physician if you are pregnant, if you are planning to have a child, or if you become pregnant while you are taking this medication.
3. Inform your physician if you are nursing.
4. Until you experience how this medication affects you, do not drive a car or operate potentially dangerous machinery, etc.
5. Do not increase the dose even if you think the medication "does not work anymore" without consulting your physician. Benzodiazepines, even when used as recommended, may produce emotional and/or physical dependence.
6. Do not stop taking this medication abruptly or decrease the dose without consulting your physician, since withdrawal symptoms can occur.
7. Some patients may find it very difficult to discontinue treatment with XANAX XR due to severe emotional and physical dependence. Discontinuation symptoms, including possible seizures, may occur following discontinuation from any dose, but the risk may be increased with extended use at doses greater than 4 mg/day, especially if discontinuation is too abrupt. It is important that you seek advice from your physician to discontinue treatment in a careful and safe manner. Proper discontinuation will help to decrease the possibility of withdrawal reactions that can range from mild reactions to severe reactions such as seizure.

Laboratory Tests
Laboratory tests are not ordinarily required in otherwise healthy patients. However, when treatment is protracted, periodic blood counts, urinalysis, and blood chemistry analyses are advisable in keeping with good medical practice.

Drug Interactions
Use with Other CNS Depressants
If XANAX XR Tablets are to be combined with other psychotropic agents or anticonvulsant drugs, careful consideration should be given to the pharmacology of the agents to be employed, particularly with compounds which might potentiate the action of benzodiazepines. The benzodiazepines, including alprazolam, produce additive CNS depressant effects when coadministered with other psychotropic medications, anticonvulsants, antihistaminics, ethanol and other drugs which themselves produce CNS depression.

Use with Imipramine and Desipramine
The steady state plasma concentrations of imipramine and desipramine have been reported to be increased an average of 31% and 20%, respectively, by the concomitant administration of XANAX Tablets in doses up to 4 mg/day. The clinical significance of these changes is unknown.

Drugs that inhibit alprazolam metabolism via cytochrome P450 3A
The initial step in alprazolam metabolism is hydroxylation catalyzed by cytochrome P450 3A (CYP3A). Drugs which inhibit this metabolic pathway may have a profound effect on the clearance of alprazolam (see CONTRAINDICATIONS and WARNINGS for additional drugs of this type).

Drugs demonstrated to be CYP3A inhibitors of possible clinical significance on the basis of clinical studies involving alprazolam (caution is recommended during coadministration with alprazolam)

Fluoxetine—Coadministration of fluoxetine with alprazolam increased the maximum plasma concentration of alprazolam by 46%, decreased clearance by 21%, increased half-life by 17%, and decreased measured psychomotor performance.

Propoxyphene—Coadministration of propoxyphene decreased the maximum plasma concentration of alprazolam by 6%, decreased clearance by 38%, and increased half-life by 58%.

Oral Contraceptives—Coadministration of oral contraceptives increased the maximum plasma concentration of alprazolam by 18%, decreased clearance by 22%, and increased half-life by 29%.

Drugs and other substances demonstrated to be CYP3A inhibitors on the basis of clinical studies involving benzodiazepines metabolized similarly to alprazolam or on the basis of in vitro studies with alprazolam or other benzodiazepines (caution is recommended during coadministration with alprazolam)

Available data from clinical studies of benzodiazepines other than alprazolam suggest a possible drug interaction with alprazolam for the following: diltiazem, isoniazid, macrolide antibiotics such as erythromycin and clarithromycin, and grapefruit juice. Data from in vitro studies of alprazolam suggest a possible drug interaction with alprazolam for the following: sertraline and paroxetine. Data from in vitro studies of benzodiazepines other than alprazolam suggest a possible drug interaction for the following: ergotamine, cyclosporine, amiodarone, nicardipine, and nifedipine. Caution is recommended during the coadministration of any of these with alprazolam (see WARNINGS).

Drugs demonstrated to be inducers of CYP3A
Carbamazepine can increase alprazolam metabolism and therefore can decrease plasma levels of alprazolam.

Drug/Laboratory Test Interactions
Although interactions between benzodiazepines and commonly employed clinical laboratory tests have occasionally been reported, there is no consistent pattern for a specific drug or specific test.

Carcinogenesis, Mutagenesis, Impairment of Fertility
No evidence of carcinogenic potential was observed during 2-year bioassay studies of alprazolam in rats at doses up to 30 mg/kg/day (150 times the maximum recommended daily human dose of 10 mg/day) and in mice at doses up to 10 mg/kg/day (50 times the maximum recommended daily human dose).

Alprazolam was not mutagenic in the rat micronucleus test at doses up to 100 mg/kg, which is 500 times the maximum recommended daily human dose of 10 mg/day. Alprazolam also was not mutagenic in vitro in the DNA Damage/Alkaline Elution Assay or the Ames Assay.

Alprazolam produced no impairment of fertility in rats at doses up to 5 mg/kg/day, which is 25 times the maximum recommended daily human dose of 10 mg/day.

Pregnancy
Teratogenic Effects: Pregnancy Category D: (see WARNINGS section).

Nonteratogenic Effects: It should be considered that the child born of a mother who is receiving benzodiazepines may be at some risk for withdrawal symptoms from the drug during the postnatal period. Also, neonatal flaccidity and respiratory problems have been reported in children born of mothers who have been receiving benzodiazepines.

Labor and Delivery
Alprazolam has no established use in labor or delivery.

Nursing Mothers
Benzodiazepines are known to be excreted in human milk. It should be assumed that alprazolam is as well. Chronic

Continued on next page

Xanax XR—Cont.

administration of diazepam to nursing mothers has been reported to cause their infants to become lethargic and to lose weight. As a general rule, nursing should not be undertaken by mothers who must use alprazolam.

Pediatric Use
Safety and effectiveness of alprazolam in individuals below 18 years of age have not been established.

Geriatric Use
The elderly may be more sensitive to the effects of benzodiazepines. They exhibit higher plasma alprazolam concentrations due to reduced clearance of the drug as compared with a younger population receiving the same doses. The smallest effective dose of alprazolam should be used in the elderly to preclude the development of ataxia and oversedation (see CLINICAL PHARMACOLOGY and DOSAGE AND ADMINISTRATION).

ADVERSE REACTIONS

The information included in the subsection on Adverse Events Observed in Short-Term, Placebo-Controlled Trials with XANAX XR Tablets is based on pooled data of five 6- and 8-week placebo-controlled clinical studies in panic disorder.

Adverse event reports were elicited either by general inquiry or by checklist, and were recorded by clinical investigators using terminology of their own choosing. The stated frequencies of adverse events represent the proportion of individuals who experienced, at least once, a treatment-emergent adverse event of the type listed. An event was considered treatment emergent if it occurred for the first time or worsened during therapy following baseline evaluation. In the tables and tabulations that follow, standard MedDRA terminology (version 4.0) was used to classify reported adverse events.

Adverse Events Observed in Short-Term, Placebo-Controlled Trials of XANAX XR

Adverse Events Reported as Reasons for Discontinuation of Treatment in Placebo-Controlled Trials

Approximately 17% of the 531 patients who received XANAX XR in placebo-controlled clinical trials for panic disorder had at least one adverse event that led to discontinuation compared to 8% of 349 placebo-treated patients. The most common events leading to discontinuation and considered to be drug-related (ie, leading to discontinuation in at least 1% of the patients treated with XANAX XR at a rate at least twice that of placebo) are shown in the following table.

Common Adverse Events Leading to Discontinuation of Treatment in Placebo-Controlled Trials

System Organ Class/Adverse Event	Percentage of Patients Discontinuing Due to Adverse Events	
	XANAX XR (n=531)	Placebo (n=349)
Nervous system disorders		
Sedation	7.5	0.6
Somnolence	3.2	0.3
Dysarthria	2.1	0
Coordination abnormal	1.9	0.3
Memory impairment	1.7	0.3
General disorders/ administration site conditions		
Fatigue	1.7	0.6
Psychiatric disorders		
Depression	2.5	1.2

Adverse Events Occurring at an Incidence of 1% or More Among Patients Treated with XANAX XR

The prescriber should be aware that adverse event incidence cannot be used to predict the incidence of adverse events in the course of usual medical practice where patient characteristics and other factors differ from those which prevailed in the clinical trials. Similarly, the cited frequencies cannot be compared with event incidence obtained from other clinical investigations involving different treatments, uses, and investigators. The cited values, however, do provide the prescribing physician with some basis for estimating the relative contribution of drug and non-drug factors to the adverse event incidence rate in the population studied. The following table shows the incidence of treatment-emergent adverse events that occurred during 6- to 8-week placebo-controlled trials in 1% or more of patients treated with XANAX XR where the incidence in patients treated with XANAX XR was greater than the incidence in placebo-treated patients. The most commonly observed adverse events in panic disorder patients treated with XANAX XR (incidence of 5% or greater and at least twice the incidence in placebo patients) were: sedation, somnolence, memory impairment, dysarthria, coordination abnormal, ataxia, libido decreased (see table).

Treatment-Emergent Adverse Events: Incidence in Short-Term, Placebo-Controlled Clinical Trials with XANAX XR

System Organ Class/Adverse Event	Percentage of Patients Reporting Adverse Event	
	XANAX XR (n=531)	Placebo (n=349)
Nervous system disorders		
Sedation	45.2	22.6
Somnolence	23.0	6.0
Memory impairment	15.4	6.9
Dysarthria	10.9	2.6
Coordination abnormal	9.4	0.9
Mental impairment	7.2	5.7
Ataxia	7.2	3.2
Disturbance in attention	3.2	0.6
Balance impaired	3.2	0.6
Paresthesia	2.4	1.7
Dyskinesia	1.7	1.4
Hypoesthesia	1.3	0.3
Hypersomnia	1.3	0
General disorders/ administration site conditions		
Fatigue	13.9	9.2
Lethargy	1.7	0.6
Infections and infestations		
Influenza	2.4	2.3
Upper respiratory tract infections	1.9	1.7
Psychiatric disorders		
Depression	12.1	9.2
Libido decreased	6.0	2.3
Disorientation	1.5	0
Confusion	1.5	0.9
Depressed mood	1.3	0.3
Anxiety	1.1	0.6
Metabolism and nutrition disorders		
Appetite decreased	7.3	7.2
Appetite increased	7.0	6.0
Anorexia	1.5	0
Gastrointestinal disorders		
Dry mouth	10.2	9.7
Constipation	8.1	4.3
Nausea	6.0	3.2
Pharyngolaryngeal pain	3.2	2.6
Investigations		
Weight increased	5.1	4.3
Weight decreased	4.3	3.7
Injury, poisoning, and procedural complications		
Road traffic accident	1.5	0
Reproductive system and breast disorders		
Dysmenorrhea	3.6	2.9
Sexual dysfunction	2.4	1.1
Premenstrual syndrome	1.7	0.6
Musculoskeletal and connective tissue disorders		
Arthralgia	2.4	0.6
Myalgia	1.5	1.1
Pain in limb	1.1	0.3
Vascular disorders		
Hot flushes	1.5	1.4
Respiratory, thoracic, and mediastinal disorders		
Dyspnea	1.5	0.3
Rhinitis allergic	1.1	0.6
Skin and subcutaneous tissue disorders		
Pruritis	1.1	0.9

Other Adverse Events Observed During the Premarketing Evaluation of XANAX XR Tablets

Following is a list of MedDRA terms that reflect treatment-emergent adverse events reported by 531 patients with panic disorder treated with XANAX XR. All potentially important reported events are included except those already listed in the above table or elsewhere in labeling, those events for which a drug cause was remote, those event terms that were so general as to be uninformative, and those events that occurred at rates similar to background rates in the general population. It is important to emphasize that, although the events reported occurred during treatment with XANAX XR, they were not necessarily caused by the drug. Events are further categorized by body system and listed in order of decreasing frequency according to the following definitions: frequent adverse events are those occurring on 1 or more occasions in at least 1/100 patients; infrequent adverse events are those occurring in less than 1/100 patients but at least 1/1000 patients; rare events are those occurring in fewer than 1/1000 patients.

Cardiac disorders: Frequent: palpitation; *Infrequent:* sinus tachycardia
Ear and Labyrinth disorders: Frequent: Vertigo; *Infrequent:* tinnitus, ear pain
Eye disorders: Frequent: blurred vision; *Infrequent:* mydriasis, photophobia
Gastrointestinal disorders: Frequent: diarrhea, vomiting, dyspepsia, abdominal pain; *Infrequent:* dysphagia, salivary hypersecretion
General disorders and administration site conditions: Frequent: malaise, weakness, chest pains; *Infrequent:* fall, pyrexia, thirst, feeling hot and cold, edema, feeling jittery, sluggishness, asthenia, feeling drunk, chest tightness, increased energy, feeling of relaxation, hangover, loss of control of legs, rigors
Musculoskeletal and connective tissue disorders: Frequent: back pain, muscle cramps, muscle twitching
Nervous system disorders: Frequent: headache, dizziness, tremor; *Infrequent:* amnesia, clumsiness, syncope, hypotonia, seizures, depressed level of consciousness, sleep apnea syndrome, sleep talking, stupor
Psychiatric system disorders: Frequent: irritability, insomnia, nervousness, derealization, libido increased, restlessness, agitation, depersonalization, nightmare; *Infrequent:* abnormal dreams, apathy, aggression, anger, bradyphrenia, euphoric mood, logorrhea, mood swings, dysphonia, hallucination, homicidal ideation, mania, hypomania, impulse control, psychomotor retardation, suicidal ideation
Renal and urinary disorders: Frequent: difficulty in micturition; *Infrequent:* urinary frequency, urinary incontinence
Respiratory, thoracic, and mediastinal disorders: Frequent: nasal congestion, hyperventilation; *Infrequent:* choking sensation, epistaxis, rhinorrhea
Skin and subcutaneous tissue disorders: Frequent: sweating increased; *Infrequent:* clamminess, rash, urticaria
Vascular disorders: Infrequent: hypotension

The categories of adverse events reported in the clinical development program for XANAX Tablets in the treatment of panic disorder differ somewhat from those reported for XANAX XR Tablets because the clinical trials with XANAX Tablets and XANAX XR Tablets used different standard medical nomenclature for reporting the adverse events. Nevertheless, the types of adverse events reported in the clinical trials with XANAX Tablets were generally the same as those reported in the clinical trials with XANAX XR Tablets.

Discontinuation-Emergent Adverse Events Occurring at an Incidence of 5% or More Among Patients Treated with XANAX XR

The following table shows the incidence of discontinuation-emergent adverse events that occurred during short-term, placebo-controlled trials in 5% or more of patients treated with XANAX XR where the incidence in patients treated with XANAX XR was two times greater than the incidence in placebo-treated patients.

Discontinuation-Emergent Symptoms: Incidence in Short-Term, Placebo-Controlled Trials with XANAX XR

System Organ Class/Adverse Event	Percentage of Patients Reporting Adverse Event	
	XANAX XR (n=422)	Placebo (n=261)
Nervous system disorders		
Tremor	28.2	10.7
Headache	26.5	12.6
Hypoesthesia	7.8	2.3
Paresthesia	7.1	2.7
Psychiatric disorders		
Insomnia	24.2	9.6
Nervousness	21.8	8.8
Depression	10.9	5.0
Derealization	8.0	3.8
Anxiety	7.8	2.7
Depersonalization	5.7	1.9
Gastrointestinal disorders		
Diarrhea	12.1	3.1
Respiratory, thoracic and mediastinal disorders		
Hyperventilation	8.5	2.7
Metabolism and nutrition disorders		
Appetite decreased	9.5	3.8
Musculoskeletal and connective tissue disorders		
Muscle twitching	7.4	2.7
Vascular disorders		
Hot flushes	5.9	2.7

There have also been reports of withdrawal seizures upon rapid decrease or abrupt discontinuation of alprazolam (see WARNINGS).

To discontinue treatment in patients taking XANAX XR Tablets, the dosage should be reduced slowly in keeping with good medical practice. It is suggested that the daily dosage of XANAX XR Tablets be decreased by no more than 0.5 mg every three days (see DOSAGE AND ADMINISTRATION). Some patients may benefit from an even slower dosage reduction. In a controlled postmarketing discontinuation study of panic disorder patients which compared this recommended taper schedule with a slower taper schedule, no difference was observed between the groups in the proportion of patients who tapered to zero dose; however, the slower schedule was associated with a reduction in symptoms associated with a withdrawal syndrome.

As with all benzodiazepines, paradoxical reactions such as stimulation, increased muscle spasticity, sleep disturbances, hallucinations, and other adverse behavioral effects such as agitation, rage, irritability, and aggressive or hostile behavior have been reported rarely. In many of the spontaneous case reports of adverse behavioral effects, patients were receiving other CNS drugs concomitantly and/or were described as having underlying psychiatric conditions. Should any of the above events occur, alprazolam should be discontinued. Isolated published reports involving small numbers of patients have suggested that patients who have borderline personality disorder, a prior history of violent or aggressive behavior, or alcohol or substance abuse may be at risk for such events. Instances of irritability, hostility, and intrusive thoughts have been reported during discontinuation of alprazolam in patients with posttraumatic stress disorder.

Post Introduction Reports
Various adverse drug reactions have been reported in association with the use of XANAX Tablets since market introduction. The majority of these reactions were reported through the medical event voluntary reporting system. Because of the spontaneous nature of the reporting of medical events and the lack of controls, a causal relationship to the use of XANAX Tablets cannot be readily determined. Reported events include: liver enzyme elevations, hepatitis, hepatic failure, Stevens-Johnson syndrome, hyperprolactinemia, gynecomastia, and galactorrhea.

DRUG ABUSE AND DEPENDENCE
Physical and Psychological Dependence
Withdrawal symptoms similar in character to those noted with sedative/hypnotics and alcohol have occurred following discontinuance of benzodiazepines, including alprazolam. The symptoms can range from mild dysphoria and insomnia to a major syndrome that may include abdominal and muscle cramps, vomiting, sweating, tremors, and convulsions. Distinguishing between withdrawal emergent signs and symptoms and the recurrence of illness is often difficult in patients undergoing dose reduction. The long-term strategy for treatment of these phenomena will vary with their cause and the therapeutic goal. When necessary, immediate management of withdrawal symptoms requires re-institution of treatment at doses of alprazolam sufficient to suppress symptoms. There have been reports of failure of other benzodiazepines to fully suppress these withdrawal symptoms. These failures have been attributed to incomplete cross-tolerance but may also reflect the use of an inadequate dosing regimen of the substituted benzodiazepine or the effects of concomitant medications.

While it is difficult to distinguish withdrawal and recurrence for certain patients, the time course and the nature of the symptoms may be helpful. A withdrawal syndrome typically includes the occurrence of new symptoms, tends to appear toward the end of taper or shortly after discontinuation, and will decrease with time. In recurring panic disorder, symptoms similar to those observed before treatment may recur either early or late, and they will persist.

While the severity and incidence of withdrawal phenomena appear to be related to dose and duration of treatment, withdrawal symptoms, including seizures, have been reported after only brief therapy with alprazolam at doses within the recommended range for the treatment of anxiety (eg, 0.75 to 4 mg/day). Signs and symptoms of withdrawal are often more prominent after rapid decrease of dosage or abrupt discontinuance.The risk of withdrawal seizures may be increased at doses above 4 mg/day (see WARNINGS).

Patients, especially individuals with a history of seizures or epilepsy, should not be abruptly discontinued from any CNS depressant agent, including alprazolam. It is recommended that all patients on alprazolam who require a dosage reduction be gradually tapered under close supervision (see WARNINGS and DOSAGE AND ADMINISTRATION).

Psychological dependence is a risk with all benzodiazepines, including alprazolam. The risk of psychological dependence may also be increased at doses greater than 4 mg/day and with longer term use, and this risk is further increased in patients with a history of alcohol or drug abuse. Some patients have experienced considerable difficulty in tapering and discontinuing from alprazolam, especially those receiving higher doses for extended periods. Addiction-prone individuals should be under careful surveillance when receiving alprazolam. As with all anxiolytics, repeat prescriptions should be limited to those who are under medical supervision.

Controlled Substance Class
Alprazolam is a controlled substance under the Controlled Substance Act by the Drug Enforcement Administration and XANAX XR Tablets have been assigned to Schedule IV.

OVERDOSAGE
Clinical Experience
Overdosage reports with XANAX Tablets are limited. Manifestations of alprazolam overdosage include somnolence, confusion, impaired coordination, diminished reflexes, and coma. Death has been reported in association with overdoses of alprazolam by itself, as it has with other benzodiazepines. In addition, fatalities have been reported in patients who have overdosed with a combination of a single benzodiazepine, including alprazolam, and alcohol; alcohol levels seen in some of these patients have been lower than those usually associated with alcohol-induced fatality.

Animal experiments have suggested that forced diuresis or hemodialysis are probably of little value in treating overdosage.

General Treatment of Overdose
As in all cases of drug overdosage, respiration, pulse rate, and blood pressure should be monitored. General supportive measures should be employed, along with immediate gastric lavage. Intravenous fluids should be administered and an adequate airway maintained. If hypotension occurs, it may be combated by the use of vasopressors. Dialysis is of limited value. As with the management of intentional overdosing with any drug, it should be borne in mind that multiple agents may have been ingested.

Flumazenil, a specific benzodiazepine receptor antagonist, is indicated for the complete or partial reversal of the sedative effects of benzodiazepines and may be used in situations when an overdose with a benzodiazepine is known or suspected. Prior to the administration of flumazenil, necessary measures should be instituted to secure airway, ventilation, and intravenous access. Flumazenil is intended as an adjunct to, not as a substitute for, proper management of benzodiazepine overdose. Patients treated with flumazenil should be monitored for re-sedation, respiratory depression, and other residual benzodiazepine effects for an appropriate period after treatment. **The prescriber should be aware of a risk of seizure in association with flumazenil treatment, particularly in long-term benzodiazepine users and in cyclic antidepressant overdose.** The complete flumazenil package insert including CONTRAINDICATIONS, WARNINGS, and PRECAUTIONS should be consulted prior to use.

DOSAGE AND ADMINISTRATION
XANAX XR Tablets may be administered once daily, preferably in the morning. The tablets should be taken intact; they should not be chewed, crushed, or broken.

The suggested total daily dose ranges between 3 to 6 mg/day. Dosage should be individualized for maximum beneficial effect. While the suggested total daily dosages given will meet the needs of most patients, there will be some patients who require doses greater than 6 mg/day. In such cases, dosage should be increased cautiously to avoid adverse effects.

Dosing in Special Populations
In elderly patients, in patients with advanced liver disease, or in patients with debilitating disease, the usual starting dose of XANAX XR is 0.5 mg once daily. This may be gradually increased if needed and tolerated (see Dose Titration). The elderly may be especially sensitive to the effects of benzodiazepines.

Dose Titration
Treatment with XANAX XR may be initiated with a dose of 0.5 mg to 1 mg once daily. Depending on the response, the dose may be increased at intervals of 3 to 4 days in increments of no more than 1 mg/day. Slower titration to the dose levels may be advisable to allow full expression of the pharmacodynamic effect of XANAX XR.

Generally, therapy should be initiated at a low dose to minimize the risk of adverse responses in patients especially sensitive to the drug. Dose should be advanced until an acceptable therapeutic response (ie, a substantial reduction in or total elimination of panic attacks) is achieved, intolerance occurs, or the maximum recommended dose is attained.

Dose Maintenance
In controlled trials conducted to establish the efficacy of XANAX XR Tablets in panic disorder, doses in the range of 1 to 10 mg/day were used. Most patients showed efficacy in the dose range of 3 to 6 mg/day. Occasional patients required as much as 10 mg/day to achieve a successful response.

The necessary duration of treatment for panic disorder patients responding to XANAX XR is unknown. However, periodic reassessment is advised. After a period of extended freedom from attacks, a carefully supervised tapered discontinuation may be attempted, but there is evidence that this may often be difficult to accomplish without recurrence of symptoms and/or the manifestation of withdrawal phenomena.

Dose Reduction
Because of the danger of withdrawal, abrupt discontinuation of treatment should be avoided (see WARNINGS, PRECAUTIONS, DRUG ABUSE AND DEPENDENCE).

In all patients, dosage should be reduced gradually when discontinuing therapy or when decreasing the daily dosage. Although there are no systematically collected data to support a specific discontinuation schedule, it is suggested that the daily dosage be decreased by no more than 0.5 mg every three days. Some patients may require an even slower dosage reduction.

In any case, reduction of dose must be undertaken under close supervision and must be gradual. If significant withdrawal symptoms develop, the previous dosing schedule should be reinstituted and, only after stabilization, should a less rapid schedule of discontinuation be attempted. In a controlled postmarketing discontinuation study of panic disorder patients which compared this recommended taper schedule with a slower taper schedule, no difference was observed between the groups in the proportion of patients who tapered to zero dose; however, the slower schedule was associated with a reduction in symptoms associated with a withdrawal syndrome. It is suggested that the dose be reduced by no more than 0.5 mg every three days, with the understanding that some patients may benefit from an even more gradual discontinuation. Some patients may prove resistant to all discontinuation regimens.

Switch from XANAX (immediate-release) Tablets to XANAX XR (extended-release) Tablets
Patients who are currently being treated with divided doses of XANAX (immediate-release) Tablets, for example 3 to 4 times a day, may be switched to XANAX XR Tablets at the same total daily dose taken once daily. If the therapeutic response after switching is inadequate, the dosage may be titrated as outlined above.

HOW SUPPLIED
XANAX XR (extended-release) Tablets are available as follows:

0.5 mg (white, pentagonal-shaped tablets debossed with an "X" on one side and "0.5" on the other side)
    Bottles of 60   NDC 0009-0057-07

1 mg (yellow, square-shaped tablets debossed with an "X" on one side and "1" on the other side)
    Bottles of 60   NDC 0009-0059-07

2 mg (blue, round-shaped tablets debossed with an "X" on one side and "2" on the other side)
    Bottles of 60   NDC 0009-0066-07

3 mg (green, triangular-shaped tablets debossed with an "X" on one side and "3" on the other side)
    Bottles of 60   NDC 0009-0068-07

Store at 25°C (77°F); excursions permitted to 15–30°C (59–86°F) [see USP Controlled Room Temperature].

℞ only

ANIMAL STUDIES
When rats were treated with alprazolam at 3, 10, and 30 mg/kg/day (15 to 150 times the maximum recommended human dose) orally for 2 years, a tendency for a dose related increase in the number of cataracts was observed in females and a tendency for a dose related increase in corneal vascularization was observed in males. These lesions did not appear until after 11 months of treatment.

Pharmacia & Upjohn Company
A subsidiary of Pharmacia Corporation
Kalamazoo, Michigan 49001, USA
January 2003   819 612 000
                                         692842

Roche Pharmaceuticals
Roche Laboratories Inc.
340 Kingsland Street
Nutley, NJ 07110-1199

For Medical Information:
(Including routine inquiries, adverse drug events and product complaints)
Call: (800) 526-6367
In Emergencies: 24-hour service
For the Medical Needs Program:
Call: (800) 285-4484
Write: Professional Product Information

COPEGUS™   ℞
[cō pĕg' ŭs]
(ribavirin, USP)
TABLETS

> **COPEGUS (ribavirin) monotherapy is not effective for the treatment of chronic hepatitis C virus infection and should not be used alone for this indication (see WARNINGS).**
>
> **The primary clinical toxicity of ribavirin is hemolytic anemia. The anemia associated with ribavirin therapy may result in worsening of cardiac disease that has led to fatal and nonfatal myocardial infarctions. Patients with a history of significant or unstable cardiac disease should not be treated with ribavirin (see WARNINGS, ADVERSE REACTIONS, and DOSAGE AND ADMINISTRATION).**
>
> **Significant teratogenic and/or embryocidal effects have been demonstrated in all animal species exposed to ribavirin. In addition, ribavirin has a multiple dose half-life of 12 days, and it may persist in non-plasma compartments for as long as 6 months. Ribavirin therapy is contraindicated in women who are pregnant and in the male partners of women who are pregnant. Extreme care must be taken to avoid pregnancy during therapy and for 6 months after completion of treatment in both female patients and in female partners of male patients who are taking ribavirin therapy. At least two reliable forms of effective contraception must be utilized during treatment and during the 6-month post-**

Continued on next page

Copegus—Cont.

treatment follow-up period (see CONTRAINDICATIONS, WARNINGS, and PRECAUTIONS: Information for Patients, and Pregnancy: Category X).

DESCRIPTION

COPEGUS, the Hoffmann-La Roche brand name for ribavirin, is a nucleoside analogue with antiviral activity. The chemical name of ribavirin is 1-β-D-ribofuranosyl-1*H*-1,2,4-triazole-3-carboxamide.

The empirical formula of ribavirin is $C_8H_{12}N_4O_5$ and the molecular weight is 244.2. Ribavirin is a white to off-white powder. It is freely soluble in water and slightly soluble in anhydrous alcohol.

COPEGUS (ribavirin) is available as a light pink to pink colored, flat, oval-shaped, film-coated tablet for oral administration. Each tablet contains 200 mg of ribavirin and the following inactive ingredients: pregelatinized starch, microcrystalline cellulose, sodium starch glycolate, corn starch, and magnesium stearate. The coating of the tablet contains Chromatone-P® or Opadry® Pink (made by using hydroxypropyl methyl cellulose, talc, titanium dioxide, synthetic yellow iron oxide, and synthetic red iron oxide), ethyl cellulose (ECD-30), and triacetin.

Mechanism of Action

Ribavirin is a synthetic nucleoside analogue. The mechanism by which the combination of ribavirin and an interferon product exerts its effects against the hepatitis C virus has not been fully established.

CLINICAL PHARMACOLOGY

Pharmacokinetics

Multiple dose ribavirin pharmacokinetic data are available for HCV patients who received ribavirin in combination with peginterferon alfa-2a. Following administration of 1200 mg/day with food for 12 weeks mean±SD (n=39; body weight >75 kg) $AUC_{0\text{-}12hr}$ was 25,361±7110 ng•hr/mL and C_{max} was 2748±818 ng/mL. The average time to reach C_{max} was 2 hours. Trough ribavirin plasma concentrations following 12 weeks of dosing with food were 1662±545 ng/mL in HCV infected patients who received 800 mg/day (n=89), and 2112±810 ng/mL in patients who received 1200 mg/day (n=75; body weight >75 kg).

The terminal half-life of ribavirin following administration of a single oral dose of COPEGUS is about 120 to 170 hours. The total apparent clearance following administration of a single oral dose of COPEGUS is about 26 L/h. There is extensive accumulation of ribavirin after multiple dosing (twice daily) such that the C_{max} at steady state was four-fold higher than that of a single dose.

Effect of Food on Absorption of Ribavirin

Bioavailability of a single oral dose of ribavirin was increased by co-administration with a high-fat meal. The absorption was slowed (T_{max} was doubled) and the $AUC_{0\text{-}192h}$ and C_{max} increased by 42% and 66%, respectively, when COPEGUS was taken with a high-fat meal compared with fasting conditions (see **PRECAUTIONS** and **DOSAGE AND ADMINISTRATION**).

Elimination and Metabolism

The contribution of renal and hepatic pathways to ribavirin elimination after administration of COPEGUS is not known. In vitro studies indicate that ribavirin is not a substrate of CYP450 enzymes.

Special Populations

Race

There were insufficient numbers of non-Caucasian subjects studied to adequately determine potential pharmacokinetic differences between populations.

Renal Dysfunction

The pharmacokinetics of ribavirin following administration of COPEGUS have not been studied in patients with renal impairment and there are limited data from clinical trials on administration of COPEGUS in patients with creatinine clearance <50 mL/min. Therefore, patients with creatinine clearance <50 mL/min should not be treated with COPEGUS (see **WARNINGS** and **DOSAGE AND ADMINISTRATION**).

Hepatic Impairment

The effect of hepatic impairment on the pharmacokinetics of ribavirin following administration of COPEGUS has not been evaluated. The clinical trials of COPEGUS were restricted to patients with Child-Pugh class A disease.

Pediatric Patients

Pharmacokinetic evaluations in pediatric patients have not been performed.

Elderly Patients

Pharmacokinetic evaluations in elderly patients have not been performed.

Gender

Ribavirin pharmacokinetics, when corrected for weight, are similar in male and female patients.

Drug Interactions

In vitro studies indicate that ribavirin does not inhibit CYP450 enzymes.

Nucleoside Analogues

Ribavirin has been shown in vitro to inhibit phosphorylation of zidovudine and stavudine which could lead to decreased antiretroviral activity. Exposure to didanosine or its active metabolite (dideoxyadenosine 5'-triphosphate) is increased when didanosine is co-administered with ribavirin, which could cause or worsen clinical toxicities (see **PRECAUTIONS: Drug Interactions**).

Clinical Studies

The safety and effectiveness of PEGASYS in combination with COPEGUS for the treatment of hepatitis C virus infection were assessed in two randomized controlled clinical trials. All patients were adults, had compensated liver disease, detectable hepatitis C virus, liver biopsy diagnosis of chronic hepatitis, and were previously untreated with interferon. Approximately 20% of patients in both studies had compensated cirrhosis (Child-Pugh class A).

In study NV15801 (described as study 4 in the PEGASYS Package Insert), patients were randomized to receive either PEGASYS 180 μg sc once weekly (qw) with an oral placebo, PEGASYS 180 μg qw with COPEGUS 1000 mg po (body weight <75 kg) or 1200 mg po (body weight ≥75 kg) or REBETRON™ (interferon alfa-2b 3 MIU sc tiw plus ribavirin 1000 mg or 1200 mg po). All patients received 48 weeks of therapy followed by 24 weeks of treatment-free follow-up. COPEGUS or placebo treatment assignment was blinded. PEGASYS in combination with COPEGUS resulted in a higher SVR (defined as undetectable HCV RNA at the end of the 24-week treatment-free follow-up period) compared to PEGASYS alone or interferon alfa-2b and ribavirin (Table 1). In all treatment arms, patients with viral genotype 1, regardless of viral load, had a lower response rate to PEGASYS in combination with COPEGUS compared to patients with other viral genotypes.

Table 1 Sustained Virologic Response (SVR) to Combination Therapy (Study NV15801*)

	Interferon alfa-2b+ Ribavirin 1000 mg or 1200 mg	PEGASYS + placebo	PEGASYS + COPEGUS 1000 mg or 1200 mg
All patients	197/444 (44%)	65/224 (29%)	241/453 (53%)
Genotype 1	103/285 (36%)	29/145 (20%)	132/298 (44%)
Genotypes 2-6	94/159 (59%)	36/79 (46%)	109/155 (70%)

Difference in overall treatment response (PEGASYS/COPEGUS–Interferon alfa-2b/ribavirin) was 9% (95% CI 2.3, 15.3).

* Described as study 4 in the PEGASYS Package Insert.

In study NV15942 (described as study 5 in the PEGASYS Package Insert), all patients received PEGASYS 180 μg sc qw and were randomized to treatment for either 24 or 48 weeks and to a COPEGUS dose of either 800 mg or 1000 mg/1200 mg (for body weight <75 kg/≥75 kg). Assignment to the four treatment arms was stratified by viral genotype and baseline HCV viral titer. Patients with genotype 1 and high viral titer (defined as $>2 \times 10^6$ HCV RNA copies/mL serum) were preferentially assigned to treatment for 48 weeks.

Genotype 1

Irrespective of baseline viral titer, treatment for 48 weeks with PEGASYS and 1000 mg or 1200 mg of COPEGUS resulted in higher SVR (defined as undetectable HCV RNA at the end of the 24-week treatment-free follow-up period) compared to shorter treatment (24 weeks) and/or 800 mg COPEGUS.

Genotype non-1

Irrespective of baseline viral titer, treatment for 24 weeks with PEGASYS and 800 mg of COPEGUS resulted in a similar SVR compared to longer treatment (48 weeks) and/or 1000 mg or 1200 mg of COPEGUS (see Table 2).

[See table 2 below]

Among the 36 patients with genotype 4, response rates were similar to those observed in patients with genotype 1 (data not shown). The numbers of patients with genotype 5 and 6 were too few to allow for meaningful assessment.

Treatment Response in Patient Subgroups

Treatment response rates are lower in patients with poor prognostic factors receiving pegylated interferon alpha therapy. In studies NV15801 and NV15942, treatment response rates were lower in patients older than 40 years (50% vs 66%), in patients with cirrhosis (47% vs 59%), in patients weighing over 85 kg (49% vs 60%), and in patients with genotype 1 with high vs low viral load (43% vs 56%). African American patients had lower response rates compared to Caucasians.

Paired liver biopsies were performed on approximately 20% of patients in studies NV15801 and NV15942. Modest reductions in inflammation compared to baseline were seen in all treatment groups.

In studies NV15801 and NV15942, lack of early virologic response at 12 weeks (defined as HCV RNA undetectable or $>2\log_{10}$ lower than baseline) was grounds for discontinuation of treatment. Of patients who lacked an early viral response at 12 weeks and completed a recommended course of therapy despite a protocol-defined option to discontinue therapy, 5/39 (13%) achieved an SVR. Of patients who lacked an early viral response at 24 weeks, nineteen completed a full course of therapy and none achieved an SVR.

INDICATIONS AND USAGE

COPEGUS in combination with PEGASYS (peginterferon alfa-2a) is indicated for the treatment of adults with chronic hepatitis C virus infection who have compensated liver disease and have not been previously treated with interferon alpha. Patients in whom efficacy was demonstrated included patients with compensated liver disease and histological evidence of cirrhosis (Child-Pugh class A).

CONTRAINDICATIONS

COPEGUS (ribavirin) is contraindicated in:

- Patients with known hypersensitivity to COPEGUS or to any component of the tablet.
- Women who are pregnant.
- Men whose female partners are pregnant.
- Patients with hemoglobinopathies (eg, thalassemia major or sickle-cell anemia).

COPEGUS and PEGASYS combination therapy is contraindicated in patients with:

- Autoimmune hepatitis.
- Hepatic decompensation (Child-Pugh class B and C) before or during treatment.

WARNINGS

COPEGUS must not be used alone because ribavirin monotherapy is not effective for the treatment of chronic hepatitis C virus infection. The safety and efficacy of COPEGUS have only been established when used together with PEGASYS (pegylated interferon alfa-2a, recombinant).

COPEGUS and PEGASYS should be discontinued in patients who develop evidence of hepatic decompensation during treatment.

There are significant adverse events caused by COPEGUS/PEGASYS therapy, including severe depression and suicidal ideation, hemolytic anemia, suppression of bone marrow function, autoimmune and infectious disorders, pulmonary dysfunction, pancreatitis, and diabetes. The PEGASYS package insert and MEDICATION GUIDE should be reviewed in their entirety prior to initiation of combination treatment for additional safety information.

General

Treatment with COPEGUS and PEGASYS should be administered under the guidance of a qualified physician and may lead to moderate to severe adverse experiences requiring dose reduction, temporary dose cessation or discontinuation of therapy.

Pregnancy

Ribavirin may cause birth defects and/or death of the exposed fetus. Extreme care must be taken to avoid pregnancy in female patients and in female partners of male patients. Ribavirin has demonstrated significant teratogenic and/or embryocidal effects in all animal species in which adequate studies have been conducted. These effects occurred at doses as low as one twentieth of the recommended human dose of ribavirin. COPEGUS THERAPY SHOULD NOT BE STARTED UNLESS A REPORT OF A NEGATIVE PREGNANCY TEST HAS BEEN OBTAINED IMMEDIATELY PRIOR TO PLANNED INITIATION OF THERAPY. Patients should be instructed to use at least two forms of effective contraception during treatment and for at least six months after treatment has been stopped. Pregnancy testing should occur monthly during COPEGUS therapy and for six months after therapy has stopped (see CONTRAINDICATIONS and PRECAUTIONS: Information for Patients and Pregnancy: Category X).

Anemia

The primary toxicity of ribavirin is hemolytic anemia (hemoglobin <10 g/dL), which was observed in approximately

Table 2 Sustained Virologic Response as a Function of Genotype (Study NV15942*)

	24 Weeks Treatment		48 Weeks Treatment	
	PEGASYS + COPEGUS 800 mg (N=207)	PEGASYS + COPEGUS 1000 mg or 1200 mg** (N=280)	PEGASYS + COPEGUS 800 mg (N=361)	PEGASYS + COPEGUS 1000 mg or 1200 mg** (N=436)
Genotype 1	29/101 (29%)	48/118 (41%)	99/250 (40%)	138/271 (51%)
Gentoype 2-3	79/96 (82%)	116/144 (81%)	75/99 (76%)	117/153 (76%)

* Described as study 5 in the PEGASYS Package Insert.

** 1000 mg for body weight <75 kg; 1200 mg for body weight ≥75 kg.

13% of COPEGUS and PEGASYS treated patients in clinical trials (see PRECAUTIONS: Laboratory Tests). The anemia associated with COPEGUS occurs within 1 to 2 weeks of initiation of therapy. BECAUSE THE INITIAL DROP IN HEMOGLOBIN MAY BE SIGNIFICANT, IT IS ADVISED THAT HEMOGLOBIN OR HEMATOCRIT BE OBTAINED PRETREATMENT AND AT WEEK 2 AND WEEK 4 OF THERAPY OR MORE FREQUENTLY IF CLINICALLY INDICATED. Patients should then be followed as clinically appropriate.

Fatal and nonfatal myocardial infarctions have been reported in patients with anemia caused by ribavirin. Patients should be assessed for underlying cardiac disease before initiation of ribavirin therapy. Patients with pre-existing cardiac disease should have electrocardiograms administered before treatment, and should be appropriately monitored during therapy. If there is any deterioration of cardiovascular status, therapy should be suspended or discontinued (see DOSAGE AND ADMINISTRATION: COPEGUS Dosage Modification Guidelines). Because cardiac disease may be worsened by drug induced anemia, patients with a history of significant or unstable cardiac disease should not use COPEGUS (see ADVERSE REACTIONS).

Pulmonary
Pulmonary symptoms, including dyspnea, pulmonary infiltrates, pneumonitis and occasional cases of fatal pneumonia, have been reported during therapy with ribavirin and interferon. In addition, sarcoidosis or the exacerbation of sarcoidosis has been reported. If there is evidence of pulmonary infiltrates or pulmonary function impairment, the patient should be closely monitored, and if appropriate, combination COPEGUS/PEGASYS treatment should be discontinued.

Other
COPEGUS and PEGASYS therapy should be suspended in patients with signs and symptoms of pancreatitis, and discontinued in patients with confirmed pancreatitis.

COPEGUS should not be used in patients with creatinine clearance <50 mL/min (see CLINICAL PHARMACOLOGY: Special Populations).

COPEGUS must be discontinued immediately and appropriate medical therapy instituted if an acute hypersensitivity reaction (eg, urticaria, angioedema, bronchoconstriction, anaphylaxis) develops. Transient rashes do not necessitate interruption of treatment.

PRECAUTIONS
The safety and efficacy of COPEGUS and PEGASYS therapy for the treatment of HIV infection, adenovirus, RSV, parainfluenza or influenza infections have not been established. COPEGUS should not be used for these indications. Ribavirin for inhalation has a separate package insert, which should be consulted if ribavirin inhalation therapy is being considered.

The safety and efficacy of COPEGUS and PEGASYS therapy have not been established in liver or other organ transplant patients, patients with decompensated liver disease due to hepatitis C virus infection, patients who are nonresponders to interferon therapy or patients co-infected with HBV or HIV.

Information for Patients
Patients must be informed that ribavirin may cause birth defects and/or death of the exposed fetus. COPEGUS therapy must not be used by women who are pregnant or by men whose female partners are pregnant. Extreme care must be taken to avoid pregnancy in female patients and in female partners of male patients taking COPEGUS therapy and for 6 months posttherapy. COPEGUS therapy should not be initiated until a report of a negative pregnancy test has been obtained immediately prior to initiation of therapy. Patients must perform a pregnancy test monthly during therapy and for 6 months posttherapy.

Female patients of childbearing potential and male patients with female partners of childbearing potential must be advised of the teratogenic/embryocidal risks and must be instructed to practice effective contraception during COPEGUS therapy and for 6 months posttherapy. Patients should be advised to notify the physician immediately in the event of a pregnancy (see CONTRAINDICATIONS and WARNINGS).

To monitor maternal-fetal outcomes of pregnant women exposed to COPEGUS, the COPEGUS Pregnancy Registry has been established. Physicians and patients are strongly encouraged to register by calling 1-800-526-6367.

The most common adverse event associated with ribavirin is anemia, which may be severe (see ADVERSE REACTIONS). Patients should be advised that laboratory evaluations are required prior to starting COPEGUS therapy and periodically thereafter (see Laboratory Tests). It is advised that patients be well hydrated, especially during the initial stages of treatment.

Patients who develop dizziness, confusion, somnolence, and fatigue should be cautioned to avoid driving or operating machinery.

Patients should be informed regarding the potential benefits and risks attendant to the use of COPEGUS. Instructions on appropriate use should be given, including review of the contents of the enclosed MEDICATION GUIDE, which is not a disclosure of all or possible adverse effects. Patients should be advised to take COPEGUS with food.

Laboratory Tests
Before beginning COPEGUS therapy, standard hematological and biochemical laboratory tests must be conducted for all patients. Pregnancy screening for women of childbearing potential must be done.

After initiation of therapy, hematological tests should be performed at 2 weeks and 4 weeks and biochemical tests should be performed at 4 weeks. Additional testing should be performed periodically during therapy. Monthly pregnancy testing should be done during combination therapy and for 6 months after discontinuing therapy.

The entrance criteria used for the clinical studies of COPEGUS and PEGASYS combination therapy may be considered as a guideline to acceptable baseline values for initiation of treatment:
- Platelet count ≥90,000 cells/mm^3
- Absolute neutrophil count (ANC) ≥1500 cells/mm^3
- TSH and T$_4$ within normal limits or adequately controlled thyroid function
- ECG (see WARNINGS)

The maximum drop in hemoglobin usually occurred during the first 8 weeks of initiation of COPEGUS therapy. Because of this initial acute drop in hemoglobin, it is advised that a complete blood count should be obtained pretreatment and at week 2 and week 4 of therapy or more frequently if clinically indicated. Additional testing should be performed periodically during therapy. Patients should then be followed as clinically appropriate.

Drug Interactions
Results from a pharmacokinetic sub-study demonstrated no pharmacokinetic interaction between PEGASYS (peginterferon alfa-2a) and ribavirin.

Nucleoside Analogues
Didanosine
Co-administration of COPEGUS and didanosine is not recommended. Reports of fatal hepatic failure, as well as peripheral neuropathy, pancreatitis, and symptomatic hyperlactatemia/lactic acidosis have been reported in clinical trials (see CLINICAL PHARMACOLOGY: Drug Interactions).

Stavudine and Zidovudine
Ribavirin can antagonize the in vitro antiviral activity of stavudine and zidovudine against HIV. Therefore, concomitant use of ribavirin with either of these drugs should be avoided (see CLINICAL PHARMACOLOGY: Drug Interactions).

Carcinogenesis, Mutagenesis, Impairment of Fertility
Carcinogenesis
The carcinogenic potential of ribavirin has not been fully determined. In a p53 (+/−) mouse carcinogenicity study at doses up to the maximum tolerated dose of 100 mg/kg/day, ribavirin was not oncogenic. However, on a body surface area basis, this dose was 0.5 times maximum recommended human 24-hour dose of ribavirin. A study to assess the carcinogenic potential of ribavirin in rats is ongoing.

Mutagenesis
Ribavirin demonstrated mutagenic activity in the in vitro mouse lymphoma assay. No clastogenic activity was observed in an in vivo mouse micronucleus assay at doses up to 2000 mg/kg. However, results from studies published in the literature show clastogenic activity in the in vivo mouse micronucleus assay at oral doses up to 2000 mg/kg. A dominant lethal assay in rats was negative, indicating that if mutations occurred in rats they were not transmitted through male gametes. However, potential carcinogenic risk to humans cannot be excluded.

Impairment of Fertility
In a fertility study in rats, ribavirin showed a marginal reduction in sperm counts at the dose of 100 mg/kg/day with no effect on fertility. Upon cessation of treatment, total recovery occurred after 1 spermatogenesis cycle. Abnormalities in sperm were observed in studies in mice designed to evaluate the time course and reversibility of ribavirin-induced testicular degeneration at doses of 15 to 150 mg/kg/day (approximately 0.1–0.8 times the maximum recommended human 24-hour dose of ribavirin) administered for 3 to 6 months. Upon cessation of treatment, essentially total recovery from ribavirin-induced testicular toxicity was apparent within 1 or 2 spermatogenic cycles.

Female patients of childbearing potential and male patients with female partners of childbearing potential should not receive COPEGUS unless the patient and his/her partner are using effective contraception (two reliable forms). Based on a multiple dose half-life ($t_{1/2}$) of ribavirin of 12 days, effective contraception must be utilized for 6 months posttherapy (ie, 15 half-lives of clearance for ribavirin).

No reproductive toxicology studies have been performed using PEGASYS in combination with COPEGUS. However, peginterferon alfa-2a and ribavirin when administered separately, each has adverse effects on reproduction. It should be assumed that the effects produced by either agent alone would also be caused by the combination of the two agents.

Pregnancy
Pregnancy: Category X (see CONTRAINDICATIONS)
Ribavirin produced significant embryocidal and/or teratogenic effects in all animal species in which adequate studies have been conducted. Malformations of the skull, palate, eye, jaw, limbs, skeleton, and gastrointestinal tract were noted. The incidence and severity of teratogenic effects increased with escalation of the drug dose. Survival of fetuses and offspring was reduced.

In conventional embryotoxicity/teratogenicity studies in rats and rabbits, observed no-effect dose levels were well below those for proposed clinical use (0.3 mg/kg/day for both the rat and rabbit; approximately 0.06 times the recommended human 24-hour dose of ribavirin). No maternal toxicity or effects on offspring were observed in a peri/postnatal toxicity study in rats dosed orally at up to 1 mg/kg/day (approximately 0.01 times the maximum recommended human 24-hour dose of ribavirin).

Treatment and Posttreatment: Potential Risk to the Fetus
Ribavirin is known to accumulate in intracellular components from where it is cleared very slowly. It is not known whether ribavirin is contained in sperm, and if so, will exert a potential teratogenic effect upon fertilization of the ova. In a study in rats, it was concluded that dominant lethality was not induced by ribavirin at doses up to 200 mg/kg for 5 days (up to 1.7 times the maximum recommended human dose of ribavirin). However, because of the potential human teratogenic effects of ribavirin, male patients should be advised to take every precaution to avoid risk of pregnancy for their female partners.

COPEGUS should not be used by pregnant women or by men whose female partners are pregnant. Female patients of childbearing potential and male patients with female partners of childbearing potential should not receive COPEGUS unless the patient and his/her partner are using effective contraception (two reliable forms) during therapy and for 6 months posttherapy.

To monitor maternal-fetal outcomes of pregnant women exposed to COPEGUS, the COPEGUS Pregnancy Registry has been established. Physicians and patients are strongly encouraged to register by calling 1-800-526-6367.

Animal Toxicology
Long-term study in the mouse and rat (18–24 months; dose 20–75 and 10–40 mg/kg/day, respectively, approximately 0.1–0.4 times the maximum human daily dose of ribavirin) have demonstrated a relationship between chronic ribavirin exposure and an increased incidence of vascular lesions (microscopic hemorrhages) in mice. In rats, retinal degeneration occurred in controls, but the incidence was increased in ribavirin-treated rats.

Nursing Mothers
It is not known whether ribavirin is excreted in human milk. Because many drugs are excreted in human milk and to avoid any potential for serious adverse reactions in nursing infants from ribavirin, a decision should be made either to discontinue nursing or therapy with COPEGUS, based on the importance of the therapy to the mother.

Pediatric Use
Safety and effectiveness of COPEGUS have not been established in patients below the age of 18.

Geriatric Use
Clinical studies of COPEGUS and PEGASYS did not include sufficient numbers of subjects aged 65 or over to determine whether they respond differently from younger subjects. Specific pharmacokinetic evaluations for ribavirin in the elderly have not been performed. The risk of toxic reactions to this drug may be greater in patients with impaired renal function. COPEGUS should not be administered to patients with creatinine clearance <50 mL/min. (see CLINICAL PHARMACOLOGY: Special Populations).

Effect of Gender
No clinically significant differences in the pharmacokinetics of ribavirin were observed between male and female subjects.

ADVERSE REACTIONS
PEGASYS in combination with COPEGUS causes a broad variety of serious adverse reactions (see BOXED WARNING and WARNINGS). In all studies, one or more serious adverse reactions occurred in 10% of patients receiving PEGASYS in combination with COPEGUS.

The most common life-threatening or fatal events induced or aggravated by PEGASYS and COPEGUS were depression, suicide, relapse of drug abuse/overdose, and bacterial infections; each occurred at a frequency of <1%.

Nearly all patients in clinical trials experienced one or more adverse events. The most commonly reported adverse reactions were psychiatric reactions, including depression, irritability, anxiety, and flu-like symptoms such as fatigue, pyrexia, myalgia, headache and rigors.

Ten percent of patients receiving 48 weeks of therapy with PEGASYS in combination with COPEGUS discontinued therapy. The most common reasons for discontinuation of therapy were psychiatric, flu-like syndrome (eg, lethargy, fatigue, headache), dermatologic and gastrointestinal disorders.

The most common reason for dose modification in patients receiving combination therapy was for laboratory abnormalities; neutropenia (20%) and thrombocytopenia (4%) for PEGASYS and anemia (22%) for COPEGUS.

PEGASYS dose was reduced in 12% of patients receiving 1000 mg to 1200 mg COPEGUS for 48 weeks and in 7% of patients receiving 800 mg COPEGUS for 24 weeks. COPEGUS dose was reduced in 21% of patients receiving 1000 mg to 1200 mg COPEGUS for 48 weeks and 12% in patients receiving 800 mg COPEGUS for 24 weeks.

Because clinical trials are conducted under widely varying and controlled conditions, adverse reaction rates observed in clinical trials of a drug cannot be directly compared to rates in the clinical trials of another drug. Also, the adverse event rates listed here may not predict the rates observed in a broader patient population in clinical practice.

Continued on next page

Copegus—Cont.

Table 3 Adverse Reactions Occurring in ≥5% of Patients in Hepatitis C Clinical Trials (Study NV15801*)

Body System	PEGASYS 180 μg + 1000 mg or 1200 mg COPEGUS 48 wk	Intron A + 1000 mg or 1200 mg REBETOL® 48 wk
	N=451	N=443
	%	%
Application Site Disorders		
Injection site reaction	23	16
Endocrine Disorders		
Hypothyroidism	4	5
Flu-like Symptoms and Signs		
Fatigue/Asthenia	65	68
Pyrexia	41	55
Rigors	25	37
Pain	10	9
Gastrointestinal		
Nausea/vomiting	25	29
Diarrhea	11	10
Abdominal pain	8	9
Dry mouth	4	7
Dyspepsia	6	5
Hematologic**		
Lymphopenia	14	12
Anemia	11	11
Neutropenia	27	8
Thrombocytopenia	5	<1
Metabolic and Nutritional		
Anorexia	24	26
Weight decrease	10	10
Musculoskeletal, Connective Tissue and Bone		
Myalgia	40	49
Arthralgia	22	23
Back pain	5	5
Neurological		
Headache	43	49
Dizziness (excluding vertigo)	14	14
Memory impairment	6	5
Psychiatric		
Irritability/Anxiety/Nervousness	33	38
Insomnia	30	37
Depression	20	28
Concentration impairment	10	13
Mood alteration	5	6
Resistance Mechanism Disorders		
Overall	12	10
Respiratory, Thoracic and Mediastinal		
Dyspnea	13	14
Cough	10	7
Dyspnea exertional	4	7
Skin and Subcutaneous Tissue		
Alopecia	28	33
Pruritus	19	18
Dermatitis	16	13
Dry Skin	10	13
Rash	8	5
Sweating Increased	6	5
Eczema	5	4
Visual Disorders		
Vision Blurred	5	2

* Described as study 4 in the PEGASYS Package Insert.
** Severe hematologic abnormalities.

Patients treated for 24 weeks with PEGASYS and 800 mg COPEGUS were observed to have lower incidence of serious adverse events (3% vs 10%), hemoglobin <10 g/dL (3% vs 15%), dose modification of PEGASYS (30% vs 36%) and COPEGUS (19% vs 38%) and of withdrawal from treatment (5% vs 15%) compared to patients treated for 48 weeks with PEGASYS and 1000 mg or 1200 mg COPEGUS. On the other hand the overall incidence of adverse events appeared to be similar in the two treatment groups.

The most common serious adverse event (3%) was bacterial infection (eg, sepsis, osteomyelitis, endocarditis, pyelonephritis, pneumonia). Other SAEs occurred at a frequency of <1% and included: suicide, suicidal ideation, psychosis, aggression, anxiety, drug abuse and drug overdose, angina, hepatic dysfunction, fatty liver, cholangitis, arrhythmia, diabetes mellitus, autoimmune phenomena (eg, hyperthyroidism, hypothyroidism, sarcoidosis, systemic lupus erythematosis, rheumatoid arthritis) peripheral neuropathy, aplastic anemia, peptic ulcer, gastrointestinal bleeding, pancreatitis, colitis, corneal ulcer, pulmonary embolism, coma, myositis, and cerebral hemorrhage.

Laboratory Test Values

Anemia due to hemolysis is the most significant toxicity of ribavirin therapy. Anemia (hemoglobin <10 g/dL) was observed in 13% of COPEGUS and PEGASYS combination-treated patients in clinical trials. The maximum drop in hemoglobin occurred during the first 8 weeks of initiation of ribavirin therapy (see **DOSAGE AND ADMINISTRATION: Dose Modifications**).

OVERDOSAGE

No cases of overdose with COPEGUS have been reported in clinical trials.

DOSAGE AND ADMINISTRATION

The recommended dose of COPEGUS tablets is provided in Table 4. The recommended duration of treatment for patients previously untreated with ribavirin and interferon is 24 to 48 weeks.

The daily dose of COPEGUS is 800 mg to 1200 mg administered orally in two divided doses. The dose should be individualized to the patient depending on baseline disease characteristics (eg, genotype), response to therapy, and tolerability of the regimen (see Table 4).

In the pivotal clinical trials, patients were instructed to take COPEGUS with food; therefore, patients are advised to take COPEGUS with food.

[See table 4 above]

Dose Modifications

If severe adverse reactions or laboratory abnormalities develop during combination COPEGUS/PEGASYS therapy, the dose should be modified or discontinued, if appropriate, until the adverse reactions abate. If intolerance persists after dose adjustment, COPEGUS/PEGASYS therapy should be discontinued.

COPEGUS should be administered with caution to patients with pre-existing cardiac disease (see Table 5). Patients should be assessed before commencement of therapy and should be appropriately monitored during therapy. If there is any deterioration of cardiovascular status, therapy should be stopped (see **WARNINGS**).

Table 5 COPEGUS Dosage Modification Guidelines

Laboratory Values	Reduce Only COPEGUS Dose to 600 mg/day* if:	Discontinue COPEGUS if:
Hemoglobin in patients with no cardiac disease	<10 g/dL	<8.5 g/dL
Hemoglobin in patients with history of stable cardiac disease	≥2 g/dL decrease in hemoglobin during any 4 week period treatment	<12 g/dL despite 4 weeks at reduced dose

*One 200 mg tablet in the morning and two 200 mg tablets in the evening.

Once COPEGUS has been withheld due to either a laboratory abnormality or clinical manifestation, an attempt may be made to restart COPEGUS at 600 mg daily and further increase the dose to 800 mg daily depending upon the physician's judgment. However, it is not recommended that COPEGUS be increased to its original assigned dose (1000 mg to 1200 mg).

Renal Impairment

COPEGUS should not be used in patients with creatinine clearance <50 mL/min (see **WARNINGS** and **CLINICAL PHARMACOLOGY: Special Populations**).

HOW SUPPLIED

COPEGUS™ (ribavirin) is available as tablets for oral administration. Each tablet contains 200 mg of ribavirin and is light pink to pink colored, flat, oval-shaped, film-coated, and engraved with RIB 200 on one side and ROCHE on the other side. They are packaged as bottle of 168 tablets (NDC 0004-0086-94).

Storage Conditions

Store the COPEGUS Tablets bottle at 25°C (77°F); excursions are permitted between 15° and 30°C (59° and 86°F) [see USP Controlled Room Temperature]. Keep bottle tightly closed.

REBETRON™ is a trademark of Schering Corporation.

Issued: December 2002

Table 4 PEGASYS and COPEGUS Dosing Recommendations

Genotype	PEGASYS Dose	COPEGUS Dose	Duration
Genotype 1, 4	180 μg	<75 kg = 1000 mg ≥75 kg = 1200 mg	48 weeks 48 weeks
Genotype 2, 3	180 μg	800 mg	24 weeks

Genotypes non-1 showed no increased response to treatment beyond 24 weeks (see Table 2).
Data on genotypes 5 and 6 are insufficient for dosing recommendations.

FUZEON™   ℞
[fūe'zē-ŏn]
(enfuvirtide)
for Injection
℞ only

DESCRIPTION

FUZEON (enfuvirtide) is an inhibitor of the fusion of HIV-1 with CD4+ cells. Enfuvirtide is a linear 36-amino acid synthetic peptide with the N-terminus acetylated and the C-terminus is a carboxamide. It is composed of naturally occurring L-amino acid residues.

Enfuvirtide is a white to off-white amorphous solid. It has negligible solubility in pure water and the solubility increases in aqueous buffers (pH 7.5) to 85-142 g/100 mL. The empirical formula of enfuvirtide is $C_{204}H_{301}N_{51}O_{64}$, and the molecular weight is 4492. It has the following primary amino acid sequence:

CH_3CO-Tyr-Thr-Ser-Leu-Ile-His-Ser-Leu-Ile-Glu-Glu-Ser-Gln-Asn-Gln-Gln-Glu-Lys-Asn-Glu-Gln-Glu-Leu-Leu-Glu-Leu-Asp-Lys-Trp-Ala-Ser-Leu-Trp-Asn-Trp-Phe-NH_2.

The drug product, FUZEON (enfuvirtide) for Injection, is a white to off-white, sterile, lyophilized powder. Each single-use vial contains 108 mg of enfuvirtide for the delivery of 90 mg. Prior to subcutaneous administration, the contents of the vial are reconstituted with 1.1 mL of Sterile Water for Injection giving a volume of approximately 1.2 mL to provide the delivery of 1 mL of the solution. Each 1 mL of the reconstituted solution contains approximately 90 mg of enfuvirtide with approximate amounts of the following excipients: 22.55 mg of mannitol, 2.39 mg of sodium carbonate (anhydrous), and sodium hydroxide and hydrochloric acid for pH adjustment as needed. The reconstituted solution has an approximate pH of 9.0.

MICROBIOLOGY

Mechanism of Action

Enfuvirtide interferes with the entry of HIV-1 into cells by inhibiting fusion of viral and cellular membranes. Enfuvirtide binds to the first heptad-repeat (HR1) in the gp41 subunit of the viral envelope glycoprotein and prevents the conformational changes required for the fusion of viral and cellular membranes.

Antiviral Activity In Vitro

The in vitro antiviral activity of enfuvirtide was assessed by infecting different CD4+ cell types with laboratory and clinical isolates of HIV-1. The IC_{50} (50% inhibitory concentration) for enfuvirtide in laboratory and primary isolates representing HIV-1 clades A to G ranged from 4 to 280 nM (18 to 1260 ng/mL). The IC_{50} for baseline clinical isolates ranged from 0.089 to 107 nM (0.4 to 480 ng/mL) by the cMAGI assay (n=130) and from 1.56 to 1680 nM (7 to 7530 ng/mL) by a recombinant phenotypic entry assay (n=612). Enfuvirtide was similarly active in vitro against R5, X4, and dual tropic viruses. Enfuvirtide has no activity against HIV-2.

Enfuvirtide exhibited additive to synergistic effects in cell culture assays when combined with individual members of various antiretroviral classes, including zidovudine, lamivudine, nelfinavir, indinavir, and efavirenz.

Drug Resistance

HIV-1 isolates with reduced susceptibility to enfuvirtide have been selected in vitro. Genotypic analysis of the in vitro-selected resistant isolates showed mutations that resulted in amino acid substitutions at the enfuvirtide binding HR1 domain positions 36 to 38 of the HIV-1 envelope glycoprotein gp41. Phenotypic analysis of site-directed mutants in positions 36 to 38 in an HIV-1 molecular clone showed a 5-fold to 684-fold decrease in susceptibility to enfuvirtide.

In clinical trials, HIV-1 isolates with reduced susceptibility to enfuvirtide have been recovered from subjects treated with FUZEON in combination with other antiretroviral agents. Posttreatment HIV-1 virus from 185 subjects exhibited decreases in susceptibility to enfuvirtide ranging from 4-fold to 422-fold relative to their respective baseline virus and exhibited genotypic changes in gp41 amino acids 36 to 45. Substitutions in this region were observed with decreasing frequency at amino acid positions 38, 43, 36, 40, 42, and 45.

Cross-resistance

HIV-1 clinical isolates resistant to nucleoside analogue reverse transcriptase inhibitors (NRTI), non-nucleoside analogue reverse transcriptase inhibitors (NNRTI), and protease inhibitors (PI) were susceptible to enfuvirtide in cell culture.

CLINICAL PHARMACOLOGY
Pharmacokinetics
The pharmacokinetic properties of enfuvirtide were evaluated in HIV-1 infected adult and pediatric patients.

Absorption
Following a 90-mg single subcutaneous injection of FUZEON into the abdomen in 12 HIV-1 infected subjects, the mean (±SD) C_{max} was 4.59 ± 1.5 µg/mL, AUC was 55.8 ± 12.1 µg•h/mL and the median T_{max} was 8 hours (ranged from 3 to 12 h). The absolute bioavailability (using a 90-mg intravenous dose as a reference) was 84.3% ± 15.5%. Following 90-mg bid dosing of FUZEON subcutaneously in combination with other antiretroviral agents in 11 HIV-1 infected subjects, the mean (±SD) steady-state C_{max} was 5.0 ± 1.7 µg/mL, C_{trough} was 3.3 ± 1.6 µg/mL, AUC_{0-12h} was 48.7 ± 19.1 µg•h/mL, and the median T_{max} was 4 hours (ranged from 4 to 8 h).

Absorption of the 90-mg dose was comparable when injected into the subcutaneous tissue of the abdomen, thigh or arm.

Distribution
The mean (±SD) steady-state volume of distribution after intravenous administration of a 90-mg dose of FUZEON (N=12) was 5.5 ± 1.1 L.

Enfuvirtide is approximately 92% bound to plasma proteins in HIV-infected plasma over a concentration range of 2 to 10 µg/mL. It is bound predominantly to albumin and to a lower extent to α-1 acid glycoprotein.

Metabolism/Elimination
As a peptide, enfuvirtide is expected to undergo catabolism to its constituent amino acids, with subsequent recycling of the amino acids in the body pool.

Mass balance studies to determine elimination pathway(s) of enfuvirtide have not been performed in humans.

In vitro studies with human microsomes and hepatocytes indicate that enfuvirtide undergoes hydrolysis to form a deamidated metabolite at the C-terminal phenylalanine residue, M3. The hydrolysis reaction is not NADPH dependent. The M3 metabolite is detected in human plasma following administration of enfuvirtide, with an AUC ranging from 2.4% to 15% of the enfuvirtide AUC.

Following a 90-mg single subcutaneous dose of enfuvirtide (N=12) the mean ±SD elimination half-life of enfuvirtide is 3.8 ± 0.6 h and the mean ±SD apparent clearance was 24.8 ± 4.1 mL/h/kg. Following 90-mg bid dosing of FUZEON subcutaneously in combination with other antiretroviral agents in 11 HIV-1 infected subjects, the mean ±SD apparent clearance was 30.6 ± 10.6 mL/h/kg.

Special Populations
Hepatic Insufficiency
Formal pharmacokinetic studies of enfuvirtide have not been conducted in patients with hepatic impairment.

Renal Insufficiency
Formal pharmacokinetic studies of enfuvirtide have not been conducted in patients with renal insufficiency. However, analysis of plasma concentration data from subjects in clinical trials indicated that the clearance of enfuvirtide is not affected in patients with creatinine clearance greater than 35 mL/min. The effect of creatinine clearance less than 35 mL/min on enfuvirtide clearance is unknown.

Gender and Weight
GENDER
Analysis of plasma concentration data from subjects in clinical trials indicated that the clearance of enfuvirtide is 20% lower in females than males after adjusting for body weight.
WEIGHT
Enfuvirtide clearance decreases with decreased body weight irrespective of gender. Relative to the clearance of a 70-kg male, a 40-kg male will have 20% lower clearance and a 110-kg male will have a 26% higher clearance. Relative to a 70-kg male, a 40-kg female will have a 36% lower clearance and a 110-kg female will have the same clearance.

No dose adjustment is recommended for weight or gender.

Race
Analysis of plasma concentration data from subjects in clinical trials indicated that the clearance of enfuvirtide was not different in Blacks compared to Caucasians. Other pharmacokinetic studies suggest no difference between Asians and Caucasians after adjusting for body weight.

Pediatric Patients
The pharmacokinetics of enfuvirtide have been studied in 18 pediatric subjects aged 6 through 16 years at a dose of 2 mg/kg. Enfuvirtide pharmacokinetics were determined in the presence of concomitant medications including antiretroviral agents. A dose of 2 mg/kg bid (maximum 90 mg bid) provided enfuvirtide plasma concentrations similar to those obtained in adult patients receiving 90 mg bid.

In the 18 pediatric subjects receiving the 2 mg/kg bid dose, the mean ±SD steady-state AUC was 53.6 ± 21.4 µg•h/mL, C_{max} was 5.9 ± 2.2 µg/mL, C_{trough} was 3.0 ± 1.5 µg/mL, and apparent clearance was 40 ± 14 mL/h/kg.

Geriatric Patients
The pharmacokinetics of enfuvirtide have not been studied in patients over 65 years of age.

Drug Interactions
Influence of FUZEON on the Metabolism of Concomitant Drugs
Based on the results from an in vitro human microsomal study, enfuvirtide is not an inhibitor of CYP450 enzymes. In an in vivo human metabolism study (N=12), FUZEON at the recommended dose of 90 mg bid did not alter the metabolism of CYP3A4, CYP2D6, CYP1A2, CYP2C19 or CYP2E1 substrates.

Influence of Concomitant Drugs on the Metabolism of Enfuvirtide
In separate pharmacokinetic interaction studies, coadministration of ritonavir (N=12), saquinavir/ritonavir (N=12), and rifampin (N=12) did not result in clinically significant pharmacokinetic interactions with FUZEON (see Table 1). [See table 1 above]

INDICATIONS AND USAGE
FUZEON in combination with other antiretroviral agents is indicated for the treatment of HIV-1 infection in treatment-experienced patients with evidence of HIV-1 replication despite ongoing antiretroviral therapy.

This indication is based on analyses of plasma HIV-1 RNA levels and CD4 cell counts in controlled studies of FUZEON of 24 weeks duration. Subjects enrolled were treatment-experienced adults; many had advanced disease. There are no studies of FUZEON in antiretroviral naive patients. There are no results from controlled trials evaluating the effect of FUZEON on clinical progression of HIV-1.

Description of Clinical Studies
Studies in Antiretroviral Experienced Patients
Studies T20-301 and T20-302 are ongoing, randomized, controlled, open-label, multicenter trials in HIV-1 infected subjects. Subjects were required to have either (1) viremia despite 3 to 6 months prior therapy with a nucleoside reverse transcriptase inhibitor (NRTI), non-nucleoside reverse transcriptase inhibitor (NNRTI), and protease inhibitor (PI) or (2) viremia and documented resistance or intolerance to at least one member in each of the NRTI, NNRTI, and PI classes.

All subjects received an individualized background regimen consisting of 3 to 5 antiretroviral agents selected on the basis of the subject's prior treatment history and baseline genotypic and phenotypic viral resistance measurements. Subjects were then randomized at a 2:1 ratio to FUZEON 90 mg bid with background regimen or background regimen alone. Demographic characteristics for studies T20-301 and T20-302 are shown in Table 2. Subjects had prior exposure to a median of 12 antiretrovirals for a median of 7 years.

Table 1 Effect of Ritonavir, Saquinavir/Ritonavir, and Rifampin on the Steady-State Pharmacokinetics of Enfuvirtide (90 mg bid)*

Coadministered Drug	Dose of Coadministered Drug	N	% Change of Enfuvirtide Pharmacokinetic Parameters[†] (90% CI)		
			C_{max}	AUC	C_{trough}
Ritonavir	200 mg, q12h, 4 days	12	↑24 (↑9 to ↑41)	↑22 (↑8 to ↑37)	↑14 (↑2 to ↑28)
Saquinavir/Ritonavir	1000/100 mg, q12h, 4 days	12	⇔	↑14 (↑5 to ↑24)	↑26 (↑17 to ↑35)
Rifampin	600 mg, qd, 10 days	12	⇔	⇔	↓15 (↓22 to ↓7)

* All studies were performed in HIV-1+ subjects using a sequential crossover design.
[†] ↑ = Increase; ↓ = Decrease; ⇔ = No Effect (↑ or ↓ <10%)

Table 2 T20-301 and T20-302 Pooled Subject Demographics

	FUZEON + Background Regimen	Background Regimen
	N=661	N=334
Sex		
Male	90%	90%
Female	10%	10%
Race		
White	89%	89%
Black	8%	7%
Mean Age (yr) (range)	43 (16-67)	43 (24-82)
Median Baseline HIV-1 RNA (log_{10} copies/mL)	5.2 (3.5-6.7)	5.1 (3.7-7.1)
Median Baseline CD4 Cell Count (cells/mm³)	88 (1-994)	97 (1-847)

The change in plasma HIV-1 RNA from baseline to week 24 was -1.52 log_{10} copies/mL for subjects receiving FUZEON plus background regimen compared to -0.73 log_{10} copies/mL for subjects receiving the background regimen only (see Table 3).

Subjects with two or more active drugs in their background regimen were more likely to achieve a HIV-1 RNA of <400 copies/mL.

Table 3 Outcomes of Randomized Treatment at Week 24 (Pooled Studies T20-301 and T20-302)

Outcomes	FUZEON + Background Regimen 90 mg bid	Background Regimen
	N=661	N=334
HIV-1 RNA Log Change from Baseline (log_{10} copies/mL)*	-1.52	-0.73
CD4+ cell count Change from Baseline (cells/mm³)#	+71	+35
HIV RNA ≥1 log below Baseline	342 (52%)	86 (26%)
HIV RNA <400 copies/mL	247 (37%)	54 (16%)
HIV RNA <50 copies/mL	151 (23%)	30 (9%)
Discontinued due to adverse reactions/labs [†]	40 (6%)	12 (4%)
Discontinued due to injection site reactions[†]	20 (3%)	N/A
Discontinued due to other reasons[†φ§]	36 (5%)	14 (4%)

* Based on results from pooled data of T20-301 and T20-302 on ITT population (week 24 viral load for subjects who were lost to follow-up, discontinued therapy, or switched from their original randomization, is replaced by their baseline value).
# Last value carried forward
[†] Percentages based on safety population FUZEON+background (N=663) and background (N=337).
φ As per the judgment of the investigator.
§ Includes discontinuations from loss to follow-up, treatment refusal, and other reasons.

CONTRAINDICATIONS
FUZEON is contraindicated in patients with known hypersensitivity to FUZEON or any of its components (see WARNINGS).

WARNINGS
Local Injection Site Reactions
The most common adverse events associated with FUZEON use are local injection site reactions. Manifestations may include pain and discomfort, induration, erythema, nodules and cysts, pruritus, and ecchymosis. Nine percent of patients had local reactions that required analgesics or limited usual activities (see ADVERSE REACTIONS). Reactions are often present at more than one injection site. Patients must be familiar with the FUZEON *Injection Instructions* in order to know how to inject FUZEON appropriately and how to monitor carefully for signs or symptoms of cellulitis or local infection.

Pneumonia
An increased rate of bacterial pneumonia was observed in subjects treated with FUZEON in the Phase 3 clinical trials compared to the control arm (see ADVERSE REACTIONS). It is unclear if the increased incidence of pneumonia is related to FUZEON use. However, because of this finding, patients with HIV infection should be carefully monitored for signs and symptoms of pneumonia, especially if they have underlying conditions which may predispose them to pneumonia. Risk factors for pneumonia included low initial CD4 cell count, high initial viral load, intravenous drug use, smoking, and a prior history of lung disease (see ADVERSE REACTIONS).

Hypersensitivity Reactions
Hypersensitivity reactions have been associated with FUZEON therapy and may recur on re-challenge. Hypersensitivity reactions have included individually and in combination: rash, fever, nausea and vomiting, chills, rigors, hypotension, and elevated serum liver transaminases. Other

Continued on next page

Fuzeon—Cont.

adverse events that may be immune mediated and have been reported in subjects receiving FUZEON include primary immune complex reaction, respiratory distress glomerulonephritis, and Guillain-Barre syndrome. Patients developing signs and symptoms suggestive of a systemic hypersensitivity reaction should discontinue FUZEON and should seek medical evaluation immediately. Therapy with FUZEON should not be restarted following systemic signs and symptoms consistent with a hypersensitivity reaction. Risk factors that may predict the occurrence or severity of hypersensitivity to FUZEON have not been identified (see ADVERSE REACTIONS).

PRECAUTIONS
Non-HIV Infected Individuals
There is a theoretical risk that FUZEON use may lead to the production of anti-enfuvirtide antibodies which cross react with HIV gp41. This could result in a false positive HIV test with an ELISA assay; a confirmatory western blot test would be expected to be negative. FUZEON has not been studied in non-HIV infected individuals.

Information for Patients
To assure safe and effective use of FUZEON, the following information and instructions should be given to patients:
- Patients should be informed that injection site reactions occur commonly. Patients must be familiar with the FUZEON *Injection Instructions* for instructions on how to appropriately inject FUZEON and how to carefully monitor for signs or symptoms of cellulitis or local infection. Patients should be instructed when to contact their healthcare provider about these reactions.
- Patients should be made aware that an increased rate of bacterial pneumonia was observed in subjects treated with FUZEON in Phase 3 clinical trials compared to the control arm. Patients should be advised to seek medical evaluation immediately if they develop signs or symptoms suggestive of pneumonia (cough with fever, rapid breathing, shortness of breath) (see WARNINGS).
- Patients should be advised of the possibility of a hypersensitivity reaction to FUZEON. Patients should be advised to discontinue therapy and immediately seek medical evaluation if they develop signs/symptoms of hypersensitivity (see WARNINGS).
- FUZEON is not a cure for HIV-1 infection and patients may continue to contract illnesses associated with HIV-1 infection. The long-term effects of FUZEON are unknown at this time. FUZEON therapy has not been shown to reduce the risk of transmitting HIV-1 to others through sexual contact or blood contamination.
- FUZEON must be taken as part of a combination antiretroviral regimen. Use of FUZEON alone may lead to rapid development of virus resistant to FUZEON and possibly other agents of the same class.
- Patients and caregivers must be instructed in the use of aseptic technique when administering FUZEON in order to avoid injection site infections. Appropriate training for FUZEON reconstitution and self-injection must be given by a healthcare provider, including a careful review of the FUZEON Patient Package Insert and FUZEON *Injection Instructions*. The first injection should be performed under the supervision of an appropriately qualified healthcare provider. It is recommended that the patient and/or caregiver's understanding and use of aseptic self-injection techniques and procedures be periodically re-evaluated.
- Patients should contact their healthcare provider for any questions regarding the administration of FUZEON. Patients should be told not to reuse needles or syringes, and be instructed in safe disposal procedures including the use of a puncture-resistant container for disposal of used needles and syringes. Patients must be instructed on the safe disposal of full containers as per local requirements. Caregivers who experience an accidental needlestick after patient injection should contact a healthcare provider immediately.
- Patients should inform their healthcare provider if they are pregnant, plan to become pregnant or become pregnant while taking this medication.
- Patients should inform their healthcare provider if they are breast-feeding.
- Patients should not change the dose or dosing schedule of FUZEON or any antiretroviral medication without consulting their healthcare provider.
- Patients should contact their healthcare provider immediately if they stop taking FUZEON or any other drug in their antiretroviral regimen.
- Patients should be told that they can obtain more information on the self-administration of FUZEON at www.FUZEON.com or by calling 1-877-4-FUZEON (1-877-438-9366).

Patients should be advised that no studies have been conducted on the ability to drive or operate machinery while taking FUZEON. If patients experience dizziness while taking FUZEON, they should be advised to talk to their healthcare provider before driving or operating machinery.

Drug Interactions
CYP450 Metabolized Drugs
Results from in vitro and in vivo studies suggest that enfuvirtide is unlikely to have significant drug interactions with concomitantly administered drugs metabolized by CYP450 enzymes (see CLINICAL PHARMACOLOGY).
Antiretroviral Agents
No drug interactions with other antiretroviral medications have been identified that would warrant alteration of either the enfuvirtide dose or the dose of the other antiretroviral medication.

Table 4 Summary of Individual Signs/Symptoms Characterizing Local Injection Site Reactions to Enfuvirtide in Studies T20-301 and T20-302 Combined (% of Subjects)

Event Category	N=663		
	Any Severity Grade	% of Events Comprising Grade 3 Reactions	% of Events Comprising Grade 4 Reactions
Pain/Discomfort[a]	95%	9%	0%
Induration[b]	89%	41%	16%
Erythema[c]	89%	22%	10%
Nodules and Cysts[d]	76%	26%	0%
Pruritus[e]	62%	4%	NA
Ecchymosis[f]	48%	8%	5%

[a] Grade 3 = severe pain requiring analgesics (or narcotic analgesics for ≤72 hours) and/or limiting usual activities; Grade 4 = severe pain requiring hospitalization or prolongation of hospitalization, resulting in death, or persistent or significant disability/incapacity, or life-threatening, or medically significant.
[b] Grade 3 = ≥25 mm but <50 mm; Grade 4 = ≥50 mm average diameter.
[c] Grade 3 = ≥50 mm but <85 mm average diameter; Grade 4 = ≥85 mm average diameter.
[d] Grade 3 = ≥3 cm; Grade 4 = if draining.
[e] Grade 3 = refractory to topical treatment or requiring oral or parenteral treatment; Grade 4 = not applicable.
[f] Grade 3 = >3 cm but ≤ 5 cm; Grade 4 = >5 cm.

Table 5 Percentage of Patients With Selected Treatment-Emergent Adverse Events* Reported in ≥2% of Adult Patients and Occurring More Frequently in Patients Treated With FUZEON (Pooled Studies T20-301/T20-302 at 24 Weeks)

Adverse Event (by System Organ Class)	FUZEON + Background Regimen	Background Regimen
	N=663	N=334
Nervous System Disorders		
Peripheral Neuropathy	8.9%	6.3%
Taste Disturbance	2.4%	1.5%
Psychiatric Disorders		
Insomnia	11.3%	8.7%
Depression	8.6%	7.2%
Anxiety	5.7%	3.0%
Respiratory, Thoracic, and Mediastinal Disorders		
Cough	7.4%	5.4%
Infections		
Sinusitis	6.2%	2.1%
Herpes Simplex	5.0%	3.9%
Skin Papilloma	4.2%	1.5%
Influenza	3.9%	1.8%
General		
Weight Decreased	6.5%	5.1%
Appetite Decreased	6.3%	2.4%
Asthenia	5.7%	4.2%
Anorexia	2.6%	1.8%
Influenza-like Illness	2.3%	0.9%
Skin and Subcutaneous Tissue Disorders		
Pruritus Nos	5.1%	4.2%
Musculoskeletal, Connective, Tissue, and Bone Disorders		
Myalgia	5.0%	2.4%
Gastrointestinal Disorders		
Constipation	3.9%	2.7%
Abdominal Pain Upper	3.0%	2.7%
Pancreatitis	2.4%	0.9%
Eye Disorders		
Conjunctivitis	2.4%	0.9%
Blood and Lymphatic System Disorders		
Lymphadenopathy	2.3%	0.3%

*Excludes Injection Site Reactions

Carcinogenesis, Mutagenesis, Impairment of Fertility
Carcinogenesis
Long-term animal carcinogenicity studies of enfuvirtide have not been conducted.
Mutagenesis
Enfuvirtide was neither mutagenic nor clastogenic in a series of in vivo and in vitro assays including the Ames bacterial reverse mutation assay, a mammalian cell forward gene mutation assay in AS52 Chinese Hamster ovary cells or an in vivo mouse micronucleus assay.
Impairment of Fertility
Enfuvirtide produced no adverse effects on fertility in male or female rats at doses of up to 30 mg/kg/day administered by subcutaneous injection (1.6 times the maximum recommended adult human daily dose on a m^2 basis).
Pregnancy
Pregnancy Category B. Reproduction studies have been performed in rats and rabbits at doses up to 27 times and 3.2 times the adult human dose on a m^2 basis. The animal studies revealed no evidence of harm to the fetus from enfuvirtide. There are no adequate and well-controlled studies in pregnant women. Because animal reproduction studies are not always predictive of human response, this drug should be used during pregnancy only if clearly needed.
Antiretroviral Pregnancy Registry
To monitor maternal-fetal outcomes of pregnant women exposed to FUZEON and other antiretroviral drugs, an Antiretroviral Pregnancy Registry has been established. Physicians are encouraged to register patients by calling 1-800-258-4263.
Nursing Mothers
The Centers for Disease Control and Prevention recommends that HIV- infected mothers not breast-feed their infants to avoid the risk of postnatal transmission of HIV. It is not known whether enfuvirtide is excreted in human milk. Because of both the potential for HIV transmission and the

potential for serious adverse reactions in nursing infants, mothers should be instructed not to breast-feed if they are receiving FUZEON.
Studies where radio-labeled ³H-enfuvirtide was administered to lactating rats indicated that radioactivity was present in the milk. It is not known whether the radioactivity in the milk was from radio-labeled enfuvirtide or from radio-labeled metabolites of enfuvirtide (ie, amino acids and peptide fragments).

Pediatric Use
The safety and pharmacokinetics of FUZEON have not been established in pediatric subjects below 6 years of age. Limited efficacy data is available in pediatric subjects 6 years of age and older.
Thirty-five HIV-1 infected pediatric subjects ages 6 through 16 years have received FUZEON in two open-label, single-arm clinical trials. Adverse experiences were similar to those observed in adult patients.
Study T20-204 was an open-label, multicenter trial that evaluated the safety, and antiviral activity of FUZEON in treatment-experienced pediatric subjects. Eleven subjects from 6 to 12 years were enrolled (median age of 9 years). Median baseline CD4 cell count was 509 cells/µL and the median baseline HIV-1 RNA was 4.5 $\log_{10}$ copies/mL.
Ten of the 11 study subjects completed 48 weeks of chronic therapy. By week 48, 6/11 (55%) subjects had ≥1 $\log_{10}$ decline in HIV-1 RNA and 4/11 (36%) subjects were below 400 copies/mL of HIV-1 RNA. The median changes from baseline in HIV-1 RNA and CD4 cell count were -1.48 $\log_{10}$ copies/mL and 122 cells/µL, respectively.
Study T20-310 is an ongoing, open-label, multicenter trial evaluating the pharmacokinetics, safety, and antiviral activity of FUZEON in treatment-experienced pediatric subjects and adolescents. Twenty-four subjects from 6 through 16 years were enrolled (median age of 13 years). Median baseline CD4 cell count was 143 cells/µL and the median baseline HIV-1 RNA was 5.0 $\log_{10}$ copies/mL. The evaluation of the antiviral activity is ongoing.

Geriatric Use
Clinical studies of FUZEON did not include sufficient numbers of subjects aged 65 and over to determine whether they respond differently from younger subjects.

ADVERSE REACTIONS
The overall safety profile of FUZEON is based on 1188 subjects who received at least 1 dose of FUZEON during various clinical trials. This includes 1153 adults, 608 of whom received the recommended dose for greater than 24 weeks, and 35 pediatric subjects.
Assessment of treatment-emergent adverse events is based on the pooled data from the two Phase 3 studies T20-301 and T20-302.

Local Injection Site Reactions
Local injection site reactions were the most frequent adverse events associated with the use of FUZEON. In Phase 3 clinical studies (T20-301 and T20-302), 98% of subjects had at least 1 local injection site reaction (ISR). Three percent of subjects discontinued treatment with FUZEON because of ISRs. Eighty-six percent of subjects experienced their first ISR during the initial week of treatment. The majority of ISRs were associated with mild to moderate pain at the injection site, erythema, induration, and the presence of nodules or cysts. For most subjects the severity of signs and symptoms associated with ISRs did not change during the 24 weeks of treatment. In 17% of subjects an individual ISR lasted for longer than 7 days. Because of the frequency and duration of individual ISRs, 23% of subjects had six or more ongoing ISRs at any given time. Individual signs and symptoms characterizing local ISRs are summarized in Table 4. Infection at the injection site (including abscess and cellulitis) was reported in 1% of subjects.
[See table 4 at top of previous page]

Other Adverse Events
Hypersensitivity reactions have been attributed to FUZEON (≤ 1%) and in some cases have recurred upon rechallenge (see WARNINGS).
The events most frequently reported in subjects receiving FUZEON+background regimen, excluding injection site reactions, were diarrhea (26.8%), nausea (20.1%), and fatigue (16.1%). These events were also commonly observed in subjects that received background regimen alone: diarrhea (33.5%), nausea (23.7%), and fatigue (17.4%).
Treatment-emergent adverse events (% of subjects), excluding ISRs, from Phase 3 studies are summarized for adult subjects, regardless of severity and causality, in Table 5. Only events occurring in ≥2% of subjects and at a higher rate in subjects treated with FUZEON are summarized in Table 5; events that occurred at a higher rate in the control arms are not displayed.
[See table 5 at top of previous page]
An increased rate of bacterial pneumonia was observed in subjects treated with FUZEON in the Phase 3 clinical trials compared to the control arm (4.68 pneumonia events per 100 patient-years versus 0.61 events per 100 patient-years, respectively). Approximately half of the study subjects with pneumonia required hospitalization. One subject death in the FUZEON arm was attributed to pneumonia. Risk factors for pneumonia included low initial CD4 lymphocyte count, high initial viral load, intravenous drug use, smoking, and a prior history of lung disease. It is unclear if the increased incidence of pneumonia was related to FUZEON use. However, because of this finding patients with HIV infection should be carefully monitored for signs and symptoms of pneumonia, especially if they have underlying conditions which may predispose them to pneumonia (see WARNINGS).

Less Common Events
The following adverse events have been reported in 1 or more subjects; however, a causal relationship to FUZEON has not been established.
Immune System Disorders: worsening abacavir hypersensitivity reaction
Renal and Urinary Disorders: renal insufficiency (glomerulonephritis); renal failure
Blood and Lymphatic Disorders: thrombocytopenia; neutropenia, and fever
Endocrine and Metabolic: hyperglycemia
Infections and Infestations: pneumonia
Nervous System Disorders: Guillain-Barre syndrome (fatal); sixth nerve palsy

Laboratory Abnormalities
Table 6 shows the treatment-emergent laboratory abnormalities that occurred in at least 2% of subjects and more frequently in those receiving FUZEON+background regimen than background regimen alone from studies T20-301 and T20-302.
[See table 6 above]

Adverse Events in Pediatric Patients
FUZEON has been studied in 35 pediatric subjects 6 through 16 years of age with duration of FUZEON exposure ranging from 1 dose to 48 weeks. Adverse experiences seen during clinical trials were similar to those observed in adult subjects.

OVERDOSAGE
There are no reports of human experience of acute overdose with FUZEON. The highest dose administered to 12 subjects in a clinical trial was 180 mg as a single dose subcutaneously. There is no specific antidote for overdose with FUZEON. Treatment of overdose should consist of general supportive measures.

Continued on next page

Table 6 Percentage of Treatment-Emergent Laboratory Abnormalities That Occurred in ≥2% of Adult Patients and More Frequently in Patients Receiving FUZEON (Pooled Studies T20-301 and T20-302 at 24 Weeks)

Laboratory Parameters	Grading	FUZEON + Background Regimen N=663	Background Regimen N=334
Eosinophilia			
1-2 X ULN (0.7×10^9/L)	0.7-1.4×10^9/L	8.3%	1.5%
>2 X ULN (0.7×10^9/L)	>1.4×10^9/L	1.8%	0.9%
Amylase (U/L)			
Gr. 3	>2-5 × ULN	6.2%	3.6%
Gr. 4	>5 × ULN or clinical pancreatitis	0.9%	0.6%
Lipase (U/L)			
Gr. 3	>2-5 × ULN	5.9%	3.6%
Gr. 4	>5 × ULN	2.3%	1.8%
Triglycerides (mmol/L)			
Gr. 3	>1000 mg/dL	8.9%	7.2%
ALT			
Gr. 3	>5-10 × ULN	3.5%	2.1%
Gr. 4	>10 × ULN	0.9%	0.6%
AST			
Gr. 3	>5-10 × ULN	3.6%	3.0%
Gr. 4	>10 × ULN	1.2%	0.6%
Creatine Phosphokinase (U/L)			
Gr. 3	>5-10 × ULN	5.9%	3.6%
Gr. 4	>10 × ULN	2.3%	3.6%
GGT (U/L)			
Gr. 3	>5-10 × ULN	3.5%	3.3%
Gr. 4	>10 × ULN	2.4%	1.8%
Hemoglobin (g/dL)			
Gr. 3	6.5-7.9 g/dL	1.5%	0.9%
Gr. 4	<6.5 g/dL	0.6%	0.6%

Table 7 Pediatric Dosing Guidelines

Weight		Dose per bid Injection (mg/dose)	Injection Volume (90 mg enfuvirtide per mL)
Kilograms (kg)	Pounds (lbs)		
11.0 to 15.5	24 to 34	27	0.3 mL
15.6 to 20.0	>34 to 44	36	0.4 mL
20.1 to 24.5	>44 to 54	45	0.5 mL
24.6 to 29.0	>54 to 64	54	0.6 mL
29.1 to 33.5	>64 to 74	63	0.7 mL
33.6 to 38.0	>74 to 84	72	0.8 mL
38.1 to 42.5	>84 to 94	81	0.9 mL
≥42.6	>94	90	1.0 mL

Fuzeon—Cont.

DOSAGE AND ADMINISTRATION
Adults
The recommended dose of FUZEON is 90 mg (1 mL) twice daily injected subcutaneously into the upper arm, anterior thigh or abdomen. Each injection should be given at a site different from the preceding injection site, and only where there is no current injection site reaction from an earlier dose. FUZEON should not be injected into moles, scar tissue, bruises or the navel. Additional detailed information regarding the administration of FUZEON is described in the FUZEON *Injection Instructions*.

Pediatric Patients
No data are available to establish a dose recommendation of FUZEON in pediatric patients below the age of 6 years. In pediatric patients 6 years through 16 years of age, the recommended dosage of FUZEON is 2 mg/kg twice daily up to a maximum dose of 90 mg twice daily injected subcutaneously into the upper arm, anterior thigh or abdomen. Each injection should be given at a site different from the preceding injection site and only where there is no current injection site reaction from an earlier dose. FUZEON should not be injected into moles, scar tissue, bruises or the navel. Table 7 contains dosing guidelines for FUZEON based on body weight. Weight should be monitored periodically and the FUZEON dose adjusted accordingly.
[See table 7 at top of previous page]

Directions for Use
For more detailed instructions, see FUZEON *Injection Instructions*.
Subcutaneous Administration
FUZEON must only be reconstituted with 1.1 mL of Sterile Water for Injection. After adding sterile water, the vial should be gently tapped for 10 seconds and then gently rolled between the hands to avoid foaming and to ensure all particles of drug are in contact with the liquid and no drug remains on the vial wall. The vial should then be allowed to stand until the powder goes completely into solution, which could take up to 45 minutes. Reconstitution time can be reduced by gently rolling the vial between the hands until the product is completely dissolved. Before the solution is withdrawn for administration, the vial should be inspected visually to ensure that the contents are fully dissolved in solution, and that the solution is clear, colorless and without bubbles or particulate matter. If there is evidence of particulate matter, the vial must not be used and should be returned to the pharmacy.

FUZEON contains no preservatives. Once reconstituted, FUZEON should be injected immediately or kept refrigerated in the original vial until use. Reconstituted FUZEON must be used within 24 hours. The subsequent dose of FUZEON can be reconstituted in advance and must be stored in the refrigerator in the original vial and used within 24 hours. Refrigerated reconstituted solution should be brought to room temperature before injection and the vial should be inspected visually again to ensure that the contents are fully dissolved in solution and that the solution is clear, colorless, and without bubbles or particulate matter.

The reconstituted solution should be injected subcutaneously in the upper arm, abdomen or anterior thigh. The injection should be given at a site different from the preceding injection site and only where there is no current injection site reaction. Also, do not inject into moles, scar tissue, bruises or the navel. A vial is suitable for single use only; unused portions must be discarded (see FUZEON *Injection Instructions*).

Patients should contact their healthcare provider for any questions regarding the administration of FUZEON. Information about the self-administration of FUZEON may also be obtained by calling the toll-free number 1-877-4-FUZEON (1-877-438-9366) or at the FUZEON website, www.FUZEON.com. Patients should be taught to recognize the signs and symptoms of injection site reactions and instructed when to contact their healthcare provider about these reactions.

HOW SUPPLIED
FUZEON (enfuvirtide) for Injection is a white to off-white, sterile, lyophilized powder and it is packaged in a single-use clear glass vial containing 108 mg of enfuvirtide for the delivery of approximately 90 mg/1 mL when reconstituted with 1.1 mL of Sterile Water for Injection.
FUZEON is available in a Convenience Kit containing 60 single-use vials (2 cartons of 30 each) of FUZEON (90 mg strength), 60 vials (2 cartons of 30 each) of Sterile Water for Injection (1.1 mL per vial), 60 reconstitution syringes (3 cc), 60 administration syringes (1 cc), alcohol wipes, Package Insert, Patient Package Insert, and Injection Instruction Guide (NDC 0004-0380-39).

Storage Conditions
Store at 25°C (77°F); excursions permitted to 15° to 30°C (59° to 86°F) [See USP Controlled Room Temperature].
Reconstituted solution should be stored under refrigeration at 2° to 8°C (36° to 46°F) and used within 24 hours.
Roche and FUZEON are trademarks of Hoffmann-La Roche Inc.
FUZEON has been jointly developed by Trimeris, Inc. and Hoffmann-La Roche Inc. FUZEON is manufactured by Hoffmann-La Roche Inc.

Distributed by:
Roche Pharmaceuticals
Roche Laboratories Inc.
340 Kingsland Street
Nutley, New Jersey 07110-1199
www.rocheusa.com
Licensed from:
Trimeris, Inc.
4727 University Drive
Durham, North Carolina 27707
www.trimeris.com

Issued: March 2003

PEGASYS®
[pĕg' ă sŭs]
(peginterferon alfa-2a)

℞

> Alpha interferons, including PEGASYS (peginterferon alfa-2a), may cause or aggravate fatal or life-threatening neuropsychiatric, autoimmune, ischemic, and infectious disorders. Patients should be monitored closely with periodic clinical and laboratory evaluations. Therapy should be withdrawn in patients with persistently severe or worsening signs or symptoms of these conditions. In many, but not all cases, these disorders resolve after stopping PEGASYS therapy (see **WARNINGS** and **ADVERSE REACTIONS**).
>
> Use with Ribavirin. Ribavirin, including COPEGUS™, may cause birth defects and/or death of the fetus. Extreme care must be taken to avoid pregnancy in female patients and in female partners of male patients. Ribavirin causes hemolytic anemia. The anemia associated with ribavirin therapy may result in a worsening of cardiac disease. Ribavirin is genotoxic and mutagenic and should be considered a potential carcinogen (see COPEGUS Package Insert for additional information and other **WARNINGS**).

DESCRIPTION
PEGASYS, peginterferon alfa-2a, is a covalent conjugate of recombinant alfa-2a interferon (approximate molecular weight [MW] 20,000 daltons) with a single branched bis-monomethoxy polyethylene glycol (PEG) chain (approximate MW 40,000 daltons). The PEG moiety is linked at a single site to the interferon alfa moiety via a stable amide bond to lysine. Peginterferon alfa-2a has an approximate molecular weight of 60,000 daltons. Interferon alfa-2a is produced using recombinant DNA technology in which a cloned human leukocyte interferon gene is inserted into and expressed in *Escherichia coli*.

Each vial contains approximately 1.2 mL of solution to deliver 1.0 mL of drug product. Subcutaneous (sc) administration of 1.0 mL delivers 180 µg of drug product (expressed as the amount of interferon alfa-2a), 8.0 mg sodium chloride, 0.05 mg polysorbate 80, 10.0 mg benzyl alcohol, 2.62 mg sodium acetate trihydrate, and 0.05 mg acetic acid. The solution is colorless to light yellow and the pH is 6.0 ± 0.01.

CLINICAL PHARMACOLOGY
Pharmacodynamics
Interferons bind to specific receptors on the cell surface initiating intracellular signaling via a complex cascade of protein-protein interactions leading to rapid activation of gene transcription. Interferon-stimulated genes modulate many biological effects including the inhibition of viral replication in infected cells, inhibition of cell proliferation, and immunomodulation. The clinical relevance of these in vitro activities is not known.
PEGASYS stimulates the production of effector proteins such as serum neopterin and 2', 5'-oligoadenylate synthetase.

Pharmacokinetics
Maximal serum concentrations (C_{max}) occur between 72 to 96 hours post-dose. The C_{max} and AUC measurements of PEGASYS increase in a dose-related manner. Week 48 mean trough concentrations (16 ng/mL; range 4 to 28) at 168 hours post-dose are approximately 2-fold higher than week 1 mean trough concentrations (8 ng/mL; range 0 to 15). Steady-state serum levels are reached within 5 to 8 weeks of once weekly dosing. The peak to trough ratio at week 48 is approximately 2.0.
The mean systemic clearance in healthy subjects given PEGASYS was 94 mL/h, which is approximately 100-fold lower than that for interferon alfa-2a (ROFERON®-A). The mean terminal half-life after sc dosing in patients with chronic hepatitis C was 80 hours (range 50 to 140 hours) compared to 5.1 hours (range 3.7 to 8.5 hours) for ROFERON®-A.

Special Populations
Gender and Age
PEGASYS administration yielded similar pharmacokinetics in male and female healthy subjects. The AUC was increased from 1295 to 1663 ng·h/mL in subjects older than 62 years taking 180 µg PEGASYS, but peak concentrations were similar (9 vs 10 ng/mL) in those older and younger than 62 years.
Pediatric Patients
The pharmacokinetics of PEGASYS have not been adequately studied in pediatric patients.

Renal Dysfunction
In patients with end stage renal disease undergoing hemodialysis, there is a 25% to 45% reduction in PEGASYS clearance (see **PRECAUTIONS: Renal Impairment**).
The pharmacokinetics of ribavirin following administration of COPEGUS have not been studied in patients with renal impairment and there are limited data from clinical trials on administration of COPEGUS in patients with creatinine clearance <50 mL/min. Therefore, patients with creatinine clearance <50 mL/min should not be treated with COPEGUS (see **WARNINGS** and **DOSAGE AND ADMINISTRATION**).
Effect of Food on Absorption of Ribavirin
Bioavailability of a single oral dose of ribavirin was increased by co-administration with a high-fat meal. The absorption was slowed (T_{max} was doubled) and the AUC_{0-192h} and C_{max} increased by 42% and 66%, respectively, when COPEGUS was taken with a high-fat meal compared with fasting conditions (see **DOSAGE AND ADMINISTRATION**).
Drug Interactions
Nucleoside Analogues
Ribavirin has been shown in vitro to inhibit phosphorylation of zidovudine and stavudine which could lead to decreased anti-retroviral activity. Exposure to didanosine or its active metabolite (dideoxyadenosine 5'-triphosphate) is increased when didanosine is co-administered with ribavirin (see **PRECAUTIONS: Drug Interactions**).

CLINICAL STUDIES
PEGASYS Monotherapy (Studies 1, 2, and 3)
The safety and effectiveness of PEGASYS for the treatment of hepatitis C virus infection were assessed in three randomized, open-label, active-controlled clinical studies. All patients were adults, had compensated liver disease, detectable hepatitis C virus (HCV), liver biopsy diagnosis of chronic hepatitis, and were previously untreated with interferon. All patients received therapy by sc injection for 48 weeks, and were followed for an additional 24 weeks to assess the durability of response. In studies 1 and 2, approximately 20% of subjects had cirrhosis or bridging fibrosis. Study 3 enrolled patients with a histological diagnosis of cirrhosis (78%) or bridging fibrosis (22%).

In study 1 (n=630), patients received either ROFERON-A (interferon alfa-2a) 3 MIU three times/week (tiw), PEGASYS 135 µg once each week (qw) or PEGASYS 180 µg qw. In study 2 (n=526), patients received either ROFERON-A 6 MIU tiw for 12 weeks followed by 3 MIU tiw for 36 weeks or PEGASYS 180 µg qw. In study 3 (n=269), patients received ROFERON-A 3 MIU tiw, PEGASYS 90 µg qw or PEGASYS 180 µg once each week.

In all three studies, treatment with PEGASYS 180 µg resulted in significantly more patients who experienced a sustained response (defined as undetectable HCV RNA and normalization of ALT on or after study week 68) compared to treatment with ROFERON-A. In study 1, response to PEGASYS 135 µg was not different from response to 180 µg. In study 3, response to PEGASYS 90 µg was intermediate between PEGASYS 180 µg and ROFERON-A.
[See table 1 at top of next page]

Matched pre- and post-treatment liver biopsies were obtained in approximately 70% of patients. Similar modest reductions in inflammation compared to baseline were observed in all treatment groups.

Of the patients who did not demonstrate either undetectable HCV RNA or at least a $2\log_{10}$ drop in HCV RNA titer from baseline by 12 weeks of PEGASYS 180 µg therapy, 2% (3/156) achieved a sustained virologic response (see **DOSAGE AND ADMINISTRATION**).

Averaged over study 1, study 2, and study 3, response rates to PEGASYS were 23% among patients with viral genotype 1 and 48% in patients with other viral genotypes. The treatment response rates were similar in men and women.

PEGASYS/COPEGUS Combination Therapy (Studies 4 and 5)
The safety and effectiveness of PEGASYS in combination with COPEGUS for the treatment of hepatitis C virus infection were assessed in two randomized controlled clinical trials. All patients were adults, had compensated liver disease, detectable hepatitis C virus, liver biopsy diagnosis of chronic hepatitis, and were previously untreated with interferon. Approximately 20% of patients in both studies had compensated cirrhosis (Child-Pugh class A).

In study 4, patients were randomized to receive either PEGASYS 180 µg sc once weekly (qw) with an oral placebo, PEGASYS 180 µg qw with COPEGUS 1000 mg po (body weight <75 kg) or 1200 mg po (body weight ≥ 75 kg) or REBETRON™ (interferon alfa-2b 3 MIU sc tiw plus ribavirin 1000 mg or 1200 mg po). All patients received 48 weeks of therapy followed by 24 weeks of treatment-free follow-up. COPEGUS or placebo treatment assignment was blinded. PEGASYS in combination with COPEGUS resulted in a higher SVR (defined as undetectable HCV RNA at the end of the 24-week treatment-free follow-up period) compared to PEGASYS alone or interferon alfa-2b and ribavirin (Table 2). In all treatment arms, patients with viral genotype 1 regardless of viral load, had a lower response rate.
[See table 2 at bottom of next page]

In study 5, all patients received PEGASYS 180 µg sc qw and were randomized to treatment for either 24 or 48 weeks and to a COPEGUS dose of either 800 mg or 1000 mg/1200 mg (for body weight <75 kg / ≥75 kg). Assignment to the four treatment arms was stratified by viral genotype and base-

Table 1 Sustained Response to Monotherapy Treatment

	Study 1			Study 2			Study 3		
	ROFERON-A 3 MIU (N=207)	PEGASYS 180 µg (N=208)	DIFF* (95% CI)	ROFERON-A 6/3 MIU (N=261)	PEGASYS 180 µg (N=265)	DIFF* (95% CI)	ROFERON-A 3 MIU (N=86)	PEGASYS 180 µg (N=87)	DIFF* (95% CI)
Combined Virologic and Biologic Sustained Response	11%	24%	13 (6, 20)	17%	35%	18 (11, 25)	7%	23%	16 (6, 26)
Sustained Virologic Response**	11%	26%	15 (8, 23)	19%	38%	19 (11, 26)	8%	30%	22 (11, 33)

* Percent difference between PEGASYS and Roferon-A treatment
** COBAS AMPLICOR® HCV Test, version 2.0

line HCV viral titer. Patients with genotype 1 and high viral titer (defined as $>2 \times 10^6$ HCV RNA copies/mL serum) were preferentially assigned to treatment for 48 weeks.

Genotype 1
Irrespective of baseline viral titer, treatment for 48 weeks with PEGASYS and 1000 mg or 1200 mg of COPEGUS resulted in higher SVR (defined as undetectable HCV RNA at the end of the 24-week treatment-free follow-up period) compared to shorter treatment (24 weeks) and/or 800 mg COPEGUS.

Genotype non-1
Irrespective of baseline viral titer, treatment for 24 weeks with PEGASYS and 800 mg of COPEGUS resulted in a similar SVR compared to longer treatment (48 weeks) and/or 1000 mg or 1200 mg of COPEGUS (see Table 3).
[See table 3 below]
Among the 36 patients with genotype 4, response rates were similar to those observed in patients with genotype 1 (data not shown). The numbers of patients with genotype 5 and 6 were too few to allow for meaningful assessment.

Treatment Response in Patient Subgroups
Treatment response rates are lower in patients with poor prognostic factors receiving pegylated interferon alpha therapy. In studies 4 and 5, treatment response rates were lower in patients older than 40 years (50% vs 66%), in patients with cirrhosis (47% vs 59%), in patients weighing over 85 kg (49% vs 60%), and in patients with genotype 1 with high vs low viral load (43% vs 56%). African American patients had lower response rates compared to Caucasians.
Paired liver biopsies were performed on approximately 20% of patients in studies 4 and 5. Modest reductions in inflammation compared to baseline were seen in all treatment groups.
In studies 4 and 5, lack of early virologic response at 12 weeks (defined as HCV RNA undetectable or $>2\log_{10}$ lower than baseline) was grounds for discontinuation of treatment. Of patients who lacked an early viral response at 12 weeks and completed a recommended course of therapy despite a protocol-defined option to discontinue therapy, 5/39 (13%) achieved an SVR. Of patients who lacked an early viral response at 24 weeks, nineteen completed a full course of therapy and none achieved an SVR.

INDICATIONS AND USAGE
PEGASYS, peginterferon alfa-2a, alone or in combination with COPEGUS, is indicated for the treatment of adults with chronic hepatitis C virus infection who have compensated liver disease and have not been previously treated with interferon alpha. Patients in whom efficacy was demonstrated included patients with compensated liver disease and histological evidence of cirrhosis (Child-Pugh class A).

CONTRAINDICATIONS
PEGASYS is contraindicated in patients with:
- hypersensitivity to PEGASYS or any of its components
- autoimmune hepatitis
- hepatic decompensation (Child-Pugh class B and C) before or during treatment

PEGASYS is contraindicated in neonates and infants because it contains benzyl alcohol. Benzyl alcohol is associated with an increased incidence of neurologic and other complications in neonates and infants, which are sometimes fatal. PEGASYS and COPEGUS combination therapy is additionally contraindicated in:
- Patients with known hypersensitivity to COPEGUS or to any component of the tablet.
- Women who are pregnant.
- Men whose female partners are pregnant.
- Patients with hemoglobinopathies (eg, thalassemia major, sickle-cell anemia).

WARNINGS
General
Patients should be monitored for the following serious conditions, some of which may become life threatening. Patients with persistently severe or worsening signs or symptoms should have their therapy withdrawn (see **BOXED WARNING**).

Neuropsychiatric
Life-threatening or fatal neuropsychiatric reactions may manifest in patients receiving therapy with PEGASYS and include suicide, suicidal ideation, depression, relapse of drug addiction, and drug overdose. These reactions may occur in patients with and without previous psychiatric illness.
PEGASYS should be used with extreme caution in patients who report a history of depression. Neuropsychiatric adverse events observed with alpha interferon treatment include aggressive behavior, psychoses, hallucinations, bipolar disorders, and mania. Physicians should monitor all patients for evidence of depression and other psychiatric symptoms. Patients should be advised to report any sign or symptom of depression or suicidal ideation to their prescribing physicians. In severe cases, therapy should be stopped immediately and psychiatric intervention instituted (see **ADVERSE REACTIONS** and **DOSAGE AND ADMINISTRATION**).

Infections
Serious and severe bacterial infections, some fatal, have been observed in patients treated with alpha interferons including PEGASYS. Some of the infections have been associated with neutropenia. PEGASYS should be discontinued in patients who develop severe infections and appropriate antibiotic therapy instituted.

Bone Marrow Toxicity
PEGASYS suppresses bone marrow function and may result in severe cytopenias. Ribavirin may potentiate the neutropenia and lymphopenia induced by alpha interferons including PEGASYS. Very rarely alpha interferons may be associated with aplastic anemia. It is advised that complete blood counts (CBC) be obtained pre-treatment and monitored routinely during therapy (see **PRECAUTIONS: Laboratory Tests**).
PEGASYS and COPEGUS should be used with caution in patients with baseline neutrophil counts <1500 cells/mm³, with baseline platelet counts <90,000 cells/mm³ or baseline hemoglobin <10 g/dL. PEGASYS therapy should be discontinued, at least temporarily, in patients who develop severe decreases in neutrophil and/or platelet counts (see **DOSAGE AND ADMINISTRATION: Dose Modifications**).

Cardiovascular Disorders
Hypertension, supraventricular arrhythmias, chest pain, and myocardial infarction have been observed in patients treated with PEGASYS.
PEGASYS should be administered with caution to patients with preexisting cardiac disease. Because cardiac disease may be worsened by ribavirin-induced anemia, patients with a history of significant or unstable cardiac disease should not use COPEGUS (see **WARNING: Anemia** and **COPEGUS Package Insert**).

Hypersensitivity
Severe acute hypersensitivity reactions (eg, urticaria, angioedema, bronchoconstriction, anaphylaxis) have been rarely observed during alpha interferon and ribavirin therapy. If such reaction occurs, therapy with PEGASYS and COPEGUS should be discontinued and appropriate medical therapy immediately instituted.

Endocrine Disorders
PEGASYS causes or aggravates hypothyroidism and hyperthyroidism. Hyperglycemia, hypoglycemia, and diabetes mellitus have been observed to develop in patients treated with PEGASYS. Patients with these conditions at baseline who cannot be effectively treated by medication should not begin PEGASYS therapy. Patients who develop these conditions during treatment and cannot be controlled with medication may require discontinuation of PEGASYS therapy.

Autoimmune Disorders
Development or exacerbation of autoimmune disorders including myositis, hepatitis, ITP, psoriasis, rheumatoid arthritis, interstitial nephritis, thyroiditis, and systemic lupus erythematosus have been reported in patients receiving alpha interferon. PEGASYS should be used with caution in patients with autoimmune disorders.

Pulmonary Disorders
Dyspnea, pulmonary infiltrates, pneumonia, bronchiolitis obliterans, interstitial pneumonitis and sarcoidosis, some resulting in respiratory failure and/or patient deaths, may be induced or aggravated by PEGASYS or alpha interferon therapy. Patients who develop persistent or unexplained pulmonary infiltrates or pulmonary function impairment should discontinue treatment with PEGASYS.

Colitis
Ulcerative, and hemorrhagic/ischemic colitis, sometimes fatal, have been observed within 12 weeks of starting alpha interferon treatment. Abdominal pain, bloody diarrhea, and fever are the typical manifestations of colitis. PEGASYS should be discontinued immediately if these symptoms develop. The colitis usually resolves within 1 to 3 weeks of discontinuation of alpha interferon.

Pancreatitis
Pancreatitis, sometimes fatal, has occurred during alpha interferon and ribavirin treatment. PEGASYS and COPEGUS should be suspended if symptoms or signs suggestive of pancreatitis are observed. PEGASYS and COPEGUS should be discontinued in patients diagnosed with pancreatitis.

Ophthalmologic Disorders
Decrease or loss of vision, retinopathy including macular edema, retinal artery or vein thrombosis, retinal hemorrhages and cotton wool spots, optic neuritis, and papilledema are induced or aggravated by treatment with PEGASYS or other alpha interferons. All patients should receive an eye examination at baseline. Patients with pre-existing ophthalmologic disorders (eg, diabetic or hypertensive retinopathy) should receive periodic ophthalmologic exams during interferon alpha treatment. Any patient who develops ocular symptoms should receive a prompt and complete eye examination. PEGASYS treatment should be discontinued in patients who develop new or worsening ophthalmologic disorders.

Use With Ribavirin (Also, see COPEGUS Package Insert.)
Ribavirin may cause birth defects and/or death of the exposed fetus. Extreme care must be taken to avoid pregnancy in female patients and in female partners of male patients taking PEGASYS and COPEGUS combination therapy. COPEGUS THERAPY SHOULD NOT BE STARTED UNLESS A REPORT OF A NEGATIVE PREGNANCY TEST HAS BEEN OBTAINED IMMEDIATELY PRIOR TO INITIATION OF THERAPY. Women of childbearing potential and men must use two forms of effective contraception during treatment and for at least six months after treatment has concluded. Routine monthly pregnancy tests must be performed during this time (see BOXED WARNING, CON-

Table 2 Sustained Virologic Response to Combination Therapy (Study 4)

	Interferon alfa-2b + Ribavirin 1000 mg or 1200 mg	PEGASYS + placebo	PEGASYS + COPEGUS 1000 mg or 1200 mg
All patients	197/444 (44%)	65/224 (29%)	241/453 (53%)
Genotype 1	103/285 (36%)	29/145 (20%)	132/298 (44%)
Genotypes 2-6	94/159 (59%)	36/79 (46%)	109/155 (70%)

Difference in overall treatment response (PEGASYS/COPEGUS − Interferon alfa-2b/ribavirin) was 9% (95% CI 2.3, 15.3).

Table 3 Sustained Virologic Response as a Function of Genotype (Study 5)

	24 Weeks Treatment		48 Weeks Treatment	
	PEGASYS + COPEGUS 800 mg (N=207)	PEGASYS + COPEGUS 1000 mg or 1200 mg* (N=280)	PEGASYS + COPEGUS 800 mg (N=361)	PEGASYS + COPEGUS 1000 mg or 1200 mg* (N=436)
Genotype 1	29/101 (29%)	48/118 (41%)	99/250 (40%)	138/271 (51%)
Genotype 2-3	79/96 (82%)	116/144 (81%)	75/99 (76%)	117/153 (76%)

*1000 mg for body weight <75 kg; 1200 mg for body weight ≥75 kg.

Continued on next page

Pegasys—Cont.

TRAINDICATIONS, PRECAUTIONS: Information for Patients, and COPEGUS Package Insert).

Anemia
The primary toxicity of ribavirin is hemolytic anemia. Hemoglobin <10 g/dL was observed in approximately 13% of COPEGUS and PEGASYS treated patients in clinical trials (see **PRECAUTIONS: Laboratory Tests**). The anemia associated with COPEGUS occurs within 1 to 2 weeks of initiation of therapy with maximum drop in hemoglobin observed during the first eight weeks. BECAUSE THE INITIAL DROP IN HEMOGLOBIN MAY BE SIGNIFICANT, IT IS ADVISED THAT HEMOGLOBIN OR HEMATOCRIT BE OBTAINED PRETREATMENT AND AT WEEK 2 AND WEEK 4 OF THERAPY OR MORE FREQUENTLY IF CLINICALLY INDICATED. Patients should then be followed as clinically appropriate.

Fatal and nonfatal myocardial infarctions have been reported in patients with anemia caused by ribavirin. Patients should be assessed for underlying cardiac disease before initiation of ribavirin therapy. Patients with pre-existing cardiac disease should have electrocardiograms administered before treatment, and should be appropriately monitored during therapy. If there is any deterioration of cardiovascular status, therapy should be suspended or discontinued (see **DOSAGE AND ADMINISTRATION: COPEGUS Dosage Modification Guidelines**). Because cardiac disease may be worsened by drug-induced anemia, patients with a history of significant or unstable cardiac disease should not use COPEGUS (see **COPEGUS Package Insert**).

Renal
It is recommended that renal function be evaluated in all patients started on COPEGUS. COPEGUS should not be administered to patients with creatinine clearance <50 mL/minute (see **CLINICAL PHARMACOLOGY: Special Populations**).

PRECAUTIONS

General
The safety and efficacy of PEGASYS alone or in combination with COPEGUS for the treatment of hepatitis C have not been established in:
- Patients who have failed other alpha interferon treatments
- Liver or other organ transplant recipients
- Patients co-infected with human immunodeficiency virus (HIV) or hepatitis B virus (HBV)

Renal Impairment
A 25% to 45% higher exposure to PEGASYS is seen in subjects undergoing hemodialysis. In patients with impaired renal function, signs and symptoms of interferon toxicity should be closely monitored. Doses of PEGASYS should be adjusted accordingly. PEGASYS should be used with caution in patients with creatinine clearance <50 mL/min (see **DOSAGE AND ADMINISTRATION: Dose Modifications**).

Information for Patients
Patients receiving PEGASYS alone or in combination with COPEGUS should be directed in its appropriate use, informed of the benefits and risks associated with treatment, and referred to the PEGASYS and, if applicable, COPEGUS (ribavirin) MEDICATION GUIDES.

PEGASYS and COPEGUS combination therapy must not be used by women who are pregnant or by men whose female partners are pregnant. COPEGUS therapy should not be initiated until a report of a negative pregnancy test has been obtained immediately before starting therapy. Female patients of childbearing potential and male patients with female partners of childbearing potential must be advised of the teratogenic/embryocidal risks and must be instructed to practice effective contraception during COPEGUS therapy and for 6 months post-therapy. Patients should be advised to notify the physician immediately in the event of a pregnancy (see **CONTRAINDICATIONS** and **WARNINGS**).

Women of childbearing potential and men must use two forms of effective contraception during treatment and during the 6 months after treatment has concluded; routine monthly pregnancy tests must be performed during this time (see **CONTRAINDICATIONS** and **COPEGUS Package Insert**).

If pregnancy does occur during treatment or during 6 months post-therapy, the patient must be advised of the significant teratogenic risk of COPEGUS therapy to the fetus. To monitor maternal-fetal outcomes of pregnant women exposed to COPEGUS, the COPEGUS Pregnancy Registry has been established. Physicians and patients are strongly encouraged to register by calling 1-800-526-6367.

Patients should be advised that laboratory evaluations are required before starting therapy and periodically thereafter (see **Laboratory Tests**). Patients should be instructed to remain well hydrated, especially during the initial stages of treatment. Patients should be advised to take COPEGUS with food.

Patients should be informed that it is not known if therapy with PEGASYS alone or in combination with COPEGUS will prevent transmission of HCV infection to others or prevent cirrhosis, liver failure or liver cancer that might result from HCV infection. Patients who develop dizziness, confusion, somnolence, and fatigue should be cautioned to avoid driving or operating machinery.

If home use is prescribed, a puncture-resistant container for the disposal of used needles and syringes should be supplied to the patients. Patients should be thoroughly instructed in the importance of proper disposal and cautioned against any reuse of any needles and syringes. The full container should be disposed of according to the directions provided by the physician (see **MEDICATION GUIDE**).

Laboratory Tests
Before beginning PEGASYS or PEGASYS and COPEGUS combination therapy, standard hematological and biochemical laboratory tests are recommended for all patients. Pregnancy screening for women of childbearing potential must be performed.

After initiation of therapy, hematological tests should be performed at 2 weeks and 4 weeks and biochemical tests should be performed at 4 weeks. Additional testing should be performed periodically during therapy. In the clinical studies, the CBC (including hemoglobin level and white blood cell and platelet counts) and chemistries (including liver function tests and uric acid) were measured at 1, 2, 4, 6, and 8, and then every 4 weeks or more frequently if abnormalities were found. Thyroid stimulating hormone (TSH) was measured every 12 weeks. Monthly pregnancy testing should be performed during combination therapy and for 6 months after discontinuing therapy.

The entrance criteria used for the clinical studies of PEGASYS may be considered as a guideline to acceptable baseline values for initiation of treatment:
- Platelet count ≥90,000 cells/mm^3 (as low as 75,000 cells/mm^3 in patients with cirrhosis)
- Caution should be exercised in initiating treatment in any patient with baseline risk of severe anemia (eg, spherocytosis, history of GI bleeding).
- Absolute neutrophil count (ANC) ≥1500 cells/mm^3
- Serum creatinine concentration <1.5 × upper limit of normal
- TSH and T$_4$ within normal limits or adequately controlled thyroid function

Table 4 Adverse Reactions Occurring in ≥5% of Patients in Hepatitis C Clinical Trials (Pooled Studies 1, 2, 3, and Study 4)

Body System	PEGASYS 180 μg 48 week†	ROFERON-A*†	PEGASYS 180 μg + 1000 mg or 1200 mg COPEGUS 48 week**	Intron A + 1000 mg or 1200 mg REBETOL® 48 week**
	N=559	N=554	N=451	N=443
	%	%	%	%
Application Site Disorders				
Injection site reaction	22	18	23	16
Endocrine Disorders				
Hypothyroidism	3	2	4	5
Flu-like Symptoms and Signs				
Fatigue/Asthenia	56	57	65	68
Pyrexia	37	41	41	55
Rigors	35	44	25	37
Pain	11	12	10	9
Gastrointestinal				
Nausea/Vomiting	24	33	25	29
Diarrhea	16	16	11	10
Abdominal pain	15	15	8	9
Dry mouth	6	3	4	7
Dyspepsia	<1	1	6	5
Hematologic‡				
Lymphopenia	3	5	14	12
Anemia	2	1	11	11
Neutropenia	21	8	27	8
Thrombocytopenia	5	2	5	<1
Metabolic and Nutritional				
Anorexia	17	17	24	26
Weight decrease	4	3	10	10
Musculoskeletal, Connective Tissue and Bone				
Myalgia	37	38	40	49
Arthralgia	28	29	22	23
Back pain	9	10	5	5
Neurological				
Headache	54	58	43	49
Dizziness (excluding vertigo)	16	12	14	14
Memory impairment	5	4	6	5
Psychiatric				
Irritability/Anxiety/Nervousness	19	22	33	38
Insomnia	19	23	30	37
Depression	18	19	20	28
Concentration impairment	8	10	10	13
Mood alteration	3	2	5	6
Resistance Mechanism Disorders				
Overall	10	6	12	10
Respiratory, Thoracic and Mediastinal				
Dyspnea	4	2	13	14
Cough	4	3	10	7
Dyspnea exertional	<1	<1	4	7
Skin and Subcutaneous Tissue				
Alopecia	23	30	28	33
Pruritus	12	8	19	18
Dermatitis	8	3	16	13
Dry skin	4	3	10	13
Rash	5	4	8	5
Sweating increased	6	7	6	5
Eczema	1	1	5	4
Visual Disorders				
Vision blurred	4	2	5	2

† Pooled studies 1, 2, and 3
* Either 3 MIU or 6/3 MIU of ROFERON-A
** Study 4
‡ Severe hematologic abnormalities

Table 5 PEGASYS and COPEGUS Dosing Recommendations

Genotype	PEGASYS Dose	COPEGUS Dose	Duration
Genotype 1, 4	180 μg	<75 kg = 1000 mg ≥75 kg = 1200 mg	48 weeks 48 weeks
Genotype 2, 3	180 μg	800 mg	24 weeks

Genotypes 2 & 3 showed no increased response to treatment beyond 24 weeks (see Table 3). Data on genotypes 5 and 6 are insufficient for dosing recommendations.

Table 6 PEGASYS Hematological Dose Modification Guidelines

Laboratory Values	PEGASYS Dose Reduction	Discontinue PEGASYS if:
ANC <750/mm^3	135 μg	ANC <500/mm^3, treatment should be suspended until ANC values return to more than 1000/mm^3. Reinstitute at 90 μg and monitor ANC
Platelet <50,000/mm^3	90 μg	Platelet count <25,000/mm^3

PEGASYS treatment was associated with decreases in WBC, ANC, lymphocytes and platelet counts often starting within the first 2 weeks of treatment (see **ADVERSE REACTIONS**). Dose reduction is recommended in patients with hematologic abnormalities (see **DOSAGE AND ADMINISTRATION: Dose Modifications**).

While fever is commonly caused by PEGASYS therapy, other causes of persistent fever must be ruled out, particularly in patients with neutropenia (see **WARNINGS: Infections**).

Transient elevations in ALT (2-fold to 5-fold above baseline) were observed in some patients receiving PEGASYS, and were not associated with deterioration of other liver function tests. When the increase in ALT levels is progressive despite dose reduction or is accompanied by increased bilirubin, PEGASYS therapy should be discontinued (see **DOSAGE AND ADMINISTRATION: Dose Modifications**).

Drug Interactions

Treatment with PEGASYS once weekly for 4 weeks in healthy subjects was associated with an inhibition of P450 1A2 and a 25% increase in theophylline AUC. Theophylline serum levels should be monitored and appropriate dose adjustments considered for patients given both theophylline and PEGASYS (see **PRECAUTIONS**). There was no effect on the pharmacokinetics of representative drugs metabolized by CYP 2C9, CYP 2C19, CYP 2D6 or CYP 3A4. In patients with chronic hepatitis C treated with PEGASYS in combination with COPEGUS, PEGASYS treatment did not affect ribavirin distribution or clearance.

Nucleoside Analogues

Didanosine

Co-administration of COPEGUS and didanosine is not recommended. Reports of fatal hepatic failure, as well as peripheral neuropathy, pancreatitis, and symptomatic hyperlactatemia/lactic acidosis have been reported in clinical trials (see **CLINICAL PHARMACOLOGY: Drug Interactions**).

Stavudine and Zidovudine

Ribavirin can antagonize the in vitro antiviral activity of stavudine and zidovudine against HIV. Therefore, concomitant use of ribavirin with either of these drugs should be avoided.

Carcinogenesis, Mutagenesis, Impairment of Fertility

Carcinogenesis

PEGASYS has not been tested for its carcinogenic potential.

Mutagenesis

PEGASYS did not cause DNA damage when tested in the Ames bacterial mutagenicity assay and in the in vitro chromosomal aberration assay in human lymphocytes, either in the presence or absence of metabolic activation.

Use With Ribavirin

Ribavirin is genotoxic and mutagenic. The carcinogenic potential of ribavirin has not been fully determined. In a p53 (+/-) mouse carcinogenicity study at doses up to the maximum tolerated dose of 100 mg/kg/day ribavirin was not oncogenic. However, on a body surface area basis, this dose was 0.5 times maximum recommended human 24-hour dose of ribavirin. A study in rats to assess the carcinogenic potential of ribavirin is ongoing.

Mutagenesis (see **COPEGUS Package Insert**)

Impairment of Fertility

PEGASYS may impair fertility in women. Prolonged menstrual cycles and/or amenorrhea were observed in female cynomolgus monkeys given sc injections of 600 μg/kg/dose (7200 μg/m^2/dose) of PEGASYS every other day for one month, at approximately 180 times the recommended weekly human dose for a 60 kg person (based on body surface area). Menstrual cycle irregularities were accompanied by both a decrease and delay in the peak 17β-estradiol and progesterone levels following administration of PEGASYS to female monkeys. A return to normal menstrual rhythm followed cessation of treatment. Every other day dosing with 100 μg/kg (1200 μg/m^2) PEGASYS (equivalent to approximately 30 times the recommended human dose) had no effects on cycle duration or reproductive hormone status.

The effects of PEGASYS on male fertility have not been studied. However, no adverse effects on fertility were observed in male Rhesus monkeys treated with non-pegylated interferon alfa-2a for 5 months at doses up to 25 × 10^6 IU/kg/day (see **COPEGUS Package Insert**).

Pregnancy

Pregnancy: Category C

PEGASYS has not been studied for its teratogenic effect. Non-pegylated interferon alfa-2a treatment of pregnant Rhesus monkeys at approximately 20 to 500 times the human weekly dose resulted in a statistically significant increase in abortions. No teratogenic effects were seen in the offspring delivered at term. PEGASYS should be assumed to have abortifacient potential. There are no adequate and well-controlled studies of PEGASYS in pregnant women. PEGASYS is to be used during pregnancy only if the potential benefit justifies the potential risk to the fetus. PEGASYS is recommended for use in women of childbearing potential only when they are using effective contraception during therapy.

Pregnancy: Category X: Use With Ribavirin (see CONTRAINDICATIONS)

Significant teratogenic and/or embryocidal effects have been demonstrated in all animal species exposed to ribavirin. COPEGUS therapy is contraindicated in women who are pregnant and in the male partners of women who are pregnant (see CONTRAINDICATIONS, WARNINGS, and COPEGUS Package Insert).

If pregnancy occurs in a patient or partner of a patient during treatment or during the 6 months after treatment cessation, such cases should be reported to the COPEGUS Pregnancy Registry at 1-800-526-6367.

Nursing Mothers

It is not known whether peginterferon or ribavirin or its components are excreted in human milk. The effect of orally ingested peginterferon or ribavirin from breast milk on the nursing infant has not been evaluated. Because of the potential for adverse reactions from the drugs in nursing infants, a decision must be made whether to discontinue nursing or discontinue PEGASYS and COPEGUS treatment.

Pediatric Use

The safety and effectiveness of PEGASYS, alone or in combination with COPEGUS in patients below the age of 18 years have not been established.

PEGASYS contains benzyl alcohol. Benzyl alcohol has been reported to be associated with an increased incidence of neurological and other complications in neonates and infants, which are sometimes fatal (see **CONTRAINDICATIONS**).

Geriatric Use

Younger patients have higher virologic response rates than older patients. Clinical studies of PEGASYS alone or in combination with COPEGUS did not include sufficient numbers of subjects aged 65 or over to determine whether they respond differently from younger subjects. Adverse reactions related to alpha interferons, such as CNS, cardiac, and systemic (eg, flu-like) effects may be more severe in the elderly and caution should be exercised in the use of PEGASYS in this population. PEGASYS and COPEGUS are excreted by the kidney, and the risk of toxic reactions to this therapy may be greater in patients with impaired renal function. Because elderly patients are more likely to have decreased renal function, care should be taken in dose selection and it may be useful to monitor renal function. PEGASYS should be used with caution in patients with creatinine clearance <50 mL/min and COPEGUS should not be administered to patients with creatinine clearance <50 mL/min.

ADVERSE REACTIONS

PEGASYS alone or in combination with COPEGUS causes a broad variety of serious adverse reactions (see **BOXED WARNING** and **WARNINGS**). In all studies, one or more serious adverse reactions occurred in 10% of patients receiving PEGASYS alone or in combination with COPEGUS.

The most common life-threatening or fatal events induced or aggravated by PEGASYS and COPEGUS were depression, suicide, relapse of drug abuse/overdose, and bacterial infections; each occurred at a frequency of <1%.

Nearly all patients in clinical trials experienced one or more adverse events. The most commonly reported adverse reactions were psychiatric reactions, including depression, irritability, anxiety, and flu-like symptoms such as fatigue, pyrexia, myalgia, headache, and rigors.

Overall 11% of patients receiving 48 weeks of therapy with PEGASYS either alone (7%) or in combination with COPEGUS (10%) discontinued therapy. The most common reasons for discontinuation of therapy were psychiatric, flu-like syndrome (eg, lethargy, fatigue, headache), dermatologic, and gastrointestinal disorders.

The most common reason for dose modification in patients receiving combination therapy was for laboratory abnormalities; neutropenia (20%) and thrombocytopenia (4%) for PEGASYS and anemia (22%) for COPEGUS.

PEGASYS dose was reduced in 12% of patients receiving 1000 mg to 1200 mg COPEGUS for 48 weeks and in 7% of patients receiving 800 mg COPEGUS for 24 weeks. COPEGUS dose was reduced in 21% of patients receiving 1000 mg to 1200 mg COPEGUS for 48 weeks and 12% in patients receiving 800 mg COPEGUS for 24 weeks.

Because clinical trials are conducted under widely varying and controlled conditions, adverse reaction rates observed in clinical trials of a drug cannot be directly compared to rates in the clinical trials of another drug. Also, the adverse event rates listed here may not predict the rates observed in a broader patient population in clinical practice.

[See table 4 at bottom of previous page]

Patients treated for 24 weeks with PEGASYS and 800 mg COPEGUS were observed to have lower incidence of serious adverse events (3% vs 10%), Hgb <10 g/dL (3% vs 15%), dose modification of PEGASYS (30% vs 36%) and COPEGUS (19% vs 38%) and of withdrawal from treatment (5% vs 15%) compared to patients treated for 48 weeks with PEGASYS and 1000 mg or 1200 mg COPEGUS. On the other hand the overall incidence of adverse events appeared to be similar in the two treatment groups.

The most common serious adverse event (3%) was bacterial infection (eg, sepsis, osteomyelitis, endocarditis, pyelonephritis, pneumonia). Other SAEs occurred at a frequency of <1% and included: suicide, suicidal ideation, psychosis, aggression, anxiety, drug abuse and drug overdose, angina, hepatic dysfunction, fatty liver, cholangitis, arrhythmia, diabetes mellitus, autoimmune phenomena (eg, hyperthyroidism, hypothyroidism, sarcoidosis, systemic lupus erythematosus, rheumatoid arthritis), peripheral neuropathy, aplastic anemia, peptic ulcer, gastrointestinal bleeding, pancreatitis, colitis, corneal ulcer, pulmonary embolism, coma, myositis, and cerebral hemorrhage.

Laboratory Test Values

Hemoglobin

The hemoglobin concentration decreased below 12 g/dL in 17% (median Hgb drop = 2.2 g/dL) of monotherapy and 52% (median Hgb drop = 3.7 g/dL) of combination therapy patients. Severe anemia (Hgb <10 g/dL) was encountered in 13% of patients receiving combination therapy and 2% of monotherapy recipients. Dose modification for anemia was required in 22% of ribavirin recipients treated for 48 weeks. Hemoglobin decreases in PEGASYS monotherapy were generally mild and did not require dose modification (see **DOSAGE AND ADMINISTRATION: Dose Modifications**).

Neutrophils

Decreases in neutrophil count below normal were observed in 95% of patients treated with PEGASYS either alone or in combination with COPEGUS. Severe potentially life-threatening neutropenia (ANC <0.5×10^9/L) occurred in approximately 5% of patients receiving PEGASYS either alone or in combination with COPEGUS. Seventeen percent of patients receiving PEGASYS monotherapy and 20% to 24% of patients receiving PEGASYS/COPEGUS combination therapy required modification of interferon dosage for neutropenia. Two percent of patients required permanent reductions of PEGASYS dosage and <1% required permanent discontinuation. Median neutrophil counts return to pretreatment levels 4 weeks after cessation of therapy (see **DOSAGE AND ADMINISTRATION: Dose Modifications**).

Lymphocytes

Decreases in lymphocyte count are induced by interferon alpha therapy. Lymphopenia was observed during both monotherapy (86%) and combination therapy with PEGASYS and COPEGUS (94%). Severe lymphopenia (<0.5×10^9/L) occurred in approximately 5% of monotherapy patients and 14% of combination PEGASYS and COPEGUS therapy recipients. Dose adjustments were not required by protocol. Median lymphocyte counts return to pre-treatment levels after 4 to 12 weeks of the cessation of therapy. The clinical significance of the lymphopenia is not known.

Platelets

Platelet counts decreased in 52% of patients treated with PEGASYS alone (median drop 45% from baseline), 33% of patients receiving combination with COPEGUS (median drop 30% from baseline). Median platelet counts return to pretreatment levels 4 weeks after the cessation of therapy.

Triglycerides

Triglyceride levels are elevated in patients receiving alfa interferon therapy and were elevated in the majority of patients participating in clinical studies receiving either PEGASYS alone or in combination with COPEGUS. Random levels higher ≥400 mg/dL were observed in about 20% of patients.

ALT Elevations

Less than 1% of patients experienced marked elevations (5- to 10-fold above baseline) in ALT levels during treatment. These transaminase elevations were on occasion associated with hyperbilirubinemia and were managed by dose reduction or discontinuation of study treatment. Liver function test abnormalities were generally transient. One case was attributed to autoimmune hepatitis, which persisted beyond study medication discontinuation (see **DOSAGE AND ADMINISTRATION: Dose Modifications**).

Continued on next page

Pegasys—Cont.

Thyroid Function
PEGASYS alone or in combination with COPEGUS was associated with the development of abnormalities in thyroid laboratory values, some with associated clinical manifestations. Hypothyroidism or hyperthyroidism requiring treatment, dose modification or discontinuation occurred in 4% and 1% of PEGASYS treated patients and 4% and 2% of PEGASYS and COPEGUS treated patients, respectively. Approximately half of the patients, who developed thyroid abnormalities during PEGASYS treatment, still had abnormalities during the follow-up period (see **PRECAUTIONS: Laboratory Tests**).

Immunogenicity
Nine percent (71/834) of patients treated with PEGASYS with or without COPEGUS developed binding antibodies to interferon alfa-2a, as assessed by an ELISA assay. Three percent of patients (25/835) receiving PEGASYS with or without COPEGUS, developed low-titer neutralizing antibodies (using an assay of a sensitivity of 100 INU/mL).
The clinical and pathological significance of the appearance of serum neutralizing antibodies is unknown. No apparent correlation of antibody development to clinical response or adverse events was observed. The percentage of patients whose test results were considered positive for antibodies is highly dependent on the sensitivity and specificity of the assays.
Additionally, the observed incidence of antibody positivity in these assays may be influenced by several factors including sample timing and handling, concomitant medications, and underlying disease. For these reasons, comparison of the incidence of antibodies to PEGASYS with the incidence of antibodies to these products may be misleading.

OVERDOSAGE
There is limited experience with overdosage. The maximum dose received by any patient was 7 times the intended dose of PEGASYS (180 μg/day for 7 days). There were no serious reactions attributed to overdosages. Weekly doses of up to 630 μg have been administered to patients with cancer. Dose-limiting toxicities were fatigue, elevated liver enzymes, neutropenia, and thrombocytopenia. There is no specific antidote for PEGASYS. Hemodialysis and peritoneal dialysis are not effective.

DOSAGE AND ADMINISTRATION
There are no safety and efficacy data on treatment for longer than 48 weeks. Consideration should be given to discontinuing therapy after 12 to 24 weeks of therapy if the patient has failed to demonstrate an early virologic response (see **CLINICAL STUDIES**).

PEGASYS
The recommended dose of PEGASYS monotherapy is 180 μg (1.0 mL) once weekly for 48 weeks by subcutaneous administration in the abdomen or thigh.

PEGASYS and COPEGUS COMBINATION
The recommended dose of PEGASYS when used in combination with ribavirin is 180 μg (1.0 mL) once weekly. The recommended dose of COPEGUS and duration for PEGASYS/COPEGUS therapy is based on viral genotype (see Table 5).

The daily dose of COPEGUS is 800 mg to 1200 mg administered orally in two divided doses. The dose should be individualized to the patient depending on baseline disease characteristics (eg, genotype), response to therapy, and tolerability of the regimen.
Since COPEGUS absorption increases when administered with a meal, patients are advised to take COPEGUS with food.
[See table at top of previous page]
A patient should self-inject PEGASYS only if the physician determines that it is appropriate and the patient agrees to medical follow-up as necessary and training in proper injection technique has been provided to him/her (see illustrated PEGASYS **MEDICATION GUIDE** for directions on injection site preparation and injection instructions).
PEGASYS should be inspected visually for particulate matter and discoloration before administration, and not used if particulate matter is visible or product is discolored. Vials with particulate matter or discoloration should be returned to the pharmacist.

Dose Modifications
If severe adverse reactions or laboratory abnormalities develop during combination COPEGUS/PEGASYS therapy, the dose should be modified or discontinued, if appropriate, until the adverse reactions abate. If intolerance persists after dose adjustment, COPEGUS/PEGASYS therapy should be discontinued.

PEGASYS
General
When dose modification is required for moderate to severe adverse reactions (clinical and/or laboratory), initial dose reduction to 135 μg (0.75 mL) is generally adequate. However, in some cases, dose reduction to 90 μg (0.5 mL) may be needed. Following improvement of the adverse reaction, re-escalation of the dose may be considered (see **WARNINGS, PRECAUTIONS**, and **ADVERSE REACTIONS**).

Hematological
[See table 6 at top of previous page]
Psychiatric: Depression
[See table 7 below]
Renal Function
In patients with end-stage renal disease requiring hemodialysis, dose reduction to 135 μg PEGASYS is recommended. Signs and symptoms of interferon toxicity should be closely monitored.
Liver Function
In patients with progressive ALT increases above baseline values, the dose of PEGASYS should be reduced to 135 μg. If ALT increases are progressive despite dose reduction or accompanied by increased bilirubin or evidence of hepatic decompensation, therapy should be immediately discontinued.

COPEGUS
[See table 8 below]
Once COPEGUS has been withheld due to a laboratory abnormality or clinical manifestation, an attempt may be made to restart COPEGUS at 600 mg daily and further increase the dose to 800 mg daily depending upon the physician's judgment. However, it is not recommended that COPEGUS be increased to the original dose (1000 mg or 1200 mg).

Renal Impairment
COPEGUS should not be used in patients with creatinine clearance <50 mL/min (see **WARNINGS** and **COPEGUS** Package Insert).

HOW SUPPLIED
Single Dose Vial
Each PEGASYS (peginterferon alfa-2a) 180 μg single use, clear glass vial provides 1.0 mL containing 180 μg peginterferon alfa-2a for sc injection. Each package contains 1 vial (NDC 0004-0350-09).
Monthly Convenience Pack
Four vials of PEGASYS (peginterferon alfa-2a), 180 μg single use, in a box with 4 syringes and 8 alcohol swabs (NDC 0004-0350-39). Each syringe is a 1 mL (1 cc) volume syringe supplied with a 27 gauge, ½ inch needle with needle-stick protection device.
Storage
Store in the refrigerator at 36° to 46°F (2° to 8°C). Do not freeze or shake. Protect from light. Vials are for single use only. Discard any unused portion.
REBETRON™ is a trademark of Schering Corporation.

Revised: December 2002

Romark Pharmaceuticals
A Division Of Romark Laboratories L.C.
6200 COURTNEY CAMPBELL CAUSEWAY
SUITE 880
TAMPA, FL 33607

For Medical Information:
Telephone: (813) 282-8544
Fax: (813) 282-4910

ALINIA™ ℞
(nitazoxanide)
for Oral Suspension
Rx Only

DESCRIPTION
Alinia™ for Oral Suspension contains the active ingredient, nitazoxanide, a synthetic antiprotozoal agent for oral administration. Nitazoxanide is a light yellow crystalline powder. It is poorly soluble in ethanol and practically insoluble in water. Chemically, nitazoxanide is 2-acetyloxy-N-(5-nitro-2-thiazolyl)benzamide. The molecular formula is $C_{12}H_9N_3O_5S$ and the molecular weight is 307.3. The structural formula is:

Alinia™ for Oral Suspension, after reconstitution, contains 100 mg nitazoxanide per 5 mL and the following inactive ingredients: sodium benzoate, sucrose, xanthan gum, microcrystalline cellulose and carboxymethylcellulose sodium, anhydrous citric acid, sodium citrate dihydrate, acacia gum, sugar syrup, FD&C Red #40 and natural strawberry flavoring.

CLINICAL PHARMACOLOGY
Absorption: Following oral administration of Alinia™ for Oral Suspension, maximum plasma concentrations of the active metabolites tizoxanide and tizoxanide glucuronide are observed within 1–4 hours. The parent nitazoxanide is not detected in plasma. Pharmacokinetic parameters of tizoxanide and tizoxanide glucuronide are shown in Table 1 below.
[See table 1 at top of next page]
No studies have been conducted to determine if the pharmacokinetics of tizoxanide and tizoxanide glucuronide differ in fasted versus fed subjects following administration of Alinia™ for Oral Suspension.
Distribution: In plasma, more than 99% of tizoxanide is bound to proteins.
Metabolism: Following oral administration in humans, nitazoxanide is rapidly hydrolyzed to an active metabolite, tizoxanide (desacetyl-nitazoxanide). Tizoxanide then undergoes conjugation, primarily by glucuronidation.
Elimination: Tizoxanide is excreted in the urine, bile and feces, and tizoxanide glucuronide is excreted in urine and bile.
Special Populations
Patients with Impaired Hepatic and/or Renal Function: The pharmacokinetics of nitazoxanide in patients with impaired hepatic and/or renal function has not been studied.
Pediatric Patients: The pharmacokinetics of nitazoxanide in pediatric patients less than one year of age has not been studied.

MICROBIOLOGY
Mechanism of action: The antiprotozoal activity of nitazoxanide is believed to be due to interference with the pyruvate:ferredoxin oxidoreductase (PFOR) enzyme-dependent electron transfer reaction which is essential to anaer-

---

Table 7 Guidelines for Modification or Discontinuation of PEGASYS and for Scheduling Visits for Patients with Depression

Depression Severity	Initial Management (4–8 weeks)		Depression		
	Dose modification	Visit schedule	Remains stable	Improves	Worsens
Mild	No change	Evaluate once weekly by visit and/or phone	Continue weekly visit schedule	Resume normal visit schedule	(See moderate or severe depression)
Moderate	Decrease PEGASYS dose to 135 μg (in some cases dose reduction to 90 μg may be needed)	Evaluate once weekly (office visit at least every other week)	Consider psychiatric consultation. Continue reduced dosing	If symptoms improve and are stable for 4 weeks, may resume normal visit schedule. Continue reduced dosing or return to normal dose	(See severe depression)
Severe	Discontinue PEGASYS permanently	Obtain immediate psychiatric consultation	Psychiatric therapy necessary		

Table 8 COPEGUS Dosage Modification Guidelines

Laboratory Values	Reduce Only COPEGUS Dose to 600 mg/day* if:	Discontinue COPEGUS if:
Hemoglobin in patients with no cardiac disease	<10 g/dL	<8.5 g/dL
Hemoglobin in patients with history of stable cardiac disease	≥2 g/dL decrease in hemoglobin during any 4 week period treatment	<12 g/dL despite 4 weeks at reduced dose

* One 200 mg tablet in the morning and two 200 mg tablets in the evening.

obic energy metabolism. Studies have shown that the PFOR enzyme from *Giardia lamblia* directly reduces nitazoxanide by transfer of electrons in the absence of ferredoxin. The DNA-derived PFOR protein sequence of *Cryptosporidium parvum* appears to be similar to that of *Giardia lamblia*. Interference with the PFOR enzyme-dependent electron transfer reaction may not be the only pathway by which nitazoxanide exhibits antiprotozoal activity.

Activity *in vitro* and *in vivo*

Nitazoxanide and its metabolite, tizoxanide, are active in vitro in inhibiting the growth of (i) sporozoites and oocysts of *Cryptosporidium parvum* and (ii) trophozoites of *Giardia lamblia*.

Alinia™ for Oral Suspension is effective in pediatric patients with *Cryptosporidium parvum* or *Giardia lamblia* infection (see INDICATIONS AND USAGE and CLINICAL STUDIES).

Drug Resistance

A potential for development of resistance by *Cryptosporidium parvum* or *Giardia lamblia* to nitazoxanide has not been examined.

Susceptibility Tests

For protozoa such as *Cryptosporidium parvum* and *Giardia lamblia*, standardized tests for use in clinical microbiology laboratories are not available.

INDICATIONS AND USAGE

Alinia™ for Oral Suspension is indicated for the treatment of diarrhea caused by *Cryptosporidium parvum* and *Giardia lamblia* in pediatric patients 1 through 11 years of age. Safety and effectiveness of Alinia™ for Oral Suspension have not been established in HIV-positive patients or patients with immunodeficiency. (See CLINICAL STUDIES). Safety and effectiveness of Alinia™ for Oral Suspension in pediatric patients less than one year of age, pediatric patients greater than 11 years of age and adults have not been studied.

CONTRAINDICATIONS

Nitazoxanide is contraindicated in patients with a prior hypersensitivity to nitazoxanide.

PRECAUTIONS

General: The pharmacokinetics of nitazoxanide in patients with compromised renal or hepatic function have not been studied. Therefore, nitazoxanide must be administered with caution to patients with hepatic and biliary disease, to patients with renal disease and to patients with combined renal and hepatic disease.

Information for Patients

Alinia™ for Oral Suspension should be taken with food. Diabetic patients and caregivers should be aware that the oral suspension contains 1.48 grams of sucrose per 5 mL.

Drug Interactions

Tizoxanide is highly bound to plasma protein (>99.9%). Therefore, caution should be used when administering nitazoxanide concurrently with other highly plasma protein-bound drugs with narrow therapeutic indices, as competition for binding sites may occur.

No interactions with other medicinal products have been reported by patients using nitazoxanide. However, no clinical studies have been conducted to specifically exclude the possibility of interactions between nitazoxanide and other medicinal products.

Carcinogenesis, Mutagenesis, Impairment of Fertility

Long-term carcinogenicity studies have not been conducted. Nitazoxanide was not genotoxic in the Chinese hamster ovary (CHO) cell chromosomal aberration assay or the mouse micronucleus assay. Nitazoxanide was genotoxic in one tester strain (TA 100) in the Ames bacterial mutagenicity assay.

Nitazoxanide did not adversely affect male or female fertility in the rat at 2400 mg/kg/day (approximately 66 times the recommended dose of patients 11 years of age, adjusted for body surface area).

Pregnancy

Teratogenic Effects

Pregnancy Category B:

Reproduction studies have been performed at doses up to 3200 mg/kg/day in rats (approximately 48 times the clinical dose adjusted for body surface area) and 100 mg/kg/day in rabbits (approximately 3 times the clinical dose adjusted for body surface area) and have revealed no evidence of impaired fertility or harm to the fetus due to nitazoxanide. There are, however, no adequate and well-controlled studies in pregnant women.

Nursing Mothers

It is not known whether nitazoxanide is excreted in human milk. Because many drugs are excreted in human milk, caution should be exercised when nitazoxanide is administered to a nursing woman.

Pediatric Use

Safety and effectiveness of Alinia™ for Oral Suspension in pediatric patients less than one year of age or greater than 11 years of age have not been studied.

Adults and Geriatrics

Safety and effectiveness of Alinia™ for Oral Suspension in adult and geriatric patients have not been studied.

HIV-Positive Patients

Safety and effectiveness of Alinia™ for Oral Suspension in HIV-positive patients have not been established.

Immunodeficient Patients

Safety and effectiveness of Alinia™ for Oral Suspension in immunodeficient patients have not been established.

Table 1. Mean (±SD) plasma pharmacokinetic parameter values following administration of a single dose of Alinia™ for Oral Suspension with food to pediatric subjects

		Tizoxanide			Tizoxanide glucuronide		
Age	Dose*	C_{max} (μg/mL)	T_{max}** (hr)	AUC_{inf} (μg•hr/mL)	C_{max} (μg/mL)	T_{max} (hr)	AUC_{inf} (μg•hr/mL)
12–47 months	100mg	3.11 (2.0)	3.5 (2–4)	11.7 (4.46)	3.64 (1.16)	4.0 (3–4)	19.0 (5.03)
4–11 years	200mg	3.00 (0.99)	2.0 (1–4)	13.5 (3.3)	2.84 (0.97)	4.0 (2–4)	16.9 (5.00)

*Dose: 100 mg/5 mL nitazoxanide, 200 mg/10 mL nitazoxanide

**T_{max} is given as Mean (Range)

Pediatric Patients with Diarrhea Caused by *Cryptosporidium parvum* Clinical Response Rates 3 to 7 Days Post-therapy, Intent-to-Treat Analyses

% (Number of Successes/Total)

Population	Nitazoxanide*	Placebo
Outpatient Study, age 1–11 years	88% (21/24)	38% (9/24)
Inpatient Study, Malnourished¶ age 12–35 months	56% (14/25)	23% (5/22)

*Clinical response rates statistically significantly higher compared to placebo.

¶60% considered severely underweight, 19% moderately underweight, 17% mild underweight.

Pediatric Patients with Diarrhea Caused by *Giardia lamblia* Clinical Response Rates 7 to 10 Days Following Initiation of Therapy Intent-to-Treat and Per Protocol Analyses

% (Number of Successes/Total) [95% Confidence Interval]

Population	Nitazoxanide (3 days)	Metronidazole (5 days)	95% *CI* Diff§
Intent-to-treat analysis†	85% (47/55)	80% (44/55)	[−9%, 20%]
Per protocol analysis¶	90% (43/48)	83% (39/47)	[−8%, 21%]

†Intent-to-treat analysis includes all patients randomized with patients not completing the study treated as failures.

¶Per protocol analysis includes only patients who took all of their medication and completed the study. Seven patients in each treatment group missed at least one dose of medication and one in the metronidazole treatment group was lost to follow-up.

§95% Confidence Interval on the difference in response rates (nitazoxanide-metronidazole).

ADVERSE REACTIONS

In controlled and uncontrolled clinical studies of 613 HIV-negative pediatric patients who received Alinia™ for Oral Suspension, the most frequent adverse events reported regardless of causality assessment were: abdominal pain (7.8%), diarrhea (2.1%), vomiting (1.1%) and headache (1.1%). These were typically mild and transient in nature. In placebo-controlled clinical trials, the rates of occurrence of these events did not differ significantly from those of the placebo. None of the 613 pediatric patients discontinued therapy because of adverse events.

Adverse events occurring in less than 1% of the patients participating in clinical trials are listed below:

Digestive System: nausea, anorexia, flatulence, appetite increase, enlarged salivary glands.

Body as a Whole: fever, infection, malaise.

Metabolic & Nutrition: increased creatinine, increased SGPT.

Skin: pruritus, sweat.

Special Senses: eye discoloration (pale yellow).

Respiratory System: rhinitis.

Nervous System: dizziness.

Urogenital System: discolored urine.

OVERDOSAGE

Information on nitazoxanide overdosage is not available. In acute studies in rodents and dogs, the oral LD_{50} was higher than 10,000 mg/kg. Single oral doses of up to 4000 mg nitazoxanide in a tablet formulation have been administered to healthy adult volunteers without significant adverse effects. In the event of overdose, gastric lavage may be appropriate soon after oral administration. Patients should be carefully observed and given symptomatic and supportive treatment.

DOSAGE & ADMINISTRATION

Age 12–47 months: 5 mL (100 mg nitazoxanide) every 12 hours for 3 days.

Age 4–11 years: 10 mL (200 mg nitazoxanide) every 12 hours for 3 days.

The oral suspension should be taken with food.

DIRECTIONS FOR MIXING ALINIA™ FOR ORAL SUSPENSION

Prepare a suspension at time of dispensing as follows: The amount of water required for preparation of the suspension is 48 mL. Tap bottle until all powder flows freely. Add approximately one-half of the total amount of water required for reconstitution and shake vigorously to suspend powder. Add remainder of water and again shake vigorously.

The container should be kept tightly closed, and the suspension should be shaken well before each administration. The suspension may be stored for 7 days, after which any unused portion must be discarded.

HOW SUPPLIED

Alinia™ for Oral Suspension is a pink-colored powder formulation that, when reconstituted as directed, contains 100 mg nitazoxanide/5 mL. The reconstituted suspension has a pink color and strawberry flavor. Alinia™ for Oral Suspension is available as: 60 mL bottle. **NDC 67546-212-21**

Storage and Stability: Store the unsuspended powder and the reconstituted oral suspension at 25°C (77°F); excursions permitted to 15–30°C (59–86°F). [See USP Controlled Room Temperature]

CLINICAL STUDIES

Cryptosporidium parvum

In two double-blind, controlled studies in pediatric patients with diarrhea caused by *Cryptosporidium parvum*, a three-day course of treatment with nitazoxanide (100 mg BID in pediatric patients ages 12–47 months, 200 mg BID in pediatric patients ages 4 through 11 years) was compared with a placebo. One study was conducted in Egypt in outpatients ages 1 through 11 years with diarrhea caused by *C. parvum*. Another study was conducted in Zambia in malnourished pediatric patients admitted to the hospital with diarrhea caused by *C. parvum*. Clinical response was evaluated 3 to 7 days post-therapy with a 'well' response defined as 'no symptoms, no watery stools and no more than 2 soft stools with no hematochezia within the past 24 hours' or 'no symptoms and no unformed stools within the past 48 hours.' The following clinical response rates were obtained:

[See second table above]

Another double-blind, placebo-controlled study was conducted in hospitalized, severely malnourished pediatric patients with acquired immune deficiency syndrome (AIDS) in Zambia. In this study, a three-day course of nitazoxanide suspension (100 mg BID in pediatric patients ages 12–47 months, 200 mg BID in pediatric patients ages 4 through 11 years) did not produce clinical cure rates that were significantly different from the placebo control.

Giardia lamblia

In a randomized, controlled study conducted in Peru in 110 pediatric patients with diarrhea caused by *Giardia lamblia*, a three-day course of treatment with nitazoxanide (100 mg BID in pediatric patients ages 24–47 months, 200 mg BID in pediatric patients ages 4 through 11 years) was compared to a five-day course of treatment with metronidazole (125 mg BID in pediatric patients ages 2 through 5 years, 250 mg BID in pediatric patients ages 6 through 11 years). Clinical response was evaluated 7 to 10 days following initiation of treatment with a 'well' response defined as 'no symptoms, no watery stools and no more than 2 soft stools with no hematochezia within the past 24 hours' or 'no symptoms and no unformed stools within the past 48 hours.' The following clinical cure rates were obtained:

[See third table above]

DATE OF ISSUANCE November 2002

Romark Pharmaceuticals

A Division of Romark Laboratories, L.C.

Tampa, FL 33607 USA

US Patents No. 5,578,621; 6,020,353; 5,968,961; 5,387,598; 6,117,894; 5,856,348; 5,859,138; 5,886,013; 5,965,590.

To keep your **PDR** up to date throughout the year, note these revisions on the corresponding pages of the annual volume. Simply write **"See Supplement A"** next to the product heading.

Schering Corporation
a wholly-owned subsidiary of Schering-Plough Corporation
2000 GALLOPING HILL ROAD
KENILWORTH, NJ 07033

Direct Inquiries to:
(908) 298-4000
CUSTOMER SERVICE:
(800) 222-7579
FAX: (908) 820-6400

For Medical Information Contact:
Schering Laboratories
Drug Information Services
2000 Galloping Hill Road
Kenilworth, NJ 07033
(800) 526-4099
FAX: (908) 298-2188

IMDUR® ℞
[*ĭm′dûr*]
(isosorbide mononitrate)
Extended Release Tablets

DESCRIPTION
Isosorbide mononitrate (ISMN), an organic nitrate and the major biologically active metabolite of isosorbide dinitrate (ISDN), is a vasodilator with effects on both arteries and veins.
IMDUR® Tablets contain 30 mg, 60 mg, or 120 mg of isosorbide mononitrate in an extended-release formulation. The inactive ingredients are aluminum silicate, colloidal silicon dioxide, hydroxypropyl cellulose, hydroxypropyl methylcellulose, iron oxide, magnesium stearate, paraffin wax, polyethylene glycol, titanium dioxide, and trace amounts of ethanol.
The chemical name for ISMN is 1,4:3,6-dianhydro-, D-glucitol 5-nitrate; the compound has the following structural formula:

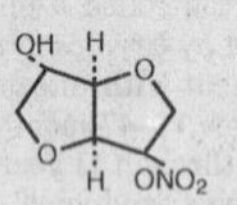

ISMN is a white, crystalline, odorless compound which is stable in air and in solution, has a melting point of about 90°C, and an optical rotation of +144° (2% in water, 20°C). Isosorbide mononitrate is freely soluble in water, ethanol, methanol, chloroform, ethyl acetate, and dichloromethane.

CLINICAL PHARMACOLOGY
Mechanism of Action: The IMDUR product is an oral extended-release formulation of ISMN, the major active metabolite of isosorbide dinitrate; most of the clinical activity of the dinitrate is attributable to the mononitrate.
The principal pharmacological action of ISMN and all organic nitrates in general is relaxation of vascular smooth muscle, producing dilatation of peripheral arteries and veins, especially the latter. Dilatation of the veins promotes peripheral pooling of blood and decreases venous return to the heart, thereby reducing left ventricular end-diastolic pressure and pulmonary capillary wedge pressure (preload). Arteriolar relaxation reduces systemic vascular resistance, and systolic arterial pressure and mean arterial pressure (afterload). Dilatation of the coronary arteries also occurs. The relative importance of preload reduction, afterload reduction, and coronary dilatation remains undefined.
Pharmacodynamics:
Dosing regimens for most chronically used drugs are designed to provide plasma concentrations that are continuously greater than a minimally effective concentration. This strategy is inappropriate for organic nitrates. Several well-controlled clinical trials have used exercise testing to assess the antianginal efficacy of continuously delivered nitrates. In the large majority of these trials, active agents were indistinguishable from placebo after 24 hours (or less) of continuous therapy. Attempts to overcome tolerance by dose escalation, even to doses far in excess of those used acutely, have consistently failed. Only after nitrates have been absent from the body for several hours has their antianginal efficacy been restored. IMDUR Tablets during long-term use over 42 days dosed at 120 mg once daily continued to improve exercise performance at 4 hours and at 12 hours after dosing, but its effects (although better than placebo) are less than or, at best, equal to the effects of the first dose of 60 mg.
Pharmacokinetics and Metabolism:
After oral administration of ISMN as a solution or immediate-release tablets, maximum plasma concentrations of ISMN are achieved in 30 to 60 minutes, with an absolute bioavailability of approximately 100%. After intravenous administration, ISMN is distributed into total body water in about 9 minutes with a volume of distribution of approximately 0.6 to 0.7 L/kg. Isosorbide mononitrate is approximately 5% bound to human plasma proteins and is distributed into blood cells and saliva. Isosorbide mononitrate is primarily metabolized by the liver, but unlike oral isosorbide dinitrate, it is not subject to first-pass metabolism. Isosorbide mononitrate is cleared by denitration to isosorbide and glucuronidation as the mononitrate, with 96% of the administered dose excreted in the urine within 5 days and only about 1% eliminated in the feces. At least six different compounds have been detected in urine, with about 2% of the dose excreted as the unchanged drug and at least five metabolites. The metabolites are not pharmacologically active. Renal clearance accounts for only about 4% of total body clearance. The mean plasma elimination half-life of ISMN is approximately 5 hours.
The disposition of ISMN in patients with various degrees of renal insufficiency, liver cirrhosis, or cardiac dysfunction was evaluated and found to be similar to that observed in healthy subjects. The elimination half-life of ISMN was not prolonged, and there was no drug accumulation in patients with chronic renal failure after multiple oral dosing.
The pharmacokinetics and/or bioavailability of IMDUR Tablets have been studied in both normal volunteers and patients following single- and multiple-dose administration. Data from these studies suggest that the pharmacokinetics of ISMN administered as IMDUR Tablets are similar between normal healthy volunteers and patients with angina pectoris. In single- and multiple-dose studies, the pharmacokinetics of ISMN were dose proportional between 30 mg and 240 mg.
In a multiple-dose study, the effect of age on the pharmacokinetic profile of IMDUR 60 mg and 120 mg (2 × 60 mg) Tablets was evaluated in subjects ≥45 years. The results of that study indicate that there are no significant differences in any of the pharmacokinetic variables of ISMN between elderly (≥65 years) and younger individuals (45-64 years) for the IMDUR 60-mg dose. The administration of IMDUR Tablets 120 mg (2 × 60 mg tablets every 24 hours for 7 days) produced a dose-proportional increase in C_{max} and AUC, without changes in T_{max} or the terminal half-life. The older group (65-74 years) showed 30% lower apparent oral clearance (Cl/F) following the higher dose, ie, 120 mg, compared to the younger group (45-64 years); Cl/F was not different between the two groups following the 60-mg regimen. While Cl/F was independent of dose in the younger group, the older group showed slightly lower Cl/F following the 120-mg regimen compared to the 60-mg regimen. Differences between the two age groups, however, were not statistically significant. In the same study, females showed a slight (15%) reduction in clearance when the dose was increased. Females showed higher AUCs and C_{max} compared to males, but these differences were accounted for by differences in body weight between the two groups. When the data were analyzed using age as a variable, the results indicated that there were no significant differences in any of the pharmacokinetic variables of ISMN between older (≥65 years) and younger individuals (45-64 years). The results of this study, however, should be viewed with caution due to the small numbers of subjects in each age subgroup and consequently the lack of sufficient statistical power.
The following table summarizes key pharmacokinetic parameters of ISMN after single- and multiple-dose administration of ISMN as an oral solution or IMDUR Tablets:
[See table below]
Food Effects:
The influence of food on the bioavailability of ISMN after single-dose administration of IMDUR Tablets 60 mg was evaluated in three different studies involving either a "light" breakfast or a high-calorie, high-fat breakfast. Results of these studies indicate that concomitant food intake may decrease the rate (increase in T_{max}) but not the extent (AUC) of absorption of ISMN.

CLINICAL TRIALS
Controlled trials with IMDUR Tablets have demonstrated antianginal activity following acute and chronic dosing. Administration of IMDUR Tablets once daily, taken early in the morning on arising, provided at least 12 hours of antianginal activity.
In a placebo-control parallel study, 30, 60, 120, and 240 mg of IMDUR Tablets were administered once daily for up to 6 weeks. Prior to randomization, all patients completed a 1- to 3-week single-blind placebo phase to demonstrate nitrate responsiveness and total exercise treadmill time reproducibility. Exercise tolerance tests using the Bruce Protocol were conducted prior to and at 4 and 12 hours after the morning dose on days 1, 7, 14, 28, and 42 of the double-blind period. IMDUR Tablets 30 and 60 mg (only doses evaluated acutely) demonstrated a significant increase from baseline in total treadmill time relative to placebo at 4 and 12 hours after the administration of the first dose. At day 42, the 120- and 240-mg dose of IMDUR Tablets demonstrated a significant increase in total treadmill time at 4 and 12 hours post-dosing, but by day 42, the 30- and 60-mg doses no longer were differentiable from placebo. Throughout chronic dosing, rebound was not observed in any IMDUR treatment group.
Pooled data from two other trials, comparing IMDUR Tablets 60 mg once daily, ISDN 30 mg QID, and placebo QID in patients with chronic stable angina using a randomized, double-blind, three-way crossover design found statistically significant increases in exercise tolerance times for IMDUR Tablets compared to placebo at hours 4, 8, and 12 and to ISDN at hour 4. The increases in exercise tolerance on day 14, although statistically significant compared to placebo, were about half of that seen on day 1 of the trial.

INDICATIONS AND USAGE
IMDUR Tablets are indicated for the prevention of angina pectoris due to coronary artery disease. The onset of action of oral isosorbide mononitrate is not sufficiently rapid for this product to be useful in aborting an acute anginal episode.

CONTRAINDICATIONS
IMDUR Tablets are contraindicated in patients who have shown hypersensitivity or idiosyncratic reactions to other nitrates or nitrites.

WARNINGS
Amplification of the vasodilatory effects of IMDUR by sildenafil can result in severe hypotension. The time course and dose dependence of this interaction have not been studied. Appropriate supportive care has not been studied, but it seems reasonable to treat this as a nitrate overdose, with elevation of the extremities and with central volume expansion.
The benefits of ISMN in patients with acute myocardial infarction or congestive heart failure have not been established. Because the effects of isosorbide mononitrate are difficult to terminate rapidly, this drug is not recommended in these settings.
If isosorbide mononitrate is used in these conditions, careful clinical or hemodynamic monitoring must be used to avoid the hazards of hypotension and tachycardia.

PRECAUTIONS
General: Severe hypotension, particularly with upright posture, may occur with even small doses of isosorbide mononitrate. This drug should therefore be used with caution in patients who may be volume depleted or who, for whatever reason, are already hypotensive. Hypotension induced by isosorbide mononitrate may be accompanied by paradoxical bradycardia and increased angina pectoris.
Nitrate therapy may aggravate the angina caused by hypertrophic cardiomyopathy.
In industrial workers who have had long-term exposure to unknown (presumably high) doses of organic nitrates, tolerance clearly occurs. Chest pain, acute myocardial infarction, and even sudden death have occurred during temporary withdrawal of nitrates from these workers, demonstrating the existence of true physical dependence. The importance of these observations to the routine, clinical use of oral isosorbide mononitrate is not known.
Information for Patients:
Patients should be told that the antianginal efficacy of IMDUR Tablets can be maintained by carefully following the prescribed schedule of dosing. For most patients, this can be accomplished by taking the dose on arising.
As with other nitrates, daily headaches sometimes accompany treatment with isosorbide mononitrate. In patients who get these headaches, the headaches are a marker of the activity of the drug. Patients should resist the temptation to avoid headaches by altering the schedule of their treatment with isosorbide mononitrate, since loss of headache may be associated with simultaneous loss of antianginal efficacy. Aspirin or acetaminophen often successfully relieves isosorbide mononitrate-induced headaches with no deleterious effect on isosorbide mononitrate's antianginal efficacy.
Treatment with isosorbide mononitrate may be associated with light-headedness on standing, especially just after rising from a recumbent or seated position. This effect may be more frequent in patients who have also consumed alcohol.
Drug Interactions:
The vasodilating effects of isosorbide mononitrate may be additive with those of other vasodilators. Alcohol, in particular, has been found to exhibit additive effects of this variety.
Marked symptomatic orthostatic hypotension has been reported when calcium channel blockers and organic nitrates were used in combination. Dose adjustments of either class of agents may be necessary.
Drug/Laboratory Test Interactions:
Nitrates and nitrites may interfere with the Zlatkis-Zak color reaction, causing falsely low readings in serum cholesterol determinations.

	SINGLE-DOSE STUDIES		MULTIPLE-DOSE STUDIES	
PARAMETER	ISMN 60 mg	IMDUR 60 mg	IMDUR 60 mg	IMDUR 120 mg
C_{max} (ng/mL)	1242-1534	424-541	557-572	1151-1180
T_{max} (hr)	0.6-0.7	3.1-4.5	2.9-4.2	3.1-3.2
AUC (ng•hr/mL)	8189-8313	5990-7452	6625-7555	14241-16800
$t_{1/2}$ (hr)	4.8-5.1	6.3-6.6	6.2-6.3	6.2-6.4
Cl/F (mL/min)	120-122	151-187	132-151	119-140

Carcinogenesis, Mutagenesis, Impairment of Fertility:
No evidence of carcinogenicity was observed in rats exposed to isosorbide mononitrate in their diets at doses of up to 900 mg/kg/day for the first 6 months and 500 mg/kg/day for the remaining duration of a study in which males were dosed for up to 121 weeks and females were dosed for up to 137 weeks. No evidence of carcinogenicity was observed in mice exposed to isosorbide mononitrate in their diets for up to 104 weeks at doses of up to 900 mg/kg/day.
Isosorbide mononitrate did not produce gene mutations (Ames test, mouse lymphoma test) or chromosome aberrations (human lymphocyte and mouse micronucleus tests) at biologically relevant concentrations.
No effects on fertility were observed in a study in which male and female rats were administered doses of up to 750 mg/kg/day beginning, in males, 9 weeks prior to mating, and in females, 2 weeks prior to mating.

Pregnancy Teratogenic Effects:
Pregnancy Category B In studies designed to detect effects of isosorbide mononitrate on embryo-fetal development, doses of up to 240 or 248 mg/kg/day, administered to pregnant rats and rabbits, were unassociated with evidence of such effects. These animal doses are about 100 times the maximum recommended human dose (120 mg in a 50-kg woman) when comparison is based on body weight; when comparison is based on body surface area, the rat dose is about 17 times the human dose and the rabbit dose is about 38 times the human dose. There are, however, no adequate and well-controlled studies in pregnant women. Because animal reproduction studies are not always predictive of human response, IMDUR Tablets should be used during pregnancy only if clearly needed.

Nonteratogenic Effects:
Neonatal survival and development and incidence of stillbirths were adversely affected when pregnant rats were administered oral doses of 750 (but not 300) mg isosorbide mononitrate/kg/day during late gestation and lactation. This dose (about 312 times the human dose when comparison is based on body weight and 54 times the human dose when comparison is based on body surface area) was associated with decreases in maternal weight gain and motor activity and evidence of impaired lactation.

Nursing Mothers:
It is not known whether this drug is excreted in human milk. Because many drugs are excreted in human milk, caution should be exercised when ISMN is administered to a nursing mother.

Pediatric Use:
The safety and effectiveness of ISMN in pediatric patients have not been established.

Geriatric Use:
Clinical studies of IMDUR Tablets did not include sufficient information on patients age 65 and over to determine if they respond differently from younger patients. Other reported clinical experience for IMDUR has not identified differences in response between elderly and younger patients. Clinical experience for organic nitrates reported in the literature identified a potential for severe hypotension and increased sensitivity to nitrates in the elderly. In general, dose selection for an elderly patient should be cautious, usually starting at the low end of the dosing range, reflecting the greater frequency of decreased hepatic, renal, or cardiac function, and of concomitant disease or other drug therapy.
Elderly patients may have reduced baroreceptor function and may develop severe orthostatic hypotension when vasodilators are used. IMDUR should therefore be used with caution in elderly patients who may be volume depleted, on multiple medications, or who, for whatever reason, are already hypotensive. Hypotension induced by isosorbide mononitrate may be accompanied by paradoxical bradycardia and increased angina pectoris.
Elderly patients may be more susceptible to hypotension and may be at a greater risk of falling at therapeutic doses of nitroglycerin.
Nitrate therapy may aggravate the angina caused by hypertrophic cardiomyopathy, particularly in the elderly.

ADVERSE REACTIONS
The table below shows the frequencies of the adverse events that occurred in >5% of the subjects in three placebo-controlled North American studies in which patients in the active treatment arm received 30 mg, 60 mg, 120 mg, or 240 mg of isosorbide mononitrate as IMDUR Tablets once daily. In parentheses, the same table shows the frequencies with which these adverse events were associated with the discontinuation of treatment. Overall, 8% of the patients who received 30 mg, 60 mg, 120 mg, or 240 mg of isosorbide mononitrate in the three placebo-controlled North American studies discontinued treatment because of adverse events. Most of these discontinued because of headache. Dizziness was rarely associated with withdrawal from these studies. Since headache appears to be a dose-related adverse effect and tends to disappear with continued treatment, it is recommended that IMDUR treatment be initiated at low doses for several days before being increased to desired levels.

FREQUENCY AND ADVERSE EVENTS (DISCONTINUED)*

Three Controlled North American Studies

Dose	Placebo	30 mg	60 mg	120 mg**	240 mg**
Patients	96	60	102	65	65
Headache	15% (0%)	38% (5%)	51% (8%)	42% (5%)	57% (8%)
Dizziness	4% (0%)	8% (0%)	11% (1%)	9% (2%)	9% (2%)

* Some individuals discontinued for multiple reasons.
** Patients were started on 60 mg and titrated to their final dose.

In addition, the three North American trials were pooled with 11 controlled trials conducted in Europe. Among the 14 controlled trials, a total of 711 patients were randomized to IMDUR Tablets. When the pooled data were reviewed, headache and dizziness were the only adverse events that were reported by >5% of patients. Other adverse events, each reported by ≤5% of exposed patients, and in many cases of uncertain relation to drug treatment, were:
Autonomic Nervous System Disorders: dry mouth, hot flushes.
Body as a Whole: asthenia, back pain, chest pain, edema, fatigue, fever, flu-like symptoms, malaise, rigors.
Cardiovascular Disorders, General: cardiac failure, hypertension, hypotension.
Central and Peripheral Nervous System Disorders: dizziness, headache, hypoesthesia, migraine, neuritis, paresis, paresthesia, ptosis, tremor, vertigo.
Gastrointestinal System Disorders: abdominal pain, constipation, diarrhea, dyspepsia, flatulence, gastric ulcer, gastritis, glossitis, hemorrhagic gastric ulcer, hemorrhoids, loose stools, melena, nausea, vomiting.
Hearing and Vestibular Disorders: earache, tinnitus, tympanic membrane perforation.
Heart Rate and Rhythm Disorders: arrhythmia, arrhythmia atrial, atrial fibrillation, bradycardia, bundle branch block, extrasystole, palpitation, tachycardia, ventricular tachycardia.
Liver and Biliary System Disorders: SGOT increase, SGPT increase.
Metabolic and Nutritional Disorders: hyperuricemia, hypokalemia.
Musculoskeletal System Disorders: arthralgia, frozen shoulder, muscle weakness, musculoskeletal pain, myalgia, myositis, tendon disorder, torticollis.
Myo-, Endo-, Pericardial, and Valve Disorders: angina pectoris aggravated, heart murmur, heart sound abnormal, myocardial infarction, Q wave abnormality.
Platelet, Bleeding, and Clotting Disorders: purpura, thrombocytopenia.
Psychiatric Disorders: anxiety, concentration impaired, confusion, decreased libido, depression, impotence, insomnia, nervousness, paroniria, somnolence.
Red Blood Cell Disorder: hypochromic anemia.
Reproductive Disorders, Female: atrophic vaginitis, breast pain.
Resistance Mechanism Disorders: bacterial infection, moniliasis, viral infection.
Respiratory System Disorders: bronchitis, bronchospasm, coughing, dyspnea, increased sputum, nasal congestion, pharyngitis, pneumonia, pulmonary infiltration, rales, rhinitis, sinusitis.
Skin and Appendages Disorders: acne, hair texture abnormal, increased sweating, pruritus, rash, skin nodule.
Urinary System Disorders: polyuria, renal calculus, urinary tract infection.
Vascular (Extracardiac) Disorders: flushing, intermittent claudication, leg ulcer, varicose vein.
Vision Disorders: conjunctivitis, photophobia, vision abnormal.
In addition, the following spontaneous adverse event has been reported during the marketing of isosorbide mononitrate: syncope.

OVERDOSAGE
Hemodynamic Effects: The ill effects of isosorbide mononitrate overdose are generally the results of isosorbide mononitrate's capacity to induce vasodilatation, venous pooling, reduced cardiac output, and hypotension. These hemodynamic changes may have protean manifestations, including increased intracranial pressure, with any or all of persistent throbbing headache, confusion, and moderate fever; vertigo; palpitations; visual disturbances; nausea and vomiting (possibly with colic and even bloody diarrhea); syncope (especially in the upright posture); air hunger and dyspnea, later followed by reduced ventilatory effort; diaphoresis, with the skin either flushed or cold and clammy; heart block and bradycardia; paralysis; coma; seizures; and death. Laboratory determinations of serum levels of isosorbide mononitrate and its metabolites are not widely available, and such determinations have, in any event, no established role in the management of isosorbide mononitrate overdose. There are no data suggesting what dose of isosorbide mononitrate is likely to be life threatening in humans. In rats and mice, there is significant lethality at doses of 2000 mg/kg and 3000 mg/kg, respectively.
No data are available to suggest physiological maneuvers (eg, maneuvers to change the pH of the urine) that might accelerate elimination of isosorbide mononitrate. In particular, dialysis is known to be ineffective in removing isosorbide mononitrate from the body.
No specific antagonist to the vasodilator effects of isosorbide mononitrate is known, and no intervention has been subject to controlled study as a therapy of isosorbide mononitrate overdose. Because the hypotension associated with isosorbide mononitrate overdose is the result of venodilatation and arterial hypovolemia, prudent therapy in this situation should be directed toward an increase in central fluid volume. Passive elevation of the patient's legs may be sufficient, but intravenous infusion of normal saline or similar fluid may also be necessary.
The use of epinephrine or other arterial vasoconstrictors in this setting is likely to do more harm than good.
In patients with renal disease or congestive heart failure, therapy resulting in central volume expansion is not without hazard. Treatment of isosorbide mononitrate overdose in these patients may be subtle and difficult, and invasive monitoring may be required.

Methemoglobinemia:
Methemoglobinemia has been reported in patients receiving other organic nitrates, and it probably could also occur as a side effect of isosorbide mononitrate. Certainly, nitrate ions liberated during metabolism of isosorbide mononitrate can oxidize hemoglobin into methemoglobin. Even in patients totally without cytochrome b_5 reductase activity, however, and even assuming that the nitrate moiety of isosorbide mononitrate is quantitatively applied to oxidation of hemoglobin, about 2 mg/kg of isosorbide mononitrate should be required before any of these patients manifest clinically significant (≥10%) methemoglobinemia. In patients with normal reductase function, significant production of methemoglobin should require even larger doses of isosorbide mononitrate. In one study in which 36 patients received 2 to 4 weeks of continuous nitroglycerin therapy at 3.1 to 4.4 mg/hr (equivalent, in total administered dose of nitrate ions, to 7.8-11.1 mg of isosorbide mononitrate per hour), the average methemoglobin level measured was 0.2%; this was comparable to that observed in parallel patients who received placebo.
Notwithstanding these observations, there are case reports of significant methemoglobinemia in association with moderate overdoses of organic nitrates. None of the affected patients had been thought to be unusually susceptible.
Methemoglobin levels are available from most clinical laboratories. The diagnosis should be suspected in patients who exhibit signs of impaired oxygen delivery despite adequate cardiac output and adequate arterial pO_2. Classically, methemoglobinemic blood is described as chocolate brown, without color change on exposure to air.
When methemoglobinemia is diagnosed, the treatment of choice is methylene blue, 1 to 2 mg/kg intravenously.

DOSAGE AND ADMINISTRATION
The recommended starting dose of IMDUR Tablets is 30 mg (given as a single 30-mg tablet or as ½ of a 60-mg tablet) or 60 mg (given as a single tablet) once daily. After several days, the dosage may be increased to 120 mg (given as a single 120-mg tablet or as two 60-mg tablets) once daily. Rarely, 240 mg may be required. The daily dose of IMDUR Tablets should be taken in the morning on arising. IMDUR Extended Release Tablets should not be chewed or crushed and should be swallowed together with a half-glassful of fluid.

HOW SUPPLIED
IMDUR Extended Release Tablets
30 mg: rose-colored tablets, scored on both sides and branded with the tradename ("IMDUR") on one side and the strength on the other.
Bottles of 100   NDC 0085-3306-03
Unit Dose 100 (10 × 10 blister strips)   NDC 0085-3306-01
60 mg: yellow-colored tablets, scored on both sides and branded with the tradename ("IMDUR") on one side and the strength on the other.
Bottles of 100   NDC 0085-4110-03
Unit Dose 100 (10 × 10 blister strips)   NDC 0085-4110-01
120 mg: white-colored tablets, branded with the tradename ("IMDUR") on one side and the strength on the other.
Bottles of 100   NDC 0085-1153-03
Unit Dose 100 (10 × 10 blister strips)   NDC 0085-1153-04
Store at controlled room temperature 20°-25°C (68°-77°F) [see USP].
Protect unit dose from excessive moisture.
Manufactured for Key Pharmaceuticals, Inc., Kenilworth, NJ 07033 by AstraZeneca PLC, Sweden.
Copyright © 1993, 1996, 1997, 1998, 2002, Key Pharmaceuticals, Inc. All rights reserved.
Rev. 7/02

B-23629321
18692953T

ZETIA™   ℞
[zĕt'ē-ă]
(EZETIMIBE)
TABLETS

DESCRIPTION
ZETIA (ezetimibe) is in a class of lipid-lowering compounds that selectively inhibits the intestinal absorption of cholesterol and related phytosterols. The chemical name of ezetimibe is 1-(4-fluorophenyl)-3(R)-[3-(4-fluorophenyl)-3(S)-hydroxypropyl]-4(S)-(4-hydroxyphenyl)-2-azetidinone. The empirical formula is $C_{24}H_{21}F_2NO_3$. Its molecular weight is 409.4 and its structural formula is:
[See chemical structure at top of next page]
Ezetimibe is a white, crystalline powder that is freely to very soluble in ethanol, methanol, and acetone and practically insoluble in water. Ezetimibe has a melting point of

Continued on next page

Zetia—Cont.

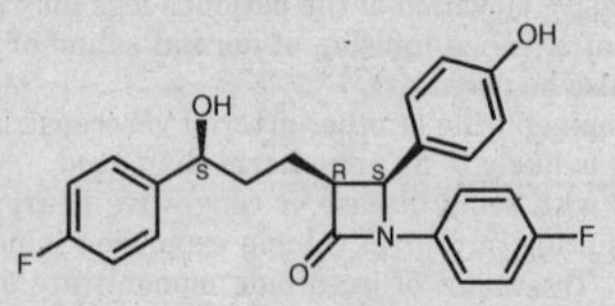

about 163°C and is stable at ambient temperature. ZETIA is available as a tablet for oral administration containing 10 mg of ezetimibe and the following inactive ingredients: croscarmellose sodium NF, lactose monohydrate NF, magnesium stearate NF, microcrystalline cellulose NF, povidone USP, and sodium lauryl sulfate NF.

CLINICAL PHARMACOLOGY

Background

Clinical studies have demonstrated that elevated levels of total cholesterol (total-C), low density lipoprotein cholesterol (LDL-C) and apolipoprotein B (Apo B), the major protein constituent of LDL, promote human atherosclerosis. In addition, decreased levels of high density lipoprotein cholesterol (HDL-C) are associated with the development of atherosclerosis. Epidemiologic studies have established that cardiovascular morbidity and mortality vary directly with the level of total-C and LDL-C and inversely with the level of HDL-C. Like LDL, cholesterol-enriched triglyceride-rich lipoproteins, including very-low-density lipoproteins (VLDL), intermediate-density lipoproteins (IDL), and remnants, can also promote atherosclerosis. The independent effect of raising HDL-C or lowering triglycerides (TG) on the risk of coronary and cardiovascular morbidity and mortality has not been determined.

ZETIA reduces total-C, LDL-C, Apo B, and TG, and increases HDL-C in patients with hypercholesterolemia. Administration of ZETIA with an HMG-CoA reductase inhibitor is effective in improving serum total-C, LDL-C, Apo B, TG, and HDL-C beyond either treatment alone. The effects of ezetimibe given either alone or in addition to an HMG-CoA reductase inhibitor on cardiovascular morbidity and mortality have not been established.

Mode of Action

Ezetimibe reduces blood cholesterol by inhibiting the absorption of cholesterol by the small intestine. In a 2-week clinical study in 18 hypercholesterolemic patients, ZETIA inhibited intestinal cholesterol absorption by 54%, compared with placebo. ZETIA had no clinically meaningful effect on the plasma concentrations of the fat-soluble vitamins A, D, and E (in a study of 113 patients), and did not impair adrenocortical steroid hormone production (in a study of 118 patients).

The cholesterol content of the liver is derived predominantly from three sources. The liver can synthesize cholesterol, take up cholesterol from the blood from circulating lipoproteins, or take up cholesterol absorbed by the small intestine. Intestinal cholesterol is derived primarily from cholesterol secreted in the bile and from dietary cholesterol.

Ezetimibe has a mechanism of action that differs from those of other classes of cholesterol-reducing compounds (HMG-CoA reductase inhibitors, bile acid sequestrants [resins], fibric acid derivatives, and plant stanols).

Ezetimibe does not inhibit cholesterol synthesis in the liver, or increase bile acid excretion. Instead, ezetimibe localizes and appears to act at the brush border of the small intestine and inhibits the absorption of cholesterol, leading to a decrease in the delivery of intestinal cholesterol to the liver. This causes a reduction of hepatic cholesterol stores and an increase in clearance of cholesterol from the blood; this distinct mechanism is complementary to that of HMG-CoA reductase inhibitors (see CLINICAL STUDIES).

Pharmacokinetics

Absorption

After oral administration, ezetimibe is absorbed and extensively conjugated to a pharmacologically active phenolic glucuronide (ezetimibe-glucuronide). After a single 10-mg dose of ZETIA to fasted adults, mean ezetimibe peak plasma concentrations (C_{max}) of 3.4 to 5.5 ng/mL were attained within 4 to 12 hours (T_{max}). Ezetimibe-glucuronide mean C_{max} values of 45 to 71 ng/mL were achieved between 1 and 2 hours (T_{max}). There was no substantial deviation from dose proportionality between 5 and 20 mg. The absolute bioavailability of ezetimibe cannot be determined, as the compound is virtually insoluble in aqueous media suitable for injection. Ezetimibe has variable bioavailability; the coefficient of variation, based on inter-subject variability, was 35 to 60% for AUC values.

Effect of Food on Oral Absorption

Concomitant food administration (high fat or non-fat meals) had no effect on the extent of absorption of ezetimibe when administered as ZETIA 10-mg tablets. The C_{max} value of ezetimibe was increased by 38% with consumption of high fat meals. ZETIA can be administered with or without food.

Distribution

Ezetimibe and ezetimibe-glucuronide are highly bound (>90%) to human plasma proteins.

Metabolism and Excretion

Ezetimibe is primarily metabolized in the small intestine and liver via glucuronide conjugation (a phase II reaction) with subsequent biliary and renal excretion. Minimal oxidative metabolism (a phase I reaction) has been observed in all species evaluated.

In humans, ezetimibe is rapidly metabolized to ezetimibe-glucuronide. Ezetimibe and ezetimibeglucuronide are the major drug-derived compounds detected in plasma, constituting approximately 10 to 20% and 80 to 90% of the total drug in plasma, respectively. Both ezetimibe and ezetimibe-glucuronide are slowly eliminated from plasma with a half-life of approximately 22 hours for both ezetimibe and ezetimibe-glucuronide. Plasma concentration-time profiles exhibit multiple peaks, suggesting enterohepatic recycling. Following oral administration of ^{14}C-ezetimibe (20 mg) to human subjects, total ezetimibe (ezetimibe + ezetimibe-glucuronide) accounted for approximately 93% of the total radioactivity in plasma. After 48 hours, there were no detectable levels of radioactivity in the plasma.

Approximately 78% and 11% of the administered radioactivity were recovered in the feces and urine, respectively, over a 10-day collection period. Ezetimibe was the major component in feces and accounted for 69% of the administered dose, while ezetimibe-glucuronide was the major component in urine and accounted for 9% of the administered dose.

Special Populations

Geriatric Patients

In a multiple dose study with ezetimibe given 10 mg once daily for 10 days, plasma concentrations for total ezetimibe were about 2-fold higher in older (≥65 years) healthy subjects compared to younger subjects.

Pediatric Patients

In a multiple dose study with ezetimibe given 10 mg once daily for 7 days, the absorption and metabolism of ezetimibe were similar in adolescents (10 to 18 years) and adults. Based on total ezetimibe, there are no pharmacokinetic differences between adolescents and adults. Pharmacokinetic data in the pediatric population <10 years of age are not available.

Gender

In a multiple dose study with ezetimibe given 10 mg once daily for 10 days, plasma concentrations for total ezetimibe were slightly higher (<20%) in women than in men.

Race

Based on a meta-analysis of multiple-dose pharmacokinetic studies, there were no pharmacokinetic differences between Blacks and Caucasians. There were too few patients in other racial or ethnic groups to permit further pharmacokinetic comparisons.

Hepatic Insufficiency

After a single 10-mg dose of ezetimibe, the mean area under the curve (AUC) for total ezetimibe was increased approximately 1.7-fold in patients with mild hepatic insufficiency (Child-Pugh score 5 to 6), compared to healthy subjects. The mean AUC values for total ezetimibe and ezetimibe were increased approximately 3-4 fold and 5-6 fold, respectively, in patients with moderate (Child-Pugh score 7 to 9) or severe hepatic impairment (Child-Pugh score 10 to 15). In a 14-day, multiple-dose study (10 mg daily) in patients with moderate hepatic insufficiency, the mean AUC values for total ezetimibe and ezetimibe were increased approximately 4-fold on Day 1 and Day 14 compared to healthy subjects. Due to the unknown effects of the increased exposure to ezetimibe in patients with moderate or severe hepatic insufficiency, ZETIA is not recommended in these patients (see CONTRAINDICATIONS and PRECAUTIONS, *Hepatic Insufficiency*).

Renal Insufficiency

After a single 10-mg dose of ezetimibe in patients with severe renal disease (n=8; mean CrCl ≤30 mL/min/1.73 m^2), the mean AUC values for total ezetimibe, ezetimibe-glucuronide, and ezetimibe were increased approximately 1.5-fold, compared to healthy subjects (n=9).

Drug Interactions (See also PRECAUTIONS, *Drug Interactions*)

ZETIA had no significant effect on a series of probe drugs (caffeine, dextromethorphan, tolbutamide, and IV midazolam) known to be metabolized by cytochrome P450 (1A2, 2D6, 2C8/9 and 3A4) in a "cocktail" study of twelve healthy adult males. This indicates that ezetimibe is neither an inhibitor nor an inducer of these cytochrome P450 isozymes, and it is unlikely that ezetimibe will affect the metabolism of drugs that are metabolized by these enzymes.

Warfarin: Concomitant administration of ezetimibe (10 mg once daily) had no significant effect on bioavailability of warfarin and prothrombin time in a study of twelve healthy adult males.

Digoxin: Concomitant administration of ezetimibe (10 mg once daily) had no significant effect on the bioavailability of digoxin and the ECG parameters (HR, PR, QT, and QTc intervals) in a study of twelve healthy adult males.

Gemfibrozil: In a study of twelve healthy adult males, concomitant administration of gemfibrozil (600 mg twice daily) significantly increased the oral bioavailability of total ezetimibe by a factor of 1.7. Ezetimibe (10 mg once daily) did not significantly affect the bioavailability of gemfibrozil.

Oral Contraceptives: Co-administration of ezetimibe (10 mg once daily) with oral contraceptives had no significant effect on the bioavailability of ethinyl estradiol or levonorgestrel in a study of eighteen healthy adult females.

Cimetidine: Multiple doses of cimetidine (400 mg twice daily) had no significant effect on the oral bioavailability of ezetimibe and total ezetimibe in a study of twelve healthy adults.

Antacids: In a study of twelve healthy adults, a single dose of antacid (Supralox™ 20 mL) administration had no significant effect on the oral bioavailability of total ezetimibe, ezetimibe-glucuronide, or ezetimibe based on AUC values. The C_{max} value of total ezetimibe was decreased by 30%.

Glipizide: In a study of twelve healthy adult males, steady-state levels of ezetimibe (10 mg once daily) had no significant effect on the pharmacokinetics and pharmacodynamics of glipizide. A single dose of glipizide (10 mg) had no significant effect on the exposure to total ezetimibe or ezetimibe.

HMG-CoA reductase inhibitors: In studies of healthy hypercholesterolemic (LDL-C ≥130 mg/dl) adult subjects, concomitant administration of ezetimibe (10 mg once daily) had no significant effect on the bioavailability of either lovastatin, simvastatin, pravastatin, atorvastatin, or fluvastatin. No significant effect on the bioavailability of total ezetimibe and ezetimibe was demonstrated by either lovastatin (20 mg once daily), pravastatin (20 mg once daily), atorvastatin (10 mg once daily), or fluvastatin (20 mg once daily).

Fenofibrate: In a study of thirty-two healthy hypercholesterolemic (LDL-C ≥130 mg/dl) adult subjects, concomitant fenofibrate (200 mg once daily) administration increased the mean C_{max} and AUC values of total ezetimibe approximately 64% and 48%, respectively. Pharmacokinetics of fenofibrate were not significantly affected by ezetimibe (10 mg once daily).

Cholestyramine: In a study of forty healthy hypercholesterolemic (LDL-C ≥130 mg/dl) adult subjects, concomitant cholestyramine (4 g twice daily) administration decreased the mean AUC values of total ezetimibe and ezetimibe approximately 55% and 80%, respectively.

Table 1
Response to ZETIA in Patients with Primary Hypercholesterolemia
(Mean[a] % Change from Untreated Baseline[b])

	Treatment group	N	Total-C	LDL-C	Apo B	TG[a]	HDL-C
Study 1[c]	Placebo	205	+1	+1	-1	-1	-1
	Ezetimibe	622	-12	-18	-15	-7	+1
Study 2[c]	Placebo	226	+1	+1	-1	+2	-2
	Ezetimibe	666	-12	-18	-16	-9	+1
Pooled Data[c] (Studies 1 & 2)	Placebo	431	0	+1	-2	0	-2
	Ezetimibe	1288	-13	-18	-16	-8	+1

[a] For triglycerides, median % change from baseline
[b] Baseline - on no lipid-lowering drug
[c] ZETIA significantly reduced total-C, LDL-C, Apo B, and TG, and increased HDL-C compared to placebo.

Table 2
Response to Addition of ZETIA to On-going HMG-CoA Reductase Inhibitor Therapy[a] in Patients with Hypercholesterolemia
(Mean[b] % Change from Treated Baseline[c])

Treatment (Daily Dose)	N	Total-C	LDL-C	Apo B	TG[b]	HDL-C
On-going HMG-CoA reductase inhibitor + Placebo[d]	390	-2	-4	-3	-3	+1
On-going HMG-CoA reductase inhibitor + ZETIA[d]	379	-17	-25	-19	-14	+3

[a] Patients receiving each HMG-CoA reductase inhibitor: 40% atorvastatin, 31% simvastatin, 29% others (pravastatin, fluvastatin, cerivastatin, lovastatin)
[b] For triglycerides, median % change from baseline
[c] Baseline - on an HMG-CoA reductase inhibitor alone.
[d] ZETIA + HMG-CoA reductase inhibitor significantly reduced total-C, LDL-C, Apo B, and TG, and increased HDL-C compared to HMG-CoA reductase inhibitor alone.

ANIMAL PHARMACOLOGY

The hypocholesterolemic effect of ezetimibe was evaluated in cholesterol-fed Rhesus monkeys, dogs, rats, and mouse models of human cholesterol metabolism. Ezetimibe was found to have an ED_{50} value of 0.5 µg/kg/day for inhibiting the rise in plasma cholesterol levels in monkeys. The ED_{50} values in dogs, rats, and mice were 7, 30, and 700 µg/kg/day, respectively. These results are consistent with ZETIA being a potent cholesterol absorption inhibitor.

In a rat model, where the glucuronide metabolite of ezetimibe (SCH 60663) was administered intraduodenally, the metabolite was as potent as the parent compound (SCH 58235) in inhibiting the absorption of cholesterol, suggesting that the glucuronide metabolite had activity similar to the parent drug.

In 1-month studies in dogs given ezetimibe (0.03-300 mg/kg/day), the concentration of cholesterol in gallbladder bile increased ~2- to 4-fold. However, a dose of 300 mg/kg/day administered to dogs for one year did not result in gallstone formation or any other adverse hepatobiliary effects. In a 14-day study in mice given ezetimibe (0.3-5 mg/kg/day) and fed a low-fat or cholesterol-rich diet, the concentration of cholesterol in gallbladder bile was either unaffected or reduced to normal levels, respectively.

A series of acute preclinical studies was performed to determine the selectivity of ZETIA for inhibiting cholesterol absorption. Ezetimibe inhibited the absorption of C14 cholesterol with no effect on the absorption of triglycerides, fatty acids, bile acids, progesterone, ethyl estradiol, or the fat-soluble vitamins A and D.

In 4- to 12-week toxicity studies in mice, ezetimibe did not induce cytochrome P450 drug metabolizing enzymes. In toxicity studies, a pharmacokinetic interaction of ezetimibe with HMG-CoA reductase inhibitors (parents or their active hydroxy acid metabolites) was seen in rats, dogs, and rabbits.

CLINICAL STUDIES

Primary Hypercholesterolemia
ZETIA reduces total-C, LDL-C, Apo B, and TG, and increases HDL-C in patients with hypercholesterolemia. Maximal to near maximal response is generally achieved within 2 weeks and maintained during chronic therapy.

ZETIA is effective in patients with hypercholesterolemia, in men and women, in younger and older patients, alone or administered with an HMG-CoA reductase inhibitor. Experience in pediatric and adolescent patients (ages 9 to 17) has been limited to patients with homozygous familial hypercholesterolemia (HoFH) or sitosterolemia.

Experience in non-Caucasians is limited and does not permit a precise estimate of the magnitude of the effects of ZETIA.

Monotherapy
In two, multicenter, double-blind, placebo-controlled, 12-week studies in 1719 patients with primary hypercholesterolemia, ZETIA significantly lowered total-C, LDL-C, Apo B, and TG, and increased HDL-C compared to placebo (see Table 1). Reduction in LDL-C was consistent across age, sex, and baseline LDL-C.
[See table 1 at top of previous page]

Combination with HMG-CoA Reductase Inhibitors
ZETIA Added to On-going HMG-CoA Reductase Inhibitor Therapy
In a multicenter, double-blind, placebo-controlled, 8-week study, 769 patients with primary hypercholesterolemia, known coronary heart disease or multiple cardiovascular risk factors who were already receiving HMG-CoA reductase inhibitor monotherapy, but who had not met their NCEP ATP II target LDL-C goal were randomized to receive either ZETIA or placebo in addition to their on-going HMG-CoA reductase inhibitor therapy.

ZETIA, added to on-going HMG-CoA reductase inhibitor therapy, significantly lowered total-C, LDL-C, Apo B, and TG, and increased HDL-C compared with an HMG-CoA reductase inhibitor administered alone (see Table 2). LDL-C reductions induced by ZETIA were generally consistent across all HMG-CoA reductase inhibitors.
[See table 2 at top of previous page]

ZETIA Initiated Concurrently with an HMG-CoA Reductase Inhibitor
In four, multicenter, double-blind, placebo-controlled, 12-week trials, in 2382 hypercholesterolemic patients, ZETIA or placebo was administered alone or with various doses of atorvastatin, simvastatin, pravastatin, or lovastatin.

When all patients receiving ZETIA with an HMG-CoA reductase inhibitor were compared to all those receiving the corresponding HMG-CoA reductase inhibitor alone, ZETIA significantly lowered total-C, LDL-C, Apo B, and TG, and, with the exception of pravastatin, increased HDL-C compared to the HMG-CoA reductase inhibitor administered alone. LDL-C reductions induced by ZETIA were generally consistent across all HMG-CoA reductase inhibitors. (See footnote c, Tables 3 to 6.)
[See table 3 above]
[See table 4 above]
[See table 5 at top of next page]
[See table 6 at top of next page]

Homozygous Familial Hypercholesterolemia (HoFH)
A study was conducted to assess the efficacy of ZETIA in the treatment of HoFH. This double-blind, randomized, 12-week study enrolled 50 patients with a clinical and/or genotypic diagnosis of HoFH, with or without concomitant LDL apheresis, already receiving atorvastatin or simvastatin (40 mg). Patients were randomized to one of three treatment groups, atorvastatin or simvastatin (80 mg), ZETIA administered with atorvastatin or simvastatin (40 mg), or ZETIA administered with atorvastatin or simvastatin (80 mg). Due to decreased bioavailability of ezetimibe in patients concomitantly receiving cholestyramine (see PRECAUTIONS), ezetimibe was dosed at least 4 hours before or after administration of resins. Mean baseline LDL-C was 341 mg/dL in those patients randomized to atorvastatin 80 mg or simvastatin 80 mg alone and 316 mg/dL in the group randomized to ZETIA plus atorvastatin 40 or 80 mg or simvastatin 40 or 80 mg. ZETIA, administered with atorvastatin or simvastatin (40 and 80 mg statin groups, pooled), significantly reduced LDL-C (21%) compared with increasing the dose of simvastatin or atorvastatin monotherapy from 40 to 80 mg (7%). In those treated with ZETIA plus 80 mg atorvastatin or with ZETIA plus 80 mg simvastatin, LDL-C was reduced by 27%.

Homozygous Sitosterolemia (Phytosterolemia)
A study was conducted to assess the efficacy of ZETIA in the treatment of homozygous sitosterolemia. In this multicenter, double-blind, placebo-controlled, 8-week trial, 37 patients with homozygous sitosterolemia with elevated plasma sitosterol levels (>5 mg/dL) on their current therapeutic regimen (diet, bile-acid-binding resins, HMG-CoA reductase inhibitors, ileal bypass surgery and/or LDL apheresis), were randomized to receive ZETIA (n=30) or placebo (n=7). Due to decreased bioavailability of ezetimibe in patients concomitantly receiving cholestyramine (see PRECAUTIONS), ezetimibe was dosed at least 2 hours before or 4 hours after resins were administered. Excluding the one subject receiving LDL-apheresis, ZETIA significantly lowered plasma sitosterol and campesterol, by 21% and 24% from baseline, respectively. In contrast, patients who received placebo had increases in sitosterol and campesterol of 4% and 3% from baseline, respectively. For patients treated with ZETIA, mean plasma levels of plant sterols were reduced progressively over the course of the study. The effects of reducing plasma sitosterol and campesterol on reducing the risks of cardiovascular morbidity and mortality have not been established.

Reductions in sitosterol and campesterol were consistent between patients taking ZETIA concomitantly with bile acid sequestrants (n=8) and patients not on concomitant bile acid sequestrant therapy (n=21).

INDICATIONS AND USAGE

Primary Hypercholesterolemia
Monotherapy
ZETIA, administered alone is indicated as adjunctive therapy to diet for the reduction of elevated total-C, LDL-C, and Apo B in patients with primary (heterozygous familial and non-familial) hypercholesterolemia.

Combination therapy with HMG-CoA reductase inhibitors
ZETIA, administered in combination with an HMG-CoA reductase inhibitor, is indicated as adjunctive therapy to diet

Continued on next page

Table 3
Response to ZETIA and Atorvastatin Initiated Concurrently in Patients with Primary Hypercholesterolemia
(Mean[a] % Change from Untreated Baseline[b])

Treatment (Daily Dose)	N	Total-C	LDL-C	Apo B	TG[a]	HDL-C
Placebo	60	+4	+4	+3	-6	+4
ZETIA	65	-14	-20	-15	-5	+4
Atorvastatin 10 mg	60	-26	-37	-28	-21	+6
ZETIA + Atorvastatin 10 mg	65	-38	-53	-43	-31	+9
Atorvastatin 20 mg	60	-30	-42	-34	-23	+4
ZETIA + Atorvastatin 20 mg	62	-39	-54	-44	-30	+9
Atorvastatin 40 mg	66	-32	-45	-37	-24	+4
ZETIA + Atorvastatin 40 mg	65	-42	-56	-45	-34	+5
Atorvastatin 80 mg	62	-40	-54	-46	-31	+3
ZETIA + Atorvastatin 80 mg	63	-46	-61	-50	-40	+7
Pooled data (All Atorvastatin Doses)[c]	248	-32	-44	-36	-24	+4
Pooled data (All ZETIA + Atorvastatin Doses)[c]	255	-41	-56	-45	-33	+7

[a] For triglycerides, median % change from baseline
[b] Baseline - on no lipid-lowering drug
[c] ZETIA + all doses of atorvastatin pooled (10-80 mg) significantly reduced total-C, LDL-C, Apo B, and TG, and increased HDL-C compared to all doses of atorvastatin pooled (10-80 mg).

Table 4
Response to ZETIA and Simvastatin Initiated Concurrently in Patients with Primary Hypercholesterolemia
(Mean[a] % Change from Untreated Baseline[b])

Treatment (Daily Dose)	N	Total-C	LDL-C	Apo B	TG[a]	HDL-C
Placebo	70	-1	-1	0	+2	+1
ZETIA	61	-13	-19	-14	-11	+5
Simvastatin 10 mg	70	-18	-27	-21	-14	+8
ZETIA + Simvastatin 10 mg	67	-32	-46	-35	-26	+9
Simvastatin 20 mg	61	-26	-36	-29	-18	+6
ZETIA + Simvastatin 20 mg	69	-33	-46	-36	-25	+9
Simvastatin 40 mg	65	-27	-38	-32	-24	+6
ZETIA + Simvastatin 40 mg	73	-40	-56	-45	-32	+11
Simvastatin 80 mg	67	-32	-45	-37	-23	+8
ZETIA + Simvastatin 80 mg	65	-41	-58	-47	-31	+8
Pooled data (All Simvastatin Doses)[c]	263	-26	-36	-30	-20	+7
Pooled data (All ZETIA + Simvastatin Doses)[c]	274	-37	-51	-41	-29	+9

[a] For triglycerides, median % change from baseline
[b] Baseline - on no lipid-lowering drug
[c] ZETIA + all doses of simvastatin pooled (10-80 mg) significantly reduced total-C, LDL-C, Apo B, and TG, and increased HDL-C compared to all doses of simvastatin pooled (10-80 mg).

Zetia—Cont.

for the reduction of elevated total-C, LDL-C, and Apo B in patients with primary (heterozygous familial and non-familial) hypercholesterolemia.

Homozygous Familial Hypercholesterolemia (HoFH)
The combination of ZETIA and atorvastatin or simvastatin, is indicated for the reduction of elevated total-C and LDL-C levels in patients with HoFH, as an adjunct to other lipid-lowering treatments (e.g., LDL apheresis) or if such treatments are unavailable.

Homozygous Sitosterolemia
ZETIA is indicated as adjunctive therapy to diet for the reduction of elevated sitosterol and campesterol levels in patients with homozygous familial sitosterolemia.

Therapy with lipid-altering agents should be a component of multiple risk-factor intervention in individuals at increased risk for atherosclerotic vascular disease due to hypercholesterolemia. Lipidaltering agents should be used in addition to an appropriate diet (including restriction of saturated fat and cholesterol) and when the response to diet and other non-pharmacological measures has been inadequate. (See NCEP Adult Treatment Panel (ATP) III Guidelines, summarized in Table 7.)

[See table 7 at top of next page]

Prior to initiating therapy with ZETIA, secondary causes for dyslipidemia (i.e., diabetes, hypothyroidism, obstructive liver disease, chronic renal failure, and drugs that increase LDL-C and decrease HDL-C [progestins, anabolic steroids, and corticosteroids]), should be excluded or, if appropriate, treated. A lipid profile should be performed to measure total-C, LDL-C, HDL-C and TG. For TG levels >400 mg/dL (>4.5 mmol/L), LDL-C concentrations should be determined by ultracentrifugation.

At the time of hospitalization for an acute coronary event, lipid measures should be taken on admission or within 24 hours. These values can guide the physician on initiation of LDL-lowering therapy before or at discharge.

CONTRAINDICATIONS
Hypersensitivity to any component of this medication.
The combination of ZETIA with an HMG-CoA reductase inhibitor is contraindicated in patients with active liver disease or unexplained persistent elevations in serum transaminases.

All HMG-CoA reductase inhibitors are contraindicated in pregnant and nursing women. When ZETIA is administered with an HMG-CoA reductase inhibitor in a woman of child-bearing potential, refer to the pregnancy category and product labeling for the HMG-CoA reductase inhibitor. (See PRECAUTIONS, Pregnancy.)

PRECAUTIONS
Concurrent administration of ZETIA with a specific HMG-CoA reductase inhibitor should be in accordance with the product labeling for that HMG-CoA reductase inhibitor.

Liver Enzymes
In controlled clinical monotherapy studies, the incidence of consecutive elevations (≥3 × the upper limit of normal [ULN]) in serum transaminases was similar between ZETIA (0.5%) and placebo (0.3%).
In controlled clinical combination studies of ZETIA initiated concurrently with an HMG-CoA reductase inhibitor, the incidence of consecutive elevations (≥3 × ULN) in serum transaminases was 1.3% for patients treated with ZETIA administered with HMG-CoA reductase inhibitors and 0.4% for patients treated with HMG-CoA reductase inhibitors alone. These elevations in transaminases were generally asymptomatic, not associated with cholestasis, and returned to baseline after discontinuation of therapy or with continued treatment. When ZETIA is co-administered with an HMG-CoA reductase inhibitor, liver function tests should be performed at initiation of therapy and according to the recommendations of the HMG-CoA reductase inhibitor.

Skeletal Muscle
In clinical trials, there was no excess of myopathy or rhabdomyolysis associated with ZETIA compared with the relevant control arm (placebo or HMG-CoA reductase inhibitor alone). However, myopathy and rhabdomyolysis are known adverse reactions to HMG-CoA reductase inhibitors and other lipid-lowering drugs. In clinical trials, the incidence of CPK >10 × ULN was 0.2% for ZETIA vs 0.1% for placebo, and 0.1% for ZETIA co-administered with an HMG-CoA reductase inhibitor vs 0.4% for HMG-CoA reductase inhibitors alone.

Hepatic Insufficiency
Due to the unknown effects of the increased exposure to ezetimibe in patients with moderate or severe hepatic insufficiency, ZETIA is not recommended in these patients. (See CLINICAL PHARMACOLOGY, *Special Populations*.)

Drug Interactions (See also CLINICAL PHARMACOLOGY, *Drug Interactions*.)
Cholestyramine: Concomitant cholestyramine administration decreased the mean AUC of total ezetimibe approximately 55%. The incremental LDL-C reduction due to adding ezetimibe to cholestyramine may be reduced by this interaction.
Fibrates: The safety and effectiveness of ezetimibe administered with fibrates have not been established.
Fibrates may increase cholesterol excretion into the bile, leading to cholelithiasis. In a preclinical study in dogs, ezetimibe increased cholesterol in the gallbladder bile (see ANIMAL PHARMACOLOGY). Co-administration of ZETIA with fibrates is not recommended until use in patients is studied.

Fenofibrate: In a pharmacokinetic study, concomitant fenofibrate administration increased total ezetimibe concentrations approximately 1.5-fold.
Gemfibrozil: In a pharmacokinetic study, concomitant gemfibrozil administration increased total ezetimibe concentrations approximately 1.7-fold.
HMG-CoA reductase inhibitors: No clinically significant pharmacokinetic interactions were seen when ezetimibe was co-administered with atorvastatin, simvastatin, pravastatin, lovastatin, or fluvastatin.
Cyclosporine: The total ezetimibe level increased 12-fold in one renal transplant patient receiving multiple medications, including cyclosporine. Patients who take both ezetimibe and cyclosporine should be carefully monitored.

Carcinogenesis, Mutagenesis, Impairment of Fertility
A 104-week dietary carcinogenicity study with ezetimibe was conducted in rats at doses up to 1500 mg/kg/day (males) and 500 mg/kg/day (females) (~20 times the human exposure at 10 mg daily based on AUC_{0-24hr} for total ezetimibe). A 104-week dietary carcinogenicity study with ezetimibe was also conducted in mice at doses up to 500 mg/kg/day (>150 times the human exposure at 10 mg daily based on AUC_{0-24hr} for total ezetimibe). There were no statistically significant increases in tumor incidences in drug-treated rats or mice.
No evidence of mutagenicity was observed in vitro in a microbial mutagenicity (Ames) test with *Salmonella typhimurium* and *Escherichia coli* with or without metabolic activation. No evidence of clastogenicity was observed *in vitro* in a chromosomal aberration assay in human peripheral blood lymphocytes with or without metabolic activation. In addition, there was no evidence of genotoxicity in the *in vivo* mouse micronucleus test.
In oral (gavage) fertility studies of ezetimibe conducted in rats, there was no evidence of reproductive toxicity at doses up to 1000 mg/kg/day in male or female rats (~7 times the human exposure at 10 mg daily based on AUC_{0-24hr} for total ezetimibe).

Pregnancy
Pregnancy Category: C
There are no adequate and well-controlled studies of ezetimibe in pregnant women. Ezetimibe should be used during pregnancy only if the potential benefit justifies the risk to the fetus.
In oral (gavage) embryo-fetal development studies of ezetimibe conducted in rats and rabbits during organogenesis, there was no evidence of embryolethal effects at the doses tested (250, 500, 1000 mg/kg/day). In rats, increased incidences of common fetal skeletal findings (extra pair of thoracic ribs, unossified cervical vertebral centra, shortened ribs) were observed at 1000 mg/kg/day (~10 times the human exposure at 10 mg daily based on AUC_{0-24hr} for total ezetimibe). In rabbits treated with ezetimibe, an increased incidence of extra thoracic ribs was observed at 1000 mg/kg/day (150 times the human exposure at 10 mg daily based on AUC_{0-24hr} for total ezetimibe). Ezetimibe crossed the placenta when pregnant rats and rabbits were given multiple oral doses.
Multiple dose studies of ezetimibe given in combination with HMG-CoA reductase inhibitors (statins) in rats and rabbits during organogenesis result in higher ezetimibe and statin exposures. Reproductive findings occur at lower doses in combination therapy compared to monotherapy.

All HMG-CoA reductase inhibitors are contraindicated in pregnant and nursing women. When ZETIA is administered with an HMG-CoA reductase inhibitor in a woman of child-bearing potential, refer to the pregnancy category and package labeling for the HMG-CoA reductase inhibitor. (See CONTRAINDICATIONS.)

Labor and Delivery
The effects of ZETIA on labor and delivery in pregnant women are unknown.

Table 5
Response to ZETIA and Pravastatin Initiated Concurrently in Patients with Primary Hypercholesterolemia
(Mean[a] % Change from Untreated Baseline[b])

Treatment (Daily Dose)	N	Total-C	LDL-C	Apo B	TG[a]	HDL-C
Placebo	65	0	-1	-2	-1	+2
ZETIA	64	-13	-20	-15	-5	+4
Pravastatin 10 mg	66	-15	-21	-16	-14	+6
ZETIA + Pravastatin 10 mg	71	-24	-34	-27	-23	+8
Pravastatin 20 mg	69	-15	-23	-18	-8	+8
ZETIA + Pravastatin 20 mg	66	-27	-40	-31	-21	+8
Pravastatin 40 mg	70	-22	-31	-26	-19	+6
ZETIA + Pravastatin 40 mg	67	-30	-42	-32	-21	+8
Pooled data (All Pravastatin Doses)[c]	205	-17	-25	-20	-14	+7
Pooled data (All ZETIA + Pravastatin Doses)[c]	204	-27	-39	-30	-21	+8

[a] For triglycerides, median % change from baseline
[b] Baseline - on no lipid-lowering drug
[c] ZETIA + all doses of pravastatin pooled (10-40 mg) significantly reduced total-C, LDL-C, Apo B, and TG compared to all doses of pravastatin pooled (10-40 mg).

Table 6
Response to ZETIA and Lovastatin Initiated Concurrently in Patients with Primary Hypercholesterolemia
(Mean[a] % Change from Untreated Baseline[b])

Treatment (Daily Dose)	N	Total-C	LDL-C	Apo B	TG[a]	HDL-C
Placebo	64	+1	0	+1	+6	0
ZETIA	72	-13	-19	-14	-5	+3
Lovastatin 10 mg	73	-15	-20	-17	-11	+5
ZETIA + Lovastatin 10 mg	65	-24	-34	-27	-19	+8
Lovastatin 20 mg	74	-19	-26	-21	-12	+3
ZETIA + Lovastatin 20 mg	62	-29	-41	-34	-27	+9
Lovastatin 40 mg	73	-21	-30	-25	-15	+5
ZETIA + Lovastatin 40 mg	65	-33	-46	-38	-27	+9
Pooled data (All Lovastatin Doses)[c]	220	-18	-25	-21	-12	+4
Pooled data (All ZETIA + Lovastatin Doses)[c]	192	-29	-40	-33	-25	+9

[a] For triglycerides, median % change from baseline
[b] Baseline - on no lipid-lowering drug
[c] ZETIA + all doses of lovastatin pooled (10-40 mg) significantly reduced total-C, LDL-C, Apo B, and TG, and increased HDL-C compared to all doses of lovastatin pooled (10-40 mg).

Nursing Mothers
In rat studies, exposure to total ezetimibe in nursing pups was up to half of that observed in maternal plasma. It is not known whether ezetimibe is excreted into human breast milk; therefore, ZETIA should not be used in nursing mothers unless the potential benefit justifies the potential risk to the infant.

Pediatric Use
The pharmacokinetics of ZETIA in adolescents (10 to 18 years) have been shown to be similar to that in adults. Treatment experience with ZETIA in the pediatric population is limited to 4 patients (9 to 17 years) in the sitosterolemia study and 5 patients (11 to 17 years) in the HoFH study. Treatment with ZETIA in children (<10 years) is not recommended. (See CLINICAL PHARMACOLOGY, *Special Populations*.)

Geriatric Use
Of the patients who received ZETIA in clinical studies, 948 were 65 and older (this included 206 who were 75 and older). The effectiveness and safety of ZETIA were similar between these patients and younger subjects. Greater sensitivity of some older individuals cannot be ruled out. (See CLINICAL PHARMACOLOGY, *Special Populations* and ADVERSE REACTIONS.)

ADVERSE REACTIONS
ZETIA has been evaluated for safety in more than 4700 patients in clinical trials. Clinical studies of ZETIA (administered alone or with an HMG-CoA reductase inhibitor) demonstrated that ZETIA was generally well tolerated. The overall incidence of adverse events reported with ZETIA was similar to that reported with placebo, and the discontinuation rate due to adverse events was also similar for ZETIA and placebo.

Monotherapy
Adverse experiences reported in ≥2% of patients treated with ZETIA and at an incidence greater than placebo in placebo-controlled studies of ZETIA, regardless of causality assessment, are shown in Table 8.

Table 8*
Clinical Adverse Events Occurring in ≥2% of Patients Treated with ZETIA and at an Incidence Greater than Placebo, Regardless of Causality

Body System/Organ Class Adverse Event	Placebo (%) n = 795	ZETIA 10 mg (%) n = 1691
Body as a whole - general disorders		
Fatigue	1.8	2.2
Gastro-intestinal system disorders		
Abdominal pain	2.8	3.0
Diarrhea	3.0	3.7
Infection and infestations		
Infection viral	1.8	2.2
Pharyngitis	2.1	2.3
Sinusitis	2.8	3.6
Musculo-skeletal system disorders		
Arthralgia	3.4	3.8
Back pain	3.9	4.1
Respiratory system disorders		
Coughing	2.1	2.3

*Includes patients who received placebo or ZETIA alone reported in Table 9.

The frequency of less common adverse events was comparable between ZETIA and placebo.

Combination with an HMG-CoA reductase Inhibitor
ZETIA has been evaluated for safety in combination studies in more than 2000 patients.

In general, adverse experiences were similar between ZETIA administered with HMG-CoA reductase inhibitors and HMG-CoA reductase inhibitors alone. However, the frequency of increased transaminases was slightly higher in patients receiving ZETIA administered with HMG-CoA reductase inhibitors than in patients treated with HMG-CoA reductase inhibitors alone. (See PRECAUTIONS, *Liver Enzymes*.)

Clinical adverse experiences reported in ≥2% of patients and at an incidence greater than placebo in four placebo-controlled trials where ZETIA was administered alone or initiated concurrently with various HMG-CoA reductase inhibitors, regardless of causality assessment, are shown in Table 9.
[See table 9 above]

OVERDOSAGE
No cases of overdosage with ZETIA have been reported. Administration of ezetimibe, 50 mg/day, to 15 subjects for up to 14 days was generally well tolerated. In the event of an overdose, symptomatic and supportive measures should be employed.

DOSAGE AND ADMINISTRATION
The patient should be placed on a standard cholesterol-lowering diet before receiving ZETIA and should continue on this diet during treatment with ZETIA.
The recommended dose of ZETIA is 10 mg once daily. ZETIA can be administered with or without food.
ZETIA may be administered with an HMG-CoA reductase inhibitor for incremental effect. For convenience, the daily dose of ZETIA may be taken at the same time as the HMG-CoA reductase inhibitor, according to the dosing recommendations for the HMG-CoA reductase inhibitor.

Patients with Hepatic Insufficiency
No dosage adjustment is necessary in patients with mild hepatic insufficiency (see PRECAUTIONS, *Hepatic Insufficiency*).

Patients with Renal Insufficiency
No dosage adjustment is necessary in patients with renal insufficiency (see CLINICAL PHARMACOLOGY, *Special Populations*).

Geriatric Patients
No dosage adjustment is necessary in geriatric patients (see CLINICAL PHARMACOLOGY, *Special Populations*).

Co-administration with Bile Acid Sequestrants
Dosing of ZETIA should occur either ≥2 hours before or ≥4 hours after administration of a bile acid sequestrant (see PRECAUTIONS, *Drug Interactions*).

HOW SUPPLIED
No. 3861-Tablets ZETIA, 10 mg, are white to off-white, capsule-shaped tablets debossed with "414" on one side. They are supplied as follows:
NDC 66582-414-31 bottles of 30
NDC 66582-414-54 bottles of 90
NDC 66582-414-74 bottles of 500
NDC 66582-414-28 unit dose packages of 100.

Storage
Store at 25°C (77°F); excursions permitted to 15-30°C (59-86°F). [See USP Controlled Room Temperature.] Protect from moisture.

MERCK/Schering-Plough Pharmaceuticals
Manufactured for: Merck/Schering-Plough Pharmaceuticals, North Wales, PA 19454, USA
By: Schering Corporation, Kenilworth, NJ 07033, USA
Issued October 2002   B-26723809
REV 00   25751809T

Table 7
Summary of NCEP ATP III Guidelines

Risk Category	LDL Goal (mg/dL)	LDL Level at Which to Initiate Therapeutic Lifestyle Changes[a] (mg/dL)	LDL level at Which to Consider Drug Therapy (mg/dL)
CHD or CHD risk equivalents[b] (10-year risk >20%)[c]	<100	≥100	≥130 (100–129: drug optional)[d]
2+ Risk factors[e] (10-year risk ≤20%)[c]	<130	≥130	10-year risk 10–20%: ≥130[c] 10-year risk <10%: ≥160[c]
0-1 Risk factor[f]	<160	≥160	≥190 (160–189: LDL-lowering drug optional)

[a] Therapeutic lifestyle changes include: 1) dietary changes: reduced intake of saturated fats (<7% of total calories) and cholesterol (<200 mg per day), and enhancing LDL lowering with plant stanols/sterols (2g/d) and increased viscous (soluble) fiber (10-25 g/d), 2) weight reduction, and 3) increased physical activity.
[b] CHD risk equivalents comprise: diabetes, multiple risk factors that confer a 10-year risk for CHD >20%, and other clinical forms of atherosclerotic disease (peripheral arterial disease, abdominal aortic aneurysm and symptomatic carotid artery disease).
[c] Risk assessment for determining the 10-year risk for developing CHD is carried out using the Framingham risk scoring. Refer to JAMA, May 16, 2001; 285 (19): 2486-2497, or the NCEP website (http://www.nhlbi.nih.gov) for more details.
[d] Some authorities recommend use of LDL-lowering drugs in this category if an LDL cholesterol <100 mg/dL cannot be achieved by therapeutic lifestyle changes. Others prefer use of drugs that primarily modify triglycerides and HDL, e.g., nicotinic acid or fibrate. Clinical judgment also may call for deferring drug therapy in this subcategory.
[e] Major risk factors (exclusive of LDL cholesterol) that modify LDL goals include cigarette smoking, hypertension (BP ≥140/90 mm Hg or on anti-hypertensive medication), low HDL cholesterol (<40 mg/dL), family history of premature CHD (CHD in male first-degree relative <55 years; CHD in female first-degree relative <65 years), age (men ≥45 years; women ≥55 years). HDL cholesterol ≥60 mg/dL counts as a "negative" risk factor; its presence removes one risk factor from the total count.
[f] Almost all people with 0-1 risk factor have a 10-year risk <10%; thus, 10-year risk assessment in people with 0-1 risk factor is not necessary.

Table 9*
Clinical Adverse Events Occurring in ≥2% of Patients and at an Incidence Greater than Placebo, Regardless of Causality, in ZETIA/Statin Combination Studies

Body System/Organ Class Adverse Event	Placebo (%) n=259	ZETIA 10 mg (%) n=262	All Statins** (%) n=936	ZETIA + All Statins** (%) n=925
Body as a whole - general disorders				
Chest pain	1.2	3.4	2.0	1.8
Dizziness	1.2	2.7	1.4	1.8
Fatigue	1.9	1.9	1.4	2.8
Headache	5.4	8.0	7.3	6.3
Gastro-intestinal system disorders				
Abdominal pain	2.3	2.7	3.1	3.5
Diarrhea	1.5	3.4	2.9	2.8
Infection and infestations				
Pharyngitis	1.9	3.1	2.5	2.3
Sinusitis	1.9	4.6	3.6	3.5
Upper respiratory tract infection	10.8	13.0	13.6	11.8
Musculo-skeletal system disorders				
Arthralgia	2.3	3.8	4.3	3.4
Back pain	3.5	3.4	3.7	4.3
Myalgia	4.6	5.0	4.1	4.5

* Includes four placebo-controlled combination studies in which ZETIA was initiated concurrently with an HMG-CoA reductase inhibitor.
**All Statins = all doses of all HMG-CoA reductase inhibitors.

COPYRIGHT © Merck/Schering-Plough Pharmaceuticals, 2001, 2002. All rights reserved. Printed in USA.

Patient Information about ZETIA
Read this information carefully before you start taking ZETIA and each time you get more ZETIA. There may be new information. This information does not take the place of talking with your doctor about your medical condition or your treatment. If you have any questions about ZETIA, ask your doctor. Only your doctor can determine if ZETIA is right for you.

What is ZETIA?
ZETIA is a medicine used to lower levels of total cholesterol and LDL (bad) cholesterol in the blood. It is used for patients who cannot control their cholesterol levels by diet alone. It can be used by itself or with other medicines to treat high cholesterol. You should stay on a cholesterol-lowering diet while taking this medicine.
ZETIA works to reduce the amount of cholesterol your body absorbs. ZETIA does not help you lose weight.
For more information about cholesterol, see the "What should I know about high cholesterol?" section that follows.

Who should not take ZETIA?
- Do not take ZETIA if you are allergic to ezetimibe, the active ingredient in ZETIA, or to the inactive ingredients. For a list of inactive ingredients, see the "Inactive ingredients" section that follows.
- If you have active liver disease, do not take ZETIA while taking cholesterol-lowering medicines called statins.
- If you are pregnant or breast-feeding, do not take ZETIA while taking a statin.

What should I tell my doctor before and while taking ZETIA?
Tell your doctor about any prescription and non-prescription medicines you are taking or plan to take, including natural or herbal remedies.

Continued on next page

Zetia—Cont.

Tell your doctor about all your medical conditions including allergies.
Tell your doctor if you:
- ever had liver problems. ZETIA may not be right for you.
- are pregnant or plan to become pregnant. Your doctor will decide if ZETIA is right for you.
- are breast-feeding. We do not know if ZETIA can pass to your baby through your milk. Your doctor will decide if ZETIA is right for you.
- experience unexplained muscle pain, tenderness, or weakness.

How should I take ZETIA?
- Take ZETIA once a day, with or without food. It may be easier to remember to take your dose if you do it at the same time every day, such as with breakfast, dinner, or at bedtime. If you also take another medicine to reduce your cholesterol, ask your doctor if you can take them at the same time.
- If you forget to take ZETIA, take it as soon as you remember. However, do not take more than one dose of ZETIA a day.
- Continue to follow a cholesterol-lowering diet while taking ZETIA. Ask your doctor if you need diet information.
- Keep taking ZETIA unless your doctor tells you to stop. It is important that you keep taking ZETIA even if you do not feel sick.

See your doctor regularly to check your cholesterol level and to check for side effects. Your doctor may do blood tests to check your liver before you start taking ZETIA with a statin and during treatment.

What are the possible side effects of ZETIA?
Patients reported few side effects while taking ZETIA. Tell your doctor if you are having stomach pain, are feeling tired, or have any other medical problems while on ZETIA. For a complete list of side effects, ask your doctor or pharmacist.

What should I know about high cholesterol?
Cholesterol is a type of fat found in your blood. Your total cholesterol is made up of LDL and HDL cholesterol.
LDL cholesterol is called "bad" cholesterol because it can build up in the wall of your arteries and form plaque. Over time, plaque build-up can cause a narrowing of the arteries. This narrowing can slow or block blood flow to your heart, brain, and other organs. High LDL cholesterol is a major cause of heart disease and stroke.
HDL cholesterol is called "good" cholesterol because it keeps the bad cholesterol from building up in the arteries.
Triglycerides also are fats found in your blood.

General information about ZETIA
Medicines are sometimes prescribed for conditions that are not mentioned in patient information leaflets. Do not use ZETIA for a condition for which it was not prescribed. Do not give ZETIA to other people, even if they have the same condition you have. It may harm them.
This summarizes the most important information about ZETIA. If you would like more information, talk with your doctor. You can ask your pharmacist or doctor for information about ZETIA that is written for health professionals.

Inactive ingredients:
Croscarmellose sodium, lactose monohydrate, magnesium stearate, microcrystalline cellulose, povidone, and sodium lauryl sulfate.

MERCK/Schering Plough Pharmaceuticals
Manufactured for:
Merck/Schering-Plough Pharmaceuticals
North Wales, PA 19454, USA
By:
Schering Corporation Kenilworth, NJ 07033, USA
Issued October 2002

26723809
REV 00   25751701T
COPYRIGHT © Merck/Schering-Plough Pharmaceuticals, 2001, 2002.
All rights reserved.

In the PDR annual,
the **Brand and Generic Name Index**
(PINK section)
alphabetizes drugs under both
brand and generic names.

Stiefel Laboratories, Inc.
**255 ALHAMBRA CIRCLE
CORAL GABLES, FL 33134**

Direct Inquiries to:
Professional Services Department
1-888-STIEFEL

DUAC™ ℞
Topical Gel
[dū'ăk]
(clindamycin, 1% - benzoyl peroxide, 5%)
For Dermatological Use Only.
Not for Ophthalmic Use.

DESCRIPTION
Duac™ Topical Gel contains clindamycin phosphate, (7(S)-chloro-7-deoxylincomycin-2-phosphate), equivalent to 1% clindamycin, and 5% benzoyl peroxide.
Clindamycin phosphate is a water soluble ester of the semi-synthetic antibiotic produced by a 7(S)-chloro-substitution of the 7(R)-hydroxyl group of the parent antibiotic lincomycin.
Clindamycin phosphate is $C_{18}H_{34}ClN_2O_8PS$. The structural formula for clindamycin phosphate is represented below:

Clindamycin phosphate has a molecular weight of 504.97 and its chemical name is methyl 7-chloro-6,7,8-trideoxy-6-(1-methyl-*trans*-4-propyl-L-2-pyrrolidinecarboxamido)-1-thio-L-*threo*-α-D-*galacto*-octopyranoside 2-(dihydrogen phosphate).
Benzoyl peroxide is $C_{14}H_{10}O_4$. It has the following structural formula:

Benzoyl peroxide has a molecular weight of 242.23.
Each gram of Duac Topical Gel contains 10 mg (1%) clindamycin, as phosphate, and 50 mg (5%) benzoyl peroxide in a base consisting of carbomer 940, dimethicone, disodium lauryl sulfosuccinate, edetate disodium, glycerin, silicon dioxide, methylparaben, poloxamer, purified water, and sodium hydroxide.

CLINICAL PHARMACOLOGY
A comparative study of the pharmacokinetics of Duac Topical Gel and 1% clindamycin solution alone in 78 patients indicated that mean plasma clindamycin levels during the four week dosing period were < 0.5 ng/ml for both treatment groups.
Benzoyl peroxide has been shown to be absorbed by the skin where it is converted to benzoic acid. Less than 2% of the dose enters systemic circulation as benzoic acid.
Microbiology:
Mechanism of Action
Clindamycin binds to the 50S ribosomal subunits of susceptible bacteria and prevents elongation of peptide chains by interfering with peptidyl transfer, thereby suppressing protein synthesis.
Benzoyl peroxide is a potent oxidizing agent.
In Vivo **Activity**
No microbiology studies were conducted in the clinical trials with this product.
In Vitro **Activity**
The clindamycin and benzoyl peroxide components individually have been shown to have *in vitro* activity against *Propionibacterium acnes*, an organism which has been associated with acne vulgaris; however, the clinical significance of this is not known.
Drug Resistance
There are reports of an increase of *P. acnes* resistance to clindamycin in the treatment of acne. In patients with *P. acnes* resistant to clindamycin, the clindamycin component may provide no additional benefit beyond benzoyl peroxide alone.

CLINICAL STUDIES
In five randomized, double-blind clinical studies of 1,319 patients, 397 used Duac, 396 used benzoyl peroxide, 349 used clindamycin and 177 used vehicle. Duac applied once daily for 11 weeks was significantly more effective than vehicle, benzoyl peroxide, and clindamycin in the treatment of inflammatory lesions of moderate to moderately severe facial acne vulgaris in three of the five studies (Studies 1, 2, and 5).
Patients were evaluated and acne lesions counted at each clinical visit: weeks 2, 5, 8, 11. The primary efficacy measures were the lesion counts and the investigator's global assessment evaluated at week 11. Patients were instructed to wash the face, wait 10 to 20 minutes, and then apply medication to the entire face, once daily, in the evening before retiring. Percent reductions in inflammatory lesion counts after treatment for 11 weeks in these five studies are shown in the following table:
[See table below]
The Duac group showed greater overall improvement in the investigator's global assessment than the benzoyl peroxide, clindamycin and vehicle groups in three of the five studies (Studies 1, 2, and 5).
Clinical studies have not adequately demonstrated the effectiveness of Duac versus benzoyl peroxide alone in the treatment of non-inflammatory lesions of acne.

INDICATIONS AND USAGE
Duac Topical Gel is indicated for the topical treatment of inflammatory acne vulgaris.
Duac Topical Gel has not been demonstrated to have any additional benefit when compared to benzoyl peroxide alone in the same vehicle when used for the treatment of non-inflammatory acne.

CONTRAINDICATIONS
Duac Topical Gel is contraindicated in those individuals who have shown hypersensitivity to any of its components or to lincomycin. It is also contraindicated in those having a history of regional enteritis, ulcerative colitis, pseudomembranous colitis, or antibiotic-associated colitis.

WARNINGS
ORALLY AND PARENTERALLY ADMINISTERED CLINDAMYCIN HAS BEEN ASSOCIATED WITH SEVERE COLITIS WHICH MAY RESULT IN PATIENT DEATH. USE OF THE TOPICAL FORMULATION OF CLINDAMYCIN RESULTS IN ABSORPTION OF THE ANTIBIOTIC FROM THE SKIN SURFACE. DIARRHEA, BLOODY DIARRHEA, AND COLITIS (INCLUDING PSEUDOMEMBRANOUS COLITIS) HAVE BEEN REPORTED WITH THE USE OF TOPICAL AND SYSTEMIC CLINDAMYCIN. STUDIES INDICATE A TOXIN(S) PRODUCED BY CLOSTRIDIA IS ONE PRIMARY CAUSE OF ANTIBIOTIC-ASSOCIATED COLITIS. THE COLITIS IS USUALLY CHARACTERIZED BY SEVERE PERSISTENT DIARRHEA AND SEVERE ABDOMINAL CRAMPS AND MAY BE ASSOCIATED WITH THE PASSAGE OF BLOOD AND MUCUS. ENDOSCOPIC EXAMINATION MAY REVEAL PSEUDOMEMBRANOUS COLITIS. STOOL CULTURE FOR *Clostridium difficile* AND STOOL ASSAY FOR *Clostridium difficile* TOXIN MAY BE HELPFUL DIAGNOSTICALLY. WHEN SIGNIFICANT DIARRHEA OCCURS, THE DRUG SHOULD BE DISCONTINUED. LARGE BOWEL ENDOSCOPY SHOULD BE CONSIDERED TO ESTABLISH A DEFINITIVE DIAGNOSIS IN CASES OF SEVERE DIARRHEA. ANTIPERISTALTIC AGENTS SUCH AS OPIATES AND DIPHENOXYLATE WITH ATROPINE MAY PROLONG AND/OR WORSEN THE CONDITION. DIARRHEA, COLITIS AND PSEUDOMEMBRANOUS COLITIS HAVE BEEN OBSERVED TO BEGIN UP TO SEVERAL WEEKS FOLLOWING CESSATION OF ORAL AND PARENTERAL THERAPY WITH CLINDAMYCIN.
Mild cases of pseudomembranous colitis usually respond to drug discontinuation alone. In moderate to severe cases, consideration should be given to management with fluids and electrolytes, protein supplementation and treatment with an antibacterial drug clinically effective against *Clostridium difficile* colitis.

PRECAUTIONS
General: For dermatological use only; not for ophthalmic use. Concomitant topical acne therapy should be used with caution because a possible cumulative irritancy effect may occur, especially with the use of peeling, desquamating, or abrasive agents.

Mean percent reduction in inflammatory lesion counts					
	Study 1 (n=120)	Study 2 (n=273)	Study 3 (n=280)	Study 4 (n=288)	Study 5 (n=358)
Duac	65%	56%	42%	57%	52%
Benzoyl Peroxide	36%	37%	32%	57%	41%
Clindamycin	34%	30%	38%	49%	33%
Vehicle	19%	-0.4%	29%		29%

Local reactions with use of Duac Topical Gel
% of patients using Duac Topical Gel with symptom present
Combined results from 5 studies (n = 397)

	Baseline			During Treatment		
	Mild	Moderate	Severe	Mild	Moderate	Severe
Erythema	28%	3%	0	26%	5%	0
Peeling	6%	<1%	0	17%	2%	0
Burning	3%	<1%	0	5%	<1%	0
Dryness	6%	<1%	0	15%	1%	0

(Percentages derived by # subjects with symptom score/# enrolled Duac subjects, n = 397).

The use of antibiotic agents may be associated with the overgrowth of nonsusceptible organisms, including fungi. If this occurs, discontinue use of this medication and take appropriate measures.
Avoid contact with eyes and mucous membranes.
Clindamycin and erythromycin containing products should not be used in combination. *In vitro* studies have shown antagonism between these two antimicrobials. The clinical significance of this *in vitro* antagonism is not known.
Information for Patients: Patients using Duac Topical Gel should receive the following information and instructions:
1. Duac Topical Gel is to be used as directed by the physician. It is for external use only. Avoid contact with eyes, and inside the nose, mouth, and all mucous membranes, as this product may be irritating.
2. This medication should not be used for any disorder other than that for which it was prescribed.
3. Patients should not use any other topical acne preparation unless otherwise directed by their physician.
4. Patients should report any signs of local adverse reactions to their physician.
5. Duac Topical Gel may bleach hair or colored fabric.
6. Duac Topical Gel can be stored at room temperature up to 25°C (77°F) for up to 2 months. Do not freeze. Keep tube tightly closed. Keep out of the reach of small children. Discard any unused product after 2 months.
7. Before applying Duac Topical Gel to affected areas, wash the skin gently, rinse with warm water, and pat dry.
8. Excessive or prolonged exposure to sunlight should be limited. To minimize exposure to sunlight, a hat or other clothing should be worn.

Carcinogenesis, Mutagenesis, Impairment of Fertility: Benzoyl peroxide has been shown to be a tumor promoter and progression agent in a number of animal studies. The clinical significance of this is unknown.
Benzoyl peroxide in acetone at doses of 5 and 10 mg administered twice per week induced squamous cell skin tumors in transgenic TgAC mice in a study using 20 weeks of topical treatment.
Genotoxicity studies were not conducted with Duac Topical Gel. Clindamycin phosphate was not genotoxic in *Salmonella typhimurium* or in a rat micronucleus test. Benzoyl peroxide has been found to cause DNA strand breaks in a variety of mammalian cell types, to be mutagenic in *Salmonella typhimurium* tests by some but not all investigators, and to cause sister chromatid exchanges in Chinese hamster ovary cells. Studies have not been performed with Duac Topical Gel or benzoyl peroxide to evaluate the effect on fertility. Fertility studies in rats treated orally with up to 300 mg/kg/day of clindamycin (approximately 120 times the amount of clindamycin in the highest recommended adult human dose of 2.5 g Duac Topical Gel, based on mg/m^2) revealed no effects on fertility or mating ability.
Pregnancy: Teratogenic Effects: Pregnancy Category C: Animal reproduction studies have not been conducted with Duac Topical Gel or benzoyl peroxide. It is also not known whether Duac Topical Gel can cause fetal harm when administered to a pregnant woman or can affect reproduction capacity. Duac Topical Gel should be given to a pregnant woman only if clearly needed.
Developmental toxicity studies performed in rats and mice using oral doses of clindamycin up to 600 mg/kg/day (240 and 120 times the amount of clindamycin in the highest recommended adult human dose based on mg/m^2, respectively) or subcutaneous doses of clindamycin up to 250 mg/kg/day (100 and 50 times the amount of clindamycin in the highest recommended adult human dose based on mg/m^2, respectively) revealed no evidence of teratogenicity.
Nursing Women: It is not known whether Duac Topical Gel is secreted into human milk after topical application. However, orally and parenterally administered clindamycin has been reported to appear in breast milk. Because of the potential for serious adverse reactions in nursing infants, a decision should be made whether to discontinue nursing or to discontinue the drug, taking into account the importance of the drug to the mother.
Pediatric Use: Safety and effectiveness of this product in pediatric patients below the age of 12 have not been established.

ADVERSE REACTIONS
During clinical trials, all patients were graded for facial erythema, peeling, burning, and dryness on the following scale: 0 = absent, 1 = mild, 2 = moderate, and 3 = severe. The percentage of patients that had symptoms present at baseline and during treatment were as follows:
[See table above]

DOSAGE AND ADMINISTRATION
Duac Topical Gel should be applied once daily, in the evening or as directed by the physician, to affected areas after the skin is gently washed, rinsed with warm water and patted dry.

HOW SUPPLIED
Duac™ (clindamycin, 1% - benzoyl peroxide, 5%) Topical Gel is available in a 45 gram tube - NDC 0145-2371-05.
Store in a cold place, preferably in a refrigerator, between 2°C and 8°C (36°F and 46°F). Do not freeze.
To the Pharmacist: Dispense with a 60 day expiration date and specify "Store at room temperature up to 25°C (77°F). Do not freeze."
Keep tube tightly closed. Keep out of the reach of small children.
U.S. Patent Nos. 5,466,446, 5,446,028, 5,767,098, and 6,013,637
Patent Pending

**Watson Pharma, Inc.
A Subsidiary of Watson Pharmaceuticals, Inc.**
311 BONNIE CIRCLE
CORONA, CA 92880

Address Inquiries to:
Customer Service Department
Telephone: 800/272-5525
FAX: 973-355-8594

OXYTROL™   ℞
[ŏks-ē-trōl]
Oxybutynin Transdermal System
Rx only

DESCRIPTION
OXYTROL, oxybutynin transdermal system, is designed to deliver oxybutynin continuously and consistently over a 3- to 4-day interval after application to intact skin. OXYTROL is available as a 39 cm^2 system containing 36 mg of oxybutynin. OXYTROL has a nominal *in vivo* delivery rate of 3.9 mg oxybutynin per day through skin of average permeability (interindividual variation in skin permeability is approximately 20%).
Oxybutynin is an antispasmodic, anticholinergic agent. Oxybutynin is administered as a racemate of R- and S-isomers. Chemically, oxybutynin is d, l (racemic) 4-diethylamino-2-butynyl phenylcyclohexylglycolate. The empirical formula of oxybutynin is $C_{22}H_{31}NO_3$. Its structural formula is:

Oxybutynin is a white powder with a molecular weight of 357. It is soluble in alcohol, but relatively insoluble in water.
Transdermal System Components
OXYTROL is a matrix-type transdermal system composed of three layers as illustrated in Figure 1 below. Layer 1 (Backing Film) is a thin flexible polyester/ethylene-vinyl acetate film that provides the matrix system with occlusivity and physical integrity and protects the adhesive/drug layer. Layer 2 (Adhesive/Drug Layer) is a cast film of acrylic adhesive containing oxybutynin and triacetin, USP. Layer 3 (Release Liner) is two overlapped siliconized polyester strips that are peeled off and discarded by the patient prior to applying the matrix system.
[See figure 1 at top of next column]

CLINICAL PHARMACOLOGY
The free base form of oxybutynin is pharmacologically equivalent to oxybutynin hydrochloride. Oxybutynin acts as a competitive antagonist of acetylcholine at postganglionic muscarinic receptors, resulting in relaxation of bladder smooth muscle. In patients with conditions characterized by involuntary detrusor contractions, cystometric studies have demonstrated that oxybutynin increases maximum urinary bladder capacity and increases the volume to first detrusor contraction. Oxybutynin thus decreases urinary urgency and the frequency of both incontinence episodes and voluntary urination.
Oxybutynin is a racemic (50:50) mixture of R- and S-isomers. Antimuscarinic activity resides predominantly in the R-isomer. The active metabolite, N-desethyloxybutynin, has pharmacological activity on the human detrusor muscle that is similar to that of oxybutynin in *in vitro* studies.
Pharmacokinetics
Absorption
Oxybutynin is transported across intact skin and into the systemic circulation by passive diffusion across the stratum corneum. The average daily dose of oxybutynin absorbed from the 39 cm^2 OXYTROL system is 3.9 mg. The average (SD) nominal dose, 0.10 (0.02) mg oxybutynin per cm^2 surface area, was obtained from analysis of residual oxybutynin content of systems worn over a continuous 4-day period during 303 separate occasions in 76 healthy volunteers. Following application of the first OXYTROL 3.9 mg/day system, oxybutynin plasma concentration increases for approximately 24 to 48 hours, reaching average maximum concentrations of 3 to 4 ng/mL. Thereafter, steady concentrations are maintained for up to 96 hours. Absorption of oxybutynin is bioequivalent when OXYTROL is applied to the abdomen, buttocks, or hip. Average plasma concentrations measured during a randomized, crossover study of the three recommended application sites in 24 healthy men and women are shown in Figure 2.

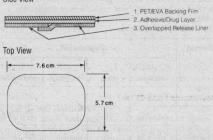

Figure 1: Side and top views of the OXYTROL system. (Not to scale)

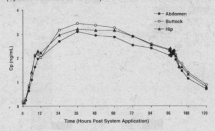

Figure 2: Average plasma oxybutynin concentrations (Cp) in 24 healthy male and female volunteers during single-dose application of OXYTROL 3.9 mg/day to the abdomen, buttock, and hip (System removal at 96 hours).

Steady-state conditions are reached during the second OXYTROL application. Average steady-state plasma concentrations were 3.1 ng/mL for oxybutynin and 3.8 ng/mL for N-desethyloxybutynin (Figure 3). Table 1 provides a summary of pharmacokinetic parameters of oxybutynin in healthy volunteers after single and multiple applications of OXYTROL.

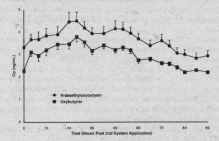

Figure 3: Average (SEM) steady-state oxybutynin and N-desethyloxybutynin plasma concentrations (Cp) measured in 13 healthy volunteers following the second transdermal system application in a multiple-dose, randomized, crossover study.

Continued on next page

Oxytrol—Cont.

Table 1: Mean (SD) oxybutynin pharmacokinetic parameters from single and multiple dose studies in healthy men and women volunteers after application of **OXYTROL** on the abdomen.

Dosing	Oxybutynin			
	C_{max}(SD) (ng/mL)	T_{max}[1] (hr)	C_{avg} (SD) (ng/mL)	AUC (SD) (ng/mLxh)
Single	3.0 (0.8)	48	—	245 (59)[2]
	3.4 (1.1)	36	—	279 (99)[2]
Multiple	6.6 (2.4)	10	4.2 (1.1)	408 (108)[3]
	4.2 (1.0)	28	3.1 (0.7)	259 (57)[4]

[1] T_{max} given as median
[2] AUC_{inf}
[3] AUC_{0-96}
[4] AUC_{0-84}

Distribution
Oxybutynin is widely distributed in body tissues following systemic absorption. The volume of distribution was estimated to be 193 L after intravenous administration of 5 mg oxybutynin chloride.

Metabolism
Oxybutynin is metabolized primarily by the cytochrome P450 enzyme systems, particularly CYP3A4, found mostly in the liver and gut wall. Metabolites include phenylcyclohexylglycolic acid, which is pharmacologically inactive, and N-desethyloxybutynin, which is pharmacologically active. After oral administration of oxybutynin, pre-systemic first-pass metabolism results in an oral bioavailability of approximately 6% and higher plasma concentration of the N-desethyl metabolite compared to oxybutynin (see Figure 4). The plasma concentration AUC ratio of N-desethyl metabolite to parent compound following a single 5 mg oral dose of oxybutynin chloride was 11.9:1.

Transdermal administration of oxybutynin bypasses the first-pass gastrointestinal and hepatic metabolism, reducing the formation of the N-desethyl metabolite (see Figure 4). Only small amounts of CYP3A4 are found in skin, limiting pre-systemic metabolism during transdermal absorption. The resulting plasma concentration AUC ratio of N-desethyl metabolite to parent compound following multiple **OXYTROL** applications was 1.3:1.

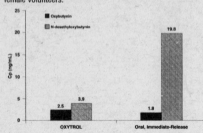

Figure 4: Average plasma concentrations (Cp) measured after a single, 96-hour application of the **OXYTROL** 3.9 mg/day system (AUC_{inf}/96) and a single, 5 mg, oral immediate-release dose of oxybutynin chloride (AUC_{inf}/8) in 16 healthy male and female volunteers.

Following intravenous administration, the elimination half-life of oxybutynin is approximately 2 hours. Following removal of **OXYTROL**, plasma concentrations of oxybutynin and N-desethyloxybutynin decline with an apparent half-life of approximately 7 to 8 hours.

Excretion
Oxybutynin is extensively metabolized by the liver, with less than 0.1% of the administered dose excreted unchanged in the urine. Also, less than 0.1% of the administered dose is excreted as the metabolite N-desethyloxybutynin.

Special Populations
Geriatric: The pharmacokinetics of oxybutynin and N-desethyloxybutynin were similar in all patients studied.
Pediatric: The pharmacokinetics of oxybutynin and N-desethyloxybutynin were not evaluated in individuals younger than 18 years of age. See **PRECAUTIONS: Pediatric Use**.
Gender: There were no significant differences in the pharmacokinetics of oxybutynin in healthy male and female volunteers following application of **OXYTROL**.
Race: Available data suggest that there are no significant differences in the pharmacokinetics of oxybutynin based on race in healthy volunteers following administration of **OXYTROL**. Japanese volunteers demonstrated a somewhat lower metabolism of oxybutynin to N-desethyloxybutynin compared to Caucasian volunteers.
Renal Insufficiency: There is no experience with the use of **OXYTROL** in patients with renal insufficiency.
Hepatic Insufficiency: There is no experience with the use of **OXYTROL** in patients with hepatic insufficiency.
Drug-Drug Interactions: See **PRECAUTIONS: Drug Interactions**.

Adhesion
Adhesion was periodically evaluated during the Phase 3 studies. Of the 4,746 **OXYTROL** evaluations in the Phase 3 trials, 20 (0.4%) were observed at clinic visits to have become completely detached and 35 (0.7%) became partially detached during routine clinic use. Similar to the pharmacokinetic studies, > 98% of the systems evaluated in the Phase 3 studies were assessed as being ≥ 75% attached and thus would be expected to perform as anticipated.

Clinical Studies
The efficacy and safety of **OXYTROL** were evaluated in patients with urge urinary incontinence in two Phase 3 controlled studies and one open-label extension. Study 1 was a Phase 3, placebo controlled study, comparing the safety and efficacy of **OXYTROL** at dose levels of 1.3, 2.6, and 3.9 mg/day to placebo in 520 patients. Open-label treatment was available for patients completing the study. Study 2 was a Phase 3 study, comparing the safety and efficacy of **OXYTROL** 3.9 mg/day versus active and placebo controls in 361 patients.

Study 1 was a randomized, double-blind, placebo-controlled, parallel group study of three dose levels of **OXYTROL** conducted in 520 patients. The 12-week double-blind treatment included **OXYTROL** doses of 1.3, 2.6, and 3.9 mg/day with matching placebo. An open-label, dose titration treatment extension allowed continued treatment for up to an additional 40 weeks for patients completing the double-blind period. The majority of patients were Caucasian (91%) and female (92%) with a mean age of 61 years (range, 20 to 88 years). Entry criteria required that patients have urge or mixed incontinence (with a predominance of urge), urge incontinence episodes of ≥ 10 per week, and ≥ 8 micturitions per day. The patient's medical history and a urinary diary during the treatment-free baseline period confirmed the diagnosis of urge incontinence. Approximately 80% of patients had no prior pharmacological treatment for incontinence. Reductions in weekly incontinence episodes, urinary frequency, and urinary void volume between placebo and active treatment groups are summarized in Table 2.

Table 2: Mean and median change from baseline to end of treatment (Week 12 or last observation carried forward) in incontinence episodes, urinary frequency, and urinary void volume in patients treated with **OXYTROL** 3.9 mg/day or placebo for 12 weeks (Study 1).

Parameter	Placebo (N=127)		OXYTROL 3.9 mg/day (N=120)	
	Mean (SD)	Median	Mean (SD)	Median
Weekly Incontinence Episodes				
Baseline	37.7 (24.0)	30	34.3 (18.2)	31
Reduction	19.2 (21.4)	15	21.0 (17.1)	19
p value vs. placebo	—		0.0265*	
Daily Urinary Frequency				
Baseline	12.3 (3.5)	11	11.8 (3.1)	11
Reduction	1.6 (3.0)	1	2.2 (2.5)	2
p value vs. placebo	—		0.0313*	
Urinary Void Volume (mL)				
Baseline	175.9 (69.5)	166.5	171.6 (65.1)	168
Increase	10.5 (56.9)	5.5	31.6 (65.6)	26
p value vs. placebo	—		0.0009**	

*Comparison significant if p < 0.05
**Comparison significant if p ≤ 0.0167

Study 2 was a randomized, double-blind, double-dummy, study of **OXYTROL** 3.9 mg/day versus active and placebo controls conducted in 361 patients. The 12-week double-blind treatment included an **OXYTROL** dose of 3.9 mg/day, an active comparator, and placebo. The majority of patients were Caucasian (95%) and female (93%) with a mean age of 64 years (range, 18 to 89 years). Entry criteria required that all patients have urge or mixed incontinence (with a predominance of urge) and had achieved a beneficial response from the anticholinergic treatment they were using at the time of study entry. The average duration of prior pharmacological treatment was greater than 2 years. The patient's medical history and a urinary diary during the treatment-free baseline period confirmed the diagnosis of urge incontinence. Reductions in daily incontinence episodes, urinary frequency, and urinary void volume between placebo and active treatment groups are summarized in Table 3.

Table 3: Mean and median change from baseline to end of treatment (Week 12 or last observation carried forward) in incontinence episodes, urinary frequency, and urinary void volume in patients treated with **OXYTROL** 3.9 mg/day or placebo for 12 weeks (Study 2).

Parameter	Placebo (N=117)		OXYTROL 3.9 mg/day (N=121)	
	Mean (SD)	Median	Mean (SD)	Median
Daily Incontinence Episodes				
Baseline	5.0 (3.2)	4	4.7 (2.9)	4
Reduction	2.1 (3.0)	2	2.9 (3.0)	3
p value vs. placebo	—		0.0137*	
Daily Urinary Frequency				
Baseline	12.3 (3.3)	12	12.4 (2.9)	12
Reduction	1.4 (2.7)	1	1.9 (2.7)	2
p value vs. placebo	—		0.1010*	
Urinary Void Volume (mL)				
Baseline	175.0 (68.0)	171.0	164.8 (62.3)	160
Increase	9.3 (63.1)	5.5	32.0 (55.2)	24
p value vs. placebo	—		0.0010*	

*Comparison significant if p < 0.05

INDICATIONS AND USAGE
OXYTROL is indicated for the treatment of overactive bladder with symptoms of urge urinary incontinence, urgency, and frequency.

CONTRAINDICATIONS
OXYTROL is contraindicated in patients with urinary retention, gastric retention, or uncontrolled narrow-angle glaucoma and in patients who are at risk for these conditions.
OXYTROL is also contraindicated in patients who have demonstrated hypersensitivity to oxybutynin or other components of the product.

PRECAUTIONS
General
OXYTROL should be used with caution in patients with hepatic or renal impairment.
Urinary Retention: **OXYTROL** should be administered with caution to patients with clinically significant bladder outflow obstruction because of the risk of urinary retention (see **CONTRAINDICATIONS**).
Gastrointestinal Disorders: **OXYTROL** should be administered with caution to patients with gastrointestinal obstructive disorders because of the risk of gastric retention (see **CONTRAINDICATIONS**).
OXYTROL, like other anticholinergic drugs, may decrease gastrointestinal motility and should be used with caution in patients with conditions such as ulcerative colitis, intestinal atony, and myasthenia gravis. **OXYTROL** should be used with caution in patients who have gastroesophageal reflux and/or who are concurrently taking drugs (such as bisphosphonates) that can cause or exacerbate esophagitis.

Information for Patients
Patients should be informed that heat prostration (fever and heat stroke due to decreased sweating) can occur when anticholinergics such as oxybutynin are used in a hot environment. Because anticholinergic agents such as oxybutynin may produce drowsiness (somnolence) or blurred vision, patients should be advised to exercise caution. Patients should be informed that alcohol may enhance the drowsiness caused by anticholinergic agents such as oxybutynin.

OXYTROL should be applied to dry, intact skin on the abdomen, hip, or buttock. A new application site should be selected with each new system to avoid re-application to the same site within 7 days. Details on use of the system are explained in the patient information leaflet that should be dispensed with the product.

Drug Interactions
The concomitant use of oxybutynin with other anticholinergic drugs or with other agents that produce dry mouth, constipation, somnolence, and/or other anticholinergic-like effects may increase the frequency and/or severity of such effects. Anticholinergic agents may potentially alter the absorption of some concomitantly administered drugs due to anticholinergic effects on gastrointestinal motility. Pharmacokinetic studies have not been performed with patients concomitantly receiving cytochrome P450 enzyme inhibitors, such as antimycotic agents (e.g. ketoconazole, itraconazole, and miconazole) or macrolide antibiotics (e.g. erythromycin and clarithromycin). No specific drug-drug interaction studies have been performed with **OXYTROL**.

Carcinogenesis, Mutagenesis, Impairment of Fertility

A 24-month study in rats at dosages of oxybutynin chloride of 20, 80 and 160 mg/kg showed no evidence of carcinogenicity. These doses are approximately 6, 25 and 50 times the maximum exposure in humans taking an oral dose based on body surface area.

Oxybutynin chloride showed no increase of mutagenic activity when tested in *Schizosaccharomyces pompholiciformis*, *Saccharomyces cerevisiae*, and *Salmonella typhimurium* test systems. Reproduction studies with oxybutynin chloride in the mouse, rat, hamster, and rabbit showed no definite evidence of impaired fertility.

Pregnancy: Teratogenic Effects
Pregnancy Category B

Reproduction studies with oxybutynin chloride in the mouse, rat, hamster, and rabbit showed no definite evidence of impaired fertility or harm to the animal fetus. Subcutaneous administration to rats at doses up to 25 mg/kg (approximately 50 times the human exposure based on surface area) and to rabbits at doses up to 0.4 mg/kg (approximately 1 times the human exposure) revealed no evidence of harm to the fetus due to oxybutynin chloride. The safety of OXYTROL administration to women who are or who may become pregnant has not been established. Therefore, OXYTROL should not be given to pregnant women unless, in the judgment of the physician, the probable clinical benefits outweigh the possible hazards.

Nursing Mothers

It is not known whether oxybutynin is excreted in human milk. Because many drugs are excreted in human milk, caution should be exercised when OXYTROL is administered to a nursing woman.

Pediatric Use

The safety and efficacy of OXYTROL in pediatric patients have not been established.

Geriatric Use

Of the total number of patients in the clinical studies of OXYTROL, 49% were 65 and over. No overall differences in safety or effectiveness were observed between these subjects and younger subjects, and other reported clinical experience has not identified differences in response between elderly and younger patients, but greater sensitivity of some older individuals cannot be ruled out (see CLINICAL PHARMACOLOGY, Pharmacokinetics, *Special Populations: Geriatric*).

ADVERSE REACTIONS

The safety of OXYTROL was evaluated in a total of 417 patients who participated in two Phase 3 clinical efficacy and safety studies and an open-label extension. Additional safety information was collected in Phase 1 and Phase 2 trials. In the two pivotal studies, a total of 246 patients received OXYTROL during the 12-week treatment periods. A total of 411 patients entered the open-label extension and of those, 65 patients and 52 patients received OXYTROL for at least 24 weeks and at least 36 weeks, respectively.

No deaths were reported during treatment. No serious adverse events related to treatment were reported.

Adverse events reported in the pivotal trials are summarized in Tables 4 and 5 below.

Table 4: Number (%) of adverse events occurring in ≥ 2% of OXYTROL-treated patients and greater in OXYTROL group than in placebo group (Study 1).

Adverse Event*	Placebo (N=132) N	%	OXYTROL (3.9 mg/day) (N=125) N	%
Application site pruritus	8	6.1%	21	16.8%
Dry mouth	11	8.3%	12	9.6%
Application site erythema	3	2.3%	7	5.6%
Application site vesicles	0	0.0%	4	3.2%
Diarrhea	3	2.3%	4	3.2%
Dysuria	0	0.0%	3	2.4%

*includes adverse events judged by the investigator as possibly, probably or definitely treatment-related.

Table 5: Number (%) of adverse events occurring in ≥ 2% of OXYTROL-treated patients and greater in OXYTROL group than in placebo group (Study 2).

Adverse Event*	Placebo (N=117) N	%	OXYTROL (3.9 mg/day) (N=121) N	%
Application site pruritus	5	4.3%	17	14.0%
Application site erythema	2	1.7%	10	8.3%
Dry mouth	2	1.7%	5	4.1%
Constipation	0	0.0%	4	3.3%
Application site rash	1	0.9%	4	3.3%
Application site macules	0	0.0%	3	2.5%
Abnormal vision	0	0.0%	3	2.5%

*includes adverse events judged by the investigator as possibly, probably or definitely treatment-related.

Other adverse events reported by > 1% of OXYTROL-treated patients, and judged by the investigator to be possibly, probably or definitely related to treatment include: abdominal pain, nausea, flatulence, fatigue, somnolence, headache, flushing, rash, application site burning and back pain.

Most treatment-related adverse events were described as mild or moderate in intensity. Severe application site reactions were reported by 6.4% of OXYTROL-treated patients in Study 1 and by 5.0% of OXYTROL-treated patients in Study 2.

Treatment-related adverse events that resulted in discontinuation were reported by 11.2% of OXYTROL-treated patients in Study 1 and 10.7% of OXYTROL-treated patients in Study 2. Most of these were secondary to application site reaction. In the two pivotal studies, no patient discontinued OXYTROL treatment due to dry mouth.

In the open-label extension, the most common treatment-related adverse events were: application site pruritus, application site erythema and dry mouth.

OVERDOSAGE

Plasma concentration of oxybutynin declines within 1 to 2 hours after removal of transdermal system(s). Patients should be monitored until symptoms resolve. Overdosage with oxybutynin has been associated with anticholinergic effects including CNS excitation, flushing, fever, dehydration, cardiac arrhythmia, vomiting, and urinary retention. Ingestion of 100 mg oral oxybutynin chloride in association with alcohol has been reported in a 13 year old boy who experienced memory loss, and in a 34 year old woman who developed stupor, followed by disorientation and agitation on awakening, dilated pupils, dry skin, cardiac arrhythmia, and retention of urine. Both patients recovered fully with symptomatic treatment.

DOSAGE AND ADMINISTRATION

OXYTROL should be applied to dry, intact skin on the abdomen, hip, or buttock. A new application site should be selected with each new system to avoid re-application to the same site within 7 days.

The dose of OXYTROL is one 3.9 mg/day system applied twice weekly (every 3 to 4 days).

HOW SUPPLIED

OXYTROL 3.9 mg/day (oxybutynin transdermal system). Each 39 cm^2 system imprinted with OXYTROL 3.9 mg/day contains 36 mg oxybutynin for nominal delivery of 3.9 mg oxybutynin per day when dosed in a twice weekly regimen.
NDC 52544-920-08   Patient Calendar Box of 8 Systems

Storage
Store at 25°C (77°F); excursions permitted to 15–30°C (59–86°F). Protect from moisture and humidity. Do not store outside the sealed pouch. Apply immediately after removal from the protective pouch. Discard used OXYTROL in household trash in a manner that prevents accidental application or ingestion by children, pets, or others.

WATSON Pharma, Inc.
A Subsidiary of Watson Pharmaceuticals, Inc.
Corona, CA 92880 USA
DATE OF ISSUANCE: FEBRUARY 2003
U.S. Patent Nos. 5,601,839 and 5,834,010

REVISED INFORMATION

As new research data and clinical findings become available, the product information in *PDR* is revised accordingly. Revisions submitted since the 2003 edition went to press can be found below. To remind yourself of a revision, write "See Supplement A" next to the product's heading in the book.

Abbott Laboratories
Pharmaceutical Products Division
NORTH CHICAGO, IL 60064, U.S.A.

Pharmaceutical Products Division—
Direct Inquiries to:
Customer Service:
(800) 255-5162
Technical Services:
(800) 441-4987
For Medical Information Contact:
Generally:
(800) 633-9110
Adverse Drug Experiences:
(800) 633-9110
Sales and Ordering:
(800) 255-5162

Hospital Products Division—
Direct Inquiries to:
Customer Service
(800) 222-6883
For Medical Information Contact:
(800) 633-9110
Sales and Ordering:
(800) 222-6883

DEPAKOTE® ER ℞
[dĕp' ă-kōte]
DIVALPROEX SODIUM
EXTENDED-RELEASE TABLETS
Rx Only

Prescribing information for this product, which appears on pages 437–441 of the 2003 PDR, has been completely revised as follows. Please write "See Supplement A" next to the product heading.

BOX WARNING:
HEPATOTOXICITY:
HEPATIC FAILURE RESULTING IN FATALITIES HAS OCCURRED IN PATIENTS RECEIVING VALPROIC ACID AND ITS DERIVATIVES. EXPERIENCE HAS INDICATED THAT CHILDREN UNDER THE AGE OF TWO YEARS ARE AT A CONSIDERABLY INCREASED RISK OF DEVELOPING FATAL HEPATOTOXICITY, ESPECIALLY THOSE ON MULTIPLE ANTICONVULSANTS, THOSE WITH CONGENITAL METABOLIC DISORDERS, THOSE WITH SEVERE SEIZURE DISORDERS ACCOMPANIED BY MENTAL RETARDATION, AND THOSE WITH ORGANIC BRAIN DISEASE. WHEN DEPAKOTE IS USED IN THIS PATIENT GROUP, IT SHOULD BE USED WITH EXTREME CAUTION AND AS A SOLE AGENT. THE BENEFITS OF THERAPY SHOULD BE WEIGHED AGAINST THE RISKS. ABOUT THIS AGE GROUP, EXPERIENCE IN EPILEPSY HAS INDICATED THAT THE INCIDENCE OF FATAL HEPATOTOXICITY DECREASES CONSIDERABLY IN PROGRESSIVELY OLDER PATIENT GROUPS.
THESE INCIDENTS USUALLY HAVE OCCURRED DURING THE FIRST SIX MONTHS OF TREATMENT. SERIOUS OR FATAL HEPATOTOXICITY MAY BE PRECEDED BY NON-SPECIFIC SYMPTOMS SUCH AS MALAISE, WEAKNESS, LETHARGY, FACIAL EDEMA, ANOREXIA, AND VOMITING. IN PATIENTS WITH EPILEPSY, A LOSS OF SEIZURE CONTROL MAY ALSO OCCUR. PATIENTS SHOULD BE MONITORED CLOSELY FOR APPEARANCE OF THESE SYMPTOMS. LIVER FUNCTION TESTS SHOULD BE PERFORMED PRIOR TO THERAPY AND AT FREQUENT INTERVALS THEREAFTER, ESPECIALLY DURING THE FIRST SIX MONTHS.

TERATOGENICITY:
VALPROATE CAN PRODUCE TERATOGENIC EFFECTS SUCH AS NEURAL TUBE DEFECTS (E.G., SPINA BIFIDA). ACCORDINGLY, THE USE OF DEPAKOTE TABLETS IN WOMEN OF CHILDBEARING POTENTIAL REQUIRES THAT THE BENEFITS OF ITS USE BE WEIGHED AGAINST THE RISK OF INJURY TO THE FETUS. THIS IS ESPECIALLY IMPORTANT WHEN THE TREATMENT OF A SPONTANEOUSLY REVERSIBLE CONDITION NOT ORDINARILY ASSOCIATED WITH PERMANENT INJURY OR RISK OF DEATH (E.G., MIGRAINE) IS CONTEMPLATED. SEE WARNINGS, INFORMATION FOR PATIENTS.
AN INFORMATION SHEET DESCRIBING THE TERATOGENIC POTENTIAL OF VALPROATE IS AVAILABLE FOR PATIENTS.

PANCREATITIS:
CASES OF LIFE-THREATENING PANCREATITIS HAVE BEEN REPORTED IN BOTH CHILDREN AND ADULTS RECEIVING VALPROATE. SOME OF THE CASES HAVE BEEN DESCRIBED AS HEMORRHAGIC WITH A RAPID PROGRESSION FROM INITIAL SYMPTOMS TO DEATH. CASES HAVE BEEN REPORTED SHORTLY AFTER INITIAL USE AS WELL AS AFTER SEVERAL YEARS OF USE. PATIENTS AND GUARDIANS SHOULD BE WARNED THAT ABDOMINAL PAIN, NAUSEA, VOMITING, AND/OR ANOREXIA CAN BE SYMPTOMS OF PANCREATITIS THAT REQUIRE PROMPT MEDICAL EVALUATION. IF PANCREATITIS IS DIAGNOSED, VALPROATE SHOULD ORDINARILY BE DISCONTINUED. ALTERNATIVE TREATMENT FOR THE UNDERLYING MEDICAL CONDITION SHOULD BE INITIATED AS CLINICALLY INDICATED. (See **WARNINGS** and **PRECAUTIONS**.)

DESCRIPTION
Divalproex sodium is a stable co-ordination compound comprised of sodium valproate and valproic acid in a 1:1 molar relationship and formed during the partial neutralization of valproic acid with 0.5 equivalent of sodium hydroxide. Chemically it is designated as sodium hydrogen bis(2-propylpentanoate). Divalproex sodium has the following structure:

$$\left(\begin{array}{c} CH_3CH_2CH_2-CH-CH_2CH_2CH_3 \\ HO-C=O \quad Na^{\oplus} \\ O=C-O^{\ominus} \\ CH_3CH_2CH_2-CH-CH_2CH_2CH_3 \end{array} \right)_n$$

Divalproex sodium occurs as a white powder with a characteristic odor.
DEPAKOTE ER 250 and 500 mg tablets are for oral administration. DEPAKOTE ER tablets contain divalproex sodium in a once-a-day extended-release formulation equivalent to 250 and 500 mg of valproic acid.

Inactive Ingredients
DEPAKOTE ER 250 and 500 mg tablets: FD&C Blue No. 1, hypromellose, lactose, microcrystalline cellulose, polyethylene glycol, potassium sorbate, propylene glycol, silicon dioxide, titanium dioxide, and triacetin.
In addition, 500 mg tablets contain iron oxide and polydextrose.

CLINICAL PHARMACOLOGY
Pharmacodynamics
Divalproex sodium dissociates to the valproate ion in the gastrointestinal tract. The mechanisms by which valproate exerts its therapeutic effects have not been established. It has been suggested that its activity in epilepsy is related to increased brain concentrations of gamma-aminobutyric acid (GABA).

Pharmacokinetics
Absorption/Bioavailability
The absolute bioavailability of DEPAKOTE ER tablets administered as a single dose after a meal was approximately 90% relative to intravenous infusion.
When given in equal total daily doses, the bioavailability of DEPAKOTE ER is less than that of DEPAKOTE (divalproex sodium delayed-release tablets). In five multiple-dose studies in healthy subjects (N=82) and in subjects with epilepsy (N=86), when administered under fasting and nonfasting conditions, DEPAKOTE ER given once daily produced an average bioavailability of 89% relative to an equal total daily dose of DEPAKOTE given BID, TID, or QID. The median time to maximum plasma valproate concentrations (C_{max}) after DEPAKOTE ER administration ranged from 4 to 17 hours. After multiple once-daily dosing of DEPAKOTE ER, the peak-to-trough fluctuation in plasma valproate concentrations was 10–20% lower than that of regular DEPAKOTE given BID, TID, or QID.
Conversion from DEPAKOTE to DEPAKOTE ER:
When DEPAKOTE ER is given in doses 8 to 20% higher than the total daily dose of DEPAKOTE, the two formulations are bioequivalent. In two randomized, crossover studies, multiple daily doses of DEPAKOTE were compared to 8 to 20% higher once-daily doses of DEPAKOTE ER. In these two studies, DEPAKOTE ER and DEPAKOTE regimens were equivalent with respect to area under the curve (AUC; a measure of the extent of bioavailability). Additionally, valproate C_{max} was lower, and C_{min} was either higher or not different, for DEPAKOTE ER relative to DEPAKOTE regimens (see following table).
[See first table at top of next page]
Concomitant antiepilepsy drugs (topiramate, phenobarbital, carbamazepine, phenytoin, and lamotrigine were evaluated) that induce the cytochrome P450 isozyme system did not significantly alter valproate bioavailability when converting between DEPAKOTE and DEPAKOTE ER.

Distribution
Protein Binding:
The plasma protein binding of valproate is concentration dependent and the free fraction increases from approximately 10% at 40 µg/mL to 18.5% at 130 µg/mL. Protein binding of valproate is reduced in the elderly, in patients with chronic hepatic diseases, in patients with renal impairment, and in the presence of other drugs (e.g., aspirin). Conversely, valproate may displace certain protein-bound drugs (e.g., phenytoin, carbamazepine, warfarin, and tolbutamide) (see **PRECAUTIONS, Drug Interactions** for more detailed information on the pharmacokinetic interactions of valproate with other drugs).

CNS Distribution:
Valproate concentrations in cerebrospinal fluid (CSF) approximate unbound concentrations in plasma (about 10% of total concentration).

Metabolism
Valproate is metabolized almost entirely by the liver. In adult patients on monotherapy, 30-50% of an administered dose appears in urine as a glucuronide conjugate. Mitochondrial β-oxidation is the other major metabolic pathway, typically accounting for over 40% of the dose. Usually, less than 15-20% of the dose is eliminated by other oxidative mechanisms. Less than 3% of an administered dose is excreted unchanged in urine.
The relationship between dose and total valproate concentration is nonlinear; concentration does not increase proportionally with the dose, but rather, increases to a lesser extent due to saturable plasma protein binding. The kinetics of unbound drug are linear.

Elimination
Mean plasma clearance and volume of distribution for total valproate are 0.56 L/hr/1.73 m² and 11 L/1.73 m², respectively. Mean plasma clearance and volume of distribution

Continued on next page

Depakote ER—Cont.

for free valproate are 4.6 L/hr/1.73 m^2 and 92 L/1.73 m^2. Mean terminal half-life for valproate monotherapy ranged from 9 to 16 hours following oral dosing regimens of 250 to 1000 mg.

The estimates cited apply primarily to patients who are not taking drugs that affect hepatic metabolizing enzyme systems. For example, patients taking enzyme-inducing antiepileptic drugs (carbamazepine, phenytoin, and phenobarbital) will clear valproate more rapidly.

Special Populations

Elderly - The capacity of elderly patients (age range: 68 to 89 years) to eliminate valproate has been shown to be reduced compared to younger adults (age range: 22 to 26 years). Intrinsic clearance is reduced by 39%; the free fraction is increased by 44%. Accordingly, the initial dosage should be reduced in the elderly (see **DOSAGE AND ADMINISTRATION**).

Effect of Gender:

There are no differences in the body surface area adjusted unbound clearance between males and females (4.8±0.17 and 4.7±0.07 L/hr per 1.73 m^2, respectively).

Effect of Race:

The effects of race on the kinetics of valproate have not been studied.

Effect of Disease:

Liver Disease - (see **BOXED WARNING, CONTRAINDICATIONS**, and **WARNINGS**). Liver disease impairs the capacity to eliminate valproate. In one study, the clearance of free valproate was decreased by 50% in 7 patients with cirrhosis and by 16% in 4 patients with acute hepatitis, compared with 6 healthy subjects. In that study, the half-life of valproate was increased from 12 to 18 hours. Liver disease is also associated with decreased albumin concentrations and larger unbound fractions (2 to 2.6 fold increase) of valproate. Accordingly, monitoring of total concentrations may be misleading since free concentrations may be substantially elevated in patients with hepatic disease whereas total concentrations may appear to be normal.

Renal Disease - A slight reduction (27%) in the unbound clearance of valproate has been reported in patients with renal failure (creatinine clearance < 10 mL/minute); however, hemodialysis typically reduces valproate concentrations by about 20%. Therefore, no dosage adjustment appears to be necessary in patients with renal failure. Protein binding in these patients is substantially reduced; thus, monitoring total concentrations may be misleading.

Plasma Levels and Clinical Effect

The relationship between plasma concentration and clinical response is not well documented. One contributing factor is the nonlinear, concentration dependent protein binding of valproate which affects the clearance of the drug. Thus, monitoring of total serum valproate cannot provide a reliable index of the bioactive valproate species.

For example, because the plasma protein binding of valproate is concentration dependent, the free fraction increases from approximately 10% at 40 µg/mL to 18.5% at 130 µg/mL. Higher than expected free fractions occur in the elderly, in hyperlipidemic patients, and in patients with hepatic and renal diseases.

Epilepsy:

The therapeutic range in epilepsy is commonly considered to be 50 to 100 µg/mL of total valproate, although some patients may be controlled with lower or higher plasma concentrations.

Clinical Trials

Migraine

The results of a multicenter, randomized, double-blind, placebo-controlled, parallel-group clinical trial demonstrated the effectiveness of DEPAKOTE ER in the prophylactic treatment of migraine headache. This trial recruited patients with a history of migraine headaches with or without aura occurring on average twice or more a month for the preceding three months. Patients with cluster or chronic daily headaches were excluded. Women of childbearing potential were allowed in the trail if they were deemed to be practicing an effective method of contraception.

Patients who experienced ≥2 migraine headaches in the 4-week baseline period were randomized in a 1:1 ratio to DEPAKOTE ER or placebo and treated for 12 weeks. Patients initiated treatment on 500 mg once daily for one week, and were then increased to 1000 mg once daily with an option to permanently decrease the dose back to 500 mg once daily during the second week of treatment if intolerance occurred. Ninety-eight of 114 DEPAKOTE ER-treated patients (86%) and 100 of 110 placebo-treated patients (91%) treated at least two weeks maintained the 1000 mg once daily dose for the duration of their treatment periods. Treatment outcome was assessed on the basis of reduction in 4-week migraine headache rate in the treatment period compared to the baseline period.

Patients (50 male, 187 female) ranging in age from 16 to 69 were treated with DEPAKOTE ER (N=122) or placebo (N=115). Four patients were below the age of 18 and 3 were above the age of 65. Two hundred and two patients (101 in each treatment group) completed the treatment period. The mean reduction in 4-week migraine headache rate was 1.2 from a baseline mean of 4.4 in the DEPAKOTE ER group, versus 0.6 from a baseline mean of 4.2 in the placebo group.

Bioavailability of DEPAKOTE ER Tablets Relative to DEPAKOTE When DEPAKOTE ER Dose is 8 to 20% Higher

Study Population	Regimens DEPAKOTE ER vs. DEPAKOTE	Relative Bioavailability		
		AUC$_{24}$	C$_{max}$	C$_{min}$
Healthy Volunteers (N=35)	1000 & 1500 mg DEPAKOTE ER vs. 875 & 1250 mg DEPAKOTE	1.059	0.882	1.173
Patients with epilepsy on concomitant enzyme-inducing antiepilepsy drugs (N=64)	1000 to 5000 mg DEPAKOTE ER vs. 875 to 4250 mg DEPAKOTE	1.008	0.899	1.022

Adjunctive Therapy Study
Median Incidence of CPS per 8 Weeks

Add-on Treatment	Number of Patients	Baseline Incidence	Experimental Incidence
DEPAKOTE	75	16.0	8.9*
Placebo	69	14.5	11.5

*Reduction from baseline statistically significantly greater for DEPAKOTE than placebo at p ≤0.05 level.

The treatment difference was statistically significant (see Figure 1).

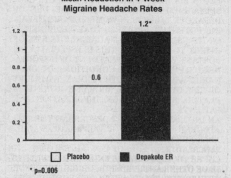

Figure 1
Mean Reduction In 4-Week Migraine Headache Rates
* p=0.006

Epilepsy

The efficacy of DEPAKOTE in reducing the incidence of complex partial seizures (CPS) that occur in isolation or in association with other seizure types was established in two controlled trials using DEPAKOTE (divalproex sodium delayed-release tablets).

In one, multiclinic, placebo controlled study employing an add-on design, (adjunctive therapy) using DEPAKOTE, 144 patients who continued to suffer eight or more CPS per 8 weeks during an 8 week period of monotherapy with doses of either carbamazepine or phenytoin sufficient to assure plasma concentrations within the "therapeutic range" were randomized to receive, in addition to their original antiepilepsy drug (AED), either DEPAKOTE or placebo. Randomized patients were to be followed for a total of 16 weeks. The following table presents the findings.

[See second table above]

Figure 2 presents the proportion of patients (X axis) whose percentage reduction from baseline in complex partial seizure rates was at least as great as that indicated on the Y axis in the adjunctive therapy study. A positive percent reduction indicates an improvement (i.e., a decrease in seizure frequency), while a negative percent reduction indicates worsening. Thus, in a display of this type, the curve for an effective treatment is shifted to the left of the curve for placebo. This figure shows that the proportion of patients achieving any particular level of improvement was consistently higher for DEPAKOTE than for placebo. For example, 45% of the patients treated with DEPAKOTE had a ≥50% reduction in complex partial seizure rate compared to 23% of patients treated with placebo.

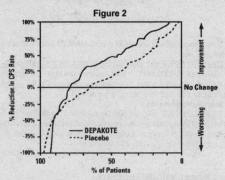

Figure 2

The second study assessed the capacity of DEPAKOTE to reduce the incidence of CPS when administered as the sole AED. The study compared the incidence of CPS among patients randomized to either a high or low dose treatment arm. Patients qualified for entry into the randomized comparison phase of this study only if 1) they continued to experience 2 or more CPS per 4 weeks during an 8 to 12 week long period of monotherapy with adequate doses of an AED (i.e., phenytoin, carbamazepine, phenobarbital, or primidone) and 2) they made a successful transition over a two week interval to DEPAKOTE. Patients entering the randomized phase were then brought to their assigned target dose, gradually tapered off their concomitant AED and followed for an interval as long as 22 weeks. Less than 50% of the patients randomized, however, completed the study. In patients converted to DEPAKOTE monotherapy, the mean total valproate concentrations during monotherapy were 71 and 123 µg/mL in the low dose and high dose groups, respectively.

The following table presents the findings for all patients randomized who had at least one post-randomization assessment.

[See table at bottom of next page]

Figure 3 presents the proportion of patients (X axis) whose percentage reduction from baseline in complex partial seizure rates was at least as great as that indicated on the Y axis in the monotherapy study. A positive percent reduction indicates an improvement (i.e., a decrease in seizure frequency), while a negative percent reduction indicates worsening. Thus, in a display of this type, the curve for a more effective treatment is shifted to the left of the curve for a less effective treatment. This figure shows that the proportion of patients achieving any particular level of reduction was consistently higher for high dose DEPAKOTE than for low dose DEPAKOTE. For example, when switching from carbamazepine, phenytoin, phenobarbital or primidone monotherapy to high dose DEPAKOTE monotherapy, 63% of patients experienced no change or a reduction in complex partial seizure rates compared to 54% of patients receiving low dose DEPAKOTE.

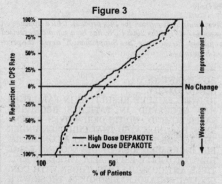

Figure 3

INDICATIONS AND USAGE

Migraine

DEPAKOTE ER is indicated for prophylaxis of migraine headaches in adults. There is no evidence that DEPAKOTE ER is useful in the acute treatment of migraine headaches. Because valproic acid may be a hazard to the fetus, DEPAKOTE ER should be considered for women of childbearing potential only after this risk has been thoroughly discussed with the patient and weighed against the potential benefits of treatment (see **WARNINGS - Usage In Pregnancy, PRECAUTIONS - Information for Patients**).

Epilepsy

DEPAKOTE ER is indicated as monotherapy and adjunctive therapy in the treatment of adult patients with complex partial seizures that occur either in isolation or in association with other types of seizures. DEPAKOTE ER is also indicated for use as sole and adjunctive therapy in the treatment of simple and complex absence seizures in adult patients, and adjunctively in adult patients with multiple seizure types that include absence seizures.

Simple absence is defined as very brief clouding of the sensorium or loss of consciousness accompanied by certain generalized epileptic discharges without other detectable clinical signs. Complex absence is the term used when other signs are also present. SEE **WARNINGS** FOR STATEMENT REGARDING FATAL HEPATIC DYSFUNCTION.

CONTRAINDICATIONS

DIVALPROEX SODIUM SHOULD NOT BE ADMINISTERED TO PATIENTS WITH HEPATIC DISEASE OR SIGNIFICANT HEPATIC DYSFUNCTION.

Divalproex sodium is contraindicated in patients with known hypersensitivity to the drug.

Divalproex sodium is contraindicated in patients with known urea cycle disorders (see **WARNINGS**).

WARNINGS
Hepatotoxicity

Hepatic failure resulting in fatalities has occurred in patients receiving valproic acid. These incidents usually have occurred during the first six months of treatment. Serious or fatal hepatotoxicity may be preceded by non-specific symptoms such as malaise, weakness, lethargy, facial edema, anorexia, and vomiting. Patients should be monitored closely for appearance of these symptoms. Liver function tests should be performed prior to therapy and at frequent intervals thereafter, especially during the first six months. However, physicians should not rely totally on serum biochemistry since these tests may not be abnormal in all instances, but should also consider the results of careful interim medical history and physical examination. Caution should be observed when administering DEPAKOTE products to patients with a prior history of hepatic disease. Patients on multiple anticonvulsants, children, those with congenital metabolic disorders, those with severe seizure disorders accompanied by mental retardation, and those with organic brain disease may be at particular risk. Experience has indicated that **children under the age of two years are at a considerably increased risk of developing fatal hepatotoxicity, especially those with the aforementioned conditions.** Above this age group, experience in epilepsy has indicated that the incidence of fatal hepatotoxicity decreases considerably in progressively older patient groups. **The use of DEPAKOTE ER in children is not recommended (see PRECAUTIONS - Pediatric Use).**

The drug should be discontinued immediately in the presence of significant hepatic dysfunction, suspected or apparent. In some cases, hepatic dysfunction has progressed in spite of discontinuation of drug.

Pancreatitis

Cases of life-threatening pancreatitis have been reported in both children and adults receiving valproate. Some of the cases have been described as hemorrhagic with rapid progression from initial symptoms to death. Some cases have occurred shortly after initial use as well as after several years of use. The rate based upon the reported cases exceeds that expected in the general population and there have been cases in which pancreatitis recurred after rechallenge with valproate. In clinical trials, there were 2 cases of pancreatitis without alternative etiology in 2416 patients, representing 1044 patient-years experience. Patients and guardians should be warned that abdominal pain, nausea, vomiting, and/or anorexia can be symptoms of pancreatitis that require prompt medical evaluation. If pancreatitis is diagnosed, valproate should ordinarily be discontinued. Alternative treatment for the underlying medical condition should be initiated as clinically indicated (see **BOXED WARNING**).

Urea Cycle Disorders (UCD)

Divalproex sodium is contraindicated in patients with known urea cycle disorders.

Hyperammonemic encephalopathy, sometimes fatal, has been reported following initiation of valproate therapy in patients with urea cycle disorders, a group of uncommon genetic abnormalities, particularly ornithine transcarbamylase deficiency. Prior to the initiation of valproate therapy, evaluation for UCD should be considered in the following patients: 1) those with a history of unexplained encephalopathy or coma, encephalopathy associated with a protein load, pregnancy-related or postpartum encephalopathy, unexplained mental retardation, or history of elevated plasma ammonia or glutamine; 2) those with cyclical vomiting and lethargy, episodic extreme irritability, ataxia, low BUN, or protein avoidance; 3) those with a family history of UCD or a family history of unexplained infant deaths (particularly males); 4) those with other signs or symptoms of UCD. Patients who develop symptoms of unexplained hyperammonemic encephalopathy while receiving valproate therapy should receive prompt treatment (including discontinuation of valproate therapy) and be evaluated for underlying urea cycle disorders (see **CONTRAINDICATIONS and PRECAUTIONS**).

Somnolence in the Elderly

In a double-blind, multicenter trial of valproate in elderly patients with dementia (mean age = 83 years), doses were increased by 125 mg/day to a target dose of 20 mg/kg/day. A significantly higher proportion of valproate patients had somnolence compared to placebo, and although not statistically significant, there was a higher proportion of patients with dehydration. Discontinuations for somnolence were also significantly higher than with placebo. In some patients with somnolence (approximately one-half), there was associated reduced nutritional intake and weight loss. There was a trend for the patients who experienced these events to have a lower baseline albumin concentration, lower valproate clearance, and a higher BUN. In elderly patients, dosage should be increased more slowly and with regular monitoring for fluid and nutritional intake, dehydration, somnolence, and other adverse events. Dose reductions or discontinuation of valproate should be considered in patients with decreased food or fluid intake and in patients with excessive somnolence (see **DOSAGE AND ADMINISTRATION**).

Thrombocytopenia

The frequency of adverse effects (particularly elevated liver enzymes and thrombocytopenia [see **PRECAUTIONS**]) may be dose-related. In a clinical trial of DEPAKOTE (divalproex sodium) as monotherapy in patients with epilepsy, 34/126 patients (27%) receiving approximately 50 mg/kg/day on average, had at least one value of platelets $\leq 75 \times 10^9$/L. Approximately half of these patients had treatment discontinued, with return of platelet counts to normal. In the remaining patients, platelet counts normalized with continued treatment. In this study, the probability of thrombocytopenia appeared to increase significantly at total valproate concentrations of ≥ 110 µg/mL (females) or ≥ 135 µg/mL (males). The therapeutic benefit which may accompany the higher doses should therefore be weighed against the possibility of a greater incidence of adverse effects.

Usage In Pregnancy

ACCORDING TO PUBLISHED AND UNPUBLISHED REPORTS, VALPROIC ACID MAY PRODUCE TERATOGENIC EFFECTS IN THE OFFSPRING OF HUMAN FEMALES RECEIVING THE DRUG DURING PREGNANCY. THE DATA DESCRIBED BELOW WERE GAINED ALMOST EXCLUSIVELY FROM WOMEN WHO RECEIVED VALPROATE TO TREAT EPILEPSY. THERE ARE MULTIPLE REPORTS IN THE CLINICAL LITERATURE WHICH INDICATE THAT THE USE OF ANTIEPILEPTIC DRUGS DURING PREGNANCY RESULTS IN AN INCREASED INCIDENCE OF BIRTH DEFECTS IN THE OFFSPRING. ALTHOUGH DATA ARE MORE EXTENSIVE WITH RESPECT TO TRIMETHADIONE, PARAMETHADIONE, PHENYTOIN, AND PHENOBARBITAL, REPORTS INDICATE A POSSIBLE SIMILAR ASSOCIATION WITH THE USE OF OTHER ANTIEPILEPTIC DRUGS. THEREFORE, ANTIEPILEPSY DRUGS SHOULD BE ADMINISTERED TO WOMEN OF CHILDBEARING POTENTIAL ONLY IF THEY ARE CLEARLY SHOWN TO BE ESSENTIAL IN THE MANAGEMENT OF THEIR SEIZURES.

THE INCIDENCE OF NEURAL TUBE DEFECTS IN THE FETUS MAY BE INCREASED IN MOTHERS RECEIVING VALPROATE DURING THE FIRST TRIMESTER OF PREGNANCY. THE CENTERS FOR DISEASE CONTROL (CDC) HAS ESTIMATED THE RISK OF VALPROIC ACID EXPOSED WOMEN HAVING CHILDREN WITH SPINA BIFIDA TO BE APPROXIMATELY 1 TO 2%.

OTHER CONGENITAL ANOMALIES (EG, CRANIOFACIAL DEFECTS, CARDIOVASCULAR MALFORMATIONS AND ANOMALIES INVOLVING VARIOUS BODY SYSTEMS), COMPATIBLE AND INCOMPATIBLE WITH LIFE, HAVE BEEN REPORTED. SUFFICIENT DATA TO DETERMINE THE INCIDENCE OF THESE CONGENITAL ANOMALIES IS NOT AVAILABLE.

THE HIGHER INCIDENCE OF CONGENITAL ANOMALIES IN ANTIEPILEPTIC DRUG-TREATED WOMEN WITH SEIZURE DISORDERS CANNOT BE REGARDED AS A CAUSE AND EFFECT RELATIONSHIP. THERE ARE INTRINSIC METHODOLOGIC PROBLEMS IN OBTAINING ADEQUATE DATA ON DRUG TERATOGENICITY IN HUMANS; GENETIC FACTORS OR THE EPILEPTIC CONDITION ITSELF, MAY BE MORE IMPORTANT THAN DRUG THERAPY IN CONTRIBUTING TO CONGENITAL ANOMALIES.

PATIENTS TAKING VALPROATE MAY DEVELOP CLOTTING ABNORMALITIES. A PATIENT WHO HAD LOW FIBRINOGEN WHEN TAKING MULTIPLE ANTICONVULSANTS INCLUDING VALPROATE GAVE BIRTH TO AN INFANT WITH AFIBRINOGENEMIA WHO SUBSEQUENTLY DIED OF HEMORRHAGE. IF VALPROATE IS USED IN PREGNANCY, THE CLOTTING PARAMETERS SHOULD BE MONITORED CAREFULLY.

HEPATIC FAILURE, RESULTING IN THE DEATH OF A NEWBORN AND OF AN INFANT, HAVE BEEN REPORTED FOLLOWING THE USE OF VALPROATE DURING PREGNANCY.

Animal studies have demonstrated valproate-induced teratogenicity. Increased frequencies of malformations, as well as intrauterine growth retardation and death, have been observed in mice, rats, rabbits, and monkeys following prenatal exposure to valproate. Malformations of the skeletal system are the most common structural abnormalities produced in experimental animals, but neural tube closure defects have been seen in mice exposed to maternal plasma valproate concentrations exceeding approximately 230 µg/mL (2.3 times the upper limit of the human therapeutic range for epilepsy) during susceptible periods of embryonic development. Administration of an oral dose of 200 mg/kg/day or greater (50% of the maximum human daily dose or greater on a mg/m^2 basis) to pregnant rats during organogenesis produced malformations (skeletal, cardiac, and urogenital) and growth retardation in the offspring. These doses resulted in peak maternal plasma valproate levels of approximately 340 µg/mL or greater (3.4 times the upper limit of the human therapeutic range for epilepsy or greater). Behavioral deficits have been reported in the offspring of rats given a dose of 200 mg/kg/day throughout most of pregnancy. An oral dose of 350 mg/kg/day (approximately 2 times the maximum human daily dose on a mg/m^2 basis) produced skeletal and visceral malformations in rabbits exposed during organogenesis. Skeletal malformations, growth retardation, and death were observed in rhesus monkeys following administration of an oral dose of 200 mg/kg/day (equal to the maximum human daily dose on a mg/m^2 basis) during organogenesis. This dose resulted in peak maternal plasma valproate levels of approximately 280 µg/mL (2.8 times the upper limit of the human therapeutic range for epilepsy).

The prescribing physician will wish to weigh the benefits of therapy against the risks in treating or counseling women of childbearing potential. If this drug is used during pregnancy, or if the patient becomes pregnant while taking this drug, the patient should be apprised of the potential hazard to the fetus.

Antiepileptic drugs should not be discontinued abruptly in patients in whom the drug is administered to prevent major seizures because of the strong possibility of precipitating status epilepticus with attendant hypoxia and threat to life. In individual cases where the severity and frequency of the seizure disorder are such that the removal of medication does not pose a serious threat to the patient, discontinuation of the drug may be considered prior to and during pregnancy, although it cannot be said with any confidence that even minor seizures do not pose some hazard to the developing embryo or fetus.

Tests to detect neural tube and other defects using current accepted procedures should be considered a part of routine prenatal care in childbearing women receiving valproate.

PRECAUTIONS
Hepatic Dysfunction

See **BOXED WARNING, CONTRAINDICATIONS** and **WARNINGS**.

Pancreatitis

See **BOXED WARNING** and **WARNINGS**.

Hyperammonemia

Hyperammonemia has been reported in association with valproate therapy and may be present despite normal liver function tests. In patients who develop unexplained lethargy and vomiting or changes in mental status, hyperammonemic encephalopathy should be considered and an ammonia level should be measured. If ammonia is increased, valproate therapy should be discontinued. Appropriate interventions for treatment of hyperammonemia should be initiated, and such patients should undergo investigation for underlying urea cycle disorders (see **CONTRAINDICATIONS and WARNINGS - Urea Cycle Disorders**).

Asymptomatic elevations of ammonia are more common and when present, require close monitoring of plasma ammonia levels. If the elevation persists, discontinuation of valproate therapy should be considered.

General

Because of reports of thrombocytopenia (see **WARNINGS**), inhibition of the secondary phase of platelet aggregation, and abnormal coagulation parameters, (e.g., low fibrinogen), platelet counts and coagulation tests are recommended before initiating therapy and at periodic intervals. It is recommended that patients receiving DEPAKOTE be monitored for platelet count and coagulation parameters prior to planned surgery. In a clinical trial of DEPAKOTE as monotherapy in patients with epilepsy, 34/126 patients (27%) receiving approximately 50 mg/kg/day on average, had at least one value of platelets $\leq 75 \times 10^9$/L. Approximately half of these patients had treatment discontinued, with return of platelet counts to normal. In the remaining patients, platelet counts normalized with continued treatment. In this study, the probability of thrombocytopenia appeared to increase significantly at total valproate concentrations of ≥ 110 µg/mL (females) or ≥ 135 µg/mL (males). Evidence of hemorrhage, bruising, or a disorder of hemostasis/coagulation is an indication for reduction of the dosage or withdrawal of therapy.

Since DEPAKOTE may interact with concurrently administered drugs which are capable of enzyme induction, periodic plasma concentration determinations of valproate and concomitant drugs are recommended during the early course of therapy where clinically appropriate (see **PRECAUTIONS - Drug Interactions**).

	Monotherapy Study Median Incidence of CPS per 8 Weeks		
Treatment	Number of Patients	Baseline Incidence	Randomized Phase Incidence
High dose DEPAKOTE	131	13.2	10.7*
Low dose DEPAKOTE	134	14.2	13.8

*Reduction from baseline statistically significantly greater for high dose than low dose at p ≤ 0.05 level.

Continued on next page

Depakote ER—Cont.

Valproate is partially eliminated in the urine as a ketometabolite which may lead to a false interpretation of the urine ketone test.

There have been reports of altered thyroid function tests associated with valproate. The clinical significance of these is unknown.

There are *in vitro* studies that suggest valproate stimulates the replication of the HIV and CMV viruses under certain experimental conditions. The clinical consequence, if any, is not known. Additionally, the relevance of these *in vitro* findings is uncertain for patients receiving maximally suppressive antiretroviral therapy. Nevertheless, these data should be borne in mind when interpreting the results from regular monitoring of the viral load in HIV infected patients receiving valproate or when following CMV infected patients clinically.

Information for Patients
Patients and guardians should be warned that abdominal pain, nausea, vomiting, and/or anorexia can be symptoms of pancreatitis and, therefore, require further medical evaluation promptly.

Patients should be informed of the signs and symptoms associated with hyperammonemic encephalopathy (see **PRECAUTIONS - Hyperammonemia**) and be told to inform the prescriber if any of these symptoms occur.

Since DEPAKOTE products may produce CNS depression, especially when combined with another CNS depressant (eg, alcohol), patients should be advised not to engage in hazardous activities, such as driving an automobile or operating dangerous machinery, until it is known that they do not become drowsy from the drug.

Since DEPAKOTE has been associated with certain types of birth defects, female patients of child-bearing age considering the use of DEPAKOTE ER for the prevention of migraine should be advised to read the **Patient Information Leaflet**, which appears as the last section of the labeling.

Drug Interactions
Effects of Co-Administered Drugs on Valproate Clearance
Drugs that affect the level of expression of hepatic enzymes, particularly those that elevate levels of glucuronosyltransferases, may increase the clearance of valproate. For example, phenytoin carbamazepine, and phenobarbital (or primidone) can double the clearance of valproate. Thus, patients on monotherapy will generally have longer half-lives and higher concentrations than patients receiving polytherapy with antiepilepsy drugs.

In contrast, drugs that are inhibitors of cytochrome P450 isozymes, e.g., antidepressants, may be expected to have little effect on valproate clearance because cytochrome P450 microsomal mediated oxidation is a relatively minor secondary metabolic pathway compared to glucuronidation and beta-oxidation.

Because of these changes in valproate clearance, monitoring of valproate and concomitant drug concentrations should be increased whenever enzyme inducing drugs are introduced or withdrawn.

The following list provides information about the potential for an influence of several commonly prescribed medications on valproate pharmacokinetics. The list is not exhaustive nor could it be, since new interactions are continuously being reported.

Drugs for which a potentially important interaction has been observed:
Aspirin - A study involving the co-administration of aspirin at antipyretic doses (11 to 16 mg/kg) with valproate to pediatric patients (n=6) revealed a decrease in protein binding and an inhibition of metabolism of valproate. Valproate free fraction was increased 4-fold in the presence of aspirin compared to valproate alone. The β-oxidation pathway consisting of 2-E-valproic acid, 3-OH-valproic acid, and 3-keto valproic acid was decreased from 25% of total metabolites excreted on valproate alone to 8.3% in the presence of aspirin. Whether or not the interaction observed in this study applies to adults is unknown, but caution should be observed if valproate and aspirin are to be co-administered.
Felbamate - A study involving the co-administration of 1200 mg/day of felbamate with valproate to patients with epilepsy (n=10) revealed an increase in mean valproate peak concentration by 35% (from 86 to 115 μg/mL) compared to valproate alone. Increasing the felbamate dose to 2400 mg/day increased the mean valproate peak concentration to 133 μg/mL (another 16% increase). A decrease in valproate dosage may be necessary when felbamate therapy is initiated.
Rifampin - A study involving the administration of a single dose of valproate (7 mg/kg) 36 hours after 5 nights of daily dosing with rifampin (600 mg) revealed a 40% increase in the oral clearance of valproate. Valproate dosage adjustment may be necessary when it is co-administered with rifampin.

Drugs for which either no interaction or a likely clinically unimportant interaction has been observed:
Antacids - A study involving the co-administration of valproate 500 mg with commonly administered antacids (Maalox, Trisogel, and Titralac - 160 mEq doses) did not reveal any effect on the extent of absorption of valproate.
Chlorpromazine - A study involving the administration of 100 to 300 mg/day of chlorpromazine to schizophrenic patients already receiving valproate (200 mg BID) revealed a 15% increase in trough plasma levels of valproate.

Haloperidol - A study involving the administration of 6 to 10 mg/day of haloperidol to schizophrenic patients already receiving valproate (200 mg BID) revealed no significant changes in valproate trough plasma levels.
Cimetidine and Ranitidine - Cimetidine and ranitidine do not affect the clearance of valproate.
Effects of Valproate on Other Drugs
Valproate has been found to be a weak inhibitor of some P450 isozymes, epoxide hydrase, and glucuronyltransferases.
The following list provides information about the potential for an influence of valproate co-administration on the pharmacokinetics or pharmacodynamics of several commonly prescribed medications. The list is not exhaustive, since new interactions are continuously being reported.
Drugs for which a potentially important valproate interaction has been observed:
Amitriptyline/Nortriptyline - Administration of a single oral 50 mg dose of amitriptyline to 15 normal volunteers (10 males and 5 females) who received valproate (500 mg BID) resulted in a 21% decrease in plasma clearance of amitriptyline and a 34% decrease in the net clearance of nortriptyline. Rare postmarketing reports of concurrent use of valproate and amitriptyline resulting in an increased amitriptyline level have been received. Concurrent use of valproate and amitriptyline has rarely been associated with toxicity. Monitoring of amitriptyline levels should be considered for patients taking valproate concomitantly with amitriptyline. Consideration should be given to lowering the dose of amitriptyline/nortriptyline in the presence of valproate.
Carbamazepine/carbamazepine-10,11-Epoxide - Serum levels of carbamazepine (CBZ) decreased 17% while that of carbamazepine-10,11-epoxide (CBZ-E) increased by 45% upon co-administration of valproate and CBZ to epileptic patients.
Clonazepam - The concomitant use of valproic acid and clonazepam may induce absence status in patients with a history of absence type seizures.
Diazepam - Valproate displaces diazepam from its plasma albumin binding sites and inhibits its metabolism. Co-administration of valproate (1500 mg daily) increased the free fraction of diazepam (10 mg) by 90% in healthy volunteers (n=6). Plasma clearance and volume of distribution for free diazepam were reduced by 25% and 20%, respectively, in the presence of valproate. The elimination half-life of diazepam remained unchanged upon addition of valproate.
Ethosuximide - Valproate inhibits the metabolism of ethosuximide. Administration of a single ethosuximide dose of 500 mg with valproate (800 to 1600 mg/day) to healthy volunteers (n=6) was accompanied by a 25% increase in elimination half-life of ethosuximide and a 15% decrease in its total clearance as compared to ethosuximide alone. Patients receiving valproate and ethosuximide, especially along with other anticonvulsants, should be monitored for alterations in serum concentrations of both drugs.
Lamotrigine - In a steady-state study involving 10 healthy volunteers, the elimination half-life of lamotrigine increased from 26 to 70 hours with valproate coadministration (a 165% increase). The dose of lamotrigine should be reduced when co-administered with valproate.
Phenobarbital - Valproate was found to inhibit the metabolism of phenobarbital. Co-administration of valproate (250 mg BID for 14 days) with phenobarbital to normal subjects (n=6) resulted in a 50% increase in half-life and a 30% decrease in plasma clearance of phenobarbital (60 mg single-dose). The fraction of phenobarbital dose excreted unchanged increased by 50% in presence of valproate.
There is evidence for severe CNS depression, with or without significant elevations of barbiturate or valproate serum concentrations. All patients receiving concomitant barbiturate therapy should be closely monitored for neurological toxicity. Serum barbiturate concentrations should be obtained, if possible, and the barbiturate dosage decreased, if appropriate.
Primidone, which is metabolized to a barbiturate, may be involved in a similar interaction with valproate.
Phenytoin - Valproate displaces phenytoin from its plasma albumin binding sites and inhibits its hepatic metabolism. Co-administration of valproate (400 mg TID) with phenytoin (250 mg) in normal volunteers (n=7) was associated with a 60% increase in the free fraction of phenytoin. Total plasma clearance and apparent volume of distribution of phenytoin increased 30% in the presence of valproate. Both the clearance and apparent volume of distribution of free phenytoin were reduced by 25%.
In patients with epilepsy, there have been reports of breakthrough seizures occurring with the combination of valproate and phenytoin. The dosage of phenytoin should be adjusted as required by the clinical situation.
Tolbutamide - From *in vitro* experiments, the unbound fraction of tolbutamide was increased from 20% to 50% when added to plasma samples taken from patients treated with valproate. The clinical relevance of this displacement is unknown.
Warfarin - In an *in vitro* study, valproate increased the unbound fraction of warfarin by up to 32.6% The therapeutic relevance of this is unknown; however, coagulation tests should be monitored if DEPAKOTE therapy is instituted in patients taking anticoagulants.
Zidovudine - In six patients who were seropositive for HIV, the clearance of zidovudine (100 mg q8h) was decreased by 38% after administration of valproate (250 to 500 mg q8h); the half-life of zidovudine was unaffected.

Drugs for which either no interaction or a likely clinically unimportant interaction has been observed:
Acetaminophen - Valproate had no effect on any of the pharmacokinetic parameters of acetaminophen when it was concurrently administered to three epileptic patients.
Clozapine - In psychotic patients (n=11), no interaction was observed when valproate was co-administered with clozapine.
Lithium - Co-administration of valproate (500 mg BID) and lithium carbonate (300 mg TID) to normal male volunteers (n=16) had no effect on the steady-state kinetics of lithium.
Lorazepam - Concomitant administration of valproate (500 mg BID) and lorazepam (1 mg BID) in normal male volunteers (n=9) was accompanied by a 17% decrease in the plasma clearance of lorazepam.
Oral Contraceptive Steroids - Administration of a single-dose of ethinyloestradiol (50 μg)/levonorgestrel (250 μg) to 6 women on valproate (200 mg BID) therapy for 2 months did not reveal any pharmacokinetic interaction.
Carcinogenesis, Mutagenesis, Impairment of Fertility
Carcinogenesis
Valproic acid was administered orally to Sprague Dawley rats and ICR (HA/ICR) mice at doses of 80 and 170 mg/kg/day (approximately 10 to 50% of the maximum human daily dose on a mg/m^2 basis) for two years. A variety of neoplasms were observed in both species. The chief findings were a statistically significant increase in the incidence of subcutaneous fibrosarcomas in high dose male rats receiving valproic acid and a statistically significant dose-related trend for benign pulmonary adenomas in male mice receiving valproic acid. The significance of these findings for humans is unknown.
Mutagenesis
Valproate was not mutagenic in an *in vitro* bacterial assay (Ames test), did not produce dominant lethal effects in mice, and did not increase chromosome aberration frequency in an *in vivo* cytogenetic study in rats. Increased frequencies of sister chromatid exchange (SCE) have been reported in a study of epileptic children taking valproate, but this association was not observed in another study conducted in adults. There is some evidence that increased SCE frequencies may be associated with epilepsy. The biological significance of an increase in SCE frequency is not known.
Fertility
Chronic toxicity studies in juvenile and adult rats and dogs demonstrated reduced spermatogenesis and testicular atrophy at oral doses of 400 mg/kg/day or greater in rats (approximately equivalent to or greater than the maximum human daily dose on a mg/m^2 basis) and 150 mg/kg/day or greater in dogs (approximately 1.4 times the maximum human daily dose or greater on a mg/m^2 basis). Segment I fertility studies in rats have shown oral doses up to 350 mg/kg/day (approximately equal to the maximum human daily dose on a mg/m^2 basis) for 60 days to have no effect on fertility. THE EFFECT OF VALPROATE ON TESTICULAR DEVELOPMENT AND ON SPERM PRODUCTION AND FERTILITY IN HUMANS IS UNKNOWN.
Pregnancy
Pregnancy Category D: see **WARNINGS**.
Nursing Mothers
Valproate is excreted in breast milk. Concentrations in breast milk have been reported to be 1-10% of serum concentrations. It is not known what effect this would have on a nursing infant. Consideration should be given to discontinuing nursing when divalproex sodium is administered to a nursing woman.
Pediatric Use
The safety and effectiveness of Depakote ER for the prophylaxis of migraine headaches and for the treatment of epilepsy (see **INDICATIONS AND USAGE** for specific seizure types) in pediatric patients has not been established.
Experience has indicated that pediatric patients under the age of two years are at a considerably increased risk of developing fatal hepatotoxicity, especially those with the aforementioned conditions (see **BOXED WARNING**). Above the age of 2 years, experience in epilepsy has indicated that the incidence of fatal hepatotoxicity decreases considerably in progressively older patient groups.
The basic toxicology and pathologic manifestations of valproate sodium in neonatal (4-day old) and juvenile (14-day old) rats are similar to those seen in young adult rats. However, additional findings, including renal alterations in juvenile rats and renal alterations and retinal dysplasia in neonatal rats, have been reported. These findings occurred at 240 mg/kg/day, a dosage approximately equivalent to the human maximum recommended daily dose on a mg/m^2 basis. They were not seen at 90 mg/kg, or 40% of the maximum human daily dose on a mg/m^2 basis.
Geriatric Use
Safety and effectiveness of DEPAKOTE ER in the prophylaxis of migraine patients over 65 have not been established.
No patients above the age of 65 years were enrolled in double-blind prospective clinical trials of mania associated with bipolar illness using DEPAKOTE (divalproex sodium delayed-release tablets). In a case review study of 583 patients using various valproate products, 72 patients (12%) were greater than 65 years of age. A higher percentage of patients above 65 years of age reported accidental injury, infection, pain, somnolence, and tremor. Discontinuation of valproate was occasionally associated with the latter two events. It is not clear whether these events indicate additional risk or whether they result from preexisting medical illness and concomitant medication use among these patients.

A study of elderly patients with dementia revealed drug related somnolence and discontinuation for somnolence (see **WARNINGS—Somnolence in the Elderly**). The starting dose should be reduced in these patients, and dosage reductions or discontinuation should be considered in patients with excessive somnolence (see **DOSAGE AND ADMINISTRATION**).

ADVERSE REACTIONS
Migraine
Based on the results of one multicenter, randomized, double-blind, placebo-controlled clinical trial, DEPAKOTE ER was well tolerated in the prophylactic treatment of migraine headache. Of the 122 patients exposed to DEPAKOTE ER in the placebo-controlled study, 8% discontinued for adverse events, compared to 9% for the 115 placebo patients.

Based on two placebo-controlled clinical trials and their long term extension, DEPAKOTE (divalproex sodium delayed-release tablets) was generally well tolerated with most adverse events rated as mild to moderate in severity. Of the 202 patients exposed to DEPAKOTE in the placebo-controlled trials, 17% discontinued for intolerance. This is compared to a rate of 5% for the 81 placebo patients. Including the long term extension study, the adverse events reported as the primary reason for discontinuation by ≥1% of 248 DEPAKOTE-treated patients were alopecia (6%), nausea and/or vomiting (5%), weight gain (2%), tremor (2%), somnolence (1%), elevated SGOT and/or SGPT (1%), and depression (1%).

Table 1 includes those adverse events reported for patients in the placebo-controlled trial where the incidence rate in the DEPAKOTE ER-treated group was greater than 5% and was greater than that for placebo patients.

Table 1
Adverse Events Reported by >5% of DEPAKOTE ER-Treated Patients During the Migraine Placebo-Controlled Trial with a Greater Incidence than Patients Taking Placebo[1]

Body System Event	Depakote ER (N=122)	Placebo (N=115)
Gastrointestinal System		
Nausea	15%	9%
Dyspepsia	7%	4%
Diarrhea	7%	3%
Vomiting	7%	2%
Abdominal Pain	7%	5%
Nervous System		
Somnolence	7%	2%
Other		
Infection	15%	14%

[1]The following adverse events occurred in greater than 5% of DEPAKOTE ER-treated patients and at a greater incidence for placebo than for DEPAKOTE ER: asthenia and flu syndrome.

The following additional adverse events were reported by greater than 1% but not more than 5% of DEPAKOTE ER-treated patients and with a greater incidence than placebo in the placebo-controlled clinical trial for migraine prophylaxis:

Body as a Whole: Accidental injury, viral infection.
Digestive System: Increased appetite, tooth disorder.
Metabolic and Nutritional Disorders: Edema, weight gain.
Nervous System: Abnormal gait, dizziness, hypertonia, insomnia, nervousness, tremor, vertigo.
Respiratory System: Pharyngitis, rhinitis.
Skin and Appendages: Rash.
Special Senses: Tinnitus.

Table 2 includes those adverse events reported for patients in the placebo-controlled trials where the incidence rate in the DEPAKOTE-treated group was greater than 5% and was greater than that for placebo patients.

Table 2
Adverse Events Reported by >5% of DEPAKOTE-Treated Patients During Migraine Placebo-Controlled Trials with a Greater Incidence than Patients Taking Placebo[1]

Body System Event	Depakote (N=202)	Placebo (N=81)
Gastrointestinal System		
Nausea	31%	10%
Dyspepsia	13%	9%
Diarrhea	12%	7%
Vomiting	11%	1%
Abdominal Pain	9%	4%
Increased Appetite	6%	4%
Nervous System		
Asthenia	20%	9%
Somnolence	17%	5%
Dizziness	12%	6%
Tremor	9%	0%
Other		
Weight Gain	8%	2%
Back Pain	8%	6%
Alopecia	7%	1%

[1]The following adverse events occurred in greater than 5% of DEPAKOTE-treated patients and at a greater incidence for placebo than for DEPAKOTE: flu syndrome and pharyngitis.

The following additional adverse events not referred to above were reported by greater than 1% but not more than 5% of DEPAKOTE-treated patients and with a greater incidence than placebo in the placebo-controlled clinical trials:

Body as a Whole: Chest pain.
Cardiovascular System: Vasodilatation.
Digestive System: Constipation, dry mouth, flatulence, stomatitis.
Hemic and Lymphatic System: Ecchymosis.
Metabolic and Nutritional Disorders: Peripheral edema.
Musculoskeletal System: Leg cramps.
Nervous System: Abnormal dreams, confusion, paresthesia, speech disorder, thinking abnormalities.
Respiratory System: Dyspnea sinusitis.
Skin and Appendages: Pruritus.
Urogenital System: Metrorrhagia.

Epilepsy
Based on a placebo-controlled trial of adjunctive therapy for treatment of complex partial seizures, DEPAKOTE was generally well tolerated with most adverse events rated as mild to moderate in severity. Intolerance was the primary reason for discontinuation in the DEPAKOTE-treated patients (6%), compared to 1% of placebo-treated patients.

Table 3 lists treatment-emergent adverse events which were reported by ≥5% of DEPAKOTE-treated patients and for which the incidence was greater than in the placebo group, in the placebo-controlled trial of adjunctive therapy for treatment of complex partial seizures. Since patients were also treated with other antiepilepsy drugs, it is not possible, in most cases, to determine whether the following adverse events can be ascribed to DEPAKOTE alone, or the combination of DEPAKOTE and other antiepilepsy drugs.

Table 3
Adverse Events Reported by ≥ 5% of Patients Treated with DEPAKOTE During Placebo-Controlled Trial of Adjunctive Therapy for Complex Partial Seizures

Body System/Event	Depakote (%) (n = 77)	Placebo (%) (n = 70)
Body as a Whole		
Headache	31	21
Asthenia	27	7
Fever	6	4
Gastrointestinal System		
Nausea	48	14
Vomiting	27	7
Abdominal Pain	23	6
Diarrhea	13	6
Anorexia	12	0
Dyspepsia	8	4
Constipation	5	1
Nervous System		
Somnolence	27	11
Tremor	25	6
Dizziness	25	13
Diplopia	16	9
Amblyopia/Blurred Vision	12	9
Ataxia	8	1
Nystagmus	8	1
Emotional Lability	6	4
Thinking Abnormal	6	0
Amnesia	5	1
Respiratory System		
Flu Syndrome	12	9
Infection	12	6
Bronchitis	5	2
Rhinitis	5	4
Other		
Alopecia	6	1
Weight Loss	6	0

Table 4 lists treatment-emergent adverse events which were reported by ≥5% of patients in the high dose DEPAKOTE group, and for which the incidence was greater than in the low dose group, in a controlled trial of DEPAKOTE monotherapy treatment of complex partial seizures. Since patients were being titrated off another antiepilepsy drug during the first portion of the trial, it is not possible, in many cases, to determine whether the following adverse events can be ascribed to DEPAKOTE alone, or the combination of DEPAKOTE and other antiepilepsy drugs.

Table 4
Adverse Events Reported by ≥ 5% of Patients in the High Dose Group in the Controlled Trial of DEPAKOTE Monotherapy for Complex Partial Seizures[1]

Body System/Event	High Dose (%) (n = 131)	Low Dow (%) (n = 134)
Body as a Whole		
Asthenia	21	10
Digestive System		
Nausea	34	26
Diarrhea	23	19
Vomiting	23	15
Abdominal Pain	12	9
Anorexia	11	4
Dyspepsia	11	10
Hemic/Lymphatic System		
Thrombocytopenia	24	1
Ecchymosis	5	4
Metabolic/Nutritional		
Weight Gain	9	4
Peripheral Edema	8	3
Nervous System		
Tremor	57	19
Somnolence	30	18
Dizziness	18	13
Insomnia	15	9
Nervousness	11	7
Amnesia	7	4
Nystagmus	7	1
Depression	5	4
Respiratory System		
Infection	20	13
Pharyngitis	8	2
Dyspnea	5	1
Skin and Appendages		
Alopecia	24	13
Special Senses		
Amblyopia/Blurred Vision	8	4
Tinnitus	7	1

[1]Headache was the only adverse event that occurred in ≥ 5% of patients in the high dose group and at an equal or greater incidence in the low dose group.

The following additional adverse events were reported by greater than 1% but less than 5% of the 358 patients treated with DEPAKOTE in the controlled trials of complex partial seizures:

Body as a Whole: Back pain, chest pain, malaise.
Cardiovascular System: Tachycardia, hypertension, palpitation.
Digestive System: Increased appetite, flatulence, hematemesis, eructation, pancreatitis, periodontal abscess.
Hemic and Lymphatic System: Petechia.
Metabolic and Nutritional Disorders: SGOT increased, SGPT increased.
Musculoskeletal System: Myalgia, twitching, arthralgia, leg cramps, myasthenia.
Nervous System: Anxiety, confusion, abnormal gait, paresthesia, hypertonia, incoordination, abnormal dreams, personality disorder.
Respiratory System: Sinusitis, cough increased, pneumonia, epistaxis.
Skin and Appendages: Rash, pruritus, dry skin.
Special Senses: Taste perversion, abnormal vision, deafness, otitis media.
Urogenital System: Urinary incontinence, vaginitis, dysmenorrhea, amenorrhea, urinary frequency.

Other Patient Populations
The following adverse events not listed previously were reported by greater than 1% of DEPAKOTE-treated patients and with a greater incidence than placebo in placebo-controlled trials of manic episodes associated with bipolar disorder:

Body as a Whole: Chills, chills and fever, drug level increased, neck rigidity.
Cardiovascular System: Arrhythmia, hypotension, postural hypotension.
Digestive System: Dysphagia, fecal incontinence, gastroenteritis, glossitis, gum hemorrhage, mouth ulceration.
Hemic and Lymphatic System: Anemia, bleeding time increased, leukopenia.
Metabolic and Nutritional Disorders: Hypoproteinemia.
Musculoskeletal System: Arthrosis.
Nervous System: Agitation, catatonic reaction, dysarthria, hallucinations, hypokinesia, psychosis, reflexes increased, sleep disorder, tardive dyskinesia.
Respiratory System: Hiccup.
Skin and Appendages: Discoid lupus erythematosis, erythema nodosum, furunculosis, maculopapular rash, seborrhea, sweating, vesiculobullous rash.
Special Senses: Conjunctivitis, dry eyes, eye disorder, eye pain, photophobia, taste perversion.
Urogenital System: Cystitis, menstrual disorder.

Adverse events that have been reported with all dosage forms of valproate from epilepsy trials, spontaneous reports, and other sources are listed below by body system.
Gastrointestinal: The most commonly reported side effects at the initiation of therapy are nausea, vomiting, and indigestion. These effects are usually transient and rarely require discontinuation of therapy. Diarrhea, abdominal cramps, and constipation have been reported. Both anorexia with some weight loss and increased appetite with weight gain have also been reported. In some patients, many of whom have functional or anatomic (including ileostomy or colostomy) gastrointestinal disorders with shortened GI transit times, there have been postmarketing reports of DEPAKOTE ER tablets in the stool.
CNS Effects: Sedative effects have occurred in patients receiving valproate alone but occur most often in patients receiving combination therapy. Sedation usually abates upon reduction of other antiepileptic medication. Tremor (may be dose-related), hallucinations, ataxia, headache, nystagmus, diplopia, asterixis, "spots before eyes", dysarthria, dizziness, confusion, hypesthesia, vertigo, incoordination, and parkinsonism have been reported with the use of valproate.

Continued on next page

Depakote ER—Cont.

Rare cases of coma have occurred in patients receiving valproate alone or in conjunction with phenobarbital. In rare instances encephalopathy with or without fever has developed shortly after the introduction of valproate monotherapy without evidence of hepatic dysfunction or inappropriately high plasma valproate levels. Although recovery has been described following drug withdrawal, there have been fatalities in patients with hyperammonemic encephalopathy, particularly in patients with underlying urea cycle disorders (see **WARNINGS - Urea Cycle Disorders** and **PRECAUTIONS**). Several reports have noted reversible cerebral atrophy and dementia in association with valproate therapy.

Dermatologic: Transient hair loss, skin rash, photosensitivity, generalized pruritus, erythema multiforme, and Stevens-Johnson syndrome. Rare cases of toxic epidermal necrolysis have been reported including a fatal case in a 6 month old infant taking valproate and several other concomitant medications. An additional case of toxic epidermal necrosis resulting in death was reported in a 35 year old patient with AIDS taking several concomitant medications and with a history of multiple cutaneous drug reactions.

Psychiatric: Emotional upset, depression, psychosis, aggression, hyperactivity, hostility, and behavioral deterioration.

Musculoskeletal: Weakness.

Hematologic: Thrombocytopenia and inhibition of the secondary phase of platelet aggregation may be reflected in altered bleeding time, petechiae, bruising, hematoma formation, epistaxis, and frank hemorrhage (see **PRECAUTIONS - General and Drug Interactions**). Relative lymphocytosis, macrocytosis, hypofibrinogenemia, leukopenia, eosinophilia, anemia including macrocytic with or without folate deficiency, bone marrow suppression, pancytopenia, aplastic anemia, and acute intermittent porphyria.

Hepatic: Minor elevations of transaminases (eg, SGOT and SGPT) and LDH are frequent and appear to be dose-related. Occasionally, laboratory test results include increases in serum bilirubin and abnormal changes in other liver function tests. These results may reflect potentially serious hepatotoxicity (see **WARNINGS**).

Endocrine: Irregular menses, secondary amenorrhea, breast enlargement, galactorrhea, and parotid gland swelling. Abnormal thyroid function tests (see **PRECAUTIONS**).

There have been rare spontaneous reports of polycystic ovary disease. A cause and effect relationship has not been established.

Pancreatic: Acute pancreatitis including fatalities (see **WARNINGS**).

Metabolic: Hyperammonemia (see **PRECAUTIONS**), hyponatremia, and inappropriate ADH secretion.

There have been rare reports of Fanconi's syndrome occurring chiefly in children.

Decreased carnitine concentrations have been reported although the clinical relevance is undetermined.

Hyperglycinemia has occurred and was associated with a fatal outcome in a patient with preexistent nonketotic hyperglycinemia.

Genitourinary: Enuresis and urinary tract infection.

Special Senses: Hearing loss, either reversible or irreversible, has been reported; however, a cause and effect relationship has not been established. Ear pain has also been reported.

Other: Anaphylaxis, edema of the extremities, lupus erythematosus, bone pain, cough increased, pneumonia, otitis media, bradycardia, cutaneous vasculitis, and fever.

OVERDOSAGE

Overdosage with valproate may result in somnolence, heart block, and deep coma. Fatalities have been reported; however patients have recovered from valproate levels as high as 2120 µg/mL.

In overdose situations, the fraction of drug not bound to protein is high and hemodialysis or tandem hemodialysis plus hemoperfusion may result in significant removal of drug. The benefit of gastric lavage or emesis will vary with the time since ingestion. General supportive measures should be applied with particular attention to the maintenance of adequate urinary output.

Naloxone has been reported to reverse the CNS depressant effects of valproate overdosage. Because naloxone could theoretically also reverse the antiepileptic effects of valproate, it should be used with caution in patients with epilepsy.

DOSAGE AND ADMINISTRATION

DEPAKOTE ER is an extended-release product intended for once-a-day oral administration. DEPAKOTE ER tablets should be swallowed whole and should not be crushed or chewed.

Migraine

The recommended starting dose is 500 mg once daily for 1 week, thereafter increasing to 1000 mg once daily. Although doses other than 1000 mg once daily of DEPAKOTE ER have not been evaluated in patients with migraine, the effective dose range of DEPAKOTE (divalproex sodium delayed-release tablets) in these patients is 500-1000 mg/day. As with other valproate products, doses of DEPAKOTE ER should be individualized and dose adjustment may be necessary. If a patient requires smaller dose adjustments than that available with DEPAKOTE ER, DEPAKOTE should be used instead.

Epilepsy

DEPAKOTE ER is indicated as monotherapy and adjunctive therapy in complex partial seizures in adult patients, and in simple and complex absence seizures in adult patients. As the DEPAKOTE ER dosage is titrated upward, concentrations of phenobarbital, carbamazepine, and/or phenytoin may be affected (see **PRECAUTIONS - Drug Interactions**).

Complex Partial Seizures for adult patients:

Monotherapy (Initial Therapy): DEPAKOTE ER has not been systematically studied as initial therapy. Patients should initiate therapy at 10 to 15 mg/kg/day. The dosage should be increased by 5 to 10 mg/kg/week to achieve optimal clinical response. Ordinarily, optimal clinical response is achieved at daily doses below 60 mg/kg/day. If satisfactory clinical response has not been achieved, plasma levels should be measured to determine whether or not they are in the usually accepted therapeutic range (50 to 100 µg/mL). No recommendation regarding the safety of valproate for use at doses above 60 mg/kg/day can be made.

The probability of thrombocytopenia increases significantly at total trough valproate plasma concentrations above 110 µg/mL in females and 135 µg/mL in males. The benefit of improved seizure control with higher doses should be weighed against the possibility of a greater incidence of adverse reactions.

Conversion to Monotherapy: Patients should initiate therapy at 10 to 15 mg/kg/day. The dosage should be increased by 5 to 10 mg/kg/week to achieve optimal clinical response. Ordinarily, optimal clinical response is achieved at daily doses below 60 mg/kg/day. If satisfactory clinical response has not been achieved, plasma levels should be measured to determine whether or not they are in the usually accepted therapeutic range (50-100 µg/mL). No recommendation regarding the safety of valproate for use at doses above 60 mg/kg/day can be made. Concomitant antiepilepsy drug (AED) dosage can ordinarily be reduced by approximately 25% every 2 weeks. This reduction may be started at initiation of DEPAKOTE ER therapy, or delayed by 1 to 2 weeks if there is a concern that seizures are likely to occur with a reduction. The speed and duration of withdrawal of the concomitant AED can be highly variable, and patients should be monitored closely during this period for increased seizure frequency.

Adjunctive Therapy: DEPAKOTE ER may be added to the patient's regimen at a dosage of 10 to 15 mg/kg/day. The dosage may be increased by 5 to 10 mg/kg/week to achieve optimal clinical response. Ordinarily, optimal clinical response is achieved at daily doses below 60 mg/kg/day. If satisfactory clinical response has not been achieved, plasma levels should be measured to determine whether or not they are in the usually accepted therapeutic range (50 to 100 µg/mL). No recommendation regarding the safety of valproate for use at doses above 60 mg/kg/day can be made.

In a study of adjunctive therapy for complex partial seizures in which patients were receiving either carbamazepine or phenytoin in addition to DEPAKOTE, no adjustment of carbamazepine or phenytoin dosage was needed (see **CLINICAL STUDIES**). However, since valproate may interact with these or other concurrently administered AEDs as well as other drugs (see **Drug Interactions**), periodic plasma concentration determinations of concomitant AEDs are recommended during the early course of therapy (see **PRECAUTIONS - Drug Interactions**).

Simple and Complex Absence Seizures for adult patients:

The recommended initial dose is 15 mg/kg/day, increasing at one week intervals by 5 to 10 mg/kg/day until seizures are controlled or side effects preclude further increases. The maximum recommended dosage is 60 mg/kg/day.

A good correlation has not been established between daily dose, serum concentrations, and therapeutic effect. However, therapeutic valproate serum concentrations for most patients with absence seizures is considered to range from 50 to 100 µg/mL. Some patients may be controlled with lower or higher serum concentrations (see **CLINICAL PHARMACOLOGY**).

As the DEPAKOTE ER dosage is titrated upward, blood concentrations of phenobarbital and/or phenytoin may be affected (see **PRECAUTIONS**).

Antiepilepsy drugs should not be abruptly discontinued in patients in whom the drug is administered to prevent major seizures because of the strong possibility of precipitating status epilepticus with attendant hypoxia and threat to life.

Conversion from DEPAKOTE to DEPAKOTE ER:
In adult patients with epilepsy previously receiving DEPAKOTE, DEPAKOTE ER should be administered once-daily using a dose 8 to 20% higher than the total daily dose of DEPAKOTE (Table 5). For patients whose DEPAKOTE total daily dose can not be directly converted to DEPAKOTE ER, consideration may be given at the clinician's discretion to increase the patient's DEPAKOTE total daily dose to the next higher dosage before converting to the appropriate total daily dose of DEPAKOTE ER.

Table 5
Dose Conversion

DEPAKOTE Total Daily Dose (mg)	DEPAKOTE ER (mg)
500*–625	750
750*–875	1000
1000*–1125	1250
1250–1375	1500
1500–1625	1750
1750	2000
1875–2000	2250
2125–2250	2500
2375	2750
2500–2750	3000
2875	3250
3000–3125	3500

*These total daily doses of DEPAKOTE cannot be directly converted to an 8 to 20% higher total daily dose of DEPAKOTE ER because the required dosing strengths of DEPAKOTE ER are not available. Consideration may be given at the clinician's discretion to increase the patient's DEPAKOTE total daily dose to the next higher dosage before converting to the appropriate total daily dose of DEPAKOTE ER.

There is insufficient data to allow a conversion factor recommendation for patients with DEPAKOTE doses above 3125 mg/day.

Plasma valproate C_{min} concentrations for DEPAKOTE ER on average are equivalent to DEPAKOTE, but may vary across patients after conversion. If satisfactory clinical response has not been achieved, plasma levels should be measured to determine whether or not they are in the usually accepted therapeutic range (50 to 100 µg/mL) (see **Pharmacokinetics - Absorption/Bioavailability**).

General Dosing Advice

Dosing in Elderly Patients - Due to a decrease in unbound clearance of valproate and possibly a greater sensitivity to somnolence in the elderly, the starting dose should be reduced in these patients. Starting doses in the elderly lower than 250 mg can only be achieved by the use of DEPAKOTE. Dosage should be increased more slowly and with regular monitoring for fluid and nutritional intake, dehydration, somnolence, and other adverse events. Dose reductions or discontinuation of valproate should be considered in patients with decreased food or fluid intake and in patients with excessive somnolence. The ultimate therapeutic dose should be achieved on the basis of both tolerability and clinical response (see **WARNINGS**).

Dose-Related Adverse Events - The frequency of adverse effects (particularly elevated liver enzymes and thrombocytopenia) may be dose-related. The probability of thrombocytopenia appears to increase significantly at total valproate concentrations of $\geq$ 110 µg/mL (females) or $\geq$ 135 µg/mL (males) (see **PRECAUTIONS**). The benefit of improved therapeutic effect with higher doses should be weighed against the possibility of a greater incidence of adverse reactions.

G.I. Irritation - Patients who experience G.I. irritation may benefit from administration of the drug with food or by initiating therapy with a lower dose of DEPAKOTE.

Compliance - Patients should be informed to take DEPAKOTE ER every day as prescribed. If a dose is missed it should be taken as soon as possible, unless it is almost time for the next dose. If a dose is skipped, the patient should not double the next dose.

HOW SUPPLIED

DEPAKOTE ER 250 mg is available as white ovaloid tablets with the corporate logo ⊇, and the Abbo-Code HF. Each DEPAKOTE ER tablet contains divalproex sodium equivalent to 250 mg of valproic acid in the following package sizes:

Bottles of 60 .... (**NDC** 0074-3826-60).
Bottles of 100 .... (**NDC** 0074-3826-13).
Bottles of 500 .... (**NDC** 0074-3826-53).
ABBO-PAC unit dose packages
of 100 .... (**NDC** 0074-3826-11).

DEPAKOTE ER 500 mg is available as gray ovaloid tablets with the corporate logo ⊇, and the Abbo-Code HC. Each DEPAKOTE ER tablet contains divalproex sodium equivalent to 500 mg of valproic acid in the following packaging sizes:

Bottles of 100 .... (**NDC** 0074-7126-13).
Bottles of 500 .... (**NDC** 0074-7126-53).
ABBO-PAC unit dose packages
of 100 .... (**NDC** 0074-7126-11).

Recommended storage: Store tablets at 25°C (77°F); excursions permitted to 15-30°C (59-86°F) [see USP Controlled Room Temperature].

Revised: January, 2003

Manufactured by:
ABBOTT LABORATORIES
NORTH CHICAGO, IL 60064, U.S.A.

Patient Information Leaflet

Important Information for Women Who Could Become Pregnant About the Use of DEPAKOTE® ER (divalproex sodium) Tablets for Migraine

Please read this leaflet carefully before you take DEPAKOTE® ER (divalproex sodium) tablets. The leaflet provides a summary of important information about taking DEPAKOTE ER for migraine to women who could become pregnant. DEPAKOTE ER may also be prescribed for uses other than those discussed in this leaflet. If you have any questions or concerns, or want more information about DEPAKOTE ER, contact your doctor or pharmacist.

Information For Women Who Could Become Pregnant

DEPAKOTE ER is used to prevent or reduce the number of migraines you experience. DEPAKOTE ER can be obtained only by prescription from your doctor. The decision to use

DEPAKOTE ER for the prevention of migraine is one that you and your doctor should make together, taking into account your individual needs and medical condition.

Before using DEPAKOTE ER, women who can become pregnant should consider the fact the DEPAKOTE has been associated with birth defects, in particular, with spina bifida and other defects related to failure of the spinal canal to close normally. Although the incidence is unknown in migraine patients treated with DEPAKOTE, approximately 1 to 2% of children born to women with epilepsy taking DEPAKOTE in the first 12 weeks of pregnancy had these defects (based on data from the Centers for Disease Control, a U.S. agency based in Atlanta). The incidence in the general population is 0.1 to 0.2%.

Information For Women Who Are Planning To Get Pregnant

- Women taking DEPAKOTE ER for the prevention of migraine who are planning to get pregnant should discuss with their doctor temporarily stopping DEPAKOTE ER, before and during their pregnancy.

Information For Women Who Become Pregnant While Taking DEPAKOTE ER

- If you become pregnant while taking DEPAKOTE ER for the prevention of migraine, you should contact your doctor immediately.

Other Important Information About DEPAKOTE ER Tablets

- DEPAKOTE ER tablets should be taken exactly as it is prescribed by your doctor to get the most benefits from DEPAKOTE ER and reduce the risk of side effects.
- If you have taken more than the prescribed dose of DEPAKOTE ER, contact your hospital emergency room or local poison center immediately.
- This medication was prescribed for your particular condition. Do not use it for another condition or give the drug to others.

Facts About Birth Defects

It is important to know that birth defects may occur even in children of individuals not taking any medications or without any additional risk factors.

Facts About Migraine

About 23 million Americans suffer from migraine headaches. About 75% of migraine sufferers are women. A migraine is described as a throbbing headache that gets worse with activity. Migraine may also include nausea and/or vomiting as well as sensitivity to light and sound. Migraine usually happens about once a month, but some people may have them as often as once or twice a week. Often, the symptoms from a migraine can cause people to miss work or school.

If you have frequent migraines, or if acute treatment is not working for you, your doctor may prescribe a preventative therapy. Preventative (prophylactic) treatment is used to prevent attacks and reduce the frequency and severity of headache events.

This summary provides important information about the use of DEPAKOTE ER for migraine to women who could become pregnant. If you would like more information about the other potential risks and benefits of DEPAKOTE ER, ask your doctor or pharmacist to let you read the professional labeling and then discuss it with them. If you have any questions or concerns about taking DEPAKOTE ER, you should discuss them with your doctor.

Ref. 03-5235-R4
Revised: January, 2003
Manufactured by:
ABBOTT LABORATORIES
NORTH CHICAGO, IL 60064, U.S.A.
02L-730-5576-1

AstraZeneca LP

WILMINGTON, DE 19850-5437

For Medical Information,
Adverse Drug Experiences,
and Customer Service
Contact: (800) 236-9933

ASTRAMORPH/PF™ ℞

[*ăs'-trâ-mŏrf'*]
(morphine sulfate injection, USP)
Preservative-Free
Rx only

Prescribing information for this product, which appears on pages 593–594 of the 2003 PDR, has been completely revised as follows. Please write "See Supplement A" next to the product heading.

DESCRIPTION

Morphine is the most important alkaloid of opium and is a phenanthrene derivative. It is available as the sulfate salt, having the following structural formula:

[See chemical structure at top of next column]

7,8-Didehydro-4,5-epoxy-17-methyl-(5α,6α)-morphinan-3,6-diol sulfate (2:1) (salt), pentahydrate

$(C_{17}H_{19}NO_3)_2 \cdot H_2SO_4 \cdot 5H_2O$ Molecular weight is 758.83

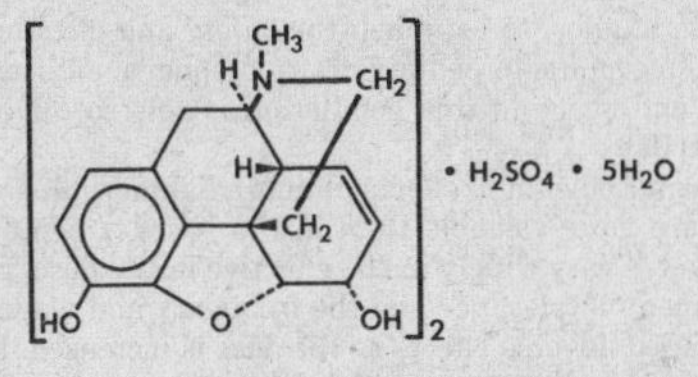

Preservative-free ASTRAMORPH/PF (Morphine Sulfate Injection, USP) is a sterile, nonpyrogenic isobaric solution of morphine sulfate free of antioxidants, preservatives or other potentially neurotoxic additives, and is intended for intravenous, epidural or intrathecal administration as a narcotic analgesic. Each milliliter contains morphine sulfate 0.5 mg or 1 mg and sodium chloride 9 mg in Water for Injection. pH range is 2.5–6.5. Ampules and vials are sealed under nitrogen. Each ampule and vial is intended for **SINGLE USE ONLY**. *Discard any unused portion.* DO NOT HEAT-STERILIZE.

CLINICAL PHARMACOLOGY

Morphine produces a wide spectrum of pharmacologic effects including analgesia, dysphoria, euphoria, somnolence, respiratory depression, diminished gastrointestinal motility and physical dependence. Opiate analgesia involves at least three anatomical areas of the central nervous system: the periaqueductal-periventricular gray matter, the ventromedial medulla and the spinal cord. A systemically administered opiate may produce analgesia by acting at any, all or some combination of these distinct regions. Morphine interacts predominantly with the μ-receptor. The μ-binding sites of opioids are very discretely distributed in the human brain, with high densities of sites found in the posterior amygdala, hypothalamus, thalamus, nucleus caudatus, putamen and certain cortical areas. They are also found on the terminal axons of primary afferents within laminae I and II (substantia gelatinosa) of the spinal cord and in the spinal nucleus of the trigeminal nerve.

Morphine has an apparent volume of distribution ranging from 1.0 to 4.7 L/kg after *intravenous* dosage. Protein binding is low, about 36%, and muscle tissue binding is reported as 54%. A blood-brain barrier exists, and when morphine is introduced outside of the CNS (eg. *intravenously*), plasma concentrations of morphine remain higher than the corresponding CSF morphine levels. Conversely, when morphine is injected into the *intrathecal* space, it diffuses out into the systemic circulation slowly, accounting for the long duration of action of morphine administered by this route.

Morphine has a total plasma clearance which ranges from 0.9 to 1.2 L/kg/h (liters/kilogram/hour) in postoperative patients, but shows considerable interindividual variation. The major pathway of clearance is hepatic glucuronidation to morphine-3-glucuronide, which is pharmacologically inactive. The major excretion path of the conjugate is through the kidneys, with about 10% in the feces. Morphine is also eliminated by the kidneys, 2 to 12% being excreted unchanged in the urine. Terminal half-life is commonly reported to vary from 1.5 to 4.5 hours, although the longer half-lives were obtained when morphine levels were monitored over protracted periods with very sensitive radioimmunoassay methods. The accepted elimination half-life in normal subject is 1.5 to 2 hours.

"Selective" blockade of pain sensation is possible by neuraxial application of morphine. In addition, duration of analgesia may be much longer by this route compared to systemic administration. However, CNS effects, associated with systemic administration, are still seen. These include respiratory depression, sedation, nausea and vomiting, pruritus and urinary retention. In particular, both early and late respiratory depression (up to 24 hours post dosing) have been reported following neuraxial administration. Circulation of the spinal fluid may also result in high concentrations of morphine reaching the brain stem directly.

The incidence of unwanted CNS effects, including delayed respiratory depression, associated with neuraxial application of morphine, is related to the circulatory dynamics of the epidural venous plexus and the spinal fluid. The lipid solubility and degree of ionization of morphine plays an important part in both the onset and duration of analgesia and the CNS effects. Morphine has a pK_a 7.9, with an octanol/water partition coefficient of 1.42 at pH 7.4. At this pH, the tertiary amino group in each of the opioids is mostly ionized, making the molecule water-soluble. Morphine, with additional hydroxyl groups on the molecule, is significantly more water-soluble than any other opioid in clinical use.

Morphine, injected into the *epidural space*, is rapidly absorbed into the general circulation. Absorption is so rapid that the plasma concentration-time profiles closely resemble those obtained after intravenous or intramuscular administration. Peak plasma concentrations averaging 33–40 ng/mL (range 5–62 ng/mL) are achieved within 10 to 15 minutes after administration of 3 mg of morphine. Plasma concentrations decline in a multi exponential fashion. The terminal half-life is reported to range from 39 to 249 minutes (mean of 90±34.3 min) and, though somewhat shorter, is similar in magnitude as values reported after intravenous and intramuscular administration (1.5–4.5 h). CSF concentrations of morphine, after epidural doses of 2 to 6 mg in postoperative patients, have been reported to be 50 to 250 times higher than corresponding plasma concentrations. The CSF levels of morphine exceed those in plasma after only 15 minutes and are detectable for as long as 20 hours after the injection of 2 mg of epidural morphine. Approximately 4% of the dose injected epidurally reaches the CSF. This corresponds to the relative minimum effective epidural and intrathecal doses of 5 mg and 0.25 mg, respectively. The disposition of morphine in the CSF follows a biphasic pattern, with an early half-life of 1.5 h and a late phase half-life of about 6 h. Morphine crosses the dura slowly, with an absorption half-life across the dura averaging 22 minutes. Maximum CSF concentrations are seen 60–90 minutes after injection. Minimum effective CSF concentrations for postoperative analgesia average 150 ng/mL (range <1–380 ng/mL).

The *intrathecal route* of administration circumvents meningeal diffusion barriers and, therefore, lower doses of morphine produce comparable analgesia to that induced by the epidural route. After intrathecal bolus injection of morphine, there is a rapid initial distribution phase lasting 15–30 minutes and a half-life in the CSF of 42–136 min (mean 90±16 min). Derived from limited data, it appears that the disposition of morphine in the CSF, from 15 minutes postintrathecal administration to the end of a six-hour observation period, represents a combination of the distribution and elimination phases. Morphine concentrations in the CSF averaged 332±137 ng/mL at 6 hours, following a bolus dose of 0.3 mg of morphine. The apparent volume of distribution of morphine in the intrathecal space is about 22±8 mL.

Time-to-peak plasma concentrations, however, are similar (5–10 min) after either epidural or intrathecal bolus administration of morphine. Maximum plasma morphine concentrations after 0.3 mg intrathecal morphine have been reported from <1 to 7.8 ng/mL. The minimum analgesic morphine plasma concentration during Patient-Controlled Analgesia (PCA) has been reported as 20–40 ng/mL, suggesting that any analgesic contribution from systemic redistribution would be minimal after the first 30–60 minutes with epidural administration and virtually absent with intrathecal administration of morphine.

INDICATIONS AND USAGE

Astramorph/PF is a systemic narcotic analgesic for administration by the intravenous, epidural or intrathecal routes. It is used for the management of pain not responsive to non-narcotic analgesics. Astramorph/PF, administered epidurally or intrathecally, provides pain relief for extended periods without attendant loss of motor, sensory or sympathetic function.

CONTRAINDICATIONS

Astramorph/PF is contraindicated in those medical conditions which would preclude the administration of opioids by the intravenous route—allergy to morphine or other opiates, acute bronchial asthma, upper airway obstruction.

WARNINGS

Morphine sulfate may be habit forming (see DRUG ABUSE AND DEPENDENCE).

Astramorph/PF administration should be limited to use by those familiar with the management of respiratory depression. Rapid intravenous administration may result in chest wall rigidity.

Prior to any epidural or intrathecal drug administration, the physician should be familiar with patient conditions (such as infection at the injection site, bleeding diathesis, anticoagulant therapy, etc.) which call for special evaluation of the benefit versus risk potential.

In the case of epidural or intrathecal administration, Astramorph/PF should be administered by or under the direction of a physician experienced in the techniques and familiar with the patient management problems associated with epidural or intrathecal drug administration. Because epidural administration has been associated with less potential for immediate or late adverse effects than intrathecal administration, the epidural route should be used whenever possible. SEVERE RESPIRATORY DEPRESSION UP TO 24 HOURS FOLLOWING EPIDURAL OR INTRATHECAL ADMINISTRATION HAS BEEN REPORTED.

BECAUSE OF THE RISK OF SEVERE ADVERSE EFFECTS WHEN THE EPIDURAL OR INTRATHECAL ROUTE OF ADMINISTRATION IS EMPLOYED, PATIENTS MUST BE OBSERVED IN A FULLY EQUIPPED AND STAFFED ENVIRONMENT FOR AT LEAST 24 HOURS AFTER THE INITIAL DOSE.

THE FACILITY MUST BE EQUIPPED TO RESUSCITATE PATIENTS WITH SEVERE OPIATE OVERDOSAGE, AND THE PERSONNEL MUST BE FAMILIAR WITH THE USE AND LIMITATIONS OF SPECIFIC NARCOTIC ANTAGONISTS (NALOXONE, NALTREXONE) IN SUCH CASES.

Tolerance and Myoclonic Activity

PATIENTS SOMETIMES MANIFEST UNUSUAL ACCELERATION OF NEURAXIAL MORPHINE REQUIREMENTS, WHICH MAY CAUSE CONCERN REGARDING SYSTEMIC ABSORPTION AND THE HAZARDS OF LARGE DOSES; THESE PATIENTS MAY BENEFIT FROM HOSPITALIZATION AND DETOXIFICATION. TWO CASES OF MYOCLONIC-LIKE SPASM OF THE LOWER EXTREMITIES HAVE BEEN REPORTED IN PATIENTS RECEIVING MORE THAN 20 MG/DAY OF INTRATHECAL MORPHINE. AFTER DETOXIFICATION, IT MIGHT BE POSSIBLE TO RESUME TREATMENT AT LOWER DOSES, AND SOME PATIENTS HAVE BEEN SUCCESSFULLY CHANGED FROM CONTINUOUS EPIDURAL MORPHINE TO CONTINUOUS INTRATHECAL MORPHINE. REPEAT DETOXIFICATION MAY BE INDICATED AT A LATER DATE. THE UPPER DAILY DOSAGE LIMIT FOR EACH PATIENT DURING CONTINUING TREATMENT MUST BE INDIVIDUALIZED.

Continued on next page

Astramorph/PF—Cont.

PRECAUTIONS

General

Control of pain by neuraxial opiate delivery is always accompanied by considerable risk to the patients and requires a high level of skill to be successfully accomplished. The task of treating these patients must be undertaken by experienced clinical teams, well-versed in patient selection, evolving technology and emerging standards of care. For safety reasons, it is recommended that administration of Astramorph/PF by the epidural or intrathecal routes be limited to the lumbar area. Intrathecal use has been associated with a higher incidence of respiratory depression than epidural use.

Seizures may result from high doses. Patients with known seizure disorders should be carefully observed for evidence of morphine-induced seizure activity.

Use in Patients with Increased Intracranial Pressure or Head Injury

Astramorph/PF should be used with extreme caution in patients with head injury or increased intracranial pressure. Pupillary changes (miosis) from morphine may obscure the existence, extent and course of intracranial pathology. High doses of neuraxial morphine may produce myoclonic events (see WARNINGS and ADVERSE REACTIONS). Clinicians should maintain a high index of suspicion for adverse drug reactions when evaluating altered mental status or movement abnormalities in patients receiving this modality of treatment.

Use in Chronic Pulmonary Disease

Care is urged in using this drug in patients who have a decreased respiratory reserve (eg., emphysema, severe obesity, kyphoscoliosis or paralysis of the phrenic nerve). Astramorph/PF should not be given in cases of chronic asthma, upper airway obstruction or in any other chronic pulmonary disorder without due consideration of the known risk of acute respiratory failure following morphine administration in such patients.

Use in Hepatic or Renal Disease

The elimination half-life of morphine may be prolonged in patients with reduced metabolic rates and with hepatic and/or renal dysfunction. Hence, care should be exercised in administering Astramorph/PF epidurally to patients with these conditions, since high blood morphine levels, due to reduced clearance, may take several days to develop.

Use in Biliary Surgery or Disorders of the Biliary Tract

As significant morphine is released into the systemic circulation from neuraxial administration, the ensuring smooth muscle hypertonicity may result in biliary colic.

Use with Disorders of the Urinary System

Initiation of neuraxial opiate analgesia is frequently associated with disturbances of micturition, especially in males with prostatic enlargement. Early recognition of difficulty in urination and prompt intervention in cases of urinary retention is indicated.

Use in Ambulatory Patients

Patients with reduced circulating blood volume, impaired myocardial function or on sympatholytic drugs should be monitored for the possible occurrence of orthostatic hypotension, a frequent complication in single-dose neuraxial morphine analgesia.

Use with Other Central Nervous System Depressants

The depressant effects of morphine are potentiated by the presence of other CNS depressants such as alcohol, sedatives, antihistaminics or psychotropic drugs. Use of neuroleptics in conjunction with neuraxial morphine may increase the risk of respiratory depression.

Carcinogenesis, Mutagenesis, Impairment of Fertility

Morphine is without known carcinogenic or mutagenic effects and is not known to impair fertility at non-narcotic doses in animals, but studies of the carcinogenic and mutagenic potential or the effect on fertility of Astramorph/PF have not been conducted.

Pregnancy

Teratogenic Effects—Pregnancy Category C. Morphine sulfate is not teratogenic in rats at 35 mg/kg/day (thirty-five times the usual human dose) but does result in increased pup mortality and growth retardation at doses that narcotize the animal (>10 mg/kg/day, ten times the usual human dose). Astramorph/PF should only be given to pregnant women when no other method of controlling pain is available and means are at hand to manage the delivery and perinatal care of the opiate-dependent infant.

Nonteratogenic Effects. Infants born to mothers who have been taking morphine chronically may exhibit withdrawal symptoms.

Labor and Delivery

Intravenous morphine readily passes into the fetal circulation and may result in respiratory depression in the neonate. Naloxone and resuscitative equipment should be available for reversal of narcotic-induced respiratory depression in the neonate. In addition, intravenous morphine may reduce the strength, duration and frequency of uterine contraction resulting in prolonged labor.

Epidurally and *intrathecally* administered morphine readily passes into the fetal circulation and may result in respiratory depression of the neonate. Controlled clinical studies have shown that *epidural* administration has little or no effect on the relief of labor pain.

Nursing Mothers

Morphine is excreted in maternal milk. Effect on the nursing infant is not known.

Pediatric Use

Adequate studies, to establish the safety and effectiveness of spinal morphine in pediatric patients, have not been performed, and usage in this population is not recommended.

Geriatric Use

The pharmacodynamic effects of neuraxial morphine in the elderly are more variable than in the younger population. Patients will vary widely in the effective initial dose, rate of development of tolerance and the frequency and magnitude of associated adverse effects as the dose is increased. Initial doses should be based on careful clinical observation following "test doses", after making due allowances for the effects of the patient's age and infirmity on his/her ability to clear the drug, particularly in patients receiving epidural morphine.

Elderly patients may be more susceptible to respiratory depression and/or respiratory arrest following administration of morphine.

ADVERSE REACTIONS

The most serious adverse experience encountered during administration of Astramorph/PF is respiratory depression and/or respiratory arrest. This depression and/or respiratory arrest may be severe and could require intervention (see WARNINGS and OVERDOSAGE). Because of delay in maximum CNS effect with intravenously administered drug (30 min), rapid administration may result in overdosing. Single-dose neuraxial administration may result in acute or delayed respiratory depression for periods at least as long as 24 hours.

Tolerance and Myoclonus: See **WARNINGS** for discussion of these and related hazards.

While low doses of intravenously administered morphine have little effect on cardiovascular stability, high doses are excitatory, resulting from **sympathetic hyperactivity** and increase in circulating catecholamines. Excitation of the central nervous system, resulting in **convulsions**, may accompany high doses of morphine given intravenously. **Dysphoric reactions** may occur after any size dose and **toxic psychoses** have been reported.

Pruritus: Single-dose epidural or intrathecal administration is accompanied by a high incidence of **pruritus** that is dose-related but not confined to the site of administration. Pruritus, following continuous infusion of epidural or intrathecal morphine, is occasionally reported in the literature; these reactions are poorly understood as to their cause.

Urinary Retention: Urinary retention, which may persist 10 to 20 hours following single epidural or intrathecal administration, is a frequent side effect and must be anticipated primarily in male patients, with a somewhat lower incidence in females. Also frequently reported in the literature is the occurrence of urinary retention during the first several days of hospitalization for the initiation of continuous intrathecal or epidural morphine therapy. Patients who develop urinary retention have responded to cholinomimetic treatment and/or judicious use of catheters (see PRECAUTIONS).

Constipation: Constipation is frequently encountered during continuous infusion of morphine; this can usually be managed by conventional therapy.

Headache: Lumbar puncture-type headache is encountered in a significant minority of cases for several days following intrathecal catheter implantation; this, generally, responds to bed rest and/or other conventional therapy.

Other: Other adverse experiences reported following morphine therapy include—**Dizziness, euphoria, anxiety, depression of cough reflex, interference with thermal regulation** and **oliguria**. Evidence of histamine release such as **urticaria, wheals** and/or **local tissue** irritation may occur. **Nausea** and **vomiting** are frequently seen in patients following morphine administration.

Pruritus, nausea/vomiting and urinary retention, if associated with continuous infusion therapy, may respond to intravenous administration of a low dose of naloxone (0.2 mg). The risks of using narcotic antagonists in patients chronically receiving narcotic therapy should be considered.

In general, side effects are amenable to reversal by narcotic antagonists.

NALOXONE INJECTION AND RESUSCITATIVE EQUIPMENT SHOULD BE IMMEDIATELY AVAILABLE FOR ADMINISTRATION IN CASE OF LIFE-THREATENING OR INTOLERABLE SIDE EFFECTS AND WHENEVER ASTRAMORPH/PF THERAPY IS BEING INITIATED.

DRUG ABUSE AND DEPENDENCE

Controlled Substance

Morphine sulfate is a Schedule II narcotic under the United States Controlled Substance Act (21 U.S.C. 801-886).

Morphine is the most commonly cited prototype for narcotic substances that possess an addiction-forming or addiction-sustaining liability. A patient may be at risk for developing a dependence to morphine if used improperly or for overly long periods of time. As with all potent opioids which are μ-agonists, tolerance as well as psychological and physical dependence to morphine may develop irrespective of the route of administration (intravenous, intramuscular, intrathecal, epidural or oral). Individuals with a prior history of opioid or other substance abuse or dependence, being more apt to respond to the euphorogenic and reinforcing properties of morphine, would be considered to be at greater risk. Care must be taken to avert withdrawal in patients who have been maintained on parenteral/oral narcotics when epidural or intrathecal administration is considered. Withdrawal symptoms may occur when morphine is discontinued abruptly or upon administration of a narcotic antagonist.

OVERDOSAGE

PARENTERAL ADMINISTRATION OF NARCOTICS IN PATIENTS RECEIVING EPIDURAL OR INTRATHECAL MORPHINE MAY RESULT IN OVERDOSAGE.

Overdosage of morphine is characterized by respiratory depression, with or without concomitant CNS depression. Since respiratory arrest may result either through direct depression of the respiratory center or as the result of hypoxia, primary attention should be given to the establishment of adequate respiratory exchange through provision of a patent airway and institution of assisted, or controlled, ventilation. The narcotic antagonist, naloxone, is a specific antidote. An initial dose of 0.4 to 2 mg of naloxone should be administered intravenously, simultaneously with respiratory resuscitation. If the desired degree of counteraction and improvement in respiratory function is not obtained, naloxone may be repeated at 2- to 3-minute intervals. If no response is observed after 10 mg of naloxone has been administered, the diagnosis of narcotic-induced, or partial narcotic-induced, toxicity should be questioned. Intramuscular or subcutaneous administration may be used if the intravenous route is not available.

As the duration of effect of naloxone is considerably shorter than that of epidural or intrathecal morphine, repeated administration may be necessary. Patients should be closely observed for evidence of renarcotization.

DOSAGE AND ADMINISTRATION

Astramorph/PF is intended for intravenous, epidural or intrathecal administration.

Intravenous Administration

Dosage

The initial dose of morphine sulfate should be 2 mg to 10 mg/70 kg of body weight. No information is available regarding the use of Astramorph/PF in patients under the age of 18.

Geriatric Use: Administer with extreme caution (see PRECAUTIONS).

Epidural Administration

ASTRAMORPH/PF SHOULD BE ADMINISTERED EPIDURALLY BY OR UNDER THE DIRECTION OF A PHYSICIAN EXPERIENCED IN THE TECHNIQUE OF EPIDURAL ADMINISTRATION AND WHO IS THOROUGHLY FAMILIAR WITH THE LABELING. IT SHOULD BE ADMINISTERED ONLY IN SETTINGS WHERE ADEQUATE PATIENT MONITORING IS POSSIBLE. RESUSCITATIVE EQUIPMENT AND A SPECIFIC ANTAGONIST (NALOXONE INJECTION) SHOULD BE IMMEDIATELY AVAILABLE FOR THE MANAGEMENT OF RESPIRATORY DEPRESSION AS WELL AS COMPLICATIONS WHICH MIGHT RESULT FROM INADVERTENT INTRATHECAL OR INTRAVASCULAR INJECTION. (NOTE: INTRATHECAL DOSAGE IS USUALLY 1/10 THAT OF EPIDURAL DOSAGE.) **PATIENT MONITORING SHOULD BE CONTINUED FOR AT LEAST 24 HOURS AFTER EACH DOSE, SINCE DELAYED RESPIRATORY DEPRESSION MAY OCCUR.**

Proper placement of a needle or catheter in the epidural space should be verified before Astramorph/PF is injected. Acceptable techniques for verifying proper placement include: a) aspiration to check for absence of blood or cerebrospinal fluid, or b) administration of 5 mL (3 mL in obstetric patients) of 1.5% PRESERVATIVE-FREE Lidocaine and Epinephrine (1:200,000) Injection and then observe the patient for lack of tachycardia (this indicates that vascular injection has *not* been made) and lack of sudden onset of segmental anesthesia (this indicates that intrathecal injection has *not* been made).

Epidural Adult Dosage

Initial injection of 5 mg in the lumbar region may provide satisfactory pain relief for up to 24 hours. If adequate pain relief is not achieved within one hour, careful administration of incremental doses of 1 to 2 mg at intervals sufficient to assess effectiveness may be given. No more than 10 mg/24 hr should be administered.

Thoracic administration has been shown to dramatically increase the incidence of early and late respiratory depression even at doses of 1 to 2 mg.

For continuous infusion an initial dose of 2 to 4 mg/24 hours is recommended. Further doses of 1 to 2 mg may be given if pain relief is not achieved initially.

Geriatric Use—Administer with extreme caution (see PRECAUTIONS).

Epidural Pediatric Use

No information on use in pediatric patients is available. (See PRECAUTIONS).

Intrathecal Administration

NOTE: INTRATHECAL DOSAGE IS USUALLY 1/10 THAT OF EPIDURAL DOSAGE.

ASTRAMORPH/PF SHOULD BE ADMINISTERED INTRATHECALLY BY OR UNDER THE DIRECTION OF A PHYSICIAN EXPERIENCED IN THE TECHNIQUE OF INTRATHECAL ADMINISTRATION AND WHO IS THOROUGHLY FAMILIAR WITH THE LABELING. IT SHOULD BE ADMINISTERED ONLY IN SETTINGS WHERE ADEQUATE PATIENT MONITORING IS POSSIBLE. RESUSCITATIVE EQUIPMENT AND A SPECIFIC ANTAGONIST (NALOXONE INJECTION) SHOULD BE IMMEDIATELY AVAILABLE FOR THE MANAGEMENT OF RESPIRATORY DEPRESSION AS WELL AS COMPLICATIONS

WHICH MIGHT RESULT FROM INADVERTENT INTRAVASCULAR INJECTION. **PATIENT MONITORING SHOULD BE CONTINUED FOR AT LEAST 24 HOURS AFTER EACH DOSE, SINCE DELAYED RESPIRATORY DEPRESSION MAY OCCUR.** RESPIRATORY DEPRESSON (BOTH EARLY AND LATE ONSET) HAS OCCURRED MORE FREQUENTLY FOLLOWING INTRATHECAL ADMINISTRATION.

Intrathecal Adult Dosage

A single injection of 0.2 to 1 mg may provide satisfactory pain relief for up to 24 hours. (CAUTION: THIS IS ONLY 0.4 TO 2 ML OF THE 5 MG/10ML AMPULE/VIAL OR 0.2 TO 1 ML OF THE 10 MG/10 ML AMPULE/VIAL OF ASTRAMORPH/PF.) DO NOT INJECT INTRATHECALLY MORE THAN 2 ML OF THE 5 MG/10 ML AMPULE/VIAL OR 1 ML OF THE 10 MG/10ML AMPULE/VIAL. USE IN THE LUMBAR AREA ONLY IS RECOMMENDED. Repeated intrathecal injections of Astramorph/PF are not recommended. A constant intravenous infusion of naloxone, 0.6 mg/hr, for 24 hours after intrathecal injection may be used to reduce the incidence of potential side effects.

Geriatric Use—Administer with extreme caution (see PRECAUTIONS).

Repeat Dosage

If pain recurs, alternative routes of administration should be considered, since experience with repeated doses of morphine by the intrathecal route is limited.

Intrathecal Pediatric Use

No information on use in pediatric patients is available. (See PRECAUTIONS).

SAFETY AND HANDLING INSTRUCTIONS

Astramorph/PF is supplied in sealed ampules and vials. Accidental dermal exposure should be treated by the removal of any contaminated clothing and rinsing the affected area with water.

Each ampule/vial of Astramorph/PF contains a potent narcotic which has been associated with abuse and dependence among health care providers. **Due to the limited indications for this product, the risk of overdosage and the risk of its diversion and abuse, it is recommended that special measures be taken to control this product within the hospital or clinic. *Astramorph/PF should be subject to rigid accounting, rigorous control of wastage and restricted access.***

Parenteral drug products should be inspected for particulate matter and discoloration prior to administration, whenever solution and container permit. DO NOT USE IF COLOR IS DARKER THAN PALE YELLOW, IF IT IS DISCOLORED IN ANY OTHER WAY OR IF IT CONTAINS A PRECIPITATE.

HOW SUPPLIED

Preservative-free ASTRAMORPH/PF (Morphine Sulfate Injection, USP) is available in ampules and single dose vial for intravenous, epidural, or intrathecal administration:

0.5 mg/mL

NDC 0186-1159-03 2 mL (1 mg) Ampule, Boxes of 10
NDC 0186-1150-02 10 mL (5 mg) Ampule, Boxes of 5
NDC 0186-1152-12 10 mL (5 mg) Single Dose Vial, Boxes of 5 E-Z OFF vial closures

1 mg/mL

NDC 0186-1160-03 2 mL (2 mg) Ampule, Boxes of 10
NDC 0186-1151-02 10 mL (10 mg) Ampule, Boxes of 5
NDC 0186-1153-12 10 mL (10 mg) Single Dose Vial, Boxes of 5 E-Z OFF vial closures

Storage

Protect from light. Store in carton at controlled room temperature, 15 to 30°C (59 to 86°F) until ready to use. DO NOT FREEZE. Astramorph/PF contains no preservative or antioxidant. DISCARD ANY UNUSED PORTION. DO NOT HEAT-STERILIZE.

All trademarks are the property of the AstraZeneca group
© AstraZeneca 2002

AstraZeneca LP, Wilmington, DE 19850
721865-06 Rev. 07/02

ATACAND® ℞

[ăt'ă-kănd]

(CANDESARTAN CILEXETIL)
TABLETS

Prescribing information for this product, which appears on pages 594–596 of the 2003 PDR, has been completely revised as follows. Please write "See Supplement A" next to the product heading.

USE IN PREGNANCY

When used in pregnancy during the second and third trimesters, drugs that act directly on the renin-angiotensin system can cause injury and even death to the developing fetus. When pregnancy is detected, ATACAND should be discontinued as soon as possible. See WARNINGS, Fetal/Neonatal Morbidity and Mortality.

DESCRIPTION

ATACAND (candesartan cilexetil), a prodrug, is hydrolyzed to candesartan during absorption from the gastrointestinal tract. Candesartan is a selective AT_1 subtype angiotensin II receptor antagonist.

Candesartan cilexetil, a nonpeptide, is chemically described as (±)-1-[[(cyclohexyloxy)carbonyl]oxy]ethyl 2-ethoxy-1-[[2'-(1H- tetrazol-5-yl) [1,1'-biphenyl]-4-yl]methyl]-1H-benzimidazole-7-carboxylate.

Its empirical formula is $C_{33}H_{34}N_6O_6$, and its structural formula is

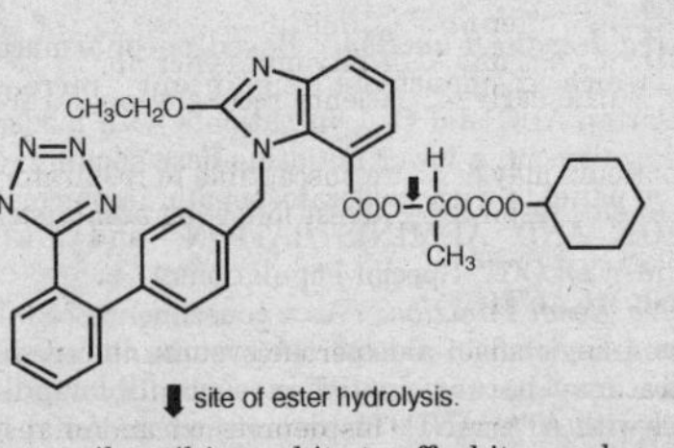

Candesartan cilexetil is a white to off-white powder with a molecular weight of 610.67. It is practically insoluble in water and sparingly soluble in methanol. Candesartan cilexetil is a racemic mixture containing one chiral center at the cyclohexyloxycarbonyloxy ethyl ester group. Following oral administration, candesartan cilexetil undergoes hydrolysis at the ester link to form the active drug, candesartan, which is achiral.

ATACAND is available for oral use as tablets containing either 4 mg, 8 mg, 16 mg, or 32 mg of candesartan cilexetil and the following inactive ingredients: hydroxypropyl cellulose, polyethylene glycol, lactose, corn starch, carboxymethylcellulose calcium, and magnesium stearate. Ferric oxide (reddish brown) is added to the 8-mg, 16-mg, and 32-mg tablets as a colorant.

CLINICAL PHARMACOLOGY

Mechanism of Action

Angiotensin II is formed from angiotensin I in a reaction catalyzed by angiotensin-converting enzyme (ACE, kininase II). Angiotensin II is the principal pressor agent of the renin-angiotensin system, with effects that include vasoconstriction, stimulation of synthesis and release of aldosterone, cardiac stimulation, and renal reabsorption of sodium. Candesartan blocks the vasoconstrictor and aldosterone-secreting effects of angiotensin II by selectively blocking the binding of angiotensin II to the AT_1 receptor in many tissues, such as vascular smooth muscle and the adrenal gland. Its action is, therefore, independent of the pathways for angiotensin II synthesis.

There is also an AT_2 receptor found in many tissues, but AT_2 is not known to be associated with cardiovascular homeostasis. Candesartan has much greater affinity (>10,000-fold) for the AT_1 receptor than for the AT_2 receptor.

Blockade of the renin-angiotensin system with ACE inhibitors, which inhibit the biosynthesis of angiotensin II from angiotensin I, is widely used in the treatment of hypertension. ACE inhibitors also inhibit the degradation of bradykinin, a reaction also catalyzed by ACE. Because candesartan does not inhibit ACE (kininase II), it does not affect the response to bradykinin. Whether this difference has clinical relevance is not yet known. Candesartan does not bind to or block other hormone receptors or ion channels known to be important in cardiovascular regulation.

Blockade of the angiotensin II receptor inhibits the negative regulatory feedback of angiotensin II on renin secretion, but the resulting increased plasma renin activity and angiotensin II circulating levels do not overcome the effect of candesartan on blood pressure.

Pharmacokinetics

General

Candesartan cilexetil is rapidly and completely bioactivated by ester hydrolysis during absorption from the gastrointestinal tract to candesartan, a selective AT_1 subtype angiotensin II receptor antagonist. Candesartan is mainly excreted unchanged in urine and feces (via bile). It undergoes minor hepatic metabolism by O-deethylation to an inactive metabolite. The elimination half-life of candesartan is approximately 9 hours. After single and repeated administration, the pharmacokinetics of candesartan are linear for oral doses up to 32 mg of candesartan cilexetil. Candesartan and its inactive metabolite do not accumulate in serum upon repeated once-daily dosing.

Following administration of candesartan cilexetil, the absolute bioavailability of candesartan was estimated to be 15%. After tablet ingestion, the peak serum concentration (C_{max}) is reached after 3 to 4 hours. Food with a high fat content does not affect the bioavailability of candesartan after candesartan cilexetil administration.

Metabolism and Excretion

Total plasma clearance of candesartan is 0.37 mL/min/kg, with a renal clearance of 0.19 mL/min/kg. When candesartan is administered orally, about 26% of the dose is excreted unchanged in urine. Following an oral dose of ^{14}C-labeled candesartan cilexetil, approximately 33% of radioactivity is recovered in urine and approximately 67% in feces. Following an intravenous dose of ^{14}C-labeled candesartan, approximately 59% of radioactivity is recovered in urine and approximately 36% in feces. Biliary excretion contributes to the elimination of candesartan.

Distribution

The volume of distribution of candesartan is 0.13 L/kg. Candesartan is highly bound to plasma proteins (>99%) and does not penetrate red blood cells. The protein binding is constant at candesartan plasma concentrations well above the range achieved with recommended doses. In rats, it has been demonstrated that candesartan crosses the blood-brain barrier poorly, if at all. It has also been demonstrated in rats that candesartan passes across the placental barrier and is distributed in the fetus.

Special Populations

Pediatric: The pharmacokinetics of candesartan cilexetil have not been investigated in patients <18 years of age.

Geriatric and Gender: The pharmacokinetics of candesartan have been studied in the elderly (≥65 years) and in both sexes. The plasma concentration of candesartan was higher in the elderly (C_{max} was approximately 50% higher, and AUC was approximately 80% higher) compared to younger subjects administered the same dose. The pharmacokinetics of candesartan were linear in the elderly, and candesartan and its inactive metabolite did not accumulate in the serum of these subjects upon repeated, once-daily administration. No initial dosage adjustment is necessary. (See DOSAGE AND ADMINISTRATION.) There is no difference in the pharmacokinetics of candesartan between male and female subjects.

Renal Insufficiency: In hypertensive patients with renal insufficiency, serum concentrations of candesartan were elevated. After repeated dosing, the AUC and C_{max} were approximately doubled in patients with severe renal impairment (creatinine clearance <30 mL/min/1.73m^2) compared to patients with normal kidney function. The pharmacokinetics of candesartan in hypertensive patients undergoing hemodialysis are similar to those in hypertensive patients with severe renal impairment. Candesartan cannot be removed by hemodialysis. No initial dosage adjustment is necessary in patients with renal insufficiency. (See DOSAGE AND ADMINISTRATION.)

Hepatic Insufficiency: The pharmacokinetics of candesartan were compared in patients with mild and moderate hepatic impairment to matched healthy volunteers following a single oral dose of 16 mg candesartan cilexetil. The increase in AUC for candesartan was 30% in patients with mild hepatic impairment (Child-Pugh A) and 145% in patients with moderate hepatic impairment (Child-Pugh B). The increase in C_{max} for candesartan was 56% in patients with mild hepatic impairment and 73% in patients with moderate hepatic impairment. The pharmacokinetics after candesartan cilexetil administration have not been investigated in patients with severe hepatic impairment. No initial dosage adjustment is necessary in patients with mild hepatic impairment. In patients with moderate hepatic impairment, consideration should be given to initiation of ATACAND at a lower dose. (See DOSAGE AND ADMINISTRATION.)

Drug Interactions

See PRECAUTIONS, Drug Interactions.

Pharmacodynamics

Candesartan inhibits the pressor effects of angiotensin II infusion in a dose-dependent manner. After 1 week of once-daily dosing with 8 mg of candesartan cilexetil, the pressor effect was inhibited by approximately 90% at peak with approximately 50% inhibition persisting for 24 hours.

Plasma concentrations of angiotensin I and angiotensin II, and plasma renin activity (PRA), increased in a dose-dependent manner after single and repeated administration of candesartan cilexetil to healthy subjects and hypertensive patients. ACE activity was not altered in healthy subjects after repeated candesartan cilexetil administration. The once-daily administration of up to 16 mg of candesartan cilexetil to healthy subjects did not influence plasma aldosterone concentrations, but a decrease in the plasma concentration of aldosterone was observed when 32 mg of candesartan cilexetil was administered to hypertensive patients. In spite of the effect of candesartan cilexetil on aldosterone secretion, very little effect on serum potassium was observed.

In multiple-dose studies with hypertensive patients, there were no clinically significant changes in metabolic function, including serum levels of total cholesterol, triglycerides, glucose, or uric acid. In a 12-week study of 161 patients with non-insulin-dependent (type 2) diabetes mellitus and hypertension, there was no change in the level of HbA_{1c}.

Clinical Trials

The antihypertensive effects of ATACAND were examined in 14 placebo-controlled trials of 4- to 12-weeks duration, primarily at daily doses of 2 to 32 mg per day in patients with baseline diastolic blood pressures of 95 to 114 mm Hg. Most of the trials were of candesartan cilexetil as a single agent, but it was also studied as add-on to hydrochlorothiazide and amlodipine. These studies included a total of 2350 patients randomized to one of several doses of candesartan cilexetil and 1027 to placebo. Except for a study in diabetics, all studies showed significant effects, generally dose related, of 2 to 32 mg on trough (24 hour) systolic and diastolic pressures compared to placebo, with doses of 8 to 32 mg giving effects of about 8–12/4–8 mm Hg. There were no exaggerated first-dose effects in these patients. Most of the antihypertensive effect was seen within 2 weeks of initial dosing, and the full effect in 4 weeks. With once-daily dosing, blood pressure effect was maintained over 24 hours, with trough to peak ratios of blood pressure effect generally over 80%. Candesartan cilexetil had an additional blood pressure lowering effect when added to hydrochlorothiazide.

The antihypertensive effects of candesartan cilexetil and losartan potassium at their highest recommended doses ad-

Continued on next page

Atacand—Cont.

ministered once-daily were compared in two randomized, double-blind trials. In a total of 1268 patients with mild to moderate hypertension who were not receiving other antihypertensive therapy, candesartan cilexetil 32 mg lowered systolic and diastolic blood pressure by 2 to 3 mm Hg on average more than losartan potassium 100 mg, when measured at the time of either peak or trough effect. The antihypertensive effects of twice daily dosing of either candesartan cilexetil or losartan potassium were not studied.
The antihypertensive effect was similar in men and women and in patients older and younger than 65. Candesartan was effective in reducing blood pressure regardless of race, although the effect was somewhat less in blacks (usually a low-renin population). This has been generally true for angiotensin II antagonists and ACE inhibitors.
In long-term studies of up to 1 year, the antihypertensive effectiveness of candesartan cilexetil was maintained, and there was no rebound after abrupt withdrawal.
There were no changes in the heart rate of patients treated with candesartan cilexetil in controlled trials.

INDICATIONS AND USAGE

ATACAND is indicated for the treatment of hypertension. It may be used alone or in combination with other antihypertensive agents.

CONTRAINDICATIONS

ATACAND is contraindicated in patients who are hypersensitive to any component of this product.

WARNINGS

Fetal/Neonatal Morbidity and Mortality

Drugs that act directly on the renin-angiotensin system can cause fetal and neonatal morbidity and death when administered to pregnant women. Several dozen cases have been reported in the world literature in patients who were taking angiotensin-converting enzyme inhibitors. When pregnancy is detected, ATACAND should be discontinued as soon as possible.
The use of drugs that act directly on the renin-angiotensin system during the second and third trimesters of pregnancy has been associated with fetal and neonatal injury, including hypotension, neonatal skull hypoplasia, anuria, reversible or irreversible renal failure, and death. Oligohydramnios has also been reported, presumably resulting from decreased fetal renal function; oligohydramnios in this setting has been associated with fetal limb contractures, craniofacial deformation, and hypoplastic lung development. Prematurity, intrauterine growth retardation, and patent ductus arteriosus have also been reported, although it is not clear whether these occurrences were due to exposure to the drug.
These adverse effects do not appear to have resulted from intrauterine drug exposure that has been limited to the first trimester. Mothers whose embryos and fetuses are exposed to an angiotensin II receptor antagonist only during the first trimester should be so informed. Nonetheless, when patients become pregnant, physicians should have the patient discontinue the use of ATACAND as soon as possible. Rarely (probably less often than once in every thousand pregnancies), no alternative to a drug acting on the renin-angiotensin system will be found. In these rare cases, the mothers should be apprised of the potential hazards to their fetuses, and serial ultrasound examinations should be performed to assess the intra-amniotic environment.
If oligohydramnios is observed, ATACAND should be discontinued unless it is considered life saving for the mother. Contraction stress testing (CST), a nonstress test (NST), or biophysical profiling (BPP) may be appropriate, depending upon the week of pregnancy. Patients and physicians should be aware, however, that oligohydramnios may not appear until after the fetus has sustained irreversible injury.
Infants with histories of *in utero* exposure to an angiotensin II receptor antagonist should be closely observed for hypotension, oliguria, and hyperkalemia. If oliguria occurs, attention should be directed toward support of blood pressure and renal perfusion. Exchange transfusion or dialysis may be required as means of reversing hypotension and/or substituting for disordered renal function.
There is no clinical experience with the use of ATACAND in pregnant women. Oral doses ≥10 mg of candesartan cilexetil/kg/day administered to pregnant rats during late gestation and continued through lactation were associated with reduced survival and an increased incidence of hydronephrosis in the offspring. The 10-mg/kg/day dose in rats is approximately 2.8 times the maximum recommended daily human dose (MRHD) of 32 mg on a mg/m^2 basis (comparison assumes human body weight of 50 kg). Candesartan cilexetil given to pregnant rabbits at an oral dose of 3 mg/kg/day (approximately 1.7 times the MRHD on a mg/m^2 basis) caused maternal toxicity (decreased body weight and death) but, in surviving dams, had no adverse effects on fetal survival, fetal weight, or external, visceral, or skeletal development. No maternal toxicity or adverse effects on fetal development were observed when oral doses up to 1000 mg of candesartan cilexetil/kg/day (approximately 138 times the MRHD on a mg/m^2 basis) were administered to pregnant mice.

Hypotension in Volume- and Salt-Depleted Patients

In patients with an activated renin-angiotensin system, such as volume- and/or salt-depleted patients (eg, those being treated with diuretics), symptomatic hypotension may occur. These conditions should be corrected prior to administration of ATACAND, or the treatment should start under close medical supervision. (See DOSAGE AND ADMINISTRATION.)
If hypotension occurs, the patients should be placed in the supine position and, if necessary, given an intravenous infusion of normal saline. A transient hypotensive response is not a contraindication to further treatment which usually can be continued without difficulty once the blood pressure has stabilized.

PRECAUTIONS

General

Impaired Hepatic Function: Based on pharmacokinetic data which demonstrate significant increases in candesartan AUC and C_{max} in patients with moderate hepatic impairment, a lower initiating dose should be considered for patients with moderate hepatic impairment. (See DOSAGE AND ADMINISTRATION, and CLINICAL PHARMACOLOGY, Special Populations.)
Impaired Renal Function: As a consequence of inhibiting the renin-angiotensin-aldosterone system, changes in renal function may be anticipated in susceptible individuals treated with ATACAND. In patients whose renal function may depend upon the activity of the renin-angiotensin-aldosterone system (eg, patients with severe congestive heart failure), treatment with angiotensin-converting enzyme inhibitors and angiotensin receptor antagonists has been associated with oliguria and/or progressive azotemia and (rarely) with acute renal failure and/or death. Similar results may be anticipated in patients treated with ATACAND. (See CLINICAL PHARMACOLOGY, Special Populations.)
In studies of ACE inhibitors in patients with unilateral or bilateral renal artery stenosis, increases in serum creatinine or blood urea nitrogen (BUN) have been reported. There has been no long-term use of ATACAND in patients with unilateral or bilateral renal artery stenosis, but similar results may be expected.

Information for Patients

Pregnancy: Female patients of childbearing age should be told about the consequences of second- and third-trimester exposure to drugs that act on the renin-angiotensin system, and they should also be told that these consequences do not appear to have resulted from intrauterine drug exposure that has been limited to the first trimester. These patients should be asked to report pregnancies to their physicians as soon as possible.

Drug Interactions

No significant drug interactions have been reported in studies of candesartan cilexetil given with other drugs such as glyburide, nifedipine, digoxin, warfarin, hydrochlorothiazide, and oral contraceptives in healthy volunteers. Because candesartan is not significantly metabolized by the cytochrome P450 system and at therapeutic concentrations has no effects on P450 enzymes, interactions with drugs that inhibit or are metabolized by those enzymes would not be expected.

Carcinogenesis, Mutagenesis, Impairment of Fertility

There was no evidence of carcinogenicity when candesartan cilexetil was orally administered to mice and rats for up to 104 weeks at doses up to 100 and 1000 mg/kg/day, respectively. Rats received the drug by gavage, whereas mice received the drug by dietary administration. These (maximally-tolerated) doses of candesartan cilexetil provided systemic exposures to candesartan (AUCs) that were, in mice, approximately 7 times and, in rats, more than 70 times the exposure in man at the maximum recommended daily human dose (32 mg).
Candesartan and its O-deethyl metabolite tested positive for genotoxicity in the *in vitro* Chinese hamster lung (CHL) chromosomal aberration assay. Neither compound tested positive in the Ames microbial mutagenesis assay or the *in vitro* mouse lymphoma cell assay. Candesartan (but not its O-deethyl metabolite) was also evaluated *in vivo* in the mouse micronucleus test and *in vitro* in the Chinese hamster ovary (CHO) gene mutation assay, in both cases with negative results. Candesartan cilexetil was evaluated in the Ames test, the *in vitro* mouse lymphoma cell and rat hepatocyte unscheduled DNA synthesis assays and the *in vivo* mouse micronucleus test, in each case with negative results. Candesartan cilexetil was not evaluated in the CHL chromosomal aberration or CHO gene mutation assay.
Fertility and reproductive performance were not affected in studies with male and female rats given oral doses of up to 300 mg/kg/day (83 times the maximum daily human dose of 32 mg on a body surface area basis).

Pregnancy

Pregnancy Categories C (first trimester) *and D* (second and third trimesters). See WARNINGS, Fetal/Neonatal Morbidity and Mortality.

Nursing Mothers

It is not known whether candesartan is excreted in human milk, but candesartan has been shown to be present in rat milk. Because of the potential for adverse effects on the nursing infant, a decision should be made whether to discontinue nursing or discontinue the drug, taking into account the importance of the drug to the mother.

Pediatric Use

Safety and effectiveness in pediatric patients have not been established.

Geriatric Use

Of the total number of subjects in clinical studies of ATACAND, 21% (683/3260) were 65 and over, while 3% (87/3260) were 75 and over. No overall differences in safety or effectiveness were observed between these subjects and younger subjects, and other reported clinical experience has not identified differences in responses between the elderly and younger patients, but greater sensitivity of some older individuals cannot be ruled out. In a placebo-controlled trial of about 200 elderly hypertensive patients (ages 65 to 87 years), administration of candesartan cilexetil was well tolerated and lowered blood pressure by about 12/6 mm Hg more than placebo.

ADVERSE REACTIONS

ATACAND has been evaluated for safety in more than 3600 patients/subjects, including more than 3200 patients treated for hypertension. About 600 of these patients were studied for at least 6 months and about 200 for at least 1 year. In general, treatment with ATACAND was well tolerated. The overall incidence of adverse events reported with ATACAND was similar to placebo.
The rate of withdrawals due to adverse events in all trials in patients (7510 total) was 3.3% (ie, 108 of 3260) of patients treated with candesartan cilexetil as monotherapy and 3.5% (ie, 39 of 1106) of patients treated with placebo. In placebo-controlled trials, discontinuation of therapy due to clinical adverse events occurred in 2.4% (ie, 57 of 2350) of patients treated with ATACAND and 3.4% (ie, 35 of 1027) of patients treated with placebo.
The most common reasons for discontinuation of therapy with ATACAND were headache (0.6%) and dizziness (0.3%).
The adverse events that occurred in placebo-controlled clinical trials in at least 1% of patients treated with ATACAND and at a higher incidence in candesartan cilexetil (n=2350) than placebo (n=1027) patients included back pain (3% vs 2%), dizziness (4% vs 3%), upper respiratory tract infection (6% vs 4%), pharyngitis (2% vs 1%), and rhinitis (2% vs 1%).
The following adverse events occurred in placebo-controlled clinical trials at a more than 1% rate but at about the same or greater incidence in patients receiving placebo compared to candesartan cilexetil: fatigue, peripheral edema, chest pain, headache, bronchitis, coughing, sinusitis, nausea, abdominal pain, diarrhea, vomiting, arthralgia, albuminuria.
Other potentially important adverse events that have been reported, whether or not attributed to treatment, with an incidence of 0.5% or greater from the 3260 patients worldwide treated in clinical trials with ATACAND are listed below. It cannot be determined whether these events were causally related to ATACAND. **Body as a Whole:** asthenia, fever; **Central and Peripheral Nervous System:** paresthesia, vertigo; **Gastrointestinal System Disorder:** dyspepsia, gastroenteritis; **Heart Rate and Rhythm Disorders:** tachycardia, palpitation; **Metabolic and Nutritional Disorders:** creatine phosphokinase increased, hyperglycemia, hypertriglyceridemia, hyperuricemia; **Musculoskeletal System Disorders:** myalgia; **Platelet/Bleeding-Clotting Disorders:** epistaxis; **Psychiatric Disorders:** anxiety, depression, somnolence; **Respiratory System Disorders:** dyspnea; **Skin and Appendages Disorders:** rash, sweating increased; **Urinary System Disorders:** hematuria.
Other reported events seen less frequently included angina pectoris, myocardial infarction, and angioedema.
Adverse events occurred at about the same rates in men and women, older and younger patients, and black and nonblack patients.

Post-Marketing Experience

The following have been very rarely reported in post-marketing experience:
Digestive: Abnormal hepatic function and hepatitis.
Hematologic: Neutropenia, leukopenia, and agranulocytosis.
Skin and Appendages Disorders: Pruritis and urticaria.

Laboratory Test Findings

In controlled clinical trials, clinically important changes in standard laboratory parameters were rarely associated with the administration of ATACAND.
Creatinine, Blood Urea Nitrogen: Minor increases in blood urea nitrogen (BUN) and serum creatinine were observed infrequently.
Hyperuricemia: Hyperuricemia was rarely found (19 or 0.6% of 3260 patients treated with candesartan cilexetil and 5 or 0.5% of 1106 patients treated with placebo).
Hemoglobin and Hematocrit: Small decreases in hemoglobin and hematocrit (mean decreases of approximately 0.2 grams/dL and 0.5 volume percent, respectively) were observed in patients treated with ATACAND alone but were rarely of clinical importance. Anemia, leukopenia, and thrombocytopenia were associated with withdrawal of one patient each from clinical trials.
Potassium: A small increase (mean increase of 0.1 mEq/L) was observed in patients treated with ATACAND alone but was rarely of clinical importance. One patient from a congestive heart failure trial was withdrawn for hyperkalemia (serum potassium = 7.5 mEq/L). This patient was also receiving spironolactone.
Liver Function Tests: Elevations of liver enzymes and/or serum bilirubin were observed infrequently. Five patients assigned to candesartan cilexetil in clinical trials were withdrawn because of abnormal liver chemistries. All had elevated transaminases. Two had mildly elevated total bilirubin, but one of these patients was diagnosed with Hepatitis A.

OVERDOSAGE

No lethality was observed in acute toxicity studies in mice, rats, and dogs given single oral doses of up to 2000 mg/kg of candesartan cilexetil. In mice given single oral doses of the primary metabolite, candesartan, the minimum lethal dose was greater than 1000 mg/kg but less than 2000 mg/kg.

The most likely manifestation of overdosage with ATACAND would be hypotension, dizziness, and tachycardia; bradycardia could occur from parasympathetic (vagal) stimulation. If symptomatic hypotension should occur, supportive treatment should be instituted.
Candesartan cannot be removed by hemodialysis.
Treatment: To obtain up-to-date information about the treatment of overdose, consult your Regional Poison Control Center. Telephone numbers of certified poison control centers are listed in the *Physicians' Desk Reference (PDR).* In managing overdose, consider the possibilities of multiple-drug overdoses, drug-drug interactions, and altered pharmacokinetics in your patient.

DOSAGE AND ADMINISTRATION

Dosage must be individualized. Blood pressure response is dose related over the range of 2 to 32 mg. The usual recommended starting dose of ATACAND is 16 mg once daily when it is used as monotherapy in patients who are not volume depleted. ATACAND can be administered once or twice daily with total daily doses ranging from 8 mg to 32 mg. Larger doses do not appear to have a greater effect, and there is relatively little experience with such doses. Most of the antihypertensive effect is present within 2 weeks, and maximal blood pressure reduction is generally obtained within 4 to 6 weeks of treatment with ATACAND.
No initial dosage adjustment is necessary for elderly patients, for patients with mildly impaired renal function, or for patients with mildly impaired hepatic function. (See CLINICAL PHARMACOLOGY, Special Populations.) In patients with moderate hepatic impairment, consideration should be given to initiation of ATACAND at a lower dose. (See CLINICAL PHARMACOLOGY, Special Populations.)
For patients with possible depletion of intravascular volume (eg, patients treated with diuretics, particularly those with impaired renal function), ATACAND should be initiated under close medical supervision and consideration should be given to administration of a lower dose. (See WARNINGS, Hypotension in Volume- and Salt-Depleted Patients.)
ATACAND may be administered with or without food.
If blood pressure is not controlled by ATACAND alone, a diuretic may be added. ATACAND may be administered with other antihypertensive agents.

HOW SUPPLIED

No. 3782 — Tablets ATACAND, 4 mg, are white to off-white, circular/biconvex-shaped, non-film-coated tablets, coded ACF on one side and 004 on the other. They are supplied as follows:
NDC 0186-0004-31 unit of use bottles of 30.
No. 3780 — Tablets ATACAND, 8 mg, are light pink, circular/biconvex-shaped, non-film-coated tablets, coded ACG on one side and 008 on the other. They are supplied as follows:
NDC 0186-0008-31 unit of use bottles of 30.
No. 3781 — Tablets ATACAND, 16 mg, are pink, circular/biconvex-shaped, non-film-coated tablets, coded ACH on one side and 016 on the other. They are supplied as follows:
NDC 0186-0016-31 unit of use bottles of 30
NDC 0186-0016-54 unit of use bottles of 90
NDC 0186-0016-28 unit dose packages of 100.
No. 3791 — Tablets ATACAND, 32 mg, are pink, circular/biconvex-shaped, non-film-coated tablets, coded ACL on one side and 032 on the other. They are supplied as follows:
NDC 0186-0032-31 unit of use bottles of 30
NDC 0186-0032-54 unit of use bottles of 90
NDC 0186-0032-28 unit dose packages of 100.

Storage

Store at 25°C (77°F); excursions permitted to 15–30°C (59–86°F) [see USP Controlled Room Temperature]. Keep container tightly closed.
ATACAND is a trademark of the AstraZeneca group

Manufactured under the license
from Takeda Chemical Industries, Ltd.
by: AstraZeneca AB, S-151 85 Södertälje, Sweden
for: AstraZeneca LP, Wilmington, DE 19850
9174308
610002-08 Rev. 09/02

LEXXEL® ℞
(enalapril maleate-felodipine ER)
TABLETS

Prescribing information for this product, which appears on pages 608–612 of the 2003 PDR, has been completely revised as follows. Please write "See Supplement A" next to the product heading.

USE IN PREGNANCY
When used in pregnancy during the second and third trimesters, ACE inhibitors can cause injury and even death to the developing fetus. When pregnancy is detected, LEXXEL should be discontinued as soon as possible. See WARNINGS, Fetal/Neonatal Morbidity and Mortality.

DESCRIPTION

LEXXEL (enalapril maleate-felodipine ER) is a combination product, consisting of an outer layer of enalapril maleate surrounding a core tablet of an extended-release felodipine formulation.
Enalapril maleate is the maleate salt of enalapril, the ethyl ester of a long-acting angiotensin converting enzyme inhibitor, enalaprilat. Enalapril maleate is chemically described as (S)-1-[N-[1-(ethoxycarbonyl)-3-phenylpropyl]-L-alanyl]-L-proline, (Z)-2-butenedioate salt (1:1). Its empirical formula is $C_{20}H_{28}N_2O_5 \bullet C_4H_4O_4$, and its structural formula is:

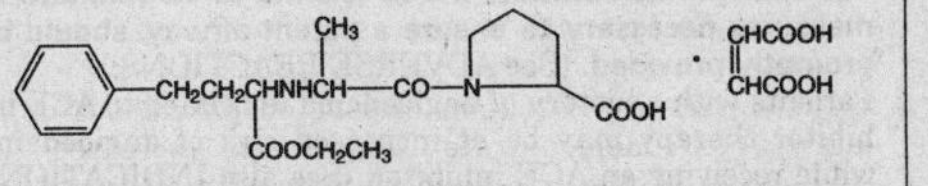

Enalapril maleate is a white to off-white, crystalline powder with a molecular weight of 492.53. It is sparingly soluble in water, soluble in ethanol, and freely soluble in methanol.
Felodipine, a calcium channel blocker, is a dihydropyridine derivative that is chemically described as ± ethyl methyl 4-(2,3-dichlorophenyl)-1,4-dihydro-2,6-dimethyl-3,5-pyridinedicarboxylate. Its empirical formula is $C_{18}H_{19}Cl_2NO_4$ and its structural formula is:

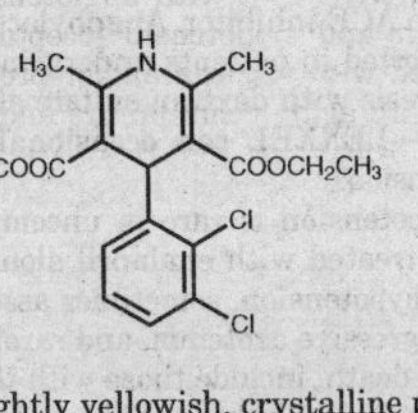

Felodipine is a slightly yellowish, crystalline powder with a molecular weight of 384.26. It is insoluble in water and is freely soluble in dichloromethane and ethanol. Felodipine is a racemic mixture; however, S-felodipine is the more biologically active enantiomer.
LEXXEL is available for oral use in two tablet combinations of enalapril maleate with felodipine as an extended-release formulation: LEXXEL 5-2.5, containing 5 mg of enalapril maleate and 2.5 mg of felodipine ER and LEXXEL 5-5, containing 5 mg of enalapril maleate and 5 mg of felodipine ER. Inactive ingredients include: propyl gallate, polyoxyl 40 hydrogenated castor oil, cellulose compounds, lactose, aluminum silicate, sodium stearyl fumarate, carnauba wax, and iron oxides. The tablets are imprinted with an ink of synthetic red iron oxide (LEXXEL 5-2.5) or synthetic black iron oxide (LEXXEL 5-5) which contains pharmaceutical glaze in SD-45, n-butyl alcohol, propylene glycol, isopropyl alcohol, ammonium hydroxide, and simethicone (LEXXEL 5-2.5) and methyl alcohol (LEXXEL 5-5).

CLINICAL PHARMACOLOGY

Mechanism of Action

The two components of LEXXEL have complementary antihypertensive actions. **Enalapril** is a pro-drug; following oral administration, it is bioactivated by hydrolysis of the ethyl ester to enalaprilat, which is the active angiotensin converting enzyme (ACE) inhibitor. Enalaprilat inhibits angiotensin-converting enzyme in humans and animals. ACE is a peptidyl dipeptidase that catalyzes the conversion of angiotensin I to the vasoconstrictor substance, angiotensin II. Angiotensin II also stimulates aldosterone secretion by the adrenal cortex. The beneficial effects of enalapril in hypertension appear to result primarily from suppression of the renin-angiotensin-aldosterone system.
Inhibition of ACE results in decreased plasma angiotensin II, which leads to decreased vasopressor activity and to decreased aldosterone secretion. Although the latter decrease is small, it results in small increases of serum potassium. In hypertensive patients treated with enalapril maleate alone for up to 48 weeks, mean increases in serum potassium of approximately 0.2 mEq/L were observed. In patients treated with enalapril maleate plus a thiazide diuretic, there was essentially no change in serum potassium. (See PRECAUTIONS.) Removal of angiotensin II negative feedback on renin secretion leads to increased plasma renin activity.
ACE is identical to kininase, an enzyme that degrades bradykinin. Whether increased levels of bradykinin, a potent vasodepressor peptide, play a role in the therapeutic effects of enalapril maleate remains to be elucidated.
While the mechanism through which enalapril lowers blood pressure is believed to be primarily suppression of the renin-angiotensin-aldosterone system, enalapril is antihypertensive even in patients with low-renin hypertension. Although enalapril was antihypertensive in all races studied, black hypertensive patients (usually a low-renin hypertensive population) had a smaller average response to enalapril monotherapy than non-black patients. **Felodipine** is a dihydropyridine calcium channel blocker that reduces the influx of Ca^{++} by an effect on the voltage dependent L-channels in vascular smooth muscle and cultured rabbit atrial cells, and blocks potassium-induced contracture of the rat portal vein. Pharmacologic studies show that the effects of felodipine on contractile processes are selective, with greater effects on vascular smooth muscle than cardiac muscle. Negative inotropic effects can be detected *in vitro*, but such effects have not been seen in intact animals.
The consequences of vasodilation produced by felodipine include a modest, short-lived reflex increase in heart rate. A mild diuretic effect is seen in several animal species and man, but most of the effects of felodipine are accounted for by its effects on peripheral vascular resistance.

Pharmacokinetics and Metabolism

Concomitant administration of enalapril and felodipine as an extended-release formulation has little effect on the bioavailability of either compound. The rate and extent of absorption of enalapril from LEXXEL is not significantly different from that of enalapril in VASOTEC* (enalapril maleate). The rate and extent of absorption of felodipine from LEXXEL has not been directly compared to the extended-release formulation of felodipine in PLENDIL** (felodipine).
Following oral administration of LEXXEL, peak concentrations of enalapril occur within about one hour. Enalapril is hydrolyzed to enalaprilat, which is a more potent angiotensin converting enzyme inhibitor than enalapril. Peak serum concentrations of enalaprilat occur about three hours after an oral dose of LEXXEL. Based on urinary recovery, the extent of absorption of enalapril is approximately 60%.
Peak concentrations of the isomers of felodipine are generally seen at 3–6 hours after administration of LEXXEL. Following oral administration, felodipine is almost completely absorbed and undergoes extensive first-pass metabolism; the systemic bioavailability of felodipine ER is approximately 20%.
When LEXXEL is taken with food (a substantial meal of 650 kcal or greater), some of the pharmacokinetics of its components are changed. Although the $AUC_{(0-48\ hr)}$ of felodipine is not changed, the peak concentration of its isomers is almost doubled, and the trough concentration is approximately halved. The bioavailability of enalapril, as measured by total urinary recovery of enalaprilat, is slightly reduced. As with other dihydropyridine calcium channel blockers, the bioavailability of felodipine was increased when taken with grapefruit juice, compared to when taken with water or orange juice.
The systemic plasma clearance of felodipine in young healthy subjects is about 0.8 L/min, and the apparent volume of distribution is 10 L/kg. Approximately 99% of felodipine is bound to plasma proteins.

* Registered trademark of Merck & Co., Inc.
**Trademark of the AstraZeneca Group

Following administration of ^{14}C-labeled intravenous or immediate-release oral felodipine in man, about 70% of the dose of radioactivity was recovered in urine and 10% in the feces. A negligible amount of intact felodipine was recovered in the urine and feces (<0.5%). Six metabolites, which account for 23% of the oral dose, have been identified; none has significant vasodilating activity. Following oral administration of the immediate-release formulation, the plasma levels of felodipine declined polyexponentially with a mean terminal half-life of 11 to 16 hours.
Excretion of enalaprilat and enalapril is primarily renal. Approximately 94% of the dose is recovered in the urine and feces as enalaprilat or enalapril. The principal components in urine are enalaprilat, accounting for about 40% of the dose, and intact enalapril. There is no evidence of metabolites of enalapril, other than enalaprilat. The serum concentration profile of enalaprilat exhibits a prolonged terminal phase, apparently representing a small fraction of the administered dose that has been bound to ACE. The amount bound does not increase with dose, indicating a saturable site of binding. The effective half-life for accumulation of enalaprilat following multiple doses of enalapril maleate is 11 hours.
The disposition of enalapril and enalaprilat in patients with renal insufficiency is similar to that in patients with normal renal function until the glomerular filtration rate is reduced to 30 mL/min or less. With glomerular filtration rate ≤30 mL/min, peak and trough enalaprilat levels increase, time to peak concentration increases, and time to steady state may be delayed. The effective half-life of enalaprilat following multiple doses of enalapril maleate is prolonged at this level of renal insufficiency. Enalaprilat is dialyzable at a rate of 62 mL/min.
Plasma concentrations of felodipine, after a single dose and at steady state, increase with age. Mean clearance of felodipine in elderly hypertensives (mean age 74) was only 45% of that for young volunteers (mean age 26). At steady state, the mean AUC for young patients was 39% of that for the elderly. Data for intermediate age ranges suggest that the AUCs fall between the extremes of the young and the elderly.
In patients with hepatic disease, the clearance of felodipine was reduced to about 60% of that seen in normal young volunteers.
Blood Brain Barrier and Blood Placental Barrier—Animal studies have shown that felodipine crosses the blood brain barrier. The plasma to brain concentration ratio of felodipine is about 20:1. Felodipine crosses the placenta. Fetal plasma levels of felodipine are similar to maternal plasma levels. Studies in dogs indicate that enalapril crosses the blood brain barrier poorly, if at all; enalaprilat does not enter the brain. Multiple doses of enalapril maleate in rats do not result in accumulation in any tissues. Milk of lactating rats contains radioactivity following administration of ^{14}C enalapril maleate. Radioactivity was found to cross the placenta following administration of labeled drug to pregnant hamsters.

Pharmacodynamics

Administration of **enalapril** maleate to patients with hypertension of severity ranging from mild to severe results in a reduction of both supine and standing blood pressure, usu-

Continued on next page

Lexxel—Cont.

ally with no orthostatic component. Symptomatic postural hypotension is infrequent with enalapril alone, although it might be anticipated in volume-depleted patients. (See WARNINGS.) In most patients studied, after oral administration of a single dose of enalapril, onset of antihypertensive activity was seen at one hour, with peak reduction of blood pressure achieved by 4 to 6 hours. At recommended doses, antihypertensive effects have been maintained for at least 24 hours. In some patients the effects may diminish toward the end of the dosing interval.

In most patients, achievement of optimal blood pressure reduction may require several weeks of therapy. The antihypertensive effects of enalapril have continued during long-term therapy. Abrupt withdrawal of enalapril has not been associated with a rapid increase in blood pressure. In hemodynamic studies in patients with essential hypertension, blood pressure reduction was accompanied by a reduction in peripheral arterial resistance with an increase in cardiac output and little or no change in heart rate. Following administration of enalapril maleate, there is an increase in renal blood flow; glomerular filtration rate is usually unchanged. The effects appear to be similar in patients with renovascular hypertension.

In a clinical pharmacology study, indomethacin or sulindac was administered to hypertensive patients receiving enalapril. In this study there was no evidence of a blunting of the antihypertensive action of enalapril. (See PRECAUTIONS, Drug Interactions.)

The effect of **felodipine** on blood pressure is principally a consequence of a dose-related decrease in peripheral vascular resistance. Blood pressure response following administration of felodipine ER to hypertensive patients is correlated with dose and plasma concentrations of felodipine. A reduction in blood pressure generally occurs within 2 to 5 hours. During chronic administration, substantial blood pressure control lasts for 24 hours, with trough reductions in diastolic blood pressure approximately 40–50% of peak reductions. A reflex increase in heart rate frequently occurs during the first week of therapy; this increase attenuates over time. Heart rate increases of 5–10 beats per minute may be seen during chronic dosing. The increase is inhibited by beta-blocking agents.

Felodipine has no significant effect on cardiac conduction (P-R, P-Q, and H-V intervals). In clinical trials in hypertensive patients without clinical evidence of left ventricular dysfunction, no symptoms suggestive of a negative inotropic effect were noted; however, none would be expected in this population.

In an 8-week, fixed-dose, parallel-group, double-blind study, 707 hypertensive patients were randomized among all possible combinations of enalapril (0, 5, or 20 mg), and extended-release felodipine (0, 2.5, 5, or 10 mg), both taken once daily. Each of the non-placebo combinations was significantly more effective than placebo in reducing seated systolic and diastolic blood pressure at peak (3 to 5 hours after dosing) and trough (24 hours after dosing). Enalapril and felodipine contributed additively to the effect, so that each active-active combination was significantly more effective than either of its component monotherapies. Most of the drug effect seen at peak was still present at trough. The efficacy of combination therapy relative to monotherapy was not significantly affected by race, sex, or age.

During chronic dosing with LEXXEL, the maximum reduction in blood pressure is generally achieved after one to two weeks. The antihypertensive effects of LEXXEL have continued during chronic therapy for at least one year.

INDICATIONS AND USAGE

LEXXEL is indicated for the treatment of hypertension.
This fixed combination drug is not indicated for the initial therapy of hypertension. (See DOSAGE AND ADMINISTRATION.)

In using LEXXEL, consideration should be given to the fact that another angiotensin converting enzyme inhibitor, captopril, has caused agranulocytosis, particularly in patients with renal impairment or collagen vascular disease, and that available data are insufficient to show that enalapril (a component of LEXXEL) does not have a similar risk. (See WARNINGS, Neutropenia/Agranulocytosis.)

In considering use of LEXXEL, it should be noted that black patients receiving ACE inhibitors have been reported to have a higher incidence of angioedema compared to non-blacks. (See WARNINGS, Angioedema.)

CONTRAINDICATIONS

LEXXEL is contraindicated in patients who are hypersensitive to any component of this product. Because of the enalapril component, LEXXEL is contraindicated in patients with a history of angioedema related to previous treatment with an angiotensin converting enzyme inhibitor and in patients with hereditary or idiopathic angioedema.

WARNINGS

Anaphylactoid and Possibly Related Reactions—Presumably because angiotensin-converting enzyme inhibitors affect the metabolism of eicosanoids and polypeptides, including endogenous bradykinin, patients receiving ACE inhibitors (including LEXXEL) may be subject to a variety of adverse reactions, some of them serious.

Angioedema: Angioedema of the face, extremities, lips, tongue, glottis, and/or larynx has been reported in patients treated with angiotensin converting enzyme inhibitors, including enalapril. This may occur at any time during treatment. In such cases LEXXEL should be promptly discontinued, and appropriate therapy and monitoring should be provided until complete and sustained resolution of signs and symptoms has occurred. In instances where swelling has been confined to the face and lips the condition has generally resolved without treatment, although antihistamines have been useful in relieving symptoms. Angioedema associated with laryngeal edema may be fatal. **Where there is involvement of the tongue, glottis or larynx, likely to cause airway obstruction, appropriate therapy, e.g., subcutaneous epinephrine solution 1:1000 (0.3 mL to 0.5 mL) and/or measures necessary to ensure a patent airway, should be promptly provided.** (See ADVERSE REACTIONS.)

Patients with a history of angioedema unrelated to ACE inhibitor therapy may be at increased risk of angioedema while receiving an ACE inhibitor. (See also INDICATIONS AND USAGE and CONTRAINDICATIONS.)

Anaphylactoid Reactions During Desensitization: Two patients undergoing desensitizing treatment with hymenoptera venom while receiving ACE inhibitors sustained life-threatening anaphylactoid reactions. In the same patients, these reactions were avoided when ACE inhibitors were temporarily withheld, but they reappeared upon inadvertent rechallenge.

Anaphylactoid Reactions During Membrane Exposure: Anaphylactoid reactions have been reported in patients dialyzed with high-flux membranes and treated concomitantly with an ACE inhibitor. Anaphylactoid reactions have also been reported in patients undergoing low-density lipoprotein apheresis with dextran sulfate absorption.

Hypotension—LEXXEL can occasionally cause symptomatic hypotension.

Excessive hypotension is rare in uncomplicated hypertensive patients treated with enalapril alone. Patients at risk for excessive hypotension, sometimes associated with oliguria and/or progressive azotemia, and rarely with acute renal failure and/or death, include those with the following conditions or characteristics: heart failure, hyponatremia, high dose diuretic therapy, recent intensive diuresis or increase in diuretic dose, renal dialysis, or severe volume and/or salt depletion of any etiology. It may be advisable to eliminate the diuretic (except in patients with heart failure), reduce the diuretic dose or increase salt intake cautiously before initiating therapy with enalapril maleate in patients at risk for excessive hypotension who are able to tolerate such adjustments. (See PRECAUTIONS, Drug Interactions and ADVERSE REACTIONS.) In patients at risk for excessive hypotension, therapy should be started under very close medical supervision and such patients should be followed closely for the first 2 weeks of treatment and whenever the dose of enalapril and/or diuretic is increased. Similar considerations may apply to patients with ischemic heart or cerebrovascular disease, in whom an excessive fall in blood pressure could result in a myocardial infarction or cerebrovascular accident.

If excessive hypotension occurs, the patient should be placed in the supine position and, if necessary, receive an intravenous infusion of normal saline. A transient hypotensive response is not a contraindication to further doses of enalapril maleate, which usually can be given without difficulty once the blood pressure has stabilized. If symptomatic hypotension develops, a dose reduction or discontinuation of enalapril or diuretic may be necessary.

Felodipine, like other calcium channel blockers, may occasionally precipitate significant hypotension and rarely syncope. It may lead to reflex tachycardia which in susceptible individuals may precipitate angina pectoris. (See ADVERSE REACTIONS.)

Neutropenia/Agranulocytosis—Another angiotensin converting enzyme inhibitor, captopril, has been shown to cause agranulocytosis and bone marrow depression, rarely in uncomplicated patients but more frequently in patients with renal impairment, especially if they also have a collagen vascular disease. Available data from clinical trials of enalapril are insufficient to show that enalapril does not cause agranulocytosis at similar rates. Marketing experience has revealed cases of neutropenia or agranulocytosis in which a causal relationship to enalapril cannot be excluded. Periodic monitoring of white blood cell counts in patients with collagen vascular disease and renal disease should be considered.

Hepatic Failure—Rarely, ACE inhibitors have been associated with a syndrome that starts with cholestatic jaundice and progresses to fulminant hepatic necrosis and (sometimes) death. The mechanism of this syndrome is not understood. Patients receiving ACE inhibitors who develop jaundice or marked elevations of hepatic enzymes should discontinue the ACE inhibitor and receive appropriate medical follow-up.

Fetal/Neonatal Morbidity and Mortality—ACE inhibitors can cause fetal and neonatal morbidity and death when administered to pregnant women. Several dozen cases have been reported in the world literature. When pregnancy is detected, LEXXEL should be discontinued as soon as possible.

The use of ACE inhibitors during the second and third trimesters of pregnancy has been associated with fetal and neonatal injury, including hypotension, neonatal skull hypoplasia, anuria, reversible or irreversible renal failure, and death. Oligohydramnios has also been reported, presumably resulting from decreased fetal renal function; oligohydramnios in this setting has been associated with fetal limb contractures, craniofacial deformation, and hypoplastic lung development. Prematurity, intrauterine growth retardation, and patent ductus arteriosus have also been reported, although it is not clear whether these occurrences were due to the ACE-inhibitor exposure.

These adverse effects do not appear to have resulted from intrauterine ACE-inhibitor exposure that has been limited to the first trimester. Mothers whose embryos and fetuses are exposed to ACE inhibitors only during the first trimester should be so informed. Nonetheless, when patients become pregnant, physicians should make every effort to discontinue the use of LEXXEL as soon as possible.

Rarely (probably less often than once in every thousand pregnancies), no alternative to ACE inhibitors will be found. In these rare cases, the mothers should be apprised of the potential hazards to their fetuses, and serial ultrasound examinations should be performed to assess the intra-amniotic environment.

If oligohydramnios is observed, LEXXEL should be discontinued unless it is considered lifesaving for the mother. Contraction stress testing (CST), a non-stress test (NST), or biophysical profiling (BPP) may be appropriate, depending upon the week of pregnancy. Patients and physicians should be aware, however, that oligohydramnios may not appear until after the fetus has sustained irreversible injury.

Infants with histories of *in utero* exposure to ACE inhibitors should be closely observed for hypotension, oliguria, and hyperkalemia. If oliguria occurs, attention should be directed toward support of blood pressure and renal perfusion. Exchange transfusion or dialysis may be required as means of reversing hypotension and/or substituting for disordered renal function. Enalapril, which crosses the placenta, has been removed from neonatal circulation by peritoneal dialysis with some clinical benefit, and theoretically may be removed by exchange transfusion, although there is no experience with the latter procedure.

No teratogenic effects of enalapril were seen in studies of pregnant rats and rabbits. On a body surface area basis, the doses used were 57 times and 12 times, respectively, the maximum recommended human daily dose (MRHDD).

In rats administered the combination of enalapril and felodipine (enalapril [E]=1.9-felodipine [F]=2.5 mg/kg/day), an increased incidence of fetuses with dilated renal pelvis/ureter was observed. However, there was no evidence of this effect in the offspring postweaning. In mice, with doses of E=23, F=30 mg/kg/day or greater, there was an increased incidence of both early and late *in utero* deaths. Other than a transient and slight decrease in body weight gain in the first generation offspring, there were no adverse effects in offspring with regard to sexual maturation, behavioral development, fertility or fecundity.

Enalapril-felodipine given to pregnant mice (enalapril 20.8, felodipine 27 mg/kg/day) and rats (enalapril =17.3, felodipine =22.5 mg/kg/day) produced plasma levels (C_{max} and AUC values) of enalapril/enalaprilat that were 76 to 418-fold greater and plasma levels of felodipine that were 151 to 433-fold greater than those expected in humans (non-pregnant) at the dose to be used in humans.

PRECAUTIONS

General

Aortic Stenosis/Hypertrophic Cardiomyopathy—As with all vasodilators, enalapril should be given with caution to patients with obstruction in the outflow tract of the left ventricle.

Impaired Renal Function—As a consequence of inhibiting the renin-angiotensin-aldosterone system, changes in renal function may be anticipated in susceptible individuals treated with enalapril. In patients with severe heart failure whose renal function may depend on the activity of the renin-angiotensin-aldosterone system, treatment with angiotensin converting enzyme inhibitors, including enalapril, may be associated with oliguria and/or progressive azotemia and rarely with acute renal failure and/or death.

In clinical studies in hypertensive patients with unilateral or bilateral renal artery stenosis, increases in blood urea nitrogen and serum creatinine were observed in 20% of patients treated with enalapril. These increases were almost always reversible upon discontinuation of enalapril and/or diuretic therapy. In such patients, renal function should be monitored during the first few weeks of therapy.

Some enalapril-treated patients with hypertension or heart failure, with no apparent pre-existing renal vascular disease, have developed increases in blood urea and serum creatinine, usually minor and transient, especially when enalapril has been given concomitantly with a diuretic. This is more likely to occur in patients with pre-existing renal impairment. Dosage reduction of enalapril or discontinuation of the diuretic may be required.

Evaluation of the hypertensive patient should always include assessment of renal function.

Hyperkalemia—Elevated serum potassium (greater than 5.7 mEq/L) was observed in approximately 1% of hypertensive patients in clinical trials treated with enalapril alone. In most cases these were isolated values which resolved despite continued therapy. Hyperkalemia was a cause of discontinuation of therapy in 0.28% of hypertensive patients. In clinical trials in heart failure, hyperkalemia was observed in 3.8% of patients but was not a cause for discontinuation.

Risk factors for the development of hyperkalemia include renal insufficiency, diabetes mellitus, and the concomitant use of potassium-sparing diuretics, potassium supplements and/or potassium-containing salt substitutes, which should be used cautiously, if at all, with enalapril. (See Drug Interactions.)

Elderly Patients or Patients with Impaired Liver Function—Patients over 65 years of age or patients with impaired liver function may have elevated plasma concentrations of felodipine. (See DOSAGE AND ADMINISTRATION.)

Cough—Presumably due to the inhibition of the degradation of endogenous bradykinin, persistent nonproductive cough has been reported with all ACE inhibitors, always resolving after discontinuation of therapy. ACE inhibitor-induced cough should be considered in the diagnosis of cough.

Surgery/Anesthesia—In patients undergoing major surgery or during anesthesia with agents that produce hypotension, enalapril may block angiotensin II formation secondary to compensatory renin release. If hypotension occurs and is considered to be due to this mechanism, it can be corrected by volume expansion.

Peripheral Edema—Peripheral edema, generally mild and not associated with generalized fluid retention, was the most common adverse event in the felodipine clinical trials. The incidence of peripheral edema was both dose and age dependent. This adverse event generally occurs within 2-3 weeks of the initiation of treatment.

Information for Patients

Patients should be instructed to take LEXXEL whole and not to divide, crush or chew the tablet.

All patients should be advised to consult their physician if they experience any of the following conditions:

Angioedema—Angioedema, including laryngeal edema, may occur at any time during treatment with angiotensin converting enzyme inhibitors, including enalapril. Patients should be so advised and told to report immediately any signs or symptoms suggesting angioedema (swelling of face, extremities, eyes, lips, tongue, difficulty in swallowing or breathing) and to take no more drug until they have consulted with the prescribing physician.

Hypotension—Patients should be cautioned to report lightheadedness especially during the first few days of therapy. If actual syncope occurs, the patients should be told to discontinue LEXXEL until they have consulted with the prescribing physician. All patients should be cautioned that excessive perspiration and dehydration may lead to an excessive fall in blood pressure because of reduction in fluid volume. Other causes of volume depletion, such as vomiting or diarrhea, may also lead to a fall in blood pressure; patients should be advised to consult with the physician.

Hyperkalemia—Patients should be told not to use salt substitutes containing potassium without consulting their physician.

Neutropenia—Patients should be told to report promptly any indication of infection (eg, sore throat, fever) which may be a sign of neutropenia.

Pregnancy—Female patients of childbearing age should be told about the consequences of second- and third-trimester exposure to ACE inhibitors, and they should also be told that these consequences do not appear to have resulted from intrauterine ACE-inhibitor exposure that has been limited to the first trimester. These patients should be asked to report pregnancies to their physicians as soon as possible.

Gingival Hyperplasia—Patients should be told that mild gingival hyperplasia (gum swelling) has been reported. Good dental hygiene decreases its incidence and severity.

Note: As with many other drugs, certain advice to patients being treated with LEXXEL is warranted. This information is intended to aid in the safe and effective use of this medication. It is not a disclosure of all possible adverse or intended effects.

Drug Interactions

Hypotension—Patients on Diuretic Therapy: Patients on diuretics, and especially those in whom diuretic therapy was recently instituted, may occasionally experience an excessive reduction of blood pressure after initiation of therapy with enalapril. The possibility of hypotensive effects with enalapril can be minimized by either discontinuing the diuretic or increasing the salt intake prior to initiation of treatment with enalapril. If it is necessary to continue the diuretic, provide close medical supervision after the initial dose for at least two hours and until blood pressure has stabilized for at least an additional hour. (See WARNINGS and DOSAGE AND ADMINISTRATION.)

Agents Causing Renin Release—The antihypertensive effect of enalapril is augmented by antihypertensive agents that cause renin release (eg, diuretics).

Non-steroidal Anti-inflammatory Agents—In some patients with compromised renal function who are being treated with non-steroidal anti-inflammatory drugs, the coadministration of enalapril may result in a further deterioration of renal function. These effects are usually reversible.

In a clinical pharmacology study, indomethacin or sulindac was administered to hypertensive patients receiving VASOTEC. In this study there was no evidence of a blunting of the antihypertensive action of VASOTEC. However, reports suggest that NSAIDs may diminish the antihypertensive effect of ACE-inhibitors. This interaction should be given consideration in patients taking NSAIDs concomitantly with ACE-inhibitors.

Agents Increasing Serum Potassium—Enalapril attenuates potassium loss caused by thiazide-type diuretics. Potassium-sparing diuretics (eg, spironolactone, triamterene, or amiloride), potassium supplements, or potassium-containing salt substitutes may lead to significant increases in serum potassium. Therefore, if concomitant use of these agents is indicated because of demonstrated hypokalemia, they should be used with caution and with frequent monitoring of serum potassium.

Lithium—Lithium toxicity has been reported in patients receiving lithium concomitantly with drugs which cause elimination of sodium, including ACE inhibitors. A few cases of lithium toxicity have been reported in patients receiving concomitant enalapril and lithium and were reversible upon discontinuation of both drugs. It is recommended that serum lithium levels be monitored frequently if enalapril is administered concomitantly with lithium.

CYP3A4 Inhibitors—Felodipine is metabolized by CYP3A4. Co-administration of CYP3A4 inhibitors (eg, ketoconazole, itraconazole, erythromycin, grapefruit juice, cimetidine) with felodipine may lead to several-fold increases in the plasma levels of felodipine, either due to an increase in bioavailability or due to a decrease in metabolism. These increases in concentration may lead to increased effects, (lower blood pressure and increased heart rate). These effects have been observed with co-administration of itraconazole (a potent CYP3A4 inhibitor). Caution should be used when CYP3A4 inhibitors are co-administered with felodipine. A conservative approach to dosing felodipine should be taken. The following specific interactions have been reported:

Itraconazole—Co-administration of another extended release formulation of felodipine with itraconazole resulted in approximately 8-fold increase in the AUC, more than 6-fold increase in the C_{max}, and 2-fold prolongation in the half-life of felodipine.

Erythromycin—Co-administration of felodipine (PLENDIL) with erythromycin resulted in approximately 2.5-fold increase in the AUC and C_{max}, and about 2-fold prolongation in the half-life of felodipine.

Grapefruit juice—Co-administration of felodipine with grapefruit juice resulted in more than 2-fold increase in the AUC and C_{max}, but no prolongation in the half-life of felodipine.

Cimetidine—Co-administration of felodipine with cimetidine (a non-specific CYP-450 inhibitor) resulted in an increase of approximately 50% in the AUC and the C_{max}, of felodipine.

Beta-Blocking Agents—Enalapril has been used concomitantly with beta adrenergic-blocking agents without evidence of clinically significant adverse interactions.

A pharmacokinetic study of felodipine in conjunction with metoprolol demonstrated no significant effects on the pharmacokinetics of felodipine. The AUC and C_{max} of metoprolol, however, were increased approximately 31% and 38%, respectively. In controlled clinical trials, however, beta blockers including metoprolol were concurrently administered with felodipine and were well tolerated.

Digoxin—Enalapril has been used concomitantly with digoxin without evidence of clinically significant adverse interactions.

When given concomitantly with felodipine ER, the pharmacokinetics of digoxin in patients with heart failure were not significantly altered.

Anticonvulsants—In a pharmacokinetic study, maximum plasma concentrations of felodipine were considerably lower in epileptic patients on long-term anticonvulsant therapy (eg, phenytoin, carbamazepine, or phenobarbital) than in healthy volunteers. In such patients, the mean area under the felodipine plasma concentration-time curve was also reduced to approximately 6% of that observed in healthy volunteers. Since a clinically significant interaction may be anticipated, alternative antihypertensive therapy should be considered in these patients.

Other Concomitant Therapy—In healthy subjects, there were no clinically significant interactions when felodipine was given concomitantly with indomethacin or spironolactone.

Enalapril has been used concomitantly with methyldopa, nitrates, hydralazine, and prazosin without evidence of clinically significant adverse interactions.

Carcinogenesis, Mutagenesis, Impairment of Fertility

No long-term carcinogenicity tests have been performed with the combination. Enalapril-felodipine was not mutagenic with or without metabolic activation *in vitro* in the Ames microbial mutation assay, the V-79 mammalian cell forward mutation assay, the alkaline elution assay with rat hepatocytes or the CHO mammalian cell cytogenetics assay. An *in vivo* mouse bone marrow cytogenetics assay was also negative.

In rats given enalapril-felodipine, there was no effect on fertility in males at doses up to 6.9/9 mg/kg/day, and in females at doses up to 17.3/22.5 mg/kg/day.

There was no evidence of a tumorigenic effect when enalapril was administered for 106 weeks to male and female rats at doses up to 90 mg/kg/day or for 94 weeks to male and female mice at doses up to 90 and 180 mg/kg/day, respectively. These doses are 26 times (in rats and female mice) and 13 times (in male mice) the maximum recommended human daily dose (MRHDD) when compared on a body surface area basis.

Neither enalapril maleate nor the active diacid was mutagenic in the Ames microbial mutagen test with or without metabolic activation. Enalapril was also negative in the following genotoxicity studies: rec-assay, reverse mutation assay with *E. coli*, sister chromatid exchange with cultured mammalian cells, and the micronucleus test with mice, as well as in an *in vivo* cytogenic study using mouse bone marrow.

There were no adverse effects on reproductive performance of male and female rats treated with up to 90 mg/kg/day of enalapril (26 times the MRHDD when compared on a body surface area basis).

In a 2-year carcinogenicity study in rats fed felodipine at doses of 7.7, 23.1 or 69.3 mg/kg/day (up to 61 times† the maximum recommended human dose on a mg/m² basis), a dose-related increase in the incidence of benign interstitial cell tumors of the testes (Leydig cell tumors) was observed in treated male rats. These tumors were not observed in a similar study in mice at doses up to 138.6 mg/kg/day (61 times† the maximum recommended human dose on a mg/m² basis). Felodipine, at the doses employed in the 2-year rat study, has been shown to lower testicular testosterone and to produce a corresponding increase in serum luteinizing hormone in rats. The Leydig cell tumor development is possibly secondary to these hormonal effects which have not been observed in man.

In this same rat study, a dose-related increase in the incidence of focal squamous cell hyperplasia, compared to control, was observed in the esophageal groove of male and female rats in all dose groups. No other drug-related esophageal or gastric pathology was observed in the rats or with chronic administration in mice and dogs. The latter species, like man, has no anatomical structure comparable to the esophageal groove.

Felodipine was not carcinogenic when fed to mice at doses of up to 138.6 mg/kg/day (61 times† the maximum recommended human dose on a mg/m² basis) for periods of up to 80 weeks in males and 99 weeks in females.

Felodipine did not display any mutagenic activity *in vitro* in the Ames microbial mutagenicity test or in the mouse lymphoma forward mutation assay. No clastogenic potential was seen *in vivo* in the mouse micronucleus test at oral doses up to 2500 mg/kg (1100 times† the maximum recommended human dose on a mg/m² basis) or *in vitro* in a human lymphocyte chromosome aberration assay.

A fertility study in which male and female rats were administered doses of 3.8, 9.6, or 26.9 mg/kg/day (up to 24 times† the maximum recommended human dose on a mg/m² basis) showed no significant effect of felodipine on reproductive performance.

Pregnancy

Pregnancy Categories C (first trimester) *and D* (second and third trimesters). See WARNINGS, Fetal/Neonatal Morbidity and Mortality.

Teratogenic Effects—Studies in pregnant rabbits administered doses of felodipine 0.46, 1.2, 2.3, and 4.6 mg/kg/day (from 0.8 to 8 times† the maximum recommended human dose on a mg/m² basis) showed digital anomalies consisting of reduction in size and degree of ossification of the terminal phalanges in the fetuses. The frequency and severity of the changes appeared dose-related and were noted even at the lowest dose. These changes have been shown to occur with other members of the dihydropyridine class and are possibly a result of compromised uterine blood flow. Similar fetal anomalies were not observed in rats given felodipine.

In a teratology study in cynomolgus monkeys, no reduction in the size of the terminal phalanges was observed, but an abnormal position of the distal phalanges was noted in about 40% of the fetuses.

Nonteratogenic Effects—A prolongation of parturition with difficult labor and an increased frequency of fetal and early postnatal deaths were observed in rats administered felodipine doses of 9.6 mg/kg/day (8 times† the maximum human dose on a mg/m² basis) and above.

Significant enlargement of the mammary glands, in excess of the normal enlargement for pregnant rabbits, was found with doses greater than or equal to 1.2 mg/kg/day (2.1 times the maximum human dose on a mg/m² basis). This effect occurred only in pregnant rabbits and regressed during lactation. Similar changes in the mammary glands were not observed in rats or monkeys.

---

†Based on patient weight of 50 kg

There are no adequate and well-controlled studies with felodipine in pregnant women. If felodipine is used during pregnancy, or if the patient becomes pregnant while taking this drug, she should be apprised of the potential hazard to the fetus, possible digital anomalies of the infant, and the potential effects of felodipine on labor and delivery, and on the mammary glands of pregnant females.

Nursing Mothers

Enalapril and enalaprilat are detected in human breast milk. It is not known whether felodipine administered as monotherapy is secreted in human milk; studies of the combination of enalapril and felodipine in rats indicate that felodipine concentrates in milk to a level almost ten-fold that found in plasma.

Because of the potential for serious adverse reactions from enalapril and felodipine in the infant, a decision should be made either to discontinue nursing or to discontinue the drug, taking into account the importance of the drug to the mother. Therefore, caution should be exercised when LEXXEL is given to a nursing mother.

Pediatric Use

Safety and effectiveness in pediatric patients have not been established.

ADVERSE REACTIONS

In a factorial study, combinations of enalapril at doses of 0, 5, and 20 mg and felodipine ER at doses of 0, 2.5, 5, and 10 mg were evaluated for safety in more than 700 patients with hypertension. In addition more than 500 patients received various combinations of enalapril (5 or 10 mg) and felodipine ER (2.5, 5, or 10 mg) with or without hydrochlorothiazide (12.5 mg) in an open-labeled study up to 52 weeks (mean 33 weeks). Adverse events were similar to those described with the individual components.

In general, treatment with enalapril maleate-felodipine ER was well tolerated and adverse events were mild and transient in nature. In the placebo-controlled, double-blind trial,

Continued on next page

Lexxel—Cont.

discontinuation of therapy due to adverse events considered related (possibly, probably or definitely) occurred in 2.8% vs 1.3% of patients treated with the combination or placebo, respectively. The most frequently observed clinical adverse events considered related to treatment with the combination were headache, edema or swelling, and dizziness.
Clinical adverse events considered related (possibly, probably, or definitely) to treatment with enalapril-felodipine ER that occurred with an incidence of 1% or greater with the combination during the placebo-controlled, double-blind trial are compared to individual components and placebo in the table below:
[See table above]

Percent of Patients with Adverse Events in the Double-Blind Trial
(Percent discontinuation shown in parentheses)

Body System Adverse Event	Enalapril[a] Felodipine ER[b] N=319	Enalapril[a] N=133	Felodipine ER[b] N=176	Placebo N=79
Body as a Whole				
Edema/Swelling	4.1(0.3)	2.3(0.0)	10.8(1.7)	1.3(0.0)
Asthenia/Fatigue	1.9(0.0)	2.3(0.8)	0.6(0.6)	3.8(0.0)
Nervous/Psychiatric				
Headache	10.3(0.6)	3.8(0.0)	10.2(1.1)	7.6(1.3)
Dizziness	4.4(0.3)	1.5(0.0)	2.8(0.6)	0.0(0.0)
Respiratory				
Cough	2.2(0.6)	2.3(0.0)	0.6(0.0)	0.0(0.0)
Skin				
Flushing	1.6(0.3)	0.0(0.0)	2.3(1.1)	0.0(0.0)

[a]Combination of dose of 5 and 20 mg daily
[b]Combination of dose 2.5, 5 and 10 mg daily

Other clinical adverse events considered related (possibly, probably, or definitely) to treatment with enalapril-felodipine ER that occurred with an incidence of less than 1% in the placebo-controlled, double-blind trial are listed below. These events are listed in order of decreasing frequency within each category. *Body as a Whole:* Syncope, facial edema, orthostatic effects, chest pain; *Cardiovascular:* Palpitation, hypotension, bradycardia, premature ventricular contraction, increased blood pressure; *Digestive:* Dry mouth, constipation, dyspepsia, flatulence, acid regurgitation, vomiting, diarrhea, nausea, anal/rectal pain; *Metabolic:* Gout; *Musculoskeletal:* Neck pain, joint swelling; *Nervous/Psychiatric:* Insomnia, nervousness, somnolence, ataxia, agitation, paresthesia, tremor; *Respiratory:* Dyspnea, respiratory congestion, pharyngeal discomfort, dry throat; *Skin:* Rash, angioedema, pruritus, alopecia, dry skin; *Special Senses:* Increased intraocular pressure; *Urogenital:* Impotence, hot flashes.

Other infrequently reported adverse events were seen in clinical trials with enalapril-felodipine ER (causal relationship unknown). These included: *Body as a Whole:* Abdominal pain, fever; *Digestive:* Dental pain; *Metabolic:* Increased ALT and AST, hyperglycemia; *Musculoskeletal:* Back pain, myalgia, foot pain, knee pain, shoulder pain, tendinitis; *Respiratory:* Upper respiratory infection, sinusitis, pharyngitis, bronchitis, nasal congestion, influenza, sinus disorder; *Special Senses:* Conjunctivitis; *Urogenital:* Proteinuria, pyuria, urinary tract infection.

Enalapril Maleate
Other adverse events that have been reported with enalapril, without regard to causality, are listed (in decreasing severity) below:
Angioedema—Angioedema has been reported in patients receiving enalapril maleate, with an incidence higher in black than in non-black patients. Angioedema associated with laryngeal edema may be fatal. If angioedema of the face, extremities, lips, tongue, glottis and/or larynx occurs, treatment with LEXXEL should be discontinued and appropriate therapy instituted immediately. (See WARNINGS.)
Body as a Whole: Anaphylactoid reactions (see WARNINGS, Anaphylactoid and Possibly Related Reactions); *Cardiovascular:* Cardiac arrest, myocardial infarction or cerebrovascular accident, possibly secondary to excessive hypotension in high risk patients (see WARNINGS, Hypotension), orthostatic hypotension, pulmonary embolism and infarction, pulmonary edema, rhythm disturbances including atrial tachycardia and bradycardia, atrial fibrillation, angina pectoris; *Digestive:* Ileus, pancreatitis, hepatic failure, hepatitis (hepatocellular [proven on rechallenge] or cholestatic jaundice) (see WARNINGS, Hepatic Failure), melena, anorexia, glossitis, stomatitis; *Hematologic:* Rare cases of neutropenia, thrombocytopenia and bone marrow depression; *Musculoskeletal:* Muscle cramps; *Nervous/Psychiatric:* Depression, confusion, peripheral neuropathy (eg, paresthesia, dysesthesia), vertigo; *Respiratory:* Bronchospasm, rhinorrhea, sore throat and hoarseness, asthma, pneumonia, pulmonary infiltrates, eosinophilic pneumonitis; *Skin:* Exfoliative dermatitis, toxic epidermal necrolysis, Stevens-Johnson syndrome, pemphigus, herpes zoster, erythema multiforme, urticaria, diaphoresis, photosensitivity; *Special Senses:* Blurred vision, taste alteration, anosmia, tinnitus, dry eyes, tearing; *Urogenital:* Renal failure, oliguria, renal dysfunction (see PRECAUTIONS), flank pain, gynecomastia; *Miscellaneous:* A symptom complex has been reported which may include a positive ANA, an elevated erythrocyte sedimentation rate, arthralgia/arthritis, myalgia/myositis, fever, serositis, vasculitis, leukocytosis, eosinophilia, photosensitivity rash and other dermatologic manifestations; *Fetal/Neonatal Morbidity and Mortality:* See WARNINGS, Fetal/Neonatal Morbidity and Mortality.

Felodipine as an Extended-Release Formulation
Other adverse events that have been reported with felodipine ER, without regard to causality, are listed (in decreasing severity) below:
Body as a Whole: Flu-like illness; *Cardiovascular:* Myocardial infarction, angina pectoris, arrhythmia, tachycardia, premature beats; *Digestive:* Gingival hyperplasia; *Endocrine:* Gynecomastia; *Hematologic:* Anemia; *Musculoskeletal:* Arthralgia, leg pain, muscle cramps, arm pain, hip pain; *Nervous/Psychiatric:* Depression, anxiety disorders, irritability, decreased libido; *Respiratory:* Upper respiratory infection, rhinorrhea, sneezing, pharyngitis, influenza, epistaxis, respiratory infection; *Skin:* Angioedema, contusion, erythema, urticaria, leukocytoclastic vasculitis; *Special Senses:* Visual disturbances; *Urogenital:* Urinary frequency, urinary urgency, dysuria, polyuria.

Laboratory Test Findings
In controlled clinical trials with enalapril-felodipine ER, clinically important changes in standard laboratory parameters associated with administration of LEXXEL were rare. No changes peculiar to the combination treatment were observed.
Serum Electrolytes—See PRECAUTIONS.
Creatinine—Minor reversible increases in serum creatinine were observed in patients treated with LEXXEL. Increases in creatinine are more likely to occur in patients with renal insufficiency or those pretreated with a diuretic and based on experience with other ACE inhibitors, would be expected to be especially likely in patients with renal artery stenosis. (See PRECAUTIONS.)
Other—Minor reversible increases or decreases in serum potassium were infrequently observed in patients treated with LEXXEL; rarely were these measurements outside the normal range.

OVERDOSAGE
Limited data are available in regard to enalapril overdosage in humans. In a suicide attempt, one patient took 150 mg felodipine together with 15 tablets each of atenolol and spironolactone and 20 tablets of nitrazepam. The patient's blood pressure and heart rate were normal on admission to hospital; he subsequently recovered without significant sequelae.
Human overdoses with any combination of enalapril and felodipine ER have not been reported.
Single oral doses of enalapril above 1000 mg/kg and ≥1775 mg/kg were associated with lethality in mice and rats, respectively. Oral doses of felodipine at 240 mg/kg and 264 mg/kg in male and female mice, respectively, and 2390 mg/kg and 2250 mg/kg in male and female rats, respectively, caused significant lethality.
In interaction studies on the acute oral toxicity of the combination in mice, pretreatment with felodipine (50 mg/kg) for one hour led to an increase in mortality at doses of enalapril maleate that exceeded 1000 mg/kg. Significant lethality with felodipine was not increased by pretreatment of mice for one hour with 100 mg/kg of enalapril maleate.
Treatment: To obtain up-to-date information about the treatment of overdose, consult your Regional Poison-Control Center. Telephone numbers of certified poison-control centers are listed in the *Physicians' Desk Reference (PDR)*. In managing overdose, consider the possibilities of multiple-drug overdoses, drug-drug interactions, and unusual drug kinetics in your patient.
The most likely effect of overdose with LEXXEL is vasodilation, with consequent hypotension and tachycardia. Repletion of central fluid volume (Trendelenburg positioning, infusion of crystalloids) may be sufficient therapy, but pressor agents (norepinephrine or high-dose dopamine) may be required.
Enalaprilat may be removed from general circulation by hemodialysis at a rate of 62 mL/min and has been removed from neonatal circulation by peritoneal dialysis. (See WARNINGS, Anaphylactoid reactions during membrane exposure.) It has not been established whether felodipine can be removed from the circulation by hemodialysis.

DOSAGE AND ADMINISTRATION
LEXXEL is an effective treatment for hypertension. This fixed combination drug is not indicated for initial therapy of hypertension.
The recommended initial dose of enalapril maleate for hypertension in patients not receiving diuretics is 5 mg once a day. The usual dosage range of enalapril maleate for hypertension is 10–40 mg per day administered in a single dose or two divided doses. In some patients treated once daily with enalapril, the antihypertensive effect may diminish toward the end of the dosing interval. In such patients, an increase in dosage or twice daily administration should be considered. The recommended initial dose of felodipine ER is 5 mg once a day with a usual dosage range of 2.5 mg–10 mg once a day. In elderly or hepatically impaired patients, the recommended initial dose of felodipine is 2.5 mg. When LEXXEL is taken with food, the peak concentration of felodipine is almost doubled, and the trough (24-hour) concentration is approximately halved. (See CLINICAL PHARMACOLOGY, Pharmacokinetics and Metabolism.)
In clinical trials of enalapril-felodipine ER combination therapy using enalapril doses of 5–20 mg and felodipine ER doses of 2.5–10 mg once daily, the antihypertensive effects increased with increasing doses of each component in all patient groups.
The hazards (see WARNINGS and ADVERSE REACTIONS) of enalapril are generally independent of dose; those of felodipine are a mixture of dose-dependent phenomena (primarily peripheral edema) and dose-independent phenomena, the former much more common than the latter. Therapy with any combination of enalapril and felodipine will thus be associated with both sets of dose-independent hazards.
Rarely, the dose-independent hazards associated with enalapril or felodipine are serious. To minimize dose-independent hazards, it is usually appropriate to begin therapy with LEXXEL only after a patient has failed to achieve the desired antihypertensive effect with one or the other monotherapy.
Replacement Therapy: Although the felodipine component of LEXXEL has not been shown to be bioequivalent to the available extended-release felodipine (PLENDIL), patients receiving enalapril and felodipine from separate tablets once a day may instead wish to receive the tablets of LEXXEL containing the same component doses.
Therapy Guided By Clinical Effect: A patient whose blood pressure is not adequately controlled with felodipine (or another dihydropyridine) or enalapril (or another ACE inhibitor) alone may be switched to combination therapy with LEXXEL, initially one tablet daily, usually LEXXEL 5-5. If blood pressure control is inadequate after a week or two, the dose may be increased to 2 tablets LEXXEL 5-5 administered once daily. The next incremental effect can be achieved with 4 tablets LEXXEL 5-2.5 administered once daily. If control remains unsatisfactory, consider addition of a thiazide diuretic.
Use in Patients with Metabolic Impairments: Regimens of therapy with LEXXEL need not be adjusted for renal function as long as the patient's creatinine clearance is >30 mL/min/1.73m^2 (serum creatinine roughly ≤3 mg/dL or 265 μmol/L). In patients with more severe renal impairment, the recommended initial dose of enalapril is 2.5 mg. LEXXEL should regularly be taken either without food or with a light meal (see CLINICAL PHARMACOLOGY, Pharmacokinetics and Metabolism). LEXXEL should be swallowed whole and not divided, crushed or chewed.

HOW SUPPLIED
No. 3771—Tablets LEXXEL, 5-2.5 are white, round/biconvex-shaped, film-coated tablets, coded LEXXEL 2, 5-2.5 on one side and no markings on the other. Each tablet contains 5 mg of enalapril maleate and 2.5 mg of felodipine as an extended-release formulation. They are supplied as follows:
NDC 0186-0002-31 unit of use bottles of 30 (with desiccants)
No. 3661—Tablets LEXXEL, 5-5 are white, round/biconvex-shaped, film-coated tablets, coded LEXXEL 1, 5-5 on one side and no markings on the other. Each tablet contains 5 mg of enalapril maleate and 5 mg of felodipine as an extended-release formulation. They are supplied as follows:
NDC 0186-0001-31 unit of use bottles of 30 (with desiccants)
NDC 0186-0001-68 bottles of 100 (with desiccants)
Storage
Store at 25°C (77°F); excursions permitted between 15°C and 30°C (59°F and 86°F) [See USP Controlled Room Temperature]. Keep container tightly closed. Protect from moisture and light. Dispense in a tight container, if product package is subdivided.
Revised 08/02
LEXXEL is a trademark of the AstraZeneca group
© AstraZeneca 2002

Manufactured for: AstraZeneca LP
Wilmington, DE 19850
By: Merck & Co., Inc., Whitehouse Station, NJ 08889, USA
9176507
620008-07

NEXIUM® ℞
[*nĕ k's ē'əm*]
(esomeprazole magnesium)
DELAYED RELEASE CAPSULES

Prescribing information for this product, which appears on pages 619–623 of the 2003 PDR, has been revised as follows. Please write "See Supplement A" next to the product heading.

Prescribing information for this product, which appears in the 2003 PDR has had revisions made to the **ADVERSE REACTIONS** *section.*
The new text appears as the eighth paragraph and reads:
Postmarketing Reports – There have been spontaneous reports of adverse events with postmarketing use of esomeprazole. These reports have included rare cases of anaphylactic reaction.

- Item number to 620514-03 and 9346603
- Copyright statement to 2003
- Rev date 02/03
- CLINICAL PHARMACOLOGY, Pharmacokinetics, Absorption, 2nd paragraph, 1st sentence, revise to read: "...is decreased by 43–53% after food intake..."
- CLINICAL PHARMACOLOGY, Pharmacodynamics, Mechanism of Action, 1st paragraph, 2nd sentence, revise to read: "The S- and R-isomers of omeprazole are protonated..."
- PRECAUTIONS, Drug Interactions, 2nd paragraph, add as the last 3 sentences: "Postmarketing reports of changes in prothrombin measures have been received among patients on concomitant warfarin and esomeprazole therapy. Increases in INR and prothrombin time may lead to abnormal bleeding and even death. Patients treated with proton pump inhibitors and warfarin concomitantly may need to be monitored for increases in INR and prothrombin time.
- OVERDOSAGE, 2nd paragraph, 1st sentence, revise to read: "There have been some reports of overdosage..."

PRILOSEC® ℞
[*prī-lō-sĕk*]
(OMEPRAZOLE)
DELAYED-RELEASE CAPSULES

Prescribing information for this product, which appears on pages 627–632 of the 2003 PDR, has been completely revised as follows. Please write "See Supplement A" next to the product heading.

DESCRIPTION

The active ingredient in PRILOSEC (omeprazole) Delayed-Release Capsules is a substituted benzimidazole, 5-methoxy-2-[[(4-methoxy-3, 5-dimethyl-2-pyridinyl) methyl] sulfinyl]-1*H*-benzimidazole, a compound that inhibits gastric acid secretion. Its empirical formula is $C_{17}H_{19}N_3O_3S$, with a molecular weight of 345.42. The structural formula is:

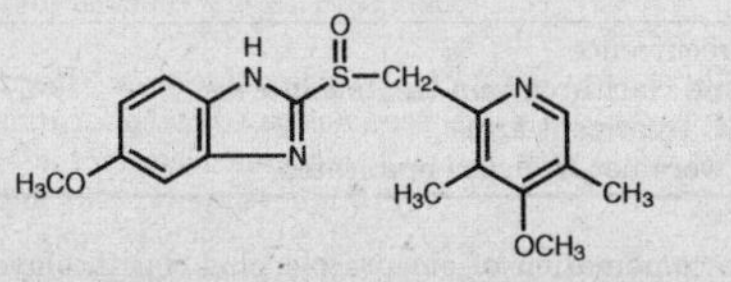

Omeprazole is a white to off-white crystalline powder which melts with decomposition at about 155°C. It is a weak base, freely soluble in ethanol and methanol, and slightly soluble in acetone and isopropanol and very slightly soluble in water. The stability of omeprazole is a function of pH; it is rapidly degraded in acid media, but has acceptable stability under alkaline conditions.
PRILOSEC is supplied as delayed-release capsules for oral administration. Each delayed-release capsule contains either 10 mg, 20 mg or 40 mg of omeprazole in the form of enteric-coated granules with the following inactive ingredients: cellulose, disodium hydrogen phosphate, hydroxypropyl cellulose, hydroxypropyl methylcellulose, lactose, mannitol, sodium lauryl sulfate and other ingredients. The capsule shells have the following inactive ingredients: gelatin-NF, FD&C Blue #1, FD&C Red #40, D&C Red #28, titanium dioxide, synthetic black iron oxide, isopropanol, butyl alcohol, FD&C Blue #2, D&C Red #7 Calcium Lake, and, in addition, the 10 mg and 40 mg capsule shells also contain D&C Yellow #10.

CLINICAL PHARMACOLOGY

Pharmacokinetics and Metabolism: Omeprazole

PRILOSEC Delayed-Release Capsules contain an enteric-coated granule formulation of omeprazole (because omeprazole is acid-labile), so that absorption of omeprazole begins only after the granules leave the stomach. Absorption is rapid, with peak plasma levels of omeprazole occurring within 0.5 to 3.5 hours. Peak plasma concentrations of omeprazole and AUC are approximately proportional to doses up to 40 mg, but because of a saturable first-pass effect, a greater than linear response in peak plasma concentration and AUC occurs with doses greater than 40 mg. Absolute bioavailability (compared to intravenous administration) is about 30–40% at doses of 20–40 mg, due in large part to presystemic metabolism. In healthy subjects the plasma half-life is 0.5 to 1 hour, and the total body clearance is 500–600 mL/min. Protein binding is approximately 95%. The bioavailability of omeprazole increases slightly upon repeated administration of PRILOSEC Delayed-Release Capsules.
Following single dose oral administration of a buffered solution of omeprazole, little if any unchanged drug was excreted in urine. The majority of the dose (about 77%) was eliminated in urine as at least six metabolites. Two were identified as hydroxyomeprazole and the corresponding carboxylic acid. The remainder of the dose was recoverable in feces. This implies a significant biliary excretion of the metabolites of omeprazole. Three metabolites have been identified in plasma — the sulfide and sulfone derivatives of omeprazole, and hydroxyomeprazole. These metabolites have very little or no antisecretory activity.
In patients with chronic hepatic disease, the bioavailability increased to approximately 100% compared to an I.V. dose, reflecting decreased first-pass effect, and the plasma half-life of the drug increased to nearly 3 hours compared to the half-life in normals of 0.5–1 hour. Plasma clearance averaged 70 mL/min, compared to a value of 500–600 mL/min in normal subjects.
In patients with chronic renal impairment, whose creatinine clearance ranged between 10 and 62 mL/min/1.73 m^2, the disposition of omeprazole was very similar to that in healthy volunteers, although there was a slight increase in bioavailability. Because urinary excretion is a primary route of excretion of omeprazole metabolites, their elimination slowed in proportion to the decreased creatinine clearance.
The elimination rate of omeprazole was somewhat decreased in the elderly, and bioavailability was increased. Omeprazole was 76% bioavailable when a single 40 mg oral dose of omeprazole (buffered solution) was administered to healthy elderly volunteers, versus 58% in young volunteers given the same dose. Nearly 70% of the dose was recovered in urine as metabolites of omeprazole and no unchanged drug was detected. The plasma clearance of omeprazole was 250 mL/min (about half that of young volunteers) and its plasma half-life averaged one hour, about twice that of young healthy volunteers.
In pharmacokinetic studies of single 20 mg omeprazole doses, an increase in AUC of approximately four-fold was noted in Asian subjects compared to Caucasians.
Dose adjustment, particularly where maintenance of healing of erosive esophagitis is indicated, for the hepatically impaired and Asian subjects should be considered.
PRILOSEC Delayed-Release Capsule 40 mg was bioequivalent when administered with and without applesauce. However, PRILOSEC Delayed-Release Capsule 20 mg was not bioequivalent when administered with and without applesauce. When administered with applesauce, a mean 25% reduction in C_{max} was observed without a significant change in AUC for PRILOSEC Delayed-Release Capsule 20 mg. The clinical relevance of this finding is unknown.
The pharmacokinetics of omeprazole have been investigated in pediatric patients of different ages.

Pharmacokinetic Parameters of Omeprazole Following Single and Repeated Oral Administration in Pediatric Populations Compared to Adults

Single or Repeated Oral Dosing/ Parameter	Children† < 20 kg 2–5 years 10 mg	Children† > 20 kg 6–16 years 20 mg	Adults‡ (mean 76 kg) 23–29 years (n=12)
	Single Dosing		
C_{max}* (ng/mL)	288 (n=10)	495 (n=49)	668
AUC* (ng h/mL)	511 (n=7)	1140 (n=32)	1220
	Repeated Dosing		
C_{max}* (ng/mL)	539 (n=4)	851 (n=32)	1458
AUC* (ng h/mL)	1179 (n=2)	2276 (n=23)	3352

Note: * = plasma concentration adjusted to an oral dose of 1 mg/kg.
† Data from single and repeated dose studies
‡ Data from a single and repeated dose study
Doses of 10, 20 and 40 mg Omeprazole as Enteric-Coated Granules

Following comparable mg/kg doses of omeprazole, younger children (2–5 years) have lower AUCs than children 6–16 years or adults; AUCs of the latter two groups did not differ, (see DOSAGE AND ADMINISTRATION, Pediatric Patients).

Pharmacokinetics: Combination Therapy with Antimicrobials

Omeprazole 40 mg daily was given in combination with clarithromycin 500 mg every 8 hours to healthy adult male subjects. The steady state plasma concentrations of omeprazole were increased (C_{max}, AUC_{0-24}, and $T_{1/2}$ increases of 30%, 89% and 34% respectively) by the concomitant administration of clarithromycin. The observed increases in omeprazole plasma concentration were associated with the following pharmacological effects. The mean 24-hour gastric pH value was 5.2 when omeprazole was administered alone and 5.7 when co-administered with clarithromycin.
The plasma levels of clarithromycin and 14-hydroxy-clarithromycin were increased by the concomitant administration of omeprazole. For clarithromycin, the mean C_{max} was 10% greater, the mean C_{min} was 27% greater, and the mean AUC_{0-8} was 15% greater when clarithromycin was administered with omeprazole than when clarithromycin was administered alone. Similar results were seen for 14-hydroxy-clarithromycin, the mean C_{max} was 45% greater, the mean C_{min} was 57% greater, and the mean AUC_{0-8} was 45% greater. Clarithromycin concentrations in the gastric tissue and mucus were also increased by concomitant administration of omeprazole.

Clarithromycin Tissue Concentrations 2 hours after Dose[1]

Tissue	Clarithromycin	Clarithromycin + Omeprazole
Antrum	10.48 ± 2.01 (n = 5)	19.96 ± 4.71 (n = 5)
Fundus	20.81 ± 7.64 (n = 5)	24.25 ± 6.37 (n = 5)
Mucus	4.15 ± 7.74 (n = 4)	39.29 ± 32.79 (n = 4)

[1]Mean ± SD (μg/g)

For information on clarithromycin pharmacokinetics and microbiology, consult the clarithromycin package insert, CLINICAL PHARMACOLOGY section.
The pharmacokinetics of omeprazole, clarithromycin, and amoxicillin have not been adequately studied when all three drugs are administered concomitantly.
For information on amoxicillin pharmacokinetics and microbiology, see the amoxicillin package insert, ACTIONS, PHARMACOLOGY and MICROBIOLOGY sections.

Pharmacodynamics

Mechanism of Action
Omeprazole belongs to a new class of antisecretory compounds, the substituted benzimidazoles, that do not exhibit anticholinergic or H_2 histamine antagonistic properties, but that suppress gastric acid secretion by specific inhibition of the H^+/K^+ ATPase enzyme system at the secretory surface of the gastric parietal cell. Because this enzyme system is regarded as the acid (proton) pump within the gastric mucosa, omeprazole has been characterized as a gastric acid-pump inhibitor, in that it blocks the final step of acid production. This effect is dose-related and leads to inhibition of both basal and stimulated acid secretion irrespective of the stimulus. Animal studies indicate that after rapid disappearance from plasma, omeprazole can be found within the gastric mucosa for a day or more.
Antisecretory Activity
After oral administration, the onset of the antisecretory effect of omeprazole occurs within one hour, with the maximum effect occurring within two hours. Inhibition of secretion is about 50% of maximum at 24 hours and the duration of inhibition lasts up to 72 hours. The antisecretory effect thus lasts far longer than would be expected from the very short (less than one hour) plasma half-life, apparently due to prolonged binding to the parietal H^+/K^+ ATPase enzyme. When the drug is discontinued, secretory activity returns gradually, over 3 to 5 days. The inhibitory effect of omeprazole on acid secretion increases with repeated once-daily dosing, reaching a plateau after four days.
Results from numerous studies of the antisecretory effect of multiple doses of 20 mg and 40 mg of omeprazole in normal volunteers and patients are shown below. The "max" value represents determinations at a time of maximum effect (2–6 hours after dosing), while "min" values are those 24 hours after the last dose of omeprazole.

Range of Mean Values from Multiple Studies of the Mean Antisecretory Effects of Omeprazole After Multiple Daily Dosing

Parameter	Omeprazole 20 mg Max	Omeprazole 20 mg Min	Omeprazole 40 mg Max	Omeprazole 40 mg Min
% Decrease in Basal Acid Output	78*	58–80	94*	80–93
% Decrease in Peak Acid Output	79*	50–59	88*	62–68
% Decrease in 24-hr. Intragastric Acidity		80–97		92–94

*Single Studies

Single daily oral doses of omeprazole ranging from a dose of 10 mg to 40 mg have produced 100% inhibition of 24-hour intragastric acidity in some patients.
Enterochromaffin-like (ECL) Cell Effects
In 24-month carcinogenicity studies in rats, a dose-related significant increase in gastric carcinoid tumors and ECL cell hyperplasia was observed in both male and female animals (see PRECAUTIONS, Carcinogenesis, Mutagenesis, Impairment of Fertility). Carcinoid tumors have also been observed in rats subjected to fundectomy or long-term treatment with other proton pump inhibitors or high doses of H_2-receptor antagonists.
Human gastric biopsy specimens have been obtained from more than 3000 patients treated with omeprazole in long-term clinical trials. The incidence of ECL cell hyperplasia in these studies increased with time; however, no case of ECL cell carcinoids, dysplasia, or neoplasia has been found in these patients (see CLINICAL PHARMACOLOGY, Pathological Hypersecretory Conditions). However, these studies are of insufficient duration and size to rule out

Continued on next page

Prilosec—Cont.

the possible influence of long-term administration of omeprazole on the development of any premalignant or malignant conditions.

Serum Gastrin Effects
In studies involving more than 200 patients, serum gastrin levels increased during the first 1 to 2 weeks of once-daily administration of therapeutic doses of omeprazole in parallel with inhibition of acid secretion. No further increase in serum gastrin occurred with continued treatment. In comparison with histamine H_2-receptor antagonists, the median increases produced by 20 mg doses of omeprazole were higher (1.3 to 3.6 fold vs. 1.1 to 1.8 fold increase). Gastrin values returned to pretreatment levels, usually within 1 to 2 weeks after discontinuation of therapy.

Other Effects
Systemic effects of omeprazole in the CNS, cardiovascular and respiratory systems have not been found to date. Omeprazole, given in oral doses of 30 or 40 mg for 2 to 4 weeks, had no effect on thyroid function, carbohydrate metabolism, or circulating levels of parathyroid hormone, cortisol, estradiol, testosterone, prolactin, cholecystokinin or secretin.

No effect on gastric emptying of the solid and liquid components of a test meal was demonstrated after a single dose of omeprazole 90 mg. In healthy subjects, a single I.V. dose of omeprazole (0.35 mg/kg) had no effect on intrinsic factor secretion. No systematic dose-dependent effect has been observed on basal or stimulated pepsin output in humans. However, when intragastric pH is maintained at 4.0 or above, basal pepsin output is low, and pepsin activity is decreased.

As do other agents that elevate intragastric pH, omeprazole administered for 14 days in healthy subjects produced a significant increase in the intragastric concentrations of viable bacteria. The pattern of the bacterial species was unchanged from that commonly found in saliva. All changes resolved within three days of stopping treatment.

The course of Barrett's esophagus in 106 patients was evaluated in a U.S. double-blind controlled study of PRILOSEC 40 mg b.i.d. for 12 months followed by 20 mg b.i.d. for 12 months or ranitidine 300 mg b.i.d. for 24 months. No clinically significant impact on Barrett's mucosa by antisecretory therapy was observed. Although neosquamous epithelium developed during antisecretory therapy, complete elimination of Barrett's mucosa was not achieved. No significant difference was observed between treatment groups in development of dysplasia in Barrett's mucosa and no patient developed esophageal carcinoma during treatment. No significant differences between treatment groups were observed in development of ECL cell hyperplasia, corpus atrophic gastritis, corpus intestinal metaplasia, or colon polyps exceeding 3 mm in diameter (see CLINICAL PHARMACOLOGY, Enterochromaffin-like (ECL) Cell Effects).

Clinical Studies
Duodenal Ulcer Disease
Active Duodenal Ulcer—In a multicenter, double-blind, placebo-controlled study of 147 patients with endoscopically documented duodenal ulcer, the percentage of patients healed (per protocol) at 2 and 4 weeks was significantly higher with PRILOSEC 20 mg once a day than with placebo ($p \leq 0.01$).

Treatment of Active Duodenal Ulcer
% of Patients Healed

	PRILOSEC 20 mg a.m. (n = 99)	Placebo a.m. (n = 48)
Week 2	*41	13
Week 4	*75	27

*($p \leq 0.01$)

Complete daytime and nighttime pain relief occurred significantly faster ($p \leq 0.01$) in patients treated with PRILOSEC 20 mg than in patients treated with placebo. At the end of the study, significantly more patients who had received PRILOSEC had complete relief of daytime pain ($p \leq 0.05$) and nighttime pain ($p \leq 0.01$).

In a multicenter, double-blind study of 293 patients with endoscopically documented duodenal ulcer, the percentage of patients healed (per protocol) at 4 weeks was significantly higher with PRILOSEC 20 mg once a day than with ranitidine 150 mg b.i.d. ($p < 0.01$).

Treatment of Active Duodenal Ulcer
% of Patients Healed

	PRILOSEC 20 mg a.m. (n = 145)	Ranitidine 150 mg b.i.d. (n = 148)
Week 2	42	34
Week 4	*82	63

*($p < 0.01$)

Healing occurred significantly faster in patients treated with PRILOSEC than in those treated with ranitidine 150 mg b.i.d. ($p < 0.01$).

In a foreign multinational randomized, double-blind study of 105 patients with endoscopically documented duodenal ulcer, 20 mg and 40 mg of PRILOSEC were compared to 150 mg b.i.d. of ranitidine at 2, 4 and 8 weeks. At 2 and 4 weeks both doses of PRILOSEC were statistically superior (per protocol) to ranitidine, but 40 mg was not superior to 20 mg of PRILOSEC, and at 8 weeks there was no significant difference between any of the active drugs.

Treatment of Active Duodenal Ulcer
% of Patients Healed

	PRILOSEC 20 mg (n = 34)	PRILOSEC 40 mg (n = 36)	Ranitidine 150 mg b.i.d. (n = 35)
Week 2	*83	*83	53
Week 4	*97	*100	82
Week 8	100	100	94

*($p \leq 0.01$)

H. pylori Eradication in Patients with Duodenal Ulcer Disease Triple Therapy (PRILOSEC/clarithromycin/amoxicillin)—Three U.S., randomized, double-blind clinical studies in patients with H. pylori infection and duodenal ulcer disease (n = 558) compared PRILOSEC plus clarithromycin plus amoxicillin to clarithromycin plus amoxicillin. Two studies (126 and 127) were conducted in patients with an active duodenal ulcer, and the other study (M96-446) was conducted in patients with a history of a duodenal ulcer in the past 5 years but without an ulcer present at the time of enrollment. The dose regimen in the studies was PRILOSEC 20 mg b.i.d. plus clarithromycin 500 mg b.i.d. plus amoxicillin 1 g b.i.d. for 10 days; or clarithromycin 500 mg b.i.d. plus amoxicillin 1 g b.i.d. for 10 days. In studies 126 and 127, patients who took the omeprazole regimen also received an additional 18 days of PRILOSEC 20 mg q.d. Endpoints studied were eradication of H. pylori and duodenal ulcer healing (studies 126 and 127 only). H. pylori status was determined by CLOtest®, histology and culture in all three studies. For a given patient, H. pylori was considered eradicated if at least two of these tests were negative, and none was positive.

Per-Protocol and Intent-to-Treat H. pylori Eradication Rates
% of Patients Cured [95% Confidence Interval]

	PRILOSEC +clarithromycin +amoxicillin		Clarithromycin +amoxicillin	
	Per-Protocol†	Intent-to-Treat‡	Per-Protocol†	Intent-to-Treat‡
Study 126	*77 [64, 86] (n = 64)	*69 [57, 79] (n = 80)	43 [31, 56] (n = 67)	37 [27, 48] (n = 84)
Study 127	*78 [67, 88] (n = 65)	*73 [61, 82] (n = 77)	41 [29, 54] (n = 68)	36 [26, 47] (n = 83)
Study M96-446	*90 [80, 96] (n = 69)	*83 [74, 91] (n = 84)	33 [24, 44] (n = 93)	32 [23, 42] (n = 99)

†Patients were included in the analysis if they had confirmed duodenal ulcer disease (active ulcer, studies 126 and 127; history of ulcer within 5 years, study M96-446) and H. pylori infection at baseline defined as at least two of three positive endoscopic tests from CLOtest®, histology, and/or culture. Patients were included in the analysis if they completed the study. Additionally, if patients dropped out of the study due to an adverse event related to the study drug, they were included in the analysis as failures of therapy. The impact of eradication on ulcer recurrence has not been assessed in patients with a past history of ulcer.
‡Patients were included in the analysis if they had documented H. pylori infection at baseline and had confirmed duodenal ulcer disease. All dropouts were included as failures of therapy.
*($p < 0.05$) versus clarithromycin plus amoxicillin.

H. pylori Eradication Rates (Per-Protocol Analysis at 4 to 6 Weeks)
% of Patients Cured [95% Confidence Interval]

	PRILOSEC + Clarithromycin	PRILOSEC	Clarithromycin
U.S. Studies			
Study M93-067	74 [60, 85]†‡ (n = 53)	0 [0, 7] (n = 54)	31 [18, 47] (n = 42)
Study M93-100	64 [51, 76]†‡ (n = 61)	0 [0, 6] (n = 59)	39 [24, 55] (n = 44)
Non U.S. Studies			
Study M92-812b	83 [71, 92]‡ (n = 60)	1 [0, 7] (n = 74)	N/A
Study M93-058	74 [64, 83]‡ (n = 86)	1 [0, 6] (n = 90)	N/A

†Statistically significantly higher than clarithromycin monotherapy ($p < 0.05$)
‡Statistically significantly higher than omeprazole monotherapy ($p < 0.05$)

Duodenal Ulcer Recurrence Rates by H. pylori Eradication Status
% of Patients with Ulcer Recurrence

	H. pylori eradicated#	H. pylori not eradicated#
U.S. Studies†		
6 months post-treatment		
Study M93-067	*35 (n = 49)	60 (n = 88)
Study M93-100	*8 (n = 53)	60 (n = 106)
Non U.S. Studies‡		
6 months post-treatment		
Study M92-812b	*5 (n = 43)	46 (n = 78)
Study M93-058	*6 (n = 53)	43 (n = 107)
12 months post-treatment		
Study M92-812b	*5 (n = 39)	68 (n = 71)

H. pylori eradication status assessed at same timepoint as ulcer recurrence
† Combined results for PRILOSEC + clarithromycin, PRILOSEC, and clarithromycin treatment arms
‡ Combined results for PRILOSEC + clarithromycin and PRILOSEC treatment arms
*($p \leq 0.01$) versus proportion with duodenal ulcer recurrence who were not H. pylori eradicated

The combination of omeprazole plus clarithromycin plus amoxicillin was effective in eradicating H. pylori. [See first table above]

Dual Therapy (PRILOSEC/clarithromycin)—Four randomized, double-blind, multicenter studies (M93-067, M93-100, M92-812b, and M93-058) evaluated PRILOSEC 40 mg q.d. plus clarithromycin 500 mg t.i.d. for 14 days, followed by PRILOSEC 20 mg q.d. (M93-067, M93-100, M93-058) or by PRILOSEC 40 mg q.d. (M92-812b) for an additional 14 days in patients with active duodenal ulcer associated with H. pylori. Studies M93-067 and M93-100 were conducted in the U.S. and Canada and enrolled 242 and 256 patients, respectively. H. pylori infection and duodenal ulcer were confirmed in 219 patients in Study M93-067 and 228 patients in Study M93-100. These studies compared the combination regimen to PRILOSEC and clarithromycin monotherapies. Studies M92-812b and M93-058 were conducted in Europe and enrolled 154 and 215 patients, respectively. H. pylori infection and duodenal ulcer were confirmed in 148 patients in study M92-812b and 208 patients in Study M93-058. These studies compared the combination regimen to omeprazole monotherapy. The results for the efficacy analyses for these studies are described below. H. pylori eradication was defined as no positive test (culture or histology) at 4 weeks following the end of treatment, and two negative tests were required to be considered eradicated of H. pylori. In the per-protocol analysis, the following patients were excluded: dropouts, patients with missing H. pylori tests post-treatment, and patients that were not assessed for H. pylori eradication because they were found to have an ulcer at the end of treatment.

The combination of omeprazole and clarithromycin was effective in eradicating H. pylori.
[See second table at top of previous page]
Ulcer healing was not significantly different when clarithromycin was added to omeprazole therapy compared to omeprazole therapy alone.
The combination of omeprazole and clarithromycin was effective in eradicating H. pylori and reduced duodenal ulcer recurrence.
[See third table at top of previous page]

Gastric Ulcer
In a U.S. multicenter, double-blind, study of omeprazole 40 mg once a day, 20 mg once a day, and placebo in 520 patients with endoscopically diagnosed gastric ulcer, the following results were obtained.

Treatment of Gastric Ulcer
% of Patients Healed
(All Patients Treated)

	PRILOSEC 20 mg q.d. (n = 202)	PRILOSEC 40 mg q.d. (n = 214)	Placebo (n = 104)
Week 4	47.5**	55.6**	30.8
Week 8	74.8**	82.7**,+	48.1

**(p < 0.01) PRILOSEC 40 mg or 20 mg versus placebo
+(p < 0.05) PRILOSEC 40 mg versus 20 mg

For the stratified groups of patients with ulcer size less than or equal to 1 cm, no difference in healing rates between 40 mg and 20 mg was detected at either 4 or 8 weeks. For patients with ulcer size greater than 1 cm, 40 mg was significantly more effective than 20 mg at 8 weeks.

In a foreign, multinational, double-blind study of 602 patients with endoscopically diagnosed gastric ulcer, omeprazole 40 mg once a day, 20 mg once a day, and ranitidine 150 mg twice a day were evaluated.

Treatment of Gastric Ulcer
% of Patients Healed
(All Patients Treated)

	PRILOSEC 20 mg q.d. (n = 200)	PRILOSEC 40 mg q.d. (n = 187)	Ranitidine 150 mg b.i.d. (n = 199)
Week 4	63.5	78.1**,++	56.3
Week 8	81.5	91.4**,++	78.4

**(p < 0.01) PRILOSEC 40 mg versus ranitidine
++(p < 0.01) PRILOSEC 40 mg versus 20 mg

Gastroesophageal Reflux Disease (GERD)
Symptomatic GERD
A placebo controlled study was conducted in Scandinavia to compare the efficacy of omeprazole 20 mg or 10 mg once daily for up to 4 weeks in the treatment of heartburn and other symptoms in GERD patients without erosive esophagitis. Results are shown below.

% Successful Symptomatic Outcome[a]

	PRILOSEC 20 mg a.m.	PRILOSEC 10 mg a.m.	Placebo a.m.
All patients	46*,† (n = 205)	31† (n = 199)	13 (n = 105)
Patients with confirmed GERD	56*,† (n = 115)	36† (n = 109)	14 (n = 59)

[a] Defined as complete resolution of heartburn
*(p < 0.005) versus 10 mg
†(p < 0.005) versus placebo

Erosive Esophagitis
In a U.S. multicenter double-blind placebo controlled study of 20 mg or 40 mg of PRILOSEC Delayed-Release Capsules in patients with symptoms of GERD and endoscopically diagnosed erosive esophagitis of grade 2 or above, the percentage healing rates (per protocol) were as follows:

Week	20 mg PRILOSEC (n = 83)	40 mg PRILOSEC (n = 87)	Placebo (n = 43)
4	39**	45**	7
8	74**	75**	14

**(p < 0.01) PRILOSEC versus placebo.

In this study, the 40 mg dose was not superior to the 20 mg dose of PRILOSEC in the percentage healing rate. Other controlled clinical trials have also shown that PRILOSEC is effective in severe GERD. In comparisons with histamine H2-receptor antagonists in patients with erosive esophagitis, grade 2 or above, PRILOSEC in a dose of 20 mg was significantly more effective than the active controls. Complete daytime and nighttime heartburn relief occurred significantly faster (p < 0.01) in patients treated with PRILOSEC than in those taking placebo or histamine H2-receptor antagonists.

In this and five other controlled GERD studies, significantly more patients taking 20 mg omeprazole (84%) reported complete relief of GERD symptoms than patients receiving placebo (12%).

Long Term Maintenance Treatment of Erosive Esophagitis
In a U.S. double-blind, randomized, multicenter, placebo controlled study, two dose regimens of PRILOSEC were studied in patients with endoscopically confirmed healed esophagitis. Results to determine maintenance of healing of erosive esophagitis are shown below.

Life Table Analysis

	PRILOSEC 20 mg q.d. (n = 138)	PRILOSEC 20 mg 3 days per week (n = 137)	Placebo (n = 131)
Percent in endoscopic remission at 6 months	*70	34	11

*(p < 0.01) PRILOSEC 20 mg q.d. versus PRILOSEC 20 mg 3 consecutive days per week or placebo.

In an international multicenter double-blind study, PRILOSEC 20 mg daily and 10 mg daily were compared to ranitidine 150 mg twice daily in patients with endoscopically confirmed healed esophagitis. The table below provides the results of this study for maintenance of healing of erosive esophagitis.

Life Table Analysis

	PRILOSEC 20 mg q.d. (n = 131)	PRILOSEC 10 mg q.d. (n = 133)	Ranitidine 150 mg b.i.d. (n = 128)
Percent in endoscopic remission at 12 months	*77	‡58	46

*(p = 0.01) PRILOSEC 20 mg q.d. versus PRILOSEC 10 mg q.d. or Ranitidine.
‡(p = 0.03) PRILOSEC 10 mg q.d. versus Ranitidine.

In patients who initially had grades 3 or 4 erosive esophagitis, for maintenance after healing 20 mg daily of PRILOSEC was effective, while 10 mg did not demonstrate effectiveness.

Pathological Hypersecretory Conditions
In open studies of 136 patients with pathological hypersecretory conditions, such as Zollinger-Ellison (ZE) syndrome with or without multiple endocrine adenomas, PRILOSEC Delayed-Release Capsules significantly inhibited gastric acid secretion and controlled associated symptoms of diarrhea, anorexia, and pain. Doses ranging from 20 mg every other day to 360 mg per day maintained basal acid secretion below 10 mEq/hr in patients without prior gastric surgery, and below 5 mEq/hr in patients with prior gastric surgery. Initial doses were titrated to the individual patient need, and adjustments were necessary with time in some patients (see DOSAGE AND ADMINISTRATION). PRILOSEC was well tolerated at these high dose levels for prolonged periods (> 5 years in some patients). In most ZE patients, serum gastrin levels were not modified by PRILOSEC. However, in some patients serum gastrin increased to levels greater than those present prior to initiation of omeprazole therapy. At least 11 patients with ZE syndrome on long-term treatment with PRILOSEC developed gastric carcinoids. These findings are believed to be a manifestation of the underlying condition, which is known to be associated with such tumors, rather than the result of the administration of PRILOSEC (see ADVERSE REACTIONS).

Microbiology
Omeprazole and clarithromycin dual therapy and omeprazole, clarithromycin and amoxicillin triple therapy have been shown to be active against most strains of *Helicobacter pylori* in vitro and in clinical infections as described in the INDICATIONS AND USAGE section.
Helicobacter
Helicobacter pylori
Pretreatment Resistance
Clarithromycin pretreatment resistance rates were 3.5% (4/113) in the omeprazole/clarithromycin dual therapy studies (M93-067, M93-100) and 9.3% (41/439) in omeprazole/clarithromycin/amoxicillin triple therapy studies (126, 127, M96-446).

Clarithromycin Susceptibility Test Results and Clinical/Bacteriological Outcomes

Clarithromycin Susceptibility Test Results and Clinical/Bacteriological Outcomes[a]

Clarithromycin Pretreatment Results	Clarithromycin Post-treatment Results				
	H. pylori negative - eradicated	H. pylori positive - not eradicated Post-treatment susceptibility results			
		S[b]	I[b]	R[b]	No MIC
Dual Therapy - (omeprazole 40 mg q.d./clarithromycin 500 mg t.i.d. for 14 days followed by omeprazole 20 mg q.d. for another 14 days) (Studies M93-067, M93-100)					
Susceptible[b] 108	72	1		26	9
Intermediate[b] 1				1	
Resistant[b] 4				4	
Triple Therapy - (omeprazole 20 mg b.i.d./clarithromycin 500 mg b.i.d./amoxicillin 1 g b.i.d. for 10 days - Studies 126, 127, M96-446; followed by omeprazole 20 mg q.d. for another 18 days - Studies 126, 127)					
Susceptible[b] 171	153	7		3	8
Intermediate[b]					
Resistant[b] 14	4	1		6	3

[a] Includes only patients with pretreatment clarithromycin susceptibility test results
[b] Susceptible (S) MIC ≤ 0.25 μg/mL, Intermediate (I) MIC 0.5 – 1.0 μg/mL, Resistant (R) MIC ≥ 2 μg/mL

Amoxicillin pretreatment susceptible isolates (≤ 0.25 μg/mL) were found in 99.3% (436/439) of the patients in the omeprazole/clarithromycin/amoxicillin triple therapy studies (126, 127, M96-446). Amoxicillin pretreatment minimum inhibitory concentrations (MICs) > 0.25 μg/mL occurred in 0.7% (3/439) of the patients, all of whom were in the clarithromycin and amoxicillin study arm. One patient had an unconfirmed pretreatment amoxicillin minimum inhibitory concentration (MIC) of > 256 μg/mL by Etest®.
[See table above]

Patients not eradicated of H. pylori following omeprazole/clarithromycin/amoxicillin triple therapy or omeprazole/clarithromycin dual therapy will likely have clarithromycin resistant H. pylori isolates. Therefore, clarithromycin susceptibility testing should be done, if possible. Patients with clarithromycin resistant H. pylori should not be treated with any of the following: omeprazole/clarithromycin dual therapy, omeprazole/clarithromycin/amoxicillin triple therapy, or other regimens which include clarithromycin as the sole antimicrobial agent.

Amoxicillin Susceptibility Test Results and Clinical/Bacteriological Outcomes
In the triple therapy clinical trials, 84.9% (157/185) of the patients in the omeprazole/clarithromycin/amoxicillin treatment group who had pretreatment amoxicillin susceptible MICs (≤ 0.25 μg/mL) were eradicated of H. pylori and 15.1% (28/185) failed therapy. Of the 28 patients who failed triple therapy, 11 had no post-treatment susceptibility test results and 17 had post-treatment H. pylori isolates with amoxicillin susceptible MICs. Eleven of the patients who failed triple therapy also had post-treatment H. pylori isolates with clarithromycin resistant MICs.

Susceptibility Test for *Helicobacter pylori*
The reference methodology for susceptibility testing of H. pylori is agar dilution[1]. One to three microliters of an inoculum equivalent to a No. 2 McFarland standard (1 × 10^7 – 1 × 10^8 CFU/mL for H. pylori) are inoculated directly onto freshly prepared antimicrobial containing Mueller-Hinton agar plates with 5% aged defibrinated sheep blood (≥ 2 weeks old). The agar dilution plates are incubated at 35°C in a microaerobic environment produced by a gas generating system suitable for campylobacters. After 3 days of incubation, the MICs are recorded as the lowest concentration of antimicrobial agent required to inhibit growth of the organism. The clarithromycin and amoxicillin MIC values should be interpreted according to the following criteria:

Clarithromycin MIC (μg/mL)[a]	Interpretation	
≤ 0.25	Susceptible	(S)
0.5	Intermediate	(I)
≥ 1.0	Resistant	(R)
Amoxicillin MIC (μg/mL)[a,b]	Interpretation	
≤ 0.25	Susceptible	(S)

[a] These are tentative breakpoints for the agar dilution methodology and they should not be used to interpret results obtained using alternative methods.
[b] There have not been enough organisms with MICs > 0.25 μg/mL to determine a resistance breakpoint.

Standardized susceptibility test procedures require the use of laboratory control microorganisms to control the technical aspects of the laboratory procedures. Standard clarithromycin and amoxicillin powders should provide the following MIC values:

Continued on next page

Prilosec—Cont.

Microorganism	Antimicrobial Agent	MIC (µg/mL)[a]
H. pylori ATCC 43504	Clarithromycin	0.016–0.12 (µg/mL)
H. pylori ATCC 43504	Amoxicillin	0.016–0.12 (µg/mL)

[a] These are quality control ranges for the agar dilution methodology and they should not be used to control test results obtained using alternative methods.

INDICATIONS AND USAGE
Duodenal Ulcer
PRILOSEC Delayed-Release Capsules are indicated for short-term treatment of active duodenal ulcer. Most patients heal within four weeks. Some patients may require an additional four weeks of therapy.
PRILOSEC Delayed-Release Capsules, in combination with clarithromycin and amoxicillin, are indicated for treatment of patients with H. pylori infection and duodenal ulcer disease (active or up to 1-year history) to eradicate H. pylori.
PRILOSEC Delayed-Release Capsules, in combination with clarithromycin, are indicated for treatment of patients with H. pylori infection and duodenal ulcer disease to eradicate H. pylori.
Eradication of H. pylori has been shown to reduce the risk of duodenal ulcer recurrence (see CLINICAL PHARMACOLOGY, Clinical Studies and DOSAGE AND ADMINISTRATION).
Among patients who fail therapy, PRILOSEC with clarithromycin is more likely to be associated with the development of clarithromycin resistance as compared with triple therapy. In patients who fail therapy, susceptibility testing should be done. If resistance to clarithromycin is demonstrated or susceptibility testing is not possible, alternative antimicrobial therapy should be instituted. (See Microbiology section, and the clarithromycin package insert, MICROBIOLOGY section.)

Gastric Ulcer
PRILOSEC Delayed-Release Capsules are indicated for short-term treatment (4–8 weeks) of active benign gastric ulcer (see CLINICAL PHARMACOLOGY, Clinical Studies, Gastric Ulcer).

Treatment of Gastroesophageal Reflux Disease (GERD)
Symptomatic GERD
PRILOSEC Delayed-Release Capsules are indicated for the treatment of heartburn and other symptoms associated with GERD.

Erosive Esophagitis
PRILOSEC Delayed-Release Capsules are indicated for the short-term treatment (4–8 weeks) of erosive esophagitis which has been diagnosed by endoscopy (see CLINICAL PHARMACOLOGY, Clinical Studies).
The efficacy of PRILOSEC used for longer than 8 weeks in these patients has not been established. In the rare instance of a patient not responding to 8 weeks of treatment, it may be helpful to give up to an additional 4 weeks of treatment. If there is recurrence of erosive esophagitis or GERD symptoms (eg, heartburn), additional 4–8 week courses of omeprazole may be considered.

Maintenance of Healing of Erosive Esophagitis
PRILOSEC Delayed-Release Capsules are indicated to maintain healing of erosive esophagitis.
Controlled studies do not extend beyond 12 months.

Pathological Hypersecretory Conditions
PRILOSEC Delayed-Release Capsules are indicated for the long-term treatment of pathological hypersecretory conditions (eg, Zollinger-Ellison syndrome, multiple endocrine adenomas and systemic mastocytosis).

CONTRAINDICATIONS
Omeprazole
PRILOSEC Delayed-Release Capsules are contraindicated in patients with known hypersensitivity to any component of the formulation.

Clarithromycin
Clarithromycin is contraindicated in patients with a known hypersensitivity to any macrolide antibiotic.
Concomitant administration of clarithromycin with cisapride, pimozide, or terfenadine is contraindicated. There have been post-marketing reports of drug interactions when clarithromycin and/or erythromycin are co-administered with cisapride, pimozide, or terfenadine resulting in cardiac arrhythmias (QT prolongation, ventricular tachycardia, ventricular fibrillation, and torsades de pointes) most likely due to inhibition of hepatic metabolism of these drugs by erythromycin and clarithromycin. Fatalities have been reported. (Please refer to full prescribing information for clarithromycin before prescribing.)

Amoxicillin
Amoxicillin is contraindicated in patients with a history of allergic reaction to any of the penicillins. (Please refer to full prescribing information for amoxicillin before prescribing.)

WARNINGS
Clarithromycin
CLARITHROMYCIN SHOULD NOT BE USED IN PREGNANT WOMEN EXCEPT IN CLINICAL CIRCUMSTANCES WHERE NO ALTERNATIVE THERAPY IS APPROPRIATE. IF PREGNANCY OCCURS WHILE TAKING CLARITHROMYCIN, THE PATIENT SHOULD BE APPRISED OF THE POTENTIAL HAZARD TO THE FETUS. (See WARNINGS in prescribing information for clarithromycin.)

Amoxicillin
SERIOUS AND OCCASIONALLY FATAL HYPERSENSITIVITY (anaphylactic) REACTIONS HAVE BEEN REPORTED IN PATIENTS ON PENICILLIN THERAPY. THESE REACTIONS ARE MORE LIKELY TO OCCUR IN INDIVIDUALS WITH A HISTORY OF PENICILLIN HYPERSENSITIVITY AND/OR A HISTORY OF SENSITIVITY TO MULTIPLE ALLERGENS. BEFORE INITIATING THERAPY WITH AMOXICILLIN, CAREFUL INQUIRY SHOULD BE MADE CONCERNING PREVIOUS HYPERSENSITIVITY REACTIONS TO PENICILLINS, CEPHALOSPORINS OR OTHER ALLERGENS. IF AN ALLERGIC REACTION OCCURS, AMOXICILLIN SHOULD BE DISCONTINUED AND APPROPRIATE THERAPY INSTITUTED. SERIOUS ANAPHYLACTIC REACTIONS REQUIRE IMMEDIATE EMERGENCY TREATMENT WITH EPINEPHRINE. OXYGEN, INTRAVENOUS STEROIDS AND AIRWAY MANAGEMENT, INCLUDING INTUBATION, SHOULD ALSO BE ADMINISTERED AS INDICATED. (See WARNINGS in prescribing information for amoxicillin.)

Antimicrobials
Pseudomembranous colitis has been reported with nearly all antibacterial agents and may range in severity from mild to life-threatening. Therefore, it is important to consider this diagnosis in patients who present with diarrhea subsequent to the administration of antibacterial agents. (See WARNINGS in prescribing information for clarithromycin and amoxicillin.)
Treatment with antibacterial agents alters the normal flora of the colon and may permit overgrowth of clostridia. Studies indicate that a toxin produced by *Clostridium difficile* is a primary cause of "antibiotic-associated colitis."
After the diagnosis of pseudomembranous colitis has been established, therapeutic measures should be initiated. Mild cases of pseudomembranous colitis usually respond to discontinuation of the drug alone. In moderate to severe cases, consideration should be given to management with fluids and electrolytes, protein supplementation, and treatment with an antibacterial drug clinically effective against *Clostridium difficile* colitis.

PRECAUTIONS
General
Symptomatic response to therapy with omeprazole does not preclude the presence of gastric malignancy.
Atrophic gastritis has been noted occasionally in gastric corpus biopsies from patients treated long-term with omeprazole.

Information for Patients
PRILOSEC Delayed-Release Capsules should be taken before eating. Patients should be cautioned that the PRILOSEC Delayed-Release Capsule should not be opened, chewed or crushed, and should be swallowed whole.
For patients who have difficulty swallowing capsules, the contents of a PRILOSEC Delayed-Release Capsule can be added to applesauce. One tablespoon of applesauce should be added to an empty bowl and the capsule should be opened. All of the pellets inside the capsule should be carefully emptied on the applesauce. The pellets should be mixed with the applesauce and then swallowed immediately with a glass of cool water to ensure complete swallowing of the pellets. The applesauce used should not be hot and should be soft enough to be swallowed without chewing. The pellets should not be chewed or crushed. The pellets/applesauce mixture should not be stored for future use.

Drug Interactions
Other
Omeprazole can prolong the elimination of diazepam, warfarin and phenytoin, drugs that are metabolized by oxidation in the liver. Although in normal subjects no interaction with theophylline or propranolol was found, there have been clinical reports of interaction with other drugs metabolized via the cytochrome P-450 system (eg, cyclosporine, disulfiram, benzodiazepines). Patients should be monitored to determine if it is necessary to adjust the dosage of these drugs when taken concomitantly with PRILOSEC.
Because of its profound and long lasting inhibition of gastric acid secretion, it is theoretically possible that omeprazole may interfere with absorption of drugs where gastric pH is an important determinant of their bioavailability (eg, ketoconazole, ampicillin esters, and iron salts). In the clinical trials, antacids were used concomitantly with the administration of PRILOSEC.

Combination Therapy with Clarithromycin
Co-administration of omeprazole and clarithromycin have resulted in increases in plasma levels of omeprazole, clarithromycin, and 14-hydroxy-clarithromycin (see also CLINICAL PHARMACOLOGY, Pharmacokinetics: Combination Therapy with Antimicrobials).
Concomitant administration of clarithromycin with cisapride, pimozide, or terfenadine is contraindicated.
There have been reports of an interaction between erythromycin and astemizole resulting in QT prolongation and torsades de pointes. Concomitant administration of erythromycin and astemizole is contraindicated. Because clarithromycin is also metabolized by cytochrome P450, concomitant administration of clarithromycin with astemizole is not recommended. (see also CONTRAINDICATIONS, Clarithromycin, above. Please refer to full prescribing information for clarithromycin before prescribing.)

Carcinogenesis, Mutagenesis, Impairment of Fertility
In two 24-month carcinogenicity studies in rats, omeprazole at daily doses of 1.7, 3.4, 13.8, 44.0 and 140.8 mg/kg/day (approximately 4 to 352 times the human dose, based on a patient weight of 50 kg and a human dose of 20 mg) produced gastric ECL cell carcinoids in a dose-related manner in both male and female rats; the incidence of this effect was markedly higher in female rats, which had higher blood levels of omeprazole. Gastric carcinoids seldom occur in the untreated rat. In addition, ECL cell hyperplasia was present in all treated groups of both sexes. In one of these studies, female rats were treated with 13.8 mg omeprazole/kg/day (approximately 35 times the human dose) for one year, then followed for an additional year without the drug. No carcinoids were seen in these rats. An increased incidence of treatment-related ECL cell hyperplasia was observed at the end of one year (94% treated vs 10% controls). By the second year the difference between treated and control rats was much smaller (46% vs 26%) but still showed more hyperplasia in the treated group. An unusual primary malignant tumor in the stomach was seen in one rat (2%). No similar tumor was seen in male or female rats treated for two years. For this strain of rat no similar tumor has been noted historically, but a finding involving only one tumor is difficult to interpret. A 78-week mouse carcinogenicity study of omeprazole did not show increased tumor occurrence, but the study was not conclusive. A 26-week p53+/- transgenic mouse carcinogenicity study was not positive.
Omeprazole was not mutagenic in an *in vitro* Ames *Salmonella typhimurium* assay, an *in vitro* mouse lymphoma cell assay and an *in vivo* rat liver DNA damage assay. A mouse micronucleus test at 625 and 6250 times the human dose gave a borderline result, as did an *in vivo* bone marrow chromosome aberration test. A second mouse micronucleus study at 2000 times the human dose, but with different (suboptimal) sampling times, was negative.
In a rat fertility and general reproductive performance test, omeprazole in a dose range of 13.8 to 138.0 mg/kg/day (approximately 35 to 345 times the human dose) was not toxic or deleterious to the reproductive performance of parental animals.

Pregnancy
Omeprazole
Pregnancy Category C
Teratology studies conducted in pregnant rats at doses up to 138 mg/kg/day (approximately 345 times the human dose) and in pregnant rabbits at doses up to 69 mg/kg/day (approximately 172 times the human dose) did not disclose any evidence for a teratogenic potential of omeprazole.
In rabbits, omeprazole in a dose range of 6.9 to 69.1 mg/kg/day (approximately 17 to 172 times the human dose) produced dose-related increases in embryo-lethality, fetal resorptions and pregnancy disruptions. In rats, dose-related embryo/fetal toxicity and postnatal developmental toxicity were observed in offspring resulting from parents treated with omeprazole 13.8 to 138.0 mg/kg/day (approximately 35 to 345 times the human dose). There are no adequate or well-controlled studies in pregnant women. Sporadic reports have been received of congenital abnormalities occurring in infants born to women who have received omeprazole during pregnancy. Omeprazole should be used during pregnancy only if the potential benefit justifies the potential risk to the fetus.

Clarithromycin
Pregnancy Category C. See WARNINGS (above) and full prescribing information for clarithromycin before using in pregnant women.

Nursing Mothers
It is not known whether omeprazole is excreted in human milk. In rats, omeprazole administration during late gestation and lactation at doses of 13.8 to 138 mg/kg/day (35 to 345 times the human dose) resulted in decreased weight gain in pups. Because many drugs are excreted in human milk, because of the potential for serious adverse reactions in nursing infants from omeprazole, and because of the potential for tumorigenicity shown for omeprazole in rat carcinogenicity studies, a decision should be made whether to discontinue nursing or to discontinue the drug, taking into account the importance of the drug to the mother.

Pediatric Use
The safety and effectiveness of PRILOSEC have been established in the age group 2 years to 16 years for the treatment of acid-related gastrointestinal diseases, including the treatment of symptomatic GERD, treatment of erosive esophagitis, and the maintenance of healing of erosive esophagitis. The safety and effectiveness of PRILOSEC have not been established for pediatric patients less than 2 years of age. Use of PRILOSEC in the age group 2 years to 16 years is supported by evidence from adequate and well-controlled studies of PRILOSEC in adults with additional clinical, pharmacokinetic, and safety studies performed in pediatric patients (see CLINICAL PHARMACOLOGY, Pharmacokinetics and Metabolism: Omeprazole).

Treatment of Gastroesophageal Reflux Disease (GERD)
Symptomatic GERD
In an uncontrolled, open-label study of patients aged 2 years to 16 years with a history of symptoms suggestive of nonerosive GERD, 113 patients were assigned to receive a single daily dose of omeprazole (10 mg or 20 mg, based on body weight) either as an intact capsule or as an open capsule in applesauce. Results showed success rates of 60% (10 mg omeprazole) and 59% (20 mg omeprazole) in reducing the number and intensity of either pain-related symptoms or vomiting/regurgitation episodes.

Erosive Esophagitis
In an uncontrolled, open-label dose-titration study, healing of erosive esophagitis in pediatric patients aged 1 to 16 years required doses that ranged from 0.7 to 3.5 mg/kg/day (80 mg/day). Doses were initiated at 0.7 mg/kg/day. Doses were increased in increments of 0.7 mg/kg/day (if intraesophageal pH showed a pH of < 4 for less than 6% of a 24-hour study). After titration, patients remained on treatment for 3 months. Forty-four percent of the patients were healed on a dose of 0.7 mg/kg body weight; most of the remaining patients were healed with 1.4 mg/kg after an additional 3 months' treatment. Erosive esophagitis was healed in 51 of 57 (90%) children who completed the first course of treatment in the healing phase of the study. In addition, after 3 months of treatment, 33% of the children had no overall symptoms, 57% had mild reflux symptoms, and 40% had less frequent regurgitation/vomiting.

Maintenance of Healing of Erosive Esophagitis
In an uncontrolled, open-label study of maintenance of healing of erosive esophagitis in 46 pediatric patients, 54% of patients required half the healing dose. The remaining patients increased the healing dose (0.7 to a maximum of 2.8 mg/kg/day) either for the entire maintenance period, or returned to half the dose before completion. Of the 46 patients who entered the maintenance phase, 19 (41%) had no relapse. In addition, maintenance therapy in erosive esophagitis patients resulted in 63% of patients having no overall symptoms.

Safety
The safety of PRILOSEC Delayed-Release Capsules has been assessed in 310 pediatric patients aged 0 to 16 years and 62 physiologically normal volunteers aged 2 years to 16 years. Of the 310 pediatric patients with acid-related disease, a group of 46 who had documented healing of erosive esophagitis after 3 months of treatment continued on maintenance therapy for up to 749 days.

PRILOSEC Delayed-Release Capsules administered to pediatric patients was generally well tolerated with an adverse event profile resembling that in adults. Unique to the pediatric population, however, adverse events of the respiratory system were most frequently reported in both the 0 to 2 year and 2 to 16 year age groups (46.2% and 18.5%, respectively). Similarly, otitis media was frequently reported in the 0 to 2 year age group (22.6%), and accidental injuries were reported frequently in the 2 to 16 year age group (3.8%).

Geriatric Use
Omeprazole was administered to over 2000 elderly individuals (≥ 65 years of age) in clinical trials in the US and Europe. There were no differences in safety and effectiveness between the elderly and younger subjects. Other reported clinical experience has not identified differences in response between the elderly and younger subjects, but greater sensitivity of some older individuals cannot be ruled out.

Pharmacokinetic studies have shown the elimination rate was somewhat decreased in the elderly and bioavailability was increased. The plasma clearance of omeprazole was 250 mL/min (about half that of young volunteers) and its plasma half-life averaged one hour, about twice that of young healthy volunteers. However, no dosage adjustment is necessary in the elderly (see CLINICAL PHARMACOLOGY).

ADVERSE REACTIONS
PRILOSEC Delayed-Release Capsules were generally well tolerated during domestic and international clinical trials in 3096 patients.

In the U.S. clinical trial population of 465 patients (including duodenal ulcer, Zollinger-Ellison syndrome and resistant ulcer patients), the following adverse experiences were reported to occur in 1% or more of patients on therapy with PRILOSEC. Numbers in parentheses indicate percentages of the adverse experiences considered by investigators as possibly, probably or definitely related to the drug:

	Omeprazole (n = 465)	Placebo (n = 64)	Ranitidine (n = 195)
Headache	6.9 (2.4)	6.3	7.7 (2.6)
Diarrhea	3.0 (1.9)	3.1 (1.6)	2.1 (0.5)
Abdominal Pain	2.4 (0.4)	3.1	2.1
Nausea	2.2 (0.9)	3.1	4.1 (0.5)
URI	1.9	1.6	2.6
Dizziness	1.5 (0.6)	0.0	2.6 (1.0)
Vomiting	1.5 (0.4)	4.7	1.5 (0.5)
Rash	1.5 (1.1)	0.0	0.0
Constipation	1.1 (0.9)	0.0	0.0
Cough	1.1	0.0	1.5
Asthenia	1.1 (0.2)	1.6 (1.6)	1.5 (1.0)
Back Pain	1.1	0.0	0.5

The following adverse reactions which occurred in 1% or more of omeprazole-treated patients have been reported in international double-blind, and open-label, clinical trials in which 2,631 patients and subjects received omeprazole.

Incidence of Adverse Experiences ≥ 1%
Causal Relationship not Assessed

	Omeprazole (n = 2631)	Placebo (n = 120)
Body as a Whole, site unspecified		
Abdominal pain	5.2	3.3
Asthenia	1.3	0.8
Digestive System		
Constipation	1.5	0.8
Diarrhea	3.7	2.5
Flatulence	2.7	5.8
Nausea	4.0	6.7
Vomiting	3.2	10.0
Acid regurgitation	1.9	3.3
Nervous System/Psychiatric		
Headache	2.9	2.5

Additional adverse experiences occurring in < 1% of patients or subjects in domestic and/or international trials, or occurring since the drug was marketed, are shown below within each body system. In many instances, the relationship to PRILOSEC was unclear.

Body as a Whole: Allergic reactions, including, rarely, anaphylaxis (see also *Skin* below), fever, pain, fatigue, malaise, abdominal swelling
Cardiovascular: Chest pain or angina, tachycardia, bradycardia, palpitation, elevated blood pressure, peripheral edema
Gastrointestinal: Pancreatitis (some fatal), anorexia, irritable colon, flatulence, fecal discoloration, esophageal candidiasis, mucosal atrophy of the tongue, dry mouth. During treatment with omeprazole, gastric fundic gland polyps have been noted rarely. These polyps are benign and appear to be reversible when treatment is discontinued.
Gastro-duodenal carcinoids have been reported in patients with ZE syndrome on long-term treatment with PRILOSEC. This finding is believed to be a manifestation of the underlying condition, which is known to be associated with such tumors.
Hepatic: Mild and, rarely, marked elevations of liver function tests [ALT (SGPT), AST (SGOT), γ-glutamyl transpeptidase, alkaline phosphatase, and bilirubin (jaundice)]. In rare instances, overt liver disease has occurred, including hepatocellular, cholestatic, or mixed hepatitis, liver necrosis (some fatal), hepatic failure (some fatal), and hepatic encephalopathy.
Metabolic/Nutritional: Hyponatremia, hypoglycemia, weight gain
Musculoskeletal: Muscle cramps, myalgia, muscle weakness, joint pain, leg pain
Nervous System/Psychiatric: Psychic disturbances including depression, aggression, hallucinations, confusion, insomnia, nervousness, tremors, apathy, somnolence, anxiety, dream abnormalities; vertigo; paresthesia; hemifacial dysesthesia
Respiratory: Epistaxis, pharyngeal pain
Skin: Rash and, rarely, cases of severe generalized skin reactions including toxic epidermal necrolysis (TEN; some fatal), Stevens-Johnson syndrome, and erythema multiforme (some severe); purpura and/or petechiae (some with rechallenge); skin inflammation, urticaria, angioedema, pruritus, alopecia, dry skin, hyperhidrosis
Special Senses: Tinnitus, taste perversion
Urogenital: Interstitial nephritis (some with positive rechallenge), urinary tract infection, microscopic pyuria, urinary frequency, elevated serum creatinine, proteinuria, hematuria, glycosuria, testicular pain, gynecomastia
Hematologic: Rare instances of pancytopenia, agranulocytosis (some fatal), thrombocytopenia, neutropenia, anemia, leucocytosis, and hemolytic anemia have been reported.
The incidence of clinical adverse experiences in patients greater than 65 years of age was similar to that in patients 65 years of age or less.

Combination Therapy for *H. pylori* Eradication
In clinical trials using either dual therapy with PRILOSEC and clarithromycin, or triple therapy with PRILOSEC, clarithromycin, and amoxicillin, no adverse experiences peculiar to these drug combinations have been observed. Adverse experiences that have occurred have been limited to those that have been previously reported with omeprazole, clarithromycin, or amoxicillin.
Triple Therapy (PRILOSEC/clarithromycin/amoxicillin) — The most frequent adverse experiences observed in clinical trials using combination therapy with PRILOSEC, clarithromycin, and amoxicillin (n = 274) were diarrhea (14%), taste perversion (10%), and headache (7%). None of these occurred at a higher frequency than that reported by patients taking the antimicrobial drugs alone.
For more information on clarithromycin or amoxicillin, refer to the respective package inserts, ADVERSE REACTIONS sections.
Dual Therapy (PRILOSEC/clarithromycin) — Adverse experiences observed in controlled clinical trials using combination therapy with PRILOSEC and clarithromycin (n = 346) which differed from those previously described for omeprazole alone were: Taste perversion (15%), tongue discoloration (2%), rhinitis (2%), pharyngitis (1%) and flu syndrome (1%).
For more information on clarithromycin, refer to the clarithromycin package insert, ADVERSE REACTIONS section.

OVERDOSAGE
Reports have been received of overdosage with omeprazole in humans. Doses ranged up to 2400 mg (120 times the usual recommended clinical dose). Manifestations were variable, but included confusion, drowsiness, blurred vision, tachycardia, nausea, vomiting, diaphoresis, flushing, headache, dry mouth, and other adverse reactions similar to those seen in normal clinical experience (see ADVERSE REACTIONS). Symptoms were transient, and no serious clinical outcome has been reported when PRILOSEC was taken alone. No specific antidote for omeprazole overdosage is known. Omeprazole is extensively protein bound and is, therefore, not readily dialyzable. In the event of overdosage, treatment should be symptomatic and supportive.

As with the management of any overdose, the possibility of multiple drug ingestion should be considered. For current information on treatment of any drug overdose, a certified Regional Poison Control Center should be contacted. Telephone numbers are listed in the Physicians' Desk Reference (PDR) or local telephone book.

Single oral doses of omeprazole at 1350, 1339, and 1200 mg/kg were lethal to mice, rats, and dogs, respectively. Animals given these doses showed sedation, ptosis, tremors, convulsions, and decreased activity, body temperature, and respiratory rate and increased depth of respiration.

DOSAGE AND ADMINISTRATION
Short-Term Treatment of Active Duodenal Ulcer
The recommended adult oral dose of PRILOSEC is 20 mg once daily. Most patients heal within four weeks. Some patients may require an additional four weeks of therapy (see INDICATIONS AND USAGE).

H. pylori **Eradication for the Reduction of the Risk of Duodenal Ulcer Recurrence**
Triple Therapy (PRILOSEC/clarithromycin/amoxicillin) — The recommended adult oral regimen is PRILOSEC 20 mg plus clarithromycin 500 mg plus amoxicillin 1000 mg each given twice daily for 10 days. In patients with an ulcer present at the time of initiation of therapy, an additional 18 days of PRILOSEC 20 mg once daily is recommended for ulcer healing and symptom relief.
Dual Therapy (PRILOSEC/clarithromycin) — The recommended adult oral regimen is PRILOSEC 40 mg once daily plus clarithromycin 500 mg t.i.d. for 14 days. In patients with an ulcer present at the time of initiation of therapy, an additional 14 days of PRILOSEC 20 mg once daily is recommended for ulcer healing and symptom relief.
Please refer to clarithromycin full prescribing information for CONTRAINDICATIONS and WARNINGS, and for information regarding dosing in elderly and renally impaired patients (see PRECAUTIONS: General, PRECAUTIONS: Geriatric Use and PRECAUTIONS: Drug Interactions).
Please refer to amoxicillin full prescribing information for CONTRAINDICATIONS and WARNINGS.

Gastric Ulcer
The recommended adult oral dose is 40 mg once a day for 4–8 weeks (see CLINICAL PHARMACOLOGY, Clinical Studies, Gastric Ulcer, and INDICATIONS AND USAGE, Gastric Ulcer).

Gastroesophageal Reflux Disease (GERD)
The recommended adult oral dose for the treatment of patients with symptomatic GERD and no esophageal lesions is 20 mg daily for up to 4 weeks. The recommended adult oral dose for the treatment of patients with erosive esophagitis and accompanying symptoms due to GERD is 20 mg daily for 4 to 8 weeks (see INDICATIONS AND USAGE).

Maintenance of Healing of Erosive Esophagitis
The recommended adult oral dose is 20 mg daily (see CLINICAL PHARMACOLOGY, Clinical Studies).

Pathological Hypersecretory Conditions
The dosage of PRILOSEC in patients with pathological hypersecretory conditions varies with the individual patient. The recommended adult oral starting dose is 60 mg once a day. Doses should be adjusted to individual patient needs and should continue for as long as clinically indicated. Doses up to 120 mg t.i.d. have been administered. Daily dosages of greater than 80 mg should be administered in divided doses. Some patients with Zollinger-Ellison syndrome have been treated continuously with PRILOSEC for more than 5 years.

Pediatric Patients
For the treatment of GERD or other acid-related disorders, the recommended dose for pediatric patients 2 years of age and older is as follows:

Patient Weight	Omeprazole Dose
< 20 kg	10 mg
≥ 20 kg	20 mg

On a per kg basis, the doses of omeprazole required to heal erosive esophagitis are greater than those for adults.
For pediatric patients unable to swallow an intact capsule, see Alternative Administration Options subsection below.

Alternative Administration Options
For patients who have difficulty swallowing capsules, the contents of a PRILOSEC Delayed-Release Capsule can be added to applesauce. One tablespoon of applesauce should be added to an empty bowl and the capsule should be opened. All of the pellets inside the capsule should be carefully emptied on the applesauce. The pellets should be mixed with the applesauce and then swallowed immediately with a glass of cool water to ensure complete swallowing of the pellets. The applesauce used should not be hot and should be soft enough to be swallowed without chewing. The pellets should not be chewed or crushed. The pellets/applesauce mixture should not be stored for future use.

No dosage adjustment is necessary for patients with renal impairment or for the elderly.
PRILOSEC Delayed-Release Capsules should be taken before eating. In the clinical trials, antacids were used concomitantly with PRILOSEC.

Continued on next page

Prilosec—Cont.

Patients should be cautioned that the PRILOSEC Delayed-Release Capsule should not be opened, chewed or crushed, and should be swallowed whole.

HOW SUPPLIED

No. 3426 — PRILOSEC Delayed-Release Capsules, 10 mg, are opaque, hard gelatin, apricot and amethyst colored capsules, coded 606 on cap and PRILOSEC 10 on the body. They are supplied as follows:
NDC 0186-0606-31 unit of use bottles of 30
NDC 0186-0606-68 bottles of 100
NDC 0186-0606-28 unit dose packages of 100
NDC 0186-0606-82 bottles of 1000.
No. 3440 — PRILOSEC Delayed-Release Capsules, 20 mg, are opaque, hard gelatin, amethyst colored capsules, coded 742 on cap and PRILOSEC 20 on body. They are supplied as follows:
NDC 0186-0742-31 unit of use bottles of 30
NDC 0186-0742-28 unit dose package of 100
NDC 0186-0742-82 bottles of 1000.
No. 3428 — PRILOSEC Delayed-Release Capsules, 40 mg, are opaque, hard gelatin, apricot and amethyst colored capsules, coded 743 on cap and PRILOSEC 40 on the body. They are supplied as follows:
NDC 0186-0743-31 unit of use bottles of 30
NDC 0186-0743-68 bottles of 100
NDC 0186-0743-28 unit dose packages of 100
NDC 0186-0743-82 bottles of 1000.

Storage

Store PRILOSEC Delayed-Release Capsules in a tight container protected from light and moisture. Store between 15°C and 30°C (59°F and 86°F).

REFERENCES

1. National Committee for Clinical Laboratory Standards. Methods for Dilution Antimicrobial Susceptibility Tests for Bacteria That Grow Aerobically—Fifth Edition. Approved Standard NCCLS Document M7-A5, Vol, 20, No. 2, NCCLS, Wayne, PA, January 2000.

All trademarks are the property of the AstraZeneca group
©AstraZeneca 2002

Manufactured for: AstraZeneca LP, Wilmington, DE 19850
By: Merck & Co., Inc., Whitehouse Station, NJ 08889, USA
9194137
640004-37 Rev. 07/02

PULMICORT RESPULES® ℞

[*pŭl-mĭ-cōrt*]
(budesonide inhalation suspension)
0.25 mg and 0.5 mg
℞ only

Prescribing information for this product, which appears on pages 632–636 of the 2003 PDR, has been completely revised as follows. Please write "See Supplement A" next to the product heading.

For inhalation use via compressed air driven jet nebulizers only (not for use with ultrasonic devices). Not for injection. Read patient instructions before using.

DESCRIPTION

Budesonide, the active component of PULMICORT RESPULES®, is a corticosteroid designated chemically as (RS)-11β, 16α, 17, 21-tetrahydroxypregna-1, 4-diene-3, 20-dione cyclic 16, 17-acetal with butyraldehyde. Budesonide is provided as a mixture of two epimers (22R and 22S). The empirical formula of budesonide is $C_{25}H_{34}O_6$ and its molecular weight is 430.5. Its structural formula is:

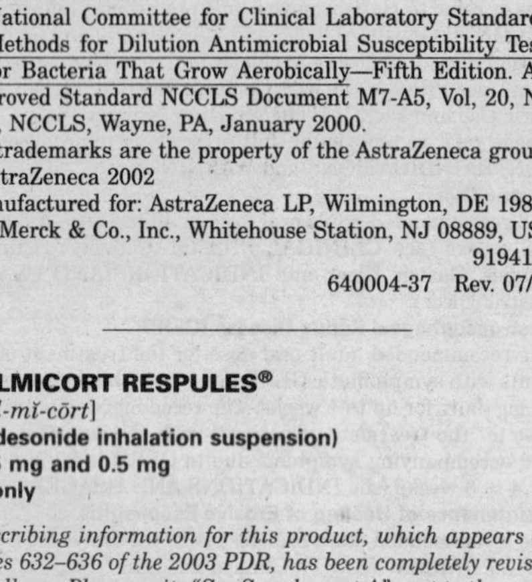

Budesonide is a white to off-white, tasteless, odorless powder that is practically insoluble in water and in heptane, sparingly soluble in ethanol, and freely soluble in chloroform. Its partition coefficient between octanol and water at pH 7.4 is 1.6×10^3.

PULMICORT RESPULES is a sterile suspension for inhalation via jet nebulizer and contains the active ingredient budesonide (micronized), and the inactive ingredients disodium edetate, sodium chloride, sodium citrate, citric acid, polysorbate 80, and Water for Injection. Two dose strengths are available in single-dose ampules (Respules™ ampules): 0.25 mg and 0.5 mg per 2 mL RESPULE ampule. For PULMICORT RESPULES, like all other nebulized treatments, the amount delivered to the lungs will depend on patient factors, the jet nebulizer utilized, and compressor performance. Using the Pari-LC-Jet Plus Nebulizer/Pari Master compressor system, under *in vitro* conditions, the mean delivered dose at the mouthpiece (% nominal dose) was approximately 17% at a mean flow rate of 5.5 L/min. The mean nebulization time was 5 minutes or less. PULMICORT RESPULES should be administered from jet nebulizers at adequate flow rates, via face masks or mouthpieces (see DOSAGE AND ADMINISTRATION).

CLINICAL PHARMACOLOGY

Mechanism of Action

Budesonide is an anti-inflammatory corticosteroid that exhibits potent glucocorticoid activity and weak mineralocorticoid activity. In standard *in vitro* and animal models, budesonide has approximately a 200-fold higher affinity for the glucocorticoid receptor and a 1000-fold higher topical anti-inflammatory potency than cortisol (rat croton oil ear edema assay). As a measure of systemic activity, budesonide is 40 times more potent than cortisol when administered subcutaneously and 25 times more potent when administered orally in the rat thymus involution assay.

The precise mechanism of corticosteroid actions on inflammation in asthma is not well known. Corticosteroids have been shown to have a wide range of inhibitory activities against multiple cell types (eg, mast cells, eosinophils, neutrophils, macrophages, and lymphocytes) and mediators (eg, histamine, eicosanoids, leukotrienes, and cytokines) involved in allergic- and non-allergic-mediated inflammation. The anti-inflammatory actions of corticosteroids may contribute to their efficacy in asthma.

Studies in asthmatic patients have shown a favorable ratio between topical anti-inflammatory activities and systemic corticosteroid effects over a wide dose range of inhaled budesonide in a variety of formulations and delivery systems including Pulmicort Turbuhaler® (an inhalation-driven, multi-dose dry powder inhaler) and the inhalation suspension for nebulization. This is explained by a combination of a relatively high local anti-inflammatory effect, extensive first pass hepatic degradation of orally absorbed drug (85–95%) and the low potency of metabolites (see below).

Pharmacokinetics

The activity of PULMICORT RESPULES is due to the parent drug, budesonide. In glucocorticoid receptor affinity studies, the 22R form was two times as active as the 22S epimer. *In vitro* studies indicated that the two forms of budesonide do not interconvert.

Budesonide is primarily cleared by the liver. In asthmatic children 4–6 years of age, the terminal half-life of budesonide after nebulization is 2.3 hours, and the systemic clearance is 0.5 L/min, which is approximately 50% greater than in healthy adults after adjustment for differences in weight.

After a single dose of 1 mg budesonide, a peak plasma concentration of 2.6 nmol/L was obtained approximately 20 minutes after nebulization in asthmatic children 4–6 years of age. The exposure (AUC) of budesonide following administration of a single 1 mg dose of budesonide by nebulization to asthmatic children 4–6 years of age is comparable to healthy adults given a single 2 mg dose by nebulization.

Absorption: In asthmatic children 4–6 years of age, the total absolute bioavailability (ie, lung + oral) following administration of PULMICORT RESPULES via jet nebulizer was approximately 6% of the labeled dose.

The peak plasma concentration of budesonide occurred 10–30 minutes after start of nebulization.

Distribution: In asthmatic children 4–6 years of age, the volume of distribution at steady-state of budesonide was 3 L/kg, approximately the same as in healthy adults. Budesonide is 85–90% bound to plasma proteins, the degree of binding being constant over the concentration range (1–100 nmol/L) achieved with, and exceeding, recommended doses. Budesonide showed little or no binding to corticosteroid-binding globulin. Budesonide rapidly equilibrated with red blood cells in a concentration independent manner with a blood/plasma ratio of about 0.8.

Metabolism: In vitro studies with human liver homogenates have shown that budesonide is rapidly and extensively metabolized. Two major metabolites formed via cytochrome P450 (CYP) isoenzyme 3A4 (CYP3A4) catalyzed biotransformation have been isolated and identified as 16α-hydroxyprednisolone and 6β-hydroxybudesonide. The corticosteroid activity of each of these two metabolites is less than 1% of that of the parent compound. No qualitative difference between the *in vitro* and *in vivo* metabolic patterns has been detected. Negligible metabolic inactivation was observed in human lung and serum preparations.

Excretion: Budesonide is excreted in urine and feces in the form of metabolites. In adults, approximately 60% of an intravenous radiolabeled dose was recovered in the urine. No unchanged budesonide was detected in the urine.

Special Populations: No differences in pharmacokinetics due to race, gender, or age have been identified.

Hepatic Insufficiency: Reduced liver function may affect the elimination of corticosteroids. The pharmacokinetics of budesonide were affected by compromised liver function as evidenced by a doubled systemic availability after oral ingestion. The intravenous pharmacokinetics of budesonide were, however, similar in cirrhotic patients and in healthy adults.

Pharmacodynamics

The therapeutic effects of conventional doses of orally inhaled budesonide are largely explained by its direct local action on the respiratory tract. To confirm that systemic absorption is not a significant factor in the clinical efficacy of inhaled budesonide, a clinical study in adult patients with asthma was performed comparing 400 mcg budesonide administered via a pressurized metered dose inhaler with a tube spacer to 1400 mcg of oral budesonide and placebo. The study demonstrated the efficacy of inhaled budesonide but not orally ingested budesonide despite comparable systemic levels.

Improvement in the control of asthma symptoms following inhalation of PULMICORT RESPULES can occur within 2–8 days of beginning treatment, although maximum benefit may not be achieved for 4–6 weeks.

Budesonide administered via Turbuhaler® has been shown in various challenge models (including histamine, methacholine, sodium metabisulfite, and adenosine monophosphate) to decrease bronchial hyperresponsiveness in asthmatic patients. The clinical relevance of these models is not certain.

Pre-treatment with budesonide administered via TURBUHALER 1600 mcg daily (800 mcg twice daily) for 2 weeks reduced the acute (early-phase reaction) and delayed (late-phase reaction) decrease in FEV_1 following inhaled allergen challenge.

The effects of PULMICORT RESPULES on the hypothalamic-pituitary-adrenal (HPA) axis were studied in three, 12-week, double-blind, placebo-controlled studies in 293 pediatric patients, 6 months to 8 years of age, with persistent asthma. For most patients, the ability to increase cortisol production in response to stress, as assessed by the short cosyntropin (ACTH) stimulation test, remained intact with PULMICORT RESPULES treatment at recommended doses. In the subgroup of children age 6 months to 2 years (n=21) receiving a total daily dose of PULMICORT RESPULES equivalent to 0.25 mg (n=5), 0.5 mg (n=5), 1 mg (n=8), or placebo (n=3), the mean change from baseline in ACTH-stimulated cortisol levels showed a decline in peak stimulated cortisol at 12 weeks compared to an increase in the placebo group. These mean differences were not statistically significant compared to placebo. Another 12-week study in 141 pediatric patients 6 to 12 months of age with mild to moderate asthma or recurrent/persistent wheezing was conducted. All patients were randomized to receive either 0.5 mg or 1 mg of PULMICORT RESPULES or placebo once daily. A total of 28, 17, and 31 patients in the PULMICORT RESPULES 0.5 mg, 1 mg, and placebo arms respectively, had an evaluation of serum cortisol levels post-ACTH stimulation both at baseline and at the end of the study. The mean change from baseline to Week 12 ACTH-stimulated minus basal plasma cortisol levels did not indicate adrenal suppression in patients treated with PULMICORT RESPULES versus placebo. However, 7 patients in this study (4 of whom received PULMICORT RESPULES 0.5 mg, 2 of whom received PULMICORT RESPULES 1 mg and 1 of whom received placebo) showed a shift from normal baseline stimulated cortisol level (≥500 nmol/L) to a subnormal level (<500 nmol/L) at Week 12. In 4 of these patients receiving PULMICORT RESPULES, the cortisol values were near the cutoff value of 500 nmol/L.

The effects of PULMICORT RESPULES at doses of 0.5 mg twice daily, and 1 mg and 2 mg twice daily (2 times and 4 times the highest recommended total daily dose, respectively) on 24-hour urinary cortisol excretion were studied in 18 patients between 6 to 15 years of age with persistent asthma in a cross-over study design (4 weeks of treatment per dose level). There was a dose-related decrease in urinary cortisol excretion at 2 and 4 times the recommended daily dose. The two higher doses of PULMICORT RESPULES (1 and 2 mg twice daily) showed statistically significantly reduced (43–52%) urinary cortisol excretion compared to the run-in period. The highest recommended dose of PULMICORT RESPULES, 1 mg total daily dose, did not show statistically significantly reduced urinary cortisol excretion compared to the run-in period.

PULMICORT RESPULES, like other inhaled corticosteroid products, may impact the HPA axis, especially in susceptible individuals, in younger children, and in patients given high doses for prolonged periods.

CLINICAL TRIALS

Three double-blind, placebo-controlled, parallel group, randomized U.S. clinical trials of 12-weeks duration each were conducted in 1018 pediatric patients, 6 months to 8 years of age, with persistent asthma of varying disease duration (2 to 107 months) and severity. Doses of 0.25 mg, 0.5 mg, and 1 mg administered either once or twice daily were compared to placebo to provide information about appropriate dosing to cover a range of asthma severity. A Pari-LC-Jet Plus Nebulizer (with a face mask or mouthpiece) connected to a Pari Master compressor was used to deliver PULMICORT RESPULES to patients in the 3 U.S. controlled clinical trials. The co-primary endpoints were nighttime and daytime asthma symptom scores (0–3 scale). Each of the five doses discussed below were studied in one or two, but not all three of the U.S. studies.

Results of the 3 controlled clinical trials for recommended dosages of budesonide inhalation suspension (0.25 mg to 0.5 mg once or twice daily, or 1 mg once daily, up to a total daily dose of 1 mg) in 946 patients, 12 months to 8 years of age, are presented below. Compared to placebo, PULMICORT RESPULES significantly decreased both nighttime and daytime symptom scores of asthma at doses of 0.25 mg once daily (one study), 0.25 mg twice daily, and 0.5 mg twice daily. PULMICORT RESPULES significantly decreased either nighttime or daytime symptom scores, but not both, at doses of 1 mg once daily, and 0.5 mg once daily (one study). Symptom reduction in response to PULMICORT RESPULES occurred across gender and age. PULMICORT RESPULES significantly reduced the need for bronchodilator therapy at all the doses studied.

Improvements in lung function were associated with PULMICORT RESPULES in the subgroup of patients capable of performing lung function testing. Significant improvements were seen in FEV_1 [PULMICORT RESPULES

0.5 mg once daily and 1 mg once daily (one study); 0.5 mg twice daily] and morning PEF [PULMICORT RESPULES 1 mg once daily (one study); 0.25 mg twice daily; 0.5 mg twice daily] compared to placebo.

A numerical reduction in nighttime and daytime symptom scores (0–3 scale) of asthma was observed within 2–8 days, although maximum benefit was not achieved for 4–6 weeks after starting treatment. The reduction in nighttime and daytime asthma symptom scores was maintained throughout the 12 weeks of the double-blind trials.

Patients Not Receiving Inhaled Corticosteroid Therapy
The efficacy of PULMICORT RESPULES at doses of 0.25 mg, 0.5 mg, and 1 mg once daily was evaluated in 344 pediatric patients, 12 months to 8 years of age, with mild to moderate persistent asthma (mean baseline nighttime asthma symptom scores of the treatment groups ranged from 1.07 to 1.34) who were not well controlled by bronchodilators alone. The changes from baseline to Weeks 0–12 in nighttime asthma symptom scores are shown in Figure 1. Nighttime asthma symptom scores improved significantly in the patients treated with PULMICORT RESPULES compared to placebo. Similar improvements were also observed for daytime asthma symptom scores.
[See figure 1 above]

Patients Previously Maintained on Inhaled Corticosteroids
The efficacy of PULMICORT RESPULES at doses of 0.25 mg and 0.5 mg twice daily was evaluated in 133 pediatric asthma patients, 4 to 8 years of age, previously maintained on inhaled corticosteroids (mean FEV_1 79.5% predicted; mean baseline nighttime asthma symptom scores of the treatment groups ranged from 1.04 to 1.18; mean baseline dose of beclomethasone dipropionate of 265 mcg/day, ranging between 42 to 1008 mcg/day; mean baseline dose of triamcinolone acetonide of 572 mcg/day, ranging between 200 to 1200 mcg/day). The changes from baseline to Weeks 0–12 in nighttime asthma symptom scores are shown in Figure 2. Nighttime asthma symptom scores were significantly improved in patients treated with PULMICORT RESPULES compared to placebo. Similar improvements were also observed for daytime asthma symptom scores.
PULMICORT RESPULES at a dose of 0.5 mg twice daily significantly improved FEV_1, and both doses (0.25 mg and 0.5 mg twice daily) significantly increased morning PEF, compared to placebo.
[See figure 2 above]

Patients Receiving Once-Daily or Twice-Daily Dosing
The efficacy of PULMICORT RESPULES at doses of 0.25 mg once daily, 0.25 mg twice daily, 0.5 mg twice daily, and 1 mg once daily, was evaluated in 469 pediatric patients 12 months to 8 years of age (mean baseline nighttime asthma symptom scores of the treatment groups ranged from 1.13 to 1.31). Approximately 70% were not previously receiving inhaled corticosteroids. The changes from baseline to Weeks 0–12 in nighttime asthma symptom scores are shown in Figure 3. PULMICORT RESPULES at doses of 0.25 mg and 0.5 mg twice daily, and 1 mg once daily, significantly improved nighttime asthma symptom scores compared to placebo. Similar improvements were also observed for daytime asthma symptom scores.
PULMICORT RESPULES at a dose of 0.5 mg twice daily significantly improved FEV_1, and at doses of 0.25 mg and 0.5 mg twice daily and 1 mg once daily significantly improved morning PEF, compared to placebo.
The evidence supports the efficacy of the same nominal dose of PULMICORT RESPULES administered on either a once-daily or twice-daily schedule. However, when all measures are considered together, the evidence is stronger for twice-daily dosing (see DOSAGE AND ADMINISTRATION).
[See figure 3 above]

INDICATIONS
PULMICORT RESPULES is indicated for the maintenance treatment of asthma and as prophylactic therapy in children 12 months to 8 years of age.
PULMICORT RESPULES is NOT indicated for the relief of acute bronchospasm.

CONTRAINDICATIONS
PULMICORT RESPULES is contraindicated as the primary treatment of status asthmaticus or other acute episodes of asthma where intensive measures are required.
Hypersensitivity to budesonide or any of the ingredients of this preparation contraindicates the use of PULMICORT RESPULES.

WARNINGS
Particular care is needed for patients who are transferred from systemically active corticosteroids to inhaled corticosteroids because deaths due to adrenal insufficiency have occurred in asthmatic patients during and after transfer from systemic corticosteroids to less systemically available inhaled corticosteroids. After withdrawal from systemic corticosteroids, a number of months are required for recovery of HPA-axis function.
Patients who have been previously maintained on 20 mg or more per day of prednisone (or its equivalent) may be most susceptible, particularly when their systemic corticosteroids have been almost completely withdrawn.
During this period of HPA-axis suppression, patients may exhibit signs and symptoms of adrenal insufficiency when exposed to trauma, surgery, infection (particularly gastroenteritis) or other conditions associated with severe electrolyte loss. Although PULMICORT RESPULES may provide control of asthma symptoms during these episodes, in recommended doses it supplies less than normal physiological

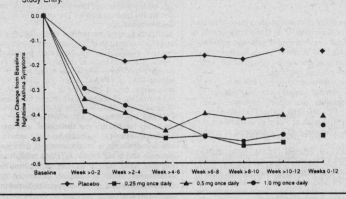

Figure 1: A 12-Week Trial in Pediatric Patients Not on Inhaled Corticosteroid Therapy Prior to Study Entry.

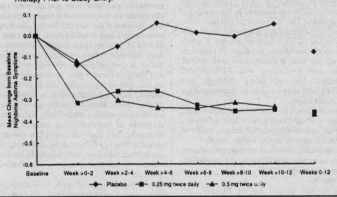

Figure 2: A 12-Week Trial in Pediatric Patients Previously Maintained on Inhaled Corticosteroid Therapy Prior to Study Entry.

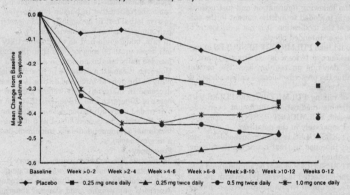

Figure 3: A 12-Week Trial in Pediatric Patients Either Maintained on Bronchodilators Alone or Inhaled Corticosteroid Therapy Prior to Study Entry.

amounts of corticosteroid systemically and does NOT provide the mineralocorticoid activity that is necessary for coping with these emergencies.
During periods of stress or a severe asthma attack, patients who have been withdrawn from systemic corticosteroids should be instructed to resume oral corticosteroids (in large doses) immediately and to contact their physicians for further instructions. These patients should also be instructed to carry a warning card indicating that they may need supplementary systemic corticosteroids during periods of stress or a severe asthma attack.
Transfer of patients from systemic corticosteroid therapy to PULMICORT RESPULES may unmask allergic conditions previously suppressed by the systemic corticosteroid therapy, eg, rhinitis, conjunctivitis, and eczema (see DOSAGE AND ADMINISTRATION).
Patients who are on drugs which suppress the immune system are more susceptible to infection than healthy individuals. Chicken pox and measles, for example, can have a more serious or even fatal course in susceptible pediatric patients or adults on immunosuppressant doses of corticosteroids. In pediatric or adult patients who have not had these diseases, or who have not been properly vaccinated, particular care should be taken to avoid exposure. How the dose, route, and duration of corticosteroid administration affects the risk of developing a disseminated infection is not known. The contribution of the underlying disease and/or prior corticosteroid treatment to the risk is also not known. If exposed, therapy with varicella zoster immune globulin (VZIG) or pooled intravenous immunoglobulin (IVIG), as appropriate, may be indicated. If exposed to measles, prophylaxis with pooled intramuscular immunoglobulin (IG) may be indicated. (See the respective package inserts for complete VZIG and IG prescribing information.) If chicken pox develops, treatment with antiviral agents may be considered.

PULMICORT RESPULES is not a bronchodilator and is not indicated for the rapid relief of acute bronchospasm or other acute episodes of asthma.
As with other inhaled asthma medications, bronchospasm, with an immediate increase in wheezing, may occur after dosing. If acute bronchospasm occurs following dosing with PULMICORT RESPULES, it should be treated immediately with a fast-acting inhaled bronchodilator. Treatment with PULMICORT RESPULES should be discontinued and alternate therapy instituted.
Patients should be instructed to contact their physician immediately when episodes of asthma not responsive to their usual doses of bronchodilators occur during treatment with PULMICORT RESPULES.

PRECAUTIONS
General
Inhaled corticosteroids may cause a reduction in growth velocity when administered to pediatric patients (see PRECAUTIONS, Pediatric Use).
During withdrawal from oral corticosteroids, some patients may experience symptoms of systemically active corticosteroid withdrawal, eg, joint and/or muscular pain, lassitude, and depression, despite maintenance or even improvement of respiratory function.
Because budesonide is absorbed into the circulation and may be systemically active, particularly at higher doses, suppression of HPA function may be associated when PULMICORT RESPULES is administered at doses exceeding those recommended (see DOSAGE AND ADMINISTRATION), or when the dose is not titrated to the lowest effective dose. Since individual sensitivity to effects on cortisol production exists, physicians should consider this information when prescribing PULMICORT RESPULES.

Continued on next page

Pulmicort—Cont.

Because of the possibility of systemic absorption of inhaled corticosteroids, patients treated with these drugs should be observed carefully for any evidence of systemic corticosteroid effects. Particular care should be taken in observing patients post-operatively or during periods of stress for evidence of inadequate adrenal response.

It is possible that systemic corticosteroid effects such as hypercorticism and adrenal suppression may appear in a small number of patients, particularly at higher doses. If such changes occur, PULMICORT RESPULES should be reduced slowly, consistent with accepted procedures for management of asthma symptoms and for tapering of systemic corticosteroids.

Although patients in clinical trials have received PULMICORT RESPULES on a continuous basis for periods of up to 1 year, the long-term local and systemic effects of PULMICORT RESPULES in human subjects are not completely known. In particular, the effects resulting from chronic use of PULMICORT RESPULES on developmental or immunological processes in the mouth, pharynx, trachea, and lung are unknown.

In clinical trials with PULMICORT RESPULES, localized infections with *Candida albicans* occurred in the mouth and pharynx in some patients. The incidences of localized infections of *Candida albicans* were similar between the placebo and PULMICORT RESPULES treatment groups. If symptomatic oropharyngeal candidiasis develops, it should be treated with appropriate local or systemic (ie, oral) antifungal therapy while still continuing with PULMICORT RESPULES therapy, but at times therapy with PULMICORT RESPULES may need to be interrupted under close medical supervision.

Inhaled corticosteroids should be used with caution, if at all, in patients with active or quiescent tuberculosis infection of the respiratory tract, untreated systemic fungal, bacterial, viral, or parasitic infections; or ocular herpes simplex.

Rare instances of glaucoma, increased intraocular pressure, and cataracts have been reported following the inhaled administration of corticosteroids.

Information for Patients

For instructions on the proper use of PULMICORT RESPULES and to attain the maximum improvement in asthma symptoms, the patient or the parent/guardian of the patient should receive, read, and follow the accompanying patient information and instructions carefully. In addition, patients being treated with PULMICORT RESPULES should receive the following information and instructions. This information is intended to aid the patient in the safe and effective use of the medication. It is not a disclosure of all possible adverse or intended effects.

- Patients should take PULMICORT RESPULES at regular intervals once or twice a day as directed, since its effectiveness depends on regular use. The patient should not alter the prescribed dosage unless advised to do so by the physician.
- The effects of mixing PULMICORT RESPULES with other nebulizable medications have not been adequately assessed. PULMICORT RESPULES should be administered separately in the nebulizer.
- PULMICORT RESPULES is not a bronchodilator, and its use is not intended to treat acute life-threatening episodes of asthma.
- PULMICORT RESPULES should be administered with a jet nebulizer connected to a compressor with an adequate air flow, equipped with a mouthpiece or suitable face mask. The face mask should be properly adjusted to optimize delivery and to avoid exposing the eyes to the nebulized medication (see DOSAGE AND ADMINISTRATION).
- Ultrasonic nebulizers are not suitable for the adequate administration of PULMICORT RESPULES and, therefore, are not recommended (see DOSAGE AND ADMINISTRATION).
- Rinsing the mouth with water after each treatment may decrease the risk of development of local candidiasis. Corticosteroid effects on the skin can be avoided if the face is washed after the use of a face mask.
- Improvement in asthma control following treatment with PULMICORT RESPULES can occur within 2–8 days of beginning treatment, although maximum benefit may not be achieved for 4–6 weeks after starting treatment. If the asthma symptoms do not improve in that time frame, or if the condition worsens, the patient or the patient's parent/guardian should be instructed to contact the physician.
- Care should be taken to avoid exposure to chicken pox and measles. If exposure occurs, and the child has not had chicken pox or been properly vaccinated, a physician should be consulted without delay.
- PULMICORT RESPULES should be stored upright at controlled room temperature 20–25°C (68–77°F) and protected from light. PULMICORT RESPULES should not be refrigerated or frozen.
- When an aluminum foil envelope has been opened, the shelf life of the unused RESPULES ampules is two weeks when protected from light. The date the envelope was opened should be recorded on the back of the envelope in the space provided.
- After opening the aluminum foil envelope, the unused RESPULES ampules should be returned to the envelope to protect them from light. Any individually opened RESPULES ampules must be used promptly.
- For proper usage of PULMICORT RESPULES and to attain maximum improvement, the accompanying Patient's Instructions for Use should be read and followed.

Drug Interactions

In clinical studies, concurrent administration of budesonide and other drugs commonly used in the treatment of asthma has not resulted in an increased frequency of adverse events. The main route of metabolism of budesonide, as well as other corticosteroids, is via cytochrome P450 (CYP) isoenzyme 3A4 (CYP3A4). After oral administration of ketoconazole, a potent inhibitor of CYP3A4, the mean plasma concentration of orally administered budesonide increased. Concomitant administration of other known inhibitors of CYP3A4 (eg, itraconazole, clarithromycin, erythromycin, etc.) may inhibit the metabolism of, and increase the systemic exposure to, budesonide. Care should be exercised when budesonide is coadministered with long-term ketoconazole and other known CYP3A4 inhibitors. Omeprazole did not have effects on the pharmacokinetics of oral budesonide, while cimetidine, primarily an inhibitor of CYP1A2, caused a slight decrease in budesonide clearance and a corresponding increase in its oral bioavailability.

Carcinogenesis, Mutagenesis, Impairment of Fertility

In a two-year study in Sprague-Dawley rats, budesonide caused a statistically significant increase in the incidence of gliomas in male rats at an oral dose of 50 mcg/kg (less than the maximum recommended daily inhalation dose in adults and children on a mcg/m^2 basis). No tumorigenicity was seen in male and female rats at respective oral doses up to 25 and 50 mcg/kg (less than the maximum recommended daily inhalation dose in adults and children on a mcg/m^2 basis). In two additional two-year studies in male Fischer and Sprague-Dawley rats, budesonide caused no gliomas at an oral dose of 50 mcg/kg (less than the maximum recommended daily inhalation dose in adults and children on a mcg/m^2 basis). However, in the male Sprague-Dawley rats, budesonide caused a statistically significant increase in the incidence of hepatocellular tumors at an oral dose of 50 mcg/kg (less than the maximum recommended daily inhalation dose in adults and children on a mcg/m^2 basis). The concurrent reference corticosteroids (prednisolone and triamcinolone acetonide) in these two studies showed similar findings.

In a 91-week study in mice, budesonide caused no treatment-related carcinogenicity at oral doses up to 200 mcg/kg (less than the maximum recommended daily inhalation dose in adults and children on a mcg/m^2 basis).

Budesonide was not mutagenic or clastogenic in six different test systems: Ames *Salmonella*/microsome plate test, mouse micronucleus test, mouse lymphoma test, chromosome aberration test in human lymphocytes, sex-linked recessive lethal test in *Drosophila melanogaster*, and DNA repair analysis in rat hepatocyte culture.

In rats, budesonide had no effect on fertility at subcutaneous doses up to 80 mcg/kg (less than the maximum recommended daily inhalation dose in adults on a mcg/m^2 basis). However, it caused a decrease in prenatal viability and viability in the pups at birth and during lactation, along with a decrease in maternal body-weight gain, at subcutaneous doses of 20 mcg/kg and above (less than the maximum recommended daily inhalation dose in adults on a mcg/m^2 basis). No such effects were noted at 5 mcg/kg (less than the maximum recommended daily inhalation dose in adults on a mcg/m^2 basis).

Pregnancy

Teratogenic Effects: Pregnancy Category B—As with other corticosteroids, budesonide was teratogenic and embryocidal in rabbits and rats. Budesonide produced fetal loss, decreased pup weights, and skeletal abnormalities at subcutaneous doses of 25 mcg/kg in rabbits (less than the maximum recommended daily inhalation dose in adults on a mcg/m^2 basis) and 500 mcg/kg in rats (approximately 4 times the maximum recommended daily inhalation dose in adults on a mcg/m^2 basis). In another study in rats, no teratogenic or embryocidal effects were seen at inhalation doses up to 250 mcg/kg (approximately 2 times the maximum recommended daily inhalation dose in adults on a mcg/m^2 basis).

Experience with oral corticosteroids since their introduction in pharmacologic, as opposed to physiologic, doses suggests that rodents are more prone to teratogenic effects from corticosteroids than humans. In addition, because there is a natural increase in corticosteroid production during pregnancy, most women will require a lower exogenous corticosteroid dose and many will not need corticosteroid treatment during pregnancy.

Studies of pregnant women, however, have not shown that inhaled budesonide increases the risk of abnormalities when administered during pregnancy. The results from a large population-based prospective cohort epidemiological study reviewing data from three Swedish registries covering approximately 99% of the pregnancies from 1995–1997 (ie, Swedish Medical Birth Registry; Registry of Congenital Malformations; Child Cardiology Registry) indicate no increased risk for congenital malformations from the use of inhaled budesonide during early pregnancy. Congenital malformations were studied in 2014 infants born to mothers reporting the use of inhaled budesonide for asthma in early pregnancy (usually 10–12 weeks after the last menstrual period), the period when most major organ malformations occur. The rate of recorded congenital malformations was similar compared to the general population rate (3.8% vs. 3.5%, respectively). In addition, after exposure to inhaled budesonide, the number of infants born with orofacial clefts was similar to the expected number in the normal population (4 children vs. 3.3, respectively).

These same data were utilized in a second study bringing the total to 2534 infants whose mothers were exposed to inhaled budesonide. In this study, the rate of congenital malformations among infants whose mothers were exposed to inhaled budesonide during early pregnancy was not different from the rate for all newborn babies during the same period (3.6%).

Despite the animal findings, it would appear that the possibility of fetal harm is remote if the drug is used during pregnancy. Nevertheless, because the studies in humans cannot rule out the possibility of harm, PULMICORT RESPULES should be used during pregnancy only if clearly needed.

Non-teratogenic Effects: Hypoadrenalism may occur in infants born of mothers receiving corticosteroids during pregnancy. Such infants should be carefully observed.

Nursing Mothers

It is not known whether budesonide is excreted in human milk. Because other corticosteroids are excreted in human milk, caution should be exercised if budesonide is administered to nursing women.

Pediatric Use

Safety in children six months to 12 months of age has been evaluated. Safety and effectiveness in children 12 months to 8 years of age have been established (see CLINICAL PHARMACOLOGY, Pharmacodynamics, CLINICAL TRIALS and ADVERSE REACTIONS).

A 12-week study in 141 pediatric patients 6 to 12 months of age with mild to moderate asthma or recurrent/persistent wheezing was conducted. All patients were randomized to receive either 0.5 mg or 1 mg of PULMICORT RESPULES or placebo once daily. Adrenal axis function was assessed with an ACTH stimulation test at the beginning and end of the study, and mean changes from baseline in this variable did not indicate adrenal suppression in patients who received PULMICORT RESPULES versus placebo. However, on an individual basis, 7 patients in this study (6 in the PULMICORT RESPULES treatment arms and 1 in the placebo arm) experienced a shift from having a normal baseline stimulated cortisol level to having a subnormal level at Week 12 (see CLINICAL PHARMACOLOGY, Pharmacodynamics). Pneumonia was observed more frequently in patients treated with PULMICORT RESPULES than in patients treated with placebo, (N = 2, 1, and 0) in the PULMICORT RESPULES 0.5 mg, 1 mg, and placebo groups, respectively.

A dose dependent effect on growth was also noted in this 12-week trial. Infants in the placebo arm experienced an average growth of 3.7 cm over 12 weeks compared with 3.5 cm and 3.1 cm in the PULMICORT RESPULES 0.5 mg and 1 mg arms respectively. This corresponds to estimated mean (95% CI) reductions in 12-week growth velocity between placebo and PULMICORT RESPULES 0.5 mg of 0.2 cm (−0.6 to 1.0) and between placebo and PULMICORT RESPULES 1 mg of 0.6 cm (−0.2 to 1.4). These findings support that the use of PULMICORT RESPULES in infants 6 to 12 months of age may result in systemic effects and are consistent with findings of growth suppression in other studies with inhaled corticosteroids.

Controlled clinical studies have shown that inhaled corticosteroids may cause a reduction in growth velocity in pediatric patients. In these studies, the mean reduction in growth velocity was approximately one centimeter per year (range 0.3 to 1.8 cm per year) and appears to be related to dose and duration of exposure. This effect has been observed in the absence of laboratory evidence of hypothalamic-pituitary-adrenal (HPA)-axis suppression, suggesting that growth velocity is a more sensitive indicator of systemic corticosteroid exposure in pediatric patients than some commonly used tests of HPA-axis function. The long-term effects of this reduction in growth velocity associated with inhaled corticosteroids, including the impact on final adult height, are unknown. The potential for "catch up" growth following discontinuation of treatment with inhaled corticosteroids has not been adequately studied. The growth of pediatric patients receiving inhaled corticosteroids, including PULMICORT RESPULES, should be monitored routinely (eg, via stadiometry). The potential growth effects of prolonged treatment should be weighed against clinical benefits obtained and the risks associated with alternative therapies. To minimize the systemic effects of inhaled corticosteroids, including PULMICORT RESPULES, each patient should be titrated to his/her lowest effective dose.

Geriatric Use

Of the 215 patients in 3 clinical trials of PULMICORT RESPULES in adult patients, 65 (30%) were 65 years of age or older, while 22 (10%) were 75 years of age or older. No overall differences in safety were observed between these patients and younger patients, and other reported clinical or medical surveillance experience has not identified differences in responses between the elderly and younger patients.

ADVERSE REACTIONS

The following adverse reactions were reported in pediatric patients treated with PULMICORT RESPULES.

The incidence of common adverse reactions is based on three double-blind, placebo-controlled, U.S. clinical trials in which 945 patients, 12 months to 8 years of age, (98 patients ≥12 months and <2 years of age; 225 patients ≥2 and <4 years of age; and 622 patients ≥4 and ≤8 years of age) were treated with PULMICORT RESPULES (0.25 to 1 mg total daily dose for 12 weeks) or vehicle placebo. The incidence and nature of adverse events reported for PULMICORT RESPULES was comparable to that reported for placebo. The following table shows the incidence of adverse events in U.S. controlled clinical trials, regardless of relationship to treatment, in patients previously receiving bronchodilators and/or inhaled corticosteroids. This population included a total of 605 male and 340 female patients. [See first table at top of next page]

The table above shows all adverse events with an incidence of 3% or more in at least one active treatment group where the incidence was higher with PULMICORT RESPULES than with placebo.

The following adverse events occurred with an incidence of 3% or more in at least one PULMICORT RESPULES group where the incidence was equal to or less than that of the placebo group: fever, sinusitis, pain, pharyngitis, bronchospasm, bronchitis, and headache.

Incidence 1% to ≤3% (by body system)
The information below includes all adverse events with an incidence of 1 to ≤3%, in at least one PULMICORT RESPULES treatment group where the incidence was higher with PULMICORT RESPULES than with placebo, regardless of relationship to treatment.
Body as a whole: allergic reaction, chest pain, fatigue, flu-like disorder
Respiratory system: stridor
Resistance mechanisms: herpes simplex, external ear infection, infection
Central & peripheral nervous system: dysphonia, hyperkinesia
Skin & appendages: eczema, pustular rash, pruritus
Hearing & vestibular: earache
Vision: eye infection
Psychiatric: anorexia, emotional lability
Musculoskeletal system: fracture, myalgia
Application site: contact dermatitis
Platelet, bleeding & clotting: purpura
White cell and resistance: cervical lymphadenopathy

The incidence of reported adverse events was similar between the 447 PULMICORT RESPULES-treated (mean total daily dose 0.5 to 1 mg) and 223 conventional therapy-treated pediatric asthma patients followed for one year in three open-label studies.

Cases of growth suppression have been reported for inhaled corticosteroids including post-marketing reports for PULMICORT RESPULES (see PRECAUTIONS, Pediatric Use).

Less frequent adverse events (<1%) reported in the published literature, long-term, open-label clinical trials, or from marketing experience for inhaled budesonide include: immediate and delayed hypersensitivity reactions including rash, contact dermatitis, angioedema, and bronchospasm; symptoms of hypocorticism and hypercorticism; psychiatric symptoms including depression, aggressive reactions, irritability, anxiety, and psychosis; and bone disorders including avascular necrosis of the femoral head and osteoporosis.

OVERDOSAGE
The potential for acute toxic effects following overdose of PULMICORT RESPULES is low. If inhaled corticosteroids are used at excessive doses for prolonged periods, systemic corticosteroid effects such as hypercorticism or growth suppression may occur (see PRECAUTIONS).

In mice the minimal lethal inhalation dose was 100 mg/kg (approximately 410 or 120 times, respectively, the maximum recommended daily inhalation dose in adults or children on a mg/m^2 basis). In rats there were no deaths at an inhalation dose of 68 mg/kg (approximately 550 or 160 times, respectively, the maximum recommended daily inhalation dose in adults or children on a mg/m^2 basis). In mice the minimal oral lethal dose was 200 mg/kg (approximately 810 or 240 times, respectively, the maximum recommended daily inhalation dose in adults or children on a mg/m^2 basis). In rats, the minimal oral lethal dose was less than 100 mg/kg (approximately 810 or 240 times, respectively, the maximum recommended daily inhalation dose in adults or children on a mg/m^2 basis).

DOSAGE AND ADMINISTRATION
PULMICORT RESPULES is indicated for use in asthmatic patients 12 months to 8 years of age. PULMICORT RESPULES should be administered by the inhaled route via jet nebulizer connected to an air compressor. Individual patients will experience a variable onset and degree of symptom relief. Improvement in asthma control following inhaled administration of PULMICORT RESPULES can occur within 2–8 days of initiation of treatment, although maximum benefit may not be achieved for 4–6 weeks. The safety and efficacy of PULMICORT RESPULES when administered in excess of recommended doses have not been established. In all patients, it is desirable to downward-titrate to the lowest effective dose once asthma stability is achieved. The recommended starting dose and highest recommended dose of PULMICORT RESPULES, based on prior asthma therapy, are listed in the following table.
[See second table at right]

In symptomatic children not responding to non-steroidal therapy, a starting dose of 0.25 mg once daily of PULMICORT RESPULES may also be considered.

If once-daily treatment with PULMICORT RESPULES does not provide adequate control of asthma symptoms, the total daily dose should be increased and/or administered as a divided dose.

Patients Not Receiving Systemic (Oral) Corticosteroids
Patients who require maintenance therapy of their asthma may benefit from treatment with PULMICORT RESPULES at the doses recommended above. Once the desired clinical effect is achieved, consideration should be given to tapering to the lowest effective dose. For the patients who do not respond adequately to the starting dose, consideration should be given to administering the total daily dose as a divided dose, if a once-daily dosing schedule was followed. If necessary, higher doses, up to the maximum recommended doses, may provide additional asthma control.

Adverse Events with ≥ 3% Incidence Reported by Patients on PULMICORT RESPULES

Adverse Events	Vehicle Placebo (n=227) %	PULMICORT RESPULES Total Daily Dose		
		0.25 mg (n=178) %	0.5 mg (n=223) %	1 mg (n=317) %
Respiratory System Disorder				
Respiratory Infection	36	34	35	38
Rhinitis	9	7	11	12
Coughing	5	5	9	8
Resistance Mechanism Disorders				
Otitis Media	11	12	11	9
Viral Infection	3	4	5	3
Moniliasis	2	4	3	4
Gastrointestinal System Disorders				
Gastroenteritis	4	5	5	5
Vomiting	3	2	4	4
Diarrhea	2	4	4	2
Abdominal Pain	2	3	2	3
Hearing and Vestibular Disorders				
Ear Infection	4	2	4	5
Platelet, Bleeding, and Clotting Disorders				
Epistaxis	1	2	4	3
Vision Disorders				
Conjunctivitis	2	<1	4	2
Skin and Appendages Disorders				
Rash	3	<1	4	2

Previous Therapy	Recommended Starting Dose	Highest Recommended Dose
Bronchodilators alone	0.5 mg total daily dose administered either once daily or twice daily in divided doses	0.5 mg total daily dose
Inhaled Corticosteroids	0.5 mg total daily dose administered either once daily or twice daily in divided doses	1 mg total daily dose
Oral Corticosteroids	1 mg total daily dose administered either as 0.5 mg twice daily or 1 mg once daily	1 mg total daily dose

Patients Maintained on Chronic Oral Corticosteroids
Initially, PULMICORT RESPULES should be used concurrently with the patient's usual maintenance dose of systemic corticosteroid. After approximately one week, gradual withdrawal of the systemic corticosteroid may be initiated by reducing the daily or alternate daily dose. Further incremental reductions may be made after an interval of one or two weeks, depending on the response of the patient. Generally, these decrements should not exceed 25% of the prednisone dose or its equivalent. A slow rate of withdrawal is strongly recommended. During reduction of oral corticosteroids, patients should be carefully monitored for asthma instability, including objective measures of airway function, and for adrenal insufficiency (see WARNINGS). During withdrawal, some patients may experience symptoms of systemic corticosteroid withdrawal, eg, joint and/or muscular pain, lassitude, and depression, despite maintenance or even improvement in pulmonary function. Such patients should be encouraged to continue with PULMICORT RESPULES but should be monitored for objective signs of adrenal insufficiency. If evidence of adrenal insufficiency occurs, the systemic corticosteroid doses should be increased temporarily and thereafter withdrawal should continue more slowly. During periods of stress or a severe asthma attack, transfer patients may require supplementary treatment with systemic corticosteroids.

A Pari-LC-Jet Plus Nebulizer (with face mask or mouthpiece) connected to a Pari Master compressor was used to deliver PULMICORT RESPULES to each patient in 3 U.S. controlled clinical studies. The safety and efficacy of PULMICORT RESPULES delivered by other nebulizers and compressors have not been established.

PULMICORT RESPULES should be administered via jet nebulizer connected to an air compressor with an adequate air flow, equipped with a mouthpiece or suitable face mask. Ultrasonic nebulizers are not suitable for the adequate administration of PULMICORT RESPULES and, therefore, are NOT recommended.

The effects of mixing PULMICORT RESPULES with other nebulizable medications have not been adequately assessed.

PULMICORT RESPULES should be administered separately in the nebulizer (see PRECAUTIONS, Information for Patients).

Directions for Use
Illustrated *Patient's Instructions for Use* accompany each package of PULMICORT RESPULES.

HOW SUPPLIED
PULMICORT RESPULES is supplied in sealed aluminum foil envelopes containing one plastic strip of five single-dose RESPULES ampules together with patient instructions for use. There are 30 RESPULES ampules in a carton. Each single-dose RESPULE ampule contains 2 mL of sterile liquid suspension.

PULMICORT RESPULES is available in two strengths, each containing 2 mL:

NDC 0186-1988-04	0.25 mg/2 mL
NDC 0186-1989-04	0.5 mg/2 mL

Storage
PULMICORT RESPULES should be stored upright at controlled room temperature 20–25°C (68–77°F) [see USP], and protected from light. When an envelope has been opened, the shelf life of the unused RESPULES ampules is 2 weeks when protected. After opening the aluminum foil envelope, the unused RESPULES ampules should be returned to the aluminum foil envelope to protect them from light. Any opened RESPULE ampule must be used promptly. Gently shake the RESPULE ampule using a circular motion before use. Keep out of reach of children. Do not freeze.

All trademarks are the property of the AstraZeneca group
© AstraZeneca 2001, 2003

Continued on next page

Pulmicort—Cont.

AstraZeneca LP, Wilmington, DE 19850
721851-03
Rev. 03/03

TOPROL-XL® ℞

[*tō'prōl*]
(metoprolol succinate)
EXTENDED-RELEASE TABLETS
Tablets: 25 MG, 50 MG, 100 MG, AND 200 MG

Prescribing information for this product, which appears on pages 645–648 of the 2003 PDR, has been completely revised as follows. Please write "See Supplement A" next to the product heading.

DESCRIPTION

TOPROL-XL, metoprolol succinate, is a $beta_1$-selective (cardioselective) adrenoceptor blocking agent, for oral administration, available as extended release tablets. TOPROL-XL has been formulated to provide a controlled and predictable release of metoprolol for once-daily administration. The tablets comprise a multiple unit system containing metoprolol succinate in a multitude of controlled release pellets. Each pellet acts as a separate drug delivery unit and is designed to deliver metoprolol continuously over the dosage interval. The tablets contain 23.75, 47.5, 95 and 190 mg of metoprolol succinate equivalent to 25, 50, 100 and 200 mg of metoprolol tartrate, USP, respectively. Its chemical name is (±)1-(isopropylamino)-3-[p-(2-methoxyethyl) phenoxy]-2-propanol succinate (2:1) (salt). Its structural formula is:

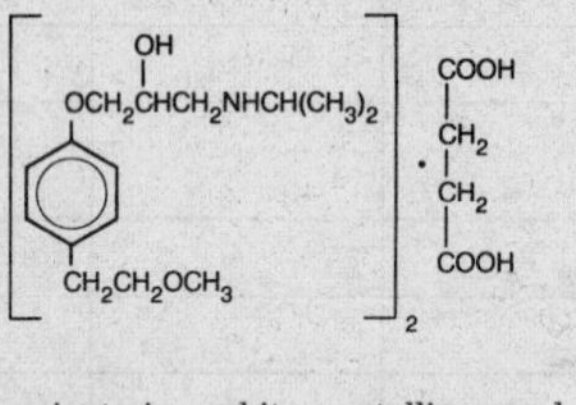

Metoprolol succinate is a white crystalline powder with a molecular weight of 652.8. It is freely soluble in water; soluble in methanol; sparingly soluble in ethanol; slightly soluble in dichloromethane and 2-propanol; practically insoluble in ethylacetate, acetone, diethylether and heptane. Inactive ingredients: silicon dioxide, cellulose compounds, sodium stearyl fumarate, polyethylene glycol, titanium dioxide, paraffin.

CLINICAL PHARMACOLOGY

General

Metoprolol is a $beta_1$-selective (cardioselective) adrenergic receptor blocking agent. This preferential effect is not absolute, however, and at higher plasma concentrations, metoprolol also inhibits $beta_2$-adrenoreceptors, chiefly located in the bronchial and vascular musculature. Metoprolol has no intrinsic sympathomimetic activity, and membrane-stabilizing activity is detectable only at plasma concentrations much greater than required for beta-blockade. Animal and human experiments indicate that metoprolol slows the sinus rate and decreases AV nodal conduction.

Clinical pharmacology studies have confirmed the beta-blocking activity of metoprolol in man, as shown by (1) reduction in heart rate and cardiac output at rest and upon exercise, (2) reduction of systolic blood pressure upon exercise, (3) inhibition of isoproterenol-induced tachycardia, and (4) reduction of reflex orthostatic tachycardia.

The relative $beta_1$-selectivity of metoprolol has been confirmed by the following: (1) In normal subjects, metoprolol is unable to reverse the $beta_2$-mediated vasodilating effects of epinephrine. This contrasts with the effect of nonselective beta-blockers, which completely reverse the vasodilating effects of epinephrine. (2) In asthmatic patients, metoprolol reduces FEV_1 and FVC significantly less than a nonselective beta-blocker, propranolol, at equivalent $beta_1$-receptor blocking doses.

In five controlled studies in normal healthy subjects, the same daily doses of TOPROL-XL and immediate release metoprolol were compared in terms of the extent and duration of $beta_1$-blockade produced. Both formulations were given in a dose range equivalent to 100–400 mg of immediate release metoprolol per day. In these studies, TOPROL-XL was administered once a day and immediate release metoprolol was administered once to four times a day. A sixth controlled study compared the $beta_1$-blocking effects of a 50 mg daily dose of the two formulations. In each study, $beta_1$-blockade was expressed as the percent change from baseline in exercise heart rate following standardized submaximal exercise tolerance tests at steady state. TOPROL-XL administered once a day, and immediate release metoprolol administered once to four times a day, provided comparable total $beta_1$-blockade over 24 hours (area under the $beta_1$-blockade versus time curve) in the dose range 100–400 mg. At a dosage of 50 mg once daily, TOPROL-XL produced significantly higher total $beta_1$-blockade over 24 hours than immediate release metoprolol. For TOPROL-XL, the percent reduction in exercise heart rate was relatively stable throughout the entire dosage interval and the level of $beta_1$-blockade increased with increasing doses from 50 to 300 mg daily. The effects at peak/trough (ie, at 24-hours post-dosing) were: 14/9, 16/10, 24/14, 27/22 and 27/20% reduction in exercise heart rate for doses of 50, 100, 200, 300 and 400 mg TOPROL-XL once a day, respectively. In contrast to TOPROL-XL, immediate release metoprolol given at a dose of 50–100 mg once a day produced a significantly larger peak effect on exercise tachycardia, but the effect was not evident at 24 hours. To match the peak to trough ratio obtained with TOPROL-XL over the dosing range of 200 to 400 mg, a t.i.d. to q.i.d. divided dosing regimen was required for immediate release metoprolol. A controlled cross-over study in heart failure patients compared the plasma concentrations and $beta_1$-blocking effects of 50 mg immediate release metoprolol administered t.i.d., 100 mg and 200 mg TOPROL-XL once daily. A 50 mg dose of immediate release metoprolol t.i.d. produced a peak plasma level of metoprolol similar to the peak level observed with 200 mg of TOPROL-XL. A 200 mg dose of TOPROL-XL produced a larger effect on suppression of exercise-induced and Holter-monitored heart rate over 24 hours compared to 50 mg t.i.d. of immediate release metoprolol.

The relationship between plasma metoprolol levels and reduction in exercise heart rate is independent of the pharmaceutical formulation. Using the E_{max} model, the maximal $beta_1$-blocking effect has been estimated to produce a 30% reduction in exercise heart rate. $Beta_1$-blocking effects in the range of 30–80% of the maximal effect (corresponding to approximately 8–23% reduction in exercise heart rate) are expected to occur at metoprolol plasma concentrations ranging from 30–540 nmol/L. The concentration-effect curve begins reaching a plateau between 200–300 nmol/L, and higher plasma levels produce little additional $beta_1$-blocking effect. The relative $beta_1$-selectivity of metoprolol diminishes and blockade of $beta_2$-adrenoceptors increases at higher plasma concentrations.

Although beta-adrenergic receptor blockade is useful in the treatment of angina, hypertension, and heart failure there are situations in which sympathetic stimulation is vital. In patients with severely damaged hearts, adequate ventricular function may depend on sympathetic drive. In the presence of AV block, beta-blockade may prevent the necessary facilitating effect of sympathetic activity on conduction. $Beta_2$-adrenergic blockade results in passive bronchial constriction by interfering with endogenous adrenergic bronchodilator activity in patients subject to bronchospasm and may also interfere with exogenous bronchodilators in such patients.

In other studies, treatment with TOPROL-XL produced an improvement in left ventricular ejection fraction. TOPROL-XL was also shown to delay the increase in left ventricular end-systolic and end-diastolic volumes after 6 months of treatment.

Hypertension

The mechanism of the antihypertensive effects of beta-blocking agents has not been elucidated. However, several possible mechanisms have been proposed: (1) competitive antagonism of catecholamines at peripheral (especially cardiac) adrenergic neuron sites, leading to decreased cardiac output; (2) a central effect leading to reduced sympathetic outflow to the periphery; and (3) suppression of renin activity.

Clinical Trials

In controlled clinical studies, an immediate release dosage form of metoprolol has been shown to be an effective antihypertensive agent when used alone or as concomitant therapy with thiazide-type diuretics at dosages of 100–450 mg daily. TOPROL-XL, in dosages of 100 to 400 mg once daily, has been shown to possess comparable β_1-blockade as conventional metoprolol tablets administered two to four times daily. In addition, TOPROL-XL administered at a dose of 50 mg once daily has been shown to lower blood pressure 24-hours post-dosing in placebo-controlled studies. In controlled, comparative, clinical studies, immediate release metoprolol appeared comparable as an antihypertensive agent to propranolol, methyldopa, and thiazide-type diuretics, and affected both supine and standing blood pressure. Because of variable plasma levels attained with a given dose and lack of a consistent relationship of antihypertensive activity to drug plasma concentration, selection of proper dosage requires individual titration.

Angina Pectoris

By blocking catecholamine-induced increases in heart rate, in velocity and extent of myocardial contraction, and in blood pressure, metoprolol reduces the oxygen requirements of the heart at any given level of effort, thus making it useful in the long-term management of angina pectoris.

Clinical Trials

In controlled clinical trials, an immediate release formulation of metoprolol has been shown to be an effective antianginal agent, reducing the number of angina attacks and increasing exercise tolerance. The dosage used in these studies ranged from 100 to 400 mg daily. TOPROL-XL, in dosages of 100 to 400 mg once daily, has been shown to possess beta-blockade similar to conventional metoprolol tablets administered two to four times daily.

Heart Failure

The precise mechanism for the beneficial effects of beta-blockers in heart failure has not been elucidated.

Clinical Trials

MERIT-HF was a double-blind, placebo-controlled study of TOPROL-XL conducted in 14 countries including the US. It randomized 3991 patients (1990 to TOPROL-XL) with ejection fraction ≤ 0.40 and NYHA Class II-IV heart failure attributable to ischemia, hypertension, or cardiomyopathy. The protocol excluded patients with contraindications to beta-blocker use, those expected to undergo heart surgery, and those within 28 days of myocardial infarction or unstable angina. The primary endpoints of the trial were (1) all-cause mortality plus all-cause hospitalization (time to first event) and (2) all-cause mortality. Patients were stabilized on optimal concomitant therapy for heart failure, including diuretics, ACE inhibitors, cardiac glycosides, and nitrates. At randomization, 41% of patients were NYHA Class II, 55% NYHA Class III; 65% of patients had heart failure attributed to ischemic heart disease; 44% had a history of hypertension; 25% had diabetes mellitus; 48% had a history of myocardial infarction. Among patients in the trial, 90% were on diuretics, 89% were on ACE inhibitors, 64% were on digitalis, 27% were on a lipid-lowering agent, 37% were on an oral anticoagulant, and the mean ejection fraction was 0.28. The mean duration of follow-up was one year. At the end of the study, the mean daily dose of TOPROL-XL was 159 mg.

The trial was terminated early for a statistically significant reduction in all-cause mortality (34%, nominal p= 0.00009). The risk of all-cause mortality plus all-cause hospitalization was reduced by 19% (p= 0.00012). The trial also showed improvements in heart failure-related mortality and heart failure-related hospitalizations, and NYHA functional class. The table below shows the principal results for the overall study population. The figure below illustrates principal results for a wide variety of subgroup comparisons, including US vs. non-US populations (the latter of which was not prespecified). The combined endpoints of all-cause mortality

Clinical Endpoints in the MERIT-HF Study

Clinical Endpoint	Number of Patients: Placebo n=2001	Number of Patients: TOPROL-XL n=1990	Relative Risk (95% CI)	Risk Reduction with TOPROL-XL	Nominal P-value
All-cause mortality plus all-cause hospitalization†	767	641	0.81 (0.73–0.90)	19%	0.00012
All-cause mortality	217	145	0.66 (0.53–0.81)	34%	0.00009
All-cause mortality plus heart failure hospitalization†	439	311	0.69 (0.60–0.80)	31%	0.0000008
Cardiovascular mortality	203	128	0.62 (0.50–0.78)	38%	0.000022
Sudden death	132	79	0.59 (0.45–0.78)	41%	0.0002
Death due to worsening heart failure	58	30	0.51 (0.33–0.79)	49%	0.0023
Hospitalizations due to worsening heart failure‡	451	317	N/A	N/A	0.0000076
Cardiovascular hospitalization‡	773	649	N/A	N/A	0.00028

† Time to first event
‡ Comparison of treatment groups examines the number of hospitalizations (Wilcoxon test); relative risk and risk reduction are not applicable.

plus all-cause hospitalization and of mortality plus heart failure hospitalization showed consistent effects in the overall study population and the subgroups, including women and the US population. However, in the US subgroup (n=1071) and women (n=898), overall mortality and cardiovascular mortality appeared less affected. Analyses of female and US patients were carried out because they each represented about 25% of the overall population. Nonetheless, subgroup analyses can be difficult to interpret and it is not known whether these represent true differences or chance effects.
[See table at top of previous page]
[See figure above]

Pharmacokinetics
In man, absorption of metoprolol is rapid and complete. Plasma levels following oral administration of conventional metoprolol tablets, however, approximate 50% of levels following intravenous administration, indicating about 50% first-pass metabolism. Metoprolol crosses the blood-brain barrier and has been reported in the CSF in a concentration 78% of the simultaneous plasma concentration.
Plasma levels achieved are highly variable after oral administration. Only a small fraction of the drug (about 12%) is bound to human serum albumin. Metoprolol is a racemic mixture of R- and S-enantiomers, and is primarily metabolized by CYP2D6. When administered orally, it exhibits stereoselective metabolism that is dependent on oxidation phenotype. Elimination is mainly by biotransformation in the liver, and the plasma half-life ranges from approximately 3 to 7 hours. Less than 5% of an oral dose of metoprolol is recovered unchanged in the urine; the rest is excreted by the kidneys as metabolites that appear to have no beta-blocking activity. Following intravenous administration of metoprolol, the urinary recovery of unchanged drug is approximately 10%. The systemic availability and half-life of metoprolol in patients with renal failure do not differ to a clinically significant degree from those in normal subjects. Consequently, no reduction in dosage is usually needed in patients with chronic renal failure.
Metoprolol is metabolized predominantly by CYP2D6, an enzyme that is absent in about 8% of Caucasians (poor metabolizers) and about 2% of most other populations. CYP2D6 can be inhibited by a number of drugs. Concomitant use of inhibiting drugs in poor metabolizers will increase blood levels of metoprolol several-fold, decreasing metoprolol's cardioselectivity (see PRECAUTIONS, Drug Interactions).
In comparison to conventional metoprolol, the plasma metoprolol levels following administration of TOPROL-XL are characterized by lower peaks, longer time to peak and significantly lower peak to trough variation. The peak plasma levels following once-daily administration of TOPROL-XL average one-fourth to one-half the peak plasma levels obtained following a corresponding dose of conventional metoprolol, administered once daily or in divided doses. At steady state the average bioavailability of metoprolol following administration of TOPROL-XL, across the dosage range of 50 to 400 mg once daily, was 77% relative to the corresponding single or divided doses of conventional metoprolol. Nevertheless, over the 24-hour dosing interval, ß₁-blockade is comparable and dose-related (see CLINICAL PHARMACOLOGY). The bioavailability of metoprolol shows a dose-related, although not directly proportional, increase with dose and is not significantly affected by food following TOPROL-XL administration.

INDICATIONS AND USAGE
Hypertension
TOPROL-XL is indicated for the treatment of hypertension. It may be used alone or in combination with other antihypertensive agents.
Angina Pectoris
TOPROL-XL is indicated in the long-term treatment of angina pectoris.
Heart Failure
TOPROL-XL is indicated for the treatment of stable, symptomatic (NYHA Class II or III) heart failure of ischemic, hypertensive, or cardiomyopathic origin. It was studied in patients already receiving ACE inhibitors, diuretics, and, in the majority of cases, digitalis. In this population, TOPROL-XL decreased the rate of mortality plus hospitalization, largely through a reduction in cardiovascular mortality and hospitalizations for heart failure.

CONTRAINDICATIONS
TOPROL-XL is contraindicated in severe bradycardia, heart block greater than first degree, cardiogenic shock, decompensated cardiac failure, sick sinus syndrome (unless a permanent pacemaker is in place) (see WARNINGS) and in patients who are hypersensitive to any component of this product.

WARNINGS

Ischemic Heart Disease: Following abrupt cessation of therapy with certain beta-blocking agents, exacerbations of angina pectoris and, in some cases, myocardial infarction have occurred. When discontinuing chronically administered TOPROL-XL, particularly in patients with ischemic heart disease, the dosage should be gradually reduced over a period of 1-2 weeks and the patient should be carefully monitored. If angina markedly worsens or acute coronary insufficiency develops, TOPROL-XL administration should be reinstated promptly, at least temporarily, and other measures appropriate for the management of unstable angina should be taken. Patients should be warned against interruption or discontinuation of therapy without the physician's advice. Because coronary artery disease is common and may be unrecognized, it may be prudent not to discontinue TOPROL-XL therapy abruptly even in patients treated only for hypertension.

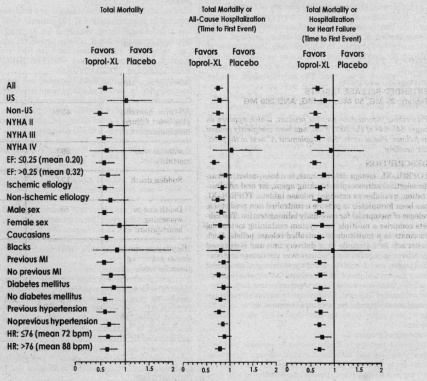

Results for Subgroups in MERIT-HF

US = United States; NYHA = New York Heart Association; EF = ejection fraction; MI = myocardial infarction; HR = heart rate.

Bronchospastic Diseases: PATIENTS WITH BRONCHOSPASTIC DISEASES SHOULD, IN GENERAL, NOT RECEIVE BETA-BLOCKERS. Because of its relative beta₁-selectivity, however, TOPROL-XL may be used with caution in patients with bronchospastic disease who do not respond to, or cannot tolerate, other antihypertensive treatment. Since beta₁-selectivity is not absolute, a beta₂-stimulating agent should be administered concomitantly, and the lowest possible dose of TOPROL-XL should be used (see DOSAGE AND ADMINISTRATION).
Major Surgery: The necessity or desirability of withdrawing beta-blocking therapy prior to major surgery is controversial; the impaired ability of the heart to respond to reflex adrenergic stimuli may augment the risks of general anesthesia and surgical procedures.
TOPROL-XL, like other beta-blockers, is a competitive inhibitor of beta-receptor agonists, and its effects can be reversed by administration of such agents, eg, dobutamine or isoproterenol. However, such patients may be subject to protracted severe hypotension. Difficulty in restarting and maintaining the heart beat has also been reported with beta-blockers.
Diabetes and Hypoglycemia: TOPROL-XL should be used with caution in diabetic patients if a beta-blocking agent is required. Beta-blockers may mask tachycardia occurring with hypoglycemia, but other manifestations such as dizziness and sweating may not be significantly affected.
Thyrotoxicosis: Beta-adrenergic blockade may mask certain clinical signs (eg, tachycardia) of hyperthyroidism. Patients suspected of developing thyrotoxicosis should be managed carefully to avoid abrupt withdrawal of beta-blockade, which might precipitate a thyroid storm.
Peripheral Vascular Disease: Beta-blockers can precipitate or aggravate symptoms of arterial insufficiency in patients with peripheral vascular disease. Caution should be exercised in such individuals.
Calcium Channel Blockers: Because of significant inotropic and chronotropic effects in patients treated with beta-blockers and calcium channel blockers of the verapamil and diltiazem type, caution should be exercised in patients treated with these agents concomitantly.

PRECAUTIONS
General
TOPROL-XL should be used with caution in patients with impaired hepatic function. In patients with pheochromocytoma, an alpha-blocking agent should be initiated prior to the use of any beta-blocking agent.
Worsening cardiac failure may occur during up-titration of TOPROL-XL. If such symptoms occur, diuretics should be increased and the dose of TOPROL-XL should not be advanced until clinical stability is restored (see DOSAGE AND ADMINISTRATION). It may be necessary to lower the dose of TOPROL-XL or temporarily discontinue it. Such episodes do not preclude subsequent successful titration of TOPROL-XL.
Information for Patients
Patients should be advised to take TOPROL-XL regularly and continuously, as directed, preferably with or immediately following meals. If a dose should be missed, the patient should take only the next scheduled dose (without doubling it). Patients should not interrupt or discontinue TOPROL-XL without consulting the physician.
Patients should be advised (1) to avoid operating automobiles and machinery or engaging in other tasks requiring alertness until the patient's response to therapy with TOPROL-XL has been determined; (2) to contact the physician if any difficulty in breathing occurs; (3) to inform the physician or dentist before any type of surgery that he or she is taking TOPROL-XL.
Heart failure patients should be advised to consult their physician if they experience signs or symptoms of worsening heart failure such as weight gain or increasing shortness of breath.
Laboratory Tests
Clinical laboratory findings may include elevated levels of serum transaminase, alkaline phosphatase, and lactate dehydrogenase.
Drug Interactions
Catecholamine-depleting drugs (eg, reserpine, mono amine oxidase (MAO) inhibitors) may have an additive effect when given with beta-blocking agents. Patients treated with TOPROL-XL plus a catecholamine depletor should therefore be closely observed for evidence of hypotension or marked bradycardia, which may produce vertigo, syncope, or postural hypotension.
Drugs that inhibit CYP2D6 such as quinidine, fluoxetine, paroxetine, and propafenone are likely to increase metoprolol concentration. In healthy subjects with CYP2D6 extensive metabolizer phenotype, coadministration of quinidine 100 mg and immediate release metoprolol 200 mg tripled the concentration of S-metoprolol and doubled the metoprolol elimination half-life. In four patients with cardiovascular disease, coadministration of propafenone 150 mg t.i.d. with immediate release metoprolol 50 mg t.i.d. resulted in two- to five-fold increases in the steady-state concentration of metoprolol. These increases in plasma concentration would decrease the cardioselectivity of metoprolol.
Beta-blockers may exacerbate the rebound hypertension which can follow the withdrawal of clonidine. If the two drugs are coadministered, the beta blocker should be withdrawn several days before the gradual withdrawal of clonidine. If replacing clonidine by beta-blocker therapy, the introduction of beta-blockers should be delayed for several days after clonidine administration has stopped.

Continued on next page

Toprol-XL—Cont.

Carcinogenesis, Mutagenesis, Impairment of Fertility
Long-term studies in animals have been conducted to evaluate the carcinogenic potential of metoprolol tartrate. In 2-year studies in rats at three oral dosage levels of up to 800 mg/kg/day (41 times, on a mg/m^2 basis, the daily dose of 200 mg for a 60-kg patient), there was no increase in the development of spontaneously occurring benign or malignant neoplasms of any type. The only histologic changes that appeared to be drug related were an increased incidence of generally mild focal accumulation of foamy macrophages in pulmonary alveoli and a slight increase in biliary hyperplasia. In a 21-month study in Swiss albino mice at three oral dosage levels of up to 750 mg/kg/day (18 times, on a mg/m^2 basis, the daily dose of 200 mg for 60-kg patient), benign lung tumors (small adenomas) occurred more frequently in female mice receiving the highest dose than in untreated control animals. There was no increase in malignant or total (benign plus malignant) lung tumors, nor in the overall incidence of tumors or malignant tumors. This 21-month study was repeated in CD-1 mice, and no statistically or biologically significant differences were observed between treated and control mice of either sex for any type of tumor.

All genotoxicity tests performed on metoprolol tartrate (a dominant lethal study in mice, chromosome studies in somatic cells, a *Salmonella*/mammalian-microsome mutagenicity test, and a nucleus anomaly test in somatic interphase nuclei) and metoprolol succinate (a *Salmonella*/mammalian-microsome mutagenicity test) were negative.

No evidence of impaired fertility due to metoprolol tartrate was observed in a study performed in rats at doses up to 22 times, on a mg/m^2 basis, the daily dose of 200 mg in a 60-kg patient.

Pregnancy Category C
Metoprolol tartrate has been shown to increase post-implantation loss and decrease neonatal survival in rats at doses up to 22 times, on a mg/m^2 basis, the daily dose of 200 mg in a 60-kg patient. Distribution studies in mice confirm exposure of the fetus when metoprolol tartrate is administered to the pregnant animal. These studies have revealed no evidence of impaired fertility or teratogenicity. There are no adequate and well-controlled studies in pregnant women. Because animal reproduction studies are not always predictive of human response, this drug should be used during pregnancy only if clearly needed.

Nursing Mothers
Metoprolol is excreted in breast milk in very small quantities. An infant consuming 1 liter of breast milk daily would receive a dose of less than 1 mg of the drug. Caution should be exercised when TOPROL-XL is administered to a nursing woman.

Pediatric Use
Safety and effectiveness in pediatric patients have not been established.

Geriatric Use
Clinical studies of TOPROL-XL in hypertension did not include sufficient numbers of subjects aged 65 and over to determine whether they respond differently from younger subjects. Other reported clinical experience in hypertensive patients has not identified differences in responses between elderly and younger patients.

Of the 1,990 patients with heart failure randomized to TOPROL-XL in the MERIT-HF trial, 50% (990) were 65 years of age and older and 12% (238) were 75 years of age and older. There were no notable differences in efficacy or the rate of adverse events between older and younger patients.

In general, dose selection for an elderly patient should be cautious, usually starting at the low end of the dosing range, reflecting greater frequency of decreased hepatic, renal, or cardiac function, and of concomitant disease or other drug therapy.

Risk of Anaphylactic Reactions
While taking beta-blockers, patients with a history of severe anaphylactic reactions to a variety of allergens may be more reactive to repeated challenge, either accidental, diagnostic, or therapeutic. Such patients may be unresponsive to the usual doses of epinephrine used to treat allergic reaction.

ADVERSE REACTIONS

Hypertension and Angina
Most adverse effects have been mild and transient. The following adverse reactions have been reported for immediate release metoprolol tartrate.

Central Nervous System: Tiredness and dizziness have occurred in about 10 of 100 patients. Depression has been reported in about 5 of 100 patients. Mental confusion and short-term memory loss have been reported. Headache, somnolence, nightmares, and insomnia have also been reported.

Cardiovascular: Shortness of breath and bradycardia have occurred in approximately 3 of 100 patients. Cold extremities; arterial insufficiency, usually of the Raynaud type; palpitations; congestive heart failure; peripheral edema; syncope; chest pain; and hypotension have been reported in about 1 of 100 patients (see CONTRAINDICATIONS, WARNINGS, and PRECAUTIONS).

Respiratory: Wheezing (bronchospasm) and dyspnea have been reported in about 1 of 100 patients (see WARNINGS).

Gastrointestinal: Diarrhea has occurred in about 5 of 100 patients. Nausea, dry mouth, gastric pain, constipation, flatulence, digestive tract disorders, and heartburn have been reported in about 1 of 100 patients.

Hypersensitive Reactions: Pruritus or rash have occurred in about 5 of 100 patients. Worsening of psoriasis has also been reported.

Miscellaneous: Peyronie's disease has been reported in fewer than 1 of 100,000 patients. Musculoskeletal pain, blurred vision, decreased libido and tinnitus have also been reported.

There have been rare reports of reversible alopecia, agranulocytosis, and dry eyes. Discontinuation of the drug should be considered if any such reaction is not otherwise explicable. The oculomucocutaneous syndrome associated with the beta-blocker practolol has not been reported with metoprolol.

Potential Adverse Reactions
A variety of adverse reactions not listed above have been reported with other beta-adrenergic blocking agents and should be considered potential adverse reactions to TOPROL-XL.

Central Nervous System: Reversible mental depression progressing to catatonia; an acute reversible syndrome characterized by disorientation for time and place, short-term memory loss, emotional lability, slightly clouded sensorium, and decreased performance on neuropsychometrics.

Cardiovascular: Intensification of AV block (see CONTRAINDICATIONS).

Hematologic: Agranulocytosis, nonthrombocytopenic purpura, thrombocytopenic purpura.

Hypersensitive Reactions: Fever combined with aching and sore throat, laryngospasm, and respiratory distress.

Heart Failure
In the MERIT-HF study, serious adverse events and adverse events leading to discontinuation of study medication were systematically collected. In the MERIT-HF study comparing TOPROL-XL in daily doses up to 200 mg (mean dose 159 mg once-daily) (n=1990) to placebo (n=2001), 10.3% of TOPROL-XL patients discontinued for adverse events vs. 12.2% of placebo patients.

The table below lists adverse events in the MERIT-HF study that occurred at an incidence of equal to or greater than 1% in the TOPROL-XL group and greater than placebo by more than 0.5%, regardless of the assessment of causality.

Adverse Events Occurring in the MERIT-HF Study at an Incidence ≥ 1% in the TOPROL-XL Group and Greater Than Placebo by More Than 0.5%

	TOPROL-XL N=1990 % of patients	Placebo N=2001 % of patients
Dizziness/vertigo	1.8	1.0
Bradycardia	1.5	0.4
Accident and/or injury	1.4	0.8

Other adverse events with an incidence of > 1% on TOPROL-XL and as common on placebo (within 0.5%) included myocardial infarction, pneumonia, cerebrovascular disorder, chest pain, dyspnea/dyspnea aggravated, syncope, coronary artery disorder, ventricular tachycardia/arrhythmia aggravated, hypotension, diabetes mellitus/diabetes mellitus aggravated, abdominal pain, and fatigue.

Post-Marketing Experience
The following adverse reactions have been reported with TOPROL-XL in worldwide post-marketing use, regardless of causality:

Cardiovascular: 2nd and 3rd degree heart block.
Gastrointestinal: hepatitis, vomiting.
Hematologic: thrombocytopenia.
Musculoskeletal: arthralgia.
Nervous System/Psychiatric: anxiety/nervousness, hallucinations, paresthesia.
Reproductive, male: impotence.
Skin: increased sweating, photosensitivity.
Special Sense Organs: taste disturbances.

OVERDOSAGE

Acute Toxicity
There have been a few reports of overdosage with TOPROL-XL and no specific overdosage information was obtained with this drug, with the exception of animal toxicology data. However, since TOPROL-XL (metoprolol succinate salt) contains the same active moiety, metoprolol, as conventional metoprolol tablets (metoprolol tartrate salt), the recommendations on overdosage for metoprolol conventional tablets are applicable to TOPROL-XL.

Signs and Symptoms
Overdosage of TOPROL-XL may lead to severe hypotension, sinus bradycardia, atrioventricular block, heart failure, cardiogenic shock, cardiac arrest, bronchospasm, impairment of consciousness/coma, nausea, vomiting, and cyanosis.

Treatment
In general, patients with acute or recent myocardial infarction or congestive heart failure may be more hemodynamically unstable than other patients and should be treated accordingly. When possible the patient should be treated under intensive care conditions. On the basis of the pharmacologic actions of metoprolol, the following general measures should be employed:

Elimination of the Drug: Gastric lavage should be performed.
Bradycardia: Atropine should be administered. If there is no response to vagal blockade, isoproterenol should be administered cautiously.
Hypotension: A vasopressor should be administered, eg, levarterenol or dopamine.
Bronchospasm: A beta$_2$-stimulating agent and/or a theophylline derivative should be administered.
Cardiac Failure: A digitalis glycoside and diuretics should be administered. In shock resulting from inadequate cardiac contractility, administration of dobutamine, isoproterenol, or glucagon may be considered.

DOSAGE AND ADMINISTRATION

TOPROL-XL is an extended release tablet intended for once-a-day administration. When switching from immediate release metoprolol tablet to TOPROL-XL, the same total daily dose of TOPROL-XL should be used.

As with immediate release metoprolol, dosages of TOPROL-XL should be individualized and titration may be needed in some patients.

TOPROL-XL tablets are scored and can be divided; however, the whole or half tablet should be swallowed whole and not chewed or crushed.

Hypertension
The usual initial dosage is 50 to 100 mg daily in a single dose, whether used alone or added to a diuretic. The dosage may be increased at weekly (or longer) intervals until optimum blood pressure reduction is achieved. In general, the maximum effect of any given dosage level will be apparent after 1 week of therapy. Dosages above 400 mg per day have not been studied.

Angina Pectoris
The dosage of TOPROL-XL should be individualized. The usual initial dosage is 100 mg daily, given in a single dose. The dosage may be gradually increased at weekly intervals until optimum clinical response has been obtained or there is a pronounced slowing of the heart rate. Dosages above 400 mg per day have not been studied. If treatment is to be discontinued, the dosage should be reduced gradually over a period of 1–2 weeks (see WARNINGS).

Heart Failure
Dosage must be individualized and closely monitored during up-titration. Prior to initiation of TOPROL-XL, the dosing of diuretics, ACE inhibitors, and digitalis (if used) should be stabilized. The recommended starting dose of TOPROL-XL is 25 mg once daily for two weeks in patients with NYHA class II heart failure and 12.5 mg once daily in patients with more severe heart failure. The dose should then be doubled every two weeks to the highest dosage level tolerated by the patient or up to 200 mg of TOPROL-XL. If transient worsening of heart failure occurs, it may be treated with increased doses of diuretics, and it may also be necessary to lower the dose of TOPROL-XL or temporarily discontinue it. The dose of TOPROL-XL should not be increased until symptoms of worsening heart failure have been stabilized. Initial difficulty with titration should not preclude later attempts to introduce TOPROL-XL. If heart failure patients experience symptomatic bradycardia, the dose of TOPROL-XL should be reduced.

HOW SUPPLIED

Tablets containing metoprolol succinate equivalent to the indicated weight of metoprolol tartrate, USP, are white, biconvex, film-coated, and scored.
[See table below]
Store at 25°C (77°F). Excursions permitted to 15–30°C (59–86°F). (See USP Controlled Room Temperature.)
All trademarks are the property of the AstraZeneca group
© AstraZeneca 2002
Manufactured for: AstraZeneca LP
Wilmington, DE 19850
By: AstraZeneca AB
S-151 85 Södertälje, Sweden
Made in Sweden
64200-00
Rev. 11/02

Tablet	Shape	Engraving	Bottle of 100 NDC 0186-	Unit Dose Packages of 100 NDC 0186-
25 mg*	Oval	A B	1088-05	1088-39
50 mg	Round	A mo	1090-05	1090-39
100 mg	Round	A ms	1092-05	1092-39
200 mg	Oval	A my	1094-05	N/A

* The 25 mg tablet is scored on both sides.

XYLOCAINE® FOR VENTRICULAR ARRHYTHMIAS
[zī'lo-caine]
(lidocaine HCl Injection, USP)

℞

Prescribing information for this product, which appears on pages 648–650 of the 2003 PDR, has been revised as follows. Please write "See Supplement A" next to the product heading.

DOSAGE AND ADMINISTRATION
The following text was added as a new second paragraph:
Continuous Intravenous Infusion
Following bolus administration, intravenous infusions of Xylocaine may be initiated at the rate of 1 to 4 mg/min of lidocaine hydrochloride (0.014 to 0.057 mg/kg/min; 0.006 to 0.026 mg/lb/min). The rate of intravenous infusions should be reassessed as soon as the patient's basic cardiac rhythm appears to be stable or at the earliest signs of toxicity. It should rarely be necessary to continue intravenous infusions for lidocaine for prolonged periods.
New Revision number 721679-05 Rev. 08/02.

AstraZeneca Pharmaceuticals LP
1800 CONCORD PIKE
WILMINGTON, DE 19850-5437 USA

For Product and Business Information, and Adverse Drug Experiences:
Information Center
1-800-236-9933

For Product Ordering:
Trade Customer Service
1-800-842-9920

Internet: www.astrazeneca-us.com

TABLETS

ARIMIDEX®   ℞
[ă-rĭ-mĭ-děx]
Anastrozole

Prescribing information for this product, which appears on pages 653–656 of the 2003 PDR, has been completely revised as follows. Please write "See Supplement A" next to the product heading.

DESCRIPTION
ARIMIDEX® (anastrozole) tablets for oral administration contain 1 mg of anastrozole, a non-steroidal aromatase inhibitor. It is chemically described as 1,3-Benzenediacetonitrile, $\alpha, \alpha, \alpha', \alpha'$-tetramethyl-5-(1H-1,2,4-triazol-1-ylmethyl). Its molecular formula is $C_{17}H_{19}N_5$ and its structural formula is:

Anastrozole is an off-white powder with a molecular weight of 293.4. Anastrozole has moderate aqueous solubility (0.5 mg/mL at 25°C); solubility is independent of pH in the physiological range. Anastrozole is freely soluble in methanol, acetone, ethanol, and tetrahydrofuran, and very soluble in acetonitrile.

Each tablet contains as inactive ingredients: lactose, magnesium stearate, hydroxypropylmethylcellulose, polyethylene glycol, povidone, sodium starch glycolate, and titanium dioxide.

CLINICAL PHARMACOLOGY
Mechanism of Action
Many breast cancers have estrogen receptors and growth of these tumors can be stimulated by estrogen. In postmenopausal women, the principal source of circulating estrogen (primarily estradiol) is conversion of adrenally-generated androstenedione to estrone by aromatase in peripheral tissues, such as adipose tissue, with further conversion of estrone to estradiol. Many breast cancers also contain aromatase; the importance of tumor-generated estrogens is uncertain.

Treatment of breast cancer has included efforts to decrease estrogen levels, by ovariectomy premenopausally and by use of anti-estrogens and progestational agents both pre- and post-menopausally; and these interventions lead to decreased tumor mass or delayed progression of tumor growth in some women.

Anastrozole is a potent and selective non-steroidal aromatase inhibitor. It significantly lowers serum estradiol concentrations and has no detectable effect on formation of adrenal corticosteroids or aldosterone.

Table 1 - Demographic and Baseline Characteristics for ATAC Trial

Demographic Characteristic	ARIMIDEX 1 mg (*N=3125)	Tamoxifen 20 mg (*N=3116)	ARIMIDEX 1 mg plus Tamoxifen 20 mg (*N=3125)
Mean Age (yrs.)	64.1	64.1	64.3
Age Range (yrs.)	38.1–92.8	32.8–94.9	37.0–92.2
Age Distribution (%)			
<45 yrs.	0.7	0.4	0.5
45-60 yrs.	34.6	35.0	34.5
>60 <70 yrs.	38.0	37.1	37.7
>70 yrs.	26.7	27.4	27.3
Mean Weight (kg)	70.8	71.1	71.3
Receptor Status (%)			
Positive[1]	83.5	83.1	83.8
Negative[2]	7.4	8.0	7.0
Other[3]	8.8	8.6	9.1
Other Treatment (%) prior to Randomization			
Mastectomy	47.8	47.3	48.1
Breast conservation[4]	52.3	52.8	52
Axillary surgery	95.5	95.7	95.2
Radiotherapy	63.3	62.5	62.0
Chemotherapy	22.3	20.8	20.8
Neoadjuvant Tamoxifen	1.6	1.6	1.7
Primary Tumor Size (%)			
T1 (≤2 cm)	63.9	62.9	64.1
T2 (>2 cm and ≤5 cm)	32.6	34.2	32.9
T3 (>5 cm)	2.7	2.2	2.3
Nodal Status (%)			
Node positive	34.9	33.6	33.5
1-3 (# of nodes)	24.4	24.4	24.3
4-9	7.5	6.4	6.8
>9	2.9	2.7	2.3
Tumor Grade (%)			
Well-differentiated	20.8	20.5	21.2
Moderately differentiated	46.8	47.8	46.6
Poorly/undifferentiated	23.7	23.3	23.7
Not assessed/recorded	8.7	8.4	8.5

[1] Includes patients who were estrogen receptor (ER) positive or progesterone receptor (PgR) positive, or both positive
[2] Includes patients with both ER negative and PgR negative receptor status
[3] Includes all other combinations of ER and PgR receptor status unknown
[4] Among the patients who had breast conservation, radiotherapy was administered to 95.0% of patients in the ARIMIDEX arm, 94.1% in the tamoxifen arm and 94.5% in the ARIMIDEX plus tamoxifen arm.
*N=Number of patients randomized to the treatment

Pharmacokinetics
Inhibition of aromatase activity is primarily due to anastrozole, the parent drug. Studies with radiolabeled drug have demonstrated that orally administered anastrozole is well absorbed into the systemic circulation with 83 to 85% of the radiolabel recovered in urine and feces. Food does not affect the extent of absorption. Elimination of anastrozole is primarily via hepatic metabolism (approximately 85%) and to a lesser extent, renal excretion (approximately 11%), and anastrozole has a mean terminal elimination half-life of approximately 50 hours in postmenopausal women. The major circulating metabolite of anastrozole, triazole, lacks pharmacologic activity. The pharmacokinetic parameters are similar in patients and in healthy postmenopausal volunteers. The pharmacokinetics of anastrozole are linear over the dose range of 1 to 20 mg and do not change with repeated dosing. Consistent with the approximately 2-day terminal elimination half-life, plasma concentrations approach steady-state levels at about 7 days of once daily dosing and steady-state levels are approximately three- to four-fold higher than levels observed after a single dose of ARIMIDEX. Anastrozole is 40% bound to plasma proteins in the therapeutic range.

Metabolism and Excretion
Studies in postmenopausal women demonstrated that anastrozole is extensively metabolized with about 10% of the dose excreted in the urine as unchanged drug within 72 hours of dosing, and the remainder (about 60% of the dose) is excreted in urine as metabolites. Metabolism of anastrozole occurs by N-dealkylation, hydroxylation and glucuronidation. Three metabolites of anastrozole have been identified in human plasma and urine. The known metabolites are triazole, a glucuronide conjugate of hydroxyanastrozole, and a glucuronide of anastrozole itself. Several minor (less than 5% of the radioactive dose) metabolites have not been identified.

Because renal elimination is not a significant pathway of elimination, total body clearance of anastrozole is unchanged even in severe (creatinine clearance less than 30 mL/min/1.73m^2) renal impairment, dosing adjustment in patients with renal dysfunction is not necessary (see Special Populations and DOSAGE AND ADMINISTRATION sections). Dosage adjustment is also unnecessary in patients with stable hepatic cirrhosis (see Special Populations and DOSAGE AND ADMINISTRATION sections).

Special Populations
Geriatric
Anastrozole pharmacokinetics have been investigated in postmenopausal female volunteers and patients with breast cancer. No age related effects were seen over the range <50 to >80 years.

Continued on next page

Arimidex—Cont.

Race
Estradiol and estrone sulfate levels were similar between Japanese and Caucasian postmenopausal women who received 1 mg of anastrozole daily for 16 days. Anastrozole mean steady-state minimum plasma concentrations in Caucasian and Japanese postmenopausal women were 25.7 and 30.4 ng/mL, respectively.

Renal Insufficiency
Anastrozole pharmacokinetics have been investigated in subjects with renal insufficiency. Anastrozole renal clearance decreased proportionally with creatinine clearance and was approximately 50% lower in volunteers with severe renal impairment (creatinine clearance <30 mL/min/1.73m^2) compared to controls. Since only about 10% of anastrozole is excreted unchanged in the urine, the reduction in renal clearance did not influence the total body clearance (see DOSAGE AND ADMINISTRATION).

Hepatic Insufficiency
Hepatic metabolism accounts for approximately 85% of anastrozole elimination. Anastrozole pharmacokinetics have been investigated in subjects with hepatic cirrhosis related to alcohol abuse. The apparent oral clearance (CL/F) of anastrozole was approximately 30% lower in subjects with stable hepatic cirrhosis than in control subjects with normal liver function. However, plasma anastrozole concentrations in the subjects with hepatic cirrhosis were within the range of concentrations seen in normal subjects across all clinical trials (see DOSAGE AND ADMINISTRATION), so that no dosage adjustment is needed.

Drug-Drug Interactions
Anastrozole inhibited reactions catalyzed by cytochrome P450 1A2, 2C8/9, and 3A4 *in vitro* with Ki values which were approximately 30 times higher than the mean steady-state C_{max} values observed following a 1 mg daily dose. Anastrozole had no inhibitory effect on reactions catalyzed by cytochrome P450 2A6 or 2D6 *in vitro*. Administration of a single 30 mg/kg or multiple 10 mg/kg doses of anastrozole to healthy subjects had no effect on the clearance of antipyrine or urinary recovery of antipyrine metabolites. Based on these *in vitro* and *in vivo* results, it is unlikely that co-administration of ARIMIDEX 1 mg with other drugs will result in clinically significant inhibition of cytochrome P450 mediated metabolism.

In a study conducted in 16 male volunteers, anastrozole did not alter the pharmacokinetics as measured by C_{max} and AUC, and anticoagulant activity as measured by prothrombin time, activated partial thromboplastine time, and thrombin time of both R- and S-warfarin.

Co-administration of anastrozole and tamoxifen in breast cancer patients reduced anastrozole plasma concentration by 27% compared to those achieved with anastrozole alone; however, the co-administration did not affect the pharmacokinetics of tamoxifen or N-desmethyltamoxifen (see **PRECAUTIONS—Drug Interactions**).

Pharmacodynamics
Effect on Estradiol: Mean serum concentrations of estradiol were evaluated in multiple daily dosing trials with 0.5, 1, 3, 5, and 10 mg of ARIMIDEX in postmenopausal women with advanced breast cancer. Clinically significant suppression of serum estradiol was seen with all doses. Doses of 1 mg and higher resulted in suppression of mean serum concentrations of estradiol to the lower limit of detection (3.7 pmol/L). The recommended daily dose, ARIMIDEX 1 mg, reduced estradiol by approximately 70% within 24 hours and by approximately 80% after 14 days of daily dosing. Suppression of serum estradiol was maintained for up to 6 days after cessation of daily dosing with ARIMIDEX 1 mg.

Effect on Corticosteroids: In multiple daily dosing trials with 3, 5, and 10 mg, the selectivity of anastrozole was assessed by examining effects on corticosteroid synthesis. For all doses, anastrozole did not affect cortisol or aldosterone secretion at baseline or in response to ACTH. No glucocorticoid or mineralocorticoid replacement therapy is necessary with anastrozole.

Other Endocrine Effects: In multiple daily dosing trials with 5 and 10 mg, thyroid stimulating hormone (TSH) was measured; there was no increase in TSH during the administration of ARIMIDEX. ARIMIDEX does not possess direct progestogenic, androgenic, or estrogenic activity in animals, but does perturb the circulating levels of progesterone, androgens, and estrogens.

Clinical Studies

Adjuvant Treatment of Breast Cancer in Postmenopausal Women: A multicenter, double-blind trial (ATAC) randomized 9,366 postmenopausal women with operable breast cancer to adjuvant treatment with ARIMIDEX 1 mg daily, tamoxifen 20 mg daily, or a combination of the two treatments for five years or until recurrence of the disease. At the time of the efficacy analysis, women had received a median of 31 months of treatment and had been followed for recurrence-free survival for a median of 33 months.

The primary endpoint of the trial is recurrence-free survival, ie, time to occurrence of a distant or local recurrence, or contralateral breast primary or death from any cause. Time to distant recurrence and the incidence of contralateral breast primaries were analyzed.

Demographic and other baseline characteristics were similar among the three treatment groups (see Table 1).

[See table 1 at top of previous page]

The recommended duration of tamoxifen therapy is five years; continued benefit of tamoxifen after 3 years has been documented. The results of the ATAC trial in a patient population treated for a median 31 months, thus allow only a preliminary comparison of ARIMIDEX and tamoxifen therapy. At this time, recurrence-free survival was improved in the ARIMIDEX arm compared to the tamoxifen arm: Hazard Ratio (HR) = 0.83, 95% CI 0.71-0.96, p=0.0144. Results were essentially the same in the hormone receptor positive patients (about 84% of the patients): HR = 0.78, 95% CI 0.65-0.93.

Recurrence-free survival in the combination treatment arm was similar to that in the tamoxifen group.

Duration of follow-up in this ongoing trial is too short to permit a mature survival analysis. The duration of therapy on the study arms and frequency of individual events comprising recurrence are described in Table 2.

[See table 2 above]

First Line Therapy in Postmenopausal Women with Advanced Breast Cancer: Two double-blind, well-controlled clinical studies of similar design (0030, a North American study and 0027, a predominately European study) were conducted to assess the efficacy of ARIMIDEX compared with tamoxifen as first-line therapy for hormone receptor positive or hormone receptor unknown locally advanced or metastatic breast cancer in postmenopausal women. A total of 1021 patients between the ages of 30 and 92 years old were randomized to receive trial treatment. Patients were randomized to receive 1 mg of ARIMIDEX once daily or 20 mg of tamoxifen once daily. The primary end points for both trials were time to tumor progression, objective tumor response rate, and safety.

Demographics and other baseline characteristics, including patients who had measurable and no measurable disease, patients who were given previous adjuvant therapy, the site of metastatic disease and ethnic origin were similar for the two treatment groups for both trials. The following table summarizes the hormone receptor status at entry for all randomized patients in trials 0030 and 0027.

[See table 3 above]

For the primary endpoints, trial 0030 showed ARIMIDEX was at least as effective as tamoxifen for objective tumor response rate. ARIMIDEX had a statistically significant advantage over tamoxifen (p=0.006) for time to tumor progression (see Table 4 and Figure 1). Trial 0027 showed ARIMIDEX was at least as effective as tamoxifen for objective tumor response rate and time to tumor progression (see Table 4 and Figure 2).

Table 2—ATAC Endpoint Summary

	ARIMIDEX 1 mg (N=3125)	Tamoxifen 20 mg (N=3116)	ARIMIDEX 1 mg plus Tamoxifen 20 mg (N=3125)
Median Duration of Therapy (mo.)[1]	30.9	30.7	30.4
Range Duration of Therapy (mo.)	<1 to 55.3	<1 to 55.7	<1 to 54.5
Median Efficacy Follow-Up (mo.)	33.6	33.2	32.9
Range Follow-Up (mo.)	<1 to 55.2	<1 to 55.7	<1 to 54.4
Recurrence-Free Survival			
First Event (n,%)	318 (10.2)	379 (12.2)	383 (12.3)
Locoregional[2]	67 (2.1)	83 (2.7)	81 (2.6)
Distant	157 (5.0)	181 (5.8)	202 (6.5)
New Contralateral Primaries	14 (0.4)	33 (1.1)	28 (0.9)
Invasive	9 (0.3)	30 (1.0)	23 (0.7)
Ductal carcinoma in situ	5 (0.2)	3 (<0.1)	5 (0.2)
Deaths[3]			
Death — breast cancer	4 (0.12)	1 (0.03)	0 (0.00)
Death — other reason	76 (2.4)	81 (2.6)	72 (2.3)

[1] Based on treatment received
[2] Includes new primary ipsilateral breast cancer (including DCIS), and recurrences at the chest wall, axillary and other regional lymph nodes
[3] Includes only deaths that were first events

Table 3
Number (%) of subjects

	Trial 0030		Trial 0027	
	ARIMIDEX 1 mg (n=171)	Tamoxifen 20 mg (n=182)	ARIMIDEX 1 mg (n=340)	Tamoxifen 20 mg (n=328)
Receptor status				
ER+ and/or PgR+	151 (88.3)	162 (89.0)	154 (45.3)	144 (43.9)
ER unknown, PgR unknown	19 (11.1)	20 (11.0)	185 (54.4)	183 (55.8)

ER = Estrogen receptor
PgR = Progesterone receptor

Table 4

End point	Trial 0030		Trial 0027	
	ARIMIDEX 1 mg (n=171)	Tamoxifen 20 mg (n=182)	ARIMIDEX 1 mg (n=340)	Tamoxifen 20 mg (n=328)
Time to progression (TTP)				
Median TTP (months)	11.1	5.6	8.2	8.3
Number (%) of subjects who progressed	114 (67%)	138 (76%)	249 (73%)	247 (75%)
Hazard ratio (LCL)[1]	1.42 (1.15)		1.01 (0.87)	
2-sided 95% CI	(1.11, 1.82)		(0.85, 1.20)	
p-value[2]	0.006		0.920	
Best objective response rate				
Number (%) of subjects with CR + PR	36 (21.1%)	31 (17.0%)	112 (32.9%)	107 (32.6%)
Odds Ratio (LCL)[3]	1.30 (0.83)		1.01 (0.77)	

CR = Complete Response
PR = Partial Response
CI = Confidence Interval
LCL = Lower Confidence Limit
[1] Tamoxifen:ARIMIDEX
[2] Two-sided Log Rank
[3] ARIMIDEX:Tamoxifen

Table 4 below summarizes the results of trial 0030 and trial 0027 for the primary efficacy endpoints.
[See table 4 at top of previous page]

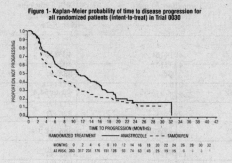

Figure 1- Kaplan-Meier probability of time to disease progression for all randomized patients (intent-to-treat) in Trial 0030

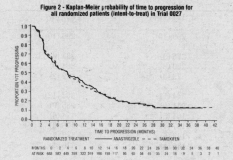

Figure 2 - Kaplan-Meier probability of time to progression for all randomized patients (intent-to-treat) in Trial 0027

Results from the secondary endpoints of time to treatment failure, duration of tumor response, and duration of clinical benefit were supportive of the results of the primary efficacy endpoints. There were too few deaths occurring across treatment groups of both trials to draw conclusions on overall survival differences.

Second Line Therapy in Postmenopausal Women with Advanced Breast Cancer who had Disease Progression following Tamoxifen Therapy: Anastrozole was studied in two well-controlled clinical trials (0004, a North American study; 0005, a predominately European study) in postmenopausal women with advanced breast cancer who had disease progression following tamoxifen therapy for either advanced or early breast cancer. Some of the patients had also received previous cytotoxic treatment. Most patients were ER-positive; a smaller fraction were ER-unknown or ER-negative; the ER-negative patients were eligible only if they had had a positive response to tamoxifen. Eligible patients with measurable and non-measurable disease were randomized to receive either a single daily dose of 1 mg or 10 mg of ARIMIDEX or megestrol acetate 40 mg four times a day. The studies were double-blinded with respect to ARIMIDEX. Time to progression and objective response (only patients with measurable disease could be considered partial responders) rates were the primary efficacy variables. Objective response rates were calculated based on the Union Internationale Contre le Cancer (UICC) criteria. The rate of prolonged (more than 24 weeks) stable disease, the rate of progression, and survival were also calculated.

Both trials included over 375 patients; demographics and other baseline characteristics were similar for the three treatment groups in each trial. Patients in the 0005 trial had responded better to prior tamoxifen treatment. Of the patients entered who had prior tamoxifen therapy for advanced disease (58% in Trial 0004; 57% in Trial 0005), 18% of these patients in Trial 0004 and 42% in Trial 0005 were reported by the primary investigator to have responded. In Trial 0004, 81% of patients were ER-positive, 13% were ER-unknown, and 6% were ER-negative. In Trial 0005, 58% of patients were ER-positive, 37% were ER-unknown, and 5% were ER-negative. In Trial 0004, 62% of patients had measurable disease compared to 79% in Trial 0005. The sites of metastatic disease were similar among treatment groups for each trial. On average, 40% of the patients had soft tissue metastases; 60% had bone metastases; and 40% had visceral (15% liver) metastases.

As shown in the table below, similar results were observed among treatment groups and between the two trials. None of the within-trial differences were statistically significant.
[See table 5 above]

More than 1/3 of the patients in each treatment group in both studies had either an objective response or stabilization of their disease for greater than 24 weeks. Among the 263 patients who received ARIMIDEX 1 mg, there were 11 complete responders and 22 partial responders. In patients who had an objective response, more than 80% were still responding at 6 months from randomization and more than 45% were still responding at 12 months from randomization.

When data from the two controlled trials are pooled, the objective response rates and median times to progression and death were similar for patients randomized to ARIMIDEX 1 mg and megestrol acetate. There is, in this data, no indication that ARIMIDEX 10 mg is superior to ARIMIDEX 1 mg.
[See table 6 above]

Objective response rates and median times to progression and death for ARIMIDEX 1 mg were similar to megestrol acetate for women over or under 65. There were too few non-white patients studied to draw conclusions about racial differences in response.

Table 5

	ARIMIDEX 1 mg	ARIMIDEX 10 mg	Megestrol Acetate 160 mg
Trial 0004 (N. America)	(n=128)	(n=130)	(n=128)
Median Follow-up (months)*	31.3	30.9	32.9
Median Time to Death (months)	29.6	25.7	26.7
2 Year Survival Probability (%)	62.0	58.0	53.1
Median Time to Progression (months)	5.7	5.3	5.1
Objective Response (all patients) (%)	12.5	10.0	10.2
Stable Disease for >24 weeks (%)	35.2	29.2	32.8
Progression (%)	86.7	85.4	90.6
Trial 0005 (Europe, Australia, S. Africa)	(n=135)	(n=118)	(n=125)
Median Follow-up (months)*	31.0	30.9	31.5
Median Time to Death (months)	24.3	24.8	19.8
2 Year Survival Probability (%)	50.5	50.9	39.1
Median Time to Progression (months)	4.4	5.3	3.9
Objective Response (all patients) (%)	12.6	15.3	14.4
Stable Disease for >24 weeks (%)	24.4	25.4	23.2
Progression (%)	91.9	89.8	92.0

*Surviving Patients

Table 6

Trials 0004 & 0005 (Pooled Data)	ARIMIDEX 1 mg N=263	ARIMIDEX 10 mg N=248	Megestrol Acetate 160 mg N=253
Median Time to Death (months)	26.7	25.5	22.5
2 Year Survival Probability (%)	56.1	54.6	46.3
Median Time to Progression (months)	4.8	5.3	4.6
Objective Response (all patients) (%)	12.5	12.5	12.3

INDICATIONS AND USAGE

ARIMIDEX is indicated for adjuvant treatment of postmenopausal women with hormone receptor positive early breast cancer.

The effectiveness of ARIMIDEX in early breast cancer is based on an analysis of recurrence-free survival in patients treated for a median of 31 months (see **CLINICAL PHARMACOLOGY—Clinical Studies** subsection). Further follow-up of study patients will be required to determine long-term outcomes.

ARIMIDEX is indicated for the first-line treatment of postmenopausal women with hormone receptor positive or hormone receptor unknown locally advanced or metastatic breast cancer.

ARIMIDEX is indicated for the treatment of advanced breast cancer in postmenopausal women with disease progression following tamoxifen therapy. Patients with ER-negative disease and patients who did not respond to previous tamoxifen therapy rarely responded to ARIMIDEX.

CONTRAINDICATIONS

ARIMIDEX is contraindicated in any patient who has shown a hypersensitivity reaction to the drug or to any of the excipients.

WARNINGS

ARIMIDEX can cause fetal harm when administered to a pregnant woman. Anastrozole has been found to cross the placenta following oral administration of 0.1 mg/kg in rats and rabbits (about 1 and 1.9 times the recommended human dose, respectively, on a mg/m^2 basis). Studies in both rats and rabbits at doses equal to or greater than 0.1 and 0.02 mg/kg/day, respectively (about 1 and 1/3, respectively, the recommended human dose on a mg/m^2 basis), administered during the period of organogenesis showed that anastrozole increased pregnancy loss (increased pre- and/or post-implantation loss, increased resorption, and decreased numbers of live fetuses); effects were dose related in rats. Placental weights were significantly increased in rats at doses of 0.1 mg/kg/day or more.

Evidence of fetotoxicity, including delayed fetal development (i.e., incomplete ossification and depressed fetal body weights), was observed in rats administered doses of 1 mg/kg/day (which produced plasma anastrozole C_{ssmax} and AUC$_{0-24 hr}$ that were 19 times and 9 times higher than the respective values found in postmenopausal volunteers at the recommended dose). There was no evidence of teratogenicity in rats administered doses up to 1.0 mg/kg/day. In rabbits, anastrozole caused pregnancy failure at doses equal to or greater than 1.0 mg/kg/day (about 16 times the recommended human dose on a mg/m^2 basis); there was no evidence of teratogenicity in rabbits administered 0.2 mg/kg/day (about 3 times the recommended human dose on a mg/m^2 basis).

There are no adequate and well-controlled studies in pregnant women using ARIMIDEX. If ARIMIDEX is used during pregnancy, or if the patient becomes pregnant while receiving this drug, the patient should be apprised of the potential hazard to the fetus or potential risk for loss of the pregnancy.

PRECAUTIONS

General

Before starting treatment with ARIMIDEX, pregnancy must be excluded (see WARNINGS). ARIMIDEX should be administered under the supervision of a qualified physician experienced in the use of anticancer agents.

Laboratory Tests

During the ATAC trial, more patients receiving ARIMIDEX were reported to have an elevated serum cholesterol compared to patients receiving tamoxifen (7% versus 3%, respectively).

Drug Interactions

(See **CLINICAL PHARMACOLOGY**) Anastrozole inhibited *in vitro* metabolic reactions catalyzed by cytochromes P450 1A2, 2C8/9, and 3A4 but only at relatively high concentrations. Anastrozole did not inhibit P450 2A6 or the polymorphic P450 2D6 in human liver microsomes. Anastrozole did not alter the pharmacokinetics of antipyrine. Although there have been no formal interaction studies other than with antipyrine, based on these *in vivo* and *in vitro* studies, it is unlikely that co-administration of a 1 mg dose of ARIMIDEX with other drugs will result in clinically significant drug inhibition of cytochrome P450-mediated metabolism of the other drugs.

An interaction study with warfarin showed no clinically significant effect of anastrozole on warfarin pharmacokinetics or anticoagulant activity.

Clinical and pharmacokinetic results from the ATAC trial suggest that tamoxifen should not be administered with anastrozole (see **CLINICAL PHARMACOLOGY — Drug Interactions and Clinical Studies** subsections). Co-administration of anastrozole and tamoxifen resulted in a reduction of anastrozole plasma levels by 27% compared with those achieved with anastrozole alone.

Estrogen-containing therapies should not be used with ARIMIDEX as they may diminish its pharmacologic action.

Drug/Laboratory Test Interactions

No clinically significant changes in the results of clinical laboratory tests have been observed.

Carcinogenesis

A conventional carcinogenesis study in rats at doses of 1.0 to 25 mg/kg/day (about 10 to 243 times the daily maximum recommended human dose on a mg/m^2 basis) administered by oral gavage for up to 2 years revealed an increase in the incidence of hepatocellular adenoma and carcinoma and uterine stromal polyps in females and thyroid adenoma in males at the high dose. A dose related increase was observed in the incidence of ovarian and uterine hyperplasia in females. At 25 mg/kg/day, plasma AUC$_{0-24hr}$ levels in rats were 110 to 125 times higher than the level exhibited in postmenopausal volunteers at the recommended dose. A separate carcinogenesis study in mice at oral doses of 5 to 50 mg/kg/day (about 24 to 243 times the daily maximum recommended human dose on a mg/m^2 basis) for up to 2 years produced an increase in the incidence of benign ovarian stromal, epithelial and granulosa cell tumors at all dose levels. A dose related increase in the incidence of ovarian hyperplasia was also observed in female mice. These ovar-

Continued on next page

Arimidex—Cont.

ian changes are considered to be rodent-specific effects of aromatase inhibition and are of questionable significance to humans. The incidence of lymphosarcoma was increased in males and females at the high dose. At 50 mg/kg/day, plasma AUC levels in mice were 35 to 40 times higher than the level exhibited in postmenopausal volunteers at the recommended dose.

Mutagenesis
ARIMIDEX has not been shown to be mutagenic in *in vitro* tests (Ames and E. coli bacterial tests, CHO-K1 gene mutation assay) or clastogenic either *in vitro* (chromosome aberrations in human lymphocytes) or *in vivo* (micronucleus test in rats).

Impairment of Fertility
Oral administration of anastrozole to female rats (from 2 weeks before mating to pregnancy day 7) produced significant incidence of infertility and reduced numbers of viable pregnancies at 1 mg/kg/day (about 10 times the recommended human dose on a mg/m^2 basis and 9 times higher than the AUC_{0-24hr} found in postmenopausal volunteers at the recommended dose). Pre-implantation loss of ova or fetus was increased at doses equal to or greater than 0.02 mg/kg/day (about one-fifth the recommended human dose on a mg/m^2 basis). Recovery of fertility was observed following a 5-week non-dosing period which followed 3 weeks of dosing. It is not known whether these effects observed in female rats are indicative of impaired fertility in humans.

Multiple-dose studies in rats administered anastrozole for 6 months at doses equal to or greater than 1 mg/kg/day (which produced plasma anastrozole C_{ssmax} and AUC_{0-24hr} that were 19 and 9 times higher than the respective values found in postmenopausal volunteers at the recommended dose) resulted in hypertrophy of the ovaries and the presence of follicular cysts. In addition, hyperplastic uteri were observed in 6-month studies in female dogs administered doses equal to or greater than 1 mg/kg/day (which produced plasma anastrozole C_{ssmax} and AUC_{0-24hr} that were 22 times and 16 times higher than the respective values found in postmenopausal women at the recommended dose). It is not known whether these effects on the reproductive organs of animals are associated with impaired fertility in premenopausal women.

Pregnancy
Pregnancy Category D (See **WARNINGS**)

Nursing Mothers
It is not known if anastrozole is excreted in human milk. Because many drugs are excreted in human milk, caution should be exercised when ARIMIDEX is administered to a nursing woman (see WARNINGS and PRECAUTIONS).

Pediatric Use
The safety and efficacy of ARIMIDEX in pediatric patients have not been established.

Geriatric Use
In studies 0030 and 0027 about 50% of patients were 65 or older. Patients ≥ 65 years of age had moderately better tumor response and time to tumor progression than patients < 65 years of age regardless of randomized treatment. In studies 0004 and 0005 50% of patients were 65 or older. Response rates and time to progression were similar for the over 65 and younger patients. In the ATAC adjuvant study, 35% of patients were < 60 years of age; 38% were ≥ 60 to ≤ 70 years of age; and 27% were > 70 years of age. The number of events by age group was insufficient to perform a subset efficacy analysis.

ADVERSE REACTIONS
Adjuvant Therapy
The median duration of adjuvant treatment for safety evaluation was 37.3 months, 36.9 months, and 36.5 months for patients receiving ARIMIDEX 1 mg, tamoxifen 20 mg, and the combination of ARIMIDEX 1 mg plus tamoxifen 20 mg, respectively.

Adverse events occurring with an incidence of at least 5% in any treatment group during treatment or within 14 days of the end of treatment are presented in Table 7.
[See table 7 above]

Non-pathologic fractures were reported more frequently in the ARIMIDEX-treated patients (219 [7%]) than in the tamoxifen-treated patients (137 [4%]).

Certain adverse events and combinations of adverse events were prospectively specified for analysis, based on the known pharmacologic properties and side effect profiles of the two drugs (see table 8). Patients receiving ARIMIDEX had an increase in musculoskeletal events and fractures (including fractures of spine, hip and wrist) compared with patients receiving tamoxifen. Patients receiving ARIMIDEX had a decrease in hot flashes, vaginal bleeding, vaginal discharge, endometrial cancer, venous thromboembolic events (including deep venous thrombosis) and ischemic cerebrovascular events compared with patients receiving tamoxifen.
[See table 8 above]

Angina pectoris was reported more frequently in the ARIMIDEX-treated patients (52 [1.7%]) than in the tamoxifen-treated patients (30 [1.0%]); the incidence of myocardial infarction was comparable (ARIMIDEX 24 patients [0.8%]; tamoxifen 25 patients [0.8%]).

Table 7 — Adverse events occurring with an incidence of at least 5% in any treatment group during treatment, or within 14 days of the end of treatment

Body system and adverse event by COSTART-preferred term*	ARIMIDEX 1 mg (N = 3092)	Tamoxifen 20 mg (N = 3093)	ARIMIDEX 1 mg plus Tamoxifen 20 mg (N = 3098)
Body as a whole			
Asthenia	512 (17)	491 (16)	468 (15)
Pain	461 (15)	435 (14)	407 (13)
Back pain	256 (8)	255 (8)	258 (8)
Headache	277 (9)	216 (7)	214 (7)
Abdominal pain	227 (7)	228 (7)	219 (7)
Infection	223 (7)	225 (7)	211 (7)
Accidental injury	221 (7)	221 (7)	226 (7)
Flu syndrome	154 (5)	170 (5)	170 (5)
Chest pain	164 (5)	122 (4)	152 (5)
Cardiovascular			
Vasodilatation	1082 (35)	1246 (40)	1261 (41)
Hypertension	292 (9)	252 (8)	270 (9)
Digestive			
Nausea	307 (10)	298 (10)	324 (10)
Constipation	201 (7)	214 (7)	232 (7)
Diarrhea	227 (7)	186 (6)	193 (6)
Dyspepsia	166 (5)	137 (4)	156 (5)
Gastrointestinal disorder	155 (5)	122 (4)	127 (4)
Hemic and lymphatic			
Lymphoedema	267 (9)	299 (10)	296 (10)
Metabolic and nutritional			
Peripheral edema	255 (8)	275 (9)	281 (9)
Weight gain	253 (8)	250 (8)	264 (9)
Hypercholesteremia	210 (7)	79 (3)	72 (2)
Musculoskeletal			
Arthritis	431 (14)	344 (11)	364 (12)
Arthralgia	390 (13)	251 (8)	265 (9)
Osteoporosis	229 (7)	161 (5)	174 (6)
Fracture	219 (7)	137 (4)	178 (6)
Bone pain	165 (5)	149 (5)	143 (5)
Arthrosis	179 (6)	136 (4)	119 (4)
Nervous system			
Depression	348 (11)	341 (11)	342 (11)
Insomnia	266 (9)	245 (8)	227 (7)
Dizziness	198 (6)	207 (7)	190 (6)
Anxiety	168 (5)	157 (5)	140 (5)
Paraesthesia	195 (6)	116 (4)	120 (4)
Respiratory			
Pharyngitis	376 (12)	359 (12)	350 (11)
Cough increased	212 (7)	237 (8)	203 (7)
Dyspnea	186 (6)	185 (6)	175 (6)
Skin and appendages			
Rash	300 (10)	331 (11)	326 (11)
Sweating	121 (4)	165 (5)	142 (5)
Urogenital			
Leukorrhea	75 (2)	265 (9)	277 (9)
Urinary tract infection	192 (6)	252 (8)	228 (7)
Breast pain	205 (7)	136 (4)	182 (6)
Vulvovaginitis	180 (6)	134 (4)	134 (4)

COSTART Coding Symbols for Thesaurus of Adverse Reaction Terms.
N = Number of patients receiving the treatment.
*A patient may have had more than 1 adverse event, including more than 1 adverse event in the same body system.

Table 8 — Number (%) of patients with Pre-specified Adverse Event in ATAC Trial

	ARIMIDEX N=3092 (%)	Tamoxifen N=3093 (%)	Odds-ratio	95% CI
All Fractures	224 (7)	145 (5)	1.59	1.28 – 1.97
Fractures of Spine, Hip, Wrist	89 (3)	62 (2)	1.45	1.04 – 2.04
Musculo-skeletal disorders[1]	940 (30)	737 (24)	1.41	1.28 – 1.55
Ischemic Cardiovascular Disease	92 (3)	74 (2)	1.25	0.91 – 1.72
Asthenia	513 (17)	491 (16)	1.05	0.93 – 1.20
Nausea and Vomiting	348 (11)	342 (11)	1.02	0.88 – 1.19
Mood Disturbances	521 (17)	511 (17)	1.02	0.90 – 1.16
Cataracts	128 (4)	140 (5)	0.91	0.71 – 1.17
Hot Flashes	1082 (35)	1246 (40)	0.80	0.73 – 0.87
Venous Thromboembolic events	73 (2)	120 (4)	0.60	0.44 – 0.81
Deep Venous Thromboembolic Events	40 (1)	60 (2)	0.66	0.43 – 1.00
Ischemic Cerebrovascular Event	40 (1)	74 (2)	0.53	0.35 – 0.80
Vaginal Bleeding	147 (5)	270 (9)	0.52	0.42 – 0.64
Vaginal Discharge	94 (3)	378 (12)	0.23	0.18 – 0.28
Endometrial Cancer	3 (0.1)	15 (0.5)	0.20	0.04 – 0.70

[1]Refers to joint symptoms, including arthritis, arthrosis and arthralgia.

Preliminary results from the ATAC trial bone substudy demonstrated that patients receiving ARIMIDEX had a mean decrease in both lumbar spine and total hip bone mineral density (BMD) compared to baseline. Patients receiving tamoxifen had a mean increase in both lumbar spine and total hip BMD compared to baseline.

First Line Therapy

ARIMIDEX was generally well tolerated in two well-controlled clinical trials (ie, Trials 0030 and 0027). Adverse events occurring with an incidence of at least 5% in either treatment group of trials 0030 and 0027 during or within 2 weeks of the end of treatment are shown in Table 9.

Table 9

Body system Adverse event[a]	Number (%) of subjects ARIMIDEX (n=506)	Tamoxifen (n=511)
Whole body		
Asthenia	83 (16)	81 (16)
Pain	70 (14)	73 (14)
Back pain	60 (12)	68 (13)
Headache	47 (9)	40 (8)
Abdominal pain	40 (8)	38 (7)
Chest pain	37 (7)	37 (7)
Flu syndrome	35 (7)	30 (6)
Pelvic pain	23 (5)	30 (6)
Cardiovascular		
Vasodilation	128 (25)	106 (21)
Hypertension	25 (5)	36 (7)
Digestive		
Nausea	94 (19)	106 (21)
Constipation	47 (9)	66 (13)
Diarrhea	40 (8)	33 (6)
Vomiting	38 (8)	36 (7)
Anorexia	26 (5)	46 (9)
Metabolic and nutritional		
Peripheral edema	51 (10)	41 (8)
Musculoskeletal		
Bone pain	54 (11)	52 (10)
Nervous		
Dizziness	30 (6)	22 (4)
Insomnia	30 (6)	38 (7)
Depression	23 (5)	32 (6)
Hypertonia	16 (3)	26 (5)
Respiratory		
Cough increased	55 (11)	52 (10)
Dyspnea	51 (10)	47 (9)
Pharyngitis	49 (10)	68 (13)
Skin and appendages		
Rash	38 (8)	34 (8)
Urogenital		
Leukorrhea	9 (2)	31 (6)

[a] A patient may have had more than 1 adverse event.

Less frequent adverse experiences reported in patients receiving ARIMIDEX 1 mg in either Trial 0030 or Trial 0027 were similar to those reported for second-line therapy.

Based on results from second-line therapy and the established safety profile of tamoxifen, the incidences of 9 prespecified adverse event categories potentially causally related to one or both of the therapies because of their pharmacology were statistically analyzed. No significant differences were seen between treatment groups.

Table 10
Number (n) and Percentage of Patients

Adverse Event Group[a]	ARIMIDEX 1 mg (n = 506) n	(%)	NOLVADEX 20 mg (n = 511) n	(%)
Depression	23	(5)	32	(6)
Tumor Flare	15	(3)	18	(4)
Thromboembolic Disease[a]	18	(4)	33	(6)
Venous[b]	5		15	
Coronary and Cerebral[c]	13		19	
Gastrointestinal Disturbance	170	(34)	196	(38)
Hot Flushes	134	(26)	118	(23)
Vaginal Dryness	9	(2)	3	(1)
Lethargy	6	(1)	15	(3)
Vaginal Bleeding	5	(1)	11	(2)
Weight Gain	11	(2)	8	(2)

[a] A patient may have had more than 1 adverse event

[b] Includes pulmonary embolus, thrombophlebitis, retinal vein thrombosis

[c] Includes myocardial infarction, myocardial ischemia, angina pectoris, cerebrovascular accident, cerebral ischemia and cerebral infarct

Despite the lack of estrogenic activity for ARIMIDEX, there was no increase in myocardial infarction or fracture when compared with tamoxifen.

Second Line Therapy

ARIMIDEX was generally well tolerated in two well-controlled clinical trials (ie, Trials 0004 and 0005), with less than 3.3% of the ARIMIDEX-treated patients and 4.0% of the megestrol acetate-treated patients withdrawing due to an adverse event.

The principal adverse event more common with ARIMIDEX than megestrol acetate was diarrhea. Adverse events reported in greater than 5% of the patients in any of the treatment groups in these two well-controlled clinical trials, regardless of causality, are presented below:

Table 11
Number (n) and Percentage of Patients with Adverse Event†

Adverse Event	ARIMIDEX 1 mg (n = 262) n	%	ARIMIDEX 10 mg (n = 246) n	%	Megestrol Acetate 160 mg (n = 253) n	%
Asthenia	42	(16)	33	(13)	47	(19)
Nausea	41	(16)	48	(20)	28	(11)
Headache	34	(13)	44	(18)	24	(9)
Hot Flashes	32	(12)	29	(11)	21	(8)
Pain	28	(11)	38	(15)	29	(11)
Back Pain	28	(11)	26	(11)	19	(8)
Dyspnea	24	(9)	27	(11)	53	(21)
Vomiting	24	(9)	26	(11)	16	(6)
Cough Increased	22	(8)	18	(7)	19	(8)
Diarrhea	22	(8)	18	(7)	7	(3)
Constipation	18	(7)	18	(7)	21	(8)
Abdominal Pain	18	(7)	14	(6)	18	(7)
Anorexia	18	(7)	19	(8)	11	(4)
Bone Pain	17	(6)	26	(12)	19	(8)
Pharyngitis	16	(6)	23	(9)	15	(6)
Dizziness	16	(6)	12	(5)	15	(6)
Rash	15	(6)	15	(6)	19	(8)
Dry Mouth	15	(6)	11	(4)	13	(5)
Peripheral Edema	14	(5)	21	(9)	28	(11)
Pelvic Pain	14	(5)	17	(7)	13	(5)
Depression	14	(5)	6	(2)	5	(2)
Chest Pain	13	(5)	18	(7)	13	(5)
Paresthesia	12	(5)	15	(6)	9	(4)
Vaginal Hemorrhage	6	(2)	4	(2)	13	(5)
Weight Gain	4	(2)	9	(4)	30	(12)
Sweating	4	(2)	3	(1)	16	(6)
Increased Appetite	0	(0)	1	(0)	13	(5)

†A patient may have more than one adverse event.

Other less frequent (2% to 5%) adverse experiences reported in patients receiving ARIMIDEX 1 mg in either Trial 0004 or Trial 0005 are listed below. These adverse experiences are listed by body system and are in order of decreasing frequency within each body system regardless of assessed causality.

Body as a Whole: Flu syndrome; fever; neck pain; malaise; accidental injury; infection

Cardiovascular: Hypertension; thrombophlebitis

Hepatic: Gamma GT increased; SGOT increased; SGPT increased

Hematologic: Anemia; leukopenia

Metabolic and Nutritional: Alkaline phosphatase increased; weight loss

Mean serum total cholesterol levels increased by 0.5 mmol/L among patients receiving ARIMIDEX. Increases in LDL cholesterol have been shown to contribute to these changes.

Musculoskeletal: Myalgia; arthralgia; pathological fracture

Nervous: Somnolence; confusion; insomnia; anxiety; nervousness

Respiratory: Sinusitis; bronchitis; rhinitis

Skin and Appendages: Hair thinning; pruritus

Urogenital: Urinary tract infection; breast pain

The incidences of the following adverse event groups potentially causally related to one or both of the therapies because of their pharmacology, were statistically analyzed: weight gain, edema, thromboembolic disease, gastrointestinal disturbance, hot flushes, and vaginal dryness. These six groups, and the adverse events captured in the groups, were prospectively defined. The results are shown in the table below.

Table 12
Number (n) and Percentage of Patients

Adverse Event Group	ARIMIDEX 1 mg (n = 262) n	(%)	ARIMIDEX 10 mg (n = 246) n	(%)	Megestrol Acetate 160 mg (n = 253) n	(%)
Gastrointestinal Disturbance	77	(29)	81	(33)	54	(21)
Hot Flushes	33	(13)	29	(12)	35	(14)
Edema	19	(7)	28	(11)	35	(14)
Thromboembolic Disease	9	(3)	4	(2)	12	(5)
Vaginal Dryness	5	(2)	3	(1)	2	(1)
Weight Gain	4	(2)	10	(4)	30	(12)

More patients treated with megestrol acetate reported weight gain as an adverse event compared to patients treated with ARIMIDEX 1 mg ($p<0.0001$). Other differences were not statistically significant.

An examination of the magnitude of change in weight in all patients was also conducted. Thirty-four percent (87/253) of the patients treated with megestrol acetate experienced weight gain of 5% or more and 11% (27/253) of the patients treated with megestrol acetate experienced weight gain of 10% or more. Among patients treated with ARIMIDEX 1 mg, 13% [33/262] experienced weight gain of 5% or more and 3% [6/262] experienced weight gain of 10% or more. On average, this 5 to 10% weight gain represented between 6 and 12 pounds.

No patients receiving ARIMIDEX or megestrol acetate discontinued treatment due to drug-related weight gain.

Vaginal bleeding has been reported infrequently, mainly in patients during the first few weeks after changing from existing hormonal therapy to treatment with ARIMIDEX. If bleeding persists, further evaluation should be considered.

During clinical trials and postmarketing experience joint pain/stiffness has been reported in association with the use of ARIMIDEX.

ARIMIDEX may also be associated with rash including very rare cases of mucocutaneous disorders such as erythema multiforme and Stevens-Johnson syndrome.

OVERDOSAGE

Clinical trials have been conducted with ARIMIDEX, up to 60 mg in a single dose given to healthy male volunteers and up to 10 mg daily given to postmenopausal women with advanced breast cancer; these dosages were well tolerated. A single dose of ARIMIDEX that results in life-threatening symptoms has not been established. In rats, lethality was observed after single oral doses that were greater than 100 mg/kg (about 800 times the recommended human dose on a mg/m^2 basis) and was associated with severe irritation to the stomach (necrosis, gastritis, ulceration, and hemorrhage).

In an oral acute toxicity study in the dog the median lethal dose was greater than 45 mg/kg/day.

There is no specific antidote to overdosage and treatment must be symptomatic. In the management of an overdose, consider that multiple agents may have been taken. Vomiting may be induced if the patient is alert. Dialysis may be helpful because ARIMIDEX is not highly protein bound. General supportive care, including frequent monitoring of vital signs and close observation of the patient, is indicated.

DOSAGE AND ADMINISTRATION

The dose of ARIMIDEX is one 1 mg tablet taken once a day. For patients with advanced breast cancer, ARIMIDEX should be continued until tumor progression.

For adjuvant treatment of early breast cancer in postmenopausal women, the optimal duration of therapy is unknown. The median duration of therapy at the time of data analysis was 31 months; the ongoing ATAC trial is planned for five years of treatment.

Patients with Hepatic Impairment

(See **CLINICAL PHARMACOLOGY**) Hepatic metabolism accounts for approximately 85% of anastrozole elimination. Although clearance of anastrozole was decreased in patients with cirrhosis due to alcohol abuse, plasma anastrozole concentrations stayed in the usual range seen in patients without liver disease. Therefore, no changes in dose are recommended for patients with mild-to-moderate hepatic impairment, although patients should be monitored for side effects. ARIMIDEX has not been studied in patients with severe hepatic impairment.

Patients with Renal Impairment

No changes in dose are necessary for patients with renal impairment.

Use in the Elderly

No dosage adjustment is necessary.

HOW SUPPLIED

White, biconvex, film-coated tablets containing 1 mg of anastrozole. The tablets are impressed on one side with a logo consisting of a letter "A" (upper case) with an arrowhead attached to the foot of the extended right leg of the "A" and on the reverse with the tablet strength marking "Adx 1". These tablets are supplied in bottles of 30 tablets (NDC 0310-0201-30).

Storage

Store at controlled room temperature, 20–25°C (68–77°F) [see USP].

AstraZeneca Pharmaceuticals LP
Wilmington, DE 19850

All trademarks are the property of the AstraZeneca group
© AstraZeneca 2002

Revised Rev 09-02 (ATAC) SIC No. 64206-00

FASLODEX® ℞

[fās'lō-dĕks]

fulvestrant injection

Prescribing information for this product, which appears on pages 668–670 of the 2003 PDR, has been completely revised as follows. Please write "See Supplement A" next to the product heading.

DESCRIPTION

FASLODEX® (fulvestrant) Injection for intramuscular administration is an estrogen receptor antagonist without known agonist effects. The chemical name is 7-alpha-[9-(4,4,5,5,5-penta fluoropentylsulphinyl) nonyl]estra-1,3,5-

Continued on next page

Faslodex—Cont.

(10)- triene-3,17-beta-diol. The molecular formula is $C_{32}H_{47}F_5O_3S$ and its structural formula is:

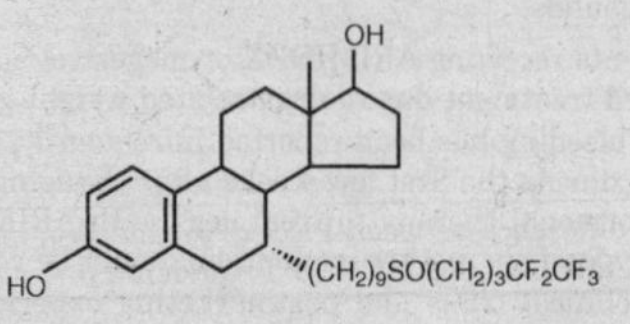

Fulvestrant is a white powder with a molecular weight of 606.77. The solution for injection is a clear, colorless to yellow, viscous liquid.

Each injection contains as inactive ingredients: Alcohol, USP, Benzyl Alcohol, NF, and Benzyl Benzoate, USP, as co-solvents, and Castor Oil, USP as a co-solvent and release rate modifier.

FASLODEX is supplied in sterile single patient pre-filled syringes containing 50-mg/mL fulvestrant either as a single 5 mL or two concurrent 2.5 mL injections to deliver the required monthly dose. FASLODEX is administered as an intramuscular injection of 250 mg once monthly.

CLINICAL PHARMACOLOGY

Mechanism of Action

Many breast cancers have estrogen receptors (ER), and the growth of these tumors can be stimulated by estrogen. Fulvestrant is an estrogen receptor antagonist that binds to the estrogen receptor in a competitive manner with affinity comparable to that of estradiol. Fulvestrant down regulates the ER protein in human breast cancer cells.

In a clinical study in postmenopausal women with primary breast cancer treated with single doses of FASLODEX 15–22 days prior to surgery, there was evidence of increasing down regulation of ER with increasing dose. This was associated with a dose-related decrease in the expression of the progesterone receptor, an estrogen-regulated protein. These effects on the ER pathway were also associated with a decrease in Ki67 labeling index, a marker of cell proliferation.

In vitro studies demonstrated that fulvestrant is a reversible inhibitor of the growth of tamoxifen-resistant, as well as estrogen-sensitive human breast cancer (MCF-7) cell lines. In *in vivo* tumor studies, fulvestrant delayed the establishment of tumors from xenografts of human breast cancer MCF-7 cells in nude mice. Fulvestrant inhibited the growth of established MCF-7 xenografts and of tamoxifen-resistant breast tumor xenografts. Fulvestrant resistant breast tumor xenografts may also be cross-resistant to tamoxifen.

Fulvestrant showed no agonist-type effects in *in vivo* uterotropic assays in immature or ovariectomized mice and rats. In *in vivo* studies in immature rats and ovariectomized monkeys, fulvestrant blocked the uterotrophic action of estradiol. In postmenopausal women, the absence of changes in plasma concentrations of FSH and LH in response to fulvestrant treatment (250 mg monthly) suggests no peripheral steroidal effects.

Pharmacokinetics

Following intravenous administration, fulvestrant is rapidly cleared at a rate approximating hepatic blood flow (about 10.5 mL plasma/min/Kg). After an intramuscular injection plasma concentrations are maximal at about 7 days and are maintained over a period of at least one month, with trough concentration about one-third of C_{max}. The apparent half-life was about 40 days. After administration of 250 mg of fulvestrant intramuscularly every month, plasma levels approach steady-state after 3 to 6 doses, with an average 2.5 fold increase in plasma AUC, compared to single dose AUC and trough levels about equal to the single dose C_{max} (see **Table 1**).

[See table 1 above]

Table 1: Summary of fulvestrant pharmacokinetic parameters in postmenopausal advanced breast cancer patients after intramuscular administration of a 250 mg dose (Mean ± SD)

	C_{max} ng/mL	C_{min} ng/mL	AUC ng.d/mL	$t_{1/2}$ days	CL mL/min
Single dose	8.5 ± 5.4	2.6 ± 1.1	131 ± 62	40 ± 11	690 ± 226
Multiple dose steady state	15.8 ± 2.4	7.4 ± 1.7	328 ± 48		

Fulvestrant was subject to extensive and rapid distribution. The apparent volume of distribution at steady state was approximately 3 to 5 L/kg. This suggests that distribution is largely extravascular. Fulvestrant was highly (99%) bound to plasma proteins; VLDL, LDL and HDL lipoprotein fractions appear to be the major binding components. The role of sex hormone-binding globulin, if any, could not be determined.

Metabolism and Excretion

Biotransformation and disposition of fulvestrant in humans have been determined following intramuscular and intravenous administration of ^{14}C-labeled fulvestrant. Metabolism of fulvestrant appears to involve combinations of a number of possible biotransformation pathways analogous to those of endogenous steroids, including oxidation, aromatic hydroxylation, conjugation with glucuronic acid and/or sulphate at the 2, 3 and 17 positions of the steroid nucleus, and oxidation of the side chain sulphoxide. Identified metabolites are either less active or exhibit similar activity to fulvestrant in antiestrogen models. Studies using human liver preparations and recombinant human enzymes indicate that cytochrome P-450 3A4 (CYP 3A4) is the only P-450 isoenzyme involved in the oxidation of fulvestrant; however, the relative contribution of P-450 and non-P-450 routes *in vivo* is unknown.

Fulvestrant was rapidly cleared by the hepatobiliary route, with excretion primarily via the feces (approximately 90%). Renal elimination was negligible (less than 1%).

Table 2: Study Population Demographics

Parameter	North American Trial FASLODEX 250 mg	North American Trial Anastrozole 1 mg	European Trial FASLODEX 250 mg	European Trial Anastrozole 1 mg
No. of Participants	206	194	222	229
Median Age (yrs)	64	61	64	65
Age Range (yrs)	33–89	36–94	35–86	33–89
Receptor Status # (%)				
ER Positive	170 (83%)	156 (80%)	156 (70%)	173 (76%)
ER/PgR Positive	179 (87%)	169 (87%)	163 (73%)	183 (80%)
ER/PgR Unknown	13 (6%)	15 (8%)	51 (23%)	37 (16%)
Previous Therapy				
Tamoxifen	196 (95%)	187 (96%)	215 (97%)	225 (98%)
Adjuvant antiestrogen only	94 (46%)	94 (48%)	95 (43%)	100 (44%)
Antiestrogen for advanced disease +/- adjuvant use	110 (53%)	97 (50%)	126 (57%)	129 (56%)
Cytotoxic Chemotherapy	129 (63%)	122 (63%)	94 (42%)	98 (43%)
Site of Metastases				
Visceral only*	39 (19%)	45 (23%)	30 (14%)	41 (18%)
Visceral Liver involvement	47 (23%)	45 (23%)	48 (22%)	56 (24%)
Visceral Lung involvement	63 (31%)	60 (31%)	56 (25%)	60 (26%)
Bone only	47 (23%)	43 (22%)	38 (17%)	40 (17%)
Soft Tissue only	12 (6%)	13 (7%)	11 (5%)	8 (3%)
Skin and soft tissue	43 (21%)	41 (21%)	40 (18%)	35 (15%)

*Defined as liver or lung metastatic, or recurrent, disease
ER/PgR Positive defined as ER positive or PgR positive
ER/PgR Unknown defined as ER unknown and PgR unknown

Special Populations

Geriatric: In patients with breast cancer, there was no difference in fulvestrant pharmacokinetic profile related to age (range 33 to 89 years).

Gender: Following administration of a single intravenous dose, there were no pharmacokinetic differences between men and women or between premenopausal and postmenopausal women. Similarly, there were no differences between men and postmenopausal women after intramuscular administration.

Race: In the advanced breast cancer treatment trials, the potential for pharmacokinetic differences due to race have been evaluated in 294 women including 87.4% Caucasian, 7.8% Black, and 4.4% Hispanic. No differences in fulvestrant plasma pharmacokinetics were observed among these groups. In a separate trial, pharmacokinetic data from postmenopausal ethnic Japanese women were similar to those obtained in non-Japanese patients.

Renal Impairment: Negligible amounts of fulvestrant are eliminated in urine; therefore, a study in patients with renal impairment was not conducted. In the advanced breast cancer trials, fulvestrant concentrations in women with estimated creatinine clearance as low as 30 mL/min were similar to women with normal creatinine.

Hepatic Impairment: Fulvestrant is metabolized primarily in the liver. In clinical trials in patients with locally advanced or metastatic breast cancer, pharmacokinetic data were obtained following administration of a 250 mg dose of FASLODEX to 261 patients classified as having normal liver function and to 24 patients with mild impairment. Mild impairment was defined as an alanine aminotransferase concentration (at any visit) greater than the upper limit of the normal (ULN) reference range, but less than 2 times the ULN; or if any 2 of the following 3 parameters were between 1- and 2-times the ULN: aspartate aminotransferase, alkaline phosphatase, or total bilirubin.

There was no clear relationship between fulvestrant clearance and hepatic impairment and the safety profile in patients with mild hepatic impairment was similar to that seen in patients with no hepatic impairment. Safety and efficacy have not been evaluated in patients with moderate to severe hepatic impairment (see **PRECAUTIONS-Hepatic Impairment** and **DOSAGE AND ADMINISTRATION-Hepatic Impairment** sections).

Pediatric: The pharmacokinetics of fulvestrant have not been evaluated in pediatric patients.

Drug-Drug Interactions

There are no known drug-drug interactions. Fulvestrant does not significantly inhibit any of the major CYP isoenzymes, including CYP 1A2, 2C9, 2C19, 2D6, and 3A4 *in vitro*, and studies of co-administration of fulvestrant with midazolam indicate that therapeutic doses of fulvestrant have no inhibitory effects on CYP 3A4 or alter blood levels of drug metabolized by that enzyme. Also, although fulvestrant is partly metabolized by CYP 3A4, a clinical study with rifampin, an inducer of CYP 3A4, showed no effect on the pharmacokinetics of fulvestrant. Clinical studies of the effect of strong CYP 3A4 inhibitors on the pharmacokinetics of fulvestrant have not been performed.

Clinical Studies

Efficacy of FASLODEX was established by comparison to the selective aromatase inhibitor anastrozole in two randomized, controlled clinical trials (one conducted in North America, the other in predominately Europe) in postmenopausal women with locally advanced or metastatic breast cancer. All patients had progressed after previous therapy with an antiestrogen or progestin for breast cancer in the adjuvant or advanced disease setting. The majority of patients in these trials had ER+ and/or PgR+ tumors. Patients who had ER-/PgR- or unknown disease must have shown prior response to endocrine therapy.

In both trials, eligible patients with measurable and/or evaluable disease were randomized to receive either FASLODEX 250 mg intramuscularly once a month (28 days ± 3 days) or anastrozole 1 mg orally once a day. All patients were assessed monthly for the first three months and every three months thereafter. The North American trial was a double-blind, randomized trial in 400 postmenopausal women. The European trial was an open, randomized trial conducted in 451 patients. Patients on the FASLODEX arm of the North American trial received two separate injections (2 x 2.5 mL), whereas FASLODEX patients received a single injection (1 x 5 mL) in the European trial. In both trials, patients were initially randomized to a 125 mg per month dose as well, but interim analysis showed a very low response rate and low dose groups were dropped.

The effectiveness endpoints were response rates (RR), based on the Union Internationale Contre le Cancer (UICC) criteria, and time to progression (TTP). Survival time was also determined. Confidence intervals (95.4%) were calculated for the difference in RR between the FASLODEX and anastrozole groups. The hazard ratio for an unfavorable event, (such as disease progression or death) between FASLODEX and anastrozole groups was also determined.

Table 2 provides the demographics and baseline characteristics of the postmenopausal women randomized to FASLODEX 250 mg or anastrozole 1 mg.

[See table 2 above]

Results of the trials, after a minimum follow-up duration of 14.6 months, are summarized in Table 3. The effectiveness of FASLODEX 250 mg was determined by comparing RR and TTP results to anastrozole 1 mg, the active control. With respect to response rate, the two studies ruled out (by one-sided 97.7% confidence limit) inferiority of FASLODEX to anastrozole of 6.3% and 1.4%.

[See table 3 at top of next page]

There are no efficacy data for the use of FASLODEX in premenopausal women with advanced breast cancer (women with functioning ovaries as evidenced by menstruation and/or premenopausal LH, FSH and estradiol levels).

INDICATIONS AND USAGE

FASLODEX is indicated for the treatment of hormone receptor positive metastatic breast cancer in postmenopausal women with disease progression following antiestrogen therapy.

CONTRAINDICATIONS

FASLODEX is contraindicated in pregnant women, and in patients with a known hypersensitivity to the drug or to any of its components.

WARNINGS

Women of childbearing potential should be advised not to become pregnant while receiving FASLODEX. FASLODEX can cause fetal harm when administered to a pregnant woman and has been shown to cross the placenta following single intramuscular doses in rats and in rabbits. In studies in the pregnant rat, intramuscular doses of fulvestrant 100 times lower than the maximum recommended human dose (based on body surface area [BSA]), caused an increased incidence of fetal abnormalities and death. Similarly, rabbits failed to maintain pregnancy and the fetuses showed an increased incidence of skeletal variations when fulvestrant was administered at one-half the recommended human dose (based on BSA).

There are no studies in pregnant women using FASLODEX. If FASLODEX is used during pregnancy or if the patient becomes pregnant while receiving this drug, the patient should be apprised of the potential hazard to the fetus, or potential risk for loss of the pregnancy. See **Pregnancy** section of **PRECAUTIONS**.

Because FASLODEX is administered intramuscularly, it should not be used in patients with bleeding diatheses, thrombocytopenia or in patients on anticoagulants.

PRECAUTIONS

General

Before starting treatment with FASLODEX, pregnancy must be excluded (see **WARNINGS**).

Hepatic Impairment

Safety and efficacy have not been evaluated in patients with moderate to severe hepatic impairment (see **CLINICAL PHARMACOLOGY-Hepatic Impairment** and **DOSAGE AND ADMINISTRATION-Hepatic Impairment** sections).

Drug Interactions

Fulvestrant is metabolized by CYP 3A4 *in vitro*. Clinical studies of the effect of strong CYP 3A4 inhibitors on the pharmacokinetics of fulvestrant have not been performed (see **CLINICAL PHARMACOLOGY-Drug-Drug Interactions**).

Carcinogenesis, Mutagenesis and Impairment of Fertility

A two-year carcinogenesis study was conducted in female and male rats, at intramuscular doses of 15 mg/kg/30 days, 10 mg/rat/30 days and 10 mg/rat/15 days. These doses correspond to approximately 1-, 3-, and 5-fold (in females) and 1.3-, 1.3-, and 1.6-fold (in males) the systemic exposure [$AUC_{0-30\ days}$] achieved in women receiving the recommended dose of 250 mg/month. An increased incidence of benign ovarian granulosa cell tumors and testicular Leydig cell tumors was evident, in females dosed at 10 mg/rat/15 days and males dosed at 15 mg/rat/30 days, respectively. Induction of such tumors is consistent with the pharmacology-related endocrine feedback alterations in gonadotropin levels caused by an antiestrogen.

Fulvestrant was not mutagenic or clastogenic in multiple *in vitro* tests with and without the addition of a mammalian liver metabolic activation factor (bacterial mutation assay in strains of Salmonella typhimurium and Escherichia coli, in vitro cytogenetics study in human lymphocytes, mammalian cell mutation assay in mouse lymphoma cells and *in vivo* micronucleus test in rat).

In female rats, fulvestrant administered at doses ≥ 0.01 mg/kg/day (approximately one-hundredth of the human recommended dose based on body surface area [BSA], for 2 weeks prior to and for 1 week following mating, caused a reduction in fertility and embryonic survival). No adverse effects on female fertility and embryonic survival were evident in female animals dosed at 0.001 mg/kg/day (approximately one-thousandth of the human dose based on BSA). Restoration of female fertility to values similar to controls was evident following a 29-day withdrawal period after dosing at 2 mg/kg/day (twice the human dose based on BSA). The effects of fulvestrant on the fertility of female rats appear to be consistent with its antiestrogenic activity. The potential effects of fulvestrant on the fertility of male animals were not studied but, in a 6-month toxicology study, male rats treated with intramuscular doses of 15 mg/kg/30 days, 10 mg/rat/30 days, or 10 mg/rat/15 days fulvestrant showed a loss of spermatozoa from the seminiferous tubules, seminiferous tubular atrophy, and degenerative changes in the epididymides. Changes in the testes and epididymides had not recovered 20 weeks after cessation of dosing. These fulvestrant doses correspond to approximately 2-, 3-, and 3-fold the systemic exposure [$AUC_{0-30\ days}$] achieved in women.

Pregnancy

Pregnancy Category D: (See **WARNINGS**).

In studies in female rats at doses ≥ 0.01 mg/kg/day (IM; approximately one-hundredth of the human recommended dose based on body surface area [BSA]), fulvestrant caused a reversible reduction in female fertility, as well as effects on embryo/fetal development consistent with its antiestrogenic activity. Fulvestrant caused an increased incidence of fetal abnormalities in rats (tarsal flexure of the hind paw at 2 mg/kg/day IM; twice the human dose on BSA) and non-ossification of the odontoid and ventral tubercle of the first cervical vertebra at doses ≥ 0.1 mg/kg/day IM (approximately one-tenth of the human dose on BSA) when administered during the period of organogenesis. Rabbits failed to maintain pregnancy when dosed with 1 mg/kg/day fulvestrant IM (twice the human dose on BSA) during the period of organogenesis. Further, in rabbits dosed at 0.25 mg/kg/day (about one-half the h man dose on BSA), increases in placental weight and post-implantation loss were observed but, there were no observed effects on fetal development. Fulvestrant was associated with an increased incidence of fetal variations in rabbits (backwards displacement of the pelvic girdle, and 27 pre-sacral vertebrae at 0.25 mg/kg/day IM; one-half the human dose on BSA) when administered during the period of organogenesis. Because pregnancy could not be maintained in the rabbit following doses of fulvestrant of 1 mg/kg/day and above, this study was inadequate to fully define the possible adverse effects on fetal development at clinically relevant exposures.

Nursing Mothers

Fulvestrant is found in rat milk at levels significantly higher (approximately 12-fold) than plasma after administration of 2 mg/kg. Drug exposure in rodent pups from fulvestrant-treated lactating dams was estimated as 10% of the administered dose. It is not known if fulvestrant is excreted in human milk. Because many drugs are excreted in human milk, and because of the potential for serious adverse reactions from FASLODEX in nursing infants, a decision should be made whether to discontinue nursing or to discontinue the drug taking into account the importance of the drug to the mother.

Table 3: Efficacy Results

Endpoint	North American Trial: FASLODEX 250 mg (n=206)	North American Trial: Anastrozole 1 mg (n=194)	European Trial: FASLODEX 250 mg (n=222)	European Trial: Anastrozole 1 mg (n=229)
Objective tumor response				
Number (%) of subjects with CR + PR	35 (17.0)	33 (17.0)	45 (20.3)	34 (14.9)
% Difference in Tumor Response Rate				
(FAS-ANA)	0.0		5.4	
2-sided 95.4% CI	(−6.3, 8.9)		(−1.4, 14.8)	
Time to progression (TTP)				
Median TTP (days)	165	103	166	156
Hazard ratio (FAS/ANA)	0.9		1.0	
2-sided 95.4% CI	(0.7, 1.1)		(0.8, 1.2)	
Stable Disease for ≥24 weeks (%)	26.7	19.1	24.3	30.1
Survival Time				
Died n (%)	109 (52.9%)	92 (47.4%)	125 (56.3%)	130 (56.8%)
Median Survival (days)	837	901	803	742
Hazard ratio	1.1		1.0	
2-sided 95% CI	(0.8, 1.5)		(0.8, 1.3)	

CR = Complete Response; PR = Partial Response; CI = Confidence Interval; FAS = FASLODEX; ANA = anastrazole

Pediatric Use

The safety and efficacy of FASLODEX in pediatric patients have not been established.

Geriatric Use

When tumor response was considered by age, objective responses were seen in 24% and 22% of patients under 65 years of age and in 16% and 11% of patients 65 years of age and older, who were treated with FASLODEX in the European and North American trials, respectively.

ADVERSE REACTIONS

The most commonly reported adverse experiences in the FASLODEX and anastrozole treatment groups, regardless of the investigator's assessment of causality, were gastrointestinal symptoms (including nausea, vomiting, constipation, diarrhea and abdominal pain), headache, back pain, vasodilatation (hot flushes), and pharyngitis.

Injection site reactions with mild transient pain and inflammation were seen with FASLODEX and occurred in 7% of patients (1% of treatments) given the single 5 mL injection (predominately European Trial) and in 27% of patients (4.6% of treatments) given the 2 x 2.5 mL injections (North American Trial).

Table 4 lists adverse experiences reported with an incidence of 5% or greater, regardless of assessed causality, from the two controlled clinical trials comparing the administration of FASLODEX 250 mg intramuscularly once a month with anastrozole 1 mg orally once a day.

Table 4: Combined Trials Adverse Events ≥ 5%

Body system and adverse event[a]	FASLODEX 250 mg N=423 (%)	Anastrozole 1 mg N=423 (%)
Body as a whole	68.3	67.6
Asthenia	22.7	27.0
Pain	18.9	20.3
Headache	15.4	16.8
Back pain	14.4	13.2
Abdominal pain	11.8	11.6
Injection site pain*	10.9	6.6
Pelvic pain	9.9	9.0
Chest pain	7.1	5.0
Flu syndrome	7.1	6.4
Fever	6.4	6.4
Accidental injury	4.5	5.7
Cardiovascular system	30.3	27.9
Vasodilatation	17.7	17.3
Digestive system	51.5	48.0
Nausea	26.0	25.3
Vomiting	13.0	11.8
Constipation	12.5	10.6
Diarrhea	12.3	12.8
Anorexia	9.0	10.9
Hemic and lymphatic systems	13.7	13.5
Anemia	4.5	5.0
Metabolic and Nutritional disorders	18.2	17.7
Peripheral edema	9.0	10.2
Musculoskeletal system	25.5	27.9
Bone pain	15.8	13.7
Arthritis	2.8	6.1
Nervous system	34.3	33.8
Dizziness	6.9	6.6
Insomnia	6.9	8.5
Paresthesia	6.4	7.6
Depression	5.7	6.9
Anxiety	5.0	3.8
Respiratory system	38.5	33.6
Pharyngitis	16.1	11.6
Dyspnea	14.9	12.3
Cough increased	10.4	10.4
Skin and appendages	22.2	23.4
Rash	7.3	8.0
Sweating	5.0	5.2
Urogenital system	18.2	14.9
Urinary tract infection	6.1	3.5

[a] A patient may have more than one adverse event.

* All patients on FASLODEX received injections, but only those anastrozole patients who were in the North American study received placebo injections.

Other adverse events reported as drug-related and seen infrequently (<1%) include thromboembolic phenomena, myalgia, vertigo, and leukopenia.

Vaginal bleeding has been reported infrequently (<1%), mainly in patients during the first 6 weeks after changing from existing hormonal therapy to treatment with FASLODEX. If bleeding persists, further evaluation should be considered.

OVERDOSAGE

Animal studies have shown no effects other than those related directly or indirectly to antiestrogen activity with intramuscular doses of fulvestrant higher than the recommended human dose. There is no clinical experience with overdosage in humans. No adverse effects were seen in healthy male and female volunteers who received intravenous fulvestrant, which resulted in peak plasma concentrations at the end of the infusion, that were approximately 10 to 15 times those seen after intramuscular injection.

DOSAGE AND ADMINISTRATION

Adults (including the elderly): The recommended dose is 250 mg to be administered intramuscularly into the buttock at intervals of one month as either a single 5 mL injection or two concurrent 2.5 mL injections (see **HOW SUPPLIED**). The injection should be administered slowly.

Patients with Hepatic Impairment

FASLODEX has not been studied in patients with moderate or severe hepatic compromise. No dosage adjustment is recommended in patients with mild hepatic impairment (see **CLINICAL PHARMACOLOGY-Hepatic Impairment** and **PRECAUTIONS-Hepatic Impairment** sections).

Instructions for Intramuscular use, handling and disposal

1. Remove glass syringe barrel from tray and check that it is not damaged.
2. Remove perforated patient record label from syringe.
3. Peel open the safety needle (SafetyGlide™) outer packaging. For complete SafetyGlide™ instructions refer below to the "Directions for Use of SafetyGlide™."
4. Break the seal of the white plastic cover on the syringe luer connector to remove the cover with the attached rubber tip cap (see Figure 1).
5. Twist to lock the needle to the luer connector.
6. Remove needle sheath.
7. Remove excess gas from the syringe (a small gas bubble may remain).
8. Administer intramuscularly slowly in the buttock.
9. Immediately activate needle protection device upon withdrawal from patient by pushing lever arm completely forward until needle tip is fully covered (see Figure 2).
10. Visually confirm that the lever arm has fully advanced and the needle tip is covered. If unable to activate, discard immediately into an approved sharps collector.
11. Repeat steps 1 through 10 for second syringe.

For the 2 x 2.5 mL syringe package only, both syringes must be administered to receive the 250 mg recommended monthly dose.

SAFETYGLIDE™ INSTRUCTIONS FROM BECTON DICKINSON

SafetyGlide™ is a trademark of Becton Dickinson and Company

Reorder number 305917

CAUTION CONCERNING SAFETYGLIDE™

Federal (USA) law restricts this device to sale by or on the order of a physician. To help avoid HIV (AIDS), HBV (Hepatitis), and other infectious diseases due to accidental needlesticks, contaminated needles should not be recapped or removed, unless there is no alternative or that such action is required by a specific medical procedure.

Continued on next page

Faslodex—Cont.

WARNING CONCERNING SAFETYGLIDE™

Do not autoclave SafetyGlide™ Needle before use. Hands must remain behind the needle at all times during use and disposal.

DIRECTIONS FOR USE OF SAFETYGLIDE™

Peel apart packaging of the SafetyGlide™, break the seal of the white plastic cover on the syringe Luer connector and attach the SafetyGlide™ needle to the Luer Lock of the syringe by twisting.

Transport filled syringe to point of administration.

Pull shield straight off needle to avoid damaging needle point.

Administer injection following package instruction.

For user convenience, the needle 'bevel up' position is orientated to the lever arm, as shown in Figure 3.

Immediately activate needle protection device upon withdrawal from patient by pushing lever arm completely forward until needle tip is fully covered (Figure 2).

Visually confirm that the lever arm has fully advanced and the needle tip is covered. If unable to activate, discard immediately into an approved sharps collector.

Activation of the protective mechanism may cause minimal splatter of fluid that may remain on the needle after injection.

For greatest safety, use a one-handed technique and activate away from self and others.

After single use, discard in an approved sharps collector in accordance with applicable regulations and institutional policy.

Becton Dickinson guarantees the contents of their unopened or undamaged packages to be sterile, nontoxic and nonpyrogenic.

Figure 1

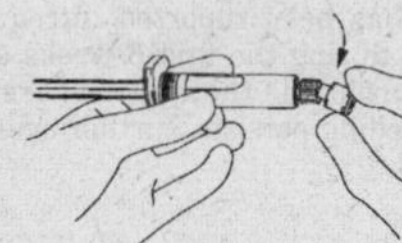

Figure 2

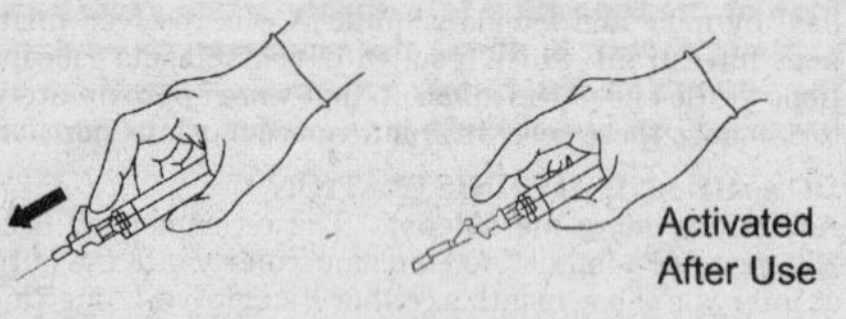

Figure 3

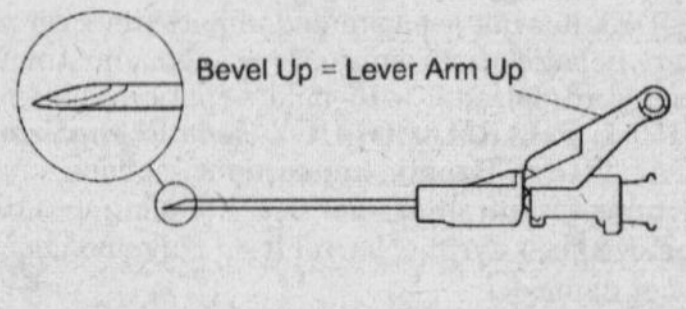

HOW SUPPLIED

One 5 mL clear neutral glass (Type 1) barrel containing 250 mg/5 mL (50 mg/mL) FASLODEX Injection for intramuscular injection and fitted with a tamper evident closure. The syringe is presented in a tray with polystyrene plunger rod and a safety needle (SafetyGlide™) for connection to the barrel.

NDC 0310-0720-50 One 5 mL Prefilled Syringe

Two 5 mL clear neutral glass (Type 1) barrels, each containing 125 mg/2.5 mL (50 mg/mL) of FASLODEX Injection for intramuscular injection and fitted with a tamper-evident closure. The syringes are presented in a tray with polystyrene plunger rod and safety needles (SafetyGlide™) for connection to the barrels.

NDC 0310-0720-25 Two 5 mL Prefilled Syringes each containing 125 mg/2.5 mL

Storage

REFRIGERATE, 2°–8°C (36°–46°F). TO PROTECT FROM LIGHT, STORE IN THE ORIGINAL CARTON UNTIL TIME OF USE.

SafetyGlide™ is a trademark of Becton Dickinson and Company

All other trademarks are the property of the AstraZeneca group

Distributed by:
AstraZeneca Pharmaceuticals LP
Wilmington, DE 19850
Manufactured for:
AstraZeneca UK Ltd.
Macclesfield, England
By: Vetter Pharma-Fertigung GmbH & Co. KG
Ravensburg, Germany
22073-00
Rev 07/02

ZOMIG® ℞

[zō'mig]

(zolmitriptan) TABLETS

ZOMIG-ZMT®

(zolmitriptan) Orally Disintegrating Tablets

Prescribing information for this product, which appears on pages 701–704 of the 2003 PDR, has been completely revised as follows. Please write "See Supplement A" next to the product heading.

DESCRIPTION

ZOMIG® (zolmitriptan) Tablets and ZOMIG-ZMT® (zolmitriptan) Orally Disintegrating Tablets contain zolmitriptan, which is a selective 5-hydroxytryptamine 1B/1D (5-$HT_{1B/1D}$) receptor agonist. Zolmitriptan is chemically designated as (S)-4-[[3-[2-(dimethylamino)ethyl]-1H-indol-5-yl]methyl]-2-oxazolidinone and has the following chemical structure:

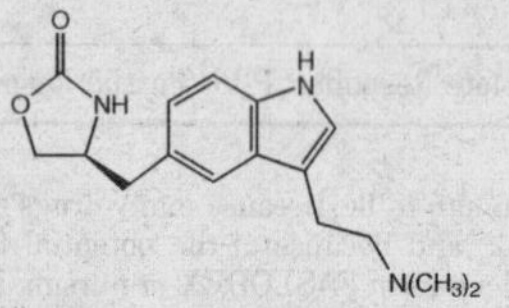

The empirical formula is $C_{16}H_{21}N_3O_2$, representing a molecular weight of 287.36. Zolmitriptan is a white to almost white powder that is readily soluble in water. ZOMIG Tablets are available as 2.5 mg (yellow) and 5 mg (pink) film coated tablets for oral administration. The film coated tablets contain anhydrous lactose NF, microcrystalline cellulose NF, sodium starch glycolate NF, magnesium stearate NF, hydroxypropyl methylcellulose USP, titanium dioxide USP, polyethylene glycol 400 NF, yellow iron oxide NF (2.5 mg tablet), red iron oxide NF (5 mg tablet), and polyethylene glycol 8000 NF.

ZOMIG-ZMT® Orally Disintegrating Tablets are available as 2.5 mg and 5.0 mg white uncoated tablets for oral administration. The orally disintegrating tablets contain mannitol USP, microcrystalline cellulose NF, crospovidone NF, aspartame NF, sodium bicarbonate USP, citric acid anhydrous USP, colloidal silicon dioxide NF, magnesium stearate NF and orange flavor SN 027512.

CLINICAL PHARMACOLOGY

Mechanism of Action

Zolmitriptan binds with high affinity to human recombinant 5-HT_{1D} and 5-HT_{1B} receptors. Zolmitriptan exhibits modest affinity for 5-HT_{1A} receptors, but has no significant affinity (as measured by radioligand binding assays) or pharmacological activity at 5-HT_2, 5-HT_3, 5-HT_4, $alpha_1$-, $alpha_2$- or $beta_1$-adrenergic; H_1, H_2, histaminic; muscarinic; $dopamine_1$, or $dopamine_2$ receptors. The N-desmethyl metabolite also has high affinity for 5-$HT_{1B/1D}$ and modest affinity for 5-HT_{1A} receptors.

Current theories proposed to explain the etiology of migraine headache suggest that symptoms are due to local cranial vasodilatation and/or to the release of sensory neuropeptides (vasoactive intestinal peptide, substance P and calcitonin gene-related peptide) through nerve endings in the trigeminal system. The therapeutic activity of zolmitriptan for the treatment of migraine headache can most likely be attributed to the agonist effects at the 5-$HT_{1B/1D}$ receptors on intracranial blood vessels (including the arterio-venous anastomoses) and sensory nerves of the trigeminal system which result in cranial vessel constriction and inhibition of pro-inflammatory neuropeptide release.

Clinical Pharmacokinetics and Bioavailability:

Zolmitriptan is well absorbed after oral administration for both the conventional tablets and the orally disintegrating tablets. Zolmitriptan displays linear kinetics over the dose range of 2.5 to 50 mg.

The AUC and C_{max} of zolmitriptan are similar following administration of ZOMIG Tablets and ZOMIG-ZMT Orally Disintegrating Tablets, but the T_{max} is somewhat later with ZOMIG-ZMT, with a median T_{max} of 3 hours for the orally disintegrating tablet compared with 1.5 hours for the conventional tablet. The AUC, C_{max}, and T_{max} for the active N-desmethyl metabolite are similar for the two formulations.

During a moderate to severe migraine attack, mean $AUC_{0\text{-}4}$ and C_{max} for zolmitriptan, dosed as a conventional tablet, were decreased by 40% and 25%, respectively, and mean T_{max} was delayed by one-half hour compared to the same patients during a migraine free period.

Food has no significant effect on the bioavailability of zolmitriptan. No accumulation occurred on multiple dosing.

Distribution:

Mean absolute bioavailability is approximately 40%. The mean apparent volume of distribution is 7.0 L/kg. Plasma protein binding of zolmitriptan is 25% over the concentration range of 10–1000ng/mL.

Metabolism:

Zolmitriptan is converted to an active N-desmethyl metabolite such that the metabolite concentrations are about two-thirds that of zolmitriptan. Because the 5$HT_{1B/1D}$ potency of the metabolite is 2 to 6 times that of the parent, the metabolite may contribute a substantial portion of the overall effect after zolmitriptan administration.

Elimination:

Total radioactivity recovered in urine and feces was 65% and 30% of the administered dose, respectively. About 8% of the dose was recovered in the urine as unchanged zolmitriptan. Indole acetic acid metabolite accounted for 31% of the dose, followed by N-oxide (7%) and N-desmethyl (4%) metabolites. The indole acetic acid and N-oxide metabolites are inactive.

Mean total plasma clearance is 31.5mL/min/kg, of which one-sixth is renal clearance. The renal clearance is greater than the glomerular filtration rate suggesting renal tubular secretion.

Special Populations:

Age: Zolmitriptan pharmacokinetics in healthy elderly non-migraineur volunteers (age 65–76 yrs) were similar to those in younger non-migraineur volunteers (age 18–39 yrs).

Gender: Mean plasma concentrations of zolmitriptan were up to 1.5-fold higher in females than males.

Renal Impairment: Clearance of zolmitriptan was reduced by 25% in patients with severe renal impairment (Clcr ≥ 5 ≤ 25 mL/min) compared to the normal group (Clcr > = 70 mL/min); no significant change in clearance was observed in the moderately renally impaired group (Clcr ≥ 26 ≤ 50 mL/min).

Hepatic Impairment: In severely hepatically impaired patients, the mean C_{max}, T_{max}, and $AUC_{0\text{-}\infty}$ of zolmitriptan were increased 1.5, 2 (2 vs 4 hr), and 3-fold, respectively, compared to normals. Seven out of 27 patients experienced 20 to 80 mm Hg elevations in systolic and/or diastolic blood pressure after a 10 mg dose. Zolmitriptan should be administered with caution in subjects with liver disease, generally using doses less than 2.5 mg (see WARNINGS and PRECAUTIONS).

Hypertensive Patients: No differences in the pharmacokinetics of zolmitriptan or its effects on blood pressure were seen in mild to moderate hypertensive volunteers compared to normotensive controls.

Race: Retrospective analysis of pharmacokinetic data between Japanese and Caucasians revealed no significant differences.

Drug Interactions

All drug interaction studies were performed in healthy volunteers using a single 10 mg dose of zolmitriptan and a single dose of the other drug except where otherwise noted.

Fluoxetine: The pharmacokinetics of zolmitriptan, as well as its effect on blood pressure, were unaffected by 4 weeks of pretreatment with oral fluoxetine (20 mg/day).

MAO Inhibitors: Following one week of administration of 150 mg bid moclobemide, a specific MAO-A inhibitor, there was an increase of about 25% in both C_{max} and AUC for zolmitriptan and a 3-fold increase in the C_{max} and AUC of the active N-desmethyl metabolite of zolmitriptan (see CONTRAINDICATIONS and PRECAUTIONS).

Selegiline, a selective MAO-B inhibitor, at a dose of 10 mg/day for 1 week, had no effect on the pharmacokinetics of zolmitriptan and its metabolite.

Propranolol: C_{max} and AUC of zolmitriptan increased 1.5-fold after one week of dosing with propranolol (160 mg/day). C_{max} and AUC of the N-desmethyl metabolite were reduced by 30% and 15%, respectively. There were no interactive effects on blood pressure or pulse rate following administration of propranolol with zolmitriptan.

Acetaminophen: A single 1 g dose of acetaminophen does not alter the pharmacokinetics of zolmitriptan and its N-desmethyl metabolite. However, zolmitriptan delayed the T_{max} of acetaminophen by one hour.

Metoclopramide: A single 10 mg dose of metoclopramide had no effect on the pharmacokinetics of zolmitriptan or its metabolites.

Oral Contraceptives: Retrospective analysis of pharmacokinetic data across studies indicated that mean plasma concentrations of zolmitriptan were generally higher in females taking oral contraceptives compared to those not taking oral contraceptives. Mean C_{max} and AUC of zolmitriptan were found to be higher by 30% and 50%, respectively, and T_{max} was delayed by one-half hour in females taking oral contraceptives. The effect of zolmitriptan on the pharmacokinetics of oral contraceptives has not been studied.

Cimetidine: Following the administration of cimetidine, the half-life and AUC of a 5 mg dose of zolmitriptan and its active metabolite were approximately doubled (see PRECAUTIONS).

Clinical Studies

The efficacy of ZOMIG Tablets in the acute treatment of migraine headaches was demonstrated in five randomized, double-blind, placebo controlled studies, of which 2 utilized the 1 mg dose, 2 utilized the 2.5 mg dose and 4 utilized the 5 mg dose; all studies used the marketed formulation. In study 1, patients treated their headaches in a clinic setting. In the other studies, patients treated their headaches as outpatients. In study 4, patients who had previously used sumatriptan were excluded, whereas in the other studies no such exclusion was applied. Patients enrolled in these 5 studies were predominantly female (82%) and Caucasian (97%) with a mean age of 40 years (range 12–65). Patients were instructed to treat a moderate to severe headache. Headache response, defined as a reduction in headache severity from moderate or severe pain to mild or no pain, was assessed at 1, 2, and, in most studies, 4 hours after dosing. Associated symptoms such as nausea, photophobia, and phonophobia were also assessed. Maintenance of response was assessed for up to 24 hours postdose. A second dose of ZOMIG Tablets or other medication was allowed 2 to 24 hours after the initial treatment for persistent and recurrent headache. The frequency and time to use of these additional treatments were also recorded. In all studies, the effect of zolmitriptan was compared to placebo in the treatment of a single migraine attack.

In all five studies, the percentage of patients achieving headache response 2 hours after treatment was significantly greater among patients receiving ZOMIG Tablets at all doses (except for the 1 mg dose in the smallest study) compared to those who received placebo. In the two studies that evaluated the 1 mg dose, there was a statistically significant greater percentage of patients with headache response at 2 hours in the higher dose groups (2.5 and/or 5 mg) compared to the 1 mg dose group. There were no statistically significant differences between the 2.5 and 5 mg dose groups (or of doses up to 20 mg) for the primary end point of headache response at 2 hours in any study. The results of these controlled clinical studies are summarized in Table 1.

Comparisons of drug performance based upon results obtained in different clinical trials are never reliable. Because studies are conducted at different times, with different samples of patients, by different investigators, employing different criteria and/or different interpretations of the same criteria, under different conditions (dose, dosing regimen, etc.), quantitative estimates of treatment response and the timing of response may be expected to vary considerably from study to study.

Table 1:
Percentage of Patients with Headache Response (Mild or no Headache) 2 Hours Following Treatment (n=number of patients randomized)

	Placebo	ZOMIG 1.0 mg	ZOMIG 2.5 mg	ZOMIG 5 mg
Study 1[a]	16% (n=19)	27% (n=22)	NA	60%*# (n=20)
Study 2	19% (n=88)	NA	NA	66%* (n=179)
Study 3	34% (n=121)	50%* (n=140)	65%*# (n=260)	67%*# (n=245)
Study 4[b]	44% (n=55)	NA	NA	59%* (n=491)
Study 5	36% (n=92)	NA NA	62%* (n=178)	NA

* $p<0.05$ in comparison with placebo.
\# $p<0.05$ in comparison with 1 mg.
a This was the only study in which patients treated the headache in a clinic setting.
b This was the only study where patients were excluded who had previously used sumatriptan.
NA - not applicable

The estimated probability of achieving an initial headache response by 4 hours following treatment is depicted in Figure 1.

Figure 1: Estimated probability of achieving initial headache response within 4 hours*

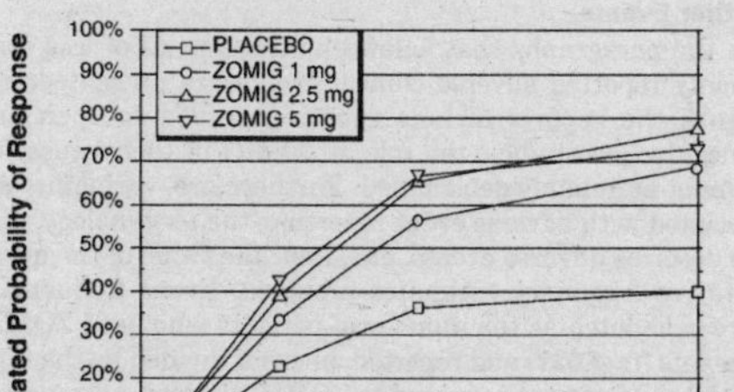

*Figure 1 shows the Kaplan-Meier plot of the probability over time of obtaining headache response (no or mild pain) following treatment with zolmitriptan. The averages displayed are based on pooled data from 3 placebo controlled, outpatient trials providing evidence of efficacy (Trials 2, 3 and 5). Patients not achieving headache response or taking additional treatment prior to 4 hours were censored to 4 hours.

For patients with migraine associated photophobia, phonophobia, and nausea at baseline, there was a decreased incidence of these symptoms following administration of ZOMIG as compared to placebo.

Two to 24 hours following the initial dose of study treatment, patients were allowed to use additional treatment for pain relief in the form of a second dose of study treatment or other medication. The estimated probability of patients taking a second dose or other medication for migraine over the 24 hours following the initial dose of study treatment is summarized in Figure 2.

[See figure 2 at top of next column]

*This Kaplan-Meier plot is based on data obtained in 3 placebo controlled clinical trials (Study 2, 3 and 5). Patients not using additional treatments were censored at 24 hours. The plot includes both patients who had headache response at 2 hours and those who had no response to the initial dose. It should be noted that the protocols did not allow remedication within 2 hours postdose.

Figure 2: The Estimated Probability Of Patients Taking A Second Dose Or Other Medication For Migraines Over The 24 Hours Following The Initial Dose Of Study Treatment *

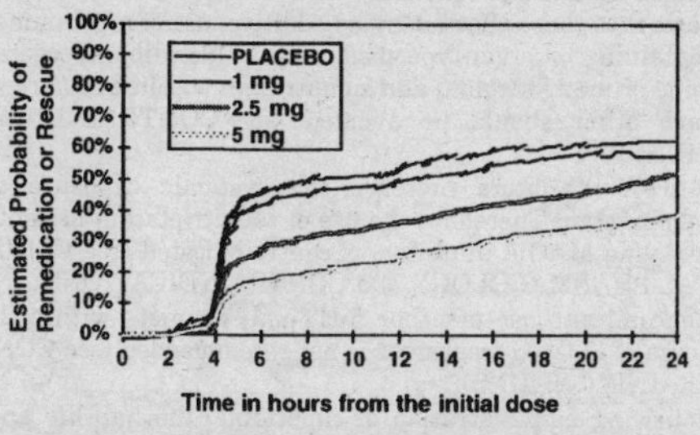

The efficacy of ZOMIG was unaffected by presence of aura; duration of headache prior to treatment; relationship to menses; gender, age, or weight of the patient; pretreatment nausea, or concomitant use of common migraine prophylactic drugs.

ZOMIG-ZMT Orally Disintegrating Tablets

The efficacy of ZOMIG-ZMT 2.5 mg was demonstrated in a randomized, placebo-controlled trial that was similar in design to the trials of ZOMIG Tablets. Patients were instructed to treat a moderate to severe headache. Of the 471 patients treated in the study, 87% were female and 97% were Caucasian, with a mean age of 41 years (range 18–62). At 2 hours post-dosing response rates in patients treated with ZOMIG-ZMT 2.5 mg were 63% compared to 22% in the placebo group. The difference was statistically significant. The estimated probability of achieving an initial headache response by 2 hours following treatment with ZOMIG-ZMT Tablets is depicted in Figure 3.

Figure 3: Estimated Probability of Achieving Initial Headache Response by 2 Hours

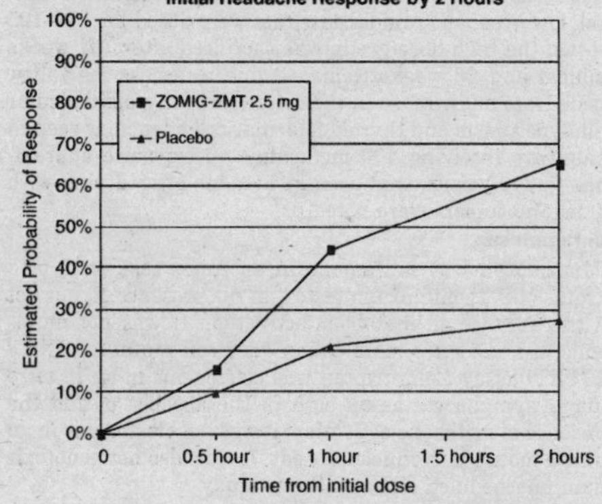

Figure 3 shows the Kaplan-Meier plot of the probability over time of obtaining headache response (no or mild pain) following treatment with ZOMIG-ZMT Tablets or placebo. Patients taking additional treatment or not achieving headache response prior to 2 hours were censored at 2 hours.

For patients with migraine-associated photophobia, phonophobia and nausea at baseline, there was a decreased incidence of these symptoms following administration of ZOMIG-ZMT as compared to placebo.

Two to 24 hours following the initial dose of study treatment, patients were allowed to use additional treatment in the form of a second dose of study treatment or other medication. The estimated probability of patients taking a second dose or other medication for migraine over the 24 hours following the initial dose of study treatment is summarized in Figure 4.

Figure 4: The Estimated Probability of Patients Taking a Second Dose or Medication for Migraines Over the 24 Hours Following the Intitial Dose of Study Treatment

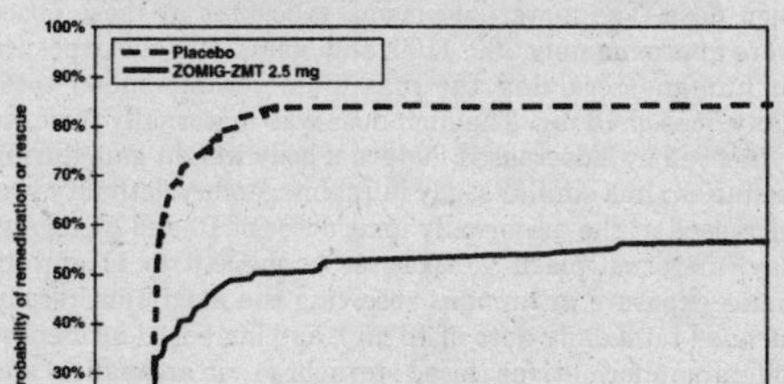

In this Kaplan-Meier plot, patients not using additional treatments were censored at 24 hours. The plot includes both patients who had headache response at 2 hours and those who had no response to the initial dose. Remedication was allowed 2 hours post-dose, and unlike the conventional tablet, remedication prior to 4 hours was not discouraged.

INDICATIONS AND USAGE

ZOMIG is indicated for the acute treatment of migraine with or without aura in adults.

ZOMIG is not intended for the prophylactic therapy of migraine or for use in the management of hemiplegic or basilar migraine (see CONTRAINDICATIONS). Safety and effectiveness of ZOMIG have not been established for cluster headache, which is present in an older, predominantly male population.

CONTRAINDICATIONS

ZOMIG should not be given to patients with ischemic heart disease (angina pectoris, history of myocardial infarction, or documented silent ischemia) or to patients who have symptoms or findings consistent with ischemic heart disease, coronary artery vasospasm, including Prinzmetal's variant angina, or other significant underlying cardiovascular disease (see WARNINGS).

Because ZOMIG may increase blood pressure, it should not be given to patients with uncontrolled hypertension (see WARNINGS).

ZOMIG should not be used within 24 hours of treatment with another 5-HT$_1$ agonist, or an ergotamine-containing or ergot-type medication like dihydroergotamine or methysergide.

ZOMIG should not be administered to patients with hemiplegic or basilar migraine.

Concurrent administration of MAO-A inhibitors or use of zolmitriptan within 2 weeks of discontinuation of MAO-A inhibitor therapy is contraindicated (see CLINICAL PHARMACOLOGY: Drug Interactions and PRECAUTIONS: Drug Interactions).

ZOMIG is contraindicated in patients who are hypersensitive to zolmitriptan or any of its inactive ingredients.

WARNINGS

ZOMIG should only be used where a clear diagnosis of migraine has been established.

Risk of Myocardial Ischemia and/or Infarction and Other Adverse Cardiac Events: ZOMIG should not be given to patients with documented ischemic or vasospastic coronary artery disease (see CONTRAINDICATIONS). It is strongly recommended that zolmitriptan not be given to patients in whom unrecognized coronary artery disease (CAD) is predicted by the presence of risk factors (e.g., hypertension, hypercholesterolemia, smoker, obesity, diabetes, strong family history of CAD, female with surgical or physiological menopause, or male over 40 years of age) unless a cardiovascular evaluation provides satisfactory clinical evidence that the patient is reasonably free of coronary artery and ischemic myocardial disease or other significant underlying cardiovascular disease. The sensitivity of cardiac diagnostic procedures to detect cardiovascular disease or predisposition to coronary artery vasospasm is modest, at best. If, during the cardiovascular evaluation, the patient's medical history, electrocardiographic or other investigations reveal findings indicative of, or consistent with, coronary artery vasospasm or myocardial ischemia, zolmitriptan should not be administered (see CONTRAINDICATIONS). For patients with risk factors predictive of CAD, who are determined to have a satisfactory cardiovascular evaluation, it is strongly recommended that administration of the first dose of zolmitriptan take place in the setting of a physician's office or similar medically staffed and equipped facility unless the patient has previously received zolmitriptan. Because cardiac ischemia can occur in the absence of clinical symptoms, consideration should be given to obtaining on the first occasion of use an electrocardiogram (ECG) during the interval immediately following ZOMIG, in these patients with risk factors.

It is recommended that patients who are intermittent long-term users of ZOMIG and who have or acquire risk factors predictive of CAD, as described above, undergo periodic interval cardiovascular evaluation as they continue to use ZOMIG.

The systematic approach described above is intended to reduce the likelihood that patients with unrecognized cardiovascular disease will be inadvertently exposed to zolmitriptan.

Cardiac Events and Fatalities:

Serious adverse cardiac events, including acute myocardial infarction, have been reported within a few hours following administration of zolmitriptan. Life-threatening disturbances of cardiac rhythm, and death have been reported within a few hours following the administration of other 5-HT$_1$ agonists. Considering the extent of use of 5-HT$_1$ agonists in patients with migraine, the incidence of these events is extremely low.

ZOMIG can cause coronary vasospasm; at least one of these events occurred in a patient with no cardiac disease history and with documented absence of coronary artery disease. Because of the close proximity of the events to ZOMIG use, a causal relationship cannot be excluded. In the cases where there has been known underlying coronary artery disease, the relationship is uncertain.

Patients with symptomatic Wolff-Parkinson-White syndrome or arrhythmias associated with other cardiac accessory conduction pathway disorders should not receive ZOMIG.

Premarketing experience with zolmitriptan:

Among the more than 2,500 patients with migraine who participated in premarketing controlled clinical trials of ZOMIG Tablets, no deaths or serious cardiac events were reported.

Postmarketing experience with zolmitriptan:

Serious cardiovascular events have been reported in association with the use of ZOMIG Tablets, and in very rare cases,

Continued on next page

Zomig—Cont.

these events have occurred in the absence of known cardiovascular disease. The uncontrolled nature of postmarketing surveillance, however, makes it impossible to determine definitively the proportion of the reported cases that were actually caused by zolmitriptan or to reliably assess causation in individual cases.

Cerebrovascular Events and Fatalities with 5-HT$_1$ agonists:
Cerebral hemorrhage, subarachnoid hemorrhage, stroke, and other cerebrovascular events have been reported in patients treated with 5-HT$_1$ agonists; and some have resulted in fatalities. In a number of cases, it appears possible that the cerebrovascular events were primary, the agonist having been administered in the incorrect belief that the symptoms experienced were a consequence of migraine, when they were not. It should be noted that patients with migraine may be at increased risk of certain cerebrovascular events (eg, stroke, hemorrhage, transient ischemic attack).

Other Vasospasm-Related Events:
5-HT$_1$ agonists may cause vasospastic reactions other than coronary artery vasospasm such as peripheral and gastrointestinal vascular ischemia. As with other serotonin 5HT$_1$ agonists, very rare gastrointestinal ischemic events including ischemic colitis and gastrointestinal infarction or necrosis have been reported with ZOMIG Tablets; these may present as bloody diarrhea or abdominal pain.

Increase in Blood Pressure:
As with other 5-HT$_1$ agonists, significant elevations in systemic blood pressure have been reported on rare occasions with ZOMIG Tablet use, in patients with and without a history of hypertension; very rarely these increases in blood pressure have been associated with significant clinical events. Zolmitriptan is contraindicated in patients with uncontrolled hypertension. In volunteers, an increase of 1 and 5 mm Hg in the systolic and diastolic blood pressure, respectively, was seen at 5 mg. In the headache trials, vital signs were measured only in the small inpatient study and no effect on blood pressure was seen. In a study of patients with moderate to severe liver disease, 7 of 27 experienced 20 to 80 mm Hg elevations in systolic and/or diastolic blood pressure after a dose of 10 mg of zolmitriptan (see CONTRAINDICATIONS).

An 18% increase in mean pulmonary artery pressure was seen following dosing with another 5-HT$_1$ agonist in a study evaluating subjects undergoing cardiac catheterization.

PRECAUTIONS

General
As with other 5-HT$_{1B/1D}$ agonists, sensations of tightness, pain, pressure, and heaviness have been reported after treatment with ZOMIG Tablets in the precordium, throat, neck, and jaw. Because zolmitriptan may cause coronary artery vasospasm, patients who experience signs or symptoms suggestive of angina following dosing should be evaluated for the presence of CAD or a predisposition to Prinzmetal's variant angina before receiving additional doses of medication, and should be monitored electrocardiographically if dosing is resumed and similar symptoms recur. Similarly, patients who experience other symptoms or signs suggestive of decreased arterial flow, such as ischemic bowel syndrome or Raynaud's syndrome following the use of any 5-HT$_1$ agonist are candidates for further evaluation (see WARNINGS).

Zolmitriptan should also be administered with caution to patients with diseases that may alter the absorption, metabolism, or excretion of drugs, such as impaired hepatic function (see CLINICAL PHARMACOLOGY).

For a given attack, if a patient does not respond to the first dose of zolmitriptan, the diagnosis of migraine headache should be reconsidered before administration of a second dose.

Binding to Melanin-Containing Tissues:
When pigmented rats were given a single oral dose of 10 mg/kg of radiolabeled zolmitriptan, the radioactivity in the eye after 7 days, the latest time point examined, was still 75% of the value measured after 4 hours. This suggests that zolmitriptan and/or its metabolites may bind to the melanin of the eye. Because there could be accumulation in melanin rich tissues over time, this raises the possibility that zolmitriptan could cause toxicity in these tissues after extended use. However, no effects on the retina related to treatment with zolmitriptan were noted in any of the toxicity studies. Although no systematic monitoring of ophthalmologic function was undertaken in clinical trials, and no specific recommendations for ophthalmologic monitoring are offered, prescribers should be aware of the possibility of long-term ophthalmologic effects.

Phenylketonurics:
Phenylketonuric patients should be informed that ZOMIG-ZMT contain phenylalanine (a component of aspartame). Each 2.5 mg orally disintegrating tablet contains 2.81 mg phenylalanine. Each 5 mg orally disintegrating tablet contains 5.62 mg phenylalanine.

Information for Patients
See PATIENT INFORMATION at the end of this labeling for the text of the separate leaflet provided for patients.

ZOMIG-ZMT Orally Disintegrating Tablets
The orally disintegrating tablet is packaged in a blister. Patients should be instructed not to remove the tablet from the blister until just prior to dosing. The blister pack should then be peeled open, and the orally disintegrating tablet placed on the tongue, where it will dissolve and be swallowed with the saliva.

Laboratory Tests:
No monitoring of specific laboratory tests is recommended.

Drug Interactions
Ergot-containing drugs have been reported to cause prolonged vasospastic reactions. Because there is a theoretical basis that these effects may be additive, use of ergotamine-containing or ergot-type medications (like dihydroergotamine or methysergide) and zolmitriptan within 24 hours of each other should be avoided (see CONTRAINDICATIONS).

MAO-A inhibitors increase the systemic exposure of zolmitriptan. Therefore, the use of zolmitriptan in patients receiving MAO-A inhibitors is contraindicated (see CLINICAL PHARMACOLOGY and CONTRAINDICATIONS).

Concomitant use of other 5-HT$_{1B/1D}$ agonists within 24 hours of ZOMIG treatment is not recommended (see CONTRAINDICATIONS).

Following administration of cimetidine, the half-life and AUC of zolmitriptan and its active metabolites were approximately doubled (see CLINICAL PHARMACOLOGY).

Selective serotonin reuptake inhibitors (SSRIs) (eg, fluoxetine, fluvoxamine, paroxetine, sertraline) have been reported, rarely, to cause weakness, hyperreflexia, and incoordination when coadministered with 5-HT$_1$ agonists. If concomitant treatment with zolmitriptan and an SSRI is clinically warranted, appropriate observation of the patient is advised.

Drug/Laboratory Test Interactions:
Zolmitriptan is not known to interfere with commonly employed clinical laboratory tests.

Carcinogenesis, Mutagenesis, Impairment of Fertility Carcinogenesis:
Carcinogenicity studies by oral gavage were carried out in mice and rats at doses up to 400 mg/kg/day. Mice were dosed for 85 weeks (males) and 92 weeks (females). The exposure (plasma AUC of parent drug) at the highest dose level was approximately 800 times that seen in humans after a single 10 mg dose (the maximum recommended total daily dose). There was no effect of zolmitriptan on tumor incidence. Control, low dose, and middle dose rats were dosed for 104–105 weeks; the high dose group was sacrificed after 101 weeks (males) and 86 weeks (females) due to excess mortality. Aside from an increase in the incidence of thyroid follicular cell hyperplasia and thyroid follicular cell adenomas seen in male rats receiving 400 mg/kg/day, an exposure approximately 3000 times that seen in humans after dosing with 10 mg, no tumors were noted.

Mutagenesis:
Zolmitriptan was mutagenic in an Ames test, in 2 of 5 strains of S. typhimurium tested, in the presence of, but not in the absence of, metabolic activation. It was not mutagenic in an in vitro mammalian gene cell mutation (CHO/HGPRT) assay. Zolmitriptan was clastogenic in an in vitro human lymphocyte assay both in the absence of and the presence of metabolic activation; it was not clastogenic in an in vivo mouse micronucleus assay. It was also not genotoxic in an unscheduled DNA synthesis study.

Impairment of Fertility:
Studies of male and female rats administered zolmitriptan prior to and during mating and up to implantation have shown no impairment of fertility at doses up to 400 mg/kg/day. Exposure at this dose was approximately 3000 times exposure at the maximum recommended human dose of 10 mg/day.

Pregnancy
Pregnancy Category C
There are no adequate and well controlled studies in pregnant women; therefore, zolmitriptan should be used during pregnancy only if the potential benefit justifies the potential risk to the fetus.

In reproductive toxicity studies in rats and rabbits, oral administration of zolmitriptan to pregnant animals was associated with embryolethality and fetal abnormalities. When pregnant rats were administered oral zolmitriptan during the period of organogenesis at doses of 100, 400, and 1200 mg/kg/day, there was a dose-related increase in embryolethality which became statistically significant at the high dose. The maternal plasma exposures at these doses were approximately 280, 1100, and 5000 times the exposure in humans receiving the maximum recommended total daily dose of 10 mg. The high dose was maternally toxic, as evidenced by a decreased maternal body weight gain during gestation. In a similar study in rabbits, embryolethality was increased at the maternally toxic doses of 10 and 30 mg/kg/day (maternal plasma exposures equivalent to 11 and 42 times exposure in humans receiving the maximum recommended total daily dose of 10 mg), and increased incidences of fetal malformations (fused sternebrae, rib anomalies) and variations (major blood vessel variations, irregular ossification pattern of ribs) were observed at 30 mg/kg/day. Three mg/kg/day was a no effect dose (equivalent to human exposure at a dose of 10 mg). When female rats were given zolmitriptan during gestation, parturition, and lactation, an increased incidence of hydronephrosis was found in the offspring at the maternally toxic dose of 400 mg/kg/day (1100 times human exposure).

Nursing Mothers
It is not known whether zolmitriptan is excreted in human milk. Because many drugs are excreted in human milk, caution should be exercised when zolmitriptan is administered to a nursing woman. Lactating rats dosed with zolmitriptan had milk levels equivalent to maternal plasma levels at 1 hour and 4 times higher than plasma levels at 4 hours.

Pediatric Use
Safety and effectiveness of ZOMIG in pediatric patients have not been established therefore, ZOMIG is not recommended for use in patients under 18 years of age.
Postmarketing experience with other triptans includes a limited number of reports that describe pediatric patients who have experienced clinically serious adverse events that are similar in nature to those reported rarely in adults.

Geriatric Use
Although the pharmacokinetic disposition of the drug in the elderly is similar to that seen in younger adults, there is no information about the safety and effectiveness of zolmitriptan in this population because patients over age 65 were excluded from the controlled clinical trials (see CLINICAL PHARMACOLOGY: Special Populations).

ADVERSE REACTIONS

Serious cardiac events, including myocardial infarction, have occurred following the use of ZOMIG Tablets. These events are extremely rare and most have been reported in patients with risk factors predictive of CAD. Events reported, in association with drugs of this class, have included coronary artery vasospasm, transient myocardial ischemia, myocardial infarction, ventricular tachycardia, and ventricular fibrillation (see CONTRAINDICATIONS, WARNINGS, and PRECAUTIONS).

Incidence in Controlled Clinical Trials:
Among 2,633 patients treated with ZOMIG Tablets in the active and placebo controlled trials, no patients withdrew for reasons related to adverse events, but as patients treated a single headache in these trials, the opportunity for discontinuation was limited. In a long-term, open label study where patients were allowed to treat multiple migraine attacks for up to 1 year, 8% (167 out of 2,058) withdrew from the trial because of adverse experience. The most common events were paresthesia, asthenia, nausea, dizziness, pain, chest or neck tightness or heaviness, somnolence, and warm sensation.

Table 2 lists the adverse events that occurred in ≥ 2% of the 2,074 patients in any one of the ZOMIG 1 mg, ZOMIG 2.5 mg or ZOMIG 5 mg Tablets dose groups of the controlled clinical trials. Only events that were more frequent in a ZOMIG Tablets group compared to the placebo groups are included. The events cited reflect experience gained under closely monitored conditions of clinical trials in a highly selected patient population. In actual clinical practice or in other clinical trials, these frequency estimates may not apply, as the conditions of use, reporting behavior, and the kinds of patients treated may differ.

Several of the adverse events appear dose related, notably paresthesia, sensation of heaviness or tightness in chest, neck, jaw, and throat, dizziness, somnolence, and possibly asthenia and nausea.

[See table 2 at bottom of next page]

ZOMIG is generally well tolerated. Across all doses, most adverse reactions were mild and transient and did not lead to long-lasting effects. The incidence of adverse events in controlled clinical trials was not affected by gender, weight, or age of the patients; use of prophylactic medications; or presence of aura. There were insufficient data to assess the impact of race on the incidence of adverse events.

Other Events
In the paragraphs that follow, the frequencies of less commonly reported adverse clinical events are presented. Because the reports include events observed in open and uncontrolled studies, the role of ZOMIG in their causation cannot be reliably determined. Furthermore, variability associated with adverse event reporting, the terminology used to describe adverse events, etc., limit the value of the quantitative frequency estimates provided. Event frequencies are calculated as the number of patients who used ZOMIG Tablets (n=4,027) and reported an event divided by the total number of patients exposed to ZOMIG Tablets. All reported events are included except those already listed in the previous table, those too general to be informative, and those not reasonably associated with the use of the drug. Events are further classified within body system categories and enumerated in order of decreasing frequency using the following definitions: infrequent adverse events are those occurring in 1/100 to 1/1,000 patients and rare adverse events are those occurring in fewer than 1/1,000 patients.

Atypical sensation: Infrequent was hyperesthesia.
General: Infrequent were allergy reaction, chills, facial edema, fever, malaise, and photosensitivity.
Cardiovascular: Infrequent were arrhythmias, hypertension, and syncope. Rare were bradycardia, extrasystoles, postural hypotension, QT prolongation, tachycardia, and thrombophlebitis.
Digestive: Infrequent were increased appetite, tongue edema, esophagitis, gastroenteritis, liver function abnormality, and thirst. Rare were anorexia, constipation, gastritis, hematemesis, pancreatitis, melena, and ulcer.
Hemic: Infrequent was ecchymosis. Rare were cyanosis, thrombocytopenia, eosinophilia, and leukopenia.
Metabolic: Infrequent was edema. Rare were hyperglycemia and alkaline phosphatase increased.
Musculoskeletal: Infrequent were back pain, leg cramps, and tenosynovitis. Rare were arthritis, asthenia, tetany, and twitching.
Neurological: Infrequent were agitation, anxiety, depression, emotional lability, and insomnia; Rare were akathisia, amnesia, apathy, ataxia, dystonia, euphoria, hallucinations, cerebral ischemia, hyperkinesia, hypotonia, hypertonia, and irritability.

Respiratory: Infrequent were bronchitis, bronchospasm, epistaxis, hiccup, laryngitis, and yawn. Rare were apnea and voice alteration.
Skin: Infrequent were pruritus, rash, and urticaria.
Special Senses: Infrequent were dry eye, eye pain, hyperacusis, ear pain, parosmia, and tinnitus. Rare were diplopia and lacrimation.
Urogenital: Infrequent were hematuria, cystitis, polyuria, urinary frequency, urinary urgency. Rare were miscarriage and dysmenorrhea.
The adverse experiences profile seen with ZOMIG-ZMT Tablets was similar to that seen with ZOMIG Tablets.

Postmarketing Experience with ZOMIG Tablets
The following section enumerates potentially important adverse events that have occurred in clinical practice and which have been reported spontaneously to various surveillance systems. The events enumerated represent reports arising from both domestic and non-domestic use of oral zolmitriptan. The events enumerated include all except those already listed in the ADVERSE REACTIONS section above or those too general to be informative. Because the reports cite events reported spontaneously from worldwide postmarketing experience, frequency of events and the role of zolmitriptan in their causation cannot be reliably determined.

Cardiovascular
Coronary artery vasospasm; transient myocardial ischemia, angina pectoris, and myocardial infarction.
Digestive
Very rare gastrointestinal ischemic events including ischemic colitis and gastrointestinal infarction or necrosis have been reported; these may present as bloody diarrhea or abdominal pain. (See WARNINGS).
Neurological: As with other acute migraine treatments including other $5HT_1$ agonists, there have been rare reports of headache.
General
As with other $5\text{-}HT_{1B/1D}$ agonists, there have been very rare reports of anaphylaxis or anaphylactoid reactions in patients receiving ZOMIG. There have been rare reports of hypersensitivity reactions, including angioedema.

DRUG ABUSE AND DEPENDENCE
The abuse potential of ZOMIG has not been assessed in clinical trials.

OVERDOSAGE
There is no experience with clinical overdose. Volunteers receiving single 50 mg oral doses of zolmitriptan commonly experienced sedation.
The elimination half-life of ZOMIG is 3 hours (see CLINICAL PHARMACOLOGY), and therefore monitoring of patients after overdose with ZOMIG should continue for at least 15 hours or while symptoms or signs persist.
There is no specific antidote to zolmitriptan. In cases of severe intoxication, intensive care procedures are recommended, including establishing and maintaining a patent airway, ensuring adequate oxygenation and ventilation, and monitoring and support of the cardiovascular system.
It is unknown what effect hemodialysis or peritoneal dialysis has on the plasma concentrations of zolmitriptan.

DOSAGE AND ADMINISTRATION
ZOMIG Tablets
In controlled clinical trials, single doses of 1, 2.5 and 5 mg of ZOMIG Tablets were effective for the acute treatment of migraines in adults. A greater proportion of patients had headache response following a 2.5 or 5 mg dose than following a 1 mg dose (see Table 1). In the only direct comparison of 2.5 and 5 mg, there was little added benefit from the larger dose but side effects are generally increased at 5 mg (see Table 2). Patients should, therefore, be started on 2.5 mg or lower. A dose lower than 2.5 mg can be achieved by manually breaking the scored 2.5 mg tablet in half.
If the headache returns, the dose may be repeated after 2 hours, not to exceed 10 mg within a 24-hour period. Controlled trials have not adequately established the effectiveness of a second dose if the initial dose is ineffective.
The safety of treating an average of more than three headaches in a 30-day period has not been established.

ZOMIG-ZMT Orally Disintegrating Tablets
In a controlled clinical trial, a single dose of 2.5 mg of ZOMIG-ZMT Tablets was effective for the acute treatment of migraines in adults.
If the headache returns, the dose may be repeated after 2 hours, not to exceed 10 mg within a 24-hour period. Controlled trials have not adequately established the effectiveness of a second dose if the initial dose is ineffective.
The safety of treating an average of more than three headaches in a 30-day period has not been established.
Administration with liquid is not necessary. The orally disintegrating tablet is packaged in a blister. Patients should be instructed not to remove the tablet from the blister until just prior to dosing. The blister pack should then be peeled open, and the orally disintegrating tablet placed on the tongue, where it will dissolve and be swallowed with the saliva. It is not recommended to break the orally disintegrating tablet.

Hepatic Impairment
Patients with moderate to severe hepatic impairment have decreased clearance of zolmitriptan and significant elevation in blood pressure was observed in some patients. Use of a low dose with blood pressure monitoring is recommended (see CLINICAL PHARMACOLOGY and WARNINGS).

HOW SUPPLIED
2.5 mg Tablets - Yellow, biconvex, round film-coated, scored tablets containing 2.5 mg of zolmitriptan identified with "ZOMIG" and "2.5" debossed on one side are supplied in cartons containing a blister pack of 6 tablets (NDC 0310-0210-20).
2.5 mg Orally Disintegrating Tablets - White, flat faced, uncoated, bevelled tablet containing 2.5 mg of zolmitriptan identified with a debossed "Z" on one side are supplied in cartons containing a blister pack of 6 tablets (NDC 0310-209-20).
5 mg Tablets - Pink, biconvex, film-coated tablets containing 5 mg of zolmitriptan identified with "ZOMIG" and "5" debossed on one side are supplied in cartons containing a blister pack of 3 tablets (NDC 0310-0211-25).
5 mg Orally Disintegrating Tablets - White, flat faced, round, uncoated, bevelled tablet containing 5.0 mg of zolmitriptan identified with a debossed "Z" and "5" on one side and plain on the other are supplied in cartons containing a blister pack of 3 tablets (NDC 0310-0213-21).

Storage
Store both ZOMIG Tablets and ZOMIG-ZMT Tablets at controlled room temperature, 20–25°C (68–77°F) [see USP]. Protect from light and moisture.

ZOMIG®
(zolmitriptan) TABLETS
ZOMIG-ZMT®
(ZOLMITRIPTAN) Orally Disintegrating Tablets
PATIENT INFORMATION
The following wording is contained in a separate leaflet provided for patients.
ZOMIG® (zolmitriptan) Tablets
ZOMIG-ZMT® (zolmitriptan) Orally Disintegrating Tablets
Patient Information about ZOMIG (Zo-mig) for Migraines
Generic Name: zolmitriptan (zol-mi-trip-tan)

Information for the Consumer on ZOMIG (zolmitriptan) Tablets
Please read this leaflet carefully before you administer ZOMIG Tablets. This provides a summary of the information available on your medicine. Please do not throw away this leaflet until you have finished your medicine. You may need to read this leaflet again. This leaflet does not contain all the information on ZOMIG Tablets. For further information or advice, ask your doctor or pharmacist.

Information About Your Medicine
The name of your medicine is ZOMIG Tablets. It can be obtained only by prescription from your doctor. The decision to use ZOMIG Tablets is one that you and your doctor should make jointly, taking into account your individual preferences and medical circumstances. If you have risk factors for heart disease (such as high blood pressure, high cholesterol, obesity, diabetes, smoking, strong family history of heart disease, or you are postmenopausal or a male over the age of 40), you should tell your doctor, who should evaluate you for heart disease in order to determine if ZOMIG Tablets are appropriate for you.

1. The Purpose of Your Medicine: ZOMIG Tablets are intended to relieve your migraine, but not to prevent or reduce the number of attacks you experience. Use ZOMIG Tablets only to treat an actual migraine attack.

2. Important Questions to Consider Before Using ZOMIG Tablets: If the answer to any of the following questions is YES or if you do not know the answer, then you must discuss it with your doctor before you use ZOMIG Tablets.

Do you have any chest pain, heart disease, shortness of breath, or irregular heartbeats? Have you had a heart attack?

Do you have risk factors for heart disease (such as high blood pressure, high cholesterol, obesity, diabetes, smoking, strong family history of heart disease, or you are postmenopausal or a male over the age of 40)?

Do you have high blood pressure?

Are you pregnant? Do you think you might be pregnant? Are you trying to become pregnant? Are you not using adequate contraception? Are you breast feeding an infant?

If you are taking ZOMIG-ZMT®, are you sensitive to phenylalanine (a component of the artificial sweetener aspartame)?

Have you ever had to stop taking this or any other medication because of an allergy or other problems?

Are you taking any other migraine medications, including $5\text{-}HT_1$ agonists (triptans) or migraine medications containing ergotamine, dihydroergotamine, or methysergide?

Are you taking any medication for depression (monoamine oxidase inhibitors or selective serotonin reuptake inhibitors [SSRIs])?

Are you taking cimetidine for gastrointestinal symptoms?

Have you had, or do you have, any disease of the liver or kidney?

Have you had, or do you have, epilepsy or seizures?

Is this headache different from your usual migraine attacks?

Remember, if you answered YES to any of the above questions, then you must discuss it with your doctor.

3. The Use of ZOMIG Tablets During Pregnancy: Do not use ZOMIG Tablets if you are pregnant, think you might be pregnant, are trying to become pregnant, or are not using adequate contraception unless you have discussed this with your doctor.

4. How to Use ZOMIG Tablets and ZOMIG-ZMT Orally Disintegrating Tablets: Adults should be started on a 2.5 mg dose or lower administered by mouth. A dose lower than 2.5 mg can be achieved by manually breaking the conventional film-coated, scored 2.5 mg tablet in half. It is not recommended to break the ZOMIG-ZMT Tablet. If your headache comes back after your initial dose, a second dose may be administered anytime after 2 hours of administering the dose. For any attack where you have no response to the first dose, do not take a second dose without first consulting with your doctor. Do not administer more than a total of 10 mg of ZOMIG in any 24-hour period. Discard any unused tablets or its portion that have been removed from the blister packaging. Do not take ZOMIG with any other drug in the same class (triptans) within 24 hours or within 24 hours of taking ergotamine-type medications such as ergotamine, dihydroergotamine or methysergide to treat your migraine.

Additionally for ZOMIG-ZMT Tablets, the blister pack should be peeled open and the orally disintegrating tablet placed on the tongue, where it will dissolve and be swallowed with the saliva.

5. Side Effects to Watch for: Some patients experience pain or tightness in the chest or throat, including muscle aches and pains, when using ZOMIG. If this happens to you, then discuss it with your doctor before using any more ZOMIG. If the chest pain is severe or does not go away, call your doctor immediately. As with other drugs in this class (triptans), there have been very rare reports of heart attack occurring in patients with and without risk factors for heart and blood vessel disease.

Some people experience; alterations of heart rate; temporary increase in blood pressure; sudden and severe stomach pain.

Shortness of breath; wheeziness; heart throbbing; swelling of eyelids, face, or lips; or a skin rash, skin lumps, or hives

Continued on next page

Table 2:
Adverse Experience Incidence in Five Placebo-Controlled Migraine Clinical Trials:
Events Reported By ≥ 2% Patients Treated With ZOMIG Tablets

Adverse Event Type	Placebo (n=401)	ZOMIG 1 mg (n=163)	ZOMIG 2.5 mg (n=498)	ZOMIG 5 mg (n=1012)
ATYPICAL SENSATIONS	6%	12%	12%	18%
Hypesthesia	1%	1%	1%	2%
Paresthesia (all types)	2%	5%	7%	9%
Sensation warm/cold	4%	6%	5%	7%
PAIN AND PRESSURE SENSATIONS	7%	13%	14%	22%
Chest - pain/tightness/pressure and/or heaviness	1%	2%	3%	4%
Neck/throat/jaw - pain/tightness/pressure	3%	4%	7%	10%
Heaviness other than chest or neck	1%	1%	2%	5%
Pain – location specified	1%	2%	2%	3%
Other – Pressure/tightness/heaviness	0%	2%	2%	2%
DIGESTIVE	8%	11%	16%	14%
Dry mouth	2%	5%	3%	3%
Dyspepsia	1%	3%	2%	1%
Dysphagia	0%	0%	0%	2%
Nausea	4%	4%	9%	6%
NEUROLOGICAL	10%	11%	17%	21%
Dizziness	4%	6%	8%	10%
Somnolence	3%	5%	6%	8%
Vertigo	0%	0%	0%	2%
OTHER				
Asthenia	3%	5%	3%	9%
Palpitations	1%	0%	<1%	2%
Myalgia	<1%	1%	1%	2%
Myasthenia	<1%	0%	1%	2%
Sweating	1%	0%	2%	3%

Zomig—Cont.

happens rarely. If it happens to you, then tell your doctor immediately. Do not take any more ZOMIG unless your doctor tells you to do so.
Some people may have feelings of dry mouth, tingling, heat, heaviness, or pressure after treatment with ZOMIG. A few people may feel drowsy, dizzy, tired, or sick. Tell your doctor immediately if you have symptoms that you do not understand.

6. What to Do if an Overdose is Taken: If you have taken more medication than you have been told, contact either your doctor, hospital emergency department, or nearest poison control center immediately. This medicine was prescribed for your particular condition and should not be used by others or for any other condition.

7. Storing Your Medicine: Keep your medicine in a safe place where children cannot reach it. It may be harmful to children. Store your medication away from light and moisture, and at a controlled room temperature. If your medication has expired (the expiration date is printed on the treatment pack), throw it away as instructed. If your doctor decides to stop your treatment, do not keep any leftover medicine unless your doctor tells you to. Throw away your medicine as instructed. Be sure that discarded tablets are out of the reach of children.

All trademarks are the property of the AstraZeneca group
© AstraZeneca 2002
ZOMIG(zolmitriptan) Tablets
Manufactured for:
AstraZeneca Pharmaceuticals LP
Wilmington, Delaware 19850
By: IPR Pharmaceuticals, Inc.
Carolina, Puerto Rico 00984-1967
ZOMIG-ZMT (zolmitriptan) Orally Disintegrating Tablets
Manufactured for:
AstraZeneca Pharmaceuticals LP
Wilmington, Delaware 19850
By: CIMA Labs, Inc.
Eden Prairie, Minnesota 55344
Rev 10/02

Aventis Pharmaceuticals Inc.
300 SOMERSET CORPORATE BOULEVARD
BRIDGEWATER, NJ 08807-2854

Direct Inquiries to:
Customer Service
300 Somerset Corporate Boulevard
Bridgewater, NJ 08807-2854
(800) 207-8049

For Medical Information Contact:
Generally:
Medical Information Services
300 Somerset Corporate Boulevard
Bridgewater, NJ 08807-2854
(800) 633-1610
For Oncology Medical Information call (866) 662-6411

LOVENOX® ℞
[lō'və-nŏks]
(enoxaparin sodium injection)
Rx only

Prescribing information for this product, which appears on pages 739–744 of the 2003 PDR has been completely revised as follows. Please write "See Supplement A" next to the product heading.

SPINAL / EPIDURAL HEMATOMAS
When neuraxial anesthesia (epidural/spinal anesthesia) or spinal puncture is employed, patients anticoagulated or scheduled to be anticoagulated with low molecular weight heparins or heparinoids for prevention of thromboembolic complications are at risk of developing an epidural or spinal hematoma which can result in long-term or permanent paralysis.
The risk of these events is increased by the use of indwelling epidural catheters for administration of analgesia or by the concomitant use of drugs affecting hemostasis such as non steroidal anti-inflammatory drugs (NSAIDs), platelet inhibitors, or other anticoagulants. The risk also appears to be increased by traumatic or repeated epidural or spinal puncture.
Patients should be frequently monitored for signs and symptoms of neurological impairment. If neurologic compromise is noted, urgent treatment is necessary.
The physician should consider the potential benefit versus risk before neuraxial intervention in patients anticoagulated or to be anticoagulated for thromboprophylaxis (see also **WARNINGS, Hemorrhage,** and **PRECAUTIONS, Drug Interactions**).

DESCRIPTION
Lovenox Injection is a sterile aqueous solution containing enoxaparin sodium, a low molecular weight heparin.

Lovenox Injection is available in two concentrations:
1. 100 mg per mL
—*Prefilled Syringes*   30 mg / 0.3 mL, 40 mg / 0.4 mL
—*Graduated Prefilled Syringes*   60 mg / 0.6 mL, 80 mg / 0.8 mL, 100 mg / 1 mL
—*Ampules*   30 mg / 0.3 mL
—*Multiple-Dose Vials*   300 mg / 3.0 mL

Lovenox Injection 100 mg/mL Concentration contains 10 mg enoxaparin sodium (approximate anti-Factor Xa activity of 1000 IU [with reference to the W.H.O. First International Low Molecular Weight Heparin Reference Standard]) per 0.1 mL Water for Injection.

2. 150 mg per mL
—*Graduated Prefilled Syringes*   120 mg / 0.8 mL, 150 mg / 1 mL

Lovenox Injection 150 mg/mL Concentration contains 15 mg enoxaparin sodium (approximate anti-Factor Xa activity of 1500 IU [with reference to the W.H.O. First International Low Molecular Weight Heparin Reference Standard]) per 0.1 mL Water for Injection.

The Lovenox prefilled syringes, graduated prefilled syringes, and ampules are preservative-free and intended for use only as a single-dose injection. The multiple-dose vial contains 15 mg/1.0 mL benzyl alcohol as a preservative. (See **DOSAGE AND ADMINISTRATION** and **HOW SUPPLIED** for dosage unit descriptions.) The pH of the injection is 5.5 to 7.5.

Enoxaparin sodium is obtained by alkaline degradation of heparin benzyl ester derived from porcine intestinal mucosa. Its structure is characterized by a 2-O-sulfo-4-enepyranosuronic acid group at the nonreducing end and a 2-N,6-O-disulfo-D-glucosamine at the reducing end of the chain. The drug substance is the sodium salt. The average molecular weight is about 4500 daltons. The molecular weight distribution is:

<2000 daltons	≤20%
2000 to 8000 daltons	≥68%
>8000 daltons	≤18%

STRUCTURAL FORMULA

CLINICAL PHARMACOLOGY
Enoxaparin is a low molecular weight heparin which has antithrombotic properties. In humans, enoxaparin given at a dose of 1.5 mg/kg subcutaneously (SC) is characterized by a higher ratio of anti-Factor Xa to anti-Factor IIa activity (mean±SD, 14.0±3.1) (based on areas under anti-Factor activity versus time curves) compared to the ratios observed for heparin (mean±SD, 1.22±0.13). Increases of up to 1.8 times the control values were seen in the thrombin time (TT) and the activated partial thromboplastin time (aPTT). Enoxaparin at a 1 mg/kg dose (100 mg / mL concentration), administered SC every 12 hours to patients in a large clinical trial resulted in aPTT values of 45 seconds or less in the majority of patients (n = 1607).

Pharmacodynamics (conducted using 100 mg / mL concentration): Maximum anti-Factor Xa and anti-thrombin (anti-Factor IIa) activities occur 3 to 5 hours after SC injection of enoxaparin. Mean peak anti-Factor Xa activity was 0.16 IU/mL (1.58 μg/mL) and 0.38 IU/mL (3.83 μg/mL) after the 20 mg and the 40 mg clinically tested SC doses, respectively. Mean (n = 46) peak anti-Factor Xa activity was 1.1 IU/mL at steady state in patients with unstable angina receiving 1mg/kg SC every 12 hours for 14 days. Mean absolute bioavailability of enoxaparin, given SC, based on anti-Factor Xa activity is 92% in healthy volunteers. The volume of distribution of anti-Factor Xa activity is about 6 L. Following intravenous (i.v.) dosing, the total body clearance of enoxaparin is 26 mL/min. After i.v. dosing of enoxaparin labeled with the gamma-emitter, ^{99m}Tc, 40% of radioactivity and 8 to 20% of anti-Factor Xa activity were recovered in urine in 24 hours. Elimination half-life based on anti-Factor Xa activity was 4.5 hours after SC administration. Following a 40 mg SC once a day dose, significant anti-Factor Xa activity persists in plasma for about 12 hours.

Following SC dosing, the apparent clearance (CL/F) of enoxaparin is approximately 15 mL/min. Apparent clearance and A_{max} derived from anti-Factor Xa values following single SC dosing (40 mg and 60 mg) were slightly higher in males than in females. The source of the gender difference in these parameters has not been conclusively identified, however, body weight may be a contributing factor.

Apparent clearance and A_{max} derived from anti-Factor Xa values following single and multiple SC dosing in elderly subjects were close to those observed in young subjects. Following once a day SC dosing of 40 mg enoxaparin, the Day 10 mean area under anti-Factor Xa activity versus time curve (AUC) was approximately 15% greater than the mean Day 1 AUC value. In subjects with moderate renal impairment (creatinine clearance 30 to 80 mL/min), anti-Factor Xa CL/F values were similar to those in healthy subjects. However, mean CL/F values of subjects with severe renal impairment (creatinine clearance <30 mL/min), were approximately 30% lower than the mean CL/F value of control group subjects. (See **PRECAUTIONS**.)

Although not studied clinically, the 150 mg/mL concentration of enoxaparin sodium is projected to result in anticoagulant activities similar to those of 100 mg/mL and 200 mg/mL concentrations at the same enoxaparin dose. When a daily 1.5 mg/kg SC injection of enoxaparin sodium was given to 25 healthy male and female subjects using a 100 mg/mL or a 200 mg/mL concentration the following pharmacokinetic profiles were obtained (see table below):
[See table above]

CLINICAL TRIALS
Prophylaxis of Deep Vein Thrombosis Following Abdominal Surgery in Patients at Risk for Thromboembolic Complications: Abdominal surgery patients at risk include those who are over 40 years of age, obese, undergoing surgery under general anesthesia lasting longer than 30 minutes or who have additional risk factors such as malignancy or a history of deep vein thrombosis or pulmonary embolism.

In a double-blind, parallel group study of patients undergoing elective cancer surgery of the gastrointestinal, urological, or gynecological tract, a total of 1116 patients were enrolled in the study, and 1115 patients were treated. Patients ranged in age from 32 to 97 years (mean age 67 years) with 52.7% men and 47.3% women. Patients were 98% Caucasian, 1.1% Black, 0.4% Oriental, and 0.4% others. Lovenox Injection 40 mg SC, administered once a day, beginning 2 hours prior to surgery and continuing for a maximum of 12 days after surgery, was comparable to heparin 5000 U every 8 hours SC in reducing the risk of deep vein thrombosis (DVT). The efficacy data are provided below.

Pharmacokinetic Parameters* After 5 Days of 1.5 mg/kg SC Once Daily Doses of Enoxaparin Sodium Using 100 mg/mL or 200 mg/mL Concentrations

	Concentration	Anti-Xa	Anti-IIa	Heptest	aPTT
A_{max} (IU/mL or Δ sec)	100 mg/mL	1.37 (±0.23)	0.23 (±0.05)	104.5 (±16.6)	19.3 (±4.7)
	200 mg/mL	1.45 (±0.22)	0.26 (±0.05)	110.9 (±17.1)	22 (±6.7)
	90% CI	102–110%		102–111%	
tmax** (h)	100 mg/mL	3 (2–6)	4 (2–5)	2.5 (2–4.5)	3 (2–4.5)
	200 mg/mL	3.5 (2–6)	4.5 (2.5–6)	3.3 (2–5)	3 (2–5)
AUC (ss) (h*IU/mL or h* Δ sec)	100 mg/mL	14.26 (±2.93)	1.54 (±0.61)	1321 (±219)	
	200 mg/mL	15.43 (±2.96)	1.77 (±0.67)	1401 (±227)	
	90% CI	105–112%		103–109%	

*Means ± SD at Day 5 and 90% Confidence Interval (CI) of the ratio
**Median (range)

Efficacy of Lovenox Injection in the Prophylaxis of Deep Vein Thrombosis Following Abdominal Surgery

	Dosing Regimen	
Indication	**Lovenox Inj.** 40 mg q.d. SC n (%)	**Heparin** 5000 U q8h SC n (%)
All Treated Abdominal Surgery Patients	555 (100)	560 (100)
Treatment Failures		
Total VTE[1] (%)	56 (10.1) (95% CI[2]: 8 to 13)	63 (11.3) (95% CI: 9 to 14)
DVT Only (%)	54 (9.7) (95% CI: 7 to 12)	61 (10.9) (95% CI: 8 to 13)

[1] VTE = Venous thromboembolic events which included DVT, PE, and death considered to be thromboembolic in origin.
[2] CI = Confidence Interval

In a second double-blind, parallel group study, Lovenox Injection 40 mg SC once a day was compared to heparin 5000 U every 8 hours SC in patients undergoing colorectal surgery (one-third with cancer). A total of 1347 patients were randomized in the study and all patients were treated. Patients ranged in age from 18 to 92 years (mean age 50.1 years) with 54.2% men and 45.8% women. Treatment was initiated approximately 2 hours prior to surgery and continued for approximately 7 to 10 days after surgery. The efficacy data are provided below.

Efficacy of Lovenox Injection in the Prophylaxis of Deep Vein Thrombosis Following Colorectal Surgery

Indication	Dosing Regimen	
	Lovenox Inj. 40 mg q.d. SC n (%)	Heparin 5000 U q8h SC n (%)
All Treated Colorectal Surgery Patients	673 (100)	674 (100)
Treatment Failures Total VTE[1] (%)	47 (7.1) (95% CI[2]: 5 to 9)	45 (6.7) (95% CI: 5 to 9)
DVT Only (%)	47 (7.0) (95% CI: 5 to 9)	44 (6.5) (95% CI: 5 to 8)

[1] VTE = Venous thromboembolic events which included DVT, PE, and death considered to be thromboembolic in origin.
[2] CI = Confidence Interval

Prophylaxis of Deep Vein Thrombosis Following Hip or Knee Replacement Surgery: Lovenox Injection has been shown to reduce the risk of post-operative deep vein thrombosis (DVT) following hip or knee replacement surgery.
In a double-blind study, Lovenox Injection 30 mg every 12 hours SC was compared to placebo in patients with hip replacement. A total of 100 patients were randomized in the study and all patients were treated. Patients ranged in age from 41 to 84 years (mean age 67.1 years) with 45% men and 55% women. After hemostasis was established, treatment was initiated 12 to 24 hours after surgery and was continued for 10 to 14 days after surgery. The efficacy data are provided below.

Efficacy of Lovenox Injection in the Prophylaxis of Deep Vein Thrombosis Following Hip Replacement Surgery

Indication	Dosing Regimen	
	Lovenox Inj. 30 mg q12h SC n (%)	Placebo q12h SC n (%)
All Treated Hip Replacement Patients	50 (100)	50 (100)
Treatment Failures Total DVT (%)	5 (10)[1]	23 (46)
Proximal DVT (%)	1 (2)[2]	11 (22)

[1] p value versus placebo = 0.0002
[2] p value versus placebo = 0.0134

A double-blind, multicenter study compared three dosing regimens of Lovenox Injection in patients with hip replacement. A total of 572 patients were randomized in the study and 568 patients were treated. Patients ranged in age from 31 to 88 years (mean age 64.7 years) with 63% men and 37% women. Patients were 93% Caucasian, 6% Black, <1% Oriental, and 1% others. Treatment was initiated within two days after surgery and was continued for 7 to 11 days after surgery. The efficacy data are provided below.
[See table below]
There was no significant difference between the 30 mg every 12 hours and 40 mg once a day regimens. In a double-blind study, Lovenox Injection 30 mg every 12 hours SC was compared to placebo in patients undergoing knee replacement surgery. A total of 132 patients were randomized in the study and 131 patients were treated, of which 99 had total knee replacement and 32 had either unicompartmental knee replacement or tibial osteotomy. The 99 patients with total knee replacement ranged in age from 42 to 85 years (mean age 70.2 years) with 36.4% men and 63.6% women. After hemostasis was established, treatment was initiated 12 to 24 hours after surgery and was continued up to 15 days after surgery. The incidence of proximal and total DVT after surgery was significantly lower for Lovenox Injection compared to placebo. The efficacy data are provided below.

Efficacy of Lovenox Injection in the Prophylaxis of Deep Vein Thrombosis Following Total Knee Replacement Surgery

Indication	Dosing Regimen	
	Lovenox Inj. 30 mg q12h SC n (%)	Placebo q12h SC n (%)
All Treated Total Knee Replacement Patients	47 (100)	52 (100)
Treatment Failures Total DVT (%)	5 (11)[1] (95% CI[2]: 1 to 21)	32 (62) (95% CI: 47 to 76)
Proximal DVT (%)	0 (0)[3] (95% Upper CL[4]: 5)	7 (13) (95% CI: 3 to 24)

[1] p value versus placebo = 0.0001
[2] CI = Confidence Interval
[3] p value versus placebo = 0.013
[4] CL = Confidence Limit

Additionally, in an open-label, parallel group, randomized clinical study, Lovenox Injection 30 mg every 12 hours SC in patients undergoing elective knee replacement surgery was compared to heparin 5000 U every 8 hours SC. A total of 453 patients were randomized in the study and all were treated. Patients ranged in age from 38 to 90 years (mean age 68.5 years) with 43.7% men and 56.3% women. Patients were 92.5% Caucasian, 5.3% Black, 0.2% Oriental, and 0.4% others. Treatment was initiated after surgery and continued up to 14 days. The incidence of deep vein thrombosis was significantly lower for Lovenox Injection compared to heparin.
Extended Prophylaxis of Deep Vein Thrombosis Following Hip Replacement Surgery: In a study of extended prophylaxis for patients undergoing hip replacement surgery, patients were treated, while hospitalized, with Lovenox Injection 40 mg SC, initiated up to 12 hours prior to surgery for the prophylaxis of post-operative DVT. At the end of the peri-operative period, all patients underwent bilateral venography. In a double-blind design, those patients with no venous thromboembolic disease were randomized to a post-discharge regimen of either Lovenox Injection 40 mg (n = 90) once a day SC or to placebo (n = 89) for 3 weeks. A total of 179 patients were randomized in the double-blind phase of the study and all patients were treated. Patients ranged in age from 47 to 87 years (mean age 69.4 years) with 57% men and 43% women. In this population of patients, the incidence of DVT during extended prophylaxis was significantly lower for Lovenox Injection compared to placebo. The efficacy data are provided below.

Efficacy of Lovenox Injection in the Extended Prophylaxis of Deep Vein Thrombosis Following Hip Replacement Surgery

Indication (Post-Discharge)	Post-Discharge Dosing Regimen	
	Lovenox Inj. 40 mg q.d. SC n (%)	Placebo q.d. SC n (%)
All Treated Extended Prophylaxis Patients	90 (100)	89 (100)
Treatment Failures Total DVT (%)	6 (7)[1] (95% CI[2]: 3 to 14)	18 (20) (95% CI: 12 to 30)
Proximal DVT (%)	5 (6)[3] (95% CI: 2 to 13)	7 (8) (95% CI: 3 to 16)

[1] p value versus placebo = 0.008

[2] CI= Confidence Interval
[3] p value versus placebo = 0.537
In a second study, patients undergoing hip replacement surgery were treated, while hospitalized, with Lovenox Injection 40 mg SC, initiated up to 12 hours prior to surgery. All patients were examined for clinical signs and symptoms of venous thromboembolic (VTE) disease. In a double-blind design, patients without clinical signs and symptoms of VTE disease were randomized to a post-discharge regimen of either Lovenox Injection 40 mg (n = 131) once a day SC or to placebo (n = 131) for 3 weeks. A total of 262 patients were randomized in the study double-blind phase and all patients were treated. Patients ranged in age from 44 to 87 years (mean age 68.5 years) with 43.1% men and 56.9% women. Similar to the first study the incidence of DVT during extended prophylaxis was significantly lower for Lovenox Injection compared to placebo, with a statistically significant difference in both total DVT (Lovenox Injection 21 [16%] versus placebo 45 [34%]; p = 0.001) and proximal DVT (Lovenox Injection 8 [6%] versus placebo 28 [21%]; p = <0.001).
Prophylaxis of Deep Vein Thrombosis (DVT) In Medical Patients with Severely Restricted Mobility During Acute Illness: In a double blind multicenter, parallel group study, Lovenox Injection 20 mg or 40 mg once a day SC was compared to placebo in the prophylaxis of DVT in medical patients with severely restricted mobility during acute illness (defined as walking distance of <10 meters for ≤ 3 days). This study included patients with heart failure (NYHA Class III or IV); acute respiratory failure or complicated chronic respiratory insufficiency (not requiring ventilatory support); acute infection (excluding septic shock); or acute rheumatic disorder [acute lumbar or sciatic pain, vertebral compression (due to osteoporosis or tumor), acute arthritic episodes of the lower extremities]. A total of 1102 patients were enrolled in the study, and 1073 patients were treated. Patients ranged in age from 40 to 97 years (mean age 73 years) with equal proportions of men and women. Treatment continued for a maximum of 14 days (median duration 7 days). When given at a dose of 40 mg once a day SC, Lovenox Injection significantly reduced the incidence of DVT as compared to placebo. The efficacy data are provided below.
[See first table at top of next page]
At approximately 3 months following enrollment, the incidence of venous thromboembolism remained significantly lower in the Lovenox Injection 40 mg treatment group versus the placebo treatment group.
Prophylaxis of Ischemic Complications in Unstable Angina and Non-Q-Wave Myocardial Infarction: In a multicenter, double-blind, parallel group study, patients who recently experienced unstable angina or non-Q-wave myocardial infarction were randomized to either Lovenox Injection 1 mg/kg every 12 hours SC or heparin i.v. bolus (5000 U) followed by a continuous infusion (adjusted to achieve an aPTT of 55 to 85 seconds). A total of 3171 patients were enrolled in the study, and 3107 patients were treated. Patients ranged in age from 25–94 years (median age 64 years), with 33.4% of patients female and 66.6% male. Race was distributed as follows: 89.8% Caucasian, 4.8% Black, 2.0% Oriental, and 3.5% other. **All** patients were also treated with aspirin 100 to 325 mg per day. Treatment was initiated within 24 hours of the event and continued until clinical stabilization, revascularization procedures, or hospital discharge, with a maximal duration of 8 days of therapy. The combined incidence of the triple endpoint of death, myocardial infarction, or recurrent angina was lower for Lovenox Injection compared with heparin therapy at 14 days after initiation of treatment. The lower incidence of the triple endpoint was sustained up to 30 days after initiation of treatment. These results were observed in an analysis of both all-randomized and all-treated patients. The efficacy data are provided below.
[See second table at top of next page]
The combined incidence of death or myocardial infarction at all time points was lower for Lovenox Injection compared to standard heparin therapy, but did not achieve statistical significance. The efficacy data are provided below.
[See third table at top of next page]
In a survey one year following treatment, with information available for 92% of enrolled patients, the combined incidence of death, myocardial infarction, or recurrent angina remained lower for Lovenox Injection versus heparin (32.0% vs 35.7%).
Urgent revascularization procedures were performed less frequently in the Lovenox Injection group as compared to the heparin group, 6.3% compared to 8.2% at 30 days (p = 0.047).
Treatment of Deep Vein Thrombosis (DVT) with or without Pulmonary Embolism (PE): In a multicenter, parallel group study, 900 patients with acute lower extremity DVT with or without PE were randomized to an inpatient (hospital) treatment of either (i) Lovenox Injection 1.5 mg/kg once a day SC, (ii) Lovenox Injection 1 mg/kg every 12 hours SC, or (iii) heparin i.v. bolus (5000 IU) followed by a continuous infusion (administered to achieve an aPTT of 55 to 85 seconds). A total of 900 patients were randomized in the study and all patients were treated. Patients ranged in age from 18 to 92 years (mean age 60.7 years) with 54.7% men and 45.3% women. All patients also received warfarin sodium (dose adjusted according to PT to achieve an International Normalization Ratio [INR] of 2.0 to 3.0), commencing

Efficacy of Lovenox Injection in the Prophylaxis of Deep Vein Thrombosis Following Hip Replacement Surgery

Indication	Dosing Regimen		
	10 mg q.d. SC n (%)	30 mg q12h SC n (%)	40 mg q.d. SC n (%)
All Treated Hip Replacement Patients	161 (100)	208 (100)	199 (100)
Treatment Failures Total DVT (%)	40 (25)	22 (11)[1]	27 (14)
Proximal DVT (%)	17 (11)	8 (4)[2]	9 (5)

[1] p value versus Lovenox 10 mg once a day = 0.0008
[2] p value versus Lovenox 10 mg once a day = 0.0168

Continued on next page

Lovenox—Cont.

within 72 hours of initiation of Lovenox Injection or standard heparin therapy, and continuing for 90 days. Lovenox Injection or standard heparin therapy was administered for a minimum of 5 days and until the targeted warfarin sodium INR was achieved. Both Lovenox Injection regimens were equivalent to standard heparin therapy in reducing the risk of recurrent venous thromboembolism (DVT and/or PE). The efficacy data are provided below.
[See fourth table above]
Similarly, in a multicenter, open-label, parallel group study, patients with acute proximal DVT were randomized to Lovenox Injection or heparin. Patients who could not receive outpatient therapy were excluded from entering the study. Outpatient exclusion criteria included the following: inability to receive outpatient heparin therapy because of associated co-morbid conditions or potential for non-compliance and inability to attend follow-up visits as an outpatient because of geographic inaccessibility. Eligible patients could be treated in the hospital, but ONLY Lovenox Injection patients were permitted to go home on therapy (72%). A total of 501 patients were randomized in the study and all patients were treated. Patients ranged in age from 19 to 96 years (mean age 57.8 years) with 60.5% men and 39.5% women. Patients were randomized to either Lovenox Injection 1 mg/kg every 12 hours SC or heparin i.v. bolus (5000 IU) followed by a continuous infusion administered to achieve an aPTT of 60 to 85 seconds (in-patient treatment). All patients also received warfarin sodium as described in the previous study. Lovenox Injection or standard heparin therapy was administered for a minimum of 5 days. Lovenox Injection was equivalent to standard heparin therapy in reducing the risk of recurrent venous thromboembolism. The efficacy data are provided below.

Efficacy of Lovenox Injection in Treatment of Deep Vein Thrombosis

	Dosing Regimen[1]	
Indication	Lovenox Inj. 1 mg/kg q12h SC n (%)	Heparin aPTT Adjusted i.v. Therapy n (%)
All Treated DVT Patients	247 (100)	254 (100)
Patient Outcome Total VTE[2] (%)	13 (5.3)[3]	17 (6.7)
DVT Only (%)	11 (4.5)	14 (5.5)
Proximal DVT (%)	10 (4.0)	12 (4.7)
PE (%)	2 (0.8)	3 (1.2)

[1] All patients were also treated with warfarin sodium commencing on the evening of the second day of Lovenox Injection or standard heparin therapy.
[2] VTE = venous thromboembolic event (deep vein thrombosis [DVT] and/or pulmonary embolism [PE]).
[3] The 95% Confidence Intervals for the treatment difference for total VTE was: Lovenox Injection versus heparin (-5.6 to 2.7).

INDICATIONS AND USAGE

- Lovenox Injection is indicated for the prophylaxis of deep vein thrombosis, which may lead to pulmonary embolism:
  - in patients undergoing abdominal surgery who are at risk for thromboembolic complications;
  - in patients undergoing hip replacement surgery, during and following hospitalization;
  - in patients undergoing knee replacement surgery;
  - in medical patients who are at risk for thromboembolic complications due to severely restricted mobility during acute illness.
- Lovenox Injection is indicated for the prophylaxis of ischemic complications of unstable angina and non-Q-wave myocardial infarction, when concurrently administered with aspirin.
- Lovenox Injection is indicated for:
  - the **inpatient treatment** of acute deep vein thrombosis **with or without pulmonary embolism**, when administered in conjunction with warfarin sodium;
  - the **outpatient treatment** of acute deep vein thrombosis **without pulmonary embolism** when administered in conjunction with warfarin sodium.

See **DOSAGE AND ADMINISTRATION: Adult Dosage** for appropriate dosage regimens.

CONTRAINDICATIONS

Lovenox Injection is contraindicated in patients with active major bleeding, in patients with thrombocytopenia associated with a positive *in vitro* test for anti-platelet antibody in the presence of enoxaparin sodium, or in patients with hypersensitivity to enoxaparin sodium.
Patients with known hypersensitivity to heparin, or pork products should not be treated with Lovenox Injection or any of its constituents.

WARNINGS

Lovenox Injection is not intended for intramuscular administration.

Efficacy of Lovenox Injection in the Prophylaxis of Deep Vein Thrombosis in Medical Patients With Severely Restricted Mobility During Acute Illness

	Dosing Regimen		
Indication	Lovenox Inj. 20 mg q.d. SC n (%)	Lovenox Inj. 40 mg q.d. SC n (%)	Placebo n (%)
All Treated Medical Patients During Acute Illness	351 (100)	360 (100)	362 (100)
Treatment Failure[1] Total VTE[2] (%)	43 (12.3)	16 (4.4)	43 (11.9)
Total DVT (%)	43 (12.3) (95% CI[3] 8.8 to 15.7)	16 (4.4) (95% CI[3] 2.3 to 6.6)	41 (11.3) (95% CI[3] 8.1 to 14.6)
Proximal DVT (%)	13 (3.7)	5 (1.4)	14 (3.9)

[1] Treatment failures during therapy, between Days 1 and 14.
[2] VTE = Venous thromboembolic events which included DVT, PE, and death considered to be thromboembolic in origin.
[3] CI = Confidence Interval

Efficacy of Lovenox Injection in the Prophylaxis of Ischemic Complications in Unstable Angina and Non-Q-Wave Myocardial Infarction (Combined Endpoint of Death, Myocardial Infarction, or Recurrent Angina)

	Dosing Regimen[1]			
Indication	Lovenox Inj. 1 mg/kg q12h SC n (%)	Heparin aPTT Adjusted i.v. Therapy n (%)	Reduction (%)	p Value
All Treated Unstable Angina and Non-Q-Wave MI Patients	1578 (100)	1529 (100)		
Timepoint[2] 48 Hours	96 (6.1)	112 (7.3)	1.2	0.120
14 Days	261 (16.5)	303 (19.8)	3.3	0.017
30 Days	313 (19.8)	358 (23.4)	3.6	0.014

[1] All patients were also treated with aspirin 100 to 325 mg per day.
[2] Evaluation timepoints are after initiation of treatment. Therapy continued for up to 8 days (median duration 2.6 days).

Efficacy of Lovenox Injection in the Prophylaxis of Ischemic Complications in Unstable Angina and Non-Q-Wave Myocardial Infarction (Combined Endpoint of Death or Myocardial Infarction)

	Dosing Regimen[1]			
Indication	Lovenox Inj. 1 mg/kg q12h SC n (%)	Heparin aPTT Adjusted i.v. Therapy n (%)	Reduction (%)	p Value
All Treated Unstable Angina and Non-Q-Wave MI Patients	1578 (100)	1529 (100)		
Timepoint[2] 48 Hours	16 (1.0)	20 (1.3)	0.3	0.126
14 Days	76 (4.8)	93 (6.1)	1.3	0.115
30 Days	96 (6.1)	118 (7.7)	1.6	0.069

[1] All patients were also treated with aspirin 100 to 325 mg per day.
[2] Evaluation timepoints are after initiation of treatment. Therapy continued for up to 8 days (median duration 2.6 days).

Efficacy of Lovenox Injection in Treatment of Deep Vein Thrombosis With or Without Pulmonary Embolism

	Dosing Regimen[1]		
Indication	Lovenox Inj. 1.5 mg/kg q.d. SC n (%)	Lovenox Inj. 1 mg/kg q12h SC n (%)	Heparin aPTT Adjusted i.v. Therapy n (%)
All Treated DVT Patients with or without PE	298 (100)	312 (100)	290 (100)
Patient Outcome Total VTE[2] (%)	13 (4.4)[3]	9 (2.9)[3]	12 (4.1)
DVT Only (%)	11 (3.7)	7 (2.2)	8 (2.8)
Proximal DVT (%)	9 (3.0)	6 (1.9)	7 (2.4)
PE (%)	2 (0.7)	2 (0.6)	4 (1.4)

[1] All patients were also treated with warfarin sodium commencing within 72 hours of Lovenox Injection or standard heparin therapy.
[2] VTE = venous thromboembolic event (DVT and/or PE).
[3] The 95% Confidence Intervals for the treatment differences for total VTE were:
Lovenox Injection once a day versus heparin (-3.0 to 3.5)
Lovenox Injection every 12 hours versus heparin (-4.2 to 1.7).

Lovenox Injection cannot be used interchangeably (unit for unit) with heparin or other low molecular weight heparins as they differ in manufacturing process, molecular weight distribution, anti-Xa and anti-IIa activities, units, and dosage. Each of these medicines has its own instructions for use.

Lovenox Injection should be used with extreme caution in patients with a history of heparin-induced thrombocytopenia.

Hemorrhage: Lovenox Injection, like other anticoagulants, should be used with extreme caution in conditions with increased risk of hemorrhage, such as bacterial endocarditis, congenital or acquired bleeding disorders, active ulcerative and angiodysplastic gastrointestinal disease, hemorrhagic stroke, or shortly after brain, spinal, or ophthalmological surgery, or in patients treated concomitantly with platelet inhibitors.

Cases of epidural or spinal hematomas have been reported with the associated use of Lovenox Injection and spinal/epidural anesthesia or spinal puncture resulting in long-term or permanent paralysis. The risk of these events is higher with the use of post-operative indwelling epidural catheters or by the concomitant use of additional drugs affecting hemostasis such as NSAIDs (see boxed WARNING; ADVERSE REACTIONS, Ongoing Safety Surveillance; and PRECAUTIONS, Drug Interactions).

Major hemorrhages including retroperitoneal and intracranial bleeding have been reported. Some of these cases have been fatal.

Bleeding can occur at any site during therapy with Lovenox Injection. An unexplained fall in hematocrit or blood pressure should lead to a search for a bleeding site.

Thrombocytopenia: Thrombocytopenia can occur with the administration of Lovenox Injection.

Moderate thrombocytopenia (platelet counts between 100,000/mm^3 and 50,000/mm^3) occurred at a rate of 1.3% in patients given Lovenox Injection, 1.2% in patients given heparin, and 0.7% in patients given placebo in clinical trials.

Platelet counts less than 50,000/mm^3 occurred at a rate of 0.1% in patients given Lovenox Injection, in 0.2% of patients given heparin, and 0.4% of patients given placebo in the same trials.

Thrombocytopenia of any degree should be monitored closely. If the platelet count falls below 100,000/mm^3, Lovenox Injection should be discontinued. Cases of heparin-induced thrombocytopenia with thrombosis have also been observed in clinical practice. Some of these cases were complicated by organ infarction, limb ischemia, or death.

Prosthetic Heart Valves: The use of Lovenox Injection is not recommended for thromboprophylaxis in patients with prosthetic heart valves. Cases of prosthetic heart valve thrombosis have been reported in patients with prosthetic valves who have received enoxaparin for thromboprophylaxis. Some of these cases were pregnant women in whom thrombosis led to maternal deaths and fetal deaths. Pregnant women with prosthetic heart valves may be at higher risk for thromboembolism (see **PRECAUTIONS: Pregnancy**).

Miscellaneous: Lovenox multiple-dose vials contain benzyl alcohol as a preservative. The administration of medications containing benzyl alcohol as a preservative to premature neonates has been associated with a fatal "Gasping Syndrome". Because benzyl alcohol may cross the placenta, Lovenox multiple-dose vials, preserved with benzyl alcohol, should be used with caution in pregnant women and only if clearly needed (see **PRECAUTIONS, Pregnancy**).

PRECAUTIONS

General: Lovenox Injection should not be mixed with other injections or infusions.

Lovenox Injection should be used with care in patients with a bleeding diathesis, uncontrolled arterial hypertension or a history of recent gastrointestinal ulceration, diabetic retinopathy, and hemorrhage. Elderly patients and patients with renal insufficiency may show delayed elimination of enoxaparin. Lovenox Injection should be used with care in these patients. Adjustment of enoxaparin sodium dose may be considered for low weight (<45 kg) patients and/or for patients with severe renal impairment (creatinine clearance <30 mL/min).

If thromboembolic events occur despite Lovenox Injection prophylaxis, appropriate therapy should be initiated.

Laboratory Tests: Periodic complete blood counts, including platelet count, and stool occult blood tests are recommended during the course of treatment with Lovenox Injection. When administered at recommended prophylaxis doses, routine coagulation tests such as Prothrombin Time (PT) and Activated Partial Thromboplastin Time (aPTT) are relatively insensitive measures of Lovenox Injection activity and, therefore, unsuitable for monitoring. Anti-Factor Xa may be used to monitor the anticoagulant effect of Lovenox Injection in patients with significant renal impairment. If during Lovenox Injection therapy abnormal coagulation parameters or bleeding should occur, anti-Factor Xa levels may be used to monitor the anticoagulant effects of Lovenox Injection (see **CLINICAL PHARMACOLOGY: Pharmacodynamics**).

Drug Interactions: Unless really needed, agents which may enhance the risk of hemorrhage should be discontinued prior to initiation of Lovenox Injection therapy. These agents include medications such as: anticoagulants, platelet inhibitors including acetylsalicylic acid, salicylates, NSAIDs (including ketorolac tromethamine), dipyridamole, or sulfinpyrazone. If co-administration is essential, conduct close clinical and laboratory monitoring (see **PRECAUTIONS: Laboratory Tests**).

Carcinogenesis, Mutagenesis, Impairment of Fertility: No long-term studies in animals have been performed to evaluate the carcinogenic potential of enoxaparin. Enoxaparin was not mutagenic in in vitro tests, including the Ames test, mouse lymphoma cell forward mutation test, and human lymphocyte chromosomal aberration test, and the in vivo rat bone marrow chromosomal aberration test. Enoxaparin was found to have no effect on fertility or reproductive performance of male and female rats at SC doses up to 20 mg/kg/day or 141 mg/m^2/day. The maximum human dose in clinical trials was 2.0 mg/kg/day or 78 mg/m^2/day (for an average body weight of 70 kg, height of 170 cm, and body surface area of 1.8 m^2).

Pregnancy: *Teratogenic Effects:* Pregnancy Category B: Teratology studies have been conducted in pregnant rats and rabbits at SC doses of enoxaparin up to 30 mg/kg/day or 211 mg/m^2/day and 410 mg/m^2/day, respectively. There was no evidence of teratogenic effects or fetotoxicity due to enoxaparin. There are, however, no adequate and well-controlled studies in pregnant women. Because animal reproduction studies are not always predictive of human response, this drug should be used during pregnancy only if clearly needed.

There have been reports of congenital anomalies in infants born to women who received enoxaparin during pregnancy including cerebral anomalies, limb anomalies, hypospadias, peripheral vascular malformation, fibrotic dysplasia, and cardiac defect. A cause and effect relationship has not been established nor has the incidence been shown to be higher than in the general population.

Non-teratogenic Effects: There have been post-marketing reports of fetal death when pregnant women received Lovenox Injection. Causality for these cases has not been determined. Pregnant women receiving anti-coagulants, including enoxaparin, are at increased risk for bleeding. Hemorrhage can occur at any site and may lead to death of mother and/or fetus. Pregnant women receiving enoxaparin should be carefully monitored. Pregnant women and women of child-bearing potential should be apprised of the potential hazard to the fetus and the mother if enoxaparin is administered during pregnancy.

In a clinical study of pregnant women with prosthetic heart valves given enoxaparin (1 mg/kg bid) to reduce the risk of thromboembolism, 2 of 7 women developed clots resulting in blockage of the valve and leading to maternal and fetal death. There are postmarketing reports of prosthetic valve thrombosis in pregnant women with prosthetic heart valves while receiving enoxaparin for thromboprophylaxis. These events resulted in maternal death or surgical interventions. The use of Lovenox Injection is not recommended for thromboprophylaxis in pregnant women with prosthetic heart valves (see **WARNINGS: Prosthetic Heart Valves**).

Cases of "Gasping Syndrome" have occurred in premature infants when large amounts of benzyl alcohol have been administered (99-405 mg/kg/day). The multiple-dose vial of Lovenox solution contains 15 mg/1.0 mL benzyl alcohol as a preservative (see **WARNINGS, Miscellaneous**).

Nursing Mothers: It is not known whether this drug is excreted in human milk. Because many drugs are excreted in human milk, caution should be exercised when Lovenox Injection is administered to nursing women.

Pediatric Use: Safety and effectiveness of Lovenox Injection in pediatric patients have not been established.

Geriatric Use: Over 2800 patients, 65 years and older, have received Lovenox Injection in pivotal clinical trials. The efficacy of Lovenox Injection in the elderly (≥65 years) was similar to that seen in younger patients (<65 years). The incidence of bleeding complications was similar between elderly and younger patients when 30 mg every 12 hours or 40 mg once a day doses of Lovenox Injection were employed. The incidence of bleeding complications was higher in elderly patients as compared to younger patients when Lovenox Injection was administered at doses of 1.5 mg/kg once a day or 1 mg/kg every 12 hours. The risk of Lovenox Injection-associated bleeding increased with age. Serious adverse events increased with age for patients receiving Lovenox Injection. Other clinical experience (including postmarketing surveillance and literature reports) has not revealed additional differences in the safety of Lovenox Injection between elderly and younger patients. Careful attention to dosing intervals and concomitant medications (especially antiplatelet medications) is advised. Monitoring of geriatric patients with low body weight (<45 kg) and those predisposed to decreased renal function should be considered. (see **CLINICAL PHARMACOLOGY** and **General** and **Laboratory Tests** subsections of **PRECAUTIONS**)

ADVERSE REACTIONS

Hemorrhage: The incidence of major hemorrhagic complications during Lovenox Injection treatment has been low. The following rates of major bleeding events have been reported during clinical trials with Lovenox Injection.

Major Bleeding Episodes Following Abdominal and Colorectal Surgery[1]

Indications	Dosing Regimen	
	Lovenox Inj. 40 mg q.d. SC	Heparin 5000 U q8h SC
Abdominal Surgery	n = 555 23 (4%)	n = 560 16 (3%)
Colorectal Surgery	n = 673 28 (4%)	n = 674 21 (3%)

[1] Bleeding complications were considered major: (1) if the hemorrhage caused a significant clinical event, or (2) if accompanied by a hemoglobin decrease ≥2 g/dL or transfusion of 2 or more units of blood products. Retroperitoneal, intraocular, and intracranial hemorrhages were always considered major.

Major Bleeding Episodes Following Hip or Knee Replacement Surgery[1]

Indications	Dosing Regimen		
	Lovenox Inj. 40 mg q.d. SC	Lovenox Inj. 30 mg q12h SC	Heparin 15,000 U/24h SC
Hip Replacement Surgery Without Extended Prophylaxis[2]		n = 786 31 (4%)	n = 541 32 (6%)
Hip Replacement Surgery With Extended Prophylaxis			
Peri-operative Period[3]	n = 288 4 (2%)		
Extended Prophylaxis Period[4]	n = 221 0 (0%)		
Knee Replacement Surgery Without Extended Prophylaxis[2]		n = 294 3 (1%)	n = 225 3 (1%)

[1] Bleeding complications were considered major: (1) if the hemorrhage caused a significant clinical event, or (2) if accompanied by a hemoglobin decrease ≥ 2 g/dL or transfusion of 2 or more units of blood products. Retroperitoneal and intracranial hemorrhages were always considered major. In the knee replacement surgery trials, intraocular hemorrhages were also considered major hemorrhages.
[2] Lovenox Injection 30 mg every 12 hours SC initiated 12 to 24 hours after surgery and continued for up to 14 days after surgery.
[3] Lovenox Injection 40 mg SC once a day initiated up to 12 hours prior to surgery and continued for up to 7 days after surgery.
[4] Lovenox Injection 40 mg SC once a day for up to 21 days after discharge.

NOTE: At no time point were the 40 mg once a day pre-operative and the 30 mg every 12 hours post-operative hip replacement surgery prophylactic regimens compared in clinical trials.

Injection site hematomas during the extended prophylaxis period after hip replacement surgery occurred in 9% of the Lovenox Injection patients versus 1.8% of the placebo patients.

Major Bleeding Episodes in Medical Patients With Severely Restricted Mobility During Acute Illness[1]

Indications	Dosing Regimen		
	Lovenox Inj.[2] 20 mg q.d. SC	Lovenox Inj.[2] 40 mg q.d. SC	Placebo[2]
Medical Patients During Acute Illness	n = 351 1 (<1%)	n = 360 3 (<1%)	n = 362 2 (<1%)

[1] Bleeding complications were considered major: (1) if the hemorrhage caused a significant clinical event, (2) if the hemorrhage caused a decrease in hemoglobin of ≥ 2 g/dL or transfusion of 2 or more units of blood products. Retroperitoneal and intracranial hemorrhages were always considered major although none were reported during the trial.
[2] The rates represent major bleeding on study medication up to 24 hours after last dose.

Major Bleeding Episodes in Unstable Angina and Non-Q-Wave Myocardial Infarction

Indication	Dosing Regimen	
	Lovenox Inj.[1] 1 mg/kg q12h SC	Heparin[1] aPTT Adjusted i.v. Therapy
Unstable Angina and Non-Q-Wave MI[2,3]	n = 1578 17 (1%)	n = 1529 18 (1%)

[1] The rates represent major bleeding on study medication up to 12 hours after dose.
[2] Aspirin therapy was administered concurrently (100 to 325 mg per day).
[3] Bleeding complications were considered major: (1) if the hemorrhage caused a significant clinical event, or (2) if accompanied by a hemoglobin decrease by ≥ 3 g/dL or trans-

Continued on next page

Lovenox—Cont.

fusion of 2 or more units of blood products. Intraocular, retroperitoneal, and intracranial hemorrhages were always considered major.

Major Bleeding Episodes in Deep Vein Thrombosis With or Without Pulmonary Embolism Treatment[1]

	Dosing Regimen[2]		
Indication	Lovenox Inj. 1.5 mg/kg q.d. SC	Lovenox Inj. 1 mg/kg q12h SC	Heparin aPTT Adjusted i.v. Therapy
Treatment of DVT and PE	n = 298 5 (2%)	n = 559 9 (2%)	n = 554 9 (2%)

[1] Bleeding complications were considered major: (1) if the hemorrhage caused a significant clinical event, or (2) if accompanied by a hemoglobin decrease ≥2 g/dL or transfusion of 2 or more units of blood products. Retroperitoneal, intraocular, and intracranial hemorrhages were always considered major.
[2] All patients also received warfarin sodium (dose-adjusted according to PT to achieve an INR of 2.0 to 3.0) commencing within 72 hours of Lovenox Injection or standard heparin therapy and continuing for up to 90 days.

Thrombocytopenia: see **WARNINGS: Thrombocytopenia.**
Elevations of Serum Aminotransferases: Asymptomatic increases in aspartate (AST [SGOT]) and alanine (ALT [SGPT]) aminotransferase levels greater than three times the upper limit of normal of the laboratory reference range have been reported in up to 6.1% and 5.9% of patients, respectively, during treatment with Lovenox Injection. Similar significant increases in aminotransferase levels have also been observed in patients and healthy volunteers treated with heparin and other low molecular weight heparins. Such elevations are fully reversible and are rarely associated with increases in bilirubin.

Since aminotransferase determinations are important in the differential diagnosis of myocardial infarction, liver disease, and pulmonary emboli, elevations that might be caused by drugs like Lovenox Injection should be interpreted with caution.

Local Reactions: Mild local irritation, pain, hematoma, ecchymosis, and erythema may follow SC injection of Lovenox Injection.

Other: Other adverse effects that were thought to be possibly or probably related to treatment with Lovenox Injection, heparin, or placebo in clinical trials with patients undergoing hip or knee replacement surgery, abdominal or colorectal surgery, or treatment for DVT and that occurred at a rate of at least 2% in the Lovenox Injection group, are provided below.

Adverse Events Occurring at ≥2% Incidence in Lovenox Injection Treated Patients[1] Undergoing Abdominal or Colorectal Surgery

	Dosing Regimen			
	Lovenox Inj. 40 mg q.d. SC n = 1228		Heparin 5000 U q8h SC n = 1234	
Adverse Event	Severe	Total	Severe	Total
Hemorrhage	<1%	7%	<1%	6%
Anemia	<1%	3%	<1%	3%
Ecchymosis	0%	3%	0%	3%

[1] Excluding unrelated adverse events.
[See first table above]

Adverse Events Occurring at ≥2% Incidence in Lovenox Injection Treated Medical Patients[1] With Severely Restricted Mobility During Acute Illness

	Dosing Regimen	
	Lovenox Inj. 40 mg q.d. SC n = 360 (%)	Placebo q.d. SC n = 362 (%)
Adverse Event		
Dyspnea	3.3	5.2
Thrombocytopenia	2.8	2.8
Confusion	2.2	1.1
Diarrhea	2.2	1.7
Nausea	2.5	1.7

[1] Excluding unrelated and unlikely adverse events.

Adverse Events in Lovenox Injection Treated Patients With Unstable Angina or Non-Q-Wave Myocardial Infarction: Non-hemorrhagic clinical events reported to be related to Lovenox Injection therapy occurred at an incidence of ≤ 1%.

Adverse Events Occurring at ≥2% Incidence in Lovenox Injection Treated Patients[1] Undergoing Hip or Knee Replacement Surgery

	Dosing Regimen							
	Lovenox Inj. 40 mg q.d. SC				Lovenox Inj. 30 mg q12h SC		Heparin 15,000 U/24h SC		Placebo q12h SC	
	Peri-operative Period n = 288[2]		Extended Prophylaxis Period n = 131[3]		n = 1080		n = 766		n = 115	
Adverse Event	Severe	Total	Severe	Total	Severe	Total	Severe	Total	Severe	Total
Fever	0%	8%	0%	0%	<1%	5%	<1%	4%	0%	3%
Hemorrhage	<1%	13%	0%	5%	<1%	4%	1%	4%	0%	3%
Nausea					<1%	3%	<1%	2%	0%	2%
Anemia	0%	16%	0%	<2%	<1%	2%	2%	5%	<1%	7%
Edema					<1%	2%	<1%	2%	0%	2%
Peripheral edema	0%	6%	0%	0%	<1%	3%	<1%	4%	0%	3%

[1] Excluding unrelated adverse events.
[2] Data represents Lovenox Injection 40 mg SC once a day initiated up to 12 hours prior to surgery in 288 hip replacement surgery patients who received Lovenox Injection peri-operatively in an unblinded fashion in one clinical trial.
[3] Data represents Lovenox Injection 40 mg SC once a day given in a blinded fashion as extended prophylaxis at the end of the peri-operative period in 131 of the original 288 hip replacement surgery patients for up to 21 days in one clinical trial.

Adverse Events Occurring at ≥2% Incidence in Lovenox Injection Treated Patients[1] Undergoing Treatment of Deep Vein Thrombosis With or Without Pulmonary Embolism

	Dosing Regimen					
	Lovenox Inj. 1.5 mg/kg q.d. SC n = 298		Lovenox Inj. 1 mg/kg q12h SC n = 559		Heparin aPTT Adjusted i.v. Therapy n = 544	
Adverse Event	Severe	Total	Severe	Total	Severe	Total
Injection Site Hemorrhage	0%	5%	0%	3%	<1%	<1%
Injection Site Pain	0%	2%	0%	2%	0%	0%
Hematuria	0%	2%	0%	<1%	<1%	2%

[1] Excluding unrelated adverse events.

100 mg/mL Concentration

Dosage Unit/Strength[1]	Anti-Xa Activity[2]	Package Size (per carton)	Label Color	NDC # 0075-
Ampules 30 mg / 0.3 mL	3000 IU	10 ampules	Medium Blue	0624-03
Prefilled Syringes[3] 30 mg / 0.3 mL	3000 IU	10 syringes	Medium Blue	0624-30
40 mg / 0.4 mL	4000 IU	10 syringes	Yellow	0620-40
Graduated Prefilled Syringes[3] 60 mg / 0.6 mL	6000 IU	10 syringes	Orange	0621-60
80 mg / 0.8 mL	8000 IU	10 syringes	Brown	0622-80
100 mg / 1 mL	10,000 IU	10 syringes	Black	0623-00
Multiple-Dose Vial[4] 300 mg / 3.0 mL	30,000 IU	1 vial	Red	0626-03

[1] Strength represents the number of milligrams of enoxaparin sodium in Water for Injection. **Lovenox Injection** ampules, 30 and 40 mg prefilled syringes, and 60, 80, and 100 mg graduated prefilled syringes each contain **10 mg enoxaparin sodium per 0.1 mL Water for Injection.**
[2] Approximate anti-Factor Xa activity based on reference to the W.H.O. First International Low Molecular Weight Heparin Reference Standard.
[3] Each **Lovenox Injection** syringe is affixed with a 27 gauge × 1/2 inch needle.
[4] Each Lovenox multiple-dose vial contains 15 mg / 1.0 mL of benzyl alcohol as a preservative.

Non-major hemorrhagic episodes, primarily injection site ecchymoses and hematomas, were more frequently reported in patients treated with SC Lovenox Injection than in patients treated with i.v. heparin.
Serious adverse events with Lovenox Injection or heparin in a clinical trial in patients with unstable angina or non-Q-wave myocardial infarction that occurred at a rate of at least 0.5% in the Lovenox Injection group, are provided below (irrespective of relationship to drug therapy).

Serious Adverse Events Occurring at ≥0.5% Incidence in Lovenox Injection Treated Patients With Unstable Angina or Non-Q-Wave Myocardial Infarction

	Dosing Regimen	
	Lovenox Inj. 1 mg/kg q12h SC n = 1578 n (%)	Heparin aPTT Adjusted i.v. Therapy n = 1529 n (%)
Adverse Event		
Atrial fibrillation	11 (0.70)	3 (0.20)
Heart failure	15 (0.95)	11 (0.72)
Lung edema	11 (0.70)	11 (0.72)
Pneumonia	13 (0.82)	9 (0.59)

[See second table above]

Ongoing Safety Surveillance: Since 1993, there have been over 80 reports of epidural or spinal hematoma formation with concurrent use of Lovenox Injection and spinal/epidural anesthesia or spinal puncture. The majority of patients had a post-operative indwelling epidural catheter placed for analgesia or received additional drugs affecting hemostasis such as NSAIDs. Many of the epidural or spinal hematomas caused neurologic injury, including long-term or permanent paralysis. Because these events were reported voluntarily from a population of unknown size, estimates of frequency cannot be made.

Other Ongoing Safety Surveillance Reports: local reactions at the injection site (i.e., skin necrosis, nodules, inflammation, oozing), systemic allergic reactions (i.e., pruritus, urticaria, anaphylactoid reactions), vesiculobullous rash, purpura, thrombocytosis, and thrombocytopenia with thrombosis (see **WARNINGS, Thrombocytopenia**). Very rare cases of hyperlipidemia have been reported, with one case of hyperlipidemia, with marked hypertriglyceridemia, reported in a diabetic pregnant woman; causality has not been determined.

OVERDOSAGE

Symptoms/Treatment: Accidental overdosage following administration of Lovenox Injection may lead to hemorrhagic complications. Injected Lovenox Injection may be largely neutralized by the slow i.v. injection of protamine sulfate (1% solution). The dose of protamine sulfate should be equal to the dose of Lovenox Injection injected: 1 mg protamine sulfate should be administered to neutralize 1 mg Lovenox Injection. A second infusion of 0.5 mg protamine sulfate per 1 mg of Lovenox Injection may be administered if the aPTT measured 2 to 4 hours after the first infusion remains prolonged. However, even with higher doses of protamine, the aPTT may remain more prolonged than under normal conditions found following administration of heparin. In all cases, the anti-Factor Xa activity is never completely neutralized (maximum about 60%). Particular care should be taken to avoid overdosage with protamine sulfate. Administration of protamine sulfate can cause severe hypotensive and anaphylactoid reactions. Because fatal reactions, often resembling anaphylaxis, have been reported with protamine sulfate, it should be given only when resuscitation techniques and treatment of anaphylactic shock are readily available. For additional information consult the labeling of Protamine Sulfate Injection, USP, products.

A single SC dose of 46.4 mg/kg enoxaparin was lethal to rats. The symptoms of acute toxicity were ataxia, decreased motility, dyspnea, cyanosis, and coma.

DOSAGE AND ADMINISTRATION

All patients should be evaluated for a bleeding disorder before administration of Lovenox Injection, unless the medication is needed urgently. Since coagulation parameters are unsuitable for monitoring Lovenox Injection activity, routine monitoring of coagulation parameters is not required (see **PRECAUTIONS, Laboratory Tests**).

Note: Lovenox Injection is available in two concentrations:
1. **100 mg/mL Concentration:** 30 mg / 0.3 mL ampules, 30 mg / 0.3 mL and 40 mg / 0.4 mL prefilled single-dose syringes, 60 mg / 0.6 mL, 80 mg / 0.8 mL, and 100 mg / 1 mL prefilled, graduated, single-dose syringes, 300 mg / 3.0 mL multiple-dose vials.
2. **150 mg/mL Concentration:** 120 mg / 0.8 mL and 150 mg / 1 mL prefilled, graduated, single-dose syringes.

Adult Dosage:

Abdominal Surgery: In patients undergoing abdominal surgery who are at risk for thromboembolic complications, the recommended dose of Lovenox Injection is **40 mg once a day** administered by SC injection with the initial dose given 2 hours prior to surgery. The usual duration of administration is 7 to 10 days; up to 12 days administration has been well tolerated in clinical trials.

Hip or Knee Replacement Surgery: In patients undergoing hip or knee replacement surgery, the recommended dose of Lovenox Injection is **30 mg every 12 hours** administered by SC injection. Provided that hemostasis has been established, the initial dose should be given 12 to 24 hours after surgery. For hip replacement surgery, a dose of **40 mg once a day** SC, given initially 12 ($\pm$3) hours prior to surgery, may be considered. Following the initial phase of thromboprophylaxis in hip replacement surgery patients, continued prophylaxis with Lovenox Injection 40 mg once a day administered by SC injection for 3 weeks is recommended. The usual duration of administration is 7 to 10 days; up to 14 days administration has been well tolerated in clinical trials.

Medical Patients During Acute Illness: In medical patients at risk for thromboembolic complications due to severely restricted mobility during acute illness, the recommended dose of Lovenox Injection is **40 mg once a day** administered by SC injection. The usual duration of administration is 6 to 11 days; up to 14 days of Lovenox Injection has been well tolerated in the controlled clinical trial.

Unstable Angina and Non-Q-Wave Myocardial Infarction: In patients with unstable angina or non-Q-wave myocardial infarction, the recommended dose of Lovenox Injection is **1 mg/kg** administered SC **every 12 hours** in conjunction with oral aspirin therapy (100 to 325 mg once daily). Treatment with Lovenox Injection should be prescribed for a minimum of 2 days and continued until clinical stabilization. To minimize the risk of bleeding following vascular instrumentation during the treatment of unstable angina, adhere precisely to the intervals recommended between Lovenox Injection doses. The vascular access sheath for instrumentation should remain in place for 6 to 8 hours following a dose of Lovenox Injection. The next scheduled dose should be given no sooner than 6 to 8 hours after sheath removal. The site of the procedure should be observed for signs of bleeding or hematoma formation. The usual duration of treatment is 2 to 8 days; up to 12.5 days of Lovenox Injection has been well tolerated in clinical trials.

Treatment of Deep Vein Thrombosis With or Without Pulmonary Embolism: In **outpatient treatment**, patients with acute deep vein thrombosis without pulmonary embolism who can be treated at home, the recommended dose of Lovenox Injection is **1 mg/kg every 12 hours** administered SC. In **inpatient (hospital) treatment**, patients with acute deep vein thrombosis with pulmonary embolism or patients with acute deep vein thrombosis without pulmonary embolism (who are not candidates for outpatient treatment), the recommended dose of Lovenox Injection is **1 mg/kg every 12 hours** administered SC **or 1.5 mg/kg once a day** administered SC at the same time every day. In both outpatient and inpatient (hospital) treatments, warfarin sodium therapy should be initiated when appropriate (usually within 72 hours of Lovenox Injection). Lovenox Injection should be continued for a minimum of 5 days and until a therapeutic oral anticoagulant effect has been achieved (International Normalization Ratio 2.0 to 3.0). The average duration of administration is 7 days; up to 17 days of Lovenox Injection administration has been well tolerated in controlled clinical trials.

Administration: Lovenox Injection is a clear, colorless to pale yellow sterile solution, and as with other parenteral drug products, should be inspected visually for particulate matter and discoloration prior to administration.

The use of a tuberculin syringe or equivalent is recommended when using Lovenox ampules or multiple-dose vials to assure withdrawal of the appropriate volume of drug.

Lovenox Injection is administered by SC injection. It must not be administered by intramuscular injection. Lovenox Injection is intended for use under the guidance of a physician. Patients may self-inject only if their physician determines that it is appropriate and with medical follow-up, as necessary. Proper training in subcutaneous injection technique (with or without the assistance of an injection device) should be provided.

Subcutaneous Injection Technique: Patients should be lying down and Lovenox Injection administered by deep SC injection. To avoid the loss of drug when using the 30 and 40 mg prefilled syringes, do not expel the air bubble from the syringe before the injection. Administration should be alternated between the left and right anterolateral and left and right posterolateral abdominal wall. The whole length of the needle should be introduced into a skin fold held between the thumb and forefinger; the skin fold should be held throughout the injection. To minimize bruising, do not rub the injection site after completion of the injection. Lovenox Injection prefilled syringes and graduated prefilled syringes are available with a system that shields the needle after injection.

- Remove the needle shield by pulling it straight off the syringe. If adjusting the dose is required, the dose adjustment must be done prior to injecting the prescribed dose to the patient.

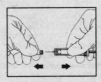

- Inject using standard technique, pushing the plunger to the bottom of the syringe.

- Remove the syringe from the injection site keeping your finger on the plunger rod.

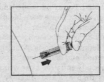

- Orienting the needle away from you and others, activate the safety system by firmly pushing the plunger rod. The protective sleeve will automatically cover the needle and an audible "click" will be heard to confirm shield activation.

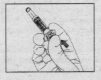

- Immediately dispose of the syringe in the nearest sharps container.

NOTE:
- The safety system can only be activated once the syringe has been emptied.
- Activation of the safety system must be done only after removing the needle from the patient's skin.
- Do not replace the needle shield after injection.
- The safety system should not be sterilized.
- Activation of the safety system may cause minimal splatter of fluid. For optimal safety activate the system while orienting it downwards away from yourself and others.

Directions for use of One Point Cut (OPC) ampules for Lovenox Injection:

Use aseptic technique throughout the process. Prior to starting, gently tap the top of the ampule to assist the flow of the solution from the upper portion of the ampule to the lower portion.

1. Locate the yellow dot on the upper portion of the ampule. Below this dot is a small score on the neck of the ampule. Hold the ampule with the yellow dot **facing away from you.** *Do not try to break the ampule at the colored rings*, which are identification marks used only in manufacturing.
2. Cover yellow dot with your index finger and position your thumb opposite yellow dot.
3. Apply pressure to the top and bottom portions of the ampule to snap the ampule open away from you.

HOW SUPPLIED

Lovenox® (enoxaparin sodium injection) is available in two concentrations:

[See third table at top of previous page]

[See table above]

Dosage Unit/Strength[1]	Anti-Xa Activity[2]	Package Size (per carton)	Syringe Label Color	NDC # 0075-
Graduated Prefilled Syringes[3]				
120 mg / 0.8 mL	12,000 IU	10 syringes	Purple	2912-01
150 mg / 1 mL	15,000 IU	10 syringes	Navy Blue	2915-01

150 mg/mL Concentration

[1] Strength represents the number of milligrams of enoxaparin sodium in Water for Injection. **Lovenox Injection** 120 and 150 mg graduated prefilled syringes contain **15 mg enoxaparin sodium per 0.1 mL** Water for Injection.
[2] Approximate anti-Factor Xa activity based on reference to the W.H.O. First International Low Molecular Weight Heparin Reference Standard.
[3] Each **Lovenox Injection** graduated prefilled syringe is affixed with a 27 gauge × 1/2 inch needle.

Store at 25°C (77°F); excursions permitted to 15-30°C (59-86°F) [see USP Controlled Room Temperature].

Keep out of the reach of children.

Lovenox Injection prefilled and graduated prefilled syringes manufactured by:
Aventis Pharma Specialties
94700 Maisons-Alfort
France
And
Aventis Pharma
Boulevard Industriel
76580 Le Trait
France
Lovenox Injection ampules manufactured by:
Aventis Pharma LTD
Dagenham Essex RM10 7XS
United Kingdom
Lovenox multiple-dose vials manufactured by:
DSM Pharmaceuticals, Inc.
Greenville, NC 27835
Manufactured for:
Aventis Pharmaceuticals Inc.
Bridgewater, NJ 08807
©2002 Aventis Pharmaceuticals Inc.
Rev. January 2003
lovp0103p

To keep your **PDR** up to date throughout the year, note these revisions on the corresponding pages of the annual volume. Simply write **"See Supplement A"** next to the product heading.

Biogen, Inc.
14 CAMBRIDGE CENTER
CAMBRIDGE, MA 02142

Direct Inquiries to:
Customer Service (800) 456-2255
Fax (617) 679-3100

AVONEX® ℞
[ă'vŏn-eks]
(Interferon beta-1a)

Prescribing information for this product, which appears on pages 1006–1010 of the 2003 PDR, has been completely revised as follows. Please write "See Supplement A" next to the product heading.

DESCRIPTION

AVONEX® (Interferon beta-1a) is a 166 amino acid glycoprotein with a predicted molecular weight of approximately 22,500 daltons. It is produced by recombinant DNA technology using genetically engineered Chinese Hamster Ovary cells into which the human interferon beta gene has been introduced. The amino acid sequence of AVONEX® is identical to that of natural human interferon beta.

Using the World Health Organization (WHO) natural interferon beta standard, Second International Standard for Interferon, Human Fibroblast (Gb-23-902-531), AVONEX® has a specific activity of approximately 200 million international units (IU) of antiviral activity per mg of Interferon beta-1a determined specifically by an *in vitro* cytopathic effect bioassay using lung carcinoma cells (A549) and Encephalomyocarditis virus (ECM). AVONEX® 30 mcg contains approximately 6 million IU of antiviral activity using this method. The activity against other standards is not known. Comparison of the activity of AVONEX® with other Interferon betas is not appropriate, because of differences in the reference standards and assays used to measure activity.

AVONEX® is formulated as a sterile, white to off-white lyophilized powder for intramuscular injection after reconstitution with supplied diluent (Sterile Water for Injection, USP).

Each 1.0 mL of reconstituted AVONEX® contains 30 mcg of Interferon beta-1a; 15 mg Albumin Human, USP; 5.8 mg Sodium Chloride, USP; 5.7 mg Dibasic Sodium Phosphate, USP; and 1.2 mg Monobasic Sodium Phosphate, USP, at a pH of approximately 7.3.

CLINICAL PHARMACOLOGY
General

Interferons are a family of naturally occurring proteins and glycoproteins that are produced by eukaryotic cells in response to viral infection and other biological inducers. Interferon beta, one member of this family, is produced by various cell types including fibroblasts and macrophages. Natural interferon beta and Interferon beta-1a are glycosylated, with each containing a single N-linked complex carbohydrate moiety. Glycosylation of other proteins is known to affect their stability, activity, aggregation, biodistribution, and half-life in blood. However, the effects of glycosylation of interferon beta on these properties have not been fully defined.

Biologic Activities

Interferons are cytokines that mediate antiviral, antiproliferative and immunomodulatory activities in response to viral infection and other biological inducers. Three major interferons have been distinguished: alpha, beta, and gamma. Interferons alpha and beta form the Type I class of interferons, and interferon gamma is a Type II interferon. These interferons have overlapping but clearly distinct biological activities.

Interferon beta exerts its biological effects by binding to specific receptors on the surface of human cells. This binding initiates a complex cascade of intracellular events that leads to the expression of numerous interferon-induced gene products and markers. These include 2', 5'-oligoadenylate synthetase, β_2-microglobulin, and neopterin. These products have been measured in the serum and cellular fractions of blood collected from patients treated with AVONEX®.

The specific interferon-induced proteins and mechanisms by which AVONEX® exerts its effects in multiple sclerosis have not been fully defined. Clinical studies conducted in multiple sclerosis patients showed that interleukin 10 (IL-10) levels in cerebrospinal fluid were increased in patients treated with AVONEX® compared to placebo. Serum IL-10 levels were increased 48 hours after intramuscular (IM) injection of AVONEX® and remained elevated for 1 week. However, no relationship has been established between absolute levels of IL-10 and clinical outcome in multiple sclerosis.

Pharmacokinetics

Pharmacokinetics of AVONEX® in multiple sclerosis patients have not been evaluated. The pharmacokinetic and pharmacodynamic profiles of AVONEX® in healthy subjects following doses of 30 mcg through 75 mcg have been investigated. Serum levels of AVONEX® as measured by antiviral activity are slightly above detectable limits following a 30 mcg IM dose, and increase with higher doses.

After an IM dose, serum levels of AVONEX® typically peak between 3 and 15 hours and then decline at a rate consistent with a 10 hour elimination half-life. Serum levels of AVONEX® may be sustained after IM administration due to prolonged absorption from the IM site. Systemic exposure, as determined by AUC and C_{max} values, is greater following IM than subcutaneous (SC) administration.

Subcutaneous administration of AVONEX® should not be substituted for intramuscular administration. Subcutaneous and intramuscular administration have been observed to have non-equivalent pharmacokinetic and pharmacodynamic parameters following administration to healthy volunteers.

Biological response markers (e.g., neopterin and β_2-microglobulin) are induced by AVONEX® following parenteral doses of 15 mcg through 75 mcg in healthy subjects and treated patients. Biological response marker levels increase within 12 hours of dosing and remain elevated for at least 4 days. Peak biological response marker levels are typically observed 48 hours after dosing. The relationship of serum AVONEX® levels or levels of these induced biological response markers to the mechanisms by which AVONEX® exerts its effects in multiple sclerosis is unknown.

Clinical Studies

The clinical effects of AVONEX® in multiple sclerosis were studied in two randomized, multicenter, double-blind, placebo-controlled studies in patients with multiple sclerosis.[1,2] Safety and efficacy of treatment with AVONEX® beyond 3 years is not known.

In Study 1, 301 patients received either 30 mcg of AVONEX® (n=158) or placebo (n=143) by IM injection once weekly. Patients were entered into the trial over a 2½ year period, received injections for up to 2 years, and continued to be followed until study completion. Two hundred eighty-two patients completed 1 year on study, and 172 patients completed 2 years on study. There were 144 patients treated with AVONEX® for more than 1 year, 115 patients for more than 18 months and 82 patients for 2 years.

All patients had a definite diagnosis of multiple sclerosis of at least 1 year duration and had at least 2 exacerbations in the 3 years prior to study entry (or 1 per year if the duration of disease was less than 3 years). At entry, study participants were without exacerbation during the prior 2 months and had Kurtzke Expanded Disability Status Scale (EDSS[3]) scores ranging from 1.0 to 3.5. Patients with chronic progressive multiple sclerosis were excluded from this study.

The primary outcome assessment was time to progression in disability, measured as an increase in the EDSS score of at least 1.0 point that was sustained for at least 6 months. An increase in EDSS score reflects accumulation of disability. This endpoint was used to ensure that progression reflected permanent increase in disability rather than a transient effect due to an exacerbation.

Secondary outcomes included exacerbation frequency and results of magnetic resonance imaging (MRI) scans including gadolinium (Gd)-enhanced lesion number and volume and T2-weighted (proton density) lesion volume. Additional secondary endpoints included 2 upper limb (tested in both arms) and 3 lower limb function tests.

Twenty-three of the 301 patients (8%) discontinued treatment prematurely. Of these, 1 patient treated with placebo (1%) and 6 patients treated with AVONEX® (4%) discontinued treatment due to adverse events. Thirteen of these 23 patients remained on study and were evaluated for clinical endpoints.

Table 1
Clinical and MRI Endpoints in Study 1

Endpoint	Placebo	AVONEX®	P-Value
PRIMARY ENDPOINT:			
Time to sustained progression in disability (N: 143, 158)[1]	–See Figure 1–		0.02[2]
Percentage of patients progressing in disability at 2 years (Kaplan-Meier estimate)[1]	34.9%	21.9%	
SECONDARY ENDPOINTS:			
DISABILITY			
Mean confirmed change in EDSS from study entry to end of study (N: 136, 150)	0.50	0.20	0.006[3]
EXACERBATIONS			
Number of exacerbations in subset completing 2 years (N: 87, 85)			0.03[3]
0	26%	38%	
1	30%	31%	
2	11%	18%	
3	14%	7%	
≥4	18%	7%	
Percentage of patients exacerbation-free in subset completing 2 years (N: 87, 85)	26%	38%	0.10[4]
Annual exacerbation rate (N: 143, 158)[1]	0.82	0.67	0.04[5]
MRI			
Number of Gd-enhanced lesions:			
At study entry (N: 132, 141)			
Mean (Median)	2.3 (1.0)	3.2 (1.0)	
Range	0-23	0-56	
Year 1 (N: 123, 134)			
Mean (Median)	1.6 (0)	1.0 (0)	0.02[3]
Range	0-22	0-28	
Year 2 (N: 82, 83)			
Mean (Median)	1.6 (0)	0.8 (0)	0.05[3]
Range	0-34	0-13	
T2 lesion volume:			
Percentage change from study entry to Year 1 (N: 116, 123)			
Median	-3.3%	-13.1%	0.02[3]
Percentage change from study entry to Year 2 (N: 83, 81)			
Median	-6.5%	-13.2%	0.36[3]

Note: (N: ,) denotes the number of evaluable placebo and AVONEX® patients, respectively.
[1] Patient data included in this analysis represent variable periods of time on study.
[2] Analyzed by Mantel-Cox (logrank) test.
[3] Analyzed by Mann-Whitney rank-sum test.
[4] Analyzed by Cochran-Mantel-Haenszel test.
[5] Analyzed by likelihood ratio test.

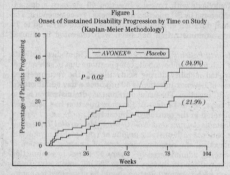

Figure 1
Onset of Sustained Disability Progression by Time on Study
(Kaplan-Meier Methodology)

Note: Disability progression represents at least a 1.0 point increase in EDSS score sustained for at least 6 months.

Time to onset of sustained progression in disability was significantly longer in patients treated with AVONEX® than in patients receiving placebo (p = 0.02). The Kaplan-Meier plots of these data are presented in Figure 1. The Kaplan-Meier estimate of the percentage of patients progressing by the end of 2 years was 34.9% for placebo-treated patients and 21.9% for AVONEX®-treated patients, indicating a slowing of the disease process. This represents a 37% relative reduction in the risk of accumulating disability in the AVONEX®-treated group compared to the placebo-treated group.

[See figure 2 at top of next column]

The distribution of confirmed EDSS change from study entry (baseline) to the end of the study is shown in Figure 2. There was a statistically significant difference between treatment groups in confirmed change for patients with at least 2 scheduled visits (136 placebo-treated and 150 AVONEX®-treated patients; p = 0.006; see Table 1).

The rate and frequency of exacerbations were determined as secondary outcomes. For all patients included in the

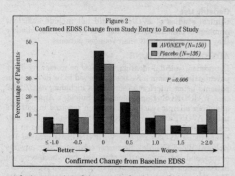

Figure 2
Confirmed EDSS Change from Study Entry to End of Study

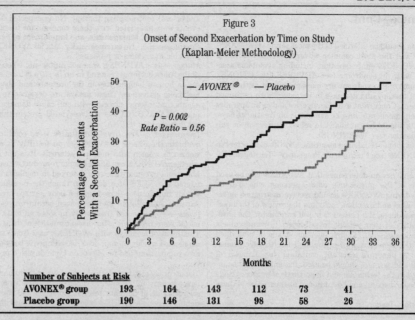

Figure 3
Onset of Second Exacerbation by Time on Study
(Kaplan-Meier Methodology)

study, irrespective of time on study, the annual exacerbation rate was 0.67 per year in the AVONEX®-treated group and 0.82 per year in the placebo-treated group (p = 0.04). AVONEX® treatment significantly decreased the frequency of exacerbations in the subset of patients who were enrolled in the study for at least 2 years (87 placebo-treated patients and 85 AVONEX®-treated patients; p = 0.03; see Table 1). Gd-enhanced and T2-weighted (proton density) MRI scans of the brain were obtained in most patients at baseline and at the end of 1 and 2 years of treatment. Gd-enhancing lesions seen on brain MRI scans represent areas of breakdown of the blood brain barrier thought to be secondary to inflammation. Patients treated with AVONEX® demonstrated significantly lower Gd-enhanced lesion number after 1 and 2 years of treatment (p ≤ 0.05; see Table 1). The volume of Gd-enhanced lesions was also analyzed, and showed similar treatment effects (p ≤ 0.03). Percentage change in T2-weighted lesion volume from study entry to Year 1 was significantly lower in AVONEX®-treated than placebo-treated patients (p = 0.02). A significant difference in T2-weighted lesion volume change was not seen between study entry and Year 2.

The exact relationship between MRI findings and the clinical status of patients is unknown. The prognostic significance of MRI findings in these studies have not been evaluated.

Of the limb function tests, only 1 demonstrated a statistically significant difference between treatment groups (favoring AVONEX®). A summary of the effects of AVONEX® on the clinical and MRI endpoints of this study is presented in Table 1.

[See table 1 at top of previous page]

In Study 2, 383 patients who had recently experienced an isolated demyelinating event involving the optic nerve, spinal cord, or brainstem/cerebellum, and who had lesions typical of multiple sclerosis on brain MRI, received either 30 mcg AVONEX® (n = 193) or placebo (n = 190) by IM injection once weekly. All patients received intravenous steroid treatment for the initiating clinical exacerbation. Patients were enrolled into the study over a two-year period and followed for up to three years or until they developed a second clinical exacerbation in an anatomically distinct region of the central nervous system. Sixteen percent of subjects on AVONEX® and 14% of subjects on placebo withdrew from the study for a reason other than the development of a second exacerbation[2]. Of these early withdrawal patients, 20% treated with placebo and 32% treated with AVONEX® withdrew due to adverse events.

The primary outcome measure was time to development of a second exacerbation in an anatomically distinct region of the central nervous system. Secondary outcomes were brain MRI measures, including the cumulative increase in the number of new or enlarging T2 lesions, T2 lesion volume compared to baseline at 18 months, and the number of Gd-enhancing lesions at 6 months.

Time to development of a second exacerbation was significantly delayed in patients treated with AVONEX® compared to placebo (p = 0.002). The Kaplan-Meier estimates of the percentage of patients developing an exacerbation within 24 months were 38.6% in the placebo group and 21.1% in the AVONEX® group (Figure 3). The relative rate of developing a second exacerbation in the AVONEX® group was 0.56 of the rate in the placebo group (95% confidence interval 0.38 to 0.81). The brain MRI findings are described in Table 2.

[See figure 3 above]
[See table 2 above]

INDICATIONS AND USAGE

AVONEX® (Interferon beta-1a) is indicated for the treatment of patients with relapsing forms of multiple sclerosis to slow the accumulation of physical disability and decrease the frequency of clinical exacerbations. Patients with multiple sclerosis in whom efficacy has been demonstrated include patients who have experienced a first clinical episode and have MRI features consistent with multiple sclerosis. Safety and efficacy in patients with chronic progressive multiple sclerosis have not been established.

CONTRAINDICATIONS

AVONEX® is contraindicated in patients with a history of hypersensitivity to natural or recombinant interferon beta, human albumin, or any other component of the formulation.

WARNINGS

Depression and Suicide
AVONEX® should be used with caution in patients with depression or other mood disorders, conditions that are common with multiple sclerosis. Depression and suicide have been reported to occur with increased frequency in patients receiving interferon compounds, including AVONEX®. Patients treated with AVONEX® should be advised to report immediately any symptoms of depression and/or suicidal ideation to their prescribing physicians. If a patient develops depression or other severe psychiatric symptoms, cessation of AVONEX® therapy should be considered. In Study 2, AVONEX®-treated patients were more likely to experience depression than placebo-treated patients. An equal incidence of depression was seen in the placebo-treated and AVONEX®-treated patients in Study 1. Additionally, there have been post-marketing reports of depression, suicidal ideation and/or development of new or worsening of preexisting other psychiatric disorders, including psychosis. Some of these patients improved upon cessation of AVONEX® dosing.

Anaphylaxis
Anaphylaxis has been reported as a rare complication of AVONEX® use. Other allergic reactions have included dyspnea, orolingual edema, skin rash and urticaria (see ADVERSE REACTIONS).

Decreased Peripheral Blood Counts
Decreased peripheral blood counts in all cell lines, including rare pancytopenia and thrombocytopenia, have been reported from post-marketing experience (see ADVERSE REACTIONS). Some cases of thrombocytopenia have had nadirs below 10,000/μL. Some cases reoccur with rechallenge (see ADVERSE REACTIONS). Patients should be monitored for signs of these disorders (see Precautions: Laboratory Tests).

Albumin (Human)
This product contains albumin, a derivative of human blood. Based on effective donor screening and product manufacturing processes, it carries an extremely remote risk for transmission of viral diseases. A theoretical risk for transmission of Creutzfeldt-Jakob disease (CJD) also is considered extremely remote. No cases of transmission of viral diseases or CJD have been identified for albumin.

PRECAUTIONS
Seizures
Caution should be exercised when administering AVONEX® to patients with pre-existing seizure disorders. In the two placebo-controlled studies in multiple sclerosis, 4 patients receiving AVONEX® experienced seizures, while no seizures occurred in the placebo group. Three of these 4 patients had no prior history of seizure (see ADVERSE REACTIONS). It is not known whether these events were related to the effects of multiple sclerosis alone, to AVONEX®, or to a combination of both. The effect of AVONEX® administration on the medical management of patients with seizure disorder is unknown.

Cardiomyopathy and Congestive Heart Failure
Patients with cardiac disease, such as angina, congestive heart failure, or arrhythmia, should be closely monitored for worsening of their clinical condition during initiation and continued treatment with AVONEX®. While AVONEX® does not have any known direct-acting cardiac toxicity, during the post-marketing period infrequent cases of congestive heart failure, cardiomyopathy, and cardiomyopathy with congestive heart failure have been reported in patients without known predisposition to these events, and without other known etiologies being established. In rare cases, these events have been temporally related to the administration of AVONEX®. In some of these instances recurrence upon rechallenge was observed.

Autoimmune Disorders
Autoimmune disorders of multiple target organs have been reported post-marketing including idiopathic thrombocytopenia, hyper- and hypothyroidism, and rare cases of autoimmune hepatitis have also been reported. Patients should be monitored for signs of these disorders (see Precautions: Laboratory Tests) and appropriate treatment implemented when observed.

Hepatic Injury
Hepatic injury including elevated serum hepatic enzyme levels and hepatitis, some of which have been severe, has been reported post-marketing. In some patients a recurrence of elevated serum levels of hepatic enzymes has occurred upon AVONEX® rechallenge. In some cases, these events have occurred in the presence of other drugs that have been associated with hepatic injury. The potential of additive effects from multiple drugs or other hepatotoxic agents (e.g., alcohol) has not been determined. Patients should be monitored for signs of hepatic injury (see Precautions: Laboratory Tests) and caution exercised when AVONEX® is used concomitantly with other drugs associated with hepatic injury.

Information to Patients
All patients should be instructed to read the AVONEX® Medication Guide supplied to them. Patients should be cautioned not to change the dosage or the schedule of administration without medical consultation.

Continued on next page

Table 2
Brain MRI Data According to Treatment Group

	AVONEX®	Placebo
CHANGE IN T2 VOLUME @18 MONTHS:	N = 119	N = 109
Actual Change (mm^3)[1]*		
Median (25th%, 75th%)	28 (-576, 397)	313 (5, 1140)
Percentage Change[1]*		
Median (25th%, 75th%)	1 (-24, 29)	16 (0, 53)
NUMBER OF NEW OR ENLARGING	N = 132	N = 119
T2 LESIONS @ 18 MONTHS[1]*:	N (%)	N (%)
0	62 (47)	22 (18)
1–3	41 (31)	47 (40)
≥4	29 (22)	50 (42)
Mean (SD)	2.13 (3.19)	4.97 (7.71)
NUMBER OF GD-ENHANCING	N = 165	N = 152
LESIONS @ 6 MONTHS[2]*:	N (%)	N (%)
0	115 (70)	93 (61)
1	27 (16)	16 (11)
>1	23 (14)	43 (28)
Mean (SD)	0.87 (2.28)	1.49 (3.14)

[1]P value <0.001
[2]P value <0.03
*P value from a Mann-Whitney rank-sum test

Avonex—Cont.

Patients should be informed of the most serious (see WARNINGS) and the most common adverse events associated with AVONEX® administration, including symptoms associated with flu syndrome (see ADVERSE REACTIONS). Symptoms of flu syndrome are most prominent at the initiation of therapy and decrease in frequency with continued treatment. Concurrent use of analgesics and/or antipyretics may help ameliorate flu-like symptoms on treatment days. Patients should be cautioned to report depression or suicidal ideation (see WARNINGS).

Patients should be advised about the abortifacient potential of AVONEX® (see Precautions: Pregnancy—Teratogenic Effects).

When a physician determines that AVONEX® can be used outside of the physician's office, persons who will be administering AVONEX® should receive instruction in reconstitution and injection, including the review of the injection procedures. If a patient is to self-administer, the physical ability of that patient to self-inject intramuscularly should be assessed. The first injection should be performed under the supervision of a qualified health care professional. A puncture-resistant container for disposal of needles and syringes should be used. Patients should be instructed in the technique and importance of proper syringe and needle disposal and be cautioned against reuse of these items.

Laboratory Tests

In addition to those laboratory tests normally required for monitoring patients with multiple sclerosis, complete blood and differential white blood cell counts, platelet counts, and blood chemistries, including liver function tests, are recommended during AVONEX® therapy (see WARNINGS: Decreased Peripheral Blood Counts and PRECAUTIONS: Cardiomyopathy and Congestive Heart Failure, and Autoimmune Disorders). During the placebo-controlled studies in multiple sclerosis, these tests were performed at least every 6 months. There were no significant differences between the placebo and AVONEX® groups in the incidence of liver enzyme elevation, leukopenia, or thrombocytopenia. However, these are known to be dose-related laboratory abnormalities associated with the use of interferons. Patients with myelosuppression may require more intensive monitoring of complete blood cell counts, with differential and platelet counts. Thyroid function should be monitored periodically. If patients have or develop symptoms of thyroid dysfunction (hypo- or hyperthyroidism), thyroid function tests should be performed according to standard medical practice.

Drug Interactions

No formal drug interaction studies have been conducted with AVONEX®. In the placebo-controlled studies in multiple sclerosis, corticosteroids or ACTH were administered for treatment of exacerbations in some patients concurrently receiving AVONEX®. In addition, some patients receiving AVONEX® were also treated with anti-depressant therapy and/or oral contraceptive therapy. No unexpected adverse events were associated with these concomitant therapies.

Carcinogenesis, Mutagenesis, and Impairment of Fertility

Carcinogenesis: No carcinogenicity data for AVONEX® are available in animals or humans.

Mutagenesis: AVONEX® was not mutagenic when tested in the Ames bacterial test and in an *in vitro* cytogenetic assay in human lymphocytes in the presence and absence of metabolic activation. These assays are designed to detect agents that interact directly with and cause damage to cellular DNA. AVONEX® is a glycosylated protein that does not directly bind to DNA.

Impairment of Fertility: No studies were conducted to evaluate the effects of AVONEX® on fertility in normal women or women with multiple sclerosis. It is not known whether AVONEX® can affect human reproductive capacity. Menstrual irregularities were observed in monkeys administered AVONEX® at a dose 100 times the recommended weekly human dose (based upon a body surface area comparison). Anovulation and decreased serum progesterone levels were also noted transiently in some animals. These effects were reversible after discontinuation of drug.

Treatment of monkeys with AVONEX® at 2 times the recommended weekly human dose (based upon a body surface area comparison) had no effects on cycle duration or ovulation.

The accuracy of extrapolating animal doses to human doses is not known. In the placebo-controlled studies in multiple sclerosis, 5% of patients receiving placebo and 6% of patients receiving AVONEX® experienced menstrual disorder. If menstrual irregularities occur in humans, it is not known how long they will persist following treatment.

Pregnancy—Teratogenic Effects

Pregnancy Category C: The reproductive toxicity of AVONEX® has not been studied in animals or humans. In pregnant monkeys given AVONEX® at 100 times the recommended weekly human dose (based upon a body surface area comparison), no teratogenic or other adverse effects on fetal development were observed. Abortifacient activity was evident following 3 to 5 doses at this level. No abortifacient effects were observed in monkeys treated at 2 times the recommended weekly human dose (based upon a body surface area comparison). Although no teratogenic effects were seen in these studies, it is not known if teratogenic effects would be observed in humans. There are no adequate and well-controlled studies with interferons in pregnant women. If a woman becomes pregnant or plans to become pregnant while taking AVONEX®, she should be informed of the potential hazards to the fetus, and discontinuation of AVONEX® therapy should be considered.

Nursing Mothers

It is not known whether AVONEX® is excreted in human milk. Because of the potential of serious adverse reactions in nursing infants, a decision should be made to either discontinue nursing or to discontinue AVONEX®.

Pediatric Use

Safety and effectiveness of AVONEX® in pediatric patients below the age of 18 years have not been evaluated.

Geriatric Use

Clinical studies of AVONEX® did not include sufficient numbers of patients aged 65 and over to determine whether they respond differently than younger patients.

ADVERSE REACTIONS

Depression, suicidal ideation, and new or worsening other psychiatric disorders have been observed to be increased in patients using interferon compounds including AVONEX® (see WARNINGS: Depression and Suicide). Anaphylaxis and other allergic reactions have been reported in patients using AVONEX® (see WARNINGS: Anaphylaxis). Decreased peripheral blood counts have been reported in patients using AVONEX® (see WARNINGS: Decreased Peripheral Blood Counts). Seizures, cardiovascular adverse events, and autoimmune disorders also have been reported in association with the use of AVONEX® (see Precautions).

The adverse reactions most commonly reported in patients associated with the use of AVONEX® were flu-like and other symptoms occurring within hours to days following an injection. Symptoms can include myalgia, fever, fatigue, headaches, chills, nausea, and vomiting. Some patients have experienced paresthesias, hypertonia and myasthenia.

The most frequently reported adverse reactions resulting in clinical intervention (e.g., discontinuation of AVONEX®, or the need for concomitant medication to treat an adverse reaction symptom) were flu-like symptoms and depression.

Because clinical trials are conducted under widely varying conditions, adverse reaction rates observed in the clinical trials of AVONEX® cannot be directly compared to rates in clinical trials of other drugs and may not reflect the rates observed in practice.

The data described below reflect exposure to AVONEX® in 351 patients, including 319 patients exposed for 6 months, and 288 patients exposed for greater than one year in placebo-controlled trials. The mean age of patients receiving AVONEX® was 35 years, 74% were women and 89% were Caucasian. Patients received either 30 mcg AVONEX® or placebo.

Table 3 enumerates adverse events and selected laboratory abnormalities that occurred at an incidence of at least 2% higher frequency in AVONEX®-treated subjects than was observed in the placebo group. Reported adverse events have been classified using standard COSTART terms.

[See table 3 below]

No AVONEX®-treated patients attempted suicide in the two placebo-controlled studies. In Study 2, AVONEX®-treated patients were more likely to experience depression than placebo-treated patients (20% in AVONEX® group vs. 13% in placebo group). The incidences of depression in the placebo-treated and AVONEX®-treated patients in Study 1 were similar. In Study 1, suicidal tendency was seen more frequently in AVONEX®-treated patients (4% in AVONEX® group vs. 1% in placebo group) (see WARNINGS).

Seizures

Seizures have been reported in 4 of 351 AVONEX®-treated patients in the placebo-controlled studies, compared to none in the placebo-treated patients (see Precautions: Seizures).

Post-Marketing Experience

The following adverse events have been identified and reported during post-approval use of AVONEX®: New or worsening other psychiatric disorders, and anaphylaxis (see WARNINGS). Autoimmune disorders including autoimmune hepatitis, idiopathic thrombocytopenia, hyper- and hypothyroidism, and seizures in patients without prior history (see Precautions).

Infrequent reports of congestive heart failure, cardiomyopathy, and cardiomyopathy with congestive heart failure with rare cases being temporally related to the administration of AVONEX® (see Precautions: Cardiomyopathy and Congestive Heart Failure).

Decreased peripheral blood counts in all cell lines, including rare pancytopenia and thrombocytopenia (see WARNINGS: Decreased Peripheral Blood Counts). Some cases of thrombocytopenia have had nadirs below 10,000/µL. Some of these cases reoccur upon rechallenge.

Hepatic injury including elevated serum hepatic enzyme levels and hepatitis, some of which have been severe, has been reported post-marketing (see Precautions: Hepatic Injury).

Meno- and metrorrhagia have also been reported in post-marketing experience.

Because reports of these reactions are voluntary and the population is of an uncertain size, it is not always possible to reliably estimate the frequency of the event or establish a causal relationship to drug exposure.

Adverse Reactions Associated with Subcutaneous Use

AVONEX® has also been evaluated in 290 patients with diseases other than multiple sclerosis, primarily chronic viral hepatitis B and C, in which the doses studied ranged from 15 mcg to 75 mcg, given SC, 3 times a week, for up to 6 months. Inflammation at the site of the subcutaneous injection was observed in 52% of treated patients in these studies. Subcutaneous injections were also associated with the following local reactions: injection site necrosis, injection site atrophy, injection site edema and injection site hemorrhage. None of the above was observed in the multiple sclerosis patients participating in Study 1. Injection site edema and injection site hemorrhage were observed in multiple sclerosis patients participating in Study 2.

Immunogenicity

As with all therapeutic proteins, there is a potential for immunogenicity. In recent studies assessing immunogenicity in multiple sclerosis patients administered AVONEX® for at least 1 year, 5% (13 of 261 patients) showed the presence of

Table 3
Adverse Events and Selected Laboratory Abnormalities in the Placebo-Controlled Studies

Adverse Event	Placebo (N = 333)	AVONEX® (N = 351)
Body as a Whole		
Headache	55%	58%
Flu-like symptoms (otherwise unspecified)	29%	49%
Pain	21%	23%
Asthenia	18%	24%
Fever	9%	20%
Chills	5%	19%
Abdominal pain	6%	8%
Injection site pain	6%	8%
Infection	4%	7%
Injection site inflammation	2%	6%
Chest pain	2%	5%
Injection site reaction	1%	3%
Toothache	1%	3%
Nervous System		
Depression	14%	18%
Dizziness	12%	14%
Resipiratory System		
Upper respiratory tract infection	12%	14%
Sinusitis	12%	14%
Bronchitis	5%	8%
Digestive System		
Nausea	19%	23%
Musculoskeletal System		
Myalgia	22%	29%
Arthralgia	6%	9%
Urogenital		
Urinary tract infection	15%	17%
Urine constituents abnormal	0%	3%
Skin and Appendages		
Alopecia	2%	4%
Special Senses		
Eye disorder	2%	4%
Hemic and Lymphatic System		
Injection site ecchymosis	4%	6%
Anemia	1%	4%
Cardiovascular System		
Migraine	3%	5%
Vasodilation	0%	2%

neutralizing antibodies at one or more times. The clinical significance of neutralizing antibodies to AVONEX® is unknown.

These data reflect the percentage of patients whose test results were considered positive for antibodies to AVONEX® using a two-tiered assay (ELISA binding assay followed by an antiviral cytopathic effect assay), and are highly dependent on the sensitivity and specificity of the assay. Additionally, the observed incidence of neutralizing activity in an assay may be influenced by several factors including sample handling, timing of sample collection, concomitant medications, and underlying disease. For these reasons, comparison of the incidence of antibodies to AVONEX® with the incidence of antibodies to other products may be misleading. Anaphylaxis has been reported as a rare complication of AVONEX® use. Other allergic reactions have included dyspnea, orolingual edema, skin rash and urticaria (see WARNINGS: Anaphylaxis).

DRUG ABUSE AND DEPENDENCE

There is no evidence that abuse or dependence occurs with AVONEX® therapy. However, the risk of dependence has not been systematically evaluated.

OVERDOSAGE

Safety of doses higher than 60 mcg once a week have not been adequately evaluated. The maximum amount of AVONEX® that can be safely administered has not been determined.

DOSAGE AND ADMINISTRATION

The recommended dosage of AVONEX® (Interferon beta-1a) is 30 mcg injected intramuscularly once a week.

AVONEX® is intended for use under the guidance and supervision of a physician. Patients may self-inject only if their physician determines that it is appropriate and with medical follow-up, as necessary, after proper training in intramuscular injection technique.

Use appropriate aseptic technique during the preparation of AVONEX®. To reconstitute lyophilized AVONEX®, use a sterile syringe and MICRO PIN® to inject 1.1 mL of the supplied diluent, Sterile Water for Injection, USP, into the AVONEX® vial. Gently swirl the vial of AVONEX® to dissolve the drug completely. **DO NOT SHAKE.** The reconstituted solution should be clear to slightly yellow and without particles. Inspect the reconstituted product visually prior to use. Discard the product if it contains particulate matter or is discolored. Each vial of reconstituted solution contains 30 mcg Interferon beta-1a.

Withdraw 1.0 mL of reconstituted solution from the vial into a sterile syringe fitted with a 23 gauge, 1¼ inch needle and inject the solution intramuscularly. Sites for injection include the thigh or upper arm. The AVONEX® and diluent vials are for single-use only; unused portions should be discarded. (See Medication Guide for self-injection procedure.)

HOW SUPPLIED

AVONEX® is supplied as a lyophilized powder in a single-use vial containing 33 mcg (6.6 million IU) of Interferon beta-1a; 16.5 mg Albumin Human, USP; 6.4 mg Sodium Chloride, USP; 6.3 mg Dibasic Sodium Phosphate, USP; and 1.3 mg Monobasic Sodium Phosphate, USP, and is preservative-free. Diluent is supplied in a single-use vial (Sterile Water for Injection, USP).

AVONEX® is available in the following package configuration (NDC 59627-001-03): Package (Administration Pack) containing four Administration Dose Packs (each containing one vial of AVONEX®, one 10 mL diluent vial, two alcohol wipes, one gauze pad, one 3 mL syringe, one Micro Pin®* vial access pin, one 23 gauge, 1¼ inch needle, and one adhesive bandage).

Stability and Storage

Vials of AVONEX® must be stored in a 2-8°C (36-46°F) refrigerator. Should refrigeration be unavailable, AVONEX® can be stored at 25°C (77°F) for a period of up to 30 days. DO NOT EXPOSE TO HIGH TEMPERATURES. DO NOT FREEZE. Do not use beyond the expiration date stamped on the vial. Following reconstitution, it is recommended the product be used as soon as possible within 6 hours stored at 2-8°C (36-46°F). DO NOT FREEZE RECONSTITUTED AVONEX®.

REFERENCES

1. Jacobs LD, et al. Intramuscular interferon beta-1a for disease progression in relapsing multiple sclerosis. Ann Neurol 1996; 39(3):285-294.
2. Jacobs LD, et al. Intramuscular interferon beta-1a initiated during a first demyelinating event in multiple sclerosis. NEJM 2000;343:898-904.
3. Kurtzke JF. Rating neurologic impairment in multiple sclerosis: an expanded disability status scale (EDSS). Neurology 1983; 33:1444-1452.

AVONEX® (Interferon beta-1a)
Manufactured by:
BIOGEN, INC.
14 Cambridge Center
Cambridge, MA 02142 USA
©2003 Biogen, Inc. All rights reserved.
1-800-456-2255
U.S. Patent Pending
I63005-4 (Revised 02/2003)
*Micro Pin® is the trademark of B. Braun Medical Inc.
℞ only

MEDICATION GUIDE

AVONEX®
Interferon beta-1a
Please read this guide carefully before you start to use AVONEX® (a-vuh-necks) and each time your prescription is refilled since there may be new information. The information in this guide does not take the place of talking with your doctor or healthcare professional.

What is the most important information I should know about AVONEX®?

AVONEX® will not cure multiple sclerosis (MS) but it has been shown to decrease the number of flare-ups and slow the occurrence of some of the physical disability that is common in people with MS. AVONEX® can cause serious side effects, so before you start taking AVONEX®, you should talk with your doctor about the possible benefits of AVONEX® and its possible side effects to decide if AVONEX® is right for you. Potential serious side effects include:

- **Depression**—Some people treated with interferons, including AVONEX®, have become depressed (feeling sad, feeling low or feeling bad about oneself). Some people have had thoughts about killing themselves and a few have committed suicide. Depression is common in people with MS. If you are noticeably sadder or feeling more hopeless, you should tell a family member or friend right away and call your doctor as soon as possible. You should tell the doctor if you have ever had any mental illness, including depression, and if you take any medicines for depression.
- **Risk to pregnancy**—If you become pregnant while taking AVONEX®, you should stop using AVONEX® immediately and call your doctor. AVONEX® may cause you to lose your baby (miscarry) or may cause harm to your unborn child. You and your doctor will need to decide whether the potential benefit of taking AVONEX® is greater than the risks are to your unborn child.
- **Allergic reactions**—Some patients taking AVONEX® have had severe allergic reactions leading to difficulty breathing. Allergic reactions can happen after your first dose or may not happen until after you have taken AVONEX® many times. Less severe allergic reactions such as rash, itching, skin bumps or swelling of the mouth and tongue can also happen. If you think you are having an allergic reaction, stop using AVONEX® immediately and call your doctor.
- **Blood problems**—You may have a drop in the levels of infection-fighting blood cells, red blood cells or cells that help to form blood clots. If the drop in levels are severe, they can lessen your ability to fight infections, make you feel tired or sluggish or cause you to bruise or bleed easily.
- **Seizures**—Some patients have had seizures while taking AVONEX®, including some patients who have never had seizures before. It is not known whether the seizures were related to the effects of their MS, to AVONEX®, or to a combination of both. If you have a seizure while taking AVONEX®, you should stop taking AVONEX® and call your doctor right away.
- **Heart problems**—While AVONEX® is not known to have direct effects on the heart, a few patients who did not have a history of heart problems developed heart muscle problems or congestive heart failure after taking AVONEX®. Some of the symptoms of heart problems are swollen ankles, shortness of breath, decreased ability to exercise, fast heartbeat, tightness in chest, increased need to urinate at night, and not being able to lay flat in bed. If you develop these symptoms or any heart problems while taking AVONEX®, you should call your doctor right away.

For more information on possible side effects with AVONEX®, please read the section on **"What are the possible side effects of AVONEX®?"** in this Medication Guide.

What is AVONEX®?

AVONEX® is a form of a protein called beta interferon that occurs naturally in the body. It is used to treat relapsing forms of multiple sclerosis. It will not cure your MS but may decrease the number of flare-ups of the disease and slow the occurrence of some of the physical disability that is common in people with MS. MS is a life-long disease that affects your nervous system by destroying the protective covering (myelin) that surrounds your nerve fibers. The way AVONEX® works in MS is not known.

Who should not take AVONEX®?

Do not take AVONEX® if you:
- have had an allergic reaction (difficulty breathing, itching, flushing or skin bumps spread widely over the body) to interferon beta or to human albumin

If you have ever had any of the following conditions or serious medical problems, you should tell your doctor before taking AVONEX®:
- Depression (sinking feeling or sadness), anxiety (feeling uneasy or fearful for no reason), or trouble sleeping
- Problems with your thyroid gland
- Blood problems such as bleeding or bruising easily and anemia (low red blood cells) or low white blood cells
- Seizures (for example, epilepsy)
- Heart problems
- Liver disease
- Are planning to become pregnant

You should tell your doctor if you are taking any other prescription or nonprescription medicines. This includes any vitamin or mineral supplements, or herbal products.

How should I take AVONEX®?

AVONEX® is given by injection into the muscle (intramuscular injection) once a week, on the same day (for example, every Monday right before bedtime). If you miss a dose, you should take your next dose as soon as you remember. You should continue your regular schedule the following week. **Do not take AVONEX® on two consecutive days.** Take only the dose your doctor has prescribed for you. Do not change your dose unless you are told to by your doctor. If you take more than your prescribed dose, call your healthcare provider right away. Your doctor may want to monitor you more closely.

You should always follow your doctor's instructions and advice about how to take this medication. If your doctor feels that you, or a family member or friend, may give you the injections, then you and/or the other person should be instructed by your doctor or other healthcare provider in how to prepare and inject your dose of AVONEX®. Do not try to give yourself injections at home until you are sure that you (or the person who will be giving you the injections) fully understands and is comfortable with how to prepare and inject the product. At the end of this guide there are detailed instructions on how to prepare and give yourself an injection of AVONEX® that will help remind you of the instructions from your doctor or healthcare provider.

Always use a new, unopened vial and syringe of AVONEX® for each injection. Never reuse vials or syringes.

It is important that you change your injection site each week. You should always avoid injecting AVONEX® into an area of skin that is sore, red, infected, or otherwise damaged.

What should I avoid while taking AVONEX®?

- **Pregnancy**—You should avoid becoming pregnant while taking AVONEX® until you have talked with your doctor. AVONEX® can cause you to lose your baby (miscarry).
- **Breast-feeding**—You should talk to your doctor if you are breast-feeding an infant. It is not known if the interferon in AVONEX® gets into the breast milk, or if it could harm your nursing baby.

What are the possible side effects of AVONEX®?

- **Flu-like symptoms**—Most people who take AVONEX® have flu-like symptoms (fever, chills, sweating, muscle aches, and tiredness) early during the course of therapy. Usually, these symptoms last for a day after the injection. You may be able to manage these flu-like symptoms by injecting your AVONEX® dose at bedtime and taking over-the-counter pain and fever reducers. For many people, these symptoms lessen or go away over time. Talk to your doctor if these symptoms continue longer than the first few months of therapy, or if they are difficult to manage.
- **Depression**—Some patients taking interferons have become severely depressed and/or anxious. If you feel sad or hopeless you should tell a friend or family member right away and call your doctor immediately. Your doctor or healthcare provider may ask that you stop taking AVONEX®, and/or may recommend that you take a medication to treat your depression. **(See "What is the most important information I should know about AVONEX®?")**
- **Blood problems**—A drop in the levels of white (infection-fighting) blood cells, red blood cells, or a part of your blood that helps to form blood clots (platelets) can happen. If this drop in blood levels is severe, it can lessen your ability to fight infections, make you feel very tired or sluggish, or cause you to bruise or bleed easily. Your doctor may ask you to have periodic blood tests. **(See "What is the most important information I should know about AVONEX®?")**
- **Liver problems**—Your liver function may be affected. Symptoms of changes in your liver include yellowing of the skin and whites of the eyes and easy bruising.
- **Thyroid problems**—Some people taking AVONEX® develop changes in the function of their thyroid. Symptoms of these changes include feeling cold or hot all the time, a change in your weight (gain or loss) without a change in your diet or amount of exercise you get, or feeling emotional.
- **Seizures**—Some patients have had seizures while taking AVONEX®, including patients who have never had seizures before. It is not known whether the seizures were related to the effects of their MS, to AVONEX®, or to a combination of both. If you have a seizure while taking AVONEX®, you should call your doctor right away. **(See "What is the most important information I should know about AVONEX®?")**
- **Heart problems**—While AVONEX® is not known to have any direct effects on the heart, a few patients who did not have a history of heart problems developed heart muscle problems or congestive heart failure after taking AVONEX®. Some of the symptoms of heart problems are swollen ankles, shortness of breath, decreased ability to exercise, fast heartbeat, tightness in chest, increased need to urinate at night, and not being able to lay flat in bed. If you develop these symptoms or any heart problems while taking AVONEX®, you should call your doctor right away. **(See "What is the most important information I should know about AVONEX®?")**

If you get any of the symptoms listed in this section or any listed in the section **"What is the most important information I should know about AVONEX®?"**, you should call your doctor right away. Whether you experience any side effects or not, you and your doctor should periodically discuss your general health. Your doctor may want to monitor you more closely or may ask you to have blood tests more frequently.

Storing AVONEX®

Prior to use, AVONEX® should be refrigerated (36-46°F or 2-8°C) but can be kept for up to 30 days at room temperature (77°F or 25°C). You should avoid exposing AVONEX® to

Continued on next page

Avonex—Cont.

high temperatures and freezing. After mixing, AVONEX® solution should be used immediately, within 6 hours when stored refrigerated at 36-46°F or 2-8°C. Do not freeze the AVONEX® solution.

General advice about prescription medicines
Medicines are sometimes prescribed for purposes other than those listed in a Medication Guide. This medication has been prescribed for your particular condition. Do not use it for another condition or give this drug to anyone else. If you have questions you should speak with your doctor or healthcare professional. You may also ask your doctor or pharmacist for a copy of the information provided to them with the product.

Keep this and all drugs out of the reach of children.

How do I prepare and inject a dose of AVONEX®?
Find a well-lit, clean, flat work surface like a table and collect all the supplies you will need to give yourself or receive an injection. You may want to take one AVONEX® Administration Dose Pack out of the refrigerator about 30 minutes before you plan on injecting your dose to allow it to reach room temperature. A room temperature solution is more comfortable to inject.

You will need the following supplies:
- vial of AVONEX® (white to off-white powder or cake)
- vial of diluent, single-use (Sterile Water for Injection, USP)
- 3 mL syringe
- blue MICRO PIN® (vial access pin)
- sterile needle
- alcohol wipes
- gauze pad
- adhesive bandage
- a puncture resistant container for disposal of used syringes, needles, and MICRO PINS®.

Preparing the AVONEX® solution
It is important to keep your work area, your hands, and your injection site clean to minimize risk of infection. You should wash your hands prior to preparing the medication.

1. Check the expiration date on the AVONEX® vial and the vial of diluent; do not use if the medication or diluent is expired.
2. Remove the caps from the vial of AVONEX® and the vial of diluent, and clean the rubber stopper on the top of each vial with an alcohol wipe.

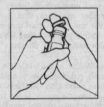

3. Remove the small light blue protective cover from the end of the syringe barrel with a counterclockwise turn.

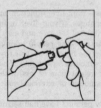

4. Attach the blue MICRO PIN® to the syringe by turning clockwise until secure.
   NOTE: Over-tightening can make the MICRO PIN® difficult to remove.

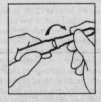

5. Pull the MICRO PIN® cover straight off; do not twist. Save the cover for later use.

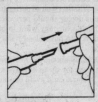

6. Pull back the syringe plunger to the 1.1 mL mark.

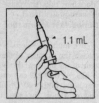

7. Firmly push the MICRO PIN® down through the **center** of the rubber stopper of the diluent vial.

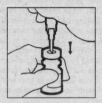

8. Inject the air in the syringe into the diluent vial by pushing down on the plunger until it cannot be pushed any further.
9. Keeping the MICRO PIN® in the vial, turn the diluent vial and syringe upside down.
10. While keeping the MICRO PIN® in the fluid, slowly pull back on the plunger to withdraw 1.1 mL of diluent into the syringe.

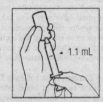

11. Gently tap the syringe with your finger to make any air bubbles rise to the top. If bubbles are present, slowly press the plunger in (to push just the bubbles out through the needle). Make sure there is still 1.1 mL of diluent in the syringe.

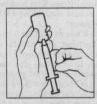

12. Slowly pull the MICRO PIN® out of the diluent vial.
13. Carefully insert the MICRO PIN® through the **center** of the rubber stopper of the vial of AVONEX®. *NOTE: Off-center punctures can push the stopper into the vial. If the stopper falls into the vial, do not use.*
14. **Slowly** inject the diluent into the vial of AVONEX®. DO NOT aim the stream of diluent directly on the AVONEX® powder. Too direct or forceful a stream of diluent onto the powder may cause foaming, and make it difficult to withdraw AVONEX®.

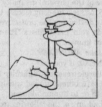

15. Without removing the syringe, **gently** swirl the vial until the AVONEX® is dissolved. **DO NOT SHAKE.**

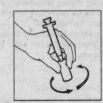

16. Check to see that all of the AVONEX® is dissolved. Check the solution in the vial of AVONEX®. It should be clear to slightly yellow in color and should not have any particles. Do not use the vial if the solution is cloudy, has particles in it or is a color other than clear to slightly yellow.
17. Turn the vial and syringe upside down. Slowly pull back on the plunger to withdraw 1.0 mL of AVONEX®. If bubbles appear, push solution slowly back into the vial and withdraw the solution again.

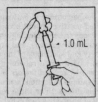

18. With the vial still upside down, tap the syringe **gently** to make any air bubbles rise to the top. Then press the plunger in until the AVONEX® is at the top of the syringe. Check the volume (should be 1.0 mL) and withdraw more medication if necessary. Withdraw the MICRO PIN® and syringe from the vial.
19. Replace the cover on the MICRO PIN® and remove from the syringe with a counterclockwise turn.
20. Attach the sterile needle for injection to the syringe turning clockwise until the needle is secure. A secure attachment will prevent leakage during the injection.

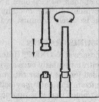

Selecting an injection site
The best sites for intramuscular injection are the thigh and upper arm:
- thigh

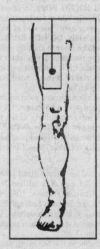

- upper arm
[See figure at top of next column]

You should rotate injection sites each week. This can be as simple as switching between thighs (if you are always injecting yourself). If another person is helping you, you can rotate among your thighs and upper arms. Make sure that the site you choose is free from any skin irritations.

Injecting the AVONEX® dose
1. Use a new alcohol wipe to clean the skin at one of the recommended intramuscular injection sites. Then, pull the protective cover **straight** off the needle; do not twist the cover off.
2. With one hand, stretch the skin out around the injection site. Hold the syringe like a pencil with the other hand, and using a quick motion insert the needle at a 90° angle, through the skin and into the muscle.
3. Once the needle is in, let go of the skin and use that hand to gently pull back slightly on the plunger. If you see

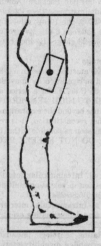

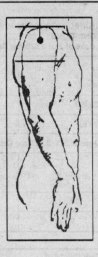

blood come into the syringe, withdraw the needle from the injection site and put pressure on the site with a gauze pad. You will need to replace the needle and choose and clean a new site for an injection.

4. If no blood came into the syringe, slowly push the plunger in until the syringe is empty.

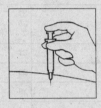

5. Hold a gauze pad near the needle at the injection site and pull the needle straight out. Use the pad to apply pressure to the site for a few seconds or rub gently in a circular motion.

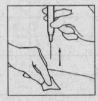

6. If there is bleeding at the site, wipe it off and, if necessary, apply an adhesive bandage.
7. Dispose of the used syringe, needle and blue MICRO PIN® in your puncture resistant container. DO NOT USE a syringe, MICRO PIN®, or needle more than once. The AVONEX® and diluent vials should be put in the trash.

Disposal of syringes and needles
There may be special state and/or local laws for disposing of used needles and syringes. Your doctor, nurse or pharmacist should provide you with instructions on how to dispose of your used needles and syringes. DO NOT throw used needles and syringes into the household trash and DO NOT RECYCLE.

This Medication Guide has been approved by the U.S. Food and Drug Administration.
Manufactured by:
Biogen, Inc.
14 Cambridge Center
Cambridge, MA 02142 USA
©2003 Biogen, Inc. All rights reserved.
1-800-456-2255
I63005-4 (02/2003)

In the PDR annual,
the **Brand and Generic Name Index**
(PINK section)
alphabetizes drugs under both
brand and generic names.

Duramed Pharmaceuticals, Inc.
5040 DURAMED DR.
CINCINNATI, OHIO 45213

Direct Inquiries to:
877-405-0369

CENESTIN® ℞
[sĕ'nĕ"stĭn]
(synthetic conjugated estrogens, A)
Tablets
℞ only

Prescribing information for this product, which appears on pages 1237–1240 of the 2003 PDR, has been completely revised as follows. Please write "See Supplement A" next to the product heading.

ESTROGENS INCREASE THE RISK OF ENDOMETRIAL CANCER
Close clinical surveillance of all women taking estrogens is important. Adequate diagnostic measures, including endometrial sampling when indicated, should be undertaken to rule out malignancy in all cases of undiagnosed persistent or recurring abnormal vaginal bleeding. There is no evidence that the use of "natural" estrogens results in a different endometrial risk profile than synthetic estrogens at equivalent estrogen doses.

CARDIOVASCULAR AND OTHER RISKS
Estrogens with and without progestins should not be used for the prevention of cardiovascular disease.
The Women's Health Initiative (WHI) study reported increased risks of myocardial infarction, stroke, invasive breast cancer, pulmonary emboli, and deep vein thrombosis in postmenopausal women during 5 years of treatment with conjugated equine estrogens (CEE 0.625mg) combined with medroxyprogesterone acetate (MPA 2.5mg) relative to placebo (**see CLINICAL PHARMACOLOGY, Clinical Studies**). Other doses of conjugated estrogens with medroxyprogesterone, and other combinations of estrogens and progestins were not studied in the WHI and, in the absence of comparable data, these risks should be assumed to be similar. Because of these risks, estrogens with or without progestins should be prescribed at the lowest effective doses and for the shortest duration consistent with treatment goals and risks for the individual woman.

DESCRIPTION
Synthetic conjugated estrogens, A tablets contain a blend of nine (9) synthetic estrogenic substances. The estrogenic substances are sodium estrone sulfate, sodium equilin sulfate, sodium 17α-dihydroequilin sulfate, sodium 17α-estradiol sulfate, sodium 17β-dihydroequilin sulfate, sodium 17α-dihydroequilenin sulfate, sodium 17β-dihydroequilenin sulfate, sodium equilenin sulfate and sodium 17β-estradiol sulfate.
The structural formulae for these estrogens are:

$C_{18}H_{21}NaO_5S$
372.42
Sodium Estrone Sulfate

$C_{18}H_{21}NaO_5S$
372.42
Sodium 17α-Dihydroequilin Sulfate

$C_{18}H_{23}NaO_5S$
374.44
Sodium 17α-Estradiol Sulfate

$C_{18}H_{17}NaO_5S$
368.39
Sodium Equilenin Sulfate

$C_{18}H_{19}NaO_5S$
370.41
Sodium 17β-Dihydroequilenin Sulfate

$C_{18}H_{19}NaO_5S$
370.41
Sodium Equilin Sulfate

$C_{18}H_{21}NaO_5S$
372.42
Sodium 17β-Dihydroequilin Sulfate

$C_{18}H_{23}NaO_5S$
374.44
Sodium 17β-Estradiol Sulfate

$C_{18}H_{19}NaO_5S$
370.41
Sodium 17α-Dihydroequilenin Sulfate

Tablets for oral administration, are available in 0.3 mg, 0.625 mg, 0.9 mg and 1.25 mg strengths of synthetic conjugated estrogens, A. Tablets also contain the following inactive ingredients: ethylcellulose, hydroxypropyl methylcellulose, lactose monohydrate, magnesium stearate, polyethylene glycol, polysorbate 80, pregelatinized starch, titanium dioxide, and triethyl citrate.
— 0.3 mg tablets also contain: FD&C Blue No. 2 aluminum lake and D&C Yellow No. 10 aluminum lake.
— 0.625 mg tablets also contain: FD&C Red No. 40 aluminum lake.
— 0.9 mg tablets do not contain any color additives.
— 1.25 mg tablets also contain FD&C Blue No. 2 aluminum lake.

CLINICAL PHARMACOLOGY
Endogenous estrogens are largely responsible for the development and maintenance of the female reproductive system and secondary sexual characteristics. Although circulating estrogens exist in a dynamic equilibrium of metabolic interconversions, estradiol is the principal intracellular human estrogen and is substantially more potent than its metabolites, estrone and estriol, at the receptor level.
The primary source of estrogen in normally cycling adult women is the ovarian follicle, which secretes 70 to 500 mcg of estradiol daily, depending on the phase of the menstrual cycle. After menopause, most endogenous estrogen is produced by conversion of androstenedione, secreted by the adrenal cortex, to estrone by peripheral tissues. Thus, estrone and the sulfate conjugated form, estrone sulfate, are the most abundant circulating estrogens in postmenopausal women.

Continued on next page

Cenestin—Cont.

Estrogens act through binding to nuclear receptors in estrogen-responsive tissues. To date, two estrogen receptors have been identified. These vary in proportion from tissue to tissue.

Circulating estrogens modulate the pituitary secretion of the gonadotropins, luteinizing hormone (LH) and follicle stimulating hormone (FSH), through a negative feed-back mechanism. Estrogens act to reduce the elevated levels of these hormones seen in postmenopausal women.

Pharmacokinetics
Absorption
Synthetic conjugated estrogens, A are soluble in water and are well absorbed from the gastrointestinal tract after release from the drug formulation. The Cenestin tablet releases the synthetic conjugated estrogens, A slowly over a period of several hours. The effect of food on the bioavailability of synthetic conjugated estrogens, A from Cenestin has not been studied.
[See table 1 above]

Table 1
PHARMACOKINETIC PARAMETERS FOR UNCONJUGATED AND CONJUGATED ESTROGENS IN HEALTHY POSTMENOPAUSAL WOMEN UNDER FASTING CONDITIONS

Pharmacokinetic Parameters of Unconjugated Estrogens Following a Dose of 2 × 0.625 mg Cenestin

Drug	C_{max} (pg/mL) CV%	t_{max} (h) CV%	AUC_{0-72h} (pg•hr/mL) CV%
Baseline-corrected estrone	84.5 (41.7)	8.25 (35.6)	1749 (43.8)
Equilin	45.6 (47.3)	7.78 (28.8)	723 (67.9)

Pharmacokinetic Parameters of Conjugated Estrogens Following a Dose of 2 × 0.625 mg Cenestin

Drug	C_{max} (ng/mL) CV%	t_{max} (h) CV%	$t_{½}$ (h) CV%	AUC_{0-72h} (ng•hr/mL) CV%
Baseline-corrected estrone	4.43 (40.4)	7.7 (30.3)	10.6 (25.4)	69.89 (39.2)
Equilin	3.27 (43.5)	5.8 (31.1)	9.7 (23.0)	46.46 (47.5)

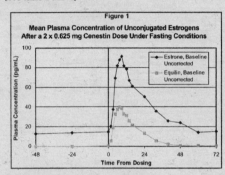

Figure 1
Mean Plasma Concentration of Unconjugated Estrogens After a 2 × 0.625 mg Cenestin Dose Under Fasting Conditions

Distribution
The distribution of exogenous estrogens is similar to that of endogenous estrogens. Estrogens are widely distributed in the body and are generally found in higher concentrations in the sex hormone target organs. Estrogens circulate in the blood largely bound to sex hormone binding globulin (SHBG) and albumin.

Metabolism
Exogenous estrogens are metabolized in the same manner as endogenous estrogens. Circulating estrogens exist in a dynamic equilibrium of metabolic interconversions. These transformations take place mainly in the liver. Estradiol is converted reversibly to estrone, and both can be converted to estriol, which is the major urinary metabolite. Estrogens also undergo enterohepatic recirculation via sulfate and glucuronide conjugation in the liver, biliary secretion of conjugates into the intestine, and hydrolysis in the gut followed by reabsorption. In postmenopausal women, a significant portion of the circulating estrogens exist as sulfate conjugates, especially estrone sulfate, which serves as a circulating reservoir for the formation of more active estrogens.

Excretion
Estradiol, estrone, and estriol are excreted in the urine along with glucuronide and sulfate conjugates.

Drug Interactions
In vitro and *in vivo* studies have shown that estrogens are metabolized partially by cytochrome P450 3A4 (CYP3A4). Therefore, inducers or inhibitors of CYP3A4 may affect estrogen drug metabolism. Inducers of CYP3A4 such as St. John's Wort preparations (Hypericum perforatum), phenobarbital, carbamazepine, and rifampin may reduce plasma concentrations of estrogens, possibly resulting in a decrease in therapeutic effects and/or changes in the uterine bleeding profile. Inhibitors of CYP3A4 such as erythromycin, clarithromycin, ketoconazole, itraconazole, ritonavir and grapefruit juice may increase plasma concentrations of estrogens and may result in side effects.

Clinical Studies
Women's Health Initiative Studies.
The Women's Health Initiative (WHI) enrolled a total of 27,000 predominantly healthy postmenopausal women to assess the risks and benefits of either the use of 0.625 mg conjugated equine estrogens (CEE) per day alone or the use of 0.625 mg conjugated equine estrogens plus 2.5 mg medroxyprogesterone acetate (MPA) per day compared to placebo in the prevention of certain chronic diseases. The primary endpoint was the incidence of coronary heart disease (CHD) (nonfatal myocardial infarction and CHD death), with invasive breast cancer as the primary adverse outcome studied. A "global index" included the earliest occurrence of CHD, invasive breast cancer, stroke, pulmonary embolism (PE), endometrial cancer, colorectal cancer, hip fracture, or death due to other cause. The study did not evaluate the effects of CEE or CEE/MPA on menopausal symptoms.

The CEE-only substudy is continuing and results have not been reported. The CEE/MPA substudy was stopped early because, according to the predefined stopping rule, the increased risk of breast cancer and cardiovascular events exceeded the specified benefits included in the "global index." Results of the CEE/MPA substudy, which included 16,608 women (average age of 63 years, range 50 to 79; 83.9% White, 6.5% Black, 5.5% Hispanic), after an average follow-up of 5.2 years are presented in Table 2 below:
[See table 2 above]

For those outcomes included in the "global index," absolute excess risks per 10,000 person-years in the group treated

Table 2. RELATIVE AND ABSOLUTE RISK SEEN IN THE CEE/MPA SUBSTUDY OF WHI[a]

Event[c]	Relative Risk CEE/MPA vs placebo at 5.2 years (95% CI*)	Placebo n = 8102	CEE/MPA n = 8506
		Absolute Risk per 10,000 Person-years	
CHD events	1.29 (1.02–1.63)	30	37
Non-fatal MI	1.32 (1.02–1.72)	23	30
CHD death	1.18 (0.70–1.97)	6	7
Invasive breast cancer[b]	1.26 (1.00–1.59)	30	38
Stroke	1.41 (1.07–1.85)	21	29
Pulmonary embolism	2.13 (1.39–3.25)	8	16
Colorectal cancer	0.63 (0.43–0.92)	16	10
Endometrial cancer	0.83 (0.47–1.47)	6	5
Hip fracture	0.66 (0.45–0.98)	15	10
Death due to causes other than the events above	0.92 (0.74–1.14)	40	37
Global index[c]	1.15 (1.03–1.28)	151	170
Deep vein thrombosis[d]	2.07 (1.49–2.87)	13	26
Vertebral fractures[d]	0.66 (0.44–0.98)	15	9
Other osteoporotic fractures[d]	0.77 (0.69–0.86)	170	131

[a]adapted from JAMA, 2002, 288:321–333
[b]includes metastatic and non-metastatic breast cancer with the exception of in situ breast cancer
[c]a subset of the events was combined in a "global index", defined as the earliest occurrence of CHD events, invasive breast cancer, stroke, pulmonary embolism, endometrial cancer, colorectal cancer, hip fracture, or death due to other causes
[d]not included in Global Index
*nominal confidence intervals unadjusted for multiple looks and multiple comparisons

with CEE/MPA were 7 more CHD events, 8 more strokes, 8 more PEs, and 8 more invasive breast cancers, while absolute risk reductions per 10,000 person-years were 6 fewer colorectal cancers and 5 fewer hip fractures. The absolute excess risk of events included in the "global index" was 19 per 10,000 person-years. There was no difference between the groups in terms of all-cause mortality. (**See BOXED WARNINGS, WARNINGS, and PRECAUTIONS.**)

Effects on vasomotor symptoms
A randomized, placebo-controlled multicenter clinical study was conducted evaluating the effectiveness of Cenestin for the treatment of vasomotor symptoms in 120 menopausal women. Patients were randomized to receive either placebo or 0.625 mg Cenestin daily for 12 weeks. Dose titration was allowed after one week of treatment. The starting dose was either doubled (2 × 0.625 mg Cenestin or placebo taken daily) or reduced (0.3 mg Cenestin or placebo taken daily), if necessary. Efficacy was assessed at 4, 8 and 12 weeks of treatment. By Week 12, 10% of the study participants remained on a single 0.625 mg Cenestin tablet daily while 77% required two (0.625 mg) tablets daily. The results in Table 3 indicate that compared to placebo, Cenestin produced a reduction in moderate-to-severe vasomotor symptoms at all time points (4, 8, and 12 weeks).

Table 3
Clinical Response*
Mean Change in Reduction of Vasomotor Symptoms

	Cenestin (n=70)	Placebo (n=47)	Difference
Baseline			
Mean # (SD)	96.8 (42.6)	94.1 (33.9)	–
Week 4			
Mean # (SD)	28.7 (28.8)	45.7 (36.8)	–
Mean Change	−68.1 (43.9)	−48.4 (46.2)	−19.9
Week 8			
Mean # (SD)	18.6 (25.0)	39.8 (39.1)	–
Mean Change	−78.3 (49.0)	−54.3 (49.2)	−24.6
Week 12			
Mean # (SD)	16.5 (25.7)	37.8 (38.7)	–
Mean Change	−80.3 (50.3)	−56.3 (48.0)	−24.7

Mean = Arithmetic Mean, SD = Standard Deviation
Difference = Difference between treatment LSMeans (Cenestin − Placebo).
*Intent-to-treat population = 117

Effects on vulvar and vaginal atrophy
The effect of Cenestin on vulvar and vaginal atrophy was confirmed in a 16-week, randomized, placebo-controlled, multicenter clinical study in 72 postmenopausal women. Patients were randomized to receive either placebo or 0.3 mg Cenestin daily for 16 weeks. Efficacy was assessed at weeks 12 and 16 for vaginal wall cytology and week 16 for vaginal pH. Results for percent of superficial cells from a maturation index of the vaginal mucosa are shown in Figure 2. Mean vaginal pH decreased from a baseline of 6.20 to 5.14 for Cenestin and increased to 6.15 from a baseline of 6.03 for placebo.

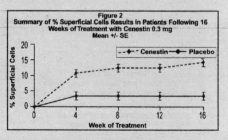

Figure 2
Summary of % Superficial Cells Results in Patients Following 16 Weeks of Treatment with Cenestin 0.3 mg
Mean +/- SE

Effects on Lipids
The effect of Cenestin 0.3 mg on lipid parameters was evaluated in a 16-week placebo-controlled trial of healthy postmenopausal women at low risk for cardiovascular disease

reporting vulvar and vaginal atrophy. Results are shown in Table 4.
[See table 4 above]

INDICATIONS AND USAGE
Cenestin is indicated for the:
1. Treatment of moderate-to-severe vasomotor symptoms associated with the menopause.
   - 0.625 mg Cenestin
   - 0.9 mg Cenestin
   - 1.25 mg Cenestin
2. Treatment of moderate to severe symptoms of vulvar and vaginal atrophy associated with the menopause.
   - 0.3 mg Cenestin

CONTRAINDICATIONS
Cenestin should not be used in individuals with any of the following conditions:
1. Undiagnosed abnormal genital bleeding.
2. Known, suspected, or history of cancer of the breast except in appropriately selected patients being treated for metastatic disease.
3. Known or suspected estrogen-dependent neoplasia.
4. Active deep vein thrombosis, pulmonary embolism or a history of these conditions.
5. Active or recent (e.g., within the past year) arterial thromboembolic disease (e.g., stroke, myocardial infarction).
6. Cenestin should not be used in patients with known hypersensitivity to its ingredients.
7. Known or suspected pregnancy. There is no indication for Cenestin in pregnancy. There appears to be little or no increased risk of birth defects in women who have used estrogens and progestins from oral contraceptives inadvertently during early pregnancy (see PRECAUTIONS).

WARNINGS
See BOXED WARNINGS.
The use of unopposed estrogens in women who have a uterus is associated with an increased risk of endometrial cancer.

1. Cardiovascular disorders.
Estrogen and estrogen/progestin therapy have been associated with an increased risk of cardiovascular events such as myocardial infarction and stroke, as well as venous thrombosis and pulmonary embolism (venous thromboembolism or VTE). Should any of these occur or be suspected, estrogens should be discontinued immediately.

Risk factors for cardiovascular disease (e.g., hypertension, diabetes mellitus, tobacco use, hypercholesterolemia, and obesity) should be managed appropriately.

a. Coronary heart disease and stroke
In the Women's Health Initiative study (WHI), an increase in the number of myocardial infarctions and strokes has been observed in women receiving CEE compared to placebo. These observations are preliminary, and the study is continuing. (See CLINICAL PHARMACOLOGY, Clinical Studies.)

In the CEE/MPA substudy of WHI an increased risk of coronary heart disease (CHD) events (defined as non-fatal myocardial infarction and CHD death) was observed in women receiving CEE/MPA compared to women receiving placebo (37 vs 30 per 10,000 person years). The increase in risk was observed in year one and persisted.

In the same substudy of WHI, an increased risk of stroke was observed in women receiving CEE/MPA compared to women receiving placebo (29 vs 21 per 10,000 person-years). The increase in risk was observed after the first year and persisted.

In postmenopausal women with documented heart disease (n = 2,763, average age 66.7 years) a controlled clinical trial of secondary prevention of cardiovascular disease (Heart and Estrogen/Progestin Replacement Study; HERS) treatment with CEE/MPA-0.625mg/2.5mg per day demonstrated no cardiovascular benefit. During an average follow-up of 4.1 years, treatment with CEE/MPA did not reduce the overall rate of CHD events in postmenopausal women with established coronary heart disease. There were more CHD events in the CEE/MPA-treated group than in the placebo group in year 1, but not during the subsequent years. Two thousand three hundred and twenty one women from the original HERS trial agreed to participate in an open label extension of HERS, HERS II. Average follow-up in HERS II was an additional 2.7 years, for a total of 6.8 years overall. Rates of CHD events were comparable among women in the CEE/MPA group and the placebo group in HERS, HERS II, and overall.

Large doses of estrogen (5 mg conjugated estrogens per day), comparable to those used to treat cancer of the prostate and breast, have been shown in a large prospective clinical trial in men to increase the risks of nonfatal myocardial infarction, pulmonary embolism, and thrombophlebitis.

b. Venous thromboembolism (VTE)
In the Women's Health Initiative study (WHI), an increase in VTE has been observed in women receiving CEE compared to placebo. These observations are preliminary, and the study is continuing. (See CLINICAL PHARMACOLOGY, Clinical Studies.)

In the CEE/MPA substudy of WHI, a 2-fold greater rate of VTE, including deep venous thrombosis and pulmonary embolism, was observed in women receiving CEE/MPA compared to women receiving placebo. The rate of VTE was 34 per 10,000 woman-years in the CEE/MPA group compared to 16 per 10,000 woman-years in the placebo group. The increase in VTE risk was observed during the first year and persisted.

Table 4
Effects on Lipids Following Treatment with Cenestin 0.3 mg at 16 Weeks

	Cenestin 0.3 mg N=34	Placebo N=29	Treatment Differences
	Mean (SD)	Mean (SD)	Mean
Total Cholesterol (mg/dL)	−16.6 (20.6)	−0.3 (20.4)	−7.6%
HDL Cholesterol (mg/dL)	4.2 (6.0)	0.7 (7.3)	4.9%
LDL Cholesterol (mg/dL)	−15.4 (14.0)	1.6 (14.0)	−17.1%
Triglycerides (mg/dL)	6.6 (38.6)	−2.7 (38.2)	7.7%
Total/HDL Cholesterol	−0.5 (0.5)	−0.04 (0.62)	−11.9%
LDL/HDL Cholesterol	−0.5 (0.5)	−0.02 (0.5)	−21.0%

If feasible, estrogens should be discontinued at least 4 to 6 weeks before surgery of the type associated with an increased risk of thromboembolism, or during periods of prolonged immobilization.

2. Malignant neoplasms
a. Endometrial cancer
The use of unopposed estrogens in women with intact uteri has been associated with an increased risk of endometrial cancer. The reported endometrial cancer risk among unopposed estrogen users is about 2- to 12-fold greater than in non-users, and appears dependent on duration of treatment and on estrogen dose. Most studies show no significant increased risk associated with use of estrogens for less than one year. The greatest risk appears associated with prolonged use, with increased risks of 15- to 24-fold for five to ten years or more and this risk has been shown to persist for at least 8 to 15 years after estrogen therapy is discontinued. Clinical surveillance of all women taking estrogen/progestin combinations is important. Adequate diagnostic measures, including endometrial sampling when indicated, should be undertaken to rule out malignancy in all cases of undiagnosed persistent or recurring abnormal vaginal bleeding. There is no evidence that the use of natural estrogens results in a different endometrial risk profile than synthetic estrogens of equivalent estrogen dose. Adding a progestin to estrogen therapy has been shown to reduce the risk of endometrial hyerplasia, which may be a precursor to endometrial cancer.

b. Breast cancer
Estrogen and estrogen/progestin therapy in postmenopausal women has been associated with an increased risk of breast cancer. In the CEE/MPA substudy of the Women's Health Initiative study (WHI), a 26% increase of invasive breast cancer (38 vs 30 per 10,000 woman-years) after an average of 5.2 years of treatment was observed in women receiving CEE/MPA compared to women receiving placebo. The increased risk of breast cancer became apparent after 4 years on CEE/MPA. The women reporting prior postmenopausal use of estrogen and/or estrogen with progestin had a higher relative risk for breast cancer associated with CEE/MPA than those who had never used these hormones. (See CLINICAL PHARMACOLOGY, Clinical Studies.)

In the WHI, no increased risk of breast cancer in CEE-treated women compared to placebo was reported after an average of 5.2 years of therapy. These data are preliminary and that substudy of WHI is continuing.

Epidemiologic studies have reported an increase risk of breast cancer in association with increasing duration of postmenopausal treatment with estrogens with or without a progestin. This association was reanalyzed in original data from 51 studies that involved various doses and types of estrogens, with and without progestins. In the reanalysis, an increased risk of having breast cancer diagnosed became apparent after about 5 years of continued treatment, and subsided after treatment had been discontinued for 5 years or longer. Some later studies have suggested that postmenopausal treatment with estrogens and progestin increase the risk of breast cancer more than treatment with estrogen alone.

A postmenopausal woman without a uterus who requires estrogen should receive estrogen-alone therapy, and should not be exposed unnecessarily to progestins. All postmenopausal women should receive yearly breast exams by a health care provider and perform monthly self-examinations. In addition, mammography examinations should be scheduled based on patient age and risk factors.

3. Gallbladder disease
A 2- to 4-fold increase in the risk of gallbladder disease requiring surgery in post-menopausal women receiving estrogens has been reported.

4. Hypercalcemia
Estrogen administration may lead to severe hypercalcemia in patients with breast cancer and bone metastases. If hypercalcemia occurs, use of the drug should be stopped and appropriate measures taken to reduce the serum calcium level.

5. Visual abnormalities
Retinal vascular thrombosis has been reported in patients receiving estrogens. Discontinue medication pending examination if there is sudden partial or complete loss of vision, or a sudden onset of proptosis, diplopia, or migraine. If examination reveals papilledema or renal vascular lesions, estrogens should be discontinued.

PRECAUTIONS
A. GENERAL
1. Addition of a progestin when a woman has not had a hysterectomy
Studies of the addition of a progestin for 10 or more days of a cycle of estrogen administration, or daily with estrogen in a continuous regimen, have reported a lowered incidence of endometrial hyperplasia than would be induced by estrogen treatment alone. Endometrial hyperplasia may be a precursor to endometrial cancer.

There are, however, possible risks that may be associated with the use of progestins with estrogens compared to estrogen-alone regimens. These include:
a. A possible increased risk of breast cancer
b. Adverse effects on lipoprotein metabolism (e.g., lowering HDL, raising LDL)
c. Impairment of glucose tolerance

2. Elevated blood pressure
In a small number of case reports, substantial increases in blood pressure have been attributed to idiosyncratic reactions to estrogens. In a large, randomized, placebo-controlled clinical trial, a generalized effect of estrogen therapy on blood pressure was not seen. Blood pressure should be monitored at regular intervals with estrogen use.

3. Familial hyperlipoproteinemia
In patients with familial defects of lipoprotein metabolism, estrogen therapy may be associated with elevations of plasma triglycerides leading to pancreatitis and other complications.

4. Impaired liver function
Estrogens may be poorly metabolized in patients with impaired liver function. For patients with a history of cholestatic jaundice associated with past estrogen use or with pregnancy, caution should be exercised and in the case of recurrence, medication should be discontinued.

5. Hypothyroidism
Estrogen administration leads to increased thyroid-binding globulin (TBG) levels. Patients with normal thyroid function can compensate for the increased TBG by making more thyroid hormone, thus maintaining free T_4 and T_3 serum concentrations in the normal range. Patients dependent on thyroid hormone replacement therapy who are also receiving estrogens may require increased doses of their thyroid replacement therapy. These patients should have their thyroid function monitored in order to maintain their free thyroid hormone levels in an acceptable range.

6. Fluid retention
Because estrogens may cause some degree of fluid retention, patients with conditions that might be influenced by this factor, such as a cardiac or renal dysfunction, warrant careful observation when estrogens are prescribed.

7. Hypocalcemia
Estrogens should be used with caution in individuals with severe hypocalcemia.

8. Ovarian cancer
Use of estrogen-only products, in particular for ten or more years, has been associated with an increased risk of ovarian cancer in some epidemiological studies. Other studies did not show a significant association. Data are insufficient to determine whether there is an increased risk with estrogen/progestin combination therapy in postmenopausal women.

9. Exacerbation of endometriosis
Endometriosis may be exacerbated with administration of estrogens.

10. Exacerbation of other conditions
Estrogens may cause an exacerbation of asthma, diabetes mellitus, epilepsy, migraine or porphyria and should be used with caution in women with these conditions.

B. PATIENT INFORMATION
Physicians are advised to discuss the PATIENT INFORMATION leaflet with patients for whom they prescribe Cenestin.

C. LABORATORY TESTS
Estrogen administration should be initiated at the lowest dose for the approved indication and then guided by clinical response, rather than by serum hormone levels (e.g., estradiol, FSH).

D. DRUG/LABORATORY TEST INTERACTIONS
1. Accelerated prothrombin time, partial thromboplastin time, and platelet aggregation time; increased platelet count; increased factors II, VII antigen, VIII antigen, VIII coagulant activity, IX, X, XII, VII-X complex, II-VII-X complex, and beta-thromboglobulin; decreased levels of antifactor Xa and antithrombin III, decreased antithrombin III activity; increased levels of fibrinogen and fibrinogen activity; increased plasminogen antigen and activity.
2. Increased thyroid-binding globulin (TBG) levels leading to increased circulating total thyroid hormone levels as measured by protein-bound iodine (PBI), T_4 levels (by column or by radioimmunoassay) or T_3 levels by radioimmunoassay. T_3 resin uptake is decreased, reflecting the elevated TBG. Free T_4 and free T_3 concentrations are unaltered. Patients on thyroid replacement therapy may require higher doses of thyroid hormone.

Continued on next page

Cenestin—Cont.

3. Other binding proteins may be elevated in serum (i.e., corticosteroid binding globulin (CBG), sex hormone-binding globulin (SHBG)) leading to increased circulating corticosteroids and sex steroids, respectively. Free or biologically active hormone concentrations are unchanged. Other plasma proteins may be increased (angiotensinogen/renin substrate, alpha-1-antitrypsin, ceruloplasmin).
4. Increased plasma HDL and HDL_2 subfraction concentrations, reduced LDL cholesterol concentration, increased triglycerides levels.
5. Impaired glucose tolerance.
6. Reduced response to metyrapone test.

E. CARCINOGENESIS, MUTAGENESIS, AND IMPAIRMENT OF FERTILITY
Long-term continuous administration of natural and synthetic estrogens in certain animal species increases the frequency of carcinomas of the breast, uterus, cervix, vagina, testis, and liver. (See BOXED WARNINGS, CONTRAINDICATIONS, and WARNINGS.)

F. PREGNANCY
Cenestin should not be used during pregnancy. (See CONTRAINDICATIONS.)

G. NURSING MOTHERS
Estrogen administration to nursing mothers has been shown to decrease the quantity and quality of the milk. Detectable amounts of estrogens have been identified in the milk of mothers receiving this drug. Caution should be exercised when Cenestin is administered to a nursing woman.

ADVERSE REACTIONS
See BOXED WARNINGS, WARNINGS, and PRECAUTIONS.
Because clinical trials are conducted under widely varying conditions, adverse reaction rates observed in the clinical trials of a drug cannot be directly compared to rates in the clinical trials of another drug and may not reflect the rates observed in practice. The adverse reaction information from clinical trials does, however, provide a basis for identifying the adverse events that appear to be related to drug use and for approximating rates.
In a 12-week clinical trial that included 72 women treated with Cenestin and 48 women treated with placebo, adverse events that occurred at a rate of ≥ 2% are summarized in Table 5.
[See table 5 below]

The following additional adverse reactions have been reported with estrogens:

1. Genitourinary system
Changes in vaginal bleeding pattern and abnormal withdrawal bleeding or flow; breakthrough bleeding; spotting; increase in size of uterine leiomyomata; vaginitis, including vaginal candidiasis; change in amount of cervical secretion; changes in cervical ectropion; ovarian cancer; endometrial hyperplasia; endometrial cancer.

2. Breasts
Tenderness, enlargement, pain, nipple discharge, galactorrhea; fibrocystic breast changes; breast cancer.

3. Cardiovascular
Deep and superficial venous thrombosis; pulmonary embolism; thrombophlebitis; myocardial infarction; stroke; increase in blood pressure.

4. Gastrointestinal
Nausea, vomiting; abdominal cramps, bloating; cholestatic jaundice; increased incidence of gallbladder disease; pancreatitis.

5. Skin
Chloasma or melasma, which may persist when drug is discontinued; erythema multiforme; erythema nodosum; hemorrhagic eruption; loss of scalp hair; hirsutism; pruritus, rash.

6. Eyes
Retinal vascular thrombosis; steepening of corneal curvature; intolerance to contact lenses.

7. Central nervous system
Headache; migraine; dizziness; mental depression; chorea; nervousness; mood disturbances; irritability; exacerbation of epilepsy.

8. Miscellaneous
Increase or decrease in weight; reduced carbohydrate tolerance; aggravation of porphyria; edema; arthalgias; leg cramps; changes in libido; anaphylactoid/anaphylactic reactions including urticaria and angioedema; hypocalcemia; exacerbation of asthma; increased triglycerides.

DOSAGE AND ADMINISTRATION
1. For treatment of moderate-to-severe vasomotor symptoms associated with the menopause, the lowest dose and regimen of Cenestin that will control symptoms should be chosen and Cenestin should be discontinued as promptly as possible. An initial dose of 0.625 mg daily is recommended with titration up to 1.25 mg. Attempts to discontinue or taper Cenestin should be made at 3 to 6 month intervals
2. For treatment of vulvar and vaginal atrophy—0.3 mg daily.

When estrogen is prescribed for a postmenopausal woman with a uterus, progestin should also be initiated to reduce the risk of endometrial cancer. A woman without a uterus does not need progestin. Use of estrogen, alone or in combination with a progestin, should be limited to the shortest duration consistent with treatment goals and risks for the individual woman. Patients should be reevaluated periodically as clinically appropriate (e.g., 3-month to 6-month intervals) to determine if treatment is still necessary (See BOXED WARNINGS and WARNINGS.) For women who have a uterus, adequate diagnostic measures, such as endometrial sampling, when indicated, should be undertaken to rule out malignancy in cases of undiagnosed persistent or recurring abnormal vaginal bleeding.

HOW SUPPLIED
Cenestin (synthetic conjugated estrogens, A) Tablets,
— 0.3 mg tablets are available in containers of 30 (NDC 51285-441-30), 100 (NDC 51285-441-02), and 1000 (NDC 51285-441-05).
Tablets are round, green, film-coated, and are debossed with letters, ⏁, and number, 41.
— 0.625 mg tablets are available in containers of 30 (NDC 51285-442-30), 100 (NDC 51285-442-02), and 1000 (NDC 51285-442-05).
Tablets are round, red, film-coated, and are debossed with letters, ⏁, and number, 42.
— 0.9 mg tablets are available in containers of 30 (NDC 51285-443-30), 100 (NDC 51285-443-02), and 1000 (NDC 51285-443-05).

Table 5
Number (%) of Patients with Adverse Events With ≥2% Occurrence Rate By Body System and Treatment Group

Body System / Adverse Event	Cenestin n (%)	Placebo n (%)	Total n (%)
Number of Patients Who Received Medication	72 (100)	48 (100)	120 (100)
Number of Patients With Adverse Events	68 (94)	43 (90)	111 (93)
Number of Patients Without Any Adverse Events	4 (6)	5 (10)	9 (8)
Body As A Whole			
Abdominal Pain	20 (28)	11 (23)	31 (26)
Allergic Reaction	0 (0)	1 (2)	1 (1)
Asthenia	24 (33)	20 (42)	44 (37)
Back Pain	10 (14)	6 (13)	16 (13)
Chest Pain	1 (1)	1 (2)	2 (2)
Chills	0 (0)	1 (2)	1 (1)
Fever	1 (1)	3 (6)	4 (3)
Flu Syndrome	3 (4)	1 (2)	4 (3)
Headache	49 (68)	32 (67)	81 (68)
Infection	10 (14)	5 (10)	15 (13)
Neck Pain	2 (3)	1 (2)	3 (3)
Neck Rigitity	1 (1)	1 (2)	2 (2)
Pain	8 (11)	9 (19)	17 (14)
Cardiovascular System			
Cardiovascular Disorder	0 (0)	1 (2)	1 (1)
Migraine	0 (0)	1 (2)	1 (1)
Palpitation	15 (21)	13 (27)	28 (23)
Vasodilation	1 (1)	2 (4)	3 (3)
Digestive System			
Constipation	4 (6)	2 (4)	6 (5)
Diarrhea	4 (6)	0 (0)	4 (3)
Dyspepsia	7 (10)	3 (6)	10 (8)
Flatulence	21 (29)	14 (29)	35 (29)
Gastrointestinal Disorder	0 (0)	1 (2)	1 (1)
Mouth Ulceration	0 (0)	1 (2)	1 (1)
Nausea	13 (18)	9 (19)	22 (18)
Periodontal Abscess	0 (0)	1 (2)	1 (1)
Vomiting	5 (7)	1 (2)	6 (5)
Hemic and Lymphatic System			
Ecchymosis	0 (0)	1 (2)	1 (1)
Metabolic and Nutritional			
Generalized Edema	3 (4)	2 (4)	5 (4)
Peripheral Edema	7 (10)	6 (13)	13 (11)
Weight Gain	0 (0)	1 (2)	1 (1)
Musculoskeletal System			
Arthralgia	18 (25)	13 (27)	31 (26)
Bone Pain	0 (0)	1 (2)	1 (1)
Joint Disorder	0 (0)	1 (2)	1 (1)
Myalgia	20 (28)	15 (31)	35 (29)
Nervous System			
Agitation	0 (0)	1 (2)	1 (1)
Confusion	0 (0)	1 (2)	1 (1)
Depression	20 (28)	18 (38)	38 (32)
Dizziness	8 (11)	5 (10)	13 (11)
Emotional Lability	1 (1)	2 (4)	3 (3)
Hypertension	2 (3)	2 (4)	4 (3)
Hypertonia	4 (6)	0 (0)	4 (3)
Hypesthesia	2 (3)	1 (2)	3 (3)
Insomnia	30 (42)	23 (48)	53 (44)
Leg Cramps	7 (10)	3 (6)	10 (8)
Nervousness	20 (28)	20 (42)	40 (33)
Paresthesia	24 (33)	15 (31)	39 (33)
Somnolence	2 (3)	0 (0)	2 (2)
Vasodilation	0 (0)	1 (2)	1 (1)
Vertigo	12 (17)	12 (25)	24 (20)
Respiratory System			
Bronchitis	2 (3)	1 (2)	3 (3)
Cough Increased	4 (6)	1 (2)	5 (4)
Dyspnea	2 (3)	0 (0)	2 (2)
Laryngitis	0 (0)	1 (2)	1 (1)
Lung Function Decreased	0 (0)	1 (2)	1 (1)
Pharyngitis	6 (8)	4 (8)	10 (8)
Rhinitis	6 (8)	7 (15)	13 (11)
Sinusitis	2 (3)	0 (0)	2 (2)
Skin and Appendages			
Alopecia	2 (3)	1 (2)	3 (3)
Pruritus	2 (3)	2 (4)	4 (3)
Rash	3 (4)	3 (6)	6 (5)
Subcutaneous Nodule	1 (1)	1 (2)	2 (2)
Special Senses			
Abnormal Vision	0 (0)	1 (2)	1 (1)
Conjunctivitis	0 (0)	1 (2)	1 (1)
Dry Eyes	0 (0)	1 (2)	1 (1)
Ear Pain	0 (0)	2 (4)	2 (2)
Lacrimation Disorder	0 (0)	1 (2)	1 (1)
Urogenital System			
Breast Neoplasm	1 (1)	1 (2)	2 (2)
Breast Pain	21 (29)	7 (15)	28 (23)
Dysmenorrhea	4 (6)	3 (6)	7 (6)
Metrorrhagia	10 (14)	3 (6)	13 (11)
Urinary Frequency	0 (0)	1 (2)	1 (1)

Tablets are round, white, film-coated, and are debossed with letters, ȸ, and number, 43.

— 1.25 mg tablets are available in containers of 30 (NDC 51285-444-30), 100 (NDC 51285-444-02), and 1000 (NDC 51285-444-05).

Tablets are round, blue, film-coated, and are debossed with letters, ȸ, and number, 44.

Store at 25°C (77°F); excursions are permitted to 15°-30°C (59°-86°F) [See USP Controlled Room Temperature]

Dispense in tight container as defined in USP.

Dispense in child-resistant packaging.

Dispenser: Include one "Information for the patient" leaflet with each package dispensed.

PATIENT INFORMATION

Cenestin®

(synthetic conjugated estrogens, A) Tablets

Read this PATIENT INFORMATION before you start taking Cenestin and read what you get each time you refill Cenestin. There may be new information. This information does not take the place of talking to your health care provider about your medical condition or your treatment.

What is the most important information I should know about Cenestin synthetic estrogen hormones?

- Estrogens increase the chances of getting cancer of the uterus.

Report any unusual vaginal bleeding right away while you are taking estrogens. Vaginal bleeding after menopause may be a warning sign of cancer of the uterus (womb). Your health care provider should check any unusual vaginal bleeding to find out the cause.

- Do not use estrogens with or without progestins to prevent heart disease, heart attacks, or strokes.

Using estrogens with or without progestins may increase your chances of getting heart attack, strokes, breast cancer, and blood clots. You and your healthcare provider should talk regularly about whether you still need treatment with Cenestin.

What is Cenestin?

Cenestin is a medicine that contains a mixture of synthetic estrogen hormones made from a plant source.

What is Cenestin used for?

Cenestin is used after menopause to:

- **reduce moderate to severe hot flashes.** Estrogens are hormones made by a woman's ovaries. The ovaries normally stop making estrogens when a woman is between 45 to 55 years old. This drop in body estrogen levels causes the "change of life" or menopause (the end of monthly menstrual periods). Sometimes, both ovaries are removed during an operation before natural menopause takes place. The sudden drop in estrogen levels causes "surgical menopause."

  When the estrogen levels begin dropping, some women develop very uncomfortable symptoms, such as feelings of warmth in the face, neck, and chest, or sudden strong feelings of heat and sweating ("hot flashes" or "hot flushes"). In some women, the symptoms are mild, and they will not need estrogens. In other women, symptoms can be more severe. You and your health care provider should talk regularly about whether you still need treatment with Cenestin.
- **treat moderate to severe dryness, itching, and burning in or around the vagina.**

  You and your health care provider should talk regularly about whether you still need treatment with Cenestin to control these problems.

Who Should Not Take Cenestin?

Do not start taking Cenestin if you:

- **have unusual vaginal bleeding.**
- **currently have or have had certain cancers.** Estrogens may increase the chances of getting certain types of cancers, including cancer of the breast or uterus. If you have or had cancer, talk with your health care provider about whether you should take Cenestin.
- **had a stroke or heart attack in the past year.**
- **currently have or have had blood clots.**
- **are allergic to Cenestin or any of its ingredients.** See the end of this leaflet for a list of ingredients in Cenestin.
- **are pregnant or think you may be pregnant.**

Tell your health care provider:

- **if you are breastfeeding.** The synthetic estrogen hormones in Cenestin can pass into your milk.
- **about all of your medical problems.** Your health care provider may need to check you more carefully if you have certain conditions, such as asthma (wheezing), epilepsy (seizures), migraine, endometriosis, or problems with your heart, liver, thyroid, kidneys, or have high calcium levels in your blood.
- **about all the medicines you take,** including prescription and nonprescription medicines, vitamins, and herbal supplements. Some medicines may affect how Cenestin works. Cenestin may also affect how your other medicines work.
- **if you are going to have surgery or will be on bed rest.** You may need to stop taking estrogens.

How Should I Take Cenestin?

Take one Cenestin tablet each day at about the same time. Estrogens should be used only as long as needed. You and your health care provider should talk regularly (for example every 3 to 6 months) about whether you still need treatment with Cenestin. If you miss a dose, take it as soon as you remember. However, if it is almost time for your next dose, skip the missed dose and take only your next regularly scheduled dose. Do not take two doses at the same time.

It is important to keep taking Cenestin for as long as your healthcare provider recommends it. Your length of treatment with Cenestin may be different than someone else's and will depend on why you are taking Cenestin.

What are the possible side effects of Cenestin?

Less common but serious side effects include:

- Breast cancer
- Cancer of the uterus
- Stroke
- Heart attack
- Blood clots
- Gallbladder disease
- Ovarian cancer

These are some of the warning signs of serious side effects:

- Breast lumps
- Unusual vaginal bleeding
- Dizziness and faintness
- Changes in speech
- Severe headaches
- Chest pain
- Shortness of breath
- Pains in your legs
- Changes in vision
- Vomiting

Call your health care provider right away if you get any of these warning signs, or any other unusual symptom that concerns you.

Common side effects include:

- Headache
- Breast pain
- Irregular vaginal bleeding or spotting
- Stomach/abdominal cramps, bloating
- Nausea and vomiting
- Hair loss

Other side effects include:

- High blood pressure
- Liver problems
- High blood sugar
- Fluid retention
- Enlargement of benign tumors of the uterus ("fibroids")
- Vaginal yeast infection

These are not all the possible side effects of Cenestin. For more information, ask your health care provider or pharmacist.

What can I do to lower my chances of a serious side effect with Cenestin?

- Talk with your health care provider regularly about whether you should continue taking Cenestin.
- See your health care provider right away if you get vaginal bleeding while taking Cenestin.
- Have a breast exam and mammogram (breast X-ray) every year unless your health care provider tells you something else. If members of your family have had breast cancer or if you have ever had breast lumps or an abnormal mammogram, you may need to have breast exams more often.
- If you have high blood pressure, high cholesterol (fat in the blood), diabetes, are overweight, or if you use tobacco, you may have higher chances for getting heart disease. Ask your health care provider for ways to lower your chances for getting heart disease.

General information about safe and effective use of Cenestin.

Medicines are sometimes prescribed for conditions that are not mentioned in patient information leaflets. Do not take Cenestin for conditions for which it was not prescribed. Do not give Cenestin to other people, even if they have the same symptoms you have. It may harm them. **Keep Cenestin out of the reach of children.**

This leaflet provides a summary of the most important information about Cenestin. If you would like more information, talk with your health care provider or pharmacist. You can ask for information about Cenestin that is written for health professionals. You can get more information by calling the toll free number 877-405-0369.

What are the ingredients in Cenestin?

Tablets for oral administration, are available in 0.3 mg, 0.625 mg, 0.9 mg and 1.25 mg strengths of synthetic conjugated estrogens, A. Tablets also contain the following inactive ingredients: ethylcellulose, hydroxypropyl methylcellulose, lactose monohydrate, magnesium stearate, polyethylene glycol, polysorbate 80, pregelatinized starch, titanium dioxide, and triethyl citrate.

— 0.3 mg tablets also contain: FD&C Blue No. 2 aluminum lake and D&C Yellow No. 10 aluminum lake.

— 0.625 mg tablets also contain: FD&C Red No. 40 aluminum lake.

— 0.9 mg tablets do not contain any color additives.

— 1.25 mg tablets also contain FD&C Blue No. 2 aluminum lake.

Manufactured by:
Duramed Pharmaceuticals, Inc.
Subsidiary of Barr Laboratories, Inc.
Pomona, NY 10970
Revised JANUARY 2003
11000422504
BR - 41, 42, 43, 44

Forest Pharmaceuticals, Inc.

(Subsidiary of Forest Laboratories, Inc.)
13600 SHORELINE DRIVE
ST. LOUIS, MO 63045

Direct Inquiries to:
Professional Affairs Department
13600 Shoreline Drive
St. Louis, MO 63045
(800) 678-1605

CELEXA™ ℞
[*sĕ-lĕ\s\ă*]
(citalopram hydrobromide)
Tablets/Oral Solution

Prescribing information for this product, which appears on pages 1344–1347 of the 2003 PDR, has been revised as follows. Please write "See Supplement A" next to the product heading.

The heading of the product was revised to include **Tablets/ Oral Solution.**

The **ADVERSE REACTIONS** *subsection* Other Events Observed During the Postmarketing Evaluation of Celexa (citalopram HBr) *was revised to:*

Other Events Observed During the Postmarketing Evaluation of Celexa (citalopram HBr)

It is estimated that over 30 million patients have been treated with Celexa since market introduction. Although no causal relationship to Celexa treatment has been found, the following adverse events have been reported to be temporally associated with Celexa treatment, and have not been described elsewhere in labeling: acute renal failure, akathisia, allergic reaction, anaphylaxis, angioedema, choreoathetosis, chest pain, delirium, dyskinesia, ecchymosis, epidermal necrolysis, erythema multiforme, gastrointestinal hemorrhage, grand mal convulsions, hemolytic anemia, hepatic necrosis, myoclonus, neuroleptic malignant syndrome, nystagmus, pancreatitis, priapism, prolactinemia, prothrombin decreased, QT prolonged, rhabdomyolysis, serotonin syndrome, spontaneous abortion, thrombocytopenia, thrombosis, ventricular arrhythmia, Torsades de pointes, and withdrawal syndrome.

LEXAPRO™ ℞
[*lĕks'ă-prō*]
(escitalopram oxalate)
TABLETS/ORAL SOLUTION
Rx only

Prescribing information for this product, which appears on pages 3532–3535 of the 2003 PDR, has been completely revised as follows. Please write "See Supplement A" next to the product heading.

DESCRIPTION

LEXAPRO™ (escitalopram oxalate) is an orally administered selective serotonin reuptake inhibitor (SSRI). Escitalopram is the pure S-enantiomer (single isomer) of the racemic bicyclic phthalane derivative citalopram. Escitalopram oxalate is designated S-(+)-1-[3-(dimethylamino)propyl]-1-(*p*-fluorophenyl)-5-phthalancarbonitrile oxalate with the following structural formula:

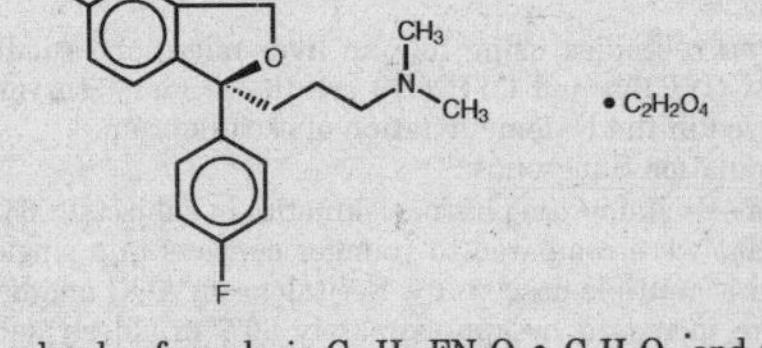

The molecular formula is $C_{20}H_{21}FN_2O \cdot C_2H_2O_4$ and the molecular weight is 414.40.

Escitalopram oxalate occurs as a fine white to slightly yellow powder and is freely soluble in methanol and dimethyl sulfoxide (DMSO), soluble in isotonic saline solution, sparingly soluble in water and ethanol, slightly soluble in ethyl acetate, and insoluble in heptane.

LEXAPRO (escitalopram oxalate) is available as tablets or as an oral solution.

LEXAPRO tablets are film coated, round tablets containing escitalopram oxalate in strengths equivalent to 10 mg and 20 mg escitalopram base. The 10 and 20 mg tablets are scored. The tablets also contain the following inactive ingredients: talc, croscarmellose sodium, microcrystalline cellulose/colloidal silicon dioxide, and magnesium stearate. The film coating contains hydroxypropyl methyl cellulose, titanium dioxide, and polyethylene glycol.

LEXAPRO oral solution contains escitalopram oxalate equivalent to 1 mg/mL escitalopram base. It also contains the following inactive ingredients: sorbitol, purified water, citric acid, sodium citrate, malic acid, glycerin, propylene glycol, methylparaben, propylparaben, and natural peppermint flavor.

Continued on next page

Lexapro—Cont.

CLINICAL PHARMACOLOGY
Pharmacodynamics
The mechanism of antidepressant action of escitalopram, the S-enantiomer of racemic citalopram, is presumed to be linked to potentiation of serotonergic activity in the central nervous system resulting from its inhibition of CNS neuronal reuptake of serotonin (5-HT). In vitro and in vivo studies in animals suggest that escitalopram is a highly selective serotonin reuptake inhibitor (SSRI) with minimal effects on norepinephrine and dopamine neuronal reuptake. Escitalopram is at least 100 fold more potent than the R-enantiomer with respect to inhibition of 5-HT reuptake and inhibition of 5-HT neuronal firing rate. Tolerance to a model of antidepressant effect in rats was not induced by long-term (up to 5 weeks) treatment with escitalopram. Escitalopram has no or very low affinity for serotonergic (5-HT$_{1-7}$) or other receptors including alpha- and beta-adrenergic, dopamine (D$_{1-5}$), histamine (H$_{1-3}$), muscarinic (M$_{1-5}$), and benzodiazepine receptors. Escitalopram also does not bind to or has low affinity for various ion channels including Na$^+$, K$^+$, Cl$^-$ and Ca^{++} channels. Antagonism of muscarinic, histaminergic and adrenergic receptors has been hypothesized to be associated with various anticholinergic, sedative and cardiovascular side effects of other psychotropic drugs.

Pharmacokinetics
The single- and multiple-dose pharmacokinetics of escitalopram are linear and dose-proportional in a dose range of 10 to 30 mg/day. Biotransformation of escitalopram is mainly hepatic, with a mean terminal half-life of about 27-32 hours. With once daily dosing, steady state plasma concentrations are achieved within approximately one week. At steady state, the extent of accumulation of escitalopram in plasma in young healthy subjects was 2.2-2.5 times the plasma concentrations observed after a single dose. The tablet and the oral solution dosage forms of escitalopram oxalate are bioequivalent.

Absorption and Distribution
Following a single oral dose (20 mg tablet or solution) of escitalopram, peak blood levels occur at about 5 hours. Absorption of escitalopram is not affected by food.
The absolute bioavailability of citalopram is about 80% relative to an intravenous dose, and the volume of distribution of citalopram is about 12 L/kg. Data specific on escitalopram are unavailable.
The binding of escitalopram to human plasma proteins is approximately 56%.

Metabolism and Elimination
Following oral administrations of escitalopram, the fraction of drug recovered in the urine as escitalopram and S-demethylcitalopram (S-DCT) is about 8% and 10%, respectively. The oral clearance of escitalopram is 600 mL/min, with approximately 7% of that due to renal clearance.
Escitalopram is metabolized to S-DCT and S-didemethylcitalopram (S-DDCT). In humans, unchanged escitalopram is the predominant compound in plasma. At steady state, the concentration of the escitalopram metabolite S-DCT in plasma is approximately one-third that of escitalopram. The level of S-DDCT was not detectable in most subjects. In vitro studies show that escitalopram is at least 7 and 27 times more potent than S-DCT and S-DDCT, respectively, in the inhibition of serotonin reuptake, suggesting that the metabolites of escitalopram do not contribute significantly to the antidepressant actions of escitalopram. S-DCT and S-DDCT also have no or very low affinity for serotonergic (5-HT$_{1-7}$) or other receptors including alpha- and beta-adrenergic, dopamine (D$_{1-5}$), histamine (H$_{1-3}$), muscarinic (M$_{1-5}$), and benzodiazepine receptors. S-DCT and S-DDCT also do not bind to various ion channels including Na$^+$, K$^+$, Cl$^-$ and Ca^{++} channels.
In vitro studies using human liver microsomes indicated that CYP3A4 and CYP2C19 are the primary isozymes involved in the N-demethylation of escitalopram.

Population Subgroups
Age - Escitalopram pharmacokinetics in subjects ≥ 65 years of age were compared to younger subjects in a single-dose and a multiple-dose study. Escitalopram AUC and half-life were increased by approximately 50% in elderly subjects, and C$_{max}$ was unchanged. 10 mg is the recommended dose for elderly patients (see Dosage and Administration).
Gender - In a multiple-dose study of escitalopram (10 mg/day for 3 weeks) in 18 male (9 elderly and 9 young) and 18 female (9 elderly and 9 young) subjects, there were no differences in AUC, C$_{max}$ and half-life between the male and female subjects. No adjustment of dosage on the basis of gender is needed.
Reduced hepatic function - Citalopram oral clearance was reduced by 37% and half-life was doubled in patients with reduced hepatic function compared to normal subjects. 10mg is the recommended dose of escitalopram for most hepatically impaired patients (see Dosage and Administration).
Reduced renal function - In patients with mild to moderate renal function impairment, oral clearance of citalopram was reduced by 17% compared to normal subjects. No adjustment of dosage for such patients is recommended. No information is available about the pharmacokinetics of escitalopram in patients with severely reduced renal function (creatinine clearance < 20 mL/min).

Drug-Drug Interactions
In vitro enzyme inhibition data did not reveal an inhibitory effect of escitalopram on CYP3A4, -1A2, -2C9, -2C19, and -2E1. Based on in vitro data, escitalopram would be expected to have little inhibitory effect on in vivo metabolism mediated by these cytochromes. While in vivo data to address this question are limited, results from drug interaction studies suggest that escitalopram, at a dose of 20 mg, has no 3A4 inhibitory effect and a modest 2D6 inhibitory effect. See Drug Interactions under Precautions for more detailed information on available drug interaction data.

Clinical Efficacy Trials
The efficacy of LEXAPRO as a treatment for major depressive disorder has been established, in part, on the basis of extrapolation from the established effectiveness of racemic citalopram, of which escitalopram is the active isomer. In addition, the efficacy of escitalopram was shown in an 8-week fixed dose study that compared 10 mg/day LEXAPRO and 20 mg/day LEXAPRO to placebo and 40 mg/day citalopram, in outpatients between 18 and 65 years of age who met DSM-IV criteria for major depressive disorder. The 10 mg/day and 20 mg/day LEXAPRO treatment groups showed significantly greater mean improvement compared to placebo on the Montgomery Asberg Depression Rating Scale (MADRS). The 10 mg and 20 mg LEXAPRO groups were similar in mean improvement on the MADRS score.
Analyses of the relationship between treatment outcome and age, gender, and race did not suggest any differential responsiveness on the basis of these patient characteristics.
In a longer-term trial, 274 patients meeting (DSM-IV) criteria for major depressive disorder, who had responded during an initial 8-week open label treatment phase with LEXAPRO 10 or 20 mg/day, were randomized to continuation of LEXAPRO at their same dose, or to placebo, for up to 36 weeks of observation for relapse. Response during the open label phase was defined by having a decrease of the MADRS total score to ≤12. Relapse during the double-blind phase was defined as an increase of the MADRS total score to ≥22, or discontinuation due to insufficient clinical response. Patients receiving continued LEXAPRO experienced a significantly longer time to relapse over the subsequent 36 weeks compared to those receiving placebo.

INDICATIONS AND USAGE
LEXAPRO (escitalopram) is indicated for the treatment of major depressive disorder.
The efficacy of LEXAPRO in the treatment of major depressive disorder was established, in part, on the basis of extrapolation from the established effectiveness of racemic citalopram, of which escitalopram is the active isomer. In addition, the efficacy of escitalopram was shown in an 8-week controlled trial of outpatients whose diagnoses corresponded most closely to the DSM-IV category of major depressive disorder (see Clinical Pharmacology).
A major depressive episode (DSM-IV) implies a prominent and relatively persistent (nearly every day for at least 2 weeks) depressed or dysphoric mood that usually interferes with daily functioning, and includes at least five of the following nine symptoms: depressed mood, loss of interest in usual activities, significant change in weight and/or appetite, insomnia or hypersomnia, psychomotor agitation or retardation, increased fatigue, feelings of guilt or worthlessness, slowed thinking or impaired concentration, a suicide attempt or suicidal ideation.
The efficacy of LEXAPRO in hospitalized patients with major depressive disorders has not been adequately studied.
The efficacy of LEXAPRO in maintaining a response, in patients with major depressive disorder who responded during an 8-week acute treatment phase while taking LEXAPRO and were then observed for relapse during a period of up to 36 weeks, was demonstrated in a placebo-controlled trial (see Clinical Efficacy Trials, under Clinical Pharmacology). Nevertheless, the physician who elects to use LEXAPRO for extended periods should periodically re-evaluate the long-term usefulness of the drug for the individual patient (see Dosage and Administration).

CONTRAINDICATIONS
Concomitant use in patients taking monoamine oxidase inhibitors (MAOIs) is contraindicated (see Warnings).
LEXAPRO is contraindicated in patients with a hypersensitivity to escitalopram or citalopram or any of the inactive ingredients in LEXAPRO.

WARNINGS
Potential for Interaction with Monoamine Oxidase Inhibitors
In patients receiving serotonin reuptake inhibitor drugs in combination with a monoamine oxidase inhibitor (MAOI), there have been reports of serious, sometimes fatal, reactions including hyperthermia, rigidity, myoclonus, autonomic instability with possible rapid fluctuations of vital signs, and mental status changes that include extreme agitation progressing to delirium and coma. These reactions have also been reported in patients who have recently discontinued SSRI treatment and have been started on a MAOI. Some cases presented with features resembling neuroleptic malignant syndrome. Furthermore, limited animal data on the effects of combined use of SSRIs and MAOIs suggest that these drugs may act synergistically to elevate blood pressure and evoke behavioral excitation. Therefore, it is recommended that LEXAPRO should not be used in combination with a MAOI, or within 14 days of discontinuing treatment with a MAOI. Similarly, at least 14 days should be allowed after stopping LEXAPRO before starting a MAOI.

PRECAUTIONS
General
Hyponatremia
One case of hyponatremia has been reported in association with LEXAPRO treatment. Several cases of hyponatremia or SIADH (syndrome of inappropriate antidiuretic hormone secretion) have been reported in association with racemic citalopram. All patients with these events have recovered with discontinuation of escitalopram or citalopram and/or medical intervention. Hyponatremia and SIADH have also been reported in association with other marketed drugs effective in the treatment of major depressive disorder.

Activation of Mania/Hypomania
In placebo-controlled trials of LEXAPRO, activation of mania/hypomania was reported in one (0.1%) of 715 patients treated with LEXAPRO and in none of the 592 patients treated with placebo. Activation of mania/hypomania has also been reported in a small proportion of patients with major affective disorders treated with racemic citalopram and other marketed drugs effective in the treatment of major depressive disorder. As with all drugs effective in the treatment of major depressive disorder, LEXAPRO should be used cautiously in patients with a history of mania.

Seizures
Although anticonvulsant effects of racemic citalopram have been observed in animal studies, LEXAPRO has not been systematically evaluated in patients with a seizure disorder. These patients were excluded from clinical studies during the product's premarketing testing. In clinical trials of LEXAPRO, no seizures occurred in subjects exposed to LEXAPRO. Like other drugs effective in the treatment of major depressive disorder, LEXAPRO should be introduced with care in patients with a history of seizure disorder.

Suicide
The possibility of a suicide attempt is inherent in major depressive disorder and may persist until significant remission occurs. Close supervision of high risk patients should accompany initial drug therapy. As with all drugs effective in the treatment of major depressive disorder, prescriptions for LEXAPRO should be written for the smallest quantity of tablets consistent with good patient management, in order to reduce the risk of overdose.

Interference with Cognitive and Motor Performance
In studies in normal volunteers, racemic citalopram in doses of 40 mg/day did not produce impairment of intellectual function or psychomotor performance. Because any psychoactive drug may impair judgment, thinking, or motor skills, however, patients should be cautioned about operating hazardous machinery, including automobiles, until they are reasonably certain that LEXAPRO therapy does not affect their ability to engage in such activities.

Use in Patients with Concomitant Illness
Clinical experience with LEXAPRO in patients with certain concomitant systemic illnesses is limited. Caution is advisable in using LEXAPRO in patients with diseases or conditions that produce altered metabolism or hemodynamic responses.
LEXAPRO has not been systematically evaluated in patients with a recent history of myocardial infarction or unstable heart disease. Patients with these diagnoses were generally excluded from clinical studies during the product's premarketing testing.
In subjects with hepatic impairment, clearance of racemic citalopram was decreased and plasma concentrations were increased. The recommended dose of LEXAPRO in hepatically impaired patients is 10 mg/day (see Dosage and Administration).
Because escitalopram is extensively metabolized, excretion of unchanged drug in urine is a minor route of elimination. Until adequate numbers of patients with severe renal impairment have been evaluated during chronic treatment with LEXAPRO, however, it should be used with caution in such patients (see Dosage and Administration).

Information for Patients
Physicians are advised to discuss the following issues with patients for whom they prescribe LEXAPRO.
In studies in normal volunteers, racemic citalopram in doses of 40 mg/day did not impair psychomotor performance. The effect of LEXAPRO on psychomotor coordination, judgment, or thinking has not been systematically examined in controlled studies. Because psychoactive drugs may impair judgment, thinking or motor skills, patients should be cautioned about operating hazardous machinery, including automobiles, until they are reasonably certain that LEXAPRO therapy does not affect their ability to engage in such activities.
Patients should be told that, although citalopram has not been shown in experiments with normal subjects to increase the mental and motor skill impairments caused by alcohol, the concomitant use of LEXAPRO and alcohol in depressed patients is not advised.
Patients should be made aware that escitalopram is the active isomer of Celexa (citalopram hydrobromide) and that the two medications should not be taken concomitantly.
Patients should be advised to inform their physician if they are taking, or plan to take, any prescription or over-the-counter drugs, as there is a potential for interactions.
Patients should be advised to notify their physician if they become pregnant or intend to become pregnant during therapy.
Patients should be advised to notify their physician if they are breast feeding an infant.
While patients may notice improvement with LEXAPRO therapy in 1 to 4 weeks, they should be advised to continue therapy as directed.

Laboratory Tests
There are no specific laboratory tests recommended.
Concomitant Administration with Racemic Citalopram
Citalopram - Since escitalopram is the active isomer of racemic citalopram (Celexa), the two agents should not be coadministered.
Drug Interactions
CNS Drugs - Given the primary CNS effects of escitalopram, caution should be used when it is taken in combination with other centrally acting drugs.
Alcohol - Although racemic citalopram did not potentiate the cognitive and motor effects of alcohol in a clinical trial, as with other psychotropic medications, the use of alcohol by patients taking LEXAPRO is not recommended.
Monoamine Oxidase Inhibitors (MAOIs) - See Contraindications and Warnings.
Cimetidine - In subjects who had received 21 days of 40 mg/day racemic citalopram, combined administration of 400 mg/day cimetidine for 8 days resulted in an increase in citalopram AUC and C_{max} of 43% and 39%, respectively. The clinical significance of these findings is unknown.
Digoxin - In subjects who had received 21 days of 40 mg/day racemic citalopram, combined administration of citalopram and digoxin (single dose of 1 mg) did not significantly affect the pharmacokinetics of either citalopram or digoxin.
Lithium - Coadministration of racemic citalopram (40 mg/day for 10 days) and lithium (30 mmol/day for 5 days) had no significant effect on the pharmacokinetics of citalopram or lithium. Nevertheless, plasma lithium levels should be monitored with appropriate adjustment to the lithium dose in accordance with standard clinical practice. Because lithium may enhance the serotonergic effects of escitalopram, caution should be exercised when LEXAPRO and lithium are coadministered.
Sumatriptan - There have been rare postmarketing reports describing patients with weakness, hyperreflexia, and incoordination following the use of a selective serotonin reuptake inhibitor (SSRI) and sumatriptan. If concomitant treatment with sumatriptan and an SSRI (e.g., fluoxetine, fluvoxamine, paroxetine, sertraline, citalopram, escitalopram) is clinically warranted, appropriate observation of the patient is advised.
Theophylline - Combined administration of racemic citalopram (40 mg/day for 21 days) and the CYP1A2 substrate theophylline (single dose of 300 mg) did not affect the pharmacokinetics of theophylline. The effect of theophylline on the pharmacokinetics of citalopram was not evaluated.
Warfarin - Administration of 40 mg/day racemic citalopram for 21 days did not affect the pharmacokinetics of warfarin, a CYP3A4 substrate. Prothrombin time was increased by 5%, the clinical significance of which is unknown.
Carbamazepine - Combined administration of racemic citalopram (40 mg/day for 14 days) and carbamazepine (titrated to 400 mg/day for 35 days) did not significantly affect the pharmacokinetics of carbamazepine, a CYP3A4 substrate. Although trough citalopram plasma levels were unaffected, given the enzyme inducing properties of carbamazepine, the possibility that carbamazepine might increase the clearance of escitalopram should be considered if the two drugs are coadministered.
Triazolam - Combined administration of racemic citalopram (titrated to 40 mg/day for 28 days) and the CYP3A4 substrate triazolam (single dose of 0.25 mg) did not significantly affect the pharmacokinetics of either citalopram or triazolam.
Ketoconazole - Combined administration of racemic citalopram (40 mg) and ketoconazole (200 mg) decreased the Cmax and AUC of ketoconazole by 21% and 10%, respectively, and did not significantly affect the pharmacokinetics of citalopram.
Ritonavir - Combined administration of a single dose of ritonavir (600 mg), both a CYP3A4 substrate and a potent inhibitor of CYP3A4, and escitalopram (20 mg) did not affect the pharmacokinetics of either ritonavir or escitalopram.
CYP3A4 and -2C19 Inhibitors - In vitro studies indicated that CYP3A4 and -2C19 are the primary enzymes involved in the metabolism of escitalopram. However, coadministration of escitalopram (20 mg) and ritonavir (600 mg), a potent inhibitor of CYP3A4, did not significantly affect the pharmacokinetics of escitalopram. Because escitalopram is metabolized by multiple enzyme systems, inhibition of a single enzyme may not appreciably decrease escitalopram clearance.
Drugs Metabolized by Cytochrome P4502D6 - In vitro studies did not reveal an inhibitory effect of escitalopram on CYP2D6. In addition, steady state levels of racemic citalopram were not significantly different in poor metabolizers and extensive CYP2D6 metabolizers after multiple-dose administration of citalopram, suggesting that coadministration, with escitalopram, of a drug that inhibits CYP2D6, is unlikely to have clinically significant effects on escitalopram metabolism. However, there are limited in vivo data suggesting a modest CYP2D6 inhibitory effect for escitalopram, i.e., coadministration of escitalopram (20 mg/day for 21 days) with the tricyclic antidepressant desipramine (single dose of 50 mg), a substrate for CYP2D6, resulted in a 40% increase in C_{max} and a 100% increase in AUC of desipramine. The clinical significance of this finding is unknown. Nevertheless, caution is indicated in the coadministration of escitalopram and drugs metabolized by CYP2D6.

Metoprolol - Administration of 20 mg/day LEXAPRO for 21 days resulted in a 50% increase in C_{max} and 82% increase in AUC of the beta-adrenergic blocker metoprolol (given in a single dose of 100 mg). Increased metoprolol plasma levels have been associated with decreased cardioselectivity. Coadministration of LEXAPRO and metoprolol had no clinically significant effects on blood pressure or heart rate.
Electroconvulsive Therapy (ECT) - There are no clinical studies of the combined use of ECT and escitalopram.
Carcinogenesis, Mutagenesis, Impairment of Fertility
Carcinogenesis
Racemic citalopram was administered in the diet to NMRI/BOM strain mice and COBS WI strain rats for 18 and 24 months, respectively. There was no evidence for carcinogenicity of racemic citalopram in mice receiving up to 240 mg/kg/day. There was an increased incidence of small intestine carcinoma in rats receiving 8 or 24 mg/kg/day racemic citalopram. A no-effect dose for this finding was not established. The relevance of these findings to humans is unknown.
Mutagenesis
Racemic citalopram was mutagenic in the in vitro bacterial reverse mutation assay (Ames test) in 2 of 5 bacterial strains (Salmonella TA98 and TA1537) in the absence of metabolic activation. It was clastogenic in the in vitro Chinese hamster lung cell assay for chromosomal aberrations in the presence and absence of metabolic activation. Racemic citalopram was not mutagenic in the in vitro mammalian forward gene mutation assay (HPRT) in mouse lymphoma cells or in a coupled in vitro/in vivo unscheduled DNA synthesis (UDS) assay in rat liver. It was not clastogenic in the in vitro chromosomal aberration assay in human lymphocytes or in two in vivo mouse micronucleus assays.
Impairment of Fertility
When racemic citalopram was administered orally to male and female rats 16/24 (males/females), prior to and throughout mating and gestation at doses of 32, 48, and 72 mg/kg/day, mating was decreased at all doses, and fertility was decreased at doses ≥32 mg/kg/day. Gestation duration was increased at 48 mg/kg/day.
Pregnancy
Pregnancy Category C
In a rat embryo/fetal development study, oral administration of escitalopram (56, 112 or 150 mg/kg/day) to pregnant animals during the period of organogenesis resulted in decreased fetal body weight and associated delays in ossification at the two higher doses (approximately ≥56 times the maximum recommended human dose [MRHD] of 20 mg/day on a body surface area [mg/m²] basis). Maternal toxicity (clinical signs and decreased body weight gain and food consumption), mild at 56 mg/kg/day, was present at all dose levels. The developmental no effect dose of 56 mg/kg/day is approximately 28 times the MRHD on a mg/m² basis. No teratogenicity was observed at any of the doses tested (as high as 75 times the MRHD on a mg/m² basis).
When female rats were treated with escitalopram (6, 12, 24, or 48 mg/kg/day) during pregnancy and through weaning, slightly increased offspring mortality and growth retardation were noted at 48 mg/kg/day which is approximately 24 times the MRHD on a mg/m² basis. Slight maternal toxicity (clinical signs and decreased body weight gain and food consumption) was seen at this dose. Slightly increased offspring mortality was seen at 24 mg/kg/day. The no effect dose was 12 mg/kg/day which is approximately 6 times the MRHD on a mg/m² basis.
In animal reproduction studies, racemic citalopram has been shown to have adverse effects on embryo/fetal and postnatal development, including teratogenic effects, when administered at doses greater than human therapeutic doses.
In two rat embryo/fetal development studies, oral administration of racemic citalopram (32, 56, or 112 mg/kg/day) to pregnant animals during the period of organogenesis resulted in decreased embryo/fetal growth and survival and an increased incidence of fetal abnormalities (including cardiovascular and skeletal defects) at the high dose. This dose was also associated with maternal toxicity (clinical signs, decreased BW gain). The developmental no effect dose was 56 mg/kg/day. In a rabbit study, no adverse effects on embryo/fetal development were observed at doses of racemic citalopram of up to 16 mg/kg/day. Thus, teratogenic effects of racemic citalopram were observed at a maternally toxic dose in the rat and were not observed in the rabbit.
When female rats were treated with racemic citalopram (4.8, 12.8, or 32 mg/kg/day) from late gestation through weaning, increased offspring mortality during the first 4 days after birth and persistent offspring growth retardation were observed at the highest dose. The no effect dose was 12.8 mg/kg/day. Similar effects on offspring mortality and growth were seen when dams were treated throughout gestation and early lactation at doses ≥24 mg/kg/day. A no effect dose was not determined in that study.
There are no adequate and well-controlled studies in pregnant women; therefore, escitalopram should be used during pregnancy only if the potential benefit justifies the potential risk to the fetus.
Labor and Delivery
The effect of LEXAPRO on labor and delivery in humans is unknown.
Nursing Mothers
Racemic citalopram, like many other drugs, is excreted in human breast milk. There have been two reports of infants experiencing excessive somnolence, decreased feeding, and weight loss in association with breast feeding from a citalopram-treated mother; in one case, the infant was reported to recover completely upon discontinuation of citalopram by its mother and, in the second case, no follow up information was available. The decision whether to continue or discontinue either nursing or LEXAPRO therapy should take into account the risks of citalopram exposure for the infant and the benefits of LEXAPRO treatment for the mother.
Pediatric Use
Safety and effectiveness in pediatric patients have not been established.
Geriatric Use
Approximately 6% of the 715 patients receiving escitalopram in controlled trials of LEXAPRO in major depressive disorder were 60 years of age or older; elderly patients in these trials received daily doses of LEXAPRO between 10 and 20 mg. The number of elderly patients in these trials was insufficient to adequately assess for possible differential efficacy and safety measures on the basis of age. Nevertheless, greater sensitivity of some elderly individuals to effects of LEXAPRO cannot be ruled out.
In two pharmacokinetic studies, escitalopram half-life was increased by approximately 50% in elderly subjects as compared to young subjects and C_{max} was unchanged (see Clinical Pharmacology). 10 mg/day is the recommended dose for elderly patients (see Dosage and Administration).
Of 4422 patients in clinical studies of racemic citalopram, 1357 were 60 and over, 1034 were 65 and over, and 457 were 75 and over. No overall differences in safety or effectiveness were observed between these subjects and younger subjects, and other reported clinical experience has not identified differences in responses between the elderly and younger patients, but again, greater sensitivity of some elderly individuals cannot be ruled out.

ADVERSE REACTIONS

Adverse event information for LEXAPRO was collected from 715 patients with major depressive disorder who were exposed to escitalopram and from 592 patients who were exposed to placebo in double-blind, placebo-controlled trials. An additional 284 patients were newly exposed to escitalopram in open-label trials.
Adverse events during exposure were obtained primarily by general inquiry and recorded by clinical investigators using terminology of their own choosing. Consequently, it is not possible to provide a meaningful estimate of the proportion of individuals experiencing adverse events without first grouping similar types of events into a smaller number of standardized event categories. In the tables and tabulations that follow, standard World Health Organization (WHO) terminology has been used to classify reported adverse events.
The stated frequencies of adverse events represent the proportion of individuals who experienced, at least once, a treatment-emergent adverse event of the type listed. An event was considered treatment-emergent if it occurred for the first time or worsened while receiving therapy following baseline evaluation.
Adverse Events Associated with Discontinuation of Treatment
Among the 715 depressed patients who received LEXAPRO in placebo-controlled trials, 6% discontinued treatment due to an adverse event, as compared to 2% of 592 patients receiving placebo. In two fixed dose studies, the rate of discontinuation for adverse events in patients receiving 10 mg/day LEXAPRO was not significantly different from the rate of discontinuation for adverse events in patients receiving placebo. The rate of discontinuation for adverse events in patients assigned to a fixed dose of 20 mg/day LEXAPRO was 10% which was significantly different from the rate of discontinuation for adverse events in patients receiving 10 mg/day LEXAPRO (4%) and placebo (3%). Adverse events that were associated with the discontinuation of at least 1% of patients treated with LEXAPRO, and for which the rate was at least twice the placebo rate, were nausea (2%) and ejaculation disorder (2% of male patients).
Incidence of Adverse Events in Placebo-Controlled Clinical Trials
Table 1 enumerates the incidence, rounded to the nearest percent, of treatment emergent adverse events that occurred among 715 depressed patients who received LEXAPRO at doses ranging from 10 to 20 mg/day in placebo-controlled trials. Events included are those occurring in 2% or more of patients treated with LEXAPRO and for which the incidence in patients treated with LEXAPRO was greater than the incidence in placebo-treated patients.
The prescriber should be aware that these figures cannot be used to predict the incidence of adverse events in the course of usual medical practice where patient characteristics and other factors differ from those which prevailed in the clinical trials. Similarly, the cited frequencies cannot be compared with figures obtained from other clinical investigations involving different treatments, uses, and investigators. The cited figures, however, do provide the prescribing physician with some basis for estimating the relative contribution of drug and non-drug factors to the adverse event incidence rate in the population studied.
The most commonly observed adverse events in LEXAPRO patients (incidence of approximately 5% or greater and approximately twice the incidence in placebo patients) were insomnia, ejaculation disorder (primarily ejaculatory delay), nausea, sweating increased, fatigue, and somnolence (see TABLE 1).

Continued on next page

Lexapro—Cont.

TABLE 1
Treatment-Emergent Adverse Events:
Incidence in Placebo-Controlled Clinical Trials*

Body System/Adverse Event	LEXAPRO (N=715)	Placebo (N=592)
Autonomic Nervous System Disorders		
Dry Mouth	6%	5%
Sweating Increased	5%	2%
Central & Peripheral Nervous System Disorders		
Dizziness	5%	3%
Gastrointestinal Disorders		
Nausea	15%	7%
Diarrhea	8%	5%
Constipation	3%	1%
Indigestion	3%	1%
Abdominal Pain	2%	1%
General		
Influenza-like Symptoms	5%	4%
Fatigue	5%	2%
Psychiatric Disorders		
Insomnia	9%	4%
Somnolence	6%	2%
Appetite Decreased	3%	1%
Libido Decreased	3%	1%
Respiratory System Disorders		
Rhinitis	5%	4%
Sinusitis	3%	2%
Urogenital		
Ejaculation Disorder[1,2]	9%	<1%
Impotence[2]	3%	<1%
Anorgasmia[3]	2%	<1%

*Events reported by at least 2% of patients treated with LEXAPRO are reported, except for the following events which had an incidence on placebo ≥ LEXAPRO: headache, upper respiratory tract infection, back pain, pharyngitis, inflicted injury, anxiety.
[1] Primarily ejaculatory delay.
[2] Denominator used was for males only (N=225 LEXAPRO; N=188 placebo).
[3] Denominator used was for females only (N=490 LEXAPRO; N=404 placebo).

Dose Dependency of Adverse Events

The potential dose dependency of common adverse events (defined as an incidence rate of ≥ 5% in either the 10 mg or 20 mg LEXAPRO groups) was examined on the basis of the combined incidence of adverse events in two fixed dose trials. The overall incidence rates of adverse events in 10 mg LEXAPRO treated patients (66%) was similar to that of the placebo treated patients (61%), while the incidence rate in 20 mg/day LEXAPRO treated patients was greater (86%). Table 2 shows common adverse events that occurred in the 20 mg/day LEXAPRO group with an incidence that was approximately twice that of the 10 mg/day LEXAPRO group and approximately twice that of the placebo group.
[See table 2 below]

Male and Female Sexual Dysfunction with SSRIs

Although changes in sexual desire, sexual performance and sexual satisfaction often occur as manifestations of a psychiatric disorder, they may also be a consequence of pharmacologic treatment. In particular, some evidence suggests that selective serotonin reuptake inhibitors (SSRIs) can cause such untoward sexual experiences.
Reliable estimates of the incidence and severity of untoward experiences involving sexual desire, performance and satisfaction are difficult to obtain, however, in part because patients and physicians may be reluctant to discuss them. Accordingly, estimates of the incidence of untoward sexual experience and performance cited in product labeling are likely to underestimate their actual incidence.
Table 3 shows the incidence rates of sexual side effects in patients with major depressive disorder in placebo controlled trials.

TABLE 3
Incidence of Sexual Side Effects in Placebo-Controlled Clinical Trials

Adverse Event	LEXAPRO	Placebo
In Males Only		
	(N=225)	(N=188)
Ejaculation Disorder (primarily ejaculatory delay)	9%	<1%
Decreased Libido	4%	2%
Impotence	3%	<1%
In Females Only		
	(N=490)	(N=404)
Decreased Libido	2%	<1%
Anorgasmia	2%	<1%

There are no adequately designed studies examining sexual dysfunction with escitalopram treatment.
Priapism has been reported with all SSRIs.
While it is difficult to know the precise risk of sexual dysfunction associated with the use of SSRIs, physicians should routinely inquire about such possible side effects.

Vital Sign Changes

LEXAPRO and placebo groups were compared with respect to (1) mean change from baseline in vital signs (pulse, systolic blood pressure, and diastolic blood pressure) and (2) the incidence of patients meeting criteria for potentially clinically significant changes from baseline in these variables. These analyses did not reveal any clinically important changes in vital signs associated with LEXAPRO treatment. In addition, a comparison of supine and standing vital sign measures in subjects receiving LEXAPRO indicated that LEXAPRO treatment is not associated with orthostatic changes.

Weight Changes

Patients treated with LEXAPRO in controlled trials did not differ from placebo-treated patients with regard to clinically important change in body weight.

Laboratory Changes

LEXAPRO and placebo groups were compared with respect to (1) mean change from baseline in various serum chemistry, hematology, and urinalysis variables and (2) the incidence of patients meeting criteria for potentially clinically significant changes from baseline in these variables. These analyses revealed no clinically important changes in laboratory test parameters associated with LEXAPRO treatment.

ECG Changes

Electrocardiograms from LEXAPRO (N=625), racemic citalopram (N=351), and placebo (N=527) groups were compared with respect to (1) mean change from baseline in various ECG parameters and (2) the incidence of patients meeting criteria for potentially clinically significant changes from baseline in these variables. These analyses revealed (1) a decrease in heart rate of 2.2 bpm for LEXAPRO and 2.7 bpm for racemic citalopram, compared to an increase of 0.3 bpm for placebo and (2) an increase in QTc interval of 3.9 msec for LEXAPRO and 3.7 msec for racemic citalopram, compared to 0.5 msec for placebo. Neither LEXAPRO nor racemic citalopram were associated with the development of clinically significant ECG abnormalities.

Other Events Observed During the Premarketing Evaluation of LEXAPRO

Following is a list of WHO terms that reflect treatment-emergent adverse events, as defined in the introduction to the ADVERSE REACTIONS section, reported by the 999 patients treated with LEXAPRO for periods of up to one year in double-blind or open-label clinical trials during its premarketing evaluation. All reported events are included except those already listed in Table 1, those occurring in only one patient, event terms that are so general as to be uninformative, and those that are unlikely to be drug related. It is important to emphasize that, although the events reported occurred during treatment with LEXAPRO, they were not necessarily caused by it.
Events are further categorized by body system and listed in order of decreasing frequency according to the following definitions: frequent adverse events are those occurring on one or more occasions in at least 1/100 patients; infrequent adverse events are those occurring in less than 1/100 patients but at least 1/1000 patients.
Cardiovascular - *Frequent:* palpitation, hypertension. *Infrequent:* bradycardia, tachycardia, ECG abnormal, flushing, varicose vein.
Central and Peripheral Nervous System Disorders - *Frequent:* paresthesia, light-headed feeling, migraine, tremor, vertigo. *Infrequent:* shaking, dysequilibrium, tics, restless legs, carpal tunnel syndrome, twitching, faintness, hyperreflexia, muscle contractions involuntary, muscular tone increased.
Gastrointestinal Disorders - *Frequent:* vomiting, flatulence, heartburn, tooth ache, gastroenteritis, abdominal cramp, gastroesophageal reflux. *Infrequent:* bloating, increased stool frequency, abdominal discomfort, dyspepsia, belching, gagging, gastritis, hemorrhoids.
General - *Frequent:* allergy, pain in limb, hot flushes, fever, chest pain. *Infrequent:* edema of extremities, chills, malaise, syncope, tightness of chest, leg pain, edema, asthenia, anaphylaxis.
Hemic and Lymphatic Disorders - *Infrequent:* bruise, anemia, nosebleed, hematoma.
Metabolic and Nutritional Disorders - *Frequent:* increased weight, decreased weight. *Infrequent:* bilirubin increased, gout, hypercholesterolemia, hyperglycemia.
Musculoskeletal System Disorders - *Frequent:* arthralgia, neck/shoulder pain, muscle cramp, myalgia. *Infrequent:* jaw stiffness, muscle stiffness, arthritis, muscle weakness, arthropathy, back discomfort, joint stiffness, jaw pain.
Psychiatric Disorders - *Frequent:* dreaming abnormal, yawning, appetite increased, lethargy, irritability, concentration impaired. *Infrequent:* agitation, jitteriness, apathy, panic reaction, restlessness aggravated, nervousness, forgetfulness, suicide attempt, depression aggravated, feeling unreal, excitability, emotional lability, crying abnormal, depression, anxiety attack, depersonalization, suicidal tendency, bruxism, confusion, carbohydrate craving, amnesia, tremulousness nervous, auditory hallucination.
Reproductive Disorders/Female* - *Frequent:* menstrual cramps. *Infrequent:* menstrual disorder, menorrhagia, spotting between menses, pelvic inflammation.

*% based on female subjects only: N= 658

Respiratory System Disorders - *Frequent:* bronchitis, sinus congestion, coughing, sinus headache, nasal congestion. *Infrequent:* asthma, breath shortness, laryngitis, pneumonia, tracheitis.
Skin and Appendages Disorders - *Frequent:* rash. *Infrequent:* acne, pruritus, eczema, alopecia, dry skin, folliculitis, lipoma, furunculosis, dermatitis.
Special Senses - *Frequent:* vision blurred, ear ache, tinnitus. *Infrequent:* taste alteration, eye irritation, conjunctivitis, vision abnormal, visual disturbance, dry eyes, eye infection, pupils dilated.
Urinary System Disorders - *Frequent:* urinary tract infection, urinary frequency. *Infrequent:* kidney stone, dysuria, urinary urgency.

Events Reported Subsequent to the Marketing of Racemic Citalopram

Although no causal relationship to racemic citalopram treatment has been found, the following adverse events have been reported to be temporally associated with racemic citalopram treatment and were not observed during the premarketing evaluation of escitalopram or citalopram: acute renal failure, akathisia, allergic reaction, anaphylaxis, angioedema, choreoathetosis, delirium, dyskinesia, ecchymosis, epidermal necrolysis, erythema multiforme, gastrointestinal hemorrhage, grand mal convulsions, hemolytic anemia, hepatic necrosis, myoclonus, neuroleptic malignant syndrome, nystagmus, pancreatitis, priapism, prolactinemia, prothrombin decreased, QT prolonged, rhabdomyolysis, serotonin syndrome, spontaneous abortion, thrombocytopenia, thrombosis, Torsades de pointes, ventricular arrhythmia, and withdrawal syndrome.

TABLE 2
Incidence of Common Adverse Events* in Patients Receiving Placebo, 10 mg/day LEXAPRO, or 20 mg/day LEXAPRO

Adverse Event	Placebo (N=311)	10 mg/day LEXAPRO (N=310)	20 mg/day LEXAPRO (N=125)
Insomnia	4%	7%	14%
Diarrhea	5%	6%	14%
Dry Mouth	3%	4%	9%
Somnolence	1%	4%	9%
Dizziness	2%	4%	7%
Sweating Increased	<1%	3%	8%
Constipation	1%	3%	6%
Fatigue	2%	2%	6%
Indigestion	1%	2%	6%

*Adverse events with an incidence rate of at least 5% in either of the LEXAPRO groups and with an incidence rate in the 20 mg/day LEXAPRO group that was approximately twice that of the 10 mg/day LEXAPRO group and the placebo group.

DRUG ABUSE AND DEPENDENCE
Controlled Substance Class
LEXAPRO is not a controlled substance.
Physical and Psychological Dependence
Animal studies suggest that the abuse liability of racemic citalopram is low. LEXAPRO has not been systematically studied in humans for its potential for abuse, tolerance, or physical dependence. The premarketing clinical experience with LEXAPRO did not reveal any drug seeking behavior. However, these observations were not systematic and it is not possible to predict on the basis of this limited experience the extent to which a CNS-active drug will be misused, diverted, and/or abused once marketed. Consequently, physicians should carefully evaluate LEXAPRO patients for history of drug abuse and follow such patients closely, observing them for signs of misuse or abuse (e.g., development of tolerance, incrementations of dose, drug seeking behavior).

OVERDOSAGE
Human Experience
There have been three reports of LEXAPRO overdose involving doses of up to 600 mg. All three patients recovered and no symptoms associated with the overdoses were reported. In clinical trials of racemic citalopram, there were no reports of fatal citalopram overdose involving overdoses of up to 2000 mg. During the postmarketing evaluation of citalopram, like other SSRIs, a fatal outcome in a patient who has taken an overdose of citalopram has been rarely reported.
Postmarketing reports of drug overdoses involving citalopram have included 12 fatalities, 10 in combination with other drugs and/or alcohol and 2 with citalopram alone (3920 mg and 2800 mg), as well as non-fatal overdoses of up to 6000 mg. Symptoms most often accompanying citalopram overdose, alone or in combination with other drugs and/or alcohol, included dizziness, sweating, nausea, vomiting, tremor, somnolence, sinus tachycardia, and convulsions. In more rare cases, observed symptoms included amnesia, confusion, coma, hyperventilation, cyanosis, rhabdomyolysis, and ECG changes (including QTc prolongation, nodal rhythm, ventricular arrhythmia, and one possible case of Torsades de pointes).
Management of Overdose
Establish and maintain an airway to ensure adequate ventilation and oxygenation. Gastric evacuation by lavage and use of activated charcoal should be considered. Careful observation and cardiac and vital sign monitoring are recommended, along with general symptomatic and supportive care. Due to the large volume of distribution of escitalopram, forced diuresis, dialysis, hemoperfusion, and exchange transfusion are unlikely to be of benefit. There are no specific antidotes for LEXAPRO.
In managing overdosage, consider the possibility of multiple drug involvement. The physician should consider contacting a poison control center for additional information on the treatment of any overdose.

DOSAGE AND ADMINISTRATION
Initial Treatment
The recommended dose of LEXAPRO is 10 mg once daily. A fixed dose trial of LEXAPRO demonstrated the effectiveness of both 10 mg and 20 mg of LEXAPRO, but failed to demonstrate a greater benefit of 20 mg over 10 mg (see Clinical Efficacy Trials under Clinical Pharmacology). If the dose is increased to 20 mg, this should occur after a minimum of one week.
LEXAPRO should be administered once daily, in the morning or evening, with or without food.
Special Populations
10 mg/day is the recommended dose for most elderly patients and patients with hepatic impairment.
No dosage adjustment is necessary for patients with mild or moderate renal impairment. LEXAPRO should be used with caution in patients with severe renal impairment.
Maintenance Treatment
It is generally agreed that acute episodes of major depressive disorder require several months or longer of sustained pharmacological therapy beyond response to the acute episode. Systematic evaluation of continuing LEXAPRO 10 or 20 mg/day for periods of up to 36 weeks in patients with major depressive disorder who responded while taking LEXAPRO during an 8-week acute treatment phase demonstrated a benefit of such maintenance treatment (see Clinical Efficacy Trials, under Clinical Pharmacology). Nevertheless, patients should be periodically reassessed to determine the need for maintenance treatment.
Switching Patients To or From a Monoamine Oxidase Inhibitor
At least 14 days should elapse between discontinuation of an MAOI and initiation of LEXAPRO therapy. Similarly, at least 14 days should be allowed after stopping LEXAPRO before starting a MAOI (see Contraindications and Warnings).

HOW SUPPLIED
10 mg Tablets:
Bottle of 100   NDC # 0456-2010-01
10 x 10 Unit Dose   NDC # 0456-2010-63
White to off-white, round, scored film coated. Imprint on scored side with "F" on the left side and "L" on the right side. Imprint on the non-scored side with "10".
20 mg Tablets:
Bottle of 100   NDC # 0456-2020-01
10 x 10 Unit Dose   NDC # 0456-2020-63
White to off-white, round, scored film coated. Imprint on scored side with "F" on the left side and "L" on the right side. Imprint on the non-scored side with "20".
Oral Solution:
5 mg/5 mL, peppermint   NDC # 0456-2101-08
flavor - (240 mL)
Store at 25°C (77°F); excursions permitted to 15-30°C (59-86°F).

ANIMAL TOXICOLOGY
Retinal Changes in Rats
Pathologic changes (degeneration/atrophy) were observed in the retinas of albino rats in the 2-year carcinogenicity study with racemic citalopram. There was an increase in both incidence and severity of retinal pathology in both male and female rats receiving 80 mg/kg/day. Similar findings were not present in rats receiving 24 mg/kg/day of racemic citalopram for two years, in mice receiving up to 240 mg/kg/day of racemic citalopram for 18 months, or in dogs receiving up to 20 mg/kg/day of racemic citalopram for one year.
Additional studies to investigate the mechanism for this pathology have not been performed, and the potential significance of this effect in humans has not been established.
Cardiovascular Changes in Dogs
In a one year toxicology study, 5 of 10 beagle dogs receiving oral racemic citalopram doses of 8 mg/kg/day died suddenly between weeks 17 and 31 following initiation of treatment. Sudden deaths were not observed in rats at doses of racemic citalopram up to 120 mg/kg/day, which produced plasma levels of citalopram and its metabolites demethylcitalopram and didemethylcitalopram (DDCT) similar to those observed in dogs at 8 mg/kg/day. A subsequent intravenous dosing study demonstrated that in beagle dogs, racemic DDCT caused QT prolongation, a known risk factor for the observed outcome in dogs.
Forest Pharmaceuticals, Inc.
Subsidiary of Forest Laboratories, Inc.
St. Louis, MO 63045 USA
Licensed from H. Lundbeck A/S
Rev. 12/02
©2002 Forest Laboratories, Inc.

GlaxoSmithKline
FIVE MOORE DRIVE
RESEARCH TRIANGLE PARK, NC 27709

For Medical Emergencies, Medical Information for Healthcare Professionals, and Consumer Inquiries, Contact:
1-888-825-5249
www.druginfo.gsk.com

ADVAIR DISKUS® 100/50   ℞
[ad'vair disk'us]
(fluticasone propionate 100 mcg and salmeterol* 50 mcg inhalation powder)

ADVAIR DISKUS® 250/50   ℞
(fluticasone propionate 250 mcg and salmeterol* 50 mcg inhalation powder)

ADVAIR DISKUS® 500/50   ℞
(fluticasone propionate 500 mcg and salmeterol* 50 mcg inhalation powder)

***As salmeterol xinafoate salt 72.5 mcg, equivalent to salmeterol base 50 mcg**

FOR ORAL INHALATION ONLY

Prescribing information for these products, which appears on pages 1433–1439 of the 2003 PDR, has been revised as follows. Please write "See Supplement A" next to the product heading.
Revised the following ingredients statement in the DESCRIPTION section to include milk proteins:
Each blister on the double-foil strip within the device contains 100, 250, or 500 mcg of microfine fluticasone propionate and 72.5 mcg of microfine salmeterol xinafoate salt, equivalent to 50 mcg of salmeterol base, in 12.5 mg of formulation containing lactose (which contains milk proteins).
The black box was removed from the WARNINGS section.
The 8th paragraph of PRECAUTIONS: General was revised to:
It is possible that systemic corticosteroid effects such as hypercorticism and adrenal suppression (including adrenal crisis) may appear in a small number of patients, particularly when fluticasone propionate is administered at higher than recommended doses over prolonged periods of time. If such effects occur, the dose of fluticasone propionate should be reduced slowly, consistent with accepted procedures for reducing systemic corticosteroids and for management of asthma symptoms.
Added the following to PRECAUTIONS: Information for Patients:
2. Most patients are able to taste or feel a dose delivered from ADVAIR DISKUS. However, whether or not patients are able to sense delivery of a dose, you should instruct them not to exceed the recommended dose of 1 inhalation each morning and evening, approximately 12 hours apart. You should instruct them to contact you or the pharmacist if they have questions.
Added the following bullet to statement number 9:
• After inhalation, rinse the mouth with water without swallowing.
In the ADVERSE REACTIONS: Observed During Clinical Practice: Ear, Nose and Throat subsection, added facial and oropharyngeal edema.
Revised the ADVERSE REACTIONS: Observed During Clinical Practice: Non-Site Specific subsection to:
Immediate and delayed hypersensitivity reaction (including very rare anaphylactic reaction), pallor. Very rare anaphylactic reaction in patients with severe milk protein allergy.
Deleted the following sentence from DOSAGE AND ADMINISTRATION:
Rinsing the mouth after inhalation is advised.
GlaxoSmithKline, Research Triangle Park, NC 27709
©2003, GlaxoSmithKline. All rights reserved.
March 2003/RL-1183

AGENERASE®   ℞
[a-jin' ə-rās]
(amprenavir)
Capsules

Prescribing information for this product, which appears on pages 1439–1443 of the 2003 PDR, has been revised as follows. Please write "See Supplement A" next to the product heading.
Under CLINICAL PHARMACOLOGY: Drug Interactions, Tables 3 and 4 were revised to include data for Delavirdine, Ethinyl estradiol, Norethindrone, and Methadone and now read as follows:
[See table 3 at top of next page]
[See table 4 at top of page 159]
The following subsection was added under CLINICAL PHARMACOLOGY: Drug Interactions: Methadone: Coadministration of amprenavir and methadone can decrease plasma levels of methadone.
Coadministration of amprenavir and methadone as compared to a non-matched historical control group resulted in a 30%, 27%, and 25% decrease in serum amprenavir AUC, C_{max}, and C_{min}, respectively.
The 9th paragraph under PRECAUTIONS: Information for Patients was revised to:
Patients taking AGENERASE should be instructed **not** to use hormonal contraceptives because some birth control pills (those containing ethinyl estradiol/norethindrone) have been found to decrease the concentration of amprenavir. Therefore, patients receiving hormonal contraceptives should be instructed to use alternate contraceptive measures during therapy with AGENERASE.
Under PRECAUTIONS: Drug Interactions, Table 7 was revised to include data for Non-nucleoside Reverse Transcriptase Inhibitor: Delavirdine and Oral contraceptives: Ethinyl estradiol/norethindrone and now reads as follows:
[See table 7 on page 159]
Under PRECAUTIONS: Drug Interactions, data for Non-nucleoside Reverse Transcriptase Inhibitor: Delavirdine and Oral contraceptives: Ethinyl estradiol/norethindrone were removed from Table 8, and data for Narcotic analgesics: Methadone were added. Table 8 now reads as follows:
[See table 8 on pages 160 and 161]
The PRECAUTIONS: Carcinogenesis and Mutagenesis section was revised to:
Carcinogenesis and Mutagenesis: Amprenavir was evaluated for carcinogenic potential by oral gavage administration to mice and rats for up to 104 weeks. Daily doses of 50, 275 to 300, and 500 to 600 mg/kg/day were administered to mice and doses of 50, 190, and 750 mg/kg/day were administered to rats. Results showed an increase in the incidence of benign hepatocellular adenomas and an increase in the combined incidence of hepatocellular adenomas plus carcinoma in males of both species at the highest doses tested. Female mice and rats were not affected. These observations were made at systemic exposures equivalent to approximately 2 times (mice) and 4 times (rats) the human exposure (based on $AUC_{0-24\ hr}$ measurement) at the recommended dose of 1,200 mg twice daily. Administration of amprenavir did not cause a statistically significant increase in the incidence of any other benign or malignant neoplasm in mice or rats. It is not known how predictive the results of rodent carcinogenicity studies may be for humans. However, amprenavir was not mutagenic or genotoxic in a battery of in vitro and in vivo assays including bacterial reverse mutation (Ames), mouse lymphoma, rat micronucleus, and chromosome aberrations in human lymphocytes.
Manufactured by R.P. Scherer, Beinheim, France
for GlaxoSmithKline, Research Triangle Park, NC 27709
Licensed from Vertex Pharmaceuticals Incorporated
Cambridge, MA 02139

Continued on next page

Agenerase Capsules—Cont.

AGENERASE is a registered trademark of the GlaxoSmithKline group of companies.
©2002, GlaxoSmithKline. All rights reserved.
October 2002/RL-1148

AGENERASE® ℞
[a-jin' ə-rās]
(amprenavir)
Oral Solution

Prescribing information for this product, which appears on pages 1444–1449 of the 2003 PDR, has been revised as follows. Please write "See Supplement A" next to the product heading.

Under **CLINICAL PHARMACOLOGY: Drug Interactions**, Tables 3 and 4 were revised to include data for Delavirdine, Ethinyl estradiol, Norethindrone, and Methadone and now read as follows:
[See table 3 at bottom of page 161]
[See table 4 at top of page 162]

The following subsection was added under **CLINICAL PHARMACOLOGY: Drug Interactions:**
Methadone: Coadministration of amprenavir and methadone can decrease plasma levels of methadone. Coadministration of amprenavir and methadone as compared to a non-matched historical control group resulted in a 30%, 27%, and 25% decrease in serum amprenavir AUC, C_{max}, and C_{min}, respectively.

The 12th paragraph under **PRECAUTIONS: Information for Patients** *was revised to:*
Patients taking AGENERASE should be instructed **not** to use hormonal contraceptives because some birth control pills (those containing ethinyl estradiol/norethindrone) have been found to decrease the concentration of amprenavir. Therefore, patients receiving hormonal contraceptives should be instructed to use alternate contraceptive measures during therapy with AGENERASE.

Under **PRECAUTIONS: Drug Interactions**, Table 7 was revised to include data for Non-nucleoside Reverse Transcriptase Inhibitor: Delavirdine and Oral contraceptives: Ethinyl estradiol/norethindrone and now reads as follows:
[See table 7 on page 162]

Under **PRECAUTIONS: Drug Interactions**, data for Non-nucleoside Reverse Transcriptase Inhibitor: Delavirdine and Oral contraceptive: Ethinyl estradiol were removed from Table 8, and data for Narcotic analgesics: Methadone were added. Table 8 now reads as follows:
[See table 8 on pages 163 and 164]

The **PRECAUTIONS: Carcinogenesis and Mutagenesis** *section was revised to:*
Carcinogenesis and Mutagenesis: Amprenavir was evaluated for carcinogenic potential by oral gavage administration to mice and rats for up to 104 weeks. Daily doses of 50, 275 to 300, and 500 to 600 mg/kg/day were administered to mice and doses of 50, 190, and 750 mg/kg/day were administered to rats. Results showed an increase in the incidence of benign hepatocellular adenomas and an increase in the combined incidence of hepatocellular adenomas plus carcinoma in males of both species at the highest doses tested. Female mice and rats were not affected. These observations were made at systemic exposures equivalent to approximately 2 times (mice) and 4 times (rats) the human exposure (based on $AUC_{0-24\ hr}$ measurement) at the recommended dose of 1,200 mg twice daily. Administration of amprenavir did not cause a statistically significant increase in the incidence of any other benign or malignant neoplasm in mice or rats. It is not known how predictive the results of rodent carcinogenicity studies may be for humans. However, amprenavir was not mutagenic or genotoxic in a battery of in vitro and in vivo assays including bacterial reverse mutation (Ames), mouse lymphoma, rat micronucleus, and chromosome aberrations in human lymphocytes.
GlaxoSmithKline, Research Triangle Park, NC 27709
Licensed from Vertex Pharmaceuticals Incorporated
Cambridge, MA 02139
AGENERASE is a registered trademark of the GlaxoSmithKline group of companies.
©2002, GlaxoSmithKline. All rights reserved.
October 2002/RL-1149

AUGMENTIN® ℞
[äg-mint' in]
amoxicillin/clavulanate potassium
Powder for Oral Suspension and Chewable Tablets

Prescribing information for these products, which appears on pages 1464–1468 of the 2003 PDR, has been revised as follows. Please write "See Supplement A" next to the product heading.

Under **CLINICAL PHARMACOLOGY:** *Microbiology:* GRAM-NEGATIVE AEROBES *subsection*, 0.5 µg/mL was changed to 2 µg/mL in the following sentence: Amoxicillin/clavulanic acid exhibits *in vitro* minimal inhibitory concentrations (MICs) of 2 µg/mL or less against most (≥90%) strains of *Streptococcus pneumoniae*....

Table 3. Drug Interactions: Pharmacokinetic Parameters for Amprenavir in the Presence of the Coadministered Drug

Co-administered Drug	Dose of Coadministered Drug	Dose of AGENERASE	n	% Change in Amprenavir Pharmacokinetic Parameters* (90% CI)		
				C_{max}	AUC	C_{min}
Abacavir	300 mg b.i.d. for 3 weeks	900 mg b.i.d. for 3 weeks	4	↑47 (↓15 to ↑154)	↑29 (↓18 to ↑103)	↑27 (↓46 to ↑197)
Clarithromycin	500 mg b.i.d. for 4 days	1,200 mg b.i.d. for 4 days	12	↑15 (↑1 to ↑31)	↑18 (↑8 to ↑29)	↑39 (↑31 to ↑47)
Delavirdine	600 mg b.i.d. for 10 days	600 mg b.i.d. for 10 days	9	↑40‡	↑130‡	↑125‡
Ethinyl estradiol/ Norethindrone	0.035 mg/1 mg for 1 cycle	1,200 mg b.i.d. for 28 days	10	⇔ (↓20 to ↑3)	↓22 (↓35 to ↓8)	↓20 (↓41 to ↑8)
Indinavir	800 mg t.i.d. for 2 weeks (fasted)	750 or 800 mg t.i.d. for 2 weeks (fasted)	9	↑18 (↓13 to ↑58)	↑33 (↑2 to ↑73)	↑25 (↓27 to ↑116)
Ketoconazole	400 mg single dose	1,200 mg single dose	12	↓16 (↓25 to ↓6)	↑31 (↑20 to ↑42)	NA
Lamivudine	150 mg single dose	600 mg single dose	11	⇔ (↓17 to ↑9)	⇔ (↓15 to ↑14)	NA
Nelfinavir	750 mg t.i.d. for 2 weeks (fed)	750 or 800 mg t.i.d. for 2 weeks (fed)	6	↓14 (↓38 to ↑20)	⇔ (↓19 to ↑47)	↑189 (↑52 to ↑448)
Rifabutin	300 mg q.d. for 10 days	1,200 mg b.i.d. for 10 days	5	⇔ (↓21 to ↑10)	↓15 (↓28 to 0)	↓15 (↓38 to ↑17)
Rifampin	300 mg q.d. for 4 days	1,200 mg b.i.d. for 4 days	11	↓70 (↓76 to ↓62)	↓82 (↓84 to ↓78)	↓92 (↓95 to ↓89)
Ritonavir	100 mg b.i.d. for 2 to 4 weeks	600 mg b.i.d.	18	↓30† (↓44 to ↓14)	↑64† (↑37 to ↑97)	↑508† (↑394 to ↑649)
Ritonavir	200 mg q.d. for 2 to 4 weeks	1,200 mg q.d.	12	⇔† (↓17 to ↑30)	↑62† (↑35 to ↑94)	↑319† (↑190 to ↑508)
Saquinavir	800 mg t.i.d. for 2 weeks (fed)	750 or 800 mg t.i.d. for 2 weeks (fed)	7	↓37 (↓54 to ↓14)	↓32 (↓49 to ↓9)	↓14 (↓52 to ↑54)
Zidovudine	300 mg single dose	600 mg single dose	12	⇔ (↓5 to ↑24)	↑13 (↑2 to ↑31)	NA

*Based on total-drug concentrations.
†Compared to amprenavir 1,200 mg b.i.d. in the same patients.
‡Median percent change; confidence interval not reported.
↑ = Increase; ↓ = Decrease; ⇔ = No change (↑ or ↓ <10%); NA = C_{min} not calculated for single-dose study.

Under the **CLINICAL PHARMACOLOGY:** *Microbiology:* SUSCEPTIBILITY TESTING: Dilution Techniques *subsection, the recommended ranges for amoxicillin/clavulanic acid susceptibility testing were revised as follows:*
For *Streptococcus pneumoniae* from non-meningitis sources: Isolates should be tested using amoxicillin/clavulanic acid and the following criteria should be used:

MIC (µg/mL)	Interpretation
≤ 2/1	Susceptible (S)
4/2	Intermediate (I)
≥ 8/4	Resistant (R)

Note: These interpretive criteria are based on the recommended doses for respiratory tract infections.
GlaxoSmithKline, Research Triangle Park, NC 27709
©2002, GlaxoSmithKline. All rights reserved.
May 2002/AG:PL10

AVANDIA® ℞
[ə-van' dē-ə]
(rosiglitazone maleate)
Tablets

Prescribing information for these products, which appears on pages 1473–1477 of the 2003 PDR, has been revised as follows. Please write "See Supplement A" next to the product heading. The following subsection was added under **CLINICAL STUDIES:**
Combination With Insulin: In two 26-week randomized, double-blind, fixed-dose studies designed to assess the efficacy and safety of AVANDIA in combination with insulin, patients inadequately controlled on insulin (65 to 67 units/day, mean range at baseline) were randomized to receive AVANDIA 4 mg plus insulin (n = 206) or placebo plus insulin (n = 203). The mean duration of disease in these patients was 12 to 13 years.
Compared to insulin plus placebo, single or divided doses of AVANDIA 4 mg daily plus insulin significantly reduced FPG (mean reduction of 32 to 40 mg/dL) and HbA1c (mean reduction of 0.6% to 0.7%). Approximately 40% of all patients treated with AVANDIA reduced their insulin dose.
Under **INDICATIONS AND USAGE,** *the words "or insulin" were added to the following sentence:*
AVANDIA is also indicated for use in combination with a sulfonylurea, metformin, or insulin when diet, exercise, and a single agent do not result in adequate glycemic control.
The **WARNINGS** *section was revised to:*
WARNINGS
Cardiac Failure and Other Cardiac Effects: AVANDIA, like other thiazolidinediones, alone or in combination with other antidiabetic agents, can cause fluid retention, which may exacerbate or lead to heart failure. Patients should be observed for signs and symptoms of heart failure. In combination with insulin, thiazolidinediones may also increase the risk of other cardiovascular adverse events. AVANDIA should be discontinued if any deterioration in cardiac status occurs. Patients with New York Heart Association (NYHA) Class 3 and 4 cardiac status were not studied during the clinical trials. AVANDIA is not recommended in patients with NYHA Class 3 and 4 cardiac status.
In three 26-week trials in patients with type 2 diabetes, 216 received 4 mg of AVANDIA plus insulin, 322 received 8 mg of AVANDIA plus insulin, and 338 received insulin alone. These trials included patients with long-standing diabetes and a high prevalence of pre-existing medical conditions, including peripheral neuropathy, retinopathy, ischemic heart disease, vascular disease, and congestive heart failure. In these clinical studies an increased incidence of edema, cardiac failure, and other cardiovascular adverse events was seen in patients on AVANDIA and insulin combination therapy compared to insulin and placebo. Patients who experienced cardiovascular events were on average older and had a longer duration of diabetes. These cardiovascular events were noted at both the 4 mg and 8 mg daily doses of AVANDIA. In this population, however, it was not possible to determine specific risk factors that could be used to identify all patients at risk of heart failure and other cardiovascular events on combination therapy. Three of 10 patients who developed cardiac failure on combination therapy during the double blind part of the studies had no known prior evidence of congestive heart failure, or pre-existing cardiac condition.

Table 4. Drug Interactions: Pharmacokinetic Parameters for Coadministered Drug in the Presence of Amprenavir

Co-administered Drug	Dose of Coadministered Drug	Dose of AGENERASE	n	% Change in Pharmacokinetic Parameters of Coadministered Drug (90% CI)		
				C_{max}	AUC	C_{min}
Clarithromycin	500 mg b.i.d. for 4 days	1,200 mg b.i.d. for 4 days	12	↓10 (↓24 to ↑7)	⇔ (↓17 to ↑11)	⇔ (↓13 to ↑20)
Delavirdine	600 mg b.i.d. for 10 days	600 mg b.i.d. for 10 days	9	↓47*	↓61*	↓88*
Ethinyl estradiol	0.035 mg for 1 cycle	1,200 mg b.i.d. for 28 days	10	⇔ (↓25 to ↑15)	⇔ (↓14 to ↑38)	↑32 (↓3 to ↑79)
Norethindrone	1.0 mg for 1 cycle	1,200 mg b.i.d. for 28 days	10	⇔ (↓20 to ↑18)	↑18 (↑1 to ↑38)	↑45 (↓13 to ↑88)
Ketoconazole	400 mg single dose	1,200 mg single dose	12	↑19 (↑8 to ↑33)	↑44 (↑31 to ↑59)	NA
Lamivudine	150 mg single dose	600 mg single dose	11	⇔ (↓17 to ↑3)	⇔ (↓11 to 0)	NA
Methadone	44 to 100 mg q.d. for >30 days	1,200 mg b.i.d. for 10 days	16	R-Methadone (active)		
				↓25 (↓32 to ↓18)	↓13 (↓21 to ↓5)	↓21 (↓32 to ↓9)
				S-Methadone (inactive)		
				↓48 (↓55 to ↓40)	↓40 (↓46 to ↓32)	↓53 (↓60 to ↓43)
Rifabutin	300 mg q.d. for 10 days	1,200 mg b.i.d. for 10 days	5	↑119 (↑82 to ↑164)	↑193 (↑156 to ↑235)	↑271 (↑171 to ↑409)
Rifampin	300 mg q.d. for 4 days	1,200 mg b.i.d. for 4 days	11	⇔ (↓13 to ↑12)	⇔ (↓10 to ↑13)	ND
Zidovudine	300 mg single dose	600 mg single dose	12	↑40 (↑14 to ↑71)	↑31 (↑19 to ↑45)	NA

*Median percent change; confidence interval not reported.
↑ = Increase; ↓ = Decrease; ⇔ = No change (↑ or ↓ <10%); NA = C_{min} not calculated for single-dose study; ND = Interaction cannot be determined as C_{min} was below the lower limit of quantitation.

Table 7. Drugs That Should Not Be Coadministered with AGENERASE

Drug Class/Drug Name	Clinical Comment
Antimycobacterials: Rifampin*	May lead to loss of virologic response and possible resistance to AGENERASE or to the class of protease inhibitors.
Ergot Derivatives: Dihydroergotamine, ergonovine, ergotamine, methylergonovine	CONTRAINDICATED due to potential for serious and/or life-threatening reactions such as acute ergot toxicity characterized by peripheral vasospasm and ischemia of the extremities and other tissues.
GI Motility Agents: Cisapride	CONTRAINDICATED due to potential for serious and/or life-threatening reactions such as cardiac arrhythmias.
Herbal Products: St. John's wort (hypericum perforatum)	May lead to loss of virologic response and possible resistance to AGENERASE or to the class of protease inhibitors.
HMG Co-Reductase Inhibitors: Lovastatin, simvastatin	Potential for serious reactions such as risk of myopathy including rhabdomyolysis.
Neuroleptic: Pimozide	CONTRAINDICATED due to potential for serious and/or life-threatening reactions such as cardiac arrhythmias.
Non-nucleoside Reverse Transcriptase Inhibitor: Delavirdine*	May lead to loss of virologic response and possible resistance to delavirdine.
Oral Contraceptives: Ethinyl estradiol/norethindrone	May lead to loss of virologic response and possible resistance to AGENERASE. Alternative methods of non-hormonal contraception are recommended.
Sedatives/Hypnotics: Midazolam, triazolam	CONTRAINDICATED due to potential for serious and/or life-threatening reactions such as prolonged or increased sedation or respiratory depression.

*See CLINICAL PHARMACOLOGY for magnitude of interaction, Tables 3 and 4.

In a double-blind study in type 2 diabetes patients with chronic renal failure (112 received 4 mg or 8 mg of AVANDIA plus insulin and 108 received insulin control), there was no difference in cardiovascular adverse events with AVANDIA in combination with insulin compared to insulin control.
Patients treated with combination AVANDIA and insulin should be monitored for cardiovascular adverse events. This combination therapy should be discontinued in patients who do not respond as manifested by a reduction in HbA1c or insulin dose after 4 to 5 months of therapy or who develop any significant adverse events. (See ADVERSE REACTIONS).
The following paragraph was added under **ADVERSE REACTIONS:**
Hypoglycemia was the most frequently reported adverse event in the fixed-dose insulin combination trials, although few patients withdrew for hypoglycemia (4 of 408 for AVANDIA plus insulin and 1 of 203 for insulin alone). Rates of hypoglycemia, confirmed by capillary blood glucose concentration ≤50 mg/dL, were 6% for insulin alone and 12% (4 mg) and 14% (8 mg) for insulin in combination with AVANDIA.
The **DOSAGE AND ADMINISTRATION** *section was revised to:*
The management of antidiabetic therapy should be individualized. AVANDIA may be administered either at a starting dose of 4 mg as a single daily dose or divided and administered in the morning and evening. For patients who respond inadequately following 8 to 12 weeks of treatment, as determined by reduction in FPG, the dose may be increased to 8 mg daily as monotherapy or in combination with metformin. Reductions in glycemic parameters by dose and regimen are described under CLINICAL STUDIES. AVANDIA may be taken with or without food.
Monotherapy: The usual starting dose of AVANDIA is 4 mg administered either as a single dose once daily or in divided doses twice daily. In clinical trials, the 4 mg twice daily regimen resulted in the greatest reduction in FPG and HbA1c.
Combination Therapy: When AVANDIA is added to existing therapy, the current dose of a sulfonylurea, metformin, or insulin can be continued upon initiation of AVANDIA therapy.
Sulfonylurea: When used in combination with sulfonylurea, the recommended dose of AVANDIA is 4 mg administered as either a single dose once daily or in divided doses twice daily. If patients report hypoglycemia, the dose of the sulfonylurea should be decreased.
Metformin: The usual starting dose of AVANDIA in combination with metformin is 4 mg administered as either a single dose once daily or in divided doses twice daily. It is unlikely that the dose of metformin will require adjustment due to hypoglycemia during combination therapy with AVANDIA.
Insulin: For patients stabilized on insulin, the insulin dose should be continued upon initiation of therapy with AVANDIA. AVANDIA should be dosed at 4 mg daily. Doses of AVANDIA greater than 4 mg daily in combination with insulin are not currently indicated. It is recommended that the insulin dose be decreased by 10% to 25% if the patient reports hypoglycemia or if FPG concentrations decrease to less than 100 mg/dL. Further adjustments should be individualized based on glucose-lowering response.
Maximum Recommended Dose: The dose of AVANDIA should not exceed 8 mg daily, as a single dose or divided twice daily. The 8 mg daily dose has been shown to be safe and effective in clinical studies as monotherapy and in combination with metformin. Doses of AVANDIA greater than 4 mg daily in combination with a sulfonylurea have not been studied in adequate and well-controlled clinical trials. Doses of AVANDIA greater than 4 mg daily in combination with insulin are not currently indicated.
AVANDIA may be taken with or without food.
No dosage adjustments are required for the elderly.
No dosage adjustment is necessary when AVANDIA is used as monotherapy in patients with renal impairment. Since metformin is contraindicated in such patients, concomitant administration of metformin and AVANDIA is also contraindicated in patients with renal impairment.
Therapy with AVANDIA should not be initiated if the patient exhibits clinical evidence of active liver disease or increased serum transaminase levels (ALT >2.5X upper limit of normal at start of therapy) (see PRECAUTIONS, General, *Hepatic Effects* and CLINICAL PHARMACOLOGY, Special Populations, *Hepatic Impairment*). Liver enzyme monitoring is recommended in all patients prior to initiation of therapy with AVANDIA and periodically thereafter (see PRECAUTIONS, General, *Hepatic Effects*).
There are no data on the use of AVANDIA in patients younger than 18 years; therefore, use of AVANDIA in pediatric patients is not recommended.
GlaxoSmithKline, Research Triangle Park, NC 27709
©2003, GlaxoSmithKline. All rights reserved.
March 2003/AV:L9

BECONASE AQ® ℞
[be'kō-nāz]
(beclomethasone dipropionate, monohydrate)
Nasal Spray, 42 mcg

For Intranasal Use Only.
SHAKE WELL BEFORE USE.

Prescribing information for this product, which appears on pages 1481–1482 of the 2003 PDR, has been completely revised as follows. Please write "See Supplement A" next to the product heading.

DESCRIPTION

Beclomethasone dipropionate, monohydrate, the active component of BECONASE AQ Nasal Spray, is an anti-inflammatory steroid having the chemical name 9-chloro-11β,17,21-trihydroxy-16β-methylpregna-1,4-diene-3,20-dione 17,21-dipropionate, monohydrate.
Beclomethasone 17,21-dipropionate is a diester of beclomethasone, a synthetic halogenated corticosteroid. Beclomethasone dipropionate, monohydrate is a white to creamy-white, odorless powder with a molecular weight of 539.06. It is very slightly soluble in water, very soluble in chloroform, and freely soluble in acetone and in ethanol.
BECONASE AQ Nasal Spray is a metered-dose, manual pump spray unit containing a microcrystalline suspension of beclomethasone dipropionate, monohydrate equivalent to 42 mcg of beclomethasone dipropionate, calculated on the dried basis, in an aqueous medium containing microcrystalline cellulose, carboxymethylcellulose sodium, dextrose, benzalkonium chloride, polysorbate 80, and 0.25% v/w phenylethyl alcohol. The pH through expiry is 5.0 to 6.8.
After initial priming (6 actuations), each actuation of the

Continued on next page

Beconase AQ—Cont.

pump delivers from the nasal adapter 100 mg of suspension containing beclomethasone dipropionate, monohydrate equivalent to 42 mcg of beclomethasone dipropionate. If the pump is not used for 7 days, it should be primed until a fine spray appears. Each 25-g bottle of BECONASE AQ Nasal Spray provides 180 metered sprays.

CLINICAL PHARMACOLOGY

Mechanism of Action: Following topical administration, beclomethasone dipropionate produces anti-inflammatory and vasoconstrictor effects. The mechanisms responsible for the anti-inflammatory action of beclomethasone dipropionate are unknown. Corticosteroids have been shown to have a wide range of effects on multiple cell types (e.g., mast cells, eosinophils, neutrophils, macrophages, and lymphocytes) and mediators (e.g., histamine, eicosanoids, leukotrienes, and cytokines) involved in inflammation. The direct relationship of these findings to the effects of beclomethasone dipropionate on allergic rhinitis symptoms is not known.

Biopsies of nasal mucosa obtained during clinical studies showed no histopathologic changes when beclomethasone dipropionate was administered intranasally.

Beclomethasone dipropionate is a pro-drug with weak glucocorticoid receptor binding affinity. It is hydrolyzed via esterase enzymes to its active metabolite beclomethasone-17-monopropionate (B-17-MP), which has high topical anti-inflammatory activity.

Pharmacokinetics: *Absorption:* Beclomethasone dipropionate is sparingly soluble in water. When given by nasal inhalation in the form of an aqueous or aerosolized suspension, the drug is deposited primarily in the nasal passages. The majority of the drug is eventually swallowed. Following intranasal administration of aqueous beclomethasone dipropionate, the systemic absorption was assessed by measuring the plasma concentrations of its active metabolite B-17-MP, for which the absolute bioavailability following intranasal administration is 44% (43% of the administered dose came from the swallowed portion and only 1% of the total dose was bioavailable from the nose). The absorption of unchanged beclomethasone dipropionate following oral and intranasal dosing was undetectable (plasma concentrations <50 pg/mL).

Distribution: The tissue distribution at steady-state for beclomethasone dipropionate is moderate (20 L) but more extensive for B-17-MP (424 L). There is no evidence of tissue storage of beclomethasone dipropionate or its metabolites. Plasma protein binding is moderately high (87%).

Metabolism: Beclomethasone dipropionate is cleared very rapidly from the systemic circulation by metabolism mediated via esterase enzymes that are found in most tissues. The main product of metabolism is the active metabolite (B-17-MP). Minor inactive metabolites, beclomethasone-21-monopropionate (B-21-MP) and beclomethasone (BOH), are also formed, but these contribute little to systemic exposure.

Elimination: The elimination of beclomethasone dipropionate and B-17-MP after intravenous administration are characterized by high plasma clearance (150 and 120 L/hour) with corresponding terminal elimination half-lives of 0.5 and 2.7 hours. Following oral administration of tritiated beclomethasone dipropionate, approximately 60% of the dose was excreted in the feces within 96 hours, mainly as free and conjugated polar metabolites. Approximately 12% of the dose was excreted as free and conjugated polar metabolites in the urine. The renal clearance of beclomethasone dipropionate and its metabolites is negligible.

Pharmacodynamics: The effects of beclomethasone dipropionate on hypothalamic-pituitary-adrenal (HPA) function have been evaluated in adult volunteers by other routes of administration. Studies with beclomethasone dipropionate by the intranasal route may demonstrate that there is more or that there is less absorption by this route of administration. There was no suppression of early morning plasma cortisol concentrations when beclomethasone dipropionate was administered in a dose of 1,000 mcg/day for 1 month as an oral aerosol or for 3 days by intramuscular injection. However, partial suppression of plasma cortisol concentrations was observed when beclomethasone dipropionate was administered in doses of 2,000 mcg/day either by oral aerosol or intramuscular injection. Immediate suppression of plasma cortisol concentrations was observed after single doses of 4,000 mcg of beclomethasone dipropionate. Suppression of HPA function (reduction of early morning plasma cortisol levels) has been reported in adult patients who received 1,600-mcg daily doses of oral beclomethasone dipropionate for 1 month. In clinical studies using beclomethasone dipropionate aerosol intranasally, there was no evidence of adrenal insufficiency. The effect of BECONASE AQ Nasal Spray on HPA function was not evaluated but would not be expected to differ from intranasal beclomethasone dipropionate aerosol.

In 1 study in children with asthma, the administration of inhaled beclomethasone at recommended daily doses for at least 1 year was associated with a reduction in nocturnal cortisol secretion. The clinical significance of this finding is not clear. It reinforces other evidence, however, that topical beclomethasone may be absorbed in amounts that can have systemic effects and that physicians should be alert for evidence of systemic effects, especially in chronically treated patients (see PRECAUTIONS).

INDICATIONS AND USAGE

BECONASE AQ Nasal Spray is indicated for the relief of the symptoms of seasonal or perennial allergic and non-allergic (vasomotor) rhinitis.

Results from 2 clinical trials have shown that significant symptomatic relief was obtained within 3 days. However, symptomatic relief may not occur in some patients for as long as 2 weeks. BECONASE AQ Nasal Spray should not be continued beyond 3 weeks in the absence of significant symptomatic improvement. BECONASE AQ Nasal Spray should not be used in the presence of untreated localized infection involving the nasal mucosa.

BECONASE AQ Nasal Spray is also indicated for the prevention of recurrence of nasal polyps following surgical removal.

Clinical studies have shown that treatment of the symptoms associated with nasal polyps may have to be continued for several weeks or more before a therapeutic result can be fully assessed. Recurrence of symptoms due to polyps can occur after stopping treatment, depending on the severity of the disease.

CONTRAINDICATIONS

Hypersensitivity to any of the ingredients of this preparation contraindicates its use.

Table 8. Established and Other Potentially Significant Drug Interactions: Alteration in Dose or Regimen May Be Recommended Based on Drug Interaction Studies or Predicted Interaction

Concomitant Drug Class: Drug Name	Effect on Concentration of Amprenavir or Concomitant Drug	Clinical Comment
HIV-Antiviral Agents		
Non-nucleoside Reverse Transcriptase Inhibitors: Efavirenz, nevirapine	↓ Amprenavir	Appropriate doses of the combinations with respect to safety and efficacy have not been established.
Nucleoside Reverse Transcriptase Inhibitor: Didanosine (buffered formulation only)	↓ Amprenavir	Take AGENERASE at least 1 hour before or after the buffered formulation of didanosine.
HIV-Protease Inhibitors: Indinavir,* lopinavir/ritonavir, nelfinavir*	↑ Amprenavir Amprenavir's effect on other protease inhibitors is not well established.	Appropriate doses of the combinations with respect to safety and efficacy have not been established.
HIV-Protease Inhibitor: Ritonavir*	↑ Amprenavir	The dose of amprenavir should be reduced when used in combination with ritonavir (see Dosage and Administration). Also, see the full prescribing information for NORVIR for additional drug interaction information.
HIV-Protease Inhibitor: Saquinavir*	↓ Amprenavir Amprenavir's effect on saquinavir is not well established.	Appropriate doses of the combination with respect to safety and efficacy have not been established.
Other Agents		
Antacids	↓ Amprenavir	Take AGENERASE at least 1 hour before or after antacids.
Antiarrhythmics: Amiodarone, lidocaine (systemic), and quinidine	↑ Antiarrhythmics	Caution is warranted and therapeutic concentration monitoring is recommended for antiarrhythmics when coadministered with AGENERASE, if available.
Antiarrhythmic: Bepridil	↑ Bepridil	Use with caution. Increased bepridil exposure may be associated with life-threatening reactions such as cardiac arrhythmias.
Anticoagulant: Warfarin		Concentrations of warfarin may be affected. It is recommended that INR (international normalized ratio) be monitored.
Anticonvulsants: Carbamazepine, phenobarbital, phenytoin	↓ Amprenavir	Use with caution. AGENERASE may be less effective due to decreased amprenavir plasma concentrations in patients taking these agents concomitantly.
Antifungals: Ketoconazole, itraconazole	↑ Ketoconazole ↑ Itraconazole	Increase monitoring for adverse events due to ketoconazole or itraconazole. Dose reduction of ketoconazole or itraconazole may be needed for patients receiving more than 400 mg ketoconazole or itraconazole per day.
Antimycobacterial: Rifabutin*	↑ Rifabutin and rifabutin metabolite	A dosage reduction of rifabutin to at least half the recommended dose is required when AGENERASE and rifabutin are coadministered.* A complete blood count should be performed weekly and as clinically indicated in order to monitor for neutropenia in patients receiving amprenavir and rifabutin.
Benzodiazepines: Alprazolam, clorazepate, diazepam, flurazepam	↑ Benzodiazepines	Clinical significance is unknown; however, a decrease in benzodiazepine dose may be needed.
Calcium Channel Blockers: Diltiazem, felodipine, nifedipine, nicardipine, nimodipine, verapamil, amlodipine, nisoldipine, isradipine	↑ Calcium channel blockers	Caution is warranted and clinical monitoring of patients is recommended.
Corticosteroid: Dexamethasone	↓ Amprenavir	Use with caution. AGENERASE may be less effective due to decreased amprenavir plasma concentrations in patients taking these agents concomitantly.

(Table continued on next page)

WARNINGS

The replacement of a systemic corticosteroid with BECONASE AQ Nasal Spray can be accompanied by signs of adrenal insufficiency.

Careful attention must be given when patients previously treated for prolonged periods with systemic corticosteroids are transferred to BECONASE AQ Nasal Spray. This is particularly important in those patients who have associated asthma or other clinical conditions where too rapid a decrease in systemic corticosteroids may cause a severe exacerbation of their symptoms.

If recommended doses of intranasal beclomethasone are exceeded or if individuals which are particularly sensitive or predisposed by virtue of recent systemic steroid therapy, symptoms of hypercorticism may occur, including very rare cases of menstrual irregularities, acneiform lesions, cataracts, and cushingoid features. If such changes occur, BECONASE AQ Nasal Spray should be discontinued slowly consistent with accepted procedures for discontinuing oral steroid therapy.

Persons who are using drugs that suppress the immune system are more susceptible to infections than healthy individuals. Chickenpox and measles, for example, can have a more serious or even fatal course in susceptible children or adults using corticosteroids. In children or adults who have not had these diseases or been properly immunized, particular care should be taken to avoid exposure. How the dose, route, and duration of corticosteroid administration affect the risk of developing a disseminated infection is not known. The contribution of the underlying disease and/or prior corticosteroid treatment to the risk is also not known. If exposed to chickenpox, prophylaxis with varicella zoster immune globulin (VZIG) may be indicated. If exposed to measles, prophylaxis with pooled intramuscular immunoglobulin (IG) may be indicated. (See the respective package inserts for complete VZIG and IG prescribing information.) If chickenpox develops, treatment with antiviral agents may be considered.

Avoid spraying in eyes.

PRECAUTIONS

General: Intranasal corticosteroids may cause a reduction in growth velocity when administered to pediatric patients (see PRECAUTIONS: Pediatric Use).

During withdrawal from oral corticosteroids, some patients may experience symptoms of withdrawal, e.g., joint and/or muscular pain, lassitude, and depression.

Rarely, immediate hypersensitivity reactions may occur after the intranasal administration of beclomethasone (see ADVERSE REACTIONS).

Rare instances of nasal septum perforation have been spontaneously reported.

Rare instances of wheezing, cataracts, glaucoma, and increased intraocular pressure have been reported following the intranasal use of beclomethasone dipropionate.

In clinical studies with beclomethasone dipropionate administered intranasally, the development of localized infections of the nose and pharynx with *Candida albicans* has occurred only rarely. When such an infection develops, it may require treatment with appropriate local therapy and discontinuation of treatment with BECONASE AQ Nasal Spray.

If persistent nasopharyngeal irritation occurs, it may be an indication for stopping BECONASE AQ Nasal Spray.

Beclomethasone dipropionate is absorbed into the circulation. Use of excessive doses of BECONASE AQ Nasal Spray may suppress HPA function.

Intranasal corticosteroids should be used with caution, if at all, in patients with active or quiescent tuberculous infections of the respiratory tract, untreated local or systemic fungal or bacterial infections, systemic viral or parasitic infections, or ocular herpes simplex.

For BECONASE AQ Nasal Spray to be effective in the treatment of nasal polyps, the spray must be able to enter the nose. Therefore, treatment of nasal polyps with BECONASE AQ Nasal Spray should be considered adjunctive therapy to surgical removal and/or the use of other medications that will permit effective penetration of BECONASE AQ Nasal Spray into the nose. Nasal polyps may recur after any form of treatment.

As with any long-term treatment, patients using BECONASE AQ Nasal Spray over several months or longer should be examined periodically for possible changes in the nasal mucosa.

Because of the inhibitory effect of corticosteroids on wound healing, patients who have experienced recent nasal septal ulcers, nasal surgery, or nasal trauma should not use a nasal corticosteroid until healing has occurred.

Although systemic effects have been minimal with recommended doses, this potential increases with excessive doses. Therefore, larger than recommended doses should be avoided.

Information for Patients: Patients being treated with BECONASE AQ Nasal Spray should receive the following information and instructions. This information is intended to aid them in the safe and effective use of this medication. It is not a disclosure of all possible adverse or intended effects.

Patients should use BECONASE AQ Nasal Spray at regular intervals since its effectiveness depends on its regular use. The patient should take the medication as directed. It is not acutely effective, and the prescribed dosage should not be increased. Instead, nasal vasoconstrictors or oral antihistamines may be needed until the effects of BECONASE AQ Nasal Spray are fully manifested. One to 2 weeks may pass before full relief is obtained. The patient should contact the physician if symptoms do not improve, if the condition worsens, or if sneezing or nasal irritation occurs.

For the proper use of BECONASE AQ Nasal Spray and to attain maximum improvement, the patient should read and follow carefully the patient's instructions accompanying the product.

Persons who are using immunosuppressant doses of corticosteroids should be warned to avoid exposure to chickenpox or measles. Patients should also be advised that if they are exposed, medical advice should be sought without delay.

Table 8 (cont.). Established and Other Potentially Significant Drug Interactions: Alteration in Dose or Regimen May Be Recommended Based on Drug Interaction Studies or Predicted Interaction

Concomitant Drug Class: Drug Name	Effect on Concentration of Amprenavir or Concomitant Drug	Clinical Comment
Other Agents (continued)		
Erectile Dysfunction Agent: Sildenafil	↑ Sildenafil	Use with caution at reduced doses of 25 mg every 48 hours with increased monitoring for adverse events.
HMG-CoA Reductase Inhibitors: Atorvastatin	↑ Atorvastatin	Use lowest possible dose of atorvastatin with careful monitoring or consider other HMG-CoA reductase inhibitors such as pravastatin or fluvastatin in combination with AGENERASE.
Immunosuppressants: Cyclosporine, tacrolimus, rapamycin	↑ Immunosuppressants	Therapeutic concentration monitoring is recommended for immunosuppressant agents when coadministered with AGENERASE.
Narcotic Analgesics: Methadone*	↓ Amprenavir	AGENERASE may be less effective due to decreased amprenavir plasma concentrations in patients taking these agents concomitantly. Alternative antiretroviral therapy should be considered.
	↓ Methadone	Dosage of methadone may need to be increased when coadministered with AGENERASE.
Tricyclic Antidepressants: Amitriptyline, imipramine	↑ Tricyclics	Therapeutic concentration monitoring is recommended for tricyclic antidepressants when coadministered with AGENERASE.

*See CLINICAL PHARMACOLOGY for magnitude of interaction, Tables 3 and 4.

Table 3. Drug Interactions: Pharmacokinetic Parameters for Amprenavir in the Presence of the Coadministered Drug

Co-administered Drug	Dose of Coadministered Drug	Dose of AGENERASE	n	% Change in Amprenavir Pharmacokinetic Parameters* (90% CI)		
				C_{max}	AUC	C_{min}
Abacavir	300 mg b.i.d. for 3 weeks	900 mg b.i.d. for 3 weeks	4	↑47 (↓15 to ↑154)	↑29 (↓18 to ↑103)	↑27 (↓46 to ↑197)
Clarithromycin	500 mg b.i.d. for 4 days	1,200 mg b.i.d. for 4 days	12	↑15 (↑1 to ↑31)	↑18 (↑8 to ↑29)	↑39 (↑31 to ↑47)
Delavirdine	600 mg b.i.d. for 10 days	600 mg b.i.d. for 10 days	9	↑40‡	↑130‡	↑125‡
Ethinyl estradiol/ Norethindrone	0.035 mg/1 mg for 1 cycle	1,200 mg b.i.d. for 28 days	10	⇔ (↓20 to ↑3)	↓22 (↓35 to ↓8)	↓20 (↓41 to ↑8)
Indinavir	800 mg t.i.d. for 2 weeks (fasted)	750 or 800 mg t.i.d. for 2 weeks (fasted)	9	↑18 (↓13 to ↑58)	↑33 (↑2 to ↑73)	↑25 (↓27 to ↑116)
Ketoconazole	400 mg single dose	1,200 mg single dose	12	↓16 (↓25 to ↓6)	↑31 (↑20 to ↑42)	NA
Lamivudine	150 mg single dose	600 mg single dose	11	⇔ (↓17 to ↑9)	⇔ (↓15 to ↑14)	NA
Nelfinavir	750 mg t.i.d. for 2 weeks (fed)	750 or 800 mg t.i.d. for 2 weeks (fed)	6	↓14 (↓38 to ↑20)	⇔ (↓19 to ↑47)	↑189 (↑52 to ↑448)
Rifabutin	300 mg q.d. for 10 days	1,200 mg b.i.d. for 10 days	5	⇔ (↓21 to ↑10)	↓15 (↓28 to 0)	↓15 (↓38 to ↑17)
Rifampin	300 mg q.d. for 4 days	1,200 mg b.i.d. for 4 days	11	↓70 (↓76 to ↓62)	↓82 (↓84 to ↓78)	↓92 (↓95 to ↓89)
Ritonavir	100 mg b.i.d. for 2 to 4 weeks	600 mg b.i.d.	18	↓30† (↓44 to ↓14)	↑64† (↑37 to ↑97)	↑508† (↑394 to ↑649)
Ritonavir	200 mg q.d. for 2 to 4 weeks	1,200 mg q.d.	12	⇔† (↓17 to ↑30)	↑62† (↑35 to ↑94)	↑319† (↑190 to ↑508)
Saquinavir	800 mg t.i.d. for 2 weeks (fed)	750 or 800 mg t.i.d. for 2 weeks (fed)	7	↓37 (↓54 to ↓14)	↓32 (↓49 to ↓9)	↓14 (↓52 to ↑54)
Zidovudine	300 mg single dose	600 mg single dose	12	⇔ (↓5 to ↑24)	↑13 (↓2 to ↑31)	NA

*Based on total-drug concentrations.
†Compared to amprenavir capsules 1,200 mg b.i.d. in the same patients.
‡Median percent change; confidence interval not reported.
↑ = Increase; ↓ = Decrease; ⇔ = No change (↑ or ↓ <10%); NA = C_{min} not calculated for single-dose study.

Continued on next page

Beconase AQ—Cont.

Carcinogenesis, Mutagenesis, Impairment of Fertility: The carcinogenicity of beclomethasone dipropionate was evaluated in rats that were exposed for a total of 95 weeks, 13 weeks at inhalation doses up to 0.4 mg/kg and the remaining 82 weeks at combined oral and inhalation doses up to 2.4 mg/kg. There was no evidence of carcinogenicity in this study at the highest dose, approximately 60 times the maximum recommended daily intranasal dose in adults on a mg/m^2 basis or approximately 35 times the maximum recommended daily intranasal dose in children on a mg/m^2 basis.

Beclomethasone dipropionate did not induce gene mutation in bacterial cells or mammalian Chinese hamster ovary (CHO) cells in vitro. No significant clastogenic effect was seen in cultured CHO cells in vitro or in the mouse micronucleus test in vivo.

In rats, beclomethasone dipropionate caused decreased conception rates at an oral dose of 16 mg/kg (approximately 390 times the maximum recommended daily intranasal dose in adults on a mg/m^2 basis). There was no significant effect of beclomethasone dipropionate on fertility in rats at oral doses of 1.6 mg/kg (approximately 40 times the maximum recommended daily intranasal dose in adults on a mg/m^2 basis). Inhibition of the estrous cycle in dogs was observed following oral dosing at 0.5 mg/kg (approximately 40 times the maximum recommended daily intranasal dose in adults on a mg/m^2 basis). No inhibition of the estrous cycle in dogs was seen following 12 months' exposure at an estimated inhalation dose of 0.33 mg/kg (approximately 25 times the maximum recommended daily intranasal dose in adults on a mg/m^2 basis).

Pregnancy: *Teratogenic Effects:* Pregnancy Category C. Like other corticosteroids, beclomethasone dipropionate was teratogenic and embryocidal in the mouse and rabbit at a subcutaneous dose of 0.1 mg/kg in mice or 0.025 mg/kg in rabbits (approximately equal to the maximum recommended daily intranasal dose in adults on a mg/m^2 basis). No teratogenicity or embryocidal effects were seen in rats when exposed to an inhalation dose of 0.1 mg/kg plus oral doses of up to 10 mg/kg per day for a combined dose of 10.1 mg/kg (approximately 240 times the maximum recommended daily intranasal dose in adults on a mg/m^2 basis). There are no adequate and well-controlled studies in pregnant women. Beclomethasone dipropionate should be used during pregnancy only if the potential benefit justifies the potential risk to the fetus.

Nonteratogenic Effects: Hypoadrenalism may occur in infants born of mothers receiving corticosteroids during pregnancy. Such infants should be carefully observed.

Nursing Mothers: It is not known whether beclomethasone dipropionate is excreted in human milk. Because other corticosteroids are excreted in human milk, caution should be exercised when BECONASE AQ Nasal Spray is administered to a nursing woman.

Pediatric Use: The safety and effectiveness of BECONASE AQ Nasal Spray have been established in children aged 6 years and above through evidence from extensive clinical use in adult and pediatric patients. The safety and effectiveness of BECONASE AQ Nasal Spray in children below 6 years of age have not been established.

Controlled clinical studies have shown that intranasal corticosteroids may cause a reduction in growth velocity in pediatric patients. This effect has been observed in the absence of laboratory evidence of HPA axis suppression, suggesting that growth velocity is a more sensitive indicator of systemic corticosteroid exposure in pediatric patients than some commonly used tests of HPA axis function. The long-term effects of this reduction in growth velocity associated with intranasal corticosteroids, including the impact on final adult height, are unknown. The potential for "catch-up" growth following discontinuation of treatment with intranasal corticosteroids has not been adequately studied. The growth of pediatric patients receiving intranasal corticosteroids, including BECONASE AQ Nasal Spray, should be monitored routinely (e.g., via stadiometry). The potential growth effects of prolonged treatment should be weighed against the clinical benefits obtained and the risks/benefits of treatment alternatives. To minimize the systemic effects of intranasal corticosteroids, including BECONASE Nasal Spray, each patient should be titrated to the lowest dose that effectively controls his/her symptoms.

In a double-blind, controlled trial, 100 children between the ages of 6 and 9½ years with allergic rhinitis were randomized to receive aqueous intranasal beclomethasone dipropionate 168 mcg twice daily or placebo for 1 year. As measured by stadiometry, children who received beclomethasone dipropionate grew more slowly than those who received placebo. A difference in mean change in height was observed within 1 month of drug initiation. At the end of 12 months, the beclomethasone dipropionate-treated group had a growth velocity on average of 4.75 cm/year compared to 6.20 cm/year in the placebo group ($P<0.01$). While the placebo group had an expected distribution of growth velocity, approximately 50% of the beclomethasone dipropionate-treated children grew below the 10th percentile.

In children 7.3 years of age, the mean age of children in this study, the range for expected growth velocity is: boys – 3rd percentile = 4.1 cm/year, 50th percentile = 5.8 cm/year, and 97th percentile = 7.5 cm/year; girls – 3rd percentile = 4.3 cm/year, 50th percentile = 5.9 cm/year, and 97th percentile = 7.5 cm/year. The potential reversibility of the reduction in growth velocity was not studied. No significant differences were observed between the 2 groups for mean basal plasma cortisol or ACTH-stimulated plasma cortisol levels.

Geriatric Use: Clinical studies of BECONASE AQ Nasal Spray did not include sufficient numbers of subjects aged 65

Table 4. Drug Interactions: Pharmacokinetic Parameters for Coadministered Drug in the Presence of Amprenavir

Co-administered Drug	Dose of Co-administered Drug	Dose of AGENERASE	n	% Change in Pharmacokinetic Parameters of Coadministered Drug (90% CI)		
				C$_{max}$	AUC	C$_{min}$
Clarithromycin	500 mg b.i.d. for 4 days	1,200 mg b.i.d. for 4 days	12	↓10 (↓24 to ↑7)	⇔ (↓17 to ↑11)	⇔ (↓13 to ↑20)
Delavirdine	600 mg b.i.d. for 10 days	600 mg b.i.d. for 10 days	9	↓47*	↓61*	↓88*
Ethinyl estradiol	0.035 mg for 1 cycle	1,200 mg b.i.d. for 28 days	10	⇔ (↓25 to ↑15)	⇔ (↓14 to ↑38)	↑32 (↓3 to ↑79)
Norethindrone	1.0 mg for 1 cycle	1,200 mg b.i.d. for 28 days	10	⇔ (↓20 to ↑18)	↑18 (↑1 to ↑38)	↑45 (↑13 to ↑88)
Ketoconazole	400 mg single dose	1,200 mg single dose	12	↑19 (↑8 to ↑33)	↑44 (↑31 to ↑59)	NA
Lamivudine	150 mg single dose	600 mg single dose	11	⇔ (↓17 to ↑3)	⇔ (↓11 to 0)	NA
Methadone	44 to 100 mg q.d. for >30 days	1,200 mg b.i.d. for 10 days	16	R-Methadone (active)		
				↓25 (↓32 to ↓18)	↓13 (↓21 to ↓5)	↓21 (↓32 to ↓9)
				S-Methadone (inactive)		
				↓48 (↓55 to ↓40)	↓40 (↓46 to ↓32)	↓53 (↓60 to ↓43)
Rifabutin	300 mg q.d. for 10 days	1,200 mg b.i.d. for 10 days	5	↑119 (↑82 to ↑164)	↑193 (↑156 to ↑235)	↑271 (↑171 to ↑409)
Rifampin	300 mg q.d. for 4 days	1,200 mg b.i.d. for 4 days	11	⇔ (↓13 to ↑12)	⇔ (↓10 to ↑13)	ND
Zidovudine	300 mg single dose	600 mg single dose	12	↑40 (↑14 to ↑71)	↑31 (↑19 to ↑45)	NA

*Median percent change; confidence interval not reported.
↑ = Increase; ↓ = Decrease; ⇔ = No change (↑ or ↓ <10%); NA = C$_{min}$ not calculated for single-dose study; ND = Interaction cannot be determined as C$_{min}$ was below the lower limit of quantitation.

Table 7. Drugs That Should Not Be Coadministered with AGENERASE Oral Solution

Drug Class/Drug Name	Clinical Comment
Alcohol-Dependence Treatment: Disulfiram	CONTRAINDICATED due to potential risk of toxicity from the large amount of the excipient, propylene glycol, in AGENERASE Oral Solution.
Antibiotic: Metronidazole	CONTRAINDICATED due to potential risk of toxicity from the large amount of the excipient, propylene glycol, in AGENERASE Oral Solution.
Antimycobacterials: Rifampin*	May lead to loss of virologic response and possible resistance to AGENERASE or to the class of protease inhibitors.
Ergot Derivatives: Dihydroergotamine, ergonovine, ergotamine, methylergonovine	CONTRAINDICATED due to potential for serious and/or life-threatening reactions such as acute ergot toxicity characterized by peripheral vasospasm and ischemia of the extremities and other tissues.
GI Motility Agents: Cisapride	CONTRAINDICATED due to potential for serious and/or life-threatening reactions such as cardiac arrhythmias.
Herbal Products: St. John's wort (hypericum perforatum)	May lead to loss of virologic response and possible resistance to AGENERASE or to the class of protease inhibitors.
HIV-Protease Inhibitor: Ritonavir oral solution	Concurrent use of AGENERASE Oral Solution and NORVIR (ritonavir) Oral Solution is not recommended because the large amount of propylene glycol in AGENERASE Oral Solution and ethanol in NORVIR Oral Solution may compete for the same metabolic pathway for elimination.
HMG Co-Reductase Inhibitors: Lovastatin, simvastatin	Potential for serious reactions such as risk of myopathy including rhabdomyolysis.
Neuroleptic: Pimozide	CONTRAINDICATED due to potential for serious and/or life-threatening reactions such as cardiac arrhythmias.
Non-nucleoside Reverse Transcriptase Inhibitor: Delavirdine*	May lead to loss of virologic response and possible resistance to delavirdine.
Oral Contraceptives: Ethinyl estradiol/norethindrone	May lead to loss of virologic response and possible resistance to AGENERASE. Alternative methods of non-hormonal contraception are recommended.
Sedative/Hypnotics: Midazolam, triazolam	CONTRAINDICATED due to potential for serious and/or life-threatening reactions such as prolonged or increased sedation or respiratory depression.

*See CLINICAL PHARMACOLOGY for magnitude of interaction, Tables 3 and 4.

Table 8. Established and Other Potentially Significant Drug Interactions: Alteration in Dose or Regimen May Be Recommended Based on Drug Interaction Studies or Predicted Interaction

Concomitant Drug Class: Drug Name	Effect on Concentration of Amprenavir or Concomitant Drug	Clinical Comment
HIV-Antiviral Agents		
Non-nucleoside Reverse Transcriptase Inhibitors: Efavirenz, nevirapine	↓ Amprenavir	Appropriate doses of the combinations with respect to safety and efficacy have not been established.
Nucleoside Reverse Transcriptase Inhibitor: Didanosine (buffered formulation only)	↓ Amprenavir	Take AGENERASE at least 1 hour before or after the buffered formulation of didanosine.
HIV-Protease Inhibitors: Indinavir,* lopinavir/ritonavir, nelfinavir*	↑ Amprenavir Amprenavir's effect on other protease inhibitors is not well established.	Appropriate doses of the combinations with respect to safety and efficacy have not been established.
HIV-Protease Inhibitor: Ritonavir Capsules*	↑ Amprenavir	The dose of amprenavir should be reduced when used in combination with ritonavir capsules (see Dosage and Administration). Also, see the full prescribing information for NORVIR for additional drug interaction information. Concurrent use of AGENERASE Oral Solution and NORVIR (ritonavir) Oral Solution is not recommended because the large amount of propylene glycol in AGENERASE Oral Solution and ethanol in NORVIR Oral Solution may compete for the same metabolic pathway for elimination.
HIV-Protease Inhibitor: Saquinavir*	↓ Amprenavir Amprenavir's effect on saquinavir is not well established.	Appropriate doses of the combination with respect to safety and efficacy have not been established.
Other Agents		
Antacids	↓ Amprenavir	Take AGENERASE at least 1 hour before or after antacids.
Antiarrhythmics: Amiodarone, lidocaine (systemic), and quinidine	↑ Antiarrhythmics	Caution is warranted and therapeutic concentration monitoring is recommended for antiarrhythmics when coadministered with AGENERASE, if available.
Antiarrhythmic: Bepridil	↑ Bepridil	Use with caution. Increased bepridil exposure may be associated with life-threatening reactions such as cardiac arrhythmias.
Anticoagulant: Warfarin		Concentrations of warfarin may be affected. It is recommended that INR (international normalized ratio) be monitored.
Anticonvulsants: Carbamazepine, phenobarbital, phenytoin	↓ Amprenavir	Use with caution. AGENERASE may be less effective due to decreased amprenavir plasma concentrations in patients taking these agents concomitantly.
Antifungals: Ketoconazole, itraconazole	↑ Ketoconazole ↑ Itraconazole	Increase monitoring for adverse events due to ketoconazole or itraconazole. Dose reduction of ketoconazole or itraconazole may be needed for patients receiving more than 400 mg ketoconazole or itraconazole per day.
Antimycobacterial: Rifabutin*	↑ Rifabutin and rifabutin metabolite	A dosage reduction of rifabutin to at least half the recommended dose is required when AGENERASE and rifabutin are coadministered.* A complete blood count should be performed weekly and as clinically indicated in order to monitor for neutropenia in patients receiving amprenavir and rifabutin.
Benzodiazepines: Alprazolam, clorazepate, diazepam, flurazepam	↑ Benzodiazepines	Clinical significance is unknown; however, a decrease in benzodiazepine dose may be needed.
Calcium Channel Blockers: Diltiazem, felodipine, nifedipine, nicardipine, nimodipine, verapamil, amlodipine, nisoldipine, isradipine	↑ Calcium channel blockers	Caution is warranted and clinical monitoring of patients is recommended.
Corticosteroid: Dexamethasone	↓ Amprenavir	Use with caution. AGENERASE may be less effective due to decreased amprenavir plasma concentrations in patients taking these agents concomitantly.
Erectile Dysfunction Agent: Sildenafil	↑ Sildenafil	Use with caution at reduced doses of 25 mg every 48 hours with increased monitoring for adverse events.

(Table continued on next page)

and over to determine whether they respond differently from younger subjects. Other reported clinical experience has not identified differences in responses between the elderly and younger patients. In general, dose selection for an elderly patient should be cautious, starting at the low end of the dosing range, reflecting the greater frequency of decreased hepatic, renal, or cardiac function, and of concomitant disease or other drug therapy.

ADVERSE REACTIONS

In general, side effects in clinical studies have been primarily associated with irritation of the nasal mucous membranes.

Adverse reactions reported in controlled clinical trials and open studies in patients treated with BECONASE AQ Nasal Spray are described below.

Mild nasopharyngeal irritation following the use of beclomethasone aqueous nasal spray has been reported in up to 24% of patients treated, including occasional sneezing attacks (about 4%) occurring immediately following use of the spray. In patients experiencing these symptoms, none had to discontinue treatment. The incidence of transient irritation and sneezing was approximately the same in the group of patients who received placebo in these studies, implying that these complaints may be related to vehicle components of the formulation.

Fewer than 5 per 100 patients reported headache, nausea, or lightheadedness following the use of BECONASE AQ Nasal Spray. Fewer than 3 per 100 patients reported nasal stuffiness, nosebleeds, rhinorrhea, or tearing eyes.

Rare cases of ulceration of the nasal mucosa and instances of nasal septum perforation have been spontaneously reported (see PRECAUTIONS).

Reports of dryness and irritation of the nose and throat, and unpleasant taste and smell have been received. There are rare reports of loss of taste and smell.

Rare instances of wheezing, cataracts, glaucoma, and increased intraocular pressure have been reported following the use of intranasal beclomethasone dipropionate (see PRECAUTIONS).

Rare cases of immediate and delayed hypersensitivity reactions, including urticaria, angioedema, rash, and bronchospasm, have been reported following the oral and intranasal inhalation of beclomethasone dipropionate.

Cases of growth suppression have been reported for intranasal corticosteroids, including BECONASE AQ (see PRECAUTIONS: Pediatric Use).

OVERDOSAGE

When used at excessive doses, systemic corticosteroid effects such as hypercorticism and adrenal suppression may appear. If such changes occur, BECONASE AQ Nasal Spray should be discontinued slowly consistent with accepted procedures for discontinuing oral steroid therapy. No deaths occurred when beclomethasone dipropionate was given as single oral doses of 3,000 mg/kg to mice (approximately 36,000 times the maximum recommended daily intranasal dose in adults on a mg/m^2 basis, or approximately 21,000 times the maximum recommended daily intranasal dose in children on a mg/m^2 basis) and 2,000 mg/kg to rats (approximately 48,000 times the maximum recommended daily intranasal dose in adults or approximately 29,000 times the maximum recommended daily intranasal dose in children on a mg/m^2 basis). One bottle of BECONASE AQ Nasal Spray contains beclomethasone dipropionate, monohydrate equivalent to 10.5 mg of beclomethasone dipropionate; therefore, acute overdosage is unlikely.

DOSAGE AND ADMINISTRATION

Adults and Children 12 Years of Age and Older: The usual dosage is 1 or 2 nasal inhalations (42 to 84 mcg) in each nostril twice a day (total dose, 168 to 336 mcg/day).

Children 6 to 12 Years of Age: Patients should be started with 1 nasal inhalation in each nostril twice daily; patients not adequately responding to 168 mcg or those with more severe symptoms may use 336 mcg (2 inhalations in each nostril). Once adequate control is achieved, the dosage should be decreased to 84 mcg (1 spray in each nostril) twice daily. BECONASE AQ Nasal Spray is *not* recommended for children below 6 years of age.

The maximum total daily dosage should not exceed 2 sprays in each nostril twice daily (336 mcg/day).

In patients who respond to BECONASE AQ Nasal Spray, an improvement of the symptoms of seasonal or perennial rhinitis usually becomes apparent within a few days after the start of therapy with BECONASE AQ Nasal Spray. However, symptomatic relief may not occur in some patients for as long as 2 weeks. BECONASE AQ Nasal Spray should not be continued beyond 3 weeks in the absence of significant symptomatic improvement.

The therapeutic effects of corticosteroids, unlike those of decongestants, are not immediate. This should be explained to the patient in advance in order to ensure cooperation and continuation of treatment with the prescribed dosage regimen.

In the presence of excessive nasal mucous secretion or edema of the nasal mucosa, the drug may fail to reach the site of intended action. In such cases it is advisable to use a nasal vasoconstrictor during the first 2 to 3 days of therapy with BECONASE AQ Nasal Spray.

Directions for Use: Illustrated Patient's Instructions for Use accompany each package of BECONASE AQ Nasal Spray.

HOW SUPPLIED

BECONASE AQ Nasal Spray, 42 mcg is supplied in an amber glass bottle fitted with a metering atomizing pump and nasal adapter in a box of 1 (NDC 0173-0388-79) with pa-

Beconase AQ—Cont.

tient's instructions for use. Each bottle contains 25 g of suspension and will provide 180 metered sprays. The correct amount of medication in each spray cannot be assured after 180 sprays even though the bottle is not completely empty. The bottle should be discarded when the labeled number of actuations has been used.

Store between 15° and 30°C (59° and 86°F).

GlaxoSmithKline, Research Triangle Park, NC 27709
December 2002/RL-1175

CEFTIN® Tablets ℞

[*sĕf' tin*]
(cefuroxime axetil tablets)

CEFTIN® for Oral Suspension ℞

(cefuroxime axetil powder for oral suspension)

Prescribing information for these products, which appears on pages 1482–1486 of the 2003 PDR, has been revised as follows. Please write "See Supplement A" next to the product heading.

The 125-mg tablets are no longer marketed and have been removed from the **DESCRIPTION**, **DOSAGE AND ADMINISTRATION**, and **HOW SUPPLIED** sections.

The 250-mg Unit Dose Packs of 100 and the 500-mg Unit Dose Packs of 50 are no longer marketed, and have been removed from the **HOW SUPPLIED** section.

GlaxoSmithKline, Research Triangle Park, NC 27709
©2002, GlaxoSmithKline. All rights reserved.
November 2002/RL-1141

COMBIVIR® ℞

[*kom' bə-vir*]
(lamivudine/zidovudine)
Tablets

Prescribing information for this product, which appears on pages 1486–1489 of the 2003 PDR, has been revised as follows. Please write "See Supplement A" next to the product heading.

The following sentence was added to the end of the **PRECAUTIONS: Patients with HIV and Hepatitis B Virus Coinfection** *subsection:*

Posttreatment exacerbations of hepatitis have also been reported (see WARNINGS).

The first paragraph in the **PRECAUTIONS: Drug Interactions: *Lamivudine*** *subsection was revised to:*

Trimethoprim (TMP) 160 mg/sulfamethoxazole (SMX) 800 mg once daily has been shown to increase lamivudine exposure (AUC). The effect of higher doses of TMP/SMX on lamivudine pharmacokinetics has not been investigated (see CLINICAL PHARMACOLOGY). No data are available regarding the potential for interactions with other drugs that have renal clearance mechanisms similar to that of lamivudine.

The following paragraph was added to the **DOSAGE AND ADMINISTRATION: Dose Adjustment** *subsection:*

A reduction in the daily dose of zidovudine may be necessary in patients with mild to moderate impaired hepatic function or liver cirrhosis. Because COMBIVIR is a fixed-dose combination that cannot be adjusted for this patient population, COMBIVIR is not recommended for patients with impaired hepatic function.

GlaxoSmithKline, Research Triangle Park, NC 27709
Lamivudine is manufactured under agreement from
Shire Pharmaceuticals Group plc, Basingstoke, UK
©2003, GlaxoSmithKline. All rights reserved.
January 2003/RL-1168

COREG® ℞

[*kor' eg*]
(carvedilol)
Tablets

Prescribing information for this product, which appears on pages 1491–1496 of the 2003 PDR, has been completely revised as follows. Please write "See Supplement A" next to the product heading.

DESCRIPTION

Carvedilol is a nonselective β-adrenergic blocking agent with α_1-blocking activity. It is (±)-1-(Carbazol-4-yloxy)-3-[[2-(o-methoxyphenoxy)ethyl]amino]-2-propanol. It is a racemic mixture.

Tablets for Oral Administration:

COREG (carvedilol) is a white, oval, film-coated tablet containing 3.125 mg, 6.25 mg, 12.5 mg, or 25 mg of carvedilol. The 6.25 mg, 12.5 mg, and 25 mg tablets are TILTAB® tablets. Inactive ingredients consist of colloidal silicon dioxide, crospovidone, hypromellose, lactose, magnesium stearate, polyethylene glycol, polysorbate 80, povidone, sucrose, and titanium dioxide.

Carvedilol is a white to off-white powder with a molecular weight of 406.5 and a molecular formula of $C_{24}H_{26}N_2O_4$. It is freely soluble in dimethylsulfoxide; soluble in methylene chloride and methanol; sparingly soluble in 95% ethanol and isopropanol; slightly soluble in ethyl ether; and practically insoluble in water, gastric fluid (simulated, TS, pH 1.1), and intestinal fluid (simulated, TS without pancreatin, pH 7.5).

Table 8 *(cont.)*. Established and Other Potentially Significant Drug Interactions: Alteration in Dose or Regimen May Be Recommended Based on Drug Interaction Studies or Predicted Interaction

Concomitant Drug Class: Drug Name	Effect on Concentration of Amprenavir or Concomitant Drug	Clinical Comment
	Other Agents (continued)	
HMG-CoA Reductase Inhibitors: Atorvastatin	↑ Atorvastatin	Use lowest possible dose of atorvastatin with careful monitoring or consider other HMG-CoA reductase inhibitors such as pravastatin or fluvastatin in combination with AGENERASE.
Immunosuppressants: Cyclosporine, tacrolimus, rapamycin	↑ Immunosuppressants	Therapeutic concentration monitoring is recommended for immunosuppressant agents when coadministered with AGENERASE.
Narcotic Analgesics: Methadone*	↓ Amprenavir	AGENERASE may be less effective due to decreased amprenavir plasma concentrations in patients taking these agents concomitantly. Alternative antiretroviral therapy should be considered.
	↓ Methadone	Dosage of methadone may need to be increased when coadministered with AGENERASE.
Tricyclic Antidepressants: Amitriptyline, imipramine	↑ Tricyclics	Therapeutic concentration monitoring is recommended for tricyclic antidepressants when coadministered with AGENERASE.

*See CLINICAL PHARMACOLOGY for magnitude of interaction, Tables 3 and 4.

CLINICAL PHARMACOLOGY

COREG is a racemic mixture in which nonselective β-adrenoreceptor blocking activity is present in the S(-) enantiomer and α-adrenergic blocking activity is present in both R(+) and S(-) enantiomers at equal potency. COREG has no intrinsic sympathomimetic activity.

Pharmacokinetics: COREG is rapidly and extensively absorbed following oral administration, with absolute bioavailability of approximately 25% to 35% due to a significant degree of first-pass metabolism. Following oral administration, the apparent mean terminal elimination half-life of carvedilol generally ranges from 7 to 10 hours. Plasma concentrations achieved are proportional to the oral dose administered. When administered with food, the rate of absorption is slowed, as evidenced by a delay in the time to reach peak plasma levels, with no significant difference in extent of bioavailability. Taking COREG with food should minimize the risk of orthostatic hypotension.

Carvedilol is extensively metabolized. Following oral administration of radiolabelled carvedilol to healthy volunteers, carvedilol accounted for only about 7% of the total radioactivity in plasma as measured by area under the curve (AUC). Less than 2% of the dose was excreted unchanged in the urine. Carvedilol is metabolized primarily by aromatic ring oxidation and glucuronidation.

The oxidative metabolites are further metabolized by conjugation via glucuronidation and sulfation. The metabolites of carvedilol are excreted primarily via the bile into the feces. Demethylation and hydroxylation at the phenol ring produce three active metabolites with β-receptor blocking activity. Based on preclinical studies, the 4'-hydroxyphenyl metabolite is approximately 13 times more potent than carvedilol for β-blockade.

Compared to carvedilol, the 3 active metabolites exhibit weak vasodilating activity. Plasma concentrations of the active metabolites are about one-tenth of those observed for carvedilol and have pharmacokinetics similar to the parent.

Carvedilol undergoes stereoselective first-pass metabolism with plasma levels of R(+)-carvedilol approximately 2 to 3 times higher than S(-)-carvedilol following oral administration in healthy subjects. The mean apparent terminal elimination half-lives for R(+)-carvedilol range from 5 to 9 hours compared with 7 to 11 hours for the S(-)-enantiomer.

The primary P450 enzymes responsible for the metabolism of both R(+) and S(-)-carvedilol in human liver microsomes were CYP2D6 and CYP2C9 and to a lesser extent CYP3A4, 2C19, 1A2, and 2E1. CYP2D6 is thought to be the major enzyme in the 4'- and 5'-hydroxylation of carvedilol, with a potential contribution from 3A4. CYP2C9 is thought to be of primary importance in the O-methylation pathway of S(-)-carvedilol.

Carvedilol is subject to the effects of genetic polymorphism with poor metabolizers of debrisoquin (a marker for cytochrome P450 2D6) exhibiting 2- to 3-fold higher plasma concentrations of R(+)-carvedilol compared to extensive metabolizers. In contrast, plasma levels of S(-)-carvedilol are increased only about 20% to 25% in poor metabolizers, indicating this enantiomer is metabolized to a lesser extent by cytochrome P450 2D6 than R(+)-carvedilol. The pharmacokinetics of carvedilol do not appear to be different in poor metabolizers of S-mephenytoin (patients deficient in cytochrome P450 2C19).

Carvedilol is more than 98% bound to plasma proteins, primarily with albumin. The plasma-protein binding is independent of concentration over the therapeutic range. Carvedilol is a basic, lipophilic compound with a steady-state volume of distribution of approximately 115 L, indicating substantial distribution into extravascular tissues. Plasma clearance ranges from 500 to 700 mL/min.

Congestive Heart Failure: Steady-state plasma concentrations of carvedilol and its enantiomers increased proportionally over the 6.25 to 50 mg dose range in patients with congestive heart failure. Compared to healthy subjects, congestive heart failure patients had increased mean AUC and C_{max} values for carvedilol and its enantiomers, with up to 50% to 100% higher values observed in 6 patients with NYHA class IV heart failure. The mean apparent terminal elimination half-life for carvedilol was similar to that observed in healthy subjects

Pharmacokinetic Drug-Drug Interactions: Since carvedilol undergoes substantial oxidative metabolism, the metabolism and pharmacokinetics of carvedilol may be affected by induction or inhibition of cytochrome P450 enzymes.

Rifampin: In a pharmacokinetic study conducted in 8 healthy male subjects, rifampin (600 mg daily for 12 days) decreased the AUC and C_{max} of carvedilol by about 70%.

Cimetidine: In a pharmacokinetic study conducted in 10 healthy male subjects, cimetidine (1000 mg/day) increased the steady-state AUC of carvedilol by 30% with no change in C_{max}.

Glyburide: In 12 healthy subjects, combined administration of carvedilol (25 mg once daily) and a single dose of glyburide did not result in a clinically relevant pharmacokinetic interaction for either compound.

Hydrochlorothiazide: A single oral dose of carvedilol 25 mg did not alter the pharmacokinetics of a single oral dose of hydrochlorothiazide 25 mg in 12 patients with hypertension. Likewise, hydrochlorothiazide had no effect on the pharmacokinetics of carvedilol.

Digoxin: Following concomitant administration of carvedilol (25 mg once daily) and digoxin (0.25 mg once daily) for 14 days, steady-state AUC and trough concentrations of digoxin were increased by 14% and 16%, respectively, in 12 hypertensive patients.

Torsemide: In a study of 12 healthy subjects, combined oral administration of carvedilol 25 mg once daily and torsemide 5 mg once daily for 5 days did not result in any significant differences in their pharmacokinetics compared with administration of the drugs alone.

Warfarin: Carvedilol (12.5 mg twice daily) did not have an effect on the steady-state prothrombin time ratios and did not alter the pharmacokinetics of R(+)- and S(-)-warfarin following concomitant administration with warfarin in 9 healthy volunteers.

Special Populations: *Elderly:* Plasma levels of carvedilol average about 50% higher in the elderly compared to young subjects.

Hepatic Impairment: Compared to healthy subjects, patients with cirrhotic liver disease exhibit significantly higher concentrations of carvedilol (approximately 4- to 7-fold) following single-dose therapy (see WARNINGS, Hepatic Injury).

Renal Insufficiency: Although carvedilol is metabolized primarily by the liver, plasma concentrations of carvedilol have been reported to be increased in patients with renal impairment. Based on mean AUC data, approximately 40% to 50% higher plasma concentrations of carvedilol were observed in hypertensive patients with moderate to severe renal impairment compared to a control group of hypertensive patients with normal renal function. However, the ranges of AUC values were similar for both groups. Changes in mean peak plasma levels were less pronounced, approximately 12% to 26% higher in patients with impaired renal function. Consistent with its high degree of plasma protein-binding, carvedilol does not appear to be cleared significantly by hemodialysis.

Pharmacodynamics: *Congestive Heart Failure:*
The basis for the beneficial effects of COREG in congestive heart failure is not established.
Two placebo-controlled studies compared the acute hemodynamic effects of COREG to baseline measurements in 59 and 49 patients with NYHA class II–IV heart failure receiving diuretics, ACE inhibitors, and digitalis. There were significant reductions in systemic blood pressure, pulmonary artery pressure, pulmonary capillary wedge pressure, and heart rate. Initial effects on cardiac output, stroke volume index, and systemic vascular resistance were small and variable.
These studies measured hemodynamic effects again at 12 to 14 weeks. COREG significantly reduced systemic blood pressure, pulmonary artery pressure, right atrial pressure, systemic vascular resistance, and heart rate, while stroke volume index was increased.
Among 839 patients with NYHA class II–III heart failure treated for 26 to 52 weeks in 4 US placebo-controlled trials, average left ventricular ejection fraction (EF) measured by radionuclide ventriculography increased by 9 EF units (%) in COREG patients and by 2 EF units in placebo patients at a target dose of 25-50 mg twice daily. The effects of carvedilol on ejection fraction were related to dose. Doses of 6.25 mg twice daily, 12.5 mg twice daily, 25 mg twice daily were associated with placebo-corrected increases in EF of 5 EF units, 6 EF units, and 8 EF units, respectively; each of these effects were nominally statistically significant.

Left Ventricular Dysfunction Following Myocardial Infarction: The basis for the beneficial effects of COREG in patients with left ventricular dysfunction following an acute myocardial infarction is not established.

Hypertension: The mechanism by which β-blockade produces an antihypertensive effect has not been established. β-adrenoreceptor blocking activity has been demonstrated in animal and human studies showing that carvedilol (1) reduces cardiac output in normal subjects; (2) reduces exercise- and/or isoproterenol-induced tachycardia and (3) reduces reflex orthostatic tachycardia. Significant β-adrenoreceptor blocking effect is usually seen within 1 hour of drug administration.

α_1-adrenoreceptor blocking activity has been demonstrated in human and animal studies, showing that carvedilol (1) attenuates the pressor effects of phenylephrine; (2) causes vasodilation and (3) reduces peripheral vascular resistance. These effects contribute to the reduction of blood pressure and usually are seen within 30 minutes of drug administration.

Due to the α_1-receptor blocking activity of carvedilol, blood pressure is lowered more in the standing than in the supine position, and symptoms of postural hypotension (1.8%), including rare instances of syncope, can occur. Following oral administration, when postural hypotension has occurred, it has been transient and is uncommon when COREG is administered with food at the recommended starting dose and titration increments are closely followed (see DOSAGE AND ADMINISTRATION).

In hypertensive patients with normal renal function, therapeutic doses of COREG decreased renal vascular resistance with no change in glomerular filtration rate or renal plasma flow. Changes in excretion of sodium, potassium, uric acid, and phosphorus in hypertensive patients with normal renal function were similar after COREG and placebo.

COREG has little effect on plasma catecholamines, plasma aldosterone, or electrolyte levels, but it does significantly reduce plasma renin activity when given for at least 4 weeks. It also increases levels of atrial natriuretic peptide.

CLINICAL TRIALS
Congestive Heart Failure:
A total of 3,946 patients with mild to severe heart failure were evaluated in placebo-controlled studies of carvedilol.
In the largest study (COPERNICUS), 2,289 patients with heart failure at rest or with minimal exertion and left ventricular ejection fraction <25% (mean 20%), despite digitalis (66%), diuretics (99%), and ACE inhibitors (89%) were randomized to placebo or carvedilol. Carvedilol was titrated from a starting dose of 3.125 mg twice daily to the maximum tolerated dose or up to 25 mg twice daily over a minimum of 6 weeks. Most subjects achieved the target dose of 25 mg. The study was conducted in Eastern and Western Europe, the United States, Israel, and Canada. Similar numbers of subjects per group (about 100) withdrew during the titration period.

The primary end point of the trial was all-cause mortality, but cause-specific mortality and the risk of death or hospitalization (total, cardiovascular [CV], or congestive heart failure [CHF]) were also examined. The developing trial data were followed by a data monitoring committee, and mortality analyses were adjusted for these multiple looks. The trial was stopped after a median follow-up of 10 months because of an observed 35% reduction in mortality (from 19.7% per patient year on placebo to 12.8% on carvedilol, hazard ratio 0.65, 95% CI 0.52–0.81, p = 0.0014, adjusted) (see Figure 1). The results of COPERNICUS are shown in Table 1.
[See table 1 above]
[See figure 1 above]
The effect on mortality was principally the result of a reduction in the rate of sudden death among patients without worsening heart failure.
Patients' global assessments, in which carvedilol-treated patients were compared to placebo, were based on pre-specified, periodic patient self-assessments regarding whether clinical status post-treatment showed improvement, worsening or no change compared to baseline. Patients treated with carvedilol showed significant improvement in global assessments compared with those treated with placebo in COPERNICUS.
The protocol also specified that hospitalizations would be assessed. Fewer patients on COREG than on placebo were hospitalized for any reason (198 vs. 268, p = 0.0001), for cardiovascular reasons (246 vs. 314, p = 0.0003), or for worsening heart failure (372 vs. 432, p = 0.0029).
COREG had a consistent and beneficial effect on all-cause mortality as well as the combined end points of all-cause mortality plus hospitalization (total, CV, or for heart failure) in the overall study population and in all subgroups examined, including men and women, elderly and non-elderly, blacks and non-blacks, and diabetics and non-diabetics (see Figure 2).

Table 1. Results of COPERNICUS

End point	Placebo N = 1,133	Carvedilol N = 1,156	Hazard ratio (95% CI)	% Reduction	Nominal p value
Mortality	190	130	0.65 (0.52–0.81)	35	0.00013
Mortality + all hospitalization	507	425	0.76 (0.67–0.87)	24	0.00004
Mortality + CV hospitalization	395	314	0.73 (0.63–0.84)	27	0.00002
Mortality + CHF hospitalization	357	271	0.69 (0.59–0.81)	31	0.000004

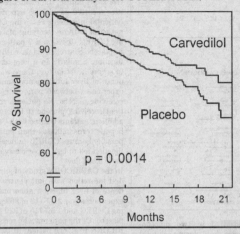

Figure 1. Survival Analysis for COPERNICUS (intent-to-treat)

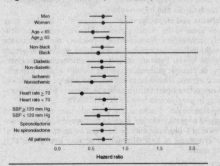

Figure 2. Effects on Mortality for Subgroups in COPERNICUS

Carvedilol was also studied in five other multicenter, placebo-controlled studies.
Four US multicenter, double-blind, placebo-controlled studies enrolled 1,094 patients (696 randomized to carvedilol) with NYHA class II–III heart failure and ejection fraction <0.35. The vast majority were on digitalis, diuretics, and an ACE inhibitor at study entry. Patients were assigned to the studies based upon exercise ability. An Australia-New Zealand double-blind, placebo-controlled study enrolled 415 patients (half randomized to carvedilol) with less severe heart failure. All protocols excluded patients expected to undergo cardiac transplantation during the 7.5 to 15 months of double-blind follow-up. All randomized patients had tolerated a 2-week course on carvedilol 6.25 mg twice daily.
In each study, there was a primary end point, either progression of heart failure (one US study) or exercise tolerance (two US studies meeting enrollment goals and the Australia-New Zealand study). There were many secondary end points specified in these studies, including NYHA classification, patient and physician global assessments, and cardiovascular hospitalization. Death was not a specified end point in any study, but it was analyzed in all studies. Other analyses not prospectively planned included the sum of deaths and total cardiovascular hospitalizations. In situations where the primary end points of a trial do not show a significant benefit of treatment, assignment of significance values to the other results is complex, and such values need to be interpreted cautiously.
The results of the US and Australia-New Zealand trials were as follows:
Slowing Progression of Heart Failure: One US multicenter study (366 subjects) had as its primary end point the sum of cardiovascular mortality, cardiovascular hospitalization, and sustained increase in heart failure medications. Heart failure progression was reduced, during an average follow-up of 7 months, by 48% (p = 0.008).
In the Australia-New Zealand study, death and total hospitalizations were reduced by about 25% over 18 to 24 months. In the three largest US studies, death and total hospitalizations were reduced by 19%, 39%, and 49%, nominally statistically significant in the last two studies. The Australia-New Zealand results were statistically borderline.
Functional Measures: None of the multicenter studies had NYHA classification as a primary end point, but all such studies had it as a secondary end point. There was at least a trend toward improvement in NYHA class in all studies. Exercise tolerance was the primary end point in 3 studies; in none was a statistically significant effect found.
Subjective Measures: Quality of life, as measured with a standard questionnaire (a primary end point in one study), was unaffected by carvedilol. However, patients' and investigators' global assessments showed significant improvement in most studies.
Mortality: Overall, in these four US trials, mortality was reduced, nominally significantly so in 2 studies.

Left Ventricular Dysfunction Following Myocardial Infarction: CAPRICORN was a double-blind study comparing carvedilol and placebo in 1,959 patients with a recent myocardial infarction (within 21 days) and left ventricular ejection fraction of ≤40%, with (47%) or without symptoms of heart failure. Patients given carvedilol received 6.25 mg twice daily, titrated as tolerated to 25 mg twice daily. Patients had to have a systolic blood pressure >90 mm Hg, a sitting heart rate >60 beats/minute, and no contraindication to β-blocker use. Treatment of the index infarction included aspirin (85%), IV or oral β-blockers (37%), nitrates (73%), heparin (64%), thrombolytics (40%), and acute angioplasty (12%). Background treatment included ACE inhibitors or angiotensin receptor blockers (97%), anticoagulants (20%), lipid-lowering agents (23%), and diuretics (34%). Baseline population characteristics included an average age of 63 years, 74% male, 95% Caucasian, mean blood pressure 121/74 mm Hg, 22% with diabetes, and 54% with a history of hypertension. Mean dosage achieved of carvedilol was 20 mg twice daily; mean duration of follow-up was 15 months.
All-cause mortality was 15% in the placebo group and 12% in the carvedilol group, indicating a 23% risk reduction in patients treated with carvedilol (95% CI 2-40%, p = 0.03), as shown in Figure 3. The effects on mortality in various subgroups are shown in Figure 4. Nearly all deaths were cardiovascular (which were reduced by 25% by carvedilol), and most of these deaths were sudden or related to pump failure (both types of death were reduced by carvedilol). Another

Continued on next page

Coreg—Cont.

study endpoint, total mortality and all-cause hospitalization, did not show a significant improvement.

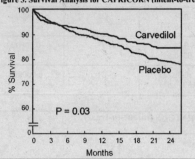

Figure 3. Survival Analysis for CAPRICORN (intent-to-treat)

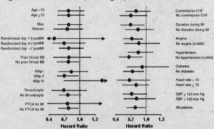

Figure 4. Effects on Mortality for Subgroups in CAPRICORN

Hypertension: COREG was studied in two placebo-controlled trials that utilized twice-daily dosing, at total daily doses of 12.5 to 50 mg. In these and other studies, the starting dose did not exceed 12.5 mg. At 50 mg per day, COREG reduced sitting trough (12-hour) blood pressure by about 9/5.5 mm Hg; at 25 mg/day the effect was about 7.5/3.5 mm Hg. Comparisons of trough to peak blood pressure showed a trough to peak ratio for blood pressure response of about 65%. Heart rate fell by about 7.5 beats/minute at 50 mg/day. In general, as is true for other β-blockers, responses were smaller in black than non-black patients. There were no age- or gender-related differences in response.

The peak antihypertensive effect occurred 1 to 2 hours after a dose. The dose-related blood pressure response was accompanied by a dose-related increase in adverse effects (see ADVERSE REACTIONS).

INDICATIONS AND USAGE
Congestive Heart Failure:
COREG is indicated for the treatment of mild to severe heart failure of ischemic or cardiomyopathic origin, usually in addition to diuretics, ACE inhibitor, and digitalis, to increase survival and, also, to reduce the risk of hospitalization (see CLINICAL TRIALS).

Left Ventricular Dysfunction Following Myocardial Infarction: COREG is indicated to reduce cardiovascular mortality in clinically stable patients who have survived the acute phase of a myocardial infarction and have a left ventricular ejection fraction of ≤40% (with or without symptomatic heart failure) (see CLINICAL TRIALS).

Hypertension: COREG is also indicated for the management of essential hypertension. It can be used alone or in combination with other antihypertensive agents, especially thiazide-type diuretics (see PRECAUTIONS, Drug Interactions).

CONTRAINDICATIONS
COREG is contraindicated in patients with bronchial asthma (2 cases of death from status asthmaticus have been reported in patients receiving single doses of COREG) or related bronchospastic conditions, second- or third-degree AV block, sick sinus syndrome or severe bradycardia (unless a permanent pacemaker is in place), or in patients with cardiogenic shock or who have decompensated heart failure requiring the use of intravenous inotropic therapy. Such patients should first be weaned from intravenous therapy before initiating COREG.

Use of COREG in patients with clinically manifest hepatic impairment is not recommended.

COREG is contraindicated in patients with hypersensitivity to the drug.

WARNINGS
Cessation of Therapy with COREG: Patients with coronary artery disease, who are being treated with COREG, should be advised against abrupt discontinuation of therapy. Severe exacerbation of angina and the occurrence of myocardial infarction and ventricular arrhythmias have been reported in angina patients following the abrupt discontinuation of therapy with β-blockers. The last two complications may occur with or without preceding exacerbation of the angina pectoris. As with other β-blockers, when discontinuation of COREG is planned, the patients should be carefully observed and advised to limit physical activity to a minimum. COREG should be discontinued over 1 to 2 weeks whenever possible. If the angina worsens or acute coronary insufficiency develops, it is recommended that COREG be promptly reinstituted, at least temporarily. Because coronary artery disease is common and may be unrecognized, it may be prudent not to discontinue COREG therapy abruptly even in patients treated only for hypertension or heart failure (See DOSAGE AND ADMINISTRATION.)

Hepatic Injury: Mild hepatocellular injury, confirmed by rechallenge, has occurred rarely with COREG therapy in the treatment of hypertension. In controlled studies of hypertensive patients, the incidence of liver function abnormalities reported as adverse experiences was 1.1% (13 of 1,142 patients) in patients receiving COREG and 0.9% (4 of 462 patients) in those receiving placebo. One patient receiving carvedilol in a placebo-controlled trial withdrew for abnormal hepatic function.

In controlled studies of primarily mild-to-moderate congestive heart failure, the incidence of liver function abnormalities reported as adverse experiences was 5.0% (38 of 765 patients) in patients receiving COREG and 4.6% (20 of 437 patients) in those receiving placebo. Three patients receiving COREG (0.4%) and 2 patients receiving placebo (0.5%) in placebo-controlled trials withdrew for abnormal hepatic function. Similarly, in a long-term, placebo-controlled trial in severe heart failure, there was no difference in the incidence of liver function abnormalities reported as adverse experiences between patients receiving COREG and those receiving placebo. No patients receiving COREG and 1 patient receiving placebo (0.09%) withdrew for hepatitis. In addition, patients treated with COREG had lower values for hepatic transaminases than patients treated with placebo, possibly because COREG-induced improvements in cardiac function led to less hepatic congestion and/or improved hepatic blood flow.

In the CAPRICORN study of survivors of an acute myocardial infarction with left ventricular dysfunction the incidence of liver function abnormalities reported as adverse experiences was 2.0% (19 of 969 patients) in patients receiving COREG and 1.5% (15 of 980 patients) in those receiving placebo. Of the patients who received carvedilol in the CAPRICORN trial, one patient (0.1%) withdrew from the study due to cholestatic jaundice.

Hepatic injury has been reversible and has occurred after short- and/or long-term therapy with minimal clinical symptomatology. No deaths due to liver function abnormalities have been reported in association with the use of COREG. At the first symptom/sign of liver dysfunction (e.g., pruritus, dark urine, persistent anorexia, jaundice, right upper quadrant tenderness, or unexplained "flu-like" symptoms), laboratory testing should be performed. If the patient has laboratory evidence of liver injury or jaundice, carvedilol should be stopped and not restarted.

Peripheral Vascular Disease: β-blockers can precipitate or aggravate symptoms of arterial insufficiency in patients with peripheral vascular disease. Caution should be exercised in such individuals.

Anesthesia and Major Surgery: If treatment with COREG is to be continued perioperatively, particular care should be taken when anesthetic agents which depress myocardial function, such as ether, cyclopropane, and trichloroethylene, are used. See OVERDOSAGE for information on treatment of bradycardia and hypertension.

Diabetes and Hypoglycemia: In general, β-blockers may mask some of the manifestations of hypoglycemia, particularly tachycardia. Nonselective β-blockers may potentiate insulin-induced hypoglycemia and delay recovery of serum glucose levels. Patients subject to spontaneous hypoglycemia, or diabetic patients receiving insulin or oral hypoglycemic agents, should be cautioned about these possibilities. In congestive heart failure patients, there is a risk of worsening hyperglycemia (see PRECAUTIONS).

Thyrotoxicosis: β-adrenergic blockade may mask clinical signs of hyperthyroidism, such as tachycardia. Abrupt withdrawal of β-blockade may be followed by an exacerbation of the symptoms of hyperthyroidism or may precipitate thyroid storm.

PRECAUTIONS
General: In clinical trials, COREG caused bradycardia in about 2% of hypertensive patients, 9% of congestive heart failure patients, and 6.5% of myocardial infarction patients with left ventricular dysfunction. If pulse rate drops below 55 beats/minute, the dosage should be reduced.

In clinical trials of primarily mild-to-moderate heart failure, hypotension and postural hypotension occurred in 9.7% and syncope in 3.4% of patients receiving COREG compared to 3.6% and 2.5% of placebo patients, respectively. The risk for these events was highest during the first 30 days of dosing, corresponding to the up-titration period and was a cause for discontinuation of therapy in 0.7% of COREG patients, compared to 0.4% of placebo patients. In a long-term, placebo-controlled trial in severe heart failure (COPERNICUS), hypotension and postural hypotension occurred in 15.1% and syncope in 2.9% of heart failure patients receiving COREG compared to 8.7% and 2.3% of placebo patients, respectively. These events were a cause for discontinuation of therapy in 1.1% of COREG patients, compared to 0.8% of placebo patients.

Postural hypotension occurred in 1.8% and syncope in 0.1% of hypertensive patients, primarily following the initial dose or at the time of dose increase and was a cause for discontinuation of therapy in 1% of patients.

In the CAPRICORN study of survivors of an acute myocardial infarction, hypotension or postural hypotension occurred in 20.2% of patients receiving COREG compared to 12.6% of placebo patients. Syncope was reported in 3.9% and 1.9% of patients, respectively. These events were a cause for discontinuation of therapy in 2.5% of patients receiving COREG, compared to 0.2% of placebo patients.

To decrease the likelihood of syncope or excessive hypotension, treatment should be initiated with 3.125 mg twice daily for congestive heart failure patients and at 6.25 mg twice daily for hypertensive patients and survivors of an acute myocardial infarction with left ventricular dysfunction. Dosage should then be increased slowly, according to recommendations in the DOSAGE AND ADMINISTRATION section, and the drug should be taken with food. During initiation of therapy, the patient should be cautioned to avoid situations such as driving or hazardous tasks, where injury could result should syncope occur.

Rarely, use of carvedilol in patients with congestive heart failure has resulted in deterioration of renal function. Patients at risk appear to be those with low blood pressure (systolic blood pressure <100 mm Hg), ischemic heart disease and diffuse vascular disease, and/or underlying renal insufficiency. Renal function has returned to baseline when carvedilol was stopped. In patients with these risk factors it is recommended that renal function be monitored during up-titration of carvedilol and the drug discontinued or dosage reduced if worsening of renal function occurs.

Worsening heart failure or fluid retention may occur during up-titration of carvedilol. If such symptoms occur, diuretics should be increased and the carvedilol dose should not be advanced until clinical stability resumes (see DOSAGE AND ADMINISTRATION). Occasionally it is necessary to lower the carvedilol dose or temporarily discontinue it. Such episodes do not preclude subsequent successful titration of, or a favorable response to, carvedilol. In a placebo-controlled trial of patients with severe heart failure, worsening heart failure during the first 3 months was reported to a similar degree with carvedilol and with placebo. When treatment was maintained beyond 3 months, worsening heart failure was reported less frequently in patients treated with carvedilol than with placebo. Worsening heart failure observed during long-term therapy is more likely to be related to the patients' underlying disease than to treatment with carvedilol.

In patients with pheochromocytoma, an α-blocking agent should be initiated prior to the use of any β-blocking agent. Although carvedilol has both α- and β-blocking pharmacologic activities, there has been no experience with its use in this condition. Therefore, caution should be taken in the administration of carvedilol to patients suspected of having pheochromocytoma.

Agents with non-selective β-blocking activity may provoke chest pain in patients with Prinzmetal's variant angina. There has been no clinical experience with carvedilol in these patients although the α-blocking activity may prevent such symptoms. However, caution should be taken in the administration of carvedilol to patients suspected of having Prinzmetal's variant angina.

In congestive heart failure patients with diabetes, carvedilol therapy may lead to worsening hyperglycemia, which responds to intensification of hypoglycemic therapy. It is recommended that blood glucose be monitored when carvedilol dosing is initiated, adjusted, or discontinued.

Risk of Anaphylactic Reaction:
While taking β-blockers, patients with a history of severe anaphylactic reaction to a variety of allergens may be more reactive to repeated challenge, either accidental, diagnostic, or therapeutic. Such patients may be unresponsive to the usual doses of epinephrine used to treat allergic reaction.

Nonallergic Bronchospasm (e.g., chronic bronchitis and emphysema):
Patients with bronchospastic disease should, in general, not receive β-blockers. COREG may be used with caution, however, in patients who do not respond to, or cannot tolerate, other antihypertensive agents. It is prudent, if COREG is used, to use the smallest effective dose, so that inhibition of endogenous or exogenous β-agonists is minimized.

In clinical trials of patients with congestive heart failure, patients with bronchospastic disease were enrolled if they did not require oral or inhaled medication to treat their bronchospastic disease. In such patients, it is recommended that carvedilol be used with caution. The dosing recommendations should be followed closely and the dose should be lowered if any evidence of bronchospasm is observed during up-titration.

Information for Patients:
Patients taking COREG should be advised of the following:
- they should not interrupt or discontinue using COREG without a physician's advice.
- congestive heart failure patients should consult their physician if they experience signs or symptoms of worsening heart failure such as weight gain or increasing shortness of breath.
- they may experience a drop in blood pressure when standing, resulting in dizziness and, rarely, fainting. Patients should sit or lie down when these symptoms of lowered blood pressure occur.
- if patients experience dizziness or fatigue, they should avoid driving or hazardous tasks.
- they should consult a physician if they experience dizziness or faintness, in case the dosage should be adjusted.
- they should take COREG with food.
- diabetic patients should report any changes in blood sugar levels to their physician.
- contact lens wearers may experience decreased lacrimation.

Drug Interactions:
(Also see CLINICAL PHARMACOLOGY, *Pharmacokinetic Drug-Drug Interactions.*)
Inhibitors of CYP2D6; poor metabolizers of debrisoquin: Interactions of carvedilol with strong inhibitors of CYP2D6 (such as quinidine, fluoxetine, paroxetine, and propafenone) have not been studied, but these drugs would be expected to increase blood levels of the R(+) enantiomer of carvedilol (see CLINICAL PHARMACOLOGY). Retrospective analysis of side effects in clinical trials showed that poor 2D6 metabolizers had a higher rate of dizziness during up-titration, presumably resulting from vasodilating effects of the higher concentrations of the α-blocking R(+) enantiomer.
Catecholamine-depleting agents: Patients taking both agents with β-blocking properties and a drug that can deplete catecholamines (e.g., reserpine and monoamine oxidase inhibitors) should be observed closely for signs of hypotension and/or severe bradycardia.
Clonidine: Concomitant administration of clonidine with agents with β-blocking properties may potentiate blood-pressure- and heart-rate-lowering effects. When concomitant treatment with agents with β-blocking properties and clonidine is to be terminated, the β-blocking agent should be discontinued first. Clonidine therapy can then be discontinued several days later by gradually decreasing the dosage.
Cyclosporine: Modest increases in mean trough cyclosporine concentrations were observed following initiation of carvedilol treatment in 21 renal transplant patients suffering from chronic vascular rejection. In about 30% of patients, the dose of cyclosporine had to be reduced in order to maintain cyclosporine concentrations within the therapeutic range, while in the remainder no adjustment was needed. On the average for the group, the dose of cyclosporine was reduced about 20% in these patients. Due to wide interindividual variability in the dose adjustment required, it is recommended that cyclosporine concentrations be monitored closely after initiation of carvedilol therapy and that the dose of cyclosporine be adjusted as appropriate.
Digoxin: Digoxin concentrations are increased by about 15% when digoxin and carvedilol are administered concomitantly. Both digoxin and COREG slow AV conduction. Therefore, increased monitoring of digoxin is recommended when initiating, adjusting, or discontinuing COREG.
Inducers and inhibitors of hepatic metabolism: Rifampin reduced plasma concentrations of carvedilol by about 70%. Cimetidine increased AUC by about 30% but caused no change in C_{max}.
Calcium channel blockers: Isolated cases of conduction disturbance (rarely with hemodynamic compromise) have been observed when COREG is co-administered with diltiazem. As with other agents with β-blocking properties, if COREG is to be administered orally with calcium channel blockers of the verapamil or diltiazem type, it is recommended that ECG and blood pressure be monitored.
Insulin or oral hypoglycemics: Agents with β-blocking properties may enhance the blood-sugar-reducing effect of insulin and oral hypoglycemics. Therefore, in patients taking insulin or oral hypoglycemics, regular monitoring of blood glucose is recommended.

Carcinogenesis, Mutagenesis, Impairment of Fertility:
In 2-year studies conducted in rats given carvedilol at doses up to 75 mg/kg/day (12 times the maximum recommended human dose [MRHD] when compared on a mg/m^2 basis) or in mice given up to 200 mg/kg/day (16 times the MRHD on a mg/m^2 basis), carvedilol had no carcinogenic effect.
Carvedilol was negative when tested in a battery of genotoxicity assays, including the Ames and the CHO/HGPRT assays for mutagenicity and the in vitro hamster micronucleus and in vivo human lymphocyte cell tests for clastogenicity.
At doses ≥200 mg/kg/day (≥32 times the MRHD as mg/m^2) carvedilol was toxic to adult rats (sedation, reduced weight gain) and was associated with a reduced number of successful matings, prolonged mating time, significantly fewer corpora lutea and implants per dam and complete resorption of 18% of the litters. The no-observed-effect dose level for overt toxicity and impairment of fertility was 60 mg/kg/day (10 times the MRHD as mg/m^2).

Pregnancy: *Teratogenic Effects.* Pregnancy Category C.
Studies performed in pregnant rats and rabbits given carvedilol revealed increased post-implantation loss in rats at doses of 300 mg/kg/day (50 times the MRHD as mg/m^2) and in rabbits at doses of 75 mg/kg/day (25 times the MRHD as mg/m^2). In the rats, there was also a decrease in fetal body weight at the maternally toxic dose of 300 mg/kg/day (50 times the MRHD as mg/m^2), which was accompanied by an elevation in the frequency of fetuses with delayed skeletal development (missing or stunted 13th rib). In rats the no-observed-effect level for developmental toxicity was 60 mg/kg/day (10 times the MRHD as mg/m^2); in rabbits it was 15 mg/kg/day (5 times the MRHD as mg/m^2). There are no adequate and well-controlled studies in pregnant women. *COREG* should be used during pregnancy only if the potential benefit justifies the potential risk to the fetus.

Nursing Mothers:
It is not known whether this drug is excreted in human milk. Studies in rats have shown that carvedilol and/or its metabolites (as well as other β-blockers) cross the placental barrier and are excreted in breast milk. There was increased mortality at one week post-partum in neonates from rats treated with 60 mg/kg/day (10 times the MRHD as mg/m^2) and above during the last trimester through day 22 of lactation. Because many drugs are excreted in human milk and because of the potential for serious adverse reactions in nursing infants from β-blockers, especially bradycardia, a decision should be made whether to discontinue nursing or to discontinue the drug, taking into account the importance of the drug to the mother. The effects of other α- and β-blocking agents have included perinatal and neonatal distress.

Pediatric Use:
Safety and efficacy in patients younger than 18 years of age have not been established.

Geriatric Use:
Of the 765 patients with congestive heart failure randomized to COREG in US clinical trials, 31% (235) were 65 years of age or older. Of the 1,156 patients randomized to COREG in a long-term, placebo-controlled trial in severe heart failure, 47% (547) were 65 years of age or older. Of 3,025 patients receiving COREG in congestive heart failure trials worldwide, 42% were 65 years of age or older. There were no notable differences in efficacy or the incidence of adverse events between older and younger patients.
Of the 975 myocardial infarction patients randomized to COREG in the CAPRICORN trial, 48% (468) were 65 years of age or older, and 11% (111) were 75 years of age or older. There were no notable differences in efficacy or the incidence of adverse events between older and younger patients.
Of the 2,065 hypertensive patients in US clinical trials of efficacy or safety who were treated with COREG, 21% (436) were 65 years of age or older. Of 3,722 patients receiving COREG in hypertension clinical trials conducted worldwide, 24% were 65 years of age or older. There were no notable differences in efficacy or the incidence of adverse events between older and younger patients. With the exception of dizziness (incidence 8.8% in the elderly vs. 6% in younger patients), there were no events for which the incidence in the elderly exceeded that in the younger population by greater than 2.0%.
Similar results were observed in a postmarketing surveillance study of 3,328 COREG patients, of whom approximately 20% were 65 years of age or older.

ADVERSE REACTIONS
Congestive Heart Failure:
COREG has been evaluated for safety in congestive heart failure in more than 3,000 patients worldwide of whom more than 2,100 participated in placebo-controlled clinical trials. Approximately 60% of the total treated population received COREG for at least 6 months and 30% received COREG for at least 12 months. The adverse experience pro-

Continued on next page

Table 2. Adverse Events (% Occurrence) Occurring More Frequently with COREG Than With Placebo in Patients With Mild-to-Moderate Heart Failure Enrolled in US Heart Failure Trials or in Patients With Severe Heart Failure in the COPERNICUS Trial (Incidence >3% in Patients Treated with Carvedilol, Regardless of Causality)

	Mild-to-Moderate HF		Severe Heart Failure	
	COREG	Placebo	COREG	Placebo
	(n = 765)	(n = 437)	(n = 1,156)	(n = 1,133)
Body as a Whole				
Asthenia	7	7	11	9
Fatigue	24	22	–	–
Pain	9	8	1	1
Digoxin level increased	5	4	2	1
Edema generalized	5	3	6	5
Edema dependent	4	2	–	–
Cardiovascular				
Bradycardia	9	1	10	3
Hypotension	9	3	14	8
Syncope	3	3	8	5
Angina Pectoris	2	3	6	4
Central Nervous System				
Dizziness	32	19	24	17
Headache	8	7	5	3
Gastrointestinal				
Diarrhea	12	6	5	3
Nausea	9	5	4	3
Vomiting	6	4	1	2
Metabolic				
Hyperglycemia	12	8	5	3
Weight increase	10	7	12	11
BUN increased	6	5	–	–
NPN increased	6	5	–	–
Hypercholesterolemia	4	3	1	1
Edema peripheral	2	1	7	6
Musculoskeletal				
Arthralgia	6	5	1	1
Respiratory				
Sinusitis	5	4	2	1
Bronchitis	5	4	5	5
Upper respiratory Infection	18	18	14	13
Cough Increased	8	9	5	4
Rales	4	4	4	2
Vision				
Vision abnormal	5	2	–	–

Coreg—Cont.

file of COREG in patients with congestive heart failure was consistent with the pharmacology of the drug and the health status of the patients. Both in US clinical trials in mild-to-moderate heart failure that compared COREG in daily doses up to 100 mg (n = 765) to placebo (n = 437), and in a multinational clinical trial in severe heart failure (COPERNICUS) that compared COREG in daily doses up to 50 mg (n = 1,156) with placebo (n = 1,133), discontinuation rates for adverse experiences were similar in carvedilol and placebo patients. In these databases, the only cause of discontinuation >1%, and occurring more often on carvedilol was dizziness (1.3% on carvedilol, 0.6% on placebo in the COPERNICUS trial).

Table 2 shows adverse events reported in patients with mild-to-moderate heart failure enrolled in US placebo-controlled clinical trials and with severe heart failure enrolled in the COPERNICUS trial. Shown are adverse events that occurred more frequently in drug-treated patients than placebo-treated patients with an incidence of >3% in patients treated with carvedilol regardless of causality. Median study medication exposure was 6.3 months for both carvedilol and placebo patients in the trials of mild-to-moderate heart failure, and 10.4 months in the trial of severe heart failure patients.

[See table 2 at top of previous page]

In addition to the events in Table 2, in these trials chest pain, injury, cardiac failure, abdominal pain, gout, insomnia, depression, anemia, viral infection, and dyspnea were also reported, but rates were equal or greater in placebo-treated patients. Rates of adverse events were generally similar across demographic subsets (men and women, elderly and non-elderly, blacks and non-blacks).

The following adverse events were reported with a frequency of >1% but ≤3% and more frequently with COREG in either the US placebo-controlled trials in patients with mild-to-moderate heart failure, or in patients with severe heart failure in the COPERNICUS trial.

Incidence >1% to ≤3%
Body as a Whole: Allergy, malaise, hypovolemia, fever, leg edema, infection, back pain.
Cardiovascular: Fluid overload, postural hypotension, aggravated angina pectoris, AV block, palpitation, hypertension.
Central and Peripheral Nervous System: Hypesthesia, vertigo, paresthesia.
Gastrointestinal: Melena, periodontitis.
Liver and Biliary System: SGPT increased, SGOT increased.
Metabolic and Nutritional: Hyperuricemia, hypoglycemia, hyponatremia, increased alkaline phosphatase, glycosuria, hypervolemia, diabetes mellitus, GGT increased, weight loss, hyperkalemia, creatinine increased.
Musculoskeletal: Muscle cramps.
Platelet, Bleeding and Clotting: Prothrombin decreased, purpura, thrombocytopenia.
Psychiatric: Somnolence.
Resistance Mechanism: Infection.
Reproductive, male: Impotence.
Special Senses: Blurred vision.
Urinary System: Renal insufficiency, albuminuria, hematuria.
Postmarketing Experience: The following adverse reaction has been reported in postmarketing experience: reports of aplastic anemia have been rare and received only when carvedilol was administered concomitantly with other medications associated with the event.

Left Ventricular Dysfunction Following Myocardial Infarction: COREG has been evaluated for safety in survivors of an acute myocardial infarction with left ventricular dysfunction in the CAPRICORN trial which involved 969 patients who received COREG and 980 who received placebo. Approximately 75% of the patients received COREG for at least 6 months and 53% received COREG for at least 12 months. Patients were treated for an average of 12.9 months and 12.8 months with COREG and placebo, respectively.

The most common adverse events reported with COREG in the CAPRICORN trial were consistent with the profile of the drug in the US heart failure trials and the COPERNICUS trial, as well as the health status of the patients. The only additional adverse events reported in CAPRICORN in >3% of the patients and more commonly on carvedilol were dyspnea, anemia, and lung edema. Hypertension and myocardial infarction were also reported, but rates were equal or greater in placebo-treated patients. The following adverse events were reported with a frequency of >1% but ≤3% and more frequently with COREG: flu syndrome, cerebrovascular accident, peripheral vascular disorder, hypotonia, depression, gastrointestinal pain, arthritis, gout and urinary tract infection. The overall rates of discontinuations due to adverse events were similar in both groups of patients. In this database, the only cause of discontinuation >1%, and occurring more often on carvedilol was hypotension (1.5% on carvedilol, 0.2% on placebo).

Hypertension: COREG has been evaluated for safety in hypertension in more than 2,193 patients in US clinical trials and in 2,976 patients in international clinical trials. Approximately 36% of the total treated population received COREG for at least 6 months. In general, COREG was well tolerated at doses up to 50 mg daily. Most adverse events reported during COREG therapy were of mild to moderate severity. In US controlled clinical trials directly comparing COREG monotherapy in doses up to 50 mg (n = 1,142) to placebo (n = 462), 4.9% of COREG patients discontinued for adverse events vs. 5.2% of placebo patients. Although there was no overall difference in discontinuation rates, discontinuations were more common in the carvedilol group for postural hypotension (1% vs. 0). The overall incidence of adverse events in US placebo-controlled trials was found to increase with increasing dose of COREG. For individual adverse events this could only be distinguished for dizziness, which increased in frequency from 2% to 5% as total daily dose increased from 6.25 mg to 50 mg.

Table 3 shows adverse events in US placebo-controlled clinical trials for hypertension that occurred with an incidence of >1% regardless of causality, and that were more frequent in drug-treated patients than placebo-treated patients.

Table 3. Adverse Events in US Placebo-Controlled Hypertension Trials Incidence ≥1%, Regardless of Causality

	Adverse Reactions	
	COREG (n = 1,142) % occurrence	Placebo (n = 462) % occurrence
Cardiovascular		
Bradycardia	2	—
Postural hypotension	2	—
Peripheral Edema	1	—
Central Nervous System		
Dizziness	6	5
Insomnia	2	1
Gastrointestinal		
Diarrhea	2	1
Hematologic		
Thrombocytopenia	1	—
Metabolic		
Hypertriglyceridemia	1	—
Resistence Mechanism		
Viral infection	2	1
Respiratory		
Pharyngitis	2	1
Urinary/Renal		
Urinary tract infection	2	1

In addition to the events in Table 3, abdominal pain, back pain, chest pain, dependent edema, dyspepsia, dyspnea, fatigue, headache, injury, nausea, pain, rhinitis, sinusitis, somnolence, and upper respiratory tract infection were also reported, but rates were equal or greater in placebo-treated patients. Rates of adverse events were generally similar across demographic subsets (men and women, elderly and non-elderly, blacks and non-blacks).

The following adverse events not described above were reported as possibly or probably related to COREG in worldwide open or controlled trials with COREG in patients with hypertension or congestive heart failure.

Incidence >0.1% to ≤1%
Cardiovascular: Peripheral ischemia, tachycardia.
Central and Peripheral Nervous System: Hypokinesia.
Gastrointestinal: Bilirubinemia, increased hepatic enzymes (0.2% of hypertension patients and 0.4% of congestive heart failure patients were discontinued from therapy because of increases in hepatic enzymes; see WARNINGS, Hepatic Injury).
Psychiatric: Nervousness, sleep disorder, aggravated depression, impaired concentration, abnormal thinking, paroniria, emotional lability.
Respiratory System: Asthma (see CONTRAINDICATIONS).
Reproductive: Male: decreased libido.
Skin and Appendages: Pruritus, rash erythematous, rash maculopapular, rash psoriaform, photosensitivity reaction.
Special Senses: Tinnitus.
Urinary System: Micturition frequency increased.
Autonomic Nervous System: Dry mouth, sweating increased.
Metabolic and Nutritional: Hypokalemia, hypertriglyceridemia.
Hematologic: Anemia, leukopenia.
The following events were reported in ≤0.1% of patients and are potentially important: complete AV block, bundle branch block, myocardial ischemia, cerebrovascular disorder, convulsions, migraine, neuralgia, paresis, anaphylactoid reaction, alopecia, exfoliative dermatitis, amnesia, GI hemorrhage, bronchospasm, pulmonary edema, decreased hearing, respiratory alkalosis, increased BUN, decreased HDL, pancytopenia, and atypical lymphocytes.
Other adverse events occurred sporadically in single patients and cannot be distinguished from concurrent disease states or medications.
COREG therapy has not been associated with clinically significant changes in routine laboratory tests in hypertensive patients. No clinically relevant changes were noted in serum potassium, fasting serum glucose, total triglycerides, total cholesterol, HDL cholesterol, uric acid, blood urea nitrogen, or creatinine.

OVERDOSAGE

The acute oral LD50 doses in male and female mice and male and female rats are over 8000 mg/kg. Overdosage may cause severe hypotension, bradycardia, cardiac insufficiency, cardiogenic shock, and cardiac arrest. Respiratory problems, bronchospasms, vomiting, lapses of consciousness, and generalized seizures may also occur.

The patient should be placed in a supine position and, where necessary, kept under observation and treated under intensive-care conditions. Gastric lavage or pharmacologically induced emesis may be used shortly after ingestion. The following agents may be administered:

for excessive bradycardia: atropine, 2 mg IV.

to support cardiovascular function: glucagon, 5 to 10 mg IV rapidly over 30 seconds, followed by a continuous infusion of 5 mg/hour; sympathomimetics (dobutamine, isoprenaline, adrenaline) at doses according to body weight and effect.

If peripheral vasodilation dominates, it may be necessary to administer adrenaline or noradrenaline with continuous monitoring of circulatory conditions. For therapy-resistant bradycardia, pacemaker therapy should be performed. For bronchospasm, β-sympathomimetics (as aerosol or IV) or aminophylline IV should be given. In the event of seizures, slow IV injection of diazepam or clonazepam is recommended.

NOTE: In the event of severe intoxication where there are symptoms of shock, treatment with antidotes must be continued for a sufficiently long period of time consistent with the 7- to 10-hour half-life of carvedilol.

Cases of overdosage with COREG alone or in combination with other drugs have been reported. Quantities ingested in some cases exceeded 1,000 milligrams. Symptoms experienced included low blood pressure and heart rate. Standard supportive treatment was provided and individuals recovered.

DOSAGE AND ADMINISTRATION

Congestive Heart Failure:
DOSAGE MUST BE INDIVIDUALIZED AND CLOSELY MONITORED BY A PHYSICIAN DURING UP-TITRATION. Prior to initiation of COREG, it is recommended that fluid retention be minimized. The recommended starting dose of COREG is 3.125 mg, twice daily for two weeks. Patients who tolerate a dose of 3.125 mg twice daily may have their dose increased to 6.25, 12.5, and 25 mg twice daily over successive intervals of at least two weeks. Patients should be maintained on lower doses if higher doses are not tolerated. A maximum dose of 50 mg twice daily has been administered to patients with mild-to-moderate heart failure weighing over 85 kg (187 lbs).

Patients should be advised that initiation of treatment and (to a lesser extent) dosage increases may be associated with transient symptoms of dizziness or lightheadedness (and rarely syncope) within the first hour after dosing. Thus during these periods they should avoid situations such as driving or hazardous tasks, where symptoms could result in injury. In addition, COREG should be taken with food to slow the rate of absorption. Vasodilatory symptoms often do not require treatment, but it may be useful to separate the time of dosing of COREG from that of the ACE inhibitor or to reduce temporarily the dose of the ACE inhibitor. The dose of COREG should not be increased until symptoms of worsening heart failure or vasodilation have been stabilized.

Fluid retention (with or without transient worsening heart failure symptoms) should be treated by an increase in the dose of diuretics.

The dose of COREG should be reduced if patients experience bradycardia (heart rate <55 beats/minute).

Episodes of dizziness or fluid retention during initiation of COREG can generally be managed without discontinuation of treatment and do not preclude subsequent successful titration of, or a favorable response to, carvedilol.

Left Ventricular Dysfunction Following Myocardial Infarction: DOSAGE MUST BE INDIVIDUALIZED AND MONITORED DURING UP-TITRATION. Treatment with COREG may be started as an inpatient or outpatient and should be started after the patient is hemodynamically stable and fluid retention has been minimized. It is recommended that COREG be started at 6.25 mg twice daily and increased after 3 to 10 days, based on tolerability to 12.5 mg twice daily, then again to the target dose of 25 mg twice daily. A lower starting dose may be used (3.125 mg twice daily) and/or, the rate of up-titration may be slowed if clinically indicated (e.g., due to low blood pressure or heart rate, or fluid retention). Patients should be maintained on lower doses if higher doses are not tolerated. The recommended dosing regimen need not be altered in patients who received treatment with an IV or oral β-blocker during the acute phase of the myocardial infarction.

Hypertension: DOSAGE MUST BE INDIVIDUALIZED. The recommended starting dose of COREG is 6.25 mg twice daily. If this dose is tolerated, using standing systolic pressure measured about 1 hour after dosing as a guide, the dose should be maintained for 7 to 14 days, and then increased to 12.5 mg twice daily if needed, based on trough blood pressure, again using standing systolic pressure one hour after dosing as a guide for tolerance. This dose should also be maintained for 7 to 14 days and can then be adjusted upward to 25 mg twice daily if tolerated and needed. The full antihypertensive effect of COREG is seen within 7 to 14 days. Total daily dose should not exceed 50 mg. COREG should be taken with food to slow the rate of absorption and reduce the incidence of orthostatic effects.

Addition of a diuretic to COREG, or COREG to a diuretic can be expected to produce additive effects and exaggerate the orthostatic component of COREG action.

Use in Patients with Hepatic Impairment: COREG should not be given to patients with severe hepatic impairment (see CONTRAINDICATIONS).

HOW SUPPLIED

Tablets: White, oval, film-coated tablets: 3.125 mg–engraved with 39 and SB, in bottles of 100; 6.25 mg–engraved with 4140 and SB, in bottles of 100; 12.5 mg–engraved with 4141 and SB, in bottles of 100; 25 mg–engraved with 4142 and SB, in bottles of 100. The 6.25 mg, 12.5 mg, and 25 mg tablets are TILTAB tablets.

Store below 30°C (86°F). Protect from moisture. Dispense in a tight, light-resistant container.

3.125 mg 100's: NDC 0007-4139-20
6.25 mg 100's: NDC 0007-4140-20
12.5 mg 100's: NDC 0007-4141-20
25 mg 100's: NDC 0007-4142-20

COREG and TILTAB are registered trademarks of GlaxoSmithKline.
GlaxoSmithKline, Research Triangle Park, NC 27709
©2003, GlaxoSmithKline. All rights reserved.
March 2003/CO:L7

CUTIVATE®
[kyoot' ə-vāt]
(fluticasone propionate ointment)
Ointment, 0.005%
For Dermatologic Use Only—
Not for Ophthalmic Use.

Prescribing information for this product, which appears on pages 1498–1499 of the 2003 PDR, has been revised as follows. Please write "See Supplement A" next to the product heading.

The **INDICATIONS AND USAGE** *section was revised to:*
CUTIVATE Ointment is a medium potency corticosteroid indicated for the relief of the inflammatory and pruritic manifestations of corticosteroid-responsive dermatoses in adult patients.

The following paragraph was moved from **PRECAUTIONS: General** *to* **PRECAUTIONS: Laboratory Tests:**
A concentrated fluticasone propionate ointment, 0.05% (10 times that of the marketed fluticasone propionate ointment, 0.005%) suppressed 24-hour urinary free cortisol levels in 2 of 6 patients when used at a dose of 30 g/day for a week in patients with psoriasis or atopic eczema. No suppression of A.M. plasma cortisol was observed. In a second study of the same concentrated formulation of fluticasone propionate ointment, 0.05%, depression of A.M. plasma cortisol levels was noted in 2 of 8 normal volunteers when applied at doses of 50 g/day for 21 days. Morning plasma levels returned to normal levels within 4 days upon discontinuation of fluticasone propionate. In this study there was no corresponding decrease in 24-hour urinary free cortisol levels.

The following paragraph was added to the end of the **PRECAUTIONS: Laboratory Tests** *section:*
In a study of 35 pediatric patients treated with fluticasone propionate ointment, 0.005% for atopic dermatitis over at least 35% of body surface area, subnormal adrenal function was observed with cosyntropin stimulation testing at the end of 3 to 4 weeks of treatment in 4 patients who had normal testing prior to treatment. It is not known if these patients had recovery of adrenal function because follow-up testing was not performed (see PRECAUTIONS: Pediatric Use and ADVERSE REACTIONS). Adrenal suppression was indicated by either a ≤5 mcg/dL prestimulation cortisol, or a cosyntropin poststimulation cortisol ≤18 mcg/dL, and/or an increase of <7 mcg/dL from the baseline cortisol level.

The **PRECAUTIONS: Pediatric Use** *subsection was revised to:*
Use of CUTIVATE Ointment in pediatric patients is not recommended.
In a study of 35 pediatric patients treated with fluticasone propionate ointment, 0.005% for atopic dermatitis over at least 35% of body surface area, subnormal adrenal function was observed with cosyntropin stimulation testing at the end of 3 to 4 weeks of treatment in 4 patients who had normal testing prior to treatment. It is not known if these patients had recovery of adrenal function because follow-up testing was not performed (see PRECAUTIONS: Laboratory Tests and ADVERSE REACTIONS). The decreased responsiveness to cosyntropin testing was not correlated to age of patient, amount of fluticasone propionate ointment used, or serum levels of fluticasone propionate. Plasma fluticasone propionate were not performed in a 6-month-old patient who demonstrated an abnormal response to cosyntropin stimulation testing.
Pediatric patients may demonstrate greater susceptibility to topical corticosteroid-induced HPA axis suppression and Cushing syndrome than mature patients because of a larger skin surface to body weight ratio.

The following paragraph was added to **ADVERSE REACTIONS:**
In a study of 35 pediatric patients treated with fluticasone propionate ointment, 0.005% for atopic dermatitis over at least 35% of body surface area, subnormal adrenal function was observed with cosyntropin stimulation testing at the end of 3 to 4 weeks of treatment in 4 patients who had normal testing prior to treatment. It is not known if these patients had recovery of adrenal function because follow-up testing was not performed (see PRECAUTIONS: Laboratory Tests and PRECAUTIONS: Pediatric Use). Telangiectasia on the face was noted in 1 patient on the eighth day of a 4-week treatment period. Facial use was discontinued and the telangiectasia resolved.

The following paragraph was added to **DOSAGE AND ADMINISTRATION:**
CUTIVATE Ointment should not be used with occlusive dressings.
GlaxoSmithKline Consumer Healthcare LP
Pittsburgh, PA 15230
©2002, GlaxoSmithKline. All rights reserved.
April 2002/RL-1080

DARAPRIM®
[dair' ə-prĭm]
(pyrimethamine)
25-mg Scored Tablets

Prescribing information for this product, which appears on pages 1499–1500 of the 2003 PDR, has been revised as follows. Please write "See Supplement A" next to the product heading.

The following **Geriatric Use** *subsection was added under* **PRECAUTIONS:**
Clinical studies of DARAPRIM did not include sufficient numbers of subjects aged 65 and over to determine whether they respond differently from younger subjects. Other reported clinical experience has not identified differences in responses between the elderly and younger patients. In general, dose selection for an elderly patient should be cautious, usually starting at the low end of the dosing range, reflecting the greater frequency of decreased hepatic, renal, or cardiac function, and of concomitant disease or other drug therapy.

Manufactured by DSM Pharmaceuticals, Inc.
Greenville, NC 27834 for
GlaxoSmithKline, Research Triangle Park, NC 27709
©2002, GlaxoSmithKline. All rights reserved.
October 2002/RL-1153

EPIVIR® Tablets
[ĕp' ə-vir]
(lamivudine tablets)
EPIVIR® Oral Solution
(lamivudine oral solution)

Prescribing information for these products, which appears on pages 1508–1512 of the 2003 PDR, has been revised as follows. Please write "See Supplement A" next to the product heading.

The second paragraph in **PRECAUTIONS: Pregnancy** *was revised to:*
In 2 clinical studies conducted in South Africa, pharmacokinetic measurements were performed on samples from pregnant women who received lamivudine beginning at week 38 of gestation (10 women who received 150 mg twice daily in combination with zidovudine and 10 who received lamivudine 300 mg twice daily without other antiretrovirals) or beginning at week 36 of gestation (16 women who received lamivudine 150 mg twice daily in combination with zidovudine). These studies were not designed or powered to provide efficacy information. Lamivudine pharmacokinetics in the pregnant women were similar to those obtained following birth and in non-pregnant adults. Lamivudine concentrations were generally similar in maternal, neonatal, and cord serum samples. In a subset of subjects from whom amniotic fluid specimens were obtained following natural rupture of membranes, amniotic fluid concentrations of lamivudine ranged from 1.2 to 2.5 mcg/mL (150 mg twice daily) and 2.1 to 5.2 mcg/mL (300 mg twice daily) and were typically greater than 2 times the maternal serum levels. See the ADVERSE REACTIONS section for the limited late-pregnancy safety information available from these studies. Lamivudine should be used during pregnancy only if the potential benefits outweigh the risks.

The second paragraph in **PRECAUTIONS: Nursing Mothers** *was revised to:*
A study in lactating rats administered 45 mg/kg of lamivudine showed that lamivudine concentrations in milk were slightly greater than those in plasma. Lamivudine is also excreted in human milk. Samples of breast milk obtained from 20 mothers receiving lamivudine monotherapy (300 mg twice daily) or combination therapy (150 mg lamivudine twice daily and 300 mg zidovudine twice daily) had measurable concentrations of lamivudine.
Because of both the potential for HIV transmission and the potential for serious adverse reactions in nursing infants, **mothers should be instructed not to breastfeed if they are receiving lamivudine.**

The following paragraph was added to the beginning of the **PRECAUTIONS: Pediatric Use:** *HIV section:*
Limited, uncontrolled pharmacokinetic and safety data are available from administration of lamivudine (and zidovudine) to 36 infants up to 1 week of age in 2 studies in South Africa. In these studies, lamivudine clearance was substantially reduced in 1-week-old neonates relative to pediatric patients (>3 months of age) studied previously. There is insufficient information to establish the time course of changes in clearance between the immediate neonatal period and the age ranges >3 months old. See the ADVERSE REACTIONS section for the limited safety information available from these studies.

The following paragraph was revised in the **PRECAUTIONS: Pediatric Use:** *HIV section:*
The safety and pharmacokinetic properties of EPIVIR in combination with antiretroviral agents other than zidovudine have not been established in pediatric patients.

The following paragraph was added immediately after Table 6 in the **ADVERSE REACTIONS** *section:*
In small, uncontrolled studies in which pregnant women were given lamivudine alone or in combination with zidovudine beginning in the last few weeks of pregnancy (see PRECAUTIONS: Pregnancy), reported adverse events included anemia, urinary tract infections, and complications of labor and delivery. In postmarketing experience, liver function abnormalities and pancreatitis have been reported in women who received lamivudine in combination with other antiretroviral drugs during pregnancy. It is not known whether risks of adverse events associated with lamivudine are altered in pregnant women compared to other HIV-infected patients.

The following was added as the third paragraph under Table 8 in the **ADVERSE REACTIONS** *section:*
Limited short-term safety information is available from 2 small, uncontrolled studies in South Africa in neonates receiving lamivudine with or without zidovudine for the first week of life following maternal treatment starting at week 38 or 36 of gestation (see PRECAUTIONS: Pediatric Use). Adverse events reported in these neonates included increased liver function tests, anemia, diarrhea, electrolyte disturbances, hypoglycemia, jaundice and hepatomegaly, rash, respiratory infections, sepsis, and syphilis; 3 neonates died (1 from gastroenteritis with acidosis and convulsions, 1 from traumatic injury, and 1 from unknown causes). Two other nonfatal gastroenteritis or diarrhea cases were reported, including 1 with convulsions; 1 infant had transient renal insufficiency associated with dehydration. The absence of control groups further limits assessments of causality, but it should be assumed that perinatally exposed infants may be at risk for adverse events comparable to those reported in pediatric and adult HIV-infected patients treated with lamivudine-containing combination regimens. Long-term effects of in utero and infant lamivudine exposure are not known.

GlaxoSmithKline, Research Triangle Park, NC 27709
Manufactured under agreement from
Shire Pharmaceuticals Group plc, Basingstoke, UK
©2002, GlaxoSmithKline. All rights reserved.
October 2002/RL-1154

FLOVENT® 44 mcg
[flō' vent]
(fluticasone propionate, 44 mcg)
Inhalation Aerosol
FLOVENT® 110 mcg
(fluticasone propionate, 110 mcg)
Inhalation Aerosol
FLOVENT® 220 mcg
(fluticasone propionate, 220 mcg)
Inhalation Aerosol

For Oral Inhalation Only

Prescribing information for these products, which appears on pages 1523–1526 of the 2003 PDR, has been revised as follows. Please write "See Supplement A" next to the product heading.

The third paragraph of the **DESCRIPTION** *section was revised to note that the lecithin is soya lecithin.*

The fourth paragraph of **PRECAUTIONS: General** *was revised to:*
It is possible that systemic corticosteroid effects such as hypercorticism and adrenal suppression (including adrenal crisis) may appear in a small number of patients, particularly when fluticasone propionate is administered at higher than recommended doses over prolonged periods of time. If such effects occur, fluticasone propionate inhalation aerosol should be reduced slowly, consistent with accepted procedures for reducing systemic corticosteroids and for management of asthma symptoms.

The following subsection was added to **ADVERSE REACTIONS: Observed During Clinical Practice:**
Non-site Specific: Very rare anaphylactic reaction.
GlaxoSmithKline, Research Triangle Park, NC 27709
©2003, GlaxoSmithKline. All rights reserved.
March 2003/RL-1184

FLOVENT® ROTADISK® 50 mcg
[flō' vent rōt' ə-dĭsk]
(fluticasone propionate inhalation powder, 50 mcg)
FLOVENT® ROTADISK® 100 mcg
(fluticasone propionate inhalation powder, 100 mcg)
FLOVENT® ROTADISK® 250 mcg
(fluticasone propionate inhalation powder, 250 mcg)

For Oral Inhalation Only
For Use With the DISKHALER® Inhalation Device

Prescribing information for these products, which appears on pages 1529–1533 of the 2003 PDR, has been revised as follows. Please write "See Supplement A" next to the product heading.

Continued on next page

Flovent Rotadisk—Cont.

Revised the following ingredients statement in the **DESCRIPTION** *section to include milk proteins:*
Each blister contains a mixture of 50, 100, or 250 mcg of microfine fluticasone propionate blended with lactose (which contains milk proteins) to a total weight of 25 mg.
The fourth paragraph of **PRECAUTIONS: General** *was revised to:*
It is possible that systemic corticosteroid effects such as hypercorticism and adrenal suppression (including adrenal crisis) may appear in a small number of patients, particularly when fluticasone propionate is administered at higher than recommended doses over prolonged periods of time. If such effects occur, fluticasone propionate inhalation powder should be reduced slowly, consistent with accepted procedures for reducing systemic corticosteroids and for management of asthma symptoms.
Added the following subsection to **ADVERSE REACTIONS: Observed During Clinical Practice:**
Non-Site Specific: Very rare anaphylactic reaction, very rare anaphylactic reaction in patients with severe milk protein allergy.
GlaxoSmithKline, Research Triangle Park, NC 27709
©2003, GlaxoSmithKline. All rights reserved.
March 2003/RL-1185

HAVRIX® ℞
[hav' rix]
Hepatitis A Vaccine, Inactivated

Prescribing information for this product, which appears on pages 1536-1538 of the 2003 PDR, has been revised as follows. Please write "See Supplement A" next to the product heading.
The following paragraph was revised in the **INDICATIONS AND USAGE** *section:*
The ACIP has issued the following recommendations regarding food handlers: "Persons who work as food handlers can contract hepatitis A and potentially transmit HAV to others. To decrease the frequency of evaluations of food handlers with hepatitis A and the need for postexposure prophylaxis of patrons, consideration may be given to vaccination of employees who work in areas where state and local health authorities or private employers determine that such vaccination is cost-effective."
The following paragraph was revised in the **DOSAGE AND ADMINISTRATION** *section:*
For individuals with clotting-factor disorders at risk of hematoma formation following intramuscular injection, the ACIP recommends that when any intramuscular vaccine is indicated for such patients, "...the vaccine should be administered intramuscularly if, in the opinion of a physician familiar with the patient's bleeding risk, the vaccine can be administered with reasonable safety by this route. If the patient receives antihemophilia or other similar therapy, intramuscular vaccinations can be scheduled shortly after such therapy is administered. A fine needle (≤23 gauge) should be used for the vaccination and firm pressure applied to the site, without rubbing, for ≥2 minutes. The patient or family should be instructed concerning the risk for hematoma from the injection."
The package of 25 prefilled disposable Tip-Lok® Syringes (packaged without needles) was deleted from the **HOW SUPPLIED** *section.*
Manufactured by GlaxoSmithKline Biologicals
Rixensart, Belgium
Distributed by GlaxoSmithKline
Research Triangle Park, NC 27709
©2002 GlaxoSmithKline. All rights reserved.
September 2002/HA:L16

HYCAMTIN® ℞
[hī-kam'tin]
brand of topotecan hydrochloride for Injection

(for intravenous use)

Prescribing information for this product, which appears on pages 1538-1541 of the 2003 PDR, has been revised as follows. Please write "See Supplement A" next to the product heading.
The following paragraph was added under **PRECAUTIONS: Drug Interactions:**
Greater myelosuppression is also likely to be seen when *Hycamtin* is used in combination with other cytotoxic agents, thereby necessitating a dose reduction. However, when combining *Hycamtin* with platinum agents (e.g., cisplatin or carboplatin), a distinct sequence-dependent interaction on myelosuppression has been reported. Coadministration of a platinum agent on day 1 of *Hycamtin* dosing required lower doses of each agent compared to coadministration on day 5 of the *Hycamtin* dosing schedule.
GlaxoSmithKline, Research Triangle Park, NC 27709
©2002, GlaxoSmithKline. All rights reserved.
November 2002/HY:L14

IMITREX® ℞
[ĭm'ĭ-trĕx]
(sumatriptan succinate)
Injection

Prescribing information for this product, which appears on pages 1542-1546 of the 2003 PDR, has been revised as follows. Please write "See Supplement A" next to the product heading.
The third paragraph under **PRECAUTIONS: General** *was revised to:*
There have been rare reports of seizure following administration of sumatriptan. Sumatriptan should be used with caution in patients with a history of epilepsy or conditions associated with a lowered seizure threshold.
GlaxoSmithKline, Research Triangle Park, NC 27709
©2003, GlaxoSmithKline. All rights reserved.
January 2003/RL-1164

IMITREX® ℞
[ĭm'ĭ-trĕx]
(sumatriptan)
Nasal Spray

Prescribing information for this product, which appears on pages 1546-1550 of the 2003 PDR, has been revised as follows. Please write "See Supplement A" next to the product heading.
The third paragraph under **PRECAUTIONS: General** *was revised to:*
There have been rare reports of seizure following administration of sumatriptan. Sumatriptan should be used with caution in patients with a history of epilepsy or conditions associated with a lowered seizure threshold.
GlaxoSmithKline, Research Triangle Park, NC 27709
©2003, GlaxoSmithKline. All rights reserved.
January 2003/RL-1165

IMITREX® ℞
[ĭm'ĭ-trĕx]
(sumatriptan succinate)
Tablets

Prescribing information for this product, which appears on pages 1550-1554 of the 2003 PDR, has been revised as follows. Please write "See Supplement A" next to the product heading.
The third paragraph under **PRECAUTIONS: General** *was revised to:*
There have been rare reports of seizure following administration of sumatriptan. Sumatriptan should be used with caution in patients with a history of epilepsy or conditions associated with a lowered seizure threshold.
GlaxoSmithKline, Research Triangle Park, NC 27709
©2002, GlaxoSmithKline. All rights reserved.
January 2003/RL-1166

INFANRIX® ℞
[in' fan-rix]
Diphtheria and Tetanus Toxoids and Acellular Pertussis Vaccine Adsorbed

Prescribing information for this product, which appears on pages 1554-1558 of the 2003 PDR, has been revised as follows. Please write "See Supplement A" next to the product heading.
The **HOW SUPPLIED** *section was revised as follows to reflect the addition of several new pack sizes:*
HOW SUPPLIED
INFANRIX is supplied as a turbid white suspension in vials and prefilled syringes containing a 0.5 mL single dose.
Single-Dose Vials
NDC 58160-840-01 (package of 1)
NDC 58160-840-11 (package of 10)
Single-Dose Prefilled Disposable Tip-Lok® Syringes (packaged without needles)
NDC 58160-840-46 (package of 5)
NDC 58160-840-50 (package of 25)
Single-Dose Prefilled Disposable Tip-Lok® Syringes with 1-inch 25-gauge BD SafetyGlide™ Needles
NDC 58160-840-56 (package of 25)
Single-Dose Prefilled Disposable Tip-Lok® Syringes with 5/8-inch 25-gauge BD SafetyGlide™ Needles
NDC 58160-840-57 (package of 25)
Manufactured by GlaxoSmithKline Biologicals
Rixensart, Belgium, US License 1090, and
Chiron Behring GmbH & Co
Marburg, Germany, US License 0097
Distributed by GlaxoSmithKline
Research Triangle Park, NC 27709
INFANRIX and TIP-LOK are registered trademarks of SmithKline Beecham.
SAFETYGLIDE is a trademark of Becton, Dickinson and Company.
©2002, GlaxoSmithKline. All rights reserved.
December 2002/IN:L8

LAMICTAL® ℞
[la-mĭk' tal]
(lamotrigine)
Tablets

LAMICTAL® ℞
(lamotrigine)
Chewable Dispersible Tablets

Prescribing information for these products, which appears on pages 1559-1566 of the 2003 PDR, has been completely revised as follows. Please write "See Supplement A" next to the product heading.

> **SERIOUS RASHES REQUIRING HOSPITALIZATION AND DISCONTINUATION OF TREATMENT HAVE BEEN REPORTED IN ASSOCIATION WITH THE USE OF LAMICTAL. THE INCIDENCE OF THESE RASHES, WHICH HAVE INCLUDED STEVENS-JOHNSON SYNDROME, IS APPROXIMATELY 0.8% (8 PER 1,000) IN PEDIATRIC PATIENTS (AGE <16 YEARS) RECEIVING LAMICTAL AS ADJUNCTIVE THERAPY AND 0.3% (3 PER 1,000) IN ADULTS. IN A PROSPECTIVELY FOLLOWED COHORT OF 1,983 PEDIATRIC PATIENTS TAKING ADJUNCTIVE LAMICTAL, THERE WAS 1 RASH-RELATED DEATH. IN WORLDWIDE POSTMARKETING EXPERIENCE, RARE CASES OF TOXIC EPIDERMAL NECROLYSIS AND/OR RASH-RELATED DEATH HAVE BEEN REPORTED IN ADULT AND PEDIATRIC PATIENTS, BUT THEIR NUMBERS ARE TOO FEW TO PERMIT A PRECISE ESTIMATE OF THE RATE.**
> **BECAUSE THE RATE OF SERIOUS RASH IS GREATER IN PEDIATRIC PATIENTS THAN IN ADULTS, IT BEARS EMPHASIS THAT LAMICTAL IS APPROVED ONLY FOR USE IN PEDIATRIC PATIENTS BELOW THE AGE OF 16 YEARS WHO HAVE SEIZURES ASSOCIATED WITH THE LENNOX-GASTAUT SYNDROME OR IN PATIENTS WITH PARTIAL SEIZURES (SEE INDICATIONS).**
> **OTHER THAN AGE, THERE ARE AS YET NO FACTORS IDENTIFIED THAT ARE KNOWN TO PREDICT THE RISK OF OCCURRENCE OR THE SEVERITY OF RASH ASSOCIATED WITH LAMICTAL. THERE ARE SUGGESTIONS, YET TO BE PROVEN, THAT THE RISK OF RASH MAY ALSO BE INCREASED BY 1) COADMINISTRATION OF LAMICTAL WITH VALPROIC ACID (VPA), 2) EXCEEDING THE RECOMMENDED INITIAL DOSE OF LAMICTAL, OR 3) EXCEEDING THE RECOMMENDED DOSE ESCALATION FOR LAMICTAL. HOWEVER, CASES HAVE BEEN REPORTED IN THE ABSENCE OF THESE FACTORS.**
> **NEARLY ALL CASES OF LIFE-THREATENING RASHES ASSOCIATED WITH LAMICTAL HAVE OCCURRED WITHIN 2 TO 8 WEEKS OF TREATMENT INITIATION. HOWEVER, ISOLATED CASES HAVE BEEN REPORTED AFTER PROLONGED TREATMENT (e.g., 6 MONTHS). ACCORDINGLY, DURATION OF THERAPY CANNOT BE RELIED UPON AS A MEANS TO PREDICT THE POTENTIAL RISK HERALDED BY THE FIRST APPEARANCE OF A RASH.**
> **ALTHOUGH BENIGN RASHES ALSO OCCUR WITH LAMICTAL, IT IS NOT POSSIBLE TO PREDICT RELIABLY WHICH RASHES WILL PROVE TO BE SERIOUS OR LIFE THREATENING. ACCORDINGLY, LAMICTAL SHOULD ORDINARILY BE DISCONTINUED AT THE FIRST SIGN OF RASH, UNLESS THE RASH IS CLEARLY NOT DRUG RELATED. DISCONTINUATION OF TREATMENT MAY NOT PREVENT A RASH FROM BECOMING LIFE THREATENING OR PERMANENTLY DISABLING OR DISFIGURING.**

DESCRIPTION
LAMICTAL (lamotrigine), an antiepileptic drug (AED) of the phenyltriazine class, is chemically unrelated to existing antiepileptic drugs. Its chemical name is 3,5-diamino-6-(2,3-dichlorophenyl)-*as*-triazine, its molecular formula is $C_9H_7N_5Cl_2$, and its molecular weight is 256.09. Lamotrigine is a white to pale cream-colored powder and has a pK_a of 5.7. Lamotrigine is very slightly soluble in water (0.17 mg/mL at 25°C) and slightly soluble in 0.1 M HCl (4.1 mg/mL at 25°C).
LAMICTAL Tablets are supplied for oral administration as 25-mg (white), 100-mg (peach), 150-mg (cream), and 200-mg (blue) tablets. Each tablet contains the labeled amount of lamotrigine and the following inactive ingredients: lactose; magnesium stearate; microcrystalline cellulose; povidone; sodium starch glycolate; FD&C Yellow No. 6 Lake (100-mg tablet only); ferric oxide, yellow (150-mg tablet only); and FD&C Blue No. 2 Lake (200-mg tablet only).
LAMICTAL Chewable Dispersible Tablets are supplied for oral administration. The tablets contain 2 mg (white), 5 mg (white), or 25 mg (white) of lamotrigine and the following inactive ingredients: blackcurrant flavor, calcium carbonate, low-substituted hydroxypropylcellulose, magnesium aluminum silicate, magnesium stearate, povidone, saccharin sodium, and sodium starch glycolate.

CLINICAL PHARMACOLOGY
Mechanism of Action: The precise mechanism(s) by which lamotrigine exerts its anticonvulsant action are unknown. In animal models designed to detect anticonvulsant activity, lamotrigine was effective in preventing seizure spread in the maximum electroshock (MES) and pentylenetetrazol (scMet) tests, and prevented seizures in the visually and electrically evoked after-discharge (EEAD) tests for antiepileptic activity. The relevance of these models to human epilepsy, however, is not known.

One proposed mechanism of action of LAMICTAL, the relevance of which remains to be established in humans, involves an effect on sodium channels. In vitro pharmacological studies suggest that lamotrigine inhibits voltage-sensitive sodium channels, thereby stabilizing neuronal membranes and consequently modulating presynaptic transmitter release of excitatory amino acids (e.g., glutamate and aspartate).

Pharmacological Properties: Although the relevance for human use is unknown, the following data characterize the performance of LAMICTAL in receptor binding assays. Lamotrigine had a weak inhibitory effect on the serotonin 5-HT_3 receptor (IC_{50} = 18 μM). It does not exhibit high affinity binding (IC_{50}>100 μM) to the following neurotransmitter receptors: adenosine A_1 and A_2; adrenergic α_1, α_2, and β; dopamine D_1 and D_2; γ-aminobutyric acid (GABA) A and B; histamine H_1; kappa opioid; muscarinic acetylcholine; and serotonin 5-HT_2. Studies have failed to detect an effect of lamotrigine on dihydropyridine-sensitive calcium channels. It had weak effects at sigma opioid receptors (IC_{50} = 145 μM). Lamotrigine did not inhibit the uptake of norepinephrine, dopamine, serotonin, or aspartic acid (IC_{50}>100 μM).

Effect of Lamotrigine on N-Methyl d-Aspartate (NMDA)-Mediated Activity: Lamotrigine did not inhibit NMDA-induced depolarizations in rat cortical slices or NMDA-induced cyclic GMP formation in immature rat cerebellum, nor did lamotrigine displace compounds that are either competitive or noncompetitive ligands at this glutamate receptor complex (CNQX, CGS, TCHP). The IC_{50} for lamotrigine effects on NMDA-induced currents (in the presence of 3 μM of glycine) in cultured hippocampal neurons exceeded 100 μM.

Folate Metabolism: In vitro, lamotrigine was shown to be an inhibitor of dihydrofolate reductase, the enzyme that catalyzes the reduction of dihydrofolate to tetrahydrofolate. Inhibition of this enzyme may interfere with the biosynthesis of nucleic acids and proteins. When oral daily doses of lamotrigine were given to pregnant rats during organogenesis, fetal, placental, and maternal folate concentrations were reduced. Significantly reduced concentrations of folate are associated with teratogenesis (see PRECAUTIONS: Pregnancy). Folate concentrations were also reduced in male rats given repeated oral doses of lamotrigine. Reduced concentrations were partially returned to normal when supplemented with folinic acid.

Accumulation in Kidneys: Lamotrigine was found to accumulate in the kidney of the male rat, causing chronic progressive nephrosis, necrosis, and mineralization. These findings are attributed to α-2 microglobulin, a species- and sex-specific protein that has not been detected in humans or other animal species.

Melanin Binding: Lamotrigine binds to melanin-containing tissues, e.g., in the eye and pigmented skin. It has been found in the uveal tract up to 52 weeks after a single dose in rodents.

Cardiovascular: In dogs, lamotrigine is extensively metabolized to a 2-N-methyl metabolite. This metabolite causes dose-dependent prolongations of the PR interval, widening of the QRS complex, and, at higher doses, complete AV conduction block. Similar cardiovascular effects are not anticipated in humans because only trace amounts of the 2-N-methyl metabolite (<0.6% of lamotrigine dose) have been found in human urine (see Drug Disposition below). However, it is conceivable that plasma concentrations of this metabolite could be increased in patients with a reduced capacity to glucuronidate lamotrigine (e.g., in patients with liver disease).

Pharmacokinetics and Drug Metabolism: The pharmacokinetics of lamotrigine have been studied in patients with epilepsy, healthy young and elderly volunteers, and volunteers with chronic renal failure. Lamotrigine pharmacokinetic parameters for adult and pediatric patients and healthy normal volunteers are summarized in Tables 1 and 2.

[See table 1 above]

Table 1. Mean* Pharmacokinetic Parameters in Adult Patients With Epilepsy or Healthy Volunteers

Adult Study Population	Number of Subjects	T_{max}: Time of Maximum Plasma Concentration (h)	$t_{½}$: Elimination Half-life (h)	Cl/F: Apparent Plasma Clearance (mL/min/kg)
Patients taking enzyme-inducing antiepileptic drugs (EIAEDs)†:				
Single-dose LAMICTAL	24	2.3 (0.5–5.0)	14.4 (6.4–30.4)	1.10 (0.51–2.22)
Multiple-dose LAMICTAL	17	2.0 (0.75–5.93)	12.6 (7.5–23.1)	1.21 (0.66–1.82)
Patients taking EIAEDs + VPA:				
Single-dose LAMICTAL	25	3.8 (1.0–10.0)	27.2 (11.2–51.6)	0.53 (0.27–1.04)
Patients taking VPA only:				
Single-dose LAMICTAL	4	4.8 (1.8–8.4)	58.8 (30.5–88.8)	0.28 (0.16–0.40)
Healthy volunteers taking VPA:				
Single-dose LAMICTAL	6	1.8 (1.0–4.0)	48.3 (31.5–88.6)	0.30 (0.14–0.42)
Multiple-dose LAMICTAL	18	1.9 (0.5–3.5)	70.3 (41.9–113.5)	0.18 (0.12–0.33)
Healthy volunteers taking no other medications:				
Single-dose LAMICTAL	179	2.2 (0.25–12.0)	32.8 (14.0–103.0)	0.44 (0.12–1.10)
Multiple-dose LAMICTAL	36	1.7 (0.5–4.0)	25.4 (11.6–61.6)	0.58 (0.24–1.15)

*The majority of parameter means determined in each study had coefficients of variation between 20% and 40% for half-life and Cl/F and between 30% and 70% for T_{max}. The overall mean values were calculated from individual study means that were weighted based on the number of volunteers/patients in each study. The numbers in parentheses below each parameter mean represent the range of individual volunteer/patient values across studies.

† Examples of EIAEDs are carbamazepine, phenobarbital, phenytoin, and primidone.

The apparent clearance of lamotrigine is affected by the coadministration of AEDs. Lamotrigine is eliminated more rapidly in patients who have been taking hepatic EIAEDs, including carbamazepine, phenytoin, phenobarbital, and primidone. Most clinical experience is derived from this population.

VPA, however, actually decreases the apparent clearance of lamotrigine (i.e., more than doubles the elimination half-life of lamotrigine). Accordingly, if lamotrigine is to be administered to a patient receiving VPA, lamotrigine must be given at a reduced dosage, less than half the dose used in patients not receiving VPA (see DOSAGE AND ADMINISTRATION and PRECAUTIONS: Drug Interactions).

Absorption: Lamotrigine is rapidly and completely absorbed after oral administration with negligible first-pass metabolism (absolute bioavailability is 98%). The bioavailability is not affected by food. Peak plasma concentrations occur anywhere from 1.4 to 4.8 hours following drug administration. The lamotrigine chewable/dispersible tablets were found to be equivalent, whether they were administered as dispersed in water, chewed and swallowed, or swallowed as whole, to the lamotrigine compressed tablets in terms of rate and extent of absorption.

Distribution: Estimates of the mean apparent volume of distribution (Vd/F) of lamotrigine following oral administration ranged from 0.9 to 1.3 L/kg. Vd/F is independent of dose and is similar following single and multiple doses in both patients with epilepsy and in healthy volunteers.

Protein Binding: Data from in vitro studies indicate that lamotrigine is approximately 55% bound to human plasma proteins at plasma lamotrigine concentrations from 1 to 10 mcg/mL (10 mcg/mL is 4 to 6 times the trough plasma concentration observed in the controlled efficacy trials). Because lamotrigine is not highly bound to plasma proteins, clinically significant interactions with other drugs through competition for protein binding sites are unlikely. The binding of lamotrigine to plasma proteins did not change in the presence of therapeutic concentrations of phenytoin, phenobarbital, or VPA. Lamotrigine did not displace other AEDs (carbamazepine, phenytoin, phenobarbital) from protein binding sites.

Drug Disposition: Lamotrigine is metabolized predominantly by glucuronic acid conjugation; the major metabolite is an inactive 2-N-glucuronide conjugate. After oral administration of 240 mg of ^{14}C-lamotrigine (15 μCi) to 6 healthy volunteers, 94% was recovered in the urine and 2% was recovered in the feces. The radioactivity in the urine consisted of unchanged lamotrigine (10%), the 2-N-glucuronide (76%), a 5-N-glucuronide (10%), a 2-N-methyl metabolite (0.14%), and other unidentified minor metabolites (4%).

Enzyme Induction: The effects of lamotrigine on specific families of mixed-function oxidase isozymes have not been systematically evaluated.

Following multiple administrations (150 mg twice daily) to normal volunteers taking no other medications, lamotrigine induced its own metabolism, resulting in a 25% decrease in $t_{½}$ and a 37% increase in Cl/F at steady state compared to values obtained in the same volunteers following a single dose. Evidence gathered from other sources suggests that self-induction by LAMICTAL may not occur when LAMICTAL is given as adjunctive therapy in patients receiving EIAEDs.

Dose Proportionality: In healthy volunteers not receiving any other medications and given single doses, the plasma concentrations of lamotrigine increased in direct proportion to the dose administered over the range of 50 to 400 mg. In 2 small studies (n = 7 and 8) of patients with epilepsy who were maintained on other AEDs, there also was a linear relationship between dose and lamotrigine plasma concentrations at steady state following doses of 50 to 350 mg twice daily.

Elimination: (see Table 1)

Special Populations: Patients With Renal Insufficiency: Twelve volunteers with chronic renal failure (mean creatinine clearance = 13 mL/min; range = 6 to 23) and another 6 individuals undergoing hemodialysis were each given a single 100-mg dose of LAMICTAL. The mean plasma half-lives determined in the study were 42.9 hours (chronic renal failure), 13.0 hours (during hemodialysis), and 57.4 hours (between hemodialysis) compared to 26.2 hours in healthy volunteers. On average, approximately 20% (range = 5.6 to 35.1) of the amount of lamotrigine present in the body was eliminated by hemodialysis during a 4-hour session.

Hepatic Disease: The pharmacokinetics of lamotrigine following a single 100-mg dose of LAMICTAL were evaluated in 24 subjects with moderate to severe hepatic dysfunction and compared with 12 subjects without hepatic impairment. The median apparent clearance of lamotrigine was 0.31, 0.24, or 0.10 mL/kg/min in patients with Grade A, B, or C (Child-Pugh Classification) hepatic impairment, respectively, compared to 0.34 mL/kg/min in the healthy controls. Median half-life of lamotrigine was 36, 60, or 110 hours in patients with Grade A, B, or C hepatic impairment, respectively, versus 32 hours in healthy controls.

Age: Pediatric Patients: The pharmacokinetics of LAMICTAL following a single 2-mg/kg dose were evaluated in 2 studies of pediatric patients (n = 29 for patients aged 10 months to 5.9 years and n = 26 for patients aged 5 to 11 years). Forty-three patients received concomitant therapy with other AEDS and 12 patients received LAMICTAL as monotherapy. Lamotrigine pharmacokinetic parameters for pediatric patients are summarized in Table 2.

Population pharmacokinetic analyses involving patients aged 2 to 18 years demonstrated that lamotrigine clearance was influenced predominantly by total body weight and concurrent AED therapy. The oral clearance of lamotrigine was higher, on a body weight basis, in pediatric patients than in adults. Weight-normalized lamotrigine clearance was higher in those subjects weighing less than 30 kg, compared with those weighing greater than 30 kg. Accordingly, patients weighing less than 30 kg may need an increase of as much as 50% in maintenance doses, based on clinical response, as compared with subjects weighing more than 30 kg being administered the same AEDs (see DOSAGE AND ADMINISTRATION). These analyses also revealed that, after accounting for body weight, lamotrigine clearance was not significantly influenced by age. Thus, the same weight-adjusted doses should be administered to children irrespective of differences in age. Concomitant AEDs which influence lamotrigine clearance in adults were found to have similar effects in children.

[See table 2 at top of next page]

Elderly: The pharmacokinetics of lamotrigine following a single 150-mg dose of LAMICTAL were evaluated in 12 elderly volunteers between the ages of 65 and 76 years (mean creatinine clearance = 61 mL/min, range = 33 to 108 mL/min). The mean half-life of lamotrigine in these subjects was 31.2 hours (range, 24.5 to 43.4 hours) and the mean clearance was 0.40 mL/min/kg (range, 0.26 to 0.48 mL/min/kg).

Gender: The clearance of lamotrigine is not affected by gender.

Race: The apparent oral clearance of lamotrigine was 25% lower in non-Caucasians than Caucasians.

CLINICAL STUDIES

The results of controlled clinical trials established the efficacy of LAMICTAL as monotherapy in adults with partial onset seizures already receiving treatment with a single enzyme-inducing antiepileptic drug (EIAED), as adjunctive therapy in adults and pediatric patients age 2 to 16 with partial seizures, and as adjunctive therapy in the generalized seizures of Lennox-Gastaut syndrome in pediatric and adult patients.

Monotherapy With LAMICTAL in Adults With Partial Seizures Already Receiving Treatment With a Single EIAED: The effectiveness of monotherapy with LAMICTAL was established in a multicenter, double-blind clinical trial enrolling 156 adult outpatients with partial seizures. The patients experienced at least 4 simple partial, complex par-

Continued on next page

Lamictal—Cont.

tial, and/or secondarily generalized seizures during each of 2 consecutive 4-week periods while receiving carbamazepine or phenytoin monotherapy during baseline. LAMICTAL (target dose of 500 mg/day) or VPA (1,000 mg/day) was added to either carbamazepine or phenytoin monotherapy over a 4-week period. Patients were then converted to monotherapy with LAMICTAL or VPA during the next 4 weeks, then continued on monotherapy for an additional 12-week period.

Study endpoints were completion of all weeks of study treatment or meeting an escape criterion. Criteria for escape relative to baseline were: (1) doubling of average monthly seizure count, (2) doubling of highest consecutive 2-day seizure frequency, (3) emergence of a new seizure type (defined as a seizure that did not occur during the 8-week baseline) that is more severe than seizure types that occur during study treatment, or (4) clinically significant prolongation of generalized-tonic-clonic (GTC) seizures. The primary efficacy variable was the proportion of patients in each treatment group who met escape criteria.

The percentage of patients who met escape criteria was 42% (32/76) in the LAMICTAL group and 69% (55/80) in the VPA group. The difference in the percentage of patients meeting escape criteria was statistically significant ($P = 0.0012$) in favor of LAMICTAL. No differences in efficacy based on age, sex, or race were detected.

Patients in the control group were intentionally treated with a relatively low dose of valproate; as such, the sole objective of this study was to demonstrate the effectiveness and safety of monotherapy with LAMICTAL, and cannot be interpreted to imply the superiority of LAMICTAL to an adequate dose of valproate.

Adjunctive Therapy With LAMICTAL in Adults With Partial Seizures: The effectiveness of LAMICTAL as adjunctive therapy (added to other AEDs) was established in 3 multicenter, placebo-controlled, double-blind clinical trials in 355 adults with refractory partial seizures. The patients had a history of at least 4 partial seizures per month in spite of receiving one or more AEDs at therapeutic concentrations and, in 2 of the studies, were observed on their established AED regimen during baselines that varied between 8 to 12 weeks. In the third, patients were not observed in a prospective baseline. In patients continuing to have at least 4 seizures per month during the baseline, LAMICTAL or placebo was then added to the existing therapy. In all 3 studies, change from baseline in seizure frequency was the primary measure of effectiveness. The results given below are for all partial seizures in the intent-to-treat population (all patients who received at least one dose of treatment) in each study, unless otherwise indicated. The median seizure frequency at baseline was 3 per week while the mean at baseline was 6.6 per week for all patients enrolled in efficacy studies.

One study (n = 216) was a double-blind, placebo-controlled, parallel trial consisting of a 24-week treatment period. Patients could not be on more than 2 other anticonvulsants and VPA was not allowed. Patients were randomized to receive placebo, a target dose of 300 mg/day of LAMICTAL, or a target dose of 500 mg/day of LAMICTAL. The median reductions in the frequency of all partial seizures relative to baseline were 8% in patients receiving placebo, 20% in patients receiving 300 mg/day of LAMICTAL, and 36% in patients receiving 500 mg/day of LAMICTAL. The seizure frequency reduction was statistically significant in the 500-mg/day group compared to the placebo group, but not in the 300-mg/day group.

A second study (n = 98) was a double-blind, placebo-controlled, randomized, crossover trial consisting of two 14-week treatment periods (the last 2 weeks of which consisted of dose tapering) separated by a 4-week washout period. Patients could not be on more than 2 other anticonvulsants and VPA was not allowed. The target dose of LAMICTAL was 400 mg/day. When the first 12 weeks of the treatment periods were analyzed, the median change in seizure frequency was a 25% reduction on LAMICTAL compared to placebo ($P<0.001$).

The third study (n = 41) was a double-blind, placebo-controlled, crossover trial consisting of two 12-week treatment periods separated by a 4-week washout period. Patients could not be on more than 2 other anticonvulsants. Thirteen patients were on concomitant VPA; these patients received 150 mg/day of LAMICTAL. The 28 other patients had a target dose of 300 mg/day of LAMICTAL. The median change in seizure frequency was a 26% reduction on LAMICTAL compared to placebo ($P<0.01$).

No differences in efficacy based on age, sex, or race, as measured by change in seizure frequency, were detected.

Adjunctive Therapy With LAMICTAL in Pediatric Patients with Partial Seizures: The effectiveness of LAMICTAL as adjunctive therapy in pediatric patients with partial seizures was established in a multicenter, double-blind, placebo-controlled trial in 199 patients aged 2 to 16 years (n = 98 on LAMICTAL, n = 101 on placebo). Following an 8-week baseline phase, patients were randomized to 18 weeks of treatment with LAMICTAL or placebo added to their current AED regimen of up to 2 drugs. Patients were dosed based on body weight and VPA use. Target doses were designed to approximate 5 mg/kg per day for patients taking VPA (maximum dose, 250 mg/day) and 15 mg/kg per day for the patients not taking VPA (maximum dose, 750 mg per day). The primary efficacy endpoint was percentage change from baseline in all partial seizures. For the intent-to-treat

Table 2. Mean Pharmacokinetic Parameters in Pediatric Patients With Epilepsy

Pediatric Study Population	Number of Subjects	T_{max} (h)	$t_{½}$ (h)	Cl/F (mL/min/kg)
Ages 10 months–5.3 years				
Patients taking EIAEDs	10	3.0 (1.0–5.9)	7.7 (5.7–11.4)	3.62 (2.44–5.28)
Patients taking AEDs with no known effect on drug-metabolizing enzymes	7	5.2 (2.9–6.1)	19.0 (12.9–27.1)	1.2 (0.75–2.42)
Patients taking VPA only	8	2.9 (1.0–6.0)	44.9 (29.5–52.5)	0.47 (0.23–0.77)
Ages 5–11 years				
Patients taking EIAEDs	7	1.6 (1.0–3.0)	7.0 (3.8–9.8)	2.54 (1.35–5.58)
Patients taking EIAEDs plus VPA	8	3.3 (1.0–6.4)	19.1 (7.0–31.2)	0.89 (0.39–1.93)
Patients taking VPA only*	3	4.5 (3.0–6.0)	65.8 (50.7–73.7)	0.24 (0.21–0.26)
Ages 13–18 years				
Patients taking EIAEDs	11	†	†	1.3
Patients taking EIAEDs plus VPA	8	†	†	0.5
Patients taking VPA only	4	†	†	0.3

*Two subjects were included in the calculation for mean T_{max}.
† Parameter not estimated.

population, the median reduction of all partial seizures was 36% in patients treated with LAMICTAL and 7% on placebo, a difference that was statistically significant ($P<0.01$).

Adjunctive Therapy With LAMICTAL in Pediatric and Adult Patients With Lennox-Gastaut Syndrome: The effectiveness of LAMICTAL as adjunctive therapy in patients with Lennox-Gastaut syndrome was established in a multicenter, double-blind, placebo-controlled trial in 169 patients aged 3 to 25 years (n = 79 on LAMICTAL, n = 90 on placebo). Following a 4-week single-blind, placebo phase, patients were randomized to 16 weeks of treatment with LAMICTAL or placebo added to their current AED regimen of up to 3 drugs. Patients were dosed on a fixed-dose regimen based on body weight and VPA use. Target doses were designed to approximate 5 mg/kg per day for patients taking VPA (maximum dose, 200 mg/day) and 15 mg/kg per day for patients not taking VPA (maximum dose, 400 mg/day). The primary efficacy endpoint was percentage change from baseline in major motor seizures (atonic, tonic, major myoclonic, and tonic-clonic seizures). For the intent-to-treat population, the median reduction of major motor seizures was 32% in patients treated with LAMICTAL and 9% on placebo, a difference that was statistically significant ($P<0.05$). Drop attacks were significantly reduced by LAMICTAL (34%) compared to placebo (9%), as were tonic-clonic seizures (36% reduction versus 10% increase for LAMICTAL and placebo, respectively).

INDICATIONS AND USAGE

Adjunctive Use: LAMICTAL is indicated as adjunctive therapy for partial seizures in adults and pediatric patients (≥2 years of age).

LAMICTAL is also indicated as adjunctive therapy for the generalized seizures of Lennox-Gastaut syndrome in adult and pediatric patients (≥2 years of age).

Monotherapy Use: LAMICTAL is indicated for conversion to monotherapy in adults with partial seizures who are receiving treatment with a single EIAED.

Safety and effectiveness of LAMICTAL have not been established 1) as initial monotherapy, 2) for conversion to monotherapy from non–enzyme-inducing AEDs (e.g., valproate), or 3) for simultaneous conversion to monotherapy from 2 or more concomitant AEDs (see DOSAGE AND ADMINISTRATION).

Safety and effectiveness in patients below the age of 16 other than those with partial seizures and the generalized seizures of Lennox-Gastaut syndrome have not been established (see BOX WARNING).

CONTRAINDICATIONS

LAMICTAL is contraindicated in patients who have demonstrated hypersensitivity to the drug or its ingredients.

WARNINGS

SEE BOX WARNING REGARDING THE RISK OF SERIOUS RASHES REQUIRING HOSPITALIZATION AND DISCONTINUATION OF LAMICTAL.

ALTHOUGH BENIGN RASHES ALSO OCCUR WITH LAMICTAL, IT IS NOT POSSIBLE TO PREDICT RELIABLY WHICH RASHES WILL PROVE TO BE SERIOUS OR LIFE THREATENING. ACCORDINGLY, LAMICTAL SHOULD ORDINARILY BE DISCONTINUED AT THE FIRST SIGN OF RASH, UNLESS THE RASH IS CLEARLY NOT DRUG RELATED. DISCONTINUATION OF TREATMENT MAY NOT PREVENT A RASH FROM BECOMING LIFE THREATENING OR PERMANENTLY DISABLING OR DISFIGURING.

Serious Rash: ***Pediatric Population:*** The incidence of serious rash associated with hospitalization and discontinuation of LAMICTAL in a prospectively followed cohort of pediatric patients receiving adjunctive therapy was approximately 0.8% (16 of 1,983). When 14 of these cases were reviewed by 3 expert dermatologists, there was considerable disagreement as to their proper classification. To illustrate, one dermatologist considered none of the cases to be Stevens-Johnson syndrome; another assigned 7 of the 14 to this diagnosis. There was one rash related death in this 1,983 patient cohort. Additionally, there have been rare cases of toxic epidermal necrolysis with and without permanent sequelae and/or death in US and foreign postmarketing experience. It bears emphasis, accordingly, that LAMICTAL is only approved for use in those patients below the age of 16 who have partial seizures or generalized seizures associated with the Lennox-Gastaut syndrome (see INDICATIONS).

There is evidence that the inclusion of VPA in a multidrug regimen increases the risk of serious, potentially life-threatening rash in pediatric patients. In pediatric patients who used VPA concomitantly, 1.2% (6 of 482) experienced a serious rash compared to 0.6% (6 of 952) patients not taking VPA.

Adult Population: Serious rash associated with hospitalization and discontinuation of LAMICTAL occurred in 0.3% (11 of 3,348) of patients who received LAMICTAL in premarketing clinical trials. No fatalities occurred among these individuals. However, in worldwide postmarketing experience, rare cases of rash-related death have been reported, but their numbers are too few to permit a precise estimate of the rate.

Among the rashes leading to hospitalization were Stevens-Johnson syndrome, toxic epidermal necrolysis, angioedema, and a rash associated with a variable number of the following systemic manifestations: fever, lymphadenopathy, facial swelling, hematologic, and hepatologic abnormalities.

There is evidence that the inclusion of VPA in a multidrug regimen increases the risk of serious, potentially life-threatening rash in adults. Specifically, of 584 patients administered LAMICTAL with VPA in clinical trials, 6 (1%) were hospitalized in association with rash; in contrast, 4 (0.16%) of 2,398 clinical trial patients and volunteers administered LAMICTAL in the absence of VPA were hospitalized.

Other examples of serious and potentially life-threatening rash that did not lead to hospitalization also occurred in premarketing development. Among these, one case was reported to be Stevens-Johnson–like.

Hypersensitivity Reactions: Hypersensitivity reactions, some fatal or life threatening, have also occurred. Some of these reactions have included clinical features of multiorgan failure/dysfunction, including hepatic abnormalities and evidence of disseminated intravascular coagulation. It is important to note that early manifestations of hypersensitivity (e.g., fever, lymphadenopathy) may be present even though a rash is not evident. If such signs or symptoms are present, the patient should be evaluated immediately. LAMICTAL should be discontinued if an alternative etiology for the signs or symptoms cannot be established.

Prior to initiation of treatment with LAMICTAL, the patient should be instructed that a rash or other signs or symptoms of hypersensitivity (e.g., fever, lymphadenopathy) may herald a serious medical event and that the patient should report any such occurrence to a physician immediately.

Acute Multiorgan Failure: Multiorgan failure, which in some cases has been fatal or irreversible, has been observed in patients receiving LAMICTAL. Fatalities associated with multiorgan failure and various degrees of hepatic failure have been reported in 2 of 3,796 adult patients and 4 of 2,435 pediatric patients who received LAMICTAL in clinical trials. Rare fatalities from multiorgan failure have also been reported in compassionate plea and postmarketing use. The majority of these deaths occurred in association with other serious medical events, including status epilepticus and overwhelming sepsis, and hantavirus making it difficult to identify the initial cause.

Additionally, 3 patients (a 45-year-old woman, a 3.5-year-old boy, and an 11-year-old girl) developed multiorgan dysfunction and disseminated intravascular coagulation 9 to 14 days after LAMICTAL was added to their AED regimens. Rash and elevated transaminases were also present in all patients and rhabdomyolysis was noted in 2 patients. Both pediatric patients were receiving concomitant therapy with VPA, while the adult patient was being treated with carbamazepine and clonazepam. All patients subsequently recovered with supportive care after treatment with LAMICTAL was discontinued.

Blood Dyscrasias: There have been reports of blood dyscrasias that may or may not be associated with the hypersensitivity syndrome. These have included neutropenia, leukopenia, anemia, thrombocytopenia, pancytopenia, and, rarely, aplastic anemia and pure red cell aplasia.

Withdrawal Seizures: As a rule, AEDs should not be abruptly discontinued because of the possibility of increasing seizure frequency. Unless safety concerns require a more rapid withdrawal, the dose of LAMICTAL should be tapered over a period of at least 2 weeks (see DOSAGE AND ADMINISTRATION).

PRECAUTIONS

Dermatological Events (see BOX WARNING, WARNINGS): Serious rashes associated with hospitalization and discontinuation of LAMICTAL have been reported. Rare deaths have been reported, but their numbers are too few to permit a precise estimate of the rate. There are suggestions, yet to be proven, that the risk of rash may also be increased by 1) coadministration of LAMICTAL with VPA, 2) exceeding the recommended initial dose of LAMICTAL, or 3) exceeding the recommended dose escalation for LAMICTAL. However, cases have been reported in the absence of these factors.

In clinical trials, approximately 10% of all patients exposed to LAMICTAL developed a rash. Rashes associated with LAMICTAL do not appear to have unique identifying features. Typically, rash occurs in the first 2 to 8 weeks following treatment initiation. However, isolated cases have been reported after prolonged treatment (e.g., 6 months). Accordingly, duration of therapy cannot be relied upon as a means to predict the potential risk heralded by the first appearance of a rash.

Although most rashes resolved even with continuation of treatment with LAMICTAL, it is not possible to predict reliably which rashes will prove to be serious or life threatening.

ACCORDINGLY, LAMICTAL SHOULD ORDINARILY BE DISCONTINUED AT THE FIRST SIGN OF RASH, UNLESS THE RASH IS CLEARLY NOT DRUG RELATED. DISCONTINUATION OF TREATMENT MAY NOT PREVENT A RASH FROM BECOMING LIFE THREATENING OR PERMANENTLY DISABLING OR DISFIGURING.

Sudden Unexplained Death in Epilepsy (SUDEP): During the premarketing development of LAMICTAL, 20 sudden and unexplained deaths were recorded among a cohort of 4,700 patients with epilepsy (5,747 patient-years of exposure).

Some of these could represent seizure-related deaths in which the seizure was not observed, e.g., at night. This represents an incidence of 0.0035 deaths per patient-year. Although this rate exceeds that expected in a healthy population matched for age and sex, it is within the range of estimates for the incidence of sudden unexplained deaths in patients with epilepsy not receiving LAMICTAL (ranging from 0.0005 for the general population of patients with epilepsy, to 0.004 for a recently studied clinical trial population similar to that in the clinical development program for LAMICTAL, to 0.005 for patients with refractory epilepsy). Consequently, whether these figures are reassuring or suggest concern depends on the comparability of the populations reported upon to the cohort receiving LAMICTAL and the accuracy of the estimates provided. Probably most reassuring is the similarity of estimated SUDEP rates in patients receiving LAMICTAL and those receiving another antiepileptic drug that underwent clinical testing in a similar population at about the same time. Importantly, that drug is chemically unrelated to LAMICTAL. This evidence suggests, although it certainly does not prove, that the high SUDEP rates reflect population rates, not a drug effect.

Status Epilepticus: Valid estimates of the incidence of treatment emergent status epilepticus among patients treated with LAMICTAL are difficult to obtain because reporters participating in clinical trials did not all employ identical rules for identifying cases. At a minimum, 7 of 2,343 adult patients had episodes that could unequivocally be described as status. In addition, a number of reports of variably defined episodes of seizure exacerbation (e.g., seizure clusters, seizure flurries, etc.) were made.

Addition of LAMICTAL to a Multidrug Regimen That Includes VPA (Dosage Reduction): Because VPA reduces the clearance of lamotrigine, the dosage of lamotrigine in the presence of VPA is less than half of that required in its absence (see DOSAGE AND ADMINISTRATION).

Use in Patients With Concomitant Illness: Clinical experience with LAMICTAL in patients with concomitant illness is limited. Caution is advised when using LAMICTAL in patients with diseases or conditions that could affect metabolism or elimination of the drug, such as renal, hepatic, or cardiac functional impairment.

Hepatic metabolism to the glucuronide followed by renal excretion is the principal route of elimination of lamotrigine (see CLINICAL PHARMACOLOGY).

A study in individuals with severe chronic renal failure (mean creatinine clearance = 13 mL/min) not receiving other AEDs indicated that the elimination half-life of unchanged lamotrigine is prolonged relative to individuals with normal renal function. Until adequate numbers of patients with severe renal impairment have been evaluated during chronic treatment with LAMICTAL, it should be used with caution in these patients, generally using a reduced maintenance dose for patients with significant impairment.

Because there is limited experience with the use of LAMICTAL in patients with impaired liver function, the use in such patients may be associated with as yet unrecognized risks (see CLINICAL PHARMACOLOGY and DOSAGE AND ADMINISTRATION).

Binding in the Eye and Other Melanin-Containing Tissues: Because lamotrigine binds to melanin, it could accumulate in melanin-rich tissues over time. This raises the possibility that lamotrigine may cause toxicity in these tissues after extended use. Although ophthalmological testing was performed in one controlled clinical trial, the testing was inadequate to exclude subtle effects or injury occurring after long-term exposure. Moreover, the capacity of available tests to detect potentially adverse consequences, if any, of lamotrigine's binding to melanin is unknown.

Accordingly, although there are no specific recommendations for periodic ophthalmological monitoring, prescribers should be aware of the possibility of long-term ophthalmologic effects.

Information for Patients: Prior to initiation of treatment with LAMICTAL, the patient should be instructed that a rash or other signs or symptoms of hypersensitivity (e.g., fever, lymphadenopathy) may herald a serious medical event and that the patient should report any such occurrence to a physician immediately. In addition, the patient should notify his or her physician if worsening of seizure control occurs.

Patients should be advised that LAMICTAL may cause dizziness, somnolence, and other symptoms and signs of central nervous system (CNS) depression. Accordingly, they should be advised neither to drive a car nor to operate other complex machinery until they have gained sufficient experience on LAMICTAL to gauge whether or not it adversely affects their mental and/or motor performance.

Patients should be advised to notify their physicians if they become pregnant or intend to become pregnant during therapy. Patients should be advised to notify their physicians if they intend to breast-feed or are breast-feeding an infant.

Patients should be informed of the availability of a patient information leaflet, and they should be instructed to read the leaflet prior to taking LAMICTAL. See PATIENT INFORMATION at the end of this labeling for the text of the leaflet provided for patients.

Laboratory Tests: The value of monitoring plasma concentrations of LAMICTAL has not been established. Because of the possible pharmacokinetic interactions between LAMICTAL and other AEDs being taken concomitantly (see Table 3), monitoring of the plasma levels of LAMICTAL and concomitant AEDs may be indicated, particularly during dosage adjustments. In general, clinical judgment should be exercised regarding monitoring of plasma levels of LAMICTAL and other anti-seizure drugs and whether or not dosage adjustments are necessary.

Drug Interactions: *Antiepileptic Drugs:* The use of AEDs in combination is complicated by the potential for pharmacokinetic interactions.

The interaction of lamotrigine with phenytoin, carbamazepine, and VPA has been studied. The net effects of these various AED combinations on individual AED plasma concentrations are summarized in Table 3.

Table 3. Summary of AED Interactions With LAMICTAL

AED	AED Plasma Concentration With Adjunctive LAMICTAL*	Lamotrigine Plasma Concentration With Adjunctive AEDs†
Phenytoin (PHT)	↔	↓
Carbamazepine (CBZ)	↔	↓
CBZ epoxide‡	?	
Valproic acid (VPA)	↓	↑
VPA + PHT and/or CBZ	NE	↔

*From adjunctive clinical trials and volunteer studies.
† Net effects were estimated by comparing the mean clearance values obtained in adjunctive clinical trials and volunteer studies.
‡ Not administered, but an active metabolite of carbamazepine.
↔ = No significant effect.
? = Conflicting data.
NE = Not evaluated.

Specific Effects of Lamotrigine on the Pharmacokinetics of Other AED Products: LAMICTAL Added to Phenytoin: LAMICTAL has no appreciable effect on steady-state phenytoin plasma concentration.

LAMICTAL Added to Carbamazepine: LAMICTAL has no appreciable effect on steady-state carbamazepine plasma concentration. Limited clinical data suggest there is a higher incidence of dizziness, diplopia, ataxia, and blurred vision in patients receiving carbamazepine with LAMICTAL than in patients receiving other EIAEDs with LAMICTAL (see ADVERSE REACTIONS). The mechanism of this interaction is unclear. The effect of lamotrigine on plasma concentrations of carbamazepine-epoxide is unclear. In a small subset of patients (n = 7) studied in a placebo-controlled trial, lamotrigine had no effect on carbamazepine-epoxide plasma concentrations, but in a small, uncontrolled study (n = 9), carbamazepine-epoxide levels were seen to increase.

LAMICTAL Added to VPA: When LAMICTAL was administered to 18 healthy volunteers receiving VPA in a pharmacokinetic study, the trough steady-state VPA concentrations in plasma decreased by an average of 25% over a 3-week period, and then stabilized. However, adding LAMICTAL to the existing therapy did not cause a change in plasma VPA concentrations in either adult or pediatric patients in controlled clinical trials.

Specific Effects of Other AED Products on the Pharmacokinetics of Lamotrigine: Phenytoin Added to LAMICTAL: The addition of phenytoin decreases lamotrigine steady-state concentrations by approximately 45% to 54% depending upon the total daily dose of phenytoin (i.e., from 100 to 400 mg).

Carbamazepine Added to LAMICTAL: The addition of carbamazepine decreases lamotrigine steady-state concentrations by approximately 40%.

Phenobarbital or Primidone Added to LAMICTAL: The addition of phenobarbital or primidone decreases lamotrigine steady-state concentrations by approximately 40%.

VPA Added to LAMICTAL: The addition of VPA increases lamotrigine steady-state concentrations in normal volunteers by slightly more than twofold.

Interactions With Drug Products Other Than AEDs: Folate Inhibitors: Lamotrigine is an inhibitor of dihydrofolate reductase. Prescribers should be aware of this action when prescribing other medications that inhibit folate metabolism.

Drug/Laboratory Test Interactions: None known.

Carcinogenesis, Mutagenesis, Impairment of Fertility: No evidence of carcinogenicity was seen in 1 mouse study or 2 rat studies following oral administration of lamotrigine for up to 2 years at maximum tolerated doses (30 mg/kg per day for mice and 10 to 15 mg/kg per day for rats, doses that are equivalent to 90 mg/m^2 and 60 to 90 mg/m^2, respectively). Steady-state plasma concentrations ranged from 1 to 4 mcg/mL in the mouse study and 1 to 10 mcg/mL in the rat study. Plasma concentrations associated with the recommended human doses of 300 to 500 mg/day are generally in the range of 2 to 5 mcg/mL, but concentrations as high as 19 mcg/mL have been recorded.

Lamotrigine was not mutagenic in the presence or absence of metabolic activation when tested in 2 gene mutation assays (the Ames test and the in vitro mammalian mouse lymphoma assay). In 2 cytogenetic assays (the in vitro human lymphocyte assay and the in vivo rat bone marrow assay), lamotrigine did not increase the incidence of structural or numerical chromosomal abnormalities.

No evidence of impairment of fertility was detected in rats given oral doses of lamotrigine up to 2.4 times the highest usual human maintenance dose of 8.33 mg/kg per day or 0.4 times the human dose on a mg/m^2 basis. The effect of lamotrigine on human fertility is unknown.

Pregnancy: Pregnancy Category C. No evidence of teratogenicity was found in mice, rats, or rabbits when lamotrigine was orally administered to pregnant animals during the period of organogenesis at doses up to 1.2, 0.5, and 1.1 times, respectively, on a mg/m^2 basis, the highest usual human maintenance dose (i.e., 500 mg/day). However, maternal toxicity and secondary fetal toxicity producing reduced fetal weight and/or delayed ossification were seen in mice and rats, but not in rabbits at these doses. Teratology studies were also conducted using bolus intravenous administration of the isethionate salt of lamotrigine in rats and rabbits. In rat dams administered an intravenous dose at 0.6 times the highest usual human maintenance dose, the incidence of intrauterine death without signs of teratogenicity was increased.

A behavioral teratology study was conducted in rats dosed during the period of organogenesis. At day 21 postpartum, offspring of dams receiving 5 mg/kg per day or higher displayed a significantly longer latent period for open field exploration and a lower frequency of rearing. In a swimming maze test performed on days 39 to 44 postpartum, time to completion was increased in offspring of dams receiving 25 mg/kg per day. These doses represent 0.1 and 0.5 times the clinical dose on a mg/m^2 basis, respectively.

Lamotrigine did not affect fertility, teratogenesis, or postnatal development when rats were dosed prior to and during mating, and throughout gestation and lactation at doses equivalent to 0.4 times the highest usual human maintenance dose on a mg/m^2 basis.

When pregnant rats were orally dosed at 0.1, 0.14, or 0.3 times the highest human maintenance dose (on a mg/m^2 basis) during the latter part of gestation (days 15 to 20), maternal toxicity and fetal death were seen. In dams, food consumption and weight gain were reduced, and the gestation period was slightly prolonged (22.6 vs. 22.0 days in the control group). Stillborn pups were found in all 3 drug-treated groups with the highest number in the high-dose group. Postnatal death was also seen, but only in the 2 highest doses, and occurred between day 1 and 20. Some of these deaths appear to be drug-related and not secondary to the maternal toxicity. A no-observed-effect level (NOEL) could not be determined for this study.

Although LAMICTAL was not found to be teratogenic in the above studies, lamotrigine decreases fetal folate concentrations in rats, an effect known to be associated with teratogenesis in animals and humans. There are no adequate and

Continued on next page

Lamictal—Cont.

well-controlled studies in pregnant women. Because animal reproduction studies are not always predictive of human response, this drug should be used during pregnancy only if the potential benefit justifies the potential risk to the fetus.

Pregnancy Exposure Registry: To facilitate monitoring fetal outcomes of pregnant women exposed to lamotrigine, physicians are encouraged to register patients, **before fetal outcome (e.g., ultrasound, results of amniocentesis, birth, etc.) is known**, and can obtain information by calling the Lamotrigine Pregnancy Registry at (800) 336-2176 (toll-free). Patients can enroll themselves in the North American Antiepileptic Drug Pregnancy Registry by calling (888) 233-2334 (toll free).

Labor and Delivery: The effect of LAMICTAL on labor and delivery in humans is unknown.

Use in Nursing Mothers: Preliminary data indicate that lamotrigine passes into human milk. Because the effects on the infant exposed to LAMICTAL by this route are unknown, breast-feeding while taking LAMICTAL is not recommended.

Pediatric Use: LAMICTAL is indicated as adjunctive therapy for partial seizures in patients above 2 years of age and for the generalized seizures of Lennox-Gastaut syndrome. Safety and effectiveness for other uses in patients below the age of 16 years have not been established (see BOX WARNING).

Geriatric Use: Clinical studies of LAMICTAL did not include sufficient numbers of subjects aged 65 and over to determine whether they respond differently from younger subjects. In general, dose selection for an elderly patient should be cautious, usually starting at the low end of the dosing range, reflecting the greater frequency of decreased hepatic, renal, or cardiac function, and of concomitant disease or other drug therapy.

ADVERSE REACTIONS

SERIOUS RASH REQUIRING HOSPITALIZATION AND DISCONTINUATION OF LAMICTAL, INCLUDING STEVENS-JOHNSON SYNDROME AND TOXIC EPIDERMAL NECROLYSIS, HAVE OCCURRED IN ASSOCIATION WITH THERAPY WITH LAMICTAL. RARE DEATHS HAVE BEEN REPORTED, BUT THEIR NUMBERS ARE TOO FEW TO PERMIT A PRECISE ESTIMATE OF THE RATE (see BOX WARNING).

Most Common Adverse Events in All Clinical Studies: *Adjunctive Therapy in Adults:* The most commonly observed (≥5%) adverse experiences seen in association with LAMICTAL during adjunctive therapy in adults and not seen at an equivalent frequency among placebo-treated patients were: dizziness, ataxia, somnolence, headache, diplopia, blurred vision, nausea, vomiting, and rash. Dizziness, diplopia, ataxia, blurred vision, nausea, and vomiting were dose related. Dizziness, diplopia, ataxia, and blurred vision occurred more commonly in patients receiving carbamazepine with LAMICTAL than in patients receiving other EIAEDs with LAMICTAL. Clinical data suggest a higher incidence of rash, including serious rash, in patients receiving concomitant VPA than in patients not receiving VPA (see WARNINGS).

Approximately 11% of the 3,378 adult patients who received LAMICTAL as adjunctive therapy in premarketing clinical trials discontinued treatment because of an adverse experience. The adverse events most commonly associated with discontinuation were rash (3.0%), dizziness (2.8%), and headache (2.5%).

In a dose response study in adults, the rate of discontinuation of LAMICTAL for dizziness, ataxia, diplopia, blurred vision, nausea, and vomiting was dose related.

Monotherapy in Adults: The most commonly observed (≥5%) adverse experiences seen in association with the use of LAMICTAL during the monotherapy phase of the controlled trial in adults not seen at an equivalent rate in the control group were vomiting, coordination abnormality, dyspepsia, nausea, dizziness, rhinitis, anxiety, insomnia, infection, pain, weight decrease, chest pain, and dysmenorrhea. The most commonly observed (≥5%) adverse experiences associated with the use of LAMICTAL during the conversion to monotherapy (add-on) period, not seen at an equivalent frequency among low-dose valproate-treated patients, were dizziness, headache, nausea, asthenia, coordination abnormality, vomiting, rash, somnolence, diplopia, ataxia, accidental injury, tremor, blurred vision, insomnia, nystagmus, diarrhea, lymphadenopathy, pruritus, and sinusitis.

Approximately 10% of the 420 adult patients who received LAMICTAL as monotherapy in premarketing clinical trials discontinued treatment because of an adverse experience. The adverse events most commonly associated with discontinuation were rash (4.5%), headache (3.1%), and asthenia (2.4%).

Adjunctive Therapy in Pediatric Patients: The most commonly observed (≥5%) adverse experiences seen in association with the use of LAMICTAL as adjunctive treatment in pediatric patients and not seen at an equivalent rate in the control group were infection, vomiting, rash, fever, somnolence, accidental injury, dizziness, diarrhea, abdominal pain, nausea, ataxia, tremor, asthenia, bronchitis, flu syndrome, and diplopia.

In 339 patients age 2 to 16 years, 4.2% of patients on LAMICTAL and 2.9% of patients on placebo discontinued due to adverse experiences. The most commonly reported adverse experiences that led to discontinuation were rash for patients treated with LAMICTAL and deterioration of seizure control for patients treated with placebo.

Approximately 11.5% of the 1,081 pediatric patients who received LAMICTAL as adjunctive therapy in premarketing clinical trials discontinued treatment because of an adverse experience. The adverse events most commonly associated with discontinuation were rash (4.4%), reaction aggravated (1.7%), and ataxia (0.6%).

Incidence in Controlled Clinical Studies: The prescriber should be aware that the figures in Tables 4, 5, 6, and 7 cannot be used to predict the frequency of adverse experiences in the course of usual medical practice where patient characteristics and other factors may differ from those prevailing during clinical studies. Similarly, the cited frequencies cannot be directly compared with figures obtained from other clinical investigations involving different treatments, uses, or investigators. An inspection of these frequencies, however, does provide the prescriber with one basis to estimate the relative contribution of drug and nondrug factors to the adverse event incidences in the population studied.

Incidence in Controlled Adjunctive Clinical Studies in Adults: Table 4 lists treatment-emergent signs and symptoms that occurred in at least 2% of adult patients with epilepsy treated with LAMICTAL in placebo-controlled trials and were numerically more common in the patients treated with LAMICTAL. In these studies, either LAMICTAL or placebo was added to the patient's current AED therapy. Adverse events were usually mild to moderate in intensity.

Table 4. Treatment-Emergent Adverse Event Incidence in Placebo-Controlled Adjunctive Trials in Adults* (Events in at least 2% of patients treated with LAMICTAL and numerically more frequent than in the placebo group.)

Body System/ Adverse Experience†	Percent of Patients Receiving Adjunctive LAMICTAL (n = 711)	Percent of Patients Receiving Adjunctive Placebo (n = 419)
Body as a whole		
Headache	29	19
Flu syndrome	7	6
Fever	6	4
Abdominal pain	5	4
Neck pain	2	1
Reaction aggravated (seizure exacerbation)	2	1
Digestive		
Nausea	19	10
Vomiting	9	4
Diarrhea	6	4
Dyspepsia	5	2
Constipation	4	3
Tooth disorder	3	2
Anorexia	2	1
Musculoskeletal		
Arthralgia	2	0
Nervous		
Dizziness	38	13
Ataxia	22	6
Somnolence	14	7
Incoordination	6	2
Insomnia	6	2
Tremor	4	1
Depression	4	3
Anxiety	4	3
Convulsion	3	1
Irritability	3	2
Speech disorder	3	0
Concentration disturbance	2	1
Respiratory		
Rhinitis	14	9
Pharyngitis	10	9
Cough increased	8	6
Skin and appendages		
Rash	10	5
Pruritus	3	2
Special Senses		
Diplopia	28	7
Blurred vision	16	5
Vision abnormality	3	1
Urogenital		
Female patients only	(n = 365)	(n = 207)
Dysmenorrhea	7	6
Vaginitis	4	1
Amenorrhea	2	1

*Patients in these adjunctive studies were receiving 1 to 3 concomitant EIAEDs in addition to LAMICTAL or placebo. Patients may have reported multiple adverse experiences during the study or at discontinuation; thus, patients may be included in more than one category.
†Adverse experiences reported by at least 2% of patients treated with LAMICTAL are included.

In a randomized, parallel study comparing placebo and 300 and 500 mg/day of LAMICTAL, some of the more common drug-related adverse events were dose related (see Table 5).

Table 5. Dose-Related Adverse Events From a Randomized, Placebo-Controlled Trial in Adults

Adverse Experience	Percent of Patients Experiencing Adverse Experiences		
	Placebo (n = 73)	LAMICTAL 300 mg (n = 71)	LAMICTAL 500 mg (n = 72)
Ataxia	10	10	28*†
Blurred vision	10	11	25*†
Diplopia	8	24*	49*†
Dizziness	27	31	54*†
Nausea	11	18	25*
Vomiting	4	11	18*

*Significantly greater than placebo group ($P<0.05$).
†Significantly greater than group receiving LAMICTAL 300 mg ($P<0.05$).

Other events that occurred in more than 1% of patients but equally or more frequently in the placebo group included: asthenia, back pain, chest pain, flatulence, menstrual disorder, myalgia, paresthesia, respiratory disorder, and urinary tract infection.

The overall adverse experience profile for LAMICTAL was similar between females and males, and was independent of age. Because the largest non-Caucasian racial subgroup was only 6% of patients exposed to LAMICTAL in placebo-controlled trials, there are insufficient data to support a statement regarding the distribution of adverse experience reports by race. Generally, females receiving either adjunctive LAMICTAL or placebo were more likely to report adverse experiences than males. The only adverse experience for which the reports on LAMICTAL were greater than 10% more frequent in females than males (without a corresponding difference by gender on placebo) was dizziness (difference = 16.5%). There was little difference between females and males in the rates of discontinuation of LAMICTAL for individual adverse experiences.

Incidence in a Controlled Monotherapy Trial in Adults With Partial Seizures: Table 6 lists treatment-emergent signs and symptoms that occurred in at least 2% of patients with epilepsy treated with monotherapy with LAMICTAL in a double-blind trial following discontinuation of either concomitant carbamazepine or phenytoin not seen at an equivalent frequency in the control group.

Table 6. Treatment-Emergent Adverse Event Incidence in Adults in a Controlled Monotherapy Trial* (Events in at least 2% of patients treated with LAMICTAL and numerically more frequent than in the valproate [VPA] group.)

Body System/ Adverse Experience†	Percent of Patients Receiving LAMICTAL Monotherapy‡ (n = 43)	Percent of Patients Receiving Low-Dose VPA§ Monotherapy (n = 44)
Body as a whole		
Pain	5	0
Infection	5	2
Chest pain	5	2
Asthenia	2	0
Fever	2	0
Digestive		
Vomiting	9	0
Dyspepsia	7	2
Nausea	7	2
Anorexia	2	0
Dry mouth	2	0
Rectal hemorrhage	2	0
Peptic ulcer	2	0
Metabolic and nutritional		
Weight decrease	5	2
Peripheral edema	2	0
Nervous		
Coordination abnormality	7	0
Dizziness	7	0
Anxiety	5	0
Insomnia	5	2
Amnesia	2	0
Ataxia	2	0
Depression	2	0
Hypesthesia	2	0
Libido increase	2	0
Decreased reflexes	2	0
Increased reflexes	2	0
Nystagmus	2	0
Irritability	2	0
Suicidal ideation	2	0
Respiratory		
Rhinitis	7	2
Epistaxis	2	0
Bronchitis	2	0
Dyspnea	2	0

Skin and appendages		
Contact dermatitis	2	0
Dry skin	2	0
Sweating	2	0
Special senses		
Vision abnormality	2	0
Urogenital (female patients only)	(n = 21)	(n = 28)
Dysmenorrhea	5	0

* Patients in these studies were converted to LAMICTAL or VPA monotherapy from adjunctive therapy with carbamazepine or phenytoin. Patients may have reported multiple adverse experiences during the study; thus, patients may be included in more than one category.
† Adverse experiences reported by at least 2% of patients are included.
‡ Up to 500 mg/day.
§ 1,000 mg/day.

Incidence in Controlled Adjunctive Trials in Pediatric Patients: Table 7 lists adverse events that occurred in at least 2% of 339 pediatric patients who received LAMICTAL up to 15 mg/kg per day or a maximum of 750 mg per day. Reported adverse events were classified using COSTART terminology.

Table 7. Treatment-Emergent Adverse Event Incidence in Placebo-Controlled Adjunctive Trials in Pediatric Patients (Events in at least 2% of patients treated with LAMICTAL and numerically more frequent than in the placebo group.)

Body System/ Adverse Experience	Percent of Patients Receiving LAMICTAL (n = 168)	Percent of Patients Receiving Placebo (n = 171)
Body as a whole		
Infection	20	17
Fever	15	14
Accidental injury	14	12
Abdominal pain	10	5
Asthenia	8	4
Flu syndrome	7	6
Pain	5	4
Facial edema	2	1
Photosensitivity	2	0
Cardiovascular		
Hemorrhage	2	1
Digestive		
Vomiting	20	16
Diarrhea	11	9
Nausea	10	2
Constipation	4	2
Dyspepsia	2	1
Tooth Disorder	2	1
Hemic and lymphatic		
Lymphadenopathy	2	1
Metabolic and nutritional		
Edema	2	0
Nervous system		
Somnolence	17	15
Dizziness	14	4
Ataxia	11	3
Tremor	10	1
Emotional lability	4	2
Gait abnormality	4	2
Thinking abnormality	3	2
Convulsions	2	1
Nervousness	2	1
Vertigo	2	1
Respiratory		
Pharyngitis	14	11
Bronchitis	7	5
Increased cough	7	6
Sinusitis	2	1
Bronchospasm	2	1
Skin		
Rash	14	12
Eczema	2	1
Pruritus	2	1
Special senses		
Diplopia	5	1
Blurred vision	4	1
Ear disorder	2	1
Visual abnormality	2	0
Urogenital		
Male and female patients		
Urinary tract infection	3	0
Male patients only	n = 93	n = 92
Penis disorder	2	0

Other Adverse Events Observed During All Clinical Trials For Adult and Pediatric Patients: LAMICTAL has been administered to 3,923 individuals for whom complete adverse event data was captured during all clinical trials, only some of which were placebo controlled. During these trials, all adverse events were recorded by the clinical investigators using terminology of their own choosing. To provide a meaningful estimate of the proportion of individuals having adverse events, similar types of events were grouped into a smaller number of standardized categories using modified COSTART dictionary terminology. The frequencies presented represent the proportion of the 3,923 individuals exposed to LAMICTAL who experienced an event of the type cited on at least one occasion while receiving LAMICTAL. All reported events are included except those already listed in the previous table, those too general to be informative, and those not reasonably associated with the use of the drug.

Events are further classified within body system categories and enumerated in order of decreasing frequency using the following definitions: *frequent* adverse events are defined as those occurring in at least 1/100 patients; *infrequent* adverse events are those occurring in 1/100 to 1/1,000 patients; *rare* adverse events are those occurring in fewer than 1/1,000 patients.

Body as a Whole: Frequent: Pain. *Infrequent:* Accidental injury, allergic reaction, back pain, chills, face edema, halitosis, infection, and malaise. *Rare:* Abdomen enlarged, abscess, photosensitivity, and suicide attempt.
Cardiovascular System: Infrequent: Flushing, hot flashes, migraine, palpitations, postural hypotension, syncope, tachycardia, and vasodilation. *Rare:* Angina pectoris, atrial fibrillation, deep thrombophlebitis, hemorrhage, hypertension, and myocardial infarction.
Dermatological: Infrequent: Acne, alopecia, dry skin, erythema, hirsutism, maculopapular rash, skin discoloration, Stevens-Johnson syndrome, sweating, urticaria, and vesiculobullous rash. *Rare:* Angioedema, erythema multiforme, fungal dermatitis, herpes zoster, leukoderma, petechial rash, pustular rash, and seborrhea.
Digestive System: Infrequent: Dry mouth, dysphagia, gingivitis, glossitis, gum hyperplasia, increased appetite, increased salivation, liver function tests abnormal, mouth ulceration, stomatitis, thirst, and tooth disorder. *Rare:* Eructation, gastritis, gastrointestinal hemorrhage, gum hemorrhage, hematemesis, hemorrhagic colitis, hepatitis, melena, stomach ulcer, and tongue edema.
Endocrine System: Rare: Goiter and hypothyroidism.
Hematologic and Lymphatic System: Infrequent: Anemia, ecchymosis, leukocytosis, leukopenia, lymphadenopathy, and petechia. *Rare:* Eosinophilia, fibrin decrease, fibrinogen decrease, iron deficiency anemia, lymphocytosis, macrocytic anemia, and thrombocytopenia.
Metabolic and Nutritional Disorders: Infrequent: Peripheral edema, weight gain, and weight loss. *Rare:* Alcohol intolerance, alkaline phosphatase increase, bilirubinemia, general edema, and hyperglycemia.
Musculoskeletal System: Infrequent: Joint disorder, myasthenia, and twitching. *Rare:* Arthritis, bursitis, leg cramps, pathological fracture, and tendinous contracture.
Nervous System: Frequent: Amnesia, confusion, hostility, memory decrease, nervousness, nystagmus, thinking abnormality, and vertigo. *Infrequent:* Abnormal dreams, abnormal gait, agitation, akathisia, apathy, aphasia, CNS depression, depersonalization, dysarthria, dyskinesia, dysphoria, emotional lability, euphoria, faintness, grand mal convulsions, hallucinations, hyperkinesia, hypertonia, hypesthesia, libido increased, mind racing, muscle spasm, myoclonus, panic attack, paranoid reaction, personality disorder, psychosis, sleep disorder, and stupor. *Rare:* Cerebrovascular accident, cerebellar syndrome, cerebral sinus thrombosis, choreoathetosis, CNS stimulation, delirium, delusions, dystonia, hemiplegia, hyperalgesia, hyperesthesia, hypoesthesia, hypokinesia, hypomania, hypotonia, libido decreased, manic depression reaction, movement disorder, neuralgia, neurosis, paralysis, and suicidal ideation.
Respiratory System: Infrequent: Dyspnea, epistaxis, and hyperventilation. *Rare:* Bronchospasm, hiccup, and sinusitis.
Special Senses: Infrequent: Abnormality of accommodation, conjunctivitis, ear pain, oscillopsia, photophobia, taste perversion, and tinnitus. *Rare:* Deafness, dry eyes, lacrimation disorder, parosmia, ptosis, strabismus, taste loss, and uveitis.
Urogenital System: Infrequent: Female lactation, hematuria, polyuria, urinary frequency, urinary incontinence, urinary retention, and vaginal moniliasis. *Rare:* Abnormal ejaculation, acute kidney failure, breast abscess, breast neoplasm, breast pain, creatinine increase, cystitis, dysuria, epididymitis, impotence, kidney failure, kidney pain, menorrhagia, and urine abnormality.

Postmarketing and Other Experience: In addition to the adverse experiences reported during clinical testing of LAMICTAL, the following adverse experiences have been reported in patients receiving marketed LAMICTAL and from worldwide noncontrolled investigational use. These adverse experiences have not been listed above, and data are insufficient to support an estimate of their incidence or to establish causation.

Blood and Lymphatic: Agranulocytosis, aplastic anemia, disseminated intravascular coagulation, hemolytic anemia, neutropenia, pancytopenia, red cell aplasia.
Gastrointestinal: Esophagitis.
Hepatobiliary Tract and Pancreas: Pancreatitis.
Immunologic: Lupus-like reaction, vasculitis.
Lower Respiratory: Apnea.
Musculoskeletal: Rhabdomyolysis has been observed in patients experiencing hypersensitivity reactions.
Neurology: Exacerbation of parkinsonian symptoms in patients with pre-existing Parkinson's disease, tics.
Non-site Specific: Hypersensitivity reaction, multiorgan failure, progressive immunosuppression.

DRUG ABUSE AND DEPENDENCE

The abuse and dependence potential of LAMICTAL have not been evaluated in human studies.

OVERDOSAGE

Human Overdose Experience: Overdoses involving quantities up to 15 g have been reported for LAMICTAL, some of which have been fatal. Overdose has resulted in ataxia, nystagmus, increased seizures, decreased level of consciousness, coma, and intraventricular conduction delay.

Management of Overdose: There are no specific antidotes for LAMICTAL. Following a suspected overdose, hospitalization of the patient is advised. General supportive care is indicated, including frequent monitoring of vital signs and close observation of the patient. If indicated, emesis should be induced or gastric lavage should be performed; usual precautions should be taken to protect the airway. It should be kept in mind that lamotrigine is rapidly absorbed (see CLINICAL PHARMACOLOGY). It is uncertain whether hemodialysis is an effective means of removing lamotrigine from the blood. In 6 renal failure patients, about 20% of the amount of lamotrigine in the body was removed by hemodialysis during a 4-hour session. A Poison Control Center should be contacted for information on the management of overdosage of LAMICTAL.

DOSAGE AND ADMINISTRATION

Adjunctive Use: LAMICTAL is indicated as adjunctive therapy for partial seizures in adults and pediatric patients (≥2 years of age). LAMICTAL is also indicated as adjunctive therapy for the generalized seizures of Lennox-Gastaut syndrome in adult and pediatric patients (≥2 years of age).

Monotherapy Use: LAMICTAL is indicated for conversion to monotherapy in adults with partial seizures who are receiving treatment with a single EIAED (e.g., carbamazepine, phenytoin, phenobarbital, etc.).

Safety and effectiveness of LAMICTAL have not been established 1) as initial monotherapy, 2) for conversion to monotherapy from non–enzyme-inducing AEDs (e.g., valproate), or 3) for simultaneous conversion to monotherapy from 2 or more concomitant AEDs.

Safety and effectiveness in pediatric patients below the age of 16 years other than those with partial seizures and the generalized seizures of Lennox-Gastaut syndrome have not been established (see BOX WARNING).

General Dosing Considerations: The risk of nonserious rash is increased when the recommended initial dose and/or the rate of dose escalation of LAMICTAL is exceeded. There are suggestions, yet to be proven, that the risk of severe, potentially life-threatening rash may be increased by 1) coadministration of LAMICTAL with valproic acid (VPA), 2) exceeding the recommended initial dose of LAMICTAL, or 3) exceeding the recommended dose escalation for LAMICTAL. However, cases have been reported in the absence of these factors (see BOX WARNING). Therefore, it is important that the dosing recommendations be followed closely.

Adjunctive Therapy With LAMICTAL: This section provides specific dosing recommendations for patients 2 to 12 years of age and patients greater than 12 years of age. Within each of these age-groups, specific dosing recommendations are provided depending upon whether or not the patient is receiving VPA (Tables 8 and 9 for patients 2 to 12 years of age, Tables 10 and 11 for patients greater than 12 years of age). In addition, the section provides a discussion of dosing for those patients receiving concomitant AEDs that have not been systematically evaluated in combination with LAMICTAL.

For dosing guidelines for LAMICTAL below, enzyme-inducing antiepileptic drugs (EIAEDs) include phenytoin, carbamazepine, phenobarbital, and primidone.

Patients 2 to 12 Years of Age: Recommended dosing guidelines for LAMICTAL added to an antiepileptic drug (AED) regimen containing VPA are summarized in Table 8. Recommended dosing guidelines for LAMICTAL added to EIAEDs are summarized in Table 9.

LAMICTAL Added to AEDs Other Than EIAEDs and VPA: The effect of AEDs other than EIAEDs and VPA on the metabolism of LAMICTAL is not currently known. Therefore, no specific dosing guidelines can be provided in that situation. Conservative starting doses and dose escalations (as with concomitant VPA) would be prudent; maintenance dosing would be expected to fall between the maintenance dose with VPA and the maintenance dose without VPA, but with an EIAED.

Note that the starting doses and dose escalations listed in Tables 8 and 9 are different than those used in clinical trials; however, the maintenance doses are the same as in clinical trials. Smaller starting doses and slower dose escalations than those used in clinical trials are recommended

Continued on next page

Lamictal—Cont.

because of the suggestions that the risk of rash may be decreased by smaller starting doses and slower dose escalations. Therefore, maintenance doses will take longer to reach in clinical practice than in clinical trials. It may take several weeks to months to achieve an individualized maintenance dose. Maintenance doses in patients weighing less than 30 kg, regardless of age or concomitant AED, may need to be increased as much as 50%, based on clinical response. **The smallest available strength of LAMICTAL Chewable Dispersible Tablets is 2 mg, and only whole tablets should be administered. If the calculated dose cannot be achieved using whole tablets, the dose should be rounded down to the nearest whole tablet (see HOW SUPPLIED and PATIENT INFORMATION for a description of the LAMICTAL Chewable Dispersible Tablet available sizes).**
[See table 8 at right]

Table 9. LAMICTAL Added to EIAEDs (Without VPA) in Patients 2 to 12 Years of Age

Weeks 1 and 2	0.6 mg/kg/day in 2 divided doses, rounded down to the nearest whole tablet.
Weeks 3 and 4	1.2 mg/kg/day in 2 divided doses, rounded down to the nearest whole tablet.

Usual maintenance dose: 5 to 15 mg/kg/day (maximum 400 mg/day in 2 divided doses). To achieve the usual maintenance dose, subsequent doses should be increased every 1 to 2 weeks as follows: calculate 1.2 mg/kg/day, round this amount down to the nearest whole tablet, and add this amount to the previously administered daily dose. Maintenance doses in patients weighing less than 30 kg may need to be increased by as much as 50%, based on clinical response.

Patients Over 12 Years of Age: Recommended dosing guidelines for LAMICTAL added to VPA are summarized in Table 10. Recommended dosing guidelines for LAMICTAL added to EIAEDs are summarized in Table 11.

LAMICTAL Added to AEDs Other Than EIAEDs and VPA: The effect of AEDs other than EIAEDs and VPA on the metabolism of LAMICTAL is not currently known. Therefore, no specific dosing guidelines can be provided in that situation. Conservative starting doses and dose escalations (as with concomitant VPA) would be prudent; maintenance dosing would be expected to fall between the maintenance dose with VPA and the maintenance dose without VPA, but with an EIAED.

Table 10. LAMICTAL Added to an AED Regimen Containing VPA in Patients Over 12 Years of Age

Weeks 1 and 2	25 mg every *other* day
Weeks 3 and 4	25 mg every day

Usual maintenance dose: 100 to 400 mg/day (1 or 2 divided doses). To achieve maintenance, doses may be increased by 25 to 50 mg/day every 1 to 2 weeks. The usual maintenance dose in patients adding LAMICTAL to VPA alone ranges from 100 to 200 mg/day.

Table 11. LAMICTAL Added to EIAEDs (Without VPA) in Patients Over 12 Years of Age

Weeks 1 and 2	50 mg/day
Weeks 3 and 4	100 mg/day in 2 divided doses

Usual maintenance dose: 300 to 500 mg/day (in 2 divided doses). To achieve maintenance, doses may be increased by 100 mg/day every 1 to 2 weeks.

Conversion From a Single EIAED to Monotherapy With LAMICTAL in Patients ≥16 Years of Age: The goal of the transition regimen is to effect the conversion to monotherapy with LAMICTAL under conditions that ensure adequate seizure control while mitigating the risk of serious rash associated with the rapid titration of LAMICTAL.
The conversion regimen involves 2 steps. In the first, LAMICTAL is titrated to the targeted dose while maintaining the dose of the EIAED at a fixed level; in the second step, the EIAED is gradually withdrawn over a period of 4 weeks.
The recommended maintenance dose of LAMICTAL as monotherapy is 500 mg/day given in 2 divided doses.
LAMICTAL should be added to an EIAED to achieve a dose of 500 mg/day according to the guidelines in Table 11 above. The regimen for the withdrawal of the concomitant EIAED is based on experience gained in the controlled monotherapy clinical trial. In that trial, the concomitant EIAED was withdrawn by 20% decrements each week over a 4-week period.
Because of an increased risk of rash, the recommended initial dose and subsequent dose escalations of LAMICTAL should not be exceeded (see BOX WARNING).
Usual Maintenance Dose: The usual maintenance doses identified in the tables above are derived from dosing regimens employed in the placebo-controlled adjunctive studies in which the efficacy of LAMICTAL was established. In patients receiving multidrug regimens employing EIAEDs **without VPA**, maintenance doses of adjunctive LAMICTAL as high as 700 mg/day have been used. In patients receiving **VPA alone**, maintenance doses of adjunctive LAMICTAL as high as 200 mg/day have been used. The advantage of using doses above those recommended in the tables above has not been established in controlled trials.

Patients With Hepatic Impairment: Experience in patients with hepatic impairment is limited. Based on a clinical pharmacology study in 24 patients with moderate to severe liver dysfunction (see CLINICAL PHARMACOLOGY), the following general recommendations can be made. Initial, escalation, and maintenance doses should generally be reduced by approximately 50% in patients with moderate (Child-Pugh Grade B) and 75% in patients with severe (Child-Pugh Grade C) hepatic impairment. Escalation and maintenance doses should be adjusted according to clinical response.

Patients With Renal Functional Impairment: Initial doses of LAMICTAL should be based on patients' AED regimen (see above); reduced maintenance doses may be effective for patients with significant renal functional impairment (see CLINICAL PHARMACOLOGY). Few patients with severe renal impairment have been evaluated during chronic treatment with LAMICTAL. Because there is inadequate experience in this population, LAMICTAL should be used with caution in these patients.

Discontinuation Strategy: For patients receiving LAMICTAL in combination with other AEDs, a reevaluation of all AEDs in the regimen should be considered if a change in seizure control or an appearance or worsening of adverse experiences is observed.
If a decision is made to discontinue therapy with LAMICTAL, a step-wise reduction of dose over at least 2 weeks (approximately 50% per week) is recommended unless safety concerns require a more rapid withdrawal (see PRECAUTIONS).
Discontinuing an EIAED should prolong the half-life of lamotrigine; discontinuing VPA should shorten the half-life of lamotrigine.

Target Plasma Levels: A therapeutic plasma concentration range has not been established for lamotrigine. Dosing of LAMICTAL should be based on therapeutic response.

Administration of LAMICTAL Chewable Dispersible Tablets: LAMICTAL Chewable Dispersible Tablets may be swallowed whole, chewed, or dispersed in water or diluted fruit juice. If the tablets are chewed, consume a small amount of water or diluted fruit juice to aid in swallowing.
To disperse LAMICTAL Chewable Dispersible Tablets, add the tablets to a small amount of liquid (1 teaspoon, or enough to cover the medication). Approximately 1 minute later, when the tablets are completely dispersed, swirl the solution and consume the entire quantity immediately. *No attempt should be made to administer partial quantities of the dispersed tablets.*

HOW SUPPLIED
LAMICTAL Tablets, 25-mg, white, scored, shield-shaped tablets debossed with "LAMICTAL" and "25", bottles of 100 (NDC 0173-0633-02).
Store at 25°C (77°F); excursions permitted to 15–30°C (59–86°F) [see USP Controlled Room Temperature] in a dry place.
LAMICTAL Tablets, 100-mg, peach, scored, shield-shaped tablets debossed with "LAMICTAL" and "100", bottles of 100 (NDC 0173-0642-55).
LAMICTAL Tablets, 150-mg, cream, scored, shield-shaped tablets debossed with "LAMICTAL" and "150", bottles of 60 (NDC 0173-0643-60).
LAMICTAL Tablets, 200-mg, blue, scored, shield-shaped tablets debossed with "LAMICTAL" and "200", bottles of 60 (NDC 0173-0644-60).
Store at 25°C (77°F); excursions permitted to 15–30°C (59–86°F) [see USP Controlled Room Temperature] in a dry place and protect from light.

Table 8. LAMICTAL Added to an AED Regimen Containing VPA in Patients 2 to 12 Years of Age

Weeks 1 and 2	0.15 mg/kg/day in 1 or 2 divided doses, rounded down to the nearest whole tablet. Only whole tablets should be used for dosing.
Weeks 3 and 4	0.3 mg/kg/day in 1 or 2 divided doses, rounded down to the nearest whole tablet.

Weight based dosing can be achieved by using the following guide:

If the patient's weight is		Give this daily dose, using the most appropriate combination of Lamictal 2 mg and 5 mg tablets.	
Greater than	And less than	Weeks 1 and 2	Weeks 3 and 4
6.7 kg	14 kg	2 mg every *other* day	2 mg every day
14.1 kg	27 kg	2 mg every day	4 mg every day
27.1 kg	34 kg	4 mg every day	8 mg every day
34.1 kg	40 kg	5 mg every day	10 mg every day

Usual maintenance dose: 1 to 5 mg/kg/day (maximum 200 mg/day in 1 or 2 divided doses). To achieve the usual maintenance dose, subsequent doses should be increased every 1 to 2 weeks as follows: calculate 0.3 mg/kg/day, round this amount down to the nearest whole tablet, and add this amount to the previously administered daily dose. The usual maintenance dose in patients adding LAMICTAL to VPA alone ranges from 1 to 3 mg/kg/day. Maintenance doses in patients weighing less than 30 kg may need to be increased by as much as 50%, based on clinical response.

LAMICTAL Chewable Dispersible Tablets, 2-mg, white to off-white, round tablets debossed with "LTG" over "2", bottles of 30 (NDC 0173-0699-00). ORDER DIRECTLY FROM GlaxoSmithKline 1-800-334-4153.
LAMICTAL Chewable Dispersible Tablets, 5-mg, white to off-white, caplet-shaped tablets debossed with "GX CL2", bottles of 100 (NDC 0173-0526-00).
LAMICTAL Chewable Dispersible Tablets, 25-mg, white, super elliptical-shaped tablets debossed with "GX CL5", bottles of 100 (NDC 0173-0527-00).
Store at 25°C (77°F); excursions permitted to 15–30°C (59–86°F) [see USP Controlled Room Temperature] in a dry place.

PATIENT INFORMATION
The following wording is contained in a separate leaflet provided for patients.

Information for the Patient
LAMICTAL® (lamotrigine) Tablets

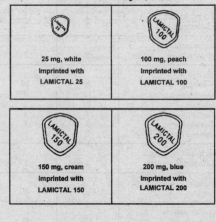

LAMICTAL® (lamotrigine)
Chewable Dispersible Tablets

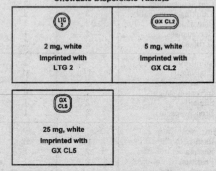

NOTE: The pictures above show actual tablet shape and size and the wording describes the color and printing that is on each strength of LAMICTAL Tablets and Chewable Dispersible Tablets. **Before taking your medicine, it is important to compare the tablets you receive from your doctor or pharmacist with these pictures to make sure you have received the correct medicine.**
Please read this leaflet carefully before you take LAMICTAL and read the leaflet provided with any refill, in case any information has changed. This leaflet provides a summary of the information about your medicine. Please do not throw away this leaflet until you have finished your

medicine. This leaflet does not contain all the information about LAMICTAL and is not meant to take the place of talking with your doctor. If you have any questions about LAMICTAL, ask your doctor or pharmacist.

Information About Your Medicine:
The name of your medicine is LAMICTAL (lamotrigine). The decision to use LAMICTAL is one that you and your doctor should make together.

1. The Purpose of Your Medicine:
Lamotrigine is intended to be used either alone or in combination with other medicines to treat seizures in people age 2 years or older. When taking lamotrigine, it is important to follow your doctor's instructions.

2. Who Should Not Take LAMICTAL:
You should not take LAMICTAL if you had an allergic reaction to it in the past.

3. Side Effects to Watch for:

- Most people who take LAMICTAL tolerate it well. The most common side effects with LAMICTAL are dizziness, headache, blurred or double vision, lack of coordination, sleepiness, nausea, vomiting, and rash.
- Although most patients who develop rash while receiving LAMICTAL have mild to moderate symptoms, some individuals may develop a serious skin reaction that requires hospitalization. Rarely, deaths have been reported. These serious skin reactions are most likely to happen within the first 8 weeks of treatment with LAMICTAL. Serious skin reactions occur more often in children than in adults.
- Rashes may be more likely to occur if you: 1) take LAMICTAL in combination with valproic acid (DEPAKENE® or DEPAKOTE®), 2) take a higher starting dose of LAMICTAL than your doctor prescribed, or 3) increase your dose of LAMICTAL faster than prescribed.
- It is not possible to predict whether a mild rash will develop into a more serious reaction.

Therefore, if you experience a skin rash, hives, fever, swollen lymph glands, painful sores in the mouth or around the eyes, or swelling of lips or tongue, tell a doctor immediately, since these symptoms may be the first signs of a serious reaction. A doctor should evaluate your condition and decide if you should continue taking LAMICTAL.

4. The Use of LAMICTAL During Pregnancy and Breast-feeding:
The effects of LAMICTAL during pregnancy are not known at this time. If you are pregnant or are planning to become pregnant, talk to your doctor. Some LAMICTAL passes into breast milk and the effects of this on infants are unknown. Therefore, if you are breast-feeding, you should discuss this with your doctor to determine if you should continue to take LAMICTAL.

5. How to Use LAMICTAL:

- It is important to take LAMICTAL exactly as instructed by your doctor. The dose of LAMICTAL must be increased slowly. It may take several weeks or months before your final dosage can be determined by your doctor, based on your response.
- Do not increase your dose of LAMICTAL or take more frequent doses than those indicated by your doctor.
- If you miss a dose of lamotrigine, do not double your next dose.
- Do NOT stop taking LAMICTAL or any of your other seizure medicines unless instructed by your doctor.
- Use caution before driving a car or operating complex, hazardous machinery until you know if LAMICTAL affects your ability to perform these tasks.
- Tell your doctor if your seizures get worse or if you have any new types of seizures.
- Always tell your doctor and pharmacist if you are taking or plan to take any other prescription or over-the-counter medicines.

6. How to Take LAMICTAL:
LAMICTAL Tablets should be swallowed whole. Chewing the tablets may leave a bitter taste.
LAMICTAL Chewable Dispersible Tablets may be swallowed whole, chewed, or mixed in water or diluted fruit juice. If the tablets are chewed, consume a small amount of water or diluted fruit juice to aid in swallowing.
To disperse LAMICTAL Chewable Dispersible Tablets, add the tablets to a small amount of liquid (1 teaspoon, or enough to cover the medication) in a glass or spoon. Approximately 1 minute later, when the tablets are completely dispersed, mix the solution and take the entire amount immediately.

7. Storing Your Medicine:
Store LAMICTAL at room temperature away from heat and light. Always keep your medicines out of the reach of children.
This medicine was prescribed for your use only to treat seizures. Do not give the drug to others.
If your doctor decides to stop your treatment, do not keep any leftover medicine unless your doctor tells you to. Throw away your medicine as instructed.

GlaxoSmithKline, Research Triangle Park, NC 27709
DEPAKENE and DEPAKOTE are registered trademarks of Abbott Laboratories.
©2003, GlaxoSmithKline. All rights reserved.
January 2003/RL-1171

NAVELBINE® ℞
[*na' vəl-bēn*]
(vinorelbine tartrate)
Injection

Prescribing information for this product, which appears on pages 1597–1600 of the 2003 PDR, has been revised as follows. Please write "See Supplement A" next to the product heading.

The **PRECAUTIONS: Pediatric Use** *subsection was revised to:*
Safety and effectiveness of NAVELBINE in pediatric patients have not been established. Data from a single-arm study in 46 patients with recurrent solid malignant tumors, including rhabdomyosarcoma/undifferentiated sarcoma, neuroblastoma, and CNS tumors, at doses similar to those used in adults, showed no meaningful clinical activity. Toxicities were similar to those reported in adults.
Manufactured by Pierre Fabre Médicament Production
64320 Idron, FRANCE
for GlaxoSmithKline, Research Triangle Park, NC 27709
Under license of Pierre Fabre Médicament -
Centre National de la Recherche Scientifique-France
©2002, GlaxoSmithKline. All rights reserved.
November 2002/RL-1157

PAXIL® ℞
[*pax'il*]
brand of paroxetine hydrochloride
tablets and oral suspension

Prescribing information for this product, which appears on pages 1603–1610 of the 2003 PDR, has been revised as follows. Please write "See Supplement A" next to the product heading.

In the **CLINICAL PHARMACOLOGY: Clinical Trials: Generalized Anxiety Disorder** *subsection, the following was added as the fifth paragraph:*
In a longer-term trial, 566 patients meeting DSM-IV criteria for Generalized Anxiety Disorder, who had responded during a single-blind, 8-week acute treatment phase with *Paxil* 20 to 50 mg/day, were randomized to continuation of *Paxil* at their same dose, or to placebo, for up to 24 weeks of observation for relapse. Response during the single-blind phase was defined by having a decrease of ≥2 points compared to baseline on the CGI-Severity of Illness scale, to a score of ≤3. Relapse during the double-blind phase was defined as an increase of ≥2 points compared to baseline on the CGI-Severity of Illness scale to a score of ≥4, or withdrawal due to lack of efficacy. Patients receiving continued *Paxil* experienced a significantly lower relapse rate over the subsequent 24 weeks compared to those receiving placebo.

In the **INDICATIONS AND USAGE: Generalized Anxiety Disorder** *subsection, the fourth paragraph was revised to:*
The efficacy of *Paxil* in maintaining a response in patients with Generalized Anxiety Disorder, who responded during an 8-week acute treatment phase while taking *Paxil* and were then observed for relapse during a period of up to 24 weeks, was demonstrated in a placebo-controlled trial (see Clinical Trials under CLINICAL PHARMACOLOGY). Nevertheless, the physician who elects to use *Paxil* for extended periods should periodically re-evaluate the long-term usefulness of the drug for the individual patient (see DOSAGE AND ADMINISTRATION).

Under **ADVERSE REACTIONS: Postmarketing Reports,** "vasculitic syndromes (such as Henoch-Schönlein purpura)" *was added.*

The **DOSAGE AND ADMINISTRATION: Generalized Anxiety Disorder: *Maintenance Therapy*** *subsection was revised to:*
Systematic evaluation of continuing *Paxil* for periods of up to 24 weeks in patients with Generalized Anxiety Disorder who had responded while taking *Paxil* during an 8-week acute treatment phase has demonstrated a benefit of such maintenance (see Clinical Trials under CLINICAL PHARMACOLOGY). Nevertheless, patients should be periodically reassessed to determine the need for maintenance treatment.
GlaxoSmithKline, Research Triangle Park, NC 27709
©2003, GlaxoSmithKline. All rights reserved.
January 2003/PX:L24

PURINETHOL® ℞
[*pur' ĭn-thawl*]
(mercaptopurine)
50-mg Scored Tablets

Prescribing information for this product, which appears on pages 1615–1617 of the 2003 PDR, has been revised as follows. Please write "See Supplement A" next to the product heading.

In **ADVERSE REACTIONS: Miscellaneous,** "transient" *was deleted from the sentence* "Transient oligospermia has been reported."

The **OVERDOSAGE** *section was revised to:*
Signs and symptoms of overdosage may be immediate such as anorexia, nausea, vomiting, and diarrhea; or delayed such as myelosuppression, liver dysfunction, and gastroenteritis. Dialysis cannot be expected to clear mercaptopurine. Hemodialysis is thought to be of marginal use due to the rapid intracellular incorporation of mercaptopurine into active metabolites with long persistence. The oral LD_{50} of mercaptopurine was determined to be 480 mg/kg in the mouse and 425 mg/kg in the rat.
There is no known pharmacologic antagonist of mercaptopurine. The drug should be discontinued immediately if unintended toxicity occurs during treatment. If a patient is seen immediately following an accidental overdosage of the drug, it may be useful to induce emesis.

The second paragraph of the **DOSAGE AND ADMINISTRATION** *section was revised to:*
The total daily dosage may be given at one time. It is calculated to the nearest multiple of 25 mg.
Manufactured by DSM Pharmaceuticals, Inc.
Greenville, NC 27834 for
GlaxoSmithKline, Research Triangle Park, NC 27709
©2002, GlaxoSmithKline. All rights reserved.
November 2002/RL-1156

RELENZA® ℞
[*ra-lin' za*]
(zanamivir for inhalation)

For Oral Inhalation Only
For Use with the DISKHALER® Inhalation Device

Prescribing information for this product, which appears on pages 1619–1621 of the 2003 PDR, has been revised as follows. Please write "See Supplement A" next to the product heading.

The phrase "(which contains milk proteins)" *was added to the following sentence in the* **DESCRIPTION** *section:*
Each RELENZA ROTADISK® contains 4 regularly spaced double-foil blisters with each blister containing a powder mixture of 5 mg of zanamivir and 20 mg of lactose (which contains milk proteins).
GlaxoSmithKline, Research Triangle Park, NC 27709
©2003, GlaxoSmithKline. All rights reserved.
March 2003/RL-1181

SEREVENT® ℞
[*ser'ə-vent*]
(salmeterol xinafoate)
Inhalation Aerosol

Bronchodilator Aerosol
For Oral Inhalation Only

Prescribing information for this product, which appears on pages 1632–1636 of the 2003 PDR, has been revised as follows. Please write "See Supplement A" next to the product heading.

The third paragraph of the **DESCRIPTION** *section was revised to note that the lecithin is* soya lecithin.
GlaxoSmithKline, Research Triangle Park, NC 27709
©2003, GlaxoSmithKline. All rights reserved.
April 2003/RL-1187

SEREVENT® DISKUS® ℞
[*ser' ə-vent disk' us*]
(salmeterol xinafoate inhalation powder)

For Oral Inhalation Only

Prescribing information for this product, which appears on pages 1636–1641 of the 2003 PDR, has been revised as follows. Please write "See Supplement A" next to the product heading.

Revised the following ingredients statement in the **DESCRIPTION** *section to include milk proteins:*
Each blister on the double-foil strip within the unit contains 50 mcg of salmeterol administered as the salmeterol xinafoate salt in 12.5 mg of formulation containing lactose (which contains milk proteins).

Added the following to **PRECAUTIONS: Information for Patients:**
2. Most patients are able to taste or feel a dose delivered from SEREVENT DISKUS. However, whether or not patients are able to sense delivery of a dose, you should instruct them not to exceed the recommended dose of 1 inhalation twice daily, morning and evening. You should instruct them to contact you or the pharmacist if they have questions.

Added the following subsection to **ADVERSE REACTIONS: Observed During Clinical Practice:**
Non-Site Specific: Very rare anaphylactic reaction in patients with severe milk protein allergy.
GlaxoSmithKline, Research Triangle Park, NC 27709
©2003, GlaxoSmithKline. All rights reserved.
March 2003/RL-1186

THORAZINE® ℞
[*thor' ə-zēn*]
brand of
chlorpromazine

Prescribing information for this product, which appears on pages 1651–1654 of the 2003 PDR, has been revised as follows. Please write "See Supplement A" next to the product heading.

The Spansule® *brand of sustained release capsules is no longer marketed and all references to it were removed from the labeling. Also, bottles of 1,000 tablets are no longer available for the 25 mg, 50 mg, and 100 mg tablets, and were removed from the* **HOW SUPPLIED** *section.*

Continued on next page

Thorazine—Cont.

GlaxoSmithKline, Research Triangle Park, NC 27709
©2002, GlaxoSmithKline. All rights reserved
April 2002/TZ:L88

TRIZIVIR®
[trī' zə-vir]
(abacavir sulfate, lamivudine, and zidovudine)
Tablets

Prescribing information for this product, which appears on pages 1664–1669 of the 2003 PDR, has been revised as follows. Please write "See Supplement A" next to the product heading.

The following paragraphs in the **ADVERSE REACTIONS:** *Abacavir:* **Hypersensitivity Reaction** *subsection were revised to:*

In clinical studies, approximately 5% of adult and pediatric patients receiving abacavir developed a hypersensitivity reaction. This reaction is characterized by the appearance of symptoms indicating multi-organ/body system involvement. Symptoms usually appear within the first 6 weeks of treatment with abacavir, although these reactions may occur at any time during therapy. Frequently observed signs and symptoms include fever, skin rash, fatigue, and gastrointestinal symptoms such as nausea, vomiting, diarrhea, or abdominal pain. Other signs and symptoms include malaise, lethargy, myalgia, myolysis, arthralgia, edema, cough, abnormal chest x-ray findings (predominantly infiltrates, which can be localized), dyspnea, headache, and paresthesia. Some patients who experienced a hypersensitivity reaction were initially thought to have acute onset or worsening respiratory disease. The diagnosis of hypersensitivity reaction should be carefully considered for patients presenting with symptoms of acute onset respiratory diseases, even if alternative respiratory diagnoses (pneumonia, bronchitis, flu-like illness) are possible.

Physical findings include lymphadenopathy, mucous membrane lesions (conjunctivitis and mouth ulcerations), and rash. The rash usually appears maculopapular or urticarial but may be variable in appearance. There have been reports of erythema multiforme. Hypersensitivity reactions have occurred without rash.

Laboratory abnormalities include elevated liver function tests, increased creatine phosphokinase or creatinine, and lymphopenia. Anaphylaxis, liver failure, renal failure, hypotension, adult respiratory distress syndrome, respiratory failure, and death have occurred in association with hypersensitivity reactions. Symptoms worsen with continued therapy but often resolve upon discontinuation of abacavir.

The following paragraphs in the **ADVERSE REACTIONS: Observed During Clinical Practice:** *Abacavir subsection were revised to:*

Suspected Stevens-Johnson syndrome (SJS) and toxic epidermal necrolysis (TEN) have been reported in patients receiving abacavir primarily in combination with medications known to be associated with SJS and TEN, respectively. Because of the overlap of clinical signs and symptoms between hypersensitivity to abacavir and SJS and TEN, and the possibility of multiple drug sensitivities in some patients, abacavir should be discontinued and not restarted in such cases.

There have also been reports of erythema multiforme with abacavir use.

GlaxoSmithKline, Research Triangle Park, NC 27709
Lamivudine is manufactured under agreement from Shire Pharmaceuticals Group plc, Basingstoke, UK
©2002, GlaxoSmithKline. All rights reserved.
August 2002/RL-1144

VALTREX®
[val' trĕx]
(valacyclovir hydrochloride)
Caplets

Prescribing information for this product, which appears on pages 1672–1674 of the 2003 PDR, has been completely revised as follows. Please write "See Supplement A" next to the product heading.

DESCRIPTION

VALTREX (valacyclovir hydrochloride) is the hydrochloride salt of L-valyl ester of the antiviral drug acyclovir (ZOVIRAX® Brand, GlaxoSmithKline).

VALTREX Caplets are for oral administration. Each caplet contains valacyclovir hydrochloride equivalent to 500 mg or 1 gram valacyclovir and the inactive ingredients carnauba wax, colloidal silicon dioxide, crospovidone, FD&C Blue No. 2 Lake, hypromellose, magnesium stearate, microcrystalline cellulose, polyethylene glycol, polysorbate 80, povidone, and titanium dioxide. The blue, film-coated caplets are printed with edible white ink.

The chemical name of valacyclovir hydrochloride is L-valine, 2-[(2-amino-1,6-dihydro-6-oxo-9H-purin-9-yl)methoxy]ethyl ester, monohydrochloride.

Valacyclovir hydrochloride is a white to off-white powder with the molecular formula $C_{13}H_{20}N_6O_4 \cdot HCl$ and a molecular weight of 360.80. The maximum solubility in water at 25°C is 174 mg/mL. The pka's for valacyclovir hydrochloride are 1.90, 7.47, and 9.43.

MICROBIOLOGY

Mechanism of Antiviral Action: Valacyclovir hydrochloride is rapidly converted to acyclovir which has demonstrated antiviral activity against herpes simplex virus types 1 (HSV-1) and 2 (HSV-2) and varicella-zoster virus (VZV) both in vitro and in vivo.

The inhibitory activity of acyclovir is highly selective due to its affinity for the enzyme thymidine kinase (TK) encoded by HSV and VZV. This viral enzyme converts acyclovir into acyclovir monophosphate, a nucleotide analogue. The monophosphate is further converted into diphosphate by cellular guanylate kinase and into triphosphate by a number of cellular enzymes. In vitro, acyclovir triphosphate stops replication of herpes viral DNA. This is accomplished in 3 ways: 1) competitive inhibition of viral DNA polymerase, 2) incorporation and termination of the growing viral DNA chain, and 3) inactivation of the viral DNA polymerase. The greater antiviral activity of acyclovir against HSV compared to VZV is due to its more efficient phosphorylation by the viral TK.

Antiviral Activities: The quantitative relationship between the in vitro susceptibility of herpesviruses to antivirals and the clinical response to therapy has not been established in humans, and virus sensitivity testing has not been standardized. Sensitivity testing results, expressed as the concentration of drug required to inhibit by 50% the growth of virus in cell culture (IC_{50}), vary greatly depending upon a number of factors. Using plaque-reduction assays, the IC_{50} against herpes simplex virus isolates ranges from 0.02 to 13.5 mcg/mL for HSV-1 and from 0.01 to 9.9 mcg/mL for HSV-2. The IC_{50} for acyclovir against most laboratory strains and clinical isolates of VZV ranges from 0.12 to 10.8 mcg/mL. Acyclovir also demonstrates activity against the Oka vaccine strain of VZV with a mean IC_{50} of 1.35 mcg/mL.

Drug Resistance: Resistance of HSV and VZV to acyclovir can result from qualitative and quantitative changes in the viral TK and/or DNA polymerase. Clinical isolates of VZV with reduced susceptibility to acyclovir have been recovered from patients with AIDS. In these cases, TK-deficient mutants of VZV have been recovered.

Resistance of HSV and VZV to acyclovir occurs by the same mechanisms. While most of the acyclovir-resistant mutants isolated thus far from immunocompromised patients have been found to be TK-deficient mutants, other mutants involving the viral TK gene (TK partial and TK altered) and DNA polymerase have also been isolated. TK-negative mutants may cause severe disease in immunocompromised patients. The possibility of viral resistance to valacyclovir (and therefore, to acyclovir) should be considered in patients who show poor clinical response during therapy.

CLINICAL PHARMACOLOGY

After oral administration, valacyclovir hydrochloride is rapidly absorbed from the gastrointestinal tract and nearly completely converted to acyclovir and L-valine by first-pass intestinal and/or hepatic metabolism.

Pharmacokinetics: The pharmacokinetics of valacyclovir and acyclovir after oral administration of VALTREX have been investigated in 14 volunteer studies involving 283 adults.

Absorption and Bioavailability: The absolute bioavailability of acyclovir after administration of VALTREX is 54.5% ± 9.1% as determined following a 1-gram oral dose of VALTREX and a 350-mg intravenous acyclovir dose to 12 healthy volunteers. Acyclovir bioavailability from the administration of VALTREX is not altered by administration with food (30 minutes after an 873 Kcal breakfast, which included 51 grams of fat).

There was a lack of dose proportionality in acyclovir maximum concentration (C_{max}) and area under the acyclovir concentration-time curve (AUC) after single-dose administration of 100 mg, 250 mg, 500 mg, 750 mg, and 1 gram of VALTREX to 8 healthy volunteers. The mean C_{max} (± SD) was 0.83 (± 0.14), 2.15 (± 0.50), 3.28 (± 0.83), 4.17 (± 1.14), and 5.65 (± 2.37) mcg/mL, respectively; and the mean AUC (± SD) was 2.28 (± 0.40), 5.76 (± 0.60), 11.59 (± 1.79), 14.11 (± 3.54), and 19.52 (± 6.04) hr•mcg/mL, respectively.

There was also a lack of dose proportionality in acyclovir C_{max} and AUC after the multiple-dose administration of 250 mg, 500 mg, and 1 gram of VALTREX administered 4 times daily for 11 days in parallel groups of 8 healthy volunteers. The mean C_{max} (± SD) was 2.11 (± 0.33), 3.69 (± 0.87), and 4.96 (± 0.64) mcg/mL, respectively, and the mean AUC (± SD) was 5.66 (± 1.09), 9.88 (± 2.01), and 15.70 (± 2.27) hr•mcg/mL, respectively.

There is no accumulation of acyclovir after the administration of valacyclovir at the recommended dosage regimens in healthy volunteers with normal renal function.

Distribution: The binding of valacyclovir to human plasma proteins ranged from 13.5% to 17.9%.

Metabolism: After oral administration, valacyclovir hydrochloride is rapidly absorbed from the gastrointestinal tract. Valacyclovir is converted to acyclovir and L-valine by first-pass intestinal and/or hepatic metabolism. Acyclovir is converted to a small extent to inactive metabolites by aldehyde oxidase and by alcohol and aldehyde dehydrogenase. Neither valacyclovir nor acyclovir is metabolized by cytochrome P450 enzymes. Plasma concentrations of unconverted valacyclovir are low and transient, generally becoming non-quantifiable by 3 hours after administration. Peak plasma valacyclovir concentrations are generally less than 0.5 mcg/mL at all doses. After single-dose administration of 1 gram of VALTREX, average plasma valacyclovir concentrations observed were 0.5, 0.4, and 0.8 mcg/mL in patients with hepatic dysfunction, renal insufficiency, and in healthy volunteers who received concomitant cimetidine and probenecid, respectively.

Elimination: The pharmacokinetic disposition of acyclovir delivered by valacyclovir is consistent with previous experience from intravenous and oral acyclovir. Following the oral administration of a single 1-gram dose of radiolabeled valacyclovir to 4 healthy subjects, 45.60% and 47.12% of administered radioactivity was recovered in urine and feces over 96 hours, respectively. Acyclovir accounted for 88.60% of the radioactivity excreted in the urine. Renal clearance of acyclovir following the administration of a single 1-gram dose of VALTREX to 12 healthy volunteers was approximately 255 ± 86 mL/min which represents 41.9% of total acyclovir apparent plasma clearance.

The plasma elimination half-life of acyclovir typically averaged 2.5 to 3.3 hours in all studies of VALTREX in volunteers with normal renal function.

End-Stage Renal Disease (ESRD): Following administration of VALTREX to volunteers with ESRD, the average acyclovir half-life is approximately 14 hours. During hemodialysis, the acyclovir half-life is approximately 4 hours. Approximately one third of acyclovir in the body is removed by dialysis during a 4-hour hemodialysis session. Apparent plasma clearance of acyclovir in dialysis patients was 86.3 ± 21.3 mL/min/1.73 m^2, compared to 679.16 ± 162.76 mL/min/1.73 m^2 in healthy volunteers.

Reduction in dosage is recommended in patients with renal impairment (see DOSAGE AND ADMINISTRATION).

Geriatrics: After single-dose administration of 1 gram of VALTREX in healthy geriatric volunteers, the half-life of acyclovir was 3.11 ± 0.51 hours, compared to 2.91 ± 0.63 hours in healthy volunteers. The pharmacokinetics of acyclovir following single- and multiple-dose oral administration of VALTREX in geriatric volunteers varied with renal function. Dose reduction may be required in geriatric patients, depending on the underlying renal status of the patient (see PRECAUTIONS and DOSAGE AND ADMINISTRATION).

Pediatrics: Valacyclovir pharmacokinetics have not been evaluated in pediatric patients.

Liver Disease: Administration of VALTREX to patients with moderate (biopsy-proven cirrhosis) or severe (with and without ascites and biopsy-proven cirrhosis) liver disease indicated that the rate but not the extent of conversion of valacyclovir to acyclovir is reduced, and the acyclovir half-life is not affected. Dosage modification is not recommended for patients with cirrhosis.

HIV Disease: In 9 patients with HIV disease and CD4 cell counts <150 cells/mm^3 who received VALTREX at a dosage of 1 gram 4 times daily for 30 days, the pharmacokinetics of valacyclovir and acyclovir were not different from that observed in healthy volunteers (see WARNINGS).

Drug Interactions: The pharmacokinetics of digoxin was not affected by coadministration of VALTREX 1 gram 3 times daily, and the pharmacokinetics of acyclovir after a single dose of VALTREX (1 gram) was unchanged by coadministration of digoxin (2 doses of 0.75 mg), single doses of antacids (Al^{3+} or Mg^{++}), or multiple doses of thiazide diuretics. Acyclovir C_{max} and AUC following a single dose of VALTREX (1 gram) increased by 8% and 32%, respectively, after a single dose of cimetidine (800 mg), or by 22% and 49%, respectively, after probenecid (1 gram), or by 30% and 78%, respectively, after a combination of cimetidine and probenecid, primarily due to a reduction in renal clearance of acyclovir. These effects are not considered to be of clinical significance in subjects with normal renal function. Therefore, no dosage adjustment is recommended when VALTREX is coadministered with digoxin, antacids, thiazide diuretics, cimetidine, or probenecid in subjects with normal renal function.

CLINICAL TRIALS

Herpes Zoster: Two randomized double-blind clinical trials in immunocompetent adults with localized herpes zoster were conducted. VALTREX was compared to placebo in patients less than 50 years of age, and to ZOVIRAX in patients greater than 50 years of age. All patients were treated within 72 hours of appearance of zoster rash. In patients less than 50 years of age, the median time to cessation of new lesion formation was 2 days for those treated with VALTREX compared to 3 days for those treated with placebo. In patients greater than 50 years of age, the median time to cessation of new lesions was 3 days in patients treated with either VALTREX or ZOVIRAX. In patients less than 50 years of age, no difference was found with respect to the duration of pain after healing (post-herpetic neuralgia) between the recipients of VALTREX and placebo. In patients greater than 50 years of age, among the 83% who reported pain after healing (post-herpetic neuralgia), the median duration of pain after healing [95% confidence interval] in days was: 40 [31, 51], 43 [36, 55], and 59 [41, 77] for 7-day VALTREX, 14-day VALTREX, and 7-day ZOVIRAX, respectively.

Genital Herpes Infections: *Initial Episode:* Six hundred and forty-three immunocompetent adults with first episode genital herpes who presented within 72 hours of symptom onset were randomized in a double-blind trial to receive 10 days of VALTREX 1 gram twice daily (n = 323) or ZOVIRAX 200 mg 5 times a day (n = 320). For both treatment groups: the median time to lesion healing was 9 days, the median time to cessation of pain was 5 days, the median time to cessation of viral shedding was 3 days.

Recurrent Episodes: Three double-blind trials (2 of them placebo-controlled) in immunocompetent adults with recurrent genital herpes were conducted. Patients self-initiated therapy within 24 hours of the first sign or symptom of a recurrent genital herpes episode.

In 1 study, patients were randomized to receive 5 days of treatment with either VALTREX 500 mg twice daily (n = 360) or placebo (n = 259). The median time to lesion healing was 4 days in the group receiving VALTREX 500 mg versus 6 days in the placebo group, and the median time to cessation of viral shedding in patients with at least 1 positive culture (42% of the overall study population) was 2 days in the group receiving VALTREX 500 mg versus 4 days in the placebo group. The median time to cessation of pain was 3 days in the group receiving VALTREX 500 mg versus 4 days in the placebo group. Results supporting efficacy were replicated in a second trial.

In a third study, patients were randomized to receive VALTREX 500 mg twice daily for 5 days (n = 398) or VALTREX 500 mg twice daily for 3 days (and matching placebo twice daily for 2 additional days) (n = 402). The median time to lesion healing was about 4½ days in both treatment groups. The median time to cessation of pain was about 3 days in both treatment groups.

Suppressive Therapy: Two clinical studies were conducted, one in immunocompetent adults and one in HIV-infected adults.

A double-blind, 12-month, placebo- and active-controlled study enrolled immunocompetent adults with a history of 6 or more recurrences per year. Outcomes for the overall study population are shown in Table 1.

[See table 1 above]

Subjects with 9 or fewer recurrences per year showed comparable results with VALTREX 500 mg once daily.

In a second study, 293 HIV-infected adults on stable antiretroviral therapy with a history of 4 or more recurrences of ano-genital herpes per year were randomized to receive either VALTREX 500 mg twice daily (n = 194) or matching placebo (n = 99) for 6 months. The median duration of recurrent genital herpes in enrolled subjects was 8 years, and the median number of recurrences in the year prior to enrollment was 5. Overall, the median prestudy HIV-1 RNA was 2.6 $\log_{10}$ copies/mL. Among patients who received VALTREX, the prestudy median CD4 cell count was 336 cells/mm^3; 11% had <100 cells/mm^3, 16% had 100 to 199 cells/mm^3, 42% had 200 to 499 cells/mm^3, and 31% had ≥500 cells/mm^3. Outcomes for the overall study population are shown in Table 2.

Table 2. Recurrence Rates in HIV-Infected Adults at 6 Months

Treatment Arm	VALTREX 500 mg b.i.d. (n = 194)	Placebo (n = 99)
Recurrence free	65%	26%
Recurrences	17%	57%
Unknowns*	18%	17%

*Includes lost to follow-up, discontinuations due to adverse events, and consent withdrawn.

Cold Sores (Herpes Labialis): Two double-blind, placebo-controlled clinical trials were conducted in 1,856 healthy adults and adolescents (≥12 years old) with a history of recurrent cold sores. Patients self-initiated therapy at the earliest symptoms and prior to any signs of a cold sore. The majority of patients initiated treatment within 2 hours of onset of symptoms. Patients were randomized to VALTREX 2 grams twice daily on Day 1 followed by placebo on Day 2, VALTREX 2 grams twice daily on Day 1 followed by 1 gram twice daily on Day 2, or placebo on Days 1 and 2.

The mean duration of cold sore episodes was about 1 day shorter in treated subjects as compared to placebo. The 2-day regimen did not offer additional benefit over the 1-day regimen.

No significant difference was observed between subjects receiving VALTREX or placebo in the prevention of progression of cold sore lesions beyond the papular stage.

INDICATIONS AND USAGE

Herpes Zoster: VALTREX is indicated for the treatment of herpes zoster (shingles).

Genital Herpes: VALTREX is indicated for the treatment or suppression of genital herpes in immunocompetent individuals and for the suppression of recurrent genital herpes in HIV-infected individuals.

Cold Sores (Herpes Labialis): VALTREX is indicated for the treatment of cold sores (herpes labialis).

CONTRAINDICATIONS

VALTREX is contraindicated in patients with a known hypersensitivity or intolerance to valacyclovir, acyclovir, or any component of the formulation.

WARNINGS

Thrombotic thrombocytopenic purpura/hemolytic uremic syndrome (TTP/HUS), in some cases resulting in death, has occurred in patients with advanced HIV disease and also in allogeneic bone marrow transplant and renal transplant recipients participating in clinical trials of VALTREX at doses of 8 grams per day.

Table 1. Recurrence Rates in Immunocompetent Adults at 6 and 12 Months

	6 Months			12 Months		
Treatment Arm	VALTREX 1 gram q.d. (n = 269)	ZOVIRAX 400 mg b.i.d. (n = 267)	Placebo (n = 134)	VALTREX 1 gram q.d. (n = 269)	ZOVIRAX 400 mg b.i.d. (n = 267)	Placebo (n = 134)
Recurrence free	55%	54%	7%	34%	34%	4%
Recurrences	35%	36%	83%	46%	46%	85%
Unknowns*	10%	10%	10%	19%	19%	10%

*Includes lost to follow-up, discontinuations due to adverse events, and consent withdrawn.

PRECAUTIONS

Dosage reduction is recommended when administering VALTREX to patients with renal impairment (see DOSAGE AND ADMINISTRATION). Acute renal failure and central nervous system symptoms have been reported in patients with underlying renal disease who have received inappropriately high doses of VALTREX for their level of renal function. Similar caution should be exercised when administering VALTREX to geriatric patients (see Geriatric Use) and patients receiving potentially nephrotoxic agents.

Given the dosage recommendations for treatment of cold sores, special attention should be paid when prescribing VALTREX for cold sores in patients who are elderly or who have impaired renal function (see DOSAGE AND ADMINISTRATION and Geriatric Use). Treatment should not exceed 1 day (2 doses of 2 grams in 24 hours). Therapy beyond 1 day does not provide additional clinical benefit.

Precipitation of acyclovir in renal tubules may occur when the solubility (2.5 mg/mL) is exceeded in the intratubular fluid. In the event of acute renal failure and anuria, the patient may benefit from hemodialysis until renal function is restored (see DOSAGE AND ADMINISTRATION).

The safety and efficacy of VALTREX have not been established in immunocompromised patients other than for the suppression of genital herpes in HIV-infected patients. The safety and efficacy of VALTREX for suppression of recurrent genital herpes in patients with advanced HIV disease (CD4 cell count <100 cells/mm^3) have not been established. The efficacy of VALTREX for the treatment of genital herpes in HIV-infected patients has not been established. The safety and efficacy of VALTREX have not been established for the treatment of disseminated herpes zoster.

Information for Patients: *Herpes Zoster:* There are no data on treatment initiated more than 72 hours after onset of the zoster rash. Patients should be advised to initiate treatment as soon as possible after a diagnosis of herpes zoster.

Genital Herpes: Patients should be informed that VALTREX is not a cure for genital herpes. There are no data evaluating whether VALTREX will prevent transmission of infection to others. Because genital herpes is a sexually transmitted disease, patients should avoid contact with lesions or intercourse when lesions and/or symptoms are present to avoid infecting partners. Genital herpes can also be transmitted in the absence of symptoms through asymptomatic viral shedding. If medical management of a genital herpes recurrence is indicated, patients should be advised to initiate therapy at the first sign or symptom of an episode.

There are no data on the effectiveness of treatment initiated more than 72 hours after the onset of signs and symptoms of a first episode of genital herpes or more than 24 hours of the onset of signs and symptoms of a recurrent episode.

There are no data on the safety or effectiveness of chronic suppressive therapy of more than 1 year's duration in otherwise healthy patients. There are no data on the safety or effectiveness of chronic suppressive therapy of more than 6 months' duration in HIV-infected patients.

Cold Sores (Herpes Labialis): Patients should be advised to initiate treatment at the earliest symptom of a cold sore (e.g., tingling, itching, or burning). There are no data on the effectiveness of treatment initiated after the development of clinical signs of a cold sore (e.g., papule, vesicle, or ulcer). Patients should be instructed that treatment for cold sores should not exceed 1 day (2 doses) and that their doses should be taken about 12 hours apart. Patients should be informed that VALTREX is not a cure for cold sores (herpes labialis).

Drug Interactions: See CLINICAL PHARMACOLOGY: Pharmacokinetics.

Carcinogenesis, Mutagenesis, Impairment of Fertility: The data presented below include references to the steady-state acyclovir AUC observed in humans treated with 1 gram VALTREX given orally 3 times a day to treat herpes zoster. Plasma drug concentrations in animal studies are expressed as multiples of human exposure to acyclovir (see CLINICAL PHARMACOLOGY: Pharmacokinetics).

Valacyclovir was noncarcinogenic in lifetime carcinogenicity bioassays at single daily doses (gavage) of up to 120 mg/kg/day for mice and 100 mg/kg/day for rats. There was no significant difference in the incidence of tumors between treated and control animals, nor did valacyclovir shorten the latency of tumors. Plasma concentrations of acyclovir were equivalent to human levels in the mouse bioassay and 1.4 to 2.3 times human levels in the rat bioassay.

Valacyclovir was tested in 5 genetic toxicity assays. An Ames assay was negative in the absence or presence of metabolic activation. Also negative were an in vitro cytogenetic study with human lymphocytes and a rat cytogenetic study at a single oral dose of 3,000 mg/kg (8 to 9 times human plasma levels).

In the mouse lymphoma assay, valacyclovir was not mutagenic in the absence of metabolic activation. In the presence of metabolic activation (76% to 88% conversion to acyclovir), valacyclovir was mutagenic.

Valacyclovir was not mutagenic in a mouse micronucleus assay at 250 mg/kg but positive at 500 mg/kg (acyclovir concentrations 26 to 51 times human plasma levels).

Valacyclovir did not impair fertility or reproduction in rats at 200 mg/kg/day (6 times human plasma levels).

Pregnancy: *Teratogenic Effects:* Pregnancy Category B. Valacyclovir was not teratogenic in rats or rabbits given 400 mg/kg (which results in exposures of 10 and 7 times human plasma levels, respectively) during the period of major organogenesis.

There are no adequate and well-controlled studies of VALTREX or ZOVIRAX in pregnant women. A prospective epidemiologic registry of acyclovir use during pregnancy was established in 1984 and completed in April 1999. There were 749 pregnancies followed in women exposed to systemic acyclovir during the first trimester of pregnancy resulting in 756 outcomes. The occurrence rate of birth defects approximates that found in the general population. However, the small size of the registry is insufficient to evaluate the risk for less common defects or to permit reliable or definitive conclusions regarding the safety of acyclovir in pregnant women and their developing fetuses. VALTREX should be used during pregnancy only if the potential benefit justifies the potential risk to the fetus.

Nursing Mothers: There is no experience with VALTREX. However, acyclovir concentrations have been documented in breast milk in 2 women following oral administration of ZOVIRAX and ranged from 0.6 to 4.1 times corresponding plasma levels. These concentrations would potentially expose the nursing infant to a dose of acyclovir as high as 0.3 mg/kg/day. VALTREX should be administered to a nursing mother with caution and only when indicated.

Pediatric Use: Safety and effectiveness of VALTREX in pre-pubertal pediatric patients have not been established.

Geriatric Use: Of the total number of subjects in clinical studies of VALTREX, 889 were 65 and over, and 350 were 75 and over. In a clinical study of herpes zoster, the duration of pain after healing (post-herpetic neuralgia) was longer in patients 65 and older compared with younger adults. Elderly patients are more likely to have reduced renal function and require dose reduction. Elderly patients are also more likely to have renal or CNS adverse events. With respect to CNS adverse events observed during clinical practice, agitation, hallucinations, confusion, delirium, and encephalopathy were reported more frequently in elderly patients (see CLINICAL PHARMACOLOGY, ADVERSE REACTIONS: Observed During Clinical Practice, and DOSAGE AND ADMINISTRATION).

ADVERSE REACTIONS

Frequently reported adverse events in clinical trials of VALTREX in healthy patients are listed in Tables 3 and 4.

Table 3. Incidence (%) of Adverse Events in Herpes Zoster Study Populations

Adverse Event	VALTREX 1 gram t.i.d. (n = 967)	Placebo (n = 195)
Nausea	15%	8%
Headache	14%	12%
Vomiting	6%	3%
Dizziness	3%	2%
Abdominal pain	3%	2%

[See table 4 at top of next page]

Laboratory abnormalities reported in clinical trials of VALTREX in otherwise healthy patients are listed in Table 5.

[See table 5 at top of next page]

Suppression of Genital Herpes in HIV-Infected Patients: In HIV-infected patients, frequently reported adverse events for VALTREX (500 mg twice daily; n = 194, median days on therapy = 172) and placebo (n = 99, median days on therapy = 59), respectively, included headache (13% vs. 8%), fatigue (8% vs. 5%), and rash (8% vs. 1%). Post-randomization laboratory abnormalities that were reported more frequently in valacyclovir subjects versus placebo included elevated alkaline phosphatase (4% vs. 2%), elevated ALT (14% vs. 10%), elevated AST (16% vs. 11%), decreased neutrophil counts (18% vs. 10%), and decreased platelet counts (3% vs. 0%).

Continued on next page

Valtrex—Cont.

Cold Sores (Herpes Labialis): In clinical studies for the treatment of cold sores, the adverse events reported by patients receiving VALTREX (n = 609) or placebo (n = 609) included headache (VALTREX 14%, placebo 10%) and dizziness (VALTREX 2%, placebo 1%). The frequencies of abnormal ALT (>2 × ULN) were 1.8% for patients receiving VALTREX compared with 0.8% for placebo. Other laboratory abnormalities (hemoglobin, white blood cells, alkaline phosphatase, and serum creatinine) occurred with similar frequencies in the 2 groups.

Observed During Clinical Practice: The following events have been identified during post-approval use of VALTREX in clinical practice. Because they are reported voluntarily from a population of unknown size, estimates of frequency cannot be made. These events have been chosen for inclusion due to either their seriousness, frequency of reporting, causal connection to VALTREX, or a combination of these factors.

General: Facial edema, hypertension, tachycardia.
Allergic: Acute hypersensitivity reactions including anaphylaxis, angioedema, dyspnea, pruritus, rash, and urticaria.
CNS Symptoms: Aggressive behavior; agitation; ataxia; coma; confusion; decreased consciousness; dysarthria; encephalopathy; mania; and psychosis, including auditory and visual hallucinations; seizures (see PRECAUTIONS).
Eye: Visual abnormalities.
Gastrointestinal: Diarrhea.
Hepatobiliary Tract and Pancreas: Liver enzyme abnormalities, hepatitis.
Renal: Elevated creatinine, renal failure.
Hematologic: Thrombocytopenia, aplastic anemia, leukocytoclastic vasculitis, TTP/HUS.
Skin: Erythema multiforme, rashes including photosensitivity, alopecia.
Renal Impairment: Renal failure and CNS symptoms have been reported in patients with renal impairment who received VALTREX or acyclovir at greater than the recommended dose. **Dose reduction is recommended in this patient population (see DOSAGE AND ADMINISTRATION).**

OVERDOSAGE

Caution should be exercised to prevent inadvertent overdose (see PRECAUTIONS). Precipitation of acyclovir in renal tubules may occur when the solubility (2.5 mg/mL) is exceeded in the intratubular fluid. In the event of acute renal failure and anuria, the patient may benefit from hemodialysis until renal function is restored (see DOSAGE AND ADMINISTRATION).

DOSAGE AND ADMINISTRATION

VALTREX Caplets may be given without regard to meals.
Herpes Zoster: The recommended dosage of VALTREX for the treatment of herpes zoster is 1 gram orally 3 times daily for 7 days. Therapy should be initiated at the earliest sign or symptom of herpes zoster and is most effective when started within 48 hours of the onset of zoster rash. No data are available on efficacy of treatment started greater than 72 hours after rash onset.
Genital Herpes: *Initial Episodes:* The recommended dosage of VALTREX for treatment of initial genital herpes is 1 gram twice daily for 10 days.
There are no data on the effectiveness of treatment with VALTREX when initiated more than 72 hours after the onset of signs and symptoms. Therapy was most effective when administered within 48 hours of the onset of signs and symptoms.
Recurrent Episodes: The recommended dosage of VALTREX for the treatment of recurrent genital herpes is 500 mg twice daily for 3 days.
If medical management of a genital herpes recurrence is indicated, patients should be advised to initiate therapy at the first sign or symptom of an episode. There are no data on the effectiveness of treatment with VALTREX when initiated more than 24 hours after the onset of signs or symptoms.
Suppressive Therapy: The recommended dosage of VALTREX for chronic suppressive therapy of recurrent genital herpes is 1 gram once daily in patients with normal immune function. In patients with a history of 9 or fewer recurrences per year, an alternative dose is 500 mg once daily. The safety and efficacy of therapy with VALTREX beyond 1 year have not been established.
In HIV-infected patients with CD4 cell count ≥100 cells/mm^3, the recommended dosage of VALTREX for chronic suppressive therapy of recurrent genital herpes is 500 mg twice daily. The safety and efficacy of therapy with VALTREX beyond 6 months in patients with HIV infection have not been established.
Cold Sores (Herpes Labialis): The recommended dosage of VALTREX for the treatment of cold sores is 2 grams twice daily for 1 day taken about 12 hours apart. Therapy should be initiated at the earliest symptom of a cold sore (e.g., tingling, itching, or burning). There are no data on the effectiveness of treatment initiated after the development of clinical signs of a cold sore (e.g., papule, vesicle, or ulcer).
Patients with Acute or Chronic Renal Impairment: In patients with reduced renal function, reduction in dosage is recommended (see Table 6).

Table 4. Incidence (%) of Adverse Events in Genital Herpes Study Populations

	Genital Herpes Treatment			Genital Herpes Suppression		
Adverse Event	VALTREX 1 gram b.i.d. (n = 1,194)	VALTREX 500 mg b.i.d. (n = 1,159)	Placebo (n = 439)	VALTREX 1 gram q.d. (n = 269)	VALTREX 500 mg q.d. (n = 266)	Placebo (n = 134)
Nausea	6%	5%	8%	11%	11%	8%
Headache	16%	15%	14%	35%	38%	34%
Vomiting	1%	<1%	<1%	3%	3%	2%
Dizziness	3%	2%	3%	4%	2%	1%
Abdominal pain	2%	1%	3%	11%	9%	6%
Dysmenorrhea	<1%	<1%	1%	8%	5%	4%
Arthralgia	<1%	<1%	<1%	6%	5%	4%
Depression	1%	0%	<1%	7%	5%	5%

Table 5. Incidence (%) of Laboratory Abnormalities in Herpes Zoster and Genital Herpes Study Populations

	Herpes Zoster		Genital Herpes Treatment			Genital Herpes Suppression		
Laboratory Abnormality	VALTREX 1 gram t.i.d.	Placebo	VALTREX 1 gram b.i.d.	VALTREX 500 mg b.i.d.	Placebo	VALTREX 1 gram q.d.	VALTREX 500 mg q.d.	Placebo
Hemoglobin (<0.8 × LLN)	0.8%	0%	0.3%	0.2%	0%	0%	0.8%	0.8%
White blood cells (<0.75 × LLN)	1.3%	0.6%	0.7%	0.6%	0.2%	0.7%	0.8%	1.5%
Platelet count (<100,000/mm^3)	1.0%	1.2%	0.3%	0.1%	0.7%	0.4%	1.1%	1.5%
AST (SGOT) (<2 × ULN)	1.0%	0%	1.0%	*	0.5%	4.1%	3.8%	3.0%
Serum creatinine (>1.5 × ULN)	0.2%	0%	0.7%	0%	0%	0%	0%	0%

*Data were not collected prospectively.
LLN = Lower limit of normal.
ULN = Upper limit of normal.

Table 6. Dosages for Patients with Renal Impairment

Indications	Normal Dosage Regimen (Creatinine Clearance ≥50)	Creatinine Clearance (mL/min)		
		30–49	10–29	<10
Herpes zoster	1 gram every 8 hours	1 gram every 12 hours	1 gram every 24 hours	500 mg every 24 hours
Genital herpes Initial treatment	1 gram every 12 hours	no reduction	1 gram every 24 hours	500 mg every 24 hours
Genital herpes Recurrent episodes	500 mg every 12 hours	no reduction	500 mg every 24 hours	500 mg every 24 hours
Genital herpes Suppressive therapy	1 gram every 24 hours	no reduction	500 mg every 24 hours	500 mg every 24 hours
	500 mg every 24 hours		500 mg every 48 hours	500 mg every 48 hours
Genital herpes Suppressive therapy in HIV-infected patients	500 mg every 12 hours	no reduction	500 mg every 24 hours	500 mg every 24 hours
Herpes labialis (cold sores) Do not exceed 1 day of treatment.	Two 2-gram doses taken about 12 hours apart	Two 1-gram doses taken about 12 hours apart	Two 500-mg doses taken about 12 hours apart	500-mg single dose

[See table 6 above]
Hemodialysis: During hemodialysis, the half-life of acyclovir after administration of VALTREX is approximately 4 hours. About one third of acyclovir in the body is removed by dialysis during a 4-hour hemodialysis session. Patients requiring hemodialysis should receive the recommended dose of VALTREX after hemodialysis.
Peritoneal Dialysis: There is no information specific to administration of VALTREX in patients receiving peritoneal dialysis. The effect of chronic ambulatory peritoneal dialysis (CAPD) and continuous arteriovenous hemofiltration/dialysis (CAVHD) on acyclovir pharmacokinetics has been studied. The removal of acyclovir after CAPD and CAVHD is less pronounced than with hemodialysis, and the pharmacokinetic parameters closely resemble those observed in patients with ESRD not receiving hemodialysis. Therefore, supplemental doses of VALTREX should not be required following CAPD or CAVHD.

HOW SUPPLIED

VALTREX Caplets (blue, film-coated, capsule-shaped tablets) containing valacyclovir hydrochloride equivalent to 500 mg valacyclovir and printed with "VALTREX 500 mg." Bottle of 30 (NDC 0173-0933-08) and unit dose pack of 100 (NDC 0173-0933-56).
VALTREX Caplets (blue, film-coated, capsule-shaped tablets) containing valacyclovir hydrochloride equivalent to 1 gram valacyclovir and printed with "VALTREX 1 gram." Bottle of 21 (NDC 0173-0565-02).

Store at 15° to 25°C (59° to 77°F).
GlaxoSmithKline, Research Triangle Park, NC 27709
©2003, GlaxoSmithKline. All rights reserved.
April 2003/RL-1195

ZIAGEN® ℞
[zī′ ə-jin]
(abacavir sulfate)
Tablets

ZIAGEN® ℞
(abacavir sulfate)
Oral Solution

Prescribing information for these products, which appears on pages 1690–1694 of the 2003 PDR, has been revised as follows. Please write "See Supplement A" next to the product heading.
The following paragraphs in the **ADVERSE REACTIONS: Abacavir: Hypersensitivity Reaction** *subsection were revised to:*
In clinical studies, approximately 5% of adult and pediatric patients receiving ZIAGEN developed a hypersensitivity reaction. This reaction is characterized by the appearance of symptoms indicating multi-organ/body system involvement. Symptoms usually appear within the first 6 weeks of treatment with ZIAGEN, although these reactions may occur at any time during therapy. Frequently observed signs and

symptoms include fever, skin rash, fatigue, and gastrointestinal symptoms such as nausea, vomiting, diarrhea, or abdominal pain. Other signs and symptoms include malaise, lethargy, myalgia, myolysis, arthralgia, edema, pharyngitis, cough, abnormal chest x-ray findings (predominantly infiltrates, which can be localized), dyspnea, headache, and paresthesia. Some patients who experienced a hypersensitivity reaction were initially thought to have acute onset or worsening respiratory disease. The diagnosis of hypersensitivity reaction should be carefully considered for patients presenting with symptoms of acute onset respiratory diseases, even if alternative respiratory diagnoses (pneumonia, bronchitis, pharyngitis, or flu-like illness) are possible.

Physical findings include lymphadenopathy, mucous membrane lesions (conjunctivitis and mouth ulcerations), and rash. The rash usually appears maculopapular or urticarial but may be variable in appearance. There have been reports of erythema multiforme. Hypersensitivity reactions have occurred without rash.

Laboratory abnormalities include elevated liver function tests, increased creatine phosphokinase or creatinine, and lymphopenia. Anaphylaxis, liver failure, renal failure, hypotension, adult respiratory distress syndrome, respiratory failure, and death have occurred in association with hypersensitivity reactions. Symptoms worsen with continued therapy but often resolve upon discontinuation of ZIAGEN.

The following subsection was added to the **ADVERSE REACTIONS: Observed during Clinical Practice** *subsection:*
Skin: Suspected Stevens-Johnson syndrome (SJS) and toxic epidermal necrolysis (TEN) have been reported in patients receiving abacavir primarily in combination with medications known to be associated with SJS and TEN, respectively. Because of the overlap of clinical signs and symptoms between hypersensitivity to abacavir and SJS and TEN, and the possibility of multiple drug sensitivities in some patients, abacavir should be discontinued and not restarted in such cases.

There have also been reports of erythema multiforme with abacavir use.

GlaxoSmithKline, Research Triangle Park, NC 27709
©2002, GlaxoSmithKline. All rights reserved.
August 2002/RL-1134

ZYBAN® ℞
[zī' ban]
(bupropion hydrochloride)
Sustained-Release Tablets

Prescribing information for this product, which appears on pages 1708–1713 of the 2003 PDR, has been revised as follows. Please write "See Supplement A" next to the product heading.

The **CLINICAL PHARMACOLOGY: Pharmacokinetics:** *Metabolism section was revised to:*
Bupropion is extensively metabolized in humans. Three metabolites have been shown to be active: hydroxybupropion, which is formed via hydroxylation of the *tert*-butyl group of bupropion, and the amino-alcohol isomers threohydrobupropion and erythrohydrobupropion, which are formed via reduction of the carbonyl group. In vitro findings suggest that cytochrome P450IIB6 (CYP2B6) is the principal isoenzyme involved in the formation of hydroxybupropion, while cytochrome P450 isoenzymes are not involved in the formation of threohydrobupropion. Oxidation of the bupropion side chain results in the formation of a glycine conjugate of meta-chlorobenzoic acid, which is then excreted as the major urinary metabolite. The potency and toxicity of the metabolites relative to bupropion have not been fully characterized. However, it has been demonstrated in an antidepressant screening test in mice that hydroxybupropion is one half as potent as bupropion, while threohydrobupropion and erythrohydrobupropion are 5-fold less potent than bupropion. This may be of clinical importance because the plasma concentrations of the metabolites are as high or higher than those of bupropion.

Because bupropion is extensively metabolized, there is the potential for drug-drug interactions, particularly with those agents that are metabolized by the cytochrome P450IIB6 (CYP2B6) isoenzyme. Although bupropion is not metabolized by cytochrome P450IID6 (CYP2D6), there is the potential for drug-drug interactions when bupropion is co-administered with drugs metabolized by this isoenzyme (see PRECAUTIONS: Drug Interactions).

Following a single dose in humans, peak plasma concentrations of hydroxybupropion occur approximately 6 hours after administration of ZYBAN Tablets. Peak plasma concentrations of hydroxybupropion are approximately 10 times the peak level of the parent drug at steady state.

The elimination half-life of hydroxybupropion is approximately 20 ($\pm$5) hours, and its AUC at steady state is about 17 times that of bupropion. The times to peak concentrations for the erythrohydrobupropion and threohydrobupropion metabolites are similar to that of the hydroxybupropion metabolite; however, their elimination half-lives are longer, 33 ($\pm$10) and 37 ($\pm$13) hours, respectively, and steady-state AUCs are 1.5 and 7 times that of bupropion, respectively.

Bupropion and its metabolites exhibit linear kinetics following chronic administration of 300 to 450 mg/day.

The **CLINICAL PHARMACOLOGY: Population Subgroups:** *Hepatic section was revised to:*

The effect of hepatic impairment on the pharmacokinetics of bupropion was characterized in 2 single-dose studies, one in patients with alcoholic liver disease and one in patients with mild to severe cirrhosis.

The first study showed that the half-life of hydroxybupropion was significantly longer in 8 patients with alcoholic liver disease than in 8 healthy volunteers (32 ± 14 hours versus 21 ± 5 hours, respectively). Although not statistically significant, the AUCs for bupropion and hydroxybupropion were more variable and tended to be greater (by 53% to 57%) in patients with alcoholic liver disease. The differences in half-life for bupropion and the other metabolites in the 2 patient groups were minimal.

The second study showed that there were no statistically significant differences in the pharmacokinetics of bupropion and its active metabolites in 9 patients with mild to moderate hepatic cirrhosis compared to 8 healthy volunteers. However, more variability was observed in some of the pharmacokinetic parameters for bupropion (AUC, C_{max}, and T_{max}) and its active metabolites ($t_{1/2}$) in patients with mild to moderate hepatic cirrhosis. In addition, in patients with severe hepatic cirrhosis, the bupropion C_{max} and AUC were substantially increased (mean difference: by approximately 70% and 3-fold, respectively) and more variable when compared to values in healthy volunteers; the mean bupropion half-life was also longer (29 hours in patients with severe hepatic cirrhosis vs. 19 hours in healthy subjects). For the metabolite hydroxybupropion, the mean C_{max} was approximately 69% lower.

For the combined amino-alcohol isomers threohydrobupropion and erythrohydrobupropion, the mean C_{max} was approximately 31% lower. The mean AUC increased by 28% for hydroxybupropion and 50% for threo/erythrohydrobupropion.

The median T_{max} was observed 19 hours later for hydroxybupropion and 21 hours later for threo/erythrohydrobupropion. The mean half-lives for hydroxybupropion and threo/erythrohydrobupropion were increased 2- and 4-fold, respectively, in patients with severe hepatic cirrhosis compared to healthy volunteers (see WARNINGS, PRECAUTIONS, and DOSAGE AND ADMINISTRATION).

The first 2 paragraphs under **WARNINGS** *were revised to:*
Patients should be made aware that ZYBAN contains the same active ingredient found in WELLBUTRIN and WELLBUTRIN SR used to treat depression, and that ZYBAN should not be used in combination with WELLBUTRIN, WELLBUTRIN SR, or any other medications that contain bupropion.

Because the use of bupropion is associated with a dose-dependent risk of seizures, clinicians should not prescribe doses over 300 mg/day for smoking cessation. The risk of seizures is also related to patient factors, clinical situation, and concurrent medications, which must be considered in selection of patients for therapy with ZYBAN. ZYBAN should be discontinued and not restarted in patients who experience a seizure while on treatment.

The **PRECAUTIONS: Drug Interactions:** *Smoking Cessation section was revised to:*
Physiological changes resulting from smoking cessation itself, with or without treatment with ZYBAN, may alter the pharmacokinetics of some concomitant medications, which may require dosage adjustment. Blood concentrations of concomitant medications that are extensively metabolized, such as theophylline and warfarin, may be expected to increase following smoking cessation due to de-induction of hepatic enzymes.

The **ADVERSE REACTIONS: Other Events Observed During the Clinical Development and Postmarketing Experience of Bupropion:** *Hemic and Lymphatic section was revised to:*
Infrequent was ecchymosis. Also observed were anemia, leukocytosis, leukopenia, lymphadenopathy, pancytopenia, and thrombocytopenia. Altered PT and/or INR, infrequently associated with hemorrhagic or thrombotic complications, were observed when bupropion was co-administered with warfarin.

Manufactured by DSM Pharmaceuticals, Inc.
Greenville, NC 27834 for
GlaxoSmithKline, Research Triangle Park, NC 27709
©2003, GlaxoSmithKline. All rights reserved.
March 2003/RL-1189

To keep your **PDR** up to date throughout the year, note these revisions on the corresponding pages of the annual volume. Simply write **"See Supplement A"** next to the product heading.

Merck & Co., Inc.
WEST POINT, PA 19486

For Medical Information Contact:
Generally:
Product and service information:
Call the Merck National Service Center, 8:00 AM to 7:00 PM (ET), Monday through Friday:
(800) NSC-MERCK
(800) 672-6372
FAX: (800) MERCK-68
FAX: (800) 637-2568

Adverse Drug Experiences:
Call the Merck National Service Center, 8:00 AM to 7:00 PM (ET), Monday through Friday:
(800) NSC-MERCK
(800) 672-6372

In Emergencies:
24-hour emergency information for healthcare professionals:
(800) NSC-MERCK
(800) 672-6372

Sales and Ordering:
For product orders and direct account inquiries only, call the Order Management Center,
8:00 AM to 7:00 PM (ET), Monday through Friday:
(800) MERCK RX
(800) 637-2579

AquaMEPHYTON® INJECTION ℞
[ă' kwă mĕ' fĭ-tŏn]
(Phytonadione)
Aqueous Colloidal Solution of Vitamin K₁

Prescribing information for this product, which appears on pages 1944–1945 of the 2003 PDR, has been revised as follows. Please write "See Supplement A" alongside product heading.

In the **PRECAUTIONS** *section, add the following subsection at the beginning:*
General
Vitamin K_1 is fairly rapidly degraded by light; therefore, always protect AquaMEPHYTON from light. Store AquaMEPHYTON in closed original carton until contents have been used. (See also HOW SUPPLIED, *Storage*.)

In the **HOW SUPPLIED** *section, replace the* **Storage** *subsection with the following:*
Store container in original carton. Always protect AquaMEPHYTON from light. Store container in closed original carton until contents have been used. (See PRECAUTIONS, *General*.)

Revisions based on 9073025, issued February 2002.

INTRAVENOUS INFUSION (not for IV Bolus Injection)
CANCIDAS® ℞
[kăn sī dəs]
(caspofungin acetate) FOR INJECTION

Prescribing information for this product, which appears on pages 1950–1953 of the 2003 PDR, has been revised as follows. Please write "See Supplement A" alongside product heading.

In the **CLINICAL PHARMACOLOGY** *section, under Pharmacokinetics, Metabolism, in the second sentence, change "5 to 20" to "≥5", change "3 to 7" to "≤7", and change "0.6 to 1.3%" to "≤1.3%".*

Also in the **CLINICAL PHARMACOLOGY** *section, under Pharmacokinetics, Excretion, replace the first sentence with* "Two single-dose radiolabeled pharmacokinetic studies were conducted. In one study, plasma, urine, and feces were collected over 27 days, and in the second study plasma was collected over 6 months." *Replace the third sentence with* "In plasma, caspofungin concentrations fell below the limit of quantitation after 6 to 8 days postdose, while radiolabel fell below the limit of quantitation at 22.3 weeks postdose."

Also in the **CLINICAL PHARMACOLOGY** *section, under Special Populations, Geriatric, replace the second sentence with* "In patients with candidemia or other *Candida* infections (intra-abdominal abscesses, peritonitis, or pleural space infections), a similar modest effect of age was seen in older patients relative to younger patients."

Also in the **CLINICAL PHARMACOLOGY** *section, under Special Populations, Renal Insufficiency, replace the third sentence with* "However, in patients with invasive aspergillosis, candidemia, or other *Candida* infections (intra-abdominal abscesses, peritonitis, or pleural space infections) who received multiple daily doses of CANCIDAS 50 mg, there was no significant effect of mild to end-stage renal impairment on caspofungin concentrations."

Continued on next page

Information on the Merck & Co., Inc., products listed on these pages is from the full prescribing information in use April 1, 2003.

Cancidas—Cont.

In the **MICROBIOLOGY** section, under Mechanism of Action, at the end of the first sentence, delete "filamentous fungi" and replace with "Aspergillus species and Candida species". In the last sentence, after "activity" and before "in regions", add "against Candida species and".

Also in the **MICROBIOLOGY** section, under Activity in vitro, replace the first two sentences with "Caspofungin exhibits in vitro activity against Aspergillus species (Aspergillus fumigatus, Aspergillus flavus, and Aspergillus terreus) and Candida species (Candida albicans, Candida glabrata, Candida guilliermondii, Candida krusei, Candida parapsilosis, and Candida tropicalis). Susceptibility testing was performed according to the National Committee for Clinical Laboratory Standards (NCCLS) method M38-A (for Aspergillus species) and M27-A (for Candida species)." In the last sentence, after "have not been established" add "for yeasts and filamentous fungi".

Also in the **MICROBIOLOGY** section, under Activity in vivo, add the following sentence at the beginning:
Caspofungin was active when parenterally administered to immunocompetent and immunosuppressed mice as long as 24 hours after disseminated infections with C. albicans, in which the endpoints were prolonged survival of infected mice and reduction of C. albicans from target organs.

Also in the **MICROBIOLOGY** section, under Drug Resistance, add the following sentence at the beginning:
A study in mice infected with C. albicans and treated with orally administered doses of caspofungin suggests that there is a potential for resistance development to occur.

Also in the **MICROBIOLOGY** section, under Drug Resistance, in the last sentence, before "Aspergillus", add "Candida and".

Also in the **MICROBIOLOGY** section, under Drug Interactions, in the first sentence, replace "A. fumigatus" with "either A. fumigatus or C. albicans".

In the **CLINICAL STUDIES** section, add the following subsections at the beginning:
Candidemia and the following other Candida infections: intra-abdominal abscesses, peritonitis and pleural space infections

In a Phase III randomized, double-blind study, patients with a proven diagnosis of invasive candidiasis received daily doses of CANCIDAS (50 mg/day following a 70-mg loading dose on Day 1) or amphotericin B deoxycholate (0.6 to 0.7 mg/kg/day for non-neutropenic patients and 0.7 to 1.0 mg/kg/day for neutropenic patients). Patients were stratified by both neutropenic status and APACHE II score. Patients with Candida endocarditis, meningitis, or osteomyelitis were excluded from this study.

Patients who met the entry criteria and received one or more doses of IV study therapy were included in the primary (modified intention-to-treat [MITT]) analysis of response at the end of IV study therapy. A favorable response at this time point required both symptom/sign resolution/improvement and microbiological clearance of the Candida infection.

Two hundred thirty-nine patients were enrolled. Patient disposition is shown in Table 1.
[See table 1 at right]
Of the 239 patients enrolled, 224 met the criteria for inclusion in the MITT population (109 treated with CANCIDAS and 115 treated with amphotericin B). Of these 224 patients, 186 patients had candidemia (92 treated with CANCIDAS and 94 treated with amphotericin B). The majority of the patients with candidemia were non-neutropenic (87%) and had an APACHE II score less than or equal to 20 (77%) in both arms. Most candidemia infections were caused by C. albicans (39%), followed by C. parapsilosis (20%), C. tropicalis (17%), C. glabrata (8%), and C. krusei (3%).

At the end of the IV study therapy, CANCIDAS was comparable to amphotericin B in the treatment of candidemia in the MITT population. For the other efficacy time points (Day 10 of IV study therapy, end of all antifungal therapy, 2-week post-therapy follow-up, and 6- to 8-week post-therapy follow-up), CANCIDAS was as effective as amphotericin B.

Outcome, relapse and mortality data are shown in Table 2.
[See table 2 at right]
In this study, the efficacy of CANCIDAS in patients with intra-abdominal abscesses, peritonitis and pleural space Candida infections was evaluated in 19 non-neutropenic patients. Two of these patients had concurrent candidemia. Candida was part of a polymicrobial infection that required adjunctive surgical drainage in 11 of these 19 patients. A favorable response was seen in 9 of 9 patients with peritonitis, 3 of 4 with abscesses (liver, parasplenic, and urinary bladder abscesses), 2 of 2 with pleural space infections, 1 of 2 with mixed peritoneal and pleural infection, 1 of 1 with mixed abdominal abscess and peritonitis, and 0 of 1 with Candida pneumonia.

Overall, across all sites of infection included in the study, the efficacy of CANCIDAS was comparable to that of amphotericin B for the primary endpoint.

In this study, the efficacy data for CANCIDAS in neutropenic patients with candidemia were limited. In a separate compassionate use study, 4 patients with hepatosplenic candidiasis received prolonged therapy with CANCIDAS following other long-term antifungal therapy; three of these patients had a favorable response.

Esophageal Candidiasis (and information on oropharyngeal candidiasis)
The safety and efficacy of CANCIDAS in the treatment of esophageal candidiasis was evaluated in one large, controlled, noninferiority, clinical trial and two smaller dose-response studies.
In all 3 studies, patients were required to have symptoms and microbiological documentation of esophageal candidiasis; most patients had advanced AIDS (with CD4 counts <50/mm³).

Of the 166 patients in the large study who had culture-confirmed esophageal candidiasis at baseline, 120 had Candida albicans and 2 had Candida tropicalis as the sole baseline pathogen whereas 44 had mixed baseline cultures containing C. albicans and one or more additional Candida species.

In the large, randomized, double-blind study comparing CANCIDAS 50 mg/day versus intravenous fluconazole 200 mg/day for the treatment of esophageal candidiasis, patients were treated for an average of 9 days (range 7-21 days). The primary endpoint was favorable overall response at 5 to 7 days following discontinuation of study therapy, which required both complete resolution of symptoms and significant endoscopic improvement. The definition of endoscopic response was based on severity of disease at baseline using a 4-grade scale and required at least a two-grade reduction from baseline endoscopic score or reduction to grade 0 for patients with a baseline score of 2 or less.
The proportion of patients with a favorable overall response for the primary endpoint was comparable for CANCIDAS and fluconazole as shown in Table 3.
[See table 3 above]
The proportion of patients with a favorable symptom response was also comparable (90.1% and 89.4% for CANCIDAS and fluconazole, respectively). In addition, the proportion of patients with a favorable endoscopic response

TABLE 1
Disposition in Candidemia and Other Candida Infections (Intra-abdominal abscesses, peritonitis, and pleural space infections)

	CANCIDAS*	Amphotericin B
Randomized patients	114	125
Patients completing study**	63 (55.3%)	69 (55.2%)
DISCONTINUATIONS OF STUDY*		
All Study Discontinuations	51 (44.7%)	56 (44.8%)
Study Discontinuations due to clinical adverse events	39 (34.2%)	43 (34.4%)
Study Discontinuations due to laboratory adverse events	0 (0%)	1 (0.8%)
DISCONTINUATIONS OF STUDY THERAPY		
All Study Therapy Discontinuations	48 (42.1%)	58 (46.4%)
Study Therapy Discontinuations due to clinical adverse events	30 (26.3%)	37 (29.6%)
Study Therapy Discontinuations due to laboratory adverse events	1 (0.9%)	7 (5.6%)
Study Therapy Discontinuations due to all drug-related*** adverse events	3 (2.6%)	29 (23.2%)

*Patients received CANCIDAS 70 mg on Day 1, then 50 mg daily for the remainder of their treatment.
**Study defined as study treatment period and 6-8 week follow-up period.
***Determined by the investigator to be possibly, probably, or definitely drug-related.

TABLE 2
Outcomes, Relapse, & Mortality in Candidemia and Other Candida Infections (Intra-abdominal abscesses, peritonitis, and pleural space infections)

	CANCIDAS*	Amphotericin B	% Difference** after adjusting for strata (Confidence Interval)***
Number of MITT† patients	109	115	
FAVORABLE OUTCOMES (MITT) AT THE END OF IV STUDY THERAPY			
All MITT patients	81/109 (74.3%)	78/115 (67.8%)	7.5 (-5.4, 20.3)
Candidemia	67/92 (72.8%)	63/94 (67%)	7.0 (-7.0, 21.1)
Neutropenic	6/14 (43%)	5/10 (50%)	
Non-neutropenic	61/78 (78%)	58/84 (69%)	
Endophthalmitis	0/1	2/3	
Multiple Sites	4/5	4/4	
Blood / Pleural	1/1	1/1	
Blood / Peritoneal	1/1	1/1	
Blood / Urine	–	1/1	
Peritoneal / Pleural	½	–	
Abdominal / Peritoneal	–	1/1	
Subphrenic / Peritoneal	1/1	–	
DISSEMINATED INFECTIONS, RELAPSES AND MORTALITY			
Disseminated Infections in neutropenic patients	4/14 (28.6%)	3/10 (30%)	
All relapses††	7/81 (8.6%)	8/78 (10.3%)	
Culture-confirmed relapse	5/81 (6%)	2/78 (3%)	
Overall study††† mortality in MITT	36/109 (33.0%)	35/115 (30.4%)	
Mortality during study therapy	18/109 (17%)	13/115 (11%)	
Mortality attributed to Candida	4/109 (4%)	7/115 (6%)	

*Patients received CANCIDAS 70 mg on Day 1, then 50 mg daily for the remainder of their treatment.
**Calculated as CANCIDAS – amphotericin B
***95% CI for candidemia, 95.6% for all patients
†Modified intention-to-treat
††Includes all patients who either developed a culture-confirmed recurrence of Candida infection or required antifungal therapy for the treatment of a proven or suspected Candida infection in the follow-up period.
†††Study defined as study treatment period and 6-8 week follow-up period.

TABLE 3
Favorable Response Rates for Patients with Esophageal Candidiasis

	CANCIDAS	Fluconazole	% Difference* (95% CI)
Day 5-7 post-treatment	66/81 (81.5%)	80/94 (85.1%)	-3.6 (-14.7, 7.5)

*calculated as CANCIDAS – fluconazole

was comparable (85.2% and 86.2% for CANCIDAS and fluconazole, respectively).
As shown in Table 4, the esophageal candidiasis relapse rates at the Day 14 post-treatment visit were similar for the two groups. At the Day 28 post-treatment visit, the group treated with CANCIDAS had a numerically higher incidence of relapse, however, the difference was not statistically significant.
[See table 4 at right]
In this trial, which was designed to establish noninferiority of CANCIDAS to fluconazole for the treatment of esophageal candidiasis, 122 (70%) patients also had oropharyngeal candidiasis. A favorable response was defined as complete resolution of all symptoms of oropharyngeal disease and all visible oropharyngeal lesions. The proportion of patients with a favorable oropharyngeal response at the 5- to 7-day post-treatment visit was numerically lower for CANCIDAS, however, the difference was not statistically significant. The results are shown in Table 5.
[See table 5 at right]
As shown in Table 6, the oropharyngeal candidiasis relapse rates at the Day 14 and the Day 28 post-treatment visits were statistically significantly higher for CANCIDAS than for fluconazole.
[See table 6 at right]
The results from the two smaller dose-ranging studies corroborate the efficacy of CANCIDAS for esophageal candidiasis that was demonstrated in the larger study.
CANCIDAS was associated with favorable outcomes in 7 of 10 esophageal *C. albicans* infections refractory to at least 200 mg of fluconazole given for 7 days, although the *in vitro* susceptibility of the infecting isolates to fluconazole was not known.
Replace the **INDICATIONS AND USAGE** *section with the following:*
CANCIDAS is indicated for the treatment of:
- Candidemia and the following *Candida* infections: intra-abdominal abscesses, peritonitis and pleural space infections. CANCIDAS has not been studied in endocarditis, osteomyelitis, and meningitis due to *Candida*.
- Esophageal Candidiasis (see CLINICAL STUDIES).
- Invasive Aspergillosis in patients who are refractory to or intolerant of other therapies (i.e., amphotericin B, lipid formulations of amphotericin B, and/or itraconazole). CANCIDAS has not been studied as initial therapy for invasive aspergillosis.
In the **WARNINGS** *section, in the second-to-last sentence, replace* "(see ADVERSE REACTIONS, *Laboratory Abnormalities*)" *with* "(see ADVERSE REACTIONS)".
In the **PRECAUTIONS** *section, under General, in the first paragraph, in the first sentence, after* "patients", *add* "with invasive aspergillosis". *After the second sentence, add* "For candidiasis, see CLINICAL STUDIES." *At the end of the third sentence, after* "adequately studied", *add* "in patients. However, CANCIDAS was generally well tolerated at a dose of 100 mg once daily for 21 days when administered to 15 healthy subjects." *In the second paragraph, change* "68 patients" *to* "112 patients"; *change* "12 patients" *to* "14 patients".
Also in the **PRECAUTIONS** *section, under Drug Interactions, in the second paragraph, in the first sentence, after* "mycophenolate,", *add* "nelfinavir,". *In the fourth paragraph, in the last sentence, change* "ADVERSE EFFECTS, *Laboratory Abnormalities*)" *to* "ADVERSE REACTIONS)".
Replace the fifth paragraph with the following:
A drug-drug interaction study with rifampin in healthy volunteers has shown a 30% decrease in caspofungin trough concentrations. Patients on rifampin should receive 70 mg of CANCIDAS daily. In addition, results from regression analyses of patient pharmacokinetic data suggest that co-administration of other inducers of drug clearance (efavirenz, nevirapine, phenytoin, dexamethasone, or carbamazepine) with CANCIDAS may result in clinically meaningful reductions in caspofungin concentrations. It is not known which drug clearance mechanism involved in caspofungin disposition may be inducible. When CANCIDAS is co-administered with inducers of drug clearance, such as efavirenz, nevirapine, phenytoin, dexamethasone, or carbamazepine, use of a daily dose of 70 mg of CANCIDAS should be considered.
Also in the **PRECAUTIONS** *section, under Patients with Hepatic Insufficiency, in the second sentence, after* "(Child-Pugh score 7 to 9),", *add* "CANCIDAS 35 mg daily is recommended. However, where recommended, a 70-mg loading dose should still be administered on Day 1 (see DOSAGE AND ADMINISTRATION)."
Also in the **PRECAUTIONS** *section, under Geriatric Use, before the last sentence, insert the following:*
A similar effect of age on pharmacokinetics was seen in patients with candidemia or other *Candida* infections (intra-abdominal abscesses, peritonitis, or pleural space infections).
In the **ADVERSE REACTIONS** *section, replace the General subsection with the following:*
Possible histamine-mediated symptoms have been reported including isolated reports of rash, facial swelling, pruritus, sensation of warmth, or bronchospasm. Anaphylaxis has been reported during administration of CANCIDAS.
Also in the **ADVERSE REACTIONS** *section, replace the Clinical Adverse Experiences subsection with the following:*

TABLE 4
Relapse Rates at 14 and 28 Days Post-Therapy in Patients with Esophageal Candidiasis at Baseline

	CANCIDAS	Fluconazole	% Difference* (95% CI)
Day 14 post-treatment	7/66 (10.6%)	6/76 (7.9%)	2.7 (-6.9, 12.3)
Day 28 post-treatment	18/64 (28.1%)	12/72 (16.7%)	11.5 (-2.5, 25.4)

*calculated as CANCIDAS – fluconazole

TABLE 5
Oropharyngeal Candidiasis Response Rates at 5 to 7 Days Post-Therapy in Patients with Oropharyngeal and Esophageal Candidiasis at Baseline

	CANCIDAS	Fluconazole	% Difference* (95% CI)
Day 5-7 post-treatment	40/56 (71.4%)	55/66 (83.3%)	-11.9 (-26.8, 3.0)

*calculated as CANCIDAS – fluconazole

TABLE 6
Oropharyngeal Candidiasis Relapse Rates at 14 and 28 Days Post-Therapy in Patients with Oropharyngeal and Esophageal Candidiasis at Baseline

	CANCIDAS	Fluconazole	% Difference* (95% CI)
Day 14 post-treatment	17/40 (42.5%)	7/53 (13.2%)	29.3 (11.5, 47.1)
Day 28 post-treatment	23/39 (59.0%)	18/51 (35.3%)	23.7 (3.4, 43.9)

*calculated as CANCIDAS – fluconazole

The overall safety of caspofungin was assessed in 876 individuals who received single or multiple doses of caspofungin acetate. There were 125 patients with candidemia and/or intra-abdominal abscesses, peritonitis, or pleural space infections, including 4 patients with chronic disseminated candidiasis; 285 patients with esophageal and/or oropharyngeal candidiasis; and 72 patients with invasive aspergillosis enrolled in phase II and phase III clinical studies. The remaining 394 individuals were enrolled in phase I studies. The majority of the patients with *Candida* infections had serious underlying medical conditions (e.g., hematologic or other malignancy, recent major surgery, HIV) requiring multiple concomitant medications. Patients in the noncomparative *Aspergillus* study often had serious predisposing medical conditions (e.g., bone marrow or peripheral stem cell transplants, hematologic malignancy, solid tumors or organ transplants) requiring multiple concomitant medications.
In the randomized, double-blinded invasive candidiasis study, patients received either CANCIDAS 50 mg/day (following a 70-mg loading dose) or amphotericin B 0.6 to 1.0 mg/kg/day. Drug-related clinical adverse experiences occurring in ≥2% of the patients in either treatment group are presented in Table 7.

TABLE 7
Drug-Related* Clinical Adverse Experiences Among Patients with Candidemia or other *Candida* Infections*
Incidence ≥2% for at least one treatment group by Body System

	CANCIDAS 50 mg*** N=114 (percent)	Amphotericin B N=125 (percent)
Body as a Whole		
Chills	5.3	26.4
Fever	7.0	23.2
Cardiovascular System		
Hypertension	1.8	6.4
Hypotension	0.9	2.4
Tachycardia	1.8	10.4
Peripheral Vascular System		
Phlebitis/thrombophlebitis	3.5	4.8
Digestive System		
Diarrhea	2.6	0.8
Jaundice	0.9	3.2
Nausea	1.8	5.6
Vomiting	3.5	8.0
Metabolic/Nutritional/Immune		
Hypokalemia	0.9	5.6
Nervous System & Psychiatric		
Tremor	1.8	2.4
Respiratory System		
Tachypnea	0.0	10.4
Skin & Skin Appendage		
Erythema	0.0	2.4
Rash	0.9	3.2
Sweating	0.9	3.2
Urogenital System		
Renal insufficiency	0.9	5.6
Renal insufficiency, acute	0.0	5.6

*Determined by the investigator to be possibly, probably, or definitely drug-related.
**Intra-abdominal abscesses, peritonitis and pleural space infections
***Patients received CANCIDAS 70 mg on Day 1, then 50 mg daily for the remainder of their treatment.

The incidence of drug-related clinical adverse experiences was significantly lower among patients treated with CANCIDAS (28.9%) than among patients treated with amphotericin B (58.4%). Also, the proportion of patients who experienced an infusion-related adverse event was significantly lower in the group treated with CANCIDAS (20.2%) than in the group treated with amphotericin B (48.8%).
Drug-related laboratory adverse experiences occurring in ≥2% of the patients in either treatment group are presented in Table 8.

TABLE 8
Drug-Related* Laboratory Adverse Experiences Among Patients with Candidemia or other *Candida* Infections*
Incidence ≥2% for at least one treatment group by Laboratory Test Category

	CANCIDAS 50 mg*** N=114 (percent)	Amphotericin B N=125 (percent)
Blood Chemistry		
ALT increased	3.7	8.1
AST increased	1.9	9.0
Blood urea increased	1.9	15.8
Direct serum bilirubin increased	3.8	8.4
Serum alkaline phosphatase increased	8.3	15.6
Serum bicarbonate decreased	0.0	3.6
Serum creatinine increased	3.7	22.6
Serum phosphate increased	0.0	2.7
Serum potassium decreased	9.9	23.4
Serum potassium increased	0.9	2.4
Total serum bilirubin increased	2.8	8.9
Hematology		
Hematocrit decreased	0.9	7.3
Hemoglobin decreased	0.9	10.5
Urinalysis		
Urine protein increased	0.0	3.7

*Determined by the investigator to be possibly, probably, or definitely drug-related.
**Intra-abdominal abscesses, peritonitis and pleural space infections
***Patients received CANCIDAS 70 mg on Day 1, then 50 mg daily for the remainder of their treatment.

The incidence of drug-related laboratory adverse experiences was signficantly lower among patients receiving

Continued on next page

Information on the Merck & Co., Inc., products listed on these pages is from the full prescribing information in use April 1, 2003.

Cancidas—Cont.

CANCIDAS (24.3%) than among patients receiving amphotericin B (54.0%).

The percentage of patients with either a drug-related clinical adverse experience or a drug-related laboratory adverse experience was significantly lower among patients receiving CANCIDAS (42.1%) than among patients receiving amphotericin B (75.2%). Furthermore, a significant difference between the two treatment groups was observed with regard to incidence of discontinuation due to drug-related clinical or laboratory adverse experience; incidences were 3/114 (2.6%) in the group treated with CANCIDAS and 29/125 (23.2%) in the group treated with amphotericin B.

To evaluate the effect of CANCIDAS and amphotericin B on renal function, nephrotoxicity was defined as doubling of serum creatinine relative to baseline or an increase of ≥1 mg/dL in serum creatinine if baseline serum creatinine was above the upper limit of the normal range. In a subgroup of patients whose baseline creatinine clearance was >30 mL/min, the incidence of nephrotoxicity was significantly lower in the group treated with CANCIDAS than in the group treated with amphotericin B.

Drug-related clinical adverse experiences occurring in ≥2% of patients with esophageal and/or oropharyngeal candidiasis are presented in Table 9.

[See table 9 at right]

Laboratory abnormalities occurring in ≥2% of patients with esophageal and/or oropharyngeal candidiasis are presented in Table 10.

[See table 10 at top of next page]

In the open-label, noncomparative aspergillosis study, in which 69 patients received CANCIDAS (70-mg loading dose on Day 1 followed by 50 mg daily), the following drug-related clinical adverse experiences were observed with an incidence of ≥2%; fever (2.9%), infused-vein complications (2.9%), nausea (2.9%), vomiting (2.9%) and flushing (2.9%). Also reported infrequently in this patient population were pulmonary edema, ARDS, and radiographic infiltrates.

Drug-related laboratory abnormalities reported with an incidence ≥2% in patients treated with CANCIDAS in the noncomparative aspergillosis study were: serum alkaline phosphatase increased (2.9%), serum potassium decreased (2.9%), eosinophils increased (3.2%), urine protein increased (4.9%), and urine RBCs increased (2.2%).

Post Marketing Experience:

The following postmarketing adverse events have been reported:
- Hepatobiliary: Rare cases of clinically significant hepatic dysfunction
- Cardiovascular: swelling and peripheral edema
- Metabolic: hypercalcemia

Concomitant Therapy

In the **OVERDOSAGE** section, in the first sentence, replace "100 mg" with "210 mg" and replace "5 patients" with "6 healthy subjects". *Replace the third sentence with* "In addition, 100 mg once daily for 21 days has been administered to 15 healthy subjects and was generally well tolerated."

In the **DOSAGE AND ADMINISTRATION** section, replace all copy preceding the "Preparation notes" box with the following:

Do not mix or co-infuse CANCIDAS with other medications, as there are no data available on the compatibility of CANCIDAS with other intravenous substances, additives, or medications. DO NOT USE DILUENTS CONTAINING DEXTROSE (α-D-GLUCOSE), as CANCIDAS is not stable in diluents containing dextrose.

Candidemia and other Candida infections (see CLINICAL STUDIES)

A single 70-mg loading dose should be administered on Day 1, followed by 50 mg daily thereafter. CANCIDAS should be administered by slow IV infusion over approximately 1 hour. Duration of treatment should be dictated by the patient's clinical and microbiological response. In general, antifungal therapy should continue for at least 14 days after the last positive culture. Patients who remain persistently neutropenic may warrant a longer course of therapy pending resolution of the neutropenia.

Esophageal Candidiasis

50 mg daily should be administered by slow IV infusion over approximately 1 hour. Because of the risk of relapse of oropharyngeal candidiasis in patients with HIV infections, suppressive oral therapy could be considered (see CLINICAL STUDIES). A 70-mg loading dose has not been studied with this indication.

Invasive Aspergillosis

A single 70-mg loading dose should be administered on Day 1, followed by 50 mg daily thereafter. CANCIDAS should be administered by slow IV infusion over approximately 1 hour. Duration of treatment should be based upon the severity of the patient's underlying disease, recovery from immunosuppression, and clincial response. The efficacy of a 70-mg dose regimen in patients who are not clinically responding to the 50-mg daily dose is not known. Limited safety data suggests that an increase in dose to 70 mg daily is well tolerated. The safety and efficacy of doses above 70 mg have not been adequately studied.

Hepatic Insufficiency

Patients with mild hepatic insufficiency (Child-Pugh score 5 to 6) do not need a dosage adjustment. For patients with moderate hepatic insufficiency (Child-Pugh score 7 to 9), CANCIDAS 35 mg daily is recommended. However, where recommended, a 70-mg loading dose should still be administered on Day 1. There is no clinical experience in patients with severe hepatic insufficiency (Child-Pugh score >9).

Concomitant Medication with Inducers of Drug Clearance

Patients on rifampin should receive 70 mg of CANCIDAS daily. Patients on nevirapine, efavirenz, carbamazepine, dexamethasone, or phenytoin may require an increase in dose to 70 mg of CANCIDAS daily (see PRECAUTIONS, *Drug Interactions*).

Preparation of CANCIDAS for use:

Do not mix or co-infuse CANCIDAS with other medications, as there are no data available on the compatibility of CANCIDAS with other intravenous substances, additives, or medications. DO NOT USE DILUENTS CONTAINING DEXTROSE (α-D-GLUCOSE), as CANCIDAS is not stable in diluents containing dextrose.

Preparation of the 70-mg infusion

1. Equilibrate the refrigerated vial of CANCIDAS to room temperature.
2. Aseptically add 10.5 mL of 0.9% Sodium Chloride Injection, Sterile Water for Injection, Bacteriostatic Water for Injection with methylparaben and propylparaben, or Bacteriostatic Water for Injection with 0.9% benzyl alcohol to the vial.[a] This reconstituted solution may be stored for up to one hour at ≤25°C (≤77°F).[b]
3. Aseptically transfer 10 mL[c] of reconstituted CANCIDAS to an IV bag (or bottle) containing 250 mL 0.9%, 0.45%, or 0.225% Sodium Chloride Injection, or Lactated Ringer's Injection. This infusion solution must be used within 24 hours if stored at ≤25°C (≤77°F) or within 48 hours if stored refrigerated at 2 to 8°C (36 to 46°F). (If a 70-mg vial is unavailable, see below: *Alternative Infusion Preparation Methods, Preparation of 70-mg Day 1 loading dose from two 50-mg vials.*)

Preparation of the daily 50-mg infusion

1. Equilibrate the refrigerated vial of CANCIDAS to room temperature.
2. Aseptically add 10.5 mL of 0.9% Sodium Chloride Injection, Sterile Water for Injection, Bacteriostatic Water for Injection with methylparaben and propylparaben, or Bacteriostatic Water for Injection with 0.9% benzyl alcohol to the vial.[a] This reconstituted solution may be stored for up to one hour at ≤25°C (≤77°F).[b]
3. Aseptically transfer 10 mL[c] of reconstituted CANCIDAS to an IV bag (or bottle) containing 250 mL 0.9%, 0.45%, or 0.225% Sodium Chloride Injection, or Lactated Ringer's Injection. This infusion solution must be used within 24 hours if stored at ≤25°C (≤77°F) or within 48 hours if stored refrigerated at 2 to 8°C (36 to 46°F). (If a reduced infusion volume is medically necessary, see below: *Alternative Infusion Preparation Methods, Preparation of 50-mg daily doses at reduced volume.*)

Alternative Infusion Preparation Methods

Preparation of 70-mg dose from two 50-mg vials

Reconstitute two 50-mg vials with 10.5 mL of diluent each (see *Preparation of the daily 50-mg infusion*). Aseptically transfer a total of 14 mL of the reconstituted CANCIDAS from the two vials to 250 mL of 0.9%, 0.45%, or 0.225% Sodium Chloride Injection, or Lactated Ringer's Injection.

Preparation of 50-mg daily doses at reduced volume

When medically necessary, the 50-mg daily doses can be prepared by adding 10 mL of reconstituted CANCIDAS to 100 mL of 0.9%, 0.45%, or 0.225% Sodium Chloride Injection, or Lactated Ringer's Injection (see *Preparation of the daily 50-mg infusion*).

Preparation of a 35-mg daily dose for patients with moderate Hepatic Insufficiency

Reconstitute one 50-mg vial (see above: *Preparation of the daily 50-mg infusion*). Aseptically transfer 7 mL of the reconstituted CANCIDAS from the vial to 250 mL or, if medically necessary, to 100 mL of 0.9%, 0.45%, or 0.225% Sodium Chloride Injection or Lactated Ringer's Injection.

In the "Preparation notes" box, delete footnote d.

TABLE 9
Drug-Related Clinical Adverse Experiences Among Patients with Esophageal and/or Oropharyngeal Candidiasis*
Incidence ≥2% for at least one treatment dose (per comparison) by Body System

	CANCIDAS 50 mg** N=83 (percent)	Fluconazole IV 200 mg** N=94 (percent)	CANCIDAS 50 mg*** N=80 (percent)	CANCIDAS 70 mg*** N=65 (percent)	Amphotericin B 0.5 mg/kg*** N=89 (percent)
Body as a Whole					
Asthenia/fatigue	0.0	0.0	0.0	0.0	6.7
Chills	0.0	0.0	2.5	1.5	75.3
Edema/swelling	0.0	0.0	0.0	0.0	5.6
Edema, facial	0.0	0.0	0.0	3.1	0.0
Fever	3.6	1.1	21.3	26.2	69.7
Flu-like illness	0.0	0.0	0.0	3.1	0.0
Malaise	0.0	0.0	0.0	0.0	5.6
Pain	0.0	0.0	1.3	4.6	5.6
Pain, abdominal	3.6	2.1	2.5	0.0	9.0
Warm sensation	0.0	0.0	0.0	1.5	4.5
Peripheral Vascular System					
Infused vein complication	12.0	8.5	2.5	1.5	0.0
Phlebitis/thrombophlebitis	15.7	8.5	11.3	13.8	22.5
Cardiovascular System					
Tachycardia	0.0	0.0	1.3	0.0	4.5
Vasculitis	0.0	0.0	0.0	0.0	3.4
Digestive System					
Anorexia	0.0	0.0	1.3	0.0	3.4
Diarrhea	3.6	2.1	1.3	3.1	11.2
Gastitis	0.0	2.1	0.0	0.0	0.0
Nausea	6.0	6.4	2.5	3.1	21.3
Vomiting	1.2	3.2	1.3	3.1	13.5
Hemic & Lymphatic System					
Anemia	0.0	0.0	3.8	0.0	9.0
Metabolic/Nutritional/Immune					
Anaphylaxis	0.0	0.0	0.0	0.0	2.2
Musculoskeletal System					
Myalgia	1.2	0.0	0.0	3.1	2.2
Pain, back	0.0	0.0	0.0	0.0	2.2
Pain, musculoskeletal	0.0	0.0	1.3	0.0	4.5
Nervous System & Psychiatric					
Dizziness	0.0	2.1	0.0	1.5	1.1
Headache	6.0	1.1	11.3	7.7	19.1
Insomnia	1.2	0.0	0.0	0.0	2.2
Paresthesia	0.0	0.0	1.3	3.1	1.1
Tremor	0.0	0.0	0.0	0.0	7.9
Respiratory System					
Tachypnea	0.0	0.0	1.3	0.0	4.5
Skin & Skin Appendage					
Erythema	1.2	0.0	1.3	1.5	7.9
Induration	0.0	0.0	0.0	3.1	6.7
Pruritus	1.2	0.0	2.5	1.5	0.0
Rash	0.0	0.0	1.3	4.6	3.4
Sweating	0.0	0.0	1.3	0.0	3.4

*Relationship to drug was determined by the investigator to be possibly, probably or definitely drug-related.
**Derived from Phase III comparator-controlled clinical study.
***Derived from Phase II comparator-controlled clinical studies.

TABLE 10
Drug-Related Laboratory Abnormalities Reported Among Patients with Esophageal and/or Oropharyngeal Candidiasis*
Incidence ≥2% (for at least one treatment dose) by Laboratory Test Category

	CANCIDAS 50 mg** N=163 (percent)	CANCIDAS 70 mg*** N=65 (percent)	Fluconazole IV 200 mg** N=94 (percent)	Amphotericin B 0.5 mg/kg*** N=89 (percent)
Blood Chemistry				
ALT increased	10.6	10.8	11.8	22.7
AST increased	13.0	10.8	12.9	22.7
Blood urea increased	0.0	0.0	1.2	10.3
Direct serum bilirubin increased	0.6	0.0	3.3	2.5
Serum albumin decreased	8.6	4.6	5.4	14.9
Serum alkaline phosphatase increased	10.5	7.7	11.8	19.3
Serum bicarbonate decreased	0.9	0.0	0.0	6.6
Serum calcium decreased	1.9	0.0	3.2	1.1
Serum creatinine increased	0.0	1.5	2.2	28.1
Serum potassium decreased	3.7	10.8	4.3	31.5
Serum potassium increased	0.6	0.0	2.2	1.1
Serum sodium decreased	1.9	1.5	3.2	1.1
Serum uric acid increased	0.6	0.0	0.0	3.4
Total serum bilirubin increased	0.0	0.0	3.2	4.5
Total serum protein decreased	3.1	0.0	3.2	3.4
Hematology				
Eosinophils increased	3.1	3.1	1.1	1.1
Hematocrit decreased	11.1	1.5	5.4	32.6
Hemoglobin decreased	12.3	3.1	5.4	37.1
Lymphocytes increased	0.0	1.6	2.2	0.0
Neutrophils decreased	1.9	3.1	3.2	1.1
Platelet count decreased	3.1	1.5	2.2	3.4
Prothrombin time increased	1.3	1.5	0.0	2.3
WBC count decreased	6.2	4.6	8.6	7.9
Urinalysis				
Urine blood increased	0.0	0.0	0.0	4.0
Urine casts increased	0.0	0.0	0.0	8.0
Urine pH increased	0.8	0.0	0.0	3.6
Urine protein increased	1.2	0.0	3.3	4.5
Urine RBCs increased	1.1	3.8	5.1	12.0
Urine WBCs increased	0.0	7.7	0.0	24.0

*Relationship to drug was determined by the investigator to be possibly, probably or definitely drug-related.
**Derived from Phase II and Phase III comparator-controlled clinical studies.
***Derived from Phase II comparator-controlled clinical studies.

Change Table 5 *to* Table 11.
In the **HOW SUPPLIED** *section, under Storage, Diluted Product, after* "24 hours" *add* "or at 2 to 8°C (36 to 46°F) for 48 hours".
Revisions based on 9344302, issued January 2003.

COZAAR® ℞

[cō 'zăr]
(losartan potassium tablets)

Prescribing information for this product, which appears on pages 1968–1970 of the 2003 PDR, has been extensively revised and should be replaced with the following. Please write "See Supplement A" alongside product heading.

USE IN PREGNANCY
When used in pregnancy during the second and third trimesters, drugs that act directly on the renin-angiotensin system can cause injury and even death to the developing fetus. When pregnancy is detected, COZAAR should be discontinued as soon as possible. See WARNINGS: *Fetal/Neonatal Morbidity and Mortality.*

DESCRIPTION

COZAAR* (losartan potassium) is an angiotensin II receptor (type AT_1) antagonist. Losartan potassium, a non-peptide molecule, is chemically described as 2-butyl-4-chloro-1-[*p*-(*o*-1*H*-tetrazol-5-ylphenyl)benzyl]imidazole-5-methanol monopotassium salt.
Its empirical formula is $C_{22}H_{22}ClKN_6O$, and its structural formula is:

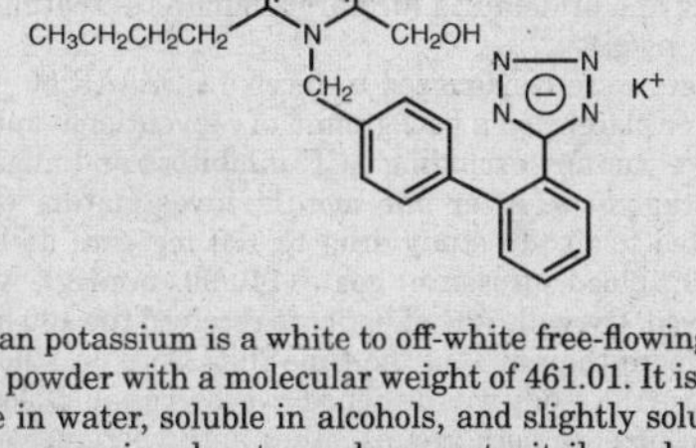

Losartan potassium is a white to off-white free-flowing crystalline powder with a molecular weight of 461.01. It is freely soluble in water, soluble in alcohols, and slightly soluble in common organic solvents, such as acetonitrile and methyl ethyl ketone. Oxidation of the 5-hydroxymethyl group on the imidazole ring results in the active metabolite of losartan.
COZAAR is available as tablets for oral administration containing either 25 mg, 50 mg or 100 mg of losartan potassium and the following inactive ingredients: microcrystalline cellulose, lactose hydrous, pregelatinized starch, magnesium stearate, hydroxypropyl cellulose, hydroxypropyl methylcellulose, titanium dioxide, D&C yellow No. 10 aluminum lake and FD&C blue No. 2 aluminum lake.
COZAAR 25 mg, 50 mg and 100 mg tablets contain potassium in the following amounts: 2.12 mg (0.054 mEq), 4.24 mg (0.108 mEq) and 8.48 mg (0.216 mEq), respectively.

*Registered trademark of E.I. du Pont de Nemours and Company, Wilmington, Delaware, USA

CLINICAL PHARMACOLOGY

Mechanism of Action
Angiotensin II [formed from angiotensin I in a reaction catalyzed by angiotensin converting enzyme (ACE, kininase II)], is a potent vasoconstrictor, the primary vasoactive hormone of the renin-angiotensin system and an important component in the pathophysiology of hypertension. It also stimulates aldosterone secretion by the adrenal cortex. Losartan and its principal active metabolite block the vasoconstrictor and aldosterone-secreting effects of angiotensin II by selectively blocking the binding of angiotensin II to the AT_1 receptor found in many tissues, (e.g., vascular smooth muscle, adrenal gland). There is also an AT_2 receptor found in many tissues but it is not known to be associated with cardiovascular homeostasis. Both losartan and its principal active metabolite do not exhibit any partial agonist activity at the AT_1 receptor and have much greater affinity (about 1000-fold) for the AT_1 receptor than for the AT_2 receptor. *In vitro* binding studies indicate that losartan is a reversible, competitive inhibitor of the AT_1 receptor. The active metabolite is 10 to 40 times more potent by weight than losartan and appears to be a reversible, non-competitive inhibitor of the AT_1 receptor.
Neither losartan nor its active metabolite inhibits ACE (kininase II, the enzyme that converts angiotensin I to angiotensin II and degrades bradykinin); nor do they bind to or block other hormone receptors or ion channels known to be important in cardiovascular regulation.
Pharmacokinetics
General
Losartan is an orally active agent that undergoes substantial first-pass metabolism by cytochrome P450 enzymes. It is converted, in part, to an active carboxylic acid metabolite that is responsible for most of the angiotensin II receptor antagonism that follows losartan treatment. The terminal half-life of losartan is about 2 hours and of the metabolite is about 6-9 hours. The pharmacokinetics of losartan and its active metabolite are linear with oral losartan doses up to 200 mg and do not change over time. Neither losartan nor its metabolite accumulate in plasma upon repeated once-daily dosing.
Following oral administration, losartan is well absorbed (based on absorption of radiolabeled losartan) and undergoes substantial first-pass metabolism; the systemic bioavailability of losartan is approximately 33%. About 14% of an orally-administered dose of losartan is converted to the active metabolite. Mean peak concentrations of losartan and its active metabolite are reached in 1 hour and in 3-4 hours, respectively. While maximum plasma concentrations of losartan and its active metabolite are approximately equal, the AUC of the metabolite is about 4 times as great as that of losartan. A meal slows absorption of losartan and decreases its C_{max} but has only minor effects on losartan AUC or on the AUC of the metabolite (about 10% decreased).
Both losartan and its active metabolite are highly bound to plasma proteins, primarily albumin, with plasma free fractions of 1.3% and 0.2%, respectively. Plasma protein binding is constant over the concentration range achieved with recommended doses. Studies in rats indicate that losartan crosses the blood-brain barrier poorly, if at all.
Losartan metabolites have been identified in human plasma and urine. In addition to the active carboxylic acid metabolite, several inactive metabolites are formed. Following oral and intravenous administration of ^{14}C-labeled losartan potassium, circulating plasma radioactivity is primarily attributed to losartan and its active metabolite. *In vitro* studies indicate that cytochrome P450 2C9 and 3A4 are involved in the biotransformation of losartan to its metabolites. Minimal conversion of losartan to the active metabolite (less than 1% of the dose compared to 14% of the dose in normal subjects) was seen in about one percent of individuals studied.
The volume of distribution of losartan is about 34 liters and of the active metabolite is about 12 liters. Total plasma clearance of losartan and the active metabolite is about 600 mL/min and 50 mL/min, respectively, with renal clearance of about 75 mL/min and 25 mL/min, respectively. When losartan is administered orally, about 4% of the dose is excreted unchanged in the urine and about 6% is excreted in urine as active metabolite. Biliary excretion contributes to the elimination of losartan and its metabolites. Following oral ^{14}C-labeled losartan, about 35% of radioactivity is recovered in the urine and about 60% in the feces. Following an intravenous dose of ^{14}C-labeled losartan, about 45% of radioactivity is recovered in the urine and 50% in the feces.
Special Populations
Pediatric: Losartan pharmacokinetics have not been investigated in patients <18 years of age.
Geriatric and Gender: Losartan pharmacokinetics have been investigated in the elderly (65-75 years) and in both genders. Plasma concentrations of losartan and its active metabolite are similar in elderly and young hypertensives. Plasma concentrations of losartan were about twice as high in female hypertensives as male hypertensives, but concentrations of the active metabolite were similar in males and females. No dosage adjustment is necessary (see DOSAGE AND ADMINISTRATION).
Race: Pharmacokinetic differences due to race have not been studied. (see also PRECAUTIONS, *Race* and CLINICAL PHARMACOLOGY, *Pharmacodynamics and Clinical Effects, Reduction in the Risk of Stroke, Race*).
Renal Insufficiency: Plasma concentrations of losartan are not altered in patients with creatinine clearance above 30 mL/min. In patients with lower creatinine clearance, AUCs are about 50% greater and they are doubled in hemodialysis patients. Plasma concentrations of the active metabolite are not significantly altered in patients with renal impairment or in hemodialysis patients. Neither losartan nor its active metabolite can be removed by hemodialysis. No dosage adjustment is necessary for patients with renal impairment unless they are volume-depleted (see WARNINGS, *Hypotension — Volume-Depleted Patients* and DOSAGE AND ADMINISTRATION).
Hepatic Insufficiency: Following oral administration in patients with mild to moderate alcoholic cirrhosis of the liver, plasma concentrations of losartan and its active metabolite were, respectively, 5-times and about 1.7-times those in young male volunteers. Compared to normal subjects the total plasma clearance of losartan in patients with hepatic insufficiency was about 50% lower and the oral bioavailability was about 2-times higher. A lower starting dose is recommended for patients with a history of hepatic impairment (see DOSAGE AND ADMINISTRATION).
Drug Interactions
Losartan, administered for 12 days, did not affect the pharmacokinetics or pharmacodynamics of a single dose of warfarin. Losartan did not affect the pharmacokinetics of oral or intravenous digoxin. Coadministration of losartan and cimetidine led to an increase of about 18% in AUC of losartan but did not affect the pharmacokinetics of its active metabolite. Coadministration of losartan and phenobarbital led to a reduction of about 20% in the AUC of losartan and that of its active metabolite. Conversion of losartan to its active metabolite after intravenous administration is not affected by ketoconazole, an inhibitor of P450 3A4. There is no pharmacokinetic interaction between losartan and hydrochlorothiazide.
Pharmacodynamics and Clinical Effects
Hypertension: Losartan inhibits the pressor effect of angiotensin II (as well as angiotensin I) infusions. A dose of 100 mg inhibits the pressor effect by about 85% at peak with 25-40% inhibition persisting for 24 hours. Removal of the negative feedback of angiotensin II causes a 2-3 fold rise in plasma renin activity and consequent rise in angiotensin II plasma concentration in hypertensive patients. Losartan

Continued on next page

Information on the Merck & Co., Inc., products listed on these pages is from the full prescribing information in use April 1, 2003.

Cozaar—Cont.

does not affect the response to bradykinin, whereas ACE inhibitors increase the response to bradykinin. Aldosterone plasma concentrations fall following losartan administration. In spite of the effect of losartan on aldosterone secretion, very little effect on serum potassium was observed.

In a single-dose study in normal volunteers, losartan had no effects on glomerular filtration rate, renal plasma flow or filtration fraction. In multiple dose studies in hypertensive patients, there were no notable effects on systemic or renal prostaglandin concentrations, fasting triglycerides, total cholesterol or HDL-cholesterol or fasting glucose concentrations. There was a small uricosuric effect leading to a minimal decrease in serum uric acid (mean decrease <0.4 mg/dL) during chronic oral administration.

The antihypertensive effects of COZAAR were demonstrated principally in 4 placebo-controlled 6-12 week trials of dosages from 10 to 150 mg per day in patients with baseline diastolic blood pressures of 95-115. The studies allowed comparisons of two doses (50-100 mg/day) as once-daily or twice-daily regimens, comparisons of peak and trough effects, and comparisons of response by gender, age, and race. Three additional studies examined the antihypertensive effects of losartan and hydrochlorothiazide in combination.

The 4 studies of losartan monotherapy included a total of 1075 patients randomized to several doses of losartan and 334 to placebo. The 10 and 25 mg doses produced some effect at peak (6 hours after dosing) but small and inconsistent trough (24 hour) responses. Doses of 50, 100 and 150 mg once daily gave statistically significant systolic/diastolic mean decreases in blood pressure, compared to placebo in the range of 5.5-10.5/3.5-7.5 mmHg, with the 150 mg dose giving no greater effect than 50-100 mg. Twice-daily dosing at 50-100 mg/day gave consistently larger trough responses than once-daily dosing at the same total dose. Peak (6 hour) effects were uniformly, but moderately, larger than trough effects, with the trough-to-peak ratio for systolic and diastolic responses 50-95% and 60-90%, respectively.

Addition of a low dose of hydrochlorothiazide (12.5 mg) to losartan 50 mg once daily resulted in placebo-adjusted blood pressure reductions of 15.5/9.2 mmHg.

Analysis of age, gender, and race subgroups of patients showed that men and women, and patients over and under 65, had generally similar responses. COZAAR was effective in reducing blood pressure regardless of race, although the effect was somewhat less in Black patients (usually a low-renin population).

The effect of losartan is substantially present within one week but in some studies the maximal effect occurred in 3-6 weeks. In long-term follow-up studies (without placebo control) the effect of losartan appeared to be maintained for up to a year. There is no apparent rebound effect after abrupt withdrawal of losartan. There was essentially no change in average heart rate in losartan-treated patients in controlled trials.

Reduction in the Risk of Stroke: The Losartan Intervention For Endpoint reduction in hypertension (LIFE) study was a multinational, double-blind study comparing COZAAR and atenolol in 9193 hypertensive patients with ECG-documented left ventricular hypertrophy. Patients with myocardial infarction or stroke within six months prior to randomization were excluded. Patients were randomized to receive once daily COZAAR 50 mg or atenolol 50 mg. If goal blood pressure (<140/90 mmHg) was not reached, hydrochlorothiazide (12.5 mg) was added first and, if needed, the dose of COZAAR or atenolol was then increased to 100 mg once daily. If necessary, other antihypertensive treatments (e.g., increase in dose of hydrochlorothiazide therapy to 25 mg or addition of other diuretic therapy, calcium channel blockers, alpha-blockers, or centrally acting agents, but not ACE inhibitors, angiotensin II antagonists, or beta-blockers) were added to the treatment regimen to reach the goal blood pressure.

Of the randomized patients, 4963 (54%) were female and 533 (6%) were Black. The mean age was 67 with 5704 (62%) age ≥65. At baseline, 1195 (13%) had diabetes, 1326 (14%) had isolated systolic hypertension, 1469 (16%) had coronary heart disease, and 728 (8%) had cerebrovascular disease. Baseline mean blood pressure was 174/98 mmHg in both treatment groups. The mean length of follow-up was 4.8 years. At the end of study or at the last visit before a primary endpoint, 77% of the group treated with COZAAR and 73% of the group treated with atenolol were still taking study medication. Of the patients still taking study medication, the mean doses of COZAAR and atenolol were both about 80 mg/day, and 15% were taking atenolol or losartan as monotherapy, while 77% were also receiving hydrochlorothiazide (at a mean dose of 20 mg/day in each group). Blood pressure reduction measured at trough was similar for both treatment groups but blood pressure was not measured at any other time of the day. At the end of study or at the last visit before a primary endpoint, the mean blood pressures were 144.1/81.3 mmHg for the group treated with COZAAR and 145.4/80.9 mmHg for the group treated with atenolol [the difference in SBP of 1.3 mmHg was significant (p<0.001), while the difference of 0.4 mmHg in DBP was not significant (p=0.098)].

The primary endpoint was the first occurrence of cardiovascular death, nonfatal stroke, or nonfatal myocardial infarction. Patients with non-fatal events remained in the trial, so that there was also an examination of the first event of each type even if it was not the first event (e.g., a stroke following an initial myocardial infarction would be counted in the analysis of stroke). Treatment with COZAAR resulted in a 13% reduction (p=0.021) in risk of the primary endpoint compared to the atenolol group (see Figure 1 and Table 1); this difference was primarily the result of an effect on fatal and nonfatal stroke. Treatment with COZAAR reduced the risk of stroke by 25% relative to atenolol (p=0.001) (see Figure 2 and Table 1).

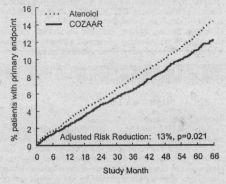

Figure 1. Kaplan-Meier estimates of the primary endpoint of time to cardiovascular death, nonfatal stroke, or nonfatal myocardial infarction in the groups treated with COZAAR and atenolol. The Risk Reduction is adjusted for baseline Framingham risk score and level of electrocardiographic left ventricular hypertrophy.

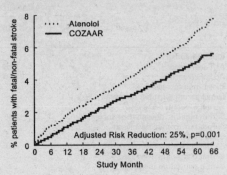

Figure 2. Kaplan-Meier estimates of the time to fatal/nonfatal stroke in the groups treated with COZAAR and atenolol. The Risk Reduction is adjusted for baseline Framingham risk score and level of electrocardiographic left ventricular hypertrophy.

Table 1 shows the results for the primary composite endpoint and the individual endpoints. The primary endpoint was the first occurrence of stroke, myocardial infarction or cardiovascular death, analyzed using an intention-to-treat (ITT) approach. The table shows the number of events for each component in two different ways. The Components of Primary Endpoint (as a first event) counts only the events that define the primary endpoint, while the Secondary Endpoints count all first events of a particular type, whether or not they were preceded by a different type of event.
[See table 1 below]

Although the LIFE study favored COZAAR over atenolol with respect to the primary endpoint (p=0.021), this result is from a single study and, therefore, is less compelling than the difference between COZAAR and placebo. Although not measured directly, the difference between COZAAR and placebo is compelling because there is evidence that atenolol is itself effective (vs. placebo) in reducing cardiovascular events, including stroke, in hypertensive patients.

Other clinical endpoints of the LIFE study were: total mortality, hospitalization for heart failure or angina pectoris, coronary or peripheral revascularization procedures, and resuscitated cardiac arrest. There were no significant differences in the rates of these endpoints between the COZAAR and atenolol groups.

For the primary endpoint and stroke, the effects of COZAAR in patient subgroups defined by age, gender, race and presence or absence of isolated systolic hypertension (ISH), diabetes, and history of cardiovascular disease (CVD) are shown in Figure 3 below. Subgroup analyses can be difficult to interpret and it is not known whether these represent true differences or chance effects.
[See figure 3 at top of next page]

Race: In the LIFE study, Black patients treated with atenolol were at lower risk of experiencing the primary composite endpoint compared with Black patients treated with COZAAR. In the subgroup of Black patients (n=533; 6% of the LIFE study patients), there were 29 primary endpoints among 263 patients on atenolol (11%, 26 per 1000 patient-years) and 46 primary endpoints among 270 patients (17%, 42 per 1000 patient-years) on COZAAR. This finding could not be explained on the basis of differences in the populations other than race or on any imbalances between treatment groups. In addition, blood pressure reductions in both treatment groups were consistent between Black and non-Black patients. Given the difficulty in interpreting subset differences in large trials, it cannot be known whether the observed difference is the result of chance. However, the LIFE study provides no evidence that the benefits of COZAAR on reducing the risk of cardiovascular events in hypertensive patients with left ventricular hypertrophy apply to Black patients.

Nephropathy in Type 2 Diabetic Patients: The Reduction of Endpoints in NIDDM with the Angiotensin II Receptor Antagonist Losartan (RENAAL) study was a randomized, placebo-controlled, double-blind, multicenter study conducted worldwide in 1513 patients with type 2 diabetes with nephropathy (defined as serum creatinine 1.3 to 3.0 mg/dl in females or males ≤60 kg and 1.5 to 3.0 mg/dl in males >60 kg and proteinuria [urinary albumin to creatinine ratio ≥300 mg/g]).

Patients were randomized to receive COZAAR 50 mg once daily or placebo on a background of conventional antihypertensive therapy excluding ACE inhibitors and angiotensin II antagonists. After one month, investigators were instructed to titrate study drug to 100 mg once daily if the trough blood pressure goal (140/90 mmHg) was not achieved. Overall, 72% of patients received the 100 mg daily dose more than 50% of the time they were on study drug. Because the study was designed to achieve equal blood pressure control in both groups, other antihypertensive agents (diuretics, calcium-channel blockers, alpha- or beta-blockers, and centrally acting agents) could be added as needed in both groups. Patients were followed for a mean duration of 3.4 years.

The study population was diverse with regard to race (Asian 16.7%, Black 15.2%, Hispanic 18.3%, White 48.6%). Overall, 63.2% of the patients were men, and 66.4% were under the

Table 1 Incidence of Primary Endpoint Events							
Primary Composite Endpoint	COZAAR		Atenolol		Risk Reduction†	95% CI	p-Value
	N (%)	Rate*	N (%)	Rate*			
	508 (11)	23.8	588 (13)	27.9	13%	2% to 23%	0.021
Components of Primary Composite Endpoint (as a first event)							
Stroke (nonfatal‡)	209 (5)		286 (6)				
Myocardial infarction (nonfatal‡)	174 (4)		168 (4)				
Cardiovascular mortality	125 (3)		134 (3)				
Secondary Endpoints (any time in study)							
Stroke (fatal/nonfatal)	232 (5)	10.8	309 (7)	14.5	25%	11% to 37%	0.001
Myocardial infarction (fatal/nonfatal)	198 (4)	9.2	188 (4)	8.7	-7%	-13% to 12%	0.491
Cardiovascular mortality	204 (4)	9.2	234 (5)	10.6	11%	-7% to 27%	0.206
Due to CHD	125 (3)	5.6	124 (3)	5.6	-3%	-32% to 20%	0.839
Due to Stroke	40 (1)	1.8	62 (1)	2.8	35%	4% to 67%	0.032
Other§	39 (1)	1.8	48 (1)	2.2	16%	-28% to 45%	0.411

*Rate per 1000 patient years of follow up
†Adjusted for baseline Framingham risk score and level of electrocardiographic left ventricular hypertrophy
‡First report of an event, in some cases the patient died subsequently to the event reported
§Death due to heart failure, non-coronary vascular disease, pulmonary embolism, or a cardiovascular cause other than stroke or coronary heart disease

age of 65 years. Almost all of the patients (96.6%) had a history of hypertension, and the patients entered the trial with a mean serum creatinine of 1.9 mg/dl and mean proteinuria (urinary albumin/creatinine) of 1808 mg/g at baseline.
The primary endpoint of the study was the time to first occurrence of any one of the following events: doubling of serum creatinine, end-stage renal disease (need for dialysis or transplantation), or death. Treatment with COZAAR resulted in a 16% risk reduction in this endpoint (see Figure 4 and Table 2). Treatment with COZAAR also reduced the occurrence of sustained doubling of serum creatinine by 25% and ESRD by 29% as separate endpoints, but had no effect on overall mortality (see Table 2).
The mean baseline blood pressures were 152/82 mmHg for COZAAR plus conventional antihypertensive therapy and 153/82 mmHg for placebo plus conventional antihypertensive therapy. At the end of the study, the mean blood pressures were 143/76 mmHg for the group treated with COZAAR and 146/77 mmHg for the group treated with placebo.

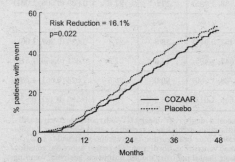

FIGURE 4: Kaplan-Meier curve for the primary composite endpoint of doubling of serum creatinine, end stage renal disease (need for dialysis or transplantation) or death.
[See table 2 at right]
The secondary endpoints of the study were change in proteinuria, change in the rate of progression of renal disease, and the composite of morbidity and mortality from cardiovascular causes (hospitalization for heart failure, myocardial infarction, revascularization, stroke, hospitalization for unstable angina, or cardiovascular death). Compared with placebo, COZAAR significantly reduced proteinuria by an average of 34%, an effect that was evident within 3 months of starting therapy, and significantly reduced the rate of decline in glomerular filtration rate during the study by 13%, as measured by the reciprocal of the serum creatinine concentration. There was no significant difference in the incidence of the composite endpoint of cardiovascular morbidity and mortality.
The favorable effects of COZAAR were seen in patients also taking other anti-hypertensive medications (angiotensin II receptor antagonists and angiotensin converting enzyme inhibitors were not allowed), oral hypoglycemic agents and lipid-lowering agents.
For the primary endpoint and ESRD, the effects of COZAAR in patient subgroups defined by age, gender and race are shown in Table 3 below. Subgroup analyses can be difficult to interpret and it is not known whether these represent true differences or chance effects.
[See table 3 at top of next page]

INDICATIONS AND USAGE

Hypertension
COZAAR is indicated for the treatment of hypertension. It may be used alone or in combination with other antihypertensive agents, including diuretics.
Hypertensive Patients with Left Ventricular Hypertrophy
COZAAR is indicated to reduce the risk of stroke in patients with hypertension and left ventricular hypertrophy, but there is evidence that this benefit does not apply to Black patients. (See PRECAUTIONS, *Race* and CLINICAL PHARMACOLOGY, *Pharmacodynamics and Clinical Effects, Reduction in the Risk of Stroke, Race*.)
Nephropathy in Type 2 Diabetic Patients
COZAAR is indicated for the treatment of diabetic nephropathy with an elevated serum creatinine and proteinuria (urinary albumin to creatinine ratio ≥300 mg/g) in patients with type 2 diabetes and a history of hypertension. In this population, COZAAR reduces the rate of progression of nephropathy as measured by the occurrence of doubling of serum creatinine or end stage renal disease (need for dialysis or renal transplantation) (see CLINICAL PHARMACOLOGY, *Pharmacodynamics and Clinical Effects*).

CONTRAINDICATIONS

COZAAR is contraindicated in patients who are hypersensitive to any component of this product.

WARNINGS

Fetal/Neonatal Morbidity and Mortality
Drugs that act directly on the renin-angiotensin system can cause fetal and neonatal morbidity and death when administered to pregnant women. Several dozen cases have been reported in the world literature in patients who were taking angiotensin converting enzyme inhibitors. When pregnancy is detected, COZAAR should be discontinued as soon as possible.

The use of drugs that act directly on the renin-angiotensin system during the second and third trimesters of pregnancy has been associated with fetal and neonatal injury, including hypotension, neonatal skull hypoplasia, anuria, reversible or irreversible renal failure, and death. Oligohydramnios has also been reported, presumably resulting from decreased fetal renal function; oligohydramnios in this setting has been associated with fetal limb contractures, craniofacial deformation, and hypoplastic lung development. Prematurity, intrauterine growth retardation, and patent ductus arteriosus have also been reported, although it is not clear whether these occurrences were due to exposure to the drug.
These adverse effects do not appear to have resulted from intrauterine drug exposure that has been limited to the first trimester.
Mothers whose embryos and fetuses are exposed to an angiotensin II receptor antagonist only during the first trimester should be so informed. Nonetheless, when patients become pregnant, physicians should have the patient discontinue the use of COZAAR as soon as possible.
Rarely (probably less often than once in every thousand pregnancies), no alternative to an angiotensin II receptor antagonist will be found. In these rare cases, the mothers should be apprised of the potential hazards to their fetuses, and serial ultrasound examinations should be performed to assess the intraamniotic environment.
If oligohydramnios is observed, COZAAR should be discontinued unless it is considered life-saving for the mother. Contraction stress testing (CST), a non-stress test (NST), or biophysical profiling (BPP) may be appropriate, depending upon the week of pregnancy. Patients and physicians should be aware, however, that oligohydramnios may not appear until after the fetus has sustained irreversible injury.
Infants with histories of *in utero* exposure to an angiotensin II receptor antagonist should be closely observed for hypotension, oliguria, and hyperkalemia. If oliguria occurs, attention should be directed toward support of blood pressure and renal perfusion. Exchange transfusion or dialysis may be required as means of reversing hypotension and/or substituting for disordered renal function.
Losartan potassium has been shown to produce adverse effects in rat fetuses and neonates, including decreased body weight, delayed physical and behavioral development, mortality and renal toxicity. With the exception of neonatal weight gain (which was affected at doses as low as 10 mg/kg/day), doses associated with these effects exceeded 25 mg/kg/day (approximately three times the maximum recommended human dose of 100 mg on a mg/m^2 basis). These findings are attributed to drug exposure in late gestation and during lactation. Significant levels of losartan and its active metabolite were shown to be present in rat fetal plasma during late gestation and in rat milk.

Hypotension — Volume-Depleted Patients
In patients who are intravascularly volume-depleted (e.g., those treated with diuretics), symptomatic hypotension may occur after initiation of therapy with COZAAR. These conditions should be corrected prior to administration of COZAAR, or a lower starting dose should be used (see DOSAGE AND ADMINISTRATION).

PRECAUTIONS

General
Hypersensitivity: Angioedema. See ADVERSE REACTIONS, *Post-Marketing Experience.*
Impaired Hepatic Function
Based on pharmacokinetic data which demonstrate significantly increased plasma concentrations of losartan in cirrhotic patients, a lower dose should be considered for patients with impaired liver function (see DOSAGE AND ADMINISTRATION and CLINICAL PHARMACOLOGY, *Pharmacokinetics*).
Impaired Renal Function
As a consequence of inhibiting the renin-angiotensin-aldosterone system, changes in renal function have been reported in susceptible individuals treated with COZAAR; in some patients, these changes in renal function were reversible upon discontinuation of therapy.
In patients whose renal function may depend on the activity of the renin-angiotensin-aldosterone system (e.g., patients with severe congestive heart failure), treatment with angiotensin converting enzyme inhibitors has been associated with oliguria and/or progressive azotemia and (rarely) with acute renal failure and/or death. Similar outcomes have been reported with COZAAR.
In studies of ACE inhibitors in patients with unilateral or bilateral renal artery stenosis, increases in serum creatinine or BUN have been reported. Similar effects have been reported with COZAAR; in some patients, these effects were reversible upon discontinuation of therapy.
Electrolyte Imbalance
Electrolyte imbalances are common in patients with renal impairment, with or without diabetes, and should be addressed. In a clinical study conducted in type 2 diabetic patients with proteinuria, the incidence of hyperkalemia was higher in the group treated with COZAAR as compared to the placebo group; however, few patients discontinued therapy due to hyperkalemia (see ADVERSE REACTIONS).

Continued on next page

Figure 3 Primary Endpoint Events† within Demographic Subgroups

	No. of Patients	Primary Composite			Stroke (Fatal/Non-fatal)		
		COZAAR Event Rate (%)	Atenolol Event Rate (%)	Hazard Ratio (95% CI)	COZAAR Event Rate (%)	Atenolol Event Rate (%)	Hazard Ratio (95% CI)
Overall Results	9193	11	13		5	7	
Age							
<65 years	3489	7	7		3	3	
≥65 years	5704	13	16		6	9	
Gender							
Female	4963	9	11		4	6	
Male	4230	14	15		6	7	
Race							
Black	533	17	11		9	5	
White	8503	11	13		5	7	
Other#	157	9	14		5	5	
ISH							
Yes	1326	11	16		5	8	
No	7867	11	12		5	6	
Diabetes							
Yes	1195	18	23		9	11	
No	7998	10	11		5	6	
History of CVD							
Yes	2307	19	21		9	11	
No	6886	8	10		4	6	

← Favors COZAAR   Favors Atenolol →

Symbols are proportional to sample size.
#Other includes Asian, Hispanic, Asiatic, Multi-race, Indian, Native American, European.
†Adjusted for baseline Framingham risk score and level of electrocardiographic left ventricular hypertrophy.

Table 2 Incidence of Primary Endpoint Events

Primary Composite Endpoint	Incidence		Risk Reduction	95% C.I.	p-Value
	Losartan	Placebo			
	43.5%	47.1%	16.1%	2.3% to 27.9%	0.022
Doubling of Serum Creatinine, ESRD and Death Occurring as a First Event					
Doubling of Serum Creatinine	21.6%	26.0%			
ESRD	8.5%	8.5%			
Death	13.4%	12.6%			
Overall Incidence of Doubling of Serum Creatinine, ESRD and Death					
Doubling of Serum Creatinine	21.6%	26.0%	25.3%	7.8% to 39.4%	0.006
ESRD	19.6%	25.5%	28.6%	11.5% to 42.4%	0.002
Death	21.0%	20.3%	-1.7%	-26.9% to 18.6%	0.884

Information on the Merck & Co., Inc., products listed on these pages is from the full prescribing information in use April 1, 2003.

Cozaar—Cont.

Information for Patients

Pregnancy: Female patients of childbearing age should be told about the consequences of second- and third-trimester exposure to drugs that act on the renin-angiotensin system, and they should also be told that these consequences do not appear to have resulted from intrauterine drug exposure that has been limited to the first trimester. These patients should be asked to report pregnancies to their physicians as soon as possible.

Potassium Supplements: A patient receiving COZAAR should be told not to use potassium supplements or salt substitutes containing potassium without consulting the prescribing physician (see PRECAUTIONS, *Drug Interactions*).

Drug Interactions

No significant drug-drug pharmacokinetic interactions have been found in interaction studies with hydrochlorothiazide, digoxin, warfarin, cimetidine and phenobarbital. (See CLINICAL PHARMACOLOGY, *Drug Interactions.*) Potent inhibitors of cytochrome P450 3A4 and 2C9 have not been studied clinically but *in vitro* studies show significant inhibition of the formation of the active metabolite by inhibitors of P450 3A4 (ketoconazole, troleandomycin, gestodene), or P450 2C9 (sulfaphenazole) and nearly complete inhibition by the combination of sulfaphenazole and ketoconazole. In humans, ketoconazole, an inhibitor of P450 3A4, did not affect the conversion of losartan to the active metabolite after intravenous administration of losartan. Inhibitors of cytochrome P450 2C9 have not been studied clinically. The pharmacodynamic consequences of concomitant use of losartan and inhibitors of P450 2C9 have not been examined.

As with other drugs that block angiotensin II or its effects, concomitant use of potassium-sparing diuretics (e.g., spironolactone, triamterene, amiloride), potassium supplements, or salt substitutes containing potassium may lead to increases in serum potassium.

As with other antihypertensive agents, the antihypertensive effect of losartan may be blunted by the non-steroidal anti-inflammatory drug indomethacin.

Carcinogenesis, Mutagenesis, Impairment of Fertility

Losartan potassium was not carcinogenic when administered at maximally tolerated dosages to rats and mice for 105 and 92 weeks, respectively. Female rats given the highest dose (270 mg/kg/day) had a slightly higher incidence of pancreatic acinar adenoma. The maximally tolerated dosages (270 mg/kg/day in rats, 200 mg/kg/day in mice) provided systemic exposures for losartan and its pharmacologically active metabolite that were approximately 160- and 90-times (rats) and 30- and 15-times (mice) the exposure of a 50 kg human given 100 mg per day.

Losartan potassium was negative in the microbial mutagenesis and V-79 mammalian cell mutagenesis assays and in the *in vitro* alkaline elution and *in vitro* and *in vivo* chromosomal aberration assays. In addition, the active metabolite showed no evidence of genotoxicity in the microbial mutagenesis, *in vitro* alkaline elution, and *in vitro* chromosomal aberration assays.

Fertility and reproductive performance were not affected in studies with male rats given oral doses of losartan potassium up to approximately 150 mg/kg/day. The administration of toxic dosage levels in females (300/200 mg/kg/day) was associated with a significant ($p<0.05$) decrease in the number of corpora lutea/female, implants/female, and live fetuses/female at C-section. At 100 mg/kg/day only a decrease in the number of corpora lutea/female was observed. The relationship of these findings to drug-treatment is uncertain since there was no effect at these dosage levels on implants/pregnant female, percent post-implantation loss, or live animals/litter at parturition. In nonpregnant rats dosed at 135 mg/kg/day for 7 days, systemic exposure (AUCs) for losartan and its active metabolite were approximately 66 and 26 times the exposure achieved in man at the maximum recommended human daily dosage (100 mg).

Pregnancy

Pregnancy Categories C (first trimester) and D (second and third trimesters). See WARNINGS, *Fetal/Neonatal Morbidity and Mortality.*

Nursing Mothers

It is not known whether losartan is excreted in human milk, but significant levels of losartan and its active metabolite were shown to be present in rat milk. Because of the potential for adverse effects on the nursing infant, a decision should be made whether to discontinue nursing or discontinue the drug, taking into account the importance of the drug to the mother.

Pediatric Use

Safety and effectiveness in pediatric patients have not been established.

Use in the Elderly

Of the total number of patients receiving COZAAR in controlled clinical studies for hypertension, 391 patients (19%) were 65 years and over, while 37 patients (2%) were 75 years and over. In a controlled clinical study for renal protection in type 2 diabetic patients with proteinuria, 248 patients (33%) were 65 years and over. In a controlled clinical study for the reduction in the combined risk of cardiovascular death, stroke and myocardial infarction in hypertensive patients with left ventricular hypertrophy, 2857 patients (62%) were 65 years and over, while 808 patients (18%) were 75 years and over. No overall differences in effectiveness or safety were observed between these patients and younger patients, but greater sensitivity of some older individuals cannot be ruled out.

Race

In the LIFE study, Black patients with hypertension and left ventricular hypertrophy had a lower risk of stroke on atenolol than on COZAAR. Given the difficulty in interpreting subset differences in large trials, it cannot be known whether the observed difference is the result of chance. However, the LIFE study does not provide evidence that the benefits of COZAAR on reducing the risk of cardiovascular events in hypertensive patients with left ventricular hypertrophy apply to Black patients. (See CLINICAL PHARMACOLOGY, *Pharmacodynamics and Clinical Effects; Reduction in the Risk of Stroke.*)

Table 3 Efficacy Outcomes within Demographic Subgroups

		Primary Composite Endpoint			ESRD		
	No. of Patients	COZAAR Event Rate %	Placebo Event Rate %	Hazard Ratio (95% CI)	COZAAR Event Rate %	Placebo Event Rate %	Hazard Ratio (95% CI)
Overall Results	1513	43.5	47.1	0.839 (0.721, 0.977)	19.6	25.5	0.714 (0.576, 0.885)
Age							
<65 years	1005	44.1	49.0	0.784 (0.653, 0.941)	21.1	28.5	0.670 (0.521, 0.863)
≥65 years	508	42.3	43.5	0.978 (0.749, 1.277)	16.5	19.6	0.847 (0.560, 1.281)
Gender							
Female	557	47.8	54.1	0.762 (0.603, 0.962)	22.8	32.8	0.601 (0.436, 0.828)
Male	956	40.9	43.3	0.892 (0.733, 1.085)	17.5	21.5	0.809 (0.605, 1.081)
Race							
Asian	252	41.9	54.8	0.655 (0.453, 0.947)	18.8	27.4	0.625 (0.367, 1.066)
Black	230	40.0	39.0	0.983 (0.647, 1.495)	17.6	21.0	0.831 (0.456, 1.516)
Hispanic	277	55.0	54.0	1.003 (0.728, 1.380)	30.0	28.5	1.024 (0.661, 1.586)
White	735	40.5	43.2	0.809 (0.645, 1.013)	16.2	23.9	0.596 (0.427, 0.831)

ADVERSE REACTIONS

Hypertension

COZAAR has been evaluated for safety in more than 3300 patients treated for essential hypertension and 4058 patients/subjects overall. Over 1200 patients were treated for over 6 months and more than 800 for over one year. In general, treatment with COZAAR was well-tolerated. The overall incidence of adverse experiences reported with COZAAR was similar to placebo.

In controlled clinical trials, discontinuation of therapy due to clinical adverse experiences was required in 2.3 percent of patients treated with COZAAR and 3.7 percent of patients given placebo.

The following table of adverse events is based on four 6-12 week placebo-controlled trials involving over 1000 patients on various doses (10-150 mg) of losartan and over 300 patients given placebo. All doses of losartan are grouped because none of the adverse events appeared to have a dose-related frequency. The adverse experiences reported in ≥1% of patients treated with COZAAR and more commonly than placebo are shown in the table below.

	Losartan (n=1075) Incidence %	Placebo (n=334) Incidence %
Musculoskeletal		
Cramp, muscle	1	0
Pain, back	2	1
Pain, leg	1	0
Nervous System/Psychiatric		
Dizziness	3	2
Respiratory		
Congestion, nasal	2	1
Infection, upper respiratory	8	7
Sinusitis	1	0

The following adverse events were also reported at a rate of 1% or greater in patients treated with losartan, but were as, or more frequent, in the placebo group: asthenia/fatigue, edema/swelling, abdominal pain, chest pain, nausea, headache, pharyngitis, diarrhea, dyspepsia, myalgia, insomnia, cough, sinus disorder.

Adverse events occurred at about the same rates in men and women, older and younger patients, and Black and non-Black patients.

A patient with known hypersensitivity to aspirin and penicillin, when treated with COZAAR, was withdrawn from study due to swelling of the lips and eyelids and facial rash, reported as angioedema, which returned to normal 5 days after therapy was discontinued.

Superficial peeling of palms and hemolysis was reported in one subject.

In addition to the adverse events above, potentially important events that occurred in at least two patients/subjects exposed to losartan or other adverse events that occurred in <1% of patients in clinical studies are listed below. It cannot be determined whether these events were causally related to losartan: *Body as a Whole:* facial edema, fever, orthostatic effects, syncope; *Cardiovascular:* angina pectoris, second degree AV block, CVA, hypotension, myocardial infarction, arrhythmias including atrial fibrillation, palpitation, sinus bradycardia, tachycardia, ventricular tachycardia, ventricular fibrillation; *Digestive:* anorexia, constipation, dental pain, dry mouth, flatulence, gastritis, vomiting; *Hematologic:* anemia; *Metabolic:* gout; *Musculoskeletal:* arm pain, hip pain, joint swelling, knee pain, musculoskeletal pain, shoulder pain, stiffness, arthralgia, arthritis, fibromyalgia, muscle weakness; *Nervous System/Psychiatric:* anxiety, anxiety disorder, ataxia, confusion, depression, dream abnormality, hypesthesia, decreased libido, memory impairment, migraine, nervousness, paresthesia, peripheral neuropathy, panic disorder, sleep disorder, somnolence, tremor, vertigo; *Respiratory:* dyspnea, bronchitis, pharyngeal discomfort, epistaxis, rhinitis, respiratory congestion; *Skin:* alopecia, dermatitis, dry skin, ecchymosis, erythema, flushing, photosensitivity, pruritus, rash, sweating, urticaria; *Special Senses:* blurred vision, burning/stinging in the eye, conjunctivitis, taste perversion, tinnitus, decrease in visual acuity; *Urogenital:* impotence, nocturia, urinary frequency, urinary tract infection.

Persistent dry cough (with an incidence of a few percent) has been associated with ACE inhibitor use and in practice can be a cause of discontinuation of ACE inhibitor therapy. Two prospective, parallel-group, double-blind, randomized, controlled trials were conducted to assess the effects of losartan on the incidence of cough in hypertensive patients who had experienced cough while receiving ACE inhibitor therapy. Patients who had typical ACE inhibitor cough when challenged with lisinopril, whose cough disappeared on placebo, were randomized to losartan 50 mg, lisinopril 20 mg, or either placebo (one study, n=97) or 25 mg hydrochlorothiazide (n=135). The double-blind treatment period lasted up to 8 weeks. The incidence of cough is shown below.

Study 1†	HCTZ	Losartan	Lisinopril
Cough	25%	17%	69%
Study 2††	Placebo	Losartan	Lisinopril
Cough	35%	29%	62%

†Demographics = (89% caucasian, 64% female)
††Demographics = (90% caucasian, 51% female)

These studies demonstrate that the incidence of cough associated with losartan therapy, in a population that all had cough associated with ACE inhibitor therapy, is similar to that associated with hydrochlorothiazide or placebo therapy.

Cases of cough, including positive re-challenges, have been reported with the use of losartan in post-marketing experience.

Hypertensive Patients with Left Ventricular Hypertrophy

In the LIFE study, adverse events with COZAAR were similar to those reported previously for patients with hypertension.

Nephropathy in Type 2 Diabetic Patients

In the RENAAL study involving 1513 patients treated with COZAAR or placebo, the overall incidences of reported adverse experiences were similar for the two groups. COZAAR was generally well tolerated as evidenced by a similar incidence of discontinuations due to side effects compared to placebo (19% for COZAAR, 24% for placebo). The adverse experiences regardless of drug relationship, reported with an incidence of ≥4% of patients treated with COZAAR and occurring more commonly than placebo, on a background of conventional antihypertensive therapy are shown in the table below.

[See table at bottom of next page]

Post-Marketing Experience

The following additional adverse reactions have been reported in post-marketing experience:

Hypersensitivity: Angioedema, including swelling of the larynx and glottis, causing airway obstruction and/or swelling of the face, lips, pharynx, and/or tongue has been reported rarely in patients treated with losartan; some of these patients previously experienced angioedema with other drugs including ACE inhibitors. Vasculitis, including Henoch-Schönlein purpura, has been reported. Anaphylactic reactions have been reported.

Digestive: Hepatitis (reported rarely).
Respiratory: Dry cough (see above).
Hyperkalemia and hyponatremia have been reported.

Laboratory Test Findings
In controlled clinical trials, clinically important changes in standard laboratory parameters were rarely associated with administration of COZAAR.

Creatinine, Blood Urea Nitrogen: Minor increases in blood urea nitrogen (BUN) or serum creatinine were observed in less than 0.1 percent of patients with essential hypertension treated with COZAAR alone (see PRECAUTIONS, *Impaired Renal Function*).

Hemoglobin and Hematocrit: Small decreases in hemoglobin and hematocrit (mean decreases of approximately 0.11 grams percent and 0.09 volume percent, respectively) occurred frequently in patients treated with COZAAR alone, but were rarely of clinical importance. No patients were discontinued due to anemia.

Liver Function Tests: Occasional elevations of liver enzymes and/or serum bilirubin have occurred. In patients with essential hypertension treated with COZAAR alone, one patient (<0.1%) was discontinued due to these laboratory adverse experiences.

OVERDOSAGE

Significant lethality was observed in mice and rats after oral administration of 1000 mg/kg and 2000 mg/kg, respectively, about 44 and 170 times the maximum recommended human dose on a mg/m^2 basis.

Limited data are available in regard to overdosage in humans. The most likely manifestation of overdosage would be hypotension and tachycardia; bradycardia could occur from parasympathetic (vagal) stimulation. If symptomatic hypotension should occur, supportive treatment should be instituted.

Neither losartan nor its active metabolite can be removed by hemodialysis.

DOSAGE AND ADMINISTRATION

COZAAR may be administered with other antihypertensive agents, and with or without food.

Hypertension
Dosing must be individualized. The usual starting dose of COZAAR is 50 mg once daily, with 25 mg used in patients with possible depletion of intravascular volume (e.g., patients treated with diuretics) (see WARNINGS, *Hypotension — Volume-Depleted Patients*) and patients with a history of hepatic impairment (see PRECAUTIONS, *General*). COZAAR can be administered once or twice daily with total daily doses ranging from 25 mg to 100 mg.

If the antihypertensive effect measured at trough using once-a-day dosing is inadequate, a twice-a-day regimen at the same total daily dose or an increase in dose may give a more satisfactory response. The effect of losartan is substantially present within one week but in some studies the maximal effect occurred in 3-6 weeks (see CLINICAL PHARMACOLOGY, *Pharmacodynamics and Clinical Effects, Hypertension*).

If blood pressure is not controlled by COZAAR alone, a low dose of a diuretic may be added. Hydrochlorothiazide has been shown to have an additive effect (see CLINICAL PHARMACOLOGY, *Pharmacodynamics and Clinical Effects, Hypertension*).

No initial dosage adjustment is necessary for elderly patients or for patients with renal impairment, including patients on dialysis.

Hypertensive Patients with Left Ventricular Hypertrophy
The usual starting dose is 50 mg of COZAAR once daily. Hydrochlorothiazide 12.5 mg daily should be added and/or the dose of COZAAR should be increased to 100 mg once daily followed by an increase in hydrochlorothiazide to 25 mg once daily based on blood pressure response (see CLINICAL PHARMACOLOGY, *Pharmacodynamics and Clinical Effects, Reduction in the Risk of Stroke*).

Nephropathy in Type 2 Diabetic Patients
The usual starting dose is 50 mg once daily. The dose should be increased to 100 mg once daily based on blood pressure response (see CLINICAL PHARMACOLOGY, *Pharmacodynamics and Clinical Effects, Nephropathy in Type 2 Diabetic Patients*). COZAAR may be administered with insulin and other commonly used hypoglycemic agents (e.g., sulfonylureas, glitazones and glucosidase inhibitors).

HOW SUPPLIED

No. 3612 — Tablets COZAAR, 25 mg, are light green, teardrop-shaped, film-coated tablets with code MRK on one side and 951 on the other. They are supplied as follows:
NDC 0006-0951-54 unit of use bottles of 90
NDC 0006-0951-58 unit of use bottles of 100
NDC 0006-0951-28 unit dose packages of 100.

No. 3613 — Tablets COZAAR, 50 mg, are green, teardrop-shaped, film-coated tablets with code MRK 952 on one side and COZAAR on the other. They are supplied as follows:
NDC 0006-0952-31 unit of use bottles of 30
NDC 0006-0952-54 unit of use bottles of 90
NDC 0006-0952-58 unit of use bottles of 100
NDC 0006-0952-28 unit dose packages of 100
NDC 0006-0952-82 bottles of 1,000.

No. 6536 — Tablets COZAAR, 100 mg, are dark green, teardrop-shaped, film-coated tablets with code 960 on one side and MRK on the other. They are supplied as follows:
NDC 0006-0960-31 unit of use bottles of 30
NDC 0006-0960-58 unit of use bottles of 100
NDC 0006-0960-28 unit dose packages of 100.

Storage
Store at 25°C (77°F); excursions permitted to 15-30°C (59-86°F) [see USP Controlled Room Temperature]. Keep container tightly closed: Protect from light.

Dist. by:
MERCK & CO., INC., Whitehouse Station, NJ 08889, USA
7882922   Issued March 2003
COPYRIGHT © MERCK & CO., Inc., 1995
Whitehouse Station, NJ, USA
All rights reserved

CRIXIVAN® Capsules   ℞
[krĭk'-sĭ-văn]
(indinavir sulfate)

Prescribing information for this product, which appears on pages 1970–1976 of the 2003 PDR has been revised as follows. Please write "See Supplement A" alongside product heading.

In the **MICROBIOLOGY** section, replace all occurrences of "HIV" with "HIV-1".

Also in the **MICROBIOLOGY** section, under Antiretroviral Activity In Vitro, move the first sentence to follow the last sentence. In the last sentence, delete "as well as with an investigational nonnucleoside (L-697,661)".

Also in the **MICROBIOLOGY** section, under Drug Resistance, in the third sentence, after "Eleven amino acid residue positions,", add "(L10I/V/R, K20I/M/R, L24I, M46I/L I54A/V, L63P, I64V, A71T/V, V82A/F/T, I84V, and L90M),". After the fourth sentence, add "No single substitution was either necessary or sufficient for measurable resistance (≥4-fold increase in IC$_{95}$)." In the fifth sentence, replace the period with a comma and add the following:
although their individual effects varied and were not additive. At least 3 amino acid substitutions must be present for phenotypic resistance to indinavir to reach measurable levels. In addition, mutations in the p7/p1 and p1/p6 gag cleavage sites were observed in some indinavir resistant HIV-1 isolates.

In vitro phenotypic susceptibilities to indinavir were determined for 38 viral isolates from 13 patients who experienced virologic rebounds during indinavir monotherapy. Pre-treatment isolates from five patients exhibited indinavir IC$_{95}$ values of 50-100 nM. At or following viral RNA rebound (after 12-76 weeks of therapy), IC$_{95}$ values ranged from 25 to >3000 nM, and the viruses carried 2 to 10 mutations in the protease gene relative to baseline.

Also in the **MICROBIOLOGY** section, under Cross-Resistance to Other Antiviral Agents, delete the first sentence. After the last sentence, add the following:
In studies with ritonavir, saquinavir, and amprenavir, the extent and spectrum of cross-resistance varied with the specific mutational patterns observed. In general, the degree of cross-resistance increased with the accumulation of resistance-associated amino acid substitutions. Within a panel of 29 viral isolates from indinavir-treated patients that exhibited measurable (≥4-fold) phenotypic resistance to indinavir, all were resistant to ritonavir. Of the indinavir resistant HIV-1 isolates, 63% showed resistance to saquinavir and 81% to amprenavir.

Revisions based on 7979824, issued September 2002.

ELSPAR®   ℞
[el'spăr]
(asparaginase)

Prescribing information for this product, which appears on pages 1993–1995 of the 2003 PDR, has been revised as follows. Please write "See Supplement A" alongside product heading.

In the **PRECAUTIONS** section, add the following subsection at the end:
Geriatric Use
Clinical studies of ELSPAR did not include sufficient numbers of subjects aged 65 and over to determine whether they respond differently from younger subjects. Other reported clinical experience has not identified differences in responses between the elderly and younger patients. In general, dose selection for an elderly patient should be cautious, usually starting at the low end of the dosing range, reflecting the greater frequency of decreased hepatic, renal, or cardiac function, and of concomitant disease or other drug therapy.

Revision based on 9463116, issued August 2002.

FOSAMAX® Tablets   ℞
[fō'să-maks]
(alendronate sodium tablets)

Prescribing information for this product, which appears on pages 1996–2003 of the 2003 PDR, has been revised as follows. Please write "See Supplement A" alongside product heading.

Continued on next page

Information on the Merck & Co., Inc., products listed on these pages is from the full prescribing information in use April 1, 2003.

	Losartan and Conventional Antihypertensive Therapy Incidence % (n=751)	Placebo and Conventional Antihypertensive Therapy Incidence % (n=762)
Body as a Whole		
Asthenia/Fatigue	14	10
Chest Pain	12	8
Fever	4	3
Infection	5	4
Influenza-like disease	10	9
Trauma	4	3
Cardiovascular		
Hypotension	7	3
Orthostatic hypotension	4	1
Digestive		
Diarrhea	15	10
Dyspepsia	4	3
Gastritis	5	4
Endocrine		
Diabetic neuropathy	4	3
Diabetic vascular disease	10	9
Eyes, Ears, Nose and Throat		
Cataract	7	5
Sinusitis	6	5
Hemic		
Anemia	14	11
Metabolic and Nutrition		
Hyperkalemia	7	3
Hypoglycemia	14	10
Weight gain	4	3
Musculoskeletal		
Back pain	12	10
Leg pain	5	4
Knee pain	5	4
Muscular weakness	7	4
Nervous System		
Hypesthesia	5	4
Respiratory		
Bronchitis	10	9
Cough	11	10
Skin		
Cellulitis	7	6
Urogenital		
Urinary tract infection	16	13

Fosamax—Cont.

In the **ADVERSE REACTIONS** section, in the Post-Marketing Experience subsection, under Special Senses, after "rarely uveitis", add ", rarely scleritis".
Revision based on 7957020, issued July 2002.

LACRISERT® Sterile Ophthalmic Insert ℞
[la-krĭ-sərt]
(hydroxypropyl cellulose ophthalmic insert)

Prescribing information for this product, which appears on pages 2021–2022 of the 2003 PDR, has been revised as follows. Please write "See Supplement A" alongside product heading.
In the **PRECAUTIONS** *section, add the following subsection at the end:*
Geriatric Use
No overall differences in safety or effectiveness have been observed between elderly and younger patients.
In the **HOW SUPPLIED** *section, replace the copy beginning with* **NDC** *with the following:*
NDC 0006-3380-60 in packages containing 60 unit doses (each wrapped in an aluminum blister), two reusable applicators, and a plastic storage container to store the applicators after use.
Also in the **HOW SUPPLIED** *section, delete the line* "(6505-01-153-4360, 5 mg 60's)."
Revisions based on 9246112, issued June 2002.

MEFOXIN® ℞
[mĕ'fŏks-ĭn]
(cefoxitin for injection)

Prescribing information for this product, which appears on pages 2029–2031 of the 2003 PDR, has been revised as follows. Please write "See Supplement A" alongside product heading.
Replace the **CLINICAL PHARMACOLOGY** *section with the following:*

CLINICAL PHARMACOLOGY
Clinical Pharmacology
Following an intravenous dose of 1 gram, serum concentrations were 110 mcg/mL at 5 minutes, declining to less than 1 mcg/mL at 4 hours. The half-life after an intravenous dose is 41 to 59 minutes. Approximately 85 percent of cefoxitin is excreted unchanged by the kidneys over a 6-hour period, resulting in high urinary concentrations. Probenecid slows tubular excretion and produces higher serum levels and increases the duration of measurable serum concentrations. Cefoxitin passes into pleural and joint fluids and is detectable in antibacterial concentrations in bile.

Microbiology
The bactericidal action of cefoxitin results from inhibition of cell wall synthesis. Cefoxitin has *in vitro* activity against a wide range of gram-positive and gram-negative organisms. The methoxy group in the 7α position provides cefoxitin with a high degree of stability in the presence of beta-lactamases, both penicillinases and cephalosporinases, of gram-negative bacteria.
Cefoxitin has been shown to be active against most strains of the following microorganisms, both *in vitro* and in clinical infections as described in the INDICATIONS AND USAGE section.

Aerobic gram-positive microorganisms
   Staphylococcus aureus[a] (including penicillinase-producing strains)
   Staphylococcus epidermidis[a]
   Streptococcus agalactiae
   Streptococcus pneumoniae
   Streptococcus pyogenes

[a] Staphylococci resistant to methicillin/oxacillin should be considered resistant to cefoxitin.
Most strains of enterococci, e.g., *Enterococcus faecalis*, are resistant.

Aerobic gram-negative microorganisms
   Escherichia coli
   Haemophilus influenzae
   Klebsiella spp. (including *K. pneumoniae*)
   Morganella morganii
   Neisseria gonorrhoeae (including penicillinase-producing strains)
   Proteus mirabilis
   Proteus vulgaris
   Providencia spp. (including *Providencia rettgeri*)

Anaerobic gram-positive microorganisms
   Clostridium spp.
   Peptococcus niger
   Peptostreptococcus spp.

Anaerobic gram-negative microorganisms
   Bacteroides distasonis
   Bacteroides fragilis
   Bacteroides ovatus
   Bacteroides thetaiotaomicron
   Bacteroides spp.

The following *in vitro* data are available, **but their clinical significance is unknown.**
Cefoxitin exhibits *in vitro* minimum inhibitory concentrations (MIC's) of 8 μg/mL or less for aerobic microorganisms and 16 μg/mL or less for anaerobic microorganisms against most (≥90%) strains of the following microorganisms; however, the safety and effectiveness of cefoxitin in treating clinical infections due to these microorganisms have not been established in adequate and well-controlled clinical trials.

Aerobic gram-negative microorganisms
   Eikenella corrodens [non-β-lactamase producers]
   Klebsiella oxytoca

Anaerobic gram-positive microorganisms
   Clostridium perfringens

Anaerobic gram-negative microorganisms
   Prevotella bivia (formerly *Bacteroides bivius*)

Cefoxitin is inactive *in vitro* against most strains of *Pseudomonas aeruginosa* and enterococci and many strains of *Enterobacter cloacae*.

Susceptibility Tests
Dilution Techniques:
Quantitative methods are used to determine antimicrobial minimum inhibitory concentrations (MIC's). These MIC's provide estimates of the susceptibility of bacteria to antimicrobial compounds. The MIC's should be determined using a standardized procedure. Standardized procedures are based on a dilution method[1] (broth or agar) or equivalent with standardized inoculum concentrations and standardized concentrations of cefoxitin powder. The MIC values should be interpreted according to the following criteria:

For testing aerobic microorganisms[a,b,c] other than *Neisseria gonorrhoeae*:

MIC (μg/mL)	Interpretation
≤ 8	Susceptible (S)
16	Intermediate (I)
≥ 32	Resistant (R)

[a] Staphylococci exhibiting resistance to methicillin/oxacillin should be reported as also resistant to cefoxitin despite apparent *in vitro* susceptibility.
[b] For testing *Haemophilus influenzae* these interpretative criteria applicable only to tests performed by broth microdilution method using Haemophilus Test Medium (HTM)[1].
[c] For testing streptococci these interpretative criteria applicable only to tests performed by broth microdilution method using cation-adjusted Mueller-Hinton broth with 2 to 5% lysed horse blood[1].

For testing *Neisseria gonorrhoeae*[d]:

MIC (μg/mL)	Interpretation
≤ 2	Susceptible (S)
4	Intermediate (I)
≥ 8	Resistant (R)

[d] Interpretative criteria applicable only to tests performed by agar dilution method using GC agar base with 1% defined growth supplement and incubated in 5% CO_2[1]. A report of "Susceptible" indicates that the pathogen is likely to be inhibited if the antimicrobial compound in the blood reaches the concentrations usually achievable. A report of "Intermediate" indicates that the result should be considered equivocal, and, if the microorganism is not fully susceptible to alternative, clinically feasible drugs, the test should be repeated. This category implies possible clinical applicability in body sites where the drug is physiologically concentrated or in situations where high dosage of drug can be used. This category also provides a buffer zone which prevents small uncontrolled technical factors from causing major discrepancies in interpretation. A report of "Resistant" indicates that the pathogen is not likely to be inhibited if the antimicrobial compound in the blood reaches the concentrations usually achievable; other therapy should be selected.

Standardized susceptibility test procedures require the use of laboratory control microorganisms to control the technical aspects of the laboratory procedures. Standard cefoxitin powder should provide the following MIC values:

Microorganism		MIC (μg/mL)
Escherichia coli	ATCC 25922	1-4
Neisseria gonorrhoeae[a]	ATCC 49226	0.5-2
Staphylococcus aureus	ATCC 29213	1-4

[a] Interpretative criteria applicable only to tests performed by agar dilution method using GC agar base with 1% defined growth supplement and incubated in 5% CO_2[1].

Diffusion Techniques:
Quantitative methods that require measurement of zone diameters also provide reproducible estimates of the susceptibility of bacteria to antimicrobial compounds. One such standardized procedure[2] requires the use of standardized inoculum concentrations. This procedure uses paper disks impregnated with 30-μg cefoxitin to test the susceptibility of microorganisms to cefoxitin.
Reports from the laboratory providing results of the standard single-disk susceptibility test with a 30-μg cefoxitin disk should be interpreted according to the following criteria:

For testing aerobic microorganisms[a,b,c] other than *Neisseria gonorrhoeae*:

Zone Diameter (mm)	Interpretation
≥ 18	Susceptible (S)
15-17	Intermediate (I)
≤ 14	Resistant (R)

[a] Staphylococci exhibiting resistance to methicillin/oxacillin should be reported as also resistant to cefoxitin despite apparent *in vitro* susceptibility.
[b] For testing *Haemophilus influenzae* these interpretative criteria applicable only to tests performed by disk diffusion method using Haemophilus Test Medium (HTM)[1].
[c] For testing streptococci these interpretative criteria applicable only to tests performed by disk diffusion method using Mueller-Hinton agar with 5% defibrinated sheep blood and incubated in 5% CO_2[2].

For testing *Neisseria gonorrhoeae*[d]:

Zone Diameter (mm)	Interpretation
≥ 28	Susceptible (S)
24-27	Intermediate (I)
≤ 23	Resistant (R)

[d] Interpretative criteria applicable only to tests performed by disk diffusion method using GC agar base with 1% defined growth supplement and incubated in 5% CO_2[2].

Interpretation should be as stated above for results using dilution techniques.
Interpretation involves correlation of the diameter obtained in the disk test with the MIC for cefoxitin.
As with standardized dilution techniques, diffusion methods require the use of laboratory control microorganisms that are used to control the technical aspects of the laboratory procedures. For the diffusion technique, the 30-μg cefoxitin disk should provide the following zone diameters in these laboratory test quality control strains:

Microorganism		Zone Diameter (mm)
Escherichia coli	ATCC 25922	23-29
Neisseria gonorrhoeae[a]	ATCC 49226	33-41
Staphylococcus aureus	ATCC 25923	23-29

[a] Interpretative criteria applicable only to tests performed by disk diffusion method using GC agar base with 1% defined growth supplement and incubated in 5% CO_2[2].

Anaerobic Techniques:
For anaerobic bacteria, the susceptibility to cefoxitin as MIC's can be determined by standardized test methods[3]. The MIC values obtained should be interpreted according to the following criteria:

MIC (μg/mL)	Interpretation
≤ 16	Susceptible (S)
32	Intermediate (I)
≥ 64	Resistant (R)

Interpretation is identical to that stated above for results using dilution techniques.
As with other susceptibility techniques, the use of laboratory control microorganisms is required to control the technical aspects of the laboratory standardized procedures. Standard cefoxitin powder should provide the following MIC values:

Using either an Agar Dilution Method[a] or Using a Broth[b] Microdilution Method:

Microorganism		MIC (μg/mL)
Bacteroides fragilis	ATCC 25285	4-16
Bacteroides thetaiotaomicron	ATCC 29741	8-32

[a] Range applicable only to tests performed using either Brucella blood or Wilkins-Chalgren agar.
[b] Range applicable only to tests performed in the broth formulation of Wilkins-Chalgren agar[3].

In the **INDICATIONS AND USAGE** *section, under Treatment, replace list points 1 through 7 with the following:*
(1) **Lower respiratory tract infections,** including pneumonia and lung abscess, caused by *Streptococcus pneumoniae*, other streptococci (excluding enterococci, e.g., *Enterococcus faecalis* [formerly *Streptococcus faecalis*]), *Staphylococcus aureus* (including penicillinase-producing strains), *Escherichia coli*, *Klebsiella* species, *Haemophilus influenzae*, and *Bacteroides* species.
(2) **Urinary tract infections** caused by *Escherichia coli*, *Klebsiella* species, *Proteus mirabilis*, *Morganella morganii*, *Proteus vulgaris* and *Providencia* species (including *P. rettgeri*).
(3) **Intra-abdominal infections,** including peritonitis and intra-abdominal abscess, caused by *Escherichia coli*, *Klebsiella* species, *Bacteroides* species including *Bacteroides fragilis*, and *Clostridium* species.
(4) **Gynecological infections,** including endometritis, pelvic cellulitis, and pelvic inflammatory disease caused by *Escherichia coli*, *Neisseria gonorrhoeae* (including penicillinase-producing strains), *Bacteroides* species including *B. fragilis*, *Clostridium* species, *Peptococcus niger*, *Peptostreptococcus* species, and *Streptococcus agalactiae*. MEFOXIN, like cephalosporins, has no activity against *Chlamydia trachomatis*. Therefore, when MEFOXIN is used in the treatment of patients with pelvic inflammatory disease and *C. trachomatis* is one of the suspected pathogens, appropriate antichlamydial coverage should be added.

(5) **Septicemia** caused by *Streptococcus pneumoniae, Staphylococcus aureus* (including penicillinase-producing strains), *Escherichia coli, Klebsiella* species, and *Bacteroides* species including *B. fragilis.*
(6) **Bone and joint infections** caused by *Staphylococcus aureus* (including penicillinase-producing strains).
(7) **Skin and skin structure infections** caused by *Staphylococcus aureus* (including penicillinase-producing strains), *Staphylococcus epidermidis, Streptococcus pyogenes* and other streptococci (excluding enterococci e.g., *Enterococcus faecalis* [formerly *Streptococcus faecalis*]), *Escherichia coli, Proteus mirabilis, Klebsiella* species, *Bacteroides* species including *B. fragilis, Clostridium* species, *Peptococcus niger,* and *Peptostreptococcus* species.

Also in the **INDICATIONS AND USAGE** *section, under Treatment, delete the footnote "***B. fragilis, B. distasonis, B. ovatus, B. thetaiotaomicron."*

In the **ADVERSE REACTIONS** *section, under Allergic Reactions, after* "toxic epidermal necrolysis),", *add* "urticaria, flushing,".

In the **DOSAGE AND ADMINISTRATION** *section, under COMPATIBILITY AND STABILITY, Vials and Bulk Packages, in the list in the second paragraph, after* "5 percent Dextrose in Lactated Ringer's Injection", *delete* "10 percent invert sugar in water" *and* "10 percent invert sugar in saline solution".

Replace the **HOW SUPPLIED** *section up to the Special storage instructions subsection with the following:*
Sterile MEFOXIN is a dry white to off-white powder supplied in vials and infusion bottles containing cefoxitin sodium as follows:
No. 3356 — 1 gram cefoxitin equivalent
NDC 0006-3356-45 in trays of 25 vials.
No. 3357 — 2 gram cefoxitin equivalent
NDC 0006-3357-53 in trays of 25 vials.
No. 3388 — 10 gram cefoxitin equivalent
NDC 0006-3388-67 in trays of 6 bulk bottles.
No. 3548 — 1 gram cefoxitin equivalent
NDC 0006-3548-45 in trays of 25 ADD-Vantage® vials.
No. 3549 — 2 gram cefoxitin equivalent
NDC 0006-3549-53 in trays of 25 ADD-Vantage® vials.

After the **CLINICAL STUDIES** *section, add the following section:*

REFERENCES

1. National Committee for Clinical Laboratory Standards. Methods for Dilution Antimicrobial Susceptibility Tests for Bacteria that Grow Aerobically - Fourth Edition. Approved Standard NCCLS Document M7-A4, Vol. 17, No. 2, NCCLS, Wayne, PA, January 1997.
2. National Committee for Clinical Laboratory Standards. Performance Standards for Antimicrobial Disk Susceptibility Tests - Sixth Edition. Approved Standard NCCLS Document M2-A6, Vol. 17, No. 1, NCCLS, Wayne, PA, January 1997.
3. National Committee for Clinical Laboratory Standards. Methods for Antimicrobial Susceptibility Testing of Anaerobic Bacteria - Fourth Edition. Approved Standard NCCLS Document M11-A4, Vol. 17, No. 22, NCCLS, Villanova, PA, December 1997.

Revisions based on 7882340, issued May 2002.

MEFOXIN® PREMIXED INTRAVENOUS SOLUTION ℞

[*mĕ'foks-ĭn*]
(cefoxitin injection)

Prescribing information for this product, which appears on pages 2031–2034 of the 2003 PDR, has been revised as follows. Please write "See Supplement A" alongside product heading.

Replace the **CLINICAL PHARMACOLOGY** *section with the following:*

CLINICAL PHARMACOLOGY

Clinical Pharmacology

Following an intravenous dose of 1 gram of cefoxitin, serum concentrations were 110 mcg/mL at 5 minutes, declining to less than 1 mcg/mL at 4 hours. The half-life after an intravenous dose is 41 to 59 minutes. Approximately 85 percent of cefoxitin is excreted unchanged by the kidneys over a 6-hour period, resulting in high urinary concentrations. Probenecid slows tubular excretion and produces higher serum levels and increases the duration of measurable serum concentrations.

Cefoxitin passes into pleural and joint fluids and is detectable in antibacterial concentrations in bile.

Microbiology

The bactericidal action of cefoxitin results from inhibition of cell wall synthesis. Cefoxitin has *in vitro* activity against a wide range of gram-positive and gram-negative organisms. The methoxy group in the 7α position provides cefoxitin with a high degree of stability in the presence of beta-lactamases, both penicillinases and cephalosporinases, of gram-negative bacteria.

Cefoxitin has been shown to be active against most strains of the following microorganisms, both in vitro and in clinical infections as described in the INDICATIONS AND USAGE section.

Aerobic gram-positive microorganisms
Staphylococcus aureus[a] (including penicillinase-producing strains)
Staphylococcus epidermidis[a]
Streptococcus agalactiae
Streptococcus pneumoniae
Streptococcus pyogenes

[a]Staphylococci resistant to methicillin/oxacillin should be considered resistant to cefoxitin.

Most strains of enterococci, e.g., *Enterococcus faecalis,* are resistant.

Aerobic gram-negative microorganisms
Escherichia coli
Haemophilus influenzae
Klebsiella spp. (including *K. pneumoniae*)
Morganella morganii
Neisseria gonorrhoeae (including penicillinase-producing strains)
Proteus mirabilis
Proteus vulgaris
Providencia spp. (including *Providencia rettgeri*)

Anaerobic gram-positive microorganisms
Clostridium spp.
Peptococcus niger
Peptostreptococcus spp.

Anaerobic gram-negative microorganisms
Bacteroides distasonis
Bacteroides fragilis
Bacteroides ovatus
Bacteroides thetaiotaomicron
Bacteroides spp.

The following *in vitro* data are available, **but their clinical significance is unknown.**

Cefoxitin exhibits *in vitro* minimum inhibitory concentrations (MIC's) of 8 µg/mL or less of aerobic microorganisms and 16 µg/mL or less for anaerobic microorganisms against most (≥90%) strains of the following microorganisms; however, the safety and effectiveness of cefoxitin in treating clinical infections due to these microorganisms have not been established in adequate and well-controlled clinical trials.

Aerobic gram-negative microorganisms
Eikenella corrodens [non-β-lactamase producers]
Klebsiella oxytoca

Anaerobic gram-positive microorganisms
Clostridium perfringens

Anaerobic gram-negative microorganisms
Prevotella bivia (formerly *Bacteroides bivius*)

Cefoxitin is inactive *in vitro* against most strains of *Pseudomonas aeruginosa* and eterococci and many strains of *Enterobacter cloacae.*

Susceptibility Tests

Dilution Techniques:

Quantitative methods are used to determine antimicrobial minimum inhibitory concentrations (MIC's). These MIC's provide estimates of the susceptibility of bacteria to antimicrobial compounds. The MIC's should be determined using a standardized procedure. Standardized procedures are based on a dilution method[1] (broth or agar) or equivalent with standardized inoculum concentrations and standardized concentrations of cefoxitin powder. The MIC values should be interpreted according to the following criteria:

For testing aerobic microorganisms[a,b,c] other than *Neisseria gonorrhoeae*:

MIC (µg/mL)	Interpretation
≤ 8	Susceptible (S)
16	Intermediate (I)
≥ 32	Resistant (R)

[a]Staphylococci exhibiting resistance to methicillin/oxacillin should be reported as also resistant to cefoxitin despite apparent *in vitro* susceptibility.
[b]For testing *Haemophilus influenzae* these interpretative criteria applicable only to tests performed by broth microdilution method using Haemophilus Test Medium (HTM)[1].
[c]For testing streptococci these interpretative criteria applicable only to tests performed by broth microdilution method using cation-adjusted Mueller-Hinton broth with 2 to 5% lysed horse blood[1].

For testing *Neisseria gonorrhoeae*[d]:

MIC (µg/mL)	Interpretation
≤ 2	Susceptible (S)
4	Intermediate (I)
≥ 8	Resistant (R)

[d]Interpretative criteria applicable only to tests performed by agar dilution method using GC agar base with 1% defined growth supplement and incubated in 5% CO_2[1]. A report of "Susceptible" indicates that the pathogen is likely to be inhibited if the antimicrobial compound in the blood reaches the concentrations usually achievable. A report of "Intermediate" indicates that the result should be considered equivocal, and, if the microorganism is not fully susceptible to alternative, clinically feasible drugs, the test should be repeated. This category implies possible clinical applicability in body sites where the drug is physiologically concentrated or in situations where high dosage of drug can be used. This category also provides a buffer zone which prevents small uncontrolled technical factors from causing major discrepancies in interpretation. A report of "Resistant" indicates that the pathogen is not likely to be inhibited if the antimicrobial compound in the blood reaches the concentrations usually achievable; other therapy should be selected.

Standardized susceptibility test procedures require the use of laboratory control microorganisms to control the technical aspects of the laboratory procedures. Standard cefoxitin powder should provide the following MIC values:

Microorganism		MIC (µg/mL)
Escherichia coli	ATCC 25922	1-4
Neisseria gonorrhoeae[a]	ATCC 49226	0.5-2
Staphylococcus aureus	ATCC 29213	1-4

[a]Interpretative criteria applicable only to tests performed by agar dilution method using GC agar base with 1% defined growth supplement and incubated in 5% CO_2[1].

Diffusion Techniques:

Quantitative methods that require measurement of zone diameters also provide reproducible estimates of the susceptibility of bacteria to antimicrobial compounds. One such standardized procedure[2] requires the use of standardized inoculum concentrations. This procedure uses paper disks impregnated with 30-µg cefoxitin to test the susceptibility of microorganisms to cefoxitin.

Reports from the laboratory providing results of the standard single-disk susceptibility test with a 30-µg cefoxitin disk should be interpreted according to the following criteria:

For testing aerobic microorganisms[a,b,c] other than *Neisseria gonorrhoeae*:

Zone Diameter (mm)	Interpretation
≥ 18	Susceptible (S)
15-17	Intermediate (I)
≤ 14	Resistant (R)

[a]Staphylococci exhibiting resistance to methicillin/oxacillin should be reported as also resistant to cefoxitin despite apparent *in vitro* susceptibility.
[b]For testing *Haemophilus influenzae* these interpretative criteria applicable only to tests performed by disk diffusion method using Haemophilus Test Medium (HTM)[1].
[c]For testing streptococci these interpretative criteria applicable only to tests performed by disk diffusion method using Mueller-Hinton agar with 5% defibrinated sheep blood and incubated in 5% CO_2[2].

For testing *Neisseria gonorrhoeae*[d]:

Zone Diameter (mm)	Interpretation
≥ 28	Susceptible (S)
24-27	Intermediate (I)
≤ 23	Resistant (R)

[d]Interpretative criteria applicable only to tests performed by disk diffusion method using GC agar base with 1% defined growth supplement and incubated in 5% CO_2[2].

Interpretation should be as stated above for results using dilution techniques.

Interpretation involves correlation of the diameter obtained in the disk test with the MIC for cefoxitin.

As with standardized dilution techniques, diffusion methods require the use of laboratory control microorganisms that are used to control the technical aspects of the laboratory procedures. For the diffusion technique, the 30-µg cefoxitin disk should provide the following zone diameters in these laboratory test quality control strains:

Microorganism		Zone Diameter (mm)
Escherichia coli	ATCC 25922	23-29
Neisseria gonorrhoeae[a]	ATCC 49226	33-41
Staphylococcus aureus	ATCC 25923	23-29

[a]Interpretative criteria applicable only to tests performed by disk diffusion method using GC agar base with 1% defined growth supplement and incubated in 5% CO_2[2].

Anaerobic Techniques:

For anaerobic bacteria, the susceptibility to cefoxitin as MIC's can be determined by standardized test methods[3]. The MIC values obtained should be interpreted according to the following criteria:

MIC (µg/mL)	Interpretation
≤ 16	Susceptible (S)
32	Intermediate (I)
≥ 64	Resistant (R)

Interpretation is identical to that stated above for results using dilution techniques.

As with other susceptibility techniques, the use of laboratory control microorganisms is required to control the technical aspects of the laboratory standardized procedures. Standard cefoxitin powder should provide the following MIC values:

Using either an Agar Dilution Method[a] or Using a Broth[b] Microdilution Method:

Microorganism		MIC (µg/mL)
Bacteroides fragilis	ATCC 25285	4-16
Bacteroides thetaiotaomicron	ATCC 29741	8-32

[a]Range applicable only to tests performed using either Brucella blood or Wilkins-Chalgren agar.
[b]Range applicable only to tests performed in the broth formulation of Wilkins-Chalgren agar[3].

Continued on next page

Information on the Merck & Co., Inc., products listed on these pages is from the full prescribing information in use April 1, 2003.

Mefoxin Premixed—Cont.

In the **INDICATIONS AND USAGE** *section, under Treatment, replace list points 1 through 7 with the following:*
(1) **Lower respiratory tract infections,** including pneumonia and lung abscess, caused by *Streptococcus pneumoniae,* other streptococci (excluding enterococci, e.g., *Enterococcus faecalis* [formerly *Streptococcus faecalis*]), *Staphylococcus aureus* (including penicillinase-producing strains), *Escherichia coli, Klebsiella* species, *Haemophilus influenzae,* and *Bacteroides* species.
(2) **Urinary tract infections** caused by *Escherichia coli, Klebsiella* species, *Proteus mirabilis, Morganella morganii, Proteus vulgaris* and *Providencia* species (including *P. rettgeri*).
(3) **Intra-abdominal infections,** including peritonitis and intra-abdominal abscess, caused by *Escherichia coli, Klebsiella* species, *Bacteroides* species including *Bacteroides fragilis,* and *Clostridium* species.
(4) **Gynecological infections,** including endometritis, pelvic cellulitis, and pelvic inflammatory disease caused by *Escherichia coli, Neisseria gonorrhoeae* (including penicillinase-producing strains), *Bacteroides* species including *B. fragilis, Clostridium* species, *Peptococcus niger, Peptostreptococcus* species, and *Streptococcus agalactiae.* MEFOXIN, like cephalosporins, has no activity against *Chlamydia trachomatis.* Therefore, when MEFOXIN is used in the treatment of patients with pelvic inflammatory disease and *C. trachomatis* is one of the suspected pathogens, appropriate anti-chlamydial coverage should be added.
(5) **Septicemia** caused by *Streptococcus pneumoniae, Staphylococcus aureus* (including penicillinase-producing strains), *Escherichia coli, Klebsiella* species, and *Bacteroides* species including *B. fragilis.*
(6) **Bone and joint infections** caused by *Staphylococcus aureus* (including penicillinase-producing strains).
(7) **Skin and skin structure infections** caused by *Staphylococcus aureus* (including penicillinase-producing strains), *Staphylococcus epidermidis, Streptococcus pyogenes* and other streptococci (excluding enterococci, e.g., *Enterococcus faecalis* [formerly *Streptococcus faecalis*]), *Escherichia coli, Proteus mirabilis, Klebsiella* species, *Bacteroides* species including *B. fragilis, Clostridium* species, *Peptococcus niger,* and *Peptostreptococcus* species.
Also in the **INDICATIONS AND USAGE** *section, under Treatment, delete the footnote "***B. fragilis, B. distasonis, B. ovatus, B. thetaiotaomicron."*
In the **ADVERSE REACTIONS** *section, under Allergic Reactions, after* "toxic epidermal necrolysis),", *add* "urticaria, flushing,".
In the **HOW SUPPLIED** *section, delete* "(6505-01-380-3410, 1 g 24's)" *and* "(6505-01-379-9245, 2 g 24's)".
After the **CLINICAL STUDIES** *section, add the following section:*

REFERENCES

1. National Committee for Clinical Laboratory Standards. Methods for Dilution Antimicrobial Susceptibility Tests for Bacteria that Grow Aerobically - Fourth Edition. Approved Standard NCCLS Document M7-A4, Vol. 17, No. 2, NCCLS, Wayne, PA, January 1997.
2. National Committee for Clinical Laboratory Standards. Performance Standards for Antimicrobial Disk Susceptibility Tests - Sixth Edition. Approved Standard NCCLS Document M2-A6, Vol. 17, No. 1, NCCLS, Wayne, PA, January 1997.
3. National Committee for Clinical Laboratory Standards. Methods for Antimicrobial Susceptibility Testing of Anaerobic Bacteria - Fourth Edition. Approved Standard NCCLS Document M11-A4, Vol. 17, No. 22, NCCLS, Villanova, PA, December 1997.

Revisions based on 7948524, issued May 2002.

MEPHYTON® ℞
[*mĕ 'fĭ-tŏn*]
(Phytonadione)
Vitamin K_1

Prescribing information for this product, which appears on page 2034 of the 2003 PDR, has been revised as follows. Please write "See Supplement A" alongside product heading.
In the **PRECAUTIONS** *section, under General, before the first paragraph, insert the following paragraph and heading:*
Vitamin K_1 is fairly rapidly degraded by light; therefore, always protect MEPHYTON from light. Store MEPHYTON in closed original carton until contents have been used. (See also HOW SUPPLIED, *Storage*).
Drug Interactions
In the **HOW SUPPLIED** *section, replace the* ***Storage*** *subsection with the following:*
Store in tightly closed original container at 25°C (77°F); excursions permitted to 15-30°C (59-86°F) [See USP Controlled Room Temperature]. Always protect MEPHYTON from light. Store in tightly closed original container and carton until contents have been used. (See PRECAUTIONS, *General.*)
Revisions based on 7918717, issued February 2002.

MEVACOR® Tablets ℞
[*mĕ'vă-kōr*]
(lovastatin)

Prescribing information for this product, which appears on pages 2036-2041 of the 2003 PDR, has been revised as follows. Please write "See Supplement A" alongside product heading.

TABLE IV
Lipid-lowering Effects of Lovastatin in Adolescent Boys with Heterozygous Familial Hypercholesterolemia
(Mean Percent Change from Baseline at week 48 in Intention-to-Treat Population)

DOSAGE	N	TOTAL-C	LDL-C	HDL-C	TG.*	Apolipoprotein B
Placebo	61	−1.1	−1.4	−2.2	−1.4	−4.4
MEVACOR	64	−19.3	−24.2	+1.1	−1.9	−21

*data presented as median percent changes

TABLE V
Lipid-lowering Effects of Lovastatin in Post-menarchal Girls with Heterozygous Familial Hypercholesterolemia
(Mean Percent Change from Baseline at Week 24 in Intention-to-Treat Population)

DOSAGE	N	TOTAL-C	LDL-C	HDL-C	TG.*	Apolipoprotein B
Placebo	18	+3.6	+2.5	+4.8	−3.0	+6.4
MEVACOR	35	−22.4	−29.2	+2.4	−22.7	−24.4

*data presented as median percent changes

NCEP Treatment Guidelines:
LDL-C Goals and Cutpoints for Therapeutic Lifestyle Changes
and Drug Therapy in Different Risk Categories

Risk Category	LDL Goal (mg/dL)	LDL Level at Which to Initiate Therapeutic Lifestyle Changes (mg/dL)	LDL Level at Which to Consider Drug Therapy (mg/dL)
CHD[†] or CHD risk equivalents (10-year risk >20%)	<100	≥100	≥130 (100-129: drug optional)[††]
2+ Risk factors (10 year risk ≤20%)	<130	≥130	10-year risk 10-20%: ≥130; 10-year risk <10%: ≥160
0-1 Risk factor[†††]	<160	≥160	≥190 (160-189: LDL-lowering drug optional)

† CHD, coronary heart disease
†† Some authorities recommend use of LDL-lowering drugs in this category if an LDL-C level of <100 mg/dL cannot be achieved by therapeutic lifestyle changes. Others prefer use of drugs that primarily modify triglycerides and HDL-C, e.g., nicotinic acid or fibrate. Clinical judgment also may call for deferring drug therapy in this subcategory.
††† Almost all people with 0-1 risk factor have a 10-year risk <10%; thus, 10-year risk assessment in people with 0-1 risk factor is not necessary.

In the **CLINICAL PHARMACOLOGY** *section, under Pharmacokinetics, before the last paragraph, add the following paragraph:*
The risk of myopathy is increased by high levels of HMG-CoA reductase inhibitory activity in plasma. Potent inhibitors of CYP3A4 can raise the plasma levels of HMG-CoA reductase inhibitory activity and increase the risk of myopathy (see WARNINGS, *Myopathy/Rhabdomyolysis* and PRECAUTIONS, *Drug Interactions*).
Also in the **CLINICAL PHARMACOLOGY** *section, add* "in Adults" *to the "Clinical Studies" subsection heading.*
Also in the **CLINICAL PHARMACOLOGY** *section, add the following subsection at the end:*
Clinical Studies in Adolescent Patients
Efficacy of Lovastatin in Adolescent Boys with Heterozygous Familial Hypercholesterolemia
In a double-blind, placebo-controlled study, 132 boys 10-17 years of age (mean age 12.7 yrs) with heterozygous familial hypercholesterolemia (heFH) were randomized to lovastatin (n=67) or placebo (n=65) for 48 weeks. Inclusion in the study required a baseline LDL-C level between 189 and 500 mg/dL and at least one parent with an LDL-C level >189 mg/dL. The mean baseline LDL-C value was 253.1 mg/dL (range: 171-379 mg/dL) in the MEVACOR group compared to 248.2 mg/dL (range 158.5-413.5 mg/dL) in the placebo group. The dosage of lovastatin (once daily in the evening) was 10 mg for the first 8 weeks, 20 mg for the second 8 weeks, and 40 mg thereafter.
MEVACOR significantly decreased plasma levels of total-C, LDL-C and apoliprotein B (see Table IV).
[See table IV above]
The mean achieved LDL-C value was 190.9 mg/dL (range: 108-336 mg/dL) in the MEVACOR group compared to 244.8 mg/dL (range: 135-404 mg/dL) in the placebo group.
Efficacy of Lovastatin in Post-menarchal Girls with Heterozygous Familial Hypercholesterolemia
In a double-blind, placebo-controlled study, 54 girls 10-17 years of age who were at least 1 year post-menarche with heFH were randomized to lovastatin (n=35) or placebo (n=19) for 24 weeks. Inclusion in the study required a baseline LDL-C level of 160-400 mg/dL and a parental history of familial hypercholesterolemia. The mean baseline LDL-C value was 218.3 mg/dL (range: 136.3-363.7 mg/dL) in the MEVACOR group compared to 198.8 mg/dL (range: 151.1-283.1 mg/dL) in the placebo group. The dosage of lovastatin (once daily in the evening) was 20 mg for the first 4 weeks, and 40 mg thereafter.
MEVACOR significantly decreased plasma levels of total-C, LDL-C, and apolipoprotein B (see Table V).
[See table V above]
The mean achieved LDL-C value was 154.5 mg/dL (range: 82-286 mg/dL) in the MEVACOR group compared to 203.5 mg/dL (range: 135-304 mg/dL) in the placebo group.
The safety and efficacy of doses above 40 mg daily have not been studied in children. The long-term efficacy of lovastatin therapy in childhood to reduce morbidity and mortality in adulthood has not been established.
In the **INDICATIONS AND USAGE** *section, after the Hypercholesterolemia subsection, add the following subsection:*
Adolescent Patients with Heterozygous Familial Hypercholesterolemia
MEVACOR is indicated as an adjunct to diet to reduce total-C, LDL-C and apolipoprotein B levels in adolescent boys and girls who are at least one year post-menarche, 10-17 years of age, with heFH if after an adequate trial of diet therapy the following findings are present:
1. LDL-C remains >189 mg/dL or
2. LDL-C remains >160 mg/dL and:
   - there is a postive family history of premature cardiovascular disease or
   - two or more other CVD risk factors are present in the adolescent patient

Also in the **INDICATIONS AND USAGE** *section, in the General Recommendations subsection, after* "The National Cholesterol Education Program (NCEP) Treatment Guidelines are summarized below:", *replace the table with the following:*
[See third table above]
After the LDL-C goal has been achieved, if the TG is still ≥200 mg/dL, non-HDL-C (total-C minus HDL-C) becomes a secondary target of therapy. Non-HDL-C goals are set 30 mg/dL higher than LDL-C goals for each risk category.
Also in the **INDICATIONS AND USAGE** *section, add the following at the end:*
The NCEP classification of cholesterol levels in pediatric patients with a familial history of hypercholesterolemia or premature cardiovascular disease is summarized below:

Category	Total-C (mg/dL)	LDL-C (mg/dL)
Acceptable	<170	<110
Borderline	170-199	110-129
High	≥200	≥130

Children treated with lovastatin in adolescence should be re-evaluated in adulthood and appropriate changes made to their cholesterol-lowering regimen to achieve adult goals for LDL-C.
In the **WARNINGS** *section, replace the Skeletal Muscle, Myopathy caused by drug interactions, and Reducing the risk of myopathy subsections with the following:*
Myopathy/Rhabdomyolysis
Lovastatin, like other inhibitors of HMG-CoA reductase, occasionally causes myopathy manifested as muscle pain, tenderness or weakness with creatine kinase (CK) above 10× the upper limit of normal (ULN). Myopathy sometimes takes the form of rhabdomyolysis with or without acute renal failure secondary to myoglobinuria, and rare fatalities have occurred. The risk of myopathy is increased by high levels of HMG-CoA reductase inhibitory activity in plasma.
- **The risk of myopathy/rhabdomyolysis is increased by concomitant use of lovastatin with the following:**
  Potent inhibitors of CYP3A4: Cyclosporine, itraconazole, ketoconazole, erythromycin, clarithromycin, HIV protease inhibitors, nefazodone, or large quantities of grapefruit juice (>1 quart daily), particularly with higher doses of lovastatin (see below; CLINICAL PHARMACOLOGY, *Pharmacokinetics*; PRECAUTIONS, *Drug Interactions, CYP3A4 Interactions*).
  Lipid-lowering drugs that can cause myopathy when given alone: Gemfibrozil, other fibrates, or lipid-lower-

ing doses (≥1 g/day) of niacin, particularly with higher doses of lovastatin (see below; CLINICAL PHARMACOLOGY, *Pharmacokinetics*; PRECAUTIONS, *Drug Interactions, Interactions with lipid-lowering drugs that can cause myopathy when given alone*).

Other drugs: The risk of myopathy/rhabdomyolysis is increased when either amiodarone or verapamil is used concomitantly with higher doses of a closely related member of the HMG-CoA reductase inhibitor class (see PRECAUTIONS, *Drug Interactions, Other drug interactions*).

• **The risk of myopathy/rhabdomyolysis is dose related.** In a clinical study (EXCEL) in which patients were carefully monitored and some interacting drugs were excluded, there was one case of myopathy among 4933 patients randomized to lovastatin 20-40 mg daily for 48 weeks, and 4 among 1649 patients randomized to 80 mg daily.

CONSEQUENTLY:

1. Use of lovastatin concomitantly with itraconazole, ketoconazole, erythromycin, clarithromycin, HIV protease inhibitors, nefazodone, or large quantities of grapefruit juice (>1 quart daily) should be avoided. If treatment with itraconazole, ketoconazole, erythromycin, or clarithromycin is unavoidable, therapy with lovastatin should be suspended during the course of treatment. Concomitant use with other medicines labeled as having a potent inhibitory effect on CYP3A4 at therapeutic doses should be avoided unless the benefits of combined therapy outweigh the increased risk.

2. The dose of lovastatin should not exceed 20 mg daily in patients receiving concomitant medication with cyclosporine, gemfibrozil, other fibrates or lipid-lowering doses (≥1 g/day) of niacin. The combined use of lovastatin with fibrates or niacin should be avoided unless the benefit of further alteration in lipid levels is likely to outweigh the increased risk of this drug combination. Addition of these drugs to lovastatin typically provides little additional reduction in LDL-C, but further reductions of TG and further increases in HDL-C may be obtained.

3. The dose of lovastatin should not exceed 40 mg daily in patients receiving concomitant medication with amiodarone or verapamil. The combined use of lovastatin at doses higher than 40 mg daily with amiodarone or verapamil should be avoided unless the clinical benefit is likely to outweigh the increased risk of myopathy.

4. All patients starting therapy with lovastatin, or whose dose of lovastatin is being increased, should be advised of the risk of myopathy and told to report promptly any unexplained muscle pain, tenderness or weakness. Lovastatin therapy should be discontinued immediately if myopathy is diagnosed or suspected. The presence of these symptoms, and/or a CK level >10 times the ULN indicates myopathy. In most cases, when patients were promptly discontinued from treatment, muscle symptoms and CK increases resolved. Periodic CK determinations may be considered in patients starting therapy with lovastatin or whose dose is being increased, but there is no assurance that such monitoring will prevent myopathy.

5. Many of the patients who have developed rhabdomyolysis on therapy with lovastatin have had complicated medical histories, including renal insufficiency usually as a consequence of long-standing diabetes mellitus. Such patients merit closer monitoring. Therapy with lovastatin should be temporarily stopped a few days prior to elective major surgery and when any major medical or surgical condition supervenes.

In the **PRECAUTIONS** *section, replace the* **Information for Patients** *subsection with the following:*

Patients should be advised about substances they should not take concomitantly with lovastatin and be advised to report promptly unexplained muscle pain, tenderness, or weakness (see list below and WARNINGS, *Myopathy/Rhabdomyolysis*). Patients should also be advised to inform other physicians prescribing a new medication that they are taking MEVACOR.

Also in the **PRECAUTIONS** *section, under Drug Interactions, replace paragraphs 1 through 4 (all paragraphs before the one beginning "Coumarin Anticoagulants") with the following:*

CYP3A4 Interactions

Lovastatin is metabolized by CYP3A4 but has no CYP3A4 inhibitory activity; therefore it is not expected to affect the plasma concentrations of other drugs metabolized by CYP3A4. Potent inhibitors of CYP3A4 (below) increase the risk of myopathy by reducing the elimination of lovastatin.

See WARNINGS, *Myopathy/Rhabdomyolysis*, and CLINICAL PHARMACOLOGY, *Pharmacokinetics*.

Itraconazole
Ketoconazole
Erythromycin
Clarithromycin
HIV protease inhibitors
Nefazodone
Cyclosporine
Large quantities of grapefruit juice (>1 quart daily)

Interactions with lipid-lowering drugs that can cause myopathy when given alone

The risk of myopathy is also increased by the following lipid-lowering drugs that are not potent CYP3A4 inhibitors, but which can cause myopathy when given alone.

See WARNINGS, *Myopathy/Rhabdomyolysis*.

Gemfibrozil
Other fibrates
Niacin (nicotinic acid) (1 g/day)

Other drug interactions

Amiodarone or Verapamil: The risk of myopathy/rhabdomyolysis is increased when either amiodarone or verapamil is used concomitantly with a closely related member of the HMG-CoA reductase inhibitor class (see WARNINGS, *Myopathy/Rhabdomyolysis*).

Also in the **PRECAUTIONS** *section, replace the Pediatric Use subsection with the following:*

Safety and effectiveness in patients 10-17 years of age with heFH have been evaluated in controlled clinical trials of 48 weeks duration in adolescent boys and controlled clinical trials of 24 weeks duration in girls who were at least 1 year post-menarche. Patients treated with lovastatin had an adverse experience profile generally similar to that of patients treated with placebo. **Doses greater than 40 mg have not been studied in this population.** In these limited controlled studies, there was no detectable effect on growth or sexual maturation in the adolescent boys or on menstrual cycle length in girls. See CLINICAL PHARMACOLOGY, *Clinical Studies in Adolescent Patients;* ADVERSE REACTIONS, *Adolescent Patients;* and DOSAGE AND ADMINISTRATION, *Adolescent Patients (10-17 years of age) with Heterozygous Familial Hypercholesterolemia.* Adolescent females should be counseled on appropriate contraceptive methods while on lovastatin therapy (see CONTRAINDICATIONS and PRECAUTIONS, *Pregnancy*).

Lovastatin has not been studied in pre-pubertal patients or patients younger than 10 years of age.

In the **ADVERSE REACTIONS** *section, under Phase III Clinical Studies, at the end of the second paragraph, after* "(see WARNINGS,", *replace "Skeletal Muscle"* with *"Myopathy/Rhabdomyolysis".*

Also in the **ADVERSE REACTIONS** *section, under Concomitant Therapy, in the first paragraph, in the fifth sentence, after* "(nicotinic acid)", *add* ". The combined use of lovastatin at doses exceeding 20 mg/day with cyclosporine, gemfibrozil, other fibrates or lipid-lowering doses (≥1 g/day) of niacin should be avoided". In the same sentence, after "(see WARNINGS,", replace *"Skeletal Muscle"* with *"Myopathy/Rhabdomyolysis".*

Also in the **ADVERSE REACTIONS** *section, add the following subsection at the end:*

Adolescent Patients (ages 10-17 years)

In a 48-week controlled study in adolescent boys with heFH (n=132) and a 24-week controlled study in girls who were at least 1 year post-menarche with heFH (n=54), the safety and tolerability profile of the groups treated with MEVACOR (10 to 40 mg daily) was generally similar to that of the groups treated with placebo (see CLINICAL PHARMACOLOGY, *Clinical Studies in Adolescent Patients* and PRECAUTIONS, *Pediatric Use*).

In the **DOSAGE AND ADMINISTRATION** *section, after the first paragraph, insert the subsection heading "Adult Patients". After the second paragraph, insert the following text and heading:*

Cholesterol levels should be monitored periodically and consideration should be given to reducing the dosage of MEVACOR if cholesterol levels fall significantly below the targeted range.

Dosage in Patients taking Cyclosporine

Also in the **DOSAGE AND ADMINISTRATION** *section, in the third paragraph, in the first sentence, after* "(see WARNINGS,", *replace "Skeletal Muscle" with "Myopathy/Rhabdomyolysis". Delete the fourth paragraph (beginning* "Cholesterol levels...").

Also in the **DOSAGE AND ADMINISTRATION** *section, after the fourth paragraph, add the following two subsections:*

Dosage in Patients taking Amiodarone or Verapamil

In patients taking amiodarone or verapamil concomitantly with MEVACOR, the dose should not exceed 40 mg/day (see WARNINGS, *Myopathy/Rhabdomyolysis* and PRECAUTIONS, *Drug Interactions, Other drug interactions*).

Adolescent Patients (10-17 years of age) with Heterozygous Familial Hypercholesterolemia

The recommended dosing range is 10-40 mg/day; the maximum recommended dose is 40 mg/day. Doses should be individualized according to the recommended goal of therapy (see NCEP Pediatric Panel Guidelines[††], CLINICAL PHARMACOLOGY, and INDICATIONS AND USAGE). Patients requiring reductions in LDL-C of 20% or more to achieve their goal should be started on 20 mg/day of MEVACOR. A starting dose of 10 mg may be considered for patients requiring smaller reductions. Adjustments should be made at intervals of 4 weeks or more.

[††]National Cholesterol Education Program (NCEP): Highlights of the Report of the Expert Panel on Blood Cholesterol Levels in Children and Adolescents. *Pediatrics.* 89(3):495–501. 1992.

Also in the **DOSAGE AND ADMINISTRATION** *section, under Concomitant Lipid-Lowering Therapy, replace the second and third sentences with the following:*

If MEVACOR is used in combination with gemfibrozil, other fibrates or lipid-lowering doses (≥1g/day) of niacin, the dose of MEVACOR should not exceed 20 mg/day (see WARNINGS, *Myopathy/Rhabdomyolysis* and PRECAUTIONS, *Drug Interactions).*

Also in the **DOSAGE AND ADMINISTRATION** *section, under Dosage in Patients with Renal Insufficiency, after* "(see CLINICAL PHARMACOLOGY and WARNINGS,", *replace "Skeletal Muscle" with "Myopathy/Rhabdomyolysis".*

Revisions based on 7825351, issued June 2002.

NOROXIN® TABLETS ℞

[nōr′oks″ĭn]
(norfloxacin)

Prescribing information for this product, which appears on pages 2050–2052 of the 2003 PDR, has been revised as follows. Please write "See Supplement A" alongside product heading.

In the **CLINICAL PHARMACOLOGY** *section, second paragraph, after the first sentence, add the following:*

Following a single 400-mg dose of norfloxacin, the mean (± SD) AUC and C_{max} of 9.8 (2.83) µg•hr/mL and 2.02 (0.77) µg/mL respectively, were observed in healthy elderly volunteers. The extent of systemic exposure was slightly higher than that seen in younger adults (AUC 6.4 µg•hr/mL and C_{max} 1.5 µg/mL).

Also in the **CLINICAL PHARMACOLOGY** *section, after the second paragraph, add the following paragraph:*

There is no information on accumulation of norfloxacin with repeated administration in elderly patients. However, no dosage adjustment is required based on age alone. In elderly patients with reduced renal function, the dosage should be adjusted as for other patients with renal impairment (see DOSAGE AND ADMINISTRATION, *Renal Impairment*).

Also in the **CLINICAL PHARMACOLOGY** *section, fourth paragraph (beginning* "Norfloxacin is eliminated..."), *add the following at the end:*

In elderly subjects (average creatinine clearance was 91 mL/min/1.73m^2) approximately 22% of the administered dose was recovered in urine and renal clearance averaged 154 mL/min.

In the **PRECAUTIONS** *section, under General, at the end, add the following paragraph:*

Some quinolones have been associated with prolongation of the QT interval on the electrocardiogram and infrequent cases of arrhythmia. During post-marketing surveillance, extremely rare cases of torsades de pointes have been reported in patients taking norfloxacin. These reports generally involve patients who had other concurrent medical conditions and the relationship to norfloxacin has not been established. Among drugs known to cause prolongation of the QT interval, the risk of arrhythmias may be reduced by avoiding use in the presence of hypokalemia, significant bradycardia, or concurrent treatment with class Ia or class III antiarrhythmic agents.

Also in the **PRECAUTIONS** *section, under Drug Interactions, after the third paragraph, add the following paragraph:*

The concomitant administration of quinolones including norfloxacin with glyburide (a sulfonylurea agent) has, on rare occasions, resulted in severe hypoglycemia. Therefore, monitoring of blood glucose is recommended when these agents are co-administered.

Also in the **PRECAUTIONS** *section, at the end, add the following subsection:*

Geriatric Use

Of the 340 subjects in one large clinical study of NOROXIN for treatment of urinary tract infections, 103 patients were 65 and older, 77 of whom were 70 and older; no overall differences in safety and effectiveness were evident between these subjects and younger subjects. In clinical practice, no difference in the type of reported adverse experiences have been observed between the elderly and younger patients; however, increased risk for adverse experiences in some older individuals cannot be ruled out (see ADVERSE REACTIONS).

This drug is known to be substantially excreted by the kidney, and the risk of toxic reactions to this drug may be greater in patients with impaired renal function. Because elderly patients are more likely to have decreased renal function, care should be taken in dose selection, and it may be useful to monitor renal function (see DOSAGE AND ADMINISTRATION).

A pharmacokinetic study of NOROXIN in elderly volunteers (65 to 75 years of age with normal renal function for their age) was carried out (see CLINICAL PHARMACOLOGY).

In the **ADVERSE REACTIONS** *section, after the Gastrointestinal subsection, add the following subsection:*

Cardiovascular

On very rare occasions, prolonged QTc interval and ventricular arrhythmia (including torsades de pointes).

Also in the **ADVERSE REACTIONS** *section, under Musculoskeletal, at the end, add* "elevated creatine kinase (CK)."

Revisions based on 7898530, issued August 2002.

PEPCID® TABLETS ℞

[pĕp-sĭd]
(famotidine)

PEPCID® FOR ORAL SUSPENSION

(famotidine)

Prescribing information for this product, which appears on pages 2055–2057 of the 2003 PDR, has been revised as follows. Please write "See Supplement A" alongside product heading.

Continued on next page

Information on the Merck & Co., Inc., products listed on these pages is from the full prescribing information in use April 1, 2003.

Pepcid Tablets—Cont.

Age (N=number of patients)	Area Under the Curve (AUC) (ng-hr/mL)	Total Clearance (Cl) (L/hr/kg)	Volume of Distribution (V_d) (L/kg)	Elimination Half-life (T½) (hours)
0-1 month[c] (N=10)	NA	0.13 ± 0.06	1.4 ± 0.4	10.5 ± 5.4
0-3 months[d] (N=6)	2688 ± 847	0.21 ± 0.06	1.8 ± 0.3	8.1 ± 3.5
>3-12 months[d] (N=11)	1160 ± 474	0.49 ± 0.17	2.3 ± 0.7	4.5 ± 1.1
1-11 yrs (N=20)	1089 ± 834	0.54 ± 0.34	2.07 ± 1.49	3.38 ± 2.60
11-15 yrs (N=6)	1140 ± 320	0.48 ± 0.14	1.5 ± 0.4	2.3 ± 0.4
Adult (N=16)	1726[b]	0.39 ± 0.14	1.3 ± 0.2	2.83 ± 0.99

Table 6
Pharmacokinetic Parameters[a] of Intravenous Famotidine

[a]Values are presented as means ± SD unless indicated otherwise.
[b]Mean value only.
[c]Single center study.
[d]Multicenter study.

Table 8

Dosage	Route	Effect[a]	Number of Patients (age range)
0.5 mg/kg, single dose	I.V.	gastric pH >4 for 19.5 hours (17.3, 21.8)[c]	11 (5-19 days)
0.3 mg/kg, single dose	I.V.	gastric pH >3.5 for 8.7 ± 4.7[b] hours	6 (2-7 years)
0.4-0.8 mg/kg	I.V.	gastric pH >4 for 6-9 hours	18 (2-69 months)
0.5 mg/kg, single dose	I.V.	a >2 pH unit increase above baseline in gastric pH for >8 hours	9 (2-13 years)
0.5 mg/kg b.i.d.	I.V.	gastric pH >5 for 13.5 ± 1.8[b] hours	4 (6-15 years)
0.5 mg/kg b.i.d.	oral	gastric pH >5 for 5.0 ± 1.1[b] hours	4 (11-15 years)

[a]Values reported in published literature.
[b]Means ± SD.
[c]Mean (95% confidence interval).

In the main heading, delete **"PEPCID RPD® (famotidine) Orally Disintegrating Tablets".**
In the **DESCRIPTION** *section, delete the fourth paragraph (beginning* "Each Orally Disintegrating Tablet..").
In the **CLINICAL PHARMACOLOGY IN ADULTS** *section, under Pharmacokinetics, replace the third sentence with the following:*
PEPCID Tablets and PEPCID for Oral Suspension are bioequivalent.
Replace the **CLINICAL PHARMACOLOGY IN PEDIATRIC PATIENTS** *section with the following:*
CLINICAL PHARMACOLOGY IN PEDIATRIC PATIENTS
Pharmacokinetics
Table 6 presents pharmacokinetic data from clinical trials and a published study in pediatric patients (<1 year of age; N=27) given famotidine I.V. 0.5 mg/kg and from published studies of small numbers of pediatric patients (1-15 years of age) given famotidine intravenously. Areas under the curve (AUCs) are normalized to a dose of 0.5 mg/kg I.V. for pediatric patients 1-15 years of age and compared with an extrapolated 40 mg intravenous dose in adults (extrapolation based on results obtained with a 20 mg I.V. adult dose).
[See table 6 at right]
Plasma clearance is reduced and elimination half-life is prolonged in pediatric patients 0-3 months of age compared to older pediatric patients. The pharmacokinetic parameters for pediatric patients, ages >3 months-15 years, are comparable to those obtained for adults.
Bioavailability studies of 8 pediatric patients (11-15 years of age) showed a mean oral bioavailability of 0.5 compared to adult values of 0.42 to 0.49. Oral doses of 0.5 mg/kg achieved AUCs of 645 ± 249 ng-hr/mL and 580 ± 60 ng-hr/mL in pediatric patients <1 year of age (N=5) and in pediatric patients 11-15 years of age, respectively, compared to 482 ± 181 ng-hr/mL in adults treated with 40 mg orally.
Pharmacodynamics
Pharmacodynamics of famotidine were evaluated in 5 pediatric patients 2-13 years of age using the sigmoid E_{max} model. These data suggest that the relationship between serum concentration of famotidine and gastric acid suppression is similar to that observed in one study of adults (Table 7).

Table 7
Pharmacodynamics of famotidine using the sigmoid E_{max} model

	EC_{50} (ng/mL)*
Pediatric Patients	26 ± 13
Data from one study	
a) healthy adult subjects	26.5 ± 10.3
b) adult patients with upper GI bleeding	18.7 ± 10.8

*Serum concentration of famotidine associated with 50% maximum gastric acid reduction. Values are presented as means ± SD.

Five published studies (Table 8) examined the effect of famotidine on gastric pH and duration of acid suppression in pediatric patients. While each study had a different design, acid suppression data over time are summarized as follows:
[See table 8 above]
The duration of effect of famotidine I.V. 0.5 mg/kg on gastric pH and acid suppression was shown in one study to be longer in pediatric patients <1 month of age than in older pediatric patients. This longer duration of gastric acid suppression is consistent with the decreased clearance in pediatric patients <3 months of age (see Table 6).
In the **PRECAUTIONS** *section, under Information for Patients, delete the second and third paragraphs (beginning* "Patients should be instructed..." *and ending* "...40 mg orally disintegrating tablet.").
Also in the **PRECAUTIONS** *section, change the Pediatric Patients subsection heading to "Pediatric Patients <1 year of age" and add the following four paragraphs and subsection heading at the beginning:*
Pediatric Patients <1 year of age
Use of PEPCID in pediatric patients <1 year of age is supported by evidence from adequate and well-controlled studies of PEPCID in adults, and by the following studies in pediatric patients <1 year of age.
Two pharmacokinetic studies in pediatric patients <1 year of age (N=48) demonstrated that clearance of famotidine in patients >3 months to 1 year of age is similar to that seen in older pediatric patients (1-15 years of age) and adults. In contrast, pediatric patients 0-3 months of age had famotidine clearance values that were 2- to 4-fold less than those in older pediatric patients and adults. These studies also show that the mean bioavailability in pediatric patients <1 year of age after oral dosing is similar to older pediatric patients and adults. Pharmacodynamic data in pediatric patients 0-3 months of age suggest that the duration of acid suppression is longer compared with older pediatric patients, consistent with the longer famotidine half-life in pediatric patients 0-3 months of age. (See CLINICAL PHARMACOLOGY IN PEDIATRIC PATIENTS, *Pharmacokinetics* and *Pharmacodynamics*.)
In a double-blind, randomized, treatment-withdrawal study, 35 pediatric patients <1 year of age who were diagnosed as having gastroesophageal reflux disease were treated for up to 4 weeks with famotidine oral suspension (0.5 mg/kg/dose or 1 mg/kg/dose). Although an intravenous famotidine formulation was available, no patients were treated with intravenous famotidine in this study. Also, caregivers were instructed to provide conservative treatment including thickened feedings. Enrolled patients were diagnosed primarily by history of vomiting (spitting up) and irritability (fussiness). The famotidine dosing regimen was once daily for patients <3 months of age and twice daily for patients ≥3 months of age. After 4 weeks of treatment, patients were randomly withdrawn from the treatment and followed an additional 4 weeks for adverse events and symptomatology. Patients were evaluated for vomiting (spitting up), irritability (fussiness) and global assessments of improvement. The study patients ranged in age at entry from 1.3 to 10.5 months (mean 5.6 ± 2.9 months), 57% were female, 91% were white and 6% were black. Most patients (27/35) continued into the treatment-withdrawal phase of the study. Two patients discontinued famotidine due to adverse events. Most patients improved during the initial treatment phase of the study. Results of the treatment-withdrawal phase were difficult to interpret because of small numbers of patients. Of the 35 patients enrolled in the study, agitation was observed in 5 patients on famotidine that resolved when the medication was discontinued; agitation was not observed in patients on placebo (see ADVERSE REACTIONS, *Pediatric Patients*).
These studies suggest that a starting dose of 0.5 mg/kg/dose of famotidine oral suspension may be of benefit for the treatment of GERD for up to 4 weeks once daily in patients <3 months of age and twice daily in patients 3 months to <1 year of age; the safety and benefit of famotidine treatment beyond 4 weeks have not been established. Famotidine should be considered for the treatment of GERD only if conservative measures (e.g., thickened feedings) are used concurrently and if the potential benefit outweighs the risk.
Pediatric Patients 1-16 years of age
Also in the **PRECAUTIONS** *section, before the Geriatric Use subsection, delete the paragraph beginning* "No pharmacokinetic...".
In the **ADVERSE REACTIONS** *section, under Other, second paragraph, delete* "and PEPCID RPD Orally Disintegrating Tablets".
Also in the **ADVERSE REACTIONS** *section, at the end, add the following subsection:*
Pediatric Patients
In a clinical study in 35 pediatric patients <1 year of age with GERD symptoms [e.g., vomiting (spitting up), irritability (fussing)], agitation was observed in 5 patients on famotidine that resolved when the medication was discontinued.
In the **DOSAGE AND ADMINISTRATION** *section, after the Gastroesophageal Reflux Disease (GERD) subsection, add the following subsection:*
Dosage for Pediatric Patients <1 year of age Gastroesophageal Reflux Disease (GERD)
See PRECAUTIONS, *Pediatric Patients <1 year of age.*
The studies described in PRECAUTIONS, *Pediatric Patients <1 year of age* suggest the following starting doses in pediatric patients <1 year of age: *Gastroesophageal Reflux Disease (GERD)* - 0.5 mg/kg/dose of famotidine oral suspension for the treatment of GERD for up to 8 weeks once daily in patients <3 months of age and 0.5 mg/kg/dose twice daily in patients 3 months to <1 year of age. Patients should also be receiving conservative measures (e.g., thickened feedings). The use of intravenous famotidine in pediatric patients <1 year of age with GERD has not been adequately studied.
Also in the **DOSAGE AND ADMINISTRATION** *section, in the Dosage for Pediatric Patients subsection, change the heading to "Dosage for Pediatric Patients 1-16 years of age". In the first two paragraphs, add "1-16 years of age" after "Pediatric Patients". In the fifth paragraph, last sentence (beginning* "Published uncontrolled..."), *add* "1-16 years of age" *after* "pediatric patients" *and delete the last paragraph.*

Also in the **DOSAGE AND ADMINISTRATION** *section, delete the Orally Disintegrating Tablets subsection.*
In the **HOW SUPPLIED** *section, delete the* No. 3553 *and* No. 3554 *items.*
Also in the **HOW SUPPLIED** *section, under Storage, first paragraph, delete* "and PEPCID RPD Orally Disintegrating Tablets".
Revisions based on 7825036, issued June 2002.

PEPCID® INJECTION PREMIXED ℞
[*pĕp-sĭd*]
(famotidine)
PEPCID® INJECTION
(famotidine)

Prescribing information for this product, which appears on pages 2057–2060 of the 2003 PDR, has been revised as follows. Please write "See Supplement A" alongside product heading.
Replace the **CLINICAL PHARMACOLOGY IN PEDIATRIC PATIENTS** *section with the following:*
CLINICAL PHARMACOLOGY IN PEDIATRIC PATIENTS
Pharmacokinetics
Table 6 presents pharmacokinetic data from clinical trials and a published study in pediatric patients (<1 year of age; N=27) given famotidine I.V. 0.5 mg/kg and from published studies of small numbers of pediatric patients (1-15 years of age) given famotidine intravenously. Areas under the curve (AUCs) are normalized to a dose of 0.5 mg/kg I.V. for pediatric patients 1-15 years of age and compared with an extrapolated 40 mg intravenous dose in adults (extrapolation based on results obtained with a 20 mg I.V. adult dose).
[See table 6 at top of next page]
Plasma clearance is reduced and elimination half-life is prolonged in pediatric patients 0-3 months of age compared to older pediatric patients. The pharmacokinetic parameters for pediatric patients, ages >3 months-15 years, are comparable to those obtained for adults.
Bioavailability studies of 8 pediatric patients (11-15 years of age) showed a mean oral bioavailability of 0.5 compared to adult values of 0.42 to 0.49. Oral doses of 0.5 mg/kg achieved AUCs of 645 ± 249 ng-hr/mL and 580 ± 60 ng-hr/mL in pediatric patients <1 year of age (N=5) and in pediatric patients 11-15 years of age, respectively, compared to 482 ± 181 ng-hr/mL in adults treated with 40 mg orally.
Pharmacodynamics
Pharmacodynamics of famotidine were evaluated in 5 pediatric patients 2-13 years of age using the sigmoid E_{max} model. These data suggest that the relationship between serum concentration of famotidine and gastric acid suppression is similar to that observed in one study of adults (Table 7).

Table 7
Pharmacodynamics of famotidine using the sigmoid E_{max} model

	EC_{50} (ng/mL)*
Pediatric Patients	26 ± 13
Data from one study	
a) healthy adult subjects	26.5 ± 10.3
b) adult patients with upper GI bleeding	18.7 ± 10.8

* Serum concentration of famotidine associated with 50% maximum gastric acid reduction. Values are presented as means ± SD.

Table 6
Pharmacokinetic Parameters[a] of Intravenous Famotidine

Age (N=number of patients)	Area Under the Curve (AUC) (ng-hr/mL)	Total Clearance (Cl) (L/hr/kg)	Volume of Distribution (V_d) (L/kg)	Elimination Half-Life ($T_{1/2}$) (hours)
0-1 month[c] (N=10)	NA	0.13 ± 0.06	1.4 ± 0.4	10.5 ± 5.4
0-3 months[d] (N=6)	2688 ± 847	0.21 ± 0.06	1.8 ± 0.3	8.1 ± 3.5
>3-12 months[d] (N=11)	1160 ± 474	0.49 ± 0.17	2.3 ± 0.7	4.5 ± 1.1
1-11 years (N=20)	1089 ± 834	0.54 ± 0.34	2.07 ± 1.49	3.38 ± 2.60
11-15 years (N=6)	1140 ± 320	0.48 ± 0.14	1.5 ± 0.4	2.3 ± 0.4
Adult (N=16)	1726[b]	0.39 ± 0.14	1.3 ± 0.2	2.83 ± 0.99

[a]Values are presented as means ± SD unless indicated otherwise.
[b]Mean value only.
[c]Single center study.
[d]Multicenter study.

Table 8

Dosage	Route	Effect[a]	Number of Patients (age range)
0.5 mg/kg, single dose	I.V.	gastric pH >4 for 19.5 hours (17.3, 21.8)[c]	11 (5-19 days)
0.3 mg/kg, single dose	I.V.	gastric pH >3.5 for 8.7 ± 4.7[b] hours	6 (2-7 years)
0.4-0.8 mg/kg	I.V.	gastric pH >4 for 6-9 hours	18 (2-69 months)
0.5 mg/kg, single dose	I.V.	a >2 pH unit increase above baseline in gastric pH for >8 hours	9 (2-13 years)
0.5 mg/kg b.i.d.	I.V.	gastric pH >5 for 13.5 ± 1.8[b] hours	4 (6-15 years)
0.5 mg/kg b.i.d.	oral	gastric pH >5 for 5.0 ± 1.1[b] hours	4 (11-15 years)

[a]Values reported in published literature.
[b]Means ± SD.
[c]Mean (95% confidence interval).

Five published studies (Table 8) examined the effect of famotidine on gastric pH and duration of acid suppression in pediatric patients. While each study had a different design, acid suppression data over time are summarized as follows:

[See table 8 above]

The duration of effect of famotidine I.V. 0.5 mg/kg on gastric pH and acid suppression was shown in one study to be longer in pediatric patients <1 month of age than in older pediatric patients. This longer duration of gastric acid suppression is consistent with the decreased clearance in pediatric patients <3 months of age (see Table 6).

In the **PRECAUTIONS** *section, change the Pediatric Patients subsection heading to "Pediatric Patients <1 year of age" and add the following four paragraphs and subsection heading at the beginning:*

Pediatric Patients <1 year of age

Use of PEPCID in pediatric patients <1 year of age is supported by evidence from adequate and well-controlled studies of PEPCID in adults, and by the following studies in pediatric patients <1 year of age.

Two pharmacokinetic studies in pediatric patients <1 year of age (N=48) demonstrated that clearance of famotidine in patients >3 months to 1 year of age is similar to that seen in older pediatric patients (1-15 years of age) and adults. In contrast, pediatric patients 0-3 months of age had famotidine clearance values that were 2- to 4-fold less than those in older pediatric patients and adults. These studies also show that the mean bioavailability in pediatric patients <1 year of age after oral dosing is similar to older pediatric patients and adults. Pharmacodynamic data in pediatric patients 0-3 months of age suggest that the duration of acid suppression is longer compared with older pediatric patients, consistent with the longer famotidine half-life in pediatric patients 0-3 months of age. (See CLINICAL PHARMACOLOGY IN PEDIATRIC PATIENTS, *Pharmacokinetics* and *Pharmacodynamics*.)

In a double-blind, randomized, treatment-withdrawal study, 35 pediatric patients <1 year of age who were diagnosed as having gastroesophageal reflux disease were treated for up to 4 weeks with famotidine oral suspension (0.5 mg/kg/dose or 1 mg/kg/dose). Although an intravenous famotidine formulation was available, no patients were treated with intravenous famotidine in this study. Also, caregivers were instructed to provide conservative treatment including thickened feedings. Enrolled patients were diagnosed primarily by history of vomiting (spitting up) and irritability (fussiness). The famotidine dosing regimen was once daily for patients <3 months of age and twice daily for patients ≥3 months of age. After 4 weeks of treatment, patients were randomly withdrawn from the treatment and followed an additional 4 weeks for adverse events and symptomatology. Patients were evaluated for vomiting (spitting up), irritability (fussiness) and global assessments of improvement. The study patients ranged in age at entry from 1.3 to 10.5 months (mean 5.6 ± 2.9 months), 57% were female, 91% were white and 6% were black. Most patients (27/35) continued into the treatment withdrawal phase of the study. Two patients discontinued famotidine due to adverse events. Most patients improved during the initial treatment phase of the study. Results of the treatment withdrawal phase were difficult to interpret because of small numbers of patients. Of the 35 patients enrolled in the study, agitation was observed in 5 patients on famotidine that resolved when the medication was discontinued; agitation was not observed in patients on placebo (see ADVERSE REACTIONS, *Pediatric Patients*).

These studies suggest that a starting dose of 0.5 mg/kg/dose of famotidine oral suspension may be of benefit for the treatment of GERD for up to 4 weeks once daily in patients <3 months of age and twice daily in patients 3 months to <1 year of age; the safety and benefit of famotidine treatment beyond 4 weeks have not been established. Famotidine should be considered for the treatment of GERD only if conservative measures (e.g., thickened feedings) are used concurrently and if the potential benefit outweighs the risk.

Pediatric Patients 1-16 years of age

Also in the **PRECAUTIONS** *section, before the Geriatric Use subsection, delete the paragraph beginning* "No pharmacokinetic. . .".

In the **ADVERSE REACTIONS** *section, at the end, add the following subsection:*

Pediatric Patients

In a clinical study in 35 pediatric patients <1 year of age with GERD symptoms [e.g., vomiting (spitting up), irritability (fussing)], agitation was observed in 5 patients on famotidine that resolved when the medication was discontinued.

In the **DOSAGE AND ADMINISTRATION** *section, after the third paragraph, add the following subsection:*

Dosage for Pediatric Patients <1 year of age Gastroesophageal Reflux Disease (GERD)

See PRECAUTIONS, *Pediatric Patients <1 year of age.*

The studies described in PRECAUTIONS, *Pediatric Patients <1 year of age* suggest the following starting doses in pediatric patients <1 year of age: *Gastroesophageal Reflux Disease (GERD)* - 0.5 mg/kg/dose of famotidine oral suspension for the treatment of GERD for up to 8 weeks once daily in patients <3 months of age and 0.5 mg/kg/dose twice daily in patients 3 months to <1 year of age. Patients should also be receiving conservative measures (e.g., thickened feedings). The use of intravenous famotidine in pediatric patients <1 year of age with GERD has not been adequately studied.

Also in the **DOSAGE AND ADMINISTRATION** *section, in the Dosage for Pediatric Patients subsection, change the heading to "Dosage for Pediatric Patients 1-16 years of age". In the first two paragraphs, add "1-16 years of age" after "Pediatric Patients". In the third paragraph, last sentence* (beginning "Published uncontrolled. . ."), *add* "1-16 years of age" *after* "pediatric patients" *and delete the last paragraph.*

Revisions based on 9042511, issued June 2002.

PROSCAR® TABLETS ℞

[*prŏ'scăr*]
(finasteride)

Prescribing information for this product, which appears on pages 2080–2083 of the 2003 PDR, has been revised as follows. Please write "See Supplement A" alongside product heading.

In the **DESCRIPTION** *section, replace the structural formula with the following:*

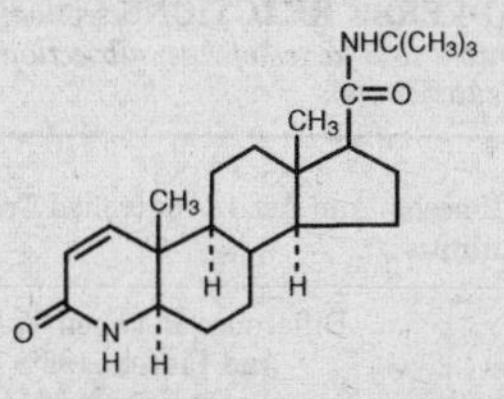

In the **HOW SUPPLIED** *section, under* "**NDC** 0006-0072-28 unit dose packages of 100", *add* "**NDC** 0006-0072-82 bottles of 1000".

Revisions based on 9132104, issued September 2002.

SINGULAIR® TABLETS AND CHEWABLE TABLETS ℞

[*sĭn gū lar*]
(montelukast sodium)

Prescribing information for this product, which appears on pages 2086–2090 of the 2003 PDR, has been revised as follows. Please write "See Supplement A" alongside product heading.

In the heading, change "**Tablets and Chewable Tablets**" *to* "**Tablets, Chewable Tablets, and Oral Granules**".

In the **DESCRIPTION** *section, fifth paragraph (beginning* "Each 10-mg film-coated..."), *before* "equivalent", *delete* "the molar", *and change* "10.0 mg of free acid" *to* "10 mg of montelukast".

Also in the **DESCRIPTION** *section, sixth paragraph, first sentence, following* "SINGULAIR tablet", *delete* "for oral administration" *and change* "the molar equivalents to 4.0 and 5.0 mg of free acid" *to* "equivalent to 4 and 5 mg of montelukast".

Also in the **DESCRIPTION** *section, at the end, add the following paragraph:*

Each packet of SINGULAIR 4-mg oral granules contains 4.2 mg montelukast sodium, which is equivalent to 4 mg of montelukast. The oral granule formulation contains the following inactive ingredients: mannitol, hydroxypropyl cellulose, and magnesium stearate.

In the **CLINICAL PHARMACOLOGY** *section, under Mechanism of Action, replace the first paragraph with the following:*

The cysteinyl leukotrienes (LTC_4, LTD_4, LTE_4) are products of arachidonic acid metabolism and are released from various cells, including mast cells and eosinophils. These eicosanoids bind to cysteinyl leukotriene (CysLT) receptors. The CysLT type-1 ($CysLT_1$) receptor is found in the human airway (including airway smooth muscle cells and airway macrophages) and on other pro-inflammatory cells (including eosinophils and certain myeloid stem cells). CysLTs have been correlated with the pathophysiology of asthma and allergic rhinitis. In asthma, leukotriene-mediated effects include airway edema, smooth muscle contraction, and altered cellular activity associated with the inflammatory process. In allergic rhinitis, CysLTs are released from the nasal mucosa after allergen exposure during both early- and late-phase reactions and are associated with symptoms of allergic rhinitis. Intranasal challenge with CysLTs has been shown to increase nasal airway resistance and symptoms of nasal obstruction. SINGULAIR has not been assessed in intranasal challenge studies. The clinical relevance of intranasal challenge studies is unknown.

Also in the **CLINICAL PHARMACOLOGY** *section, under Pharmacokinetics, Absorption, replace the fourth paragraph with the following two paragraphs:*

The 4-mg oral granule formulation is bioequivalent to the 4-mg chewable tablet when administered to adults in the fasted state. The coadministration of the oral granule formulation with applesauce did not have a clinically significant effect on the pharmacokinetics of montelukast. A high fat meal in the morning did not affect the AUC of montelukast oral granules, however, the meal decreased C_{max} by 35% and prolonged T_{max} from 2.3 ± 1.0 hours to 6.4 ± 2.9 hours.

The safety and efficacy of SINGULAIR in patients with asthma were demonstrated in clinical trials in which the 10-mg film-coated tablet and 5-mg chewable tablet formulations were administered in the evening without regard to the time of food ingestion. The safety of SINGULAIR in patients with asthma was also demonstrated in clinical trials in which the 4-mg chewable tablet and 4-mg oral granule formulations were administered in the evening without regard to the time of food ingestion. The safety and efficacy of SINGULAIR in patients with seasonal allergic rhinitis were demonstrated in clinical trials in which the 10-mg film-coated tablet was administered in the morning or evening without regard to the time of food ingestion.

Also in the **CLINICAL PHARMACOLOGY** *section, under Special Populations, replace the Adolescents and Pediatric Patients subsection with the following:*

Adolescents and Pediatric Patients: Pharmacokinetic studies evaluated the systemic exposure of the 4-mg oral granule formulation in pediatric patients 6 to 23 months of age, the 4-mg chewable tablets in pediatric patients 2 to 5 years of age, the 5-mg chewable tablets in pediatric patients 6 to 14 years of age, and the 10-mg film-coated tablets in young adults and adolescents ≥15 years of age.

The plasma concentration profile of montelukast following administration of the 10-mg film-coated tablets is similar in adolescents ≥15 years of age and young adults. The 10-mg film-coated tablet is recommended for use in patients ≥15 years of age.

The mean systemic exposure of the 4-mg chewable tablet in pediatric patients 2 to 5 years of age and the 5-mg chewable tablets in pediatric patients 6 to 14 years of age is similar to the mean systemic exposure of the 10-mg film-coated tablet in adults. The 5-mg chewable tablet should be used in pediatric patients 6 to 14 years of age and the 4-mg chewable tablet should be used in pediatric patients 2 to 5 years of age.

In children 6 to 11 months of age, the systemic exposure to montelukast and the variability of plasma montelukast concentrations were higher than those observed in adults. Based on population analyses, the mean AUC (4296 ng•hr/mL [range 1200 to 7153]) was 60% higher and the mean C_{max} (667 ng/mL [range 201 to 1058]) was 89% higher than those observed in adults (mean AUC 2689 ng•hr/mL [range 1521 to 4595]) and mean C_{max} [range 180 to 548]).

Continued on next page

Information on the Merck & Co., Inc., products listed on these pages is from the full prescribing information in use April 1, 2003.

Singulair—Cont.

The systemic exposure in children 12 to 23 months of age was less variable, but was still higher than that observed in adults. The mean AUC (3574 ng•hr/mL [range 2229 to 5408]) was 33% higher and the mean C_{max} (562 ng/mL [range 296 to 814]) was 60% higher than those observed in adults. Safety and tolerability of montelukast in a single-dose pharmacokinetic study in 26 children 6 to 23 months of age were similar to that of patients two years and above (see ADVERSE REACTIONS). The 4-mg oral granule formulation should be used for pediatric patients 12 to 23 months of age. Since the 4-mg oral granule formulation is bioequivalent to the 4-mg chewable tablet, it can also be used as an alternative formulation to the 4-mg chewable tablet in pediatric patients 2 to 5 years of age.

Also in the **CLINICAL PHARMACOLOGY** *section, under Drug Interactions, second bullet, change copy in first set of parentheses to* "(primarily a substrate of CYP 2C9, 3A4 and 1A2)"; *fourth bullet, change copy in parentheses to* "(a substrate of CYP 3A4)".

Also in the **CLINICAL PHARMACOLOGY** *section, under Pharmacodynamics, replace the second paragraph with the following:*
The effect of SINGULAIR on eosinophils in the peripheral blood was examined in clinical trials. In patients with asthma aged 2 years and older who received SINGULAIR, a decrease in mean peripheral blood eosinophil counts ranging from 9% to 15% was noted, compared with placebo, over the double-blind treatment periods. In patients with seasonal allergic rhinitis aged 15 years and older who received SINGULAIR, a mean increase of 0.2% in peripheral blood eosinophil counts was noted, compared with a mean increase of 12.5% in placebo-treated patients, over the double-blind treatment periods; this reflects a mean difference of 12.3% in favor of SINGULAIR. The relationship between these observations and the clinical benefits of montelukast noted in the clinical trials is not known (see CLINICAL PHARMACOLOGY, *Clinical Studies*).

Also in the **CLINICAL PHARMACOLOGY** *section, replace the Clinical Studies, GENERAL subsection with the following:*
Clinical Studies – Asthma and Seasonal Allergic Rhinitis
GENERAL
There have been no clinical trials in asthmatics to evaluate the relative efficacy of morning versus evening dosing. The pharmacokinetics of montelukast are similar whether dosed in the morning or evening. Efficacy has been demonstrated for asthma when montelukast was administered in the evening without regard to time of food ingestion. Efficacy was demonstrated for seasonal allergic rhinitis when montelukast was administered in the morning or the evening without regard to time of food ingestion.
Clinical Studies – Asthma
Also in the **CLINICAL PHARMACOLOGY** *section, at the end, add the following subsection:*
Clinical Studies – Seasonal Allergic Rhinitis
The efficacy of SINGULAIR tablets for the treatment of seasonal allergic rhinitis was investigated in 5 similarly designed, randomized, double-blind, parallel-group, placebo- and active-controlled (loratadine) trials conducted in North America. The 5 trials enrolled a total of 5029 patients, of whom 1799 were treated with SINGULAIR tablets. Patients were 15 to 82 years of age with a history of seasonal allergic rhinitis, a positive skin test to at least one relevant seasonal allergen, and active symptoms of seasonal allergic rhinitis at study entry.
The period of randomized treatment was 2 weeks in 4 trials and 4 weeks in one trial. The primary outcome variable was mean change from baseline in daytime nasal symptoms score (the average of individual scores of nasal congestion, rhinorrhea, nasal itching, sneezing) as assessed by patients on a 0-3 categorical scale.
Four of the five trials showed a significant reduction in daytime nasal symptoms scores with SINGULAIR 10 mg tablets compared with placebo. The efficacy results of one trial are shown below; the remaining three trials that demonstrated efficacy showed similar results. The mean changes from baseline in daytime nasal symptoms score in the treatment groups that received SINGULAIR tablets, loratadine and placebo are shown in Table 3.
[See table 3 below]

In the **INDICATIONS AND USAGE** *section, change "2 years" to "12 months" and add the following paragraph:*
SINGULAIR is indicated for the relief of symptoms of seasonal allergic rhinitis in adults and pediatric patients 2 years of age and older.
In the **PRECAUTIONS** *section, under Eosinophilic Conditions, first sentence, after "patients", add "with asthma".*
Also in the **PRECAUTIONS** *section, under Information for Patients, second bullet, change "oral tablets of SINGULAIR are" to "oral SINGULAIR is".*
Also in the **PRECAUTIONS** *section, under Carcinogenesis, Mutagenesis, Impairment of Fertility, first paragraph, change "120 times" to "90 times" and change "45 times" to "30 times".*
Also in the **PRECAUTIONS** *section, replace the Pediatric Use subsection with the following:*
Pediatric Use
Safety and efficacy of SINGULAIR have been established in adequate and well-controlled studies in pediatric patients with asthma 6 to 14 years of age. Safety and efficacy profiles in this age group are similar to those seen in adults. (See *Clinical Studies* and ADVERSE REACTIONS.)
The efficacy of SINGULAIR for the treatment of seasonal allergic rhinitis in pediatric patients 2 to 14 years of age is supported by extrapolation from the demonstrated efficacy in patients 15 years of age and older with seasonal allergic rhinitis as well as the assumption that the disease course, pathophysiology and the drug's effect are substantially similar among these populations.
The safety of SINGULAIR 4-mg chewable tablets in pediatric patients 2 to 5 years of age with asthma has been demonstrated by adequate and well-controlled data (see ADVERSE REACTIONS). Efficacy of SINGULAIR in this age group is extrapolated from the demonstrated efficacy in patients 6 years of age and older with asthma and is based on similar pharmacokinetic data, as well as the assumption that the disease course, pathophysiology and the drug's effect are substantially similar among these populations. Efficacy in this age group is supported by exploratory efficacy assessments from a large, well-controlled safety study conducted in patients 2 to 5 years of age.
The safety of SINGULAIR 4-mg oral granules in pediatric patients 12 to 23 months of age with asthma has been demonstrated in an analysis of 172 pediatric patients, 124 of whom were treated with SINGULAIR, in a 6-week, double-blind, placebo-controlled study (see ADVERSE REACTIONS). Efficacy of SINGULAIR in this age group is extrapolated from the demonstrated efficacy in patients 6 years of age and older with asthma based on similar mean systemic exposure (AUC), and that the disease course, pathophysiology and the drug's effect are substantially similar among these populations, supported by efficacy data from a safety trial in which efficacy was an exploratory assessment.
The safety of SINGULAIR 4-mg and 5-mg chewable tablets in pediatric patients aged 2 to 14 years with seasonal allergic rhinitis is supported by data from studies conducted in pediatric patients aged 2 to 14 years with asthma. A safety study in pediatric patients 2 to 14 years of age with seasonal allergic rhinitis demonstrated a similar safety profile (see ADVERSE REACTIONS).
The safety and effectiveness in pediatric patients below the age of 12 months have not been established. Long-term trials evaluating the effect of chronic administration of SINGULAIR on linear growth in pediatric patients have not been conducted.
In the **ADVERSE REACTIONS** *section, change the first subsection heading to "Adults and Adolescents 15 Years of Age and Older with Asthma".*
Also in the **ADVERSE REACTIONS** *section, in the second subsection heading Pediatric Patients 6 to 14 Years of Age, add "with Asthma".*
Also in the **ADVERSE REACTIONS** *section, under Pediatric Patients 6 to 14 Years of Age, first paragraph, first sentence, delete "also" and change "approximately 320" to "321". In the third sentence, delete "versus placebo" after "SINGULAIR".*
Also in the **ADVERSE REACTIONS** *section, in the subsection heading Pediatric Patients 2 to 5 Years of Age, add "with Asthma".*
Also in the **ADVERSE REACTIONS** *section, after the Pediatric Patients 2 to 5 Years of Age subsection, add the following three subsections:*

Pediatric Patients 12 to 23 Months of Age with Asthma
SINGULAIR has been evaluated for safety in 124 pediatric patients 12 to 23 months of age. The safety profile of SINGULAIR in a 6-week, double-blind, placebo-controlled clinical study was generally similar to the safety profile in adults and pediatric patients 2 to 14 years of age. SINGULAIR administered once daily at bedtime was generally well tolerated. In pediatric patients 12 to 23 months of age receiving SINGULAIR, the following events occurred with a frequency ≥2% and more frequently than in pediatric patients who received placebo, regardless of causality assessment: upper respiratory infection, wheezing; otitis media; pharyngitis, tonsillitis, cough; and rhinitis. The frequency of less common adverse events was comparable between SINGULAIR and placebo.
Adults and Adolescents 15 years of Age and Older with Seasonal Allergic Rhinitis
SINGULAIR has been evaluated for safety in 2199 adult and adolescent patients 15 years of age and older in clinical trials. SINGULAIR administered once daily in the morning or in the evening was generally well tolerated with a safety profile similar to that of placebo. In placebo-controlled clinical trials, the following event was reported with SINGULAIR with a frequency ≥1% and at an incidence greater than placebo, regardless of causality assessment: upper respiratory infection, 1.9% of patients receiving SINGULAIR vs. 1.5% of patients receiving placebo. In a 4-week, placebo-controlled clinical study, the safety profile was consistent with that observed in 2-week studies. The incidence of somnolence was similar to that of placebo in all studies.
Pediatric Patients 2 to 14 Years of Age with Seasonal Allergic Rhinitis
SINGULAIR has been evaluated in 280 pediatric patients 2 to 14 years of age in a 2-week, multicenter, double-blind, placebo-controlled, parallel-group, safety study. SINGULAIR administered once daily in the evening was generally well tolerated with a safety profile similar to that of placebo. In this study, the following events occurred with a frequency ≥2% and at an incidence greater than placebo, regardless of causality assessment: headache, otitis media, pharyngitis, and upper respiratory infection.
Also in the **ADVERSE REACTIONS** *section, under Post-Marketing Experience, first paragraph, first sentence, after "irritability," add "agitation, including aggressive behavior,"; after "pancreatitis;" add "arthralgia,"; after "bruising;" add "palpitations;". In the second paragraph, first sentence, after "patients" add "with asthma".*
In the **OVERDOSAGE** *section, first paragraph, change "340 times" to "250 times" and change "230 times" to "170 times".*
Replace the **DOSAGE AND ADMINISTRATION** *section with the following:*
General Information
SINGULAIR should be taken once daily. For asthma, the dose should be taken in the evening. For seasonal allergic rhinitis, the time of administration may be individualized to suit patient needs.
Patients with both asthma and seasonal allergic rhinitis should taken only one tablet daily in the evening.
Adults and Adolescents 15 Years of Age and Older with Asthma or Seasonal Allergic Rhinitis
The dosage for adults and adolescents 15 years of age and older is one 10-mg tablet daily.
Pediatric Patients 6 to 14 Years of Age with Asthma or Seasonal Allergic Rhinitis
The dosage for pediatric patients 6 to 14 years of age is one 5-mg chewable tablet daily. No dosage adjustment within this age group is necessary.
Pediatric Patients 2 to 5 Years of Age with Asthma or Seasonal Allergic Rhinitis
The dosage for pediatric patients 2 to 5 years of age is one 4-mg chewable tablet or one packet of 4-mg oral granules daily.
Pediatric Patients 12 to 23 Months of Age with Asthma
The dosage for pediatric patients 12 to 23 months of age is one packet of 4-mg oral granules daily to be taken in the evening. Safety and effectiveness in pediatric patients younger than 12 months of age have not been established.
Administration of SINGULAIR Oral Granules
SINGULAIR 4-mg oral granules can be administered either directly in the mouth, or mixed with a spoonful of cold or room temperature soft foods; based on stability studies, only applesauce, carrots, rice or ice cream should be used. The packet should not be opened until ready to use. After opening the packet, the full dose (with or without mixing with food) must be administered within 15 minutes. If mixed with food, SINGULAIR oral granules must not be stored for future use. Discard any unused portion. SINGULAIR oral granules are not intended to be dissolved in liquid for administration. However, liquids may be taken subsequent to administration. SINGULAIR oral granules can be administered without regard to the time of meals.
In the **HOW SUPPLIED** *section, add the following at the beginning:*
No. 3841—SINGULAIR Oral Granules, 4 mg, are white granules with 500 mg net weight, packed in a child-resistant foil packet. They are supplied as follows:
NDC 0006-3841-30 unit of use carton with 30 packets.
Also in the **HOW SUPPLIED** *section, under No. 3796, delete* "**NDC** 0006-0711-68...canister" *and* "**NDC** 0006-0711-74...canisters".
Also in the **HOW SUPPLIED** *section, replace the Storage subsection with the following:*

TABLE 3
Effects of SINGULAIR on Daytime Nasal Symptoms Score* in a Placebo- and Active-controlled Trial in Patients with Seasonal Allergic Rhinitis

Treatment Group (N)	Baseline Mean Score	Mean Change from Baseline	Difference Between Treatment and Placebo (95% CI) Least-Squares Mean
SINGULAIR 10 mg (344)	2.09	-0.39	-0.13‡ (-0.21, -0.06)
Placebo (351)	2.10	-0.26	N.A.
Active Control† (Loratadine 10 mg) (599)	2.06	-0.46	-0.24‡ (-0.31, -0.17)

*Average of individual scores of nasal congestion, rhinorrhea, nasal itching, sneezing as assessed by patients on a 0-3 categorical scale.
†The study was not designed for statistical comparison between SINGULAIR and the active control (loratadine).
‡Statistically different from placebo (p≤0.001).

Store SINGULAIR 4-mg oral granules, 4-mg chewable tablets, 5-mg chewable tablets and 10-mg film-coated tablets at 25°C (77°F), excursions permitted to 15-30°C (59-86°F) [see USP Controlled Room Temperature]. Protect from moisture and light. Store in original package.
Revisions based on 9088815, issued December 2002.
Replace the Patient Information with the following:
Patient Information
SINGULAIR® (SING-u-lair) Tablets, Chewable Tablets, and Oral Granules
Generic name: montelukast (mon-te-LOO-kast) sodium
Read this information before you start taking SINGULAIR®. Also, read the leaflet you get each time you refill SINGULAIR, since there may be new information in the leaflet since the last time you saw it. This leaflet does not take the place of talking with your doctor about your medical condition and/or your treatment.
What is SINGULAIR*?
- SINGULAIR is a medicine called a leukotriene receptor antagonist. It works by blocking substances in the body called leukotrienes. Blocking leukotrienes improves asthma and seasonal allergic rhinitis (also known as hay fever). SINGULAIR is not a steroid.

*Registered trademark of MERCK & CO., Inc.
SINGULAIR is prescribed for the treatment of asthma and seasonal allergic rhinitis:
1. **Asthma.**
   SINGULAIR should be used for the long-term management of asthma in adults and children ages 12 months and older.
   Do not take SINGULAIR for the immediate relief of an asthma attack. If you get an asthma attack, you should follow the instructions your doctor gave you for treating asthma attacks. (See the end of this leaflet for more information about asthma.)
2. **Seasonal Allergic Rhinitis.**
   SINGULAIR is used to help control the symptoms of seasonal allergic rhinitis (sneezing, stuffy nose, runny nose, itching of the nose) in adults and children ages 2 years and older. (See the end of this leaflet for more information about seasonal allergic rhinitis.)

Who should not take SINGULAIR?
Do not take SINGULAIR if you are allergic to SINGULAIR or any of its ingredients.
The active ingredient in SINGULAIR is montelukast sodium.
See the end of this leaflet for a list of all the ingredients in SINGULAIR.
What should I tell my doctor before I start taking SINGULAIR?
Tell your doctor about:
- **Pregnancy:** If you are pregnant or plan to become pregnant. SINGULAIR may not be right for you.
- **Breast-feeding:** If you are breast-feeding, SINGULAIR may be passed in your milk to your baby. You should consult your doctor before taking SINGULAIR if you are breast-feeding or intend to breast-feed.
- **Medical Problems or Allergies:** Talk about any medical problems or allergies you have now or had in the past.
- **Other Medicines:** Tell your doctor about all the medicines you take, including prescription and non-prescription medicines, and herbal supplements. Some medicines may affect how SINGULAIR works, or SINGULAIR may affect how your other medicines work.

How should I take SINGULAIR?
For adults or children 12 months and older with asthma:
- Take SINGULAIR once a day in the evening.
- Take SINGULAIR every day for as long as your doctor prescribes it, even if you have no asthma symptoms.
- You may take SINGULAIR with food or without food.
- If your asthma symptoms get worse, or if you need to increase the use of your inhaled rescue medicine for asthma attacks, call your doctor right away.
- **Do not take SINGULAIR for the immediate relief of an asthma attack.** If you get an asthma attack, you should follow the instructions your doctor gave you for treating asthma attacks.
- Always have your inhaled rescue medicine for asthma attacks with you.
- Do not stop taking or lower the dose of your other asthma medicines unless your doctor tells you to.
- If your doctor has prescribed a medicine for you to use before exercise, keep using that medicine unless your doctor tells you not to.

For adults and children 2 years of age and older with seasonal allergic rhinitis:
- Take SINGULAIR once a day, at about the same time each day.
- Take SINGULAIR every day for as long as your doctor prescribes it.
- You may take SINGULAIR with food or without food.

How should I give SINGULAIR oral granules to my child?
Do not open the packet until ready to use.
SINGULAIR 4-mg oral granules can be given either:
- directly in the mouth;

OR
- mixed with a spoonful of one of the following soft foods at cold or room temperature: applesauce, mashed carrots, rice, or ice cream. Be sure that the entire dose is mixed with the food and that the child is given the entire spoonful of the mixture right away (with 15 minutes).

IMPORTANT: Never store any oral granule/food mixture for use at a later time. Throw away any unused portion.
Do not put SINGULAIR oral granules in liquid drink. However, your child may drink liquids after swallowing the SINGULAIR oral granules.
What is the daily dose of SINGULAIR for asthma or seasonal allergic rhinitis?
For Asthma (Take in the evening):
- One 10-mg tablet for adults and adolescents 15 years of age and older,
- One 5-mg chewable tablet for children 6 to 14 years of age,
- One 4-mg chewable tablet or one packet of 4-mg oral granules for children 2 to 5 years of age, or
- One packet of 4-mg oral granules for children 12 to 23 months of age.

For Seasonal Allergic Rhinitis (Take at about the same time each day):
- One 10-mg tablet for adults and adolescents 15 years of age and older,
- One 5-mg chewable tablet for children 6 to 14 years of age, or
- One 4-mg chewable tablet or one packet of 4-mg oral granules for children 2 to 5 years of age.

What should I avoid while taking SINGULAIR?
If you have asthma and if your asthma is made worse by aspirin, continue to avoid aspirin or other medicines called non-steroidal anti-inflammatory drugs while taking SINGULAIR.
What are the possible side effects of SINGULAIR?
The side effects of SINGULAIR are usually mild, and generally did not cause patients to stop taking their medicine. The side effects in patients treated with SINGULAIR were similar in type and frequency to side effects in patients who were given a placebo (a pill containing no medicine).
The most common side effects with SINGULAIR include:
- stomach pain
- stomach or intestinal upset
- heartburn
- tiredness
- fever
- stuffy nose
- cough
- flu
- upper respiratory infection
- dizziness
- headache
- rash

Less common side effects that have happened with SINGULAIR include (listed alphabetically):
agitation including aggressive behavior, allergic reactions (including swelling of the face, lips, tongue, and/or throat, which may cause trouble breathing or swallowing), hives, and itching, bad/vivid dreams, increased bleeding tendency, bruising, diarrhea, hallucinations (seeing things that are not there), indigestion, inflammation of the pancreas, irritability, joint pain, muscle aches and muscle cramps, nausea, palpitations, restlessness, seizures (convulsions or fits), swelling, trouble sleeping, and vomiting.
Rarely, asthmatic patients taking SINGULAIR have experienced a condition that includes certain symptoms that do not go away or that get worse. These occur usually, but not always, in patients who were taking steroid pills by mouth for asthma and those steroids were being slowly lowered or stopped. Although SINGULAIR has not been shown to cause this condition, **you must tell your doctor right away if you get one or more of these symptoms:**
- a feeling of pins and needles or numbness of arms or legs
- a flu-like illness
- rash
- severe inflammation (pain and swelling) of the sinuses (sinusitis)

These are not all the possible side effects of SINGULAIR. For more information ask your doctor or pharmacist.
Talk to your doctor if you think you have side effects from taking SINGULAIR.
General Information about the safe and effective use of SINGULAIR
Medicines are sometimes prescribed for conditions that are not mentioned in patient information leaflets. Do not use SINGULAIR for a condition for which it was not prescribed. Do not give SINGULAIR to other people even if they have the same symptoms you have. It may harm them. **Keep SINGULAIR and all medicines out of the reach of children.**
Store SINGULAIR at 25°C (77°F). Protect from moisture and light. Store in original package.
This leaflet summarizes information about SINGULAIR. If you would like more information, talk to your doctor. You can ask your pharmacist or doctor for information about SINGULAIR that is written for health professionals.
What are the ingredients in SINGULAIR?
Active Ingredient: montelukast sodium
SINGULAIR chewable tablets contain aspartame, a source of phenylalanine.
Phenylketonurics: SINGULAIR 4-mg and 5-mg chewable tablets contain 0.674 and 0.842 mg phenylalanine, respectively.
Inactive ingredients:
- 4-mg oral granules: mannitol, hydroxypropyl cellulose, and magnesium stearate.
- 4-mg and 5-mg chewable tablets: mannitol, microcrystalline cellulose, hydroxypropyl cellulose, red ferric oxide, croscarmellose sodium, cherry flavor, aspartame, and magnesium stearate.
- 10-mg tablet: microcrystalline cellulose, lactose monohydrate, croscarmellose sodium, hydroxypropyl cellulose, magnesium stearate, hydroxypropyl methylcellulose, titanium dioxide, red ferric oxide, yellow ferric oxide, and carnauba wax.

What is asthma?
Asthma is a continuing (chronic) inflammation of the bronchial passageways which are the tubes that carry air from outside the body to the lungs.
Symptoms of asthma include:
- coughing
- wheezing
- chest tightness
- shortness of breath

What is seasonal allergic rhinitis?
- Seasonal allergic rhinitis, also known as hay fever, is an allergic response caused by pollens from trees, grasses and weeds.
- Symptoms of seasonal allergic rhinitis may include:
  - stuffy, runny, and/or itchy nose
  - sneezing

Rx Only
9094214 Issued December 2002
COPYRIGHT © MERCK & CO., Inc., 1998, 2001, 2002
All rights reserved.

STROMECTOL® TABLETS ℞
[*strō'mĕk-tōl*]
(ivermectin)

Prescribing information for this product, which appears on pages 2090–2092 of the 2003 PDR, has been revised as follows. Please write "See Supplement A" alongside product heading.
In the **PRECAUTIONS** *section, under General, second paragraph, add the following after the first sentence:*
In these patients, the following adverse experiences have also been reported: back pain, conjunctival hemorrhage, dyspnea, urinary and/or fecal incontinence, difficulty in standing, mental status changes, confusion, lethargy, stupor, or coma.
Revision based on 9032304, issued July 2002.

VAQTA® ℞
[*văk'ta*]
(Hepatitis A Vaccine, Inactivated)

Prescribing information for this product, which appears on pages 2105–2108 of the 2003 PDR, has been revised as follows. Please write "See Supplement A" alongside product heading.
In the **DESCRIPTION** *section, first paragraph, third sentence, change* "aluminum hydroxide" *to* "amorphous aluminum hydroxyphosphate sulfate".
Also in the **DESCRIPTION** *section under both* **Pediatric/Adolescent Formulation:** *and* **Adult Formulation:**, *change* "aluminum hydroxide" *to* "amorphous aluminum hydroxyphosphate sulfate".
In the **CLINICAL PHARMACOLOGY** *section, after the Clinical Trials subsection, add the following subsection:*
Post-marketing Safety Study
In a post-marketing short-term safety surveillance study, conducted at a large health maintenance organization in the United States, a total of 42,110 individuals ≥2 years of age received 1 or 2 doses of VAQTA (13,735 children/adolescent and 28,375 adult subjects). Safety was passively monitored by electronic search of the automated medical records database for emergency room and outpatient visits, hospitalizations, and deaths. Medical charts were reviewed when indicated. There was no serious, vaccine-related, adverse event identified among the 42,110 vaccine recipients in this study. Diarrhea/gastroenteritis, resulting in outpatient visits, was determined by the investigator to be the only vaccine-related nonserious adverse event in the study. There was no vaccine-related, adverse event identified that had not been reported in earlier clinical trials with VAQTA. (See ADVERSE REACTIONS, *Post-marketing Safety Study*.)
Also in the **CLINICAL PHARMACOLOGY** *section, replace Table 1 and footnotes with the following:*
[See table 1 at top of next page]
Also in the **CLINICAL PHARMACOLOGY** *section, in the Persistence subsection, third paragraph, first sentence, change* "12" months *to* "18" months. *In the second sentence, change* "or 12" *to* "to 18" months.
Also in the **CLINICAL PHARMACOLOGY** *section, replace Table 2, Table 3, and the two paragraphs following Table 3 (beginning* "In separate studies…"*) with the following:*
[See table 2 on next page]
[See table 3 on next page]
In a clinical study involving healthy children and adolescents who received two doses (~25U) of VAQTA, detectable levels of anti-HAV antibodies (≥10mIU/mL) were present in 100% of subjects for up to 6 years postvaccination. In subjects who received VAQTA at 0 and 6 months, the GMT was

Continued on next page

Information on the Merck & Co., Inc., products listed on these pages is from the full prescribing information in use April 1, 2003.

Table 1
Seroconversion Rates (%) and Geometric Mean Titers (GMT) after Vaccination with
VAQTA plus IG, VAQTA Alone, and IG Alone

Weeks	VAQTA plus IG	VAQTA	IG
		Seroconversion Rate GMT (mIU/mL)	
4	100% 42 (n=129)	96% 38 (n=135)	87% 19 (n=30)
24	92% 83 (n=125)	97%* 137* (n=132)	0% Undetectable† (n=28)
28	100% 4872 (n=114)	100% 6498 (n=128)	N/A

† Undetectable is defined as <10mIU/mL.
*The seroconversion rate and the GMT in the group receiving VAQTA alone were significantly higher than in the group receiving VAQTA plus IG (p=0.05, p<0.001, respectively).
N/A = Not Applicable

Table 2
Children/Adolescents
Seroconversion Rates (%) and Geometric Mean Titers (GMT) for Cohorts of Initially Seronegative Vaccinees at the Time of the Booster (~25U) and 4 Weeks Later

Months Following Initial ~25U Dose	Cohort* (n=960) 0 and 6 Months	Cohort* (n=35) 0 and 12 Months	Cohort* (n=39) 0 and 18 Months
	Seroconversion Rate GMT (mIU/mL) (95% CI)		
6	97% 107 (98, 117)	—	—
7	100% 10433 (9681, 11243)	—	—
12	—	91% 48 (33, 71)	—
13	—	100% 12308 (9337, 16226)	—
18	—	—	90% 50 (28, 89)
19	—	—	100% 9591 (7613, 12082)

*Blood samples were taken at prebooster and postbooster time points.

Table 3
Adults
Seroconversion Rates (%) and Geometric Mean Titers (GMT) for a Cohort of Vaccinees at the Time of the Booster (~50U) and 4 Weeks Later

Months Following Initial ~50U Dose	Cohort* (n=1201) 0 and 6 Months	Cohort* (n=91) 0 and 12 Months	Cohort* (n=84) 0 and 18 Months
	Seroconversion Rate GMT (mIU/mL) (95% CI)		
6	98% 139 (129, 149)	—	—
7	100% 5987 (5561, 6445)	—	—
12	—	93% 107 (78, 146)	—
13	—	98% 4896 (3589, 6679)	—
18	—	—	96% 120 (88, 164)
19	—	—	100% 6043 (4687, 7793)

*Blood samples were taken at prebooster and postbooster time points.

Vaqta—Cont.

819 mIU/mL (n=175) at 2.5 to 3.5 years and 505 mIU/mL (n=174) at 5 to 6 years postvaccination. In subjects who received VAQTA at 0 and 12 months, the GMT was 2224 mIU/mL (n=49) at 2.5 to 3.5 years and 1191 mIU/mL (n=47) at 5 to 6 years postvaccination. In subjects who received VAQTA at 0 and 18 months, the GMT was 2501 mIU/mL (n=53) at 2.5 to 3.5 years and 1500 mIU/mL (n=53) at 5 to 6 years postvaccination.

In studies of healthy adults who received two doses (~50U) of VAQTA at 0 and 6 months, the hepatitis A antibody response to date has been shown to persist up to 6 years. Detectable levels of anti-HAV antibodies (≥10 mIU/mL) were present in 100% (378/378) of subjects with a GMT of 1734 mIU/mL at 1 year, 99.2% (252/254) of subjects with a GMT of 687 mIU/mL at 2 to 3 years, 99.1% (219/221) of subjects with a GMT of 605 mIU/mL at 4 years, and 99.4% (170/171) of subjects with a GMT of 684 mIU/mL at 6 years postvaccination.

In the **PRECAUTIONS** section, under *Geriatric Use*, add the following after the second sentence:
In a large post-marketing safety study in 42,110 individuals, ≥2 years of age, 4769 were 65 years of age or older, 1073 of whom were 75 years of age or older. There were no adverse experiences judged by the investigator to be vaccine related in the geriatric study population.

In the **ADVERSE REACTIONS** section, add the following as the first sentence and first subsection heading:
VAQTA is generally well tolerated; adverse reactions usually are mild and transient.
Clinical Studies

Also in the **ADVERSE REACTIONS** section, in the Children/Adolescents — 2 through 18 Years of Age subsection, under LOCALIZED INJECTION-SITE REACTIONS, delete "(generally mild and transient)".

Also in the **ADVERSE REACTIONS** section, in the Adults — 19 Years of Age and Older subsection, under LOCALIZED INJECTION-SITE REACTIONS, delete "(generally mild and transient)".

Also in the **ADVERSE REACTIONS** section, at the end, add the following subsection:
Post-marketing Safety Study
In a post-marketing safety study, a total of 42,110 people ≥2 years of age received 1 or 2 doses of VAQTA. There was no serious, vaccine-related adverse event identified among the 42,110 vaccine recipients in this study. There was no vaccine-related, adverse event identified that had not been reported in earlier clinical trials with VAQTA. Diarrhea/gastroenteritis, resulting in outpatient visits (in adults), was determined by the investigator to be the only vaccine-related nonserious adverse event in the study. VAQTA was generally well tolerated in this study. (See CLINICAL PHARMACOLOGY, *Post-marketing Safety Study*.)
In the **DOSAGE AND ADMINISTRATION** section, under DOSAGE, Adult, in the first sentence, change "12" months to "18" months and add the following as the second paragraph:
For all age groups, a booster dose is recommended anytime between 6 and 18 months after the administration of the primary dose in order to elicit a high antibody titer.
In the **HOW SUPPLIED** section, under ADULT FORMULATION, Vials, at the end, add the following:
No. 4841 — VAQTA for adult use is supplied as 50U/1 mL of hepatitis A virus protein in a 1 mL single-dose vial, in a box of 10 single-dose vials, **NDC** 0006-4841-41.
At the very end, under "Manuf. And Dist. by:", after "**MERCK & CO., INC.**," change "West Point, PA 19486" to "Whitehouse Station, NJ 08889" and change "Medeva Pharma" to "Evans Vaccines" Ltd.
Revisions based on 9413403, issued December 2002.

VIOXX® ℞
[vī-ŏks]
(rofecoxib tablets and oral suspension)

Prescribing information for this product, which appears on pages 2120–2125 of the 2003 PDR, has been revised as follows. Please write "See Supplement A" alongside product heading.
In the Patient Information, under "**What are the possible side effects of VIOXX?**", *in the paragraph beginning* "In addition, the following side effects . . .", *after* "blurred vision," *add* "colitis," *and after* "low blood cell counts," *add* "menstrual disorder,".
Revision based on 9183907, issued September 2002.

Novartis Pharmaceuticals Corporation

NOVARTIS PHARMACEUTICALS CORPORATION
One Health Plaza
East Hanover, NJ 07936
(for branded products)

For Information Contact *(branded products)*:

Customer Response Department
(888) NOW-NOVARTIS [888-669-6682]

Global Internet Address:
http://www.novartis.com

ELIDEL® ℞
[ĕl-ĭ-dĕl]
(pimecrolimus) Cream 1%
FOR DERMATOLOGIC USE ONLY
NOT FOR OPHTHALMIC USE
Rx only
Prescribing Information

Prescribing information for this product, which appears on pages 2257–2260 of the 2003 PDR, has been completely revised as follows. Please write "See Supplement A" next to the product heading.

DESCRIPTION
Elidel® (pimecrolimus) Cream 1% contains the compound pimecrolimus, the 33-epi-chloro-derivative of the macrolactam ascomycin.
Chemically, pimecrolimus is (1R,9S,12S,13R,14S,17R,18E,21S,23S,24R,25S,27R)-12-[(1E)-2-[(1R,3R,4S)-4-chloro-3-methoxycyclohexyl]-1-methylvinyl]-17-ethyl-1,14-dihydroxy-23,25-dimethoxy-13,19,21,27-tetramethyl-11,28-dioxa-4-aza-tricyclo[22.3.1.0^{4,9}]octacos-18-ene-2,3,10,16-tetraone.
The compound has the empirical formula $C_{43}H_{68}ClNO_{11}$ and the molecular weight of 810.47. The structural formula is [See chemical structure at top of next column]
Pimecrolimus is a white to off-white fine crystalline powder. It is soluble in methanol and ethanol and insoluble in water.
Each gram of Elidel Cream 1% contains 10 mg of pimecrolimus in a whitish cream base of benzyl alcohol, cetyl alcohol, citric acid, mono- and di-glycerides, oleyl alcohol, propylene glycol, sodium cetostearyl sulphate, sodium hydroxide, stearyl alcohol, triglycerides, and water.

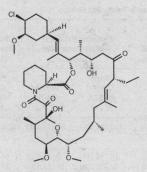

CLINICAL PHARMACOLOGY
Mechanism of Action/Pharmacodynamics
The mechanism of action of pimecrolimus in atopic dermatitis is not known. While the following have been observed, the clinical significance of these observations in atopic dermatitis is not known. It has been demonstrated that pimecrolimus binds with high affinity to macrophilin-12 (FKBP-12) and inhibits the calcium-dependent phosphatase, calcineurin. As a consequence, it inhibits T cell activation by blocking the transcription of early cytokines. In particular, pimecrolimus inhibits at nanomolar concentrations Interleukin-2 and interferon gamma (Th1-type) and Interleukin-4 and Interleukin-10 (Th2-type) cytokine synthesis in human T cells. In addition, pimecrolimus prevents the release of inflammatory cytokines and mediators from mast cells *in vitro* after stimulation by antigen/IgE.

Pharmacokinetics
Absorption
In adult patients being treated for atopic dermatitis [13%-62% Body Surface Area (BSA) involvement] for periods up to a year, blood concentrations of pimecrolimus are routinely either at or below the limit of quantification of the assay (< 0.5 ng/mL). In those subjects with detectable blood levels they are routinely < 2 ng/mL and show no sign of drug accumulation with time. Because of the low systemic absorption of pimecrolimus following topical application the calculation of standard pharmacokinetic measures such as AUC, C_{max}, $T_{1/2}$, et cetera cannot be reliably done.

Distribution
In vitro studies of the protein binding of pimecrolimus indicate that it is 74%-87% bound to plasma proteins.

Metabolism
Following the administration of a single oral radiolabeled dose of pimecrolimus numerous circulating O-demethylation metabolites were seen. Studies with human liver microsomes indicate that pimecrolimus is metabolized *in vitro* by the CYP3A sub-family of metabolizing enzymes. No evidence of skin mediated drug metabolism was identified *in vivo* using the minipig or *in vitro* using stripped human skin.

Elimination
Based on the results of the aforementioned radiolabeled study, following a single oral dose of pimecrolimus ~81% of the administered radioactivity was recovered, primarily in the feces (78.4%) as metabolites. Less than 1% of the radioactivity found in the feces was due to unchanged pimecrolimus.

Special Populations
Pediatrics
The systemic exposure to pimecrolimus from Elidel® (pimecrolimus) Cream 1% was investigated in 26 pediatric patients with atopic dermatitis (20%-69% BSA involvement) between the ages of 2-14 yrs. Following twice daily application for three weeks, blood concentrations of pimecrolimus were consistently low (< 3 ng/mL), with the majority of the blood samples being below the limit of quantification (0.5 ng/mL). However, the children (20 children out of the total 23 children investigated) had at least one detectable blood level as compared to the adults (13 adults out of the total 25 adults investigated) over a 3-week treatment period. Due to the low and erratic nature of the blood levels observed, no correlation could be made between amount of cream, degree of BSA involvement, and blood concentrations. In general, the blood concentrations measured in adult atopic dermatitis patients were comparable to those seen in the pediatric population.

In a second group of 22 pediatric patients aged 3-23 months with 10%-92% BSA involvement, a higher proportion of detectable blood levels was seen ranging from 0.1 ng/mL to 2.6 ng/mL (limit of quantification 0.1 ng/mL). This increase in the absolute number of positive blood levels may be due to the larger surface area to body mass ratio seen in these younger subjects. In addition, a higher incidence of upper respiratory symptoms/infections was also seen relative to the older age group in the PK studies. At this time a causal relationship between these findings and Elidel use cannot be ruled out. Use of Elidel in this population is not recommended *(see Pediatric Use)*.

Renal Insufficiency
The effect of renal insufficiency on the pharmacokinetics of topically administered pimecrolimus has not been evaluated. Given the very low systemic exposure of pimecrolimus via the topical route, no change in dosing is required.

Hepatic Insufficiency
The effect of hepatic insufficiency on the pharmacokinetics of topically administered pimecrolimus has not been evaluated. Given the very low systemic exposure of pimecrolimus via the topical route, no change in dosing is required.

CLINICAL STUDIES
Three randomized, double-blind, vehicle-controlled, multi-center, Phase 3 studies were conducted in 1335 pediatric patients ages 3 months-17 years old to evaluate Elidel® (pimecrolimus) Cream 1% for the treatment of mild to moderate atopic dermatitis. Two of the three trials support the use of Elidel Cream in patients 2 years and older with mild to moderate atopic dermatitis *(see Pediatric Use)*. Three other trials provided additional data regarding the safety of Elidel Cream in the treatment of atopic dermatitis. Two of these other trials were vehicle-controlled with optional sequential use of a medium potency topical corticosteroid in pediatric patients and one trial was an active comparator trial in adult patients with atopic dermatitis *(see Pediatric Use and ADVERSE REACTIONS)*.

Two identical 6-week, randomized, vehicle-controlled, multi-center, Phase 3 trials were conducted to evaluate Elidel Cream for the treatment of mild to moderate atopic dermatitis. A total of 403 pediatric patients 2-17 years old were included in the studies. The male/female ratio was approximately 50% and 29% of the patients were African American. At study entry, 59% of patients had moderate disease and the mean body surface area (BSA) affected was 26%. About 75% of patients had atopic dermatitis affecting the face and/or neck region. In these studies, patients applied either Elidel Cream or vehicle cream twice daily to 5% to 96% of their BSA for up to 6 weeks. At endpoint, based on the physician's global evaluation of clinical response, 35% of patients treated with Elidel Cream were clear or almost clear of signs of atopic dermatitis compared to only 18% of vehicle-treated patients. More Elidel patients (57%) had mild or no pruritus at 6 weeks compared to vehicle patients (34%). The improvement in pruritus occurred in conjunction with the improvement of the patients' atopic dermatitis.

In these two 6-week studies of Elidel, the combined efficacy results at endpoint are as follows:

	% Patients	
	Elidel® (N=267)	Vehicle (N=136)
Global Assessment		
Clear	28 (10%)	5 (4%)
Clear or Almost Clear	93 (35%)	25 (18%)
Clear to Mild Disease	180 (67%)	55 (40%)

In the two pediatric studies that independently support the use of Elidel Cream in mild to moderate atopic dermatitis, a significant treatment effect was seen by day 15. Of the key signs of atopic dermatitis, erythema, infiltration/papulation, lichenification, and excoriations, erythema and infiltration/papulation were reduced at day 8 when compared to vehicle.

The following graph depicts the time course of improvement in the percent body surface area affected as a result of treatment with Elidel Cream in 2-17 year olds.

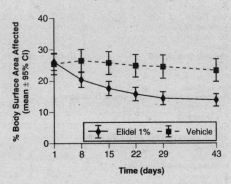

Figure 1
Body Surface Area Over Time

The following graph shows the time course of improvement in erythema as a result of treatment with Elidel Cream in 2-17 year olds.
[See figure 2 at top of next column]

INDICATIONS AND USAGE
Elidel® (pimecrolimus) Cream 1% is indicated for short-term and intermittent long-term therapy in the treatment of *mild to moderate* atopic dermatitis in non-immunocompromised patients 2 years of age and older, in whom the use of alternative, conventional therapies is deemed inadvisable because of potential risks, or in the treatment of patients who are not adequately responsive to or intolerant of alternative, conventional therapies *(see DOSAGE AND ADMINISTRATION)*.

CONTRAINDICATIONS
Elidel® (pimecrolimus) Cream 1% is contraindicated in individuals with a history of hypersensitivity to pimecrolimus or any of the components of the cream.

PRECAUTIONS
General
Elidel® (pimecrolimus) Cream 1% should not be applied to areas of active cutaneous viral infections.

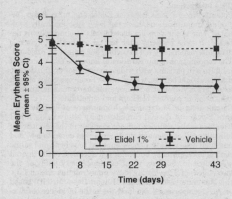

Figure 2
Mean Erythema Over Time

Studies have not evaluated the safety and efficacy of Elidel Cream in the treatment of clinically infected atopic dermatitis. Before commencing treatment with Elidel Cream, clinical infections at treatment sites should be cleared.

While patients with atopic dermatitis are predisposed to superficial skin infections including eczema herpeticum (Kaposi's varicelliform eruption), treatment with Elidel Cream may be associated with an increased risk of varicella zoster virus infection (chicken pox or shingles), herpes simplex virus infection, or eczema herpeticum. In the presence of these skin infections, the balance of risks and benefits associated with Elidel Cream use should be evaluated.

In clinical studies, 14 cases of lymphadenopathy (0.9%) were reported while using Elidel Cream. These cases of lymphadenopathy were usually related to infections and noted to resolve upon appropriate antibiotic therapy. Of these 14 cases, the majority had either a clear etiology or were known to resolve. Patients who receive Elidel Cream and who develop lymphadenopathy should have the etiology of their lymphadenopathy investigated. In the absence of a clear etiology for the lymphadenopathy, or in the presence of acute infectious mononucleosis, discontinuation of Elidel Cream should be considered. Patients who develop lymphadenopathy should be monitored to ensure that the lymphadenopathy resolves.

In clinical studies, 15 cases of skin papilloma or warts (1%) were observed in patients using Elidel Cream. The youngest patient was age 2 and the oldest was age 12. In cases where there is worsening of skin papillomas or they do not respond to conventional therapy, discontinuation of Elidel Cream should be considered until complete resolution of the warts is achieved.

The enhancement of ultraviolet carcinogenicity is not necessarily dependent on phototoxic mechanisms. Despite the absence of observed phototoxicity in humans *(see ADVERSE REACTIONS)*, Elidel Cream shortened the time to skin tumor formation in an animal photo-carcinogenicity study *(see Carcinogenesis, Mutagenesis, Impairment of Fertility)*. Therefore, it is prudent for patients to minimize or avoid natural or artificial sunlight exposure.

The use of Elidel Cream in patients with Netherton's Syndrome is not recommended due to the potential for increased systemic absorption of pimecrolimus.

There are no data to support use of Elidel in immunocompromised patients.

The use of Elidel Cream may cause local symptoms such as skin burning. Localized symptoms are most common during the first few days of Elidel Cream application and typically improve as the lesions of atopic dermatitis resolve. Most application site reactions lasted no more than 5 days, were mild to moderate in severity, and started within 1-5 days of treatment. *(See ADVERSE REACTIONS.)*

Information for Patients
Patients using Elidel should receive the following information and instructions:
- Patients should use Elidel Cream as directed by the physician. Elidel Cream is for external use on the skin only. As with any topical medication, patients or caregivers should wash hands after application if hands are not an area for treatment.
- Patients should minimize or avoid exposure to natural or artificial sunlight (tanning beds or UVA/B treatment) while using Elidel Cream.
- Patients should not use this medication for any disorder other than that for which it was prescribed.
- Patients should report any signs or symptoms of adverse reactions to their physician.
- Therapy should be discontinued after signs and symptoms of atopic dermatitis have resolved. Treatment with Elidel should be resumed at the first signs or symptoms of recurrence.
- Use of Elidel may cause reactions at the site of application such as a mild to moderate feeling of warmth and/or sensation of burning. Patients should see a physician if an application site reaction is severe or persists for more than 1 week.
- The patient should contact the physician if no improvement in the atopic dermatitis is seen following 6 weeks of treatment, or if at any time the condition worsens.

Continued on next page

Elidel—Cont.

Drug Interactions
Potential interactions between Elidel and other drugs, including immunizations, have not been systematically evaluated. Due to the very low blood levels of pimecrolimus detected in some patients after topical application, systemic drug interactions are not expected, but cannot be ruled out. The concomitant administration of known CYP3A family of inhibitors in patients with widespread and/or erythrodermic disease should be done with caution. Some examples of such drugs are erythromycin, itraconazole, ketoconazole, fluconazole, calcium channel blockers and cimetidine.

Carcinogenesis, Mutagenesis, Impairment of Fertility
In a 2-year rat dermal carcinogenicity study using Elidel Cream, a statistically significant increase in the incidence of follicular cell adenoma of the thyroid was noted in low, mid and high dose male animals compared to vehicle and saline control male animals. Follicular cell adenoma of the thyroid was noted in the dermal rat carcinogenicity study at the lowest dose of 2 mg/kg/day [0.2% pimecrolimus cream; 1.5× the Maximum Recommended Human Dose (MRHD) based on AUC comparisons]. No increase in the incidence of follicular cell adenoma of the thyroid was noted in the oral carcinogenicity study in male rats up to 10 mg/kg/day (66× MRHD based on AUC comparisons). However, oral studies may not reflect continuous exposure or the same metabolic profile as by the dermal route. In a mouse dermal carcinogenicity study using pimecrolimus in an ethanolic solution, no increase in incidence of neoplasms was observed in the skin or other organs up to the highest dose of 4 mg/kg/day (0.32% pimecrolimus in ethanol) 27× MRHD based on AUC comparisons. However, lymphoproliferative changes (including lymphoma) were noted in a 13 week repeat dose dermal toxicity study conducted in mice using pimecrolimus in an ethanolic solution at a dose of 25 mg/kg/day (47× MRHD based on AUC comparisons). No lymphoproliferative changes were noted in this study at a dose of 10 mg/kg/day (17× MRHD based on AUC comparison). However, the latency time to lymphoma formation was shortened to 8 weeks after dermal administration of pimecrolimus dissolved in ethanol at a dose of 100 mg/kg/day (179-217× MRHD based on AUC comparisons).

In a mouse oral (gavage) carcinogenicity study, a statistically significant increase in the incidence of lymphoma was noted in high dose male and female animals compared to vehicle control male and female animals. Lymphomas were noted in the oral mouse carcinogenicity study at a dose of 45 mg/kg/day (258-340× MRHD based on AUC comparisons). No drug-related tumors were noted in the mouse oral carcinogenicity study at a dose of 15 mg/kg/day (60-133× MRHD based on AUC comparisons). In an oral (gavage) rat carcinogenicity study, a statistically significant increase in the incidence of benign thymoma was noted in 10 mg/kg/day pimecrolimus treated male and female animals compared to vehicle control treated male and female animals. In addition, a significant increase in the incidence of benign thymoma was noted in another oral (gavage) rat carcinogenicity study in 5 mg/kg/day pimecrolimus treated male animals compared to vehicle control treated male animals. No drug-related tumors were noted in the rat oral carcinogenicity study at a dose of 1 mg/kg/day male animals (1.1× MRHD based on AUC comparisons) and at a dose of 5 mg/kg/day for female animals (21× MRHD based on AUC comparisons).

In a 52-week dermal photo-carcinogenicity study, the median time to onset of skin tumor formation was decreased in hairless mice following chronic topical dosing with concurrent exposure to UV radiation (40 weeks of treatment followed by 12 weeks of observation) with the Elidel Cream vehicle alone. No additional effect on tumor development beyond the vehicle effect was noted with the addition of the active ingredient, pimecrolimus, to the vehicle cream.

A battery of in vitro genotoxicity tests, including Ames assay, mouse lymphoma L5178Y assay, and chromosome aberration test in V79 Chinese hamster cells and an in vivo mouse micronucleus test revealed no evidence for a mutagenic or clastogenic potential for the drug.

An oral fertility and embryofetal developmental study in rats revealed estrus cycle disturbances, post-implantation loss and reduction in litter size at the 45 mg/kg/day dose (38× MRHD based on AUC comparisons). No effect on fertility in female rats was noted at 10 mg/kg/day (12× MRHD based on AUC comparisons). No effect on fertility in male rats was noted at 45 mg/kg/day (23× MRHD based on AUC comparisons), which was the highest dose tested in this study.

Pregnancy
Teratogenic Effects: Pregnancy Category C
There are no adequate and well-controlled studies of topically administered pimecrolimus in pregnant women. The experience with Elidel Cream when used by pregnant women is too limited to permit assessment of the safety of its use during pregnancy.

In dermal embryofetal developmental studies, no maternal or fetal toxicity was observed up to the highest practicable doses tested, 10 mg/kg/day (1% pimecrolimus cream) in rats (0.14× MRHD based on body surface area) and 10 mg/kg/day (1% pimecrolimus cream) in rabbits (0.65× MRHD based on AUC comparisons). The 1% pimecrolimus cream was administered topically for 6 hours/day during the period of organogenesis in rats and rabbits (gestational days 6-21 in rats and gestational days 6-20 in rabbits).

A combined oral fertility and embryofetal developmental study was conducted in rats and an oral embryofetal developmental study was conducted in rabbits. Pimecrolimus was administered during the period of organogenesis (2 weeks prior to mating until gestational day 16 in rats, gestational days 6-18 in rabbits) up to dose levels of 45 mg/kg/day in rats and 20 mg/kg/day in rabbits. In the absence of maternal toxicity, indicators of embryofetal toxicity (post-implantation loss and reduction in litter size) were noted at 45 mg/kg/day (38× MRHD based on AUC comparisons) in the oral fertility and embryofetal developmental study conducted in rats. No malformations in the fetuses were noted at 45 mg/kg/day (38× MRHD based on AUC comparisons) in this study. No maternal toxicity, embryotoxicity or teratogenicity were noted in the oral rabbit embryofetal developmental toxicity study at 20 mg/kg/day (3.9× MRHD based on AUC comparisons), which was the highest dose tested in this study.

An oral peri- and post-natal developmental study was conducted in rats. Pimecrolimus was administered from gestational day 6 through lactational day 21 up to a dose level of 40 mg/kg/day. Only 2 of 22 females delivered live pups at the highest dose of 40 mg/kg/day. Postnatal survival, development of the F1 generation, their subsequent maturation and fertility were not affected at 10 mg/kg/day (12× MRHD based on AUC comparisons), the highest dose evaluated in this study.

Treatment Emergent Adverse Events (≥ 1%) in Elidel® Treatment Groups

	Pediatric Patients* Vehicle-Controlled (6 weeks)		Pediatric Patients* Open-Label (20 weeks)	Pediatric Patients* Vehicle-Controlled (1 year)		Adult Active Comparator (1 year)
	Elidel® Cream (N=267) N (%)	Vehicle (N=136) N (%)	Elidel® Cream (N=335) N (%)	Elidel® Cream (N=272) N (%)	Vehicle (N=75) N (%)	Elidel® Cream (N=328) N (%)
At least 1 AE	182 (68.2%)	97 (71.3%)	240 (72.0%)	230 (84.6%)	56 (74.7%)	256 (78.0%)
Infections and Infestations						
Upper Respiratory Tract Infection NOS	38 (14.2%)	18 (13.2%)	65 (19.4%)	13 (4.8%)	6 (8.0%)	14 (4.3%)
Nasopharyngitis	27 (10.1%)	10 (7.4%)	32 (19.6%)	72 (26.5%)	16 (21.3%)	25 (7.6%)
Skin Infection NOS	8 (3.0%)	9 (5.1%)	18 (5.4%)	6 (2.2%)	3 (4.0%)	21 (6.4%)
Influenza	8 (3.0%)	1 (0.7%)	22 (6.6%)	36 (13.2%)	3 (4.0%)	32 (9.8%)
Ear Infection NOS	6 (2.2%)	2 (1.5%)	19 (5.7%)	9 (3.3%)	1 (1.3%)	2 (0.6%)
Otitis Media	6 (2.2%)	1 (0.7%)	10 (3.0%)	8 (2.9%)	4 (5.3%)	2 (0.6%)
Impetigo	5 (1.9%)	3 (2.2%)	12 (3.6%)	11 (4.0%)	4 (5.3%)	8 (2.4%)
Bacterial Infection	4 (1.5%)	3 (2.2%)	4 (1.2%)	3 (1.1%)	0	6 (1.8%)
Folliculitis	3 (1.1%)	1 (0.7%)	3 (0.9%)	6 (2.2%)	3 (4.0%)	20 (6.1%)
Sinusitis	3 (1.1%)	1 (0.7%)	11 (3.3%)	6 (2.2%)	1 (1.3%)	2 (0.6%)
Pneumonia NOS	3 (1.1%)	1 (0.7%)	5 (1.5%)	0	1 (1.3%)	1 (0.3%)
Pharyngitis NOS	2 (0.7%)	2 (1.5%)	3 (0.9%)	22 (8.1%)	2 (2.7%)	3 (0.9%)
Pharyngitis Streptococcal	2 (0.7%)	2 (1.5%)	10 (3.0%)	0	<1%	0
Molluscum Contagiosum	2 (0.7%)	0	4 (1.2%)	5 (1.8%)	0	0
Staphylococcal Infection	1 (0.4%)	5 (3.7%)	7 (2.1%)	0	<1%	3 (0.9%)
Bronchitis NOS	1 (0.4%)	3 (2.2%)	4 (1.2%)	29 (10.7%)	6 (8.0%)	8 (2.4%)
Herpes Simplex	1 (0.4%)	0	4 (1.2%)	9 (3.3%)	2 (2.7%)	13 (4.0%)
Tonsillitis NOS	1 (0.4%)	0	3 (0.9%)	17 (6.3%)	0	2 (0.6%)
Viral Infection NOS	2 (0.7%)	1 (0.7%)	1 (0.3%)	18 (6.6%)	1 (1.3%)	0
Gastroenteritis NOS	0	3 (2.2%)	2 (0.6%)	20 (7.4%)	2 (2.7%)	6 (1.8%)
Chickenpox	2 (0.7%)	0	3 (0.9%)	8 (2.9%)	3 (4.0%)	1 (0.3%)
Skin Papilloma	1 (0.4%)	0	2 (0.6%)	9 (3.3%)	<1%	0
Tonsillitis Acute NOS	0	0	0	7 (2.6%)	0	0
Upper Respiratory Tract Infection Viral NOS	1 (0.4%)	0	3 (0.9%)	4 (1.5%)	0	1 (0.3%)
Herpes Simplex Dermatitis	0	0	1 (0.3%)	4 (1.5%)	0	2 (0.6%)
Bronchitis Acute NOS	0	0	0	4 (1.5%)	0	0
Eye Infection NOS	0	0	0	3 (1.1%)	<1%	1 (0.3%)
General Disorders and Administration Site Conditions						
Application Site Burning	28 (10.4%)	17 (12.5%)	5 (1.5%)	23 (8.5%)	5 (6.7%)	85 (25.9%)
Pyrexia	20 (7.5%)	12 (8.8%)	41 (12.2%)	34 (12.5%)	4 (5.3%)	4 (1.2%)
Application Site Reaction NOS	8 (3.0%)	7 (5.1%)	7 (2.1%)	9 (3.3%)	2 (2.7%)	48 (14.6%)
Application Site Irritation	8 (3.0%)	8 (5.9%)	3 (0.9%)	1 (0.4%)	3 (4.0%)	21 (6.4%)
Influenza Like Illness	1 (0.4%)	0	2 (0.6%)	5 (1.8%)	2 (2.7%)	6 (1.8%)
Application Site Erythema	1 (0.4%)	0	0	6 (2.2%)	0	7 (2.1%)
Application Site Pruritus	3 (1.1%)	2 (1.5%)	2 (0.6%)	5 (1.8%)	0	18 (5.5%)
Respiratory, Thoracic and Mediastinal Disorders						
Cough	31 (11.6%)	11 (8.1%)	31 (9.3%)	43 (15.8%)	8 (10.7%)	8 (2.4%)
Nasal Congestion	7 (2.6%)	2 (1.5%)	6 (1.8%)	4 (1.5%)	1 (1.3%)	2 (0.6%)
Rhinorrhea	5 (1.9%)	1 (0.7%)	3 (0.9%)	1 (0.4%)	1 (1.3%)	0
Asthma Aggravated	4 (1.5%)	3 (2.2%)	13 (3.9%)	3 (1.1%)	1 (1.3%)	0
Sinus Congestion	3 (1.1%)	1 (0.7%)	2 (0.6%)	<1%	<1%	3 (0.9%)
Rhinitis	1 (0.4%)	0	5 (1.5%)	12 (4.4%)	5 (6.7%)	7 (2.1%)
Wheezing	1 (0.4%)	1 (0.7%)	4 (1.2%)	2 (0.7%)	<1%	0
Asthma NOS	2 (0.7%)	1 (0.7%)	11 (3.3%)	10 (3.7%)	2 (2.7%)	8 (2.4%)
Epistaxis	0	1 (0.7%)	0	9 (3.3%)	1 (1.3%)	1 (0.3%)
Dyspnea NOS	0	0	0	5 (1.8%)	1 (1.3%)	2 (0.6%)
Gastrointestinal Disorders						
Abdominal Pain Upper	11 (4.1%)	6 (4.4%)	10 (3.0%)	15 (5.5%)	5 (6.7%)	1 (0.3%)
Sore Throat	9 (3.4%)	5 (3.7%)	15 (5.4%)	22 (8.1%)	4 (5.3%)	12 (3.7%)
Vomiting NOS	8 (3.0%)	6 (4.4%)	14 (4.2%)	18 (6.6%)	6 (8.0%)	2 (0.6%)
Diarrhea NOS	3 (1.1%)	1 (0.7%)	2 (0.6%)	21 (7.7%)	4 (5.3%)	7 (2.1%)
Nausea	1 (0.4%)	3 (2.2%)	4 (1.2%)	11 (4.0%)	5 (6.7%)	6 (1.8%)
Abdominal Pain NOS	1 (0.4%)	1 (0.7%)	5 (1.5%)	12 (4.4%)	3 (4.0%)	1 (0.3%)
Toothache	1 (0.4%)	1 (0.7%)	2 (0.6%)	7 (2.6%)	1 (1.3%)	2 (0.6%)
Constipation	1 (0.4%)	0	2 (0.6%)	10 (3.7%)	<1%	0
Loose Stools	0	1 (0.7%)	4 (1.2%)	<1%	<1%	0
Reproductive System and Breast Disorders						
Dysmenorrhea	3 (1.1%)	0	5 (1.5%)	3 (1.1%)	1 (1.3%)	4 (1.2%)
Eye Disorders						
Conjunctivitis NEC	2 (0.7%)	1 (0.7%)	7 (2.1%)	6 (2.2%)	3 (4.0%)	10 (3.0%)
Skin & Subcutaneous Tissue Disorders						
Urticaria	3 (1.1%)	0	1 (0.3%)	1 (0.4%)	<1%	3 (0.9%)
Acne NOS	0	1 (0.7%)	1 (0.3%)	4 (1.5%)	<1%	6 (1.8%)
Immune System Disorders						
Hypersensitivity NOS	11 (4.1%)	6 (4.4%)	16 (4.8%)	14 (5.1%)	1 (1.3%)	11 (3.4%)
Injury and Poisoning						
Accident NOS	3 (1.1%)	1 (0.7%)	1 (0.3%)	<1%	1 (1.3%)	0
Laceration	2 (0.7%)	1 (0.7%)	5 (1.5%)	<1%	<1%	0
Musculoskeletal, Connective Tissue and Bone Disorders						
Back Pain	1 (0.4%)	2 (1.5%)	1 (0.3%)	<1%	0	6 (1.8%)
Arthralgias	0	0	1 (0.3%)	3 (1.1%)	1 (1.3%)	5 (1.5%)
Ear and Labyrinth Disorders						
Earache	2 (0.7%)	1 (0.7%)	0	8 (2.9%)	2 (2.7%)	0
Nervous System Disorders						
Headache	37 (13.9%)	12 (8.8%)	38 (11.3%)	69 (25.4%)	12 (16.0%)	23 (7.0%)

*Ages 2-17 years

Pimecrolimus was transferred across the placenta in oral rat and rabbit embryofetal developmental studies.

There are, however, no adequate and well-controlled studies in pregnant women. Because animal reproduction studies are not always predictive of human response, this drug should be used only if clearly needed during pregnancy.

Nursing Mothers

It is not known whether this drug is excreted in human milk. Because of the potential for serious adverse reactions in nursing infants from pimecrolimus, a decision should be made whether to discontinue nursing or to discontinue the drug, taking into account the importance of the drug to the mother.

Pediatric Use

Elidel Cream may be used in pediatric patients 2 years of age and older. Three Phase 3 pediatric studies were conducted involving 1114 patients 2-17 years of age. Two studies were 6-week randomized vehicle-controlled studies with a 20-week open-label phase and one was a vehicle-controlled long-term (up to 1 year) safety study with the option for sequential topical corticosteroid use. Of these patients 542 (49%) were 2-6 years of age. In the short-term studies, 11% of Elidel patients did not complete these studies and 1.5% of Elidel patients discontinued due to adverse events. In the one-year study, 32% of Elidel patients did not complete this study and 3% of Elidel patients discontinued due to adverse events. Most discontinuations were due to unsatisfactory therapeutic effect.

The most common local adverse event in the short-term studies of Elidel Cream in pediatric patients ages 2-17 was application site burning (10% vs. 13% vehicle); the incidence in the long-term study was 9% Elidel vs. 7% vehicle *(see ADVERSE REACTIONS)*. Adverse events that were more frequent (> 5%) in patients treated with Elidel Cream compared to vehicle were headache (14% vs. 9%) in the short-term trial. Nasopharyngitis (26% vs. 21%), influenza (13% vs. 4%), pharyngitis (8% vs. 3%), viral infection (7% vs. 1%), pyrexia (13% vs. 5%), cough (16% vs. 11%), and headache (25% vs. 16%) were increased over vehicle in the 1-year safety study *(see ADVERSE REACTIONS)*. In 843 patients ages 2-17 years treated with Elidel Cream, 9 (0.8%) developed eczema herpeticum (5 on Elidel Cream alone and 4 on Elidel Cream used in sequence with corticosteroids). In 211 patients on vehicle alone, there were no cases of eczema herpeticum. The majority of adverse events were mild to moderate in severity.

Elidel Cream is not recommended for use in pediatric patients below the age of 2 years. Two Phase 3 studies were conducted involving 436 infants age 3 months - 23 months. One 6-week randomized vehicle-controlled study with a 20-week open-label phase and one long term safety study were conducted. In the 6-week study, 11% of Elidel and 48% of vehicle patients did not complete this study; no patient in either group discontinued due to adverse events. Infants on Elidel Cream had an increased incidence of some adverse events compared to vehicle. In the 6-week vehicle-controlled study these adverse events included pyrexia (32% vs. 13% vehicle), URI (24% vs. 14%), nasopharyngitis (15% vs. 8%), gastroenteritis (7% vs. 3%), otitis media (4% vs. 0%), and diarrhea (8% vs. 0%). In the open-label phase of the study, for infants who switched to Elidel Cream from vehicle, the incidence of the above-cited adverse events approached or equaled the incidence of those patients who remained on Elidel Cream. In the 6-month safety data, 16% of Elidel and 35% of vehicle patients discontinued early and 1.5% of Elidel and 0% of vehicle patients discontinued due to adverse events. Infants on Elidel Cream had a greater incidence of some adverse events as compared to vehicle. These included pyrexia (30% vs. 20%), URI (21% vs. 17%), cough (15% vs. 9%), hypersensitivity (8% vs. 2%), teething (27% vs. 22%), vomiting (9% vs. 4%), rhinitis (13% vs. 9%), viral rash (4% vs. 0%), rhinorrhea (4% vs. 0%), and wheezing (4% vs. 0%).

The effects of Elidel Cream on the developing immune system in infants are unknown.

Geriatric Use

Nine (9) patients ≥ 65 years old received Elidel Cream in Phase 3 studies. Clinical studies of Elidel did not include sufficient numbers of patients aged 65 and over to assess efficacy and safety.

ADVERSE REACTIONS

In human dermal safety studies, Elidel® (pimecrolimus) Cream 1% did not induce contact sensitization, phototoxicity, or photoallergy, nor did it show any cumulative irritation.

In a one-year safety study in pediatric patients age 2-17 years old involving sequential use of Elidel Cream and a topical corticosteroid, 43% of Elidel patients and 68% of vehicle patients used corticosteroids during the study. Corticosteroids were used for more than 7 days by 34% of Elidel patients and 54% of vehicle patients. An increased incidence of impetigo, skin infection, superinfection (infected atopic dermatitis), rhinitis, and urticaria were found in the patients that had used Elidel Cream and topical corticosteroid sequentially as compared to Elidel Cream alone.

In 3 randomized, double-blind vehicle-controlled pediatric studies and one active-controlled adult study, 843 and 328 patients respectively, were treated with Elidel Cream. In these clinical trials, 48 (4%) of the 1171 Elidel patients and 13 (3%) of 408 vehicle-treated patients discontinued therapy due to adverse events. Discontinuations for AEs were primarily due to application site reactions, and cutaneous infections. The most common application site reaction was application site burning, which occurred in 8%-26% of patients treated with Elidel Cream.

The following table depicts the incidence of adverse events pooled across the 2 identically designed 6-week studies with their open label extensions and the 1-year safety study for pediatric patients ages 2-17. Data from the adult active-controlled study is also included in this table. Adverse events are listed regardless of relationship to study drug.

[See table at top of previous page]

OVERDOSAGE

There has been no experience of overdose with Elidel® (pimecrolimus) Cream 1%. No incidents of accidental ingestion have been reported. If oral ingestion occurs, medical advice should be sought.

DOSAGE AND ADMINISTRATION

Apply a thin layer of Elidel® (pimecrolimus) Cream 1% to the affected skin twice daily and rub in gently and completely. Elidel may be used on all skin surfaces, including the head, neck, and intertriginous areas.

Elidel should be used twice daily for as long as signs and symptoms persist. Treatment should be discontinued if resolution of disease occurs. If symptoms persist beyond 6 weeks, the patient should be re-evaluated.

The safety of Elidel Cream under occlusion, which may promote systemic exposure, has not been evaluated. **Elidel Cream should not be used with occlusive dressings.**

HOW SUPPLIED

Elidel® (pimecrolimus) Cream 1% is available in tubes of 15 grams, 30 grams, 60 grams, and 100 grams.

15 gram tube	NDC 0078-0375-40
30 gram tube	NDC 0078-0375-46
60 gram tube	NDC 0078-0375-49
100 gram tube	NDC 0078-0375-63

Store at 25°C (77°F); excursions permitted to 15°C-30°C (59°F-86°F). Do not freeze.

Manufactured by:
Novartis Pharma GmbH
Wehr, Germany
Distributed by:
Novartis Pharmaceuticals Corp.
East Hanover, NJ 07936

REV: APRIL 2003
T2003-01
89012002
492362/1 US

Ortho-McNeil Pharmaceutical

RARITAN, NJ 08869-0602

www.ortho-mcneil.com
For Medical Information Contact:
(800) 682-6532
In Emergencies:
(908) 218-7325
For Patient Education Materials Contact:
877-323-2200
For Customer Service (Sales and Ordering):
800-631-5273

LEVAQUIN® TABLETS ℞
[lĕv-ă-kwĭn]
(levofloxacin)

LEVAQUIN® INJECTION
(levofloxacin)

LEVAQUIN® INJECTION
(levofloxacin in 5% dextrose)

Prescribing information for this product, which appears on pages 2466–2472 of the 2003 PDR, has been completely revised as follows. Please write "See Supplement A" next to the product heading.

DESCRIPTION

LEVAQUIN® (levofloxacin) is a synthetic broad spectrum antibacterial agent for oral and intravenous administration. Chemically, levofloxacin, a chiral fluorinated carboxyquinolone, is the pure (-)-(S)-enantiomer of the racemic drug substance ofloxacin. The chemical name is (-)-(S)-9-fluoro-2,3-dihydro-3-methyl-10-(4-methyl-1-piperazinyl)-7-oxo-7H-pyrido[1,2,3-de]-1,4-benzoxazine-6-carboxylic acid hemihydrate.

The chemical structure is:

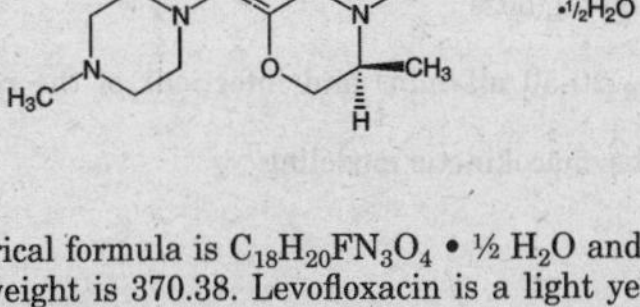

Its empirical formula is $C_{18}H_{20}FN_3O_4 \bullet \frac{1}{2} H_2O$ and its molecular weight is 370.38. Levofloxacin is a light yellowish-white to yellow-white crystal or crystalline powder. The molecule exists as a zwitterion at the pH conditions in the small intestine.

The data demonstrate that from pH 0.6 to 5.8, the solubility of levofloxacin is essentially constant (approximately 100 mg/mL). Levofloxacin is considered *soluble to freely soluble* in this pH range, as defined by USP nomenclature. Above pH 5.8, the solubility increases rapidly to its maximum at pH 6.7 (272 mg/mL) and is considered *freely soluble* in this range. Above pH 6.7, the solubility decreases and reaches a minimum value (about 50 mg/mL) at a pH of approximately 6.9.

Levofloxacin has the potential to form stable coordination compounds with many metal ions. This in vitro chelation potential has the following formation order: $Al^{+3} > Cu^{+2} > Zn^{+2} > Mg^{+2} > Ca^{+2}$.

LEVAQUIN Tablets are available as film-coated tablets and contain the following inactive ingredients:

250 mg (as expressed in the anhydrous form): hydroxypropyl methylcellulose, crospovidone, microcrystalline cellulose, magnesium stearate, polyethylene glycol, titanium dioxide, polysorbate 80 and synthetic red iron oxide.

500 mg (as expressed in the anhydrous form): hydroxypropyl methylcellulose, crospovidone, microcrystalline cellulose, magnesium stearate, polyethylene glycol, titanium dioxide, polysorbate 80 and synthetic red and yellow iron oxides.

750 mg (as expressed in the anhydrous form): hydroxypropyl methylcellulose, crospovidone, microcrystalline cellulose, magnesium stearate, polyethylene glycol, titanium dioxide, polysorbate 80.

LEVAQUIN Injection in Single-Use Vials is a sterile, preservative-free aqueous solution of levofloxacin with pH ranging from 3.8 to 5.8. LEVAQUIN Injection in Premix Flexible Containers is a sterile, preservative-free aqueous solution of levofloxacin with pH ranging from 3.8 to 5.8. The appearance of LEVAQUIN Injection may range from a clear yellow to a greenish-yellow solution. This does not adversely affect product potency.

LEVAQUIN Injection in Single-Use Vials contains levofloxacin in Water for Injection. LEVAQUIN Injection in Premix Flexible Containers is a dilute, non-pyrogenic, nearly isotonic premixed solution that contains levofloxacin in 5% Dextrose (D_5W). Solutions of hydrochloric acid and sodium hydroxide may have been added to adjust the pH.

The flexible container is fabricated from a specially formulated non-plasticized, thermoplastic copolyester (CR3). The amount of water that can permeate from the container into the overwrap is insufficient to affect the solution significantly. Solutions in contact with the flexible container can leach out certain of the container's chemical components in very small amounts within the expiration period. The suitability of the container material has been confirmed by tests in animals according to USP biological tests for plastic containers.

CLINICAL PHARMACOLOGY

The mean ±SD pharmacokinetic parameters of levofloxacin determined under single and steady state conditions following oral (p.o.) or intravenous (i.v.) doses of levofloxacin are summarized in Table 1.

Absorption

Levofloxacin is rapidly and essentially completely absorbed after oral administration. Peak plasma concentrations are usually attained one to two hours after oral dosing. The absolute bioavailability of a 500 mg tablet and a 750 mg tablet of levofloxacin are both approximately 99%, demonstrating complete oral absorption of levofloxacin. Following a single intravenous dose of levofloxacin to healthy volunteers, the mean ±SD peak plasma concentration attained was 6.2 ±1.0 µg/mL after a 500 mg dose infused over 60 minutes and 11.5 ±4.0 µg/mL after a 750 mg dose infused over 90 minutes.

Levofloxacin pharmacokinetics are linear and predictable after single and multiple oral/or i.v. dosing regimens. Steady-state conditions are reached within 48 hours following a 500 mg or 750 mg once-daily dosage regimen. The mean ±SD peak and trough plasma concentrations attained following multiple once-daily oral dosage regimens were approximately 5.7 ±1.4 and 0.5 ±0.2 µg/mL after the 500 mg doses, and 8.6 ±1.9 and 1.1 ±0.4 µg/mL after the 750 mg doses, respectively. The mean ±SD peak and trough plasma concentrations attained following multiple once-daily i.v. regimens were approximately 6.4 ±0.8 and 0.6 ±0.2 µg/mL after the 500 mg doses, and 12.1 ±4.1 and 1.3 ±0.71 µg/mL after the 750 mg doses, respectively.

Oral administration of a 500-mg LEVAQUIN tablet with food slightly prolongs the time to peak concentration by approximately 1 hour and slightly decreases the peak concentration by approximately 14%. Therefore, levofloxacin tablets can be administered without regard to food.

The plasma concentration profile of levofloxacin after i.v. administration is similar and comparable in extent of exposure (AUC) to that observed for levofloxacin tablets when equal doses (mg/mg) are administered. Therefore, the oral and i.v. routes of administration can be considered interchangeable. (See following chart.)

[See first figure at top of next column]
[See second figure at top of next column]

Distribution

The mean volume of distribution of levofloxacin generally ranges from 74 to 112 L after single and multiple 500 mg or 750 mg doses, indicating widespread distribution into body tissues. Levofloxacin reaches its peak levels in skin tissues and in blister fluid of healthy subjects at approximately 3 hours after dosing. The skin tissue biopsy to plasma AUC

Continued on next page

Levaquin—Cont.

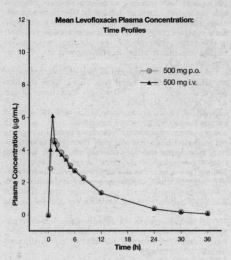

Mean Levofloxacin Plasma Concentration: Time Profiles (500 mg p.o., 500 mg i.v.)

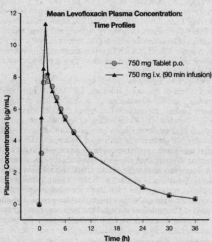

Mean Levofloxacin Plasma Concentration: Time Profiles (750 mg Tablet p.o., 750 mg i.v. (90 min infusion))

ratio is approximately 2 and the blister fluid to plasma AUC ratio is approximately 1 following multiple once-daily oral administration of 750 mg and 500 mg levofloxacin, respectively, to healthy subjects. Levofloxacin also penetrates well into lung tissues. Lung tissue concentrations were generally 2- to 5- fold higher than plasma concentrations and ranged from approximately 2.4 to 11.3 µg/g over a 24-hour period after a single 500 mg oral dose.

In vitro, over a clinically relevant range (1 to 10 µg/mL) of serum/plasma levofloxacin concentrations, levofloxacin is approximately 24 to 38% bound to serum proteins across all species studied, as determined by the equilibrium dialysis method. Levofloxacin is mainly bound to serum albumin in humans. Levofloxacin binding to serum proteins is independent of the drug concentration.

Metabolism
Levofloxacin is stereochemically stable in plasma and urine and does not invert metabolically to its enantiomer, D-ofloxacin. Levofloxacin undergoes limited metabolism in humans and is primarily excreted as unchanged drug in the urine. Following oral administration, approximately 87% of an administered dose was recovered as unchanged drug in urine within 48 hours, whereas less than 4% of the dose was recovered in feces in 72 hours. Less than 5% of an administered dose was recovered in the urine as the desmethyl and N-oxide metabolites, the only metabolites identified in humans. These metabolites have little relevant pharmacological activity.

Excretion
Levofloxacin is excreted largely as unchanged drug in the urine. The mean terminal plasma elimination half-life of levofloxacin ranges from approximately 6 to 8 hours following single or multiple doses of levofloxacin given orally or intravenously. The mean apparent total body clearance and renal clearance range from approximately 144 to 226 mL/min and 96 to 142 mL/min, respectively. Renal clearance in excess of the glomerular filtration rate suggests that tubular secretion of levofloxacin occurs in addition to its glomerular filtration. Concomitant administration of either cimetidine or probenecid results in approximately 24% and 35% reduction in the levofloxacin renal clearance, respectively, indicating that secretion of levofloxacin occurs in the renal proximal tubule. No levofloxacin crystals were found in any of the urine samples freshly collected from subjects receiving levofloxacin.

Special Populations
Geriatric: There are no significant differences in levofloxacin pharmacokinetics between young and elderly subjects when the subjects' differences in creatinine clearance are taken into consideration. Following a 500 mg oral dose of levofloxacin to healthy elderly subjects (66-80 years of age), the mean terminal plasma elimination half-life of levofloxacin was about 7.6 hours, as compared to approximately 6 hours in younger adults. The difference was attributable to the variation in renal function status of the subjects and was not believed to be clinically significant. Drug absorption appears to be unaffected by age. Levofloxacin dose adjustment based on age alone is not necessary.

Pediatric: The pharmacokinetics of levofloxacin in pediatric subjects have not been studied.

Gender: There are no significant differences in levofloxacin pharmacokinetics between male and female subjects when subjects' differences in creatinine clearance are taken into consideration. Following a 500 mg oral dose of levofloxacin to healthy male subjects, the mean terminal plasma elimination half-life of levofloxacin was about 7.5 hours, as compared to approximately 6.1 hours in female subjects. This difference was attributable to the variation in renal function status of the male and female subjects and was not believed to be clinically significant. Drug absorption appears to be unaffected by the gender of the subjects. Dose adjustment based on gender alone is not necessary.

Race: The effect of race on levofloxacin pharmacokinetics was examined through a covariate analysis performed on data from 72 subjects: 48 white and 24 nonwhite. The apparent total body clearance and apparent volume of distribution were not affected by the race of the subjects.

Renal insufficiency: Clearance of levofloxacin is substantially reduced and plasma elimination half-life is substantially prolonged in patients with impaired renal function (creatinine clearance <50 mL/min), requiring dosage adjustment in such patients to avoid accumulation. Neither hemodialysis nor continuous ambulatory peritoneal dialysis (CAPD) is effective in removal of levofloxacin from the body, indicating that supplemental doses of levofloxacin are not required following hemodialysis or CAPD. (See **PRECAUTIONS: General** and **DOSAGE AND ADMINISTRATION.**)

Hepatic insufficiency: Pharmacokinetic studies in hepatically impaired patients have not been conducted. Due to the limited extent of levofloxacin metabolism, the pharmacokinetics of levofloxacin are not expected to be affected by hepatic impairment.

Bacterial infection: The pharmacokinetics of levofloxacin in patients with serious community-acquired bacterial infections are comparable to those observed in healthy subjects.

Drug-drug interactions: The potential for pharmacokinetic drug interactions between levofloxacin and theophylline, warfarin, cyclosporine, digoxin, probenecid, cimetidine, sucralfate, and antacids has been evaluated. (See **PRECAUTIONS: Drug Interactions.**)
[See table 1 below]

MICROBIOLOGY
Levofloxacin is the L-isomer of the racemate, ofloxacin, a quinolone antimicrobial agent. The antibacterial activity of ofloxacin resides primarily in the L-isomer. The mechanism of action of levofloxacin and other fluoroquinolone antimicrobials involves inhibition of bacterial topoisomerase IV and DNA gyrase (both of which are type II topoisomerases), enzymes required for DNA replication, transcription, repair and recombination.

Levofloxacin has in vitro activity against a wide range of gram-negative and gram-positive microorganisms. Levofloxacin is often bactericidal at concentrations equal to or slightly greater than inhibitory concentrations.

Fluoroquinolones, including levofloxacin, differ in chemical structure and mode of action from aminoglycosides, macrolides and β-lactam antibiotics, including penicillins. Fluoroquinolones may, therefore, be active against bacteria resistant to these antimicrobials.

Resistance to levofloxacin due to spontaneous mutation in vitro is a rare occurrence (range: 10^{-9} to 10^{-10}). Although cross-resistance has been observed between levofloxacin and some other fluoroquinolones, some microorganisms resistant to other fluoroquinolones may be susceptible to levofloxacin.

Levofloxacin has been shown to be active against most strains of the following microorganisms both in vitro and in clinical infections as described in the **INDICATIONS AND USAGE** section:

Aerobic gram-positive microorganisms
Enterococcus faecalis (many strains are only moderately susceptible)
Staphylococcus aureus (methicillin-susceptible strains)
Staphylococcus saprophyticus
Streptococcus pneumoniae (including penicillin-resistant strains*)
Streptococcus pyogenes

*Note: penicillin-resistant *S. pneumoniae* are those strains with a penicillin MIC value of ≥2 µg/mL

Aerobic gram-negative microorganisms
Enterobacter cloacae
Escherichia coli
Haemophilus influenzae
Haemophilus parainfluenzae
Klebsiella pneumoniae
Legionella pneumophila
Moraxella catarrhalis
Proteus mirabilis
Pseudomonas aeruginosa
Serratia marcescens

As with other drugs in this class, some strains of *Pseudomonas aeruginosa* may develop resistance fairly rapidly during treatment with levofloxacin.

Other microorganisms
Chlamydia pneumoniae
Mycoplasma pneumoniae

The following in vitro data are available, **but their clinical significance is unknown**.

Levofloxacin exhibits in vitro minimum inhibitory concentrations (MIC values) of 2 µg/mL or less against most (≥90%) strains of the following microorganisms; however,

Table 1. Mean ±SD Levofloxacin PK Parameters

Regimen	C_{max} (µg/mL)	T_{max} (h)	AUC (µg·h/mL)	CL/F^1 (mL/min)	Vd/F^2 (L)	$t_{1/2}$ (h)	CL_R (mL/min)
Single dose							
250 mg p.o.[3]	2.8 ± 0.4	1.6 ± 1.0	27.2 ± 3.9	156 ± 20	ND	7.3 ± 0.9	142 ± 21
500 mg p.o.[3]*	5.1 ± 0.8	1.3 ± 0.6	47.9 ± 6.8	178 ± 28	ND	6.3 ± 0.6	103 ± 30
500 mg i.v.[3]	6.2 ± 1.0	1.0 ± 0.1	48.3 ± 5.4	175 ± 20	90 ± 11	6.4 ± 0.7	112 ± 25
750 mg p.o.[5]*	9.3 ± 1.6	1.6 ± 0.8	101 ± 20	129 ± 24	83 ± 17	7.5 ± 0.9	ND
750 mg i.v.[5]	11.5 ± 4.0[4]	ND	110 ± 40	126 ± 39	75 ± 13	7.5 ± 1.6	ND
Multiple dose							
500 mg q24h p.o.[3]	5.7 ± 1.4	1.1 ± 0.4	47.5 ± 6.7	175 ± 25	102 ± 22	7.6 ± 1.6	116 ± 31
500 mg q24h i.v.[3]	6.4 ± 0.8	ND	54.6 ± 11.1	158 ± 29	91 ± 12	7.0 ± 0.8	99 ± 28
500 mg or 250 mg q24h i.v., patients with bacterial infection[6]	8.7 ± 4.0[7]	ND	72.5 ± 51.2[7]	154 ± 72	111 ± 58	ND	ND
750 mg q24h p.o.[5]	8.6 ± 1.9	1.4 ± 0.5	90.7 ± 17.6	143 ± 29	100 ± 16	8.8 ± 1.5	116 ± 28
750 mg q24h i.v.[5]	12.1 ± 4.1[4]	ND	108 ± 34	126 ± 37	80 ± 27	7.9 ± 1.9	ND
500 mg p.o. single dose, effects of gender and age:							
Male[8]	5.5 ± 1.1	1.2 ± 0.4	54.4 ± 18.9	166 ± 44	89 ± 13	7.5 ± 2.1	126 ± 38
Female[9]	7.0 ± 1.6	1.7 ± 0.5	67.7 ± 24.2	136 ± 44	62 ± 16	6.1 ± 0.8	106 ± 40
Young[10]	5.5 ± 1.0	1.5 ± 0.6	47.5 ± 9.8	182 ± 35	83 ± 18	6.0 ± 0.9	140 ± 33
Elderly[11]	7.0 ± 1.6	1.4 ± 0.5	74.7 ± 23.3	121 ± 33	67 ± 19	7.6 ± 2.0	91 ± 29
500 mg p.o. single dose, patients with renal insufficiency:							
CL_{CR} 50–80 mL/min	7.5 ± 1.8	1.5 ± 0.5	95.6 ± 11.8	88 ± 10	ND	9.1 ± 0.9	57 ± 8
CL_{CR} 20–49 mL/min	7.1 ± 3.1	2.1 ± 1.3	182.1 ± 62.6	51 ± 19	ND	27 ± 10	26 ± 13
CL_{CR} <20 mL/min	8.2 ± 2.6	1.1 ± 1.0	263.5 ± 72.5	33 ± 8	ND	35 ± 5	13 ± 3
Hemodialysis	5.7 ± 1.0	2.8 ± 2.2	ND	ND	ND	76 ± 42	ND
CAPD	6.9 ± 2.3	1.4 ± 1.1	ND	ND	ND	51 ± 24	ND

[1] clearance/bioavailability
[2] volume of distribution/bioavailability
[3] healthy males 18-53 years of age
[4] 60 min infusion for 250 mg and 500 mg doses, 90 min infusion for 750 mg dose
[5] healthy male and female subjects 18-54 years of age
[6] 500 mg q48h for patients with moderate renal impairment (CL_{CR} 20-50 mL/min) and infections of the respiratory tract or skin
[7] dose-normalized values (to 500 mg dose), estimated by population pharmacokinetic modeling
[8] healthy males 22-75 years of age
[9] healthy females 18-80 years of age
[10] young healthy male and female subjects 18-36 years of age
[11] healthy elderly male and female subjects 66-80 years of age
* Absolute bioavailability; F = 0.99 ± 0.08 from a 500-mg tablet and F=0.99 ± 0.06 from a 750-mg tablet; ND = not determined.

the safety and effectiveness of levofloxacin in treating clinical infections due to these microorganisms have not been established in adequate and well-controlled trials.

Aerobic gram-positive microorganisms
Staphylococcus epidermidis (methicillin-susceptible strains)
Streptococcus (Group C/F)
Streptococcus (Group G)
Streptococcus agalactiae
Streptococcus milleri
Viridans group streptococci

Aerobic gram-negative microorganisms
Acinetobacter baumannii
Acinetobacter lwoffii
Bordetella pertussis
Citrobacter (diversus) koseri
Citrobacter freundii
Enterobacter aerogenes
Enterobacter sakazakii
Klebsiella oxytoca
Morganella morganii
Pantoea (Enterobacter) agglomerans
Proteus vulgaris
Providencia rettgeri
Providencia stuartii
Pseudomonas fluorescens

Anaerobic gram-positive microorganisms
Clostridium perfringens

Susceptibility Tests
Susceptibility testing for levofloxacin should be performed, as it is the optimal predictor of activity.

Dilution techniques: Quantitative methods are used to determine antimicrobial minimal inhibitory concentrations (MIC values). These MIC values provide estimates of the susceptibility of bacteria to antimicrobial compounds. The MIC values should be determined using a standardized procedure. Standardized procedures are based on a dilution method[1] (broth or agar) or equivalent with standardized inoculum concentrations and standardized concentrations of levofloxacin powder. The MIC values should be interpreted according to the following criteria:

For testing *Enterobacteriaceae*, Enterococci, *Staphylococcus* species, and *Pseudomonas aeruginosa*:

MIC (µg/mL)	Interpretation
≤2	Susceptible (S)
4	Intermediate (I)
≥8	Resistant (R)

For testing *Haemophilus influenzae* and *Haemophilus parainfluenzae*:[a]

MIC (µg/mL)	Interpretation
≤2	Susceptible (S)

[a] These interpretive standards are applicable only to broth microdilution susceptibility testing with *Haemophilus influenzae* and *Haemophilus parainfluenzae* using Haemophilus Test Medium.[1]

The current absence of data on resistant strains precludes defining any categories other than "Susceptible." Strains yielding MIC results suggestive of a "nonsusceptible" category should be submitted to a reference laboratory for further testing.

For testing *Streptococcus* spp. including *S. pneumoniae*:[b]

MIC (µg/mL)	Interpretation
≤2	Susceptible (S)
4	Intermediate (I)
≥8	Resistant (R)

[b] These interpretive standards are applicable only to broth microdilution susceptibility tests using cation-adjusted Mueller-Hinton broth with 2–5% lysed horse blood.

A report of "Susceptible" indicates that the pathogen is likely to be inhibited if the antimicrobial compound in the blood reaches the concentrations usually achievable. A report of "Intermediate" indicates that the result should be considered equivocal, and, if the microorganism is not fully susceptible to alternative, clinically feasible drugs, the test should be repeated. This category implies possible clinical applicability in body sites where the drug is physiologically concentrated or in situations where a high dosage of drug can be used. This category also provides a buffer zone which prevents small uncontrolled technical factors from causing major discrepancies in interpretation. A report of "Resistant" indicates that the pathogen is not likely to be inhibited if the antimicrobial compound in the blood reaches the concentrations usually achievable; other therapy should be selected.

Standardized susceptibility test procedures require the use of laboratory control microorganisms to control the technical aspects of the laboratory procedures. Standard levofloxacin powder should give the following MIC values:

Microorganism		MIC (µg/mL)
Enterococcus faecalis	ATCC 29212	0.25-2
Escherichia coli	ATCC 25922	0.008-0.06
Escherichia coli	ATCC 35218	0.015-0.06
Haemophilus influenzae	ATCC 49247[c]	0.008-0.03
Pseudomonas aeruginosa	ATCC 27853	0.5-4
Staphylococcus aureus	ATCC 29213	0.06-0.5
Streptococcus pneumoniae	ATCC 49619[d]	0.5-2

[c] This quality control range is applicable to only *H. influenzae* ATCC 49247 tested by a broth microdilution procedure using Haemophilus Test Medium (HTM).[1]

[d] This quality control range is applicable to only *S. pneumoniae* ATCC 49619 tested by a broth microdilution procedure using cation-adjusted Mueller-Hinton broth with 2-5% lysed horse blood.

Diffusion techniques: Quantitative methods that require measurement of zone diameters also provide reproducible estimates of the susceptibility of bacteria to antimicrobial compounds. One such standardized procedure[2] requires the use of standardized inoculum concentrations. This procedure uses paper disks impregnated with 5-µg levofloxacin to test the susceptibility of microorganisms to levofloxacin.

Reports from the laboratory providing results of the standard single-disk susceptibility test with a 5-µg levofloxacin disk should be interpreted according to the following criteria:

For testing *Enterobacteriaceae*, Enterococci, *Staphylococcus* species, and *Pseudomonas aeruginosa*:

Zone diameter (mm)	Interpretation
≥17	Susceptible (S)
14-16	Intermediate (I)
≤13	Resistant (R)

For *Haemophilus influenzae* and *Haemophilus parainfluenzae*:[e]

Zone diameter (mm)	Interpretation
≥17	Susceptible (S)

[e] These interpretive standards are applicable only to disk diffusion susceptibility testing with *Haemophilus influenzae* and *Haemophilus parainfluenzae* using Haemophilus Test Medium.

The current absence of data on resistant strains precludes defining any categories other than "Susceptible." Strains yielding zone diameter results suggestive of a "nonsusceptible" category should be submitted to a reference laboratory for further testing.

For *Streptococcus* spp. including *S. pneumoniae*:[f]

Zone diameter (mm)	Interpretation
≥17	Susceptible (S)
14-16	Intermediate (I)
≤13	Resistant (R)

[f] These zone diameter standards for *Streptococcus* spp. including *S. pneumoniae* apply only to tests performed using Mueller-Hinton agar supplemented with 5% sheep blood and incubated in 5% CO_2.

Interpretation should be as stated above for results using dilution techniques. Interpretation involves correlation of the diameter obtained in the disk test with the MIC for levofloxacin.

As with standardized dilution techniques, diffusion methods require the use of laboratory control microorganisms to control the technical aspects of the laboratory procedures. For the diffusion technique, the 5-µg levofloxacin disk should provide the following zone diameters in these laboratory test quality control strains:

Microorganism		Zone Diameter (mm)
Escherichia coli	ATCC 25922	29-37
Haemophilus influenzae	ATCC 49247[g]	32-40
Pseudomonas aeruginosa	ATCC 27853	19-26
Staphylococcus aureus	ATCC 25923	25-30
Streptococcus pneumoniae	ATCC 49619[h]	20-25

[g] This quality control range is applicable to only *H. influenzae* ATCC 49247 tested by a disk diffusion procedure using Haemophilus Test Medium (HTM).[2]

[h] This quality control range is applicable to only *S. pneumoniae* ATCC 49619 tested by a disk diffusion procedure using Mueller-Hinton agar supplemented with 5% sheep blood and incubated in 5% CO_2.

INDICATIONS AND USAGE
LEVAQUIN Tablets/Injection are indicated for the treatment of adults (≥18 years of age) with mild, moderate, and severe infections caused by susceptible strains of the designated microorganisms in the conditions listed below. LEVAQUIN Injection is indicated when intravenous administration offers a route of administration advantageous to the patient (e.g., patient cannot tolerate an oral dosage form). Please see **DOSAGE AND ADMINISTRATION** for specific recommendations.

Acute maxillary sinusitis due to *Streptococcus pneumoniae*, *Haemophilus influenzae*, or *Moraxella catarrhalis*.

Acute bacterial exacerbation of chronic bronchitis due to *Staphylococcus aureus*, *Streptococcus pneumoniae*, *Haemophilus influenzae*, *Haemophilus parainfluenzae*, or *Moraxella catarrhalis*.

Nosocomial pneumonia due to methicillin-susceptible *Staphylococcus aureus*, *Pseudomonas aeruginosa*, *Serratia marcescens*, *Escherichia coli*, *Klebsiella pneumoniae*, *Haemophilus influenzae*, or *Streptococcus pneumoniae*. Adjunctive therapy should be used as clinically indicated. Where *Pseudomonas aeruginosa* is a documented or presumptive pathogen, combination therapy with an anti-pseudomonal β-lactam is recommended. (See **CLINICAL STUDIES**.)

Community-acquired pneumonia due to *Staphylococcus aureus*, *Streptococcus pneumoniae* (including penicillin-resistant strains, MIC value for penicillin ≥2 µg/mL), *Haemophilus influenzae*, *Haemophilus parainfluenzae*, *Klebsiella pneumoniae*, *Moraxella catarrhalis*, *Chlamydia pneumoniae*, *Legionella pneumophila*, or *Mycoplasma pneumoniae*. (See **CLINICAL STUDIES**.)

Complicated skin and skin structure infections due to methicillin-susceptible *Staphylococcus aureus*, *Enterococcus faecalis*, *Streptococcus pyogenes*, or *Proteus mirabilis*.

Uncomplicated skin and skin structure infections (mild to moderate) including abscesses, cellulitis, furuncles, impetigo, pyoderma, wound infections, due to *Staphylococcus aureus* or *Streptococcus pyogenes*.

Complicated urinary tract infections (mild to moderate) due to *Enterococcus faecalis*, *Enterobacter cloacae*, *Escherichia coli*, *Klebsiella pneumoniae*, *Proteus mirabilis*, or *Pseudomonas aeruginosa*.

Acute pyelonephritis (mild to moderate) caused by *Escherichia coli*.

Uncomplicated urinary tract infections (mild to moderate) due to *Escherichia coli*, *Klebsiella pneumoniae*, or *Staphylococcus saprophyticus*.

Appropriate culture and susceptibility tests should be performed before treatment in order to isolate and identify organisms causing the infection and to determine their susceptibility to levofloxacin. Therapy with levofloxacin may be initiated before results of these tests are known; once results become available, appropriate therapy should be selected.

As with other drugs in this class, some strains of *Pseudomonas aeruginosa* may develop resistance fairly rapidly during treatment with levofloxacin. Culture and susceptibility testing performed periodically during therapy will provide information about the continued susceptibility of the pathogens to the antimicrobial agent and also the possible emergence of bacterial resistance.

CONTRAINDICATIONS
Levofloxacin is contraindicated in persons with a history of hypersensitivity to levofloxacin, quinolone antimicrobial agents, or any other components of this product.

WARNINGS

THE SAFETY AND EFFICACY OF LEVOFLOXACIN IN PEDIATRIC PATIENTS, ADOLESCENTS (UNDER THE AGE OF 18 YEARS), PREGNANT WOMEN, AND NURSING WOMEN HAVE NOT BEEN ESTABLISHED. (See **PRECAUTIONS: Pediatric Use, Pregnancy,** and **Nursing Mothers** subsections.)

In immature rats and dogs, the oral and intravenous administration of levofloxacin increased the incidence and severity of osteochondrosis. Other fluoroquinolones also produce similar erosions in the weight bearing joints and other signs of arthropathy in immature animals of various species. (See **ANIMAL PHARMACOLOGY**.)

Convulsions and toxic psychoses have been reported in patients receiving quinolones, including levofloxacin. Quinolones may also cause increased intracranial pressure and central nervous system stimulation which may lead to tremors, restlessness, anxiety, lightheadedness, confusion, hallucinations, paranoia, depression, nightmares, insomnia, and, rarely, suicidal thoughts or acts. These reactions may occur following the first dose. If these reactions occur in patients receiving levofloxacin, the drug should be discontinued and appropriate measures instituted. As with other quinolones, levofloxacin should be used with caution in patients with a known or suspected CNS disorder that may predispose to seizures or lower the seizure threshold (e.g., severe cerebral arteriosclerosis, epilepsy) or in the presence of other risk factors that may predispose to seizures or lower the seizure threshold (e.g., certain drug therapy, renal dysfunction.) (See **PRECAUTIONS: General, Information for Patients, Drug Interactions** and **ADVERSE REACTIONS**.)

Serious and occasionally fatal hypersensitivity and/or anaphylactic reactions have been reported in patients receiving therapy with quinolones, including levofloxacin. These reactions often occur following the first dose. Some reactions have been accompanied by cardiovascular collapse, hypotension/shock, seizure, loss of consciousness, tingling, angioedema (including tongue, laryngeal, throat, or facial edema/swelling), airway obstruction (including bronchospasm, shortness of breath, and acute respiratory distress), dyspnea, urticaria, itching, and other serious skin reactions. Levofloxacin should be discontinued immediately at the first appearance of a skin rash or any other sign of hypersensitivity. Serious acute hypersensitivity reactions may require treatment with epinephrine and other resuscitative measures, including oxygen, intravenous fluids, antihistamines, corticosteroids, pressor amines, and airway management, as clinically indicated. (See **PRECAUTIONS** and **ADVERSE REACTIONS**.)

Serious and sometimes fatal events, some due to hypersensitivity, and some due to uncertain etiology, have been reported rarely in patients receiving therapy with quinolones, including levofloxacin. These events may be severe and generally occur following the administration of multiple doses. Clinical manifestations may include one or more of the following: fever, rash or severe dermatologic reactions (e.g., toxic epidermal necrolysis, Stevens-Johnson Syndrome); vasculitis; arthralgia; myalgia; serum sickness; allergic pneumonitis; interstitial nephritis; acute renal insufficiency or failure; hepatitis; jaundice; acute hepatic necrosis or failure; anemia, including hemolytic and aplastic; thrombocytopenia, including thrombotic thrombocytopenic purpura;

Continued on next page

Levaquin—Cont.

leukopenia; agranulocytosis; pancytopenia; and/or other hematologic abnormalities. The drug should be discontinued immediately at the first appearance of a skin rash or any other sign of hypersensitivity and supportive measures instituted. (See **PRECAUTIONS: Information for Patients** and **ADVERSE REACTIONS**.)

Pseudomembranous colitis has been reported with nearly all antibacterial agents, including levofloxacin, and may range in severity from mild to life-threatening. Therefore, it is important to consider this diagnosis in patients who present with diarrhea subsequent to the administration of any antibacterial agent.

Treatment with antibacterial agents alters the normal flora of the colon and may permit overgrowth of clostridia. Studies indicate that a toxin produced by *Clostridium difficile* is one primary cause of "antibiotic-associated colitis."

After the diagnosis of pseudomembranous colitis has been established, therapeutic measures should be initiated. Mild cases of pseudomembranous colitis usually respond to drug discontinuation alone. In moderate to severe cases, consideration should be given to management with fluids and electrolytes, protein supplementation, and treatment with an antibacterial drug clinically effective against *C. difficile* colitis. (See **ADVERSE REACTIONS**.)

Ruptures of the shoulder, hand, or Achilles tendons that required surgical repair or resulted in prolonged disability have been reported in patients receiving quinolones, including levofloxacin. Post-marketing surveillance reports indicate that this risk may be increased in patients receiving concomitant corticosteroids, especially in the elderly. Levofloxacin should be discontinued if the patient experiences pain, inflammation, or rupture of a tendon. Patients should rest and refrain from exercise until the diagnosis of tendinitis or tendon rupture has been confidently excluded. Tendon rupture can occur during or after therapy with quinolones, including levofloxacin.

PRECAUTIONS
General

Because a rapid or bolus intravenous injection may result in hypotension, LEVOFLOXACIN INJECTION SHOULD ONLY BE ADMINISTERED BY SLOW INTRAVENOUS INFUSION OVER A PERIOD OF 60 OR 90 MINUTES DEPENDING ON THE DOSAGE. (See **DOSAGE AND ADMINISTRATION**.)

Although levofloxacin is more soluble than other quinolones, adequate hydration of patients receiving levofloxacin should be maintained to prevent the formation of a highly concentrated urine.

Administer levofloxacin with caution in the presence of renal insufficiency. Careful clinical observation and appropriate laboratory studies should be performed prior to and during therapy since elimination of levofloxacin may be reduced. In patients with impaired renal function (creatinine clearance <50 mL/min), adjustment of the dosage regimen is necessary to avoid the accumulation of levofloxacin due to decreased clearance. (See **CLINICAL PHARMACOLOGY** and **DOSAGE AND ADMINISTRATION**.)

Moderate to severe phototoxicity reactions have been observed in patients exposed to direct sunlight while receiving drugs in this class. Excessive exposure to sunlight should be avoided. However, in clinical trials with levofloxacin, phototoxicity has been observed in less than 0.1% of patients. Therapy should be discontinued if phototoxicity (e.g., a skin eruption) occurs.

As with other quinolones, levofloxacin should be used with caution in any patient with a known or suspected CNS disorder that may predispose to seizures or lower the seizure threshold (e.g., severe cerebral arteriosclerosis, epilepsy) or in the presence of other risk factors that may predispose to seizures or lower the seizure threshold (e.g., certain drug therapy, renal dysfunction). (See **WARNINGS** and **Drug Interactions**.)

As with other quinolones, disturbances of blood glucose, including symptomatic hyper- and hypoglycemia, have been reported, usually in diabetic patients receiving concomitant treatment with an oral hypoglycemic agent (e.g., glyburide/glibenclamide) or with insulin. In these patients, careful monitoring of blood glucose is recommended. If a hypoglycemic reaction occurs in a patient being treated with levofloxacin, levofloxacin should be discontinued immediately and appropriate therapy should be initiated immediately. (See **Drug Interactions** and **ADVERSE REACTIONS**.)

Some quinolones, including levofloxacin, have been associated with prolongation of the QT interval on the electrocardiogram and infrequent cases of arrhythmia. During post-marketing surveillance, rare cases of torsades de pointes have been reported in patients taking levofloxacin. These reports generally involved patients with concurrent medical conditions or concomitant medications that may have been contributory. The risk of arrhythmias may be reduced by avoiding concurrent use with other drugs that prolong the QT interval including class Ia or class III antiarrhythmic agents; in addition, use of levofloxacin in the presence of risk factors for torsades de pointes such as hypokalemia, significant bradycardia, and cardiomyopathy should be avoided.

As with any potent antimicrobial drug, periodic assessment of organ system functions, including renal, hepatic, and hematopoietic, is advisable during therapy. (See **WARNINGS** and **ADVERSE REACTIONS**.)

Information for Patients
Patients should be advised:
- to drink fluids liberally;
- that antacids containing magnesium, or aluminum, as well as sucralfate, metal cations such as iron, and multivitamin preparations with zinc or Videx® (didanosine), chewable/buffered tablets or the pediatric powder for oral solution should be taken at least two hours before or two hours after oral levofloxacin administration. (See **Drug Interactions**);
- that oral levofloxacin can be taken without regard to meals;
- that levofloxacin may cause neurologic adverse effects (e.g., dizziness, lightheadedness) and that patients should know how they react to levofloxacin before they operate an automobile or machinery or engage in other activities requiring mental alertness and coordination. (See **WARNINGS** and **ADVERSE REACTIONS**);
- to discontinue treatment and inform their physician if they experience pain, inflammation, or rupture of a tendon, and to rest and refrain from exercise until the diagnosis of tendinitis or tendon rupture has been confidently excluded;
- that levofloxacin may be associated with hypersensitivity reactions, even following the first dose, and to discontinue the drug at the first sign of a skin rash, hives or other skin reactions, a rapid heartbeat, difficulty in swallowing or breathing, any swelling suggesting angioedema (e.g., swelling of the lips, tongue, face, tightness of the throat, hoarseness), or other symptoms of an allergic reaction. (See **WARNINGS** and **ADVERSE REACTIONS**);
- to avoid excessive sunlight or artificial ultraviolet light while receiving levofloxacin and to discontinue therapy if phototoxicity (i.e., skin eruption) occurs;
- that if they are diabetic and are being treated with insulin or an oral hypoglycemic agent and a hypoglycemic reaction occurs, they should discontinue levofloxacin and consult a physician. (See **PRECAUTIONS: General** and **Drug Interactions**.);
- that concurrent administration of warfarin and levofloxacin has been associated with increases of the International Normalized Ratio (INR) or prothrombin time and clinical episodes of bleeding. Patients should notify their physician if they are taking warfarin.
- that convulsions have been reported in patients taking quinolones, including levofloxacin, and to notify their physician before taking this drug if there is a history of this condition.

Drug Interactions
Antacids, Sucralfate, Metal Cations, Multivitamins
LEVAQUIN Tablets: While the chelation by divalent cations is less marked than with other quinolones, concurrent administration of LEVAQUIN Tablets with antacids containing magnesium, or aluminum, as well as sucralfate, metal cations such as iron, and multivitamin preparations with zinc may interfere with the gastrointestinal absorption of levofloxacin, resulting in systemic levels considerably lower than desired. Tablets with antacids containing magnesium, aluminum, as well as sucralfate, metal cations such as iron, and multivitamins preparations with zinc or Videx® (didanosine), chewable/buffered tablets or the pediatric powder for oral solution may substantially interfere with the gastrointestinal absorption of levofloxacin, resulting in systemic levels considerably lower than desired. These agents should be taken at least two hours before or two hours after levofloxacin administration.
LEVAQUIN Injection: There are no data concerning an interaction of **intravenous** quinolones with **oral** antacids, sucralfate, multivitamins, Videx® (didanosine), or metal cations. However, no quinolone should be co-administered with any solution containing multivalent cations, e.g., magnesium, through the same intravenous line. (See **DOSAGE AND ADMINISTRATION**.)

Theophylline: No significant effect of levofloxacin on the plasma concentrations, AUC, and other disposition parameters for theophylline was detected in a clinical study involving 14 healthy volunteers. Similarly, no apparent effect of theophylline on levofloxacin absorption and disposition was observed. However, concomitant administration of other quinolones with theophylline has resulted in prolonged elimination half-life, elevated serum theophylline levels, and a subsequent increase in the risk of theophylline-related adverse reactions in the patient population. Therefore, theophylline levels should be closely monitored and appropriate dosage adjustments made when levofloxacin is co-administered. Adverse reactions, including seizures, may occur with or without an elevation in serum theophylline levels. (See **WARNINGS** and **PRECAUTIONS: General**.)

Warfarin: No significant effect of levofloxacin on the peak plasma concentrations, AUC, and other disposition parameters for R- and S- warfarin was detected in a clinical study involving healthy volunteers. Similarly, no apparent effect of warfarin on levofloxacin absorption and disposition was observed. There have been reports during the post-marketing experience in patients that levofloxacin enhances the effects of warfarin. Elevations of the prothrombin time in the setting of concurrent warfarin and levofloxacin use have been associated with episodes of bleeding. Prothrombin time, International Normalized Ratio (INR), or other suitable anticoagulation tests should be closely monitored if levofloxacin is administered concomitantly with warfarin. Patients should also be monitored for evidence of bleeding.

Cyclosporine: No significant effect of levofloxacin on the peak plasma concentrations, AUC, and other disposition parameters for cyclosporine was detected in a clinical study involving healthy volunteers. However, elevated serum levels of cyclosporine have been reported in the patient population when co-administered with some other quinolones. Levofloxacin C_{max} and k_e were slightly lower while T_{max} and $t_{1/2}$ were slightly longer in the presence of cyclosporine than those observed in other studies without concomitant medication. The differences, however, are not considered to be clinically significant. Therefore, no dosage adjustment is required for levofloxacin or cyclosporine when administered concomitantly.

Digoxin: No significant effect of levofloxacin on the peak plasma concentrations, AUC, and other disposition parameters for digoxin was detected in a clinical study involving healthy volunteers. Levofloxacin absorption and disposition kinetics were similar in the presence or absence of digoxin. Therefore, no dosage adjustment for levofloxacin or digoxin is required when administered concomitantly.

Probenecid and Cimetidine: No significant effect of probenecid or cimetidine on the rate and extent of levofloxacin absorption was observed in a clinical study involving healthy volunteers. The AUC and $t_{1/2}$ of levofloxacin were 27-38% and 30% higher, respectively, while CL/F and CL_R were 21-35% lower during concomitant treatment with probenecid or cimetidine compared to levofloxacin alone. Although these differences were statistically significant, the changes were not high enough to warrant dosage adjustment for levofloxacin when probenecid or cimetidine is co-administered.

Non-steroidal anti-inflammatory drugs: The concomitant administration of a non-steroidal anti-inflammatory drug with a quinolone, including levofloxacin, may increase the risk of CNS stimulation and convulsive seizures. (See **WARNINGS** and **PRECAUTIONS: General**.)

Antidiabetic agents: Disturbances of blood glucose, including hyperglycemia and hypoglycemia, have been reported in patients treated concomitantly with quinolones and an antidiabetic agent. Therefore, careful monitoring of blood glucose is recommended when these agents are co-administered.

Carcinogenesis, Mutagenesis, Impairment of Fertility
In a lifetime bioassay in rats, levofloxacin exhibited no carcinogenic potential following daily dietary administration for 2 years; the highest dose (100 mg/kg/day) was 1.4 times the highest recommended human dose (750 mg) based upon relative body surface area. Levofloxacin did not shorten the time to tumor development of UV-induced skin tumors in hairless albino (Skh-1) mice at any levofloxacin dose level and was therefore not photo-carcinogenic under conditions of this study. Dermal levofloxacin concentrations in the hairless mice ranged from 25 to 42 µg/g at the highest levofloxacin dose level (300 mg/kg/day) used in the photo-carcinogenicity study. By comparison, dermal levofloxacin concentrations in human subjects receiving 750 mg of levofloxacin averaged approximately 11.8 µg/g at Cmax.
Levofloxacin was not mutagenic in the following assays; Ames bacterial mutation assay (*S. typhimurium* and *E. coli*), CHO/HGPRT forward mutation assay, mouse micronucleus test, mouse dominant lethal test, rat unscheduled DNA synthesis assay, and the mouse sister chromatid exchange assay. It was positive in the in vitro chromosomal aberration (CHL cell line) and sister chromatid exchange (CHL/IU cell line) assays.
Levofloxacin caused no impairment of fertility or reproductive performance in rats at oral doses as high as 360 mg/kg/day, corresponding to 4.2 times the highest recommended human dose based upon relative body surface area and intravenous doses as high as 100 mg/kg/day, corresponding to 1.2 times the highest recommended human dose based upon relative body surface area.

Pregnancy: Teratogenic Effects. Pregnancy Category C.
Levofloxacin was not teratogenic in rats at oral doses as high as 810 mg/kg/day which corresponds to 9.4 times the highest recommended human dose based upon relative body surface area, or at intravenous doses as high as 160 mg/kg/day corresponding to 1.9 times the highest recommended human dose based upon relative body surface area. The oral dose of 810 mg/kg/day to rats caused decreased fetal body weight and increased fetal mortality. No teratogenicity was observed when rabbits were dosed orally as high as 50 mg/kg/day which corresponds to 1.1 times the highest recommended human dose based upon relative body surface area, or when dosed intravenously as high as 25 mg/kg/day, corresponding to 0.5 times the highest recommended human dose based upon relative body surface area.
There are, however, no adequate and well-controlled studies in pregnant women. Levofloxacin should be used during pregnancy only if the potential benefit justifies the potential risk to the fetus. (See **WARNINGS**.)

Nursing Mothers
Levofloxacin has not been measured in human milk. Based upon data from ofloxacin, it can be presumed that levofloxacin will be excreted in human milk. Because of the potential for serious adverse reactions from levofloxacin in nursing infants, a decision should be made whether to discontinue nursing or to discontinue the drug, taking into account the importance of the drug to the mother.

Pediatric Use
Safety and effectiveness in pediatric patients and adolescents below the age of 18 years have not been established. Quinolones, including levofloxacin, cause arthropathy and osteochondrosis in juvenile animals of several species. (See **WARNINGS**.)

Geriatric Use
In phase 3 clinical trials, 1,190 levofloxacin-treated patients (25%) were ≥65 years of age. Of these, 675 patients (14%)

were between the ages of 65 and 74 and 515 patients (11%) were 75 years or older. No overall differences in safety or effectiveness were observed between these subjects and younger subjects, and other reported clinical experience has not identified differences in responses between the elderly and younger patients, but greater sensitivity of some older individuals cannot be ruled out.

The pharmacokinetic properties of levofloxacin in younger adults and elderly adults do not differ significantly when creatinine clearance is taken into consideration. However since the drug is known to be substantially excreted by the kidney, the risk of toxic reactions to this drug may be greater in patients with impaired renal function. Because elderly patients are more likely to have decreased renal function, care should be taken in dose selection, and it may be useful to monitor renal function.

ADVERSE REACTIONS

The incidence of drug-related adverse reactions in patients during Phase 3 clinical trials conducted in North America was 6.2%. Among patients receiving levofloxacin therapy, 4.1% discontinued levofloxacin therapy due to adverse experiences. The overall incidence, type and distribution of adverse events was similar in patients receiving levofloxacin doses of 750 mg once daily compared to patients receiving doses from 250 mg once daily to 500 mg twice daily.

In clinical trials, the following events were considered likely to be drug-related in patients receiving levofloxacin:

nausea 1.3%, diarrhea 1.0%, vaginitis 0.7%, insomnia 0.4%, abdominal pain 0.4%, flatulence 0.3%, pruritus 0.3%, dizziness 0.3%, dyspepsia 0.3%, rash 0.3%, genital moniliasis 0.2%, taste perversion 0.2%, vomiting 0.2%, constipation 0.1%, fungal infection 0.1%, genital pruritis 0.1%, headache 0.1%, moniliasis 0.1%, nervousness 0.1%, rash erythematous 0.1%, urticaria 0.1%.

In clinical trials, the following events occurred in >3% of patients, regardless of drug relationship:

nausea 7.0%, headache 6.1%, diarrhea 5.7%, insomnia 4.5%, injection site reaction 3.5%, constipation 3.3%.

In clinical trials, the following events occurred in 1 to 3% of patients, regardless of drug relationship:

dizziness 2.6%, abdominal pain 2.5%, dyspepsia 2.3%, vomiting 2.4%, vaginitis 1.8%, injection site pain 1.7%, flatulence 1.4%, pain 1.4%, pruritus 1.3%, sinusitis 1.3%, chest pain 1.2%, fatigue 1.3%, rash 1.4%, back pain 1.1%, injection site inflammation 1.1%, rhinitis 1.0%, taste perversion 1.0%.

In clinical trials, the following events, of potential medical importance, occurred at a rate of 0.1% to 1.0%, regardless of drug relationship:

[See first table at right]

In clinical trials using multiple-dose therapy, ophthalmologic abnormalities, including cataracts and multiple punctate lenticular opacities, have been noted in patients undergoing treatment with other quinolones. The relationship of the drugs to these events is not presently established.

Crystalluria and cylindruria have been reported with other quinolones.

The following markedly abnormal laboratory values appeared in >2% of patients receiving levofloxacin. It is not known whether these abnormalities were caused by the drug or the underlying condition being treated.

Blood Chemistry: decreased glucose (2.2%)

Hematology: decreased lymphocytes (2.4%)

Post-Marketing Adverse Reactions

Additional adverse events reported from worldwide post-marketing experience with levofloxacin include:

allergic pneumonitis, anaphylactic shock, anaphylactoid reaction, dysphonia, abnormal EEG, encephalopathy, eosinophilia, erythema multiforme, hemolytic anemia, multi-system organ failure, increased International Normalized Ratio (INR)/prothrombin time, Stevens-Johnson Syndrome, tendon rupture, torsades de pointes, vasodilation.

OVERDOSAGE

Levofloxacin exhibits a low potential for acute toxicity. Mice, rats, dogs and monkeys exhibited the following clinical signs after receiving a single high dose of levofloxacin: ataxia, ptosis, decreased locomotor activity, dyspnea, prostration, tremors, and convulsions. Doses in excess of 1500 mg/kg orally and 250 mg/kg i.v. produced significant mortality in rodents. In the event of an acute overdosage, the stomach should be emptied. The patient should be observed and appropriate hydration maintained. Levofloxacin is not efficiently removed by hemodialysis or peritoneal dialysis.

DOSAGE AND ADMINISTRATION

LEVAQUIN Injection should only be administered by intravenous infusion. It is not for intramuscular, intrathecal, intraperitoneal, or subcutaneous administration.

CAUTION: RAPID OR BOLUS INTRAVENOUS INFUSION MUST BE AVOIDED. Levofloxacin Injection should be infused intravenously slowly over a period of not less than 60 or 90 minutes, depending on the dosage. (See **PRECAUTIONS.**)

Single-use vials require dilution prior to administration. (See **PREPARATION FOR ADMINISTRATION.**)

The usual dose of LEVAQUIN Tablets or Injection is 250 mg or 500 mg administered orally or by slow infusion over 60 minutes every 24 hours, or 750 mg administered orally or by slow infusion over 90 minutes every 24 hours, as indicated by infection and described in the following dosing chart. These recommendations apply to patients with normal renal function (i.e., creatinine clearance > 80 mL/min). For patients with altered renal function see the **Patients with Impaired Renal Function** subsection. Oral doses should be administered at least two hours before or two hours after antacids containing magnesium, aluminum, as well as sucralfate, metal cations such as iron, and multivitamin preparations with zinc or Videx® (didanosine), chewable/buffered tablets or the pediatric powder for oral solution.

[See second table above]

[See third table above]

When only the serum creatinine is known, the following formula may be used to estimate creatinine clearance.

Men: Creatinine Clearance (mL/min) = $\dfrac{\text{Weight (kg)} \times (140 - \text{age})}{72 \times \text{serum creatinine (mg/dL)}}$

Women: 0.85 × the value calculated for men.

The serum creatinine should represent a steady state of renal function.

Preparation of Levofloxacin Injection for Administration

LEVAQUIN Injection in Single-Use Vials: LEVAQUIN Injection is supplied in single-use vials containing a concentrated levofloxacin solution with the equivalent of 500 mg (20 mL vial) and 750 mg (30 mL vial) of levofloxacin in Water for Injection, USP. The 20 mL and 30 mL vials each contain 25 mg of levofloxacin/mL. **THESE LEVAQUIN INJECTION SINGLE-USE VIALS MUST BE FURTHER DILUTED WITH AN APPROPRIATE SOLUTION PRIOR TO INTRAVENOUS ADMINISTRATION.** (See **COMPATIBLE INTRAVENOUS SOLUTIONS.**) The concentration of the resulting diluted solution should be 5 mg/mL prior to administration. This intravenous drug product should be inspected visually for particulate matter prior to administration. Samples containing visible particles should be discarded.

Since no preservative or bacteriostatic agent is present in this product, aseptic technique must be used in preparation of the final intravenous solution. **Since the vials are for single-use only, any unused portion remaining in the vial should be discarded. When used to prepare two**

Continued on next page

Autonomic Nervous System Disorders:	Postural hypotension
Body as a Whole – General Disorders:	Asthenia, fever, malaise, rigors, substernal chest pain, syncope, enlarged abdomen, allergic reaction, headache, hot flashes, edema, influenza-like symptoms, leg pain, multiple organ failure
Cardiovascular Disorders, General:	Cardiac failure, circulatory failure, hypertension, hypotension, postural hypotension
Central and Peripheral Nervous System Disorders:	Abnormal coordination, coma, convulsions (seizures), hyperkinesia, hypertonia, hypoesthesia, involuntary muscle contractions, paresthesia, paralysis, speech disorder, stupor, tremor, vertigo, encephalopathy abnormal gait, leg cramps, intracranial hypertension
Gastro-Intestinal System Disorders:	Dry mouth, dysphagia, gastroenteritis, G.I. hemorrhage, pancreatitis, pseudomembranous colitis, tongue edema, gastritis, gastroesophageal reflux, melena, esophagitis, stomatitis
Hearing and Vestibular Disorders:	Earache, tinnitus
Heart Rate and Rhythm Disorders:	Arrhythmia, atrial fibrillation, bradycardia, cardiac arrest, palpitation, supraventricular tachycardia, ventricular tachycardia, tachycardia
Liver and Biliary System Disorders:	Elevated bilirubin, abnormal hepatic function, cholelithiasis, jaundice, hepatic failure
Metabolic and Nutritional Disorders:	Hypomagnesemia, thirst, aggravated diabetes mellitus, dehydration, hyperglycemia, hyperkalemia, hypoglycemia, hypokalemia
Musculo-Skeletal System Disorders:	Arthralgia, arthritis, arthrosis, pathological fracture, myalgia, osteomyelitis, synovitis, tendinitis
Myo, Endo, Pericardial and Valve Disorders:	Angina pectoris, myocardial infarction
Neoplasms:	Carcinoma
Other Special Senses Disorders:	Parosmia, taste perversion
Platelet, Bleeding and Clotting Disorders:	Pulmonary embolism, hematoma, epistaxis, purpura, thrombocytopenia
Psychiatric Disorders:	Abnormal dreaming, agitation, anorexia, anxiety, confusion, depression, hallucination, nervousness, paranoia, sleep disorder, somnolence
Red Blood Cell Disorders:	Anemia
Reproductive Disorders:	Dysmenorrhea, leukorrhea
Resistance Mechanism Disorders:	Abscess, herpes simplex, bacterial infection, viràl infection, moniliasis, otitis media, sepsis, fungal infection
Respiratory System Disorders:	Bronchitis, epistaxis, pharyngitis, rhinitis, upper respiratory tract infection, asthma, coughing, dyspnea, hemoptysis, hypoxia, pleural effusion, respiratory insufficiency
Skin and Appendages Disorders:	Rash, dry skin, genital pruritus, increased sweating, skin disorder, skin exfoliation, skin ulceration, urticaria
Urinary System Disorders:	Urinary tract infection, abnormal renal function, acute renal failure, hematuria
Vascular (Extracardiac) Disorders:	Cerebrovascular disorder, phlebitis, purpura, thrombophlebitis (deep)
Vision Disorders:	Abnormal vision, conjunctivitis
White Cell and RES Disorders:	Granulocytopenia, leukocytosis, lymphadenopathy, WBC abnormal (not otherwise specified)

Patients with Normal Renal Function

Infection*	Unit Dose	Freq.	Duration**	Daily Dose
Acute Bacterial Exacerbation of Chronic Bronchitis	500 mg	q24h	7 days	500 mg
Nosocomial Pneumonia	750 mg	q24h	7-14 days	750 mg
Comm. Acquired Pneumonia	500 mg	q24h	7-14 days	500 mg
Acute Maxillary Sinusitis	500 mg	q24h	10-14 days	500 mg
Complicated SSSI	750 mg	q24h	7-14 days	750 mg
Uncomplicated SSSI	500 mg	q24h	7-10 days	500 mg
Complicated UTI	250 mg	q24h	10 days	250 mg
Acute pyelonephritis	250 mg	q24h	10 days	250 mg
Uncomplicated UTI	250 mg	q24h	3 days	250 mg

* **DUE TO THE DESIGNATED PATHOGENS** (See **INDICATIONS AND USAGE.**)
** Sequential therapy (intravenous to oral) may be instituted at the discretion of the physician.

Patients with Impaired Renal Function

Renal Status	Initial Dose	Subsequent Dose
Acute Bacterial Exacerbation of Chronic Bronchitis/ Comm. Acquired Pneumonia/Acute Maxillary Sinusitis/Uncomplicated SSSI		
CL_{CR} from 50 to 80 mL/min	No dosage adjustment required	
CL_{CR} from 20 to 49 mL/min	500 mg	250 mg q24h
CL_{CR} from 10 to 19 mL/min	500 mg	250 mg q48h
Hemodialysis	500 mg	250 mg q48h
CAPD	500 mg	250 mg q48h
Complicated SSSI/Nosocomial Pneumonia		
CL_{CR} from 50 to 80 mL/min	No dosage adjustment required	
CL_{CR} from 20 to 49 mL/min	750 mg	750 mg q48h
CL_{CR} from 10 to 19 mL/min	750 mg	500 mg q48h
Hemodialysis	750 mg	500 mg q48h
CAPD	750 mg	500 mg q48h
Complicated UTI/Acute Pyelonephritis		
CL_{CR} ≥20 mL/min	No dosage adjustment required	
CL_{CR} from 10 to 19 mL/min	250 mg	250 mg q48h
Uncomplicated UTI	No dosage adjustment required	

CL_{CR}=creatinine clearances
CAPD=chronic ambulatory peritoneal dialysis

Levaquin—Cont.

250 mg doses from the 20 mL vial containing 500 mg of levofloxacin, the full content of the vial should be withdrawn at once using a single-entry procedure, and a second dose should be prepared and stored for subsequent use. (See Stability of LEVAQUIN Injection Following Dilution.)

Since only limited data are available on the compatibility of levofloxacin intravenous injection with other intravenous substances, **additives or other medications should not be added to LEVAQUIN Injection in single-use vials or infused simultaneously through the same intravenous line.** If the same intravenous line is used for sequential infusion of several different drugs, the line should be flushed before and after infusion of LEVAQUIN Injection with an infusion solution compatible with LEVAQUIN Injection and with any other drug(s) administered via this common line.

Prepare the desired dosage of levofloxacin according to the following chart:
[See table below]

For example, to prepare a 500 mg dose using the 20 mL vial (25 mg/mL), withdraw 20 mL and dilute with a compatible intravenous solution to a total volume of 100 mL.

Compatible Intravenous Solutions: Any of the following intravenous solutions may be used to prepare a 5 mg/mL levofloxacin solution with the approximate pH values:

Intravenous Fluids	Final pH of LEVAQUIN Solution
0.9% Sodium Chloride Injection, USP	4.71
5% Dextrose Injection, USP	4.58
5% Dextrose/0.9% NaCl Injection	4.62
5% Dextrose in Lactated Ringers	4.92
Plasma-Lyte® 56/5% Dextrose Injection	5.03
5% Dextrose, 0.45% Sodium Chloride, and 0.15% Potassium Chloride Injection	4.61
Sodium Lactate Injection (M/6)	5.54

LEVAQUIN Injection Premix in Single-Use Flexible Containers: LEVAQUIN Injection is also supplied in flexible containers containing a premixed, ready-to-use levofloxacin solution in D_5W for single-use. The fill volume is either 50 or 100 mL for the 100 mL flexible container or 150 mL for the 150 mL container. **NO FURTHER DILUTION OF THESE PREPARATIONS ARE NECESSARY. Consequently each 50 mL, 100 mL, and 150 mL premix flexible container already contains a dilute solution with the equivalent of 250 mg, 500 mg, and 750 mg of levofloxacin, respectively (5 mg/mL) in 5% Dextrose (D_5W).**

This parenteral drug product should be inspected visually for particulate matter prior to administration. Samples containing visible particles should be discarded.

Since the premix flexible containers are for single-use only, any unused portion should be discarded.

Since only limited data are available on the compatibility of levofloxacin intravenous injection with other intravenous substances, **additives or other medications should not be added to LEVAQUIN Injection in flexible containers or infused simultaneously through the same intravenous line.** If the same intravenous line is used for sequential infusion of several different drugs, the line should be flushed before and after infusion of LEVAQUIN Injection with an infusion solution compatible with LEVAQUIN Injection and with any other drug(s) administered via this common line.

Instructions for the Use of LEVAQUIN Injection Premix in Flexible Containers
To open:
1. Tear outer wrap at the notch and remove solution container.
2. Check the container for minute leaks by squeezing the inner bag firmly. If leaks are found, or if the seal is not intact, discard the solution, as the sterility may be compromised.
3. Do not use if the solution is cloudy or a precipitate is present.
4. Use sterile equipment.
5. **WARNING: Do not use flexible containers in series connections.** Such use could result in air embolism due to residual air being drawn from the primary container before administration of the fluid from the secondary container is complete.

Preparation for administration:
1. Close flow control clamp of administration set.
2. Remove cover from port at bottom of container.
3. Insert piercing pin of administration set into port with a twisting motion until the pin is firmly seated. **NOTE: See full directions on administration set carton.**
4. Suspend container from hanger.
5. Squeeze and release drip chamber to establish proper fluid level in chamber during infusion of LEVAQUIN Injection in Premix Flexible Containers.
6. Open flow control clamp to expel air from set. Close clamp.
7. Regulate rate of administration with flow control clamp.

Stability of LEVAQUIN Injection as Supplied
When stored under recommended conditions, LEVAQUIN Injection, as supplied in 20 mL and 30 mL vials, or 100 mL and 150 mL flexible containers, is stable through the expiration date printed on the label.

Stability of LEVAQUIN Injection Following Dilution
LEVAQUIN Injection, when diluted in a compatible intravenous fluid to a concentration of 5 mg/mL, is stable for 72 hours when stored at or below 25°C (77°F) and for 14 days when stored under refrigeration at 5°C (41°F) in plastic intravenous containers. Solutions that are diluted in a compatible intravenous solution and frozen in glass bottles or plastic intravenous containers are stable for 6 months when stored at −20°C (−4°F). **THAW FROZEN SOLUTIONS AT ROOM TEMPERATURE 25°C (77°F) OR IN A REFRIGERATOR 8°C (46°F). DO NOT FORCE THAW BY MICROWAVE IRRADIATION OR WATER BATH IMMERSION. DO NOT REFREEZE AFTER INITIAL THAWING.**

HOW SUPPLIED
LEVAQUIN Tablets
LEVAQUIN (levofloxacin) Tablets are supplied as 250, 500, and 750 mg modified rectangular, film-coated tablets. LEVAQUIN Tablets are packaged in bottles and in unit-dose blister strips in the following configurations:

250 mg tablets: color: terra cotta pink
 debossing: "LEVAQUIN" on side 1 and "250" on side 2
 bottles of 50 (NDC 0045-1520-50)
 unit-dose/100 tablets (NDC 0045-1520-10)
500 mg tablets: color: peach
 debossing: "LEVAQUIN" on side 1 and "500" on side 2
 bottles of 50 (NDC 0045-1525-50)
 unit-dose/100 tablets (NDC 0045-1525-10)
750 mg tablets: color: white
 debossing: "LEVAQUIN" on side 1 and "750" on side 2
 bottles of 50 (NDC 0045-1530-50)
 unit-dose/100 tablets (NDC 0045-1530-10)

LEVAQUIN Tablets should be stored at 15° to 30°C (59° to 86°F) in well-closed containers.

LEVAQUIN Tablets are manufactured for OMP DIVISION, ORTHO-McNEIL PHARMACEUTICAL, INC. by Janssen Ortho LLC, Gurabo, Puerto Rico 00778.

LEVAQUIN Injection
Single-Use Vials: LEVAQUIN (levofloxacin) Injection is supplied in single-use vials. Each vial contains a concentrated solution with the equivalent of 500 mg of levofloxacin in 20 mL vials and 750 mg of levofloxacin in 30 mL vials.
25 mg/mL, 20 mL vials (NDC 0045-0069-51)
25 mg/mL, 30 mL vials (NDC 0045-0065-55)
LEVAQUIN Injection in Single-Use Vials should be stored at controlled room temperature and protected from light.
LEVAQUIN Injection in Single-Use Vials is manufactured for OMP DIVISION, ORTHO-McNEIL PHARMACEUTICAL, INC. by OMJ Pharmaceuticals, Inc., San German, Puerto Rico, 00683.

Premix in Flexible Containers: LEVAQUIN (levofloxacin in 5% dextrose) Injection is supplied as a single-use, premixed solution in flexible containers. Each bag contains a dilute solution with the equivalent of 250, 500, or 750 mg of levofloxacin, respectively, in 5% Dextrose (D_5W).
5 mg/mL (250 mg), 50 mL flexible container (NDC 0045-0067-01)
5 mg/mL (500 mg), 100 mL flexible container (NDC 0045-0068-01)
5 mg/mL (750 mg), 150 mL flexible container (NDC 0045-0066-01)

LEVAQUIN Injection Premix in Flexible Containers should be stored at or below 25°C (77°F); however, brief exposure up to 40°C (104°F) does not adversely affect the product. Avoid excessive heat and protect from freezing and light.

LEVAQUIN Injection Premix in Flexible Containers is manufactured for OMP DIVISION, ORTHO-McNEIL PHARMACEUTICAL, INC. by ABBOTT Laboratories, North Chicago, IL 60064.

CLINICAL STUDIES
Nosocomial Pneumonia
Adult patients with clinically and radiologically documented nosocomial pneumonia were enrolled in a multi-center, randomized, open-label study comparing intravenous levofloxacin (750 mg once daily) followed by oral levofloxacin (750 mg once daily) for a total of 7-15 days to intravenous imipenem/cilastatin (500-1000 mg q6-8 hours daily) followed by oral ciprofloxacin (750 mg q12 hours daily) for a total of 7-15 days. Levofloxacin-treated patients received an average of 7 days of intravenous therapy (range: 1-16 days); comparator-treated patients received an average of 8 days of intravenous therapy (range: 1-19 days).

Overall, in the clinically and microbiologically evaluable population, adjunctive therapy was empirically initiated at study entry in 56 of 93 (60.2%) patients in the levofloxacin arm and 53 of 94 (56.4%) patients in the comparator arm. The average duration of adjunctive therapy was 7 days in the levofloxacin arm and 7 days in the comparator. In clinically and microbiologically evaluable patients with documented *Pseudomonas aeruginosa* infection, 15 of 17 (88.2%) received ceftazidime (N=11) or piperacillin/tazobactam (N=4) in the levofloxacin arm and 16 of 17 (94.1%) received an aminoglycoside in the comparator arm. Overall, in clinically and microbiologically evaluable patients, vancomycin was added to the treatment regimen of 37 of 93 (39.8%) patients in the levofloxacin arm and 28 of 94 (29.8%) patients in the comparator arm for suspected methicillin-resistant *S. aureus* infection.

Clinical success rates in clinically and microbiologically evaluable patients at the posttherapy visit (primary study endpoint assessed on day 3-15 after completing therapy) were 58.1% for levofloxacin and 60.6% for comparator. The 95% CI for the difference of response rates (levofloxacin minus comparator) was [-17.2, 12.0]. The microbiological eradication rates at the posttherapy visit were 66.7% for levofloxacin and 60.6% for comparator. The 95% CI for the difference of eradication rates (levofloxacin minus comparator) was [-8.3, 20.3]. Clinical success and microbiological eradication rates by pathogen were as follows:
[See table at bottom of next page]

Community-Acquired Bacterial Pneumonia
Adult inpatients and outpatients with a diagnosis of community-acquired bacterial pneumonia were evaluated in two pivotal clinical studies. In the first study, 590 patients were enrolled in a prospective, multicenter, unblinded randomized trial comparing levofloxacin 500 mg once daily orally or intravenously for 7 to 14 days to ceftriaxone 1 to 2 grams intravenously once or in equally divided doses twice daily followed by cefuroxime axetil 500 mg orally twice daily for a total of 7 to 14 days. Patients assigned to treatment with the control regimen were allowed to receive erythromycin (or doxycycline if intolerant of erythromycin) if an infection due to atypical pathogens was suspected or proven. Clinical and microbiologic evaluations were performed during treatment, 5 to 7 days posttherapy, and 3 to 4 weeks posttherapy. Clinical success (cure plus improvement) with levofloxacin at 5 to 7 days posttherapy, the primary efficacy variable in this study, was superior (95%) to the control group (83%). The 95% CI for the difference of response rates (levofloxacin minus comparator) was [-6, 19]. In the second study, 264 patients were enrolled in a prospective, multi-center, non-comparative trial of 500 mg levofloxacin administered orally or intravenously once daily for 7 to 14 days. Clinical success for clinically evaluable patients was 93%. For both studies, the clinical success rate in patients with atypical pneumonia due to *Chlamydia pneumoniae*, *Mycoplasma pneumoniae*, and *Legionella pneumophila* were 96%, 96%, and 70%, respectively. Microbiologic eradication rates across both studies were as follows:

Pathogen	No. Pathogens	Microbiologic Eradication Rate (%)
H. influenzae	55	98
S. pneumoniae	83	95
S. aureus	17	88
M. catarrhalis	18	94
H. parainfluenzae	19	95
K. pneumoniae	10	100.0

Additional studies were initiated to evaluate the utility of LEVAQUIN in community-acquired pneumonia due to *S. pneumoniae*, with particular interest in penicillin-resistant strains (MIC value for penicillin ≥2 µg/mL). In addition to the studies previously discussed, inpatients and outpatients with mild to severe community-acquired pneumonia were evaluated in six additional clinical studies; one double-blind study, two open label randomized studies, and three open label non-comparative studies. The total number of clinically evaluable patients with *S. pneumoniae* across all 8 studies was 250 for levofloxacin and 41 for comparators. The clinical success rate (cured or improved) among the 250 levofloxacin-treated patients with *S. pneumoniae* was 245/250 (98%). The clinical success rate among the 41 comparator-treated patients with *S. pneumoniae* was 39/41 (95%). Across these 8 studies, 18 levofloxacin-treated and 4 non-quinolone comparator-treated patients with community-acquired pneumonia due to penicillin-resistant *S. pneumoniae* (MIC value for penicillin ≥2 µg/mL) were identified. Of the 18 levofloxacin-treated patients, 15 were evaluable following the completion of therapy. Fifteen out of the 15 evaluable levofloxacin-treated patients with community-acquired pneumonia due to penicillin-resistant *S. pneumoniae* achieved clinical success (cure or improvement). Of these 15 patients, 6 were bacteremic and 5 were classified as having severe disease. Of the 4 comparator-treated patients with community-acquired pneumonia due to penicillin-resistant *S. pneumoniae*, 3 were evaluable for clinical efficacy. Three out of the 3 evaluable comparator-treated patients achieved clinical success. All three of the comparator-treated patients were bacteremic and had disease classified as severe.

Complicated Skin and Skin Structure Infections
Three hundred ninety-nine patients were enrolled in an open-label, randomized, comparative study for complicated skin and skin structure infections. The patients were randomized to receive either levofloxacin 750mg QD (IV followed by oral), or an approved comparator for a median of 10 ± 4.7 days. As is expected in complicated skin and skin structure infections, surgical procedures were performed in the levofloxacin and comparator groups. Surgery (incision and drainage or debridement) was performed on 45% of the levofloxacin treated patients and 44% of the comparator treated patients, either shortly before or during antibiotic treatment and formed an integral part of therapy for this indication.

Desired Dosage Strength	From Appropriate Vial, Withdraw Volume	Volume of Diluent	Infusion Time
250 mg	10 mL (20 mL Vial)	40 mL	60 min
500 mg	20 mL (20 mL Vial)	80 mL	60 min
750 mg	30 mL (30 mL Vial)	120 mL	90 min

Among those who could be evaluated clinically 2-5 days after completion of study drug, overall success rates (improved or cured) were 116/138 (84.1%) for patients treated with levofloxacin and 106/132 (80.3%) for patients treated with the comparator.

Success rates varied with the type of diagnosis ranging from 68% in patients with infected ulcers to 90% in patients with infected wounds and abscesses. These rates were equivalent to those seen with comparator drugs.

ANIMAL PHARMACOLOGY

Levofloxacin and other quinolones have been shown to cause arthropathy in immature animals of most species tested. (See **WARNINGS.**) In immature dogs (4–5 months old), oral doses of 10 mg/kg/day for 7 days and intravenous doses of 4 mg/kg/day for 14 days of levofloxacin resulted in arthropathic lesions. Administration at oral doses of 300 mg/kg/day for 7 days and intravenous doses of 60 mg/kg/day for 4 weeks produced arthropathy in juvenile rats.

When tested in a mouse ear swelling bioassay, levofloxacin exhibited phototoxicity similar in magnitude to ofloxacin, but less phototoxicity than other quinolones.

While crystalluria has been observed in some intravenous rat studies, urinary crystals are not formed in the bladder, being present only after micturition and are not associated with nephrotoxicity.

In mice, the CNS stimulatory effect of quinolones is enhanced by concomitant administration of non-steroidal anti-inflammatory drugs.

In dogs, levofloxacin administered at 6 mg/kg or higher by rapid intravenous injection produced hypotensive effects. These effects were considered to be related to histamine release.

In vitro and in vivo studies in animals indicate that levofloxacin is neither an enzyme inducer or inhibitor in the human therapeutic plasma concentration range; therefore, no drug metabolizing enzyme-related interactions with other drugs or agents are anticipated.

REFERENCES

1. National Committee for Clinical Laboratory Standards. Methods for Dilution Antimicrobial Susceptibility Tests for Bacteria That Grow Aerobically Fifth Edition. Approved Standard NCCLS Document M7-A5, Vol. 20, No. 2, NCCLS, Wayne, PA, January, 2000.
2. National Committee for Clinical Laboratory Standards. Performance Standards for Antimicrobial Disk Susceptibility Tests Seventh Edition. Approved Standard NCCLS Document M2-A7, Vol. 20, No. 1, NCCLS, Wayne, PA, January, 2000.

Patient Information About:
LEVAQUIN®
(levofloxacin) Tablets
250 mg Tablets, 500 mg Tablets, and 750 mg Tablets

This leaflet contains important information about LEVAQUIN® (levofloxacin), and should be read completely before you begin treatment. This leaflet does not take the place of discussions with your doctor or health care professional about your medical condition or your treatment. This leaflet does not list all benefits and risks of LEVAQUIN®. The medicine described here can be prescribed only by a licensed health care professional. If you have any questions about LEVAQUIN® talk to your health care professional. Only your health care professional can determine if LEVAQUIN® is right for you.

What is LEVAQUIN®?

LEVAQUIN® is a quinolone antibiotic used to treat lung, sinus, skin, and urinary tract infections caused by certain germs called bacteria. LEVAQUIN® kills many of the types of bacteria that can infect the lungs, sinuses, skin, and urinary tract and has been shown in a large number of clinical trials to be safe and effective for the treatment of bacterial infections.

Sometimes viruses rather than bacteria may infect the lungs and sinuses (for example the common cold). LEVAQUIN®, like other antibiotics, does not kill viruses.

You should contact your health care professional if you think that your condition is not improving while taking LEVAQUIN®. LEVAQUIN® Tablets are terra cotta pink for the 250 mg tablet, peach colored for the 500 mg tablet, or white for the 750 mg tablet.

How and when should I take LEVAQUIN®?

LEVAQUIN® should be taken once a day for 3, 7, 10, or 14 days depending on your prescription. It should be swallowed and may be taken with or without food. Try to take the tablet at the same time each day and drink fluids liberally.

You may begin to feel better quickly; however, in order to make sure that all bacteria are killed, you should complete the full course of medication. Do not take more than the prescribed dose of LEVAQUIN® even if you missed a dose by mistake. You should not take a double dose.

Who should not take LEVAQUIN®?

You should not take LEVAQUIN® if you have ever had a severe allergic reaction to any of the group of antibiotics known as "quinolones" such as ciprofloxacin. Serious and occasionally fatal allergic reactions have been reported in patients receiving therapy with quinolones, including LEVAQUIN®.

If you are pregnant or are planning to become pregnant while taking LEVAQUIN®, talk to your health care professional before taking this medication. LEVAQUIN® is not recommended for use during pregnancy or nursing, as the effects on the unborn child or nursing infant are unknown. LEVAQUIN® is not recommended for children.

What are possible side effects of LEVAQUIN®?

LEVAQUIN® is generally well tolerated. The most common side effects caused by LEVAQUIN®, which are usually mild, include nausea, diarrhea, itching, abdominal pain, dizziness, flatulence, rash and vaginitis in women.

You should be careful about driving or operating machinery until you are sure LEVAQUIN® is not causing dizziness.

Allergic reactions have been reported in patients receiving quinolones including LEVAQUIN®, even after just one dose. If you develop hives, skin rash or other symptoms of an allergic reaction, you should stop taking this medication and call your health care professional.

Ruptures of shoulder, hand, or Achilles tendons have been reported in patients receiving quinolones, including LEVAQUIN®. If you develop pain, swelling, or rupture of a tendon you should stop taking LEVAQUIN® and contact your health care professional.

Some quinolone antibiotics have been associated with the development of phototoxicity ("sunburns" and "blistering sunburns") following exposure to sunlight or other sources of ultraviolet light such as artificial ultraviolet light used in tanning salons. LEVAQUIN® has been infrequently associated with phototoxicity. You should avoid excessive exposure to sunlight or artificial ultraviolet light while you are taking LEVAQUIN®.

If you have diabetes and you develop a hypoglycemic reaction while on LEVAQUIN®, you should stop taking LEVAQUIN® and call your health care professional.

Convulsions have been reported in patients receiving quinolone antibiotics including LEVAQUIN®. If you have experienced convulsions in the past, be sure to let your physician know that you have a history of convulsions.

Quinolones, including LEVAQUIN®, may also cause central nervous system stimulation which may lead to tremors, restlessness, anxiety, lightheadedness, confusion, hallucinations, paranoia, depression, nightmares, insomnia, and rarely, suicidal thoughts or acts.

If you notice any side effects not mentioned in this leaflet or you have concerns about the side effects you are experiencing, please inform your health care professional.

For more complete information regarding levofloxacin, please refer to the full prescribing information, which may be obtained from your health care professional, pharmacist, or the Physicians' Desk Reference (PDR).

What about other medicines I am taking?

Taking warfarin (Coumadin®) and LEVAQUIN® together can further predispose you to the development of bleeding problems. If you take warfarin, be sure to tell your health care professional.

Many antacids and multivitamins may interfere with the absorption of LEVAQUIN® and may prevent it from working properly. You should take LEVAQUIN® either 2 hours before or 2 hours after taking these products.

It is important to let your health care professional know all of the medicines you are using.

Other information

Take your dose of LEVAQUIN® once a day.

Complete the course of medication even if you are feeling better.

Keep this medication out of the reach of children.

This information does not take the place of discussions with your doctor or health care professional about your medical condition or your treatment.

Pathogen	N	Levofloxacin No. (%) of Patients Microbiologic / Clinical Outcomes	N	Imipenem/Cilastatin No. (%) of Patients Microbiologic / Clinical Outcomes
MSSA[a]	21	14 (66.7) / 13 (61.9)	19	13 (68.4) / 15 (78.9)
P. aeruginosa[b]	17	10 (58.8) / 11 (64.7)	17	5 (29.4) / 7 (41.2)
S. marcescens	11	9 (81.8) / 7 (63.6)	7	2 (28.6) / 3 (42.9)
E. coli	12	10 (83.3) / 7 (58.3)	11	7 (63.6) / 8 (72.7)
K. pneumoniae[c]	11	9 (81.8) / 5 (45.5)	7	6 (85.7) / 3 (42.9)
H. influenzae	16	13 (81.3) / 10 (62.5)	15	14 (93.3) / 11 (73.3)
S. pneumoniae	4	3 (75.0) / 3 (75.0)	7	5 (71.4) / 4 (57.1)

[a] Methicillin-susceptible *S. aureus*.
[b] See above text for use of combination therapy.
[c] The observed differences in rates for the clinical and microbiological outcomes may reflect other factors that were not accounted for in the study.

ORTHO-McNEIL
OMP DIVISION
ORTHO-McNEIL PHARMACEUTICAL, INC.
Raritan, New Jersey, USA 08869
U.S. Patent No. 4,382,892 and U.S. Patent No. 5,053,407
7518205
 633-10-816-6
Revised November 2002

Parke-Davis

A Warner-Lambert Division
A Pfizer Company
201 TABOR ROAD
MORRIS PLAINS, NEW JERSEY 07950

For Medical Information Contact:
(800) 438-1985
24 hours a day, seven days a week.

Distribution:
1855 Shelby Oaks Drive North
Memphis, TN 38134
(901) 387-5200
Customer Service:
(800) 533-4535

EXPORT INQUIRIES:
Pfizer International Inc.
(212) 573-2323

LOPID® ℞

[lō′pĭd]
(Gemfibrozil Tablets, USP)

Prescribing information for this product, which appears on pages 2559–2563 of the 2003 PDR, has been completely revised as follows. Please write "See Supplement A" next to the product heading.

DESCRIPTION

LOPID® (gemfibrozil tablets, USP) is a lipid regulating agent. It is available as tablets for oral administration. Each tablet contains 600 mg gemfibrozil. Each also contains calcium stearate, NF; candelilla wax, FCC; microcrystalline cellulose, NF; hydroxypropyl cellulose, NF; hydroxypropylmethylcellulose, USP; methylparaben, NF; Opaspray white; polyethylene glycol, NF; polysorbate 80, NF; propylparaben, NF; colloidal silicon dioxide, NF; pregelatinized starch, NF.

The chemical name is 5-(2,5-dimethylphenoxy)-2,2-dimethylpentanoic acid, with the following structural formula:

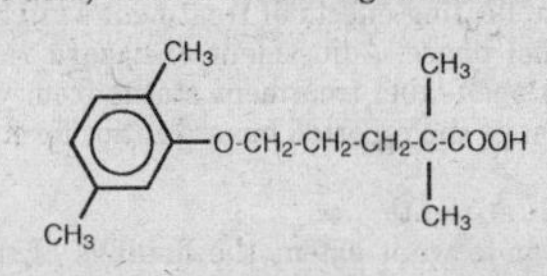
CH3
CH3
O-CH2-CH2-CH2-C-COOH
CH3
CH3

The empirical formula is $C_{15}H_{22}O_3$ and the molecular weight is 250.35; the solubility in water and acid is 0.0019% and in dilute base it is greater than 1%. The melting point is 58°-61° C. Gemfibrozil is a white solid which is stable under ordinary conditions.

CLINICAL PHARMACOLOGY

LOPID (gemfibrozil tablets, USP) is a lipid regulating agent which decreases serum triglycerides and very low density lipoprotein (VLDL) cholesterol, and increases high density lipoprotein (HDL) cholesterol. While modest decreases in total and low density lipoprotein (LDL) cholesterol may be observed with LOPID therapy, treatment of patients with elevated triglycerides due to Type IV hyperlipoproteinemia often results in a rise in LDL-cholesterol. LDL-cholesterol levels in Type IIb patients with elevations of both serum LDL-cholesterol and triglycerides are, in general, minimally affected by LOPID treatment; however, LOPID usually raises HDL-cholesterol significantly in this group. LOPID increases levels of high density lipoprotein (HDL) subfractions HDL_2 and HDL_3, as well as apolipoproteins AI and AII. Epidemiological studies have shown that both low HDL-cholesterol and high LDL-cholesterol are independent risk factors for coronary heart disease.

In the primary prevention component of the Helsinki Heart Study (refs. 1,2), in which 4081 male patients between the ages of 40 and 55 were studied in a randomized, double-blind, placebo-controlled fashion, LOPID therapy was associated with significant reductions in total plasma triglycerides and a significant increase in high density lipoprotein cholesterol. Moderate reductions in total plasma cholesterol and low density lipoprotein cholesterol were observed for the LOPID treatment group as a whole, but the lipid response was heterogeneous, especially among different Fredrickson types. The study involved subjects with serum non-HDL-cholesterol of over 200 mg/dL and no previous history of coronary heart disease. Over the five-year study period, the LOPID group experienced a 1.4% absolute (34% relative) reduction in the rate of serious coronary events (sudden cardiac deaths plus fatal and nonfatal myocardial infarctions) compared to placebo, p=0.04 (see Table I). There was a 37% relative reduction in the rate of nonfatal myocardial infarction compared to placebo, equivalent to a treat-

Continued on next page

Lopid—Cont.

ment-related difference of 13.1 events per thousand persons. Deaths from any cause during the double-blind portion of the study totaled 44 (2.2%) in the LOPID randomization group and 43 (2.1%) in the placebo group.
[See table I at right]

Among Fredrickson types, during the 5-year double-blind portion of the primary prevention component of the Helsinki Heart Study, the greatest reduction in the incidence of serious coronary events occurred in Type IIb patients who had elevations of both LDL-cholesterol and total plasma triglycerides. This subgroup of Type IIb gemfibrozil group patients had a lower mean HDL-cholesterol level at baseline than the Type IIa subgroup that had elevations of LDL-cholesterol and normal plasma triglycerides. The mean increase in HDL-cholesterol among the Type IIb patients in this study was 12.6% compared to placebo. The mean change in LDL-cholesterol among Type IIb patients was −4.1% with LOPID compared to a rise of 3.9% in the placebo subgroup. The Type IIb subjects in the Helsinki Heart Study had 26 fewer coronary events per thousand persons over five years in the gemfibrozil group compared to placebo. The difference in coronary events was substantially greater between LOPID and placebo for that subgroup of patients with the triad of LDL-cholesterol >175 mg/dL (>4.5 mmol), triglycerides >200 mg/dL (>2.2 mmol), and HDL-cholesterol <35 mg/dL (<0.90 mmol) (see Table I).

Further information is available from a 3.5 year (8.5 year cumulative) follow-up of all subjects who had participated in the Helsinki Heart Study. At the completion of the Helsinki Heart Study, subjects could choose to start, stop, or continue to receive LOPID; without knowledge of their own lipid values or double-blind treatment, 60% of patients originally randomized to placebo began therapy with LOPID and 60% of patients originally randomized to LOPID continued medication. After approximately 6.5 years following randomization, all patients were informed of their original treatment group and lipid values during the five years of the double-blind treatment. After further elective changes in LOPID treatment status, 61% of patients in the group originally randomized to LOPID were taking drug; in the group originally randomized to placebo, 65% were taking LOPID. The event rate per 1000 occurring during the open-label follow-up period is detailed in Table II.
[See table II at right]

Cumulative mortality through 8.5 years showed a 20% relative excess of deaths in the group originally randomized to LOPID versus the originally randomized placebo group and a 20% relative decrease in cardiac events in the group originally randomized to LOPID versus the originally randomized placebo group (see Table III). This analysis of the originally randomized "intent-to-treat" population neglects the possible complicating effects of treatment switching during the open-label phase. Adjustment of hazard ratios taking into account open-label treatment status from years 6.5 to 8.5 could change the reported hazard ratios for mortality toward unity.
[See table III at right]

It is not clear to what extent the findings of the primary prevention component of the Helsinki Heart Study can be extrapolated to other segments of the dyslipidemic population not studied (such as women, younger or older males, or those with lipid abnormalities limited solely to HDL-cholesterol) or to other lipid-altering drugs.

The secondary prevention component of the Helsinki Heart Study was conducted over five years in parallel and at the same centers in Finland in 628 middle-aged males excluded from the primary prevention component of the Helsinki Heart Study because of a history of angina, myocardial infarction or unexplained ECG changes (ref. 3). The primary efficacy endpoint of the study was cardiac events (the sum of fatal and non-fatal myocardial infarctions and sudden cardiac deaths). The hazard ratio (LOPID:placebo) for cardiac events was 1.47 (95% confidence limits 0.88-2.48, p=0.14). Of the 35 patients in the LOPID group who experienced cardiac events, 12 patients suffered events after discontinuation from the study. Of the 24 patients in the placebo group with cardiac events, 4 patients suffered events after discontinuation from the study. There were 17 cardiac deaths in the LOPID group and 8 in the placebo group (hazard ratio 2.18; 95% confidence limits 0.94-5.05, p=0.06). Ten of these deaths in the LOPID group and 3 in the placebo group occurred after discontinuation from therapy. In this study of patients with known or suspected coronary heart disease, no benefit from LOPID treatment was observed in reducing cardiac events or cardiac deaths. Thus, LOPID has shown benefit only in selected dyslipidemic patients without suspected or established coronary heart disease. Even in patients with coronary heart disease and the triad of elevated LDL-cholesterol, elevated triglycerides, plus low HDL-cholesterol, the possible effect of LOPID on coronary events has not been adequately studied.

No efficacy in the patients with established coronary heart disease was observed during the Coronary Drug Project with the chemically and pharmacologically related drug, clofibrate. The Coronary Drug Project was a 6-year randomized, double-blind study involving 1000 clofibrate, 1000 nicotinic acid, and 3000 placebo patients with known coronary heart disease. A clinically and statistically significant reduction in myocardial infarctions was seen in the concurrent nicotinic acid group compared to placebo; no reduction was seen with clofibrate.

The mechanism of action of gemfibrozil has not been definitely established. In man, LOPID has been shown to inhibit peripheral lipolysis and to decrease the hepatic extraction of free fatty acids, thus reducing hepatic triglyceride production. LOPID inhibits synthesis and increases clearance of VLDL carrier apolipoprotein B, leading to a decrease in VLDL production.

Animal studies suggest that gemfibrozil may, in addition to elevating HDL-cholesterol, reduce incorporation of long-chain fatty acids into newly formed triglycerides, accelerate turnover and removal of cholesterol from the liver, and increase excretion of cholesterol in the feces. LOPID is well absorbed from the gastrointestinal tract after oral administration. Peak plasma levels occur in 1 to 2 hours with a plasma half-life of 1.5 hours following multiple doses.

Gemfibrozil is completely absorbed after oral administration of LOPID tablets, reaching peak plasma concentrations 1 to 2 hours after dosing. Gemfibrozil pharmacokinetics are affected by the timing of meals relative to time of dosing. In one study (ref. 4), both the rate and extent of absorption of the drug were significantly increased when administered 0.5 hour before meals. Average AUC was reduced by 14-44% when LOPID was administered after meals compared to 0.5 hour before meals. In a subsequent study (ref. 4), rate of absorption of LOPID was maximum when administered 0.5 hour before meals with the Cmax 50-60% greater than when given either with meals or fasting. In this study, there were no significant effects on AUC of timing of dose relative to meals (see DOSAGE AND ADMINISTRATION).

LOPID mainly undergoes oxidation of a ring methyl group to successively form a hydroxymethyl and a carboxyl metabolite. Approximately seventy percent of the administered human dose is excreted in the urine, mostly as the glucuronide conjugate, with less than 2% excreted as unchanged gemfibrozil. Six percent of the dose is accounted for in the feces. Gemfibrozil is highly bound to plasma proteins and there is potential for displacement interactions with other drugs (see PRECAUTIONS).

INDICATIONS AND USAGE

LOPID (gemfibrozil tablets, USP) is indicated as adjunctive therapy to diet for:

1. Treatment of adult patients with very high elevations of serum triglyceride levels (Types IV and V hyperlipidemia) who present a risk of pancreatitis and who do not respond adequately to a determined dietary effort to control them. Patients who present such risk typically have serum triglycerides over 2000 mg/dL and have elevations of VLDL-cholesterol as well as fasting chylomicrons (Type V hyperlipidemia). Subjects who consistently have total serum or plasma triglycerides below 1000 mg/dL are unlikely to present a risk of pancreatitis. LOPID therapy may be considered for those subjects with triglyceride elevations between 1000 and 2000 mg/dL who have a history of pancreatitis or of recurrent abdominal pain typical of pancreatitis. It is recognized that some Type IV patients with triglycerides under 1000 mg/dL may, through dietary or alcoholic indiscretion, convert to a Type V pattern with massive triglyceride elevations accompanying fasting chylomicronemia, but the influence of LOPID therapy on the risk of pancreatitis in such situations has not been adequately studied. Drug therapy is not indicated for patients with Type I hyperlipoproteinemia, who have elevations of chylomicrons and plasma triglycerides, but who have normal levels of very low density lipoprotein (VLDL). Inspection of plasma refrigerated for 14 hours is helpful in distinguishing Types I, IV, and V hyperlipoproteinemia (ref. 5).

2. Reducing the risk of developing coronary heart disease **only** in Type IIb patients without history of or symptoms of existing coronary heart disease who have had an inadequate response to weight loss, dietary therapy, exercise, and other pharmacologic agents (such as bile acid sequestrants and nicotinic acid, known to reduce LDL- and raise HDL-cholesterol) **and** who have the following triad of lipid abnormalities: low HDL-cholesterol levels in addition to elevated LDL-cholesterol and elevated triglycerides (see WARNINGS, PRECAUTIONS, and CLINICAL PHARMACOLOGY). The National Cholesterol Education Program has defined a serum HDL-cholesterol value that is consistently below 35 mg/dL as constituting an independent risk factor for coronary heart disease (ref. 6). Patients with significantly elevated triglycerides should be closely observed when treated with gemfibrozil. In some patients with high triglyceride levels, treatment with gemfibrozil is associated with a significant increase in LDL-cholesterol. BECAUSE OF POTENTIAL TOXICITY SUCH AS MALIGNANCY, GALLBLADDER DISEASE, ABDOMINAL PAIN LEADING TO APPENDECTOMY AND OTHER ABDOMINAL SURGERIES, AN INCREASED INCIDENCE IN NON-CORONARY MORTALITY, AND THE 44% RELATIVE INCREASE DURING THE TRIAL PERIOD IN AGE-ADJUSTED ALL-CAUSE MORTALITY SEEN WITH THE CHEMICALLY AND PHARMACOLOGICALLY RELATED DRUG, CLOFIBRATE, THE POTENTIAL BENEFIT OF

Table I
Reduction in CHD Rates (events per 1000 patients) by Baseline Lipids[1] in the Helsinki Heart Study, Years 0–5[2]

	All Patients			LDL-C>175; HDL-C>46.4			LDL-C>175; TG>177			LDL-C>175; TG>200; HDL-C<35		
	P	L	Dif[3]	P	L	Dif	P	L	Dif	P	L	Dif
Incidence of Events[4]	41	27	14	32	29	3	71	44	27	149	64	85

[1] lipid values in mg/dL at baseline
[2] P = placebo group; L = LOPID group
[3] difference in rates between placebo and LOPID groups
[4] fatal and nonfatal myocardial infarctions plus sudden cardiac deaths (events per 1000 patients over 5 years)

Table II
Cardiac Events and All-Cause Mortality (events per 1000 patients) Occurring During the 3.5 Year Open-Label Follow-up to the Helsinki HeartStudy[1]

Group:	PDrop N=215	PN N=494	PL N=1283	LDrop N=221	LN N=574	LL N=1207
Cardiac Events	38.8	22.9	22.5	37.2	28.3	25.4
All-Cause Mortality	41.9	22.3	15.6	72.3	19.2	24.9

[1] The six open-label groups are designated first by the original randomization (P = placebo, L = LOPID) and then by the drug taken in the follow-up period (N = Attend clinic but took no drug, L = LOPID, Drop = No attendance at clinic during open-label).

Table III
Cardiac Events, Cardiac Deaths, Non-Cardiac Deaths and All-Cause Mortality in the Helsinki Heart Study, Years 0–8.5[1]

Event	LOPID at Study Start	Placebo at Study Start	LOPID:Placebo Hazard Ratio[2]	CI Hazard Ratio[3]
Cardiac Events[4]	110	131	0.80	0.62-1.03
Cardiac Deaths	36	38	0.98	0.63-1.54
Non-Cardiac Deaths	65	45	1.40	0.95-2.05
All-Cause Mortality	101	83	1.20	0.90-1.61

[1] Intention-to-Treat Analysis of originally randomized patients neglecting the open-label treatment switches and exposure to study conditions.
[2] Hazard ration for risk event in the group originally randomized to LOPID compared to the group originally randomized to placebo neglecting open-label treatment switch and exposure to study condition.
[3] 95% confidence intervals of LOPID:placebo group hazard ratio
[4] Fatal and non-fatal myocardial infarctions plus sudden cardiac deaths over the 8.5 year period.

	CAUSAL RELATIONSHIP PROBABLE	CAUSAL RELATIONSHIP NOT ESTABLISHED
General:		weight loss
Cardiac:		extrasystoles
Gastrointestinal:	cholestatic jaundice	pancreatitis hepatoma colitis
Central Nervous System:	dizziness somnolence paresthesia peripheral neuritis decreased libido depression headache	confusion convulsions syncope
Eye:	blurred vision	retinal edema
Genitourinary:	impotence	decreased male fertility renal dysfunction
Musculoskeletal:	myopathy myasthenia myalgia painful extremities arthralgia synovitis rhabdomyolysis (see WARNINGS and Drug Interactions under PRECAUTIONS)	
Clinical Laboratory:	increased creatine phosphokinase increased bilirubin increased liver transaminases (AST [SGOT], ALT [SGPT]) increased alkaline phosphatase	positive antinuclear antibody
Hematopoietic:	anemia leukopenia bone marrow hypoplasia eosinophilia	thrombocytopenia
Immunologic:	angioedema laryngeal edema urticaria	anaphylaxis Lupus-like syndrome vasculitis
Integumentary:	exfoliative dermatitis rash dermatitis pruritus	alopecia photosensitivity

GEMFIBROZIL IN TREATING TYPE IIA PATIENTS WITH ELEVATIONS OF LDL-CHOLESTEROL ONLY IS NOT LIKELY TO OUTWEIGH THE RISKS. LOPID IS ALSO NOT INDICATED FOR THE TREATMENT OF PATIENTS WITH LOW HDL-CHOLESTEROL AS THEIR ONLY LIPID ABNORMALITY.

In a subgroup analysis of patients in the Helsinki Heart Study with above-median HDL-cholesterol values at baseline (greater than 46.4 mg/dL), the incidence of serious coronary events was similar for gemfibrozil and placebo subgroups (see Table I).

The initial treatment for dyslipidemia is dietary therapy specific for the type of lipoprotein abnormality. Excess body weight and excess alcohol intake may be important factors in hypertriglyceridemia and should be managed prior to any drug therapy. Physical exercise can be an important ancillary measure, and has been associated with rises in HDL-cholesterol. Diseases contributory to hyperlipidemia such as hypothyroidism or diabetes mellitus should be looked for and adequately treated. Estrogen therapy is sometimes associated with massive rises in plasma triglycerides, especially in subjects with familial hypertriglyceridemia. In such cases, discontinuation of estrogen therapy may obviate the need for specific drug therapy of hypertriglyceridemia. The use of drugs should be considered only when reasonable attempts have been made to obtain satisfactory results with nondrug methods. If the decision is made to use drugs, the patient should be instructed that this does not reduce the importance of adhering to diet.

CONTRAINDICATIONS

1. Combination therapy of LOPID with cerivastatin due to the increased risk of myopathy and rhabdomyolysis (see WARNINGS).

2. Hepatic or severe renal dysfunction, including primary biliary cirrhosis.

3. Preexisting gallbladder disease (see WARNINGS).

4. Hypersensitivity to gemfibrozil.

WARNINGS

1. Because of chemical, pharmacological, and clinical similarities between gemfibrozil and clofibrate, the adverse findings with clofibrate in two large clinical studies may also apply to gemfibrozil. In the first of those studies, the Coronary Drug Project, 1000 subjects with previous myocardial infarction were treated for five years with clofibrate. There was no difference in mortality between the clofibrate-treated subjects and 3000 placebo-treated subjects, but twice as many clofibrate-treated subjects developed cholelithiasis and cholecystitis requiring surgery. In the other study, conducted by the World Health Organization (WHO), 5000 subjects without known coronary heart disease were treated with clofibrate for five years and followed one year beyond. There was a statistically significant, 44%, higher age-adjusted total mortality in the clofibrate-treated than in a comparable placebo-treated control group during the trial period. The excess mortality was due to a 33% increase in non-cardiovascular causes, including malignancy, post-cholecystectomy complications, and pancreatitis. The higher risk of clofibrate-treated subjects for gallbladder disease was confirmed.

Because of the more limited size of the Helsinki Heart Study, the observed difference in mortality from any cause between the LOPID and placebo group is not statistically significantly different from the 29% excess mortality reported in the clofibrate group in the separate WHO study at the nine year follow-up (see CLINICAL PHARMACOLOGY). Noncoronary heart disease related mortality showed an excess in the group originally randomized to LOPID primarily due to cancer deaths observed during the open-label extension.

During the five year primary prevention component of the Helsinki Heart Study, mortality from any cause was 44 (2.2%) in the LOPID group and 43 (2.1%) in the placebo group; including the 3.5 year follow-up period since the trial was completed, cumulative mortality from any cause was 101 (4.9%) in the LOPID group and 83 (4.1%) in the group originally randomized to placebo (hazard ratio 1:20 in favor of placebo). Because of the more limited size of the Helsinki Heart Study, the observed difference in mortality from any cause between the LOPID and placebo groups at Year-5 or at Year-8.5 is not statistically significantly different from the 29% excess mortality reported in the clofibrate group in the separate WHO study at the nine year follow-up. Noncoronary heart disease related mortality showed an excess in the group originally randomized to LOPID at the 8.5 year follow-up (65 LOPID versus 45 placebo noncoronary deaths).

The incidence of cancer (excluding basal cell carcinoma) discovered during the trial and in the 3.5 years after the trial was completed was 51 (2.5%) in both originally randomized groups. In addition, there were 16 basal cell carcinomas in the group originally randomized to LOPID and 9 in the group randomized to placebo (p=0.22). There were 30 (1.5%) deaths attributed to cancer in the group originally randomized to LOPID and 18 (0.9%) in the group originally randomized to placebo (p=0.11). Adverse outcomes, including coronary events, were higher in gemfibrozil patients in a corresponding study in men with a history of known or suspected coronary heart disease in the secondary prevention component of the Helsinki Heart Study. (See CLINICAL PHARMACOLOGY.)

A comparative carcinogenicity study was also done in rats comparing three drugs in this class: fenofibrate (10 and 60 mg/kg; 0.3 and 1.6 times the human dose), clofibrate (400 mg/kg; 1.6 times the human dose), and gemfibrozil (250 mg/kg; 1.7 times the human dose). Pancreatic acinar adenomas were increased in males and females on fenofibrate; hepatocellular carcinoma and pancreatic acinar adenomas were increased in males and hepatic neoplastic nodules in females treated with clofibrate; hepatic neoplastic nodules were increased in males and females treated with clofibrate; hepatic neoplastic nodules were increased in males and females treated with gemfibrozil while testicular interstitial cell (Leydig cell) tumors were increased in males on all three drugs.

2. A gallstone prevalence substudy of 450 Helsinki Heart Study participants showed a trend toward a greater prevalence of gallstones during the study within the LOPID treatment group (7.5% vs 4.9% for the placebo group, a 55% excess for the gemfibrozil group). A trend toward a greater incidence of gallbladder surgery was observed for the LOPID group (17 vs 11 subjects, a 54% excess). This result did not differ statistically from the increased incidence of cholecystectomy observed in the WHO study in the group treated with clofibrate. Both clofibrate and gemfibrozil may increase cholesterol excretion into the bile leading to cholelithiasis. If cholelithiasis is suspected, gallbladder studies are indicated. LOPID therapy should be discontinued if gallstones are found. Cases of cholelithiasis have been reported with gemfibrozil therapy (ref. 7).

3. Since a reduction of mortality from coronary heart disease has not been demonstrated and because liver and interstitial cell testicular tumors were increased in rats, LOPID should be administered only to those patients described in the INDICATIONS AND USAGE section. If a significant serum lipid response is not obtained, LOPID should be discontinued.

4. Concomitant Anticoagulants–Caution should be exercised when anticoagulants are given in conjunction with LOPID. The dosage of the anticoagulant should be reduced to maintain the prothrombin time at the desired level to prevent bleeding complications. Frequent prothrombin determinations are advisable until it has been definitely determined that the prothrombin level has stabilized.

5. Concomitant therapy with LOPID and an HMG-CoA reductase inhibitor is associated with an increased risk of skeletal muscle toxicity manifested as rhabdomyolysis, markedly elevated creatine kinase (CPK) levels and myoglobinuria, leading in a high proportion of cases to acute renal failure and death. **Because of an observed marked increased risk of myopathy and rhabdomyolysis, the specific combination of LOPID and cerivastatin is absolutely contraindicated (see CONTRAINDICATIONS).** IN PATIENTS WHO HAVE HAD AN UNSATISFACTORY LIPID RESPONSE TO EITHER DRUG ALONE, THE BENEFIT OF COMBINED THERAPY WITH LOPID AND HMG-CoA REDUCTASE INHIBITORS OTHER THAN CERIVASTATIN DOES NOT OUTWEIGH THE RISKS OF SEVERE MYOPATHY, RHABDOMYOLYSIS, AND ACUTE RENAL FAILURE (refs. 8, 9, 10, 11) (see Drug Interactions). The use of fibrates alone, including LOPID, may occasionally be associated with myositis. Patients receiving LOPID and complaining of muscle pain, tenderness or weakness should have prompt medical evaluation for myositis, including serum creatine–kinase level determination. If myositis is suspected or diagnosed, LOPID therapy should be withdrawn.

6. Cataracts–Subcapsular bilateral cataracts occurred in 10%, and unilateral in 6.3%, of male rats treated with gemfibrozil at 10 times the human dose.

PRECAUTIONS

1. **Initial Therapy**—Laboratory studies should be done to ascertain that the lipid levels are consistently abnormal. Before instituting LOPID therapy, every attempt should be made to control serum lipids with appropriate diet, exercise, weight loss in obese patients, and control of any medical problems such as diabetes mellitus and hypothyroidism that are contributing to the lipid abnormalities.

2. **Continued Therapy**—Periodic determination of serum lipids should be obtained, and the drug withdrawn if lipid response is inadequate after three months of therapy.

3. **Drug Interactions**—(A) **HMG-CoA reductase inhibitors:** The risk of myopathy and rhabdomyolysis is increased with combined gemfibrozil and HMG-CoA reductase inhibitor therapy (see CONTRAINDICATIONS). Myopathy or rhabdomyolysis with or without acute renal failure have been reported as early as three weeks after initiation of combined therapy or after several months (refs. 8, 9, 10, 11). (See WARNINGS.) There is no assurance that periodic monitoring of creatine kinase will prevent the occurrence of severe myopathy and kidney damage.

(B) **Anticoagulants:** CAUTION SHOULD BE EXERCISED WHEN ANTI-COAGULANTS ARE GIVEN IN CONJUNCTION WITH LOPID. THE DOSAGE OF THE ANTICOAGULANT SHOULD BE REDUCED TO MAINTAIN THE PROTHROMBIN TIME AT THE DESIRED LEVEL TO PREVENT BLEEDING COMPLICATIONS. FREQUENT PROTHROMBIN DETERMINATIONS ARE ADVISABLE UNTIL IT HAS BEEN DEFINITELY DETERMINED THAT THE PROTHROMBIN LEVEL HAS STABILIZED.

4. **Carcinogenesis, Mutagenesis, Impairment of Fertility**—Long-term studies have been conducted in rats at 0.2 and 1.3 times the human exposure (based on AUC). The incidence of benign liver nodules and liver carcinomas was significantly increased in high dose male rats. The incidence of liver carcinomas increased also in low dose males, but this increase was not statistically significant (p=0.1). Male rats had a dose-related and statistically significant increase of benign Leydig cell tumors. The higher dose female rats had a significant increase in the combined incidence of benign and malignant liver neoplasms.

Long-term studies have been conducted in mice at 0.1 and 0.7 times the human exposure (based on AUC). There were no statistically significant differences from controls in the incidence of liver tumors, but the doses tested were lower than those shown to be carcinogenic with other fibrates.

Electron microscopy studies have demonstrated a florid hepatic peroxisome proliferation following LOPID administration to the male rat. An adequate study to test for peroxisome proliferation has not been done in humans but

Continued on next page

Lopid—Cont.

changes in peroxisome morphology have been observed. Peroxisome proliferation has been shown to occur in humans with either of two other drugs of the fibrate class when liver biopsies were compared before and after treatment in the same individual.

Administration of approximately 2 times the human dose (based on surface area) to male rats for 10 weeks resulted in a dose-related decrease of fertility. Subsequent studies demonstrated that this effect was reversed after a drug-free period of about eight weeks, and it was not transmitted to the offspring.

5. **Pregnancy Category C**—LOPID has been shown to produce adverse effects in rats and rabbits at doses between 0.5 and 3 times the human dose (based on surface area). There are no adequate and well-controlled studies in pregnant women. LOPID should be used during pregnancy only if the potential benefit justifies the potential risk to the fetus.

Administration of LOPID to female rats at 2 times the human dose (based on surface area) before and throughout gestation caused a dose-related decrease in conception rate and, an increase in stillborns and a slight reduction in pup weight during lactation. There were also dose-related increased skeletal variations. Anophthalmia occurred, but rarely.

Administration of 0.6 and 2 times the human dose (based on surface area) of LOPID to female rats from gestation day 15 through weaning caused dose-related decreases in birth weight and suppressions of pup growth during lactation.

Administration of 1 and 3 times the human dose (based on surface area) of LOPID to female rabbits during organogenesis caused a dose-related decrease in litter size and, at the high dose, an increased incidence of parietal bone variations.

6. **Nursing Mothers**—It is not known whether this drug is excreted in human milk. Because many drugs are excreted in human milk and because of the potential for tumorigenicity shown for LOPID in animal studies, a decision should be made whether to discontinue nursing or to discontinue the drug, taking into account the importance of the drug to the mother.

7. **Hematologic Changes**—Mild hemoglobin, hematocrit and white blood cell decreases have been observed in occasional patients following initiation of LOPID therapy. However, these levels stabilize during long-term administration. Rarely, severe anemia, leukopenia, thrombocytopenia, and bone marrow hypoplasia have been reported. Therefore, periodic blood counts are recommended during the first 12 months of LOPID administration.

8. **Liver Function**—Abnormal liver function tests have been observed occasionally during LOPID administration, including elevations of AST (SGOT), ALT (SGPT), LDH, bilirubin, and alkaline phosphatase. These are usually reversible when LOPID is discontinued. Therefore, periodic liver function studies are recommended and LOPID therapy should be terminated if abnormalities persist.

9. **Kidney Function**—There have been reports of worsening renal insufficiency upon the addition of LOPID therapy in individuals with baseline plasma creatinine >2.0 mg/dL. In such patients, the use of alternative therapy should be considered against the risks and benefits of a lower dose of LOPID.

10. **Pediatric Use**—Safety and efficacy in pediatric patients have not been established.

ADVERSE REACTIONS

In the double-blind controlled phase of the primary prevention component of the Helsinki Heart Study, 2046 patients received LOPID for up to five years. In that study, the following adverse reactions were statistically more frequent in subjects in the LOPID group:

	LOPID (N = 2046)	PLACEBO (N = 2035)
	Frequency in percent of subjects	
Gastrointestinal reactions	34.2	23.8
Dyspepsia	19.6	11.9
Abdominal pain	9.8	5.6
Acute appendicitis (histologically confirmed in most cases where data were available)	1.2	0.6
Atrial fibrillation	0.7	0.1
Adverse events reported by more than 1% of sublects, but without a significant difference between groups:		
Diarrhea	7.2	6.5
Fatigue	3.8	3.5
Nausea/Vomiting	2.5	2.1
Eczema	1.9	1.2
Rash	1.7	1.3
Vertigo	1.5	1.3
Constipation	1.4	1.3
Headache	1.2	1.1

Gallbladder surgery was performed in 0.9% of LOPID and 0.5% of placebo subjects in the primary prevention component, a 64% excess, which is not statistically different from the excess of gallbladder surgery observed in the clofibrate compared to the placebo group of the WHO study. Gallbladder surgery was also performed more frequently in the LOPID group compared to placebo (1.9% vs 0.3%, p=0.07) in the secondary prevention component. A statistically significant increase in appendectomy in the gemfibrozil group was seen also in the secondary prevention component (6 on gemfibrozil vs 0 on placebo, p=0.014).

Nervous system and special senses adverse reactions were more common in the LOPID group. These included hypesthesia, paresthesias, and taste perversion. Other adverse reactions that were more common among LOPID treatment group subjects but where a causal relationship was not established include cataracts, peripheral vascular disease, and intracerebral hemorrhage.

From other studies it seems probable that LOPID is causally related to the occurrence of MUSCULOSKELETAL SYMPTOMS (see WARNINGS), and to ABNORMAL LIVER FUNCTION TESTS and HEMATOLOGIC CHANGES (see PRECAUTIONS).

Reports of viral and bacterial infections (common cold, cough, urinary tract infections) were more common in gemfibrozil treated patients in other controlled clinical trials of 805 patients. Additional adverse reactions that have been reported for gemfibrozil are listed below by system. These are categorized according to whether a causal relationship to treatment with LOPID is probable or not established:

[See table at top of previous page]

Additional adverse reactions that have been reported include cholecystitis and cholelithiasis (ref. 12) (see WARNINGS).

DOSAGE AND ADMINISTRATION

The recommended dose for adults is 1200 mg administered in two divided doses 30 minutes before the morning and evening meal (see CLINICAL PHARMACOLOGY).

OVERDOSAGE

There have been reported cases of overdosage with LOPID. In one case, a 7-year-old child recovered after ingesting up to 9 grams of LOPID. Symptoms reported with overdosage were abdominal cramps, abnormal liver function tests, diarrhea, increased CPK, joint and muscle pain, nausea and vomiting. Symptomatic supportive measures should be taken, should an overdose occur.

HOW SUPPLIED

LOPID (Tablet 737), white, elliptical, film-coated, scored tablets, each containing 600 mg gemfibrozil, are available as follows:

N 0071-0737-20: Bottles of 60
N 0071-0737-30: Bottles of 500
Parcode® No. 737

Store at controlled room temperature 20°-25°C (68°-77°F) [see USP]. Protect from light and humidity.

REFERENCES

1. Frick MH, Elo O, Haapa K, et al: Helsinki Heart Study: Primary prevention trial with gemfibrozil in middle-aged men with dyslipidemia. *N Engl J Med* 1987; 317:1237-1245.
2. Manninen V, Elo O, Frick MH, et al: Lipid alterations and decline in the incidence of coronary heart disease in the Helsinki Heart Study. *JAMA* 1988; 260:641-651.
3. Frick MH, Heinonen OP, et al: Efficacy of gemfibrozil in dyslipidemic subjects with suspected heart disease. An ancillary study in the Helsinki Heart Study frame population. *Annals of Medicine* 1993; 25:41-45.
4. Data on file. Parke-Davis; Morris Plains, NJ.
5. Nikkila EA: Familial lipoprotein lipase deficiency and related disorders of chylomicron metabolism. In Stanbury JB et al. (eds.): *The Metabolic Basis of Inherited Disease*, 5th ed., McGraw-Hill, 1983, Chap. 30, pp. 622-642.
6. Report of the National Cholesterol Education Program Expert Panel on Detection, Evaluation, and Treatment of High Blood Cholesterol. *Arch Int Med* 1988;148:36-69.
7. Data on file. Pfizer; NY, NY.
8. Pierce LR, Wysowski DK, Gross TP. Myopathy and rhabdomyolysis associated with lovastatin/gemfibrozil combination therapy. *JAMA* 1990;264:71-75.
9. Bermingham RP, Whitsitt TB, Smart ML et al. Rhabdomyolysis in a patient receiving the combination of cerivastatin and gemfibrozil. Am J Health-Syst Pharm 2000;57:461-464.
10. Duell PB, Connor WE, Illingworth DR. Rhabdomyolysis after taking atorvastatin with gemfibrozil. Am J Cardiol 1998;81:368-369.
11. Tal A, Rajeshawari M, Isley W. Rhabdomyolysis associated with simvastatin/gemfibrozil therapy. South Med J 1997;90:546-547.
12. Data on file. Pfizer; NY, NY.

℞ only

Revised June 2002
Manufactured by:
Pfizer Pharmaceuticals, Ltd.
Vega Baja, PR 00694
Distributed by:
Parke-Davis
Division of Pfizer Inc, NY, NY 10017

69-5829-00-2

Pfizer Inc.

235 EAST 42ND STREET
NEW YORK, NY 10017-5755

For Medical Information Contact:
(800) 438-1985
24 hours a day, seven days a week.

ARICEPT® ℞

[ă′rĭ-sĕpt]
(Donepezil Hydrochloride Tablets)

Prescribing information for this product, which appears on pages 2574–2577 of the 2003 PDR, has been completely revised as follows. Please write "See Supplement A" next to the product heading.

DESCRIPTION

ARICEPT® (donepezil hydrochloride) is a reversible inhibitor of the enzyme acetylcholinesterase, known chemically as (±)-2,3-dihydro-5,6-dimethoxy-2-[[1-(phenylmethyl)-4-piperidinyl]methyl]-1*H*-inden-1-one hydrochloride. Donepezil hydrochloride is commonly referred to in the pharmacological literature as E2020. It has an empirical formula of $C_{24}H_{29}NO_3HCl$ and a molecular weight of 415.96. Donepezil hydrochloride is a white crystalline powder and is freely soluble in chloroform, soluble in water and in glacial acetic acid, slightly soluble in ethanol and in acetonitrile and practically insoluble in ethyl acetate and in n-hexane.

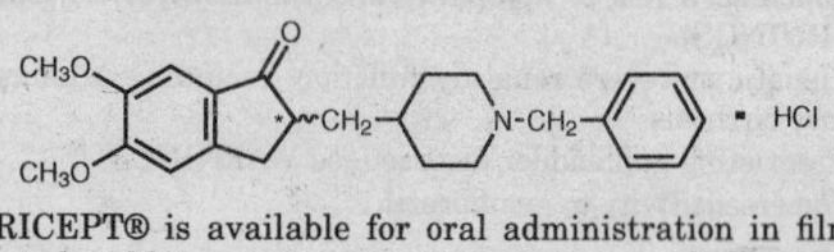

ARICEPT® is available for oral administration in film-coated tablets containing 5 or 10 mg of donepezil hydrochloride. Inactive ingredients are lactose monohydrate, corn starch, microcrystalline cellulose, hydroxypropyl cellulose, and magnesium stearate. The film coating contains talc, polyethylene glycol, hydroxypropyl methylcellulose and titanium dioxide. Additionally, the 10 mg tablet contains yellow iron oxide (synthetic) as a coloring agent.

CLINICAL PHARMACOLOGY

Current theories on the pathogenesis of the cognitive signs and symptoms of Alzheimer's Disease attribute some of them to a deficiency of cholinergic neurotransmission. Donepezil hydrochloride is postulated to exert its therapeutic effect by enhancing cholinergic function. This is accomplished by increasing the concentration of acetylcholine through reversible inhibition of its hydrolysis by acetylcholinesterase. If this proposed mechanism of action is correct, donepezil's effect may lessen as the disease process advances and fewer cholinergic neurons remain functionally intact. There is no evidence that donepezil alters the course of the underlying dementing process.

Clinical Trial Data

The effectiveness of ARICEPT® as a treatment for Alzheimer's Disease is demonstrated by the results of two randomized, double-blind, placebo-controlled clinical investigations in patients with Alzheimer's Disease (diagnosed by NINCDS and DSM III-R criteria, Mini-Mental State Examination ≥ 10 and ≤ 26 and Clinical Dementia Rating of 1 or 2). The mean age of patients participating in ARICEPT® trials was 73 years with a range of 50 to 94. Approximately 62% of patients were women and 38% were men. The racial distribution was white 95%, black 3% and other races 2%.

Study Outcome Measures: In each study, the effectiveness of treatment with ARICEPT® was evaluated using a dual outcome assessment strategy.

The ability of ARICEPT® to improve cognitive performance was assessed with the cognitive subscale of the Alzheimer's Disease Assessment Scale (ADAS-cog), a multi-item instrument that has been extensively validated in longitudinal cohorts of Alzheimer's Disease patients. The ADAS-cog examines selected aspects of cognitive performance including elements of memory, orientation, attention, reasoning, language and praxis. The ADAS-cog scoring range is from 0 to 70, with higher scores indicating greater cognitive impairment. Elderly normal adults may score as low as 0 or 1, but it is not unusual for non-demented adults to score slightly higher.

The patients recruited as participants in each study had mean scores on the Alzheimer's Disease Assessment Scale (ADAS-cog) of approximately 26 units, with a range from 4 to 61. Experience gained in longitudinal studies of ambulatory patients with mild to moderate Alzheimer's Disease suggest that they gain 6 to 12 units a year on the ADAS-cog. However, lesser degrees of change are seen in patients with very mild or very advanced disease because the ADAS-cog is not uniformly sensitive to change over the course of the disease. The annualized rate of decline in the placebo patients participating in ARICEPT® trials was approximately 2 to 4 units per year.

The ability of ARICEPT® to produce an overall clinical effect was assessed using a Clinician's Interview Based Impression of Change that required the use of caregiver information, the CIBIC plus. The CIBIC plus is not a single instrument and is not a standardized instrument like the ADAS-cog. Clinical trials for investigational drugs have used a variety of CIBIC formats, each different in terms of depth and structure.

As such, results from a CIBIC plus reflect clinical experience from the trial or trials in which it was used and cannot be compared directly with the results of CIBIC plus evaluations from other clinical trials. The CIBIC plus used in ARICEPT® trials was a semi-structured instrument that was intended to examine four major areas of patient function: General, Cognitive, Behavioral and Activities of Daily Living. It represents the assessment of a skilled clinician based upon his/her observations at an interview with the patient, in combination with information supplied by a caregiver familiar with the behavior of the patient over the interval rated. The CIBIC plus is scored as a seven point categorical rating, ranging from a score of 1, indicating "markedly improved," to a score of 4, indicating "no change" to a score of 7, indicating "markedly worse." The CIBIC plus has not been systematically compared directly to assessments not using information from caregivers (CIBIC) or other global methods.

Thirty-Week Study
In a study of 30 weeks duration, 473 patients were randomized to receive single daily doses of placebo, 5 mg/day or 10 mg/day of ARICEPT®. The 30-week study was divided into a 24-week double-blind active treatment phase followed by a 6-week single-blind placebo washout period. The study was designed to compare 5 mg/day or 10 mg/day fixed doses of ARICEPT® to placebo. However, to reduce the likelihood of cholinergic effects, the 10 mg/day treatment was started following an initial 7-day treatment with 5 mg/day doses.

Effects on the ADAS-cog:
Figure 1 illustrates the time course for the change from baseline in ADAS-cog scores for all three dose groups over the 30 weeks of the study. After 24 weeks of treatment, the mean differences in the ADAS-cog change scores for ARICEPT® treated patients compared to the patients on placebo were 2.8 and 3.1 units for the 5 mg/day and 10 mg/day treatments, respectively. These differences were statistically significant. While the treatment effect size may appear to be slightly greater for the 10 mg/day treatment, there was no statistically significant difference between the two active treatments.

Following 6 weeks of placebo washout, scores on the ADAS-cog for both the ARICEPT® treatment groups were indistinguishable from those patients who had received only placebo for 30 weeks. This suggests that the beneficial effects of ARICEPT® abate over 6 weeks following discontinuation of treatment and do not represent a change in the underlying disease. There was no evidence of a rebound effect 6 weeks after abrupt discontinuation of therapy.

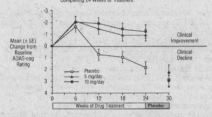

Figure 1. Time-course of the Change from Baseline in ADAS-cog Score for Patients Completing 24 Weeks of Treatment.

Figure 2 illustrates the cumulative percentages of patients from each of the three treatment groups who had attained the measure of improvement in ADAS-cog score shown on the X axis. Three change scores, (7-point and 4-point reductions from baseline or no change in score) have been identified for illustrative purposes and the percent of patients in each group achieving that result is shown in the inset table. The curves demonstrate that both patients assigned to placebo and ARICEPT® have a wide range of responses, but that the active treatment groups are more likely to show the greater improvements. A curve for an effective treatment would be shifted to the left of the curve for placebo, while an ineffective or deleterious treatment would be superimposed upon or shifted to the right of the curve for placebo, respectively.

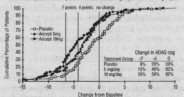

Figure 2. Cumulative Percentage of Patients Completing 24 Weeks of Double-blind Treatment with Specified Changes from Baseline ADAS-cog Scores. The Percentages of Randomized Patients who Completed the Study were: Placebo 80%, 5 mg/day 85% and 10 mg/day 68%.

Effects on the CIBIC plus:
Figure 3 is a histogram of the frequency distribution of CIBIC plus scores attained by patients assigned to each of the three treatment groups who completed 24 weeks of treatment. The mean drug-placebo differences for these groups of patients were 0.35 units and 0.39 units for 5 mg/day and 10 mg/day of ARICEPT®, respectively. These differences were statistically significant. There was no statistically significant difference between the two active treatments.
[See figure 3 at top of next column]

Fifteen-Week Study
In a study of 15 weeks duration, patients were randomized to receive single daily doses of placebo or either 5 mg/day or 10 mg/day of ARICEPT® for 12 weeks, followed by a 3-week placebo washout period. As in the 30-week study, to avoid acute cholinergic effects, the 10 mg/day treatment followed an initial 7-day treatment with 5 mg/day doses.

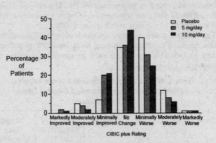

Figure 3. Frequency Distribution of CIBIC plus Scores at Week 24

Effects on the ADAS-Cog:
Figure 4 illustrates the time course of the change from baseline in ADAS-cog scores for all three dose groups over the 15 weeks of the study. After 12 weeks of treatment, the differences in mean ADAS-cog change scores for the ARICEPT® treated patients compared to the patients on placebo were 2.7 and 3.0 units each, for the 5 and 10 mg/day ARICEPT® treatment groups respectively. These differences were statistically significant. The effect size for the 10 mg/day group may appear to be slightly larger than that for 5 mg/day. However, the differences between active treatments were not statistically significant.

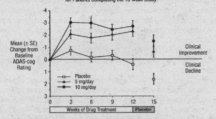

Figure 4. Time-course of the Change from Baseline in ADAS-cog Score for Patients Completing the 15-week Study.

Following 3 weeks of placebo washout, scores on the ADAS-cog for both the ARICEPT® treatment groups increased, indicating that discontinuation of ARICEPT® resulted in a loss of its treatment effect. The duration of this placebo washout period was not sufficient to characterize the rate of loss of the treatment effect, but, the 30-week study (see above) demonstrated that treatment effects associated with the use of ARICEPT® abate within 6 weeks of treatment discontinuation.

Figure 5 illustrates the cumulative percentages of patients from each of the three treatment groups who attained the measure of improvement in ADAS-cog score shown on the X axis. The same three change scores, (7-point and 4-point reductions from baseline or no change in score) as selected for the 30-week study have been used for this illustration. The percentages of patients achieving those results are shown in the inset table.

As observed in the 30-week study, the curves demonstrate that patients assigned to either placebo or to ARICEPT® have a wide range of responses, but that the ARICEPT® treated patients are more likely to show the greater improvements in cognitive performance.

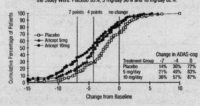

Figure 5. Cumulative Percentage of Patients with Specified Changes from Baseline ADAS-cog Scores. The Percentages of Randomized Patients Within Each Treatment Group Who Completed the Study Were: Placebo 93%, 5 mg/day 90% and 10 mg/day 82%.

Effects on the CIBIC plus:
Figure 6 is a histogram of the frequency distribution of CIBIC plus scores attained by patients assigned to each of the three treatment groups who completed 12 weeks of treatment. The differences in mean scores for ARICEPT® treated patients compared to the patients on placebo at Week 12 were 0.36 and 0.38 units for the 5 mg/day and 10 mg/day treatment groups, respectively. These differences were statistically significant.

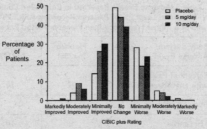

Figure 6. Frequency Distribution of CIBIC plus Scores at Week 12

In both studies, patient age, sex and race were not found to predict the clinical outcome of ARICEPT® treatment.

Clinical Pharmacokinetics
Donepezil is well absorbed with a relative oral bioavailability of 100% and reaches peak plasma concentrations in 3 to 4 hours. Pharmacokinetics are linear over a dose range of 1-10 mg given once daily. Neither food nor time of administration (morning vs. evening dose) influences the rate or extent of absorption. The elimination half life of donepezil is about 70 hours and the mean apparent plasma clearance (Cl/F) is 0.13 L/hr/kg. Following multiple dose administration, donepezil accumulates in plasma by 4-7 fold and steady state is reached within 15 days. The steady state volume of distribution is 12 L/kg. Donepezil is approximately 96% bound to human plasma proteins, mainly to albumins (about 75%) and alpha$_1$ - acid glycoprotein (about 21%) over the concentration range of 2-1000 ng/mL.

Donepezil is both excreted in the urine intact and extensively metabolized to four major metabolites, two of which are known to be active, and a number of minor metabolites, not all of which have been identified. Donepezil is metabolized by CYP 450 isoenzymes 2D6 and 3A4 and undergoes glucuronidation. Following administration of ^{14}C-labeled donepezil, plasma radioactivity, expressed as a percent of the administered dose, was present primarily as intact donepezil (53%) and as 6-O-desmethyl donepezil (11%), which has been reported to inhibit AChE to the same extent as donepezil in vitro and was found in plasma at concentrations equal to about 20% of donepezil. Approximately 57% and 15% of the total radioactivity was recovered in urine and feces, respectively, over a period of 10 days, while 28% remained unrecovered, with about 17% of the donepezil dose recovered in the urine as unchanged drug.

Special Populations:
Hepatic Disease: In a study of 10 patients with stable alcoholic cirrhosis, the clearance of ARICEPT® was decreased by 20% relative to 10 healthy age and sex matched subjects.
Renal Disease: In a study of 4 patients with moderate to severe renal impairment (Cl_{Cr} < 22 mL/min/1.73 m^2) the clearance of ARICEPT® did not differ from 4 age and sex matched healthy subjects.
Age: No formal pharmacokinetic study was conducted to examine age related differences in the pharmacokinetics of ARICEPT®. However, mean plasma ARICEPT® concentrations measured during therapeutic drug monitoring of elderly patients with Alzheimer's Disease are comparable to those observed in young healthy volunteers.
Gender and Race: No specific pharmacokinetic study was conducted to investigate the effects of gender and race on the disposition of ARICEPT®. However, retrospective pharmacokinetic analysis indicates that gender and race (Japanese and Caucasians) did not affect the clearance of ARICEPT®.

Drug-Drug Interactions
Drugs Highly Bound to Plasma Proteins: Drug displacement studies have been performed in vitro between this highly bound drug (96%) and other drugs such as furosemide, digoxin, and warfarin. ARICEPT® at concentrations of 0.3-10 µg/mL did not affect the binding of furosemide (5 µg/mL), digoxin (2 ng/mL), and warfarin (3 µg/mL) to human albumin. Similarly, the binding of ARICEPT® to human albumin was not affected by furosemide, digoxin and warfarin.

Effect of ARICEPT® on the Metabolism of Other Drugs: No in vivo clinical trials have investigated the effect of ARICEPT® on the clearance of drugs metabolized by CYP 3A4 (e.g. cisapride, terfenadine) or by CYP 2D6 (e.g. imipramine). However, in vitro studies show a low rate of binding to these enzymes (mean K_i about 50-130 µM), that, given the therapeutic plasma concentrations of donepezil (164 nM), indicates little likelihood of interference.

Whether ARICEPT® has any potential for enzyme induction is not known.

Formal pharmacokinetic studies evaluated the potential of ARICEPT® for interaction with theophylline, cimetidine, warfarin and digoxin. No significant effects on the pharmacokinetics of these drugs were observed.

Effect of Other Drugs on the Metabolism of ARICEPT®: Ketoconazole and quinidine, inhibitors of CYP450, 3A4 and 2D6, respectively, inhibit donepezil metabolism in vitro. Whether there is a clinical effect of these inhibitors is not known. Inducers of CYP 2D6 and CYP 3A4 (e.g., phenytoin, carbamazepine, dexamethasone, rifampin, and phenobarbital) could increase the rate of elimination of ARICEPT®.

Formal pharmacokinetic studies demonstrated that the metabolism of ARICEPT® is not significantly affected by concurrent administration of digoxin or cimetidine.

INDICATIONS AND USAGE
ARICEPT® is indicated for the treatment of mild to moderate dementia of the Alzheimer's type.

CONTRAINDICATIONS
ARICEPT® is contraindicated in patients with known hypersensitivity to donepezil hydrochloride or to piperidine derivatives.

WARNINGS
Anesthesia: ARICEPT®, as a cholinesterase inhibitor, is likely to exaggerate succinylcholine-type muscle relaxation during anesthesia.
Cardiovascular Conditions: Because of their pharmacological action, cholinesterase inhibitors may have vagotonic effects on the sinoatrial and atrioventricular nodes. This effect may manifest as bradycardia or heart block in patients

Continued on next page

Aricept—Cont.

both with and without known underlying cardiac conduction abnormalities. Syncopal episodes have been reported in association with the use of ARICEPT®.

Gastrointestinal Conditions: Through their primary action, cholinesterase inhibitors may be expected to increase gastric acid secretion due to increased cholinergic activity. Therefore, patients should be monitored closely for symptoms of active or occult gastrointestinal bleeding, especially those at increased risk for developing ulcers, e.g., those with a history of ulcer disease or those receiving concurrent nonsteroidal anti-inflammatory drugs (NSAIDS). Clinical studies of ARICEPT® have shown no increase, relative to placebo, in the incidence of either peptic ulcer disease or gastrointestinal bleeding.

ARICEPT®, as a predictable consequence of its pharmacological properties, has been shown to produce diarrhea, nausea and vomiting. These effects, when they occur, appear more frequently with the 10 mg/day dose than with the 5 mg/day dose. In most cases, these effects have been mild and transient, sometimes lasting one to three weeks, and have resolved during continued use of ARICEPT®.

Genitourinary: Although not observed in clinical trials of ARICEPT®, cholinomimetics may cause bladder outflow obstruction.

Neurological Conditions: Seizures: Cholinomimetics are believed to have some potential to cause generalized convulsions. However, seizure activity also may be a manifestation of Alzheimer's Disease.

Pulmonary Conditions: Because of their cholinomimetic actions, cholinesterase inhibitors should be prescribed with care to patients with a history of asthma or obstructive pulmonary disease.

PRECAUTIONS

Drug-Drug Interactions (see Clinical Pharmacology: Clinical Pharmacokinetics: Drug-drug Interactions)

Effect of ARICEPT® on the Metabolism of Other Drugs: No *in vivo* clinical trials have investigated the effect of ARICEPT® on the clearance of drugs metabolized by CYP 3A4 (e.g. cisapride, terfenadine) or by CYP 2D6 (e.g. imipramine). However, *in vitro* studies show a low rate of binding to these enzymes (mean K_i about 50-130 µM), that, given the therapeutic plasma concentrations of donepezil (164 nM), indicates little likelihood of interference.

Whether ARICEPT® has any potential for enzyme induction is not known.

Effect of Other Drugs on the Metabolism of ARICEPT®: Ketoconazole and quinidine, inhibitors of CYP450, 3A4 and 2D6, respectively, inhibit donepezil metabolism *in vitro*. Whether there is a clinical effect of these inhibitors is not known. Inducers of CYP 2D6 and CYP 3A4 (e.g., phenytoin, carbamazepine, dexamethasone, rifampin, and phenobarbital) could increase the rate of elimination of ARICEPT®.

Use with Anticholinergics: Because of their mechanism of action, cholinesterase inhibitors have the potential to interfere with the activity of anticholinergic medications.

Use with Cholinomimetics and Other Cholinesterase Inhibitors: A synergistic effect may be expected when cholinesterase inhibitors are given concurrently with succinylcholine, similar neuromuscular blocking agents or cholinergic agonists such as bethanechol.

Carcinogenesis, Mutagenesis, Impairment of Fertility
Carcinogenicity studies of donepezil have not been completed.

Donepezil was not mutagenic in the Ames reverse mutation assay in bacteria. In the chromosome aberration test in cultures of Chinese hamster lung (CHL) cells, some clastogenic effects were observed. Donepezil was not clastogenic in the *in vivo* mouse micronucleus test.

Donepezil had no effect on fertility in rats at doses up to 10 mg/kg/day (approximately 8 times the maximum recommended human dose on a mg/m² basis).

Pregnancy
Pregnancy Category C: Teratology studies conducted in pregnant rats at doses up to 16 mg/kg/day (approximately 13 times the maximum recommended human dose on a mg/m² basis) and in pregnant rabbits at doses up to 10 mg/kg/day (approximately 16 times the maximum recommended human dose on a mg/m² basis) did not disclose any evidence for a teratogenic potential of donepezil. However, in a study in which pregnant rats were given up to 10 mg/kg/day (approximately 8 times the maximum recommended human dose on a mg/m² basis) from day 17 of gestation through day 20 postpartum, there was a slight increase in still births and a slight decrease in pup survival through day 4 postpartum at this dose; the next lower dose tested was 3 mg/kg/day. There are no adequate or well-controlled studies in pregnant women. ARICEPT® should be used during pregnancy only if the potential benefit justifies the potential risk to the fetus.

Nursing Mothers
It is not known whether donepezil is excreted in human breast milk. ARICEPT® has no indication for use in nursing mothers.

Pediatric Use
There are no adequate and well-controlled trials to document the safety and efficacy of ARICEPT® in any illness occurring in children.

ADVERSE REACTIONS

Adverse Events Leading to Discontinuation
The rates of discontinuation from controlled clinical trials of ARICEPT® due to adverse events for the ARICEPT® 5 mg/day treatment groups were comparable to those of placebo-treatment groups at approximately 5%. The rate of discontinuation of patients who received 7-day escalations from 5 mg/day to 10 mg/day, was higher at 13%.

The most common adverse events leading to discontinuation, defined as those occurring in at least 2% of patients and at twice the incidence seen in placebo patients, are shown in Table 1.

Table 1. Most Frequent Adverse Events Leading to Withdrawal from Controlled Clinical Trials by Dose Group

Dose Group	Placebo	5 mg/day ARICEPT®	10 mg/day ARICEPT®
Patients Randomized	355	350	315
Event/% Discontinuing			
Nausea	1%	1%	3%
Diarrhea	0%	<1%	3%
Vomiting	<1%	<1%	2%

Most Frequent Adverse Clinical Events Seen in Association with the Use of ARICEPT®

The most common adverse events, defined as those occurring at a frequency of at least 5% in patients receiving 10 mg/day and twice the placebo rate, are largely predicted by ARICEPT®'s cholinomimetic effects. These include nausea, diarrhea, insomnia, vomiting, muscle cramp, fatigue and anorexia. These adverse events were often of mild intensity and transient, resolving during continued ARICEPT® treatment without the need for dose modification.

There is evidence to suggest that the frequency of these common adverse events may be affected by the rate of titration. An open-label study was conducted with 269 patients who received placebo in the 15 and 30-week studies. These patients were titrated to a dose of 10 mg/day over a 6-week period. The rates of common adverse events were lower than those seen in patients titrated to 10 mg/day over one week in the controlled clinical trials and were comparable to those seen in patients on 5 mg/day.

See Table 2 for a comparison of the most common adverse events following one and six week titration regimens.

Table 2. Comparison of rates of adverse events in patients titrated to 10 mg/day over 1 and 6 weeks

	No titration		One week titration	Six week titration
Adverse Event	Placebo (n=315)	5 mg/day (n=311)	10 mg/day (n=315)	10 mg/day (n=269)
Nausea	6%	5%	19%	6%
Diarrhea	5%	8%	15%	9%
Insomnia	6%	6%	14%	6%
Fatigue	3%	4%	8%	3%
Vomiting	3%	3%	8%	5%
Muscle cramps	2%	6%	8%	3%
Anorexia	2%	3%	7%	3%

Adverse Events Reported in Controlled Trials

The events cited reflect experience gained under closely monitored conditions of clinical trials in a highly selected patient population. In actual clinical practice or in other clinical trials, these frequency estimates may not apply, as the conditions of use, reporting behavior, and the kinds of patients treated may differ. Table 3 lists treatment emergent signs and symptoms that were reported in at least 2% of patients in placebo-controlled trials who received ARICEPT® and for which the rate of occurrence was greater for ARICEPT® assigned than placebo assigned patients. In general, adverse events occurred more frequently in female patients and with advancing age.

Table 3. Adverse Events Reported in Controlled Clinical Trials in at Least 2% of Patients Receiving ARICEPT® and at a Higher Frequency than Placebo-treated Patients

Body System/ Adverse Event	Placebo (n=355)	ARICEPT® (n=747)
Percent of Patients with any Adverse Event	72	74
Body as a Whole		
Headache	9	10
Pain, various locations	8	9
Accident	6	7
Fatigue	3	5
Cardiovascular System		
Syncope	1	2
Digestive System		
Nausea	6	11
Diarrhea	5	10
Vomiting	3	5
Anorexia	2	4
Hemic and Lymphatic System		
Ecchymosis	3	4
Metabolic and Nutritional Systems		
Weight Decrease	1	3
Musculoskeletal System		
Muscle Cramps	2	6
Arthritis	1	2
Nervous System		
Insomnia	6	9
Dizziness	6	8
Depression	<1	3
Abnormal Dreams	0	3
Somnolence	<1	2
Urogenital System		
Frequent Urination	1	2

Other Adverse Events Observed During Clinical Trials
ARICEPT® has been administered to over 1700 individuals during clinical trials worldwide. Approximately 1200 of these patients have been treated for at least 3 months and more than 1000 patients have been treated for at least 6 months. Controlled and uncontrolled trials in the United States included approximately 900 patients. In regards to the highest dose of 10 mg/day, this population includes 650 patients treated for 3 months, 475 patients treated for 6 months and 116 patients treated for over 1 year. The range of patient exposure is from 1 to 1214 days.

Treatment emergent signs and symptoms that occurred during 3 controlled clinical trials and two open-label trials in the United States were recorded as adverse events by the clinical investigators using terminology of their own choosing. To provide an overall estimate of the proportion of individuals having similar types of events, the events were grouped into a smaller number of standardized categories using a modified COSTART dictionary and event frequencies were calculated across all studies. These categories are used in the listing below. The frequencies represent the proportion of 900 patients from these trials who experienced that event while receiving ARICEPT®. All adverse events occurring at least twice are included, except for those already listed in Tables 2 or 3, COSTART terms too general to be informative, or events less likely to be drug caused. Events are classified by body system and listed using the following definitions: *frequent adverse events* - those occurring in at least 1/100 patients; *infrequent adverse events* - those occurring in 1/100 to 1/1000 patients. These adverse events are not necessarily related to ARICEPT® treatment and in most cases were observed at a similar frequency in placebo-treated patients in the controlled studies. No important additional adverse events were seen in studies conducted outside the United States.

Body as a Whole: *Frequent:* influenza, chest pain, toothache; *Infrequent:* fever, edema face, periorbital edema, hernia hiatal, abscess, cellulitis, chills, generalized coldness, head fullness, listlessness.
Cardiovascular System: *Frequent:* hypertension, vasodilation, atrial fibrillation, hot flashes, hypotension; *Infrequent:* angina pectoris, postural hypotension, myocardial infarction, AV block (first degree), congestive heart failure, arteritis, bradycardia, peripheral vascular disease, supraventricular tachycardia, deep vein thrombosis.
Digestive System: *Frequent:* fecal incontinence, gastrointestinal bleeding, bloating, epigastric pain; *Infrequent:* eructation, gingivitis, increased appetite, flatulence, periodontal abscess, cholelithiasis, diverticulitis, drooling, dry mouth, fever sore, gastritis, irritable colon, tongue edema, epigastric distress, gastroenteritis, increased transaminases, hemorrhoids, ileus, increased thirst, jaundice, melena, polydipsia, duodenal ulcer, stomach ulcer.
Endocrine System: *Infrequent:* diabetes mellitus, goiter.
Hemic and Lymphatic System: *Infrequent:* anemia, thrombocythemia, thrombocytopenia, eosinophilia, erythrocytopenia.

Metabolic and Nutritional Disorders: *Frequent:* dehydration; *Infrequent:* gout, hypokalemia, increased creatine kinase, hyperglycemia, weight increase, increased lactate dehydrogenase.
Musculoskeletal System: *Frequent:* bone fracture; *Infrequent:* muscle weakness, muscle fasciculation.
Nervous System: *Frequent:* delusions, tremor, irritability, paresthesia, aggression, vertigo, ataxia, increased libido, restlessness, abnormal crying, nervousness, aphasia; *Infrequent:* cerebrovascular accident, intracranial hemorrhage, transient ischemic attack, emotional lability, neuralgia, coldness (localized), muscle spasm, dysphoria, gait abnormality, hypertonia, hypokinesia, neurodermatitis, numbness (localized), paranoia, dysarthria, dysphasia, hostility, decreased libido, melancholia, emotional withdrawal, nystagmus, pacing.
Respiratory System: *Frequent:* dyspnea, sore throat, bronchitis; *Infrequent:* epistaxis, post nasal drip, pneumonia, hyperventilation, pulmonary congestion, wheezing, hypoxia, pharyngitis, pleurisy, pulmonary collapse, sleep apnea, snoring.
Skin and Appendages: *Frequent:* pruritus, diaphoresis, urticaria; *Infrequent:* dermatitis, erythema, skin discoloration, hyperkeratosis, alopecia, fungal dermatitis, herpes zoster, hirsutism, skin striae, night sweats, skin ulcer.
Special Senses: *Frequent:* cataract, eye irritation, vision blurred; *Infrequent:* dry eyes, glaucoma, earache, tinnitus, blepharitis, decreased hearing, retinal hemorrhage, otitis externa, otitis media, bad taste, conjunctival hemorrhage, ear buzzing, motion sickness, spots before eyes.
Urogenital System: *Frequent:* urinary incontinence, nocturia; *Infrequent:* dysuria, hematuria, urinary urgency, metrorrhagia, cystitis, enuresis, prostate hypertrophy, pyelonephritis, inability to empty bladder, breast fibroadenosis, fibrocystic breast, mastitis, pyuria, renal failure, vaginitis.

Postintroduction Reports

Voluntary reports of adverse events temporally associated with ARICEPT® that have been received since market introduction that are not listed above, and that there is inadequate data to determine the causal relationship with the drug include the following: abdominal pain, agitation, cholecystitis, confusion, convulsions, hallucinations, heart block (all types), hemolytic anemia, hepatitis, hyponatremia, neuroleptic malignant syndrome, pancreatitis, and rash.

OVERDOSAGE

Because strategies for the management of overdose are continually evolving, it is advisable to contact a Poison Control Center to determine the latest recommendations for the management of an overdose of any drug.

As in any case of overdose, general supportive measures should be utilized. Overdosage with cholinesterase inhibitors can result in cholinergic crisis characterized by severe nausea, vomiting, salivation, sweating, bradycardia, hypotension, respiratory depression, collapse and convulsions. Increasing muscle weakness is a possibility and may result in death if respiratory muscles are involved. Tertiary anticholinergics such as atropine may be used as an antidote for ARICEPT® overdosage. Intravenous atropine sulfate titrated to effect is recommended: an initial dose of 1.0 to 2.0 mg IV with subsequent doses based upon clinical response. Atypical responses in blood pressure and heart rate have been reported with other cholinomimetics when coadministered with quaternary anticholinergics such as glycopyrrolate. It is not known whether ARICEPT® and/or its metabolites can be removed by dialysis (hemodialysis, peritoneal dialysis, or hemofiltration).

Dose-related signs of toxicity in animals included reduced spontaneous movement, prone position, staggering gait, lacrimation, clonic convulsions, depressed respiration, salivation, miosis, tremors, fasciculation and lower body surface temperature.

DOSAGE AND ADMINISTRATION

The dosages of ARICEPT® shown to be effective in controlled clinical trials are 5 mg and 10 mg administered once per day.

The higher dose of 10 mg did not provide a statistically significantly greater clinical benefit than 5 mg. There is a suggestion, however, based upon order of group mean scores and dose trend analyses of data from these clinical trials, that a daily dose of 10 mg of ARICEPT® might provide additional benefit for some patients. Accordingly, whether or not to employ a dose of 10 mg is a matter of prescriber and patient preference.

Evidence from the controlled trials indicates that the 10 mg dose, with a one week titration, is likely to be associated with a higher incidence of cholinergic adverse events than the 5 mg dose. In open label trials using a 6 week titration, the frequency of these same adverse events was similar between the 5 mg and 10 mg dose groups. Therefore, because steady state is not achieved for 15 days and because the incidence of untoward effects may be influenced by the rate of dose escalation, treatment with a dose of 10 mg should not be contemplated until patients have been on a daily dose of 5 mg for 4 to 6 weeks.

ARICEPT® should be taken in the evening, just prior to retiring. ARICEPT® can be taken with or without food.

HOW SUPPLIED

ARICEPT® is supplied as film-coated, round tablets containing either 5 mg or 10 mg of donepezil hydrochloride.

The 5 mg tablets are white. The strength, in mg (5), is debossed on one side and ARICEPT is debossed on the other side.

The 10 mg tablets are yellow. The strength, in mg (10), is debossed on one side and ARICEPT is debossed on the other side.

5 mg (White)	Bottles of 30 (NDC# 62856-245-30)
	Bottles of 90 (NDC# 62856-245-90)
	Unit Dose Blister Package 100 (10×10) (NDC# 62856-245-41)
10 mg (Yellow)	Bottles of 30 (NDC# 62856-246-30)
	Bottles of 90 (NDC# 62856-246-90)
	Unit Dose Blister Package 100 (10×10) (NDC# 62856-246-41)

Storage: Store at controlled room temperature, 15°C to 30°C (59°F to 86°F).

℞ only

ARICEPT® is a registered trademark of Eisai Co., Ltd.

Manufactured and Marketed by Eisai Inc., Teaneck, NJ 07666

Marketed by Pfizer Inc, New York, NY 10017

200237

Revised August 2002

BEXTRA® ℞

[*bĕk'stră*]

valdecoxib tablets

Prescribing information for this product, which appears on pages 2577–2581 of the 2003 PDR, has been completely revised as follows. Please write "See Supplement A" next to the product heading.

DESCRIPTION

Valdecoxib is chemically designated as 4-(5-methyl-3-phenyl-4-isoxazolyl) benzenesulfonamide and is a diaryl substituted isoxazole. It has the following chemical structure:

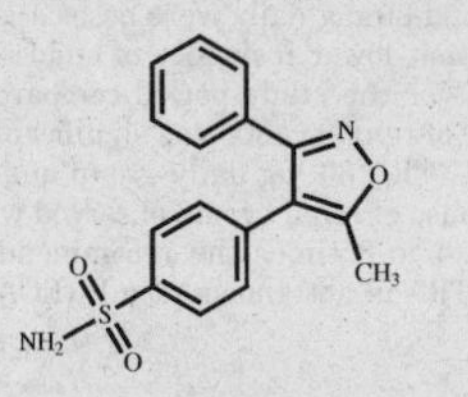

Valdecoxib

The empirical formula for valdecoxib is $C_{16}H_{14}N_2O_3S$, and the molecular weight is 314.36. Valdecoxib is a white crystalline powder that is relatively insoluble in water (10 µg/mL) at 25°C and pH 7.0, soluble in methanol and ethanol, and freely soluble in organic solvents and alkaline (pH=12) aqueous solutions.

BEXTRA Tablets for oral administration contain either 10 mg or 20 mg of valdecoxib. Inactive ingredients include lactose monohydrate, microcrystalline cellulose, pregelatinized starch, croscarmellose sodium, magnesium stearate, hydroxypropyl methylcellulose, polyethylene glycol, polysorbate 80, and titanium dioxide.

CLINICAL PHARMACOLOGY

Mechanism of Action

Valdecoxib is a nonsteroidal anti-inflammatory drug (NSAID) that exhibits anti-inflammatory, analgesic and antipyretic properties in animal models. The mechanism of action is believed to be due to inhibition of prostaglandin synthesis primarily through inhibition of cyclooxygenase-2 (COX-2). At therapeutic plasma concentrations in humans valdecoxib does not inhibit cyclooxygenase-1 (COX-1).

Pharmacokinetics

Absorption

Valdecoxib achieves maximal plasma concentrations in approximately 3 hours. The absolute bioavailability of valdecoxib is 83% following oral administration of BEXTRA compared to intravenous infusion of valdecoxib.

Dose proportionality was demonstrated after single doses (1-400 mg) of valdecoxib. With multiple doses (up to 100 mg/day for 14 days), valdecoxib exposure as measured by the AUC, increases in a more than proportional manner at doses above 10 mg BID. Steady state plasma concentrations of valdecoxib are achieved by day 4.

The steady state pharmacokinetic parameters of valdecoxib in healthy male subjects are shown in Table 1.

Table 1

Mean (SD) Steady State Pharmacokinetic Parameters

Steady State Pharmacokinetic Parameters after Valdecoxib 10 mg Once Daily for 14 Days	Healthy Male Subjects (n=8, 20 to 42 yr.)
$AUC_{(0-24hr)}$ (hr•ng/mL)	1479.0 (291.9)
C_{max} (ng/mL)	161.1 (48.1)
T_{max} (hr)	2.25 (0.71)
C_{min} (ng/mL)	21.9 (7.68)
Elimination Half-life (hr)	8.11 (1.32)

No clinically significant age or gender differences were seen in pharmacokinetic parameters that would require dosage adjustments.

Effect of Food and Antacid

BEXTRA can be taken with or without food. Food had no significant effect on either the peak plasma concentration (C_{max}) or extent of absorption (AUC) of valdecoxib when BEXTRA was taken with a high fat meal. The time to peak plasma concentration (T_{max}), however, was delayed by 1-2 hours. Administration of BEXTRA with antacid (aluminum/magnesium hydroxide) had no significant effect on either the rate or extent of absorption of valdecoxib.

Distribution

Plasma protein binding for valdecoxib is about 98% over the concentration range (21-2384 ng/mL). Steady state apparent volume of distribution (Vss/F) of valdecoxib is approximately 86 L after oral administration. Valdecoxib and its active metabolite preferentially partition into erythrocytes with a blood to plasma concentration ratio of about 2.5:1. This ratio remains approximately constant with time and therapeutic blood concentrations.

Metabolism

In humans, valdecoxib undergoes extensive hepatic metabolism involving both P450 isoenzymes (3A4 and 2C9) and non-P450 dependent pathways (i.e., glucuronidation). Concomitant administration of BEXTRA with known CYP 3A4 and 2C9 inhibitors (e.g., fluconazole and ketoconazole) can result in increased plasma exposure of valdecoxib (see PRECAUTIONS — Drug Interactions).

One active metabolite of valdecoxib has been identified in human plasma at approximately 10% the concentration of valdecoxib. This metabolite, which is a less potent COX-2 specific inhibitor than the parent, also undergoes extensive metabolism and constitutes less than 2% of the valdecoxib dose excreted in the urine and feces. Due to its low concentration in the systemic circulation, it is not likely to contribute significantly to the efficacy profile of BEXTRA.

Excretion

Valdecoxib is eliminated predominantly via hepatic metabolism with less than 5% of the dose excreted unchanged in the urine and feces. About 70% of the dose is excreted in the urine as metabolites, and about 20% as valdecoxib N-glucuronide. The apparent oral clearance (CL/F) of valdecoxib is about 6 L/hr. The mean elimination half-life ($T_{1/2}$) ranges from 8-11 hours, and increases with age.

Special Populations

Geriatric

In elderly subjects (> 65 years), weight-adjusted steady state plasma concentrations ($AUC_{(0-12hr)}$) are about 30% higher than in young subjects. No dose adjustment is needed based on age.

Pediatric

BEXTRA has not been investigated in pediatric patients below 18 years of age.

Race

Pharmacokinetic differences due to race have not been identified in clinical and pharmacokinetic studies conducted to date.

Hepatic Insufficiency

Valdecoxib plasma concentrations are significantly increased (130%) in patients with moderate (Child-Pugh Class B) hepatic impairment. In clinical trials, doses of BEXTRA above those recommended have been associated with fluid retention. Hence, treatment with BEXTRA should be initiated with caution in patients with mild to moderate hepatic impairment and fluid retention. The use of BEXTRA in patients with severe hepatic impairment (Child-Pugh Class C) is not recommended.

Renal Insufficiency

The pharmacokinetics of valdecoxib have been studied in patients with varying degrees of renal impairment. Because renal elimination of valdecoxib is not important to its disposition, no clinically significant changes in valdecoxib clearance were found even in patients with severe renal impairment or in patients undergoing renal dialysis. In patients undergoing hemodialysis the plasma clearance (CL/F) of valdecoxib was similar to the CL/F found in healthy elderly subjects (CL/F about 6 to 7 L/hr.) with normal renal function (based on creatinine clearance).

NSAIDs have been associated with worsening renal function and use in advanced renal disease is not recommended (see PRECAUTIONS – Renal Effects).

Drug Interactions

Also see **PRECAUTIONS — Drug Interactions.**

General

Valdecoxib undergoes both P450 (CYP) dependent and non-P450 dependent (glucuronidation) metabolism. In vitro studies indicate that valdecoxib is not a significant inhibitor of CYP 1A2, 3A4, or 2D6 and is only a weak inhibitor of CYP 2C9 and 2C19 at therapeutic concentrations. The P450-mediated metabolic pathway of valdecoxib predominantly involves the 3A4 and 2C9 isozymes. Using prototype inhibitors and substrates of these isozymes, the following results were obtained. Coadministration of a known inhibitor of CYP 2C9/3A4 (fluconazole) and a CYP 3A4 (ketoconazole) inhibitor enhanced the total plasma exposure (AUC) of valdecoxib. Coadministration of valdecoxib with warfarin caused a small, but statistically significant increase in plasma exposures of R-warfarin and S-warfarin, and also in the pharmacodynamic effects (International Normalized Ratio — INR) of warfarin. (See PRECAUTIONS — Drug Interactions.)

Coadministration of valdecoxib, or its injectable prodrug, with substrates of CYP 2C9 (propofol) and CYP 3A4 (midazolam, alfentanil, fentanyl) did not inhibit the metabolism of either substrate.

Continued on next page

Bextra—Cont.

Coadministration of valdecoxib with a CYP 3A4 substrate (glyburide) or a CYP 2D6 substrate (dextromethorphan) did not result in clinically important inhibition in the metabolism of these agents.

CLINICAL STUDIES

The efficacy and clinical utility of BEXTRA Tablets have been demonstrated in osteoarthritis (OA), rheumatoid arthritis (RA) and in the treatment of primary dysmenorrhea.

Osteoarthritis

BEXTRA was evaluated for treatment of the signs and symptoms of osteoarthritis of the knee or hip, in five double-blind, randomized, controlled trials in which 3918 patients were treated for 3 to 6 months. BEXTRA was shown to be superior to placebo in improvement in three domains of OA symptoms: (1) the WOMAC (Western Ontario and McMaster Universities) osteoarthritis index, a composite of pain, stiffness and functional measures in OA, (2) the overall patient assessment of pain, and (3) the overall patient global assessment. The two 3-month pivotal trials in OA generally showed changes statistically significantly different from placebo, and comparable to the naproxen control, in measures of these domains for the 10 mg/day dose. No additional benefit was seen with a valdecoxib 20-mg daily dose.

Rheumatoid Arthritis

BEXTRA demonstrated significant reduction compared to placebo in the signs and symptoms of RA, as measured by the ACR (American College of Rheumatology) 20 improvement, a composite defined as both improvement of 20% in the number of tender and number of swollen joints, and a 20% improvement in three of the following five: patient global, physician global, patient pain, patient function assessment, and C-reactive protein (CRP). BEXTRA was evaluated for treatment of the signs and symptoms of rheumatoid arthritis in four double-blind, randomized, controlled studies in which 3444 patients were treated for 3 to 6 months. The two 3-month pivotal trials compared valdecoxib to naproxen and placebo. The results for the ACR20 responses in these trials are shown below (Table 2). Trials of BEXTRA in rheumatoid arthritis allowed concomitant use of corticosteroids and/or disease-modifying anti-rheumatic drugs (DMARDs), such as methotrexate, gold salts, and hydroxychloroquine. No additional benefit was seen with a valdecoxib 20-mg daily dose.

Table 2
ACR20 Response Rate (%) in Rheumatoid Arthritis

	Study 1	Study 2
BEXTRA 10 mg/day	49%** (103/209)	46%** (103/226)
BEXTRA 20 mg/day	48%** (102/212)	47%* (103/219)
Naproxen 500 mg BID	44%* (100/225)	53%** (115/219)
Placebo	32% (70/222)	32% (71/220)

* $p<0.01$; ** $p<0.001$ compared to placebo

Primary Dysmenorrhea

BEXTRA was compared to naproxen sodium 550 mg in two placebo-controlled studies of women with moderate to severe primary dysmenorrhea. The onset of analgesia was within 60 minutes for BEXTRA 20 mg. The onset, magnitude, and duration of analgesic effect with BEXTRA 20 mg were comparable to naproxen sodium 550 mg.

Safety Studies

Gastrointestinal (GI) Endoscopy Studies with Therapeutic Doses: Scheduled upper GI endoscopic evaluations were performed with BEXTRA at doses of 10 and 20 mg daily in over 800 OA patients who were enrolled into two randomized 3-month studies using active comparators and placebo controls (Study 3 and Study 4). These studies enrolled patients free of endoscopic ulcers at baseline and compared rates of endoscopic ulcers, defined as any gastroduodenal ulcer seen endoscopically provided it was of "unequivocal depth" and at least 3 mm in diameter.

In both studies, BEXTRA 10 mg daily was associated with a statistically significant lower incidence of endoscopic gastroduodenal ulcers over the study period compared to the active comparators. Figure 1 summarizes the incidence of gastroduodenal ulcers in Studies 3 and 4 for the placebo, valdecoxib, and active control arms.

Figure 1
Incidence of Endoscopically Observed Gastroduodenal Ulcers in OA Patients

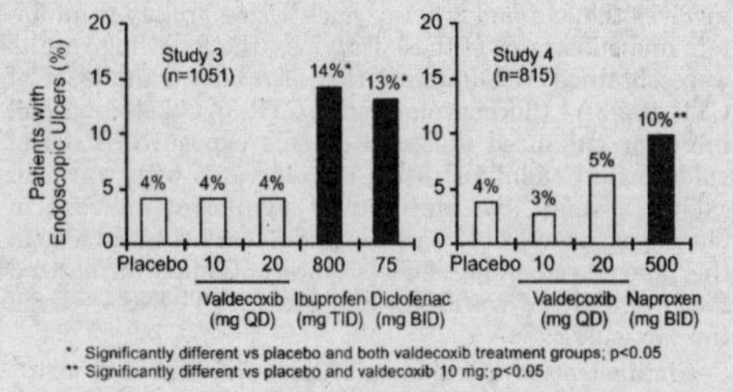

* Significantly different vs placebo and both valdecoxib treatment groups; p<0.05
** Significantly different vs placebo and valdecoxib 10 mg; p<0.05

Safety Study with Supratherapeutic Doses: Scheduled upper GI endoscopic evaluations were performed in a randomized 6-month study of 1217 patients with OA and RA comparing valdecoxib 20 mg BID (40 mg daily) and 40 mg BID (80 mg daily) (4 to 8 times the recommended therapeutic dose) to naproxen 500 mg BID (Study 5). This study also formally assessed renal events as a primary outcome with supratherapeutic doses of BEXTRA. The renal endpoint was defined as any of the following: new/increase in edema, new/increase in congestive heart failure, increase in blood pressure (BP; >20 mm Hg systolic, >10 mm Hg diastolic), new/increase in BP treatment, new/increase in diuretic therapy, creatinine increase over 30% (or >1.2 mg/dL if baseline <0.9 mg/dL), BUN increase over 200% or >50 mg/dL, 24-hr urinary protein increase to >500 mg (if baseline 0-150 mg or >750 if baseline 151-300 or >1000 if baseline 301-500), serum potassium increase to >6 mEq/L, or serum sodium decrease to <130 mEq/L.

Table 3
Incidence of Endoscopic Gastroduodenal Ulcers in Patients With and Without Selected Risk Factors

Risk Factor	Placebo-controlled Studies: Placebo	Placebo-controlled Studies: Valdecoxib (10–20 mg daily)	Active-controlled Studies: Valdecoxib (10–80 mg daily)	Ibuprofen 800 mg TID	Naproxen 500 mg BID	Diclofenac 75 mg BID
Age						
<65 yrs	3.7% (8/219)	3.5% (17/484)	3.7% (48/1306)	8.2% (9/110)	12.8% (51/397)	13.2% (34/258)
≥65 yrs	5.8% (8/137)	4.6% (12/262)	7.6% (43/568)	21.6% (16/74)	22.0% (33/150)	18.2% (25/137)
Concomitant Low Dose Aspirin Use						
no	4.4% (13/298)	3.2% (21/650)	3.8% (64/1671)	9.8% (15/153)	16.0% (75/468)	12.8% (45/351)
yes	5.2% (3/58)	8.3% (8/96)	13.3% (27/203)	32.3% (10/31)	11.4% (9/79)	31.8% (14/44)
History of Ulcer Disease						
no	4.4% (14/317)	3.4% (22/647)	4.1% (68/1666)	13.8% (22/160)	13.3% (63/475)	14.7% (52/354)
yes	5.1% (2/39)	7.1% (7/99)	11.1% (23/208)	12.5% (3/24)	29.2% (21/72)	17.1% (7/41)

No statistical conclusions can be drawn from these comparisons.

Figure 2 summarizes the incidence rates of gastroduodenal ulcers and renal events that were seen in Study 5. BEXTRA 40 mg daily and 80 mg daily were associated with a statistically significant lower incidence of endoscopic gastroduodenal ulcers over the study period compared to naproxen. The incidence of renal events was significantly different between the BEXTRA 80 mg daily group and naproxen. The clinical relevance of renal events observed with supratherapeutic doses (4 to 8 times the recommended therapeutic dose) of BEXTRA is not known (see PRECAUTIONS – Renal Effects).

Figure 2
Incidence of Endoscopic Gastroduodenal Ulcers and Renal Events in the High-dose Safety Study

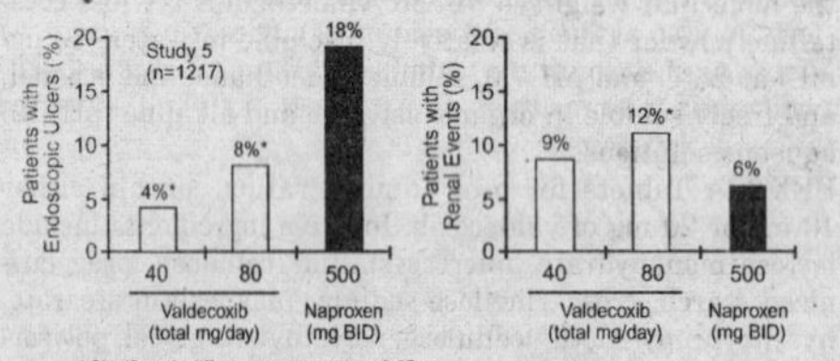

* Significantly different vs naproxen, p<0.05

Renal Safety at the Therapeutic Chronic Dose: The renal effects of valdecoxib compared with placebo and conventional NSAIDs were also assessed by prospectively designed pooled analyses of renal events data (see definition above — Supratherapeutic Doses) from five placebo- and active-controlled 12-week arthritis trials that included 995 OA or RA patients given valdecoxib 10 mg daily. The incidence of renal events observed in this analysis with valdecoxib 10 mg daily (3%), ibuprofen 800 mg TID (7%), naproxen 500 mg BID (2%) and diclofenac 75 mg BID (4%) were significantly higher than placebo-treated patients (1%). In all treatment groups, the majority of renal events were either due to the occurrence of edema or worsening BP.

Gastrointestinal Ulcers in High-Risk Patients: Subset analyses were performed of patients with risk factors (age, concomitant low-dose aspirin use, history of prior ulcer disease) enrolled in four upper GI endoscopic studies. Table 3 summarizes the trends seen.

[See table 3 above]

The correlation between findings of endoscopic studies, and the incidence of clinically significant serious upper GI events has not been established.

Platelets: In four clinical studies with young and elderly (≥65 years) subjects, single and multiple doses up to 7 days of BEXTRA 10 to 40 mg BID had no effect on platelet aggregation.

INDICATIONS AND USAGE

BEXTRA Tablets are indicated:

- For relief of the signs and symptoms of osteoarthritis and adult rheumatoid arthritis.
- For the treatment of primary dysmenorrhea.

CONTRAINDICATIONS

BEXTRA should not be given to patients who have demonstrated allergic-type reactions to sulfonamides. BEXTRA Tablets are contraindicated in patients with known hypersensitivity to valdecoxib. BEXTRA should not be given to patients who have experienced asthma, urticaria, or allergic-type reactions after taking aspirin or NSAIDs. Severe, rarely fatal, anaphylactic-like reactions to NSAIDs are possible in such patients (see WARNINGS — Anaphylactoid Reactions, and PRECAUTIONS — Preexisting Asthma).

WARNINGS

Gastrointestinal (GI) Effects — Risk of GI Ulceration, Bleeding, and Perforation

Serious gastrointestinal toxicity such as bleeding, ulceration and perforation of the stomach, small intestine or large intestine can occur at any time with or without warning symptoms in patients treated with nonsteroidal anti-inflammatory drugs (NSAIDs). Minor gastrointestinal problems such as dyspepsia are common and may also occur at any time during NSAID therapy. Therefore, physicians and patients should remain alert for ulceration and bleeding even in the absence of previous GI tract symptoms. Patients should be informed about the signs and symptoms of serious GI toxicity and the steps to take if they occur. The utility of periodic laboratory monitoring has not been demonstrated, nor has it been adequately assessed. Only one in five patients who develop a serious upper GI adverse event on NSAID therapy is symptomatic. It has been demonstrated that upper GI ulcers, gross bleeding or perforation caused by NSAIDs appear to occur in approximately 1% of patients treated for 3 to 6 months and 2-4% of patients treated for one year. These trends continue, thus increasing the likelihood of developing a serious GI event at some time during the course of therapy. However, even short-term therapy is not without risk.

NSAIDs should be prescribed with extreme caution in patients with a prior history of ulcer disease or gastrointestinal bleeding. Most spontaneous reports of fatal GI events are in elderly or debilitated patients and therefore special care should be taken in treating this population. For high risk patients, alternate therapies that do not involve NSAIDs should be considered.

Studies have shown that patients with a *prior history of peptic ulcer disease and/or gastrointestinal bleeding* and who use NSAIDs, have a greater than 10-fold higher risk for developing a GI bleed than patients with neither of these risk factors. In addition to a past history of ulcer disease, pharmacoepidemiological studies have identified several other co-therapies or co-morbid conditions that may increase the risk for GI bleeding such as: treatment with oral corticosteroids, treatment with anticoagulants, longer duration of NSAID therapy, smoking, alcoholism, older age, and poor general health status. (See CLINICAL STUDIES — Safety Studies.)

Serious Skin Reactions

Serious skin reactions, including exfoliative dermatitis, Stevens-Johnson syndrome, and toxic epidermal necrolysis, have been reported through postmarketing surveillance in patients receiving BEXTRA (see ADVERSE REACTIONS-Postmarketing Experience). As these reactions can be life-threatening, BEXTRA should be discontinued at the first appearance of skin rash or any other sign of hypersensitivity.

Anaphylactoid Reactions

In postmarketing experience, cases of hypersensitivity reactions (anaphylactic reactions and angioedema) have been reported in patients receiving BEXTRA (see ADVERSE REACTIONS-Postmarketing Experience). These cases have occurred in patients with and without a history of allergic-type reactions to sulfonamides (see CONTRAINDICATIONS). BEXTRA should not be given to patients with the aspirin triad. This symptom complex typically occurs in asthmatic patients who experience rhinitis with or without nasal polyps, or who exhibit severe, potentially fatal bronchospasm after taking aspirin or other NSAIDs (see CONTRAINDICATIONS and PRECAUTIONS — Pre-existing Asthma). Emergency help should be sought in cases where an anaphylactoid reaction occurs.

Advanced Renal Disease

No information is available regarding the safe use of BEXTRA Tablets in patients with advanced kidney disease. Therefore, treatment with BEXTRA is not recommended in these patients. If therapy with BEXTRA must be initiated, close monitoring of the patient's kidney function is advisable (see PRECAUTIONS — Renal Effects).

Pregnancy

In late pregnancy, BEXTRA should be avoided because it may cause premature closure of the ductus arteriosus.

PRECAUTIONS

General

BEXTRA Tablets cannot be expected to substitute for corticosteroids or to treat corticosteroid insufficiency. Abrupt discontinuation of corticosteroids may lead to exacerbation of corticosteroid-responsive illness. Patients on prolonged corticosteroid therapy should have their therapy tapered slowly if a decision is made to discontinue corticosteroids.

The pharmacological activity of valdecoxib in reducing fever and inflammation may diminish the utility of these diagnostic signs in detecting complications of presumed noninfectious, painful conditions.

Hepatic Effects

Borderline elevations of one or more liver tests may occur in up to 15% of patients taking NSAIDs. Notable elevations of ALT or AST (approximately three or more times the upper limit of normal) have been reported in approximately 1% of patients in clinical trials with NSAIDs. These laboratory abnormalities may progress, may remain unchanged, or may remain transient with continuing therapy. Rare cases of severe hepatic reactions, including jaundice and fatal fulminant hepatitis, liver necrosis and hepatic failure (some with fatal outcome) have been reported with NSAIDs. In controlled clinical trials of valdecoxib, the incidence of borderline (defined as 1.2- to 3.0-fold) elevations of liver tests was 8.0% for valdecoxib and 8.4% for placebo, while approximately 0.3% of patients taking valdecoxib, and 0.2% of patients taking placebo, had notable (defined as greater than 3-fold) elevations of ALT or AST.

A patient with symptoms and/or signs suggesting liver dysfunction, or in whom an abnormal liver test has occurred, should be monitored carefully for evidence of the development of a more severe hepatic reaction while on therapy with BEXTRA. If clinical signs and symptoms consistent with liver disease develop, or if systemic manifestations occur (e.g., eosinophilia, rash), BEXTRA should be discontinued.

Renal Effects

Long-term administration of NSAIDs has resulted in renal papillary necrosis and other renal injury. Renal toxicity has also been seen in patients in whom renal prostaglandins have a compensatory role in the maintenance of renal perfusion. In these patients, administration of a nonsteroidal anti-inflammatory drug may cause a dose-dependent reduction in prostaglandin formation and, secondarily, in renal blood flow, which may precipitate overt renal decompensation. Patients at greatest risk of this reaction are those with impaired renal function, heart failure, liver dysfunction, those taking diuretics and Angiotensin Converting Enzyme (ACE) inhibitors, and the elderly. Discontinuation of NSAID therapy is usually followed by recovery to the pretreatment state.

Caution should be used when initiating treatment with BEXTRA in patients with considerable dehydration. It is advisable to rehydrate patients first and then start therapy with BEXTRA. Caution is also recommended in patients with preexisting kidney disease. (See WARNINGS — Advanced Renal Disease.)

Hematological Effects

Anemia is sometimes seen in patients receiving BEXTRA. Patients on long-term treatment with BEXTRA should have their hemoglobin or hematocrit checked if they exhibit any signs or symptoms of anemia.

BEXTRA does not generally affect platelet counts, prothrombin time (PT), or activated partial thromboplastin time (APTT), and does not appear to inhibit platelet aggregation at indicated dosages (See CLINICAL STUDIES — Safety Studies — Platelets).

Fluid Retention and Edema

Fluid retention and edema have been observed in some patients taking BEXTRA (see ADVERSE REACTIONS). Therefore, BEXTRA should be used with caution in patients with fluid retention, hypertension, or heart failure.

Preexisting Asthma

Patients with asthma may have aspirin-sensitive asthma. The use of aspirin in patients with aspirin-sensitive asthma has been associated with severe bronchospasm, which can be fatal. Since cross reactivity, including bronchospasm, between aspirin and other nonsteroidal anti-inflammatory drugs has been reported in such aspirin-sensitive patients, BEXTRA should not be administered to patients with this form of aspirin sensitivity and should be used with caution in patients with preexisting asthma.

Information for Patients

BEXTRA can cause GI discomfort and, rarely, more serious GI side effects, which may result in hospitalization and even fatal outcomes. Although serious GI tract ulcerations and bleeding can occur without warning symptoms, patients should be alert for the signs and symptoms of ulcerations and bleeding, and should ask for medical advice when observing any indicative sign or symptoms. Patients should be apprised of the importance of this follow-up (see WARNINGS — Gastrointestinal (GI) Effects — Risk of GI Ulceration, Bleeding, and Perforation).

Patients should report to their physicians, signs or symptoms of gastrointestinal ulceration or bleeding, skin rash, weight gain, or edema.

Patients should be informed of the warning signs and symptoms of hepatotoxicity (e.g., nausea, fatigue, lethargy, pruritus, jaundice, right upper quadrant tenderness, and flu-like symptoms). If these occur, patients should be instructed to stop therapy and seek immediate medical attention.

Patients should also be instructed to seek immediate emergency help in the case of an anaphylactoid reaction (see WARNINGS — Anaphylactoid Reactions).

In late pregnancy, BEXTRA should be avoided because it may cause premature closure of the ductus arteriosus.

Table 4

Adverse Events with Incidence ≥ 2.0% in Valdecoxib Treatment Groups: Controlled Arthritis Trials of Three Months or Longer

		(Total Daily Dose)				
		Valdecoxib		Diclofenac	Ibuprofen	Naproxen
Adverse Event	**Placebo**	**10 mg**	**20 mg**	**150 mg**	**2400 mg**	**1000 mg**
Number Treated	973	1214	1358	711	207	766
Autonomic Nervous System Disorders						
Hypertension	0.6	1.6	2.1	2.5	2.4	1.7
Body as a Whole						
Back pain	1.6	1.6	2.7	2.8	1.4	1.0
Edema peripheral	0.7	2.4	3.0	3.2	2.9	2.1
Influenza-like symptoms	2.2	2.0	2.2	3.1	2.9	2.0
Injury accidental	2.8	4.0	3.7	3.9	3.9	3.0
Central and Peripheral Nervous System Disorders						
Dizziness	2.1	2.6	2.7	4.2	3.4	2.7
Headache	7.1	4.8	8.5	6.6	4.3	5.5
Gastrointestinal System Disorders						
Abdominal fullness	2.0	2.1	1.9	3.0	2.9	2.5
Abdominal pain	6.3	7.0	8.2	17.0	8.2	10.1
Diarrhea	4.2	5.4	6.0	10.8	3.9	4.7
Dyspepsia	6.3	7.9	8.7	13.4	15.0	12.9
Flatulence	4.1	2.9	3.5	3.1	7.7	5.4
Nausea	5.9	7.0	6.3	8.4	7.7	8.7
Musculoskeletal System Disorders						
Myalgia	1.6	2.0	1.9	2.4	2.4	1.4
Respiratory System Disorders						
Sinusitis	2.2	2.6	1.8	1.1	3.4	3.4
Upper respiratory tract infection	6.0	6.7	5.7	6.3	4.3	6.4
Skin and Appendages Disorders						
Rash	1.0	1.4	2.1	1.5	0.5	1.4

Laboratory Tests

Because serious GI tract ulcerations and bleeding can occur without warning symptoms, physicians should monitor for signs and symptoms of GI bleeding.

Drug Interactions

The drug interaction studies with valdecoxib were performed both with valdecoxib and a rapidly hydrolyzed intravenous prodrug form. The results from trials using the intravenous prodrug are reported in this section as they relate to the role of valdecoxib in drug interactions.

General: In humans, valdecoxib metabolism is predominantly mediated via CYP 3A4 and 2C9 with glucuronidation being a further (20%) route of metabolism. In vitro studies indicate that valdecoxib is a moderate inhibitor of CYP 2C19 (IC50 = 6 µg/mL), and a weak inhibitor of both 3A4 (IC50 = 44 µg/mL) and 2C9 (IC50 = 13 µg/mL). In view of the limitations of in vitro studies and the high valdecoxib IC50 values, the potential for such metabolic inhibitory effects in vivo at therapeutic doses of valdecoxib is low.

Aspirin: Concomitant administration of aspirin with valdecoxib may result in an increased risk of GI ulceration and complications compared to valdecoxib alone. Because of its lack of anti-platelet effect valdecoxib is not a substitute for aspirin for cardiovascular prophylaxis.

In a parallel group drug interaction study comparing the intravenous prodrug form of valdecoxib at 40 mg BID (n=10) vs placebo (n=9), valdecoxib had no effect on in vitro aspirin-mediated inhibition of arachidonate- or collagen-stimulated platelet aggregation.

Methotrexate: Valdecoxib 10 mg BID did not show a significant effect on the plasma exposure or renal clearance of methotrexate.

ACE-inhibitors: Reports suggest that NSAIDs may diminish the antihypertensive effect of ACE-inhibitors. This interaction should be given consideration in patients taking BEXTRA concomitantly with ACE-inhibitors.

Furosemide: Clinical studies, as well as post-marketing observations, have shown that NSAIDs can reduce the natriuretic effect of furosemide and thiazides in some patients. This response has been attributed to inhibition of renal prostaglandin synthesis.

Anticonvulsants: Anticonvulsant drug interaction studies with valdecoxib have not been conducted. As with other drugs, routine monitoring should be performed when therapy with BEXTRA is either initiated or discontinued in patients on anticonvulsant therapy.

Dextromethorphan: Dextromethorphan is primarily metabolized by CYP 2D6 and to a lesser extent by 3A4. Coadministration with valdecoxib (40 mg BID for 7 days) resulted in a significant increase in dextromethorphan plasma levels suggesting that, at these doses, valdecoxib is a weak inhibitor of 2D6. Dextromethorphan plasma concentrations in the presence of high doses of valdecoxib were almost 5-fold lower than those seen in CYP 2D6 poor metabolizers.

Lithium: Valdecoxib 40 mg BID for 7 days produced significant decreases in lithium serum clearance (25%) and renal clearance (30%) with a 34% higher serum exposure compared to lithium alone. Lithium serum concentrations should be monitored closely when initiating or changing therapy with BEXTRA in patients receiving lithium. Lithium carbonate (450 mg BID for 7 days) had no effect on valdecoxib pharmacokinetics.

Warfarin: The effect of valdecoxib on the anticoagulant effect of warfarin (1-8 mg/day) was studied in healthy subjects by coadministration of BEXTRA 40 mg BID for 7 days. Valdecoxib caused a statistically significant increase in plasma exposures of R-warfarin and S-warfarin (12% and 15%, respectively), and in the pharmacodynamic effects (prothrombin time, measured as INR) of warfarin. While mean INR values were only slightly increased with coadministration of valdecoxib, the day-to-day variability in individual INR values was increased. Anticoagulant therapy should be monitored, particularly during the first few weeks, after initiating therapy with BEXTRA in patients receiving warfarin or similar agents.

Fluconazole and Ketoconazole: Ketoconazole and fluconazole are predominantly CYP 3A4 and 2C9 inhibitors, respectively. Concomitant single dose administration of valdecoxib 20 mg with multiple doses of ketoconazole and fluconazole produced a significant increase in exposure of valdecoxib. Plasma exposure (AUC) to valdecoxib was increased 62% when coadministered with fluconazole and 38% when coadministered with ketoconazole.

Glyburide: Glyburide is a CYP 3A4 substrate. Coadministration of valdecoxib (10 mg BID for 7 days) with glyburide (5 mg QD or 10 mg BID) did not affect the pharmacokinetics (exposure) of glyburide.

Carcinogenesis, Mutagenesis, Impairment of Fertility

Valdecoxib was not carcinogenic in rats given oral doses up to 7.5 mg/kg/day for males and 1.5 mg/kg/day for females (equivalent to approximately 2- to 6-fold human exposure at 20 mg QD as measured by the $AUC_{(0-24hr)}$) or in mice given oral doses up to 25 mg/kg/day for males and 50 mg/kg/day for females (equivalent to approximately 0.6- to 2.4-fold human exposure at 20 mg QD as measured by the $AUC_{(0-24hr)}$) for two years.

Valdecoxib was not mutagenic in an Ames test or a mutation assay in Chinese hamster ovary (CHO) cells, nor was it clastogenic in a chromosome aberration assay in CHO cells or in an in vivo micronucleus test in rat bone marrow.

Valdecoxib did not impair male rat fertility at oral doses up to 9.0 mg/kg/day (equivalent to approximately 3- to 6-fold human exposure at 20 mg QD as measured by the $AUC_{(0-24hr)}$). In female rats, a decrease in ovulation with increased pre- and post-implantation loss resulted in decreased live embryos/fetuses at doses ≥2 mg/kg/day (equivalent to approximately 2-fold human exposure at 20 mg QD as measured by the $AUC_{(0-24hr)}$ for valdecoxib). The effects on female fertility were reversible. This effect is expected with inhibition of prostaglandin synthesis and is not the result of irreversible alteration of female reproductive function.

Pregnancy

Teratogenic Effects: Pregnancy Category C.

The incidence of fetuses with skeletal anomalies such as semi-bipartite thoracic vertebra centra and fused sternebrae was slightly higher in rabbits at an oral dose of 40 mg/kg/day (equivalent to approximately 72-fold human exposures at 20 mg QD as measured by the $AUC_{(0-24hr)}$) throughout organogenesis. Valdecoxib was not teratogenic in rabbits up to an oral dose of 10 mg/kg/day (equivalent to approximately 8-fold human exposures at 20 mg QD as measured by the $AUC_{(0-24hr)}$).

Valdecoxib was not teratogenic in rats up to an oral dose of 10 mg/kg/day (equivalent to approximately 19-fold human exposure at 20 mg QD as measured by the $AUC_{(0-24hr)}$). There are no studies in pregnant women. However, valdecoxib crosses the placenta in rats and rabbits. BEXTRA should be used during pregnancy only if the potential benefit justifies the potential risk to the fetus.

Non-Teratogenic Effects: Valdecoxib caused increased pre- and post-implantation loss with reduced live fetuses at oral doses ≥10 mg/kg/day (equivalent to approximately 19-fold human exposure at 20 mg QD as measured by the $AUC_{(0-24hr)}$) in rats and an oral dose of 40 mg/kg/day (equivalent to approximately 72-fold human exposure at 20 mg QD as measured by the $AUC_{(0-24hr)}$) in rabbits throughout organogenesis. In addition, reduced neonatal survival and decreased neonatal body weight when rats were treated

Continued on next page

Bextra—Cont.

with valdecoxib at oral doses ≥6 mg/kg/day (equivalent to approximately 7-fold human exposure at 20 mg QD as measured by the $AUC_{(0-24hr)}$) throughout organogenesis and lactation period. No studies have been conducted to evaluate the effect of valdecoxib on the closure of the ductus arteriosus in humans. Therefore, as with other drugs known to inhibit prostaglandin synthesis, use of BEXTRA during the third trimester of pregnancy should be avoided.

Labor and Delivery

Valdecoxib produced no evidence of delayed labor or parturition at oral doses up to 10 mg/kg/day in rats (equivalent to approximately 19-fold human exposure at 20 mg QD as measured by the $AUC_{(0-24hr)}$). The effects of BEXTRA on labor and delivery in pregnant women are unknown.

Nursing Mothers

Valdecoxib and its active metabolite are excreted in the milk of lactating rats. It is not known whether this drug is excreted in human milk. Because many drugs are excreted in human milk, and because of the potential for adverse reactions in nursing infants from BEXTRA, a decision should be made whether to discontinue nursing or to discontinue the drug, taking into account the importance of the drug to the mother and the importance of nursing to the infant.

Pediatric Use

Safety and effectiveness of BEXTRA in pediatric patients below the age of 18 years have not been evaluated.

Geriatric Use

Of the patients who received BEXTRA in arthritis clinical trials of three months duration, or greater, approximately 2100 were 65 years of age or older, including 570 patients who were 75 years or older. No overall differences in effectiveness were observed between these patients and younger patients.

ADVERSE REACTIONS

Of the patients treated with BEXTRA Tablets in controlled arthritis trials, 2665 were patients with OA, and 2684 were patients with RA. More than 4000 patients have received a chronic total daily dose of BEXTRA 10 mg or more. More than 2800 patients have received BEXTRA 10 mg/day, or more, for at least 6 months and 988 of these have received BEXTRA for at least 1 year.

Osteoarthritis and Rheumatoid Arthritis

Table 4 lists all adverse events, regardless of causality, that occurred in ≥2.0% of patients receiving BEXTRA 10 and 20 mg/day in studies of three months or longer from 7 controlled studies conducted in patients with OA or RA that included a placebo and/or a positive control group.

[See table 4 at top of previous page]

In these placebo- and active-controlled clinical trials, the discontinuation rate due to adverse events was 7.5% for arthritis patients receiving valdecoxib 10 mg daily, 7.9% for arthritis patients receiving valdecoxib 20 mg daily and 6.0% for patients receiving placebo.

In the seven controlled OA and RA studies, the following adverse events occurred in 0.1–1.9% of patients treated with BEXTRA 10–20 mg daily, regardless of causality.

Application site disorders: Cellulitis, dermatitis contact

Cardiovascular: Aggravated hypertension, aneurysm, angina pectoris, arrhythmia, cardiomyopathy, congestive heart failure, coronary artery disorder, heart murmur, hypotension

Central, peripheral nervous system: Cerebrovascular disorder, hypertonia, hypoesthesia, migraine, neuralgia, neuropathy, paresthesia, tremor, twitching, vertigo

Endocrine: Goiter

Female reproductive: Amenorrhea, dysmenorrhea, leukorrhea, mastitis, menstrual disorder, menorrhagia, menstrual bloating, vaginal hemorrhage

Gastrointestinal: Abnormal stools, constipation, diverticulosis, dry mouth, duodenal ulcer, duodenitis, eructation, esophagitis, fecal incontinence, gastric ulcer, gastritis, gastroenteritis, gastroesophageal reflux, hematemesis, hematochezia, hemorrhoids, hemorrhoids bleeding, hiatal hernia, melena, stomatitis, stool frequency increased, tenesmus, tooth disorder, vomiting

General: Allergy aggravated, allergic reaction, asthenia, chest pain, chills, cyst NOS, edema generalized, face edema, fatigue, fever, hot flushes, halitosis, malaise, pain, periorbital swelling, peripheral pain

Hearing and vestibular: Ear abnormality, earache, tinnitus

Heart rate and rhythm: Bradycardia, palpitation, tachycardia

Hemic: Anemia

Liver and biliary system: Hepatic function abnormal, hepatitis, ALT increased, AST increased

Male reproductive: Impotence, prostatic disorder

Metabolic and nutritional: Alkaline phosphatase increased, BUN increased, CPK increased, creatinine increased, diabetes mellitus, glycosuria, gout, hypercholesterolemia, hyperglycemia, hyperkalemia, hyperlipemia, hyperuricemia, hypocalcemia, hypokalemia, LDH increased, thirst increased, weight decrease, weight increase, xerophthalmia

Musculoskeletal: Arthralgia, fracture accidental, neck stiffness, osteoporosis, synovitis, tendonitis

Neoplasm: Breast neoplasm, lipoma, malignant ovarian cyst

Platelets (bleeding or clotting): Ecchymosis, epistaxis, hematoma NOS, thrombocytopenia

Psychiatric: Anorexia, anxiety, appetite increased, confusion, depression, depression aggravated, insomnia, nervousness, morbid dreaming, somnolence

Resistance mechanism disorders: Herpes simplex, herpes zoster, infection fungal, infection soft tissue, infection viral, moniliasis, moniliasis genital, otitis media

Respiratory: Abnormal breath sounds, bronchitis, bronchospasm, coughing, dyspnea, emphysema, laryngitis, pneumonia, pharyngitis, pleurisy, rhinitis

Skin and appendages: Acne, alopecia, dermatitis, dermatitis fungal, eczema, photosensitivity allergic reaction, pruritus, rash erythematous, rash maculopapular, rash psoriaform, skin dry, skin hypertrophy, skin ulceration, sweating increased, urticaria

Special senses: Taste perversion

Urinary system: Albuminuria, cystitis, dysuria, hematuria, micturition frequency increased, pyuria, urinary incontinence, urinary tract infection

Vascular: Claudication intermittent, hemangioma acquired, varicose vein

Vision: Blurred vision, cataract, conjunctival hemorrhage, conjunctivitis, eye pain, keratitis, vision abnormal

White cell and RES disorders: Eosinophilia, leukopenia, leukocytosis, lymphadenopathy, lymphangitis, lymphopenia

Other serious adverse events that were reported rarely (estimated <0.1%) in clinical trials, regardless of causality, in patients taking BEXTRA:

Autonomic nervous system disorders: Hypertensive encephalopathy, vasospasm

Cardiovascular: Abnormal ECG, aortic stenosis, atrial fibrillation, carotid stenosis, coronary thrombosis, heart block, heart valve disorders, mitral insufficiency, myocardial infarction, myocardial ischemia, pericarditis, syncope, thrombophlebitis, unstable angina, ventricular fibrillation

Central, peripheral nervous system: Convulsions

Endocrine: Hyperparathyroidism

Female reproductive: Cervical dysplasia

Gastrointestinal: Appendicitis, colitis with bleeding, dysphagia, esophageal perforation, gastrointestinal bleeding, ileus, intestinal obstruction, peritonitis

Hemic: Lymphoma-like disorder, pancytopenia

Liver and biliary system: Cholelithiasis

Metabolic: Dehydration

Musculoskeletal: Pathological fracture, osteomyelitis

Neoplasm: Benign brain neoplasm, bladder carcinoma, carcinoma, gastric carcinoma, prostate carcinoma, pulmonary carcinoma

Platelets (bleeding or clotting): Embolism, pulmonary embolism, thrombosis

Psychiatric: Manic reaction, psychosis

Renal: Acute renal failure

Resistance mechanism disorders: Sepsis

Respiratory: Apnea, pleural effusion, pulmonary edema, pulmonary fibrosis, pulmonary infarction, pulmonary hemorrhage, respiratory insufficiency

Skin: Basal cell carcinoma, malignant melanoma

Urinary system: Pyelonephritis, renal calculus

Vision: Retinal detachment

Postmarketing Eperience

The following reactions have been identified during postmarketing use of BEXTRA. These reactions have been chosen for inclusion either due to their seriousness, reporting frequency, possible causal relationship to BEXTRA, or a combination of these factors. Because these reactions were reported voluntarily from a population of uncertain size, it is not possible to reliably estimate their frequency or establish a causal relationship to drug exposure.

General: Hypersensitivity reactions (including anaphylactic reactions and angioedema)

Skin and appendages: Erythema multiforme, exfoliative dermatitis, Stevens-Johnson syndrome, toxic epidermal necrolysis

OVERDOSAGE

Symptoms following acute NSAID overdoses are usually limited to lethargy, drowsiness, nausea, vomiting, and epigastric pain, which are generally reversible with supportive care. Gastrointestinal bleeding can occur. Hypertension, acute renal failure, respiratory depression and coma may occur, but are rare.

Anaphylactoid reactions have been reported with therapeutic ingestion of NSAIDs, and may occur following an overdose.

Patients should be managed by symptomatic and supportive care following an NSAID overdose. There are no specific antidotes. Hemodialysis removed only about 2% of administered valdecoxib from the systemic circulation of 8 patients with end-stage renal disease and, based on its degree of plasma protein binding (>98%), dialysis is unlikely to be useful in overdose. Forced diuresis, alkalinization of urine, or hemoperfusion also may not be useful due to high protein binding.

DOSAGE AND ADMINISTRATION

Osteoarthritis and Adult Rheumatoid Arthritis

The recommended dose of BEXTRA Tablets for the relief of the signs and symptoms of arthritis is 10 mg once daily.

Primary Dysmenorrhea

The recommended dose of BEXTRA Tablets for treatment of primary dysmenorrhea is 20 mg twice daily, as needed.

HOW SUPPLIED

BEXTRA Tablets 10 mg are white, film-coated, and capsule-shaped, debossed "10" on one side with a four pointed star shape on the other, supplied as:

NDC Number	Size
0025-1975-31	Bottle of 100
0025-1975-51	Bottle of 500
0025-1975-34	Carton of 100 unit dose

BEXTRA Tablets 20 mg are white, film-coated, and capsule-shaped, debossed "20" on one side with a four pointed star shape on the other, supplied as:

NDC Number	Size
0025-1980-31	Bottle of 100
0025-1980-51	Bottle of 500
0025-1980-34	Carton of 100 unit dose

Store at 25°C (77°F); excursions permitted to 15-30°C (59-86°F) [See USP Controlled Room Temperature].

℞ only

Revised: October 2002

Manufactured for:
G.D. Searle LLC
A subsidiary of Pharmacia Corporation
Chicago, IL 60680, USA
Pfizer Inc
New York, NY 10017, USA
by: Searle Ltd.
Caguas, PR 00725

818 763 002 P04001-2/PS4001-2

CARDURA® ℞

[*kär'dŭră*]

(doxazosin mesylate)

Tablets

Prescribing information for this product, which appears on pages 2581–2584 of the 2003 PDR, has been completely revised as follows. Please write "See Supplement A" next to the product heading.

DESCRIPTION

CARDURA® (doxazosin mesylate) is a quinazoline compound that is a selective inhibitor of the $alpha_1$ subtype of alpha adrenergic receptors. The chemical name of doxazosin mesylate is 1-(4-amino-6,7-dimethoxy-2-quinazolinyl)-4-(1,4-benzodioxan-2-ylcarbonyl) piperazine methanesulfonate. The empirical formula for doxazosin mesylate is $C_{23}H_{25}N_5O_5 \cdot CH_4O_3S$ and the molecular weight is 547.6. It has the following structure:

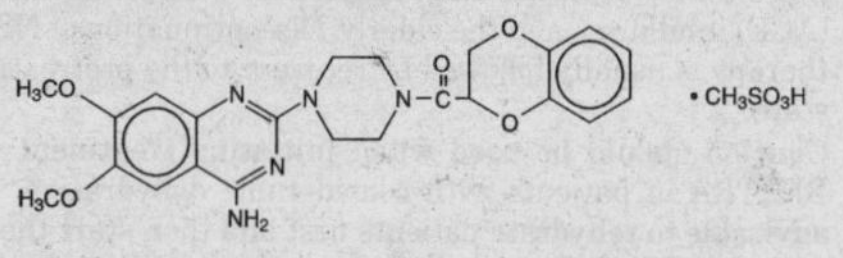

CARDURA® (doxazosin mesylate) is freely soluble in dimethylsulfoxide, soluble in dimethylformamide, slightly soluble in methanol, ethanol, and water (0.8% at 25°C), and very slightly soluble in acetone and methylene chloride. CARDURA® is available as colored tablets for oral use and contains 1 mg (white), 2 mg (yellow), 4 mg (orange) and 8 mg (green) of doxazosin as the free base.

The inactive ingredients for all tablets are: microcrystalline cellulose, lactose, sodium starch glycolate, magnesium stearate and sodium lauryl sulfate. The 2 mg tablet contains D & C yellow 10 and FD & C yellow 6; the 4 mg tablet contains FD & C yellow 6; the 8 mg tablet contains FD & C blue 10 and D & C yellow 10.

CLINICAL PHARMACOLOGY

Pharmacodynamics

A. Benign Prostatic Hyperplasia (BPH)

Benign prostatic hyperplasia (BPH) is a common cause of urinary outflow obstruction in aging males. Severe BPH may lead to urinary retention and renal damage. A static and a dynamic component contribute to the symptoms and reduced urinary flow rate associated with BPH. The static component is related to an increase in prostate size caused, in part, by a proliferation of smooth muscle cells in the prostatic stroma. However, the severity of BPH symptoms and the degree of urethral obstruction do not correlate well with the size of the prostate. The dynamic component of BPH is associated with an increase in smooth muscle tone in the prostate and bladder neck. The degree of tone in this area is mediated by the $alpha_1$ adrenoceptor, which is present in high density in the prostatic stroma, prostatic capsule and bladder neck. Blockade of the $alpha_1$ receptor decreases urethral resistance and may relieve the obstruction and BPH symptoms. In the human prostate, CARDURA® antagonizes phenylephrine ($alpha_1$ agonist)-induced contractions, *in vitro*, and binds with high affinity to the $alpha_{1c}$ adrenoceptor. The receptor subtype is thought to be the predominant functional type in the prostate. CARDURA® acts within 1–2 weeks to decrease the severity of BPH symptoms and improve urinary flow rate. Since $alpha_1$ adrenoceptors are of low density in the urinary bladder (apart from the bladder neck), CARDURA® should maintain bladder contractility.

The efficacy of CARDURA® was evaluated extensively in over 900 patients with BPH in double-blind, placebo-controlled trials. CARDURA® treatment was superior to placebo in improving patient symptoms and urinary flow rate. Significant relief with CARDURA® was seen as early as one week into the treatment regimen, with CARDURA® treated patients (N=173) showing a significant (p<0.01) increase in maximum flow rate of 0.8 mL/sec compared to a decrease of 0.5 mL/sec in the placebo group (N=41). In long-term studies improvement was maintained for up to 2 years of treatment. In 66-71% of patients, improvements above baseline were seen in both symptoms and maximum urinary flow rate.

In three placebo-controlled studies of 14-16 weeks duration obstructive symptoms (hesitation, intermittency, dribbling, weak urinary stream, incomplete emptying of the bladder) and irritative symptoms (nocturia, daytime frequency, urgency, burning) of BPH were evaluated at each visit by patient-assessed symptom questionnaires. The bothersomeness of symptoms was measured with a modified Boyarsky questionnaire. Symptom severity/frequency was assessed using a modified Boyarsky questionnaire or an AUA-based questionnaire. Uroflowmetric evaluations were performed at times of peak (2-6 hours post-dose) and/or trough (24 hours post-dose) plasma concentrations of CARDURA®.

The results from the three placebo-controlled studies (N=609) showing significant efficacy with 4 mg and 8 mg doxazosin are summarized in Table 1. In all three studies, CARDURA® resulted in statistically significant relief of obstructive and irritative symptoms compared to placebo. Statistically significant improvements of 2.3-3.3 mL/sec in maximum flow rate were seen with CARDURA® in Studies 1 and 2, compared to 0.1-0.7 mL/sec with placebo.

[See table 1 at right]

In one fixed dose study (Study 2) CARDURA® (doxazosin mesylate) therapy (4-8 mg, once daily) resulted in a significant and sustained improvement in maximum urinary flow rate of 2.3-3.3 mL/sec (Table 1) compared to placebo (0.1 mL/sec). In this study, the only study in which weekly evaluations were made, significant improvement with CARDURA® vs. placebo was seen after one week. The proportion of patients who responded with a maximum flow rate improvement of ≥ 3 mL/sec was significantly larger with CARDURA® (34-42%) than placebo (13-17%). A significantly greater improvement was also seen in average flow rate with CARDURA® (1.6 mL/sec) than with placebo (0.2 mL/sec). The onset and time course of symptom relief and increased urinary flow from Study 1 are illustrated in Figure 1.

Figure 1–Study 1

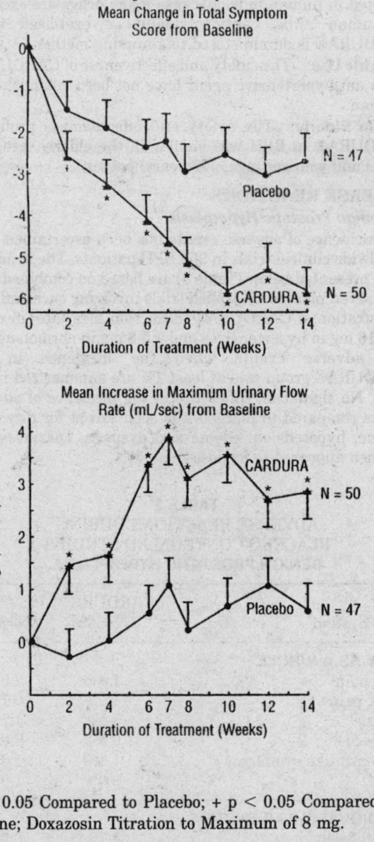

* $p < 0.05$ Compared to Placebo; + $p < 0.05$ Compared to Baseline; Doxazosin Titration to Maximum of 8 mg.

In BPH patients (N=450) treated for up to 2 years in open-label studies, CARDURA® therapy resulted in significant improvement above baseline in urinary flow rates and BPH symptoms. The significant effects of CARDURA® were maintained over the entire treatment period.

Although blockade of $alpha_1$ adrenoceptors also lowers blood pressure in hypertensive patients with increased peripheral vascular resistance, CARDURA® treatment of normotensive men with BPH did not result in a clinically significant blood pressure lowering effect (Table 2). The proportion of normotensive patients with a sitting systolic blood pressure less than 90 mmHg and/or diastolic blood pressure less than 60 mmHg at any time during treatment with CARDURA® 1-8 mg once daily was 6.7% with doxazosin and not significantly different (statistically) from that with placebo (5%).

TABLE 1
SUMMARY OF EFFECTIVENESS DATA IN PLACEBO-CONTROLLED TRIALS

	SYMPTOM SCORE[a]			MAXIMUM FLOW RATE (mL/sec)		
	N	MEAN BASELINE	MEAN[b] CHANGE	N	MEAN BASELINE	MEAN[c] CHANGE
STUDY 1 (Titration to maximum dose of 8 mg)[e]						
Placebo	47	15.6	-2.3	41	9.7	+0.7
CARDURA	49	14.5	-4.9**	41	9.8	+2.9**
STUDY 2 (Titration to fixed dose–14 weeks)[d]						
Placebo	37	20.7	-2.5	30	10.6	+0.1
CARDURA 4 mg	38	21.2	-5.0**	32	9.8	+2.3*
CARDURA 8 mg	42	19.9	-4.2*	36	10.5	+3.3**
STUDY 3 (Titration to fixed dose–12 weeks)						
Placebo	47	14.9	-4.7	44	9.9	+2.1
CARDURA 4 mg	46	16.6	-6.1*	46	9.6	+2.6

[a] AUA questionnaire (range 0-30) in studies 1 and 3.
Modified Boyarsky Questionnaire (range 7-39) in study 2.
[b] Change is to endpoint.
[c] Change is to fixed-dose efficacy phase, 22-26 hours post-dose for studies 1 and 3 and 2-6 hours post-dose for study 2.
[d] Study in hypertensives with BPH
[e] 36 patients received a dose of 8 mg CARDURA*
*(**) $p < 0.05$ (0.01) compared to placebo mean change.

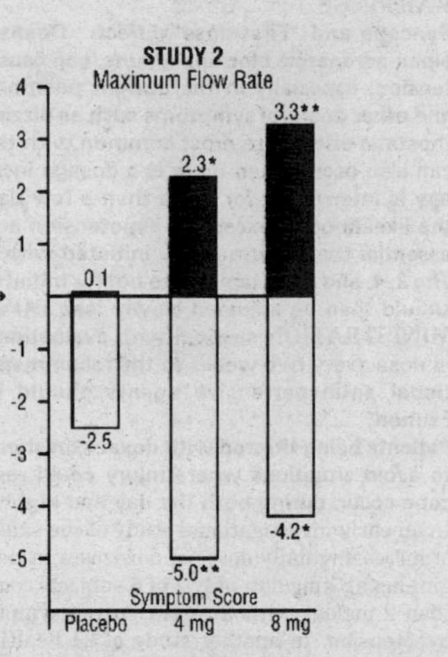

TABLE 2
Mean Changes in Blood Pressure from Baseline to the Mean of the Final Efficacy Phase in Normotensives (Diastolic BP <90 mmHg) in Two Double-blind, Placebo-controlled U.S. Studies with CARDURA® 1–8 mg once daily.

	PLACEBO (N=85)		CARDURA® (N=183)	
Sitting BP (mmHg)	**Baseline**	**Change**	**Baseline**	**Change**
Systolic	128.4	−1.4	128.8	−4.9*
Diastolic	79.2	−1.2	79.6	−2.4*
Standing BP (mmHg)	**Baseline**	**Change**	**Baseline**	**Change**
Systolic	128.5	−0.6	128.5	−5.3*
Diastolic	80.5	−0.7	80.4	−2.6*

*$p \leq 0.05$ compared to placebo

B. *Hypertension*

The mechanism of action of CARDURA® (doxazosin mesylate) is selective blockade of the $alpha_1$ (postjunctional) subtype of adrenergic receptors. Studies in normal human subjects have shown that doxazosin competitively antagonized the pressor effects of phenylephrine (an $alpha_1$ agonist) and the systolic pressor effect of norepinephrine. Doxazosin and prazosin have similar abilities to antagonize phenylephrine. The antihypertensive effect of CARDURA® results from a decrease in systemic vascular resistance. The parent compound doxazosin is primarily responsible for the antihypertensive activity. The low plasma concentrations of known active and inactive metabolites of doxazosin (2-piperazinyl, 6'- and 7'-hydroxy and 6- and 7-O-desmethyl compounds) compared to parent drug indicate that the contribution of even the most potent compound (6'-hydroxy) to the antihypertensive effect of doxazosin in man is probably small. The 6'- and 7'-hydroxy metabolites have demonstrated antioxidant properties at concentrations of 5 μM, *in vitro*.

Administration of CARDURA® results in a reduction in systemic vascular resistance. In patients with hypertension there is little change in cardiac output. Maximum reductions in blood pressure usually occur 2-6 hours after dosing and are associated with a small increase in standing heart rate. Like other $alpha_1$-adrenergic blocking agents, doxazosin has a greater effect on blood pressure and heart rate in the standing position.

In a pooled analysis of placebo-controlled hypertension studies with about 300 hypertensive patients per treatment group, doxazosin, at doses of 1-16 mg given once daily, lowered blood pressure at 24 hours by about 10/8 mmHg compared to placebo in the standing position and about 9/5 mmHg in the supine position. Peak blood pressure effects (1-6 hours) were larger by about 50-75% (i.e., trough values were about 55-70% of peak effect), with the larger peak-trough differences seen in systolic pressures. There was no apparent difference in the blood pressure response of Caucasians and blacks or of patients above and below age 65. In these predominantly normocholesterolemic patients doxazosin produced small reductions in total serum cholesterol (2-3%), LDL cholesterol (4%), and a similarly small increase in HDL/total cholesterol ratio (4%). The clinical significance of these findings is uncertain. In the same patient population, patients receiving CARDURA® gained a mean of 0.6 kg compared to a mean loss of 0.1 kg for placebo patients.

Pharmacokinetics

After oral administration of therapeutic doses, peak plasma levels of CARDURA® (doxazosin mesylate) occur at about 2–3 hours. Bioavailability is approximately 65%, reflecting first pass metabolism of doxazosin by the liver. The effect of food on the pharmacokinetics of CARDURA® was examined in a crossover study with twelve hypertensive subjects. Reductions of 18% in mean maximum plasma concentration and 12% in the area under the concentration-time curve occurred when CARDURA® was administered with food. Neither of these differences was statistically or clinically significant.

CARDURA® is extensively metabolized in the liver, mainly by O-demethylation of the quinazoline nucleus or hydroxylation of the benzodioxan moiety. Although several active metabolites of doxazosin have been identified, the pharmacokinetics of these metabolites have not been characterized. In a study of two subjects administered radiolabelled doxazosin 2 mg orally and 1 mg intravenously on two separate occasions, approximately 63% of the dose was eliminated in the feces and 9% of the dose was found in the urine. On average only 4.8% of the dose was excreted as unchanged drug in the feces and only a trace of the total radioactivity in the urine was attributed to unchanged drug. At the plasma concentrations achieved by therapeutic doses approximately 98% of the circulating drug is bound to plasma proteins.

Plasma elimination of doxazosin is biphasic, with a terminal elimination half-life of about 22 hours. Steady-state studies in hypertensive patients given doxazosin doses of 2–16 mg once daily showed linear kinetics and dose proportionality. In two studies, following the administration of 2 mg orally once daily, the mean accumulation ratios (steady-state AUC vs. first dose AUC) were 1.2 and 1.7. Enterohepatic recycling is suggested by secondary peaking of plasma doxazosin concentrations.

In a crossover study in 24 normotensive subjects, the pharmacokinetics and safety of doxazosin were shown to be similar with morning and evening dosing regimens. The area under the curve after morning dosing was, however, 11% less than that after evening dosing and the time to peak concentration after evening dosing occurred significantly later than that after morning dosing (5.6 hr vs. 3.5 hr).

The pharmacokinetics of CARDURA® (doxazosin mesylate) in young (<65 years) and elderly (≥65 years) subjects were similar for plasma half-life values and oral clearance. Pharmacokinetic studies in elderly patients and patients with renal impairment have shown no significant alterations compared to younger patients with normal renal function. Administration of a single 2 mg dose to patients with cirrhosis (Child-Pugh Class A) showed a 40% increase in exposure to doxazosin. There are only limited data on the effects of drugs known to influence the hepatic metabolism of doxazosin [e.g., cimetidine (see PRECAUTIONS)]. As with any drug wholly metabolized by the liver, use of CARDURA® in patients with altered liver function should be undertaken with caution.

In two placebo-controlled studies, of normotensive and hypertensive BPH patients, in which doxazosin was administered in the morning and the titration interval was two weeks and one week, respectively, trough plasma concentrations of CARDURA® were similar in the two populations. Linear kinetics and dose proportionality were observed.

INDICATIONS AND USAGE

A. *Benign Prostatic Hyperplasia (BPH).* CARDURA® is indicated for the treatment of both the urinary outflow obstruction and obstructive and irritative symptoms associated with BPH: obstructive symptoms (hesitation, intermittency, dribbling, weak urinary stream, incomplete emptying of the bladder) and irritative symptoms (nocturia, daytime frequency, urgency, burning). CARDURA® may be used in all BPH patients whether hypertensive or normotensive. In patients with hypertension and BPH, both conditions were effectively treated with CARDURA® monotherapy. CARDURA® provides rapid improvement in symptoms and urinary flow rate in 66-71% of patients. Sustained improvements with CARDURA® were seen in patients treated for up to 14 weeks in double-blind studies and up to 2 years in open-label studies.

B. *Hypertension.* CARDURA® (doxazosin mesylate) is also indicated for the treatment of hypertension. CARDURA® may be used alone or in combination with diuretics, beta-adrenergic blocking agents, calcium channel blockers or angiotensin-converting enzyme inhibitors.

CONTRAINDICATIONS

CARDURA® is contraindicated in patients with a known sensitivity to quinazolines (e.g., prazosin, terazosin), doxazosin, or any of the inert ingredients.

Continued on next page

Cardura—Cont.

WARNINGS

Syncope and "First-dose" Effect: Doxazosin, like other alpha-adrenergic blocking agents, can cause marked hypotension, especially in the upright position, with syncope and other postural symptoms such as dizziness. Marked orthostatic effects are most common with the first dose but can also occur when there is a dosage increase, or if therapy is interrupted for more than a few days. To decrease the likelihood of excessive hypotension and syncope, it is essential that treatment be initiated with the 1 mg dose. The 2, 4, and 8 mg tablets are not for initial therapy. Dosage should then be adjusted slowly (see DOSAGE AND ADMINISTRATION section) with evaluations and increases in dose every two weeks to the recommended dose. Additional antihypertensive agents should be added with caution.

Patients being titrated with doxazosin should be cautioned to avoid situations where injury could result should syncope occur, during both the day and night.

In an early investigational study of the safety and tolerance of increasing daily doses of doxazosin in normotensives beginning at 1 mg/day, only 2 of 6 subjects could tolerate more than 2 mg/day without experiencing symptomatic postural hypotension. In another study of 24 healthy normotensive male subjects receiving initial doses of 2 mg/day of doxazosin, seven (29%) of the subjects experienced symptomatic postural hypotension between 0.5 and 6 hours after the first dose necessitating termination of the study. In this study, 2 of the normotensive subjects experienced syncope. Subsequent trials in hypertensive patients always began doxazosin dosing at 1 mg/day resulting in a 4% incidence of postural side effects at 1 mg/day with no cases of syncope.

In multiple dose clinical trials in hypertension involving over 1500 hypertensive patients with dose titration every one to two weeks, syncope was reported in 0.7% of patients. None of these events occurred at the starting dose of 1 mg and 1.2% (8/664) occurred at 16 mg/day.

In placebo-controlled, clinical trials in BPH, 3 out of 665 patients (0.5%) taking doxazosin reported syncope. Two of the patients were taking 1 mg doxazosin, while one patient was taking 2 mg doxazosin when syncope occurred. In the open-label, long-term extension follow-up of approximately 450 BPH patients, there were 3 reports of syncope (0.7%). One patient was taking 2 mg, one patient was taking 8 mg and one patient was taking 12 mg when syncope occurred. In a clinical pharmacology study, one subject receiving 2 mg experienced syncope.

If syncope occurs, the patient should be placed in a recumbent position and treated supportively as necessary.

Priapism: Rarely (probably less frequently than once in every several thousand patients), $alpha_1$ antagonists, including doxazosin, have been associated with priapism (painful penile erection, sustained for hours and unrelieved by sexual intercourse or masturbation). Because this condition can lead to permanent impotence if not promptly treated, patients must be advised about the seriousness of the condition (see **PRECAUTIONS: Information for Patients**).

PRECAUTIONS

General:

Prostate Cancer: Carcinoma of the prostate causes many of the symptoms associated with BPH and the two disorders frequently co-exist. Carcinoma of the prostate should therefore be ruled out prior to commencing therapy with CARDURA®.

Orthostatic Hypotension: While syncope is the most severe orthostatic effect of CARDURA®, other symptoms of lowered blood pressure, such as dizziness, lightheadedness, or vertigo can occur, especially at initiation of therapy or at the time of dose increases.

a) Hypertension

These symptoms were common in clinical trials in hypertension, occurring in up to 23% of all patients treated and causing discontinuation of therapy in about 2%.

In placebo-controlled titration trials in hypertension, orthostatic effects were minimized by beginning therapy at 1 mg per day and titrating every two weeks to 2, 4, or 8 mg per day. There was an increased frequency of orthostatic effects in patients given 8 mg or more, 10%, compared to 5% at 1-4 mg and 3% in the placebo group.

b) Benign Prostatic Hyperplasia

In placebo-controlled trials in BPH, the incidence of orthostatic hypotension with doxazosin was 0.3% and did not increase with increasing dosage (to 8 mg/day). The incidence of discontinuations due to hypotensive or orthostatic symptoms was 3.3% with doxazosin and 1% with placebo. The titration interval in these studies was one to two weeks.

Patients in occupations in which orthostatic hypotension could be dangerous should be treated with particular caution. As $alpha_1$ antagonists can cause orthostatic effects, it is important to evaluate standing blood pressure two minutes after standing and patients should be advised to exercise care when arising from a supine or sitting position.

If hypotension occurs, the patient should be placed in the supine position and, if this measure is inadequate, volume expansion with intravenous fluids or vasopressor therapy may be used. A transient hypotensive response is not a contraindication to further doses of CARDURA® (doxazosin mesylate).

Information for Patients ***(See patient package insert)*****:** Patients should be made aware of the possibility of syncopal and orthostatic symptoms, especially at the initiation of therapy, and urged to avoid driving or hazardous tasks for 24 hours after the first dose, after a dosage increase, and after interruption of therapy when treatment is resumed. They should be cautioned to avoid situations where injury could result should syncope occur during initiation of doxazosin therapy. They should also be advised of the need to sit or lie down when symptoms of lowered blood pressure occur, although these symptoms are not always orthostatic, and to be careful when rising from a sitting or lying position. If dizziness, lightheadedness, or palpitations are bothersome they should be reported to the physician, so that dose adjustment can be considered. Patients should also be told that drowsiness or somnolence can occur with CARDURA® (doxazosin mesylate) or any selective $alpha_1$ adrenoceptor antagonist, requiring caution in people who must drive or operate heavy machinery.

Patients should be advised about the possibility of priapism as a result of treatment with $alpha_1$ antagonists. Patients should know that this adverse event is very rare. If they experience priapism, it should be brought to immediate medical attention for if not treated promptly it can lead to permanent erectile dysfunction (impotence).

Drug/Laboratory Test Interactions: CARDURA® does not affect the plasma concentration of prostate specific antigen in patients treated for up to 3 years. Both doxazosin, an $alpha_1$ inhibitor, and finasteride, a 5-alpha reductase inhibitor, are highly protein bound and hepatically metabolized. There is no definitive controlled clinical experience on the concomitant use of $alpha_1$ inhibitors and 5-alpha reductase inhibitors at this time.

Impaired Liver Function: CARDURA® should be administered with caution to patients with evidence of impaired hepatic function or to patients receiving drugs known to influence hepatic metabolism (see CLINICAL PHARMACOLOGY).

Leukopenia/Neutropenia: Analysis of hematologic data from hypertensive patients receiving CARDURA® in controlled hypertension clinical trials showed that the mean WBC (N=474) and mean neutrophil counts (N=419) were decreased by 2.4% and 1.0%, respectively, compared to placebo, a phenomenon seen with other alpha blocking drugs. In BPH patients the incidence of clinically significant WBC abnormalities was 0.4% (2/459) with CARDURA® and 0% (0/147) with placebo, with no statistically significant difference between the two treatment groups. A search through a data base of 2400 hypertensive patients and 665 BPH patients revealed 4 hypertensives in which drug-related neutropenia could not be ruled out and one BPH patient in which drug related leukopenia could not be ruled out. Two hypertensives had a single low value on the last day of treatment. Two hypertensives had stable, non-progressive neutrophil counts in the $1000/mm^3$ range over periods of 20 and 40 weeks. One BPH patient had a decrease from a WBC count of $4800/mm^3$ to $2700/mm^3$ at the end of the study; there was no evidence of clinical impairment. In cases where follow-up was available the WBCs and neutrophil counts returned to normal after discontinuation of CARDURA®. No patients became symptomatic as a result of the low WBC or neutrophil counts.

Drug Interactions: Most (98%) of plasma doxazosin is protein bound. *In vitro* data in human plasma indicate that CARDURA® has no effect on protein binding of digoxin, warfarin, phenytoin or indomethacin. There is no information on the effect of other highly plasma protein bound drugs on doxazosin binding. CARDURA® has been administered without any evidence of an adverse drug interaction to patients receiving thiazide diuretics, beta-blocking agents, and nonsteroidal anti-inflammatory drugs. In a placebo-controlled trial in normal volunteers, the administration of a single 1 mg dose of doxazosin on day 1 of a four-day regimen of oral cimetidine (400 mg twice daily) resulted in a 10% increase in mean AUC of doxazosin (p=0.006), and a slight but not statistically significant increase in mean C_{max} and mean half-life of doxazosin. The clinical significance of this increase in doxazosin AUC is unknown.

In clinical trials, CARDURA® tablets have been administered to patients on a variety of concomitant medications; while no formal interaction studies have been conducted, no interactions were observed. CARDURA® tablets have been used with the following drugs or drug classes: 1) analgesic/anti-inflammatory (e.g., acetaminophen, aspirin, codeine and codeine combinations, ibuprofen, indomethacin); 2) antibiotics (e.g., erythromycin, trimethoprim and sulfamethoxazole, amoxicillin); 3) antihistamines (e.g., chlorpheniramine); 4) cardiovascular agents (e.g., atenolol, hydrochlorothiazide, propranolol); 5) corticosteroids; 6) gastrointestinal agents (e.g., antacids); 7) hypoglycemics and endocrine drugs; 8) sedatives and tranquilizers (e.g., diazepam); 9) cold and flu remedies.

Cardiac Toxicity in Animals: An increased incidence of myocardial necrosis or fibrosis was displayed by Sprague-Dawley rats after 6 months of dietary administration at concentrations calculated to provide 80 mg doxazosin/kg/day and after 12 months of dietary administration at concentrations calculated to provide 40 mg doxazosin/kg/day (AUC exposure in rats 8 times the human AUC exposure with a 12 mg/day therapeutic dose). Myocardial fibrosis was observed in both rats and mice treated in the same manner with 40 mg doxazosin/kg/day for 18 months (exposure 8 times human AUC exposure in rats and somewhat equivalent to human C_{max} exposure in mice). No cardiotoxicity was observed at lower doses (up to 10 or 20 mg/kg/day, depending on the study) in either species. These lesions were not observed after 12 months of oral dosing in dogs at maximum doses of 20 mg/kg/day [maximum plasma concentrations (C_{max}) in dogs 14 times the C_{max} exposure in humans receiving a 12 mg/day therapeutic dose] and in Wistar rats at doses of 100 mg/kg/day (C_{max} exposures 15 times human C_{max} exposure with a 12 mg/day therapeutic dose). There is no evidence that similar lesions occur in humans.

Carcinogenesis, Mutagenesis, Impairment of Fertility: Chronic dietary administration (up to 24 months) of doxazosin mesylate at maximally tolerated doses of 40 mg/kg/day in rats and 120 mg/kg/day in mice revealed no evidence of carcinogenic potential. The highest doses evaluated in the rat and mouse studies are associated with AUCs (a measure of systemic exposure) that are 8 times and 4 times, respectively, the human AUC at a dose of 16 mg/day.

Mutagenicity studies revealed no drug- or metabolite-related effects at either chromosomal or subchromosomal levels.

Studies in rats showed reduced fertility in males treated with doxazosin at oral doses of 20 (but not 5 or 10) mg/kg/day, about 4 times the AUC exposures obtained with a 12 mg/day human dose. This effect was reversible within two weeks of drug withdrawal. There have been no reports of any effects of doxazosin on male fertility in humans.

Pregnancy: Teratogenic Effects, Pregnancy Category C. Studies in pregnant rabbits and rats at daily oral doses of up to 41 and 20 mg/kg, respectively (plasma drug concentrations 10 and 4 times human C_{max} and AUC exposures with a 12 mg/day therapeutic dose), have revealed no evidence of harm to the fetus. A dosage regimen of 82 mg/kg/day in the rabbit was associated with reduced fetal survival. There are no adequate and well-controlled studies in pregnant women. Because animal reproduction studies are not always predictive of human response, CARDURA® should be used during pregnancy only if clearly needed.

Radioactivity was found to cross the placenta following oral administration of labelled doxazosin to pregnant rats.

Nonteratogenic Effects: In peri-postnatal studies in rats, postnatal development at maternal doses of 40 or 50 mg/kg/day of doxazosin (8 times human AUC exposure with a 12 mg/day therapeutic dose) was delayed as evidenced by slower body weight gain and slightly later appearance of anatomical features and reflexes.

Nursing Mothers: Studies in lactating rats given a single oral dose of 1 mg/kg of [$2-^{14}C$]-CARDURA® indicate that doxazosin accumulates in rat breast milk with a maximum concentration about 20 times greater than the maternal plasma concentration. It is not known whether this drug is excreted in human milk. Because many drugs are excreted in human milk, caution should be exercised when CARDURA® is administered to a nursing mother.

Pediatric Use: The safety and effectiveness of CARDURA® as an antihypertensive agent have not been established in children.

Use in Elderly: The safety and effectiveness profile of CARDURA® in BPH was similar in the elderly (age ≥65 years) and younger (age <65 years) patients.

ADVERSE REACTIONS

A. Benign Prostatic Hyperplasia

The incidence of adverse events has been ascertained from worldwide clinical trials in 965 BPH patients. The incidence rates presented below (Table 3) are based on combined data from seven placebo-controlled trials involving once daily administration of CARDURA® (doxazosin mesylate) in doses of 1–16 mg in hypertensives and 0.5-8 mg in normotensives. The adverse events when the incidence in the CARDURA® group was at least 1% are summarized in Table 3. No significant difference in the incidence of adverse events compared to placebo was seen except for dizziness, fatigue, hypotension, edema and dyspnea. Dizziness and dyspnea appeared to be dose-related.

TABLE 3
ADVERSE REACTIONS DURING
PLACEBO-CONTROLLED STUDIES
BENIGN PROSTATIC HYPERPLASIA

Body System	CARDURA® (N=665)	PLACEBO (N=300)
BODY AS A WHOLE		
Back pain	1.8%	2.0%
Chest pain	1.2%	0.7%
Fatigue	8.0%*	1.7%
Headache	9.9%	9.0%
Influenza-like symptoms	1.1%	1.0%
Pain	2.0%	1.0%
CARDIOVASCULAR SYSTEM		
Hypotension	1.7%*	0.0%
Palpitation	1.2%	0.3%
DIGESTIVE SYSTEM		
Abdominal Pain	2.4%	2.0%
Diarrhea	2.3%	2.0%
Dyspepsia	1.7%	1.7%
Nausea	1.5%	0.7%
METABOLIC AND NUTRITIONAL DISORDERS		
Edema	2.7%*	0.7%
NERVOUS SYSTEM		
Dizziness†	15.6%*	9.0%
Mouth Dry	1.4%	0.3%
Somnolence	3.0%	1.0%

RESPIRATORY SYSTEM		
Dyspnea	2.6%*	0.3%
Respiratory Disorder	1.1%	0.7%
SPECIAL SENSES		
Vision Abnormal	1.4%	0.7%
UROGENITAL SYSTEM		
Impotence	1.1%	1.0%
Urinary Tract Infection	1.4%	2.3%
SKIN & APPENDAGES		
Sweating Increased	1.1%	1.0%
PSYCHIATRIC DISORDERS		
Anxiety	1.1%	0.3%
Insomnia	1.2%	0.3%

*$p \leq 0.05$ for treatment differences
†Includes vertigo

In these placebo-controlled studies of 665 CARDURA® patients, treated for a mean of 85 days, additional adverse reactions have been reported. These are less than 1% and not distinguishable from those that occurred in the placebo group. Adverse reactions with an incidence of less than 1% but of clinical interest are (CARDURA® vs. placebo): *Cardiovascular System:* angina pectoris (0.6% vs. 0.7%), postural hypotension (0.3% vs. 0.3%), syncope (0.5% vs. 0.0%), tachycardia (0.9% vs. 0.0%); *Urogenital System:* dysuria (0.5% vs. 1.3%), and *Psychiatric Disorders:* libido decreased (0.8% vs. 0.3%). The safety profile in patients treated for up to three years was similar to that in the placebo-controlled studies.
The majority of adverse experiences with CARDURA® were mild.

B. *Hypertension*
CARDURA® has been administered to approximately 4000 hypertensive patients, of whom 1679 were included in the hypertension clinical development program. In that program, minor adverse effects were frequent, but led to discontinuation of treatment in only 7% of patients. In placebo-controlled studies adverse effects occurred in 49% and 40% of patients in the doxazosin and placebo groups, respectively, and led to discontinuation in 2% of patients in each group. The major reasons for discontinuation were postural effects (2%), edema, malaise/fatigue, and some heart rate disturbance, each about 0.7%.
In controlled hypertension clinical trials directly comparing CARDURA® to placebo there was no significant difference in the incidence of side effects, except for dizziness (including postural), weight gain, somnolence and fatigue/malaise. Postural effects and edema appeared to be dose related. The prevalence rates presented below are based on combined data from placebo-controlled studies involving once daily administration of doxazosin at doses ranging from 1-16 mg. Table 4 summarizes those adverse experiences (possibly/probably related) reported for patients in these hypertension studies where the prevalence rate in the doxazosin group was at least 0.5% or where the reaction is of particular interest.

TABLE 4
ADVERSE REACTIONS DURING
PLACEBO-CONTROLLED STUDIES
HYPERTENSION

	DOXAZOSIN (N=339)	PLACEBO (N=336)
CARDIOVASCULAR SYSTEM		
Dizziness	19%	9%
Vertigo	2%	1%
Postural Hypotension	0.3%	0%
Edema	4%	3%
Palpitation	2%	3%
Arrhythmia	1%	0%
Hypotension	1%	0%
Tachycardia	0.3%	1%
Peripheral Ischemia	0.3%	0%
SKIN & APPENDAGES		
Rash	1%	1%
Pruritus	1%	1%
MUSCULOSKELETAL SYSTEM		
Arthralgia/Arthritis	1%	0%
Muscle Weakness	1%	0%
Myalgia	1%	0%
CENTRAL & PERIPHERAL N.S.		
Headache	14%	16%
Paresthesia	1%	1%
Kinetic Disorders	1%	0%
Ataxia	1%	0%
Hypertonia	1%	0%
Muscle Cramps	1%	0%
AUTONOMIC		
Mouth Dry	2%	2%
Flushing	1%	0%
SPECIAL SENSES		
Vision Abnormal	2%	1%
Conjunctivitis/Eye Pain	1%	1%
Tinnitus	1%	0.3%
PSYCHIATRIC		
Somnolence	5%	1%
Nervousness	2%	2%
Depression	1%	1%
Insomnia	1%	1%
Sexual Dysfunction	2%	1%
GASTROINTESTINAL		
Nausea	3%	4%
Diarrhea	2%	3%
Constipation	1%	1%
Dyspepsia	1%	1%
Flatulence	1%	1%
Abdominal Pain	0%	2%
Vomiting	0%	1%
RESPIRATORY		
Rhinitis	3%	1%
Dyspnea	1%	1%
Epistaxis	1%	0%
URINARY		
Polyuria	2%	0%
Urinary Incontinence	1%	0%
Micturition Frequency	0%	2%
GENERAL		
Fatigue/Malaise	12%	6%
Chest Pain	2%	2%
Asthenia	1%	1%
Face Edema	1%	0%
Pain	2%	2%

Additional adverse reactions have been reported, but these are, in general, not distinguishable from symptoms that might have occurred in the absence of exposure to doxazosin. The following adverse reactions occurred with a frequency of between 0.5% and 1%: syncope, hypoesthesia, increased sweating, agitation, increased weight. The following additional adverse reactions were reported by <0.5% of 3960 patients who received doxazosin in controlled or open, short- or long-term clinical studies, including international studies. *Cardiovascular System:* angina pectoris, myocardial infarction, cerebrovascular accident; *Autonomic Nervous System:* pallor; *Metabolic:* thirst, gout, hypokalemia; *Hematopoietic:* lymphadenopathy, purpura; *Reproductive System:* breast pain; *Skin Disorders:* alopecia, dry skin, eczema; *Central Nervous System:* paresis, tremor, twitching, confusion, migraine, impaired concentration; *Psychiatric:* paroniria, amnesia, emotional lability, abnormal thinking, depersonalization; *Special Senses:* parosmia, earache, taste perversion, photophobia, abnormal lacrimation; *Gastrointestinal System:* increased appetite, anorexia, fecal incontinence, gastroenteritis; *Respiratory System:* bronchospasm, sinusitis, coughing, pharyngitis; *Urinary System:* renal calculus; *General Body System:* hot flushes, back pain, infection, fever/rigors, decreased weight, influenza-like symptoms.
CARDURA® has not been associated with any clinically significant changes in routine biochemical tests. No clinically relevant adverse effects were noted on serum potassium, serum glucose, uric acid, blood urea nitrogen, creatinine or liver function tests. CARDURA® has been associated with decreases in white blood cell counts (see PRECAUTIONS).
In post-marketing experience the following additional adverse reactions have been reported: *Autonomic Nervous System:* priapism; *Central Nervous System:* hypoesthesia; *Endocrine System:* gynecomastia; *Gastrointestinal System:* vomiting; *General Body System:* allergic reaction; *Heart Rate/Rhythm:* bradycardia; *Hematopoietic:* leukopenia, thrombocytopenia; *Liver/Biliary System:* hepatitis, hepatitis cholestatic; *Respiratory System:* bronchospasm aggravated; *Skin Disorders:* urticaria; *Urinary System:* hematuria, micturition disorder, micturition frequency, nocturia.

OVERDOSAGE

Experience with CARDURA® overdosage is limited. Two adolescents who each intentionally ingested 40 mg CARDURA® with diclofenac or paracetamol, were treated with gastric lavage with activated charcoal and made full recoveries. A two-year-old child who accidently ingested 4 mg CARDURA® was treated with gastric lavage and remained normotensive during the five-hour emergency room observation period. A six-month-old child accidentally received a crushed 1 mg tablet of CARDURA® and was reported to have been drowsy. A 32-year-old female with chronic renal failure, epilepsy and depression intentionally ingested 60 mg CARDURA® (blood level 0.9 μg/mL; normal values in hypertensives=0.02 μg/mL); death was attributed to a grand mal seizure resulting from hypotension. A 39-year-old female who ingested 70 mg CARDURA®, alcohol and Dalmane® (flurazepam) developed hypotension which responded to fluid therapy.
The oral LD_{50} of doxazosin is greater than 1000 mg/kg in mice and rats. The most likely manifestation of overdosage would be hypotension, for which the usual treatment would be intravenous infusion of fluid. As doxazosin is highly protein bound, dialysis would not be indicated.

DOSAGE AND ADMINISTRATION

DOSAGE MUST BE INDIVIDUALIZED. The initial dosage of CARDURA® in patients with hypertension and/or BPH is 1 mg given once daily in the a.m. or p.m. This starting dose is intended to minimize the frequency of postural hypotension and first dose syncope associated with CARDURA®. Postural effects are most likely to occur between 2 and 6 hours after a dose. Therefore blood pressure measurements should be taken during this time period after the first dose and with each increase in dose. If CARDURA® administration is discontinued for several days, therapy should be restarted using the initial dosing regimen.

A. *BENIGN PROSTATIC HYPERPLASIA 1-8 mg once daily.* The initial dosage of CARDURA® is 1 mg, given once daily in the a.m. or p.m. Depending on the individual patient's urodynamics and BPH symptomatology, dosage may then be increased to 2 mg and thereafter to 4 mg and 8 mg once daily, the maximum recommended dose for BPH. The recommended titration interval is 1–2 weeks. Blood pressure should be evaluated routinely in these patients.

B. *HYPERTENSION 1–16 mg once daily.* The initial dosage of CARDURA® is 1 mg given once daily. Depending on the individual patient's standing blood pressure response (based on measurements taken at 2-6 hours post-dose and 24 hours post-dose), dosage may then be increased to 2 mg and thereafter if necessary to 4 mg, 8 mg and 16 mg to achieve the desired reduction in blood pressure. **Increases in dose beyond 4 mg increase the likelihood of excessive postural effects including syncope, postural dizziness/vertigo and postural hypotension. At a titrated dose of 16 mg once daily the frequency of postural effects is about 12% compared to 3% for placebo.**

HOW SUPPLIED

CARDURA® (doxazosin mesylate) is available as colored tablets for oral administration. Each tablet contains doxazosin mesylate equivalent to 1 mg (white), 2 mg (yellow), 4 mg (orange) or 8 mg (green) of the active constituent, doxazosin.
CARDURA® TABLETS (doxazosin mesylate) are available as 1 mg (white), 2 mg (yellow), 4 mg (orange) and 8 mg (green) scored tablets.

Bottles of 100:	1 mg (NDC 0049-2750-66)
	2 mg (NDC 0049-2760-66)
	4 mg (NDC 0049-2770-66)
	8 mg (NDC 0049-2780-66)
Unit Dose Packages of 100:	1 mg (NDC 0049-2750-41)
	2 mg (NDC 0049-2760-41)
	4 mg (NDC 0049-2770-41)
	8 mg (NDC 0049-2780-41)

Recommended Storage: Store below 86°F (30°C).
℞ only

Pfizer Roerig
Division of Pfizer Inc, NY, NY 10017
70-4538-00-8 Revised October 2001

CEFOBID® ℞

[*sĕf-ō-bĭd*]
(sterile cefoperazone)
Formerly known as sterile cefoperazone sodium
For Intravenous or Intramuscular Use

Prescribing information for this product, which appears on pages 2584–2586 of the 2003 PDR, has been completely revised as follows. Please write "See Supplement A" next to the product heading.

DESCRIPTION

CEFOBID® (sterile cefoperazone), formerly known as sterile cefoperazone sodium, contains cefoperazone as cefoperazone sodium. It is a semisynthetic, broad-spectrum cephalosporin antibiotic. Chemically, cefoperazone sodium is sodium (6*R*,7*R*)-7-[(*R*)-2-(4-ethyl-2,3-dioxo-1-piperazine-carboxamido)-2-(*p*-hydroxyphenyl)- acetamido-3-[[(1-methyl-1*H*-tetrazol-5-yl)thio]methyl]-8-oxo-5-thia-1-azabicyclo [4.2.0]oct-2-ene-2-carboxylate. Its molecular formula is $C_{25}H_{26}N_9NaO_8S_2$ with a molecular weight of 667.65. The structural formula is given below:

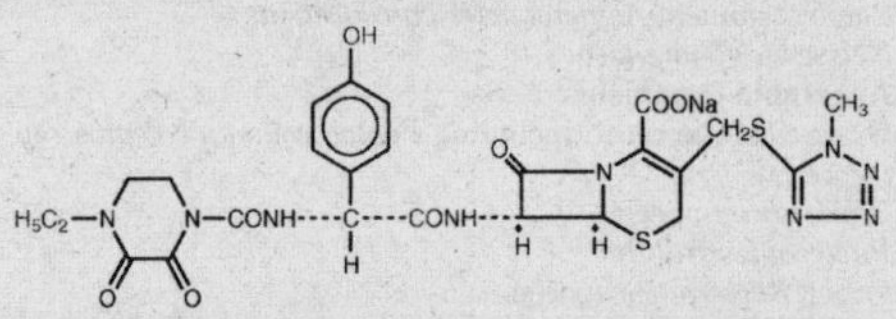

CEFOBID (sterile cefoperazone) contains 34 mg sodium (1.5 mEq) per gram. CEFOBID is a white powder which is freely soluble in water. The pH of a 25% (w/v) freshly reconstituted solution varies between 4.5–6.5 and the solution ranges from colorless to straw yellow depending on the concentration.
CEFOBID (sterile cefoperazone) in crystalline form is supplied in vials containing 1 g or 2 g cefoperazone as cefoperazone sodium for intravenous or intramuscular administration.

CLINICAL PHARMACOLOGY

High serum and bile levels of CEFOBID are attained after a single dose of the drug. Table 1 demonstrates the serum concentrations of CEFOBID in normal volunteers following either a single 15-minute constant rate intravenous infusion of 1, 2, 3 or 4 grams of the drug, or a single intramuscular injection of 1 or 2 grams of the drug.
[See table 1 at top of next page]
The mean serum half-life of CEFOBID is approximately 2.0 hours, independent of the route of administration.

Continued on next page

Cefobid IM/IV—Cont.

In vitro studies with human serum indicate that the degree of CEFOBID reversible protein binding varies with the serum concentration from 93% at 25 mcg/mL of CEFOBID to 90% at 250 mcg/mL and 82% at 500 mcg/mL.

CEFOBID achieves therapeutic concentrations in the following body tissues and fluids:

[See second table at right]

CEFOBID is excreted mainly in the bile. Maximum bile concentrations are generally obtained between one and three hours following drug administration and exceed concurrent serum concentrations by up to 100 times. Reported biliary concentrations of CEFOBID range from 66 mcg/mL at 30 minutes to as high as 6000 mcg/mL at 3 hours after an intravenous bolus injection of 2 grams.

Following a single intramuscular or intravenous dose, the urinary recovery of CEFOBID over a 12-hour period averages 20–30%. No significant quantity of metabolites has been found in the urine. Urinary concentrations greater than 2200 mcg/mL have been obtained following a 15-minute infusion of a 2 g dose. After an IM injection of 2 g, peak urine concentrations of almost 1000 mcg/mL have been obtained, and therapeutic levels are maintained for 12 hours.

Repeated administration of CEFOBID at 12-hour intervals does not result in accumulation of the drug in normal subjects. Peak serum concentrations, areas under the curve (AUC's), and serum half-lives in patients with severe renal insufficiency are not significantly different from those in normal volunteers. In patients with hepatic dysfunction, the serum half-life is prolonged and urinary excretion is increased. In patients with combined renal and hepatic insufficiencies, CEFOBID may accumulate in the serum.

CEFOBID has been used in pediatrics, but the safety and effectiveness in children have not been established. The half-life of CEFOBID in serum is 6-10 hours in low birth-weight neonates.

Microbiology

CEFOBID is active *in vitro* against a wide range of aerobic and anaerobic, gram-positive and gram-negative pathogens. The bactericidal action of CEFOBID results from the inhibition of bacterial cell wall synthesis. CEFOBID has a high degree of stability in the presence of beta-lactamases produced by most gram-negative pathogens. CEFOBID is usually active against organisms which are resistant to other beta-lactam antibiotics because of beta-lactamase production. CEFOBID is usually active against the following organisms *in vitro* and in clinical infections:

Gram-Positive Aerobes:

Staphylococcus aureus, penicillinase and non-penicillinase-producing strains
Staphylococcus epidermidis
Streptococcus pneumoniae (formerly *Diplococcus pneumoniae*)
Streptococcus pyogenes (Group A beta-hemolytic streptococci)
Streptococcus agalactiae (Group B beta-hemolytic streptococci)
Enterococcus (*Streptococcus faecalis, S. faecium* and *S. durans*)

Gram-Negative Aerobes:

Escherichia coli
Klebsiella species (including *K. pneumoniae*)
Enterobacter species
Citrobacter species
Haemophilus influenzae
Proteus mirabilis
Proteus vulgaris
Morganella morganii (formerly *Proteus morganii*)
Providencia stuartii
Providencia rettgeri (formerly *Proteus rettgeri*)
Serratia marcescens
Pseudomonas aeruginosa
Pseudomonas species
Some strains of *Acinetobacter calcoaceticus*
Neisseria gonorrhoeae

Anaerobic Organisms:

Gram-positive cocci (including *Peptococcus and Peptostreptococcus*)
Clostridium species
Bacteroides fragilis
Other *Bacteroides* species

CEFOBID is also active *in vitro* against a wide variety of other pathogens although the clinical significance is unknown. These organisms include: *Salmonella* and *Shigella* species, *Serratia liquefaciens, N. meningitidis, Bordetella pertussis, Yersinia enterocolitica, Clostridium difficile, Fusobacterium* species, *Eubacterium* species and beta-lactamase producing strains of *H. influenzae* and *N. gonorrhoeae*.

SUSCEPTIBILITY TESTING

Diffusion Technique. For the disk diffusion method of susceptibility testing, a 75 mcg CEFOBID diffusion disk should be used. Organisms should be tested with the CEFOBID 75 mcg disk since CEFOBID has been shown *in vitro* to be active against organisms which are found to be resistant to other beta-lactam antibiotics. Tests should be interpreted by the following criteria:

Zone diameter	Interpretation
Greater than or equal to 21 mm	Susceptible
16–20 mm	Moderately Susceptible
Less than or equal to 15 mm	Resistant

Quantitative procedures that require measurement of zone diameters give the most precise estimate of susceptibility. One such method which has been recommended for use with the CEFOBID 75 mcg disk is the NCCLS approved standard. (Performance Standards for Antimicrobial Disk Susceptibility Tests. Second Information Supplement Vol. 2 No. 2 pp. 49-69. Publisher–National Committee for Clinical Laboratory Standards, Villanova, Pennsylvania.)

Table 1. Cefoperazone Serum Concentrations

Dose/Route	Mean Serum Concentrations (mcg/mL) 0*	0.5 hr	1 hr	2 hr	4 hr	8 hr	12 hr
1 g IV	153	114	73	38	16	4	0.5
2 g IV	252	153	114	70	32	8	2
3 g IV	340	210	142	89	41	9	2
4 g IV	506	325	251	161	71	19	6
1 g IM	32 **	52	65	57	33	7	1
2 g IM	40 **	69	93	97	58	14	4

* Hours post-administration, with 0 time being the end of the infusion.
** Values obtained 15 minutes post-injection.

Tissue or Fluid	Dose	Concentration
Ascitic Fluid	2 g	64 mcg/mL
Cerebrospinal Fluid (in patients with inflamed meninges)	50 mg/kg	1.8 mcg/mL to 8.0 mcg/mL
Urine	2 g	3,286 mcg/mL
Sputum	3 g	6.0 mcg/mL
Endometrium	2 g	74 mcg/g
Myometrium	2 g	54 mcg/g
Palatine Tonsil	1 g	8 mcg/g
Sinus Mucous Membrane	1 g	8 mcg/g
Umbilical Cord Blood	1 g	25 mcg/mL
Amniotic Fluid	1 g	4.8 mcg/mL
Lung	1 g	28 mcg/g
Bone	2 g	40 mcg/g

A report of "susceptible" indicates that the infecting organism is likely to respond to CEFOBID therapy and a report of "resistant" indicates that the infecting organism is not likely to respond to therapy. A "moderately susceptible" report suggests that the infecting organism will be susceptible to CEFOBID if a higher than usual dosage is used or if the infection is confined to tissues and fluids (e.g., urine or bile) in which high antibiotic levels are attained.

Dilution Techniques. Broth or agar dilution methods may be used to determine the minimal inhibitory concentration (MIC) of CEFOBID. Serial twofold dilutions of CEFOBID should be prepared in either broth or agar. Broth should be inoculated to contain 5×10^5 organism/mL and agar "spotted" with 10^4 organisms.

MIC test results should be interpreted in light of serum, tissue, and body fluid concentrations of CEFOBID. Organisms inhibited by CEFOBID at 16 mcg/mL or less are considered susceptible, while organisms with MIC's of 17-63 mcg/mL are moderately susceptible. Organisms inhibited at CEFOBID concentrations of greater than or equal to 64 mcg/mL are considered resistant, although clinical cures have been obtained in some patients infected by such organisms.

INDICATIONS AND USAGE

CEFOBID is indicated for the treatment of the following infections when caused by susceptible organisms:

Respiratory Tract Infections caused by *S. pneumoniae, H. influenzae, S. aureus* (penicillinase and non-penicillinase producing strains), *S. pyogenes** (Group A beta-hemolytic streptococci), *P. aeruginosa, Klebsiella pneumoniae, E. coli, Proteus mirabilis*, and *Enterobacter* species.

Peritonitis and Other Intra-abdominal Infections caused by *E. coli, P. aeruginosa*,* and anaerobic gram-negative bacilli (including *Bacteroides fragilis*).

Bacterial Septicemia caused by *S. pneumoniae, S. agalactiae,* S. aureus, Pseudomonas aeruginosa,* E. coli, Klebsiella spp.,* Klebsiella pneumoniae,* Proteus* species* (indole-positive and indole-negative), *Clostridium* spp.* and anaerobic gram-positive cocci.*

Infections of the Skin and Skin Structures caused by *S. aureus* (penicillinase and non-penicillinase producing strains), *S. pyogenes*,* and *P. aeruginosa*.

Pelvic Inflammatory Disease, Endometritis, and Other Infections of the Female Genital Tract caused by *N. gonorrhoeae, S. epidermidis,* S. agalactiae, E. coli, Clostridium* spp.,* *Bacteroides* species (including *Bacteroides fragilis*), and anaerobic gram-positive cocci.

Urinary Tract Infections caused by *Escherichia coli* and *Pseudomonas aeruginosa*.

Enterococcal Infections: Although cefoperazone has been shown to be clinically effective in the treatment of infections caused by enterococci in cases of **peritonitis and other intra-abdominal infections, infections of the skin and skin structures, pelvic inflammatory disease, endometritis and other infections of the female genital tract, and urinary tract infections,*** the majority of clinical isolates of enterococci tested are not susceptible to cefoperazone but fall just at or in the intermediate zone of susceptibility, and are moderately resistant to cefoperazone. However, *in vitro* susceptibility testing may not correlate directly with *in vivo* results. Despite this, cefoperazone therapy has resulted in clinical cures of enterococcal infections, chiefly in polymicrobial infections. Cefoperazone should be used in enterococcal infections with care and at doses that achieve satisfactory serum levels of cefoperazone.

* Efficacy of this organism in this organ system was studied in fewer than 10 infections.

Susceptibility Testing

Before instituting treatment with CEFOBID, appropriate specimens should be obtained for isolation of the causative organism and for determination of its susceptibility to the drug. Treatment may be started before results of susceptibility testing are available.

Combination Therapy

Synergy between CEFOBID and aminoglycosides has been demonstrated with many gram-negative bacilli. However, such enhanced activity of these combinations is not predictable. If such therapy is considered, *in vitro* susceptibility tests should be performed to determine the activity of the drugs in combination, and renal function should be monitored carefully. (See PRECAUTIONS, and DOSAGE AND ADMINISTRATION sections.)

CONTRAINDICATIONS

CEFOBID is contraindicated in patients with known allergy to the cephalosporin-class of antibiotics.

WARNINGS

BEFORE THERAPY WITH CEFOBID IS INSTITUTED, CAREFUL INQUIRY SHOULD BE MADE TO DETERMINE WHETHER THE PATIENT HAS HAD PREVIOUS HYPERSENSITIVITY REACTIONS TO CEPHALOSPORINS, PENICILLINS OR OTHER DRUGS. THIS PRODUCT SHOULD BE GIVEN CAUTIOUSLY TO PENICILLIN-SENSITIVE PATIENTS. ANTIBIOTICS SHOULD BE ADMINISTERED WITH CAUTION TO ANY PATIENT WHO HAS DEMONSTRATED SOME FORM OF ALLERGY, PARTICULARLY TO DRUGS. SERIOUS ACUTE HYPERSENSITIVITY REACTIONS MAY REQUIRE THE USE OF SUBCUTANEOUS EPINEPHRINE AND OTHER EMERGENCY MEASURES.

PSEUDOMEMBRANOUS COLITIS HAS BEEN REPORTED WITH THE USE OF CEPHALOSPORINS (AND OTHER BROAD-SPECTRUM ANTIBIOTICS); THEREFORE, IT IS IMPORTANT TO CONSIDER ITS DIAGNOSIS IN PATIENTS WHO DEVELOP DIARRHEA IN ASSOCIATION WITH ANTIBIOTIC USE.

Treatment with broad-spectrum antibiotics alters normal flora of the colon and may permit overgrowth of clostridia. Studies indicate a toxin produced by *Clostridium difficile* is one primary cause of antibiotic-associated colitis. Cholestyramine and colestipol resins have been shown to bind the toxin *in vitro*.

Mild cases of colitis may respond to drug discontinuance alone.

Moderate to severe cases should be managed with fluid, electrolyte, and protein supplementation as indicated.

When the colitis is not relieved by drug discontinuance or when it is severe, oral vancomycin is the treatment of choice for antibiotic-associated pseudomembranous colitis produced by *C. difficile*. Other causes of colitis should also be considered.

PRECAUTIONS

Although transient elevations of the BUN and serum creatinine have been observed, CEFOBID alone does not appear to cause significant nephrotoxicity. However, concomitant administration of aminoglycosides and other cephalosporins has caused nephrotoxicity.

CEFOBID is extensively excreted in bile. The serum half-life of CEFOBID is increased 2–4 fold in patients with hepatic disease and/or biliary obstruction. In general, total daily dosage above 4 g should not be necessary in such patients. If higher dosages are used, serum concentrations should be monitored.

Because renal excretion is not the main route of elimination of CEFOBID (see CLINICAL PHARMACOLOGY), patients with renal failure require no adjustment in dosage when usual doses are administered. When high doses of

CEFOBID are used, concentrations of drug in the serum should be monitored periodically. If evidence of accumulation exists, dosage should be decreased accordingly.

The half-life of CEFOBID is reduced slightly during hemodialysis. Thus, dosing should be scheduled to follow a dialysis period. In patients with both hepatic dysfunction and significant renal disease, CEFOBID dosage should not exceed 1-2 g daily without close monitoring of serum concentrations.

As with other antibiotics, vitamin K deficiency has occurred rarely in patients treated with CEFOBID. The mechanism is most probably related to the suppression of gut flora which normally synthesize this vitamin. Those at risk include patients with a poor nutritional status, malabsorption states (e.g., cystic fibrosis), alcoholism, and patients on prolonged hyper-alimentation regimens (administered either intravenously or via a naso-gastric tube). Prothrombin time should be monitored in these patients and exogenous vitamin K administered as indicated.

A disulfiram-like reaction characterized by flushing, sweating, headache, and tachycardia has been reported when alcohol (beer, wine) was ingested within 72 hours after CEFOBID administration. Patients should be cautioned about the ingestion of alcoholic beverages following the administration of CEFOBID. A similar reaction has been reported with other cephalosporins.

Prolonged use of CEFOBID may result in the overgrowth of nonsusceptible organisms. Careful observation of the patient is essential. If superinfection occurs during therapy, appropriate measures should be taken.

CEFOBID should be prescribed with caution in individuals with a history of gastrointestinal disease, particularly colitis.

Drug/Laboratory Test Interactions

A false-positive reaction for glucose in the urine may occur with Benedict's or Fehling's solution.

Carcinogenesis, Mutagenesis, Impairment of Fertility

Long term studies in animals have not been performed to evaluate carcinogenic potential. The maximum duration of CEFOBID animal toxicity studies is six months. In none of the *in vivo* or *in vitro* genetic toxicology studies did CEFOBID show any mutagenic potential at either the chromosomal or subchromosomal level. CEFOBID produced no impairment of fertility and had no effects on general reproductive performance or fetal development when administered subcutaneously at daily doses up to 500 to 1000 mg/kg prior to and during mating, and to pregnant female rats during gestation. These doses are 10 to 20 times the estimated usual single clinical dose. CEFOBID had adverse effects on the testes of prepubertal rats at all doses tested. Subcutaneous administration of 1000 mg/kg per day (approximately 16 times the average adult human dose) resulted in reduced testicular weight, arrested spermatogenesis, reduced germinal cell population and vacuolation of Sertoli cell cytoplasm. The severity of lesions was dose dependent in the 100 to 1000 mg/kg per day range; the low dose caused a minor decrease in spermatocytes. This effect has not been observed in adult rats. Histologically the lesions were reversible at all but the highest dosage levels. However, these studies did not evaluate subsequent development of reproductive function in the rats. The relationship of these findings to humans is unknown.

Usage in Pregnancy

Pregnancy Category B: Reproduction studies have been performed in mice, rats, and monkeys at doses up to 10 times the human dose and have revealed no evidence of impaired fertility or harm to the fetus due to CEFOBID. There are, however, no adequate and well controlled studies in pregnant women. Because animal reproduction studies are not always predictive of human response, this drug should be used during pregnancy only if clearly needed.

Usage in Nursing Mothers

Only low concentrations of CEFOBID are excreted in human milk. Although CEFOBID passes poorly into breast milk of nursing mothers, caution should be exercised when CEFOBID is administered to a nursing woman.

Pediatric Use

Safety and effectiveness in children have not been established. For information concerning testicular changes in prepubertal rats (see Carcinogenesis, Mutagenesis, Impairment of Fertility).

Geriatric Use

Clinical studies of CEFOBID® (sterile cefoperazone sodium) did not include sufficient numbers of subjects aged 65 and over to determine whether they respond differently from younger subjects. Other reported clinical experience has not identified differences in responses between the elderly and younger patients. In general, dose selection for an elderly patient should be cautious, usually starting at the low end of the dosing range, reflecting the greater frequency of decreased hepatic, renal, or cardiac function, and of concomitant disease or other drug therapy.

ADVERSE REACTIONS

In clinical studies the following adverse effects were observed and were considered to be related to CEFOBID therapy or of uncertain etiology:

Hypersensitivity: As with all cephalosporins, hypersensitivity manifested by skin reactions (1 patient in 45), drug fever (1 in 260), or a change in Coombs' test (1 in 60) has been reported. These reactions are more likely to occur in patients with a history of allergies, particularly to penicillin.

	Final Cefoperazone Concentration	Step 1 Volume of Sterile Water	Step 2 Volume of 2% Lidocaine	Withdrawable Volume*†
1 g vial	333 mg/mL	2.0 mL	0.6 mL	3 mL
	250 mg/mL	2.8 mL	1.0 mL	4 mL
2 g vial	333 mg/mL	3.8 mL	1.2 mL	6 mL
	250 mg/mL	5.4 mL	1.8 mL	8 mL

When a diluent other than Lidocaine HCl Injection (USP) is used reconstitute as follows:

	Cefoperazone Concentration	Volume of Diluent to be Added	Withdrawable Volume*
1 g vial	333 mg/mL	2.6 mL	3 mL
	250 mg/mL	3.8 mL	4 mL
2 g vial	333 mg/mL	5.0 mL	6 mL
	250 mg/mL	7.2 mL	8 mL

* There is sufficient excess present to allow for withdrawal of the stated volume.

† Final lidocaine concentration will approximate that obtained if a 0.5% Lidocaine Hydrochloride Solution is used as diluent.

Room Temperature (15°–25°C/59°–77°F)

24 Hours	Approximate Concentrations
Bacteriostatic Water for Injection [Benzyl Alcohol or Parabens] (USP)	300 mg/mL
5% Dextrose Injection (USP)	2 mg to 50 mg/mL
5% Dextrose and Lactated Ringer's Injection	2 mg to 50 mg/mL
5% Dextrose and 0.9% Sodium Chloride Injection (USP)	2 mg to 50 mg/mL
5% Dextrose and 0.2% Sodium Chloride Injection (USP)	2 mg to 50 mg/mL
10% Dextrose Injection (USP)	2 mg to 50 mg/mL
Lactated Ringer's Injection (USP)	2 mg/mL
0.5% Lidocaine Hydrochloride Injection (USP)	300 mg/mL
0.9% Sodium Chloride Injection (USP)	2 mg to 300 mg/mL
Normosol® M and 5% Dextrose Injection	2 mg to 50 mg/mL
Normosol® R	2 mg to 50 mg/mL
Sterile Water for Injection	300 mg/mL

Reconstituted CEFOBID solutions may be stored in glass or plastic syringes, or in glass or flexible plastic parenteral solution containers.

Refrigerator Temperature (2°–8°C/36°–46°F)

5 Days	Approximate Concentrations
Bacteriostatic Water for Injection [Benzyl Alcohol or Parabens] (USP)	300 mg/mL
5% Dextrose Injection (USP)	2 mg to 50 mg/mL
5% Dextrose and 0.9% Sodium Chloride Injection (USP)	2 mg to 50 mg/mL
5% Dextrose and 0.2% Sodium Chloride Injection (USP)	2 mg to 50 mg/mL
Lactated Ringer's Injection (USP)	2 mg/mL
0.5% Lidocaine Hydrochloride Injection (USP)	300 mg/mL
0.9% Sodium Chloride Injection (USP)	2 mg to 300 mg/mL
Normosol® M and 5% Dextrose Injection	2 mg to 50 mg/mL
Normosol® R	2 mg to 50 mg/mL
Sterile Water for Injection	300 mg/mL

Reconstituted CEFOBID solutions may be stored in glass or plastic syringes, or in glass or flexible plastic parenteral solution containers.

Freezer Temperature (−20° to −10°C/−4° to 14°F)

3 Weeks	Approximate Concentrations
5% Dextrose Injection (USP)	50 mg/mL
5% Dextrose and 0.9% Sodium Chloride Injection (USP)	2 mg/mL
5% Dextrose and 0.2% Sodium Chloride Injection (USP)	2 mg/mL
5 Weeks	
0.9% Sodium Chloride Injection (USP)	300 mg/mL
Sterile Water for Injection	300 mg/mL

Reconstituted CEFOBID solutions may be stored in plastic syringes, or in flexible plastic parenteral solution containers.

Frozen samples should be thawed at room temperature before use. After thawing, unused portions should be discarded. Do not refreeze.

Hematology: As with other beta-lactam antibiotics, reversible neutropenia may occur with prolonged administration. Slight decreases in neutrophil count (1 patient in 50) have been reported. Decreased hemoglobins (1 in 20) or hematocrits (1 in 20) have been reported, which is consistent with published literature on other cephalosporins. Transient eosinophilia has occurred in 1 patient in 10.

Hepatic: Of 1285 patients treated with cefoperazone in clinical trials, one patient with a history of liver disease developed significantly elevated liver function enzymes during CEFOBID therapy. Clinical signs and symptoms of nonspecific hepatitis accompanied these increases. After CEFOBID therapy was discontinued, the patient's enzymes returned to pre-treatment levels and the symptomatology resolved. As with other antibiotics that achieve high bile levels, mild transient elevations of liver function enzymes have been observed in 5-10% of the patients receiving CEFOBID therapy. The relevance of these findings, which were not accompanied by overt signs or symptoms of hepatic dysfunction, has not been established.

Gastrointestinal: Diarrhea or loose stools has been reported in 1 in 30 patients. Most of these experiences have been mild or moderate in severity and self-limiting in nature. In all cases, these symptoms responded to symptomatic therapy or ceased when cefoperazone therapy was stopped. Nausea and vomiting have been reported rarely. Symptoms of pseudomembranous colitis can appear during or for several weeks subsequent to antibiotic therapy (see WARNINGS).

Renal Function Tests: Transient elevations of the BUN (1 in 16) and serum creatinine (1 in 48) have been noted.

Local Reactions: CEFOBID is well tolerated following intramuscular administration. Occasionally, transient pain (1 in 140) may follow administration by this route. When CEFOBID is administered by intravenous infusion some patients may develop phlebitis (1 in 120) at the infusion site.

DOSAGE AND ADMINISTRATION

The usual adult daily dose of CEFOBID (sterile cefoperazone) is 2 to 4 grams per day administered in equally divided doses every 12 hours.

In severe infections or infections caused by less sensitive organisms, the total daily dose and/or frequency may be increased. Patients have been successfully treated with a total daily dosage of 6–12 grams divided into 2, 3 or 4 administrations ranging from 1.5 to 4 grams per dose.

In a pharmacokinetic study, a total daily dose of 16 grams was administered to severely immunocompromised patients by constant infusion without complications. Steady state serum concentrations were approximately 150 mcg/mL in these patients.

When treating infections caused by *Streptococcus pyogenes*, therapy should be continued for at least 10 days.

Solutions of CEFOBID and aminoglycoside should not be directly mixed, since there is a physical incompatibility between them. If combination therapy with CEFOBID and an aminoglycoside is contemplated (see INDICATIONS) this can be accomplished by sequential intermittent intravenous infusion provided that separate secondary intravenous tubing is used, and that the primary intravenous tubing is adequately irrigated with an approved diluent between doses. It is also suggested that CEFOBID be administered prior to the aminoglycoside. *In vitro* testing of the effectiveness of drug combination(s) is recommended.

Continued on next page

Cefobid IM/IV—Cont.

RECONSTITUTION

The following solutions may be used for the initial reconstitution of CEFOBID (sterile cefoperazone).

Table 1. Solutions for Initial Reconstitution

5% Dextrose Injection (USP)
5% Dextrose and 0.9% Sodium Chloride Injection (USP)
5% Dextrose and 0.2% Sodium Chloride Injection (USP)
10% Dextrose Injection (USP)
Bacteriostatic Water for Injection [Benzyl Alcohol or Parabens] (USP)*†
0.9% Sodium Chloride Injection (USP)
Normosol® M and 5% Dextrose Injection
Normosol® R
Sterile Water for Injection*

* Not to be used as a vehicle for intravenous infusion.
† Preparations containing Benzyl Alcohol should not be used in neonates.

General Reconstitution Procedures

CEFOBID (sterile cefoperazone) for intravenous or intramuscular use may be initially reconstituted with any compatible solution mentioned above in Table 1. Solutions should be allowed to stand after reconstitution to allow any foaming to dissipate to permit visual inspection for complete solubilization. Vigorous and prolonged agitation may be necessary to solubilize CEFOBID in higher concentrations (above 333 mg cefoperazone/mL). The maximum solubility of CEFOBID (sterile cefoperazone) is approximately 475 mg cefoperazone/mL of compatible diluent.

Preparation for Intravenous Use

General. CEFOBID (sterile cefoperazone) concentrations between 2 mg/mL and 50 mg/mL are recommended for intravenous administration.

Preparation of Vials. Vials of CEFOBID (sterile cefoperazone) may be initially reconstituted with a minimum of 2.8 mL per gram of cefoperazone of any compatible reconstituting solution appropriate for intravenous administration listed above in Table 1. For ease of reconstitution the use of 5 mL of compatible solution per gram of CEFOBID is recommended. The entire quantity of the resulting solution should then be withdrawn for further dilution and administration using any of the following vehicles for intravenous infusion:

Table 2. Vehicles for Intravenous Infusion

5% Dextrose Injection (USP)
5% Dextrose and Lactated Ringer's Injection
5% Dextrose and 0.9% Sodium Chloride Injection (USP)
5% Dextrose and 0.2% Sodium Chloride Injection (USP)
10% Dextrose Injection (USP)
Lactated Ringer's Injection (USP)
0.9% Sodium Chloride Injection (USP)
Normosol® M and 5% Dextrose Injection
Normosol® R

The resulting intravenous solution should be administered in one of the following manners:

Intermittent Infusion: Solutions of CEFOBID should be administered over a 15-30 minute time period.

Continuous Infusion: CEFOBID can be used for continuous infusion after dilution to a final concentration of between 2 and 25 mg cefoperazone per mL.

Preparation for Intramuscular Injection

Any suitable solution listed above may be used to prepare CEFOBID (sterile cefoperazone) for intramuscular injection. When concentrations of 250 mg/mL or more are to be administered, a lidocaine solution should be used. These solutions should be prepared using a combination of Sterile Water for Injection and 2% Lidocaine Hydrochloride Injection (USP) that approximates a 0.5% Lidocaine Hydrochloride Solution. A two-step dilution process as follows is recommended: First, add the required amount of Sterile Water for Injection and agitate until CEFOBID powder is completely dissolved. Second, add the required amount of 2% lidocaine and mix.

[See first table at top of previous page]

STORAGE AND STABILITY

CEFOBID (sterile cefoperazone) is to be stored at or below 25°C (77°F) and protected from light prior to reconstitution. After reconstitution, protection from light is not necessary. The following parenteral diluents and approximate concentrations of CEFOBID provide stable solutions under the following conditions for the indicated time periods. (After the indicated time periods, unused portions of solutions should be discarded.)

[See second table at top of previous page]

HOW SUPPLIED

CEFOBID® (sterile cefoperazone) is available in vials containing cefoperazone sodium equivalent to 1 g cefoperazone × 10 (NDC 0049-1201-83) and 2 g cefoperazone × 10 (NDC 0049-1202-83) for intramuscular and intravenous administration.

CEFOBID® (sterile cefoperazone) is available in 10 g (NDC 0049-1219-28) Pharmacy Bulk Package for intravenous administration.

CEFOBID® is a registered trademark of Pfizer Inc.

℞ only

Distributed by:
Pfizer Roerig
Division of Pfizer Inc, NY, NY 10017
70-4169-00-8.1 Revised January 2003

CEFOBID® ℞

[sĕf-o-bĭd]

(sterile cefoperazone, USP)
Formerly known as sterile cefoperazone sodium, USP
PHARMACY BULK PACKAGE
NOT FOR DIRECT INFUSION

Prescribing information for this product, which appears on pages 2586–2589 of the 2003 PDR, has been completely revised as follows. Please write "See Supplement A" next to the product heading.

DESCRIPTION

CEFOBID® (cefoperazone), formerly known as cefoperazone sodium, is a sterile, semisynthetic, broad-spectrum, parenteral cephalosporin antibiotic for intravenous or intramuscular administration. It is the sodium salt of 7-[(*R*)-2-(4-ethyl-2,3-dioxo-1-piperazinecarboxamido)-2-(*p*-hydroxyphenyl) acetamido-3-[[(1-methyl-*H*-tetrazol-5-yl) thio]methyl]-8-oxo-5-thia-1-azabicyclo[4.2.0]oct-2-ene-2-carboxylate. Its chemical formula is $C_{25}H_{26}N_9NaO_8S_2$ with a molecular weight of 667.65. The structural formula is given below:

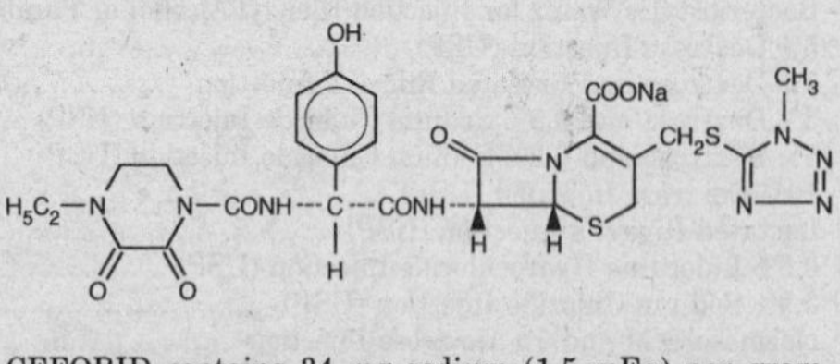

CEFOBID contains 34 mg sodium (1.5 mEq) per gram. CEFOBID is a white powder which is freely soluble in water. The pH of a 25% (w/v) freshly reconstituted solution varies between 4.5–6.5 and the solution ranges from colorless to straw yellow depending on the concentration.

CEFOBID in crystalline form is supplied in vials equivalent to 1 g or 2 g of cefoperazone. A pharmacy bulk package is a container of a sterile preparation for parenteral use that contains many single doses.

This Pharmacy Bulk Package is for use in a pharmacy admixture service; it provides many single doses of cefoperazone for addition to suitable parenteral fluids in the preparation of admixtures for intravenous infusion. (See DOSAGE AND ADMINISTRATION, and DIRECTIONS FOR PROPER USE OF PHARMACY BULK PACKAGE.)

CLINICAL PHARMACOLOGY

High serum and bile levels of CEFOBID are attained after a single dose of the drug. Table 1 demonstrates the serum concentrations of CEFOBID in normal volunteers following either a single 15-minute constant rate intravenous infusion of 1, 2, 3 or 4 grams of the drug, or a single intramuscular injection of 1 or 2 grams of the drug.

[See table 1 below]

The mean serum half-life of CEFOBID is approximately 2.0 hours, independent of the route of administration.

In vitro studies with human serum indicate that the degree of CEFOBID reversible protein binding varies with the serum concentration from 93% at 25 mcg/mL of CEFOBID to 90% at 250 mcg/mL and 82% at 500 mcg/mL.

CEFOBID achieves therapeutic concentrations in the following body tissues and fluids:

Tissue or Fluid	Dose	Concentration
Ascitic Fluid	2 g	64 mcg/mL
Cerebrospinal Fluid (in patients with inflamed meninges)	50 mg/kg	1.8 mcg/mL to 8.0 mcg/mL
Urine	2 g	3,286 mcg/mL
Sputum	3 g	6.0 mcg/mL
Endometrium	2 g	74 mcg/g
Myometrium	2 g	54 mcg/g
Palatine Tonsil	1 g	8 mcg/g
Sinus Mucous Membrane	1 g	8 mcg/g
Umbilical Cord Blood	1 g	25 mcg/mL
Amniotic Fluid	1 g	4.8 mcg/mL
Lung	1 g	28 mcg/g
Bone	2 g	40 mcg/g

CEFOBID is excreted mainly in the bile. Maximum bile concentrations are generally obtained between one and three hours following drug administration and exceed concurrent serum concentrations by up to 100 times. Reported biliary concentrations of CEFOBID range from 66 mcg/mL at 30 minutes to as high as 6000 mcg/mL at 3 hours after an intravenous bolus injection of 2 grams.

Following a single intramuscular or intravenous dose, the urinary recovery of CEFOBID over a 12-hour period averages 20–30%. No significant quantity of metabolites has been found in the urine. Urinary concentrations greater than 2200 mcg/mL have been obtained following a 15-minute infusion of a 2 g dose. After an IM injection of 2 g, peak urine concentrations of almost 1000 mcg/mL have been obtained, and therapeutic levels are maintained for 12 hours.

Repeated administration of CEFOBID at 12-hour intervals does not result in accumulation of the drug in normal subjects. Peak serum concentrations, areas under the curve (AUC's), and serum half-lives in patients with severe renal insufficiency are not significantly different from those in normal volunteers. In patients with hepatic dysfunction, the serum half-life is prolonged and urinary excretion is increased. In patients with combined renal and hepatic insufficiencies, CEFOBID may accumulate in the serum.

CEFOBID has been used in pediatrics, but the safety and effectiveness in children have not been established. The half-life of CEFOBID in serum is 6–10 hours in low birth-weight neonates.

Microbiology

CEFOBID is active *in vitro* against a wide range of aerobic and anaerobic, gram-positive and gram-negative pathogens. The bactericidal action of CEFOBID results from the inhibition of bacterial cell wall synthesis. CEFOBID has a high degree of stability in the presence of beta-lactamases produced by most gram-negative pathogens. CEFOBID is usually active against organisms which are resistant to other beta-lactam antibiotics because of beta-lactamase production. CEFOBID is usually active against the following organisms *in vitro* and in clinical infections:

Gram-Positive Aerobes:

Staphylococcus aureus, penicillinase and non-penicillinase producing strains
Staphylococcus epidermidis
Streptococcus pneumoniae (formerly *Diplococcus pneumoniae*)
Streptococcus pyogenes (Group A beta-hemolytic streptococci)
Streptococcus agalactiae (Group B beta-hemolytic streptococci)
Enterococcus (*Streptococcus faecalis, S. faecium* and *S. durans*)

Gram-Negative Aerobes:

Escherichia coli
Klebsiella species (including *K. pneumoniae*)
Enterobacter species
Citrobacter species
Haemophilus influenzae
Proteus mirabilis
Proteus vulgaris
Morganella morganii (formerly *Proteus morganii*)
Providencia stuartii
Providencia rettgeri (formerly *Proteus rettgeri*)
Serratia marcescens
Pseudomonas aeruginosa
Pseudomonas species
Some strains of *Acinetobacter calcoaceticus*
Neisseria gonorrhoeae

Anaerobic Organisms:

Gram-positive cocci (including *Peptococcus* and *Peptostreptococcus*)
Clostridium species
Bacteroides fragilis
Other *Bacteroides* species

CEFOBID is also active *in vitro* against a wide variety of other pathogens although the clinical significance is unknown. These organisms include: *Salmonella* and *Shigella* species, *Serratia liquefaciens, N. meningitidis, Bordetella pertussis, Yersinia enterocolitica, Clostridium difficile, Fusobacterium* species, *Eubacterium* species and beta-lactamase producing strains of *H. influenzae* and *N. gonorrhoeae*.

SUSCEPTIBILITY TESTING

Diffusion Technique. For the disk diffusion method of susceptibility testing, a 75 mcg CEFOBID diffusion disk should be used. Organisms should be tested with the CEFOBID 75 mcg disk since CEFOBID has been shown *in vitro* to be active against organisms which are found to be resistant to other beta-lactam antibiotics.

Tests should be interpreted by the following criteria:

Zone Diameter	Interpretation
Greater than or equal to 21 mm	Susceptible
16–20 mm	Moderately Susceptible
Less than or equal to 15 mm	Resistant

TABLE 1. Cefoperazone Serum Concentrations

Dose/Route	Mean Serum Concentrations (mcg/mL)						
	0*	0.5 hr	1 hr	2 hr	4 hr	8 hr	12 hr
1 g IV	153	114	73	38	16	4	0.5
2 g IV	252	153	114	70	32	8	2
3 g IV	340	210	142	89	41	9	2
4 g IV	506	325	251	161	71	19	6
1 g IM	32 **	52	65	57	33	7	1
2 g IM	40 **	69	93	97	58	14	4

* Hours post-administration, with 0 time being the end of the infusion.
** Values obtained 15 minutes post-injection.

Quantitative procedures that require measurement of zone diameters give the most precise estimate of susceptibility. One such method which has been recommended for use with the CEFOBID 75 mcg disk is the NCCLS approved standard. (Performance Standards for Antimicrobial Disk Susceptibility Tests. Second Information Supplement Vol. 2 No. 2 pp. 49–69. Publisher–National Committee for Clinical Laboratory Standards, Villanova, Pennsylvania.)
A report of "susceptible" indicates that the infecting organism is likely to respond to CEFOBID therapy and a report of "resistant" indicates that the infecting organism is not likely to respond to therapy. A "moderately susceptible" report suggests that the infecting organism will be susceptible to CEFOBID if a higher than usual dosage is used or if the infection is confined to tissues and fluids (e.g., urine or bile) in which high antibiotic levels are attained.
Dilution Techniques. Broth or agar dilution methods may be used to determine the minimal inhibitory concentration (MIC) of CEFOBID. Serial twofold dilutions of CEFOBID should be prepared in either broth or agar. Broth should be inoculated to contain 5×10^5 organisms/mL and agar "spotted" with 10^4 organisms.
MIC test results should be interpreted in light of serum, tissue, and body fluid concentrations of CEFOBID. Organisms inhibited by CEFOBID at 16 mcg/mL or less are considered susceptible, while organisms with MIC's of 17–63 mcg/mL are moderately susceptible. Organisms inhibited at CEFOBID concentrations of greater than or equal to 64 mcg/mL are considered resistant, although clinical cures have been obtained in some patients infected by such organisms.

INDICATIONS AND USAGE

CEFOBID is indicated for the treatment of the following infections when caused by susceptible organisms:
Respiratory Tract Infections caused by *S. pneumoniae*, *H. influenzae*, *S. aureus* (penicillinase and non-penicillinase producing strains), *S. pyogenes** (Group A beta-hemolytic streptococci), *P. aeruginosa*, *Klebsiella pneumoniae*, *E. coli*, *Proteus mirabilis*, and *Enterobacter* species.
Peritonitis and Other Intra-abdominal Infections caused by *E. coli*, *P. aeruginosa*,* and anaerobic gram-negative bacilli (including *Bacteroides fragilis*).
Bacterial Septicemia caused by *S. pneumoniae*, *S. agalactiae*,* *S. aureus*, *Pseudomonas aeruginosa*,* *E. coli*, *Klebsiella* spp.,* *Klebsiella pneumoniae*,* *Proteus* species* (indole-positive and indole-negative), *Clostridium* spp.* and anaerobic gram-positive cocci.*
Infections of the Skin and Skin Structures caused by *S. aureus* (penicillinase and non-penicillinase producing strains), *S. pyogenes*,* and *P. aeruginosa*.
Pelvic Inflammatory Disease, Endometritis, and Other Infections of the Female Genital Tract caused by *N. gonorrhoeae*, *S. epidermidis*,* *S. agalactiae*, *E. coli*, *Clostridium* spp.,* *Bacteroides* species (including *Bacteroides fragilis*), and anaerobic gram-positive cocci.
Cefobid®, like other cephalosporins, has no activity against *Chlamydia trachomatis*. Therefore, when cephalosporins are used in the treatment of patients with pelvic inflammatory disease and *C. trachomatis* is one of the suspected pathogens, appropriate anti-chlamydial coverage should be added.
Urinary Tract Infections caused by *Escherichia coli* and *Pseudomonas aeruginosa*.
Enterococcal Infections: Although cefoperazone has been shown to be clinically effective in the treatment of infections caused by enterococci in cases of **peritonitis and other intra-abdominal infections, infections of the skin and skin structures, pelvic inflammatory disease, endometritis and other infections of the female genital tract, and urinary tract infections,*** the majority of clinical isolates of enterococci tested are not susceptible to cefoperazone but fall just at or in the intermediate zone of susceptibility, and are moderately resistant to cefoperazone. However, *in vitro* susceptibility testing may not correlate directly with *in vivo* results. Despite this, cefoperazone therapy has resulted in clinical cures of enterococcal infections, chiefly in polymicrobial infections. Cefoperazone should be used in enterococcal infections with care and at doses that achieve satisfactory serum levels of cefoperazone.

* Efficacy of this organism in this organ system was studied in fewer than 10 infections.

Susceptibility Testing
Before instituting treatment with CEFOBID, appropriate specimens should be obtained for isolation of the causative organism and for determination of its susceptibility to the drug. Treatment may be started before results of susceptibility testing are available.
Combination Therapy
Synergy between CEFOBID and aminoglycosides has been demonstrated with many gram-negative bacilli. However, such enhanced activity of these combinations is not predictable. If such therapy is considered, *in vitro* susceptibility tests should be performed to determine the activity of the drugs in combination, and renal function should be monitored carefully. (See PRECAUTIONS, and DOSAGE AND ADMINISTRATION sections.)

CONTRAINDICATIONS

CEFOBID is contraindicated in patients with known allergy to the cephalosporin-class of antibiotics.

WARNINGS

BEFORE THERAPY WITH CEFOBID IS INSTITUTED, CAREFUL INQUIRY SHOULD BE MADE TO DETERMINE WHETHER THE PATIENT HAS HAD PREVIOUS HYPERSENSITIVITY REACTIONS TO CEPHALOSPORINS, PENICILLINS OR OTHER DRUGS. THIS PRODUCT SHOULD BE GIVEN CAUTIOUSLY TO PENICILLIN-SENSITIVE PATIENTS. ANTIBIOTICS SHOULD BE ADMINISTERED WITH CAUTION TO ANY PATIENT WHO HAS DEMONSTRATED SOME FORM OF ALLERGY, PARTICULARLY TO DRUGS. SERIOUS ACUTE HYPERSENSITIVITY REACTIONS MAY REQUIRE THE USE OF SUBCUTANEOUS EPINEPHRINE AND OTHER EMERGENCY MEASURES.
PSEUDOMEMBRANOUS COLITIS HAS BEEN REPORTED WITH THE USE OF CEPHALOSPORINS (AND OTHER BROAD-SPECTRUM ANTIBIOTICS); THEREFORE, IT IS IMPORTANT TO CONSIDER ITS DIAGNOSIS IN PATIENTS WHO DEVELOP DIARRHEA IN ASSOCIATION WITH ANTIBIOTIC USE.
Treatment with broad-spectrum antibiotics alters normal flora of the colon and may permit overgrowth of clostridia. Studies indicate a toxin produced by *Clostridium difficile* is one primary cause of antibiotic-associated colitis. Cholestyramine and colestipol resins have been shown to bind the toxin *in vitro*.
Mild cases of colitis may respond to drug discontinuance alone.
Moderate to severe cases should be managed with fluid, electrolyte, and protein supplementation as indicated.
When the colitis is not relieved by drug discontinuance or when it is severe, oral vancomycin is the treatment of choice for antibiotic-associated pseudomembranous colitis produced by *C. difficile*. Other causes of colitis should also be considered.

Table 1. Solutions for Initial Reconstitution

5% Dextrose Injection (USP)	0.9% Sodium Chloride Injection (USP)
5% Dextrose and 0.9% Sodium Chloride Injection (USP)	Normosol® M and 5% Dextrose Injection
5% Dextrose and 0.2% Sodium Chloride Injection (USP)	Normosol® R
10% Dextrose Injection (USP)	Sterile Water for Injection*
Bacteriostatic Water for Injection [Benzyl Alcohol or Parabens] (USP)*†	

*Not to be used as a vehicle for intravenous infusion.
†Preparations containing Benzyl Alcohol should not be used in neonates.

Table 2. Vehicles for Intravenous Infusion

5% Dextrose Injection (USP)	Lactated Ringer's Injection (USP)
5% Dextrose and Lactated Ringer's Injection	0.9% Sodium Chloride Injection (USP)
5% Dextrose and 0.9% Sodium Chloride Injection (USP)	Normosol® M and 5% Dextrose Injection
5% Dextrose and 0.2% Sodium Chloride Injection (USP)	Normosol® R
10% Dextrose Injection (USP)	

PRECAUTIONS

Although transient elevations of the BUN and serum creatinine have been observed, CEFOBID alone does not appear to cause significant nephrotoxicity. However, concomitant administration of aminoglycosides and other cephalosporins has caused nephrotoxicity.
CEFOBID is extensively excreted in bile. The serum half-life of CEFOBID is increased 2–4 fold in patients with hepatic disease and/or biliary obstruction. In general, total daily dosage above 4 g should not be necessary in such patients. If higher dosages are used, serum concentrations should be monitored.
Because renal excretion is not the main route of elimination of CEFOBID (see CLINICAL PHARMACOLOGY), patients with renal failure require no adjustment in dosage when usual doses are administered. When high doses of CEFOBID are used, concentrations of drug in the serum should be monitored periodically. If evidence of accumulation exists, dosage should be decreased accordingly.
The half-life of CEFOBID is reduced slightly during hemodialysis. Thus, dosing should be scheduled to follow a dialysis period. In patients with both hepatic dysfunction and significant renal disease, CEFOBID dosage should not exceed 1–2 g daily without close monitoring of serum concentrations.
As with other antibiotics, vitamin K deficiency has occurred rarely in patients treated with CEFOBID. The mechanism is most probably related to the suppression of gut flora which normally synthesize this vitamin. Those at risk include patients with a poor nutritional status, malabsorption states (e.g., cystic fibrosis), alcoholism, and patients on prolonged hyper-alimentation regimens (administered either intravenously or via a naso-gastric tube).
Prothrombin time should be monitored in these patients and exogenous vitamin K administered as indicated.
A disulfiram-like reaction characterized by flushing, sweating, headache, and tachycardia has been reported when alcohol (beer, wine) was ingested within 72 hours after CEFOBID administration. Patients should be cautioned about the ingestion of alcoholic beverages following the administration of CEFOBID. A similar reaction has been reported with other cephalosporins.
Prolonged use of CEFOBID may result in the overgrowth of nonsusceptible organisms. Careful observation of the patient is essential. If superinfection occurs during therapy, appropriate measures should be taken.
CEFOBID should be prescribed with caution in individuals with a history of gastrointestinal disease, particularly colitis.
Drug/Laboratory Test Interactions
A false-positive reaction for glucose in the urine may occur with Benedict's or Fehling's solution.
Carcinogenesis, Mutagenesis, Impairment of Fertility
Long-term studies in animals have not been performed to evaluate carcinogenic potential. The maximum duration of CEFOBID animal toxicity studies is six months. In none of the *in vivo* or *in vitro* genetic toxicology studies did CEFOBID show any mutagenic potential at either the chromosomal or subchromosomal level. CEFOBID produced no impairment of fertility and had no effects on general reproductive performance or fetal development when administered subcutaneously at daily doses up to 500 to 1000 mg/kg prior to and during mating, and to pregnant female rats during gestation. These doses are 10 to 20 times the estimated usual single clinical dose. CEFOBID had adverse effects on the testes of prepubertal rats at all doses tested. Subcutaneous administration of 1000 mg/kg per day (approximately 16 times the average adult human dose) resulted in reduced testicular weight, arrested spermatogenesis, reduced germinal cell population and vacuolation of Sertoli cell cytoplasm. The severity of lesions was dose dependent in the 100 to 1000 mg/kg per day range; the low dose caused a minor decrease in spermatocytes. This effect has not been observed in adult rats. Histologically the lesions were reversible at all but the highest dosage levels. However, these studies did not evaluate subsequent development of reproductive function in the rats. The relationship of these findings to humans is unknown.
Usage in Pregnancy
Pregnancy Category B: Reproduction studies have been performed in mice, rats and monkeys at doses up to 10 times the human dose and have revealed no evidence of impaired fertility or harm to the fetus due to CEFOBID. There are, however, no adequate and well controlled studies in pregnant women. Because animal reproduction studies are not always predictive of human response, this drug should be used during pregnancy only if clearly needed.
Usage in Nursing Mothers
Only low concentrations of CEFOBID are excreted in human milk. Although CEFOBID passes poorly into breast milk of nursing mothers, caution should be exercised when CEFOBID is administered to a nursing woman.
Pediatric Use
Safety and effectiveness in children have not been established. For information concerning testicular changes in prepubertal rats, see Carcinogenesis, Mutagenesis, Impairment of Fertility.
Geriatric Use
Clinical studies of CEFOBID® (sterile cefoperazone sodium) did not include sufficient numbers of subjects aged 65 and over to determine whether they respond differently from younger subjects. Other reported clinical experience has not identified differences in responses between the elderly and younger patients. In general, dose selection for an elderly patient should be cautious, usually starting at the low end of the dosing range, reflecting the greater frequency of decreased hepatic, renal, or cardiac function, and of concomitant disease or other drug therapy.

ADVERSE REACTIONS

In clinical studies the following adverse effects were observed and were considered to be related to CEFOBID therapy or of uncertain etiology:
Hypersensitivity: As with all cephalosporins, hypersensitivity manifested by skin reactions (1 patient in 45), drug fever (1 in 260), or a change in Coombs' test (1 in 60) has been reported. These reactions are more likely to occur in patients with a history of allergies, particularly to penicillin.
Hematology: As with other beta-lactam antibiotics, reversible neutropenia may occur with prolonged administration. Slight decreases in neutrophil count (1 patient in 50) have been reported. Decreased hemoglobins (1 in 20) or hematocrits (1 in 20) have been reported, which is consistent with published literature on other cephalosporins. Transient eosinophilia has occurred in 1 patient in 10.
Hepatic: Of 1285 patients treated with cefoperazone in clinical trials, one patient with a history of liver disease developed significantly elevated liver function enzymes during CEFOBID therapy. Clinical signs and symptoms of nonspecific hepatitis accompanied these increases. After CEFOBID therapy was discontinued, the patient's enzymes returned to pre-treatment levels and the symptomatology resolved. As with other antibiotics that achieve high bile levels, mild transient elevations of liver function enzymes have been ob-

Continued on next page

Cefobid Pharmacy Bulk—Cont.

served in 5–10% of the patients receiving CEFOBID therapy. The relevance of these findings, which were not accompanied by overt signs or symptoms of hepatic dysfunction, has not been established.

Gastrointestinal: Diarrhea or loose stools has been reported in 1 in 30 patients. Most of these experiences have been mild or moderate in severity and self-limiting in nature. In all cases, these symptoms responded to symptomatic therapy or ceased when cefoperazone therapy was stopped. Nausea and vomiting have been reported rarely.

Symptoms of pseudomembranous colitis can appear during or for several weeks subsequent to antibiotic therapy (see WARNINGS).

Renal Function Tests: Transient elevations of the BUN (1 in 16) and serum creatinine (1 in 48) have been noted.

Local Reactions: CEFOBID is well tolerated following intramuscular administration. Occasionally, transient pain (1 in 140) may follow administration by this route. When CEFOBID is administered by intravenous infusion some patients may develop phlebitis (1 in 120) at the infusion site.

DOSAGE AND ADMINISTRATION

Sterile cefoperazone sodium can be administered by IM or IV injection (following dilution). However, the intent of this pharmacy bulk package is for the preparation of solutions for IV infusion only.

The usual adult daily dose of CEFOBID is 2 to 4 grams per day administered in equally divided doses every 12 hours. In severe infections or infections caused by less sensitive organisms, the total daily dose and/or frequency may be increased. Patients have been successfully treated with a total daily dosage of 6–12 grams divided into 2, 3, or 4 administrations ranging from 1.5 to 4 grams per dose.

When treating infections caused by *Streptococcus pyogenes*, therapy should be continued for at least 10 days.

If *C. trachomatis* is a suspected pathogen, appropriate antichlamydial coverage should be added, because cefoperazone has no activity against this organism.

Solutions of CEFOBID and aminoglycoside should not be directly mixed, since there is a physical incompatibility between them. If combination therapy with CEFOBID and an aminoglycoside is contemplated (see INDICATIONS) this can be accomplished by sequential intermittent intravenous infusion provided that separate secondary intravenous tubing is used, and that the primary intravenous tubing is adequately irrigated with an approved diluent between doses. It is also suggested that CEFOBID be administered prior to the aminoglycoside. *In vitro* testing of the effectiveness of drug combination(s) is recommended.

In a pharmacokinetic study, a total daily dose of 16 grams was administered to severely immunocompromised patients by constant infusion without complications. Steady-state serum concentrations were approximately 150 mcg/mL in these patients.

Reconstitution

The following solutions may be used for the initial reconstitution of CEFOBID sterile powder:

[See table 1 at top of previous page]

General Reconstitution Procedures

CEFOBID sterile powder for intravenous or intramuscular use may be initially reconstituted with any compatible solution mentioned above in Table 1. Solutions should be allowed to stand after reconstitution to allow any foaming to dissipate to permit visual inspection for complete solubilization. Vigorous and prolonged agitation may be necessary to solubilize CEFOBID in higher concentrations (above 333 mg cefoperazone/mL). The maximum solubility of CEFOBID sterile powder is approximately 475 mg cefoperazone/mL of compatible diluent.

Preparation for Intravenous Use

General. CEFOBID concentrations between 2 mg/mL and 50 mg/mL are recommended for intravenous administration.

[See table 2 at top of previous page]

DIRECTIONS FOR PROPER USE OF PHARMACY BULK PACKAGE

The 10 gram vial should be reconstituted with 95 mL of sterile water for injection in two separate aliquots in a suitable work area such as a laminar flow hood. Add 45 mL of solution, shake to dissolve and add 50 mL, shake for final solution. The resulting solution will contain 100 mg/mL of cefoperazone. This closure may be penetrated only one time after reconstitution, if needed, using a suitable sterile transfer device or dispensing set which allows measured dispensing of the contents.

Discard unused solution within 24 hours of initial entry.

Reconstituted Bulk Solutions Should Not Be Used For Direct Infusion.

Although after reconstitution of the Pharmacy Bulk Package, no significant loss of potency occurs for 24 hours at room temperature and for 5 days if refrigerated, transfer individual dose to appropriate intravenous infusion solutions as soon as possible following reconstitution of the bulk package. Discard unused portions of solution held longer than these recommended periods at room temperature or under refrigeration. The stability of the solution which has been transferred into a container varies according to diluent and concentration. (See STORAGE AND STABILITY.)

The 10 gram vials may be further diluted with the parenteral diluents listed under **Table 2. Vehicles for Intravenous Infusion**. The parenteral diluents and approximate concentrations of CEFOBID that provide stable solutions are presented under STORAGE AND STABILITY.

Parenteral drug products should be inspected visually for particulate matter and discoloration prior to administration, whenever solution and container permit.

Storage and Stability

CEFOBID sterile powder is to be stored at or below 25°C (77°F) and protected from light prior to reconstitution. After reconstitution, protection from light is not necessary.

The following parenteral diluents and approximate concentrations of CEFOBID provide stable solutions under the following conditions for the indicated time periods. (After the indicated time periods, unused portions of solutions should be discarded.)

[See table below]

Controlled Room Temperature (15°–25°C/59°–77°F)	**Approximate**
24 Hours	**Concentrations**
Bacteriostatic Water for Injection [Benzyl Alcohol or Parabens] (USP)	300 mg/mL
5% Dextrose Injection (USP)	2 mg to 50 mg/mL
5% Dextrose and Lactated Ringer's Injection	2 mg to 50 mg/mL
5% Dextrose and 0.9% Sodium Chloride Injection (USP)	2 mg to 50 mg/mL
5% Dextrose and 0.2% Sodium Chloride Injection (USP)	2 mg to 50 mg/mL
10% Dextrose Injection (USP)	2 mg to 50 mg/mL
Lactated Ringer's Injection (USP)	2 mg/mL
0.5% Lidocaine Hydrochloride Injection (USP)	300 mg/mL
0.9% Sodium Chloride Injection (USP)	2 mg to 300 mg/mL
Normosol® M and 5% Dextrose Injection	2 mg to 50 mg/mL
Normosol® R	2 mg to 50 mg/mL
Sterile Water for Injection	100 mg to 300 mg/mL
Reconstituted CEFOBID solutions may be stored in glass or plastic syringes, or in glass or flexible plastic parenteral solution containers.	
Refrigerator Temperature (2°–8°C/36°–46°F)	**Approximate**
5 Days	**Concentrations**
Bacteriostatic Water for Injection [Benzyl Alcohol or Parabens] (USP)	300 mg/mL
5% Dextrose Injection (USP)	2 mg to 50 mg/mL
5% Dextrose and 0.9% Sodium Chloride Injection (USP)	2 mg to 50 mg/mL
5% Dextrose and 0.2% Sodium Chloride Injection (USP)	2 mg to 50 mg/mL
Lactated Ringer's Injection (USP)	2 mg/mL
0.5% Lidocaine Hydrochloride Injection (USP)	300 mg/mL
0.9% Sodium Chloride Injection (USP)	2 mg to 300 mg/mL
Normosol® M and 5% Dextrose Injection	2 mg to 50 mg/mL
Normosol® R	2 mg to 50 mg/mL
Sterile Water for Injection	100 mg to 300 mg/mL
Reconstituted CEFOBID solutions may be stored in glass or plastic syringes, or in glass or flexible plastic parenteral solution containers.	
Freezer Temperature (−20° to −10°C/−4° to 14°F)	**Approximate**
3 Weeks	**Concentrations**
5% Dextrose Injection (USP)	50 mg/mL
5% Dextrose and 0.9% Sodium Chloride Injection (USP)	2 mg/mL
5% Dextrose and 0.2% Sodium Chloride Injection (USP)	2 mg/mL
5 Weeks	
0.9% Sodium Chloride Injection (USP)	300 mg/mL
Sterile Water for Injection	300 mg/mL
Reconstituted CEFOBID solutions may be stored in plastic syringes, or in flexible plastic parenteral solution containers. Frozen samples should be thawed at room temperature before use. After thawing, unused portions should be discarded. Do not refreeze.	

HOW SUPPLIED

CEFOBID® sterile powder is available in Pharmacy Bulk Package containing cefoperazone sodium equivalent to 10 g cefoperazone × 1 (NDC 0049-1219-28).

Other Size Packages Available

CEFOBID® sterile powder is available in vials containing cefoperazone sodium equivalent to 1 g cefoperazone × 10 (NDC 0049-1201-83) and 2 g cefoperazone × 10 (NDC 0049-1202-83) for intramuscular and intravenous administration.

Rx only

Distributed by:

Pfizer Roerig

Division of Pfizer Inc, NY, NY 10017

70-4482-00-7 Revised January 2003

CELEBREX® ℞

[*sĕ-lĕ-brĕks*]

celecoxib capsules

Prescribing information for this product, which appears on pages 2589–2593 of the 2003 PDR, has been completely revised as follows. Please write "See Supplement A" next to the product heading.

DESCRIPTION

CELEBREX (celecoxib) is chemically designated as 4-[5-(4-methylphenyl)-3-(trifluoromethyl)-1H-pyrazol-1-yl] benzenesulfonamide and is a diaryl-substituted pyrazole. It has the following chemical structure:

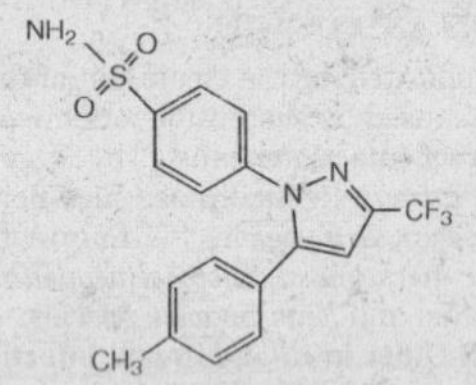

The empirical formula for celecoxib is $C_{17}H_{14}F_3N_3O_2S$, and the molecular weight is 381.38.

CELEBREX oral capsules contain either 100 mg, 200 mg or 400 mg of celecoxib.

The inactive ingredients in CELEBREX capsules include: croscarmellose sodium, edible inks, gelatin, lactose monohydrate, magnesium stearate, povidone, sodium lauryl sulfate and titanium dioxide.

CLINICAL PHARMACOLOGY

Mechanism of Action: CELEBREX is a nonsteroidal anti-inflammatory drug that exhibits anti-inflammatory, analgesic, and antipyretic activities in animal models. The mechanism of action of CELEBREX is believed to be due to inhibition of prostaglandin synthesis, primarily via inhibition of cyclooxygenase-2 (COX-2), and at therapeutic concentrations in humans, CELEBREX does not inhibit the cyclooxygenase-1 (COX-1) isoenzyme. In animal colon tumor models, celecoxib reduced the incidence and multiplicity of tumors.

Pharmacokinetics:

Absorption

Peak plasma levels of celecoxib occur approximately 3 hrs after an oral dose. Under fasting conditions, both peak plasma levels (C_{max}) and area under the curve (AUC) are roughly dose proportional up to 200 mg BID; at higher doses there are less than proportional increases in Cmax and AUC (see Food Effects). Absolute bioavailability studies have not been conducted. With multiple dosing, steady state conditions are reached on or before day 5.

The pharmacokinetic parameters of celecoxib in a group of healthy subjects are shown in Table 1.

[See table 1 at top of next page]

Food Effects

When CELEBREX capsules were taken with a high fat meal, peak plasma levels were delayed for about 1 to 2 hours with an increase in total absorption (AUC) of 10% to 20%. Under fasting conditions, at doses above 200 mg, there is less than a proportional increase in C_{max} and AUC, which is thought to be due to the low solubility of the drug in aqueous media. Coadministration of CELEBREX with an aluminum- and magnesium-containing antacid resulted in a reduction in plasma celecoxib concentrations with a decrease of 37% in Cmax and 10% in AUC. CELEBREX, at doses up to 200 mg BID can be administered without regard to the timing of meals. Higher doses (400 mg BID) should be administered with food to improve absorption.

Distribution

In healthy subjects, celecoxib is highly protein bound (~97%) within the clinical dose range. *In vitro* studies indicate that celecoxib binds primarily to albumin and, to a lesser extent, α_1-acid glycoprotein. The apparent volume of distribution at steady state (V_{ss}/F) is approximately 400 L, suggesting extensive distribution into the tissues. Celecoxib is not preferentially bound to red blood cells.

Metabolism

Celecoxib metabolism is primarily mediated via cytochrome P450 2C9. Three metabolites, a primary alcohol, the corresponding carboxylic acid and its glucuronide conjugate, have been identified in human plasma. These metabolites are inactive as COX-1 or COX-2 inhibitors. Patients who are known or suspected to be P450 2C9 poor metabolizers based on a previous history should be administered celecoxib with caution as they may have abnormally high plasma levels due to reduced metabolic clearance.

Excretion
Celecoxib is eliminated predominantly by hepatic metabolism with little (<3%) unchanged drug recovered in the urine and feces. Following a single oral dose of radiolabeled drug, approximately 57% of the dose was excreted in the feces and 27% was excreted into the urine. The primary metabolite in both urine and feces was the carboxylic acid metabolite (73% of dose) with low amounts of the glucuronide also appearing in the urine. It appears that the low solubility of the drug prolongs the absorption process making terminal half-life ($t_{1/2}$) determinations more variable. The effective half-life is approximately 11 hours under fasted conditions. The apparent plasma clearance (CL/F) is about 500 mL/min.

Special Populations
Geriatric: At steady state, elderly subjects (over 65 years old) had a 40% higher Cmax and a 50% higher AUC compared to the young subjects. In elderly females, celecoxib Cmax and AUC are higher than those for elderly males, but these increases are predominantly due to lower body weight in elderly females. Dose adjustment in the elderly is not generally necessary. However, for patients of less than 50 kg in body weight, initiate therapy at the lowest recommended dose.

Pediatric: CELEBREX capsules have not been investigated in pediatric patients below 18 years of age.

Race: Meta-analysis of pharmacokinetic studies has suggested an approximately 40% higher AUC of celecoxib in Blacks compared to Caucasians. The cause and clinical significance of this finding is unknown.

Hepatic Insufficiency: A pharmacokinetic study in subjects with mild (Child-Pugh Class A) and moderate (Child-Pugh Class B) hepatic impairment has shown that steady-state celecoxib AUC is increased about 40% and 180%, respectively, above that seen in healthy control subjects. Therefore, the daily recommended dose of CELEBREX capsules should be reduced by approximately 50% in patients with moderate (Child-Pugh Class B) hepatic impairment. Patients with severe hepatic impairment (Child-Pugh Class C) have not been studied. The use of CELEBREX in patients with severe hepatic impairment is not recommended.

Renal Insufficiency: In a cross-study comparison, celecoxib AUC was approximately 40% lower in patients with chronic renal insufficiency (GFR 35–60 mL/min) than that seen in subjects with normal renal function. No significant relationship was found between GFR and celecoxib clearance. Patients with severe renal insufficiency have not been studied. Similar to other NSAIDs, CELEBREX is not recommended in patients with severe renal insufficiency (see WARNINGS – Advanced Renal Disease).

Drug Interactions
Also see **PRECAUTIONS – Drug Interactions.**

General: Significant interactions may occur when celecoxib is administered together with drugs that inhibit P450 2C9. *In vitro* studies indicate that celecoxib is not an inhibitor of cytochrome P450 2C9, 2C19 or 3A4.

Clinical studies with celecoxib have identified potentially significant interactions with fluconazole and lithium. Experience with nonsteroidal anti-inflammatory drugs (NSAIDs) suggests the potential for interactions with furosemide and ACE inhibitors. The effects of celecoxib on the pharmacokinetics and/or pharmacodynamics of glyburide, ketoconazole, methotrexate, phenytoin, and tolbutamide have been studied *in vivo* and clinically important interactions have not been found.

CLINICAL STUDIES
Osteoarthritis (OA): CELEBREX has demonstrated significant reduction in joint pain compared to placebo. CELEBREX was evaluated for treatment of the signs and the symptoms of OA of the knee and hip in approximately 4,200 patients in placebo- and active-controlled clinical trials of up to 12 weeks duration. In patients with OA, treatment with CELEBREX 100 mg BID or 200 mg QD resulted in improvement in WOMAC (Western Ontario and McMaster Universities) osteoarthritis index, a composite of pain, stiffness, and functional measures in OA. In three 12-week studies of pain accompanying OA flare, CELEBREX doses of 100 mg BID and 200 mg BID provided significant reduction of pain within 24–48 hours of initiation of dosing. At doses of 100 mg BID or 200 mg BID the effectiveness of CELEBREX was shown to be similar to that of naproxen 500 mg BID. Doses of 200 mg BID provided no additional benefit above that seen with 100 mg BID. A total daily dose of 200 mg has been shown to be equally effective whether administered as 100 mg BID or 200 mg QD.

Rheumatoid Arthritis (RA): CELEBREX has demonstrated significant reduction in joint tenderness/pain and joint swelling compared to placebo. CELEBREX was evaluated for treatment of the signs and symptoms of RA in approximately 2,100 patients in placebo- and active-controlled clinical trials of up to 24 weeks in duration. CELEBREX was shown to be superior to placebo in these studies, using the ACR20 Responder Index, a composite of clinical, laboratory, and functional measures in RA. CELEBREX doses of 100 mg BID and 200 mg BID were similar in effectiveness and both were comparable to naproxen 500 mg BID.

Although CELEBREX 100 mg BID and 200 mg BID provided similar overall effectiveness, some patients derived additional benefit from the 200 mg BID dose. Doses of 400 mg BID provided no additional benefit above that seen with 100–200 mg BID.

Analgesia, including primary dysmenorrhea: In acute analgesic models of post-oral surgery pain, post-orthopedic surgical pain, and primary dysmenorrhea, CELEBREX relieved pain that was rated by patients as moderate to severe. Single doses (see DOSAGE AND ADMINISTRATION) of CELEBREX provided pain relief within 60 minutes.

Familial Adenomatous Polyposis (FAP): CELEBREX was evaluated to reduce the number of adenomatous colorectal polyps. A randomized double-blind placebo-controlled study was conducted in 83 patients with FAP. The study population included 58 patients with a prior subtotal or total colectomy and 25 patients with an intact colon. Thirteen patients had the attenuated FAP phenotype.

One area in the rectum and up to four areas in the colon were identified at baseline for specific follow-up, and polyps were counted at baseline and following six months of treatment. The mean reduction in the number of colorectal polyps was 28% for CELEBREX 400 mg BID, 12% for CELEBREX 100 mg BID and 5% for placebo. The reduction in polyps observed with CELEBREX 400 mg BID was statistically superior to placebo at the six-month timepoint (p=0.003). (See Figure 1.)

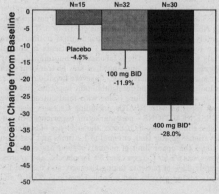

**Figure 1
Percent Change from Baseline in Number of Colorectal Polyps (FAP Patients)**

*p=0.003 versus placebo

Special Studies
Endoscopic Studies: Scheduled upper GI endoscopic evaluations were performed in over 4,500 arthritis patients who were enrolled in five controlled randomized 12-24 week trials using active comparators, two of which also included placebo controls. There was no consistent relationship between the incidence of gastroduodenal ulcers and the dose of CELEBREX over the range studied.

Table 2 summarizes the incidence of endoscopic ulcers in two 12-week studies that enrolled patients in whom baseline endoscopies revealed no ulcers.

[See table 2 above]

Table 3 summarizes data from two 12-week studies that enrolled patients in whom baseline endoscopies revealed no ulcers. Patients underwent interval endoscopies every 4 weeks to give information on ulcer risk over time.

[See table 3 above]

One randomized and double-blind 6-month study in 430 RA patients was conducted in which an endoscopic examination was performed at 6 months.

The incidence of endoscopic ulcers in patients taking CELEBREX 200 mg BID was 4% vs 15% for patients taking diclofenac SR 75 mg BID (p<0.001).

In 4 of the 5 endoscopic studies, approximately 11% of patients (440/4,000) were taking aspirin (≤325 mg/day). In the CELEBREX groups, the endoscopic ulcer rate appeared to be higher in aspirin users than in non-users. However, the increased rate of ulcers in these aspirin users was less than the endoscopic ulcer rates observed in the active comparator groups, with or without aspirin.

The correlation between findings of endoscopic studies, and the relative incidence of clinically significant serious upper GI events has not been established. Serious clinically significant upper GI bleeding has been observed in patients receiving CELEBREX in controlled and open-labeled trials, albeit infrequently (see *Use with Aspirin* and WARNINGS — Gastrointestinal (GI) Effects).

Use with Aspirin: The Celecoxib Long-Term Arthritis Safety Study (CLASS) was a prospective long-term safety outcome study conducted postmarketing in approximately 5,800 OA patients and 2,200 RA patients. Patients received CELEBREX 400 mg BID (4-fold and 2-fold the recommended OA and RA doses, respectively, and the approved dose for FAP), ibuprofen 800 mg TID or diclofenac 75 mg BID (common therapeutic doses). Median exposures for CELEBREX (n = 3,987) and diclofenac (n = 1,996) were 9 months while ibuprofen (n = 1,985) was 6 months. The Kaplan-Meier cumulative rates at 9 months are provided for all analyses. The primary endpoint of this outcome study was the incidence of *complicated ulcers* (gastrointestinal bleeding, perforation or obstruction). Patients were allowed to take concomitant low-dose (≤ 325 mg/day) aspirin (ASA) for cardiovascular prophylaxis (ASA subgroups: CELEBREX, n = 882; diclofenac, n = 445; ibuprofen, n = 412). Differences in the incidence of *complicated ulcers* between CELEBREX and the combined group of ibuprofen and diclofenac were not statistically significant. Those patients on CELEBREX and concomitant low-dose ASA experienced 4-fold higher rates of *complicated ulcers* compared to those not on ASA (see WARNINGS — Gastrointestinal (GI) Effects). The results for CELEBREX are

Continued on next page

Table 1: Summary of Single Dose (200 mg) Disposition Kinetics of CELECOXIB in Healthy Subjects[1]

Mean (%CV) PK Parameter Values				
C_{max}, ng/mL	T_{max}, hr	Effective $t_{1/2}$, hr	V_{ss}/F, L	CL/F, L/hr
705 (38)	2.8 (37)	11.2 (31)	429 (34)	27.7 (28)

[1] Subjects under fasting conditions (n=36, 19–52 yrs.)

**Table 2
Incidence of Gastroduodenal Ulcers from Endoscopic Studies in OA and RA Patients**

	3 Month Studies	
	Study 1 (n = 1108)	Study 2 (n = 1049)
Placebo	2.3% (5/217)	2.0% (4/200)
CELEBREX 50 mg BID	3.4% (8/233)	—
CELEBREX 100 mg BID	3.1% (7/227)	4.0% (9/223)
CELEBREX 200 mg BID	5.9% (13/221)	2.7% (6/219)
CELEBREX 400 mg BID	—	4.1% (8/197)
Naproxen 500 mg BID	16.2% (34/210)*	17.6% (37/210)*

*p≤0.05 vs all other treatments

**Table 3
Incidence of Gastroduodenal Ulcers from 3-Month Serial Endoscopy Studies in OA and RA Patients**

	Week 4	Week 8	Week 12	Final
Study 3 (n=523)				
CELEBREX 200 mg BID	4.0% (10/252)*	2.2% (5/227)*	1.5% (3/196)*	7.5% (20/266)*
Naproxen 500 mg BID	19.0% (47/247)	14.2% (26/182)	9.9% (14/141)	34.6% (89/257)
Study 4 (n=1062)				
CELEBREX 200 mg BID	3.9% (13/337)†	2.4% (7/296)†	1.8% (5/274)†	7.0% (25/356)†
Diclofenac 75 mg BID	5.1% (18/350)	3.3% (10/306)	2.9% (8/278)	9.7% (36/372)
Ibuprofen 800 mg TID	13.0% (42/323)	6.2% (15/241)	9.6% (21/219)	23.3% (78/334)

* p ≤0.05 CELEBREX vs. naproxen based on interval and cumulative analyses
† p ≤0.05 CELEBREX vs. ibuprofen based on interval and cumulative analyses

Celebrex—Cont.

displayed in Table 4. For *complicated and symptomatic ulcer* rates, see WARNINGS — Gastrointestinal (GI) Effects – Risk of GI Ulceration, Bleeding, and Perforation.

Table 4
Effects of Co-Administration of Low-Dose Aspirin on *Complicated Ulcer* Rates with CELEBREX 400 mg BID (Kaplan-Meier Rates at 9 months [%])

	Non-Aspirin Users n=3105	Aspirin Users n=882
Complicated Ulcers	0.32	1.12

Platelets: In clinical trials, CELEBREX at single doses up to 800 mg and multiple doses of 600 mg BID for up to 7 days duration (higher than recommended therapeutic doses) had no effect on platelet aggregation and bleeding time. Comparators (naproxen 500 mg BID, ibuprofen 800 mg TID, diclofenac 75 mg BID) significantly reduced platelet aggregation and prolonged bleeding time.
Because of its lack of platelet effects, CELEBREX is not a substitute for aspirin for cardiovascular prophylaxis.

INDICATIONS AND USAGE
CELEBREX is indicated:
1) For relief of the signs and symptoms of osteoarthritis.
2) For relief of the signs and symptoms of rheumatoid arthritis in adults.
3) For the management of acute pain in adults (see CLINICAL STUDIES).
4) For the treatment of primary dysmenorrhea.
5) To reduce the number of adenomatous colorectal polyps in familial adenomatous polyposis (FAP), as an adjunct to usual care (e.g., endoscopic surveillance, surgery). It is not known whether there is a clinical benefit from a reduction in the number of colorectal polyps in FAP patients. It is also not known whether the effects of CELEBREX treatment will persist after CELEBREX is discontinued. The efficacy and safety of CELEBREX treatment in patients with FAP beyond six months have not been studied (see CLINICAL STUDIES, WARNINGS and PRECAUTIONS sections).

CONTRAINDICATIONS
CELEBREX is contraindicated in patients with known hypersensitivity to celecoxib.
CELEBREX should not be given to patients who have demonstrated allergic-type reactions to sulfonamides.
CELEBREX should not be given to patients who have experienced asthma, urticaria, or allergic-type reactions after taking aspirin or other NSAIDs. Severe, rarely fatal, anaphylactic-like reactions to NSAIDs have been reported in such patients (see WARNINGS — Anaphylactoid Reactions, and PRECAUTIONS — Preexisting Asthma).

WARNINGS
Gastrointestinal (GI) Effects—Risk of GI Ulceration, Bleeding, and Perforation
Serious gastrointestinal toxicity such as bleeding, ulceration, and perforation of the stomach, small intestine or large intestine, can occur at any time, with or without warning symptoms, in patients treated with nonsteroidal anti-inflammatory drugs (NSAIDs). Minor upper gastrointestinal problems, such as dyspepsia, are common and may also occur at any time during NSAID therapy. Therefore, physicians and patients should remain alert for ulceration and bleeding, even in the absence of previous GI tract symptoms (see PRECAUTIONS – Hematological Effects). Patients should be informed about the signs and/or symptoms of serious GI toxicity and the steps to take if they occur. The utility of periodic laboratory monitoring has not been demonstrated, nor has it been adequately assessed. Only one in five patients who develop a serious upper GI adverse event on NSAID therapy is symptomatic. It has been demonstrated that upper GI ulcers, gross bleeding or perforation, caused by NSAIDs, appear to occur in approximately 1% of patients treated for 3–6 months, and in about 2–4% of patients treated for one year. These trends continue thus, increasing the likelihood of developing a serious GI event at some time during the course of therapy. However, even short-term therapy is not without risk.
NSAIDs should be prescribed with extreme caution in patients with a prior history of ulcer disease or gastrointestinal bleeding. Most spontaneous reports of fatal GI events are in elderly or debilitated patients and therefore special care should be taken in treating this population. **To minimize the potential risk for an adverse GI event, the lowest effective dose should be used for the shortest possible duration.** For high risk patients, alternate therapies that do not involve NSAIDs should be considered.
Studies have shown that patients with a *prior history of peptic ulcer disease and/or gastrointestinal bleeding* and who use NSAIDs, have a greater than 10-fold higher risk for developing a GI bleed than patients with neither of these risk factors. In addition to a past history of ulcer disease, pharmacoepidemiological studies have identified several other co-therapies or co-morbid conditions that may increase the risk for GI bleeding such as: treatment with oral corticosteroids, treatment with anticoagulants, longer duration of NSAID therapy, smoking, alcoholism, older age, and poor general health status.
CLASS Study: The estimated cumulative rates at 9 months of *complicated and symptomatic ulcers* (an adverse event similar but not identical to the "upper GI ulcers, gross bleeding or perforation" described in the preceding paragraphs) for patients treated with CELEBREX 400 mg BID (see Special Studies – *Use with Aspirin*) are described in Table 5. Table 5 also displays results for patients less than or greater than or equal to the age of 65 years. The differences in rates between CELEBREX alone and CELEBREX with ASA groups may be due to the higher risk for GI events in ASA users.

Table 5
***Complicated and Symptomatic Ulcer* Rates in Patients Taking CELEBREX 400 mg BID (Kaplan-Meier Rates at 9 months [%]) Based on Risk Factors**

	Complicated and Symptomatic Ulcer Rates
All Patients	
CELEBREX alone (n=3105)	0.78
CELEBREX with ASA (n=882)	2.19
Patients <65 Years	
CELEBREX alone (n=2025)	0.47
CELEBREX with ASA (n=403)	1.26
Patients ≥65 Years	
CELEBREX alone (n=1080)	1.40
CELEBREX with ASA (n=479)	3.06

In a small number of patients with a history of ulcer disease, the *complicated and symptomatic ulcer* rates in patients taking CELEBREX alone or CELEBREX with ASA were, respectively, 2.56% (n=243) and 6.85% (n=91) at 48 weeks. These results are to be expected in patients with a prior history of ulcer disease (see WARNINGS – Gastrointestinal (GI) Effects – Risk of GI Ulceration, Bleeding, and Perforation).

Anaphylactoid Reactions
As with NSAIDs in general, anaphylactoid reactions have occurred in patients without known prior exposure to CELEBREX. In post-marketing experience, rare cases of anaphylactic reactions and angioedema have been reported in patients receiving CELEBREX. CELEBREX should not be given to patients with the aspirin triad. This symptom complex typically occurs in asthmatic patients who experience rhinitis with or without nasal polyps, or who exhibit severe, potentially fatal bronchospasm after taking aspirin or other NSAIDs (see CONTRAINDICATIONS and PRECAUTIONS — Preexisting Asthma). Emergency help should be sought in cases where an anaphylactoid reaction occurs.

Advanced Renal Disease
No information is available from controlled clinical studies regarding the use of CELEBREX in patients with advanced kidney disease. Therefore, treatment with CELEBREX is not recommended in these patients with advanced kidney disease. If CELEBREX therapy must be initiated, close monitoring of the patient's kidney function is advisable (see PRECAUTIONS — Renal Effects).

Pregnancy
In late pregnancy CELEBREX should be avoided because it may cause premature closure of the ductus arteriosus.

Familial Adenomatous Polyposis (FAP): Treatment with CELEBREX in FAP has not been shown to reduce the risk of gastrointestinal cancer or the need for prophylactic colectomy or other FAP-related surgeries. Therefore, the usual care of FAP patients should not be altered because of the concurrent administration of CELEBREX. In particular, the frequency of routine endoscopic surveillance should not be decreased and prophylactic colectomy or other FAP-related surgeries should not be delayed.

PRECAUTIONS
General: CELEBREX cannot be expected to substitute for corticosteroids or to treat corticosteroid insufficiency. Abrupt discontinuation of corticosteroids may lead to exacerbation of corticosteroid-responsive illness. Patients on prolonged corticosteroid therapy should have their therapy tapered slowly if a decision is made to discontinue corticosteroids.
The pharmacological activity of CELEBREX in reducing inflammation, and possibly fever, may diminish the utility of these diagnostic signs in detecting infectious complications of presumed noninfectious, painful conditions.
Hepatic Effects: Borderline elevations of one or more liver associated enzymes may occur in up to 15% of patients taking NSAIDs, and notable elevations of ALT or AST (approximately 3 or more times the upper limit of normal) have been reported in approximately 1% of patients in clinical trials with NSAIDs. These laboratory abnormalities may progress, may remain unchanged, or may be transient with continuing therapy. Rare cases of severe hepatic reactions, including jaundice and fatal fulminant hepatitis, liver necrosis and hepatic failure (some with fatal outcome) have been reported with NSAIDs, including CELEBREX (see ADVERSE REACTIONS – post-marketing experience). In controlled clinical trials of CELEBREX, the incidence of borderline elevations (greater than or equal to 1.2 times and less than 3 times the upper limit of normal) of liver associated enzymes was 6% for CELEBREX and 5% for placebo, and approximately 0.2% of patients taking CELEBREX and 0.3% of patients taking placebo had notable elevations of ALT and AST.
A patient with symptoms and/or signs suggesting liver dysfunction, or in whom an abnormal liver test has occurred, should be monitored carefully for evidence of the development of a more severe hepatic reaction while on therapy with CELEBREX. If clinical signs and symptoms consistent with liver disease develop, or if systemic manifestations occur (e.g., eosinophilia, rash, etc.), CELEBREX should be discontinued.

Renal Effects: Long-term administration of NSAIDs has resulted in renal papillary necrosis and other renal injury. Renal toxicity has also been seen in patients in whom renal prostaglandins have a compensatory role in the maintenance of renal perfusion. In these patients, administration of a nonsteroidal anti-inflammatory drug may cause a dose-dependent reduction in prostaglandin formation and, secondarily, in renal blood flow, which may precipitate overt renal decompensation. Patients at greatest risk of this reaction are those with impaired renal function, heart failure, liver dysfunction, those taking diuretics and ACE inhibitors, and the elderly. Discontinuation of NSAID therapy is usually followed by recovery to the pretreatment state. Clinical trials with CELEBREX have shown renal effects similar to those observed with comparator NSAIDs.
Caution should be used when initiating treatment with CELEBREX in patients with considerable dehydration. It is advisable to rehydrate patients first and then start therapy with CELEBREX. Caution is also recommended in patients with preexisting kidney disease (see WARNINGS—Advanced Renal Disease).

Hematological Effects: Anemia is sometimes seen in patients receiving CELEBREX. In controlled clinical trials the incidence of anemia was 0.6% with CELEBREX and 0.4% with placebo. Patients on long-term treatment with CELEBREX should have their hemoglobin or hematocrit checked if they exhibit any signs or symptoms of anemia or blood loss. CELEBREX does not generally affect platelet counts, prothrombin time (PT), or partial thromboplastin time (PTT), and does not inhibit platelet aggregation at indicated dosages (see CLINICAL STUDIES—Special Studies—Platelets).

Fluid Retention, Edema, and Hypertension: Fluid retention and edema have been observed in some patients taking CELEBREX (see ADVERSE REACTIONS). In the CLASS study (see Special Studies – *Use with Aspirin*), the Kaplan-Meier cumulative rates at 9 months of peripheral edema in patients on CELEBREX 400 mg BID (4-fold and 2-fold the recommended OA and RA doses, respectively, and the approved dose for FAP), ibuprofen 800 mg TID and diclofenac 75 mg BID were 4.5%, 6.9% and 4.7%, respectively. The rates of hypertension in the CELEBREX, ibuprofen and diclofenac treated patients were 2.4%, 4.2% and 2.5%, respectively. As with other NSAIDs, CELEBREX should be used with caution in patients with fluid retention, hypertension, or heart failure.

Preexisting Asthma: Patients with asthma may have aspirin-sensitive asthma. The use of aspirin in patients with aspirin-sensitive asthma has been associated with severe bronchospasm which can be fatal. Since cross reactivity, including bronchospasm, between aspirin, and other nonsteroidal anti-inflammatory drugs has been reported in such aspirin-sensitive patients, CELEBREX should not be administered to patients with this form of aspirin sensitivity and should be used with caution in patients with preexisting asthma.

Information for Patients: CELEBREX can cause discomfort and, rarely, more serious side effects, such as gastrointestinal bleeding, which may result in hospitalization and even fatal outcomes. Although serious GI tract ulcerations and bleeding can occur without warning symptoms, patients should be alert for the signs and symptoms of ulcerations and bleeding, and should ask for medical advice when observing any indicative signs or symptoms. Patients should be apprised of the importance of this follow-up (see WARNINGS — Gastrointestinal (GI) Effects – Risk of Gastrointestinal Ulceration, Bleeding, and Perforation).
Patients should promptly report signs or symptoms of gastrointestinal ulceration or bleeding, skin rash, unexplained weight gain, or edema to their physicians.
Patients should be informed of the warning signs and symptoms of hepatotoxicity (e.g., nausea, fatigue, lethargy, pruritus, jaundice, right upper quadrant tenderness, and "flu-like" symptoms). If these occur, patients should be instructed to stop therapy and seek immediate medical therapy.
Patients should also be instructed to seek immediate emergency help in the case of an anaphylactoid reaction (see WARNINGS).
In late pregnancy CELEBREX should be avoided because it may cause premature closure of the ductus arteriosus.
Patients with familial adenomatous polyposis (FAP) should be informed that CELEBREX has not been shown to reduce colorectal, duodenal or other FAP-related cancers, or the need for endoscopic surveillance, prophylactic or other FAP-related surgery. Therefore, all patients with FAP should be instructed to continue their usual care while receiving CELEBREX.

Laboratory Tests: Because serious GI tract ulcerations and bleeding can occur without warning symptoms, physicians should monitor for signs or symptoms of GI bleeding. In controlled clinical trials, elevated BUN occurred more frequently in patients receiving CELEBREX compared with patients on placebo. This laboratory abnormality was also seen in patients who received comparator NSAIDs in these studies. The clinical significance of this abnormality has not been established.

Drug Interactions
General: Celecoxib metabolism is predominantly mediated via cytochrome P450 2C9 in the liver. Co-administration of celecoxib with drugs that are known to inhibit 2C9 should be done with caution.
In vitro studies indicate that celecoxib, although not a substrate, is an inhibitor of cytochrome P450 2D6. Therefore, there is a potential for an *in vivo* drug interaction with drugs that are metabolized by P450 2D6.

ACE-inhibitors: Reports suggest that NSAIDs may diminish the antihypertensive effect of Angiotensin Converting

Enzyme (ACE) inhibitors. This interaction should be given consideration in patients taking CELEBREX concomitantly with ACE-inhibitors.

Furosemide: Clinical studies, as well as post marketing observations, have shown that NSAIDs can reduce the natriuretic effect of furosemide and thiazides in some patients. This response has been attributed to inhibition of renal prostaglandin synthesis.

Aspirin: CELEBREX can be used with low-dose aspirin. However, concomitant administration of aspirin with CELEBREX increases the rate of GI ulceration or other complications, compared to use of CELEBREX alone (see CLINICAL STUDIES — Special Studies — *Use with Aspirin* and WARNINGS – Gastrointestinal (GI) Effects – Risk of GI Ulceration, Bleeding, and Perforation – CLASS Study).

Because of its lack of platelet effects, CELEBREX is not a substitute for aspirin for cardiovascular prophylaxis.

Fluconazole: Concomitant administration of fluconazole at 200 mg QD resulted in a two-fold increase in celecoxib plasma concentration. This increase is due to the inhibition of celecoxib metabolism via P450 2C9 by fluconazole (see Pharmacokinetics — Metabolism). CELEBREX should be introduced at the lowest recommended dose in patients receiving fluconazole.

Lithium: In a study conducted in healthy subjects, mean steady-state lithium plasma levels increased approximately 17% in subjects receiving lithium 450 mg BID with CELEBREX 200 mg BID as compared to subjects receiving lithium alone. Patients on lithium treatment should be closely monitored when CELEBREX is introduced or withdrawn.

Methotrexate: In an interaction study of rheumatoid arthritis patients taking methotrexate, CELEBREX did not have a significant effect on the pharmacokinetics of methotrexate.

Warfarin: Anticoagulant activity should be monitored, particularly in the first few days, after initiating or changing CELEBREX therapy in patients receiving warfarin or similar agents, since these patients are at an increased risk of bleeding complications. The effect of celecoxib on the anticoagulant effect of warfarin was studied in a group of healthy subjects receiving daily doses of 2–5 mg of warfarin. In these subjects, celecoxib did not alter the anticoagulant effect of warfarin as determined by prothrombin time. However, in post-marketing experience, bleeding events have been reported, predominantly in the elderly, in association with increases in prothrombin time in patients receiving CELEBREX concurrently with warfarin.

Carcinogenesis, mutagenesis, impairment of fertility: Celecoxib was not carcinogenic in rats given oral doses up to 200 mg/kg for males and 10 mg/kg for females (approximately 2- to 4-fold the human exposure as measured by the AUC_{0-24} at 200 mg BID) or in mice given oral doses up to 25 mg/kg for males and 50 mg/kg for females (approximately equal to human exposure as measured by the AUC_{0-24} at 200 mg BID) for two years.

Celecoxib was not mutagenic in an Ames test and a mutation assay in Chinese hamster ovary (CHO) cells, nor clastogenic in a chromosome aberration assay in CHO cells and an *in vivo* micronucleus test in rat bone marrow.

Celecoxib did not impair male and female fertility in rats at oral doses up to 600 mg/kg/day (approximately 11-fold human exposure at 200 mg BID based on the AUC_{0-24}).

Pregnancy

Teratogenic effects: Pregnancy Category C. Celecoxib at oral doses ≥150 mg/kg/day (approximately 2-fold human exposure at 200 mg BID as measured by AUC_{0-24}), caused an increased incidence of ventricular septal defects, a rare event, and fetal alterations, such as ribs fused, sternebrae fused and sternebrae misshapen when rabbits were treated throughout organogenesis. A dose-dependent increase in diaphragmatic hernias was observed when rats were given celecoxib at oral doses ≥30 mg/kg/day (approximately 6-fold human exposure based on the AUC_{0-24} at 200 mg BID) throughout organogenesis. There are no studies in pregnant women. CELEBREX should be used during pregnancy only if the potential benefit justifies the potential risk to the fetus.

Nonteratogenic effects: Celecoxib produced pre-implantation and post-implantation losses and reduced embryo/fetal survival in rats at oral dosages ≥50 mg/kg/day (approximately 6-fold human exposure based on the AUC_{0-24} at 200 mg BID). These changes are expected with inhibition of prostaglandin synthesis and are not the result of permanent alteration of female reproductive function, nor are they expected at clinical exposures. No studies have been conducted to evaluate the effect of celecoxib on the closure of the ductus arteriosus in humans. Therefore, use of CELEBREX during the third trimester of pregnancy should be avoided.

Labor and delivery: Celecoxib produced no evidence of delayed labor or parturition at oral doses up to 100 mg/kg in rats (approximately 7-fold human exposure as measured by the AUC_{0-24} at 200 mg BID). The effects of CELEBREX on labor and delivery in pregnant women are unknown.

Nursing mothers: Celecoxib is excreted in the milk of lactating rats at concentrations similar to those in plasma. It is not known whether this drug is excreted in human milk. Because many drugs are excreted in human milk and because of the potential for serious adverse reactions in nursing infants from CELEBREX, a decision should be made whether to discontinue nursing or to discontinue the drug, taking into account the importance of the drug to the mother.

Pediatric Use

Safety and effectiveness in pediatric patients below the age of 18 years have not been evaluated.

Table 6
Adverse Events Occurring in ≥2% of CELEBREX Patients From CELEBREX Premarketing Controlled Arthritis Trials

	CELEBREX (100–200 mg BID or 200 mg QD) (n=4146)	Placebo (n=1864)	Naproxen 500 mg BID (n=1366)	Diclofenac 75 mg BID (n=387)	Ibuprofen 800 mg TID (n=345)
Gastrointestinal					
Abdominal Pain	4.1%	2.8%	7.7%	9.0%	9.0%
Diarrhea	5.6%	3.8%	5.3%	9.3%	5.8%
Dyspepsia	8.8%	6.2%	12.2%	10.9%	12.8%
Flatulence	2.2%	1.0%	3.6%	4.1%	3.5%
Nausea	3.5%	4.2%	6.0%	3.4%	6.7%
Body as a whole					
Back Pain	2.8%	3.6%	2.2%	2.6%	0.9%
Peripheral edema	2.1%	1.1%	2.1%	1.0%	3.5%
Injury-accidental	2.9%	2.3%	3.0%	2.6%	3.2%
Central and peripheral nervous system					
Dizziness	2.0%	1.7%	2.6%	1.3%	2.3%
Headache	15.8%	20.2%	14.5%	15.5%	15.4%
Psychiatric					
Insomnia	2.3%	2.3%	2.9%	1.3%	1.4%
Respiratory					
Pharyngitis	2.3%	1.1%	1.7%	1.6%	2.6%
Rhinitis	2.0%	1.3%	2.4%	2.3%	0.6%
Sinusitis	5.0%	4.3%	4.0%	5.4%	5.8%
Upper respiratory tract infection	8.1%	6.7%	9.9%	9.8%	9.9%
Skin					
Rash	2.2%	2.1%	2.1%	1.3%	1.2%

Gastrointestinal:	Constipation, diverticulitis, dysphagia, eructation, esophagitis, gastritis, gastroenteritis, gastroesophageal reflux, hemorrhoids, hiatal hernia, melena, dry mouth, stomatitis, tenesmus, tooth disorder, vomiting
Cardiovascular:	Aggravated hypertension, angina pectoris, coronary artery disorder, myocardial infarction
General:	Allergy aggravated, allergic reaction, asthenia, chest pain, cyst NOS, edema generalized, face edema, fatigue, fever, hot flushes, influenza-like symptoms, pain, peripheral pain
Resistance mechanism disorders:	Herpes simplex, herpes zoster, infection bacterial, infection fungal, infection soft tissue, infection viral, moniliasis, moniliasis genital, otitis media
Central, peripheral nervous system:	Leg cramps, hypertonia, hypoesthesia, migraine, neuralgia, neuropathy, paresthesia, vertigo
Female reproductive:	Breast fibroadenosis, breast neoplasm, breast pain, dysmenorrhea, menstrual disorder, vaginal hemorrhage, vaginitis
Male reproductive:	Prostatic disorder
Hearing and vestibular:	Deafness, ear abnormality, earache, tinnitus
Heart rate and rhythm:	Palpitation, tachycardia
Liver and biliary system:	Hepatic function abnormal, SGOT increased, SGPT increased
Metabolic and nutritional:	BUN increased, CPK increased, diabetes mellitus, hypercholesterolemia, hyperglycemia, hypokalemia, NPN increase, creatinine increased, alkaline phosphatase increased, weight increase
Musculoskeletal:	Arthralgia, arthrosis, bone disorder, fracture accidental, myalgia, neck stiffness, synovitis, tendinitis
Platelets (bleeding or clotting):	Ecchymosis, epistaxis, thrombocythemia
Psychiatric:	Anorexia, anxiety, appetite increased, depression, nervousness, somnolence
Hemic:	Anemia
Respiratory:	Bronchitis, bronchospasm, bronchospasm aggravated, coughing, dyspnea, laryngitis, pneumonia
Skin and appendages:	Alopecia, dermatitis, nail disorder, photosensitivity reaction, pruritus, rash erythematous, rash maculopapular, skin disorder, skin dry, sweating increased, urticaria
Application site disorders:	Cellulitis, dermatitis contact, injection site reaction, skin nodule
Special senses:	Taste perversion
Urinary system:	Albuminuria, cystitis, dysuria, hematuria, micturition frequency, renal calculus, urinary incontinence, urinary tract infection
Vision:	Blurred vision, cataract, conjunctivitis, eye pain, glaucoma

Cardiovascular:	Syncope, congestive heart failure, ventricular fibrillation, pulmonary embolism, cerebrovascular accident, peripheral gangrene, thrombophlebitis, *vasculitis*
Gastrointestinal:	Intestinal obstruction, intestinal perforation, gastrointestinal bleeding, colitis with bleeding, esophageal perforation, pancreatitis, ileus
Liver and biliary system:	Cholelithiasis, *hepatitis, jaundice, liver failure*
Hemic and lymphatic:	Thrombocytopenia, *agranulocytosis, aplastic anemia, pancytopenia, leukopenia*
Metabolic:	Hypoglycemia, hyponatremia
Nervous system:	*Aseptic meningitis,* ataxia, suicide
Renal:	Acute renal failure, *interstitial nephritis*
Skin:	*Erythema multiforme, exfoliative dermatitis, Stevens-Johnson syndrome, toxic epidermal necrolysis*
General:	Sepsis, sudden death, *anaphylactoid reaction, angioedema*

Geriatric Use

Of the total number of patients who received CELEBREX in clinical trials, more than 3,300 were 65–74 years of age, while approximately 1,300 additional patients were 75 years and over. No substantial differences in effectiveness were observed between these subjects and younger subjects. In clinical studies comparing renal function as measured by the GFR, BUN and creatinine, and platelet function as measured by bleeding time and platelet aggregation, the results were not different between elderly and young volunteers. However, as with other NSAIDs, including those that selectively inhibit COX-2, there have been more spontaneous post-marketing reports of fatal GI events and acute renal failure in the elderly than in younger patients (see WARNINGS – Gastrointestinal (GI) Effects – Risk of GI Ulceration, Bleeding, and Perforation).

ADVERSE REACTIONS

Of the CELEBREX treated patients in the premarketing controlled clinical trials, approximately 4,250 were patients with OA, approximately 2,100 were patients with RA, and approximately 1,050 were patients with post-surgical pain. More than 8,500 patients have received a total daily dose of CELEBREX of 200 mg (100 mg BID or 200 mg QD) or more, including more than 400 treated at 800 mg (400 mg BID). Approximately 3,900 patients have received CELEBREX at these doses for 6 months or more; approximately 2,300 of these have received it for 1 year or more and 124 of these have received it for 2 years or more.

Adverse events from CELEBREX premarketing controlled arthritis trials: Table 6 lists all adverse events, regardless of causality, occurring in ≥2% of patients receiving CELEBREX from 12 controlled studies conducted in patients with OA or RA that included a placebo and/or a positive control group.

[See table 6 above]

In placebo- or active-controlled clinical trials, the discontinuation rate due to adverse events was 7.1% for patients receiving CELEBREX and 6.1% for patients receiving placebo.

Continued on next page

Celebrex—Cont.

Among the most common reasons for discontinuation due to adverse events in the CELEBREX treatment groups were dyspepsia and abdominal pain (cited as reasons for discontinuation in 0.8% and 0.7% of CELEBREX patients, respectively). Among patients receiving placebo, 0.6% discontinued due to dyspepsia and 0.6% withdrew due to abdominal pain.

The following adverse events occurred in 0.1–1.9% of patients regardless of causality.

CELEBREX
(100–200 mg BID or 200 mg QD)
[See second table on previous page]

Other serious adverse reactions which occur rarely (estimated <0.1%), regardless of causality: The following serious adverse events have occurred rarely in patients taking CELEBREX. Cases reported only in the post-marketing experience are indicated in italics.
[See third table on previous page]

Safety Data from CLASS Study:
Hematological Events:
During this study (see Special Studies – *Use with Aspirin*), the incidence of clinically significant decreases in hemoglobin (>2 g/dL) confirmed by repeat testing was lower in patients on CELEBREX 400 mg BID (4-fold and 2-fold the recommended OA and RA doses, respectively, and the approved dose for FAP) compared to patients on either diclofenac 75 mg BID or ibuprofen 800 mg TID: 0.5%, 1.3% and 1.9%, respectively. The lower incidence of events with CELEBREX was maintained with or without ASA use (see CLINICAL STUDIES – Special Studies – Platelets).
Withdrawals/Serious Adverse Events:
Kaplan-Meier cumulative rates at 9 months for withdrawals due to adverse events for CELEBREX, diclofenac and ibuprofen were 24%, 29%, and 26%, respectively. Rates for serious adverse events (i.e. those causing hospitalization or felt to be life threatening or otherwise medically significant) regardless of causality were not different across treatment groups, respectively, 8%, 7%, and 8%.
Based on Kaplan-Meier cumulative rates for investigator-reported serious cardiovascular thromboembolic adverse events*, there were no differences between the CELEBREX, diclofenac, or ibuprofen treatment groups. The rates in all patients at 9 months for CELEBREX, diclofenac, and ibuprofen were 1.2%, 1.4%, and 1.1%, respectively. The rates for non-ASA users in each of the three treatment groups were less than 1%. The rates for myocardial infarction in each of the three non-ASA treatment groups were less than 0.2%.

*includes myocardial infarction, pulmonary embolism, deep venous thrombosis, unstable angina, transient ischemic attacks or ischemic cerebrovascular accidents.

Adverse events from analgesia and dysmenorrhea studies: Approximately 1,700 patients were treated with CELEBREX in analgesia and dysmenorrhea studies. All patients in post-oral surgery pain studies received a single dose of study medication. Doses up to 600 mg/day of CELEBREX were studied in primary dysmenorrhea and post-orthopedic surgery pain studies. The types of adverse events in the analgesia and dysmenorrhea studies were similar to those reported in arthritis studies. The only additional adverse event reported was post-dental extraction alveolar osteitis (dry socket) in the post-oral surgery pain studies.

Adverse events from the controlled trial in familial adenomatous polyposis: The adverse event profile reported for the 83 patients with familial adenomatous polyposis enrolled in the randomized, controlled clinical trial was similar to that reported for patients in the arthritis controlled trials. Intestinal anastomotic ulceration was the only new adverse event reported in the FAP trial, regardless of causality, and was observed in 3 of 58 patients (one at 100 mg BID, and two at 400 mg BID) who had prior intestinal surgery.

OVERDOSAGE

No overdoses of CELEBREX were reported during clinical trials. Doses up to 2400 mg/day for up to 10 days in 12 patients did not result in serious toxicity.
Symptoms following acute NSAID overdoses are usually limited to lethargy, drowsiness, nausea, vomiting, and epigastric pain, which are generally reversible with supportive care. Gastrointestinal bleeding can occur. Hypertension, acute renal failure, respiratory depression and coma may occur, but are rare. Anaphylactoid reactions have been reported with therapeutic ingestion of NSAIDs, and may occur following an overdose.
Patients should be managed by symptomatic and supportive care following an NSAID overdose. There are no specific antidotes. No information is available regarding the removal of celecoxib by hemodialysis, but based on its high degree of plasma protein binding (>97%) dialysis is unlikely to be useful in overdose. Emesis and/or activated charcoal (60 to 100 g in adults, 1 to 2 g/kg in children) and/or osmotic cathartic may be indicated in patients seen within 4 hours of ingestion with symptoms or following a large overdose. Forced diuresis, alkalinization of urine, hemodialysis, or hemoperfusion may not be useful due to high protein binding.

DOSAGE AND ADMINISTRATION

For osteoarthritis and rheumatoid arthritis, the lowest dose of CELEBREX should be sought for each patient. These doses can be given without regard to timing of meals.
Osteoarthritis: For relief of the signs and symptoms of osteoarthritis the recommended oral dose is 200 mg per day administered as a single dose or as 100 mg twice per day.
Rheumatoid arthritis: For relief of the signs and symptoms of rheumatoid arthritis the recommended oral dose is 100 to 200 mg twice per day.
Management of Acute Pain and Treatment of Primary Dysmenorrhea: The recommended dose of CELEBREX is 400 mg initially, followed by an additional 200 mg dose if needed on the first day. On subsequent days, the recommended dose is 200 mg twice daily as needed.
Familial adenomatous polyposis (FAP): Usual medical care for FAP patients should be continued while on CELEBREX. To reduce the number of adenomatous colorectal polyps in patients with FAP, the recommended oral dose is 400 mg twice per day to be taken with food.
Special Populations
Hepatic Insufficiency: The daily recommended dose of CELEBREX capsules in patients with moderate hepatic impairment (Child-Pugh Class B) should be reduced by approximately 50% (see CLINICAL PHARMACOLOGY – Special Populations).

HOW SUPPLIED

CELEBREX 100-mg capsules are white, reverse printed white on blue band of body and cap with markings of 7767 on the cap and 100 on the body, supplied as:

NDC Number	Size
0025-1520-31	bottle of 100
0025-1520-51	bottle of 500
0025-1520-34	carton of 100 unit dose

CELEBREX 200-mg capsules are white, with reverse printed white on gold band with markings of 7767 on the cap and 200 on the body, supplied as:

NDC Number	Size
0025-1525-31	bottle of 100
0025-1525-51	bottle of 500
0025-1525-34	carton of 100 unit dose

CELEBREX 400-mg capsules are white, with reverse printed white on green band with markings of 7767 on the cap and 400 on the body, supplied as:

NDC Number	Size
0025-1530-02	bottle of 60
0025-1530-01	carton of 100 unit dose

Store at 25°C (77°F); excursions permitted to 15–30°C (59–86°F) [see USP Controlled Room Temperature]

Rx only Revised: August 2002

Manufactured for: *G.D. Searle LLC*
A subsidiary of Pharmacia Corporation
Chicago IL 60680 USA
Pfizer Inc
New York, NY 10017, USA
by: *Searle Ltd.*
Caguas, PR 00725

PHARMACIA
CELEBREX®
celecoxib capsules
A05264-9

GLUCOTROL XL® ℞

[*glū'kă-trōl*]
(glipizide)
Extended Release Tablets
For Oral Use

Prescribing information for this product, which appears on pages 2608–2610 of the 2003 PDR, has been completely revised as follows. Please write "See Supplement A" next to the product heading.

DESCRIPTION

Glipizide is an oral blood-glucose-lowering drug of the sulfonylurea class.
The Chemical Abstracts name of glipizide is 1-cyclohexyl-3-[[p-[2-(5-methylpyrazinecarboxamido)ethyl] phenyl]sulfonyl]urea. The molecular formula is $C_{21}H_{27}N_5O_4S$; the molecular weight is 445.55; the structural formula is shown below:

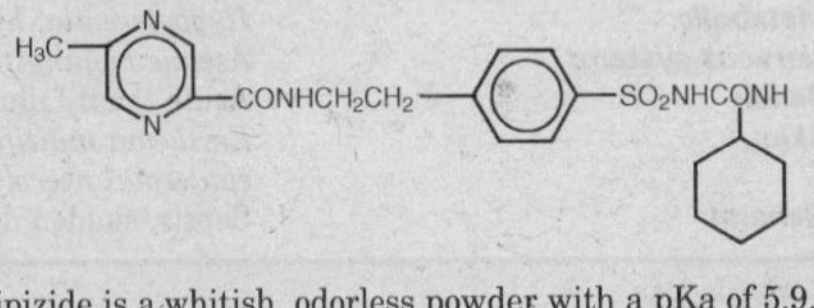

H₃C
N
N
CONHCH₂CH₂
SO₂NHCONH

Glipizide is a whitish, odorless powder with a pKa of 5.9. It is insoluble in water and alcohols, but soluble in 0.1 *N* NaOH; it is freely soluble in dimethylformamide. GLUCOTROL XL® is a registered trademark for glipizide GITS. Glipizide GITS (Gastrointestinal Therapeutic System) is formulated as a once-a-day controlled release tablet for oral use and is designed to deliver 2.5, 5, or 10 mg of glipizide.
Inert ingredients in the 2.5 mg, 5 mg and 10 mg formulations are: polyethylene oxide, hydroxypropyl methylcellulose, magnesium stearate, sodium chloride, red ferric oxide, cellulose acetate, polyethylene glycol, opadry blue (OY-LS-20921)(2.5 mg tablets), opadry white (YS-2-7063)(5 mg and 10 mg tablet) and black ink (S-1-8106).

System Components and Performance
GLUCOTROL XL Extended Release Tablet is similar in appearance to a conventional tablet. It consists, however, of an osmotically active drug core surrounded by a semipermeable membrane. The core itself is divided into two layers: an "active" layer containing the drug, and a "push" layer containing pharmacologically inert (but osmotically active) components. The membrane surrounding the tablet is permeable to water but not to drug or osmotic excipients. As water from the gastrointestinal tract enters the tablet, pressure increases in the osmotic layer and "pushes" against the drug layer, resulting in the release of drug through a small, laser-drilled orifice in the membrane on the drug side of the tablet.
The GLUCOTROL XL Extended Release Tablet is designed to provide a controlled rate of delivery of glipizide into the gastrointestinal lumen which is independent of pH or gastrointestinal motility. The function of the GLUCOTROL XL Extended Release Tablet depends upon the existence of an osmotic gradient between the contents of the bi-layer core and fluid in the GI tract. Drug delivery is essentially constant as long as the osmotic gradient remains constant, and then gradually falls to zero. The biologically inert components of the tablet remain intact during GI transit and are eliminated in the feces as an insoluble shell.

CLINICAL PHARMACOLOGY

Mechanism of Action: Glipizide appears to lower blood glucose acutely by stimulating the release of insulin from the pancreas, an effect dependent upon functioning beta cells in the pancreatic islets. Extrapancreatic effects also may play a part in the mechanism of action of oral sulfonylurea hypoglycemic drugs. Two extrapancreatic effects shown to be important in the action of glipizide are an increase in insulin sensitivity and a decrease in hepatic glucose production. However, the mechanism by which glipizide lowers blood glucose during long-term administration has not been clearly established. Stimulation of insulin secretion by glipizide in response to a meal is of major importance. The insulinotropic response to a meal is enhanced with GLUCOTROL XL administration in diabetic patients. The postprandial insulin and C-peptide responses continue to be enhanced after at least 6 months of treatment. In 2 randomized, double-blind, dose-response studies comprising a total of 347 patients, there was no significant increase in fasting insulin in all GLUCOTROL XL-treated patients combined compared to placebo, although minor elevations were observed at some doses. There was no increase in fasting insulin over the long term.
Some patients fail to respond initially, or gradually lose their responsiveness to sulfonylurea drugs, including glipizide. Alternatively, glipizide may be effective in some patients who have not responded or have ceased to respond to other sulfonylureas.

Effects on Blood Glucose
The effectiveness of GLUCOTROL XL Extended Release Tablets in type 2 diabetes at doses from 5-60 mg once daily has been evaluated in 4 therapeutic clinical trials each with long-term open extensions involving a total of 598 patients. Once daily administration of 5, 10 and 20 mg produced statistically significant reductions from placebo in hemoglobin A_{1C}, fasting plasma glucose and postprandial glucose in patients with mild to severe type 2 diabetes. In a pooled analysis of the patients treated with 5 mg and 20 mg, the relationship between dose and GLUCOTROL XL's effect of reducing hemoglobin A_{1C} was not established. However, in the case of fasting plasma glucose patients treated with 20 mg had a statistically significant reduction of fasting plasma glucose compared to the 5 mg-treated group.
The reductions in hemoglobin A_{1C} and fasting plasma glucose were similar in younger and older patients. Efficacy of GLUCOTROL XL was not affected by gender, race or weight (as assessed by body mass index). In long term extension trials, efficacy of GLUCOTROL XL was maintained in 81% of patients for up to 12 months.
In an open, two-way crossover study 132 patients were randomly assigned to either GLUCOTROL XL or Glucotrol® for 8 weeks and then crossed over to the other drug for an additional 8 weeks. GLUCOTROL XL administration resulted in significantly lower fasting plasma glucose levels and equivalent hemoglobin A_{1C} levels, as compared to Glucotrol.
Other Effects: It has been shown that GLUCOTROL XL therapy is effective in controlling blood glucose without deleterious changes in the plasma lipoprotein profiles of patients treated for type 2 diabetes.
In a placebo-controlled, crossover study in normal volunteers, glipizide had no antidiuretic activity, and, in fact, led to a slight increase in free water clearance.
Pharmacokinetics and Metabolism: Glipizide is rapidly and completely absorbed following oral administration in an immediate release dosage form. The absolute bioavailability of glipizide was 100% after single oral doses in patients with type 2 diabetes. Beginning 2 to 3 hours after administration of GLUCOTROL XL Extended Release Tablets, plasma drug concentrations gradually rise reaching maximum concentrations within 6 to 12 hours after dosing. With subsequent once daily dosing of GLUCOTROL XL Extended Release Tablets, effective plasma glipizide concentrations are maintained throughout the 24 hour dosing interval with less peak to trough fluctuation than that observed with twice daily dosing of immediate release glipizide. The mean relative bioavailability of glipizide in 21 males with type 2 diabetes after administration of 20 mg GLUCOTROL XL Extended Release Tablets, compared to immediate release Glucotrol (10 mg given twice daily), was 90% at steady-state. Steady-state plasma concentrations were achieved by at least the fifth day of dosing with GLUCOTROL XL Extended Release Tablets in 21 males with type 2 diabetes and patients younger than 65 years. Approximately 1 to 2 days longer were required to reach steady-state in 24 elderly (≥65 years) males and females with type 2 diabetes.

No accumulation of drug was observed in patients with type 2 diabetes during chronic dosing with GLUCOTROL XL Extended Release Tablets. Administration of GLUCOTROL XL with food has no effect on the 2 to 3 hour lag time in drug absorption. In a single dose, food effect study in 21 healthy male subjects, the administration of GLUCOTROL XL immediately before a high fat breakfast resulted in a 40% increase in the glipizide mean Cmax value, which was significant, but the effect on the AUC was not significant. There was no change in glucose response between the fed and fasting state. Markedly reduced GI retention times of the GLUCOTROL XL tablets over prolonged periods (e.g., short bowel syndrome) may influence the pharmacokinetic profile of the drug and potentially result in lower plasma concentrations. In a multiple dose study in 26 males with type 2 diabetes, the pharmacokinetics of glipizide were linear over the dose range of 5 to 60 mg of GLUCOTROL XL in that the plasma drug concentrations increased proportionately with dose. In a single dose study in 24 healthy subjects, four 5 mg, two 10 mg, and one 20 mg GLUCOTROL XL Extended Release Tablets were bioequivalent. In a separate single dose study in 36 healthy subjects, four 2.5-mg GLUCOTROL XL Extended Release Tablets were bioequivalent to one 10-mg GLUCOTROL XL Extended Release Tablet.

Glipizide is eliminated primarily by hepatic biotransformation: less than 10% of a dose is excreted as unchanged drug in urine and feces; approximately 90% of a dose is excreted as biotransformation products in urine (80%) and feces (10%). The major metabolites of glipizide are products of aromatic hydroxylation and have no hypoglycemic activity. A minor metabolite which accounts for less than 2% of a dose, an acetylamino-ethyl benzene derivative, is reported to have 1/10 to 1/3 as much hypoglycemic activity as the parent compound. The mean total body clearance of glipizide was approximately 3 liters per hour after single intravenous doses in patients with type 2 diabetes. The mean apparent volume of distribution was approximately 10 liters. Glipizide is 98-99% bound to serum proteins, primarily to albumin. The mean terminal elimination half-life of glipizide ranged from 2 to 5 hours after single or multiple doses in patients with type 2 diabetes. There were no significant differences in the pharmacokinetics of glipizide after single dose administration to older diabetic subjects compared to younger healthy subjects. There is only limited information regarding the effects of renal impairment on the disposition of glipizide, and no information regarding the effects of hepatic disease. However, since glipizide is highly protein bound and hepatic biotransformation is the predominant route of elimination, the pharmacokinetics and/or pharmacodynamics of glipizide may be altered in patients with renal or hepatic impairment.

In mice no glipizide or metabolites were detectable autoradiographically in the brain or spinal cord of males or females, nor in the fetuses of pregnant females. In another study, however, very small amounts of radioactivity were detected in the fetuses of rats given labelled drug.

INDICATIONS AND USAGE

GLUCOTROL XL is indicated as an adjunct to diet for the control of hyperglycemia and its associated symptomatology in patients with type 2 diabetes formerly known as non-insulin-dependent diabetes mellitus (NIDDM) or maturity-onset diabetes, after an adequate trial of dietary therapy has proved unsatisfactory. GLUCOTROL XL is indicated when diet alone has been unsuccessful in correcting hyperglycemia, but even after the introduction of the drug in the patient's regimen, dietary measures should continue to be considered as important. In 12 week, well-controlled studies there was a maximal average net reduction in hemoglobin A_{1C} of 1.7% in absolute units between placebo-treated and GLUCOTROL XL-treated patients.

In initiating treatment for type 2 diabetes, diet should be emphasized as the primary form of treatment. Caloric restriction and weight loss are essential in the obese diabetic patient. Proper dietary management alone may be effective in controlling blood glucose and symptoms of hyperglycemia. The importance of regular physical activity should also be stressed, cardiovascular risk factors should be identified, and corrective measures taken where possible.

If this treatment program fails to reduce symptoms and/or blood glucose, the use of an oral sulfonylurea should be considered. If additional reduction of symptoms and/or blood glucose is required, the addition of insulin to the treatment regimen should be considered. Use of GLUCOTROL XL must be viewed by both the physician and patient as a treatment in addition to diet, and not as a substitute for diet or as a convenient mechanism for avoiding dietary restraint. Furthermore, loss of blood-glucose control on diet alone also may be transient, thus requiring only short-term administration of glipizide.

Some patients fail to respond initially or gradually lose their responsiveness to sulfonylurea drugs, including GLUCOTROL XL. In these cases, concomitant use of GLUCOTROL XL with other oral blood-glucose-lowering agents can be considered. Other approaches that can be considered include substitution of GLUCOTROL XL therapy with that of another oral blood-glucose-lowering agent or insulin. GLUCOTROL XL should be discontinued if it no longer contributes to glucose lowering. Judgment of response to therapy should be based on regular clinical and laboratory evaluations.

In considering the use of GLUCOTROL XL in asymptomatic patients, it should be recognized that controlling blood glucose in type 2 diabetes has not been definitely established to be effective in preventing the long-term cardiovascular or neural complications of diabetes. However, in insulin-dependent diabetes mellitus controlling blood glucose has been effective in slowing the progression of diabetic retinopathy, nephropathy, and neuropathy.

CONTRAINDICATIONS

Glipizide is contraindicated in patients with:
1. Known hypersensitivity to the drug.
2. Diabetic ketoacidosis, with or without coma. This condition should be treated with insulin.

WARNINGS

SPECIAL WARNING ON INCREASED RISK OF CARDIOVASCULAR MORTALITY: The administration of oral hypoglycemic drugs has been reported to be associated with increased cardiovascular mortality as compared to treatment with diet alone or diet plus insulin. This warning is based on the study conducted by the University Group Diabetes Program (UGDP), a long-term prospective clinical trial designed to evaluate the effectiveness of glucose-lowering drugs in preventing or delaying vascular complications in patients with type 2 diabetes. The study involved 823 patients who were randomly assigned to one of four treatment groups (*Diabetes*, 19, SUPP. 2: 747-830, 1970).

UGDP reported that patients treated for 5 to 8 years with diet plus a fixed dose of tolbutamide (1.5 grams per day) had a rate of cardiovascular mortality approximately 2½ times that of patients treated with diet alone. A significant increase in total mortality was not observed, but the use of tolbutamide was discontinued based on the increase in cardiovascular mortality, thus limiting the opportunity for the study to show an increase in overall mortality. Despite controversy regarding the interpretation of these results, the findings of the UGDP study provide an adequate basis for this warning. The patient should be informed of the potential risks and advantages of glipizide and of alternative modes of therapy.

Although only one drug in the sulfonylurea class (tolbutamide) was included in this study, it is prudent from a safety standpoint to consider that this warning may also apply to other oral hypoglycemic drugs in this class, in view of their close similarities in mode of action and chemical structure.

As with any other non-deformable material, caution should be used when administering GLUCOTROL XL Extended Release Tablets in patients with preexisting severe gastrointestinal narrowing (pathologic or iatrogenic). There have been rare reports of obstructive symptoms in patients with known strictures in association with the ingestion of another drug in this non-deformable sustained release formulation.

PRECAUTIONS

General

Renal and Hepatic Disease: The pharmacokinetics and/or pharmacodynamics of glipizide may be affected in patients with impaired renal or hepatic function. If hypoglycemia should occur in such patients, it may be prolonged and appropriate management should be instituted.

GI Disease: Markedly reduced GI retention times of the GLUCOTROL XL Extended Release Tablets may influence the pharmacokinetic profile and hence the clinical efficacy of the drug.

Hypoglycemia: All sulfonylurea drugs are capable of producing severe hypoglycemia. Proper patient selection, dosage, and instructions are important to avoid hypoglycemic episodes. Renal or hepatic insufficiency may affect the disposition of glipizide and the latter may also diminish gluconeogenic capacity, both of which increase the risk of serious hypoglycemic reactions. Elderly, debilitated or malnourished patients, and those with adrenal or pituitary insufficiency are particularly susceptible to the hypoglycemic action of glucose-lowering drugs. Hypoglycemia may be difficult to recognize in the elderly, and in people who are taking beta-adrenergic blocking drugs. Hypoglycemia is more likely to occur when caloric intake is deficient, after severe or prolonged exercise, when alcohol is ingested, or when more than one glucose-lowering drug is used. Therapy with a combination of glucose-lowering agents may increase the potential for hypoglycemia.

Loss of Control of Blood Glucose: When a patient stabilized on any diabetic regimen is exposed to stress such as fever, trauma, infection, or surgery, a loss of control may occur. At such times, it may be necessary to discontinue glipizide and administer insulin.

The effectiveness of any oral hypoglycemic drug, including glipizide, in lowering blood glucose to a desired level decreases in many patients over a period of time, which may be due to progression of the severity of the diabetes or to diminished responsiveness to the drug. This phenomenon is known as secondary failure, to distinguish it from primary failure in which the drug is ineffective in an individual patient when first given. Adequate adjustment of dose and adherence to diet should be assessed before classifying a patient as a secondary failure.

Laboratory Tests: Blood and urine glucose should be monitored periodically. Measurement of hemoglobin A_{1C} may be useful.

Information for Patients: Patients should be informed that GLUCOTROL XL Extended Release Tablets should be swallowed whole. Patients should not chew, divide or crush tablets. Patients should not be concerned if they occasionally notice in their stool something that looks like a tablet. In the GLUCOTROL XL Extended Release Tablet, the medication is contained within a nonabsorbable shell that has been specially designed to slowly release the drug so the body can absorb it. When this process is completed, the empty tablet is eliminated from the body.

Patients should be informed of the potential risks and advantages of GLUCOTROL XL and of alternative modes of therapy. They should also be informed about the importance of adhering to dietary instructions, of a regular exercise program, and of regular testing of urine and/or blood glucose. The risks of hypoglycemia, its symptoms and treatment, and conditions that predispose to its development should be explained to patients and responsible family members. Primary and secondary failure also should be explained.

Drug Interactions: The hypoglycemic action of sulfonylureas may be potentiated by certain drugs including nonsteroidal anti-inflammatory agents and other drugs that are highly protein bound, salicylates, sulfonamides, chloramphenicol, probenecid, coumarins, monoamine oxidase inhibitors, and beta-adrenergic blocking agents. When such drugs are administered to a patient receiving glipizide, the patient should be observed closely for hypoglycemia. When such drugs are withdrawn from a patient receiving glipizide, the patient should be observed closely for loss of control. *In vitro* binding studies with human serum proteins indicate that glipizide binds differently than tolbutamide and does not interact with salicylate or dicumarol. However, caution must be exercised in extrapolating these findings to the clinical situation and in the use of glipizide with these drugs.

Certain drugs tend to produce hyperglycemia and may lead to loss of control. These drugs include the thiazides and other diuretics, corticosteroids, phenothiazines, thyroid products, estrogens, oral contraceptives, phenytoin, nicotinic acid, sympathomimetics, calcium channel blocking drugs, and isoniazid. When such drugs are administered to a patient receiving glipizide, the patient should be closely observed for loss of control. When such drugs are withdrawn from a patient receiving glipizide, the patient should be observed closely for hypoglycemia.

A potential interaction between oral miconazole and oral hypoglycemic agents leading to severe hypoglycemia has been reported. Whether this interaction also occurs with the intravenous, topical, or vaginal preparations of miconazole is not known. The effect of concomitant administration of Diflucan® (fluconazole) and Glucotrol has been demonstrated in a placebo-controlled crossover study in normal volunteers. All subjects received Glucotrol alone and following treatment with 100 mg of Diflucan® as a single daily oral dose for 7 days. The mean percentage increase in the Glucotrol AUC after fluconazole administration was 56.9% (range: 35 to 81%).

Carcinogenesis, Mutagenesis, Impairment of Fertility: A twenty month study in rats and an eighteen month study in mice at doses up to 75 times the maximum human dose revealed no evidence of drug-related carcinogenicity. Bacterial and *in vivo* mutagenicity tests were uniformly negative. Studies in rats of both sexes at doses up to 75 times the human dose showed no effects on fertility.

Pregnancy: Pregnancy Category C: Glipizide was found to be mildly fetotoxic in rat reproductive studies at all dose levels (5-50 mg/kg). This fetotoxicity has been similarly noted with other sulfonylureas, such as tolbutamide and tolazamide. The effect is perinatal and believed to be directly related to the pharmacologic (hypoglycemic) action of glipizide. In studies in rats and rabbits no teratogenic effects were found. There are no adequate and well controlled studies in pregnant women. Glipizide should be used during pregnancy only if the potential benefit justifies the potential risk to the fetus.

Because recent information suggests that abnormal blood-glucose levels during pregnancy are associated with a higher incidence of congenital abnormalities, many experts recommend that insulin be used during pregnancy to maintain blood-glucose levels as close to normal as possible.

Nonteratogenic Effects: Prolonged severe hypoglycemia (4 to 10 days) has been reported in neonates born to mothers who were receiving a sulfonylurea drug at the time of delivery. This has been reported more frequently with the use of agents with prolonged half-lives. If glipizide is used during pregnancy, it should be discontinued at least one month before the expected delivery date.

Nursing Mothers: Although it is not known whether glipizide is excreted in human milk, some sulfonylurea drugs are known to be excreted in human milk. Because the potential for hypoglycemia in nursing infants may exist, a decision should be made whether to discontinue nursing or to discontinue the drug, taking into account the importance of the drug to the mother. If the drug is discontinued and if diet alone is inadequate for controlling blood glucose, insulin therapy should be considered.

Pediatric Use: Safety and effectiveness in children have not been established.

Geriatric Use: Of the total number of patients in clinical studies of GLUCOTROL XL, 33 percent were 65 and over. No overall differences in effectiveness or safety were observed between these patients and younger patients, but greater sensitivity of some individuals cannot be ruled out. Approximately 1-2 days longer were required to reach steady-state in the elderly. (See CLINICAL PHARMACOLOGY and DOSAGE AND ADMINISTRATION.)

ADVERSE REACTIONS

In U.S. controlled studies the frequency of serious adverse experiences reported was very low and causal relationship has not been established.

The 580 patients from 31 to 87 years of age who received GLUCOTROL XL Extended Release Tablets in doses from 5 mg to 60 mg in both controlled and open trials were included in the evaluation of adverse experiences. All adverse experiences reported were tabulated independently of their possible causal relation to medication.

Continued on next page

Glucotrol XL—Cont.

Hypoglycemia: See PRECAUTIONS and OVERDOSAGE sections.
Only 3.4% of patients receiving GLUCOTROL XL Extended Release Tablets had hypoglycemia documented by a blood-glucose measurement <60 mg/dL and/or symptoms believed to be associated with hypoglycemia. In a comparative efficacy study of GLUCOTROL XL and Glucotrol, hypoglycemia occurred rarely with an incidence of less than 1% with both drugs.
In double-blind, placebo-controlled studies the adverse experiences reported with an incidence of 3% or more in GLUCOTROL XL-treated patients include:

Adverse Effect	GLUCOTROL XL (%) (N=278)	Placebo (%) (N=69)
Asthenia	10.1	13.0
Headache	8.6	8.7
Dizziness	6.8	5.8
Nervousness	3.6	2.9
Tremor	3.6	0.0
Diarrhea	5.4	0.0
Flatulence	3.2	1.4

The following adverse experiences occurred with an incidence of less than 3% in GLUCOTROL XL-treated patients:
Body as a whole–pain
Nervous system–insomnia, paresthesia, anxiety, depression and hypesthesia
Gastrointestinal–nausea, dyspepsia, constipation and vomiting
Metabolic–hypoglycemia
Musculoskeletal–arthralgia, leg cramps and myalgia
Cardiovascular–syncope
Skin–sweating and pruritus
Respiratory–rhinitis
Special senses–blurred vision
Urogenital–polyuria
Other adverse experiences occurred with an incidence of less than 1% in GLUCOTROL XL-treated patients:
Body as a whole–chills
Nervous system–hypertonia, confusion, vertigo, somnolence, gait abnormality and decreased libido
Gastrointestinal–anorexia and trace blood in stool
Metabolic–thirst and edema
Cardiovascular–arrhythmia, migraine, flushing and hypertension
Skin–rash and urticaria
Respiratory–pharyngitis and dyspnea
Special senses–pain in the eye, conjunctivitis and retinal hemorrhage
Urogenital–dysuria
Although these adverse experiences occurred in patients treated with GLUCOTROL XL, a causal relationship to the medication has not been established in all cases.
There have been rare reports of gastrointestinal irritation and gastrointestinal bleeding with use of another drug in this non-deformable sustained release formulation, although causal relationship to the drug is uncertain.
The following are adverse experiences reported with immediate release glipizide and other sulfonylureas, but have not been observed with GLUCOTROL XL:
Hematologic: Leukopenia, agranulocytosis, thrombocytopenia, hemolytic anemia, aplastic anemia, and pancytopenia have been reported with sulfonylureas.
Metabolic: Hepatic porphyria and disulfiram-like reactions have been reported with sulfonylureas. In the mouse, glipizide pretreatment did not cause an accumulation of acetaldehyde after ethanol administration. Clinical experience to date has shown that glipizide has an extremely low incidence of disulfiram-like alcohol reactions.
Endocrine Reactions: Cases of hyponatremia and the syndrome of inappropriate antidiuretic hormone (SIADH) secretion have been reported with glipizide and other sulfonylureas.
Laboratory Tests: The pattern of laboratory test abnormalities observed with glipizide was similar to that for other sulfonylureas. Occasional mild to moderate elevations of SGOT, LDH, alkaline phosphatase, BUN and creatinine were noted. One case of jaundice was reported. The relationship of these abnormalities to glipizide is uncertain, and they have rarely been associated with clinical symptoms.

OVERDOSAGE

There is no well-documented experience with GLUCOTROL XL overdosage in humans. There have been no known suicide attempts associated with purposeful overdosing with GLUCOTROL XL. In nonclinical studies the acute oral toxicity of glipizide was extremely low in all species tested (LD_{50} greater than 4 g/kg). Overdosage of sulfonylureas including glipizide can produce hypoglycemia. Mild hypoglycemic symptoms without loss of consciousness or neurologic findings should be treated aggressively with oral glucose and adjustments in drug dosage and/or meal patterns. Close monitoring should continue until the physician is assured that the patient is out of danger. Severe hypoglycemic reactions with coma, seizure, or other neurological impairment occur infrequently, but constitute medical emergencies requiring immediate hospitalization. If hypoglycemic coma is diagnosed or suspected, the patient should be given rapid intravenous injection of concentrated (50%) glucose solution. This should be followed by a continuous infusion of a more dilute (10%) glucose solution at a rate that will maintain the blood glucose at a level above 100 mg/dL. Patients should be closely monitored for a minimum of 24 to 48 hours since hypoglycemia may recur after apparent clinical recovery. Clearance of glipizide from plasma may be prolonged in persons with liver disease. Because of the extensive protein binding of glipizide, dialysis is unlikely to be of benefit.

DOSAGE AND ADMINISTRATION

There is no fixed dosage regimen for the management of diabetes mellitus with GLUCOTROL XL Extended Release Tablet or any other hypoglycemic agent. Glycemic control should be monitored with hemoglobin A_{1C} and/or blood-glucose levels to determine the minimum effective dose for the patient; to detect primary failure, i.e., inadequate lowering of blood glucose at the maximum recommended dose of medication; and to detect secondary failure, i.e., loss of an adequate blood-glucose-lowering response after an initial period of effectiveness. Home blood-glucose monitoring may also provide useful information to the patient and physician. Short-term administration of GLUCOTROL XL Extended Release Tablet may be sufficient during periods of transient loss of control in patients usually controlled on diet.
In general, GLUCOTROL XL should be given with breakfast.
Recommended Dosing: The usual starting dose of GLUCOTROL XL as initial therapy is 5 mg per day, given with breakfast. Those patients who may be more sensitive to hypoglycemic drugs may be started at a lower dose.
Dosage adjustment should be based on laboratory measures of glycemic control. While fasting blood-glucose levels generally reach steady-state following initiation or change in GLUCOTROL XL dosage, a single fasting glucose determination may not accurately reflect the response to therapy. In most cases, hemoglobin A_{1C} level measured at three month intervals is the preferred means of monitoring response to therapy.
Hemoglobin A_{1C} should be measured as GLUCOTROL XL therapy is initiated and repeated approximately three months later. If the result of this test suggests that glycemic control over the preceding three months was inadequate, the GLUCOTROL XL dose may be increased.
Subsequent dosage adjustments should be made on the basis of hemoglobin A_{1C} levels measured at three month intervals. If no improvement is seen after three months of therapy with a higher dose, the previous dose should be resumed. Decisions which utilize fasting blood glucose to adjust GLUCOTROL XL therapy should be based on at least two or more similar, consecutive values obtained seven days or more after the previous dose adjustment.
Most patients will be controlled with 5 mg to 10 mg taken once daily. However, some patients may require up to the maximum recommended daily dose of 20 mg. While the glycemic control of selected patients may improve with doses which exceed 10 mg, clinical studies conducted to date have not demonstrated an additional group average reduction of hemoglobin A_{1C} beyond what was achieved with the 10 mg dose.
Based on the results of a randomized crossover study, patients receiving immediate release glipizide may be switched safely to GLUCOTROL XL Extended Release Tablets once-a-day at the nearest equivalent total daily dose. Patients receiving immediate release Glucotrol also may be titrated to the appropriate dose of GLUCOTROL XL starting with 5 mg once daily. The decision to switch to the nearest equivalent dose or to titrate should be based on clinical judgment.
In elderly patients, debilitated or malnourished patients, and patients with impaired renal or hepatic function, the initial and maintenance dosing should be conservative to avoid hypoglycemic reactions (see PRECAUTIONS section).
Combination Use:
When adding other blood-glucose-lowering agents to GLUCOTROL XL for combination therapy, the agent should be initiated at the lowest recommended dose, and patients should be observed carefully for hypoglycemia. Refer to the product information supplied with the oral agent for additional information.
When adding GLUCOTROL XL to other blood-glucose-lowering agents, GLUCOTROL XL can be initiated at 5 mg. Those patients who may be more sensitive to hypoglycemic drugs may be started at a lower dose. Titration should be based on clinical judgment.
Patients Receiving Insulin: As with other sulfonylurea-class hypoglycemics, many patients with stable type 2 diabetes receiving insulin may be transferred safely to treatment with GLUCOTROL XL Extended Release Tablets. When transferring patients from insulin to GLUCOTROL XL, the following general guidelines should be considered:
For patients whose daily insulin requirement is 20 units or less, insulin may be discontinued and GLUCOTROL XL therapy may begin at usual dosages. Several days should elapse between titration steps.
For patients whose daily insulin requirement is greater than 20 units, the insulin dose should be reduced by 50% and GLUCOTROL XL therapy may begin at usual dosages. Subsequent reductions in insulin dosage should depend on individual patient response. Several days should elapse between titration steps.
During the insulin withdrawal period, the patient should test urine samples for sugar and ketone bodies at least three times daily. Patients should be instructed to contact the prescriber immediately if these tests are abnormal. In some cases, especially when the patient has been receiving greater than 40 units of insulin daily, it may be advisable to consider hospitalization during the transition period.
Patients Receiving Other Oral Hypoglycemic Agents: As with other sulfonylurea-class hypoglycemics, no transition period is necessary when transferring patients to GLUCOTROL XL Extended Release Tablets. Patients should be observed carefully (1-2 weeks) for hypoglycemia when being transferred from longer half-life sulfonylureas (e.g., chlorpropamide) to GLUCOTROL XL due to potential overlapping of drug effect.

HOW SUPPLIED

GLUCOTROL XL® (glipizide) Extended Release Tablets are supplied as 2.5 mg, 5 mg, and 10 mg round, biconvex tablets and imprinted with black ink as follows:
2.5 mg tablets are blue and imprinted with "GLUCOTROL XL 2.5" on one side.
Bottles of 30: NDC 0049-1620-30
5 mg tablets are white and imprinted with "GLUCOTROL XL 5" on one side.
Bottles of 100: NDC 0049-1550-66
Bottles of 500: NDC 0049-1550-73
10 mg tablets are white and imprinted with "GLUCOTROL XL 10" on one side.
Bottles of 100: NDC 0049-1560-66
Bottles of 500: NDC 0049-1560-73
Recommended Storage: The tablets should be protected from moisture and humidity and stored at controlled room temperature, 59° to 86°F (15° to 30°C).
℞ Only

Pfizer U.S. Pharmaceuticals
Pfizer Inc, NY, NY 10017
69-4951-00-6 Revised April 2001

LIPITOR® ℞

[lĭ'pĭ-tōr]
(Atorvastatin Calcium)
Tablets
Rx only

Prescribing information for this product, which appears on pages 2610–2613 of the 2003 PDR, has been completely revised as follows. Please write "See Supplement A" next to the product heading.

DESCRIPTION

Lipitor® (atorvastatin calcium) is a synthetic lipid-lowering agent. Atorvastatin is an inhibitor of 3-hydroxy-3-methylglutaryl-coenzyme A (HMG-CoA) reductase. This enzyme catalyzes the conversion of HMG-CoA to mevalonate, an early and rate-limiting step in cholesterol biosynthesis.
Atorvastatin calcium is [R-(R*, R*)]-2-(4-fluorophenyl)-β, δ-dihydroxy-5-(1-methylethyl)-3-phenyl-4-[(phenylamino)-carbonyl]-1H-pyrrole-1-heptanoic acid, calcium salt (2:1) trihydrate. The empirical formula of atorvastatin calcium is $(C_{33}H_{34}FN_2O_5)_2Ca \bullet 3H_2O$ and its molecular weight is 1209.42. Its structural formula is:

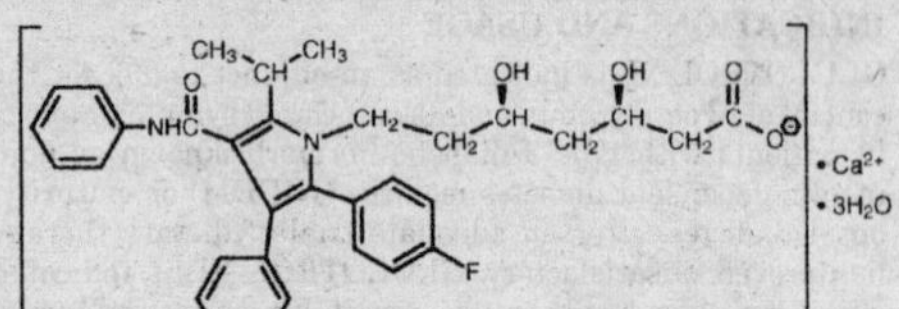

Atorvastatin calcium is a white to off-white crystalline powder that is insoluble in aqueous solutions of pH 4 and below. Atorvastatin calcium is very slightly soluble in distilled water, pH 7.4 phosphate buffer, and acetonitrile, slightly soluble in ethanol, and freely soluble in methanol.
Lipitor tablets for oral administration contain 10, 20, 40 or 80 mg atorvastatin and the following inactive ingredients: calcium carbonate, USP; candelilla wax, FCC; croscarmellose sodium, NF; hydroxypropyl cellulose, NF; lactose monohydrate, NF; magnesium stearate, NF; microcrystalline cellulose, NF; Opadry White YS-1-7040 (hydroxypropylmethylcellulose, polyethylene glycol, talc, titanium dioxide); polysorbate 80, NF; simethicone emulsion.

CLINICAL PHARMACOLOGY

Mechanism of Action
Atorvastatin is a selective, competitive inhibitor of HMG-CoA reductase, the rate-limiting enzyme that converts 3-hydroxy-3-methylglutaryl-coenzyme A to mevalonate, a precursor of sterols, including cholesterol. Cholesterol and triglycerides circulate in the bloodstream as part of lipoprotein complexes. With ultracentrifugation, these complexes separate into HDL (high-density lipoprotein), IDL (intermediate-density lipoprotein), LDL (low-density lipoprotein), and VLDL (very-low-density lipoprotein) fractions. Triglycerides (TG) and cholesterol in the liver are incorporated into VLDL and released into the plasma for delivery to peripheral tissues. LDL is formed from VLDL and is catabolized primarily through the high-affinity LDL receptor. Clinical and pathologic studies show that elevated plasma levels of total cholesterol (total-C), LDL-cholesterol (LDL-C), and apolipoprotein B (apo B) promote human atherosclerosis and are risk factors for developing cardiovascular disease, while increased levels of HDL-C are associated with a decreased cardiovascular risk.
In animal models, Lipitor lowers plasma cholesterol and lipoprotein levels by inhibiting HMG-CoA reductase and cholesterol synthesis in the liver and by increasing the number

of hepatic LDL receptors on the cell-surface to enhance uptake and catabolism of LDL; Lipitor also reduces LDL production and the number of LDL particles. Lipitor reduces LDL-C in some patients with homozygous familial hypercholesterolemia (FH), a population that rarely responds to other lipid-lowering medication(s).

A variety of clinical studies have demonstrated that elevated levels of total-C, LDL-C, and apo B (a membrane complex for LDL-C) promote human atherosclerosis. Similarly, decreased levels of HDL-C (and its transport complex, apo A) are associated with the development of atherosclerosis. Epidemiologic investigations have established that cardiovascular morbidity and mortality vary directly with the level of total-C and LDL-C, and inversely with the level of HDL-C.

Lipitor reduces total-C, LDL-C, and apo B in patients with homozygous and heterozygous FH, nonfamilial forms of hypercholesterolemia, and mixed dyslipidemia. Lipitor also reduces VLDL-C and TG and produces variable increases in HDL-C and apolipoprotein A-1. Lipitor reduces total-C, LDL-C, VLDL-C, apo B, TG, and non-HDL-C, and increases HDL-C in patients with isolated hypertriglyceridemia. Lipitor reduces intermediate density lipoprotein cholesterol (IDL-C) in patients with dysbetalipoproteinemia. The effect of Lipitor on cardiovascular morbidity and mortality has not been determined.

Like LDL, cholesterol-enriched triglyceride-rich lipoproteins, including VLDL, intermediate density lipoprotein (IDL), and remnants, can also promote atherosclerosis. Elevated plasma triglycerides are frequently found in a triad with low HDL-C levels and small LDL particles, as well as in association with non-lipid metabolic risk factors for coronary heart disease. As such, total plasma TG has not consistently been shown to be an independent risk factor for CHD. Furthermore, the independent effect of raising HDL or lowering TG on the risk of coronary and cardiovascular morbidity and mortality has not been determined.

Pharmacodynamics

Atorvastatin as well as some of its metabolites are pharmacologically active in humans. The liver is the primary site of action and the principal site of cholesterol synthesis and LDL clearance. Drug dosage rather than systemic drug concentration correlates better with LDL-C reduction. Individualization of drug dosage should be based on therapeutic response (see DOSAGE AND ADMINISTRATION).

Pharmacokinetics and Drug Metabolism

Absorption: Atorvastatin is rapidly absorbed after oral administration; maximum plasma concentrations occur within 1 to 2 hours. Extent of absorption increases in proportion to atorvastatin dose. The absolute bioavailability of atorvastatin (parent drug) is approximately 14% and the systemic availability of HMG-CoA reductase inhibitory activity is approximately 30%. The low systemic availability is attributed to presystemic clearance in gastrointestinal mucosa and/or hepatic first-pass metabolism. Although food decreases the rate and extent of drug absorption by approximately 25% and 9%, respectively, as assessed by Cmax and AUC, LDL-C reduction is similar whether atorvastatin is given with or without food. Plasma atorvastatin concentrations are lower (approximately 30% for Cmax and AUC) following evening drug administration compared with morning. However, LDL-C reduction is the same regardless of the time of day of drug administration (see DOSAGE AND ADMINISTRATION).

Distribution: Mean volume of distribution of atorvastatin is approximately 381 liters. Atorvastatin is ≥98% bound to plasma proteins. A blood/plasma ratio of approximately 0.25 indicates poor drug penetration into red blood cells. Based on observations in rats, atorvastatin is likely to be secreted in human milk (see CONTRAINDICATIONS, Pregnancy and Lactation, and PRECAUTIONS, Nursing Mothers).

Metabolism: Atorvastatin is extensively metabolized to ortho- and parahydroxylated derivatives and various beta-oxidation products. *In vitro* inhibition of HMG-CoA reductase by ortho- and parahydroxylated metabolites is equivalent to that of atorvastatin. Approximately 70% of circulating inhibitory activity for HMG-CoA reductase is attributed to active metabolites. *In vitro* studies suggest the importance of atorvastatin metabolism by cytochrome P450 3A4, consistent with increased plasma concentrations of atorvastatin in humans following coadministration with erythromycin, a known inhibitor of this isozyme (see PRECAUTIONS, Drug Interactions). In animals, the ortho-hydroxy metabolite undergoes further glucuronidation.

Excretion: Atorvastatin and its metabolites are eliminated primarily in bile following hepatic and/or extra-hepatic metabolism; however, the drug does not appear to undergo enterohepatic recirculation. Mean plasma elimination half-life of atorvastatin in humans is approximately 14 hours, but the half-life of inhibitory activity for HMG-CoA reductase is 20 to 30 hours due to the contribution of active metabolites. Less than 2% of a dose of atorvastatin is recovered in urine following oral administration.

Special Populations

Geriatric: Plasma concentrations of atorvastatin are higher (approximately 40% for Cmax and 30% for AUC) in healthy elderly subjects (age ≥65 years) than in young adults. Clinical data suggest a greater degree of LDL-lowering at any dose of drug in the elderly patient population compared to younger adults (see PRECAUTIONS section; Geriatric Use subsection).

Pediatric: Pharmacokinetic data in the pediatric population are not available.

TABLE 1. Dose-Response in Patients With Primary Hypercholesterolemia (Adjusted Mean % Change From Baseline)[a]

Dose	N	TC	LDL-C	Apo B	TG	HDL-C	Non-HDL-C/ HDL-C
Placebo	21	4	4	3	10	-3	7
10	22	-29	-39	-32	-19	6	-34
20	20	-33	-43	-35	-26	9	-41
40	21	-37	-50	-42	-29	6	-45
80	23	-45	-60	-50	-37	5	-53

[a]Results are pooled from 2 dose-response studies.

TABLE 2. Mean Percent Change From Baseline at End Point (Double-Blind, Randomized, Active-Controlled Trials)

Treatment (Daily Dose)	N	Total-C	LDL-C	Apo B	TG	HDL-C	Non-HDL-C/ HDL-C
Study 1							
Atorvastatin 10 mg	707	-27[a]	-36[a]	-28[a]	-17[a]	+7	-37[a]
Lovastatin 20 mg	191	-19	-27	-20	-6	+7	-28
95% CI for Diff[1]		-9.2, -6.5	-10.7, -7.1	-10.0, -6.5	-15.2, -7.1	-1.7, 2.0	-11.1, -7.1
Study 2							
Atorvastatin 10 mg	222	-25[b]	-35[b]	-27[b]	-17[b]	+6	-36[b]
Pravastatin 20 mg	77	-17	-23	-17	-9	+8	-28
95% CI for Diff[1]		-10.8, -6.1	-14.5, -8.2	-13.4, -7.4	-14.1, -0.7	-4.9, 1.6	-11.5, -4.1
Study 3							
Atorvastatin 10 mg	132	-29[c]	-37[c]	-34[c]	-23[c]	+7	-39[c]
Simvastatin 10 mg	45	-24	-30	-30	-15	+7	-33
95% CI for Diff[1]		-8.7, -2.7	-10.1, -2.6	-8.0, -1.1	-15.1, -0.7	-4.3, 3.9	-9.6, -1.9

[1] A negative value for the 95% CI for the difference between treatments favors atorvastatin for all except HDL-C, for which a positive value favors atorvastatin. If the range does not include 0, this indicates a statistically significant difference.
[a] Significantly different from lovastatin, ANCOVA, p ≤0.05
[b] Significantly different from pravastatin, ANCOVA, p ≤0.05
[c] Significantly different from simvastatin, ANCOVA, p ≤0.05

TABLE 3. Combined Patients With Isolated Elevated TG: Median (min, max) Percent Changes From Baseline

	Placebo (N=12)	Atorvastatin 10 mg (N=37)	Atorvastatin 20 mg (N=13)	Atorvastatin 80 mg (N=14)
Triglycerides	-12.4 (-36.6, 82.7)	-41.0 (-76.2, 49.4)	-38.7 (-62.7, 29.5)	-51.8 (-82.8, 41.3)
Total-C	-2.3 (-15.5, 24.4)	-28.2 (-44.9, -6.8)	-34.9 (-49.6, -15.2)	-44.4 (-63.5, -3.8)
LDL-C	3.6 (-31.3, 31.6)	-26.5 (-57.7, 9.8)	-30.4 (-53.9, 0.3)	-40.5 (-60.6, -13.8)
HDL-C	3.8 (-18.6, 13.4)	13.8 (-9.7, 61.5)	11.0 (-3.2, 25.2)	7.5 (-10.8, 37.2)
VLDL-C	-1.0 (-31.9, 53.2)	-48.8 (-85.8, 57.3)	-44.6 (-62.2, -10.8)	-62.0 (-88.2, 37.6)
non-HDL-C	-2.8 (-17.6, 30.0)	-33.0 (-52.1, -13.3)	-42.7 (-53.7, -17.4)	-51.5 (-72.9, -4.3)

Gender: Plasma concentrations of atorvastatin in women differ from those in men (approximately 20% higher for Cmax and 10% lower for AUC); however, there is no clinically significant difference in LDL-C reduction with Lipitor between men and women.

Renal Insufficiency: Renal disease has no influence on the plasma concentrations or LDL-C reduction of atorvastatin; thus, dose adjustment in patients with renal dysfunction is not necessary (see DOSAGE AND ADMINISTRATION).

Hemodialysis: While studies have not been conducted in patients with end-stage renal disease, hemodialysis is not expected to significantly enhance clearance of atorvastatin since the drug is extensively bound to plasma proteins.

Hepatic Insufficiency: In patients with chronic alcoholic liver disease, plasma concentrations of atorvastatin are markedly increased. Cmax and AUC are each 4-fold greater in patients with Childs-Pugh A disease. Cmax and AUC are approximately 16-fold and 11-fold increased, respectively, in patients with Childs-Pugh B disease (see CONTRAINDICATIONS).

Clinical Studies

Hypercholesterolemia (Heterozygous Familial and Nonfamilial) and Mixed Dyslipidemia (*Fredrickson* Types IIa and IIb)

Lipitor reduces total-C, LDL-C, VLDL-C, apo B, and TG, and increases HDL-C in patients with hypercholesterolemia and mixed dyslipidemia. Therapeutic response is seen within 2 weeks, and maximum response is usually achieved within 4 weeks and maintained during chronic therapy.

Lipitor is effective in a wide variety of patient populations with hypercholesterolemia, with and without hypertriglyceridemia, in men and women, and in the elderly. Experience in pediatric patients has been limited to patients with homozygous FH. In two multicenter, placebo-controlled, dose-response studies in patients with hypercholesterolemia, Lipitor given as a single dose over 6 weeks significantly reduced total-C, LDL-C, apo B, and TG (Pooled results are provided in Table 1).

[See table 1 above]

In patients with *Fredrickson* Types IIa and IIb hyperlipoproteinemia pooled from 24 controlled trials, the median (25th and 75th percentile) percent changes from baseline in HDL-C for atorvastatin 10, 20, 40, and 80 mg were 6.4 (-1.4, 14), 8.7 (0, 17), 7.8 (0, 16), and 5.1 (-2.7, 15), respectively. Additionally, analysis of the pooled data demonstrated consistent and significant decreases in total-C, LDL-C, TG, total-C/HDL-C, and LDL-C/HDL-C.

In three multicenter, double-blind studies in patients with hypercholesterolemia, Lipitor was compared to other HMG-CoA reductase inhibitors. After randomization, patients were treated for 16 weeks with either Lipitor 10 mg per day or a fixed dose of the comparative agent (Table 2).

[See table 2 above]

The impact on clinical outcomes of the differences in lipid-altering effects between treatments shown in Table 2 is not known. Table 2 does not contain data comparing the effects of atorvastatin 10 mg and higher doses of lovastatin, pravastatin, and simvastatin. The drugs compared in the studies summarized in the table are not necessarily interchangeable.

Hypertriglyceridemia (*Fredrickson* Type IV)

The response to Lipitor in 64 patients with isolated hypertriglyceridemia treated across several clinical trials is shown in the table below. For the atorvastatin-treated patients, median (min, max) baseline TG level was 565 (267-1502).

[See table 3 above]

Dysbetalipoproteinemia (*Fredrickson* Type III)

The results of an open-label crossover study of 16 patients (genotypes: 14 apo E2/E2 and 2 apo E3/E2) with dysbetalipoproteinemia (*Fredrickson* Type III) are shown in the table below.

[See table 4 at top of next page]

Homozygous Familial Hypercholesterolemia

In a study without a concurrent control group, 29 patients ages 6 to 37 years with homozygous FH received maximum daily doses of 20 to 80 mg of Lipitor. The mean LDL-C reduction in this study was 18%. Twenty-five patients with a reduction in LDL-C had a mean response of 20% (range of 7% to 53%, median of 24%); the remaining 4 patients had 7% to 24% increases in LDL-C. Five of the 29 patients had absent LDL receptor function. Of these, 2 patients also had a portacaval shunt and had no significant reduction in LDL-C. The remaining 3 receptor-negative patients had a mean LDL-C reduction of 22%.

Heterozygous Familial Hypercholesterolemia in Pediatric Patients

In a double-blind, placebo-controlled study followed by an open-label phase, 187 boys and postmenarchal girls 10–17

Continued on next page

Lipitor—Cont.

years of age (mean age 14.1 years) with heterozygous familial hypercholesterolemia (FH) or severe hypercholesterolemia were randomized to Lipitor (n=140) or placebo (n=47) for 26 weeks and then all received Lipitor for 26 weeks. Inclusion in the study required 1) a baseline LDL-C level ≥ 190 mg/dL or 2) a baseline LDL-C ≥ 160 mg/dL and positive family history of FH or documented premature cardiovascular disease in a first- or second-degree relative. The mean baseline LDL-C value was 218.6 mg/dL (range: 138.5-385.0 mg/dL) in the Lipitor group compared to 230.0 mg/dL (range: 160.0-324.5 mg/dL) in placebo group. The dosage of Lipitor (once daily) was 10 mg for the first 4 weeks and up-titrated to 20 mg if the LDL-C level was > 130 mg/dL. The number of Lipitor-treated patients who required up-titration to 20 mg after Week 4 during the double-blind phase was 80 (57.1%).

Lipitor significantly decreased plasma levels of total-C, LDL-C, triglycerides, and apolipoprotein B during the 26 week double-blind phase (see Table 5).

[See table 5 at right]

The mean achieved LDL-C value was 130.7 mg/dL (range: 70.0–242.0 mg/dL) in the Lipitor group compared to 228.5 mg/dL (range: 152.0–385.0 mg/dL) in the placebo group during the 26 week double-blind phase.

The safety and efficacy of doses above 20 mg have not been studied in controlled trials in children. The long-term efficacy of Lipitor therapy in childhood to reduce morbidity and mortality in adulthood has not been established.

INDICATIONS AND USAGE

Lipitor is indicated:

1. as an adjunct to diet to reduce elevated total-C, LDL-C, apo B, and TG levels and to increase HDL-C in patients with primary hypercholesterolemia (heterozygous familial and nonfamilial) and mixed dyslipidemia (*Fredrickson* Types IIa and IIb);
2. as an adjunct to diet for the treatment of patients with elevated serum TG levels (*Fredrickson* Type IV);
3. for the treatment of patients with primary dysbetalipoproteinemia (*Fredrickson* Type III) who do not respond adequately to diet;
4. to reduce total-C and LDL-C in patients with homozygous familial hypercholesterolemia as an adjunct to other lipid-lowering treatments (eg, LDL apheresis) or if such treatments are unavailable.
5. as an adjunct to diet to reduce total-C, LDL-C, and apo B levels in boys and postmenarchal girls, 10 to 17 years of age, with heterozygous familial hypercholesterolemia if after an adequate trial of diet therapy the following findings are present:
   a. LDL-C remains ≥ 190 mg/dL or
   b. LDL-C remains ≥ 160 mg/dL and:
      - there is a positive family history of premature cardiovascular disease or
      - two or more other CVD risk factors are present in the pediatric patient

Therapy with lipid-altering agents should be a component of multiple-risk-factor intervention in individuals at increased risk for atherosclerotic vascular disease due to hypercholesterolemia. Lipid-altering agents should be used in addition to a diet restricted in saturated fat and cholesterol only when the response to diet and other nonpharmacological measures has been inadequate (see *National Cholesterol Education Program (NCEP) Guidelines*, summarized in Table 6).

[See table 6 at right]

After the LDL-C goal has been achieved, if the TG is still ≥200 mg/dL, non HDL-C (total-C minus HDL-C) becomes a secondary target of therapy. Non-HDL-C goals are set 30 mg/dL higher than LDL-C goals for each risk category.

Prior to initiating therapy with Lipitor, secondary causes for hypercholesterolemia (eg, poorly controlled diabetes mellitus, hypothyroidism, nephrotic syndrome, dysproteinemias, obstructive liver disease, other drug therapy, and alcoholism) should be excluded, and a lipid profile performed to measure total-C, LDL-C, HDL-C, and TG. For patients with TG <400 mg/dL (<4.5 mmol/L), LDL-C can be estimated using the following equation: LDL-C = total-C - (0.20 × [TG] + HDL-C). For TG levels >400 mg/dL (>4.5 mmol/L), this equation is less accurate and LDL-C concentrations should be determined by ultracentrifugation.

Lipitor has not been studied in conditions where the major lipoprotein abnormality is elevation of chylomicrons (*Fredrickson* Types I and V).

The NCEP classification of cholesterol levels in pediatric patients with a familial history of hypercholesterolemia or premature cardiovascular disease is summarized below:

Category	Total-C (mg/dL)	LDL-C (mg/dL)
Acceptable	<170	
Borderline	170-199	
High	≥200	≥1[illegible]

CONTRAINDICATIONS

Active liver disease or unexplained persistent elevations of serum transaminases.

Hypersensitivity to any component of this medication.

Pregnancy and Lactation

Atherosclerosis is a chronic process and discontinuation of lipid-lowering drugs during pregnancy should have little impact on the outcome of long-term therapy of primary hypercholesterolemia. Cholesterol and other products of cholesterol biosynthesis are essential components for fetal development (including synthesis of steroids and cell membranes). Since HMG-CoA reductase inhibitors decrease cholesterol synthesis and possibly the synthesis of other biologically active substances derived from cholesterol, they may cause fetal harm when administered to pregnant women. Therefore, HMG-CoA reductase inhibitors are contraindicated during pregnancy and in nursing mothers. ATORVASTATIN SHOULD BE ADMINISTERED TO WOMEN OF CHILDBEARING AGE ONLY WHEN SUCH PATIENTS ARE HIGHLY UNLIKELY TO CONCEIVE AND HAVE BEEN INFORMED OF THE POTENTIAL HAZARDS. If the patient becomes pregnant while taking this drug, therapy should be discontinued and the patient apprised of the potential hazard to the fetus.

TABLE 4. Open-Label Crossover Study of 16 Patients With Dysbetalipoproteinemia (*Fredrickson* Type III)

	Median (min, max) at Baseline (mg/dL)	Median % Change (min, max) Atorvastatin 10 mg	Atorvastatin 80 mg
Total-C	442 (225, 1320)	-37 (-85, 17)	-58 (-90, -31)
Triglycerides	678 (273, 5990)	-39 (-92, -8)	-53 (-95, -30)
IDL-C + VLDL-C	215 (111, 613)	-32 (-76, 9)	-63 (-90, -8)
non-HDL-C	411 (218, 1272)	-43 (-87, -19)	-64 (-92, -36)

TABLE 5
Lipid-lowering Effects of Lipitor in Adolescent Boys and Girls with Heterozygous Familial Hypercholesterolemia or Severe Hypercholesterolemia
(Mean Percent Change from Baseline at Endpoint in Intention-to-Treat Population)

DOSAGE	N	Total-C	LDL-C	HDL-C	TG	Apolipoprotein B
Placebo	47	-1.5	-0.4	-1.9	1.0	0.7
Lipitor	140	-31.4	-39.6	2.8	-12.0	-34.0

TABLE 6. NCEP Treatment Guidelines: LDL-C Goals and Cutpoints for Therapeutic Lifestyle Changes and Drug Therapy in Different Risk Categories

Risk Category	LDL Goal (mg/dL)	LDL Level at Which to Initiate Therapeutic Lifestyle Changes (mg/dL)	LDL Level at Which to Consider Drug Therapy (mg/dL)
CHD[a] or CHD risk equivalents (10-year risk >20%)	<100	≥100	≥130 (100–129: drug optional)[b]
2+ Risk Factors (10-year risk ≤20%)	<130	≥130	10-year risk 10%–20%: ≥130 10-year risk <10%: ≥160
0-1 Risk factor[c]	<160	≥160	≥190 (160–189: LDL-lowering drug optional)

[a] CHD, coronary heart disease

[b] Some authorities recommend use of LDL-lowering drugs in this category if an LDL-C level of <100 mg/dL cannot be achieved by therapeutic lifestyle changes. Others prefer use of drugs that primarily modify triglycerides and HDL-C, e.g., nicotinic acid or fibrate. Clinical judgement also may call for deferring drug therapy in this subcategory.

[c] Almost all people with 0-1 risk factor have 10-year risk <10%; thus, 10-year risk assessment in people with 0-1 risk factor is not necessary.

WARNINGS

Liver Dysfunction

HMG-CoA reductase inhibitors, like some other lipid-lowering therapies, have been associated with biochemical abnormalities of liver function. **Persistent elevations (>3 times the upper limit of normal [ULN] occurring on 2 or more occasions) in serum transaminases occurred in 0.7% of patients who received atorvastatin in clinical trials. The incidence of these abnormalities was 0.2%, 0.2%, 0.6%, and 2.3% for 10, 20, 40, and 80 mg, respectively.**

One patient in clinical trials developed jaundice. Increases in liver function tests (LFT) in other patients were not associated with jaundice or other clinical signs or symptoms. Upon dose reduction, drug interruption, or discontinuation, transaminase levels returned to or near pretreatment levels without sequelae. Eighteen of 30 patients with persistent LFT elevations continued treatment with a reduced dose of atorvastatin.

It is recommended that liver function tests be performed prior to and at 12 weeks following both the initiation of therapy and any elevation of dose, and periodically (eg, semiannually) thereafter. Liver enzyme changes generally occur in the first 3 months of treatment with atorvastatin. Patients who develop increased transaminase levels should be monitored until the abnormalities resolve. Should an increase in ALT or AST of >3 times ULN persist, reduction of dose or withdrawal of atorvastatin is recommended.

Atorvastatin should be used with caution in patients who consume substantial quantities of alcohol and/or have a history of liver disease. Active liver disease or unexplained persistent transaminase elevations are contraindications to the use of atorvastatin (see CONTRAINDICATIONS).

Skeletal Muscle

Rare cases of rhabdomyolysis with acute renal failure secondary to myoglobinuria have been reported with atorvastatin and with other drugs in this class.

Uncomplicated myalgia has been reported in atorvastatin-treated patients (see ADVERSE REACTIONS). Myopathy, defined as muscle aches or muscle weakness in conjunction with increases in creatine phosphokinase (CPK) values >10 times ULN, should be considered in any patient with diffuse myalgias, muscle tenderness or weakness, and/or marked elevation of CPK. Patients should be advised to report promptly unexplained muscle pain, tenderness or weakness, particularly if accompanied by malaise or fever. Atorvastatin therapy should be discontinued if markedly elevated CPK levels occur or myopathy is diagnosed or suspected.

The risk of myopathy during treatment with drugs in this class is increased with concurrent administration of cyclosporine, fibric acid derivatives, erythromycin, niacin, or azole antifungals. Physicians considering combined therapy with atorvastatin and fibric acid derivatives, erythromycin, immunosuppressive drugs, azole antifungals, or lipid-lowering doses of niacin should carefully weigh the potential benefits and risks and should carefully monitor patients for any signs or symptoms of muscle pain, tenderness, or weakness, particularly during the initial months of therapy and during any periods of upward dosage titration of either drug. Periodic creatine phosphokinase (CPK) determinations may be considered in such situations, but there is no assurance that such monitoring will prevent the occurrence of severe myopathy.

Atorvastatin therapy should be temporarily withheld or discontinued in any patient with an acute, serious condition suggestive of a myopathy or having a risk factor predisposing to the development of renal failure secondary to rhabdomyolysis (eg, severe acute infection, hypotension, major surgery, trauma, severe metabolic, endocrine and electrolyte disorders, and uncontrolled seizures).

PRECAUTIONS

General

Before instituting therapy with atorvastatin, an attempt should be made to control hypercholesterolemia with appropriate diet, exercise, and weight reduction in obese patients, and to treat other underlying medical problems (see INDICATIONS AND USAGE).

Information for Patients

Patients should be advised to report promptly unexplained muscle pain, tenderness, or weakness, particularly if accompanied by malaise or fever.

Drug Interactions

The risk of myopathy during treatment with drugs of this class is increased with concurrent administration of cyclosporine, fibric acid derivatives, niacin (nicotinic acid), erythromycin, azole antifungals (see WARNINGS, Skeletal Muscle).

Antacid: When atorvastatin and Maalox® TC suspension were coadministered, plasma concentrations of atorvastatin decreased approximately 35%. However, LDL-C reduction was not altered.

Antipyrine: Because atorvastatin does not affect the pharmacokinetics of antipyrine, interactions with other drugs metabolized via the same cytochrome isozymes are not expected.

Colestipol: Plasma concentrations of atorvastatin decreased approximately 25% when colestipol and atorvastatin were coadministered. However, LDL-C reduction was greater when atorvastatin and colestipol were coadministered than when either drug was given alone.

Cimetidine: Atorvastatin plasma concentrations and LDL-C reduction were not altered by coadministration of cimetidine.

Digoxin: When multiple doses of atorvastatin and digoxin were coadministered, steady-state plasma digoxin concentrations increased by approximately 20%. Patients taking digoxin should be monitored appropriately.

Erythromycin: In healthy individuals, plasma concentrations of atorvastatin increased approximately 40% with coadministration of atorvastatin and erythromycin, a known inhibitor of cytochrome P450 3A4 (see WARNINGS, Skeletal Muscle).

Oral Contraceptives: Coadministration of atorvastatin and an oral contraceptive increased AUC values for norethindrone and ethinyl estradiol by approximately 30% and 20%. These increases should be considered when selecting an oral contraceptive for a woman taking atorvastatin.

Warfarin: Atorvastatin had no clinically significant effect on prothrombin time when administered to patients receiving chronic warfarin treatment.

Endocrine Function

HMG-CoA reductase inhibitors interfere with cholesterol synthesis and theoretically might blunt adrenal and/or gonadal steroid production. Clinical studies have shown that atorvastatin does not reduce basal plasma cortisol concentration or impair adrenal reserve. The effects of HMG-CoA reductase inhibitors on male fertility have not been studied in adequate numbers of patients. The effects, if any, on the pituitary-gonadal axis in premenopausal women are unknown. Caution should be exercised if an HMG-CoA reductase inhibitor is administered concomitantly with drugs that may decrease the levels or activity of endogenous steroid hormones, such as ketoconazole, spironolactone, and cimetidine.

CNS Toxicity

Brain hemorrhage was seen in a female dog treated for 3 months at 120 mg/kg/day. Brain hemorrhage and optic nerve vacuolation were seen in another female dog that was sacrificed in moribund condition after 11 weeks of escalating doses up to 280 mg/kg/day. The 120 mg/kg dose resulted in a systemic exposure approximately 16 times the human plasma area-under-the-curve (AUC, 0-24 hours) based on the maximum human dose of 80 mg/day. A single tonic convulsion was seen in each of 2 male dogs (one treated at 10 mg/kg/day and one at 120 mg/kg/day) in a 2-year study. No CNS lesions have been observed in mice after chronic treatment for up to 2 years at doses up to 400 mg/kg/day or in rats at doses up to 100 mg/kg/day. These doses were 6 to 11 times (mouse) and 8 to 16 times (rat) the human AUC (0-24) based on the maximum recommended human dose of 80 mg/day.

CNS vascular lesions, characterized by perivascular hemorrhages, edema, and mononuclear cell infiltration of perivascular spaces, have been observed in dogs treated with other members of this class. A chemically similar drug in this class produced optic nerve degeneration (Wallerian degeneration of retinogeniculate fibers) in clinically normal dogs in a dose-dependent fashion at a dose that produced plasma drug levels about 30 times higher than the mean drug level in humans taking the highest recommended dose.

Carcinogenesis, Mutagenesis, Impairment of Fertility

In a 2-year carcinogenicity study in rats at dose levels of 10, 30, and 100 mg/kg/day, 2 rare tumors were found in muscle in high-dose females: in one, there was a rhabdomyosarcoma and, in another, there was a fibrosarcoma. This dose represents a plasma AUC (0–24) value of approximately 16 times the mean human plasma drug exposure after an 80 mg oral dose.

A 2-year carcinogenicity study in mice given 100, 200, or 400 mg/kg/day resulted in a significant increase in liver adenomas in high-dose males and liver carcinomas in high-dose females. These findings occurred at plasma AUC (0-24) values of approximately 6 times the mean human plasma drug exposure after an 80 mg oral dose.

In vitro, atorvastatin was not mutagenic or clastogenic in the following tests with and without metabolic activation: the Ames test with *Salmonella typhimurium* and *Escherichia coli*, the HGPRT forward mutation assay in Chinese hamster lung cells, and the chromosomal aberration assay in Chinese hamster lung cells. Atorvastatin was negative in the *in vivo* mouse micronucleus test.

Studies in rats performed at doses up to 175 mg/kg (15 times the human exposure) produced no changes in fertility. There was aplasia and aspermia in the epididymis of 2 of 10 rats treated with 100 mg/kg/day of atorvastatin for 3 months (16 times the human AUC at the 80 mg dose); testis weights were significantly lower at 30 and 100 mg/kg and epididymal weight was lower at 100 mg/kg. Male rats given 100 mg/kg/day for 11 weeks prior to mating had decreased sperm motility, spermatid head concentration, and increased abnormal sperm. Atorvastatin caused no adverse effects on semen parameters, or reproductive organ histopathology in dogs given doses of 10, 40, or 120 mg/kg for two years.

TABLE 7. Adverse Events in Placebo-Controlled Studies (% of Patients)

BODY SYSTEM/ Adverse Event	Placebo N = 270	Atorvastatin 10 mg N = 863	Atorvastatin 20 mg N = 36	Atorvastatin 40 mg N = 79	Atorvastatin 80 mg N = 94
BODY AS A WHOLE					
Infection	10.0	10.3	2.8	10.1	7.4
Headache	7.0	5.4	16.7	2.5	6.4
Accidental Injury	3.7	4.2	0.0	1.3	3.2
Flu Syndrome	1.9	2.2	0.0	2.5	3.2
Abdominal Pain	0.7	2.8	0.0	3.8	2.1
Back Pain	3.0	2.8	0.0	3.8	1.1
Allergic Reaction	2.6	0.9	2.8	1.3	0.0
Asthenia	1.9	2.2	0.0	3.8	0.0
DIGESTIVE SYSTEM					
Constipation	1.8	2.1	0.0	2.5	1.1
Diarrhea	1.5	2.7	0.0	3.8	5.3
Dyspepsia	4.1	2.3	2.8	1.3	2.1
Flatulence	3.3	2.1	2.8	1.3	1.1
RESPIRATORY SYSTEM					
Sinusitis	2.6	2.8	0.0	2.5	6.4
Pharyngitis	1.5	2.5	0.0	1.3	2.1
SKIN AND APPENDAGES					
Rash	0.7	3.9	2.8	3.8	1.1
MUSCULOSKELETAL SYSTEM					
Arthralgia	1.5	2.0	0.0	5.1	0.0
Myalgia	1.1	3.2	5.6	1.3	0.0

Pregnancy

Pregnancy Category X

See CONTRAINDICATIONS

Safety in pregnant women has not been established. Atorvastatin crosses the rat placenta and reaches a level in fetal liver equivalent to that of maternal plasma. Atorvastatin was not teratogenic in rats at doses up to 300 mg/kg/day or in rabbits at doses up to 100 mg/kg/day. These doses resulted in multiples of about 30 times (rat) or 20 times (rabbit) the human exposure based on surface area (mg/m^2).

In a study in rats given 20, 100, or 225 mg/kg/day, from gestation day 7 through to lactation day 21 (weaning), there was decreased pup survival at birth, neonate, weaning, and maturity in pups of mothers dosed with 225 mg/kg/day. Body weight was decreased on days 4 and 21 in pups of mothers dosed at 100 mg/kg/day; pup body weight was decreased at birth and at days 4, 21, and 91 at 225 mg/kg/day. Pup development was delayed (rotorod performance at 100 mg/kg/day and acoustic startle at 225 mg/kg/day; pinnae detachment and eye opening at 225 mg/kg/day). These doses correspond to 6 times (100 mg/kg) and 22 times (225 mg/kg) the human AUC at 80 mg/day. Rare reports of congenital anomalies have been received following intrauterine exposure to HMG-CoA reductase inhibitors. There has been one report of severe congenital bony deformity, tracheo-esophageal fistula, and anal atresia (VATER association) in a baby born to a woman who took lovastatin with dextroamphetamine sulfate during the first trimester of pregnancy. Lipitor should be administered to women of child-bearing potential only when such patients are highly unlikely to conceive and have been informed of the potential hazards. If the woman becomes pregnant while taking Lipitor, it should be discontinued and the patient advised again as to the potential hazards to the fetus.

Nursing Mothers

Nursing rat pups had plasma and liver drug levels of 50% and 40%, respectively, of that in their mother's milk. Because of the potential for adverse reactions in nursing infants, women taking Lipitor should not breast-feed (see CONTRAINDICATIONS).

Pediatric Use

Safety and effectiveness in patients 10-17 years of age with heterozygous familial hypercholesterolemia have been evaluated in controlled clinical trials of 6 months duration in adolescent boys and postmenarchal girls. Patients treated with Lipitor had an adverse experience profile generally similar to that of patients treated with placebo, the most common adverse experiences observed in both groups, regardless of causality assessment, were infections. **Doses greater than 20 mg have not been studied in this patient population.** In this limited controlled study, there was no detectable effect on growth or sexual maturation in boys or on menstrual cycle length in girls. See CLINICAL PHARMACOLOGY, *Clinical Studies section;* ADVERSE REACTIONS, *Pediatric Patients*; and DOSAGE AND ADMINISTRATION, *Pediatric Patients (10–17 years of age) with Heterozygous Familial Hypercholesterolemia*. Adolescent females should be counseled on appropriate contraceptive methods while on Lipitor therapy (see CONTRAINDICATIONS and PRECAUTIONS, *Pregnancy*). **Lipitor has not been studied in controlled clinical trials involving prepubertal patients or patients younger than 10 years of age.**

Clinical efficacy with doses up to 80 mg/day for 1 year have been evaluated in an uncontrolled study of patients with homozygous FH including 8 pediatric patients. See CLINICAL PHARMACOLOGY, *Clinical Studies in Homozygous Familial Hypercholesterolemia*.

Geriatric Use

The safety and efficacy of atorvastatin (10-80 mg) in the geriatric population (≥65 years of age) was evaluated in the ACCESS study. In this 54-week open-label trial 1,958 patients initiated therapy with atorvastatin 10 mg. Of these, 835 were elderly (≥65 years) and 1,123 were non-elderly. The mean change in LDL-C from baseline after 6 weeks of treatment with atorvastatin 10 mg was –38.2% in the elderly patients versus –34.6% in the non-elderly group.

The rates of discontinuation due to adverse events were similar between the two age groups. There were no differences in clinically relevant laboratory abnormalities between the age groups.

ADVERSE REACTIONS

Lipitor is generally well-tolerated. Adverse reactions have usually been mild and transient. In controlled clinical studies of 2502 patients, <2% of patients were discontinued due to adverse experiences attributable to atorvastatin. The most frequent adverse events thought to be related to atorvastatin were constipation, flatulence, dyspepsia, and abdominal pain.

Clinical Adverse Experiences

Adverse experiences reported in ≥2% of patients in placebo-controlled clinical studies of atorvastatin, regardless of causality assessment, are shown in Table 7.

[See table 7 above]

The following adverse events were reported, regardless of causality assessment in patients treated with atorvastatin in clinical trials. The events in italics occurred in ≥2% of patients and the events in plain type occurred in <2% of patients.

Body as a Whole: *Chest pain*, face edema, fever, neck rigidity, malaise, photosensitivity reaction, generalized edema.

Digestive System: *Nausea*, gastroenteritis, liver function tests abnormal, colitis, vomiting, gastritis, dry mouth, rectal hemorrhage, esophagitis, eructation, glossitis, mouth ulceration, anorexia, increased appetite, stomatitis, biliary pain, cheilitis, duodenal ulcer, dysphagia, enteritis, melena, gum hemorrhage, stomach ulcer, tenesmus, ulcerative stomatitis, hepatitis, pancreatitis, cholestatic jaundice.

Respiratory System: *Bronchitis, rhinitis*, pneumonia, dyspnea, asthma, epistaxis.

Nervous System: *Insomnia, dizziness*, paresthesia, somnolence, amnesia, abnormal dreams, libido decreased, emotional lability, incoordination, peripheral neuropathy, torticollis, facial paralysis, hyperkinesia, depression, hypesthesia, hypertonia.

Musculoskeletal System: *Arthritis*, leg cramps, bursitis, tenosynovitis, myasthenia, tendinous contracture, myositis.

Skin and Appendages: Pruritus, contact dermatitis, alopecia, dry skin, sweating, acne, urticaria, eczema, seborrhea, skin ulcer.

Urogenital System: *Urinary tract infection*, urinary frequency, cystitis, hematuria, impotence, dysuria, kidney calculus, nocturia, epididymitis, fibrocystic breast, vaginal hemorrhage, albuminuria, breast enlargement, metrorrhagia, nephritis, urinary incontinence, urinary retention, urinary urgency, abnormal ejaculation, uterine hemorrhage.

Special Senses: Amblyopia, tinnitus, dry eyes, refraction disorder, eye hemorrhage, deafness, glaucoma, parosmia, taste loss, taste perversion.

Cardiovascular System: Palpitation, vasodilatation, syncope, migraine, postural hypotension, phlebitis, arrhythmia, angina pectoris, hypertension.

Metabolic and Nutritional Disorders: *Peripheral edema*, hyperglycemia, creatine phosphokinase increased, gout, weight gain, hypoglycemia.

Hemic and Lymphatic System: Ecchymosis, anemia, lymphadenopathy, thrombocytopenia, petechia.

Postintroduction Reports

Adverse events associated with Lipitor therapy reported since market introduction, that are not listed above, regardless of causality assessment, include the following: anaphylaxis, angioneurotic edema, bullous rashes (including erythema multiforme, Stevens-Johnson syndrome, and toxic epidermal necrolysis), and rhabdomyolysis.

Continued on next page

Lipitor—Cont.

Pediatric Patients (ages 10–17 years)

In a 26-week controlled study in boys and postmenarchal girls (n=140), the safety and tolerability profile of Lipitor 10 to 20 mg daily was generally similar to that of placebo (see CLINICAL PHARMACOLOGY, *Clinical Studies, section* and PRECAUTIONS, *Pediatric Use*).

OVERDOSAGE

There is no specific treatment for atorvastatin overdosage. In the event of an overdose, the patient should be treated symptomatically, and supportive measures instituted as required. Due to extensive drug binding to plasma proteins, hemodialysis is not expected to significantly enhance atorvastatin clearance.

DOSAGE AND ADMINISTRATION

The patient should be placed on a standard cholesterol-lowering diet before receiving Lipitor and should continue on this diet during treatment with Lipitor.

Hypercholesterolemia (Heterozygous Familial and Nonfamilial) and Mixed Dyslipidemia (*Fredrickson* Types IIa and IIb)

The recommended starting dose of Lipitor is 10 or 20 mg once daily. Patients who require a large reduction in LDL-C (more than 45%) may be started at 40 mg once daily. The dosage range of Lipitor is 10 to 80 mg once daily. Lipitor can be administered as a single dose at any time of the day, with or without food. The starting dose and maintenance doses of Lipitor should be individualized according to patient characteristics such as goal of therapy and response (see *NCEP Guidelines*, summarized in Table 5). After initiation and/or upon titration of Lipitor, lipid levels should be analyzed within 2 to 4 weeks and dosage adjusted accordingly.

Since the goal of treatment is to lower LDL-C, the NCEP recommends that LDL-C levels be used to initiate and assess treatment response. Only if LDL-C levels are not available, should total-C be used to monitor therapy.

Heterozygous Familial Hypercholesterolemia in Pediatric Patients (10–17 years of age)

The recommended starting dose of Lipitor is 10 mg/day; the maximum recommended dose is 20 mg/day (doses greater than 20 mg have not been studied in this patient population). Doses should be individualized according to the recommended goal of therapy (see NCEP Pediatric Panel Guidelines[1], CLINICAL PHARMACOLOGY, and INDICATIONS AND USAGE). Adjustments should be made at intervals of 4 weeks or more.

[1] National Cholesterol Education Program (NCEP): Highlights of the Report of the Expert Panel on Blood Cholesterol Levels in Children Adolescents, *Pediatrics*. 89(3):495–501. 1992.

Homozygous Familial Hypercholesterolemia

The dosage of Lipitor in patients with homozygous FH is 10 to 80 mg daily. Lipitor should be used as an adjunct to other lipid-lowering treatments (eg, LDL apheresis) in these patients or if such treatments are unavailable.

Concomitant Therapy

Atorvastatin may be used in combination with a bile acid binding resin for additive effect. The combination of HMG-CoA reductase inhibitors and fibrates should generally be avoided (see WARNINGS, Skeletal Muscle, and PRECAUTIONS, Drug Interactions for other drug-drug interactions).

Dosage in Patients With Renal Insufficiency

Renal disease does not affect the plasma concentrations nor LDL-C reduction of atorvastatin; thus, dosage adjustment in patients with renal dysfunction is not necessary (see CLINICAL PHARMACOLOGY, Pharmacokinetics).

HOW SUPPLIED

Lipitor is supplied as white, elliptical, film-coated tablets of atorvastatin calcium containing 10, 20, 40 and 80 mg atorvastatin.

10 mg tablets: coded "PD 155" on one side and "10" on the other.

N0071-0155-23 bottles of 90

N0071-0155-34 bottles of 5000

N0071-0155-40 10 × 10 unit dose blisters

20 mg tablets: coded "PD 156" on one side and "20" on the other.

N0071-0156-23 bottles of 90

N0071-0156-40 10 × 10 unit dose blisters

40 mg tablets: coded "PD 157" on one side and "40" on the other.

N0071-0157-23 bottles of 90

80 mg tablets: coded "PD 158" on one side and "80" on the other.

N0071-0158-23 bottles of 90

Storage

Store at controlled room temperature 20-25°C (68-77°F) [see USP].

Manufactured by:

Pfizer Ireland Pharmaceuticals

Dublin, Ireland

Distributed by:

Pfizer Parke-Davis

Division of Pfizer Inc, NY, NY 10017

69-5884-00-2 Revised November 2002

NAVANE® ℞

[*nah' vān*]

Thiothixene Capsules Thiothixene Hydrochloride Concentrate

Prescribing information for this product, which appears on pages 2616–2617 of the 2003 PDR, has been completely revised as follows. Please write "See Supplement A" next to the product heading.

DESCRIPTION

Navane® (thiothixene) is a thioxanthene derivative. Specifically, it is the *cis* isomer of N,N-dimethyl-9-[3-(4-methyl-1-piperazinyl)-propylidene] thioxanthene-2-sulfonamide.

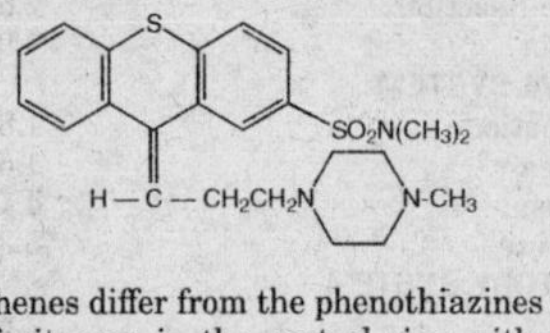

The thioxanthenes differ from the phenothiazines by the replacement of nitrogen in the central ring with a carbon-linked side chain fixed in space in a rigid structural configuration. An N,N-dimethyl sulfonamide functional group is bonded to the thioxanthene nucleus.

Inert ingredients for the capsule formulations are: hard gelatin capsules (which contain gelatin and titanium dioxide; may contain Yellow 10, Yellow 6, Blue 1, Green 3, Red 3, and other inert ingredients); lactose; magnesium stearate; sodium lauryl sulfate; starch.

Inert ingredients for the oral concentrate formulation are: alcohol; cherry flavor; dextrose; passion fruit flavor; sorbitol solution; water.

ACTIONS

Navane is an antipsychotic of the thioxanthene series. Navane possesses certain chemical and pharmacological similarities to the piperazine phenothiazines and differences from the aliphatic group of phenothiazines.

INDICATIONS

Navane is effective in the management of schizophrenia. Navane has not been evaluated in the management of behavioral complications in patients with mental retardation.

CONTRAINDICATIONS

Navane is contraindicated in patients with circulatory collapse, comatose states, central nervous system depression due to any cause, and blood dyscrasias. Navane is contraindicated in individuals who have shown hypersensitivity to the drug. It is not known whether there is a cross sensitivity between the thioxanthenes and the phenothiazine derivatives, but this possibility should be considered.

WARNINGS

Tardive Dyskinesia—Tardive dyskinesia, a syndrome consisting of potentially irreversible, involuntary, dyskinetic movements may develop in patients treated with antipsychotic drugs. Although the prevalence of the syndrome appears to be highest among the elderly, especially elderly women, it is impossible to rely upon prevalence estimates to predict, at the inception of antipsychotic treatment, which patients are likely to develop the syndrome. Whether antipsychotic drug products differ in their potential to cause tardive dyskinesia is unknown.

Both the risk of developing the syndrome and the likelihood that it will become irreversible are believed to increase as the duration of treatment and the total cumulative dose of antipsychotic drugs administered to the patient increase. However, the syndrome can develop, although much less commonly, after relatively brief treatment periods at low doses.

There is no known treatment for established cases of tardive dyskinesia, although the syndrome may remit, partially or completely, if antipsychotic treatment is withdrawn. Antipsychotic treatment, itself, however, may suppress (or partially suppress) the signs and symptoms of the syndrome and thereby may possibly mask the underlying disease process. The effect that symptomatic suppression has upon the long-term course of the syndrome is unknown.

Given these considerations, antipsychotics should be prescribed in a manner that is most likely to minimize the occurrence of tardive dyskinesia. Chronic antipsychotic treatment should generally be reserved for patients who suffer from a chronic illness that, 1) is known to respond to antipsychotic drugs, and, 2) for whom alternative, equally effective, but potentially less harmful treatments are *not* available or appropriate. In patients who do require chronic treatment, the smallest dose and the shortest duration of treatment producing a satisfactory clinical response should be sought. The need for continued treatment should be reassessed periodically.

If signs and symptoms of tardive dyskinesia appear in a patient on antipsychotics, drug discontinuation should be considered. However, some patients may require treatment despite the presence of the syndrome.

(For further information about the description of tardive dyskinesia and its clinical detection, please refer to "Information for Patients" in the PRECAUTIONS section, and to the ADVERSE REACTIONS section.)

Neuroleptic Malignant Syndrome (NMS)—A potentially fatal symptom complex sometimes referred to as Neuroleptic Malignant Syndrome (NMS) has been reported in association with antipsychotic drugs. Clinical manifestations of NMS are hyperpyrexia, muscle rigidity, altered mental status and evidence of autonomic instability (irregular pulse or blood pressure, tachycardia, diaphoresis, and cardiac dysrhythmias).

The diagnostic evaluation of patients with this syndrome is complicated. In arriving at a diagnosis, it is important to identify cases where the clinical presentation includes both serious medical illness (e.g., pneumonia, systemic infection, etc.) and untreated or inadequately treated extrapyramidal signs and symptoms (EPS). Other important considerations in the differential diagnosis include central anticholinergic toxicity, heat stroke, drug fever and primary central nervous system (CNS) pathology.

The management of NMS should include 1) immediate discontinuation of antipsychotic drugs and other drugs not essential to concurrent therapy, 2) intensive symptomatic treatment and medical monitoring, and 3) treatment of any concomitant serious medical problems for which specific treatments are available. There is no general agreement about specific pharmacological treatment regimens for uncomplicated NMS.

If a patient requires antipsychotic drug treatment after recovery from NMS, the potential reintroduction of drug therapy should be carefully considered. The patient should be carefully monitored, since recurrences of NMS have been reported.

Usage in Pregnancy—Safe use of Navane during pregnancy has not been established. Therefore, this drug should be given to pregnant patients only when, in the judgment of the physician, the expected benefits from the treatment exceed the possible risks to mother and fetus. Animal reproduction studies and clinical experience to date have not demonstrated any teratogenic effects.

In the animal reproduction studies with Navane, there was some decrease in conception rate and litter size, and an increase in resorption rate in rats and rabbits. Similar findings have been reported with other psychotropic agents. After repeated oral administration of Navane to rats (5 to 15 mg/kg/day), rabbits (3 to 50 mg/kg/day), and monkeys (1 to 3 mg/kg/day) before and during gestation, no teratogenic effects were seen.

Usage in Children—The use of Navane in children under 12 years of age is not recommended because safe conditions for its use have not been established.

As is true with many CNS drugs, Navane may impair the mental and/or physical abilities required for the performance of potentially hazardous tasks such as driving a car or operating machinery, especially during the first few days of therapy. Therefore, the patient should be cautioned accordingly.

As in the case of other CNS-acting drugs, patients receiving Navane (thiothixene) should be cautioned about the possible additive effects (which may include hypotension) with CNS depressants and with alcohol.

PRECAUTIONS

An antiemetic effect was observed in animal studies with Navane; since this effect may also occur in man, it is possible that Navane may mask signs of overdosage of toxic drugs and may obscure conditions such as intestinal obstruction and brain tumor.

In consideration of the known capability of Navane and certain other psychotropic drugs to precipitate convulsions, extreme caution should be used in patients with a history of convulsive disorders or those in a state of alcohol withdrawal, since it may lower the convulsive threshold. Although Navane potentiates the actions of the barbiturates, the dosage of the anticonvulsant therapy should not be reduced when Navane is administered concurrently.

Though exhibiting rather weak anticholinergic properties, Navane should be used with caution in patients who might be exposed to extreme heat or who are receiving atropine or related drugs.

Use with caution in patients with cardiovascular disease.

Caution as well as careful adjustment of the dosages is indicated when Navane is used in conjunction with other CNS depressants.

Also, careful observation should be made for pigmentary retinopathy and lenticular pigmentation (fine lenticular pigmentation has been noted in a small number of patients treated with Navane for prolonged periods). Blood dyscrasias (agranulocytosis, pancytopenia, thrombocytopenic purpura), and liver damage (jaundice, biliary stasis) have been reported with related drugs.

Antipsychotic drugs elevate prolactin levels; the elevation persists during chronic administration. Tissue culture experiments indicate that approximately one-third of human breast cancers are prolactin dependent *in vitro*, a factor of potential importance if the prescription of these drugs is contemplated in a patient with a previously detected breast cancer. Although disturbances such as galactorrhea, amenorrhea, gynecomastia, and impotence have been reported, the clinical significance of elevated serum prolactin levels is unknown for most patients. An increase in mammary neoplasms has been found in rodents after chronic administration of antipsychotic drugs. Neither clinical studies nor epidemiologic studies conducted to date, however, have shown an association between chronic administration of these drugs and mammary tumorigenesis; the available evidence is considered too limited to be conclusive at this time.

Information for Patients: Given the likelihood that some patients exposed chronically to antipsychotics will develop tardive dyskinesia, it is advised that all patients in whom chronic use is contemplated be given, if possible, full information about this risk. The decision to inform patients and/or their guardians must obviously take into account the clinical circumstances and the competency of the patient to understand the information provided.

ADVERSE REACTIONS

NOTE: Not all of the following adverse reactions have been reported with Navane. However, since Navane has certain chemical and pharmacologic similarities to the phenothiazines, all of the known side effects and toxicity associated with phenothiazine therapy should be borne in mind when Navane is used.

Cardiovascular Effects: Tachycardia, hypotension, lightheadedness, and syncope. In the event hypotension occurs, epinephrine should not be used as a pressor agent since a paradoxical further lowering of blood pressure may result. Nonspecific EKG changes have been observed in some patients receiving Navane. These changes are usually reversible and frequently disappear on continued Navane therapy. The incidence of these changes is lower than that observed with some phenothiazines. The clinical significance of these changes is not known.

CNS Effects: Drowsiness, usually mild, may occur although it usually subsides with continuation of Navane therapy. The incidence of sedation appears similar to that of the piperazine group of phenothiazines but less than that of certain aliphatic phenothiazines. Restlessness, agitation and insomnia have been noted with Navane. Seizures and paradoxical exacerbation of psychotic symptoms have occurred with Navane infrequently.

Hyperreflexia has been reported in infants delivered from mothers having received structurally related drugs.

In addition, phenothiazine derivatives have been associated with cerebral edema and cerebrospinal fluid abnormalities.

Extrapyramidal symptoms, such as pseudoparkinsonism, akathisia and dystonia have been reported. Management of these extra-pyramidal symptoms depends upon the type and severity. Rapid relief of acute symptoms may require the use of an injectable antiparkinson agent. More slowly emerging symptoms may be managed by reducing the dosage of Navane and/or administering an oral antiparkinson agent.

Persistent Tardive Dyskinesia: As with all antipsychotic agents, tardive dyskinesia may appear in some patients on long-term therapy or may occur after drug therapy has been discontinued. The syndrome is characterized by rhythmical involuntary movements of the tongue, face, mouth or jaw (e.g., protrusion of tongue, puffing of cheeks, puckering of mouth, chewing movements). Sometimes these may be accompanied by involuntary movements of extremities.

Since early detection of tardive dyskinesia is important, patients should be monitored on an ongoing basis. It has been reported that fine vermicular movement of the tongue may be an early sign of the syndrome. If this or any other presentation of the syndrome is observed, the clinician should consider possible discontinuation of antipsychotic medication. (See WARNINGS section.)

Hepatic Effects: Elevations of serum transaminase and alkaline phosphatase, usually transient, have been infrequently observed in some patients. No clinically confirmed cases of jaundice attributable to Navane (thiothixene) have been reported.

Hematologic Effects: As is true with certain other psychotropic drugs, leukopenia and leucocytosis, which are usually transient, can occur occasionally with Navane. Other antipsychotic drugs have been associated with agranulocytosis, eosinophilia, hemolytic anemia, thrombocytopenia and pancytopenia.

Allergic Reactions: Rash, pruritus, urticaria, photosensitivity and rare cases of anaphylaxis have been reported with Navane. Undue exposure to sunlight should be avoided. Although not experienced with Navane, exfoliative dermatitis and contact dermatitis (in nursing personnel) have been reported with certain phenothiazines.

Endocrine Disorders: Lactation, moderate breast enlargement and amenorrhea have occurred in a small percentage of females receiving Navane. If persistent, this may necessitate a reduction in dosage or the discontinuation of therapy. Phenothiazines have been associated with false positive pregnancy tests, gynecomastia, hypoglycemia, hyperglycemia and glycosuria.

Autonomic Effects: Dry mouth, blurred vision, nasal congestion, constipation, increased sweating, increased salivation and impotence have occurred infrequently with Navane therapy. Phenothiazines have been associated with miosis, mydriasis, and adynamic ileus.

Other Adverse Reactions: Hyperpyrexia, anorexia, nausea, vomiting, diarrhea, increase in appetite and weight, weakness or fatigue, polydipsia, and peripheral edema.

Although not reported with Navane, evidence indicates there is a relationship between phenothiazine therapy and the occurrence of a systemic lupus erythematosus-like syndrome.

Neuroleptic Malignant Syndrome (NMS): Please refer to the text regarding NMS in the WARNINGS section.

NOTE: Sudden deaths have occasionally been reported in patients who have received certain phenothiazine derivatives. In some cases the cause of death was apparently cardiac arrest or asphyxia due to failure of the cough reflex. In others, the cause could not be determined nor could it be established that death was due to phenothiazine administration.

DOSAGE AND ADMINISTRATION

Dosage of Navane should be individually adjusted depending on the chronicity and severity of the symptoms of schizophrenia. In general, small doses should be used initially and gradually increased to the optimal effective level, based on patient response.

Some patients have been successfully maintained on once-a-day Navane therapy.

The use of Navane in children under 12 years of age is not recommended because safe conditions for its use have not been established.

In milder conditions, an initial dose of 2 mg three times daily. If indicated, a subsequent increase to 15 mg/day total daily dose is often effective.

In more severe conditions, an initial dose of 5 mg twice daily.

The usual optimal dose is 20 to 30 mg daily. If indicated, an increase to 60 mg/day total daily dose is often effective. Exceeding a total daily dose of 60 mg rarely increases the beneficial response.

OVERDOSAGE

Manifestations include muscular twitching, drowsiness and dizziness. Symptoms of gross overdosage may include CNS depression, rigidity, weakness, torticollis, tremor, salivation, dysphagia, hypotension, disturbances of gait, or coma.

Treatment: Essentially symptomatic and supportive. Early gastric lavage is helpful. Keep patient under careful observation and maintain an open airway, since involvement of the extrapyramidal system may produce dysphagia and respiratory difficulty in severe overdosage. If hypotension occurs, the standard measures for managing circulatory shock should be used (I.V. fluids and/or vasoconstrictors).

If a vasoconstrictor is needed, levarterenol and phenylephrine are the most suitable drugs. Other pressor agents, including epinephrine, are not recommended, since phenothiazine derivatives may reverse the usual pressor action of these agents and cause further lowering of blood pressure.

If CNS depression is marked, symptomatic treatment is indicated. Extrapyramidal symptoms may be treated with antiparkinson drugs.

There are no data on the use of peritoneal or hemodialysis, but they are known to be of little value in phenothiazine intoxication.

HOW SUPPLIED

Navane® (thiothixene) Capsules

Bottles of 100's:	1 mg (NDC 0049-5710-66)
	2 mg (NDC 0049-5720-66)
	5 mg (NDC 0049-5730-66)
	10 mg (NDC 0049-5740-66)
	20 mg (NDC 0049-5770-66)

℞ only

Roerig
Division of Pfizer Inc, NY, NY 10017
69-1655-00-9 Revised May 2001

NAVANE® ℞

[*nah'vān*]

thiothixene hydrochloride
Intramuscular For Injection
STERILE

Prescribing information for this product, which appears on pages 2617–2618 of the 2003 PDR, has been completely revised as follows. Please write "See Supplement A" next to the product heading.

DESCRIPTION

Navane (thiothixene hydrochloride) is a thioxanthene derivative. Specifically, thiothixene is the *cis* isomer of N,N-dimethyl-9-[3-(4-methyl-1-piperazinyl)-propylidene] thioxanthene-2-sulfonamide.

The thioxanthenes differ from the phenothiazines by the replacement of nitrogen in the central ring with a carbon-linked side chain fixed in space in a rigid structural configuration. An N,N-dimethyl sulfonamide functional group is bonded to the thioxanthene nucleus.

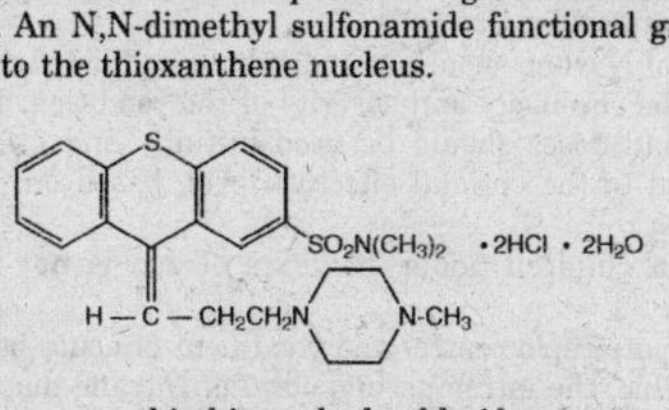

thiothixene hydrochloride

Inert ingredients for the intramuscular for injection formulation are: water; mannitol.

ACTIONS

Navane is a psychotropic agent of the thioxanthene series. Navane possesses certain chemical and pharmacological similarities to the piperazine phenothiazines and differences from the aliphatic group of phenothiazines. Navane's mode of action has not been clearly established.

INDICATIONS

Navane is effective in the management of manifestations of psychotic disorders. Navane has not been evaluated in the management of behavioral complications in patients with mental retardation.

CONTRAINDICATIONS

Navane is contraindicated in patients with circulatory collapse, comatose states, central nervous system depression due to any cause, and blood dyscrasias. Navane is contraindicated in individuals who have shown hypersensitivity to the drug. It is not known whether there is a cross sensitivity between the thioxanthenes and the phenothiazine derivatives, but this possibility should be considered.

WARNINGS

Tardive Dyskinesia—Tardive dyskinesia, a syndrome consisting of potentially irreversible, involuntary, dyskinetic movements may develop in patients treated with neuroleptic (antipsychotic) drugs. Although the prevalence of the syndrome appears to be highest among the elderly, especially elderly women, it is impossible to rely upon prevalence estimates to predict, at the inception of neuroleptic treatment, which patients are likely to develop the syndrome. Whether neuroleptic drug products differ in their potential to cause tardive dyskinesia is unknown.

Both the risk of developing the syndrome and the likelihood that it will become irreversible are believed to increase as the duration of treatment and the total cumulative dose of neuroleptic drugs administered to the patient increase. However, the syndrome can develop, although much less commonly, after relatively brief treatment periods at low doses.

There is no known treatment for established cases of tardive dyskinesia, although the syndrome may remit, partially or completely, if neuroleptic treatment is withdrawn. Neuroleptic treatment, itself, however, may suppress (or partially suppress) the signs and symptoms of the syndrome and thereby may possibly mask the underlying disease process. The effect that symptomatic suppression has upon the long-term course of the syndrome is unknown.

Given these considerations, neuroleptics should be prescribed in a manner that is most likely to minimize the occurrence of tardive dyskinesia. Chronic neuroleptic treatment should generally be reserved for patients who suffer from a chronic illness that, 1) is known to respond to neuroleptic drugs, and, 2) for whom alternative, equally effective, but potentially less harmful treatments are *not* available or appropriate. In patients who do require chronic treatment, the smallest dose and the shortest duration of treatment producing a satisfactory clinical response should be sought. The need for continued treatment should be reassessed periodically.

If signs and symptoms of tardive dyskinesia appear in a patient on neuroleptics, drug discontinuation should be considered. However, some patients may require treatment despite the presence of the syndrome

(For further information about the description of tardive dyskinesia and its clinical detection, please refer to "Information for Patients" in the PRECAUTIONS section, and to the ADVERSE REACTIONS section.)

Neuroleptic Malignant Syndrome (NMS)—A potentially fatal symptom complex sometimes referred to as Neuroleptic Malignant Syndrome (NMS) has been reported in association with antipsychotic drugs. Clinical manifestations of NMS are hyperpyrexia, muscle rigidity, altered mental status and evidence of autonomic instability (irregular pulse or blood pressure, tachycardia, diaphoresis, and cardiac dysrhythmias).

The diagnostic evaluation of patients with this syndrome is complicated. In arriving at a diagnosis, it is important to identify cases where the clinical presentation includes both serious medical illness (e.g., pneumonia, systemic infection, etc.) and untreated or inadequately treated extrapyramidal signs and symptoms (EPS). Other important considerations in the differential diagnosis include central anticholinergic toxicity, heat stroke, drug fever and primary central nervous system (CNS) pathology.

The management of NMS should include 1) immediate discontinuation of antipsychotic drugs and other drugs not essential to concurrent therapy, 2) intensive symptomatic treatment and medical monitoring, and 3) treatment of any concomitant serious medical problems for which specific treatments are available. There is no general agreement about specific pharmacological treatment regimens for uncomplicated NMS.

If a patient requires antipsychotic drug treatment after recovery from NMS, the potential reintroduction of drug therapy should be carefully considered. The patient should be carefully monitored, since recurrences of NMS have been reported.

Usage in Pregnancy—Safe use of Navane during pregnancy has not been established. Therefore, this drug should be given to pregnant patients only when, in the judgment of the physician, the expected benefits from treatment exceed the possible risks to mother and fetus. Animal reproductive studies and clinical experience to date have not demonstrated any teratogenic effects.

In the animal reproduction studies with Navane, there was some decrease in conception rate and litter size, and an increase in resorption rate in rats and rabbits, changes which have been similarly reported with other psychotropic agents. After repeated oral administration of Navane to rats (5 to 15 mg/kg/day), rabbits (3 to 50 mg/kg/day), and monkeys (1 to 3 mg/kg/day) before and during gestation, no teratogenic effects were seen. (See Precautions).

Usage in Children—The use of Navane in children under 12 years of age is not recommended because safety and efficacy in the pediatric age group have not been established.

As is true with many CNS drugs, Navane may impair the mental and/or physical abilities required for the performance of potentially hazardous tasks such as driving a car

Continued on next page

Navane IM—Cont.

or operating machinery, especially during the first few days of therapy. Therefore, the patient should be cautioned accordingly.

As in the case of other CNS-acting drugs, patients receiving Navane should be cautioned about the possible additive effects, (which may include hypotension) with CNS depressants and with alcohol.

PRECAUTIONS

General: An antiemetic effect was observed in animal studies with Navane (thiothixene hydrochloride); since this effect may also occur in man, it is possible that Navane may mask signs of overdosage of toxic drugs and may obscure conditions such as intestinal obstruction and brain tumor.

In consideration of the known capability of Navane and certain other psychotropic drugs to precipitate convulsions, extreme caution should be used in patients with a history of convulsive disorders, or those in a state of alcohol withdrawal since it may lower the convulsive threshold. Although Navane potentiates the actions of the barbiturates, the dosage of the anticonvulsant therapy should not be reduced when Navane is administered concurrently.

Caution as well as careful adjustment of the dosage is indicated when Navane is used in conjunction with other CNS depressants other than anticonvulsant drugs.

Though exhibiting rather weak anticholinergic properties, Navane should be used with caution in patients who are known or suspected to have glaucoma, or who might be exposed to extreme heat, or who are receiving atropine or related drugs.

Use with caution in patients with cardiovascular disease.

Also, careful observation should be made for pigmentary retinopathy, and lenticular pigmentation (fine lenticular pigmentation has been noted in a small number of patients treated with Navane for prolonged periods). Blood dyscrasias (agranulocytosis, pancytopenia, thrombocytopenic purpura), and liver damage (jaundice, biliary stasis), have been reported with related drugs.

Undue exposure to sunlight should be avoided. Photosensitive reactions have been reported in patients on Navane.

As with all intramuscular preparations, Navane Intramuscular For Injection should be injected well within the body of a relatively large muscle. The preferred sites are the upper outer quadrant of the buttock (i.e., gluteus maximus) and the mid-lateral thigh.

The deltoid area should be used only if well developed such as in certain adults and older children, and then only with caution to avoid radial nerve injury. Intramuscular injections should not be made into the lower and mid-thirds of the upper arm. As with all intramuscular injections, aspiration is necessary to help avoid inadvertent injection into a blood vessel.

Neuroleptic drugs elevate prolactin levels; the elevation persists during chronic administration. Tissue culture experiments indicate that approximately one-third of human breast cancers are prolactin dependent *in vitro*, a factor of potential importance if the prescription of these drugs is contemplated in a patient with a previously detected breast cancer. Although disturbances such as galactorrhea, amenorrhea, gynecomastia, and impotence have been reported, the clinical significance of elevated serum prolactin levels is unknown for most patients. An increase in mammary neoplasms has been found in rodents after chronic administration of neuroleptic drugs. Neither clinical studies nor epidemiologic studies conducted to date, however, have shown an association between chronic administration of these drugs and mammary tumorigenesis; the available evidence is considered too limited to be conclusive at this time.

Information for Patients: Given the likelihood that some patients exposed chronically to neuroleptics will develop tardive dyskinesia, it is advised that all patients in whom chronic use is contemplated be given, if possible, full information about this risk. The decision to inform patients and/or their guardians must obviously take into account the clinical circumstances and the competency of the patient to understand the information provided.

ADVERSE REACTIONS

NOTE: Not all of the following adverse reactions have been reported with Navane. However, since Navane has certain chemical and pharmacologic similarities to the phenothiazines, all of the known side effects and toxicity associated with phenothiazine therapy should be borne in mind when Navane is used.

Cardiovascular Effects: Tachycardia, hypotension, lightheadedness, and syncope. In the event hypotension occurs, epinephrine should not be used as a pressor agent since a paradoxical further lowering of blood pressure may result. Nonspecific EKG changes have been observed in some patients receiving Navane. These changes are usually reversible and frequently disappear on continued Navane therapy. The clinical significance of these changes is not known.

CNS Effects: Drowsiness, usually mild, may occur although it usually subsides with continuation of Navane therapy. The incidence of sedation appears similar to that of the piperazine group of phenothiazines, but less than that of certain aliphatic phenothiazines. Restlessness, agitation and insomnia have been noted with Navane. Seizures and paradoxical exacerbation of psychotic symptoms have occurred with Navane infrequently.

Hyperreflexia has been reported in infants delivered from mothers having received structurally related drugs.

In addition, phenothiazine derivatives have been associated with cerebral edema and cerebrospinal fluid abnormalities.

Extrapyramidal symptoms, such as pseudo-parkinsonism, akathisia, and dystonia have been reported. Management of these extrapyramidal symptoms depends upon the type and severity. Rapid relief of acute symptoms may require the use of an injectable antiparkinson agent. More slowly emerging symptoms may be managed by reducing the dosage of Navane and/or administering an oral antiparkinson agent.

Persistent Tardive Dyskinesia: As with all antipsychotic agents tardive dyskinesia may appear in some patients on long term therapy or may occur after drug therapy has been discontinued. The syndrome is characterized by rhythmical involuntary movements of the tongue, face, mouth or jaw (e.g., protrusion of tongue, puffing of cheeks, puckering of mouth, chewing movements). Sometimes these may be accompanied by involuntary movements of extremities.

Since early detection of tardive dyskinesia is important, patients should be monitored on an ongoing basis. It has been reported that fine vermicular movement of the tongue may be an early sign of the syndrome. If this or any other presentation of the syndrome is observed, the clinician should consider possible discontinuation of neuroleptic medication. (See WARNINGS section.)

Hepatic Effects: Elevations of serum transaminase and alkaline phosphatase, usually transient, have been infrequently observed in some patients. No clinically confirmed cases of jaundice attributable to Navane (thiothixene hydrochloride) have been reported.

Hematologic Effects: As is true with certain other psychotropic drugs, leukopenia and leucocytosis, which are usually transient, can occur occasionally with Navane. Other antipsychotic drugs have been associated with agranulocytosis, eosinophilia, hemolytic anemia, thrombocytopenia and pancytopenia.

Allergic Reactions: Rash, pruritus, urticaria, and rare cases of anaphylaxis have been reported with Navane. Undue exposure to sunlight should be avoided. Although not experienced with Navane, exfoliative dermatitis, contact dermatitis (in nursing personnel), have been reported with certain phenothiazines.

Endocrine Disorders: Lactation, moderate breast enlargement and amenorrhea have occurred in a small percentage of females receiving Navane. If persistent, this may necessitate a reduction in dosage or the discontinuation of therapy. Phenothiazines have been associated with false positive pregnancy tests, gynecomastia, hypoglycemia, hyperglycemia, and glycosuria.

Autonomic Effects: Dry mouth, blurred vision, nasal congestion, constipation, increased sweating, increased salivation, and impotence have occurred infrequently with Navane therapy. Phenothiazines have been associated with miosis, mydriasis, and adynamic ileus.

Other Adverse Reactions: Hyperpyrexia, anorexia, nausea, vomiting, diarrhea, increase in appetite and weight, weakness or fatigue, polydipsia and peripheral edema.

Although not reported with Navane, evidence indicates there is a relationship between phenothiazine therapy and the occurrence of a systemic lupus erythematosus-like syndrome.

Neuroleptic Malignant Syndrome (NMS): Please refer to the text regarding NMS in the WARNINGS section.

NOTE: Sudden deaths have occasionally been reported in patients who have received certain phenothiazine derivatives. In some cases the cause of death was apparently cardiac arrest or asphyxia due to failure of the cough reflex. In others, the cause could not be determined nor could it be established that death was due to phenothiazine administration.

DOSAGE AND ADMINISTRATION

Preparation

Navane (thiothixene hydrochloride) Intramuscular For Injection must be reconstituted with 2.2 ml of sterile water for injection.

For Intramuscular Use Only

Dosage of Navane should be individually adjusted depending on the chronicity and severity of the condition. In general, small doses should be used initially and gradually increased to the optimal effective level, based on patient response.

Usage in children under 12 years of age is not recommended.

Where more rapid control and treatment of acute behavior is desirable, the intramuscular form of Navane may be indicated. It is also of benefit where the very nature of the patient's symptomatology, whether acute or chronic, renders oral administration impractical or even impossible.

For treatment of acute symptomatology or in patients unable or unwilling to take oral medication, the usual dose is 4 mg of Navane Intramuscular For Injection administered 2 to 4 times daily. Dosage may be increased or decreased depending on response. Most patients are controlled on a total daily dosage of 16 to 20 mg. The maximum recommended dosage is 30 mg/day. An oral form should supplant the injectable form as soon as possible. It may be necessary to adjust the dosage when changing from the intramuscular to oral dosage forms. Dosage recommendations for Navane Capsules and Concentrate can be found in the Navane oral package insert.

OVERDOSAGE

Manifestations include muscular twitching, drowsiness, and dizziness. Symptoms of gross overdosage may include CNS depression, rigidity, weakness, torticollis, tremor, salivation, dysphagia, hypotension, disturbances of gait, or coma.

Treatment: Essentially symptomatic and supportive. Keep patient under careful observation and maintain an open airway, since involvement of the extrapyramidal system may produce dysphagia and respiratory difficulty in severe overdosage. If hypotension occurs, the standard measures for managing circulatory shock should be used (I.V. fluids and/or vasoconstrictors).

If a vasoconstrictor is needed, levarterenol and phenylephrine are the most suitable drugs. Other pressor agents, including epinephrine, are not recommended, since phenothiazine derivatives may reverse the usual pressor elevating action of these agents and cause further lowering of blood pressure.

If CNS depression is marked, symptomatic treatment is indicated. Extrapyramidal symptoms may be treated with antiparkinson drugs.

There are no data on the use of peritoneal or hemodialysis, but they are known to be of little value in phenothiazine intoxication.

HOW SUPPLIED

Navane (thiothixene hydrochloride) Intramuscular For Injection is available in amber glass vials in packages of 10 vials (NDC 0049-5765-83). When reconstituted with 2.2 ml of STERILE WATER FOR INJECTION, each ml contains thiothixene hydrochloride equivalent to 5 mg of thiothixene, and 59.6 mg of mannitol. The reconstituted solution of Navane Intramuscular For Injection may be stored for 48 hours at room temperature before discarding.

Manufactured by The Upjohn Company
Kalamazoo, Michigan 49001
Distributed by
Pfizer Roerig
A division of Pfizer Inc.
New York, New York 10017
70-4177-00-4 Revised Jan. 1988

VFEND® Tablets ℞
[*vee'fənd*]
(voriconazole)
VFEND® I.V.
(voriconazole) for Injection

Prescribing information for this product, which appears on pages 2645–2653 of the 2003 PDR, has been completely revised as follows. Please write "See Supplement A" next to the product heading.

DESCRIPTION

VFEND® (voriconazole), a triazole antifungal agent, is available as film-coated tablets for oral administration, and as a lyophilized powder for solution for intravenous infusion. The structural formula is:

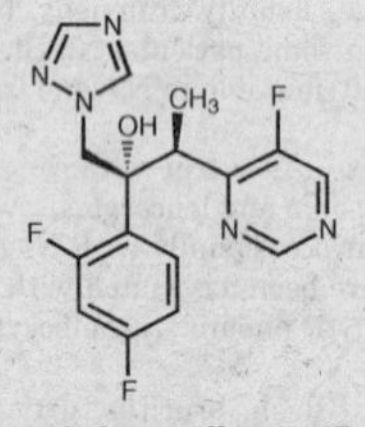

VFEND is designated chemically as (2R, 3S)-2-(2,4-difluorophenyl)-3-(5-fluoro-4-pyrimidinyl)-1-(1*H*-1,2,4-triazol-1-yl)-2-butanol with an empirical formula of $C_{16}H_{14}F_3N_5O$ and a molecular weight of 349.3.

VFEND drug substance is a white to light-colored powder.

VFEND Tablets contain 50 mg or 200 mg of voriconazole. The inactive ingredients include lactose monohydrate, pregelatinized starch, croscarmellose sodium, povidone, magnesium stearate and a coating containing hydroxypropyl methylcellulose, titanium dioxide, lactose monohydrate and triacetin.

VFEND I.V. is a white lyophilized powder containing nominally 200 mg voriconazole and 3200 mg sulfobutyl ether beta-cyclodextrin sodium in a 30 mL Type I clear glass vial.

VFEND I.V. is intended for administration by intravenous infusion. It is a single dose, unpreserved product. Vials containing 200 mg lyophilized VFEND are intended for reconstitution with Water for Injection to produce a solution containing 10 mg/mL VFEND and 160 mg/mL of sulfobutyl ether beta-cyclodextrin sodium. The resultant solution is further diluted prior to administration as an intravenous infusion (see DOSAGE AND ADMINISTRATION).

CLINICAL PHARMACOLOGY

Pharmacokinetics

General Pharmacokinetic Characteristics

The pharmacokinetics of voriconazole have been characterized in healthy subjects, special populations and patients.

The pharmacokinetics of voriconazole are non-linear due to saturation of its metabolism. The interindividual variability of voriconazole pharmacokinetics is high. Greater than proportional increase in exposure is observed with increasing dose. It is estimated that, on average, increasing the oral dose in healthy subjects from 200 mg Q12h to 300 mg Q12h leads to a 2.5-fold increase in exposure (AUC_τ) while increasing the intravenous dose from 3 mg/kg Q12h to 4 mg/kg Q12h produces a 2.3-fold increase in exposure (Table 1).

[See table 1 at right]

During oral administration of 200 mg or 300 mg twice daily for 14 days in patients at risk of aspergillosis (mainly patients with malignant neoplasms of lymphatic or hematopoietic tissue), the observed pharmacokinetic characteristics were similar to those observed in healthy subjects (Table 2).

[See table 2 at right]

Sparse plasma sampling for pharmacokinetics was conducted in the therapeutic studies in patients aged 12-18 years. In 11 adolescent patients who received a mean voriconazole maintenance dose of 4 mg/kg IV, the median of the calculated mean plasma concentrations was 1.60 µg/mL (inter-quartile range 0.28 to 2.73 µg/mL). In 17 adolescent patients for whom mean plasma concentrations were calculated following a mean oral maintenance dose of 200 mg Q12h, the median of the calculated mean plasma concentrations was 1.16 µg/mL (inter-quartile range 0.85 to 2.14 µg/mL).

When the recommended intravenous or oral loading dose regimens are administered to healthy subjects, peak plasma concentrations close to steady state are achieved within the first 24 hours of dosing. Without the loading dose, accumulation occurs during twice-daily multiple dosing with steady-state peak plasma voriconazole concentrations being achieved by day 6 in the majority of subjects (Table 3).

[See table 3 at right]

Steady state trough plasma concentrations with voriconazole are achieved after approximately 5 days of oral or intravenous dosing without a loading dose regimen. However, when an intravenous loading dose regimen is used, steady state trough plasma concentrations are achieved within one day.

Absorption

The pharmacokinetic properties of voriconazole are similar following administration by the intravenous and oral routes. Based on a population pharmacokinetic analysis of pooled data in healthy subjects (N=207), the oral bioavailability of voriconazole is estimated to be 96% (CV 13%).

Maximum plasma concentrations (C_{max}) are achieved 1-2 hours after dosing. When multiple doses of voriconazole are administered with high fat meals, the mean C_{max} and AUC_τ are reduced by 34% and 24%, respectively (see DOSAGE AND ADMINISTRATION).

In healthy subjects, the absorption of voriconazole is not affected by coadministration of oral ranitidine, cimetidine, or omeprazole, drugs that are known to increase gastric pH.

Distribution

The volume of distribution at steady state for voriconazole is estimated to be 4.6 L/kg, suggesting extensive distribution into tissues. Plasma protein binding is estimated to be 58% and was shown to be independent of plasma concentrations achieved following single and multiple oral doses of 200 mg or 300 mg (approximate range: 0.9-15 µg/mL). Varying degrees of hepatic and renal insufficiency do not affect the protein binding of voriconazole.

Metabolism

In vitro studies showed that voriconazole is metabolized by the human hepatic cytochrome P450 enzymes, CYP2C19, CYP2C9 and CYP3A4 (see CLINICAL PHARMACOLOGY—Drug Interactions).

In vivo studies indicated that CYP2C19 is significantly involved in the metabolism of voriconazole. This enzyme exhibits genetic polymorphism. For example, 15–20% of Asian populations may be expected to be poor metabolizers. For Caucasians and Blacks, the prevalence of poor metabolizers is 3–5%. Studies conducted in Caucasian and Japanese healthy subjects have shown that poor metabolizers have, on average, 4-fold higher voriconazole exposure (AUC_τ) than their homozygous extensive metabolizer counterparts. Subjects who are heterozygous extensive metabolizers have, on average, 2-fold higher voriconazole exposure than their homozygous extensive metabolizer counterparts.

The major metabolite of voriconazole is the N-oxide, which accounts for 72% of the circulating radiolabelled metabolites in plasma. Since this metabolite has minimal antifungal activity, it does not contribute to the overall efficacy of voriconazole.

Excretion

Voriconazole is eliminated via hepatic metabolism with less than 2% of the dose excreted unchanged in the urine. After administration of a single radiolabelled dose of either oral or IV voriconazole, preceded by multiple oral or IV dosing, approximately 80% to 83% of the radioactivity is recovered in the urine. The majority (>94%) of the total radioactivity is excreted in the first 96 hours after both oral and intravenous dosing.

As a result of non-linear pharmacokinetics, the terminal half-life of voriconazole is dose dependent and therefore not useful in predicting the accumulation or elimination of voriconazole.

Pharmacokinetic-pharmacodynamic Relationships

In ten clinical trials, the median values for the average and maximum voriconazole plasma concentrations in individual patients across these studies (N=1121) was 2.51 µg/mL (inter-quartile range 1.21 to 4.44 µg/mL) and 3.79 µg/mL (inter-quartile range 2.06 to 6.31 µg/mL), respectively. A pharmacokinetic-pharmacodynamic analysis of patient data from 6 of these 10 clinical trials (N=280) could not detect a positive association between mean, maximum or minimum plasma voriconazole concentration and efficacy. However, PK/PD analyses of the data from all 10 clinical trials identified positive associations between plasma voriconazole

Table 1
Population Pharmacokinetic Parameters of Voriconazole in Volunteers

	200 mg Oral Q12h	300 mg Oral Q12h	3 mg/kg IV Q12h	4 mg/kg IV Q12h
AUC_τ* (µg•h/mL) (CV%)	19.86 (94%)	50.32 (74%)	21.81 (100%)	50.40 (83%)

*Mean AUC_τ are predicted values from population pharmacokinetic analysis of data from 236 volunteers

Table 2
Pharmacokinetic Parameters of Voriconazole in Patients at Risk for Aspergillosis

	200 mg Oral Q12h (n=9)	300 mg Oral Q12h (n=9)
AUC_τ* (µg•h/mL) (CV%)	20.31 (69%)	36.51 (45%)
C_{max}* (µg/mL) (CV%)	3.00 (51%)	4.66 (35%)

*Geometric mean values on Day 14 of multiple dosing in 2 cohorts of patients

Table 3
Pharmacokinetic Parameters of Voriconazole from Loading Dose and Maintenance Dose Regimens (Individual Studies in Volunteers)

	400 mg Q12h on Day 1, 200 mg Q12h on Days 2 to 10 (n=17)		6 mg/kg IV** Q12h on Day 1, 3 mg/kg IV Q12h on Days 2 to 10 (n=9)	
	Day 1, 1st dose	Day 10	Day 1, 1st dose	Day 10
AUC_τ* (µg•h/mL) (CV%)	9.31 (38%)	11.13 (103%)	13.22 (22%)	13.25 (58%)
C_{max} (µg/mL) (CV%)	2.30 (19%)	2.08 (62%)	4.70 (22%)	3.06 (31%)

*AUC_τ values are calculated over dosing interval of 12 hours
Pharmacokinetic parameters for loading and maintenance doses summarized for same cohort of volunteers
**IV infusion over 60 minutes

concentrations and rate of both liver function test abnormalities and visual disturbances (see ADVERSE REACTIONS).

Pharmacokinetics in Special Populations

Gender

In a multiple oral dose study, the mean C_{max} and AUC_τ for healthy young females were 83% and 113% higher, respectively, than in healthy young males (18-45 years). In the same study, no significant differences in the mean C_{max} and AUC_τ were observed between healthy elderly males and healthy elderly females (≥65 years).

In the clinical program, no dosage adjustment was made on the basis of gender. The safety profile and plasma concentrations observed in male and female subjects were similar. Therefore, no dosage adjustment based on gender is necessary.

Geriatric

In an oral multiple dose study the mean C_{max} and AUC_τ in healthy elderly males (≥ 65 years) were 61% and 86% higher, respectively, than in young males (18-45 years). No significant differences in the mean C_{max} and AUC_τ were observed between healthy elderly females (≥ 65 years) and healthy young females (18–45 years).

In the clinical program, no dosage adjustment was made on the basis of age. An analysis of pharmacokinetic data obtained from 552 patients from 10 voriconazole clinical trials showed that the median voriconazole plasma concentrations in the elderly patients (>65 years) were approximately 80% to 90% higher than those in the younger patients (≤65 years) after either IV or oral administration. However, the safety profile of voriconazole in young and elderly subjects was similar and, therefore, no dosage adjustment is necessary for the elderly.

Pediatric

A population pharmacokinetic analysis was conducted on pooled data from 35 immunocompromised pediatric patients aged 2 to <12 years old who were included in two pharmacokinetic studies of intravenous voriconazole (single dose and multiple dose). Twenty-four of these patients received multiple intravenous maintenance doses of 3 mg/kg and 4 mg/kg. A comparison of the pediatric and adult population pharmacokinetic data revealed that the predicted average steady state plasma concentrations were similar at the maintenance dose of 4 mg/kg every 12 hours in children and 3 mg/kg every 12 hours in adults (medians of 1.19 µg/mL and 1.16 µg/mL in children and adults, respectively). (See PRECAUTIONS, Pediatric Use.)

Hepatic Insufficiency

After a single oral dose (200 mg) of voriconazole in 8 patients with mild (Child-Pugh Class A) and 4 patients with moderate (Child-Pugh Class B) hepatic insufficiency, the mean systemic exposure (AUC) was 3.2-fold higher than in age and weight matched controls with normal hepatic function. There was no difference in mean peak plasma concentrations (C_{max}) between the groups. When only the patients with mild (Child-Pugh Class A) hepatic insufficiency were compared to controls, there was still a 2.3-fold increase in the mean AUC in the group with hepatic insufficiency compared to controls.

In an oral multiple dose study, AUC_τ was similar in six subjects with moderate hepatic impairment (Child-Pugh Class B) given a lower maintenance dose of 100 mg twice daily compared to six subjects with normal hepatic function given the standard 200 mg twice daily maintenance dose. The mean peak plasma concentrations (C_{max}) were 20% lower in the hepatically impaired group.

It is recommended that the standard loading dose regimens be used but that the maintenance dose be halved in patients with mild to moderate hepatic cirrhosis (Child-Pugh Class A and B) receiving voriconazole. No pharmacokinetic data are available for patients with severe hepatic cirrhosis (Child-Pugh Class C) (see DOSAGE AND ADMINISTRATION).

Renal Insufficiency

In a single oral dose (200 mg) study in 24 subjects with normal renal function and mild to severe renal impairment, systemic exposure (AUC) and peak plasma concentration (C_{max}) of voriconazole were not significantly affected by renal impairment. Therefore, no adjustment is necessary for oral dosing in patients with mild to severe renal impairment.

In a multiple dose study of IV voriconazole (6 mg/kg IV loading dose × 2, then 3 mg/kg IV × 5.5 days) in 7 patients with moderate renal dysfunction (creatinine clearance 30-50 mL/min), the systemic exposure (AUC) and peak plasma concentrations (C_{max}) were not significantly different from those in 6 volunteers with normal renal function.

However, in patients with moderate renal dysfunction (creatinine clearance 30–50 mL/min), accumulation of the intravenous vehicle, SBECD, occurs. The mean systemic exposure (AUC) and peak plasma concentrations (C_{max}) of SBECD were increased by 4-fold and almost 50%, respectively, in the moderately impaired group compared to the normal control group.

Intravenous voriconazole should be avoided in patients with moderate or severe renal impairment (creatinine clearance <50 mL/min), unless an assessment of the benefit/risk to the patient justifies the use of intravenous voriconazole (see DOSAGE AND ADMINISTRATION—Dosage Adjustment).

A pharmacokinetic study in subjects with renal failure undergoing hemodialysis showed that voriconazole is dialyzed with clearance of 121 mL/min. The intravenous vehicle, SBECD, is hemodialyzed with clearance of 55 mL/min. A 4-hour hemodialysis session does not remove a sufficient amount of voriconazole to warrant dose adjustment.

Drug Interactions

Effects Of Other Drugs On Voriconazole

Voriconazole is metabolized by the human hepatic cytochrome P450 enzymes CYP2C19, CYP2C9, and CYP3A4. Results of *in vitro* metabolism studies indicate that the affinity of voriconazole is highest for CYP2C19, followed by CYP2C9, and is appreciably lower for CYP3A4. Inhibitors or inducers of these three enzymes may increase or decrease voriconazole systemic exposure (plasma concentrations), respectively.

The systemic exposure to voriconazole is significantly reduced or is expected to be reduced by the concomitant administration of the following agents and their use is contraindicated:

***Rifampin* (potent CYP450 inducer):** Rifampin (600 mg once daily) decreased the steady state C_{max} and AUC_τ of

Continued on next page

VFEND—Cont.

voriconazole (200 mg Q12h × 7 days) by an average of 93% and 96%, respectively, in healthy subjects. Doubling the dose of voriconazole to 400 mg Q12h does not restore adequate exposure to voriconazole during coadministration with rifampin. **Coadministration of voriconazole and rifampin is contraindicated** (see CONTRAINDICATIONS, PRECAUTIONS—Drug Interactions).

Carbamazepine and long acting barbiturates **(potent CYP450 inducers):** Although not studied *in vitro* or *in vivo*, carbamazepine and long acting barbiturates (e.g. phenobarbital, mephobarbital) are likely to significantly decrease plasma voriconazole concentrations. **Coadministration of voriconazole with carbamazepine or long acting barbiturates is contraindicated** (see CONTRAINDICATIONS, PRECAUTIONS—Drug Interactions).

Minor or no significant pharmacokinetic interactions that do not require dosage adjustment:

Cimetidine **(non-specific CYP450 inhibitor and increases gastric pH):** Cimetidine (400 mg Q12h × 8 days) increased voriconazole steady state C_{max} and AUC_τ by an average of 18% (90% CI: 6%, 32%) and 23% (90% CI: 13%, 33%), respectively, following oral doses of 200 mg Q12h × 7 days to healthy subjects.

Ranitidine **(increases gastric pH):** Ranitidine (150 mg Q12h) had no significant effect on voriconazole C_{max} and AUC_τ following oral doses of 200 mg Q12h × 7 days to healthy subjects.

Macrolide antibiotics: Co-administration of **erythromycin** (CYP3A4 inhibitor; 1g Q12h for 7 days) or **azithromycin** (500 mg qd for 3 days) with voriconazole 200 mg Q12h for 14 days had no significant effect on voriconazole steady state C_{max} and AUC_τ in healthy subjects. The effects of voriconazole on the pharmacokinetics of either erythromycin or azithromycin are not known.

Effects Of Voriconazole On Other Drugs

In vitro studies with human hepatic microsomes show that voriconazole inhibits the metabolic activity of the cytochrome P450 enzymes CYP2C19, CYP2C9, and CYP3A4. In these studies, the inhibition potency of voriconazole for CYP3A4 metabolic activity was significantly less than that of two other azoles, ketoconazole and itraconazole. *In vitro* studies also show that the major metabolite of voriconazole, voriconazole N-oxide, inhibits the metabolic activity of CYP2C9 and CYP3A4 to a greater extent than that of CYP2C19. Therefore, there is potential for voriconazole and its major metabolite to increase the systemic exposure (plasma concentrations) of other drugs metabolized by these CYP450 enzymes.

The systemic exposure of the following drugs is significantly increased or is expected to be significantly increased by coadministration of voriconazole and their use is contraindicated:

Sirolimus **(CYP3A4 substrate):** Repeat dose administration of oral voriconazole (400 mg Q12h for 1 day, then 200 mg Q12h for 8 days) increased the C_{max} and AUC of sirolimus (2 mg single dose) an average of 7-fold (90% CI: 5.7, 7.5) and 11-fold (90% CI: 9.9, 12.6), respectively, in healthy subjects. **Coadministration of voriconazole and sirolimus is contraindicated** (see CONTRAINDICATIONS, PRECAUTIONS—Drug Interactions).

Terfenadine, astemizole, cisapride, pimozide and quinidine **(CYP3A4 substrates):** Although not studied *in vitro* or *in vivo*, concomitant administration of voriconazole with terfenadine, astemizole, cisapride, pimozide or quinidine may result in inhibition of the metabolism of these drugs. Increased plasma concentrations of these drugs can lead to QT prolongation and rare occurrences of *torsade de pointes*. **Coadministration of voriconazole and terfenadine, astemizole, cisapride, pimozide and quinidine is contraindicated** (see CONTRAINDICATIONS, PRECAUTIONS—Drug Interactions).

Ergot alkaloids: Although not studied *in vitro* or *in vivo*, voriconazole may increase the plasma concentration of ergot alkaloids (ergotamine and dihydroergotamine) and lead to ergotism. **Coadministration of voriconazole with ergot alkaloids is contraindicated** (see CONTRAINDICATIONS, PRECAUTIONS—Drug Interactions).

Coadministration of voriconazole with the following agents results in increased exposure or is expected to result in increased exposure to these drugs. Therefore, careful monitoring and/or dosage adjustment of these drugs is needed:

Cyclosporine **(CYP3A4 substrate):** In stable renal transplant recipients receiving chronic cyclosporine therapy, concomitant administration of oral voriconazole (200 mg Q12h for 8 days) increased cyclosporine C_{max} and AUC_τ an average of 1.1 times (90% CI: 0.9, 1.41) and 1.7 times (90% CI: 1.5, 2.0), respectively, as compared to when cyclosporine was administered without voriconazole. When initiating therapy with voriconazole in patients already receiving cyclosporine, it is recommended that the cyclosporine dose be reduced to one-half of the original dose and followed with frequent monitoring of the cyclosporine blood levels. Increased cyclosporine levels have been associated with nephrotoxicity. When voriconazole is discontinued, cyclosporine levels should be frequently monitored and the dose increased as necessary (see PRECAUTIONS—Drug Interactions).

Tacrolimus **(CYP3A4 substrate):** Repeat oral dose administration of voriconazole (400 mg Q12h × 1 day then 200 mg Q12h × 6 days) increased tacrolimus (0.1 mg/kg single dose) C_{max} and AUC_τ in healthy subjects by an average of 2-fold (90% CI: 1.9, 2.5) and 3-fold (90% CI: 2.7, 3.8), respectively. When initiating therapy with voriconazole in patients already receiving tacrolimus, it is recommended that the tacrolimus dose be reduced to one-third of the original dose and followed with frequent monitoring of the tacrolimus blood levels. Increased tacrolimus levels have been associated with nephrotoxicity. When voriconazole is discontinued, tacrolimus levels should be carefully monitored and the dose increased as necessary (see PRECAUTIONS—Drug Interactions).

Warfarin **(CYP2C9 substrate):** Coadministration of voriconazole (300 mg Q12h × 12 days) with warfarin (30 mg single dose) significantly increased maximum prothrombin time by approximately 2-times that of placebo in healthy subjects. Close monitoring of prothrombin time or other suitable anti-coagulation tests is recommended if warfarin and voriconazole are coadministered and the warfarin dose adjusted accordingly (see PRECAUTIONS—Drug Interactions).

Oral Coumarin Anticoagulants **(CYP2C9, CYP3A4 substrates):** Although not studied *in vitro* or *in vivo*, voriconazole may increase the plasma concentrations of coumarin anticoagulants and therefore may cause an increase in prothrombin time. If patients receiving coumarin preparations are treated simultaneously with voriconazole, the prothrombin time or other suitable anticoagulation tests should be monitored at close intervals and the dosage of anticoagulants adjusted accordingly (see PRECAUTIONS—Drug Interactions).

Statins **(CYP3A4 substrates):** Although not studied clinically, voriconazole has been shown to inhibit lovastatin metabolism *in vitro* (human liver microsomes). Therefore, voriconazole is likely to increase the plasma concentrations of statins that are metabolized by CYP3A4. It is recommended that dose adjustment of the statin be considered during coadministration. Increased statin concentrations in plasma have been associated with rhabdomyolysis (see PRECAUTIONS—Drug Interactions).

Benzodiazepines **(CYP3A4 substrates):** Although not studied clinically, voriconazole has been shown to inhibit midazolam metabolism *in vitro* (human liver microsomes). Therefore, voriconazole is likely to increase the plasma concentrations of benzodiazepines that are metabolized by CYP3A4 (e.g., midazolam, triazolam, and alprazolam) and lead to a prolonged sedative effect. It is recommended that dose adjustment of the benzodiazepine be considered during coadministration (see PRECAUTIONS—Drug Interactions).

Calcium Channel Blockers **(CYP3A4 substrates):** Although not studied clinically, voriconazole has been shown to inhibit felodipine metabolism *in vitro* (human liver microsomes). Therefore, voriconazole may increase the plasma concentrations of calcium channel blockers that are metabolized by CYP3A4. Frequent monitoring for adverse events and toxicity related to calcium channel blockers is recommended during coadministration. Dose adjustment of the calcium channel blocker may be needed (see PRECAUTIONS—Drug Interactions).

Sulfonylureas **(CYP2C9 substrates):** Although not studied *in vitro* or *in vivo*, voriconazole may increase plasma concentrations of sulfonylureas (e.g., tolbutamide, glipizide, and glyburide) and therefore cause hypoglycemia. Frequent monitoring of blood glucose and appropriate adjustment (i.e., reduction) of the sulfonylurea dosage is recommended during coadministration (see PRECAUTIONS—Drug Interactions).

Vinca Alkaloids **(CYP3A4 substrates):** Although not studied *in vitro* or *in vivo*, voriconazole may increase the plasma concentrations of the vinca alkaloids (e.g., vincristine and vinblastine) and lead to neurotoxicity. Therefore, it is recommended that dose adjustment of the vinca alkaloid be considered.

No significant pharmacokinetic interactions were observed when voriconazole was coadministered with the following agents. Therefore, no dosage adjustment for these agents is recommended:

Prednisolone **(CYP3A4 substrate):** Voriconazole (200 mg Q12h × 30 days) increased C_{max} and AUC of prednisolone (60 mg single dose) by an average of 11% and 34%, respectively, in healthy subjects.

Digoxin **(P-glycoprotein mediated transport):** Voriconazole (200 mg Q12h × 12 days) had no significant effect on steady state C_{max} and AUC_τ of digoxin (0.25 mg once daily for 10 days) in healthy subjects.

Mycophenolic acid **(UDP-glucuronyl transferase substrate):** Voriconazole (200 mg Q12h × 5 days) had no significant effect on the C_{max} and AUC of mycophenolic acid and its major metabolite, mycophenolic acid glucuronide after administration of a 1 g single oral dose of mycophenolate mofetil.

Two-way Interactions

Concomitant use of the following agent with voriconazole is contraindicated:

Rifabutin **(potent CYP450 inducer):** Rifabutin (300 mg once daily) decreased the C_{max} and AUC_τ of voriconazole at 200 mg twice daily by an average of 67% (90% CI: 58%, 73%) and 79% (90% CI: 71%, 84%), respectively, in healthy subjects. During coadministration with rifabutin (300 mg once daily), the steady state C_{max} and AUC_τ of voriconazole following an increased dose of 400 mg twice daily were on average approximately 2-times higher, compared with voriconazole alone at 200 mg twice daily. Coadministration of voriconazole at 400 mg twice daily with rifabutin 300 mg twice daily increased the C_{max} and AUC_τ of rifabutin by an average of 3-times (90% CI: 2.2, 4.0) and 4-times (90% CI: 3.5, 5.4), respectively, compared to rifabutin given alone. **Coadministration of voriconazole and rifabutin is contraindicated.**

Significant drug interactions that may require dosage adjustment, frequent monitoring of drug levels and/or frequent monitoring of drug-related adverse events/toxicity:

Phenytoin **(CYP2C9 substrate and potent CYP450 inducer):** Repeat dose administration of phenytoin (300 mg once daily) decreased the steady state C_{max} and AUC_τ of orally administered voriconazole (200 mg Q12h × 14 days) by an average of 50% and 70%, respectively, in healthy subjects. Administration of a higher voriconazole dose (400 mg Q12h × 7 days) with phenytoin (300 mg once daily) resulted in comparable steady state voriconazole C_{max} and AUC, estimates as compared to when voriconazole was given at 200 mg Q12h without phenytoin.

Phenytoin may be coadministered with voriconazole if the maintenance dose of voriconazole is increased from 4 mg/kg to 5 mg/kg intravenously every 12 hours or from 200 mg to 400 mg orally, every 12 hours (100 mg to 200 mg orally, every 12 hours in patients less than 40 kg) (see DOSAGE AND ADMINISTRATION).

Repeat dose administration of voriconazole (400 mg Q12h × 10 days) increased the steady state C_{max} and AUC_τ of phenytoin (300 mg once daily) by an average of 70% and 80%, respectively, in healthy subjects. The increase in phenytoin C_{max} and AUC when coadministered with voriconazole may be expected to be as high as 2-times the C_{max} and AUC estimates when phenytoin is given without voriconazole. Therefore, frequent monitoring of plasma phenytoin concentrations and phenytoin-related adverse effects is recommended when phenytoin is coadministered with voriconazole (see PRECAUTIONS—Drug Interactions).

Omeprazole **(CYP2C19 inhibitor; CYP2C19 and CYP3A4 substrate):** Coadministration of omeprazole (40 mg once daily × 10 days) with oral voriconazole (400 mg Q12h × 1 day, then 200 mg Q12h × 9 days) increased the steady state C_{max} and AUC_τ of voriconazole by an average of 15% (90% CI: 5%, 25%) and 40% (90% CI: 29%, 55%), respectively, in healthy subjects. No dosage adjustment of voriconazole is recommended.

Coadministration of voriconazole (400 mg Q12h × 1 day, then 200 mg × 6 days) with omeprazole (40 mg once daily × 7 days) to healthy subjects significantly increased the steady state C_{max} and AUC_τ of omeprazole an average of 2-times (90% CI: 1.8, 2.6) and 4-times (90% CI: 3.3, 4.4), respectively, as compared to when omeprazole is given without voriconazole. When initiating voriconazole in patients already receiving omeprazole doses of 40 mg or greater, it is recommended that the omeprazole dose be reduced by one-half (see PRECAUTIONS—Drug Interactions).

The metabolism of other proton pump inhibitors that are CYP2C19 substrates may also be inhibited by voriconazole and may result in increased plasma concentrations of these drugs.

No significant pharmacokinetic interaction was seen and no dosage adjustment of these drugs is recommended:

Indinavir **(CYP3A4 inhibitor and substrate):** Repeat dose administration of indinavir (800 mg TID for 10 days) had no significant effect on voriconazole C_{max} and AUC following repeat dose administration (200 mg Q12h for 17 days) in healthy subjects.

Repeat dose administration of voriconazole (200 mg Q12h for 7 days) did not have a significant effect on steady state C_{max} and AUC_τ of indinavir following repeat dose administration (800 mg TID for 7 days) in healthy subjects.

Other Two-Way Interactions Expected to be Significant Based on *In Vitro* Findings:

Other HIV Protease Inhibitors **(CYP3A4 substrates and inhibitors):** *In vitro* studies (human liver microsomes) suggest that voriconazole may inhibit the metabolism of HIV protease inhibitors (e.g. saquinavir, amprenavir and nelfinavir). *In vitro* studies (human liver microsomes) also show that the metabolism of voriconazole may be inhibited by HIV protease inhibitors (e.g., ritonavir, saquinavir, and amprenavir). Patients should be frequently monitored for drug toxicity during the coadministration of voriconazole and HIV protease inhibitors (see PRECAUTIONS—Drug Interactions).

Non-Nucleoside Reverse Transcriptase Inhibitors (NNRTI) **(CYP3A4 substrates, inhibitors or CYP450 inducers):** *In vitro* studies (human liver microsomes) show that the metabolism of voriconazole may be inhibited by an NNRTI (e.g., delavirdine and efavirenz). Although not studied *in vitro* or *in vivo*, the metabolism of voriconazole may be induced by an NNRTI, such as efavirenz or nevirapine. *In vitro* studies (human liver microsomes) show that voriconazole may also inhibit the metabolism of an NNRTI (e.g., delavirdine). Patients should be frequently monitored for drug toxicity during the coadministration of voriconazole and an NNRTI (see PRECAUTIONS—Drug Interactions).

MICROBIOLOGY

Mechanism Of Action

Voriconazole is a triazole antifungal agent. The primary mode of action of voriconazole is the inhibition of fungal cytochrome P-450-mediated 14 alpha-lanosterol demethylation, an essential step in fungal ergosterol biosynthesis. The accumulation of 14 alpha-methyl sterols correlates with the subsequent loss of ergosterol in the fungal cell wall and may be responsible for the antifungal activity of voriconazole. Voriconazole has been shown to be more selective for fungal cytochrome P-450 enzymes than for various mammalian cytochrome P-450 enzyme systems.

Activity *In Vitro* And *In Vivo*

Voriconazole has demonstrated *in vitro* activity against *Aspergillus fumigatus* isolates as well as *A. flavus*, *A. niger* and *A. terreus*. Variable *in vitro* activity against *Scedosporium apiospermum* and *Fusarium* spp., including *Fusarium*

solani, has been seen. Most of the speciated isolates from clinical studies were *Aspergillus fumigatus* but clinical efficacy was also seen in a small number of species other than *A. fumigatus* (see INDICATIONS AND USAGE and CLINICAL STUDIES—Invasive Aspergillosis).
In vitro susceptibility testing was performed according to the National Committee for Clinical Laboratory Standards (NCCLS) proposed method (M38-P). Voriconazole breakpoints have not been established for any fungi. The relationship between clinical outcome and *in vitro* susceptibility results remains to be elucidated.
Voriconazole has demonstrated *in vivo* activity in normal and immunocompromised guinea pigs with established systemic *A. fumigatus* infections in which the endpoints were prolonged survival of infected animals and reduction of mycological burden from target organs. Activity has also been shown in immunocompromised guinea pigs with pulmonary *A. fumigatus* infections. Voriconazole demonstrated activity in immunocompromised guinea pigs with systemic infections produced by an *A. fumigatus* isolate with reduced susceptibility to itraconazole (itraconazole MIC 3.1 μg/mL). The exact mechanism of resistance was not identified for that particular isolate. In one experiment, voriconazole exhibited activity against *Scedosporium apiospermum* infections in immune competent guinea pigs.

Drug Resistance

Voriconazole drug resistance development has not been adequately studied *in vitro* against the filamentous fungi, including *Aspergillus, Scedosporium* and *Fusarium* species. The frequency of drug resistance development for the various fungi for which this drug is indicated is not known.
Fungal isolates exhibiting reduced susceptibility to fluconazole or itraconazole may also show reduced susceptibility to voriconazole, suggesting cross-resistance can occur among these azoles. The relevance of cross-resistance and clinical outcome has not been fully characterized. Clinical cases where azole cross-resistance is demonstrated may require alternative antifungal therapy.

INDICATIONS AND USAGE

VFEND is indicated for use in the treatment of the following fungal infections:
Treatment of invasive aspergillosis. In clinical trials, the majority of isolates recovered were *Aspergillus fumigatus*. There was a small number of cases of culture-proven disease due to species of *Aspergillus* other than *A. fumigatus* (see CLINICAL STUDIES and MICROBIOLOGY sections).
Treatment of serious fungal infections caused by *Scedosporium apiospermum* (asexual form of *Pseudallescheria boydii*) and *Fusarium* spp. including *Fusarium solani*, in patients intolerant of, or refractory to, other therapy.
Specimens for fungal culture and other relevant laboratory studies (including histopathology) should be obtained prior to therapy to isolate and identify causative organism(s). Therapy may be instituted before the results of the cultures and other laboratory studies are known. However, once these results become available, antifungal therapy should be adjusted accordingly.

CLINICAL STUDIES

Voriconazole, administered orally or parenterally, has been evaluated as primary or salvage therapy in 520 patients aged 12 years and older with infections caused by *Aspergillus* spp., *Fusarium* spp., and *Scedosporium* spp.

Invasive Aspergillosis

Voriconazole was studied in patients for primary therapy of invasive aspergillosis (randomized, controlled study 307/602), for primary and salvage therapy of aspergillosis (non-comparative study 304) and for treatment of patients with invasive aspergillosis who were refractory to, or intolerant of, other antifungal therapy (non-comparative study 309/604).

Study 307/602

The efficacy of voriconazole compared to amphotericin B in the primary treatment of acute invasive aspergillosis was demonstrated in 277 patients treated for 12 weeks in Study 307/602. The majority of study patients had underlying hematologic malignancies, including bone marrow transplantation. The study also included patients with solid organ transplantation, solid tumors, and AIDS. The patients were mainly treated for definite or probable invasive aspergillosis of the lungs. Other aspergillosis infections included disseminated disease, CNS infections and sinus infections. Diagnosis of definite or probable invasive aspergillosis was made according to criteria modified from those established by the National Institute of Allergy and Infectious Diseases Mycoses Study Group/European Organisation for Research and Treatment of Cancer (NIAID MSG/EORTC).
Voriconazole was administered intravenously with a loading dose of 6 mg/kg every 12 hours for the first 24 hours followed by a maintenance dose of 4 mg/kg every 12 hours for a minimum of seven days. Therapy could then be switched to the oral formulation at a dose of 200 mg Q12h. Median duration of IV voriconazole therapy was 10 days (range 2-90 days). After IV voriconazole therapy, the median duration of PO voriconazole therapy was 76 days (range 2-232 days).
Patients in the comparator group received conventional amphotericin B as a slow infusion at a daily dose of 1.0–1.5 mg/kg/day. Median duration of IV amphotericin therapy was 12 days (range 1-85 days). Treatment was then continued with other licensed antifungal therapy (OLAT), including itraconazole and lipid amphotericin B formulations. Although initial therapy with conventional amphotericin B was to be continued for at least two weeks, actual duration of therapy was at the discretion of the investigator. Patients who discontinued initial randomized 13 therapy due to toxicity or lack of efficacy were eligible to continue in the study with OLAT treatment.
A satisfactory global response at 12 weeks (complete or partial resolution of all attributable symptoms, signs, radiographic/bronchoscopic abnormalities present at baseline) was seen in 53% of voriconazole treated patients compared to 32% of amphotericin B treated patients (Table 4). A benefit of voriconazole compared to amphotericin B on patient survival at Day 84 was seen with a 71% survival rate on voriconazole compared to 58% on amphotericin B (Table 4).
Table 4 also summarizes the response (success) based on mycological confirmation and species.
[See table 4 above]

Table 4
Overall Efficacy and Success by Species in the Primary Treatment of Acute Invasive Aspergillosis Study 307/602

	Voriconazole	Ampho B[c]	Stratified Difference (95% CI)[d]
	n/N (%)	n/N (%)	
Efficacy as Primary Therapy			
Satisfactory Global Response[a]	76/144 (53)	42/133 (32)	21.8% (10.5%, 33.0%) $p<0.0001$
Survival at Day 84[b]	102/144 (71)	77/133 (58)	13.1% (2.1%, 24.2%)
Success by Species			
	Success n/N (%)		
Overall success	76/144 (53)	42/133 (32)	
Mycologically confirmed[e]	37/84 (44)	16/67 (24)	
Aspergillus spp.[f]			
A. fumigatus	28/63 (44)	12/47 (26)	
A. flavus	3/6	4/9	
A. terreus	2/3	0/3	
A. niger	1/4	0/9	
A. nidulans	1/1	0/0	

a Assessed by independent Data Review Committee (DRC)
b Proportion of subjects alive
c Amphotericin B followed by other licensed antifungal therapy
d Difference and corresponding 95% confidence interval are stratified by protocol
e Not all mycologically confirmed specimens were speciated
f Some patients had more than one species isolated at baseline

Study 304

The results of this comparative trial (Study 307/602) confirmed the results of an earlier trial in the primary and salvage treatment of patients with acute invasive aspergillosis (Study 304). In this earlier study, an overall success rate of 52% (26/50) was seen in patients treated with voriconazole for primary therapy. Success was seen in 17/29 (59%) with *Aspergillus fumigatus* infections and 3/6 (50%) patients with infections due to non-*fumigatus* species [*A. flavus* (1/1); *A. nidulans* (0/2); *A. niger* (2/2); *A. terreus* (0/1)]. Success in patients who received voriconazole as salvage therapy is presented in Table 5.

Study 309/604

Additional data regarding response rates in patients who were refractory to, or intolerant of, other antifungal agents are also provided in Table 5. Overall mycological eradication for culture-documented infections due to *fumigatus* and non-*fumigatus* species of *Aspergillus* was 36/82 (44%) and 12/30 (40%), respectively, in voriconazole treated patients. Patients had various underlying diseases and species other than *A. fumigatus* contributed to mixed infections in some cases.
For patients who were infected with a single pathogen and were refractory to, or intolerant of, other antifungal agents, the satisfactory response rates for voriconazole in studies 304 and 309/604 are presented in Table 5.

Table 5 Combined Response Data in Salvage Patients with Single Aspergillus Species (Studies 304 and 309/604)

	Success n/N
A. fumigatus	43/97 (44%)
A. flavus	5/12
A. nidulans	1/3
A. niger	4/5
A. terreus	3/8
A. versicolor	0/1

Nineteen patients had more than one species of *Aspergillus* isolated. Success was seen in 4/17 (24%) of these patients.

Other Serious Fungal Pathogens

In pooled analyses of patients, voriconazole was shown to be effective against the following additional fungal pathogens:
Scedosporium apiospermum—Successful response to voriconazole therapy was seen in 15 of 24 patients (63%). Three of these patients relapsed within 4 weeks, including 1 patient with pulmonary, skin and eye infections, 1 patient with cerebral disease, and 1 patient with skin infection. Ten patients had evidence of cerebral disease and 6 of these had a successful outcome (1 relapse). In addition, a successful response was seen in one of three patients with mixed organism infections.
Fusarium spp.—Nine of 21 (43%) patients were successfully treated with voriconazole. Of these nine patients, three had eye infections, one had an eye and blood infection, one had a skin infection, one had a blood infection alone, two had sinus infections, and one had disseminated infection (pulmonary, skin, hepatosplenic). Three of these patients (one with disseminated disease, one with an eye infection and one with a blood infection) had *Fusarium solani* and were complete successes. Two of these patients relapsed, one with a sinus infection and profound neutropenia and one post surgical patient with blood and eye infections.

CONTRAINDICATIONS

VFEND is contraindicated in patients with known hypersensitivity to voriconazole or its excipients. There is no information regarding cross-sensitivity between VFEND (voriconazole) and other azole antifungal agents. Caution should be used when prescribing VFEND to patients with hypersensitivity to other azoles.
Coadministration of the CYP3A4 substrates, terfenadine, astemizole, cisapride, pimozide or quinidine with VFEND are contraindicated since increased plasma concentrations of these drugs can lead to QT prolongation and rare occurrences of *torsade de pointes* (see CLINICAL PHARMACOLOGY—Drug Interactions, PRECAUTIONS—Drug Interactions).
Coadministration of VFEND with sirolimus is contraindicated because VFEND significantly increases sirolimus concentrations in healthy subjects (see CLINICAL PHARMACOLOGY—Drug Interactions, PRECAUTIONS—Drug Interactions).
Coadministration of VFEND with rifampin, carbamazepine and long-acting barbiturates is contraindicated since these drugs are likely to decrease plasma voriconazole concentrations significantly (see CLINICAL PHARMACOLOGY—Drug Interactions, PRECAUTIONS—Drug Interactions).
Coadministration of VFEND with rifabutin is contraindicated since VFEND significantly increases rifabutin plasma concentrations and rifabutin also significantly decreases voriconazole plasma concentrations (see CLINICAL PHARMACOLOGY—Drug Interactions, PRECAUTIONS—Drug Interactions).
Coadministration of VFEND with ergot alkaloids (ergotamine and dihydroergotamine) is contraindicated because VFEND may increase the plasma concentration of ergot alkaloids, which may lead to ergotism.

WARNINGS

VISUAL DISTURBANCES: The effect of VFEND on visual function is not known if treatment continues beyond 28

Continued on next page

VFEND—Cont.

days. If treatment continues beyond 28 days, visual function including visual acuity, visual field and color perception should be monitored (see PRECAUTIONS—Information for Patients and ADVERSE EVENTS—Visual Disturbances).

HEPATIC TOXICITY: In clinical trials, there have been uncommon cases of serious hepatic reactions during treatment with VFEND (including clinical hepatitis, cholestasis and fulminant hepatic failure, including fatalities). Instances of hepatic reactions were noted to occur primarily in patients with serious underlying medical conditions (predominantly hematological malignancy). Hepatic reactions, including hepatitis and jaundice, have occurred among patients with no other identifiable risk factors. Liver dysfunction has usually been reversible on discontinuation of therapy (see PRECAUTIONS—Laboratory Tests and ADVERSE EVENTS—Clinical Laboratory Values).

Monitoring of hepatic function: Liver function tests should be evaluated at the start of and during the course of VFEND therapy. Patients who develop abnormal liver function tests during VFEND therapy should be monitored for the development of more severe hepatic injury. Patient management should include laboratory evaluation of hepatic function (particularly liver function tests and bilirubin). Discontinuation of VFEND must be considered if clinical signs and symptoms consistent with liver disease develop that may be attributable to VFEND (see PRECAUTIONS—Laboratory Tests, DOSAGE AND ADMINISTRATION—Dosage Adjustment, ADVERSE EVENTS—Clinical Laboratory Tests).

Pregnancy Category D: Voriconazole can cause fetal harm when administered to a pregnant woman.

Voriconazole was teratogenic in rats (cleft palates, hydronephrosis/hydroureter) from 10 mg/kg (0.3 times the recommended maintenance dose (RMD) on a mg/m^2 basis) and embryotoxic in rabbits at 100 mg/kg (6 times the RMD). Other effects in rats included reduced ossification of sacral and caudal vertebrae, skull, pubic and hyoid bone, super numerary ribs, anomalies of the sternebrae and dilatation of the ureter/renal pelvis. Plasma estradiol in pregnant rats was reduced at all dose levels. Voriconazole treatment in rats produced increased gestational length and dystocia, which were associated with increased perinatal pup mortality at the 10 mg/kg dose. The effects seen in rabbits were an increased embryomortality, reduced fetal weight and increased incidences of skeletal variations, cervical ribs and extra sternebral ossification sites.

If this drug is used during pregnancy, or if the patient becomes pregnant while taking this drug, the patient should be apprised of the potential hazard to the fetus.

Galactose intolerance: VFEND tablets contain lactose and should not be given to patients with rare hereditary problems of galactose intolerance, Lapp lactase deficiency or glucose-galactose malabsorption.

PRECAUTIONS

General
(See WARNINGS, DOSAGE AND ADMINISTRATION)
Some azoles, including voriconazole, have been associated with prolongation of the QT interval on the electrocardiogram. During clinical development and post-marketing surveillance, there have been rare cases of torsade de pointes in patients taking voriconazole. These reports involved seriously ill patients with multiple confounding risk factors, such as history of cardiotoxic chemotherapy, cardiomyopathy, hypokalemia and concomitant medications that may have been contributory.

Voriconazole should be administered with caution to patients with these potentially proarryhthmic conditions.

Rigorous attempts to correct potassium, magnesium and calcium should be made before starting voriconazole.

Infusion Related Reactions
During infusion of the intravenous formulation of voriconazole in healthy subjects, anaphylactoid-type reactions, including flushing, fever, sweating, tachycardia, chest tightness, dyspnea, faintness, nausea, pruritus and rash, have occurred uncommonly. Symptoms appeared immediately upon initiating the infusion. Consideration should be given to stopping the infusion should these reactions occur.

Information For Patients
Patients should be advised:
- that VFEND Tablets should be taken at least one hour before, or one hour following, a meal.
- that they should not drive at night while taking VFEND. VFEND may cause changes to vision, including blurring and/or photophobia.
- that they should avoid potentially hazardous tasks, such as driving or operating machinery if they perceive any change in vision.
- that strong, direct sunlight should be avoided during VFEND therapy.

Laboratory Tests
Electrolyte disturbances such as hypokalemia, hypomagnesemia and hypocalcemia should be corrected prior to initiation of VFEND therapy.

Patient management should include laboratory evaluation of renal (particularly serum creatinine) and hepatic function (particularly liver function tests and bilirubin).

Drug Interactions
Tables 6 and 7 provide a summary of significant drug interactions with voriconazole that either have been studied *in vivo* (clinically) or that may be expected to occur based on results of *in vitro* metabolism studies with human liver microsomes. For more details, see CLINICAL PHARMACOLOGY—Drug Interactions.
[See table 6 above]
[See table 7 above and on next page]

Patients with Hepatic Insufficiency
It is recommended that the standard loading dose regimens be used but that the maintenance dose be halved in patients with mild to moderate hepatic cirrhosis (Child-Pugh Class A and B) receiving VFEND (see CLINICAL PHARMACOLOGY—Hepatic Insufficiency, DOSAGE and ADMINISTRATION—Hepatic Insufficiency).

VFEND has not been studied in patients with severe cirrhosis (Child-Pugh Class C). VFEND has been associated with elevations in liver function tests and clinical signs of liver damage, such as jaundice, and should only be used in pa-

Table 6 Effect of Other Drugs on Voriconazole Pharmacokinetics

Drug/Drug Class (Mechanism of Interaction by the Drug)	Voriconazole Plasma Exposure (C_{max} and AUC_τ after 200 mg Q12h)	Recommendations for Voriconazole Dosage Adjustment/Comments
Rifampin* and Rifabutin* (CYP450 Induction)	Significantly Reduced	**Contraindicated**
Carbamazepine (CYP450 Induction)	Not Studied *In Vivo* or *In Vitro*, but Likely to Result in Significant Reduction	**Contraindicated**
Long Acting Barbiturates (CYP450 Induction)	Not Studied *In Vivo* or *In Vitro*, but Likely to Result in Significant Reduction	**Contraindicated**
Phenytoin* (CYP450 Induction)	Significantly Reduced	Increase voriconazole maintenance dose from 4 mg/kg to 5 mg/kg IV every 12 hrs or from 200 mg to 400 mg orally every 12 hrs (100 mg to 200 mg orally every 12 hrs in patients weighing less than 40 kg)
HIV Protease Inhibitors (CYP3A4 Inhibition)	*In Vivo* Studies Showed No Significant Effects of Indinavir on Voriconazole Exposure. *In Vitro* Studies Demonstrate Potential for Inhibition of Voriconazole Metabolism (Increased Plasma Exposure)	No dosage adjustment in the voriconazole dosage needed when coadministered with indinavir. Frequent monitoring for adverse events and toxicity related to voriconazole when coadministered with other HIV protease inhibitors
NNRTI** (CYP3A4 Inhibition or CYP450 Induction)	*In Vitro* Studies Demonstrate Potential for Inhibition of Voriconazole Metabolism (Increased Plasma Exposure). Not Studied *In Vitro* or *In Vivo*, but Metabolism of Voriconazole May also be Induced (Decreased Plasma Exposure)	Frequent monitoring for adverse events and toxicity related to voriconazole. Careful assessment of voriconazole effectiveness

*Results based on *in vivo* clinical studies generally following repeat oral dosing with 200 mg Q12h voriconazole to healthy subjects
** Non-Nucleoside Reverse Transcriptase Inhibitors

Table 7 Effect of Voriconazole on Pharmacokinetics of Other Drugs

Drug/Drug Class (Mechanism of Interaction by Voriconazole)	Drug Plasma Exposure (C_{max} and AUC_τ)	Recommendations for Drug Dosage Adjustment/Comments
Sirolimus* (CYP3A4 Inhibition)	Significantly Increased	**Contraindicated**
Rifabutin* (CYP3A4 Inhibition)	Significantly Increased	**Contraindicated**
Terfenadine, Astemizole, Cisapride, Pimozide, Quinidine (CYP3A4 Inhibition)	Not Studied *In Vivo* or *In Vitro*, but Drug Plasma Exposure Likely to be Increased	**Contraindicated** because of potential for QT prolongation and rare occurrence of *torsade de pointes*
Ergot Alkaloids (CYP450 Inhibition)	Not Studied *In Vivo* or *In Vitro*, but Drug Plasma Exposure Likely to be Increased	**Contraindicated**
Cyclosporine* (CYP3A4 Inhibition)	AUC_τ Significantly Increased; No Significant Effect on C_{max}	When initiating therapy with VFEND in patients already receiving cyclosporine, reduce the cyclosporine dose to one-half of the starting dose and follow with frequent monitoring of cyclosporine blood levels. Increased cyclosporine levels have been associated with nephrotoxicity. When VFEND is discontinued, cyclosporine concentrations must be frequently monitored and the dose increased as necessary.
Tacrolimus* (CYP3A4 Inhibition)	Significantly Increased	When initiating therapy with VFEND in patients already receiving tacrolimus, reduce the tacrolimus dose to one-third of the starting dose and follow with frequent monitoring of tacrolimus blood levels. Increased tacrolimus levels have been associated with nephrotoxicity. When VFEND is discontinued, tacrolimus concentrations must be frequently monitored and the dose increased as necessary.
Phenytoin* (CYP2C9 Inhibition)	Significantly Increased	Frequent monitoring of phenytoin plasma concentrations and frequent monitoring of adverse effects related to phenytoin.
Warfarin* (CYP2C9 Inhibition)	Prothrombin Time Significantly Increased	Monitor PT or other suitable anticoagulation tests. Adjustment of warfarin dosage may be needed.

(Table continued on next page)

Table 7 (cont.) Effect of Voriconazole on Pharmacokinetics of Other Drugs

Drug/Drug Class (Mechanism of Interaction by Voriconazole)	Drug Plasma Exposure (C_{max} and AUC_τ)	Recommendations for Drug Dosage Adjustment/Comments
Omeprazole* (CYP2C19/3A4 Inhibition)	Significantly Increased	When initiating therapy with VFEND in patients already receiving omeprazole doses of 40 mg or greater, reduce the omeprazole dose by one-half. The metabolism of other proton pump inhibitors that are CYP2C19 substrates may also be inhibited by voriconazole and may result in increased plasma concentrations of other proton pump inhibitors.
HIV Protease Inhibitors (CYP3A4 Inhibition)	*In Vivo* Studies showed No Significant Effects on Indinavir Exposure *In Vitro* Studies Demonstrate Potential for Voriconazole to Inhibit Metabolism (Increased Plasma Exposure)	No dosage adjustment for indinavir when coadministered with VFEND Frequent monitoring for adverse events and toxicity related to other HIV protease inhibitors
NNRTI** (CYP3A4 Inhibition)	*In Vitro* Studies Demonstrate Potential for Voriconazole to Inhibit Metabolism (Increased Plasma Exposure)	Frequent monitoring for adverse events and toxicity related to NNRTI
Benzodiazepines (CYP3A4 Inhibition)	*In Vitro* Studies Demonstrate Potential for Voriconazole to Inhibit Metabolism (Increased Plasma Exposure)	Frequent monitoring for adverse events and toxicity (i.e., prolonged sedation) related to benzodiazepines metabolized by CYP3A4 (e.g., midazolam, triazolam, alprazolam). Adjustment of benzodiazepine dosage may be needed.
HMG-CoA Reductase Inhibitors (Statins) (CYP3A4 Inhibition)	*In Vitro* Studies Demonstrate Potential for Voriconazole to Inhibit Metabolism (Increased Plasma Exposure)	Frequent monitoring for adverse events and toxicity related to statins. Increased statin concentrations in plasma have been associated with rhabdomyolysis. Adjustment of the statin dosage may be needed.
Dihydropyridine Calcium Channel Blockers (CYP3A4 Inhibition)	*In Vitro* Studies Demonstrate Potential for Voriconazole to Inhibit Metabolism (Increased Plasma Exposure)	Frequent monitoring for adverse events and toxicity related to calcium channel blockers. Adjustment of calcium channel blocker dosage may be needed.
Sulfonylurea Oral Hypoglycemics (CYP2C9 Inhibition)	Not Studied *In Vivo* or *In Vitro*, but Drug Plasma Exposure Likely to be Increased	Frequent monitoring of blood glucose and for signs and symptoms of hypoglycemia. Adjustment of oral hypoglycemic drug dosage may be needed.
Vinca Alkaloids (CYP3A4 Inhibition)	Not Studied *In Vivo* or *In Vitro*, but Drug Plasma Exposure Likely to be Increased	Frequent monitoring for adverse events and toxicity (i.e., neurotoxicity) related to vinca alkaloids. Adjustment of vinca alkaloid dosage may be needed.

*Results based on *in vivo* clinical studies generally following repeat oral dosing with 200 mg BID voriconazole to healthy subjects
** Non-Nucleoside Reverse Transcriptase Inhibitors

Table 8
TREATMENT-EMERGENT ADVERSE EVENTS
Rate ≥ 1% or Adverse Events of Concern in All Therapeutic Studies Possibly Related to Therapy or Causality Unknown

	All Therapeutic Studies	Protocol 305 (oral therapy)		Protocol 307/602 (IV/oral therapy)	
	Voriconazole N = 1493	Voriconazole N = 200	Fluconazole N = 191	Voriconazole N = 196	Ampho B** N = 185
	N (%)	N (%)	N (%)	N (%)	N (%)
Special senses*					
Abnormal vision	307 (20.6)	31 (15.5)	8 (4.2)	55 (28.1)	1 (0.5)
Photophobia	36 (2.4)	5 (2.5)	2 (1.0)	7 (3.6)	0
Chromatopsia	20 (1.3)	2 (1.0)	0	2 (1.0)	0
Eye hemorrhage	3 (0.2)	0	0	0	0
Body as a Whole					
Fever	93 (6.2)	0	0	7 (3.6)	25 (13.5)
Chills	61 (4.1)	1 (0.5)	0	0	36 (19.5)
Headache	48 (3.2)	0	1 (0.5)	7 (3.6)	8 (4.3)
Abdominal pain	25 (1.7)	0	0	5 (2.6)	6 (3.2)
Chest pain	13 (0.9)	0	0	4 (2.0)	2 (1.1)

(Table continued on next page)

tients with severe hepatic insufficiency if the benefit outweighs the potential risk. Patients with hepatic insufficiency must be carefully monitored for drug toxicity.

Patients With Renal Insufficiency
In patients with moderate to severe renal dysfunction (creatinine clearance <50 mL/min), accumulation of the intravenous vehicle, SBECD, occurs. Oral voriconazole should be administered to these patients, unless an assessment of the benefit/risk to the patient justifies the use of intravenous voriconazole. Serum creatinine levels should be closely monitored in these patients, and if increases occur, consideration should be given to changing to oral voriconazole therapy (see CLINICAL PHARMACOLOGY—Renal Insufficiency, DOSAGE AND ADMINISTRATION—Renal Insufficiency).

Renal adverse events
Acute renal failure has been observed in severely ill patients undergoing treatment with VFEND. Patients being treated with voriconazole are likely to be treated concomitantly with nephrotoxic medications and have concurrent conditions that may result in decreased renal function.

Monitoring of renal function
Patients should be monitored for the development of abnormal renal function. This should include laboratory evaluation, particularly serum creatinine.

Dermatological Reactions
Patients have rarely developed serious cutaneous reactions, such as Stevens-Johnson syndrome, during treatment with VFEND. If patients develop a rash, they should be monitored closely and consideration given to discontinuation of VFEND. VFEND has been infrequently associated with photosensitivity skin reaction, especially during long-term therapy. It is recommended that patients avoid strong, direct sunlight during VFEND therapy.

Carcinogenesis, Mutagenesis, Impairment Of Fertility
Two-year carcinogenicity studies were conducted in rats and mice. Rats were given oral doses of 6, 18 or 50 mg/kg voriconazole, or 0.2, 0.6, or 1.6 times the recommended maintenance dose (RMD) on a mg/m^2 basis. Hepatocellular adenomas were detected in females at 50 mg/kg and hepatocellular carcinomas were found in males at 6 and 50 mg/kg. Mice were given oral doses of 10, 30 or 100 mg/kg voriconazole, or 0.1, 0.4, or 1.4 times the RMD on a mg/m^2 basis. In mice, hepatocellular adenomas were detected in males and females and hepatocellular carcinomas were detected in males at 1.4 times the RMD of voriconazole.
Voriconazole demonstrated clastogenic activity (mostly chromosome breaks) in human lymphocyte cultures *in vitro*. Voriconazole was not genotoxic in the Ames assay, CHO assay, the mouse micronucleus assay or the DNA repair test (Unscheduled DNA Synthesis assay).
Voriconazole produced a reduction in the pregnancy rates of rats dosed at 50 mg/kg, or 1.6 times the RMD. This was statistically significant only in the preliminary study and not in a larger fertility study.

Teratogenic Effects
Pregnancy category D. See WARNINGS

Women Of Childbearing Potential
Women of childbearing potential should use effective contraception during treatment.

Nursing Mothers
The excretion of voriconazole in breast milk has not been investigated. VFEND should not be used by nursing mothers unless the benefit clearly outweighs the risk.

Pediatric Use
Safety and effectiveness in pediatric patients below the age of 12 years have not been established.
A total of 22 patients aged 12–18 years with invasive aspergillosis were included in the therapeutic studies. Twelve out of 22 (55%) patients had successful response after treatment with a maintenance dose of voriconazole 4 mg/kg Q12h.
Sparse plasma sampling for pharmacokinetics in adolescents was conducted in the therapeutic studies (see CLINICAL PHARMACOLOGY—Pharmacokinetics, General Pharmacokinetic Characteristics).

Geriatric Use
In multiple dose therapeutic trials of voriconazole, 9.2% of patients were ≥ 65 years of age and 1.8% of patients were ≥ 75 years of age. In a study in healthy volunteers, the systemic exposure (AUC) and peak plasma concentrations (C_{max}) were increased in elderly males compared to young males. Pharmacokinetic data obtained from 552 patients from 10 voriconazole therapeutic trials showed that voriconazole plasma concentrations in the elderly patients were approximately 80% to 90% higher than those in younger patients after either IV or oral administration. However, the overall safety profile of the elderly patients was similar to that of the young so no dosage adjustment is recommended (see CLINICAL PHARMACOLOGY—Pharmacokinetics in Special Populations).

ADVERSE REACTIONS
Overview
The most frequently reported adverse events (all causalities) in the therapeutic trials were visual disturbances, fever, rash, vomiting, nausea, diarrhea, headache, sepsis, peripheral edema, abdominal pain, and respiratory disorder. The treatment-related adverse events which most often led to discontinuation of voriconazole therapy were elevated liver function tests, rash, and visual disturbances (see hepatic toxicity under WARNINGS and discussion of Clinical Laboratory Values and dermatological and visual adverse events below).

Discussion Of Adverse Reactions
The data described in the table below reflect exposure to voriconazole in 1493 patients in the therapeutic studies. This represents a heterogeneous population, including immunocompromised patients, e.g., patients with hematological malignancy or HIV and non-neutropenic patients. This subgroup does not include healthy volunteers and patients treated in the compassionate use and non-therapeutic studies. This patient population was 62% male, had a mean age of 45.1 years (range 12-90, including 49 patients aged 12-18 years), and was 81% white and 9% black. Five hundred six-

VFEND—Cont.

ty-one patients had a duration of voriconazole therapy of greater than 12 weeks, with 136 patients receiving voriconazole for over six months. Table 8 includes all adverse events which were reported in therapeutic studies at an incidence of ≥1% as well as events of concern which occurred at an incidence of <1% during voriconazole therapy. In study 307/602, 381 patients (196 on voriconazole, 185 on amphotericin B) were treated to compare voriconazole to amphotericin B followed by other licensed antifungal therapy in the primary treatment of patients with acute invasive aspergillosis. Study 305 evaluated the effects of oral voriconazole (200 patients) and oral fluconazole (191 patients) for another indication in immunocompromised (primarily HIV) patients. Laboratory test abnormalities for these studies are discussed under Clinical Laboratory Values below.

[See table 8 on previous page and at right]

VISUAL DISTURBANCES: Voriconazole treatment-related visual disturbances are common. In clinical trials, approximately 30% of patients experienced altered/enhanced visual perception, blurred vision, color vision change and/or photophobia. The visual disturbances were generally mild and rarely resulted in discontinuation. Visual disturbances may be associated with higher plasma concentrations and/or doses.

The mechanism of action of the visual disturbance is unknown, although the site of action is most likely to be within the retina. In a study in healthy volunteers investigating the effect of 28-day treatment with voriconazole on retinal function, voriconazole caused a decrease in the electroretinogram (ERG) waveform amplitude, a decrease in the visual field, and an alteration in color perception. The ERG measures electrical currents in the retina. The effects were noted early in administration of voriconazole and continued through the course of study drug dosing. Fourteen days after end of dosing, ERG, visual fields and color perception returned to normal (see WARNINGS, PRECAUTIONS—Information For Patients).

Dermatological Reactions: Dermatological reactions were common in the patients treated with voriconazole. The mechanism underlying these dermatologic adverse events remains unknown. In clinical trials, rashes considered related to therapy were reported by 6% (86/1493) of voriconazole-treated patients. The majority of rashes were of mild to moderate severity. Cases of photosensitivity reactions appear to be more likely to occur with long-term treatment. Patients have rarely developed serious cutaneous reactions, including Stevens-Johnson syndrome, toxic epidermal necrolysis and erythema multiforme during treatment with VFEND. If patients develop a rash, they should be monitored closely and consideration given to discontinuation of VFEND. It is recommended that patients avoid strong, direct sunlight during VFEND therapy.

Less Common Adverse Events

The following adverse events occurred in <1% of all voriconazole-treated patients, including healthy volunteers and patients treated under compassionate use protocols (total N = 2090). This listing includes events where a causal relationship to voriconazole cannot be ruled out or those which may help the physician in managing the risks to the patients. The list does not include events included in Table 8 above and does not include every event reported in the voriconazole clinical program.

Body as a whole: abdomen enlarged, allergic reaction, anaphylactoid reaction (see PRECAUTIONS), ascites, asthenia, back pain, cellulitis, edema, face edema, flank pain, flu syndrome, graft versus host reaction, granuloma, infection, bacterial infection, fungal infection, injection site pain, injection site infection/inflammation, mucous membrane disorder, multi-organ failure, pain, pelvic pain, peritonitis, sepsis, substernal chest pain

Cardiovascular: atrial arrhythmia, atrial fibrillation, AV block complete, bigeminy, bradycardia, bundle branch block, cardiomegaly, cardiomyopathy, cerebral hemorrhage, cerebral ischemia, cerebrovascular accident, congestive heart failure, deep thrombophlebitis, endocarditis, extrasystoles, heart arrest, myocardial infarction, nodal arrhythmia, palpitation, phlebitis, postural hypotension, pulmonary embolus, QT interval prolonged, supraventricular tachycardia, syncope, thrombophlebitis, vasodilatation, ventricular arrhythmia, ventricular fibrillation, ventricular tachycardia (including *torsade de pointes*)

Digestive: anorexia, cheilitis, cholecystitis, cholelithiasis, constipation, duodenal ulcer perforation, duodenitis, dyspepsia, dysphagia, esophageal ulcer, esophagitis, flatulence, gastroenteritis, gastrointestinal hemorrhage, GGT/LDH elevated, gingivitis, glossitis, gum hemorrhage, gum hyperplasia, hematemesis, hepatic coma, hepatic failure, hepatitis, intestinal perforation, intestinal ulcer, enlarged liver, melena, mouth ulceration, pancreatitis, parotid gland enlargement, periodontitis, proctitis, pseudomembranous colitis, rectal disorder, rectal hemorrhage, stomach ulcer, stomatitis, tongue edema

Endocrine: adrenal cortex insufficiency, diabetes insipidus, hyperthyroidism, hypothyroidism

Hemic and lymphatic: agranulocytosis, anemia (macrocytic, megaloblastic, microcytic, normocytic), aplastic anemia, hemolytic anemia, bleeding time increased, cyanosis, DIC, ecchymosis, eosinophilia, hypervolemia, lymphadenopathy, lymphangitis, marrow depression, petechia, purpura, enlarged spleen, thrombotic thrombocytopenic purpura

Metabolic and Nutritional: albuminuria, BUN increased, creatine phosphokinase increased, edema, glucose tolerance decreased, hypercalcemia, hypercholesteremia, hyperglycemia, hyperkalemia, hypermagnesemia, hypernatremia, hyperuricemia, hypocalcemia, hypoglycemia, hyponatremia, hypophosphatemia, uremia

Musculoskeletal: arthralgia, arthritis, bone necrosis, bone pain, leg cramps, myalgia, myasthenia, myopathy, osteomalacia, osteoporosis

Nervous system: abnormal dreams, acute brain syndrome, agitation, akathisia, amnesia, anxiety, ataxia, brain edema, coma, confusion, convulsion, delirium, dementia, depersonalization, depression, diplopia, encephalitis, encephalopathy, euphoria, Extrapyramidal Syndrome, grand mal convulsion, Guillain-Barré syndrome, hypertonia, hypesthesia, insomnia, intracranial hypertension, libido decreased, neuralgia, neuropathy, nystagmus, oculogyric crisis, paresthesia, psychosis, somnolence, suicidal ideation, tremor, vertigo

Respiratory system: cough increased, dyspnea, epistaxis, hemoptysis, hypoxia, lung edema, pharyngitis, pleural effusion, pneumonia, respiratory disorder, respiratory distress syndrome, respiratory tract infection, rhinitis, sinusitis, voice alteration

Skin and Appendages: alopecia, angioedema, contact dermatitis, discoid lupus erythematosis, eczema, erythema multiforme, exfoliative dermatitis, fixed drug eruption, furunculosis, herpes simplex, melanosis, photosensitivity skin reaction, psoriasis, skin discoloration, skin disorder, skin dry, Stevens-Johnson syndrome, sweating, toxic epidermal necrolysis, urticaria

Special senses: abnormality of accommodation, blepharitis, color blindness, conjunctivitis, corneal opacity, deafness, ear

Table 8 (cont.)
TREATMENT-EMERGENT ADVERSE EVENTS
Rate ≥ 1% or Adverse Events of Concern in All Therapeutic Studies Possibly Related to Therapy or Causality Unknown

	All Therapeutic Studies	Protocol 305 (oral therapy)		Protocol 307/602 (IV/oral therapy)	
	Voriconazole N = 1493	Voriconazole N = 200	Fluconazole N = 191	Voriconazole N = 196	Ampho B** N = 185
	N (%)	N (%)	N (%)	N (%)	N (%)
Cardiovascular system					
Tachycardia	37 (2.5)	0	0	5 (2.6)	5 (2.7)
Hypertension	29 (1.9)	0	0	1 (0.5)	2 (1.1)
Hypotension	26 (1.7)	1 (0.5)	0	1 (0.5)	3 (1.6)
Vasodilatation	23 (1.5)	0	0	2 (1.0)	2 (1.1)
Digestive system					
Nausea	88 (5.9)	2 (1.0)	3 (1.6)	14 (7.1)	29 (15.7)
Vomiting	71 (4.8)	2 (1.0)	1 (0.5)	11 (5.6)	18 (9.7)
Liver function tests abnormal	41 (2.7)	6 (3.0)	2 (1.0)	9 (4.6)	4 (2.2)
Diarrhea	16 (1.1)	0	0	3 (1.5)	6 (3.2)
Cholestatic jaundice	16 (1.1)	3 (1.5)	0	4 (2.0)	0
Dry mouth	15 (1.0)	0	1 (0.5)	3 (1.5)	0
Jaundice	3 (0.2)	1 (0.5)	0	0	0
Hemic and lymphatic system					
Thrombocytopenia	7 (0.5)	0	1 (0.5)	2 (1.0)	2 (1.1)
Anemia	2 (0.1)	0	0	0	5 (2.7)
Leukopenia	4 (0.3)	0	0	1 (0.5)	0
Pancytopenia	1 (0.1)	0	0	0	0
Metabolic and Nutritional Systems					
Alkaline phosphatase increased	54 (3.6)	10 (5.0)	3 (1.6)	6 (3.1)	4 (2.2)
Hepatic enzymes increased	28 (1.9)	3 (1.5)	0	7 (3.6)	5 (2.7)
SGOT increased	28 (1.9)	8 (4.0)	2 (1.0)	1 (0.5)	0
SGPT increased	27 (1.8)	6 (3.0)	2 (1.0)	3 (1.5)	1 (0.5)
Hypokalemia	24 (1.6)	0	0	1 (0.5)	36 (19.5)
Peripheral edema	16 (1.1)	1 (0.5)	0	7 (3.6)	9 (4.9)
Hypomagnesemia	16 (1.1)	0	0	2 (1.0)	10 (5.4)
Bilirubinemia	12 (0.8)	1 (0.5)	0	1 (0.5)	3 (1.6)
Creatinine increased	4 (0.3)	1 (0.5)	0	0	59 (31.9)
Nervous system					
Hallucinations	37 (2.5)	0	0	10 (5.1)	1 (0.5)
Dizziness	20 (1.3)	0	2 (1.0)	5 (2.6)	0
Skin and Appendages					
Rash	86 (5.8)	3 (1.5)	1 (0.5)	13 (6.6)	7 (3.8)
Pruritus	16 (1.1)	0	0	2 (1.0)	2 (1.1)
Maculopapular rash	17 (1.1)	3 (1.5)	0	1 (0.5)	0
Urogenital					
Kidney function abnormal	8 (0.5)	1 (0.5)	1 (0.5)	4 (2.0)	40 (21.6)
Acute kidney failure	7 (0.5)	0	0	0	11 (5.9)

* See WARNINGS—Visual Disturbances, PRECAUTIONS—Information For Patients
** Amphotericin B followed by other licensed antifungal therapy

pain, eye pain, dry eyes, keratitis, keratoconjunctivitis, mydriasis, night blindness, optic atrophy, optic neuritis, otitis externa, papilledema, retinal hemorrhage, retinitis, scleritis, taste loss, taste perversion, tinnitus, uveitis, visual field defect

Urogenital: anuria, blighted ovum, creatinine clearance decreased, dysmenorrhea, dysuria, epididymitis, glycosuria, hemorrhagic cystitis, hematuria, hydronephrosis, impotence, kidney pain, kidney tubular necrosis, metrorrhagia, nephritis, nephrosis, oliguria, scrotal edema, urinary incontinence, urinary retention, urinary tract infection, uterine hemorrhage, vaginal hemorrhage

Clinical Laboratory Values

The overall incidence of clinically significant transaminase abnormalities in the voriconazole clinical program was 13.4% (200/1493) of patients treated with voriconazole. Increased incidence of liver function test abnormalities may be associated with higher plasma concentrations and/or doses. The majority of abnormal liver function tests either resolved during treatment without dose adjustment or following dose adjustment, including discontinuation of therapy.

Voriconazole has been infrequently associated with cases of serious hepatic toxicity including cases of jaundice and rare cases of hepatitis and hepatic failure leading to death. Most of these patients had other serious underlying conditions. Liver function tests should be evaluated at the start of and during the course of VFEND therapy. Patients who develop abnormal liver function tests during VFEND therapy should be monitored for the development of more severe hepatic injury. Patient management should include laboratory evaluation of hepatic function (particularly liver function tests and bilirubin). Discontinuation of VFEND must be considered if clinical signs and symptoms consistent with liver disease develop that may be attributable to VFEND (see WARNINGS and PRECAUTIONS—Laboratory Tests). Acute renal failure has been observed in severely ill patients undergoing treatment with VFEND. Patients being treated with voriconazole are likely to be treated concomitantly with nephrotoxic medications and have concurrent conditions that may result in decreased renal function. It is recommended that patients are monitored for the development of abnormal renal function. This should include laboratory evaluation, particularly serum creatinine.

Tables 9 and 10 show the number of patients with hypokalemia and clinically significant changes in renal and liver function tests in two randomized, comparative multicenter studies. In study 305, patients were randomized to either oral voriconazole or oral fluconazole to evaluate an indication other than invasive aspergillosis in immunocompromised patients. In study 307/602, patients with definite or probable invasive aspergillosis were randomized to either voriconazole or amphotericin B therapy.
[See table 9 at right]
[See table 10 at right]

OVERDOSE

In clinical trials, there were three cases of accidental overdose. All occurred in pediatric patients who received up to five times the recommended intravenous dose of voriconazole. A single adverse event of photophobia of 10 minutes duration was reported.

There is no known antidote to voriconazole.

Voriconazole is hemodialyzed with clearance of 121 mL/min. The intravenous vehicle, SBECD, is hemodialyzed with clearance of 55 mL/min. In an overdose, hemodialysis may assist in the removal of voriconazole and SBECD from the body.

The minimum lethal oral dose in mice and rats was 300 mg/kg (equivalent to 4 and 7 times the recommended maintenance dose (RMD), based on body surface area). At this dose, clinical signs observed in both mice and rats included salivation, mydriasis, titubation (loss of balance while moving), depressed behavior, prostration, partially closed eyes, and dyspnea. Other signs in mice were convulsions, corneal opacification and swollen abdomen.

DOSAGE AND ADMINISTRATION
Administration

VFEND Tablets should be taken at least one hour before, or one hour following, a meal.

VFEND I.V. for Injection requires reconstitution to 10 mg/mL and subsequent dilution to 5 mg/mL or less prior to administration as an infusion, at a maximum rate of 3 mg/kg per hour over 1–2 hours (see Intravenous Administration).

NOT FOR IV BOLUS INJECTION

Electrolyte disturbances such as hypokalemia, hypomagnesemia and hypocalcemia should be corrected prior to initiation of VFEND therapy (see PRECAUTIONS).

Use In Adults

Therapy must be initiated with the specified loading dose regimen of intravenous VFEND to achieve plasma concentrations on Day 1 that are close to steady state. On the basis of high oral bioavailability, switching between intravenous and oral administration is appropriate when clinically indicated (see CLINICAL PHARMACOLOGY).

For the treatment of adults with invasive aspergillosis and infections due to *Fusarium* spp. and *Scedosporium apiospermum*, the recommended dosing regimen of VFEND is as follows:

Loading dose of 6 mg/kg VFEND I.V. every 12 hours for two doses, followed by a maintenance dose of 4 mg/kg VFEND I.V. every 12 hours.

Once the patient can tolerate medication given by mouth, the oral tablet form of voriconazole may be utilized. Patients who weigh more than 40 kg should receive an oral maintenance dose of 200 mg VFEND tablet every 12 hours. Adult patients who weigh less than 40 kg should receive an oral maintenance dose of 100 mg every 12 hours.

Dosage Adjustment

If patient response is inadequate, the oral maintenance dose may be increased from 200 mg every 12 hours to 300 mg every 12 hours. For adult patients weighing less than 40 kg, the oral maintenance dose may be increased from 100 mg every 12 hours to 150 mg every 12 hours.

If patients are unable to tolerate treatment, reduce the intravenous maintenance dose to 3 mg/kg every 12 hours and the oral maintenance dose by 50 mg steps to a minimum of 200 mg every 12 hours (or to 100 mg every 12 hours for adult patients weighing less than 40 kg).

Phenytoin may be coadministered with VFEND if the maintenance dose of VFEND is increased to 5 mg/kg I.V. every 12 hours, or from 200 mg to 400 mg every 12 hours orally (100 mg to 200 mg every 12 hours orally in adult patients weighing less than 40 kg) (see CLINICAL PHARMACOLOGY, PRECAUTIONS—Drug Interactions).

Duration of therapy should be based on the severity of the patient's underlying disease, recovery from immunosuppression, and clinical response.

Use In Geriatric Patients

No dose adjustment is necessary for geriatric patients.

Use In Patients With Hepatic Insufficiency

In the clinical program, patients were included who had baseline liver function tests (ALT, AST) up to 5 times the upper limit of normal. No dose adjustment is necessary in patients with this degree of abnormal liver function, but continued monitoring of liver function tests for further elevations is recommended (see WARNINGS).

Table 9
PROTOCOL 305
Clinically Significant Laboratory Test Abnormalities

	Criteria*	VORICONAZOLE n/N (%)	FLUCONAZOLE n/N (%)
T. Bilirubin	>1.5× ULN	8/185 (4.3)	7/186 (3.8)
AST	>3.0× ULN	38/187 (20.3)	15/186 (8.1)
ALT	>3.0× ULN	20/187 (10.7)	12/186 (6.5)
Alk phos	>3.0× ULN	19/187 (10.2)	14/186 (7.5)

* Without regard to baseline value
n number of patients with a clinically significant abnormality while on study therapy
N total number of patients with at least one observation of the given lab test while on study therapy
ULN upper limit of normal

Table 10
PROTOCOL 307/602
Clinically Significant Laboratory Test Abnormalities

	Criteria*	VORICONAZOLE n/N (%)	AMPHOTERICIN B** n/N (%)
T. Bilirubin	>1.5× ULN	35/180 (19.4)	46/173 (26.6)
AST	>3.0× ULN	21/180 (11.7)	18/174 (10.3)
ALT	>3.0× ULN	34/180 (18.9)	40/173 (23.1)
Alk phos	>3.0× ULN	29/181 (16.0)	38/173 (22.0)
Creatinine	>1.3× ULN	39/182 (21.4)	102/177 (57.6)
Potassium	<0.9× LLN	30/181 (16.6)	70/178 (39.3)

* Without regard to baseline value
** Amphotericin B followed by other licensed antifungal therapy
n number of patients with a clinically significant abnormality while on study therapy
N total number of patients with at least one observation of the given lab test while on study therapy
ULN upper limit of normal
LLN lower limit of normal

Table 11 Required Volumes of 10 mg/mL VFEND Concentrate

Body Weight (kg)	Volume of VFEND Concentrate (10 mg/mL) required for:		
	3 mg/kg dose (number of vials)	4 mg/kg dose (number of vials)	6 mg/kg dose (number of vials)
30	9.0 mL (1)	12 mL (1)	18 mL (1)
35	10.5 mL (1)	14 mL (1)	21 mL (2)
40	12.0 mL (1)	16 mL (1)	24 mL (2)
45	13.5 mL (1)	18 mL (1)	27 mL (2)
50	15.0 mL (1)	20 mL (1)	30 mL (2)
55	16.5 mL (1)	22 mL (2)	33 mL (2)
60	18.0 mL (1)	24 mL (2)	36 mL (2)
65	19.5 mL (1)	26 mL (2)	39 mL (2)
70	21.0 mL (2)	28 mL (2)	42 mL (3)
75	22.5 mL (2)	30 mL (2)	45 mL (3)
80	24.0 mL (2)	32 mL (2)	48 mL (3)
85	25.5 mL (2)	34 mL (2)	51 mL (3)
90	27.0 mL (2)	36 mL (2)	54 mL (3)
95	28.5 mL (2)	38 mL (2)	57 mL (3)
100	30.0 mL (2)	40 mL (2)	60 mL (3)

Continued on next page

VFEND—Cont.

It is recommended that the standard loading dose regimens be used but that the maintenance dose be halved in patients with mild to moderate hepatic cirrhosis (Child-Pugh Class A and B).
VFEND has not been studied in patients with severe hepatic cirrhosis (Child-Pugh Class C) or in patients with chronic hepatitis B or chronic hepatitis C disease. VFEND has been associated with elevations in liver function tests and clinical signs of liver damage, such as jaundice, and should only be used in patients with severe hepatic insufficiency if the benefit outweighs the potential risk. Patients with hepatic insufficiency must be carefully monitored for drug toxicity.

Use In Patients With Renal Insufficiency
The pharmacokinetics of orally administered VFEND are not significantly affected by renal insufficiency. Therefore, no adjustment is necessary for oral dosing in patients with mild to severe renal impairment (see CLINICAL PHARMACOLOGY—Special Populations).
In patients with moderate or severe renal insufficiency (creatinine clearance <50 mL/min), accumulation of the intravenous vehicle, SBECD, occurs. Oral voriconazole should be administered to these patients, unless an assessment of the benefit/risk to the patient justifies the use of intravenous voriconazole. Serum creatinine levels should be closely monitored in these patients, and, if increases occur, consideration should be given to changing to oral voriconazole therapy (see DOSAGE and ADMINISTRATION).
Voriconazole is hemodialyzed with clearance of 121 mL/min. The intravenous vehicle, SBECD, is hemodialyzed with clearance of 55 mL/min. A 4-hour hemodialysis session does not remove a sufficient amount of voriconazole to warrant dose adjustment.

Intravenous Administration
VFEND I.V. For Injection:

Reconstitution
The powder is reconstituted with 19 mL of Water For Injection to obtain an extractable volume of 20 mL of clear concentrate containing 10 mg/mL of voriconazole. It is recommended that a standard 20 mL (non-automated) syringe be used to ensure that the exact amount (19.0 mL) of water for injection is dispensed. Discard the vial if a vacuum does not pull the diluent into the vial. Shake the vial until all the powder is dissolved.

Dilution
VFEND must be infused over 1–2 hours, at a concentration of 5 mg/mL or less. Therefore, the required volume of the 10 mg/mL VFEND concentrate should be further diluted as follows (appropriate diluents listed below):

1. Calculate the volume of 10 mg/mL VFEND concentrate required based on the patient's weight (see Table 11).
2. In order to allow the required volume of VFEND concentrate to be added, withdraw and discard at least an equal volume of diluent from the infusion bag or bottle to be used. The volume of diluent remaining in the bag or bottle should be such that when the 10 mg/mL VFEND concentrate is added, the final concentration is not less than 0.5 mg/mL nor greater than 5 mg/mL.
3. Using a suitable size syringe and aseptic technique, withdraw the required volume of VFEND concentrate from the appropriate number of vials and add to the infusion bag or bottle. DISCARD PARTIALLY USED VIALS.

The final VFEND solution must be infused over 1-2 hours at a maximum rate of 3 mg/kg per hour.
[See table 11 on previous page]
VFEND is a single dose unpreserved sterile lyophile. Therefore, from a microbiological point of view, once reconstituted, the product should be used immediately. If not used immediately, in-use storage times and conditions prior to use are the responsibility of the user and should not be longer than 24 hours at 2° to 8°C (37° to 46°F). This medicinal product is for single use only and any unused solution should be discarded. Only clear solutions without particles should be used.
The reconstituted solution can be diluted with:
9 mg/mL (0.9%) Sodium Chloride USP
Lactated Ringers USP
5% Dextrose and Lactated Ringers USP
5% Dextrose and 0.45% Sodium Chloride, USP
5% Dextrose USP
5% Dextrose and 20 mEq Potassium Chloride, USP
0.45% Sodium Chloride USP
5% Dextrose and 0.9% Sodium Chloride, USP
The compatibility of VFEND I.V. with diluents other than those described above is unknown (see Incompatibilities below).
Parenteral drug products should be inspected visually for particulate matter and discoloration prior to administration, whenever solution and container permit.
Incompatibilities:
VFEND I.V. must not be infused into the same line or cannula concomitantly with other drug infusions, including parenteral nutrition, e.g., Aminofusin 10% Plus. Aminofusin 10% Plus is physically incompatible, with an increase in subvisible particulate matter after 24 hours storage at 4°C.
Infusions of blood products must not occur simultaneously with VFEND I.V.
Infusions of total parenteral nutrition can occur simultaneously with VFEND I.V.
VFEND I.V. must not be diluted with 4.2% Sodium Bicarbonate Infusion. The mildly alkaline nature of this diluent caused slight degradation of VFEND after 24 hours storage at room temperature. Although refrigerated storage is recommended following reconstitution, use of this diluent is not recommended as a precautionary measure. Compatibility with other concentrations is unknown.

Stability
VFEND Tablets: Store at controlled room temperature 15° - 30°C (59° - 86°F).
VFEND I.V. for Injection: Store at controlled room temperature 15° - 30°C (59° - 86°F).

HOW SUPPLIED

Tablets
VFEND 50 mg tablets—white, film-coated, round, debossed with "Pfizer" on one side and "VOR50" on the reverse.
Bottles of 30 (NDC 0049-3170-30)
VFEND 200 mg tablets—white, film-coated, capsule shaped, debossed with "Pfizer" on one side and "VOR200" on the reverse.
Bottles of 30 (NDC 0049-3180-30)

Powder for Solution for Injection
VFEND I.V. for Injection is supplied in a single use vial as a sterile lyophilized powder equivalent to 200 mg VFEND and 3200 mg sulfobutyl ether beta-cyclodextrin sodium (SBECD).
Individually packaged vials of 200 mg VFEND I.V.
(NDC 0049-3190-28)

Storage
VFEND Tablets should be stored at controlled room temperature 15° - 30°C (59° - 86°F).
Unreconstituted vials should be stored at controlled room temperature 15° - 30°C (59° - 86°F). VFEND is a single dose unpreserved sterile lyophile. From a microbiological point of view, following reconstitution of the lyophile with Water for Injection, the reconstituted solution should be used immediately. If not used immediately, in-use storage times and conditions prior to use are the responsibility of the user and should not be longer than 24 hours at 2° to 8°C (37° to 46°F). Chemical and physical in-use stability has been demonstrated for 24 hours at 2° to 8°C (37° to 46°F). This medicinal product is for single use only and any unused solution should be discarded. Only clear solutions without particles should be used (see DOSAGE AND ADMINISTRATION—Intravenous Administration).

REFERENCES

1. National Committee for Clinical Laboratory Standards. Reference method for broth dilution antifungal susceptibility testing of conidium-forming filamentous fungi. Approved Standard M38-P. National Committee for Clinical Laboratory Standards, Villanova, Pa.

℞ only

Distributed by
Pfizer Roerig
Division of Pfizer Inc, NY, NY 10017
69-5906-00-1 Issued January 2003

VIAGRA® ℞

[*vī-ă-grə*]
(sildenafil citrate)
Tablets

Prescribing information for this product, which appears on pages 2653–2656 of the 2003 PDR, has been completely revised as follows. Please write "See Supplement A" next to the product heading.

DESCRIPTION

VIAGRA®, an oral therapy for erectile dysfunction, is the citrate salt of sildenafil, a selective inhibitor of cyclic guanosine monophosphate (cGMP)-specific phosphodiesterase type 5 (PDE5).
Sildenafil citrate is designated chemically as 1-[[3-(6,7-dihydro-1-methyl-7-oxo-3-propyl-1*H*-pyrazolo[4,3-*d*]pyrimidin-5-yl)-4-ethoxyphenyl]sulfonyl]-4-methylpiperazine citrate and has the following structural formula:

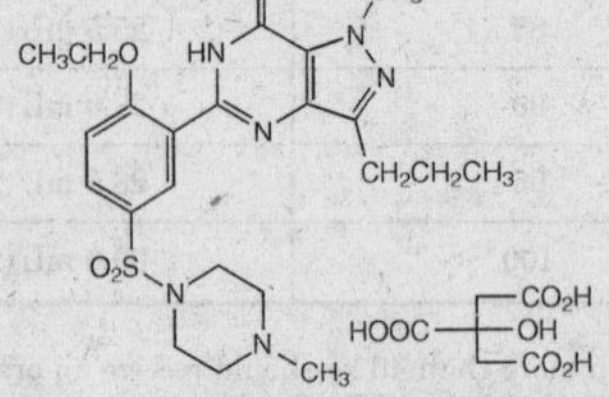

Sildenafil citrate is a white to off-white crystalline powder with a solubility of 3.5 mg/mL in water and a molecular weight of 666.7. VIAGRA (sildenafil citrate) is formulated as blue, film-coated rounded-diamond-shaped tablets equivalent to 25 mg, 50 mg and 100 mg of sildenafil for oral administration. In addition to the active ingredient, sildenafil citrate, each tablet contains the following inactive ingredients: microcrystalline cellulose, anhydrous dibasic calcium phosphate, croscarmellose sodium, magnesium stearate, hydroxypropyl methylcellulose, titanium dioxide, lactose, triacetin, and FD & C Blue #2 aluminum lake.

CLINICAL PHARMACOLOGY

Mechanism of Action
The physiologic mechanism of erection of the penis involves release of nitric oxide (NO) in the corpus cavernosum during sexual stimulation. NO then activates the enzyme guanylate cyclase, which results in increased levels of cyclic guanosine monophosphate (cGMP), producing smooth muscle relaxation in the corpus cavernosum and allowing inflow of blood. Sildenafil has no direct relaxant effect on isolated human corpus cavernosum, but enhances the effect of nitric oxide (NO) by inhibiting phosphodiesterase type 5 (PDE5), which is responsible for degradation of cGMP in the corpus cavernosum. When sexual stimulation causes local release of NO, inhibition of PDE5 by sildenafil causes increased levels of cGMP in the corpus cavernosum, resulting in smooth muscle relaxation and inflow of blood to the corpus cavernosum. Sildenafil at recommended doses has no effect in the absence of sexual stimulation.
Studies *in vitro* have shown that sildenafil is selective for PDE5. Its effect is more potent on PDE5 than on other known phosphodiesterases (10-fold for PDE6, >80-fold for PDE1, >700-fold for PDE2, PDE3, PDE4, PDE7, PDE8, PDE9, PDE10, and PDE11). The approximately 4,000-fold selectivity for PDE5 versus PDE3 is important because PDE3 is involved in control of cardiac contractility. Sildenafil is only about 10-fold as potent for PDE5 compared to PDE6, an enzyme found in the retina which is involved in the phototransduction pathway of the retina. This lower selectivity is thought to be the basis for abnormalities related to color vision observed with higher doses or plasma levels (see **Pharmacodynamics**).
In addition to human corpus cavernosum smooth muscle, PDE5 is also found in lower concentrations in other tissues including platelets, vascular and visceral smooth muscle, and skeletal muscle. The inhibition of PDE5 in these tissues by sildenafil may be the basis for the enhanced platelet antiaggregatory activity of nitric oxide observed *in vitro*, an inhibition of platelet thrombus formation *in vivo* and peripheral arterial-venous dilatation *in vivo*.

Pharmacokinetics and Metabolism
VIAGRA is rapidly absorbed after oral administration, with absolute bioavailability of about 40%. Its pharmacokinetics are dose-proportional over the recommended dose range. It is eliminated predominantly by hepatic metabolism (mainly cytochrome P450 3A4) and is converted to an active metabolite with properties similar to the parent, sildenafil. The concomitant use of potent cytochrome P450 3A4 inhibitors (e.g., erythromycin, ketoconazole, itraconazole) as well as the nonspecific CYP inhibitor, cimetidine, is associated with increased plasma levels of sildenafil (see **DOSAGE AND ADMINISTRATION**). Both sildenafil and the metabolite have terminal half lives of about 4 hours.
Mean sildenafil plasma concentrations measured after the administration of a single oral dose of 100 mg to healthy male volunteers is depicted below:

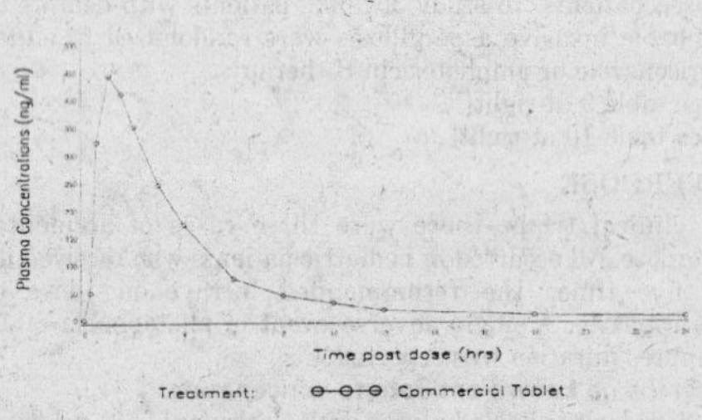

Figure 1: Mean Sildenafil Plasma Concentrations in Healthy Male Volunteers.

Absorption and Distribution: VIAGRA is rapidly absorbed. Maximum observed plasma concentrations are reached within 30 to 120 minutes (median 60 minutes) of oral dosing in the fasted state. When VIAGRA is taken with a high fat meal, the rate of absorption is reduced, with a mean delay in T_{max} of 60 minutes and a mean reduction in C_{max} of 29%. The mean steady state volume of distribution (Vss) for sildenafil is 105 L, indicating distribution into the tissues. Sildenafil and its major circulating N-desmethyl metabolite are both approximately 96% bound to plasma proteins. Protein binding is independent of total drug concentrations.
Based upon measurements of sildenafil in semen of healthy volunteers 90 minutes after dosing, less than 0.001% of the administered dose may appear in the semen of patients.
Metabolism and Excretion: Sildenafil is cleared predominantly by the CYP3A4 (major route) and CYP2C9 (minor route) hepatic microsomal isoenzymes. The major circulating metabolite results from N-desmethylation of sildenafil, and is itself further metabolized. This metabolite has a PDE selectivity profile similar to sildenafil and an *in vitro* potency for PDE5 approximately 50% of the parent drug. Plasma concentrations of this metabolite are approximately 40% of those seen for sildenafil, so that the metabolite accounts for about 20% of sildenafil's pharmacologic effects.
After either oral or intravenous administration, sildenafil is excreted as metabolites predominantly in the feces (approximately 80% of administered oral dose) and to a lesser extent in the urine (approximately 13% of the administered oral dose). Similar values for pharmacokinetic parameters were seen in normal volunteers and in the patient population, using a population pharmacokinetic approach.

Pharmacokinetics in Special Populations
Geriatrics: Healthy elderly volunteers (65 years or over) had a reduced clearance of sildenafil, with free plasma concentrations approximately 40% greater than those seen in healthy younger volunteers (18–45 years).
Renal Insufficiency: In volunteers with mild (CLcr=50-80 mL/min) and moderate (CLcr=30-49 mL/min) renal im-

pairment, the pharmacokinetics of a single oral dose of VIAGRA (50 mg) were not altered. In volunteers with severe (CLcr=<30 mL/min) renal impairment, sildenafil clearance was reduced, resulting in approximately doubling of AUC and C_{max} compared to age-matched volunteers with no renal impairment.
Hepatic Insufficiency: In volunteers with hepatic cirrhosis (Child-Pugh A and B), sildenafil clearance was reduced, resulting in increases in AUC (84%) and C_{max} (47%) compared to age-matched volunteers with no hepatic impairment.
Therefore, age >65, hepatic impairment and severe renal impairment are associated with increased plasma levels of sildenafil. A starting oral dose of 25 mg should be considered in those patients (see **DOSAGE AND ADMINISTRATION**).
Pharmacodynamics
Effects of VIAGRA on Erectile Response: In eight double-blind, placebo-controlled crossover studies of patients with either organic or psychogenic erectile dysfunction, sexual stimulation resulted in improved erections, as assessed by an objective measurement of hardness and duration of erections (RigiScan®), after VIAGRA administration compared with placebo. Most studies assessed the efficacy of VIAGRA approximately 60 minutes post dose. The erectile response, as assessed by RigiScan®, generally increased with increasing sildenafil dose and plasma concentration. The time course of effect was examined in one study, showing an effect for up to 4 hours but the response was diminished compared to 2 hours.
Effects of VIAGRA on Blood Pressure: Single oral doses of sildenafil (100 mg) administered to healthy volunteers produced decreases in supine blood pressure (mean maximum decrease in systolic/diastolic blood pressure of 8.4/5.5 mmHg). The decrease in blood pressure was most notable approximately 1-2 hours after dosing, and was not different than placebo at 8 hours. Similar effects on blood pressure were noted with 25 mg, 50 mg and 100 mg of VIAGRA, therefore the effects are not related to dose or plasma levels within this dosage range. Larger effects were recorded among patients receiving concomitant nitrates (see **CONTRAINDICATIONS**).

Figure 2: Mean Change from Baseline in Sitting Systolic Blood Pressure, Healthy Volunteers.

Effects of VIAGRA on Cardiac Parameters: Single oral doses of sildenafil up to 100 mg produced no clinically relevant changes in the ECGs of normal male volunteers.
Studies have produced relevant data on the effects of VIAGRA on cardiac output. In one small, open-label, uncontrolled, pilot study, eight patients with stable ischemic heart disease underwent Swan-Ganz catheterization. A total dose of 40 mg sildenafil was administered by four intravenous infusions.
The results from this pilot study are shown in Table 1; the mean resting systolic and diastolic blood pressures decreased by 7% and 10% compared to baseline in these patients. Mean resting values for right atrial pressure, pulmonary artery pressure, pulmonary artery occluded pressure and cardiac output decreased by 28%, 28%, 20% and 7% respectively. Even though this total dosage produced plasma sildenafil concentrations which were approximately 2 to 5 times higher than the mean maximum plasma concentrations following a single oral dose of 100 mg in healthy male volunteers, the hemodynamic response to exercise was preserved in these patients.
[See table 1 above]
In a double-blind study, 144 patients with erectile dysfunction and chronic stable angina limited by exercise, not receiving chronic oral nitrates, were randomized to a single dose of placebo or VIAGRA 100 mg 1 hour prior to exercise testing. The primary endpoint was time to limiting angina in the evaluable cohort. The mean times (adjusted for baseline) to onset of limiting angina were 423.6 and 403.7 seconds for sildenafil (N=70) and placebo, respectively. These results demonstrated that the effect of VIAGRA on the primary endpoint was statistically non-inferior to placebo.
Effects of VIAGRA on Vision: At single oral doses of 100 mg and 200 mg, transient dose-related impairment of color discrimination (blue/green) was detected using the Farnsworth-Munsell 100-hue test, with peak effects near the time of peak plasma levels. This finding is consistent with the inhibition of PDE6, which is involved in phototransduction in the retina. An evaluation of visual function at doses up to twice the maximum recommended dose revealed no effects of VIAGRA on visual acuity, intraocular pressure, or pupillometry.
Clinical Studies
In clinical studies, VIAGRA was assessed for its effect on the ability of men with erectile dysfunction (ED) to engage in sexual activity and in many cases specifically on the ability to achieve and maintain an erection sufficient for satisfactory sexual activity. VIAGRA was evaluated primarily at doses of 25 mg, 50 mg and 100 mg in 21 randomized, double-blind, placebo-controlled trials of up to 6 months in duration, using a variety of study designs (fixed dose, titration, parallel, crossover). VIAGRA was administered to more than 3,000 patients aged 19 to 87 years, with ED of various etiologies (organic, psychogenic, mixed) with a mean duration of 5 years. VIAGRA demonstrated statistically significant improvement compared to placebo in all 21 studies. The studies that established benefit demonstrated improvements in success rates for sexual intercourse compared with placebo.

The effectiveness of VIAGRA was evaluated in most studies using several assessment instruments. The primary measure in the principal studies was a sexual function questionnaire (the International Index of Erectile Function - IIEF) administered during a 4-week treatment-free run-in period, at baseline, at follow-up visits, and at the end of double-blind, placebo-controlled, at-home treatment. Two of the questions from the IIEF served as primary study endpoints; categorical responses were elicited to questions about (1) the ability to achieve erections sufficient for sexual intercourse and (2) the maintenance of erections after penetration. The patient addressed both questions at the final visit for the last 4 weeks of the study. The possible categorical responses to these questions were (0) no attempted intercourse, (1) never or almost never, (2) a few times, (3) sometimes, (4) most times, and (5) almost always or always. Also collected as part of the IIEF was information about other aspects of sexual function, including information on erectile function, orgasm, desire, satisfaction with intercourse, and overall sexual satisfaction. Sexual function data were also recorded by patients in a daily diary. In addition, patients were asked a global efficacy question and an optional partner questionnaire was administered.
The effect on one of the major end points, maintenance of erections after penetration, is shown in Figure 3, for the pooled results of 5 fixed-dose, dose-response studies of greater than one month duration, showing response according to baseline function. Results with all doses have been pooled, but scores showed greater improvement at the 50 and 100 mg doses than at 25 mg. The pattern of responses was similar for the other principal question, the ability to achieve an erection sufficient for intercourse. The titration studies, in which most patients received 100 mg, showed similar results. Figure 3 shows that regardless of the baseline levels of function, subsequent function in patients treated with VIAGRA was better than that seen in patients treated with placebo. At the same time, on-treatment function was better in treated patients who were less impaired at baseline.
[See figure 3 at top of next column]
The frequency of patients reporting improvement of erections in response to a global question in four of the randomized, double-blind, parallel, placebo-controlled fixed dose studies (1797 patients) of 12 to 24 weeks duration is shown in Figure 4. These patients had erectile dysfunction at baseline that was characterized by median categorical scores of 2 (a few times) on principal IIEF questions. Erectile dysfunction was attributed to organic (58%; generally not characterized, but including diabetes and excluding spinal cord injury), psychogenic (17%), or mixed (24%) etiologies. Sixty-three percent, 74%, and 82% of the patients on 25 mg, 50 mg and 100 mg of VIAGRA, respectively, reported an improvement in their erections, compared to 24% on placebo. In the titration studies (n=644) (with most patients eventually receiving 100 mg), results were similar.
[See figure 4 at right]
The patients in studies had varying degrees of ED. One-third to one-half of the subjects in these studies reported successful intercourse at least once during a 4-week, treatment-free run-in period.
In many of the studies, of both fixed dose and titration designs, daily diaries were kept by patients. In these studies, involving about 1600 patients, analyses of patient diaries showed no effect of VIAGRA on rates of attempted intercourse (about 2 per week), but there was clear treatment-related improvement in sexual function: per patient weekly success rates averaged 1.3 on 50–100 mg of VIAGRA vs 0.4 on placebo; similarly, group mean success rates (total successes divided by total attempts) were about 66% on VIAGRA vs about 20% on placebo.
During 3 to 6 months of double-blind treatment or longer-term (1 year), open-label studies, few patients withdrew from active treatment for any reason, including lack of effectiveness. At the end of the long-term study, 88% of patients reported that VIAGRA improved their erections. Men with untreated ED had relatively low baseline scores for all aspects of sexual function measured (again using a 5-point scale) in the IIEF. VIAGRA improved these aspects of sexual function: frequency, firmness and maintenance of erections; frequency of orgasm; frequency and level of desire; satisfaction, satisfaction and enjoyment of intercourse; and overall relationship satisfaction.
One randomized, double-blind, flexible-dose, placebo-controlled study included only patients with erectile dysfunction attributed to complications of diabetes mellitus (n=268). As in the other titration studies, patients were

TABLE 1. HEMODYNAMIC DATA IN PATIENTS WITH STABLE ISCHEMIC HEART DISEASE AFTER IV ADMINISTRATION OF 40 MG SILDENAFIL

Means ± SD	At rest				After 4 minutes of exercise			
	n	Baseline (B2)	n	Sildenafil (D1)	n	Baseline	n	Sildenafil
PAOP (mmHg)	8	8.1 ± 5.1	8	6.5 ± 4.3	8	36.0 ± 13.7	8	27.8 ± 15.3
Mean PAP (mmHg)	8	16.7 ± 4	8	12.1 ± 3.9	8	39.4 ± 12.9	8	31.7 ± 13.2
Mean RAP (mmHg)	7	5.7 ± 3.7	8	4.1 ± 3.7	–	–	–	–
Systolic SAP (mmHg)	8	150.4 ± 12.4	8	140.6 ± 16.5	8	199.5 ± 37.4	8	187.8 ± 30.0
Diastolic SAP (mmHg)	8	73.6 ± 7.8	8	65.9 ± 10	8	84.6 ± 9.7	8	79.5 ± 9.4
Cardiac output (L/min)	8	5.6 ± 0.9	8	5.2 ± 1.1	8	11.5 ± 2.4	8	10.2 ± 3.5
Heart rate (bpm)	8	67 ± 11.1	8	66.9 ± 12	8	101.9 ± 11.6	8	99.0 ± 20.4

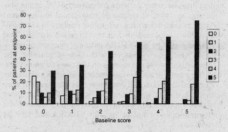

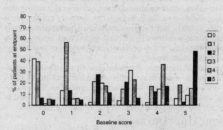

Figure 3. Effect of VIAGRA and Placebo on Maintenance of Erection by Baseline Score.

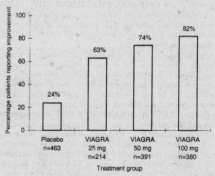

Overall treatment p<0.0001

Figure 4. Percentage of Patients Reporting an Improvement in Erections.

Continued on next page

Viagra—Cont.

started on 50 mg and allowed to adjust the dose up to 100 mg or down to 25 mg of VIAGRA; all patients, however, were receiving 50 mg or 100 mg at the end of the study. There were highly statistically significant improvements on the two principal IIEF questions (frequency of successful penetration during sexual activity and maintenance of erections after penetration) on VIAGRA compared to placebo. On a global improvement question, 57% of VIAGRA patients reported improved erections versus 10% on placebo. Diary data indicated that on VIAGRA, 48% of intercourse attempts were successful versus 12% on placebo.

One randomized, double-blind, placebo-controlled, crossover, flexible-dose (up to 100 mg) study of patients with erectile dysfunction resulting from spinal cord injury (n=178) was conducted. The changes from baseline in scoring on the two end point questions (frequency of successful penetration during sexual activity and maintenance of erections after penetration) were highly statistically significantly in favor of VIAGRA. On a global improvement question, 83% of patients reported improved erections on VIAGRA versus 12% on placebo. Diary data indicated that on VIAGRA, 59% of attempts at sexual intercourse were successful compared to 13% on placebo.

Across all trials, VIAGRA improved the erections of 43% of radical prostatectomy patients compared to 15% on placebo. Subgroup analyses of responses to a global improvement question in patients with psychogenic etiology in two fixed-dose studies (total n=179) and two titration studies (total n=149) showed 84% of VIAGRA patients reported improvement in erections compared with 26% of placebo. The changes from baseline in scoring on the two end point questions (frequency of successful penetration during sexual activity and maintenance of erections after penetration) were highly statistically significantly in favor of VIAGRA. Diary data in two of the studies (n=178) showed rates of successful intercourse per attempt of 70% for VIAGRA and 29% for placebo.

A review of population subgroups demonstrated efficacy regardless of baseline severity, etiology, race and age. VIAGRA was effective in a broad range of ED patients, including those with a history of coronary artery disease, hypertension, other cardiac disease, peripheral vascular disease, diabetes mellitus, depression, coronary artery bypass graft (CABG), radical prostatectomy, transurethral resection of the prostate (TURP) and spinal cord injury, and in patients taking antidepressants/antipsychotics and antihypertensives/diuretics.

Analysis of the safety database showed no apparent difference in the side effect profile in patients taking VIAGRA with and without antihypertensive medication. This analysis was performed retrospectively, and was not powered to detect any pre-specified difference in adverse reactions.

INDICATION AND USAGE

VIAGRA is indicated for the treatment of erectile dysfunction.

CONTRAINDICATIONS

Consistent with its known effects on the nitric oxide/cGMP pathway (see **CLINICAL PHARMACOLOGY**), VIAGRA was shown to potentiate the hypotensive effects of nitrates, and its administration to patients who are using organic nitrates, either regularly and/or intermittently, in any form is therefore contraindicated.

After patients have taken VIAGRA, it is unknown when nitrates, if necessary, can be safely administered. Based on the pharmacokinetic profile of a single 100 mg oral dose given to healthy normal volunteers, the plasma levels of sildenafil at 24 hours post dose are approximately 2 ng/mL (compared to peak plasma levels of approximately 440 ng/mL) (see **CLINICAL PHARMACOLOGY: Pharmacokinetics and Metabolism**). In the following patients: age >65, hepatic impairment (e.g., cirrhosis), severe renal impairment (e.g., creatinine clearance <30 mL/min), and concomitant use of potent cytochrome P450 3A4 inhibitors (erythromycin), plasma levels of sildenafil at 24 hours post dose have been found to be 3 to 8 times higher than those seen in healthy volunteers. Although plasma levels of sildenafil at 24 hours post dose are much lower than at peak concentration, it is unknown whether nitrates can be safely coadministered at this time point.

VIAGRA is contraindicated in patients with a known hypersensitivity to any component of the tablet.

WARNINGS

There is a potential for cardiac risk of sexual activity in patients with preexisting cardiovascular disease. Therefore, treatments for erectile dysfunction, including VIAGRA, should not be generally used in men for whom sexual activity is inadvisable because of their underlying cardiovascular status.

VIAGRA has systemic vasodilatory properties that resulted in transient decreases in supine blood pressure in healthy volunteers (mean maximum decrease of 8.4/5.5 mmHg), (see **CLINICAL PHARMACOLOGY: Pharmacodynamics**). While this normally would be expected to be of little consequence in most patients, prior to prescribing VIAGRA, physicians should carefully consider whether their patients with underlying cardiovascular disease could be affected adversely by such vasodilatory effects, especially in combination with sexual activity.

Patients with the following underlying conditions can be particularly sensitive to the actions of vasodilators including VIAGRA – those with left ventricular outflow obstruction (e.g. aortic stenosis, idiopathic hypertrophic subaortic stenosis) and those with severely impaired autonomic control of blood pressure.

There is no controlled clinical data on the safety or efficacy of VIAGRA in the following groups; if prescribed, this should be done with caution.

- Patients who have suffered a myocardial infarction, stroke, or life-threatening arrhythmia within the last 6 months;
- Patients with resting hypotension (BP <90/50) or hypertension (BP >170/110);
- Patients with cardiac failure or coronary artery disease causing unstable angina;
- Patients with retinitis pigmentosa (a minority of these patients have genetic disorders of retinal phosphodiesterases).

Prolonged erection greater than 4 hours and priapism (painful erections greater than 6 hours in duration) have been reported infrequently since market approval of VIAGRA. In the event of an erection that persists longer than 4 hours, the patient should seek immediate medical assistance. If priapism is not treated immediately, penile tissue damage and permanent loss of potency could result.

The concomitant administration of the protease inhibitor ritonavir substantially increases serum concentrations of sildenafil (**11-fold increase in AUC**). If VIAGRA is prescribed to patients taking ritonavir, caution should be used. Data from subjects exposed to high systemic levels of sildenafil are limited. Visual disturbances occurred more commonly at higher levels of sildenafil exposure. Decreased blood pressure, syncope, and prolonged erection were reported in some healthy volunteers exposed to high doses of sildenafil (200-800 mg). To decrease the chance of adverse events in patients taking ritonavir, a decrease in sildenafil dosage is recommended (see **Drug Interactions, ADVERSE REACTIONS and DOSAGE AND ADMINISTRATION**).

PRECAUTIONS

General

The evaluation of erectile dysfunction should include a determination of potential underlying causes and the identification of appropriate treatment following a complete medical assessment.

Before prescribing VIAGRA, it is important to note the following:

Patients on multiple antihypertensive medications were included in the pivotal clinical trials for VIAGRA. In a separate drug interaction study, when amlodipine, 5 mg or 10 mg, and VIAGRA, 100 mg were orally administered concomitantly to hypertensive patients mean additional blood pressure reduction of 8 mmHg systolic and 7 mmHg diastolic were noted (see **Drug Interactions**).

When the alpha blocker doxazosin (4 mg) and VIAGRA (25 mg) were administered simultaneously to patients with benign prostatic hyperplasia (BPH), mean additional reductions of supine blood pressure of 7 mmHg systolic and 7 mmHg diastolic were observed. When higher doses of VIAGRA and doxazosin (4 mg) were administered simultaneously, there were infrequent reports of patients who experienced symptomatic postural hypotension within 1 to 4 hours of dosing. Simultaneous administration of VIAGRA to patients taking alpha-blocker therapy may lead to symptomatic hypotension in some patients. Therefore, VIAGRA doses above 25 mg should not be taken within 4 hours of taking an alpha-blocker.

The safety of VIAGRA is unknown in patients with bleeding disorders and patients with active peptic ulceration.

VIAGRA should be used with caution in patients with anatomical deformation of the penis (such as angulation, cavernosal fibrosis or Peyronie's disease), or in patients who have conditions which may predispose them to priapism (such as sickle cell anemia, multiple myeloma, or leukemia).

The safety and efficacy of combinations of VIAGRA with other treatments for erectile dysfunction have not been studied. Therefore, the use of such combinations is not recommended.

In humans, VIAGRA has no effect on bleeding time when taken alone or with aspirin. *In vitro* studies with human platelets indicate that sildenafil potentiates the antiaggregatory effect of sodium nitroprusside (a nitric oxide donor). The combination of heparin and VIAGRA had an additive effect on bleeding time in the anesthetized rabbit, but this interaction has not been studied in humans.

Information for Patients

Physicians should discuss with patients the contraindication of VIAGRA with regular and/or intermittent use of organic nitrates.

Physicians should discuss with patients the potential cardiac risk of sexual activity in patients with preexisting cardiovascular risk factors. Patients who experience symptoms (e.g., angina pectoris, dizziness, nausea) upon initiation of sexual activity should be advised to refrain from further activity and should discuss the episode with their physician. Physicians should warn patients that prolonged erections greater than 4 hours and priapism (painful erections greater than 6 hours in duration) have been reported infrequently since market approval of VIAGRA. In the event of an erection that persists longer than 4 hours, the patient should seek immediate medical assistance. If priapism is not treated immediately, penile tissue damage and permanent loss of potency may result.

Physicians should advise patients that simultaneous administration of VIAGRA doses above 25 mg and an alpha-blocker may lead to symptomatic hypotension in some patients. Therefore, VIAGRA doses above 25 mg should not be taken within four hours of taking an alpha-blocker.

The use of VIAGRA offers no protection against sexually transmitted diseases. Counseling of patients about the protective measures necessary to guard against sexually transmitted diseases, including the Human Immunodeficiency Virus (HIV), may be considered.

Drug Interactions
Effects of Other Drugs on VIAGRA

In vitro **studies**: Sildenafil metabolism is principally mediated by the cytochrome P450 (CYP) isoforms 3A4 (major route) and 2C9 (minor route). Therefore, inhibitors of these isoenzymes may reduce sildenafil clearance.

In vivo **studies**: Cimetidine (800 mg), a nonspecific CYP inhibitor, caused a 56% increase in plasma sildenafil concentrations when coadministered with VIAGRA (50 mg) to healthy volunteers.

When a single 100 mg dose of VIAGRA was administered with erythromycin, a specific CYP3A4 inhibitor, at steady state (500 mg bid for 5 days), there was a 182% increase in sildenafil systemic exposure (AUC). In addition, in a study performed in healthy male volunteers, coadministration of the HIV protease inhibitor saquinavir, also a CYP3A4 inhibitor, at steady state (1200 mg tid) with VIAGRA (100 mg single dose) resulted in a 140% increase in sildenafil C_{max} and a 210% increase in sildenafil AUC. VIAGRA had no effect on saquinavir pharmacokinetics. Stronger CYP3A4 inhibitors such as ketoconazole or itraconazole would be expected to have still greater effects, and population data from patients in clinical trials did indicate a reduction in sildenafil clearance when it was coadministered with CYP3A4 inhibitors (such as ketoconazole, erythromycin, or cimetidine) (see **DOSAGE AND ADMINISTRATION**).

In another study in healthy male volunteers, coadministration with the HIV protease inhibitor ritonavir, which is a highly potent P450 inhibitor, at steady state (500 mg bid) with VIAGRA (100 mg single dose) resulted in a 300% (4-fold) increase in sildenafil C_{max} and a 1000% (11-fold) increase in sildenafil plasma AUC. At 24 hours the plasma levels of sildenafil were still approximately 200 ng/mL, compared to approximately 5 ng/mL when sildenafil was dosed alone. This is consistent with ritonavir's marked effects on a broad range of P450 substrates. VIAGRA had no effect on ritonavir pharmacokinetics (see **DOSAGE AND ADMINISTRATION**).

Although the interaction between other protease inhibitors and sildenafil has not been studied, their concomitant use is expected to increase sildenafil levels.

It can be expected that concomitant administration of CYP3A4 inducers, such as rifampin, will decrease plasma levels of sildenafil.

Single doses of antacid (magnesium hydroxide/aluminum hydroxide) did not affect the bioavailability of VIAGRA.

Pharmacokinetic data from patients in clinical trials showed no effect on sildenafil pharmacokinetics of CYP2C9 inhibitors (such as tolbutamide, warfarin), CYP2D6 inhibitors (such as selective serotonin reuptake inhibitors, tricyclic antidepressants), thiazide and related diuretics, ACE inhibitors, and calcium channel blockers. The AUC of the active metabolite, N-desmethyl sildenafil, was increased 62% by loop and potassium-sparing diuretics and 102% by nonspecific beta-blockers. These effects on the metabolite are not expected to be of clinical consequence.

Effects of VIAGRA on Other Drugs

In vitro **studies**: Sildenafil is a weak inhibitor of the cytochrome P450 isoforms 1A2, 2C9, 2C19, 2D6, 2E1 and 3A4 (IC50 >150 µM). Given sildenafil peak plasma concentrations of approximately 1 µM after recommended doses, it is unlikely that VIAGRA will alter the clearance of substrates of these isoenzymes.

In vivo **studies**: When VIAGRA 100 mg oral was coadministered with amlodipine, 5 mg or 10 mg oral, to hypertensive patients, the mean additional reduction on supine blood pressure was 8 mmHg systolic and 7 mmHg diastolic.

No significant interactions were shown with tolbutamide (250 mg) or warfarin (40 mg), both of which are metabolized by CYP2C9.

VIAGRA (50 mg) did not potentiate the increase in bleeding time caused by aspirin (150 mg).

VIAGRA (50 mg) did not potentiate the hypotensive effect of alcohol in healthy volunteers with mean maximum blood alcohol levels of 0.08%.

In a study of healthy male volunteers, sildenafil (100 mg) did not affect the steady state pharmacokinetics of the HIV protease inhibitors, saquinavir and ritonavir, both of which are CYP3A4 substrates.

Carcinogenesis, Mutagenesis, Impairment of Fertility

Sildenafil was not carcinogenic when administered to rats for 24 months at a dose resulting in total systemic drug exposure (AUCs) for unbound sildenafil and its major metabolite of 29- and 42-times, for male and female rats, respectively, the exposures observed in human males given the Maximum Recommended Human Dose (MRHD) of 100 mg. Sildenafil was not carcinogenic when administered to mice for 18–21 months at dosages up to the Maximum Tolerated Dose (MTD) of 10 mg/kg/day, approximately 0.6 times the MRHD on a mg/m² basis.

Sildenafil was negative in *in vitro* bacterial and Chinese hamster ovary cell assays to detect mutagenicity, and *in vitro* human lymphocytes and *in vivo* mouse micronucleus assays to detect clastogenicity.

There was no impairment of fertility in rats given sildenafil up to 60 mg/kg/day for 36 days to females and 102 days to males, a dose producing an AUC value of more than 25 times the human male AUC.

There was no effect on sperm motility or morphology after single 100 mg oral doses of VIAGRA in healthy volunteers.

Pregnancy, Nursing Mothers and Pediatric Use

VIAGRA is not indicated for use in newborns, children, or women.

Pregnancy Category B. No evidence of teratogenicity, embryotoxicity or fetotoxicity was observed in rats and rabbits which received up to 200 mg/kg/day during organogenesis. These doses represent, respectively, about 20 and 40 times the MRHD on a mg/m^2 basis in a 50 kg subject. In the rat pre- and postnatal development study, the no observed adverse effect dose was 30 mg/kg/day given for 36 days. In the nonpregnant rat the AUC at this dose was about 20 times human AUC. There are no adequate and well-controlled studies of sildenafil in pregnant women.

Geriatric Use: Healthy elderly volunteers (65 years or over) had a reduced clearance of sildenafil (see **CLINICAL PHARMACOLOGY: Pharmacokinetics in Special Populations**). Since higher plasma levels may increase both the efficacy and incidence of adverse events, a starting dose of 25 mg should be considered (see **DOSAGE AND ADMINISTRATION**).

ADVERSE REACTIONS

PRE-MARKETING EXPERIENCE:

VIAGRA was administered to over 3700 patients (aged 19–87 years) during clinical trials worldwide. Over 550 patients were treated for longer than one year.

In placebo-controlled clinical studies, the discontinuation rate due to adverse events for VIAGRA (2.5%) was not significantly different from placebo (2.3%). The adverse events were generally transient and mild to moderate in nature.

In trials of all designs, adverse events reported by patients receiving VIAGRA were generally similar. In fixed-dose studies, the incidence of some adverse events increased with dose. The nature of the adverse events in flexible-dose studies, which more closely reflect the recommended dosage regimen, was similar to that for fixed-dose studies.

When VIAGRA was taken as recommended (on an as-needed basis) in flexible-dose, placebo-controlled clinical trials, the following adverse events were reported:

TABLE 2. ADVERSE EVENTS REPORTED BY ≥2% OF PATIENTS TREATED WITH VIAGRA AND MORE FREQUENT ON DRUG THAN PLACEBO IN PRN FLEXIBLE-DOSE PHASE II/III STUDIES

Adverse Event	Percentage of Patients Reporting Event	
	VIAGRA N = 734	PLACEBO N = 725
Headache	16%	4%
Flushing	10%	1%
Dyspepsia	7%	2%
Nasal Congestion	4%	2%
Urinary Tract Infection	3%	2%
Abnormal Vision[†]	3%	0%
Diarrhea	3%	1%
Dizziness	2%	1%
Rash	2%	1%

[†] Abnormal Vision: Mild and transient, predominantly color tinge to vision, but also increased sensitivity to light or blurred vision. In these studies, only one patient discontinued due to abnormal vision.

Other adverse reactions occurred at a rate of >2%, but equally common on placebo: respiratory tract infection, back pain, flu syndrome, and arthralgia.

In fixed-dose studies, dyspepsia (17%) and abnormal vision (11%) were more common at 100 mg than at lower doses. At doses above the recommended dose range, adverse events were similar to those detailed above but generally were reported more frequently.

The following events occurred in <2% of patients in controlled clinical trials; a causal relationship to VIAGRA is uncertain. Reported events include those with a plausible relation to drug use; omitted are minor events and reports too imprecise to be meaningful:

Body as a whole: face edema, photosensitivity reaction, shock, asthenia, pain, chills, accidental fall, abdominal pain, allergic reaction, chest pain, accidental injury.

Cardiovascular: angina pectoris, AV block, migraine, syncope, tachycardia, palpitation, hypotension, postural hypotension, myocardial ischemia, cerebral thrombosis, cardiac arrest, heart failure, abnormal electrocardiogram, cardiomyopathy.

Digestive: vomiting, glossitis, colitis, dysphagia, gastritis, gastroenteritis, esophagitis, stomatitis, dry mouth, liver function tests abnormal, rectal hemorrhage, gingivitis.

Hemic and Lymphatic: anemia and leukopenia.

Metabolic and Nutritional: thirst, edema, gout, unstable diabetes, hyperglycemia, peripheral edema, hyperuricemia, hypoglycemic reaction, hypernatremia.

Musculoskeletal: arthritis, arthrosis, myalgia, tendon rupture, tenosynovitis, bone pain, myasthenia, synovitis.

Nervous: ataxia, hypertonia, neuralgia, neuropathy, paresthesia, tremor, vertigo, depression, insomnia, somnolence, abnormal dreams, reflexes decreased, hypesthesia.

Respiratory: asthma, dyspnea, laryngitis, pharyngitis, sinusitis, bronchitis, sputum increased, cough increased.

Skin and Appendages: urticaria, herpes simplex, pruritus, sweating, skin ulcer, contact dermatitis, exfoliative dermatitis.

Special Senses: mydriasis, conjunctivitis, photophobia, tinnitus, eye pain, deafness, ear pain, eye hemorrhage, cataract, dry eyes.

Urogenital: cystitis, nocturia, urinary frequency, breast enlargement, urinary incontinence, abnormal ejaculation, genital edema and anorgasmia.

POST-MARKETING EXPERIENCE:

Cardiovascular and cerebrovascular

Serious cardiovascular, cerebrovascular, and vascular events, including myocardial infarction, sudden cardiac death, ventricular arrhythmia, cerebrovascular hemorrhage, transient ischemic attack, hypertension, subarachnoid and intracerebral hemorrhages, and pulmonary hemorrhage have been reported post-marketing in temporal association with the use of VIAGRA. Most, but not all, of these patients had preexisting cardiovascular risk factors. Many of these events were reported to occur during or shortly after sexual activity, and a few were reported to occur shortly after the use of VIAGRA without sexual activity. Others were reported to have occurred hours to days after the use of VIAGRA and sexual activity. It is not possible to determine whether these events are related directly to VIAGRA, to sexual activity, to the patient's underlying cardiovascular disease, to a combination of these factors, or to other factors (see **WARNINGS** for further important cardiovascular information).

Other events

Other events reported post-marketing to have been observed in temporal association with VIAGRA and not listed in the pre-marketing adverse reactions section above include:

Nervous: seizure and anxiety.

Urogenital: prolonged erection, priapism (see **WARNINGS**) and hematuria.

Special Senses: diplopia, temporary vision loss/decreased vision, ocular redness or bloodshot appearance, ocular burning, ocular swelling/pressure, increased intraocular pressure, retinal vascular disease or bleeding, vitreous detachment/traction, paramacular edema and epistaxis.

OVERDOSAGE

In studies with healthy volunteers of single doses up to 800 mg, adverse events were similar to those seen at lower doses but incidence rates were increased.

In cases of overdose, standard supportive measures should be adopted as required. Renal dialysis is not expected to accelerate clearance as sildenafil is highly bound to plasma proteins and it is not eliminated in the urine.

DOSAGE AND ADMINISTRATION

For most patients, the recommended dose is 50 mg taken, as needed, approximately 1 hour before sexual activity. However, VIAGRA may be taken anywhere from 4 hours to 0.5 hour before sexual activity. Based on effectiveness and toleration, the dose may be increased to a maximum recommended dose of 100 mg or decreased to 25 mg. The maximum recommended dosing frequency is once per day.

The following factors are associated with increased plasma levels of sildenafil: age >65 (40% increase in AUC), hepatic impairment (e.g., cirrhosis, 80%), severe renal impairment (creatinine clearance <30 mL/min, 100%), and concomitant use of potent cytochrome P450 3A4 inhibitors [ketoconazole, itraconazole, erythromycin (182%), saquinavir (210%)]. Since higher plasma levels may increase both the efficacy and incidence of adverse events, a starting dose of 25 mg should be considered in these patients.

Ritonavir greatly increased the systemic level of sildenafil in a study of healthy, non-HIV infected volunteers (11-fold increase in AUC, see **Drug Interactions.**) Based on these pharmacokinetic data, it is recommended not to exceed a maximum single dose of 25 mg of VIAGRA in a 48 hour period.

VIAGRA was shown to potentiate the hypotensive effects of nitrates and its administration in patients who use nitric oxide donors or nitrates in any form is therefore contraindicated.

Simultaneous administration of VIAGRA doses above 25 mg and an alpha-blocker may lead to symptomatic hypotension in some patients. Doses of 50 mg or 100 mg of VIAGRA should not be taken within 4 hours of alpha-blocker administration. A 25 mg dose of VIAGRA may be taken at any time.

HOW SUPPLIED

VIAGRA® (sildenafil citrate) is supplied as blue, film-coated, rounded-diamond-shaped tablets containing sildenafil citrate equivalent to the nominally indicated amount of sildenafil as follows:

[See table above]

	25 mg	50 mg	100 mg
Obverse	VGR25	VGR50	VGR100
Reverse	PFIZER	PFIZER	PFIZER
Bottle of 30	NDC-0069-4200-30	NDC-0069-4210-30	NDC-0069-4220-30
Bottle of 100	N/A	NDC-0069-4210-66	NDC-0069-4220-66

Recommended Storage: Store at 25°C (77°F); excursions permitted to 15-30°C (59-86°F) [see USP Controlled Room Temperature].

℞ Only

Distributed by
Pfizer Labs
Division of Pfizer Inc, NY, NY 10017
69-5485-00-8 Revised September 2002

VIBRAMYCIN® ℞

[*vī-bră-mī-sĭn*]
Calcium
(doxycycline calcium)
oral suspension
SYRUP
Hyclate
(doxycycline hyclate)
CAPSULES
Monohydrate
(doxycycline monohydrate)
for ORAL SUSPENSION

VIBRA-TABS®

(doxycycline hyclate)
FILM COATED TABLETS

Prescribing information for this product, which appears on pages 2656–2658 of the 2003 PDR, has been completely revised as follows. Please write "See Supplement A" next to the product heading.

DESCRIPTION

Vibramycin® is a broad-spectrum antibiotic synthetically derived from oxytetracycline, and is available as Vibramycin Monohydrate (doxycycline monohydrate); Vibramycin Hyclate and Vibra-Tabs (doxycycline hydrochloride hemiethanolate hemihydrate); and Vibramycin Calcium (doxycycline calcium) for oral administration.

The structural formula of doxycycline monohydrate is

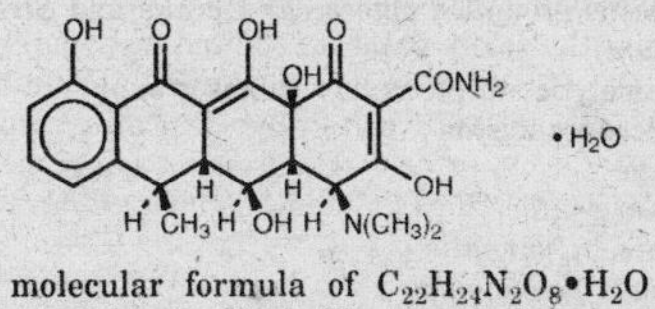

with a molecular formula of $C_{22}H_{24}N_2O_8 \bullet H_2O$ and a molecular weight of 462.46. The chemical designation for doxycycline is 4-(Dimethylamino)-1, 4, 4a, 5, 5a, 6, 11, 12a-octahydro-3, 5, 10, 12, 12a-pentahydroxy-6-methyl-1, 11-dioxo-2-naphthacenecarboxamide monohydrate. The molecular formula for doxycycline hydrochloride hemiethanolate hemihydrate is $(C_{22}H_{24}N_2O_8 \bullet HCl)_2 \bullet C_2H_6O \bullet H_2O$ and the molecular weight is 1025.89. Doxycycline is a light-yellow crystalline powder. Doxycycline hyclate is soluble in water, while doxycycline monohydrate is very slightly soluble in water.

Doxycycline has a high degree of lipoid solubility and a low affinity for calcium binding. It is highly stable in normal human serum. Doxycycline will not degrade into an epianhydro form.

Inert ingredients in the syrup formulation are: apple flavor; butylparaben; calcium chloride; carmine; glycerin; hydrochloric acid; magnesium aluminum silicate; povidone; propylene glycol; propylparaben; raspberry flavor; simethicone emulsion; sodium hydroxide; sodium metabisulfite; sorbitol solution; water.

Inert ingredients in the capsule formulations are: hard gelatin capsules (which may contain Blue 1 and other inert ingredients); magnesium stearate; microcrystalline cellulose; sodium lauryl sulfate.

Inert ingredients for the oral suspension formulation are: carboxymethylcellulose sodium; Blue 1; methylparaben; microcrystalline cellulose; propylparaben; raspberry flavor; Red 28; simethicone emulsion; sucrose.

Inert ingredients for the tablet formulation are: ethylcellulose; hydroxypropyl methylcellulose; magnesium stearate; microcrystalline cellulose; propylene glycol; sodium lauryl sulfate; talc; titanium dioxide; Yellow 6 Lake.

CLINICAL PHARMACOLOGY

Tetracyclines are readily absorbed and are bound to plasma proteins in varying degree. They are concentrated by the liver in the bile, and excreted in the urine and feces at high concentrations and in a biologically active form. Doxycycline is virtually completely absorbed after oral adminstration.

Following a 200 mg dose, normal adult volunteers averaged peak serum levels of 2.6 mcg/mL of doxycycline at 2 hours decreasing to 1.45 mcg/mL at 24 hours. Excretion of doxycycline by the kidney is about 40%/72 hours in individuals with normal function (creatinine clearance about 75 mL/min.). This percentage excretion may fall as low as 1-5%/72 hours in individuals with severe renal insufficiency (creatinine clearance below 10 mL/min.). Studies have

Continued on next page

Vibramycin—Cont.

shown no significant difference in serum half-life of doxycycline (range 18-22 hours) in individuals with normal and severely impaired renal function.
Hemodialysis does not alter serum half-life.
Results of animal studies indicate that tetracyclines cross the placenta and are found in fetal tissues.

Microbiology
The tetracyclines are primarily bacteriostatic and are thought to exert their antimicrobial effect by the inhibition of protein synthesis. The tetracyclines, including doxycycline, have a similar antimicrobial spectrum of activity against a wide range of gram-positive and gram-negative organisms. Cross-resistance of these organisms to tetracyclines is common.

Gram-Negative Bacteria
Neisseria gonorrhoeae
Calymmatobacterium granulomatis
Haemophilus ducreyi
Haemophilus influenzae
Yersinia pestis (formerly *Pasteurella pestis*)
Francisella tularensis (formerly *Pasteurella tularensis*)
Vibrio cholerae (formerly *Vibrio comma*)
Bartonella bacilliformis
Brucella species

Because many strains of the following groups of gram-negative microorganisms have been shown to be resistant to tetracyclines, culture and susceptibility testing are recommended:
Escherichia coli
Klebsiella species
Enterobacter aerogenes
Shigella species
Acinetobacter species (formerly *Mima* species and *Herellea* species)
Bacteroides species

Gram-Positive Bacteria
Because many strains of the following groups of gram-positive microorganisms have been shown to be resistant to tetracycline, culture and susceptibility testing are recommended. Up to 44 percent of strains of *Streptococcus pyogenes* and 74 percent of *Streptococcus faecalis* have been found to be resistant to tetracycline drugs. Therefore, tetracycline should not be used for streptococcal disease unless the organism has been demonstrated to be susceptible.
Streptococcus pyogenes
Streptococcus pneumoniae
Enterococcus group (*Streptococcus faecalis* and *Streptococcus faecium*)
Alpha-hemolytic streptococci (viridans group)

Other Microorganisms
Rickettsiae
Chlamydia psittaci
Chlamydia trachomatis
Mycoplasma pneumoniae
Ureaplasma urealyticum
Borrelia recurrentis
Treponema pallidum
Treponema pertenue
Clostridium species
Fusobacterium fusiforme
Actinomyces species
Bacillus anthracis
Propionibacterium acnes
Entamoeba species
Balantidium coli
Plasmodium falciparum

Doxycycline has been found to be active against the asexual erythrocytic forms of *Plasmodium falciparum* but not against the gametocytes of *P. falciparum*. The precise mechanism of action of the drug is not known.

Susceptibility tests: Diffusion techniques: Quantitative methods that require measurement of zone diameters give the most precise estimate of the susceptibility of bacteria to antimicrobial agents. One such standard procedure[1] which has been recommended for use with disks to test susceptibility of organisms to doxycycline uses the 30-mcg tetracycline-class disk or the 30-mcg doxycycline disk. Interpretation involves the correlation of the diameter obtained in the disk test with the minimum inhibitory concentration (MIC) for tetracycline or doxycycline, respectively.
Reports from the laboratory giving results of the standard single-disk susceptibility test with a 30-mcg tetracycline-class disk or the 30-mcg doxycycline disk should be interpreted according to the following criteria:

Zone Diameter (mm)		Interpretation
tetracycline	doxycycline	
≥19	≥16	Susceptible
15-18	13-15	Intermediate
≤14	≤12	Resistant

A report of "Susceptible" indicates that the pathogen is likely to be inhibited by generally achievable blood levels. A report of "Intermediate" suggests that the organism would be susceptible if a high dosage is used or if the infection is confined to tissues and fluids in which high antimicrobial levels are attained. A report of "Resistant" indicates that achievable concentrations are unlikely to be inhibitory, and other therapy should be selected.
Standardized procedures require the use of laboratory control organisms. The 30-mcg tetracycline-class disk or the 30-mcg doxycycline disk should give the following zone diameters:

Organism	Zone Diameter (mm)	
	tetracycline	doxycycline
E. coli ATCC 25922	18-25	18-24
S. aureus ATCC 25923	19-28	23-29

Dilution techniques: Use a standardized dilution method[2] (broth, agar, microdilution) or equivalent with tetracycline powder. The MIC values obtained should be interpreted according to the following criteria:

MIC (mcg/mL)	Interpretation
≤4	Susceptible
8	Intermediate
≥16	Resistant

As with standard diffusion techniques, dilution methods require the use of laboratory control organisms. Standard tetracycline powder should provide the following MIC values:

Organism	MIC (mcg/mL)
E. coli ATCC 25922	1.0-4.0
S. aureus ATCC 29213	0.25-1.0
E. faecalis ATCC 29212	8-32
P. aeruginosa ATCC 27853	8-32

INDICATIONS AND USAGE

Treatment:
Doxycycline is indicated for the treatment of the following infections:
 Rocky Mountain spotted fever, typhus fever and the typhus group, Q fever, rickettsialpox, and tick fevers caused by Rickettsiae.
 Respiratory tract infections caused by *Mycoplasma pneumoniae*.
 Lymphogranuloma venereum caused by *Chlamydia trachomatis*.
 Psittacosis (ornithosis) caused by *Chlamydia psittaci*.
 Trachoma caused by *Chlamydia trachomatis*, although the infectious agent is not always eliminated as judged by immunofluorescence.
 Inclusion conjunctivitis caused by *Chlamydia trachomatis*.
 Uncomplicated urethral, endocervical or rectal infections in adults caused by *Chlamydia trachomatis*.
 Nongonococcal urethritis caused by *Ureaplasma urealyticum*.
 Relapsing fever due to *Borrelia recurrentis*.
Doxycycline is also indicated for the treatment of infections caused by the following gram-negative microorganisms:
 Chancroid caused by *Haemophilus ducreyi*.
 Plague due to *Yersinia pestis* (formerly *Pasteurella pestis*).
 Tularemia due to *Francisella tularensis* (formerly *Pasteurella tularensis*).
 Cholera caused by *Vibrio cholerae* (formerly *Vibrio comma*).
 Campylobacter fetus infections caused by *Campylobacter fetus* (formerly *Vibrio fetus*).
 Brucellosis due to *Brucella* species (in conjunction with streptomycin).
 Bartonellosis due to *Bartonella bacilliformis*.
 Granuloma inguinale caused by *Calymmatobacterium granulomatis*.
Because many strains of the following groups of microorganisms have been shown to be resistant to doxycycline, culture and susceptibility testing are recommended.
Doxycycline is indicated for treatment of infections caused by the following gram-negative microorganisms, when bacteriologic testing indicates appropriate susceptibility to the drug:
 Escherichia coli.
 Enterobacter aerogenes (formerly *Aerobacter aerogenes*).
 Shigella species.
 Acinetobacter species (formerly *Mima* species and *Herellea* species).
 Respiratory tract infections caused by *Haemophilus influenzae*.
 Respiratory tract and urinary tract infections caused by *Klebsiella* species.
Doxycycline is indicated for treatment of infections caused by the following gram-positive microorganisms when bacteriologic testing indicates appropriate susceptibility to the drug:
 Upper respiratory infections caused by *Streptococcus pneumoniae* (formerly *Diplococcus pneumoniae*).
 Anthrax due to *Bacillus anthracis*, including inhalational anthrax (post-exposure): to reduce the incidence or progression of disease following exposure to aerosolized *Bacillus anthracis*.
When penicillin is contraindicated, doxycycline is an alternative drug in the treatment of the following infections:
 Uncomplicated gonorrhea caused by *Neisseria gonorrhoeae*.
 Syphilis caused by *Treponema pallidum*.
 Yaws caused by *Treponema pertenue*.
 Listeriosis due to *Listeria monocytogenes*.
 Vincent's infection caused by *Fusobacterium fusiforme*.
 Actinomycosis caused by *Actinomyces israelii*.
 Infections caused by *Clostridium* species.
In acute intestinal amebiasis, doxycycline may be a useful adjunct to amebicides.
In severe acne, doxycycline may be useful adjunctive therapy.

Prophylaxis:
Doxycycline is indicated for the prophylaxis of malaria due to *Plasmodium falciparum* in short-term travelers (<4 months) to areas with chloroquine and/or pyrimethamine-sulfadoxine resistant strains. See DOSAGE AND ADMINISTRATION section and Information for Patients subsection of the PRECAUTIONS section.

CONTRAINDICATIONS
This drug is contraindicated in persons who have shown hypersensitivity to any of the tetracyclines.

WARNINGS
THE USE OF DRUGS OF THE TETRACYCLINE CLASS DURING TOOTH DEVELOPMENT (LAST HALF OF PREGNANCY, INFANCY AND CHILDHOOD TO THE AGE OF 8 YEARS) MAY CAUSE PERMANENT DISCOLORATION OF THE TEETH (YELLOW-GRAY-BROWN). This adverse reaction is more common during long-term use of the drugs, but it has been observed following repeated short-term courses. Enamel hypoplasia has also been reported. TETRACYCLINE DRUGS, THEREFORE, SHOULD NOT BE USED IN THIS AGE GROUP, EXCEPT FOR ANTHRAX, INCLUDING INHALATIONAL ANTHRAX (POST-EXPOSURE), UNLESS OTHER DRUGS ARE NOT LIKELY TO BE EFFECTIVE OR ARE CONTRAINDICATED.

Pseudomembranous colitis has been reported with nearly all antibacterial agents, including doxycycline, and may range in severity from mild to life-threatening. Therefore, it is important to consider this diagnosis in patients who present with diarrhea subsequent to the administration of antibacterial agents.
Treatment with antibacterial agents alters the normal flora of the colon and may permit overgrowth of clostridia. Studies indicate that a toxin produced by *Clostridium difficile* is a primary cause of "antibiotic-associated colitis."
After the diagnosis of pseudomembranous colitis has been established, therapeutic measures should be initiated. Mild cases of pseudomembranous colitis usually respond to discontinuation of the drug alone. In moderate to severe cases, consideration should be given to management with fluids and electrolytes, protein supplementation and treatment with an antibacterial drug clinically effective against *Clostridium difficile* colitis.
All tetracyclines form a stable calcium complex in any bone-forming tissue. A decrease in fibula growth rate has been observed in prematures given oral tetracycline in doses of 25 mg/kg every 6 hours. This reaction was shown to be reversible when the drug was discontinued.
Results of animal studies indicate that tetracyclines cross the placenta, are found in fetal tissues, and can have toxic effects on the developing fetus (often related to retardation of skeletal development). Evidence of embryotoxicity has also been noted in animals treated early in pregnancy. If any tetracycline is used during pregnancy or if the patient becomes pregnant while taking this drug, the patient should be apprised of the potential hazard to the fetus.
The antianabolic action of the tetracyclines may cause an increase in BUN. Studies to date indicate that this does not occur with the use of doxycycline in patients with impaired renal function.
Photosensitivity manifested by an exaggerated sunburn reaction has been observed in some individuals taking tetracyclines. Patients apt to be exposed to direct sunlight or ultraviolet light should be advised that this reaction can occur with tetracycline drugs, and treatment should be discontinued at the first evidence of skin erythema.
Vibramycin Syrup contains sodium metabisulfite, a sulfite that may cause allergic-type reactions, including anaphylactic symptoms and life-threatening or less severe asthmatic episodes in certain susceptible people. The overall prevalence of sulfite sensitivity in the general population is unknown and probably low. Sulfite sensitivity is seen more frequently in asthmatic than in non-asthmatic people.

PRECAUTIONS
General
As with other antibiotic preparations, use of this drug may result in overgrowth of nonsusceptible organisms, including fungi. If superinfection occurs, the antibiotic should be discontinued and appropriate therapy instituted.
Bulging fontanels in infants and benign intracranial hypertension in adults have been reported in individuals receiving tetracyclines. These conditions disappeared when the drug was discontinued.
Incision and drainage or other surgical procedures should be performed in conjunction with antibiotic therapy, when indicated.
Doxycycline offers substantial but not complete suppression of the asexual blood stages of *Plasmodium* strains.
Doxycycline does not suppress *P. falciparum's* sexual blood stage gametocytes. Subjects completing this prophylactic regimen may still transmit the infection to mosquitoes outside endemic areas.

Information for Patients
Patients taking doxycycline for malaria prophylaxis should be advised:
— that no present-day antimalarial agent, including doxycycline, guarantees protection against malaria.
— to avoid being bitten by mosquitoes by using personal protective measures that help avoid contact with mosquitoes, especially from dusk to dawn (e.g., staying in well-screened areas, using mosquito nets, covering the body with clothing, and using an effective insect repellent).
— that doxycycline prophylaxis:
— should begin 1-2 days before travel to the malarious area,
— should be continued daily while in the malarious area and after leaving the malarious area,

— should be continued for 4 further weeks to avoid development of malaria after returning from an endemic area,
— should not exceed 4 months.

All patients taking doxycycline should be advised:
— to avoid excessive sunlight or artificial ultraviolet light while receiving doxycycline and to discontinue therapy if phototoxicity (e.g., skin eruption, etc.) occurs. Sunscreen or sunblock should be considered (See WARNINGS.)
— to drink fluids liberally along with doxycycline to reduce the risk of esophageal irritation and ulceration. (See ADVERSE REACTIONS.)
— that the absorption of tetracyclines is reduced when taken with foods, especially those which contain calcium. However, the absorption of doxycycline is not markedly influenced by simultaneous ingestion of food or milk. (See DRUG INTERACTIONS.)
— that the absorption of tetracyclines is reduced when taking bismuth subsalicylate (See DRUG INTERACTIONS.)
— that the use of doxycycline might increase the incidence of vaginal candidiasis.

Laboratory Tests
In venereal disease, when co-existent syphilis is suspected, dark field examinations should be done before treatment is started and the blood serology repeated monthly for at least 4 months.

In long-term therapy, periodic laboratory evaluation of organ systems, including hematopoietic, renal, and hepatic studies, should be performed.

Drug Interactions
Because tetracyclines have been shown to depress plasma prothrombin activity, patients who are on anticoagulant therapy may require downward adjustment of their anticoagulant dosage.

Since bacteriostatic drugs may interfere with the bactericidal action of penicillin, it is advisable to avoid giving tetracyclines in conjunction with penicillin.

Absorption of tetracyclines is impaired by antacids containing aluminum, calcium, or magnesium, and iron-containing preparations.

Absorption of tetracyclines is impaired by bismuth subsalicylate.

Barbiturates, carbamazepine, and phenytoin decrease the half-life of doxycycline.

The concurrent use of tetracycline and Penthrane® (methoxyflurane) has been reported to result in fatal renal toxicity.

Concurrent use of tetracycline may render oral contraceptives less effective.

Drug/Laboratory Test Interactions
False elevations of urinary catecholamine levels may occur due to interference with the fluorescence test.

Carcinogenesis, Mutagenesis, Impairment of Fertility
Long-term studies in animals to evaluate carcinogenic potential of doxycycline have not been conducted. However, there has been evidence of oncogenic activity in rats in studies with the related antibiotics, oxytetracycline (adrenal and pituitary tumors), and minocycline (thyroid tumors). Likewise, although mutagenicity studies of doxycycline have not been conducted, positive results in in vitro mammalian cell assays have been reported for related antibiotics (tetracycline, oxytetracycline).

Doxycycline administered orally at dosage levels as high as 250 mg/kg/day had no apparent effect on the fertility of female rats. Effect on male fertility has not been studied.

Pregnancy: Teratogenic Effects. Pregnancy Category D: There are no adequate and well-controlled studies on the use of doxycycline in pregnant women. The vast majority of reported experience with doxycycline during human pregnancy is short-term, first trimester exposure. There are no human data available to assess the effects of long-term therapy of doxycycline in pregnant women such as that proposed for treatment of anthrax exposure. An expert review of published data on experiences with doxycycline use during pregnancy by TERIS – the Teratogen Information System – concluded that therapeutic doses during pregnancy are unlikely to pose a substantial teratogenic risk (the quantity and quality of data were assessed as limited to fair), but the data are insufficient to state that there is no risk[a]. A case-control study (18,515 mothers of infants with congenital anomalies and 32,804 mothers of infants with no congenital anomalies) shows a weak but marginally statistically significant association with total malformations and use of doxycycline anytime during pregnancy. Sixty-three (0.19%) of the controls and fifty-six (0.30%) of the cases were treated with doxycycline. This association was not seen when the analysis was confined to maternal treatment during the period of organogenesis (i.e., in the second and third months of gestation) with the exception of a marginal relationship with neural tube defect based on only two exposed cases[b].

A small prospective study of 81 pregnancies describes 43 pregnant women treated for 10 days with doxycycline during early first trimester. All mothers reported their exposed infants were normal at 1 year of age[c].

Nonteratogenic effects: (See WARNINGS).

Labor and Delivery
The effect of tetracyclines on labor and delivery is unknown.

Nursing Mothers
Tetracyclines are excreted in human milk; however, the extent of absorption of tetracyclines, including doxycycline, by the breastfed infant is not known. Short-term use by lactating women is not necessarily contraindicated; however, the effects of prolonged exposure to doxycycline in breast milk are unknown[d]. Because of the potential for serious adverse reactions in nursing infants from doxycycline, a decision should be made whether to discontinue nursing or to discontinue the drug, taking into account the importance of the drug to the mother. (See WARNINGS.)

Pediatric Use
See WARNINGS and DOSAGE AND ADMINISTRATION.

ADVERSE REACTIONS
Due to oral doxycycline's virtually complete absorption, side effects of the lower bowel, particularly diarrhea, have been infrequent. The following adverse reactions have been observed in patients receiving tetracyclines:

Gastrointestinal: anorexia, nausea, vomiting, diarrhea, glossitis, dysphagia, enterocolitis, and inflammatory lesions (with monilial overgrowth) in the anogenital region. Hepatotoxicity has been reported rarely. These reactions have been caused by both the oral and parenteral administration of tetracyclines. Rare instances of esophagitis and esophageal ulcerations have been reported in patients receiving capsule and tablet forms of the drugs in the tetracycline class. Most of these patients took medications immediately before going to bed. (See DOSAGE AND ADMINISTRATION.)

Skin: maculopapular and erythematous rashes. Exfoliative dermatitis has been reported but is uncommon. Photosensitivity is discussed above. (See WARNINGS.)

Renal toxicity: Rise in BUN has been reported and is apparently dose related. (See WARNINGS.)

Hypersensitivity reactions: urticaria, angioneurotic edema, anaphylaxis, anaphylactoid purpura, serum sickness, pericarditis, and exacerbation of systemic lupus erythematosus.

Blood: Hemolytic anemia, thrombocytopenia, neutropenia, and eosinophilia have been reported.

Other: bulging fontanels in infants and intracranial hypertension in adults. (See PRECAUTIONS – General.)

When given over prolonged periods, tetracyclines have been reported to produce brown-black microscopic discoloration of the thyroid gland. No abnormalities of thyroid function studies are known to occur.

OVERDOSAGE
In case of overdosage, discontinue medication, treat symptomatically and institute supportive measures. Dialysis does not alter serum half-life and thus would not be of benefit in treating cases of overdosage.

DOSAGE AND ADMINISTRATION
THE USUAL DOSAGE AND FREQUENCY OF ADMINISTRATION OF DOXYCYCLINE DIFFERS FROM THAT OF THE OTHER TETRACYCLINES. EXCEEDING THE RECOMMENDED DOSAGE MAY RESULT IN AN INCREASED INCIDENCE OF SIDE EFFECTS. Adults: The usual dose of oral doxycycline is 200 mg on the first day of treatment (administered 100 mg every 12 hours) followed by a maintenance dose of 100 mg/day. The maintenance dose may be administered as a single dose or as 50 mg every 12 hours.

In the management of more severe infections (particularly chronic infections of the urinary tract), 100 mg every 12 hours is recommended.

For children above eight years of age: The recommended dosage schedule for children weighing 100 pounds or less is 2 mg/lb of body weight divided into two doses on the first day of treatment, followed by 1 mg/lb of body weight given as a single daily dose or divided into two doses, on subsequent days. For more severe infections up to 2 mg/lb of body weight may be used. For children over 100 lb the usual adult dose should be used.

The therapeutic antibacterial serum activity will usually persist for 24 hours following recommended dosage.

When used in streptococcal infections, therapy should be continued for 10 days.

Administration of adequate amounts of fluid along with capsule and tablet forms of drugs in the tetracycline class is recommended to wash down the drugs and reduce the risk of esophageal irritation and ulceration. (See ADVERSE REACTIONS.)

If gastric irritation occurs, it is recommended that doxycycline be given with food or milk. The absorption of doxycycline is not markedly influenced by simultaneous ingestion of food or milk.

Studies to date have indicated that administration of doxycycline at the usual recommended doses does not lead to excessive accumulation of the antibiotic in patients with renal impairment.

Uncomplicated gonococcal infections in adults (except anorectal infections in men): 100 mg, by mouth, twice a day for 7 days. As an alternate single visit dose, administer 300 mg stat followed in one hour by a second 300 mg dose. The dose may be administered with food, including milk or carbonated beverage, as required.

Uncomplicated urethral, endocervical, or rectal infection in adults caused by *Chlamydia trachomatis*: 100 mg by mouth twice a day for 7 days.

Nongonococcal urethritis (NGU) caused by *C. trachomatis* or *U. urealyticum*: 100 mg by mouth twice a day for 7 days.

Syphilis – early: Patients who are allergic to penicillin should be treated with doxycycline 100 mg by mouth twice a day for 2 weeks.

Syphilis of more than one year's duration: Patients who are allergic to penicillin should be treated with doxycycline 100 mg by mouth twice a day for 4 weeks.

Acute epididymo-orchitis caused by *N. gonorrhoeae*: 100 mg, by mouth, twice a day for at least 10 days.

Acute epididymo-orchitis caused by *C. trachomatis*: 100 mg, by mouth, twice a day for at least 10 days.

For prophylaxis of malaria: For adults, the recommended dose is 100 mg daily. For children over 8 years of age, the recommended dose is 2 mg/kg given once daily up to the adult dose. Prophylaxis should begin 1-2 days before travel to the malarious area. Prophylaxis should be continued daily during travel in the malarious area and for 4 weeks after the traveler leaves the malarious area.

Inhalational anthrax (post-exposure):
ADULTS: 100 mg of doxycycline, by mouth, twice a day for 60 days.
CHILDREN: weighing less than 100 lb (45 kg); 1 mg/lb (2.2 mg/kg) of body weight, by mouth, twice a day for 60 days. Children weighing 100 lb or more should receive the adult dose.

HOW SUPPLIED
Vibramycin® Hyclate (doxycycline hyclate) is available in capsules containing doxycycline hyclate equivalent to:

50 mg doxycycline
bottles of 50 (NDC 0069-0940-50)
The capsules are white and light blue and are imprinted with "VIBRA" on one half and "PFIZER 094" on the other half.

100 mg doxycycline
bottles of 50 (NDC 0069-0950-50)
The capsules are light blue and are imprinted with "VIBRA" on one half and "PFIZER 095" on the other half.

Vibra-Tabs® (doxycycline hyclate) is available in salmon colored film-coated tablets containing doxycycline hyclate equivalent to:

100 mg doxycycline
bottles of 50 (NDC 0069-0990-50)
The tablets are imprinted on one side with "VIBRA-TABS" and "PFIZER 099" on the other side.

Vibramycin® Calcium Syrup (doxycycline calcium) oral suspension is available as a raspberry-apple flavored oral suspension. Each teaspoonful (5 mL) contains doxycycline calcium equivalent to 50 mg of doxycycline: 1 pint (473 mL) bottles (NDC 0069-0971-93).

Vibramycin® Monohydrate (doxycycline monohydrate) for Oral Suspension is available as a raspberry-flavored, dry powder for oral suspension. When reconstituted, each teaspoonful (5 mL) contains doxycycline monohydrate equivalent to 25 mg of doxycycline: 2 oz (60 mL) bottles (NDC 0069-0970-65).

All products are to be stored below 86°F (30°C) and dispensed in tight, light-resistant containers (USP).

ANIMAL PHARMACOLOGY AND ANIMAL TOXICOLOGY
Hyperpigmentation of the thyroid has been produced by members of the tetracycline class in the following species: in rats by oxytetracycline, doxycycline, tetracycline PO_4, and methacycline; in minipigs by doxycycline, minocycline, tetracycline PO_4, and methacycline; in dogs by doxycycline and minocycline; in monkeys by minocycline.

Minocycline, tetracycline PO_4, methacycline, doxycycline, tetracycline base, oxytetracycline HCl, and tetracycline HCl were goitrogenic in rats fed a low iodine diet. This goitrogenic effect was accompanied by high radioactive iodine uptake. Administration of minocycline also produced a large goiter with high radioiodine uptake in rats fed a relatively high iodine diet.

Treatment of various animal species with this class of drugs has also resulted in the induction of thyroid hyperplasia in the following: in rats and dogs (minocycline); in chickens (chlortetracycline); and in rats and mice (oxytetracycline). Adrenal gland hyperplasia has been observed in goats and rats treated with oxytetracycline.

REFERENCES
1. National Committee for Clinical Laboratory Standards, *Performance Standards for Antimicrobial Disk Susceptibility Tests*, Fourth Edition. Approved Standard NCCLS Document M2-A4, Vol. 10, No. 7 NCCLS, Villanova, PA, April 1990.
2. National Committee for Clinical Laboratory Standards, *Methods for Dilution Antimicrobial Susceptibility Tests for Bacteria that Grow Aerobically*, Second Edition. Approved Standard NCCLS Document M7-A2, Vol. 10, No. 8 NCCLS, Villanova, PA, April 1990.
3. [a]Friedman JM and Polifka JE. *Teratogenic Effects of Drugs. A Resource for Clinicians (TERIS)*. Baltimore, MD: The Johns Hopkins University Press, 2000: 149-195.
[b]Cziezel AE and Rockenbauer M. Teratogenic study of doxycycline. *Obstet Gynecol* 1997; 89: 524-528.
[c]Horne HW Jr and Kundsin RB. The role of mycoplasma among 81 consecutive pregnancies: a prospective study. *Int J Fertil* 1980; 25: 315-317.
[d]Hale T. *Medications and Mothers Milk*. 9th edition. Amarillo, TX: Pharmasoft Publishing, 2000: 225-226.

©2002 Pfizer Inc.
℞ only
Pfizer Labs
Division of Pfizer Inc, NY, NY 10017
69-1680-32-7   Revised May 2002

ZITHROMAX®   ℞
(azithromycin tablets)
and
(azithromycin for oral suspension)

Prescribing information for this product, which appears on pages 2661–2667 of the 2003 PDR, has been completely revised as follows. Please write "See Supplement A" next to the product heading.

Continued on next page

Zithromax Tabs/O.S.—Cont.

DESCRIPTION

ZITHROMAX® (azithromycin tablets and azithromycin for oral suspension) contain the active ingredient azithromycin, an azalide, a subclass of macrolide antibiotics, for oral administration. Azithromycin has the chemical name (*2R,3S,4R,5R,8R, 10R,11R,12S,13S,14R*)- 13-[(2,6-dideoxy-3-*C*-methyl-3-*O*-methyl-α-*L*-*ribo*-hexopyranosyl)oxy]-2-ethyl-3,4,10-trihydroxy-3,5,6,8,10,12,14-heptamethyl-11-[[3,4,6-trideoxy-3-(dimethylamino)-β-*D*-*xylo*-hexopyranosyl]oxy]-1-oxa-6-azacyclopentadecan-15-one. Azithromycin is derived from erythromycin; however, it differs chemically from erythromycin in that a methyl-substituted nitrogen atom is incorporated into the lactone ring. Its molecular formula is $C_{38}H_{72}N_2O_{12}$, and its molecular weight is 749.00. Azithromycin has the following structural formula:

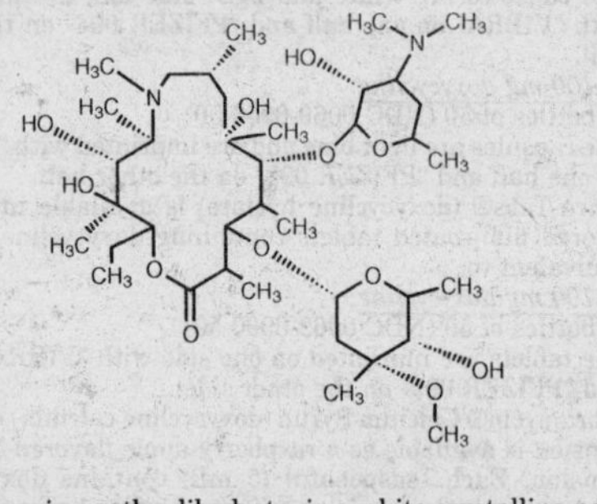

Azithromycin, as the dihydrate, is a white crystalline powder with a molecular formula of $C_{38}H_{72}N_2O_{12}•2H_2O$ and a molecular weight of 785.0.

ZITHROMAX® is supplied for oral administration as film-coated, modified capsular shaped tablets containing azithromycin dihydrate equivalent to either 250 mg or 500 mg azithromycin and the following inactive ingredients: dibasic calcium phosphate anhydrous, pregelatinized starch, sodium croscarmellose, magnesium stearate, sodium lauryl sulfate, hydroxypropyl methylcellulose, lactose, titanium dioxide, triacetin and D&C Red #30 aluminum lake. ZITHROMAX® for oral suspension is supplied in bottles containing azithromycin dihydrate powder equivalent to 300 mg, 600 mg, 900 mg, or 1200 mg azithromycin per bottle and the following inactive ingredients: sucrose; sodium phosphate, tribasic, anhydrous; hydroxypropyl cellulose; xanthan gum; FD&C Red #40; and spray dried artificial cherry, creme de vanilla and banana flavors. After constitution, each 5 mL of suspension contains 100 mg or 200 mg of azithromycin.

CLINICAL PHARMACOLOGY

Pharmacokinetics

Following oral administration of a single 500 mg dose (two 250 mg tablets) to 36 fasted healthy male volunteers, the mean (SD) pharmacokinetic parameters were AUC_{0-72} = 4.3 (1.2) μg•hr/mL; C_{max} = 0.5 (0.2) μg/mL; T_{max} = 2.2 (0.9) hours.

With a regimen of 500 mg (two 250 mg capsules*) on day 1, followed by 250 mg daily (one 250 mg capsule) on days 2 through 5, the pharmacokinetic parameters of azithromycin in plasma in healthy young adults (18-40 years of age) are portrayed in the chart below. C_{min} and C_{max} remained essentially unchanged from day 2 through day 5 of therapy.

Pharmacokinetic Parameters (Mean)	Total n=12 Day 1	Day 5
C_{max} (μg/mL)	0.41	0.24
T_{max} (h)	2.5	3.2
AUC_{0-24} (μg/•h/mL)	2.6	2.1
C_{min} (μg/mL)	0.05	0.05
Urinary Excret. (% dose)	4.5	6.5

*Azithromycin 250 mg tablets are bioequivalent to 250 mg capsules in the fasted state. Azithromycin 250 mg capsules are no longer commercially available.

In a two-way crossover study, 12 adult healthy volunteers (6 males, 6 females) received 1,500 mg of azithromycin administered in single daily doses over either 5 days (two 250 mg tablets on day 1, followed by one 250 mg tablet on days 2-5) or 3 days (500 mg per day for days 1-3). Due to limited serum samples on day 2 (3-day regimen) and days 2-4 (5-day regimen), the serum concentration-time profile of each subject was fit to a 3-compartment model and the $AUC_{0-\infty}$ for the fitted concentration profile was comparable between the 5-day and 3-day regimens.

[See first table at right]

Pharmackoinetic Parameter [mean (SD)]	3-Day Regimen Day 1	3-Day Regimen Day 3	5-Day Regimen Day 1	5-Day Regimen Day 5
C_{max} (serum, μg/mL)	0.44 (0.22)	0.54 (0.25)	0.43 (0.20)	0.24 (0.06)
Serum $AUC_{0-\infty}$(μg•hr/mL)	17.4 (6.2)*		14.9 (3.1)*	
Serum $T_{1/2}$	71.8 hr		68.9 hr	

*Total AUC for the entire 3-day and 5-day regimens

Median azithromycin exposure (AUC_{0-288}) in mononuclear (MN) and polymorphonuclear (PMN) leukocytes following either the 5-day or 3-day regimen was more than a 1000-fold and 800-fold greater than in serum, respectively. Administration of the same total dose with either the 5-day or 3-day regimen may be expected to provide comparable concentrations of azithromycin within MN and PMN leukocytes.

Two azithromycin 250 mg tablets are bioequivalent to a single 500 mg tablet.

Absorption

The absolute bioavailability of azithromycin 250 mg capsules is 38%.

In a two-way crossover study in which 12 healthy subjects received a single 500 mg dose of azithromycin (two 250 mg tablets) with or without a high fat meal, food was shown to increase C_{max} by 23% but had no effect on AUC.

When azithromycin suspension was administered with food to 28 adult healthy male subjects, C_{max} increased by 56% and AUC was unchanged.

The AUC of azithromycin was unaffected by co-administration of an antacid containing aluminum and magnesium hydroxide with azithromycin capsules; however, the C_{max} was reduced by 24%. Administration of cimetidine (800 mg) two hours prior to azithromycin had no effect on azithromycin absorption.

Distribution

The serum protein binding of azithromycin is variable in the concentration range approximating human exposure, decreasing from 51% at 0.02 μg/mL to 7% at 2 μg/mL.

Following oral administration, azithromycin is widely distributed throughout the body with an apparent steady-state volume of distribution of 31.1 L/kg. Greater azithromycin concentrations in tissues than in plasma or serum were observed. High tissue concentrations should not be interpreted to be quantitatively related to clinical efficacy. The antimicrobial activity of azithromycin is pH related and appears to be reduced with decreasing pH. However, the extensive distribution of drug to tissues may be relevant to clinical activity.

Selected tissue (or fluid) concentration and tissue (or fluid) to plasma/serum concentration ratios are shown in the following table:

[See second table above]

AZITHROMYCIN CONCENTRATIONS FOLLOWING A 500 mg DOSE (TWO 250 mg CAPSULES) IN ADULTS[1]

TISSUE OR FLUID	TIME AFTER DOSE (h)	TISSUE OR FLUID CONCENTRATION (μg/g or μg/mL)	CORRESPONSING PLASMA OR SERUM LEVEL (μg/mL)	TISSUE (FLUID) PLASMA (SERUM) RATIO
SKIN	72-96	0.4	0.012	35
LUNG	72-96	4.0	0.012	>100
SPUTUM*	2-4	1.0	0.64	2
SPUTUM**	10-12	2.9	0.1	30
TONSIL***	9-18	4.5	0.03	>100
TONSIL***	180	0.9	0.006	>100
CERVIX****	19	2.8	0.04	70

[1] Azithromycin tissue concentrations were originally determined using 250 mg capsules.
* Sample was obtained 2-4 hours after the first dose.
** Sample was obtained 10-12 hours after the first dose.
*** Dosing regimen of two doses of 250 mg each, separated by 12 hours.
**** Sample was obtained 19 hours after a single 500 mg dose.

The extensive tissue distribution was confirmed by examination of additional tissues and fluids (bone, ejaculum, prostate, ovary, uterus, salpinx, stomach, liver, and gallbladder). As there are no data from adequate and well-controlled studies of azithromycin treatment of infections in these additional body sites, the clinical importance of these tissue concentration data is unknown.

Following a regimen of 500 mg on the first day and 250 mg daily for 4 days, only very low concentrations were noted in cerebrospinal fluid (less than 0.01 μg/mL) in the presence of non-inflamed meninges.

Metabolism

In vitro and *in vivo* studies to assess the metabolism of azithromycin have not been performed.

Elimination

Plasma concentrations of azithromycin following single 500 mg oral and i.v. doses declined in a polyphasic pattern with a mean apparent plasma clearance of 630 mL/min and terminal elimination half-life of 68 hours. The prolonged terminal half-life is thought to be due to extensive uptake and subsequent release of drug from tissues.

Biliary excretion of azithromycin, predominantly as unchanged drug, is a major route of elimination. Over the course of a week, approximately 6% of the administered dose appears as unchanged drug in urine.

Special Populations

Renal Insufficiency

Azithromycin pharmacokinetics were investigated in 42 adults (21 to 85 years of age) with varying degrees of renal impairment. Following the oral administration of a single 1,000 mg dose of azithromycin, mean C_{max} and AUC_{0-120} increased by 5.1% and 4.2%, respectively in subjects with mild to moderate renal impairment (GFR 10 to 80 mL/min) compared to subjects with normal renal function (GFR >80 mL/min). The mean C_{max} and AUC_{0-120} increased 61% and 35%, respectively in subjects with severe renal impairment (GFR <10 mL/min) compared to subjects with normal renal function (GFR >80 mL/min). (See **DOSAGE AND ADMINISTRATION.**)

Hepatic Insufficiency

The pharmacokinetics of azithromycin in subjects with hepatic impairment have not been established.

Gender

There are no significant differences in the disposition of azithromycin between male and female subjects. No dosage adjustment is recommended based on gender.

Geriatric Patients

When studied in healthy elderly subjects aged 65 to 85 years, the pharmacokinetic parameters of azithromycin in elderly men were similar to those in young adults; however, in elderly women, although higher peak concentrations (increased by 30 to 50%) were observed, no significant accumulation occurred.

Pediatric Patients

In two clinical studies, azithromycin for oral suspension was dosed at 10 mg/kg on day 1, followed by 5 mg/kg on days 2 through 5 to two groups of children (aged 1-5 years and 5-15 years, respectively). The mean pharmacokinetic parameters on day 5 were C_{max}=0.216 μg/mL, T_{max}=1.9 hours, and AUC_{0-24}=1.822 μg•hr/mL for the 1- to 5-year-old group and were C_{max}=0.383 μg/mL, T_{max}=2.4 hours, and AUC_{0-24}=3.109 μg•hr/mL for the 5- to 15-year-old group.

Two clinical studies were conducted in 68 children aged 3-16 years to determine the pharmacokinetics and safety of azithromycin for oral suspension in children. Azithromycin was administered following a low-fat breakfast.

The first study consisted of 35 pediatric patients treated with 20 mg/kg/day (maximum daily dose 500 mg) for 3 days of whom 34 patients were evaluated for pharmacokinetics.

In the second study, 33 pediatric patients received doses of 12 mg/kg/day (maximum daily dose 500 mg) for 5 days of whom 31 patients were evaluated for pharmacokinetics.

In both studies, azithromycin concentrations were determined over a 24 hour period following the last daily dose. Patients weighing above 25.0 kg in the 3-day study or 41.7 kg in the 5-day study received the maximum adult daily dose of 500 mg. Eleven patients (weighing 25.0 kg or less) in the first study and 17 patients (weighing 41.7 kg or less) in the second study received a total dose of 60 mg/kg. The following table shows pharmacokinetic data in the subset of children who received a total dose of 60 mg/kg.

Pharmacokinetic Parameter [mean (SD)]	3-Day Regimen (20 mg/kg × 3 days)	5-Day Regimen (12 mg/kg × 5 days)
n	11	17
C_{max} (μg/mL)	1.1 (0.4)	0.5 (0.4)
T_{max} (hr)	2.7 (1.9)	2.2 (0.8)
AUC_{0-24} (μg•hr/mL)	7.9 (2.9)	3.9 (1.9)

The similarity of the overall exposure ($AUC_{0-\infty}$) between the 3-day and 5-day regimens in pediatric patients is unknown.

Single dose pharmacokinetics in children given doses of 30 mg/kg have not been studied. (See **DOSAGE AND ADMINISTRATION.**)

Drug-Drug Interactions

Drug interaction studies were performed with azithromycin and other drugs likely to be co-administered. The effects of co-administration of azithromycin on the pharmacokinetics of other drugs are shown in Table 1 and the effect of other drugs on the pharmacokinetics of azithromycin are shown in Table 2.

Co-administration of azithromycin at therapeutic doses had a modest effect on the pharmacokinetics of the drugs listed in Table 1. No dosage adjustment of drugs listed in Table 1 is recommended when co-administered with azithromycin. Co-administration of azithromycin with efavirenz or fluconazole had a modest effect on the pharmacokinetics of azithromycin. Nelfinavir significantly increased the C_{max} and AUC of azithromycin. No dosage adjustment of azithromycin is recommended when administered with drugs listed in Table 2. (See **PRECAUTIONS - Drug Interactions.**)

[See table 1 at right]
[See table 2 at top of next page]

Microbiology: Azithromycin acts by binding to the 50S ribosomal subunit of susceptible microorganisms and, thus, interfering with microbial protein synthesis. Nucleic acid synthesis is not affected.

Azithromycin concentrates in phagocytes and fibroblasts as demonstrated by *in vitro* incubation techniques. Using such methodology, the ratio of intracellular to extracellular concentration was >30 after one hour incubation. *In vivo* studies suggest that concentration in phagocytes may contribute to drug distribution to inflamed tissues.

Azithromycin has been shown to be active against most isolates of the following microorganisms, both *in vitro* and in clinical infections as described in the **INDICATIONS AND USAGE** section.

Aerobic and facultative gram-positive microorganisms
Staphylococcus aureus
Streptococcus agalactiae
Streptococcus pneumoniae
Streptococcus pyogenes

NOTE: Azithromycin demonstrates cross-resistance with erythromycin-resistant gram-positive strains. Most strains of *Enterococcus faecalis* and methicillin-resistant staphylococci are resistant to azithromycin.

Aerobic and facultative gram-negative microorganisms
Haemophilus ducreyi
Haemophilus influenzae
Moraxella catarrhalis
Neisseria gonorrhoeae

"Other" microorganisms
Chlamydia pneumoniae
Chlamydia trachomatis
Mycoplasma pneumoniae

Beta-lactamase production should have no effect on azithromycin activity.

The following *in vitro* data are available, **but their clinical significance is unknown.**

At least 90% of the following microorganisms exhibit an *in vitro* minimum inhibitory concentration (MIC) less than or equal to the susceptible breakpoints for azithromycin. However, the safety and effectiveness of azithromycin in treating clinical infections due to these microorganisms have not been established in adequate and well-controlled trials.

Aerobic and facultative gram-positive microorganisms
Streptococci (Groups C, F, G)
Viridans group streptococci

Aerobic and facultative gram-negative microorganisms
Bordetella pertussis
Legionella pneumophila

Anaerobic microorganisms
Peptostreptococcus species
Prevotella bivia

"Other" microorganisms
Ureaplasma urealyticum

Susceptibility Testing Methods:
When available, the results of *in vitro* susceptibility test results for antimicrobial drugs used in resident hospitals should be provided to the physician as periodic reports which describe the susceptibility profile of nosocomial and community-acquired pathogens. These reports may differ from susceptibility data obtained from outpatient use, but could aid the physician in selecting the most effective antimicrobial.

Dilution techniques:
Quantitative methods are used to determine antimicrobial minimum inhibitory concentrations (MICs). These MICs provide estimates of the susceptibility of bacteria to antimicrobial compounds. The MICs should be determined using a standardized procedure. Standardized procedures are based on a dilution method[1,3] (broth or agar) or equivalent with standardized inoculum concentrations and standardized concentrations of azithromycin powder. The MIC values should be interpreted according to criteria provided in Table 1.

Diffusion techniques:
Quantitative methods that require measurement of zone diameters also provide reproducible estimates of the susceptibility of bacteria to antimicrobial compounds. One such standardized procedure[2,3] requires the use of standardized inoculum concentrations. This procedure uses paper disks impregnated with 15-µg azithromycin to test the susceptibility of microorganisms to azithromycin. The disk diffusion interpretive criteria are provided in Table 1.

[See table 1 on next page]
No interpretive criteria have been established for testing *Neisseria gonorrhoeae*. This species is not usually tested.

A report of "susceptible" indicates that the pathogen is likely to be inhibited if the antimicrobial compound reaches the concentrations usually achievable. A report of "intermediate" indicates that the result should be considered equivocal, and, if the microorganism is not fully susceptible to alternative, clinically feasible drugs, the test should be repeated. This category implies possible clinical applicability in body sites where the drug is physiologically concentrated or in situations where high dosage of drug can be used. This category also provides a buffer zone which prevents small uncontrolled technical factors from causing major discrepancies in interpretation. A report of "resistant" indicates that the pathogen is not likely to be inhibited if the antimicrobial compound reaches the concentrations usually achievable; other therapy should be selected.

QUALITY CONTROL:
Standardized susceptibility test procedures require the use of quality control microorganisms to control the technical aspects of the test procedures. Standard azithromycin powder should provide the following range of values noted in Table 2. Quality control microorganisms are specific strains of organisms with intrinsic biological properties. QC strains are very stable strains which will give a standard and repeatable susceptibility pattern. The specific strains used for microbiological quality control are not clinically significant.
[See table 2 at top of next page]

INDICATIONS AND USAGE
ZITHROMAX® (azithromycin) is indicated for the treatment of patients with mild to moderate infections (pneumonia: see **WARNINGS**) caused by susceptible strains of the designated microorganisms in the specific conditions listed below. As recommended dosages, durations of therapy and applicable patient populations vary among these infections, please see **DOSAGE AND ADMINISTRATION** for specific dosing recommendations.

Adults:
Acute bacterial exacerbations of chronic obstructive pulmonary disease due to *Haemophilus influenzae*, *Moraxella catarrhalis* or *Streptococcus pneumoniae*.
Community-acquired pneumonia due to *Chlamydia pneumoniae*, *Haemophilus influenzae*, *Mycoplasma pneumoniae* or *Streptococcus pneumoniae* in patients appropriate for oral therapy.
NOTE: Azithromycin should not be used in patients with pneumonia who are judged to be inappropriate for oral therapy because of moderate to severe illness or risk factors such as any of the following:
   patients with cystic fibrosis,
   patients with nosocomially acquired infections,
   patients with known or suspected bacteremia,
   patients requiring hospitalization,
   elderly or debilitated patients, or
   patients with significant underlying health problems that may compromise their ability to respond to their illness (including immunodeficiency or functional asplenia).

Pharyngitis/tonsillitis caused by *Streptococcus pyogenes* as an alternative to first-line therapy in individuals who cannot use first-line therapy.

Continued on next page

Table 1. Drug Interactions: Pharmacokinetic Parameters for Co-administered Drugs in the Presence of Azithromycin

Co-administered Drug	Dose of Co-administered Drug	Dose of Azithromycin	n	Ratio (with/without azithromycin) of Co-administered Drug Pharmacokinetic Parameters (90% CI); No Effect = 1.00	
				Mean C_{max}	Mean AUC
Atrovastatin	10 mg/day × 8 days	500 mg/day PO on days 6-8	12	0.83 (0.63 to 1.08)	1.01 (0.81 to 1.25)
Carbamazepine	200 mg/day × 2 days, then 200 mg BID × 18 days	500 mg/day PO for days 16-18	7	0.97 (0.88 to 1.06)	0.96 (0.88 to 1.06)
Cetirizine	20 mg/day × 11 days	500 mg PO on day 7, then 250 mg day on days 8-11	14	1.03 (0.93 to 1.14)	1.02 (0.92 to 1.13)
Didanosine	200 mg PO BID × 21 days	1,200 mg/day PO on days 8-21	6	1.44 (0.85 to 2.43)	1.14 (0.83 to 1.57)
Efavirenz	400 mg/day × 7 days	600 mg PO on day 7	14	1.04*	0.95*
Fluconazole	200 mg PO single dose	1,200 mg PO single dose	18	1.04 (0.98 to 1.11)	1.01 (0.97 to 1.05)
Indinavir	800 mg TID × 5 days	1,200 mg PO on day 5	18	0.96 (0.86 to 1.08)	0.90 (0.81 to 1.00)
Midazolam	15 mg PO on day 3	500 mg/day PO × 3 days	12	1.27 (0.89 to 1.81)	1.26 (1.01 to 1.56)
Nelfinavir	750 mg TID × 11 days	1,200 mg PO on day 9	14	0.90 (0.81 to 1.01)	0.85 (0.78 to 0.93)
Rifabutin	300 mg/day × 10 days	500 mg PO on day 1, then 250 mg/day on days 2–10	6	See footnote below	NA
Sildenafil	100 mg on days 1 and 4	500 mg/day PO × 3 days	12	1.16 (0.86 to 1.57)	0.92 (0.75 to 1.12)
Theophylline	4 mg/kg IV on days 1, 11, 25	500 mg PO on day 7, 250 mg/day on days 8-11	10	1.19 (1.02 to 1.40)	1.02 (0.86 to 1.22)
Theophylline	300 mg PO BID × 15 days	500 mg PO on day 6, then 250 mg/day on days 7-10	8	1.09 (0.92 to 1.29)	1.08 (0.89 to 1.31)
Triazolam	0.125 mg on day 2	500 mg PO on day 1, then 250 mg/day on day 2	12	1.06*	1.02*
Trimethoprim/Sulfamethoxazole	160 mg/800 mg/day PO × 7 days	1,200 mg PO on day 7	12	0.85 (0.75 to 0.97)/ 0.90 (0.78 to 1.03)	0.87 (0.80 to 0.95)/ 0.96 (0.88 to 1.03)
Zidovudine	500 mg/day PO × 21 days	600 mg/day PO × 14 days	5	1.12 (0.42 to 3.02)	0.94 (0.52 to 1.70)
Zidovudine	500 mg/day PO × 21 days	1,200 mg/day PO × 14 days	4	1.31 (0.43 to 3.97)	1.30 (0.69 to 2.43)

NA - Not Available
* - 90% Confidence interval not reported
Mean rifabutin concentrations one-half day after the last dose of rifabutin were 60 ng/mL when co-administered with azithromycin and 71 ng/mL when co-administered with placebo.

Zithromax Tabs/O.S.—Cont.

NOTE: Penicillin by the intramuscular route is the usual drug of choice in the treatment of *Streptococcus pyogenes* infection and the prophylaxis of rheumatic fever. ZITHROMAX® is often effective in the eradication of susceptible strains of *Streptococcus pyogenes* from the nasopharynx. Because some strains are resistant to ZITHROMAX®, susceptibility tests should be performed when patients are treated with ZITHROMAX®. Data establishing efficacy of azithromycin in subsequent prevention of rheumatic fever are not available.

Uncomplicated skin and skin structure infections due to *Staphylococcus aureus, Streptococcus pyogenes*, or *Streptococcus agalactiae*. Abscesses usually require surgical drainage.

Urethritis and cervicitis due to *Chlamydia trachomatis* or *Neisseria gonorrhoeae*.

Genital ulcer disease in men due to *Haemophilus ducreyi* (chancroid). Due to the small number of women included in clinical trials, the efficacy of azithromycin in the treatment of chancroid in women has not been established.

ZITHROMAX®, at the recommended dose, should not be relied upon to treat syphilis. Antimicrobial agents used in high doses for short periods of time to treat non-gonococcal urethritis may mask or delay the symptoms of incubating syphilis. All patients with sexually-transmitted urethritis or cervicitis should have a serologic test for syphilis and appropriate cultures for gonorrhea performed at the time of diagnosis. Appropriate antimicrobial therapy and follow-up tests for these diseases should be initiated if infection is confirmed.

Appropriate culture and susceptibility tests should be performed before treatment to determine the causative organism and its susceptibility to azithromycin. Therapy with ZITHROMAX® may be initiated before results of these tests are known; once the results become available, antimicrobial therapy should be adjusted accordingly.

Children: (See **PRECAUTIONS—Pediatric Use** and **CLINICAL STUDIES IN PEDIATRIC PATIENTS.**)

Acute otitis media caused by *Haemophilus influenzae, Moraxella catarrhalis* or *Streptococcus pneumoniae*. (For specific dosage recommendation, see **DOSAGE AND ADMINISTRATION.**)

Community-acquired pneumonia due to *Chlamydia pneumoniae, Haemophilus influenzae, Mycoplasma pneumoniae* or *Streptococcus pneumoniae* in patients appropriate for oral therapy. (For specific dosage recommendation, see **DOSAGE AND ADMINISTRATION.**)

NOTE: Azithromycin should not be used in pediatric patients with pneumonia who are judged to be inappropriate for oral therapy because of moderate to severe illness or risk factors such as any of the following:

- **patients with cystic fibrosis,**
- **patients with nosocomially acquired infections,**
- **patients with known or suspected bacteremia,**
- **patients requiring hospitalization, or**
- **patients with significant underlying health problems that may compromise their ability to respond to their illness (including immunodeficiency or functional asplenia).**

Pharyngitis/tonsillitis caused by *Streptococcus pyogenes* as an alternative to first-line therapy in individuals who cannot use first-line therapy. (For specific dosage recommendation, see **DOSAGE AND ADMINISTRATION.**)

NOTE: Penicillin by the intramuscular route is the usual drug of choice in the treatment of *Streptococcus pyogenes* infection and the prophylaxis of rheumatic fever. ZITHROMAX® is often effective in the eradication of susceptible strains of *Streptococcus pyogenes* from the nasopharynx. Because some strains are resistant to ZITHROMAX®, susceptibility tests should be performed when patients are treated with ZITHROMAX®. Data establishing efficacy of azithromycin in subsequent prevention of rheumatic fever are not available.

Appropriate culture and susceptibility tests should be performed before treatment to determine the causative organism and its susceptibility to azithromycin. Therapy with ZITHROMAX® may be initiated before results of these tests are known; once the results become available, antimicrobial therapy should be adjusted accordingly.

CONTRAINDICATIONS

ZITHROMAX® is contraindicated in patients with known hypersensitivity to azithromycin, erythromycin or any macrolide antibiotic.

WARNINGS

Serious allergic reactions, including angioedema, anaphylaxis, and dermatologic reactions including Stevens Johnson Syndrome and toxic epidermal necrolysis have been reported rarely in patients on azithromycin therapy. Although rare, fatalities have been reported. (See **CONTRAINDICATIONS.**) Despite initially successful symptomatic treatment of the allergic symptoms, when symptomatic therapy was discontinued, the allergic symptoms **recurred soon thereafter in some patients without further azithromycin exposure.** These patients required prolonged periods of observation and symptomatic treatment. The relationship of these episodes to the long tissue half-life of azithromycin and subsequent prolonged exposure to antigen is unknown at present.

If an allergic reaction occurs, the drug should be discontinued and appropriate therapy should be instituted. Physicians should be aware that reappearance of the allergic symptoms may occur when symptomatic therapy is discontinued.

Table 2. Drug Interactions: Pharmacokinetic Parameters for Azithromycin in the Presence of Co-administered Drugs (See **PRECAUTIONS—Drug Interactions.**)

Co-administered Drug	Dose of Co-administered Drug	Dose of Azithromycin	n	Ratio (with/without co-administered drug) of Azithromycin Pharmacokinetic Parameters (90% CI); No Effect = 1.00	
				Mean C_{max}	Mean AUC
Efavirenz	400 mg/day × 7 days	600 mg PO on day 7	14	1.22 (1.04 to 1.42)	0.92*
Fluconazole	200 mg PO single dose	1,200 mg PO single dose	18	0.82 (0.66 to 1.02)	1.07 (0.94 to 1.22)
Nelfinavir	750 mg TID × 11 days	1,200 mg PO on day 9	14	2.36 (1.77 to 3.15)	2.12 (1.80 to 2.50)
Rifabutin	300 mg/day × 10 days	500 mg PO on day 1, then 250 mg/day on days 2-10	6	See footnote below	NA

NA – Not available
* - 90% Confidence interval not reported
Mean azithromycin concentrations one day after the last dose were 53 ng/mL when coadministered with 300 mg daily rifabutin and 49 ng/mL when coadministered with placebo.

Table 1. Susceptibility Interpretive Criteria for Azithromycin
Susceptibility Test Result Interpretive Criteria

Pathogen	Minimum Inhibitory Concentrations (μg/mL)			Disk Diffusion (zone diameters in mm)		
	S	I	R[a]	S	I	R[a]
Haemophilus spp.	≤ 4	—	—	≥ 12	—	—
Staphylococcus aureus	≤ 2	4	≥ 8	≥ 18	14-17	≤ 13
Streptococci including *S. pneumoniae*[b]	≤ 0.5	1	≥ 2	≥ 18	14-17	≤ 13

[a]The current absence of data on resistant strains precludes defining any category other than "susceptible." If strains yield MIC results other than susceptible, they should be submitted to a reference laboratory for further testing.
[b]Susceptibility of streptococci including *S. pneumoniae* to azithromycin and other macrolides can be predicted by testing erythromycin.

Table 2. Acceptable Quality Control Ranges for Azithromycin

QC Strain	Minimum Inhibitory Concentrations (μg/mL)	Disk Diffusion (zone diameters in mm)
Haemophilus influenzae ATCC 49247	1.0-4.0	13-21
Staphylococcus aureus ATCC 29213	0.5-2.0	
Staphylococcus aureus ATCC 25923		21-26
Streptococcus pneumoniae ATCC 49619	0.06-0.25	19-25

In the treatment of pneumonia, azithromycin has only been shown to be safe and effective in the treatment of community-acquired pneumonia due to *Chlamydia pneumoniae, Haemophilus influenzae, Mycoplasma pneumoniae* or *Streptococcus pneumoniae* in patients appropriate for oral therapy. Azithromycin should not be used in patients with pneumonia who are judged to be inappropriate for oral therapy because of moderate to severe illness or risk factors such as any of the following: patients with cystic fibrosis, patients with nosocomially acquired infections, patients with known or suspected bacteremia, patients requiring hospitalization, elderly or debilitated patients, or patients with significant underlying health problems that may compromise their ability to respond to their illness (including immunodeficiency or functional asplenia.)

Pseudomembranous colitis has been reported with nearly all antibacterial agents and may range in severity from mild to life-threatening. Therefore, it is important to consider this diagnosis in patients who present with diarrhea subsequent to the administration of antibacterial agents.

Treatment with antibacterial agents alters the normal flora of the colon and may permit overgrowth of clostridia. Studies indicate that a toxin produced by *Clostridium difficile* is a primary cause of "antibiotic-associated colitis."

After the diagnosis of pseudomembranous colitis has been established, therapeutic measures should be initiated. Mild cases of pseudomembranous colitis usually respond to discontinuation of the drug alone. In moderate to severe cases, consideration should be given to management with fluids and electrolytes, protein supplementation, and treatment with an antibacterial drug clinically effective against *Clostridium difficile* colitis.

PRECAUTIONS

General: Because azithromycin is principally eliminated via the liver, caution should be exercised when azithromycin is administered to patients with impaired hepatic function. Due to the limited data in subjects with GFR <10 mL/min, caution should be exercised when prescribing azithromycin in these patients. (See **CLINICAL PHARMACOLOGY—Special Populations—Renal Insufficiency.**)

The following adverse events have been reported with macrolide products: ventricular arrhythmias, including ventricular tachycardia and *torsade de pointes*, in individuals with prolonged QT intervals.

There has been a spontaneous report from the post-marketing experience of a patient with previous history of arrhythmias who experienced *torsade de pointes* and subsequent myocardial infarction following a course of azithromycin therapy.

Information for Patients:

ZITHROMAX® tablets and oral suspension can be taken with or without food.

Patients should also be cautioned not to take aluminum- and magnesium-containing antacids and azithromycin simultaneously.

The patient should be directed to discontinue azithromycin immediately and contact a physician if any signs of an allergic reaction occur.

Drug Interactions:

Co-administration of nelfinavir at steady-state with a single oral dose of azithromycin resulted in increased azithromycin serum concentrations. Although a dose adjustment of azithromycin is not recommended when administered in combination with nelfinavir, close monitoring for known side effects of azithromycin, such as liver enzyme abnormalities and hearing impairment, is warranted. (See **ADVERSE REACTIONS.**)

Azithromycin did not affect the prothrombin time response to a single dose of warfarin. However, prudent medical practice dictates careful monitoring of prothrombin time in all patients treated with azithromycin and warfarin concomitantly. Concurrent use of macrolides and warfarin in clinical practice has been associated with increased anticoagulant effects.

Drug interaction studies were performed with azithromycin and other drugs likely to be co-administered. (See **CLINICAL PHARMACOLOGY—Drug-Drug Interactions.**) When used in therapeutic doses, azithromycin had a modest effect on the pharmacokinetics of atorvastatin, carbamazepine, cetirizine, didanosine, efavirenz, fluconazole, indinavir, midazolam, rifabutin, sildenafil, theophylline (intravenous and oral), triazolam, trimethoprim/sulfamethoxazole or zidovudine. Co-administration with efavirenz, or fluconazole had a modest effect on the pharmacokinetics of azithromycin. No dosage adjustment of either drug is recommended when azithromycin is coadministered with any of the above agents.

Interactions with the drugs listed below have not been reported in clinical trials with azithromycin; however, no specific drug interaction studies have been performed to evaluate potential drug-drug interaction. Nonetheless, they have been observed with macrolide products. Until further data are developed regarding drug interactions when azithromycin and these drugs are used concomitantly, careful monitoring of patients is advised:

Digoxin–elevated digoxin concentrations.

Ergotamine or dihydroergotamine–acute ergot toxicity characterized by severe peripheral vasospasm and dysesthesia.

Terfenadine, cyclosporine, hexobarbital and phenytoin concentrations.

Laboratory Test Interactions: There are no reported laboratory test interactions.

Carcinogenesis, Mutagenesis, Impairment of Fertility: Long-term studies in animals have not been performed to evaluate carcinogenic potential. Azithromycin has shown no mutagenic potential in standard laboratory tests: mouse lymphoma assay, human lymphocyte clastogenic assay, and mouse bone marrow clastogenic assay. No evidence of impaired fertility due to azithromycin was found.

Pregnancy: Teratogenic Effects. Pregnancy Category B: Reproduction studies have been performed in rats and mice at doses up to moderately maternally toxic dose concentrations (i.e., 200 mg/kg/day). These doses, based on a mg/m^2 basis, are estimated to be 4 and 2 times, respectively, the human daily dose of 500 mg. In the animal studies, no evidence of harm to the fetus due to azithromycin was found. There are, however, no adequate and well-controlled studies in pregnant women. Because animal reproduction studies are not always predictive of human response, azithromycin should be used during pregnancy only if clearly needed.

Nursing Mothers: It is not known whether azithromycin is excreted in human milk. Because many drugs are excreted in human milk, caution should be exercised when azithromycin is administered to a nursing woman.

Pediatric Use: (See **CLINICAL PHARMACOLOGY, INDICATIONS AND USAGE**, and **DOSAGE AND ADMINISTRATION**.)

Acute Otitis Media (total dosage regimen: 30 mg/kg, see **DOSAGE AND ADMINISTRATION**): Safety and effectiveness in the treatment of children with otitis media under 6 months of age have not been established.

Community-Acquired Pneumonia (dosage regimen: 10 mg/kg on Day 1 followed by 5 mg/kg on Days 2-5): Safety and effectiveness in the treatment of children with community-acquired pneumonia under 6 months of age have not been established. Safety and effectiveness for pneumonia due to *Chlamydia pneumoniae* and *Mycoplasma pneumoniae* were documented in pediatric clinical trials. Safety and effectiveness for pneumonia due to *Haemophilus influenzae* and *Streptococcus pneumoniae* were not documented bacteriologically in the pediatric clinical trial due to difficulty in obtaining specimens. Use of azithromycin for these two microorganisms is supported, however, by evidence from adequate and well-controlled studies in adults.

Pharyngitis/Tonsillitis (dosage regimen: 12 mg/kg on Days 1-5): Safety and effectiveness in the treatment of children with pharyngitis/tonsillitis under 2 years of age have not been established.

Studies evaluating the use of repeated courses of therapy have not been conducted. (See **CLINICAL PHARMACOLOGY** and **ANIMAL TOXICOLOGY**.)

Geriatric Use: Pharmacokinetic parameters in older volunteers (65-85 years old) were similar to those in younger volunteers (18-40 years old) for the 5-day therapeutic regimen. Dosage adjustment does not appear to be necessary for older patients with normal renal and hepatic function receiving treatment with this dosage regimen. (See **CLINICAL PHARMACOLOGY**.)

In multiple-dose clinical trials of oral azithromycin, 9% of patients were at least 65 years of age (458/4949) and 3% of patients (144/4949) were at least 75 years of age. No overall differences in safety or effectiveness were observed between these subjects and younger subjects, and other reported clinical experience has not identified differences in response between the elderly and younger patients, but greater sensitivity of some older individuals cannot be ruled out.

ZITHROMAX® 250 mg tablets contain 0.9 mg of sodium per tablet.

ZITHROMAX® 500 mg tablets contain 1.8 mg of sodium per tablet.

ZITHROMAX® for oral suspension 100 mg/5 mL contains 3.7 mg of sodium per 5 mL of constituted solution.

ZITHROMAX® for oral suspension 200 mg/5 mL contains 7.4 mg of sodium per 5 mL of constituted solution.

ADVERSE REACTIONS

In clinical trials, most of the reported side effects were mild to moderate in severity and were reversible upon discontinuation of the drug. Potentially serious side effects of angioedema and cholestatic jaundice were reported rarely. Approximately 0.7% of the patients (adults and children) from the 5-day multiple-dose clinical trials discontinued ZITHROMAX® (azithromycin) therapy because of treatment-related side effects. In adults given 500 mg/day for 3 days, the discontinuation rate due to treatment-related side effects was 0.4%. In clinical trials in children given 30 mg/kg, either as a single dose or over 3 days, discontinuation from the trials due to treatment-related side effects was approximately 1%. (See **DOSAGE AND ADMINISTRATION**.) Most of the side effects leading to discontinuation were related to the gastrointestinal tract, e.g., nausea, vomiting, diarrhea, or abdominal pain. (See **CLINICAL STUDIES IN PEDIATRIC PATIENTS**.)

Dosage Regimen	Diarrhea, %	Abdominal Pain, %	Vomiting, %	Nausea, %	Rash, %
1-day	4.3%	1.4%	4.9%	1.0%	1.0%
3-day	2.6%	1.7%	2.3%	0.4%	0.6%
5-day	1.8%	1.2%	1.1%	0.5%	0.4%

Dosage Regimen	Diarrhea/Loose stools, %	Abdominal Pain, %	Vomiting, %	Nausea, %	Rash, %
5-day	5.8%	1.9%	1.9%	1.9%	1.6%

Dosage Regimen	Diarrhea, %	Abdominal Pain, %	Vomiting, %	Nausea, %	Rash, %	Headache, %
5-day	5.4%	3.4%	5.6%	1.8%	0.7%	1.1%

Clinical:
Adults:
Multiple-dose regimens: Overall, the most common treatment-related side effects in adult patients receiving multiple-dose regimens of ZITHROMAX® were related to the gastrointestinal system with diarrhea/loose stools (4-5%), nausea (3%) and abdominal pain (2-3%) being the most frequently reported.

No other treatment-related side effects occurred in patients on the multiple-dose regimens of ZITHROMAX® with a frequency greater than 1%. Side effects that occurred with a frequency of 1% or less included the following:

Cardiovascular: Palpitations, chest pain.
Gastrointestinal: Dyspepsia, flatulence, vomiting, melena and cholestatic jaundice.
Genitourinary: Monilia, vaginitis and nephritis.
Nervous System: Dizziness, headache, vertigo and somnolence.
General: Fatigue.
Allergic: Rash, pruritus, photosensitivity and angioedema.

Single 1-gram dose regimen: Overall, the most common side effects in patients receiving a single-dose regimen of 1 gram of ZITHROMAX® were related to the gastrointestinal system and were more frequently reported than in patients receiving the multiple-dose regimen.

Side effects that occurred in patients on the single one-gram dosing regimen of ZITHROMAX® with a frequency of 1% or greater included diarrhea/loose stools (7%), nausea (5%), abdominal pain (5%), vomiting (2%), dyspepsia (1%) and vaginitis (1%).

Single 2-gram dose regimen: Overall, the most common side effects in patients receiving a single 2-gram dose of ZITHROMAX® were related to the gastrointestinal system. Side effects that occurred in patients in this study with a frequency of 1% or greater included nausea (18%), diarrhea/loose stools (14%), vomiting (7%), abdominal pain (7%), vaginitis (2%), dyspepsia (1%) and dizziness (1%). The majority of these complaints were mild in nature.

Children:
Single and Multiple-dose regimens: The types of side effects in children were comparable to those seen in adults, with different incidence rates for the dosage regimens recommended in children.

Acute Otitis Media: For the recommended total dosage regimen of 30 mg/kg, the most frequent side effects (≥ 1%) attributed to treatment were diarrhea, abdominal pain, vomiting, nausea and rash. (See **DOSAGE AND ADMINISTRATION** and **CLINICAL STUDIES IN PEDIATRIC PATIENTS**.)

The incidence, based on dosing regimen, is described in the table below:
[See first table above]

Community-Acquired Pneumonia: For the recommended dosage regimen of 10 mg/kg on Day 1 followed by 5 mg/kg on Days 2-5, the most frequent side effects attributed to treatment were diarrhea/loose stools, abdominal pain, vomiting, nausea and rash.

The incidence is described in the table below:
[See second table above]

Pharyngitis/tonsillitis: For the recommended dosage regimen of 12 mg/kg on Days 1-5, the most frequent side effects attributed to treatment were diarrhea, vomiting, abdominal pain, nausea and headache.

The incidence is described in the table below:
[See third table above]

With any of the treatment regimens, no other treatment-related side effects occurred in children treated with ZITHROMAX® with a frequency greater than 1%. Side effects that occurred with a frequency of 1% or less included the following:

Cardiovascular: Chest pain.
Gastrointestinal: Dyspepsia, constipation, anorexia, enteritis, flatulence, gastritis, jaundice, loose stools and oral moniliasis.
Hematologic and Lymphatic: Anemia and leukopenia.
Nervous System: Headache (otitis media dosage), hyperkinesia, dizziness, agitation, nervousness and insomnia.
General: Fever, face edema, fatigue, fungal infection, malaise and pain.
Allergic: Rash and allergic reaction.
Respiratory: Cough increased, pharyngitis, pleural effusion and rhinitis.
Skin and Appendages: Eczema, fungal dermatitis, pruritus, sweating, urticaria and vesiculobullous rash.
Special Senses: Conjunctivitis.

Post-Marketing Experience:
Adverse events reported with azithromycin during the post-marketing period in adult and/or pediatric patients for which a causal relationship may not be established include:

Allergic: Arthralgia, edema, urticaria and angioedema.
Cardiovascular: Arrhythmias including ventricular tachycardia and hypotension.
Gastrointestinal: Anorexia, constipation, dyspepsia, flatulence, vomiting/diarrhea rarely resulting in dehydration, pseudomembranous colitis, pancreatitis, oral candidiasis and rare reports of tongue discoloration.
General: Asthenia, paresthesia, fatigue, malaise and anaphylaxis (rarely fatal).
Genitourinary: Interstitial nephritis and acute renal failure and vaginitis.
Hematopoietic: Thrombocytopenia.
Liver/Biliary: Abnormal liver function including hepatitis and cholestatic jaundice, as well as rare cases of hepatic necrosis and hepatic failure, some of which have resulted in death.
Nervous System: Convulsions, dizziness/vertigo, headache, somnolence, hyperactivity, nervousness, agitation and syncope.
Psychiatric: Aggressive reaction and anxiety.
Skin/Appendages: Pruritus, rarely serious skin reactions including erythema multiforme, Stevens Johnson Syndrome and toxic epidermal necrolysis.
Special Senses: Hearing disturbances including hearing loss, deafness and/or tinnitus and rare reports of taste perversion.

Laboratory Abnormalities:
Adults:
Clinically significant abnormalities (irrespective of drug relationship) occurring during the clinical trials were reported as follows: with an incidence of greater than 1%: decreased hemoglobin, hematocrit, lymphocytes and blood glucose; elevated serum creatine phosphokinase, potassium, ALT (SGPT), GGT, and AST (SGOT), BUN, creatinine, blood glucose, platelet count, eosinophils; with an incidence of less than 1%: leukopenia, neutropenia, decreased platelet count, elevated serum alkaline phosphatase, bilirubin, LDH and phosphate. The majority of subjects with elevated serum creatinine also had abnormal values at baseline.

When follow-up was provided, changes in laboratory tests appeared to be reversible.

In multiple-dose clinical trials involving more than 4500 patients, three patients discontinued therapy because of treatment-related liver enzyme abnormalities and one because of a renal function abnormality.

Children:
One, Three and Five Day Regimens
Laboratory data collected from comparative clinical trials employing two 3-day regimens (30 mg/kg or 60 mg/kg in divided doses over 3 days), or two 5-day regimens (30 mg/kg or 60 mg/kg in divided doses over 5 days) were similar for regimens of azithromycin and all comparators combined, with most clinically significant laboratory abnormalities occurring at incidences of 1–5%. Laboratory data for patients receiving 30 mg/kg as a single dose were collected in one single center trial. In that trial, an absolute neutrophil count between 500–1500 cells/mm^3 was observed in 10/64 patients receiving 30 mg/kg as a single dose, 9/62 patients receiving 30 mg/kg given over 3 days, and 8/63 comparator patients. No patient had an absolute neutrophil count <500 cells/mm^3. (See **DOSAGE AND ADMINISTRATION**.)

In multiple-dose clinical trials involving approximately 4700 pediatric patients, no patients discontinued therapy because of treatment-related laboratory abnormalities.

DOSAGE AND ADMINISTRATION

(See **INDICATIONS AND USAGE** and **CLINICAL PHARMACOLOGY**.)

Adults:
The recommended dose of ZITHROMAX® for the treatment of community-acquired pneumonia of mild severity, pharyngitis/tonsillitis (as second-line therapy), and uncomplicated skin and skin structure infections due to the indicated organisms is: 500 mg as a single dose on the first day followed by 250 mg once daily on Days 2 through 5. The recommended dose of ZITHROMAX® for the treatment of mild to moderate acute bacterial exacerbations of chronic obstructive pulmonary disease is: either 500 mg per day for 3 days or 500 mg as a single dose on the first day followed by 250 mg once daily on Days 2 through 5.

Continued on next page

Zithromax Tabs/O.S.—Cont.

ZITHROMAX® tablets can be taken with or without food. The recommended dose of ZITHROMAX® for the treatment of genital ulcer disease due to *Haemophilus ducreyi* (chancroid), non-gonococcal urethritis and cervicitis due to *C. trachomatis* is: a single 1 gram (1000 mg) dose of ZITHROMAX®.

The recommended dose of ZITHROMAX® for the treatment of urethritis and cervicitis due to *Neisseria gonorrhoeae* is a single 2 gram (2000 mg) dose of ZITHROMAX®.

Renal Insufficiency:
No dosage adjustment is recommended for subjects with renal impairment (GFR ≤80 mL/min). The mean AUC_{0-120} was similar in subjects with GFR 10–80 mL/min compared to subjects with normal renal function, whereas it increased 35% in subjects with GFR <10 mL/min compared to subjects with normal renal function. Caution should be exercised when azithromycin is administered to subjects with severe renal impairment. (See **CLINICAL PHARMACOLOGY, Special Populations, Renal Insufficiency**.)

Hepatic Insufficiency:
The pharmacokinetics of azithromycin in subjects with hepatic impairment have not been established. No dose adjustment recommendations can be made in patients with impaired hepatic function (See **CLINICAL PHARMACOLOGY, Special Populations, Hepatic Insufficiency**.)

No dosage adjustment is recommended based on age or gender. (See **CLINICAL PHARMACOLOGY, Special Populations**.)

Children:
ZITHROMAX® for oral suspension can be taken with or without food.

Acute Otitis Media: The recommended dose of ZITHROMAX® for oral suspension for the treatment of children with acute otitis media is 30 mg/kg given as a single dose or 10 mg/kg once daily for 3 days or 10 mg/kg as a single dose on the first day followed by 5 mg/kg/day on Days 2 through 5. (See chart below.)

Community-Acquired Pneumonia: The recommended dose of ZITHROMAX® for oral suspension for the treatment of children with community-acquired pneumonia is 10 mg/kg as a single dose on the first day followed by 5 mg/kg on Days 2 through 5. (See chart below.)

[See first table above]
[See second table above]
[See third table above]

The safety of re-dosing azithromycin in children who vomit after receiving 30 mg/kg as a single dose has not been established. In clinical studies involving 487 patients with acute otitis media given a single 30 mg/kg dose of azithromycin, eight patients who vomited within 30 minutes of dosing were re-dosed at the same total dose.

Pharyngitis/Tonsillitis: The recommended dose of ZITHROMAX® for children with pharyngitis/tonsillitis is 12 mg/kg once daily for 5 days. (See chart below.)
[See first table on next page]

Constituting instructions for ZITHROMAX® Oral Suspension, 300, 600, 900, 1200 mg bottles. The table below indicates the volume of water to be used for constitution:
[See second table on next page]

Following constitution, and for use with the oral syringe, the supplied Press in Bottle Adapter should be inserted into the neck of the bottle then sealed with the original closure. Shake well before each use. Oversized bottle provides shake space. Keep tightly closed.

Use only the dosing device provided to measure the correct amount of suspension. (See **HOW SUPPLIED**.) The dosing device may need to be filled multiple times to provide the complete dose prescribed. Rinse the device with water after the complete daily dose has been administered.

After mixing, store suspension at 5° to 30°C (41° to 86°F) and use within 10 days. Discard after full dosing is completed.

HOW SUPPLIED

ZITHROMAX® 250 mg tablets are supplied as pink modified capsular shaped, engraved, film-coated tablets containing azithromycin dihydrate equivalent to 250 mg of azithromycin. ZITHROMAX® 250 mg tablets are engraved with "PFIZER" on one side and "306" on the other. These are packaged in bottles and blister cards of 6 tablets (Z-PAKS®) as follows:

Bottles of 30	NDC 0069-3060-30
Boxes of 3 (Z-PAKS® of 6)	NDC 0069-3060-75
Unit Dose package of 50	NDC 0069-3060-86

ZITHROMAX® 500 mg tablets are supplied as pink modified capsular shaped, engraved, film-coated tablets containing azithromycin dihydrate equivalent to 500 mg of azithromycin. ZITHROMAX® 500 mg tablets are engraved with "Pfizer" on one side and "ZTM500" on the other. These are packaged in bottles and blister cards of 3 tablets (TRI-PAKS™) as follows:

Bottles of 30	NDC 0069-3070-30
Boxes of 3 (TRI-PAKS™ of 3 tablets)	NDC 0069-3070-75
Unit Dose package of 50	NDC 0069-3070-86

ZITHROMAX® tablets should be stored between 15° to 30°C (59° to 86°F).

ZITHROMAX® for oral suspension after constitution contains a flavored suspension. ZITHROMAX® for oral suspension is supplied to provide 100 mg/5 mL or 200 mg/5 mL suspension in bottles with accompanying calibrated dosing device as follows:

Azithromycin contents per bottle	NDC
300 mg	0069-3110-19
600 mg	0069-3120-19
900 mg	0069-3130-19
1200 mg	0069-3140-19

See **DOSAGE AND ADMINISTRATION** for constitution instructions with each bottle type.
Storage: Store dry powder below 30°C (86°F). Store constituted suspension between 5° to 30°C (41° to 86°F) and discard when full dosing is completed.

CLINICAL STUDIES (See **INDICATIONS AND USAGE** and **Pediatric Use**.)

Pediatric Patients
From the perspective of evaluating pediatric clinical trials, Days 11-14 were considered on-therapy evaluations because of the extended half-life of azithromycin. Day 11-14 data are provided for clinical guidance. Day 24-32 evaluations were considered the primary test of cure endpoint.

Acute Otitis Media
Safety and efficacy using azithromycin 30 mg/kg given over 5 days

Protocol 1
In a double-blind, controlled clinical study of acute otitis media performed in the United States, azithromycin (10 mg/kg on Day 1 followed by 5 mg/kg on Days 2-5) was compared to amoxicillin/clavulanate potassium (4:1). For the 553 patients who were evaluated for clinical efficacy, the clinical success rate (i.e., cure plus improvement) at the Day 11 visit was 88% for azithromycin and 88% for the control agent. For the 521 patients who were evaluated at the Day 30 visit, the clinical success rate was 73% for azithromycin and 71% for the control agent.

In the safety analysis of the above study, the incidence of treatment-related adverse events, primarily gastrointesti-

---

PEDIATRIC DOSAGE GUIDELINES FOR OTITIS MEDIA AND COMMUNITY-ACQUIRED PNEUMONIA
(Age 6 months and above, see PRECAUTIONS—Pediatric Use.)
Based on Body Weight

OTITIS MEDIA AND COMMUNITY-ACQUIRED PNEUMONIA: 5-Day Regimen*

Dosing Calculated on 10 mg/kg/day Day 1 and 5 mg/kg/day Days 2 to 5.

Weight		100 mg/5 mL		200 mg/5 mL		Total mL per Treatment Course	Total mg per Treatment Course
Kg	Lbs.	Day 1	Days 2-5	Day 1	Days 2-5		
5	11	2.5 mL (½ tsp)	1.25 mL (¼ tsp)			7.5 mL	150 mg
10	22	5 mL (1 tsp)	2.5 mL (½ tsp)			15 mL	300 mg
20	44			5 mL (1 tsp)	2.5 mL (½ tsp)	15 mL	600 mg
30	66			7.5 mL (1½ tsp)	3.75 mL (¾ tsp)	22.5 mL	900 mg
40	88			10 mL (2 tsp)	5 mL (1 tsp)	30 mL	1200 mg
50 and above	110 and above			12.5 mL (2½ tsp)	6.25 mL (1¼ tsp)	37.5 mL	1500 mg

*Effectiveness of the 3-day or 1-day regimen in children with community-acquired pneumonia has not been established.

OTITIS MEDIA: (3-Day Regimen)

Dosing Calculated on 10 mg/kg/day

Weight		100 mg/5 mL	200 mg/5 mL	Total mL per Treatment Course	Total mg per Treatment Course
Kg	Lbs.	Day 1-3	Day 1-3		
5	11	2.5 mL (½ tsp)		7.5 mL	150 mg
10	22	5 mL (1 tsp)		15 mL	300 mg
20	44		5 mL (1 tsp)	15 mL	600 mg
30	66		7.5 mL (1½ tsp)	22.5 mL	900 mg
40	88		10 mL (2 tsp)	30 mL	1200 mg
50 and above	110 and above		12.5 mL (2½ tsp)	37.5 mL	1500 mg

OTITIS MEDIA: (1-Day Regimen)

Dosing Calculated on 30 mg/kg as a single dose

Weight		200 mg/5 mL	Total mL per Treatment Course	Total mg per Treatment Course
Kg	Lbs.	Day 1		
5	11	3.75 mL (¾ tsp)	3.75 mL	150 mg
10	22	7.5 mL (1½ tsp)	7.5 mL	300 mg
20	44	15 mL (3 tsp)	15 mL	600 mg
30	66	22.5 mL (4½ tsp)	22.5 mL	900 mg
40	88	30 mL (6 tsp)	30 mL	1200 mg
50 and above	110 and above	37.5 mL (7½ tsp)	37.5 mL	1500 mg

nal, in all patients treated was 9% with azithromycin and 31% with the control agent. The most common side effects were diarrhea/loose stools (4% azithromycin vs. 20% control), vomiting (2% azithromycin vs. 7% control), and abdominal pain (2% azithromycin vs. 5% control).

Protocol 2
In a non-comparative clinical and microbiologic trial performed in the United States, where significant rates of beta-lactamase producing organisms (35%) were found, 131 patients were evaluable for clinical efficacy. The combined clinical success rate (i.e., cure and improvement) at the Day 11 visit was 84% for azithromycin. For the 122 patients who were evaluated at the Day 30 visit, the clinical success rate was 70% for azithromycin.

Microbiologic determinations were made at the pre-treatment visit. Microbiology was not reassessed at later visits. The following presumptive bacterial/clinical cure outcomes (i.e., clinical success) were obtained from the evaluable group:

Presumed Bacteriologic Eradication

	Day 11 Azithromycin	Day 30 Azithromycin
S. pneumoniae	61/74 (82%)	40/56 (71%)
H. influenzae	43/54 (80%)	30/47 (64%)
M. catarrhalis	28/35 (80%)	19/26 (73%)
S. pyogenes	11/11 (100%)	7/7
Overall	177/217 (82%)	97/137 (73%)

In the safety analysis of this study, the incidence of treatment-related adverse events, primarily gastrointestinal, in all patients treated was 9%. The most common side effect was diarrhea (4%).

Protocol 3
In another controlled comparative clinical and microbiologic study of otitis media performed in the United States, azithromycin was compared to amoxicillin/clavulanate potassium (4:1). This study utilized two of the same investigators as Protocol 2 (above), and these two investigators enrolled 90% of the patients in Protocol 3. For this reason, Protocol 3 was not considered to be an independent study. Significant rates of beta-lactamase producing organisms (20%) were found. Ninety-two (92) patients were evaluable for clinical and microbiologic efficacy. The combined clinical success rate (i.e., cure and improvement) of those patients with a baseline pathogen at the Day 11 visit was 88% for azithromycin vs. 100% for control; at the Day 30 visit, the clinical success rate was 82% for azithromycin vs. 80% for control.

Microbiologic determinations were made at the pre-treatment visit. Microbiology was not reassessed at later visits. At the Day 11 and Day 30 visits, the following presumptive bacterial/clinical cure outcomes (i.e., clinical success) were obtained from the evaluable group:
[See third table at right]

In the safety analysis of the above study, the incidence of treatment-related adverse events, primarily gastrointestinal, in all patients treated was 4% with azithromycin and 31% with the control agent. The most common side effect was diarrhea/loose stools (2% azithromycin vs. 29% control).

Safety and efficacy using azithromycin 30 mg/kg given over 3 days

Protocol 4
In a double-blind, controlled, randomized clinical study of acute otitis media in children from 6 months to 12 years of age, azithromycin (10 mg/kg per day for 3 days) was compared to amoxicillin/clavulanate potassium (7:1) in divided doses q12h for 10 days. Each child received active drug and placebo matched for the comparator.

For the 366 patients who were evaluated for clinical efficacy at the Day 12 visit, the clinical success rate (i.e., cure plus improvement) was 83% for azithromycin and 88% for the control agent. For the 362 patients who were evaluated at the Day 24–28 visit, the clinical success rate was 74% for azithromycin and 69% for the control agent.

In the safety analysis of the above study, the incidence of treatment-related adverse events, primarily gastrointestinal, in all patients treated was 10.6% with azithromycin and 20.0% with the control agent. The most common side effects were diarrhea/loose stools (5.9% azithromycin vs. 14.6% control), vomiting (2.1% azithromycin vs. 1.1% control), and rash (0.0% azithromycin vs. 4.3% control).

Safety and efficacy using azithromycin 30 mg/kg given as a single dose

Protocol 5
A double blind, controlled, randomized trial was performed at nine clinical centers. Infants and children from 6 months to 12 years of age were randomized 1:1 to treatment with either azithromycin (given at 30 mg/kg as a single dose on Day 1) or amoxicillin/clavulanate potassium (7:1) divided q12h for 10 days. Each child received active drug, and placebo matched for the comparator.

Clinical response (Cure, Improvement, Failure) was evaluated at End of Therapy (Day 12–16) and Test of Cure (Day 28–32). Safety was evaluated throughout the trial for all treated subjects. For the 321 subjects who were evaluated at End of Treatment, the clinical success rate (cure plus improvement) was 87% for azithromycin, and 88% for the comparator. For the 305 subjects who were evaluated at Test of Cure, the clinical success rate was 75% for both azithromycin and the comparator.

In the safety analysis, the incidence of treatment-related adverse events, primarily gastrointestinal, was 16.8% with azithromycin, and 22.5% with the comparator. The most common side effects were diarrhea (6.4% with azithromycin vs. 12.7% with the comparator), vomiting (4% with each agent), rash (1.7% with azithromycin vs. 5.2% with the comparator) and nausea (1.7% with azithromycin vs. 1.2% with the comparator).

Protocol 6
In a non-comparative clinical and microbiological trial, 248 patients from 6 months to 12 years of age with documented acute otitis media were dosed with a single oral dose of azithromycin (30 mg/kg on Day 1).

For the 240 patients who were evaluable for clinical modified Intent-to-Treat (MITT) analysis, the clinical success rate (i.e., cure plus improvement) at Day 10 was 89% and for the 242 patients evaluable at Day 24-28, the clinical success rate (cure) was 85%.

Presumed Bacteriologic Eradication

	Day 10	Day 24-28
S. pneumoniae	70/76 (92%)	67/76 (88%)
H. influenzae	30/42 (71%)	28/44 (64%)
M. catarrhalis	10/10 (100%)	10/10 (100%)
Overall	110/128 (86%)	105/130 (81%)

In the safety analysis of this study, the incidence of treatment-related adverse events, primarily gastrointestinal, in all the subjects treated was 12.1%. The most common side effects were vomiting (5.6%), diarrhea (3.2%), and abdominal pain (1.6%).

Pharyngitis/Tonsillitis
In three double-blind controlled studies, conducted in the United States, azithromycin (12 mg/kg once a day for 5 days) was compared to penicillin V (250 mg three times a day for 10 days) in the treatment of pharyngitis due to documented Group A β-hemolytic streptococci (GABHS or S. pyogenes). Azithromycin was clinically and microbiologically statistically superior to penicillin at Day 14 and Day 30 with the following clinical success (i.e., cure and improvement) and bacteriologic efficacy rates (for the combined evaluable patient with documented GABHS):
[See fourth table above]
Approximately 1% of azithromycin-susceptible S. pyogenes isolates were resistant to azithromycin following therapy. The incidence of treatment-related adverse events, primarily gastrointestinal, in all patients treated was 18% on azithromycin and 13% on penicillin. The most common side effects were diarrhea/loose stools (6% azithromycin vs. 2% penicillin), vomiting (6% azithromycin vs. 4% penicillin), and abdominal pain (3% azithromycin vs. 1% penicillin).

PEDIATRIC DOSAGE GUIDELINES FOR PHARYNGITIS/TONSILLITIS
(Age 2 years and above, see PRECAUTIONS—Pediatric Use.)
Based on Body Weight

PHARYNGITIS/TONSILLITIS: (5-Day Regimen)

Dosing Calculated on 12 mg/kg/day for 5 days.

Weight		200 mg/5 mL	Total mL per Treatment Course	Total mg per Treatment Course
Kg	Lbs.	Day 1–5		
8	18	2.5 mL (½ tsp)	12.5 mL	500 mg
17	37	5 mL (1 tsp)	25 mL	1000 mg
25	55	7.5 mL (1½ tsp)	37.5 mL	1500 mg
33	73	10 mL (2 tsp)	50 mL	2000 mg
40	88	12.5 mL (2½ tsp)	62.5 mL	2500 mg

Amount of water to be added	Total volume after constitution (azithromycin content)	Azithromycin concentration after constitution
9 mL (300 mg)	15 mL (300 mg)	100 mg/5 mL
9 mL (600 mg)	15 mL (600 mg)	200 mg/5 mL
12 mL (900 mg)	22.5 mL (900 mg)	200 mg/5 mL
15 mL (1200 mg)	30 mL (1200 mg)	200 mg/5 mL

Presumed Bacteriologic Eradication

	Day 11 Azithromycin	Day 11 Control	Day 30 Azithromycin	Day 30 Control
S. pneumoniae	25/29 (86%)	26/26 (100%)	22/28 (79%)	18/22 (82%)
H. influenzae	9/11 (82%)	9/9	8/10 (80%)	6/8
M. catarrhalis	7/7	5/5	5/5	2/3
S. pyogenes	2/2	5/5	2/2	4/4
Overall	43/49 (88%)	45/45 (100%)	37/45 (82%)	30/37 (81%)

Three U.S. Streptococcal Pharyngitis Studies
Azithromycin vs. Penicillin V
EFFICACY RESULTS

	Day 14	Day 30
Bacteriologic Eradication:		
Azithromycin	323/340 (95%)	255/330 (77%)
Penicillin V	242/332 (73%)	206/325 (63%)
Clinical Success (Cure plus improvement):		
Azithromycin	336/343 (98%)	310/330 (94%)
Penicillin V	284/338 (84%)	241/325 (74%)

Adult Patients
Acute Bacterial Exacerbations of Chronic Obstructive Pulmonary Disease

In a randomized, double-blind controlled clinical trial of acute exacerbation of chronic bronchitis (AECB), azithromycin (500 mg once daily for 3 days) was compared with clarithromycin (500 mg twice daily for 10 days). The primary endpoint of this trial was the clinical cure rate at Day 21-24. For the 304 patients analyzed in the modified intent to treat analysis at the Day 21-24 visit, the clinical cure rate for 3 days of azithromycin was 85% (125/147) compared to 82% (129/157) for 10 days of clarithromycin.

The following outcomes were the clinical cure rates at the Day 21-24 visit for the bacteriologically evaluable patients by pathogen:

Pathogen	Azithromycin (3 Days)	Clarithromycin (10 Days)
S. pneumoniae	29/32 (91%)	21/27 (78%)
H. influenzae	12/14 (86%)	14/16 (88%)
M. catarrhalis	11/12 (92%)	12/15 (80%)

In the safety analysis of this study, the incidence of treatment-related adverse events, primarily gastrointestinal, were comparable between treatment arms (25% with azithromycin and 29% with clarithromycin). The most common side effects were diarrhea, nausea and abdominal pain with comparable incidence rates for each symptom of 5-9% between the two treatment arms. (See **ADVERSE REACTIONS.**)

ANIMAL TOXICOLOGY

Phospholipidosis (intracellular phospholipid accumulation) has been observed in some tissues of mice, rats, and dogs given multiple doses of azithromycin. It has been demonstrated in numerous organ systems (e.g., eye, dorsal root ganglia, liver, gallbladder, kidney, spleen, and pancreas) in dogs treated with azithromycin at doses which, expressed on the basis of mg/m^2, are approximately equal to the recommended adult human dose, and in rats treated at doses approximately one-sixth of the recommended adult human dose. This effect has been shown to be reversible after cessation of azithromycin treatment. Phospholipidosis has been observed to a similar extent in the tissues of neonatal rats and dogs given daily doses of azithromycin ranging from 10 days to 30 days. Based on the pharmacokinetic

Continued on next page

Zithromax Tabs/O.S.—Cont.

data, phospholipidosis has been seen in the rat (30 mg/kg dose) at observed C_{max} value of 1.3 µg/mL (six times greater than the observed C_{max} of 0.216 µg/mL at the pediatric dose of 10 mg/kg). Similarly, it has been shown in the dog (10 mg/kg dose) at observed C_{max} value of 1.5 µg/mL (seven times greater than the observed same C_{max} and drug dose in the studied pediatric population). On a mg/m^2 basis, 30 mg/kg dose in the neonatal rat (135 mg/m^2) and 10 mg/kg dose in the neonatal dog (79 mg/m^2) are approximately 0.5 and 0.3 times, respectively, the recommended dose in the pediatric patients with an average body weight of 25 kg. Phospholipidosis, similar to that seen in the adult animals, is reversible after cessation of azithromycin treatment. The significance of these findings for animals and for humans is unknown.

REFERENCES:

1. National Committee for Clinical Laboratory Standards, *Methods for Dilution Antimicrobial Susceptibility Tests for Bacteria That Grow Aerobically* – Fifth Edition. Approved Standard NCCLS Document M7-A5, Vol. 20, No. 2 (ISBN 1-56238-394-9). NCCLS, 940 West Valley Road, Suite 1400, Wayne, PA 19087-1898, January 2000.
2. National Committee for Clinical Laboratory Standards, *Performance Standards for Antimicrobial Disk Susceptibility Tests* – Seventh Edition. Approved Standard NCCLS Document M2-A7, Vol. 20, No. 1 (ISBN 1-56238-393-0). NCCLS, 940 West Valley Road, Suite 1400, Wayne, PA 19087-1898, January 2000.
3. National Committee for Clinical Laboratory Standards. *Performance Standards for Antimicrobial Susceptibility Testing* – Eleventh Informational Supplement. NCCLS Document M100-S11, Vol. 21, No. 1 (ISBN 1-56238-426-0). NCCLS, 940 West Valley Road, Suite 1400, Wayne, PA 19087-1898, January 2001.

℞ only

Licensed from Pliva

Distributed by:
Pfizer Labs
Division of Pfizer Inc, NY, NY 10017
70-5179-00-1 Revised October 2002

ZITHROMAX® ℞

[*zi'th-rō-maks*]
(azithromycin capsules)
(azithromycin tablets)
and
(azithromycin for oral suspension)

Prescribing information for this product, which appears on pages 2667–2672 of the 2003 PDR, has been completely revised as follows. Please write "See Supplement A" next to the product heading.

DESCRIPTION

ZITHROMAX® (azithromycin capsules, azithromycin tablets and azithromycin for oral suspension) contain the active ingredient azithromycin, an azalide, a subclass of macrolide antibiotics, for oral administration. Azithromycin has the chemical name (*2R,3S,4R,5R,8R,10R,11R,12S,13S,14R*)-13-[(2,6-dideoxy-3-*C*-methyl-3-*O*-methyl-α-*L*-*ribo*-hexopyranosyl)oxy]-2-ethyl-3,4,10-trihydroxy-3,5,6,8,10,12,14-heptamethyl-11-[[3,4,6-trideoxy-3-(dimethylamino)-β-*D*-*xylo*-hexopyranosyl]oxy]-1-oxa-6-azacyclopentadecan-15-one. Azithromycin is derived from erythromycin; however, it differs chemically from erythromycin in that a methyl-substituted nitrogen atom is incorporated into the lactone ring. Its molecular formula is $C_{38}H_{72}N_2O_{12}$, and its molecular weight is 749.0. Azithromycin has the following structural formula:

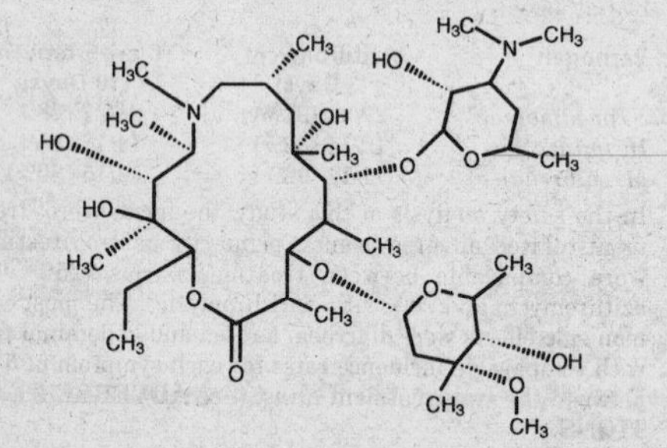

Azithromycin, as the dihydrate, is a white crystalline powder with a molecular formula of $C_{38}H_{72}N_2O_{12} \cdot 2H_2O$ and a molecular weight of 785.0.

ZITHROMAX® capsules contain azithromycin dihydrate equivalent to 250 mg of azithromycin. The capsules are supplied in red opaque hard-gelatin capsules (containing FD&C Red #40). They also contain the following inactive ingredients: anhydrous lactose, corn starch, magnesium stearate, and sodium lauryl sulfate.

ZITHROMAX® tablets contain azithromycin dihydrate equivalent to 600 mg azithromycin. The tablets are supplied as white, modified oval-shaped, film-coated tablets. They also contain the following inactive ingredients: dibasic calcium phosphate anhydrous, pregelatinized starch, sodium croscarmellose, magnesium stearate, sodium lauryl sulfate and an aqueous film coat consisting of hydroxypropyl methyl cellulose, titanium dioxide, lactose and triacetin.

MEAN (CV%) PK PARAMETER

DOSE/DOSAGE FORM (serum, except as indicated)	Subjects	Day No.	C_{max} (µg/mL)	T_{max} (hr)	C_{24} (µg/mL)	ACU (µg•hr/mL)	$T_{½}$ (hr)	Urinary Excretion (% of dose)
500 mg/250 mg capsule	12	Day 1	0.41	2.5	0.05	2.6[a]	—	4.5
and 250 mg on Days 2-5	12	Day 5	0.24	3.2	0.05	2.1[a]	—	6.5
1200 mg/600 mg tablets	12	Day 1	0.66	2.5	0.074	6.8[b]	40	—
%CV			(62%)	(79%)	(49%)	(64%)	(33%)	
600 mg tablet/day	7	1	0.33	2.0	0.039	2.4[a]		
%CV			25%	(50%)	(36%)	(19%)		
	7	22	0.55	2.1	0.14	5.8[a]	84.5	—
%CV			(18%)	(52%)	(26%)	(25%)		—
600 mg tablet/day (leukocytes)	7	22	252	10.9	146	4763[a]	82.8	—
%CV			(49%)	(28%)	(33%)	(42%)	—	—

[a]AUC_{0-24}; [b]0–last.

ZITHROMAX® for oral suspension is supplied in a single dose packet containing azithromycin dihydrate equivalent to 1 g azithromycin. It also contains the following inactive ingredients: colloidal silicon dioxide, sodium phosphate tribasic, anhydrous; spray dried artificial banana flavor, spray dried artificial cherry flavor, and sucrose.

CLINICAL PHARMACOLOGY

Pharmacokinetics: Following oral administration, azithromycin is rapidly absorbed and widely distributed throughout the body. Rapid distribution of azithromycin into tissues and high concentration within cells result in significantly higher azithromycin concentrations in tissues than in plasma or serum. The 1 g single dose packet is bioequivalent to four 250 mg capsules.

The pharmacokinetic parameters of azithromycin in plasma after dosing as per labeled recommendations in healthy young adults and asymptomatic HIV-seropositive adults (age 18-40 years old) are portrayed in the following chart:

[See table above]

In these studies (500 mg Day 1, 250 mg Days 2-5), there was no significant difference in the disposition of azithromycin between male and female subjects. Plasma concentrations of azithromycin following single 500 mg oral and i.v. doses declined in a polyphasic pattern resulting in an average terminal half-life of 68 hours. With a regimen of 500 mg on Day 1 and 250 mg/day on Days 2-5, C_{min} and C_{max} remained essentially unchanged from Day 2 through Day 5 of therapy. However, without a loading dose, azithromycin C_{min} levels required 5 to 7 days to reach steady-state.

In asymptomatic HIV-seropositive adult subjects receiving 600-mg ZITHROMAX® tablets once daily for 22 days, steady state azithromycin serum levels were achieved by Day 15 of dosing.

When azithromycin capsules were administered with food, the rate of absorption (C_{max}) of azithromycin was reduced by 52% and the extent of absorption (AUC) by 43%.

When the oral suspension of azithromycin was administered with food, the C_{max} increased by 46% and the AUC by 14%.

The absolute bioavailability of two 600 mg tablets was 34% (CV=56%). Administration of two 600 mg tablets with food increased C_{max} by 31% (CV=43%) while the extent of absorption (AUC) was unchanged (mean ratio of AUCs=1.00; CV=55%).

The AUC of azithromycin in 250 mg capsules was unaffected by coadministration of an antacid containing aluminum and magnesium hydroxide with ZITHROMAX® (azithromycin); however, the C_{max} was reduced by 24%. Administration of cimetidine (800 mg) two hours prior to azithromycin had no effect on azithromycin absorption.

When studied in healthy elderly subjects from age 65 to 85 years, the pharmacokinetic parameters of azithromycin (500 mg Day 1, 250 mg Days 2-5) in elderly men were similar to those in young adults; however, in elderly women, although higher peak concentrations (increased by 30 to 50%) were observed, no significant accumulation occurred.

The high values in adults for apparent steady-state volume of distribution (31.1 L/kg) and plasma clearance (630 mL/min) suggest that the prolonged half-life is due to extensive uptake and subsequent release of drug from tissues. Selected tissue (or fluid) concentration and tissue (or fluid) to plasma/serum concentration ratios are shown in the following table:

[See table at bottom of next page]

The extensive tissue distribution was confirmed by examination of additional tissues and fluids (bone, ejaculum, prostate, ovary, uterus, salpinx, stomach, liver, and gallbladder). As there are no data from adequate and well-controlled studies of azithromycin treatment of infections in these additional body sites, the clinical significance of these tissue concentration data is unknown.

Following a regimen of 500 mg on the first day and 250 mg daily for 4 days, only very low concentrations were noted in cerebrospinal fluid (less than 0.01 µg/mL) in the presence of non-inflamed meninges.

Following oral administration of a single 1200 mg dose (two 600 mg tablets), the mean maximum concentration in peripheral leukocytes was 140 µg/mL. Concentrations remained above 32 µg/mL for approximately 60 hr. The mean half-lives for 6 males and 6 females were 34 hr and 57 hr, respectively. Leukocyte to plasma C_{max} ratios for males and females were 258 (±77%) and 175 (±60%), respectively, and the AUC ratios were 804 (±31%) and 541 (±28%), respectively. The clinical relevance of these findings is unknown.

Following oral administration of multiple daily doses of 600 mg (1 tablet/day) to asymptomatic HIV-seropositive adults, mean maximum concentration in peripheral leukocytes was 252 µg/mL (±49%). Trough concentrations in peripheral leukocytes at steady-state averaged 146 µg/mL (±33%). The mean leukocyte to serum C_{max} ratio was 456 (±38%) and the mean leukocyte to serum AUC ratio was 816 (±31%). The clinical relevance of these findings is unknown.

The serum protein binding of azithromycin is variable in the concentration range approximating human exposure, decreasing from 51% at 0.02 µg/mL to 7% at 2 µg/mL. Biliary excretion of azithromycin, predominantly as unchanged drug, is a major route of elimination. Over the course of a week, approximately 6% of the administered dose appears as unchanged drug in urine.

There are no pharmacokinetic data available from studies in hepatically- or renally-impaired individuals.

The effect of azithromycin on the plasma levels or pharmacokinetics of theophylline administered in multiple doses adequate to reach therapeutic steady-state plasma levels is not known. (See PRECAUTIONS.)

Mechanism of Action: Azithromycin acts by binding to the 50S ribosomal subunit of susceptible microorganisms and, thus, interfering with microbial protein synthesis. Nucleic acid synthesis is not affected.

Azithromycin concentrates in phagocytes and fibroblasts as demonstrated by *in vitro* incubation techniques. Using such methodology, the ratio of intracellular to extracellular concentration was >30 after one hour incubation. *In vivo* studies suggest that concentration in phagocytes may contribute to drug distribution to inflamed tissues.

Microbiology:

Azithromycin has been shown to be active against most strains of the following microorganisms, both *in vitro* and in clinical infections as described in the INDICATIONS AND USAGE section.

Aerobic Gram-Positive Microorganisms

Staphylococcus aureus
Streptococcus agalactiae
Streptococcus pneumoniae
Streptococcus pyogenes

NOTE: Azithromycin demonstrates cross-resistance with erythromycin-resistant gram-positive strains. Most strains of *Enterococcus faecalis* and methicillin-resistant staphylococci are resistant to azithromycin.

Aerobic Gram-Negative Microorganisms

Haemophilus influenzae
Moraxella catarrhalis

"Other" Microorganisms

Chlamydia trachomatis

Beta-lactamase production should have no effect on azithromycin activity.

Azithromycin has been shown to be active *in vitro* and in the prevention and treatment of disease caused by the following microorganisms:

Mycobacteria

Mycobacterium avium complex (MAC) consisting of:
Mycobacterium avium
Mycobacterium intracellulare.

The following *in vitro* data are available, *but their clinical significance is unknown.*

Azithromycin exhibits *in vitro* minimal inhibitory concentrations (MICs) of 2.0 μg/mL or less against most (≥90%) strains of the following microorganisms; however, the safety and effectiveness of azithromycin in treating clinical infections due to these microorganisms have not been established in adequate and well-controlled trials.

Aerobic Gram-Positive Microorganisms

Streptococci (Groups C, F, G)
Viridans group streptococci

Aerobic Gram-Negative Microorganisms

Bordetella pertussis
Campylobacter jejuni
Haemophilus ducreyi
Legionella pneumophila

Anaerobic Microorganisms

Bacteroides bivius
Clostridium perfringens
Peptostreptococcus species

"Other" Microorganisms

Borrelia burgdorferi
Mycoplasma pneumoniae
Treponema pallidum
Ureaplasma urealyticum

Susceptibility Testing of Bacteria Excluding Mycobacteria

The *in vitro* potency of azithromycin is markedly affected by the pH of the microbiological growth medium during incubation. Incubation in a 10% CO_2 atmosphere will result in lowering of media pH (7.2 to 6.6) within 18 hours and in an apparent reduction of the *in vitro* potency of azithromycin. Thus, the initial pH of the growth medium should be 7.2-7.4, and the CO_2 content of the incubation atmosphere should be as low as practical.

Azithromycin can be solubilized for *in vitro* susceptibility testing by dissolving in a minimum amount of 95% ethanol and diluting to working concentration with water.

Dilution Techniques:

Quantitative methods are used to determine minimal inhibitory concentrations that provide reproducible estimates of the susceptibility of bacteria to antimicrobial compounds. One such standardized procedure uses a standardized dilution method[1] (broth, agar or microdilution) or equivalent with azithromycin powder. The MIC values should be interpreted according to the following criteria:

MIC (μg/mL)	Interpretation
≤ 2	Susceptible (S)
4	Intermediate (I)
≥ 8	Resistant (R)

A report of "Susceptible" indicates that the pathogen is likely to respond to monotherapy with azithromycin. A report of "Intermediate" indicates that the result should be considered equivocal, and, if the microorganism is not fully susceptible to alternative, clinically feasible drugs, the test should be repeated. This category also provides a buffer zone which prevents small uncontrolled technical factors from causing major discrepancies in interpretation. A report of "Resistant" indicates that usually achievable drug concentrations are unlikely to be inhibitory and that other therapy should be selected.

Measurement of MIC or MBC and achieved antimicrobial compound concentrations may be appropriate to guide therapy in some infections. (See CLINICAL PHARMACOLOGY section for further information on drug concentrations achieved in infected body sites and other pharmacokinetic properties of this antimicrobial drug product.)

Standardized susceptibility test procedures require the use of laboratory control microorganisms. Standard azithromycin powder should provide the following MIC values:

Microorganism	MIC (μg/mL)
Escherichia coli ATCC 25922	2.0-8.0
Enterococcus faecalis ATCC 29212	1.0-4.0
Staphylococcus aureus ATCC 29213	0.25-1.0

Diffusion Techniques:

Quantitative methods that require measurement of zone diameters also provide reproducible estimates of the susceptibility of bacteria to antimicrobial compounds. One such standardized procedure[2] that has been recommended for use with disks to test the susceptibility of microorganisms to azithromycin uses the 15-μg azithromycin disk. Interpretation involves the correlation of the diameter obtained in the disk test with the minimal inhibitory concentration (MIC) for azithromycin.

Reports from the laboratory providing results of the standard single-disk susceptibility test with a 15 μg azithromycin disk should be interpreted according to the following criteria:

Zone Diameter (mm)	Interpretation
≥ 18	(S) Susceptible
14-17	(I) Intermediate
≤ 13	(R) Resistant

Interpretation should be as stated above for results using dilution techniques.

As with standardized dilution techniques, diffusion methods require the use of laboratory control microorganisms. The 15-μg azithromycin disk should provide the following zone diameters in these laboratory test quality control strains:

Microorganism	Zone Diameter (mm)
Staphylococcus aureus ATCC 25923	21-26

***In Vitro* Activity of Azithromycin Against Mycobacteria.**

Azithromycin has demonstrated *in vitro* activity against *Mycobacterium avium* complex (MAC) organisms. While gene probe techniques may be used to distinguish between *M. avium* and *M. intracellulare*, many studies only reported results on *M. avium* complex (MAC) isolates. Azithromycin has also been shown to be active against phagocytized *M. avium* complex (MAC) organisms in mouse and human macrophage cell cultures as well as in the beige mouse infection model.

Various *in vitro* methodologies employing broth or solid media at different pHs, with and without oleic acid-albumin dextrose-catalase (OADC), have been used to determine azithromycin MIC values for *Mycobacterium avium* complex strains. In general, azithromycin MIC values decreased 4 to 8 fold as the pH of Middlebrook 7H11 agar media increased from 6.6 to 7.4. At pH 7.4, azithromycin MIC values determined with Mueller-Hinton agar were 4 fold higher than that observed with Middlebrook 7H12 media at the same pH. Utilization of oleic acid-albumin-dextrose-catalase (OADC) in these assays has been shown to further alter MIC values. The relationship between azithromycin and clarithromycin MIC values has not been established. In general, azithromycin MIC values were observed to be 2 to 32 fold higher than clarithromycin independent of the susceptibility method employed.

The ability to correlate MIC values and plasma drug levels is difficult as azithromycin concentrates in macrophages and tissues. (See CLINICAL PHARMACOLOGY)

Drug Resistance:

Complete cross-resistance between azithromycin and clarithromycin has been observed with *Mycobacterium avium* complex (MAC) isolates. In most isolates, a single point mutation at a position that is homologous to the *Escherichia coli* positions 2058 or 2059 on the 23S rRNA gene is the mechanism producing this cross-resistance pattern.[3,4] *Mycobacterium avium* complex (MAC) isolates exhibiting cross-resistance show an increase in azithromycin MICs to ≥128 μg/mL with clarithromycin MICs increasing to ≥32 μg/mL. These MIC values were determined employing the radiometric broth dilution susceptibility testing method with Middlebrook 7H12 medium. The clinical significance of azithromycin and clarithromycin cross-resistance is not fully understood at this time but preclinical data suggest that reduced activity to both agents will occur after *M. avium* complex strains produce the 23S rRNA mutation.

AZITHROMYCIN CONCENTRATIONS FOLLOWING TWO 250 mg (500 mg) CAPSULES IN ADULTS

TISSUE OR FLUID	TIME AFTER DOSE (h)	TISSUE OR FLUID CONCENTRATION (μg/g or μg/mL)[1]	CORRESPONDING PLASMA OR SERUM LEVEL (μg/mL)	TISSUE (FLUID) PLASMA (SERUM) RATIO[1]
SKIN	72-96	0.4	0.012	35
LUNG	72-96	4.0	0.012	>100
SPUTUM*	2–4	1.0	0.64	2
SPUTUM**	10–12	2.9	0.1	30
TONSIL***	9–18	4.5	0.03	>100
TONSIL***	180	0.9	0.006	>100
CERVIX****	19	2.8	0.04	70

[1] High tissue concentrations should not be interpreted to be quantitatively related to clinical efficacy. The antimicrobial activity of azithromycin is pH related. Azithromycin is concentrated in cell lysosomes which have a low intraorganelle pH, at which the drug's activity is reduced. However, the extensive distribution of drug to tissues may be relevant to clinical activity.

* Sample was obtained 2-4 hours after the first dose.
** Sample was obtained 10-12 hours after the first dose.
*** Dosing regimen of 2 doses of 250 mg each, separated by 12 hours.
**** Sample was obtained 19 hours after a single 500 mg dose.

Susceptibility testing for *Mycobacterium avium* complex (MAC):

The disk diffusion techniques and dilution methods for susceptibility testing against Gram-positive and Gram-negative bacteria should not be used for determining azithromycin MIC values against mycobacteria. *In vitro* susceptibility testing methods and diagnostic products currently available for determining minimal inhibitory concentration (MIC) values against *Mycobacterium avium* complex (MAC) organisms have not been standardized or validated. Azithromycin MIC values will vary depending on the susceptibility testing method employed, composition and pH of media and the utilization of nutritional supplements. Breakpoints to determine whether clinical isolates of *M. avium* or *M. intracellulare* are susceptible or resistant to azithromycin have not been established.

The clinical relevance of azithromycin *in vitro* susceptibility test results for other mycobacterial species, including *Mycobacterium tuberculosis*, using any susceptibility testing method has not been determined.

INDICATIONS AND USAGE

ZITHROMAX® (azithromycin) is indicated for the treatment of patients with mild to moderate infections (pneumonia: see WARNINGS) caused by susceptible strains of the designated microorganisms in the specific conditions listed below.

Lower Respiratory Tract:

Acute bacterial exacerbations of chronic obstructive pulmonary disease due to *Haemophilus influenzae, Moraxella catarrhalis*, or *Streptococcus pneumoniae.*

Community-acquired pneumonia of mild severity due to *Streptococcus pneumoniae* or *Haemophilus influenzae* in patients appropriate for outpatient oral therapy.

NOTE: Azithromycin should not be used in patients with pneumonia who are judged to be inappropriate for outpatient oral therapy because of moderate to severe illness or risk factors such as any of the following:

patients with nosocomially acquired infections,
patients with known or suspected bacteremia,
patients requiring hospitalization,
elderly or debilitated patients, or
patients with significant underlying health problems that may compromise their ability to respond to their illness (including immunodeficiency or functional asplenia).

Upper Respiratory Tract:

Streptococcal pharyngitis/tonsillitis—As an alternative to first line therapy of acute pharyngitis/tonsillitis due to *Streptococcus pyogenes* occurring in individuals who cannot use first line therapy.

NOTE: Penicillin is the usual drug of choice in the treatment of *Streptococcus pyogenes* infection and the prophylaxis of rheumatic fever. ZITHROMAX® is often effective in the eradication of susceptible strains of *Streptococcus pyogenes* from the nasopharynx. Data establishing efficacy of azithromycin in subsequent prevention of rheumatic fever are not available.

Skin and Skin Structure

Uncomplicated skin and skin structure infections due to *Staphylococcus aureus, Streptococcus pyogenes*, or *Streptococcus agalactiae*. Abscesses usually require surgical drainage.

Sexually Transmitted Diseases

Non-gonococcal urethritis and cervicitis due to *Chlamydia trachomatis*.

ZITHROMAX®, at the recommended dose, should not be relied upon to treat gonorrhea or syphilis. Antimicrobial agents used in high doses for short periods of time to treat non-gonococcal urethritis may mask or delay the symptoms of incubating gonorrhea or syphilis. All patients with sexually-transmitted urethritis or cervicitis should have a serologic test for syphilis and appropriate cultures for gonorrhea performed at the time of diagnosis. Appropriate antimicrobial therapy and follow-up tests for these diseases should be initiated if infection is confirmed.

Appropriate culture and susceptibility tests should be performed before treatment to determine the causative organism and its susceptibility to azithromycin. Therapy with ZITHROMAX® may be initiated before results of these tests are known; once the results become available, antimicrobial therapy should be adjusted accordingly.

Mycobacterial Infections

Prophylaxis of Disseminated *Mycobacterium avium* complex (MAC) Disease

ZITHROMAX®, taken alone or in combination with rifabutin at its approved dose, is indicated for the prevention of disseminated *Mycobacterium avium* complex (MAC) disease in persons with advanced HIV infection. (See DOSAGE AND ADMINISTRATION, CLINICAL STUDIES)

Treatment of Disseminated *Mycobacterium avium* complex (MAC) Disease

ZITHROMAX®, taken in combination with ethambutol, is indicated for the treatment of disseminated MAC infections in persons with advanced HIV infection. (See DOSAGE AND ADMINISTRATION, CLINICAL STUDIES)

CONTRAINDICATIONS

ZITHROMAX® is contraindicated in patients with known hypersensitivity to azithromycin, erythromycin, or any macrolide antibiotic.

Continued on next page

Zithromax Caps/Tabs/O.S.—Cont.

WARNINGS

Rare serious allergic reactions, including angioedema and anaphylaxis, have been reported rarely in patients on azithromycin therapy. (See **CONTRAINDICATIONS.**) Despite initially successful symptomatic treatment of the allergic symptoms, when symptomatic therapy was discontinued, the allergic symptoms **recurred soon thereafter in some patients without further azithromycin exposure.** These patients required prolonged periods of observation and symptomatic treatment. The relationship of these episodes to the long tissue half-life of azithromycin and subsequent prolonged exposure to antigen is unknown at present. If an allergic reaction occurs, the drug should be discontinued and appropriate therapy should be instituted. Physicians should be aware that reappearance of the allergic symptoms may occur when symptomatic therapy is discontinued.

In the treatment of pneumonia, azithromycin has only been shown to be safe and effective in the treatment of community-acquired pneumonia of mild severity due to *Streptococcus pneumoniae* or *Haemophilus influenzae* in patients appropriate for outpatient oral therapy. Azithromycin should not be used in patients with pneumonia who are judged to be inappropriate for outpatient oral therapy because of moderate to severe illness or risk factors such as any of the following: patients with nosocomially acquired infections, patients with known or suspected bacteremia, patients requiring hospitalization, elderly or debilitated patients, or patients with significant underlying health problems that may compromise their ability to respond to their illness (including immunodeficiency or functional asplenia).

Pseudomembranous colitis has been reported with nearly all antibacterial agents and may range in severity from mild to life-threatening. Therefore, it is important to consider this diagnosis in patients who present with diarrhea subsequent to the administration of antibacterial agents.

Treatment with antibacterial agents alters the normal flora of the colon and may permit overgrowth of clostridia. Studies indicate that a toxin produced by *Clostridium difficile* is a primary cause of "antibiotic-associated colitis."

After the diagnosis of pseudomembranous colitis has been established, therapeutic measures should be initiated. Mild cases of pseudomembranous colitis usually respond to discontinuation of the drug alone. In moderate to severe cases, consideration should be given to management with fluids and electrolytes, protein supplementation, and treatment with an antibacterial drug clinically effective against *Clostridium difficile* colitis.

PRECAUTIONS

General: Because azithromycin is principally eliminated via the liver, caution should be exercised when azithromycin is administered to patients with impaired hepatic function. There are no data regarding azithromycin usage in patients with renal impairment; thus, caution should be exercised when prescribing azithromycin in these patients.

The following adverse events have been reported with macrolide products: ventricular arrhythmias, including ventricular tachycardia and *torsades de pointes*, in individuals with prolonged QT intervals.

There has been a spontaneous report from the post-marketing experience of a patient with previous history of arrhythmias who experienced *torsades de pointes* and subsequent myocardial infarction following a course of azithromycin therapy.

Information for Patients:

Patients should be cautioned to take ZITHROMAX® capsules at least one hour prior to a meal or at least two hours after a meal. Azithromycin capsules should not be taken with food.

ZITHROMAX® tablets may be taken with or without food. However, increased tolerability has been observed when tablets are taken with food.

ZITHROMAX® for oral suspension in single 1 g packets can be taken with or without food after constitution.

Patients should also be cautioned not to take aluminum- and magnesium-containing antacids and azithromycin simultaneously.

The patient should be directed to discontinue azithromycin immediately and contact a physician if any signs of an allergic reaction occur.

Drug Interactions: Aluminum- and magnesium-containing antacids reduce the peak serum levels (rate) but not the AUC (extent) of azithromycin (500 mg) absorption.

Administration of cimetidine (800 mg) two hours prior to azithromycin had no effect on azithromycin (500 mg) absorption.

A single oral dose of 1200 mg azithromycin (2 x 600 mg ZITHROMAX® tablets) did not alter the pharmacokinetics of a single 800 mg oral dose of fluconazole in healthy adult subjects.

Total exposure (AUC) and half-life of azithromycin following the single oral tablet dose of 1200 mg were unchanged and the reduction in Cmax was not significant (mean decrease of 18%) by coadministration with 800 mg fluconazole.

A single oral dose of 1200 mg azithromycin (2 x 600 mg ZITHROMAX® tablets) had no significant effect on the pharmacokinetics of indinavir (800 mg indinavir tid for 5 days) in healthy adult subjects.

Coadministration of a single oral dose of 1200 mg azithromycin (2 x 600 mg ZITHROMAX® tablets) with steady-state nelfinavir (750 mg tid) to healthy adult subjects produced a decrease of approximately 15% in mean AUC_{0-8} of nelfinavir and its M8 metabolite. Mean Cmax of nelfinavir and its M8 metabolite were not significantly affected. No dosage adjustment of nelfinavir is required when nelfinavir is coadministered with azithromycin.

Coadministration of nelfinavir (750 mg tid) at steady state with a single oral dose of 1200 mg azithromycin increased the mean $AUC_{0-\infty}$ of azithromycin by approximately a factor of 2-times (range of up to 4 times) of that when azithromycin was given alone. The mean Cmax of azithromycin was also increased by approximately a factor of 2-times (range of up to 5 times) of that when azithromycin was given alone. Dose adjustment of azithromycin is not recommended. However, when administered in conjunction with nelfinavir, close monitoring for known side effects of azithromycin, such as liver enzyme abnormalities and hearing impairment, is warranted. (See ADVERSE REACTIONS.)

Following administration of trimethoprim/sulfamethoxazole DS (160 mg/800 mg) for 7 days to healthy adult subjects, coadministration of 1200 mg azithromycin (2 x 600 mg ZITHROMAX® tablets) on the 7th day had no significant effects on peak concentrations (C_{max}), total exposure (AUC), and the urinary excretion of either trimethoprim or sulfamethoxazole.

Coadministration of trimethoprim/sulfamethoxazole DS for 7 days had no significant effect on the peak concentration (C_{max}) and total exposure (AUC) of azithromycin following administration of the single 1200 mg tablet dose to healthy adult subjects.

Administration of a 600 mg single oral dose of azithromycin had no effect on the pharmacokinetics of efavirenz given at 400 mg doses for 7 days to healthy adult subjects.

Efavirenz, when administered at a dose of 400 mg for seven days produced a 22% increase in the C_{max} of azithromycin administered as a 600 mg single oral dose, while the AUC of azithromycin was not affected.

Azithromycin (500 mg Day 1, 250 mg Days 2-5) did not affect the plasma levels or pharmacokinetics of theophylline administered as a single intravenous dose. The effect of azithromycin on the plasma levels or pharmacokinetics of theophylline administered in multiple doses resulting in therapeutic steady-state levels of theophylline is not known. However, concurrent use of macrolides and theophylline has been associated with increases in the serum concentrations of theophylline. Therefore, until further data are available, prudent medical practice dictates careful monitoring of plasma theophylline levels in patients receiving azithromycin and theophylline concomitantly.

Azithromycin (500 mg Day 1, 250 mg Days 2-5) did not affect the prothrombin time response to a single dose of warfarin. However, prudent medical practice dictates careful monitoring of prothrombin time in all patients treated with azithromycin and warfarin concomitantly. Concurrent use of macrolides and warfarin in clinical practice has been associated with increased anticoagulant effects.

Dose adjustments are not indicated when azithromycin and zidovudine are coadministered. When zidovudine (100 mg q3h x5) was coadministered with daily azithromycin (600 mg, n=5 or 1200 mg, n=7), mean C_{max}, AUC and Clr increased by 26% (CV 54%), 10% (CV 26%) and 38% (CV 114%), respectively. The mean AUC of phosphorylated zidovudine increased by 75% (CV 95%), while zidovudine glucuronide C_{max} and AUC increased by less than 10%. In another study, addition of 1 gram azithromycin per week to a regimen of 10 mg/kg daily zidovudine resulted in 25% (CV 70%) and 13% (CV 37%) increases in zidovudine C_{max} and AUC, respectively. Zidovudine glucuronide mean C_{max} and AUC increased by 16% (CV 61%) and 8.0% (CV 32%), respectively.

Doses of 1200 mg/day azithromycin for 14 days in 6 subjects increased C_{max} of concurrently administered didanosine (200 mg *q*.12h) by 44% (54% CV) and AUC by 14% (23% CV). However, none of these changes were significantly different from those produced in a parallel placebo control group of subjects.

Preliminary data suggest that coadministration of azithromycin and rifabutin did not markedly affect the mean serum concentrations of either drug. Administration of 250 mg azithromycin daily for 10 days (500 mg on the first day) produced mean concentrations of azithromycin 1 day after the last dose of 53 ng/mL when coadministered with 300 mg daily rifabutin and 49 mg/mL when coadministered with placebo. Mean concentrations 5 days after the last dose were 23 ng/mL and 21 ng/mL in the two groups of subjects. Administration of 300 mg rifabutin for 10 days produced mean concentrations of rifabutin one half day after the last dose of 60 mg/mL when coadministered with daily 250 mg azithromycin and 71 ng/mL when coadministered with placebo. Mean concentrations 5 days after the last dose were 8.1 ng/mL and 9.2 ng/mL in the two groups of subjects.

The following drug interactions have not been reported in clinical trials with azithromycin; however, no specific drug interaction studies have been performed to evaluate potential drug-drug interaction. Nonetheless, they have been observed with macrolide products. Until further data are developed regarding drug interactions when azithromycin and these drugs are used concomitantly, careful monitoring of patients is advised:

Digoxin–elevated digoxin levels.

Ergotamine or dihydroergotamine–acute ergot toxicity characterized by severe peripheral vasospasm and dysesthesia.

Triazolam–decrease the clearance of triazolam and thus may increase the pharmacologic effect of triazolam.

Drugs metabolized by the cytochrome P^{450} system–elevations of serum carbamazepine, cyclosporine, hexobarbital, and phenytoin levels.

Laboratory Test Interactions: There are no reported laboratory test interactions.

Carcinogenesis, Mutagenesis, Impairment of Fertility: Long-term studies in animals have not been performed to evaluate carcinogenic potential. Azithromycin has shown no mutagenic potential in standard laboratory tests: mouse lymphoma assay, human lymphocyte clastogenic assay, and mouse bone marrow clastogenic assay.

Pregnancy: Teratogenic Effects. Pregnancy Category B: Reproduction studies have been performed in rats and mice at doses up to moderately maternally toxic dose levels (i.e., 200 mg/kg/day). These doses, based on a mg/m^2 basis, are estimated to be 4 and 2 times, respectively, the human daily dose of 500 mg.

With regard to the MAC treatment dose of 600 mg daily, on a mg/m^2/day basis, the doses in rats and mice are approximately 3.3 and 1.7 times the human dose, respectively.

With regard to the MAC prophylaxis dose of 1200 mg weekly, on a mg/m^2/day basis, the doses in rats and mice are approximately 2 and 1 times the human dose, respectively.

No evidence of impaired fertility or harm to the fetus due to azithromycin was found. There are, however, no adequate and well-controlled studies in pregnant women. Because animal reproduction studies are not always predictive of human response, azithromycin should be used during pregnancy only if clearly needed.

Nursing Mothers: It is not known whether azithromycin is excreted in human milk. Because many drugs are excreted in human milk, caution should be exercised when azithromycin is administered to a nursing woman.

Pediatric Use:

In controlled clinical studies, azithromycin has been administered to pediatric patients ranging in age from 6 months to 12 years. For information regarding the use of ZITHROMAX (azithromycin for oral suspension) in the treatment of pediatric patients, please refer to the INDICATIONS AND USAGE and DOSAGE AND ADMINISTRATION sections of the prescribing information for ZITHROMAX (azithromycin for oral suspension) 100 mg/5 mL and 200 mg/5 mL bottles.

Safety in HIV-Infected Pediatric Patients: Safety and efficacy of azithromycin for the prevention or treatment of MAC in HIV-infected children have not been established. Safety data are available for 72 children 5 months to 18 years of age (mean 7 years) who received azithromycin for treatment of opportunistic infections. The mean duration of therapy was 242 days (range 3–2004 days) at doses of <1 to 52 mg/kg/day (mean 12 mg/kg/day). Adverse events were similar to those observed in the adult population, most of which involved the gastrointestinal tract. Treatment related reversible hearing impairment in children was observed in 4 subjects (5.6%). Two (2.8%) children prematurely discontinued treatment due to side effects: one due to back pain and one due to abdominal pain, hot and cold flushes, dizziness, headache, and numbness. A third child discontinued due to a laboratory abnormality (eosinophilia). The protocols upon which these data are based specified a daily dose of 10–20 mg/kg/day (oral and/or i.v.) of azithromycin.

Geriatric Use: Pharmacokinetic parameters in older volunteers (65–85 years old) were similar to those in younger volunteers (18–40 years old) for the 5-day therapeutic regimen. Dosage adjustment does not appear to be necessary for older patients with normal renal and hepatic function receiving treatment with this dosage regimen. (See CLINICAL PHARMACOLOGY.)

In multiple-dose clinical trials of oral azithromycin, 9% of patients were at least 65 years of age (458/4949) and 3% of patients (144/4949) were at least 75 years of age. No overall differences in safety or effectiveness were observed between these subjects and younger subjects, and other reported clinical experience has not identified differences in responses between the elderly and younger patients, but greater sensitivity of some older individuals cannot be ruled out.

ZITHROMAX® 600 mg tablets contain 2.1 mg of sodium per tablet. ZITHROMAX® for oral suspension 1 gram single-dose packets contain 37.0 mg of sodium per packet.

Geriatric Patients with Opportunistic Infections, Including *Mycobacterium avium* complex (MAC) Disease: Safety data are available for 30 patients (65–94 years old) treated with azithromycin at doses >300 mg/day for a mean of 207 days. These patients were treated for a variety of opportunistic infections, including MAC. The side effect profile was generally similar to that seen in younger patients, except for a higher incidence of side effects relating to the gastrointestinal system and to reversible impairment of hearing. (See DOSAGE AND ADMINISTRATION.)

ADVERSE REACTIONS

In clinical trials, most of the reported side effects were mild to moderate in severity and were reversible upon discontinuation of the drug. Approximately 0.7% of the patients from the multiple-dose clinical trials discontinued ZITHROMAX® (azithromycin) therapy because of treatment-related side effects. Most of the side effects leading to discontinuation were related to the gastrointestinal tract, e.g., nausea, vomiting, diarrhea, or abdominal pain. Rarely but potentially serious side effects were angioedema and cholestatic jaundice.

Clinical:

Multiple-dose regimen:

Overall, the most common side effects in adult patients receiving a multiple-dose regimen of ZITHROMAX® were related to the gastrointestinal system with diarrhea/loose stools (5%), nausea (3%), and abdominal pain (3%) being the most frequently reported.

No other side effects occurred in patients on the multiple-dose regimen of ZITHROMAX® with a frequency greater than 1%. Side effects that occurred with a frequency of 1% or less included the following:

Cardiovascular: Palpitations, chest pain.
Gastrointestinal: Dyspepsia, flatulence, vomiting, melena, and cholestatic jaundice.
Genitourinary: Monilia, vaginitis, and nephritis.
Nervous System: Dizziness, headache, vertigo, and somnolence.
General: Fatigue.
Allergic: Rash, photosensitivity, and angioedema.

Chronic therapy with 1200 mg weekly regimen: The nature of side effects seen with the 1200 mg weekly dosing regimen for the prevention of *Mycobacterium avium* infection in severely immunocompromised HIV-infected patients were similar to those seen with short term dosing regimens. (See CLINICAL STUDIES.)

Chronic therapy with 600 mg daily regimen combined with ethambutol: The nature of side effects seen with the 600 mg daily dosing regimen for the treatment of *Mycobacterium avium* complex infection in severely immunocompromised HIV-infected patients were similar to those seen with short term dosing regimens. Five percent of patients experienced reversible hearing impairment in the pivotal clinical trial for the treatment of disseminated MAC in patients with AIDS. Hearing impairment has been reported with macrolide antibiotics, especially at higher doses. Other treatment related side effects occurring in >5% of subjects and seen at any time during a median of 87.5 days of therapy include: abdominal pain (14%), nausea (14%), vomiting (13%), diarrhea (12%), flatulence (5%), headache (5%) and abnormal vision (5%). Discontinuations from treatment due to laboratory abnormalities or side effects considered related to study drug occurred in 8/88 (9.1%) of subjects.

Single 1-gram dose regimen: Overall, the most common side effects in patients receiving a single-dose regimen of 1 gram of ZITHROMAX® were related to the gastrointestinal system and were more frequently reported than in patients receiving the multiple-dose regimen.

Side effects that occurred in patients on the single one-gram dosing regimen of ZITHROMAX® with a frequency of 1% or greater included diarrhea/loose stools (7%), nausea (5%), abdominal pain (5%), vomiting (2%), dyspepsia (1%), and vaginitis (1%).

Post-Marketing Experience:
Adverse events reported with azithromycin during the post-marketing period in adult and/or pediatric patients for which a causal relationship may not be established include:
Allergic: Arthralgia, edema, urticaria, angioedema.
Cardiovascular: Arrhythmias including ventricular tachycardia, hypotension.
Gastrointestinal: Anorexia, constipation, dyspepsia, flatulence, vomiting/diarrhea rarely resulting in dehydration, pseudomembranous colitis, pancreatitis, oral candidiasis and rare reports of tongue discoloration.
General: Asthenia, paresthesia, fatigue, malaise and anaphylaxis (rarely fatal).
Genitourinary: Interstitial nephritis and acute renal failure, vaginitis.
Hematopoietic: Thrombocytopenia.
Liver/Biliary: Abnormal liver function including hepatitis and cholestatic jaundice, as well as rare cases of hepatic necrosis and hepatic failure, some of which have resulted in death.
Nervous System: Convulsions, dizziness/vertigo, headache, somnolence, hyperactivity, nervousness, agitation and syncope.
Psychiatric: Aggressive reaction and anxiety.
Skin/Appendages: Pruritus, rarely serious skin reactions including erythema multiforme, Stevens Johnson Syndrome, and toxic epidermal necrolysis.
Special Senses: Hearing disturbances including hearing loss, deafness, and/or tinnitus, rare reports of taste perversion.

Laboratory Abnormalities:
Significant abnormalities (irrespective of drug relationship) occurring during the clinical trials were reported as follows:
With an incidence of 1–2%, elevated serum creatine phosphokinase, potassium, ALT (SGPT), GGT, and AST (SGOT).
With an incidence of less than 1%, leukopenia, neutropenia, decreased platelet count, elevated serum alkaline phosphatase, bilirubin, BUN, creatinine, blood glucose, LDH, and phosphate.

When follow-up was provided, changes in laboratory tests appeared to be reversible.

In multiple-dose clinical trials involving more than 3000 patients, 3 patients discontinued therapy because of treatment-related liver enzyme abnormalities and 1 because of a renal function abnormality.

In a phase I drug interaction study performed in normal volunteers, 1 of 6 subjects given the combination of azithromycin and rifabutin, 1 of 7 given rifabutin alone and 0 of 6 given azithromycin alone developed a clinically significant neutropenia (<500 cells/mm³).

Laboratory abnormalities seen in clinical trials for the prevention of disseminated *Mycobacterium avium* disease in severely immunocompromised HIV-infected patients are presented in the CLINICAL STUDIES section.

Chronic therapy (median duration: 87.5 days, range: 1-229 days) that resulted in laboratory abnormalities in >5% subjects with normal baseline values in the pivotal trial for treatment of disseminated MAC in severely immunocompromised HIV infected patients treated with azithromycin 600 mg daily in combination with ethambutol include: a reduction in absolute neutrophils to <50% of the lower limit of normal (10/52, 19%) and an increase to five times the upper limit of normal in alkaline phosphatase (3/35, 9%). These findings in subjects with normal baseline values are similar when compared to all subjects for analyses of neutrophil reductions (22/75 [29%]) and elevated alkaline phosphatase (16/80 [20%]). Causality of these laboratory abnormalities due to the use of study drug has not been established.

DOSAGE AND ADMINISTRATION
(See INDICATIONS AND USAGE.)

ZITHROMAX® capsules should be given at least 1 hour before or 2 hours after a meal. ZITHROMAX® capsules should not be mixed with or taken with food.

ZITHROMAX® for oral suspension (single dose 1 g packet) can be taken with or without food after constitution. Not for pediatric use. For pediatric suspension, please refer to the INDICATIONS AND USAGE and DOSAGE AND ADMINISTRATION sections of the prescribing information for ZITHROMAX (azithromycin for oral suspension) 100 mg/5 mL and 200 mg/5 mL bottles.

ZITHROMAX® tablets may be taken without regard to food. However, increased tolerability has been observed when tablets are taken with food.

The recommended dose of ZITHROMAX® or the treatment of individuals 16 years of age and older with mild to moderate acute bacterial exacerbations of chronic obstructive pulmonary disease, pneumonia, pharyngitis/tonsillitis (as second line therapy), and uncomplicated skin and skin structure infections due to the indicated organisms is: 500 mg as a single dose on the first day followed by 250 mg once daily on Days 2 through 5 for a total dose of 1.5 grams of ZITHROMAX®.

The recommended dose of ZITHROMAX® for the treatment of non-gonococcal urethritis and cervicitis due to *C. trachomatis* is: a single 1 gram (1000 mg) dose of ZITHROMAX®. This dose can be administered as four 250 mg capsules or as one single dose packet (1 g).

Prevention of Disseminated MAC Infections
The recommended dose of ZITHROMAX® for the prevention of disseminated *Mycobacterium avium* complex (MAC) disease is: 1200 mg taken once weekly. This dose of ZITHROMAX® may be combined with the approved dosage regimen of rifabutin.

Treatment of Disseminated MAC Infections
ZITHROMAX® should be taken at a daily dose of 600 mg, in combination with ethambutol at the recommended daily dose of 15 mg/kg. Other antimycobacterial drugs that have shown *in vitro* activity against MAC may be added to the regimen of azithromycin plus ethambutol at the discretion of the physician or health care provider.

DIRECTIONS FOR ADMINISTRATION OF ZITHROMAX® for oral suspension in the single dose packet (1 g): The entire contents of the packet should be mixed thoroughly with two ounces (approximately 60 mL) of water. Drink the entire contents immediately; add an additional two ounces of water, mix, and drink to assure complete consumption of dosage. **The single dose packet should not be used to administer doses other than 1000 mg of azithromycin. This packet not for pediatric use.**

HOW SUPPLIED
ZITHROMAX® capsules (imprinted with "Pfizer 305") are supplied in red opaque hard-gelatin capsules containing azithromycin dihydrate equivalent to 250 mg of azithromycin. These are packaged in bottles and blister cards of 6 capsules (Z-PAKS®) as follows:

Bottles of 50	NDC 0069-3050-50
Boxes of 3 (Z-PAKS®) of 6)	NDC 0069-3050-34
Unit Dose package of 50	NDC 0069-3050-86

Store capsules below 30°C (86°F).

ZITHROMAX® 600 mg tablets (engraved on front with "PFIZER" and on back with "308") are supplied as white, modified oval-shaped, film-coated tablets containing azithromycin dihydrate equivalent to 600 mg azithromycin. These are packaged in bottles of 30 tablets. ZITHROMAX® tablets are supplied as follows:

Bottles of 30	NDC 0069-3080-30

Tablets should be stored at or below 30°C (86°F).

ZITHROMAX® for oral suspension is supplied in single dose packets containing azithromycin dihydrate equivalent to 1 gram of azithromycin as follows:

Boxes of 10 Single Dose Packets (1 g)	NDC 0069-3051-07
Boxes of 3 Single Dose Packets (1 g)	NDC 0069-3051-75

Store single dose packets between 5° and 30°C (41° and 86°F).

CLINICAL STUDIES IN PATIENTS WITH ADVANCED HIV INFECTION FOR THE PREVENTION AND TREATMENT OF DISEASE DUE TO DISSEMINATED *MYCOBACTERIUM AVIUM* COMPLEX (MAC)
(See INDICATIONS AND USAGE):

Prevention of Disseminated MAC Disease
Two randomized, double blind clinical trials were performed in patients with CD4 counts <100 cells/μL. The first study (155) compared azithromycin (1200 mg once weekly) to placebo and enrolled 182 patients with a mean CD4 count of 35 cells/μL. The second study (174) randomized 723 patients to either azithromycin (1200 mg once weekly), rifabutin (300 mg daily) or the combination of both. The mean CD4 count was 51 cells/μL. The primary endpoint in these studies was disseminated MAC disease. Other endpoints included the incidence of clinically significant MAC disease and discontinuations from therapy for drug-related side effects.

Continued on next page

Cumulative Incidence Rate, %: Placebo (n=89)

Month	MAC Free and Alive	MAC	Adverse Experience	Lost to Follow-up
6	69.7	13.5	6.7	10.1
12	47.2	19.1	15.7	18.0
18	37.1	22.5	18.0	22.5

Cumulative Incidence Rate, %: Azithromycin (n=85)

Month	MAC Free and Alive	MAC	Adverse Experience	Lost to Follow-up
6	84.7	3.5	9.4	2.4
12	63.5	8.2	16.5	11.8
18	44.7	11.8	25.9	17.6

Cumulative Incidence Rate, %: Rifabutin (n=223)

Month	MAC Free and Alive	MAC	Adverse Experience	Lost to Follow-up
6	83.4	7.2	8.1	1.3
12	60.1	15.2	16.1	8.5
18	40.8	21.5	24.2	13.5

Cumulative Incidence Rate, %: Azithromycin (n=223)

Month	MAC Free and Alive	MAC	Adverse Experience	Lost to Follow-up
6	85.2	3.6	5.8	5.4
12	65.5	7.6	16.1	10.8
18	45.3	12.1	23.8	18.8

Cumulative Incidence Rate, %: Azithromycin/Rifabutin Combination (n=218)

Month	MAC Free and Alive	MAC	Adverse Experience	Lost to Follow-up
6	89.4	1.8	5.5	3.2
12	71.6	2.8	15.1	10.6
18	49.1	6.4	29.4	15.1

Zithromax Caps/Tabs/O.S.—Cont.

MAC bacteremia
In trial 155, 85 patients randomized to receive azithromycin and 89 patients randomized to receive placebo met study entrance criteria. Cumulative incidences at 6, 12 and 18 months of the possible outcomes are in the following table:
[See first table on previous page]
The difference in the one year cumulative incidence rates of disseminated MAC disease (placebo–azithromycin) is 10.9%. This difference is statistically significant (p=0.037) with a 95% confidence interval for this difference of (0.8%, 20.9%). The comparable number of patients experiencing adverse events and the fewer number of patients lost to follow-up on azithromycin should be taken into account when interpreting the significance of this difference.
In trial 174, 223 patients randomized to receive rifabutin, 223 patients randomized to receive azithromycin, and 218 patients randomized to receive both rifabutin and azithromycin met study entrance criteria. Cumulative incidences at 6, 12 and 18 months of the possible outcomes are recorded in the following table:
[See second table on previous page]
Comparing the cumulative one year incidence rates, azithromycin monotherapy is at least as effective as rifabutin monotherapy. The difference (rifabutin–azithromycin) in the one year rates (7.6%) is statistically significant (p=0.022) with an adjusted 95% confidence interval (0.9%, 14.3%). Additionally, azithromycin/rifabutin combination therapy is more effective than rifabutin alone. The difference (rifabutin–azithromycin/rifabutin) in the cumulative one year incidence rates (12.5%) is statistically significant (p<0.001) with an adjusted 95% confidence interval of (6.6%, 18.4%). The comparable number of patients experiencing adverse events and the fewer number of patients lost to follow-up on rifabutin should be taken into account when interpreting the significance of this difference.
In Study 174, sensitivity testing[5] was performed on all available MAC isolates from subjects randomized to either azithromycin, rifabutin or the combination. The distribution of MIC values for azithromycin from susceptibility testing of the breakthrough isolates was similar between study arms. As the efficacy of azithromycin in the treatment of disseminated MAC has not been established, the clinical relevance of these *in vitro* MICs as an indicator of susceptibility or resistance is not known.

Clinically Significant Disseminated MAC Disease
In association with the decreased incidence of bacteremia, patients in the groups randomized to either azithromycin alone or azithromycin in combination with rifabutin showed reductions in the signs and symptoms of disseminated MAC disease, including fever or night sweats, weight loss and anemia.

Discontinuations From Therapy For Drug-Related Side Effects
In Study 155, discontinuations for drug-related toxicity occurred in 8.2% of subjects treated with azithromycin and 2.3% of those given placebo (p=0.121). In Study 174, more subjects discontinued from the combination of azithromycin and rifabutin (22.7%) than from azithromycin alone (13.5%; p=0.026) or rifabutin alone (15.9%; p=0.209).

Safety
As these patients with advanced HIV disease were taking multiple concomitant medications and experienced a variety of intercurrent illnesses, it was often difficult to attribute adverse events to study medication. Overall, the nature of side effects seen on the weekly dosage regimen of azithromycin over a period of approximately one year in patients with advanced HIV disease was similar to that previously reported for shorter course therapies.
[See first table at right]
Side effects related to the gastrointestinal tract were seen more frequently in patients receiving azithromycin than in those receiving placebo or rifabutin. In Study 174, 86% of diarrheal episodes were mild to moderate in nature with discontinuation of therapy for this reason occurring in only 9/233 (3.8%) of patients.

Changes in Laboratory Values
In these immunocompromised patients with advanced HIV infection, it was necessary to assess laboratory abnormalities developing on study with additional criteria if baseline values were outside the relevant normal range.
[See second table at right]

Treatment of Disseminated MAC Disease
One randomized, double blind clinical trial (Study 189) was performed in patients with disseminated MAC. In this trial, 246 HIV infected patients with disseminated MAC received either azithromycin 250 mg qd (N=65), azithromycin 600 mg qd (N=91) or clarithromycin 500 mg bid (N=90), each administered with ethambutol 15 mg/kg qd, for 24 weeks. Patients were cultured and clinically assessed every 3 weeks through week 12 and monthly thereafter through week 24. After week 24, patients were switched to any open label therapy at the discretion of the investigator and followed every 3 months through the last follow up visit of the trial. Patients were followed from the baseline visit for a period of up to 3.7 years (median: 9 months). MAC isolates recovered during study treatment or post-treatment were obtained whenever possible.
The primary endpoint was sterilization by week 24. Sterilization was based on data from the central laboratory, and was defined as two consecutive observed negative blood cultures for MAC, independent of missing culture data between the two negative observations. Analyses were performed on all randomized patients who had a positive baseline culture for MAC.
The azithromycin 250 mg arm was discontinued after an interim analysis at 12 weeks showed a significantly lower clearance of bacteremia compared to clarithromycin 500 mg bid.
Efficacy results for the azithromycin 600 mg qd and clarithromycin 500 mg bid treatment regimens are described in the following table:

Response to therapy of patients taking ethambutol and either azithromycin 600 mg qd or clarithromycin 500 mg bid

	Azithromycin 600 mg qd	Clarithromycin 500 mg bid	**95% CI on difference
Patients with positive culture at baseline	68	57	
Week 24 Two consecutive negative blood cultures*	31/68 (46%)	32/57 (56%)	[-28, 7]
Mortality	16/68 (24%)	15/57 (26%)	[-18, 13]

*Primary endpoint

**[95% confidence interval] on difference in rates (azithromycin-clarithromycin)

The primary endpoint, rate of sterilization of blood cultures (two consecutive negative cultures) at 24 weeks, was lower in the azithromycin 600 mg qd group than in the clarithromycin 500 mg bid group.

INCIDENCE OF ONE OR MORE TREATMENT RELATED* ADVERSE EVENTS** IN HIV INFECTED PATIENTS RECEIVING PROPHYLAXIS FOR DISSEMINATED MAC OVER APPROXIMATELY 1 YEAR

	Study 155		Study 174		
	Placebo (N=91)	Azithromycin 1200 mg weekly (N=89)	Azithromycin 1200 mg weekly (N=233)	Rifabutin 300 mg daily (N=236)	Azithromycin + Rifabutin (N=224)
Mean Duration of Therapy (days)	303.8	402.9	315	296.1	344.4
Discontinuation of Therapy	2.3	8.2	13.5	15.9	22.7
Autonomic Nervous System					
Mouth Dry	0	0	0	3.0	2.7
Central Nervous System					
Dizziness	0	1.1	3.9	1.7	0.4
Headache	0	0	3.0	5.5	4.5
Gastrointestinal					
Diarrhea	15.4	52.8	50.2	19.1	50.9
Loose Stools	6.6	19.1	12.9	3.0	9.4
Abdominal Pain	6.6	27	32.2	12.3	31.7
Dyspepsia	1.1	9	4.7	1.7	1.8
Flatulence	4.4	9	10.7	5.1	5.8
Nausea	11	32.6	27.0	16.5	28.1
Vomiting	1.1	6.7	9.0	3.8	5.8
General					
Fever	1.1	0	2.1	4.2	4.9
Fatigue	0	2.2	3.9	2.1	3.1
Malaise	0	1.1	0.4	0	2.2
Musculoskeletal					
Arthralgia	0	0	3.0	4.2	7.1
Psychiatric					
Anorexia	1.1	0	2.1	2.1	3.1
Skin & Appendages					
Pruritus	3.3	0	3.9	3.4	7.6
Rash	3.2	3.4	8.1	9.4	11.1
Skin discoloration	0	0	0	2.1	2.2
Special Senses					
Tinnitus	4.4	3.4	0.9	1.3	0.9
Hearing Decreased	2.2	1.1	0.9	0.4	0
Uveitis	0	0	0.4	1.3	1.8
Taste Perversion	0	0	1.3	2.5	1.3

* Includes those events considered possibly or probably related to study drug
** >2% adverse event rates for any group (except uveitis).

Prophylaxis Against Disseminated MAC Abnormal Laboratory Values*

		Placebo		Azithromycin 1200 mg weekly		Rifabutin 300 mg daily		Azithromycin & Rifabutin	
Hemoglobin	<8 g/dl	1/51	2%	4/170	2%	4/114	4%	8/107	8%
Platelet Count	<50 × 10³/mm³	1/71	1%	4/260	2%	2/182	1%	6/181	3%
WBC Count	<1 × 10³/mm³	0/8	0%	2/70	3%	2/47	4%	0/43	0%
Neutrophils	<500/mm³	0/26	0%	4/106	4%	3/82	4%	2/78	3%
SGOT	>5 × ULN[a]	1/41	2%	8/158	5%	3/121	3%	6/114	5%
SGPT	>5 × ULN	0/49	0%	8/166	5%	3/130	2%	5/117	4%
Alk Phos	>5 × ULN	1/80	1%	4/247	2%	2/172	1%	3/164	2%

[a]=Upper Limit of Normal
*excludes subjects outside of the relevant normal range at baseline

Sterilization by Baseline Colony Count
Within both treatment groups, the sterilization rates at week 24 decreased as the range of MAC cfu/mL increased.

Groups Stratified by MAC Colony Counts at Baseline	Azithromycin 600 mg (N=68) No. (%) Subjects in Stratified Group Sterile at Week 24	Clarithromycin 500 mg bid (N=57) No. (%) Subjects in Stratified Group Sterile at Week 24
≤ 10 cfu/mL	10/15 (66.7%)	12/17 (70.6%)
11-100 cfu/mL	13/28 (46.4%)	13/19 (68.4%)
101-1,000 cfu/mL	7/19 (36.8%)	5/13 (38.5%)
1,001-10,000 cfu/mL	1/5 (20.0%)	1/5 (20%)
>10,000 cfu/mL	0/1 (0.0%)	1/3 (33.3%)

Susceptibility Pattern of MAC Isolates:
Susceptibility testing was performed on MAC isolates recovered at baseline, at the time of breakthrough on therapy or during post-therapy follow-up. The T100 radiometric broth method was employed to determine azithromycin and clarithromycin MIC values. Azithromycin MIC values ranged from <4 to >256 μg/mL and clarithromycin MICs ranged from <1 to >32 μg/mL. The individual MAC susceptibility results demonstrated that azithromycin MIC values could be 4 to 32 fold higher than clarithromycin MIC values. During study treatment and post-treatment follow up for up to 3.7 years (median: 9 months) in study 189, a total of 6/68 (9%) and 6/57 (11%) of the patients randomized to azithromycin 600 mg daily and clarithromycin 500 mg bid, respectively, developed MAC blood culture isolates that had a sharp increase in MIC values. All twelve MAC isolates had azithromycin MIC's ≥256 μg/mL and clarithromycin MIC's >32 μg/mL. These high MIC values suggest develop-

ment of drug resistance. However, at this time, specific breakpoints for separating susceptible and resistant MAC isolates have not been established for either macrolide.

ANIMAL TOXICOLOGY

Phospholipidosis (intracellular phospholipid binding) has been observed in some tissues of mice, rats, and dogs given multiple doses of azithromycin. It has been demonstrated in numerous organ systems (e.g., eye, dorsal root ganglia, liver, gallbladder, kidney, spleen, and pancreas) in dogs administered doses which, based on pharmacokinetics, are as low as 2 times greater than the recommended adult human dose and in rats at doses comparable to the recommended adult human dose. This effect has been reversible after cessation of azithromycin treatment. The significance of these findings for humans is unknown.

REFERENCES

1. National Committee for Clinical Laboratory Standards. Methods for Dilution Antimicrobial Susceptibility Tests for Bacteria that Grow Aerobically–Third Edition. Approved Standard NCCLS Document M7-A3, Vol. 13, No. 25, NCCLS, Villanova, PA, December 1993.
2. National Committee for Clinical Laboratory Standards. Performance Standards for Antimicrobial Disk Susceptibility Tests–Fifth Edition. Approved Standard NCCLS Document M2-A5, Vol. 13, No. 24, NCCLS, Villanova, PA, December 1993.
3. Dunne MW, Foulds G, Retsema JA. Rationale for the use of azithromycin as *Mycobacterium avium* chemoprophylaxis. *American J Medicine* 1997; 102(5C):37-49.
4. Meier A, Kirshner P, Springer B, et al. Identification of mutations in 23S rRNA gene of clarithromycin-resistant *Mycobacterium intracellulare*. *Antimicrob Agents Chemother*. 1994;38:381-384.
5. Methodology per Inderlied CB, et al. Determination of *In Vitro* Susceptibility of *Mycobacterium avium* Complex Isolates to Antimicrobial Agents by Various Methods. *Antimicrob Agents Chemother* 1987; 31:1697-1702.

℞ Only
Licensed from Pliva   ©2002 PFIZER INC
Distributed by:
Pfizer Labs
Division of Pfizer Inc, NY, NY 10017
69-4763-00-7   Revised October 2002

ZITHROMAX® ℞
[zī′ th-rō-maks]
(azithromycin for injection)
For IV infusion only

Prescribing information for this product, which appears on pages 2672–2675 of the 2003 PDR, has been completely revised as follows. Please write "See Supplement A" next to the product heading.

DESCRIPTION

ZITHROMAX® (azithromycin for injection) contains the active ingredient azithromycin, an azalide, a subclass of macrolide antibiotics, for intravenous injection. Azithromycin has the chemical name (2R,3S,4R,5R,8R,10R,11R,12S,13S,14R)-13-[(2,6-dideoxy-3-C-methyl-3-O-methyl-α-L-ribo-hexopyranosyl)oxy]-2-ethyl-3,4,10-trihydroxy-3,5,6,8,10,12,14-hepta-methyl-11-[[3,4,6-trideoxy-3-(dimethylamino)-β-D-xylo-hexopyranosyl]oxy]-1-oxa-6-azacyclopentadecan-15-one. Azithromycin is derived from erythromycin; however, it differs chemically from erythromycin in that a methyl-substituted nitrogen atom is incorporated into the lactone ring. Its molecular formula is $C_{38}H_{72}N_2O_{12}$, and its molecular weight is 749.00. Azithromycin has the following structural formula:

Azithromycin, as the dihydrate, is a white crystalline powder with a molecular formula of $C_{38}H_{72}N_2O_{12} \cdot 2H_2O$ and a molecular weight of 785.0.
ZITHROMAX® (azithromycin for injection) consists of azithromycin dihydrate and the following inactive ingredients: citric acid and sodium hydroxide. ZITHROMAX® (azithromycin for injection) is supplied in lyophilized form in a 10-mL vial equivalent to 500 mg of azithromycin for intravenous administration. Reconstitution, according to label directions, results in approximately 5 mL of ZITHROMAX® for intravenous injection with each mL containing azithromycin dihydrate equivalent to 100 mg of azithromycin.

CLINICAL PHARMACOLOGY

In patients hospitalized with community-acquired pneumonia receiving single daily one-hour intravenous infusions for 2 to 5 days of 500 mg azithromycin at a concentration of 2 mg/mL, the mean Cmax ± S.D. achieved was 3.63 ± 1.60 μg/mL, while the 24-hour trough level was 0.20 ± 0.15 μg/mL, and the AUC_{24} was 9.60 ± 4.80 μg·h/mL. The mean Cmax, 24-hour trough and AUC_{24} values were 1.14 ± 0.14 μg/mL, 0.18 ± 0.02 μg/mL, and 8.03 ± 0.86 μg·h/mL, respectively, in normal volunteers receiving a 3-hour intravenous infusion of 500 mg azithromycin at a concentration of 1 mg/mL. Similar pharmacokinetic values were obtained in patients hospitalized with community-acquired pneumonia that received the same 3-hour dosage regimen for 2-5 days.
[See first table above]
The average CL_t and V_d values were 10.18 mL/min/kg and 33.3 L/kg, respectively, in 18 normal volunteers receiving 1000 to 4000-mg doses given as 1 mg/mL over 2 hours.
Comparison of the plasma pharmacokinetic parameters following the 1st and 5th daily doses of 500 mg intravenous azithromycin showed only an 8% increase in C_{max} but a 61% increase in AUC_{24} reflecting a threefold rise in C_{24} trough levels.
Following single oral doses of 500 mg azithromycin to 12 healthy volunteers, C_{max}, trough level, and AUC_{24} were reported to be 0.41 μg/mL, 0.05 μg/mL, and 2.6 μg/mL, respectively. These oral values are approximately 38%, 83%, and 52% of the values observed following a single 500-mg I.V. 3-hour infusion (C_{max}: 1.08 μg/mL, trough: 0.06 μg/mL, and AUC_{24}: 5.0 μg·h/mL).
Thus, plasma concentrations are higher following the intravenous regimen throughout the 24-hour interval. The pharmacokinetic parameters on day 5 of azithromycin 250-mg capsules following a 500-mg oral loading dose to healthy young adults (age 18-40 years old) were as follows: C_{max}: 0.24 μg/mL, AUC_{24}: 2.1 μg·h/mL. Tissue levels have not been obtained following intravenous infusions of azithromycin. Selected tissue (or fluid) concentration and tissue (or fluid) to plasma/serum concentration ratios following oral administration of azithromycin are shown in the following table:
[See second table above]
Tissue levels were determined following a single oral dose of 500 mg azithromycin in 7 gynecological patients. Approximately 17 hours after dosing, azithromycin concentrations were 2.7 μg/g in ovarian tissue, 3.5 μg/g in uterine tissue, and 3.3 μg/g in salpinx. Tissue levels have not been obtained following intravenous infusion of azithromycin.
In a multiple-dose study in 12 normal volunteers utilizing a 500-mg (1 mg/mL) one-hour intravenous-dosage regimen for five days, the amount of administered azithromycin dose excreted in urine in 24 hours was about 11% after the 1st dose and 14% after the 5th dose. These values are greater than the reported 6% excreted unchanged in urine after oral administration of azithromycin. Biliary excretion is a major route of elimination for unchanged drug, following oral administration.
The serum protein binding of azithromycin is variable in the concentration range approximating human exposure decreasing from 51% at 0.02 μg/mL to 7% at 2 μg/mL.
Microbiology: Azithromycin acts by binding to the 50S ribosomal subunit of susceptible microorganisms and, thus, interfering with microbial protein synthesis. Nucleic acid synthesis is not affected.
Azithromycin concentrates in phagocytes and fibroblasts as demonstrated by *in vitro* incubation techniques. Using such methodology, the ratio of intracellular to extracellular concentration was >30 after one hour incubation. *In vivo* studies suggest that concentration in phagocytes may contribute to drug distribution to inflamed tissues.
Azithromycin has been shown to be active against most strains of the following microorganisms, both *in vitro* and in clinical infections as described in the **INDICATIONS AND USAGE** section of the package insert for ZITHROMAX® (azithromycin for injection).
Aerobic gram-positive microorganisms
Staphylococcus aureus
Streptococcus pneumoniae
NOTE: Azithromycin demonstrates cross-resistance with erythromycin-resistant gram-positive strains. Most strains of *Enterococcus faecalis* and methicillin-resistant staphylococci are resistant to azithromycin.
Aerobic gram-negative microorganisms
Haemophilus influenzae
Moraxella catarrhalis
Neisseria gonorrhoeae
"Other" microorganisms
Chlamydia pneumoniae
Chlamydia trachomatis
Legionella pneumophila
Mycoplasma hominis
Mycoplasma pneumoniae
Beta-lactamase production should have no effect on azithromycin activity.
Azithromycin has been shown to be active against most strains of the following microorganisms, both *in vitro* and in clinical infections as described in the **INDICATIONS AND USAGE** section of the package insert for ZITHROMAX® (azithromycin tablets) and ZITHROMAX® (azithromycin for oral suspension).
Aerobic gram-positive microorganisms
Staphylococcus aureus
Streptococcus agalactiae
Streptococcus pneumoniae
Streptococcus pyogenes
Aerobic gram-negative microorganisms
Haemophilus ducreyi
Haemophilus influenzae
Moraxella catarrhalis
Neisseria gonorrhoeae
"Other" microorganisms
Chlamydia pneumoniae
Chlamydia trachomatis
Mycoplasma pneumoniae
The following *in vitro* data are available, **but their clinical significance is unknown.**
Azithromycin exhibits *in vitro* minimum inhibitory concentrations (MIC's) of 0.5 μg/mL or less against most (≥90%) strains of streptococci listed below and MIC's of 2.0 μg/mL or less against most (≥90%) strains of other listed microorganisms. However, the safety and effectiveness of azithromycin in treating clinical infections due to these microorganisms have not been established in adequate and well-controlled clinical trials.

Continued on next page

Plasma concentrations (μg/mL ± S.D.) after the last daily intravenous infusion of 500 mg azithromycin

Infusion Concentration, Duration	Time after starting the infusion (hr)								
	0.5	1	2	3	4	6	8	12	24
2 mg/mL, 1 hr[a]	2.98 ±1.12	3.63 ±1.73	0.60 ±0.31	0.40 ±0.23	0.33 ±0.16	0.26 ±0.14	0.27 ±0.15	0.20 ±0.12	0.20 ±0.15
1 mg/mL, 3 hr[b]	0.91 ±0.13	1.02 ±0.11	1.14 ±0.13	1.13 ±0.16	0.32 ±0.05	0.28 ±0.04	0.27 ±0.03	0.22 ±0.02	0.18 ±0.02

a = 500 mg (2 mg/mL) for 2-5 days in Community-acquired pneumonia patients.
b = 500 mg (1 mg/mL) for 5 days in healthy subjects.

AZITHROMYCIN CONCENTRATIONS FOLLOWING TWO - 250 mg (500 mg) CAPSULES IN ADULTS

TISSUE OR FLUID	TIME AFTER DOSE (h)	TISSUE OR FLUID CONCENTRATION (μg/g or μg/mL)[1]	CORRESPONDING PLASMA OR SERUM LEVEL (μg/mL)	TISSUE (FLUID) PLASMA (SERUM) RATIO[1]
SKIN	72-96	0.4	0.012	35
LUNG	72-96	4.0	0.012	>100
SPUTUM*	2-4	1.0	0.64	2
SPUTUM**	10-12	2.9	0.1	30
TONSIL***	9-18	4.5	0.03	>100
TONSIL***	180	0.9	0.006	>100
CERVIX****	19	2.8	0.04	70

[1]High tissue concentrations should not be interpreted to be quantitatively related to clinical efficacy. The antimicrobial activity of azithromycin is pH related. Azithromycin is concentrated in cell lysosomes which have a low intraorganelle pH, at which the drug's activity is reduced. However, the extensive distribution of drug to tissues may be relevant to clinical activity.
* Sample was obtained 2-4 hours after the first dose.
** Sample was obtained 10-12 hours after the first dose.
*** Dosing regimen of 2 doses of 250 mg each, separated by 12 hours.
**** Sample was obtained 19 hours after a single 500 mg dose.

Zithromax IV—Cont.

Aerobic gram-positive microorganisms
Streptococci (Groups C, F, G)
Viridans group streptococci
Aerobic gram-negative microorganisms
Bordetella pertussis
Anaerobic microorganisms
Peptostreptococcus species
Prevotella bivia
"Other" microorganisms
Ureaplasma urealyticum
Susceptibility Tests
Azithromycin can be solubilized for *in vitro* susceptibility testing using dilution techniques by dissolving in a minimum amount of 95% ethanol and diluting to the working stock concentration with broth.
Dilution Techniques:
Quantitative methods are used to determine antimicrobial minimum inhibitory concentrations (MIC's). These MIC's provide estimates of the susceptibility of bacteria to antimicrobial compounds. The MIC's should be determined using a standardized procedure. Standardized procedures are based on a dilution method[1] (broth or agar) or equivalent with standardized inoculum concentrations and standardized concentrations of azithromycin powder. The MIC values should be interpreted according to the following criteria:
For testing aerobic microorganisms other than *Haemophilus* species, *Neisseria gonorrhoeae*, and streptococci:

MIC (μg/mL)	Interpretation
≤ 2	Susceptible (S)
4	Intermediate (I)
≥ 8	Resistant (R)

For testing *Haemophilus* species:[a]

MIC (μg/mL)	Interpretation
≤ 4	Susceptible (S)

[a] This interpretive standard is applicable only to broth microdilution susceptibility testing with *Haemophilus* species using *Haemophilus* Test Medium (HTM)[1].

The current absence of data on resistant strains precludes defining any categories other than "Susceptible". Strains yielding MIC results suggestive of a "nonsusceptible" category should be submitted to a reference laboratory for further testing.
For testing streptococci including *S. pneumoniae*:[b]

MIC (μg/mL)	Interpretation
≤ 0.5	Susceptible (S)
1	Intermediate (I)
≥ 2	Resistant (R)

[b] These interpretive standards are applicable only to broth microdilution susceptibility tests using cation-adjusted Mueller-Hinton broth with 2–5% lysed horse blood.[1]

No interpretive criteria have been established for testing *Neisseria gonorrhoeae*. This species is not usually tested.
A report of "Susceptible" indicates that the pathogen is likely to respond to monotherapy with azithromycin. A report of "Intermediate" indicates that the result should be considered equivocal, and, if the microorganism is not fully susceptible to alternative, clinically feasible drugs, the test should be repeated. This category implies possible clinical applicability in body sites where the drug is physiologically concentrated or in situations where high dosage of drug can be used. This category also provides a buffer zone which prevents small uncontrolled technical factors from causing major discrepancies in interpretation. A report of "Resistant" indicates that achievable drug concentrations are unlikely to be inhibitory; other therapy should be selected.
Standardized susceptibility test procedures require the use of laboratory control microorganisms to control the technical aspects of the laboratory procedures. Standard azithromycin powder should provide the following MIC values:

Microorganism	MIC (μg/mL)
Haemophilus influenzae ATCC 49247[a]	1.0–4.0
Staphylococcus aureus ATCC 29213	0.5–2.0
Streptococcus pneumoniae ATCC 49619[b]	0.06–0.25

[a] This quality control range is applicable to only *H. influenzae* ATCC 49247 tested by a broth microdilution procedure using *Haemophilus* Test Medium (HTM)[1].
[b] This quality control range is applicable to only *S. pneumoniae* ATCC 49619 tested by a broth microdilution procedure using cation-adjusted Mueller-Hinton broth with 2-5% lysed horse blood.[1]

Diffusion Techniques:
Quantitative methods that require measurement of zone diameters also provide reproducible estimates of the susceptibility of bacteria to antimicrobial compounds. One such standardized procedure[2] requires the use of standardized inoculum concentrations. This procedure uses paper disks impregnated with 15-μg azithromycin to test the susceptibility of microorganisms to azithromycin.
Reports from the laboratory providing results of the standard single-disk susceptibility test with a 15-μg azithromycin disk should be interpreted according to the following criteria:
For testing aerobic microorganisms (including streptococci)[a] except *Haemophilus* species and *Neisseria gonorrhoeae*:

Zone Diameter (mm)	Interpretation
≥ 18	Susceptible (S)
14–17	Intermediate (I)
≤ 13	Resistant (R)

[a] These zone diameter standards for streptococci apply only to tests performed using Mueller-Hinton agar supplemented with 5% sheep blood and incubated in 5% CO_2.[2]

For testing *Haemophilus* species:[b]

Zone Diameter (mm)	Interpretation
≥ 12	Susceptible (S)

[b] This zone diameter standard is applicable only to tests with *Haemophilus* species using *Haemophilus* Test Medium (HTM)[2].

The current absence of data on resistant strains precludes defining any categories other than "Susceptible". Strains yielding zone diameter results suggestive of a "nonsusceptible" category should be submitted to a reference laboratory for further testing.
No interpretive criteria have been established for testing *Neisseria gonorrhoeae*. This species is not usually tested.
Interpretation should be as stated above for results using dilution techniques. Interpretation involves correlation of the diameter obtained in the disk test with the MIC for azithromycin.
As with standardized dilution techniques, diffusion methods require the use of laboratory control microorganisms that are used to control the technical aspects of the laboratory procedures. For the diffusion technique, the 15-μg azithromycin disk should provide the following zone diameters in these laboratory test quality control strains:

Microorganism	Zone Diameter (mm)
Haemophilus influenzae ATCC 49247[a]	13–21
Staphylococcus aureus ATCC 25923	21–26
Streptococcus pneumoniae ATCC 49619[b]	19–25

[a] These quality control limits are applicable only to tests conducted with *H. influenzae* ATCC 49247 using *Haemophilus* Test Medium (HTM)[2].
[b] These quality control limits are applicable only to tests conducted with *S. pneumoniae* ATCC 49619 using Mueller-Hinton agar supplemented with 5% sheep blood incubated in 5% CO_2.[2]

INDICATIONS AND USAGE
ZITHROMAX® (azithromycin for injection) is indicated for the treatment of patients with infections caused by susceptible strains of the designated microorganisms in the conditions listed below. As recommended dosages, durations of therapy, and applicable patient populations vary among these infections, please see **DOSAGE AND ADMINISTRATION** for dosing recommendations.
Community-acquired pneumonia due to *Chlamydia pneumoniae*, *Haemophilus influenzae*, *Legionella pneumophila*, *Moraxella catarrhalis*, *Mycoplasma pneumoniae*, *Staphylococcus aureus*, or *Streptococcus pneumoniae* in patients who require initial intravenous therapy.
Pelvic inflammatory disease due to *Chlamydia trachomatis*, *Neisseria gonorrhoeae*, or *Mycoplasma hominis* in patients who require initial intravenous therapy. If anaerobic microorganisms are suspected of contributing to the infection, an antimicrobial agent with anaerobic activity should be administered in combination with ZITHROMAX®.
ZITHROMAX® (azithromycin for injection) should be followed by ZITHROMAX® by the oral route as required. (See **DOSAGE AND ADMINISTRATION**.)
Appropriate culture and susceptibility tests should be performed before treatment to determine the causative microorganism and its susceptibility to azithromycin. Therapy with ZITHROMAX® may be initiated before results of these tests are known; once the results become available, antimicrobial therapy should be adjusted accordingly.

CONTRAINDICATIONS
ZITHROMAX® is contraindicated in patients with known hypersensitivity to azithromycin, erythromycin, or any macrolide antibiotic.

WARNINGS
Serious allergic reactions, including angioedema, anaphylaxis, and dermatologic reactions including Stevens Johnson Syndrome and toxic epidermal necrolysis have been reported rarely in patients on azithromycin therapy. Although rare, fatalities have been reported. (See **CONTRAINDICATIONS**.) Despite initially successful symptomatic treatment of the allergic symptoms, when symptomatic therapy was discontinued, the allergic symptoms **recurred soon thereafter in some patients without further azithromycin exposure**. These patients required prolonged periods of observation and symptomatic treatment. The relationship of these episodes to the long tissue half-life of azithromycin and subsequent prolonged exposure to antigen is unknown at present.
If an allergic reaction occurs, the drug should be discontinued and appropriate therapy should be instituted. Physicians should be aware that reappearance of the allergic symptoms may occur when symptomatic therapy is discontinued.

Pseudomembranous colitis has been reported with nearly all antibacterial agents and may range in severity from mild to life-threatening. Therefore, it is important to consider this diagnosis in patients who present with diarrhea subsequent to the administration of antibacterial agents.
Treatment with antibacterial agents alters the normal flora of the colon and may permit overgrowth of clostridia. Studies indicate that a toxin produced by *Clostridium difficile* is a primary cause of "antibiotic-associated colitis."
After the diagnosis of pseudomembranous colitis has been established, therapeutic measures should be initiated. Mild cases of pseudomembranous colitis usually respond to discontinuation of the drug alone. In moderate to severe cases, consideration should be given to management with fluids and electrolytes, protein supplementation, and treatment with an antibacterial drug clinically effective against *Clostridium difficile* colitis.

PRECAUTIONS
General: Because azithromycin is principally eliminated via the liver, caution should be exercised when azithromycin is administered to patients with impaired hepatic function.
There are no data regarding azithromycin usage in patients with renal impairment; therefore, caution should be exercised when prescribing azithromycin in these patients.
ZITHROMAX® (azithromycin for injection) should be reconstituted and diluted as directed and administered as an intravenous infusion over not less than 60 minutes. (See **DOSAGE AND ADMINISTRATION**.)
Local I.V. site reactions have been reported with the intravenous administration of azithromycin. The incidence and severity of these reactions were the same when 500 mg azithromycin were given over 1 hour (2 mg/mL as 250 mL infusion) or over 3 hours (1 mg/mL as 500 mL infusion). (See **ADVERSE REACTIONS**.) All volunteers who received infusate concentrations above 2.0 mg/mL experienced local I.V. site reactions and, therefore, higher concentrations should be avoided.
The following adverse events have been reported with macrolide products: ventricular arrhythmias, including ventricular tachycardia, and *torsades de pointes*, in individuals with prolonged QT intervals.
There has been a spontaneous report from the post-marketing experience of a patient with previous history of arrhythmias who experienced *torsades de pointes* and subsequent myocardial infarction following a course of oral azithromycin therapy.
Information for Patients:
Patients should be cautioned not to take aluminum- and magnesium-containing antacids and azithromycin by the oral route simultaneously.
Patients should be directed to discontinue azithromycin and contact a physician if any signs of an allergic reaction occur.
Drug Interactions: Aluminum- and magnesium-containing antacids reduce the peak serum levels (rate) but not the AUC (extent) of orally administered azithromycin.
Administration of cimetidine (800 mg) two hours prior to orally administered azithromycin had no effect on azithromycin absorption.
Azithromycin given by the oral route did not affect the plasma levels or pharmacokinetics of theophylline administered as a single intravenous dose. The effect of azithromycin on the plasma levels or pharmacokinetics of theophylline administered in multiple doses resulting in therapeutic steady-state levels of theophylline is not known. However, concurrent use of macrolides and theophylline has been associated with increases in the serum concentrations of theophylline. Therefore, until further data are available, prudent medical practice dictates careful monitoring of plasma theophylline levels in patients receiving azithromycin and theophylline concomitantly.
Azithromycin given by the oral route did not affect the prothrombin time response to a single dose of warfarin. However, prudent medical practice dictates careful monitoring of prothrombin time in all patients treated with azithromycin and warfarin concomitantly. Concurrent use of macrolides and warfarin in clinical practice has been associated with increased anticoagulant effects.
The following drug interactions have not been reported in clinical trials with azithromycin; however, no specific drug interaction studies have been performed to evaluate potential drug-drug interaction. Nonetheless, they have been observed with macrolide products. Until further data are developed regarding drug interactions when azithromycin and these drugs are used concomitantly, careful monitoring of patients is advised:
Digoxin-elevated digoxin levels.
Ergotamine or dihydroergotamine–acute ergot toxicity characterized by severe peripheral vasospasm and dysesthesia.
Triazolam-Increased pharmacologic effect of triazolam by decreasing the clearance of triazolam.
Drugs metabolized by the cytochrome P^{450} system-elevations of serum carbamazepine, terfenadine, cyclosporine, hexobarbital, and phenytoin levels.
Laboratory Test Interactions: There are no reported laboratory test interactions.
Carcinogenesis, Mutagenesis, Impairment of Fertility: Long-term studies in animals have not been performed to evaluate carcinogenic potential. Azithromycin has shown no mutagenic potential in standard laboratory tests: mouse lymphoma assay, human lymphocyte clastogenic assay, and mouse bone marrow clastogenic assay. No evidence of impaired fertility due to azithromycin was found.

Pregnancy: Teratogenic Effects. Pregnancy Category B: Reproduction studies have been performed in rats and mice at doses up to moderately maternally toxic dose levels (i.e., 200 mg/kg/day by the oral route). These doses, based on a mg/m^2 basis, are estimated to be 4 and 2 times, respectively, the human daily dose of 500 mg by the oral route. In the animal studies, no evidence of harm to the fetus due to azithromycin was found. There are, however, no adequate and well-controlled studies in pregnant women. Because animal reproduction studies are not always predictive of human response, azithromycin should be used during pregnancy only if clearly needed.

Nursing Mothers: It is not known whether azithromycin is excreted in human milk. Because many drugs are excreted in human milk, caution should be exercised when azithromycin is administered to a nursing woman.

Pediatric Use: Safety and effectiveness of azithromycin for injection in children or adolescents under 16 years have not been established. In controlled clinical studies, azithromycin has been administered to pediatric patients (age 6 months to 16 years) by the oral route. For information regarding the use of ZITHROMAX® (azithromycin for oral suspension) in the treatment of pediatric patients, refer to the **INDICATIONS AND USAGE** and **DOSAGE AND ADMINISTRATION** sections of the prescribing information for ZITHROMAX® (azithromycin for oral suspension) 100 mg/5 mL and 200 mg/5 mL bottles.

Geriatric Use: Pharmacokinetic studies with intravenous azithromycin have not been performed in older volunteers. Pharmacokinetics of azithromycin following oral administration in older volunteers (65–85 years old) were similar to those in younger volunteers (18–40 years old) for the 5-day therapeutic regimen.

In multiple-dose clinical trials of intravenous azithromycin in the treatment of community-acquired pneumonia, 45% of patients (188/414) were at least 65 years of age and 22% of patients (91/414) were at least 75 years of age. No overall differences in safety were observed between these subjects and younger subjects in terms of adverse events, laboratory abnormalities, and discontinuations. Similar decreases in clinical response were noted in azithromycin- and comparator-treated patients with increasing age.

ZITHROMAX® (azithromycin for injection) contains 114 mg (4.96 mEq) of sodium per vial. At the usual recommended doses, patients would receive 114 mg (4.96 mEq) of sodium. The geriatric population may respond with a blunted natriuresis to salt loading. The total sodium content from dietary and non-dietary sources may be clinically important with regard to such diseases as congestive heart failure.

ADVERSE REACTIONS

In clinical trials of intravenous azithromycin for community-acquired pneumonia, in which 2-5 I.V. doses were given, most of the reported side effects were mild to moderate in severity and were reversible upon discontinuation of the drug. The majority of patients in these trials had one or more comorbid diseases and were receiving concomitant medications. Approximately 1.2% of the patients discontinued intravenous ZITHROMAX® therapy, and a total of 2.4% discontinued azithromycin therapy by either the intravenous or oral route because of clinical or laboratory side effects.

In clinical trials conducted in patients with pelvic inflammatory disease, in which 1-2 I.V. doses were given, 2% of women who received monotherapy with azithromycin and 4% who received azithromycin plus metronidazole discontinued therapy due to clinical side effects.

Clinical side effects leading to discontinuations from these studies were most commonly gastrointestinal (abdominal pain, nausea, vomiting, diarrhea), and rashes; laboratory side effects leading to discontinuation were increases in transaminase levels and/or alkaline phosphatase levels.

Clinical:

Overall, the most common side effects associated with treatment in adult patients who received I.V./P.O. ZITHROMAX® in studies of community-acquired pneumonia were related to the gastrointestinal system with diarrhea/loose stools (4.3%), nausea (3.9%), abdominal pain (2.7%), and vomiting (1.4%) being the most frequently reported. Approximately 12% of patients experienced a side effect related to the intravenous infusion; most common were pain at the injection site (6.5%) and local inflammation (3.1%).

The most common side effects associated with treatment in adult women who received I.V./P.O. ZITHROMAX® in studies of pelvic inflammatory disease were related to the gastrointestinal system. Diarrhea (8.5%) and nausea (6.6%) were most commonly reported, followed by vaginitis (2.8%), abdominal pain (1.9%), anorexia (1.9%), rash and pruritus (1.9%). When azithromycin was co-administered with metronidazole in these studies, a higher proportion of women experienced side effects of nausea (10.3%), abdominal pain (3.7%), vomiting (2.8%), application site reaction, stomatitis, dizziness, or dyspnea (all at 1.9%).

No other side effects occurred in patients on the multiple dose I.V./P.O. regimen of ZITHROMAX® in these studies with a frequency greater than 1%.

Side effects that occurred with a frequency of 1% or less included the following:

Gastrointestinal: dyspepsia, flatulence, mucositis, oral moniliasis, and gastritis

Nervous System: headache, somnolence

Allergic: bronchospasm

Special Senses: taste perversion

Post-Marketing Experience:

Adverse events reported with orally administered azithromycin during the post-marketing period in adult and/or pediatric patients for which a causal relationship could not be established include:

Allergic: arthralgia, edema, urticaria, angioedema

Cardiovascular: arrhythmias, including ventricular tachycardia, hypotension

Gastrointestinal: anorexia, constipation, dyspepsia, flatulence, vomiting/diarrhea rarely resulting in dehydration, pseudomembranous colitis, pancreatitis, oral candidiasis and rare reports of tongue discoloration

General: asthenia, paresthesia, fatigue, malaise and anaphylaxis (rarely fatal)

Genitourinary: interstitial nephritis and acute renal failure, vaginitis

Hematopoietic: thrombocytopenia

Liver/Biliary: abnormal liver function including hepatitis and cholestatic jaundice, as well as rare cases of hepatic necrosis and hepatic failure, some of which have resulted in death

Nervous System: convulsions, dizziness/vertigo, headache, somnolence, hyperactivity, nervousness, agitation and syncope

Psychiatric: aggressive reaction and anxiety

Skin/Appendages: pruritus, rarely serious skin reactions including erythema multiforme, Stevens Johnson Syndrome, and toxic epidermal necrolysis

Special Senses: hearing disturbances including hearing loss, deafness, and/or tinnitus, rare reports of taste perversion

Laboratory Abnormalities:

Significant abnormalities (irrespective of drug relationship) occurring during the clinical trials were reported as follows: with an incidence of 4–6%, elevated ALT (SGPT), AST (SGOT), creatinine

with an incidence of 1–3%, elevated LDH, bilirubin

with an incidence of less than 1%, leukopenia, neutropenia, decreased platelet count, and elevated serum alkaline phosphatase

When follow-up was provided, changes in laboratory tests appeared to be reversible.

In multiple-dose clinical trials involving more than 750 patients treated with ZITHROMAX® (I.V./P.O.), less than 2% of patients discontinued azithromycin therapy because of treatment-related liver enzyme abnormalities.

DOSAGE AND ADMINISTRATION

(See INDICATIONS AND USAGE and CLINICAL PHARMACOLOGY.)

The recommended dose of ZITHROMAX® (azithromycin for injection) for the treatment of adult patients with community-acquired pneumonia due to the indicated organisms is: 500 mg as a single daily dose by the intravenous route for at least two days. Intravenous therapy should be followed by azithromycin by the oral route at a single, daily dose of 500 mg, administered as two 250-mg tablets to complete a 7- to 10-day course of therapy. The timing of the switch to oral therapy should be done at the discretion of the physician and in accordance with clinical response.

The recommended dose of ZITHROMAX® (azithromycin) for the treatment of adult patients with pelvic inflammatory disease due to the indicated organisms is: 500 mg as a single daily dose by the intravenous route for one or two days. Intravenous therapy should be followed by azithromycin by the oral route at a single, daily dose of 250 mg to complete a 7-day course of therapy. The timing of the switch to oral therapy should be done at the discretion of the physician and in accordance with clinical response. If anaerobic microorganisms are suspected of contributing to the infection, an antimicrobial agent with anaerobic activity should be administered in combination with ZITHROMAX®.

The infusate concentration and rate of infusion for ZITHROMAX® (azithromycin for injection) should be either 1 mg/mL over 3 hours or 2 mg/mL over 1 hour.

Preparation of the solution for intravenous administration is as follows:

Reconstitution

Prepare the initial solution of ZITHROMAX® (azithromycin for injection) by adding 4.8 mL of Sterile Water For Injection to the 500 mg vial and shaking the vial until all of the drug is dissolved. Since ZITHROMAX® (azithromycin for injection) is supplied under vacuum, it is recommended that a standard 5 mL (non-automated) syringe be used to ensure that the exact amount of 4.8 mL of Sterile Water is dispensed. Each mL of reconstituted solution contains 100 mg azithromycin. Reconstituted solution is stable for 24 hours when stored below 30°C or 86°F.

Parenteral drug products should be inspected visually for particulate matter prior to administration. If particulate matter is evident in reconstituted fluids, the drug solution should be discarded.

Dilute this solution further prior to administration as instructed below.

Dilution

To provide azithromycin over a concentration range of 1.0–2.0 mg/mL, transfer 5 mL of the 100 mg/mL azithromycin solution into the appropriate amount of any of the diluents listed below:

Normal Saline (0.9% sodium chloride)
1/2 Normal Saline (0.45% sodium chloride)
5% Dextrose in Water
Lactated Ringer's Solution
5% Dextrose in 1/2 Normal Saline (0.45% sodium chloride) with 20 mEq KCl
5% Dextrose in Lactated Ringer's Solution
5% Dextrose in 1/3 Normal Saline (0.3% sodium chloride)
5% Dextrose in 1/2 Normal Saline (0.45% sodium chloride)
Normosol®-M in 5% Dextrose
Normosol®-R in 5% Dextrose

When used with the Vial-Mate™ drug reconstitution device, please reference the Vial-Mate™ instructions for assembly and reconstitution.

Final Infusion Solution Concentration (mg/mL)	Amount of Diluent (mL)
1.0 mg/mL	500 mL
2.0 mg/mL	250 mL

It is recommended that a 500-mg dose of ZITHROMAX® (azithromycin for injection), diluted as above, be infused over a period of not less than 60 minutes.

ZITHROMAX® (azithromycin for injection) should not be given as a bolus or as an intramuscular injection.

Other intravenous substances, additives, or medications should not be added to ZITHROMAX® (azithromycin for injection), or infused simultaneously through the same intravenous line.

Storage

When diluted according to the instructions (1.0 mg/mL to 2.0 mg/mL), ZITHROMAX® (azithromycin for injection) is stable for 24 hours at or below room temperature (30°C or 86°F), or for 7 days if stored under refrigeration (5°C or 41°F).

HOW SUPPLIED

ZITHROMAX® (azithromycin for injection) is supplied in lyophilized form under a vacuum in a 10-mL vial equivalent to 500 mg of azithromycin for intravenous administration. Each vial also contains sodium hydroxide and 413.6 mg citric acid.

These are packaged as follows:

10 vials of 500 mg	NDC 0069-3150-83
10 vials of 500 mg with 1 Vial-Mate™ Adaptor each	NDC 0069-3150-14

CLINICAL STUDIES

Community-Acquired Pneumonia

In a controlled study of community-acquired pneumonia performed in the U.S., azithromycin (500 mg as a single daily dose by the intravenous route for 2-5 days, followed by 500 mg/day by the oral route to complete 7-10 days therapy) was compared to cefuroxime (2250 mg/day in three divided doses by the intravenous route for 2-5 days followed by 1000 mg/day in two divided doses by the oral route to complete 7-10 days therapy), with or without erythromycin. For the 291 patients who were evaluable for clinical efficacy, the clinical outcome rates, i.e., cure, improved, and success (cure + improved) among the 277 patients seen at 10–14 days post-therapy were as follows:

Clinical Outcome	Azithromycin	Comparator
Cure	46%	44%
Improved	32%	30%
Success (Cure + Improved)	78%	74%

In a separate, uncontrolled clinical and microbiological trial performed in the U.S., 94 patients with community-acquired pneumonia who received azithromycin in the same regimen were evaluable for clinical efficacy. The clinical outcome rates, i.e., cure, improved, and success (cure + improved) among the 84 patients seen at 10–14 days post-therapy were as follows:

Clinical Outcome	Azithromycin
Cure	60%
Improved	29%
Success (Cure + Improved)	89%

Microbiological determinations in both trials were made at the pre-treatment visit and, where applicable, were reassessed at later visits. Serological testing was done on baseline and final visit specimens. The following combined presumptive bacteriological eradication rates were obtained from the evaluable groups:

Combined Bacteriological Eradication Rates for Azithromycin:

(at last completed visit)	Azithromycin
S. pneumoniae	64/67 (96%)[a]
H. influenzae	41/43 (95%)
M. catarrhalis	9/10
S. aureus	9/10

[a] Nineteen of twenty-four patients (79%) with positive blood cultures for *S. pneumoniae* were cured (intent to treat analysis) with eradication of the pathogen.

The presumed bacteriological outcomes at 10-14 days post-therapy for patients treated with azithromycin with evidence (serology and/or culture) of atypical pathogens for both trials were as follows:

Evidence of Infection	Total	Cure	Improved	Cure + Improved
Mycoplasma pneumoniae	18	11 (61%)	5 (28%)	16 (89%)
Chlamydia pneumoniae	34	15 (44%)	13 (38%)	28 (82%)
Legionella pneumophila	16	5 (31%)	8 (50%)	13 (81%)

Continued on next page

Zithromax IV—Cont.

ANIMAL TOXICOLOGY

Phospholipidosis (intracellular phospholipid accumulation) has been observed in some tissues of mice, rats, and dogs given multiple doses of azithromycin. It has been demonstrated in numerous organ systems (e.g., eye, dorsal root ganglia, liver, gallbladder, kidney, spleen, and pancreas) in dogs treated with azithromycin at doses which, expressed on a mg/kg basis, are only 2 times greater than the recommended adult human dose and in rats at doses comparable to the recommended adult human dose. This effect has been reversible after cessation of azithromycin treatment. Phospholipidosis has been observed to a similar extent in the tissues of neonatal rats and dogs given daily doses of azithromycin ranging from 10 days to 30 days. Based on the pharmacokinetic data, phospholipidosis has been seen in the rat (30 mg/kg dose) at observed C_{max} value of 1.3 μg/mL (6 times greater than the observed C_{max} of 0.216 μg/mL at the pediatric dose of 10 mg/kg). Similarly, it has been shown in the dog (10 mg/kg dose) at observed C_{max} value of 1.5 μg/mL (7 times greater than the observed same C_{max} and drug dose in the studied pediatric population). On mg/m^2 basis, 30 mg/kg dose in the rat (135 mg/m^2) and 10 mg/kg dose in the dog (79 mg/m^2) are approximately 0.4 and 0.6 times, respectively, the recommended dose in the pediatric patients with an average body weight of 25 kg. This effect, similar to that seen in the adult animals, is reversible after cessation of azithromycin treatment. The significance of these findings for animals and for humans is unknown.

REFERENCES

1. National Committee for Clinical Laboratory Standards. Methods for Dilution Antimicrobial Susceptibility Tests for Bacteria that Grow Aerobically - Third Edition. Approved Standard NCCLS Document M7-A3, Vol. 13, No. 25, NCCLS, Villanova, PA, December, 1993.

2. National Committee for Clinical Laboratory Standards. Performance Standards for Antimicrobial Disk Susceptibility Tests - Fifth Edition. Approved Standard NCCLS Document M2-A5, Vol. 13, No. 24, NCCLS, Villanova, PA, December, 1993.

℞ Only

Licensed from Pliva

©2002 PFIZER INC

Vial-Mate is a trademark of Baxter International Inc., Reg. U.S. Pat and TM Off.

Distributed by:
Pfizer Labs
Division of Pfizer Inc
NY, NY 10017
70-5191-00-7

Revised October 2002

ZOLOFT® ℞

[*zō-lŏft*]
(sertraline hydrochloride)
Tablets and Oral Concentrate

Prescribing information for this product, which appears on pages 2675–2681 of the 2003 PDR, has been completely revised as follows. Please write "See Supplement A" next to the product heading.

DESCRIPTION

ZOLOFT® (sertraline hydrochloride) is a selective serotonin reuptake inhibitor (SSRI) for oral administration. It has a molecular weight of 342.7. Sertraline hydrochloride has the following chemical name: (1S-cis)-4-(3,4-dichlorophenyl)-1,2,3,4-tetrahydro-N-methyl-1-naphthalenamine hydrochloride. The empirical formula $C_{17}H_{17}NCl_2 \bullet HCl$ is represented by the following structural formula:

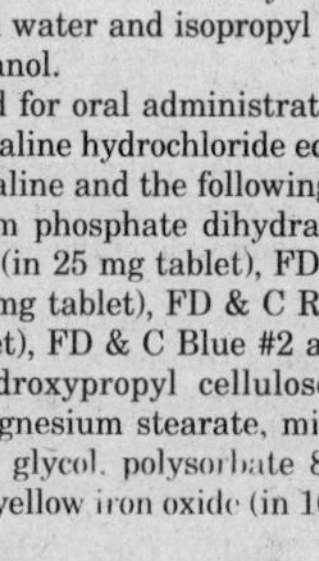

Sertraline hydrochloride is a white crystalline powder that is slightly soluble in water and isopropyl alcohol, and sparingly soluble in ethanol.

ZOLOFT is supplied for oral administration as scored tablets containing sertraline hydrochloride equivalent to 25, 50 and 100 mg of sertraline and the following inactive ingredients: dibasic calcium phosphate dihydrate, D & C Yellow #10 aluminum lake (in 25 mg tablet), FD & C Blue #1 aluminum lake (in 25 mg tablet), FD & C Red #40 aluminum lake (in 25 mg tablet), FD & C Blue #2 aluminum lake (in 50 mg tablet), hydroxypropyl cellulose, hydroxypropyl methylcellulose, magnesium stearate, microcrystalline cellulose, polyethylene glycol, polysorbate 80, sodium starch glycolate, synthetic yellow iron oxide (in 100 mg tablet), and titanium dioxide.

ZOLOFT oral concentrate is available in a multidose 60 mL bottle. Each mL of solution contains sertraline hydrochloride equivalent to 20 mg of sertraline. The solution contains the following inactive ingredients: glycerin, alcohol (12%), menthol, butylated hydroxytoluene (BHT). The oral concentrate must be diluted prior to administration (see PRECAUTIONS, Information for Patients and DOSAGE AND ADMINISTRATION).

CLINICAL PHARMACOLOGY

Pharmacodynamics

The mechanism of action of sertraline is presumed to be linked to its inhibition of CNS neuronal uptake of serotonin (5HT). Studies at clinically relevant doses in man have demonstrated that sertraline blocks the uptake of serotonin into human platelets. *In vitro* studies in animals also suggest that sertraline is a potent and selective inhibitor of neuronal serotonin reuptake and has only very weak effects on norepinephrine and dopamine neuronal reuptake. *In vitro* studies have shown that sertraline has no significant affinity for adrenergic ($alpha_1$, $alpha_2$, beta), cholinergic, GABA, dopaminergic, histaminergic, serotonergic ($5HT_{1A}$, $5HT_{1B}$, $5HT_2$), or benzodiazepine receptors; antagonism of such receptors has been hypothesized to be associated with various anticholinergic, sedative, and cardiovascular effects for other psychotropic drugs. The chronic administration of sertraline was found in animals to downregulate brain norepinephrine receptors, as has been observed with other drugs effective in the treatment of major depressive disorder. Sertraline does not inhibit monoamine oxidase.

Pharmacokinetics

Systemic Bioavailability—In man, following oral once-daily dosing over the range of 50 to 200 mg for 14 days, mean peak plasma concentrations (Cmax) of sertraline occurred between 4.5 to 8.4 hours post-dosing. The average terminal elimination half-life of plasma sertraline is about 26 hours. Based on this pharmacokinetic parameter, steady-state sertraline plasma levels should be achieved after approximately one week of once-daily dosing. Linear dose-proportional pharmacokinetics were demonstrated in a single dose study in which the Cmax and area under the plasma concentration time curve (AUC) of sertraline were proportional to dose over a range of 50 to 200 mg. Consistent with the terminal elimination half-life, there is an approximately two-fold accumulation, compared to a single dose, of sertraline with repeated dosing over a 50 to 200 mg dose range. The single dose bioavailability of sertraline tablets is approximately equal to an equivalent dose of solution.

In a relative bioavailability study comparing the pharmacokinetics of 100 mg sertraline as the oral solution to a 100 mg sertraline tablet in 16 healthy adults, the solution to tablet ratio of geometric mean AUC and Cmax values were 114.8% and 120.6%, respectively. 90% confidence intervals (CI) were within the range of 80–125% with the exception of the upper 90% CI limit for Cmax which was 126.5%.

The effects of food on the bioavailability of the sertraline tablet and oral concentrate were studied in subjects administered a single dose with and without food. For the tablet, AUC was slightly increased when drug was administered with food but the Cmax was 25% greater, while the time to reach peak plasma concentration (Tmax) decreased from 8 hours post-dosing to 5.5 hours. For the oral concentrate, Tmax was slightly prolonged from 5.9 hours to 7.0 hours with food.

Metabolism—Sertraline undergoes extensive first pass metabolism. The principal initial pathway of metabolism for sertraline is N-demethylation. N-desmethylsertraline has a plasma terminal elimination half-life of 62 to 104 hours. Both *in vitro* biochemical and *in vivo* pharmacological testing have shown N-desmethylsertraline to be substantially less active than sertraline. Both sertraline and N-desmethylsertraline undergo oxidative deamination and subsequent reduction, hydroxylation, and glucuronide conjugation. In a study of radiolabeled sertraline involving two healthy male subjects, sertraline accounted for less than 5% of the plasma radioactivity. About 40-45% of the administered radioactivity was recovered in urine in 9 days. Unchanged sertraline was not detectable in the urine. For the same period, about 40-45% of the administered radioactivity was accounted for in feces, including 12-14% unchanged sertraline.

Desmethylsertraline exhibits time-related, dose dependent increases in AUC (0-24 hour), Cmax and Cmin, with about a 5-9 fold increase in these pharmacokinetic parameters between day 1 and day 14.

Protein Binding—*In vitro* protein binding studies performed with radiolabeled ^3H-sertraline showed that sertraline is highly bound to serum proteins (98%) in the range of 20 to 500 ng/mL. However, at up to 300 and 200 ng/mL concentrations, respectively, sertraline and N-desmethylsertraline did not alter the plasma protein binding of two other highly protein bound drugs, viz., warfarin and propranolol (see PRECAUTIONS).

Pediatric Pharmacokinetics—Sertraline pharmacokinetics were evaluated in a group of 61 pediatric patients (29 aged 6-12 years, 32 aged 13-17 years) with a DSM-III-R diagnosis of major depressive disorder or obsessive-compulsive disorder. Patients included both males (N=28) and females (N=33). During 42 days of chronic sertraline dosing, sertraline was titrated up to 200 mg/day and maintained at that dose for a minimum of 11 days. On the final day of sertraline 200 mg/day, the 6-12 year old group exhibited a mean sertraline AUC (0-24 hr) of 3107 ng-hr/mL, mean Cmax of 165 ng/mL, and mean half-life of 26.2 hr. The 13-17 year old group exhibited a mean sertraline AUC (0-24 hr) of 2296 ng-hr/mL, mean Cmax of 123 ng/mL, and mean half-life of 27.8 hr. Higher plasma levels in the 6-12 year old group were largely attributable to patients with lower body weights. No gender associated differences were observed. By comparison, a group of 22 separately studied adults between 18 and 45 years of age (11 male, 11 female) received 30 days of 200 mg/day sertraline and exhibited a mean sertraline AUC (0-24 hr) of 2570 ng-hr/mL, mean Cmax of 142 ng/mL, and mean half-life of 27.2 hr. Relative to the adults, both the 6–12 year olds and the 13-17 year olds showed about 22% lower AUC (0-24 hr) and Cmax values when plasma concentration was adjusted for weight. These data suggest that pediatric patients metabolize sertraline with slightly greater efficiency than adults. Nevertheless, lower doses may be advisable for pediatric patients given their lower body weights, especially in very young patients, in order to avoid excessive plasma levels (see DOSAGE AND ADMINISTRATION).

Age—Sertraline plasma clearance in a group of 16 (8 male, 8 female) elderly patients treated for 14 days at a dose of 100 mg/day was approximately 40% lower than in a similarly studied group of younger (25 to 32 y.o.) individuals. Steady-state, therefore, should be achieved after 2 to 3 weeks in older patients. The same study showed a decreased clearance of desmethylsertraline in older males, but not in older females.

Liver Disease—As might be predicted from its primary site of metabolism, liver impairment can affect the elimination of sertraline. In patients with chronic mild liver impairment (N=10, 8 patients with Child-Pugh scores of 5-6 and 2 patients with Child-Pugh scores of 7-8) who received 50 mg sertraline per day maintained for 21 days, sertraline clearance was reduced, resulting in approximately 3-fold greater exposure compared to age-matched volunteers with no hepatic impairment (N=10). The exposure to desmethylsertraline was approximately 2-fold greater compared to age-matched volunteers with no hepatic impairment. There were no significant differences in plasma protein binding observed between the two groups. The effects of sertraline in patients with moderate and severe hepatic impairment have not been studied. The results suggest that the use of sertraline in patients with liver disease must be approached with caution. If sertraline is administered to patients with liver impairment, a lower or less frequent dose should be used (see PRECAUTIONS and DOSAGE AND ADMINISTRATION).

Renal Disease—Sertraline is extensively metabolized and excretion of unchanged drug in urine is a minor route of elimination. In volunteers with mild to moderate (CLcr=30-60 mL/min), moderate to severe (CLcr=10-29 mL/min) or severe (receiving hemodialysis) renal impairment (N=10 each group), the pharmacokinetics and protein binding of 200 mg sertraline per day maintained for 21 days were not altered compared to age-matched volunteers (N=12) with no renal impairment. Thus sertraline multiple dose pharmacokinetics appear to be unaffected by renal impairment (see PRECAUTIONS).

Clinical Trials

Major Depressive Disorder—The efficacy of ZOLOFT as a treatment for major depressive disorder was established in two placebo-controlled studies in adult outpatients meeting DSM-III criteria for major depressive disorder. Study 1 was an 8-week study with flexible dosing of ZOLOFT in a range of 50 to 200 mg/day; the mean dose for completers was 145 mg/day. Study 2 was a 6-week fixed-dose study, including ZOLOFT doses of 50, 100, and 200 mg/day. Overall, these studies demonstrated ZOLOFT to be superior to placebo on the Hamilton Depression Rating Scale and the Clinical Global Impression Severity and Improvement scales. Study 2 was not readily interpretable regarding a dose response relationship for effectiveness.

Study 3 involved depressed outpatients who had responded by the end of an initial 8-week open treatment phase on ZOLOFT 50-200 mg/day. These patients (N=295) were randomized to continuation for 44 weeks on double-blind ZOLOFT 50-200 mg/day or placebo. A statistically significantly lower relapse rate was observed for patients taking ZOLOFT compared to those on placebo. The mean dose for completers was 70 mg/day.

Analyses for gender effects on outcome did not suggest any differential responsiveness on the basis of sex.

Obsessive-Compulsive Disorder (OCD)—The effectiveness of ZOLOFT in the treatment of OCD was demonstrated in three multicenter placebo-controlled studies of adult outpatients (Studies 1-3). Patients in all studies had moderate to severe OCD (DSM-III or DSM-III-R) with mean baseline ratings on the Yale–Brown Obsessive-Compulsive Scale (YBOCS) total score ranging from 23 to 25.

Study 1 was an 8-week study with flexible dosing of ZOLOFT in a range of 50 to 200 mg/day; the mean dose for completers was 186 mg/day. Patients receiving ZOLOFT experienced a mean reduction of approximately 4 points on the YBOCS total score which was significantly greater than the mean reduction of 2 points in placebo-treated patients.

Study 2 was a 12-week fixed-dose study, including ZOLOFT doses of 50, 100, and 200 mg/day. Patients receiving ZOLOFT doses of 50 and 200 mg/day experienced mean reductions of approximately 6 points on the YBOCS total score which were significantly greater than the approximately 3 point reduction in placebo-treated patients.

Study 3 was a 12-week study with flexible dosing of ZOLOFT in a range of 50 to 200 mg/day; the mean dose for completers was 185 mg/day. Patients receiving ZOLOFT experienced a mean reduction of approximately 7 points on the YBOCS total score which was significantly greater than the mean reduction of approximately 4 points in placebo-treated patients.

Analyses for age and gender effects on outcome did not suggest any differential responsiveness on the basis of age or sex.

The effectiveness of ZOLOFT for the treatment of OCD was also demonstrated in a 12-week, multicenter, placebo-controlled, parallel group study in a pediatric outpatient population (children and adolescents, ages 6-17). Patients receiving ZOLOFT in this study were initiated at doses of either 25 mg/day (children, ages 6-12) or 50 mg/day (adolescents, ages 13-17), and then titrated over the next four weeks to a maximum dose of 200 mg/day, as tolerated. The mean dose for completers was 178 mg/day. Dosing was once a day in the morning or evening. Patients in this study had moderate to severe OCD (DSM-III-R) with mean baseline ratings on the Children's Yale-Brown Obsessive-Compulsive Scale (CYBOCS) total score of 22. Patients receiving sertraline experienced a mean reduction of approximately 7 points on the CYBOCS total score which was significantly greater than the 3 point reduction for placebo patients. Analyses for age and gender effects on outcome did not suggest any differential responsiveness on the basis of age or sex.

In a longer-term study, patients meeting DSM-III-R criteria for OCD who had responded during a 52-week single-blind trial on ZOLOFT 50-200 mg/day (n=224) were randomized to continuation of ZOLOFT or to substitution of placebo for up to 28 weeks of observation for discontinuation due to relapse or insufficient clinical response. Response during the single-blind phase was defined as a decrease in the YBOCS score of ≥ 25% compared to baseline and a CGI- I of 1 (very much improved), 2 (much improved) or 3 (minimally improved). Relapse during the double-blind phase was defined as the following conditions being met (on three consecutive visits for 1 and 2, and for visit 3 for condition 3): (1) YBOCS score increased by ≥ 5 points, to a minimum of 20, relative to baseline; (2) CGI-I increased by ≥ one point; and (3) worsening of the patient's condition in the investigator's judgment, to justify alternative treatment. Insufficient clinical response indicated a worsening of the patient's condition that resulted in study discontinuation, as assessed by the investigator. Patients receiving continued ZOLOFT treatment experienced a significantly lower rate of discontinuation due to relapse or insufficient clinical response over the subsequent 28 weeks compared to those receiving placebo. This pattern was demonstrated in male and female subjects.

Panic Disorder—The effectiveness of ZOLOFT in the treatment of panic disorder was demonstrated in three double-blind, placebo-controlled studies (Studies 1-3) of adult outpatients who had a primary diagnosis of panic disorder (DSM-III-R), with or without agoraphobia.

Studies 1 and 2 were 10-week flexible dose studies. ZOLOFT was initiated at 25 mg/day for the first week, and then patients were dosed in a range of 50-200 mg/day on the basis of clinical response and toleration. The mean ZOLOFT doses for completers to 10 weeks were 131 mg/day and 144 mg/day, respectively, for Studies 1 and 2. In these studies, ZOLOFT was shown to be significantly more effective than placebo on change from baseline in panic attack frequency and on the Clinical Global Impression Severity of Illness and Global Improvement scores. The difference between ZOLOFT and placebo in reduction from baseline in the number of full panic attacks was approximately 2 panic attacks per week in both studies.

Study 3 was a 12-week fixed-dose study, including ZOLOFT doses of 50, 100, and 200 mg/day. Patients receiving ZOLOFT experienced a significantly greater reduction in panic attack frequency than patients receiving placebo. Study 3 was not readily interpretable regarding a dose response relationship for effectiveness.

Subgroup analyses did not indicate that there were any differences in treatment outcomes as a function of age, race, or gender.

In a longer-term study, patients meeting DSM-III-R criteria for Panic Disorder who had responded during a 52-week open trial on ZOLOFT 50-200 mg/day (n=183) were randomized to continuation of ZOLOFT or to substitution of placebo for up to 28 weeks of observation for discontinuation due to relapse or insufficient clinical response. Response during the open phase was defined as a CGI-I score of 1 (very much improved) or 2 (much improved). Relapse during the double-blind phase was defined as the following conditions being met on three consecutive visits: (1) CGI-I ≥ 3; (2) meets DSM-III-R criteria for Panic Disorder; (3) number of panic attacks greater than at baseline. Insufficient clinical response indicated a worsening of the patient's condition that resulted in study discontinuation, as assessed by the investigator. Patients receiving continued ZOLOFT treatment experienced a significantly lower rate of discontinuation due to relapse or insufficient clinical response over the subsequent 28 weeks compared to those receiving placebo. This pattern was demonstrated in male and female subjects.

Posttraumatic Stress Disorder (PTSD)—The effectiveness of ZOLOFT in the treatment of PTSD was established in two multicenter placebo-controlled studies (Studies 1-2) of adult outpatients who met DSM-III-R criteria for PTSD. The mean duration of PTSD for these patients was 12 years (Studies 1 and 2 combined) and 44% of patients (169 of the 385 patients treated) had secondary depressive disorder.

Studies 1 and 2 were 12-week flexible dose studies. ZOLOFT was initiated at 25 mg/day for the first week, and patients were then dosed in the range of 50-200 mg/day on the basis of clinical response and toleration. The mean ZOLOFT dose for completers was 146 mg/day and 151 mg/day, respectively for Studies 1 and 2. Study outcome was assessed by the Clinician-Administered PTSD Scale Part 2 (CAPS) which is a multi-item instrument that measures the three PTSD diagnostic symptom clusters of reexperiencing/intrusion, avoidance/numbing, and hyperarousal as well as the patient-rated Impact of Event Scale (IES) which measures intrusion and avoidance symptoms. ZOLOFT was shown to be significantly more effective than placebo on change from baseline to endpoint on the CAPS, IES and on the Clinical Global Impressions (CGI) Severity of Illness and Global Improvement scores. In two additional placebo-controlled PTSD trials, the difference in response to treatment between patients receiving ZOLOFT and patients receiving placebo was not statistically significant. One of these additional studies was conducted in patients similar to those recruited for Studies 1 and 2, while the second additional study was conducted in predominantly male veterans.

As PTSD is a more common disorder in women than men, the majority (76%) of patients in these trials were women (152 and 139 women on sertraline and placebo versus 39 and 55 men on sertraline and placebo; Studies 1 and 2 combined). Post hoc exploratory analyses revealed a significant difference between ZOLOFT and placebo on the CAPS, IES and CGI in women, regardless of baseline diagnosis of comorbid major depressive disorder, but essentially no effect in the relatively smaller number of men in these studies. The clinical significance of this apparent gender interaction is unknown at this time. There was insufficient information to determine the effect of race or age on outcome.

In a longer-term study, patients meeting DSM-III-R criteria for PTSD who had responded during a 24-week open trial on ZOLOFT 50-200 mg/day (n=96) were randomized to continuation of ZOLOFT or to substitution of placebo for up to 28 weeks of observation for relapse. Response during the open phase was defined as a CGI-I of 1 (very much improved) or 2 (much improved), and a decrease in the CAPS-2 score of > 30% compared to baseline. Relapse during the double-blind phase was defined as the following conditions being met on two consecutive visits: (1) CGI-I ≥ 3; (2) CAPS-2 score increased by ≥ 30% and by ≥ 15 points relative to baseline; and (3) worsening of the patient's condition in the investigator's judgment. Patients receiving continued ZOLOFT treatment experienced significantly lower relapse rates over the subsequent 28 weeks compared to those receiving placebo. This pattern was demonstrated in male and female subjects.

Premenstrual Dysphoric Disorder (PMDD)—The effectiveness of ZOLOFT for the treatment of PMDD was established in two double-blind, parallel group, placebo-controlled flexible dose trials (Studies 1 and 2) conducted over 3 menstrual cycles. Patients in Study 1 met DSM-III-R criteria for Late Luteal Phase Dysphoric Disorder (LLPDD), the clinical entity now referred to as Premenstrual Dysphoric Disorder (PMDD) in DSM-IV. Patients in Study 2 met DSM-IV criteria for PMDD. Study 1 utilized daily dosing throughout the study, while Study 2 utilized luteal phase dosing for the 2 weeks prior to the onset of menses. The mean duration of PMDD symptoms for these patients was approximately 10.5 years in both studies. Patients on oral contraceptives were excluded from these trials; therefore, the efficacy of sertraline in combination with oral contraceptives for the treatment of PMDD is unknown.

Efficacy was assessed with the Daily Record of Severity of Problems (DRSP), a patient-rated instrument that mirrors the diagnostic criteria for PMDD as identified in the DSM-IV, and includes assessments for mood, physical symptoms, and other symptoms. Other efficacy assessments included the Hamilton Depression Rating Scale (HAMD-17), and the Clinical Global Impression Severity of Illness (CGI-S) and Improvement (CGI-I) scores.

In Study 1, involving n=251 randomized patients, ZOLOFT treatment was initiated at 50 mg/day and administered daily throughout the menstrual cycle. In subsequent cycles, patients were dosed in the range of 50-150 mg/day on the basis of clinical response and toleration. The mean dose for completers was 102 mg/day. ZOLOFT administered daily throughout the menstrual cycle was significantly more effective than placebo on change from baseline to endpoint on the DRSP total score, the HAMD-17 total score, and the CGI-S score, as well as the CGI-I score at endpoint.

In Study 2, involving n=281 randomized patients, ZOLOFT treatment was initiated at 50 mg/day in the late luteal phase (last 2 weeks) of each menstrual cycle and then discontinued at the onset of menses. In subsequent cycles, patients were dosed in the range of 50–100 mg/day in the luteal phase of each cycle, on the basis of clinical response and toleration. Patients who were titrated to 100 mg/day received 50 mg/day for the first 3 days of the cycle, then 100 mg/day for the remainder of the cycle. The mean ZOLOFT dose for completers was 74 mg/day. ZOLOFT administered in the late luteal phase of the menstrual cycle was significantly more effective than placebo on change from baseline to endpoint on the DRSP total score and the CGI-S score, as well as the CGI-I score at endpoint.

There was insufficient information to determine the effect of race or age on outcome in these studies.

Social Anxiety Disorder—The effectiveness of ZOLOFT in the treatment of social anxiety disorder (also known as social phobia) was established in two multicenter placebo-controlled studies (Study 1 and 2) of adult outpatients who met DSM-IV criteria for social anxiety disorder.

Study 1 was a 12-week, multicenter, flexible dose study comparing ZOLOFT (50-200 mg/day) to placebo, in which ZOLOFT was initiated at 25 mg/day for the first week. Study outcome was assessed by (a) the Liebowitz Social Anxiety Scale (LSAS), a 24-item clinician administered instrument that measures fear, anxiety and avoidance of social and performance situations, and by (b) the proportion of responders as defined by the Clinical Global Impression of Improvement (CGI-I) criterion of CGI-I ≤ 2 (very much or much improved). ZOLOFT was statistically significantly more effective than placebo as measured by the LSAS and the percentage of responders.

Study 2 was a 20-week, multicenter, flexible dose study that compared ZOLOFT (50-200 mg/day) to placebo. Study outcome was assessed by the (a) Duke Brief Social Phobia Scale (BSPS), a multi-item clinician-rated instrument that measures fear, avoidance and physiologic response to social or performance situations, (b) the Marks Fear Questionnaire Social Phobia Subscale (FQ-SPS), a 5-item patient-rated instrument that measures change in the severity of phobic avoidance and distress, and (c) the CGI-I responder criterion of ≤ 2. ZOLOFT was shown to be statistically significantly more effective than placebo as measured by the BSPS total score and fear, avoidance and physiologic factor scores, as well as the FQ-SPS total score, and to have significantly more responders than placebo as defined by the CGI-I.

Subgroup analyses did not suggest differences in treatment outcome on the basis of gender. There was insufficient information to determine the effect of race or age on outcome.

In a longer-term study, patients meeting DSM-IV criteria for social anxiety disorder who had responded while assigned to ZOLOFT (CGI-I of 1 or 2) during a 20-week placebo-controlled trial on ZOLOFT 50–200 mg/day were randomized to continuation of ZOLOFT or to substitution of placebo for up to 24 weeks of observation for relapse. Relapse was defined as ≥ 2 point increase in the Clinical Global Impression – Severity of Illness (CGI-S) score compared to baseline or study discontinuation due to lack of efficacy. Patients receiving ZOLOFT continuation treatment experienced a statistically significantly lower relapse rate over this 24-week study than patients randomized to placebo substitution.

INDICATIONS AND USAGE

Major Depressive Disorder—ZOLOFT® (sertraline hydrochloride) is indicated for the treatment of major depressive disorder.

The efficacy of ZOLOFT in the treatment of a major depressive episode was established in six to eight week controlled trials of outpatients whose diagnoses corresponded most closely to the DSM-III category of major depressive disorder (see Clinical Trials under CLINICAL PHARMACOLOGY).

A major depressive episode implies a prominent and relatively persistent depressed or dysphoric mood that usually interferes with daily functioning (nearly every day for at least 2 weeks); it should include at least 4 of the following 8 symptoms: change in appetite, change in sleep, psychomotor agitation or retardation, loss of interest in usual activities or decrease in sexual drive, increased fatigue, feelings of guilt or worthlessness, slowed thinking or impaired concentration, and a suicide attempt or suicidal ideation.

The antidepressant action of ZOLOFT in hospitalized depressed patients has not been adequately studied.

The efficacy of ZOLOFT in maintaining an antidepressant response for up to 44 weeks following 8 weeks of open-label acute treatment (52 weeks total) was demonstrated in a placebo-controlled trial. The usefulness of the drug in patients receiving ZOLOFT for extended periods should be re-evaluated periodically (see Clinical Trials under CLINICAL PHARMACOLOGY).

Obsessive-Compulsive Disorder—ZOLOFT is indicated for the treatment of obsessions and compulsions in patients with obsessive-compulsive disorder (OCD), as defined in the DSM-III-R; i.e., the obsessions or compulsions cause marked distress, are time-consuming, or significantly interfere with social or occupational functioning.

The efficacy of ZOLOFT was established in 12-week trials with obsessive-compulsive outpatients having diagnoses of obsessive-compulsive disorder as defined according to DSM-III or DSM-III-R criteria (see Clinical Trials under CLINICAL PHARMACOLOGY).

Obsessive-compulsive disorder is characterized by recurrent and persistent ideas, thoughts, impulses, or images (obsessions) that are ego-dystonic and/or repetitive, purposeful, and intentional behaviors (compulsions) that are recognized by the person as excessive or unreasonable.

The efficacy of ZOLOFT in maintaining a response, in patients with OCD who responded during a 52-week treatment phase while taking ZOLOFT and were then observed for relapse during a period of up to 28 weeks, was demonstrated in a placebo-controlled trial (see Clinical Trials under CLINICAL PHARMACOLOGY). Nevertheless, the physician who elects to use ZOLOFT for extended periods should periodically re-evaluate the long-term usefulness of the drug for the individual patient (see DOSAGE AND ADMINISTRATION).

Panic Disorder—ZOLOFT is indicated for the treatment of panic disorder, with or without agoraphobia, as defined in DSM-IV. Panic disorder is characterized by the occurrence of unexpected panic attacks and associated concern about having additional attacks, worry about the implications or consequences of the attacks, and/or a significant change in behavior related to the attacks.

The efficacy of ZOLOFT was established in three 10-12 week trials in panic disorder patients whose diagnoses corresponded to the DSM-III-R category of panic disorder (see Clinical Trials under CLINICAL PHARMACOLOGY).

Panic disorder (DSM-IV) is characterized by recurrent unexpected panic attacks, i.e., a discrete period of intense fear or discomfort in which four (or more) of the following symptoms develop abruptly and reach a peak within 10 minutes: (1) palpitations, pounding heart, or accelerated heart rate; (2) sweating; (3) trembling or shaking; (4) sensations of shortness of breath or smothering; (5) feeling of choking; (6) chest pain or discomfort; (7) nausea or abdominal distress;

Continued on next page

Zoloft—Cont.

(8) feeling dizzy, unsteady, lightheaded, or faint; (9) derealization (feelings of unreality) or depersonalization (being detached from oneself); (10) fear of losing control; (11) fear of dying; (12) paresthesias (numbness or tingling sensations); (13) chills or hot flushes.

The efficacy of ZOLOFT in maintaining a response, in patients with panic disorder who responded during a 52-week treatment phase while taking ZOLOFT and were then observed for relapse during a period of up to 28 weeks, was demonstrated in a placebo-controlled trial (see Clinical Trials under CLINICAL PHARMACOLOGY). Nevertheless, the physician who elects to use ZOLOFT for extended periods should periodically re-evaluate the long-term usefulness of the drug for the individual patient (see DOSAGE AND ADMINISTRATION).

Posttraumatic Stress Disorder (PTSD)—ZOLOFT (sertraline hydrochloride) is indicated for the treatment of posttraumatic stress disorder.

The efficacy of ZOLOFT in the treatment of PTSD was established in two 12-week placebo-controlled trials of outpatients whose diagnosis met criteria for the DSM-III-R category of PTSD (see Clinical Trials under CLINICAL PHARMACOLOGY).

PTSD, as defined by DSM-III-R/IV, requires exposure to a traumatic event that involved actual or threatened death or serious injury, or threat to the physical integrity of self or others, and a response which involves intense fear, helplessness, or horror. Symptoms that occur as a result of exposure to the traumatic event include reexperiencing of the event in the form of intrusive thoughts, flashbacks or dreams, and intense psychological distress and physiological reactivity on exposure to cues to the event; avoidance of situations reminiscent of the traumatic event, inability to recall details of the event, and/or numbing of general responsiveness manifested as diminished interest in significant activities, estrangement from others, restricted range of affect, or sense of foreshortened future; and symptoms of autonomic arousal including hypervigilance, exaggerated startle response, sleep disturbance, impaired concentration, and irritability or outbursts of anger. A PTSD diagnosis requires that the symptoms are present for at least a month and that they cause clinically significant distress or impairment in social, occupational, or other important areas of functioning.

The efficacy of ZOLOFT in maintaining a response in patients with PTSD for up to 28 weeks following 24 weeks of open-label treatment was demonstrated in a placebo-controlled trial. Nevertheless, the physician who elects to use ZOLOFT for extended periods should periodically re-evaluate the long-term usefulness of the drug for the individual patient (see DOSAGE AND ADMINISTRATION).

Premenstrual Dysphoric Disorder (PMDD)—ZOLOFT is indicated for the treatment of premenstrual dysphoric disorder (PMDD).

The efficacy of ZOLOFT in the treatment of PMDD was established in 2 placebo-controlled trials of female outpatients treated for 3 menstrual cycles who met criteria for the DSM-III-R/IV category of PMDD (see Clinical Trials under CLINICAL PHARMACOLOGY).

The essential features of PMDD include markedly depressed mood, anxiety or tension, affective lability, and persistent anger or irritability. Other features include decreased interest in activities, difficulty concentrating, lack of energy, change in appetite or sleep, and feeling out of control. Physical symptoms associated with PMDD include breast tenderness, headache, joint and muscle pain, bloating and weight gain. These symptoms occur regularly during the luteal phase and remit within a few days following onset of menses; the disturbance markedly interferes with work or school or with usual social activities and relationships with others. In making the diagnosis, care should be taken to rule out other cyclical mood disorders that may be exacerbated by treatment with an antidepressant.

The effectiveness of ZOLOFT in long-term use, that is, for more than 3 menstrual cycles, has not been systematically evaluated in controlled trials. Therefore, the physician who elects to use ZOLOFT for extended periods should periodically re-evaluate the long-term usefulness of the drug for the individual patient (see DOSAGE AND ADMINISTRATION).

Social Anxiety Disorder—ZOLOFT (sertraline hydrochloride) is indicated for the treatment of social anxiety disorder, also known as social phobia.

The efficacy of ZOLOFT in the treatment of social anxiety disorder was established in two placebo-controlled trials of outpatients with a diagnosis of social anxiety disorder as defined by DSM-IV criteria (see Clinical Trials under CLINICAL PHARMACOLOGY).

Social anxiety disorder, as defined by DSM-IV, is characterized by marked and persistent fear of social or performance situations involving exposure to unfamiliar people or possible scrutiny by others and by fears of acting in a humiliating or embarrassing way. Exposure to the feared social situation almost always provokes anxiety and feared social or performance situations are avoided or else are endured with intense anxiety or distress. In addition, patients recognize that the fear is excessive or unreasonable and the avoidance and anticipatory anxiety of the feared situation is associated with functional impairment or marked distress.

The efficacy of ZOLOFT in maintaining a response in patients with social anxiety disorder for up to 24 weeks following 20 weeks of ZOLOFT treatment was demonstrated in a placebo-controlled trial. Physicians who prescribe ZOLOFT for extended periods should periodically re-evaluate the long-term usefulness of the drug for the individual patient (see Clinical Trials under CLINICAL PHARMACOLOGY).

CONTRAINDICATIONS

All Dosage Forms of ZOLOFT:
Concomitant use in patients taking monoamine oxidase inhibitors (MAOIs) is contraindicated (see WARNINGS). Concomitant use in patients taking pimozide is contraindicated (see PRECAUTIONS).
ZOLOFT is contraindicated in patients with a hypersensitivity to sertraline or any of the inactive ingredients in ZOLOFT.
Oral Concentrate:
ZOLOFT oral concentrate is contraindicated with ANTABUSE (disulfiram) due to the alcohol content of the concentrate.

WARNINGS

Cases of serious sometimes fatal reactions have been reported in patients receiving ZOLOFT® (sertraline hydrochloride), a selective serotonin reuptake inhibitor (SSRI), in combination with a monoamine oxidase inhibitor (MAOI). Symptoms of a drug interaction between an SSRI and an MAOI include: hyperthermia, rigidity, myoclonus, autonomic instability with possible rapid fluctuations of vital signs, mental status changes that include confusion, irritability, and extreme agitation progressing to delirium and coma. These reactions have also been reported in patients who have recently discontinued an SSRI and have been started on an MAOI. Some cases presented with features resembling neuroleptic malignant syndrome. Therefore, ZOLOFT should not be used in combination with an MAOI, or within 14 days of discontinuing treatment with an MAOI. Similarly, at least 14 days should be allowed after stopping ZOLOFT before starting an MAOI.

PRECAUTIONS

General

Activation of Mania/Hypomania—During premarketing testing, hypomania or mania occurred in approximately 0.4% of ZOLOFT® (sertraline hydrochloride) treated patients.

Weight Loss—Significant weight loss may be an undesirable result of treatment with sertraline for some patients, but on average, patients in controlled trials had minimal, 1 to 2 pound weight loss, versus smaller changes on placebo. Only rarely have sertraline patients been discontinued for weight loss.

Seizure—ZOLOFT has not been evaluated in patients with a seizure disorder. These patients were excluded from clinical studies during the product's premarket testing. No seizures were observed among approximately 3000 patients treated with ZOLOFT in the development program for major depressive disorder. However, 4 patients out of approximately 1800 (220<18 years of age) exposed during the development program for obsessive-compulsive disorder experienced seizures, representing a crude incidence of 0.2%. Three of these patients were adolescents, two with a seizure disorder and one with a family history of seizure disorder, none of whom were receiving anticonvulsant medication. Accordingly, ZOLOFT should be introduced with care in patients with a seizure disorder.

Suicide—The possibility of a suicide attempt is inherent in major depressive disorder and may persist until significant remission occurs. Close supervision of high risk patients should accompany initial drug therapy. Prescriptions for ZOLOFT should be written for the smallest quantity of tablets consistent with good patient management, in order to reduce the risk of overdose.

Because of the well-established comorbidity between OCD, panic disorder, PTSD, PMDD or social anxiety disorder and major depressive disorder, the same precautions observed when treating patients with major depressive disorder should be observed when treating patients with OCD, panic disorder, PTSD, PMDD or social anxiety disorder.

Weak Uricosuric Effect—ZOLOFT® (sertraline hydrochloride) is associated with a mean decrease in serum uric acid of approximately 7%. The clinical significance of this weak uricosuric effect is unknown.

Use in Patients with Concomitant Illness—Clinical experience with ZOLOFT in patients with certain concomitant systemic illness is limited. Caution is advisable in using ZOLOFT in patients with diseases or conditions that could affect metabolism or hemodynamic responses.

ZOLOFT has not been evaluated or used to any appreciable extent in patients with a recent history of myocardial infarction or unstable heart disease. Patients with these diagnoses were excluded from clinical studies during the product's premarket testing. However, the electrocardiograms of 774 patients who received ZOLOFT in double-blind trials were evaluated and the data indicate that ZOLOFT is not associated with the development of significant ECG abnormalities.

ZOLOFT is extensively metabolized by the liver. In patients with chronic mild liver impairment, sertraline clearance was reduced, resulting in increased AUC, Cmax and elimination half-life. The effects of sertraline in patients with moderate and severe hepatic impairment have not been studied. The use of sertraline in patients with liver disease must be approached with caution. If sertraline is administered to patients with liver impairment, a lower or less frequent dose should be used (see CLINICAL PHARMACOLOGY and DOSAGE AND ADMINISTRATION).

Since ZOLOFT is extensively metabolized, excretion of unchanged drug in urine is a minor route of elimination. A clinical study comparing sertraline pharmacokinetics in healthy volunteers to that in patients with renal impairment ranging from mild to severe (requiring dialysis) indicated that the pharmacokinetics and protein binding are unaffected by renal disease. Based on the pharmacokinetic results, there is no need for dosage adjustment in patients with renal impairment (see CLINICAL PHARMACOLOGY).

Interference with Cognitive and Motor Performance—In controlled studies, ZOLOFT did not cause sedation and did not interfere with psychomotor performance. (See **Information for Patients**.)

Hyponatremia—Several cases of hyponatremia have been reported and appeared to be reversible when ZOLOFT was discontinued. Some cases were possibly due to the syndrome of inappropriate antidiuretic hormone secretion. The majority of these occurrences have been in elderly individuals, some in patients taking diuretics or who were otherwise volume depleted.

Platelet Function—There have been rare reports of altered platelet function and/or abnormal results from laboratory studies in patients taking ZOLOFT. While there have been reports of abnormal bleeding or purpura in several patients taking ZOLOFT, it is unclear whether ZOLOFT had a causative role.

Information for Patients

Physicians are advised to discuss the following issues with patients for whom they prescribe ZOLOFT:

Patients should be told that although ZOLOFT has not been shown to impair the ability of normal subjects to perform tasks requiring complex motor and mental skills in laboratory experiments, drugs that act upon the central nervous system may affect some individuals adversely. Therefore, patients should be told that until they learn how they respond to ZOLOFT they should be careful doing activities when they need to be alert, such as driving a car or operating machinery.

Patients should be told that although ZOLOFT has not been shown in experiments with normal subjects to increase the mental and motor skill impairments caused by alcohol, the concomitant use of ZOLOFT and alcohol is not advised.

Patients should be told that while no adverse interaction of ZOLOFT with over-the-counter (OTC) drug products is known to occur, the potential for interaction exists. Thus, the use of any OTC product should be initiated cautiously according to the directions of use given for the OTC product.

Patients should be advised to notify their physician if they become pregnant or intend to become pregnant during therapy.

Patients should be advised to notify their physician if they are breast feeding an infant.

ZOLOFT oral concentrate is contraindicated with ANTABUSE (disulfiram) due to the alcohol content of the concentrate.

ZOLOFT Oral Concentrate contains 20 mg/mL of sertraline (as the hydrochloride) as the active ingredient and 12% alcohol. ZOLOFT Oral Concentrate must be diluted before use. Just before taking, use the dropper provided to remove the required amount of ZOLOFT Oral Concentrate and mix with 4 oz (1/2 cup) of water, ginger ale, lemon/lime soda, lemonade or orange juice ONLY. Do not mix ZOLOFT Oral Concentrate with anything other than the liquids listed. The dose should be taken immediately after mixing. Do not mix in advance. At times, a slight haze may appear after mixing; this is normal. Note that caution should be exercised for persons with latex sensitivity, as the dropper dispenser contains dry natural rubber.

Laboratory Tests

None.

Drug Interactions

Potential Effects of Coadministration of Drugs Highly Bound to Plasma Proteins—Because sertraline is tightly bound to plasma protein, the administration of ZOLOFT® (sertraline hydrochloride) to a patient taking another drug which is tightly bound to protein (e.g., warfarin, digitoxin) may cause a shift in plasma concentrations potentially resulting in an adverse effect. Conversely, adverse effects may result from displacement of protein bound ZOLOFT by other tightly bound drugs.

In a study comparing prothrombin time AUC (0-120 hr) following dosing with warfarin (0.75 mg/kg) before and after 21 days of dosing with either ZOLOFT (50-200 mg/day) or placebo, there was a mean increase in prothrombin time of 8% relative to baseline for ZOLOFT compared to a 1% decrease for placebo (p<0.02). The normalization of prothrombin time for the ZOLOFT group was delayed compared to the placebo group. The clinical significance of this change is unknown. Accordingly, prothrombin time should be carefully monitored when ZOLOFT therapy is initiated or stopped.

Cimetidine—In a study assessing disposition of ZOLOFT (100 mg) on the second of 8 days of cimetidine administration (800 mg daily), there were significant increases in ZOLOFT mean AUC (50%), Cmax (24%) and half-life (26%) compared to the placebo group. The clinical significance of these changes is unknown.

CNS Active Drugs—In a study comparing the disposition of intravenously-administered diazepam before and after 21 days of dosing with either ZOLOFT (50 to 200 mg/day escalating dose) or placebo, there was a 32% decrease relative to baseline in diazepam clearance for the ZOLOFT group compared to a 19% decrease relative to baseline for the placebo

TABLE 1
MOST COMMON TREATMENT-EMERGENT ADVERSE EVENTS: INCIDENCE IN PLACEBO-CONTROLLED CLINICAL TRIALS

	Percentage of Patients Reporting Event													
	Major Depressive Disorder/Other*		OCD		Panic Disorder		PTSD		PMDD Daily Dosing		PMDD Luteal Phase Dosing(2)		Social Anxiety Disorder	
Body System/ Adverse Event	ZOLOFT (N=861)	Placebo (N=853)	ZOLOFT (N=533)	Placebo (N=373)	ZOLOFT (N=430)	Placebo (N=275)	ZOLOFT (N=374)	Placebo (N=376)	ZOLOFT (N=121)	Placebo (N=122)	ZOLOFT (N=136)	Placebo (N=127)	ZOLOFT (N=344)	Placebo (N=268)
Autonomic Nervous System Disorders														
Ejaculation Failure(1)	7	<1	17	2	19	1	11	1	N/A	N/A	N/A	N/A	14	—
Mouth Dry	16	9	14	9	15	10	11	6	6	3	10	3	12	4
Sweating Increased	8	3	6	1	5	1	4	2	6	<1	3	0	11	2
Centr. & Periph. Nerv. System Disorders														
Somnolence	13	6	15	8	15	9	13	9	7	<1	2	0	9	6
Tremor	11	3	8	1	5	1	5	1	2	0	<1	<1	9	3
Dizziness	12	7	17	9	10	10	8	5	6	3	7	5	14	6
General														
Fatigue	11	8	14	10	11	6	10	5	16	7	10	<1	12	6
Pain	1	2	3	1	3	3	4	6	6	<1	3	2	1	3
Malaise	<1	1	1	1	7	14	10	10	9	5	7	5	8	3
Gastrointestinal Disorders														
Abdominal Pain	2	2	5	5	6	7	6	5	7	<1	3	3	5	5
Anorexia	3	2	11	2	7	2	8	2	3	2	5	0	6	3
Constipation	8	6	6	4	7	3	3	3	2	3	1	2	5	3
Diarrhea/Loose Stools	18	9	24	10	20	9	24	15	13	3	13	7	21	8
Dyspepsia	6	3	10	4	10	8	6	6	7	2	7	3	13	5
Nausea	26	12	30	11	29	18	21	11	23	9	13	3	22	8
Psychiatric Disorders														
Agitation	6	4	6	3	6	2	5	5	2	<1	1	0	4	2
Insomnia	16	9	28	12	25	18	20	11	17	11	12	10	25	10
Libido Decreased	1	<1	11	2	7	1	7	2	11	2	4	2	9	3

(1)Primarily ejaculatory delay. Denominator used was for male patients only (N=271 ZOLOFT major depressive disorder/other*; N=271 placebo major depressive disorder/other*; N=296 ZOLOFT OCD; N=219 placebo OCD; N=216 ZOLOFT panic disorder; N=134 placebo panic disorder; N=130 ZOLOFT PTSD; N=149 placebo PTSD; No male patients in PMDD studies; N=205 ZOLOFT social anxiety disorder; N=153 placebo social anxiety disorder).
*Major depressive disorder and other premarketing controlled trials.
(2)The luteal phase and daily dosing PMDD trials were not designed for making direct comparisons between the two dosing regimens. Therefore, a comparison between the two dosing regimens of the PMDD trials of incidence rates shown in Table 1 should be avoided.

group (p<0.03). There was a 23% increase in Tmax for desmethyldiazepam in the ZOLOFT group compared to a 20% decrease in the placebo group (p<0.03). The clinical significance of these changes is unknown.

In a placebo-controlled trial in normal volunteers, the administration of two doses of ZOLOFT did not significantly alter steady-state lithium levels or the renal clearance of lithium.

Nonetheless, at this time, it is recommended that plasma lithium levels be monitored following initiation of ZOLOFT therapy with appropriate adjustments to the lithium dose.

In a controlled study of a single dose (2 mg) of pimozide, 200 mg sertraline (q.d.) co-administration to steady state was associated with a mean increase in pimozide AUC and Cmax of about 40%, but was not associated with any changes in EKG. Since the highest recommended pimozide dose (10 mg) has not been evaluated in combination with sertraline, the effect on QT interval and PK parameters at doses higher than 2 mg at this time are not known. While the mechanism of this interaction is unknown, due to the narrow therapeutic index of pimozide and due to the interaction noted at a low dose of pimozide, concomitant administration of ZOLOFT and pimozide should be contraindicated (see CONTRAINDICATIONS).

The risk of using ZOLOFT in combination with other CNS active drugs has not been systematically evaluated. Consequently, caution is advised if the concomitant administration of ZOLOFT and such drugs is required.

There is limited controlled experience regarding the optimal timing of switching from other drugs effective in the treatment of major depressive disorder, obsessive-compulsive disorder, panic disorder, posttraumatic stress disorder, premenstrual dysphoric disorder and social anxiety disorder to ZOLOFT. Care and prudent medical judgment should be exercised when switching, particularly from long-acting agents. The duration of an appropriate washout period which should intervene before switching from one selective serotonin reuptake inhibitor (SSRI) to another has not been established.

Monoamine Oxidase Inhibitors—See CONTRAINDICATIONS and WARNINGS.

Drugs Metabolized by P450 3A4—In three separate in vivo interaction studies, sertraline was co-administered with cytochrome P450 3A4 substrates, terfenadine, carbamazepine, or cisapride under steady-state conditions. The results of these studies indicated that sertraline did not increase plasma concentrations of terfenadine, carbamazepine, or cisapride. These data indicate that sertraline's extent of inhibition of P450 3A4 activity is not likely to be of clinical significance. Results of the interaction study with cisapride indicate that sertraline 200 mg (q.d.) induces the metabolism of cisapride (cisapride AUC and Cmax were reduced by about 35%).

Drugs Metabolized by P450 2D6—Many drugs effective in the treatment of major depressive disorder, e.g., the SSRIs, including sertraline, and most tricyclic antidepressant drugs effective in the treatment of major depressive disorder inhibit the biochemical activity of the drug metabolizing isozyme cytochrome P450 2D6 (debrisoquin hydroxylase), and, thus, may increase the plasma concentrations of co-administered drugs that are metabolized by P450 2D6. The drugs for which this potential interaction is of greatest concern are those metabolized primarily by 2D6 and which have a narrow therapeutic index, e.g., the tricyclic antidepressant drugs effective in the treatment of major depressive disorder and the Type 1C antiarrhythmics propafenone and flecainide. The extent to which this interaction is an important clinical problem depends on the extent of the inhibition of P450 2D6 by the antidepressant and the therapeutic index of the co-administered drug. There is variability among the drugs effective in the treatment of major depressive disorder in the extent of clinically important 2D6 inhibition, and in fact sertraline at lower doses has a less prominent inhibitory effect on 2D6 than some others in the class. Nevertheless, even sertraline has the potential for clinically important 2D6 inhibition. Consequently, concomitant use of a drug metabolized by P450 2D6 with ZOLOFT may require lower doses than usually prescribed for the other drug. Furthermore, whenever ZOLOFT is withdrawn from co-therapy, an increased dose of the co-administered drug may be required (see Tricyclic Antidepressant Drugs Effective in the Treatment of Major Depressive Disorder under PRECAUTIONS).

Sumatriptan—There have been rare postmarketing reports describing patients with weakness, hyperreflexia, and incoordination following the use of a selective serotonin reuptake inhibitor (SSRI) and sumatriptan. If concomitant treatment with sumatriptan and an SSRI (e.g., citalopram, fluoxetine, fluvoxamine, paroxetine, sertraline) is clinically warranted, appropriate observation of the patient is advised.

Tricyclic Antidepressant Drugs Effective in the Treatment of Major Depressive Disorder (TCAs)—The extent to which SSRI-TCA interactions may pose clinical problems will depend on the degree of inhibition and the pharmacokinetics of the SSRI involved. Nevertheless, caution is indicated in the co-administration of TCAs with ZOLOFT, because sertraline may inhibit TCA metabolism. Plasma TCA concentrations may need to be monitored, and the dose of TCA may need to be reduced, if a TCA is co-administered with ZOLOFT (see Drugs Metabolized by P450 2D6 under PRECAUTIONS).

Hypoglycemic Drugs—In a placebo-controlled trial in normal volunteers, administration of ZOLOFT for 22 days (including 200 mg/day for the final 13 days) caused a statistically significant 16% decrease from baseline in the clear-

Continued on next page

Zoloft—Cont.

ance of tolbutamide following an intravenous 1000 mg dose. ZOLOFT administration did not noticeably change either the plasma protein binding or the apparent volume of distribution of tolbutamide, suggesting that the decreased clearance was due to a change in the metabolism of the drug. The clinical significance of this decrease in tolbutamide clearance is unknown.

Atenolol—ZOLOFT (100 mg) when administered to 10 healthy male subjects had no effect on the beta-adrenergic blocking ability of atenolol.

Digoxin—In a placebo-controlled trial in normal volunteers, administration of ZOLOFT for 17 days (including 200 mg/day for the last 10 days) did not change serum digoxin levels or digoxin renal clearance.

Microsomal Enzyme Induction—Preclinical studies have shown ZOLOFT to induce hepatic microsomal enzymes. In clinical studies, ZOLOFT was shown to induce hepatic enzymes minimally as determined by a small (5%) but statistically significant decrease in antipyrine half-life following administration of 200 mg/day for 21 days. This small change in antipyrine half-life reflects a clinically insignificant change in hepatic metabolism.

Electroconvulsive Therapy—There are no clinical studies establishing the risks or benefits of the combined use of electroconvulsive therapy (ECT) and ZOLOFT.

Alcohol—Although ZOLOFT did not potentiate the cognitive and psychomotor effects of alcohol in experiments with normal subjects, the concomitant use of ZOLOFT and alcohol is not recommended.

Carcinogenesis—Lifetime carcinogenicity studies were carried out in CD-1 mice and Long-Evans rats at doses up to 40 mg/kg/day. These doses correspond to 1 times (mice) and 2 times (rats) the maximum recommended human dose (MRHD) on a mg/m^2 basis. There was a dose-related increase of liver adenomas in male mice receiving sertraline at 10–40 mg/kg (0.25-1.0 times the MRHD on a mg/m^2 basis). No increase was seen in female mice or in rats of either sex receiving the same treatments, nor was there an increase in hepatocellular carcinomas. Liver adenomas have a variable rate of spontaneous occurrence in the CD-1 mouse and are of unknown significance to humans. There was an increase in follicular adenomas of the thyroid in female rats receiving sertraline at 40 mg/kg (2 times the MRHD on a mg/m^2 basis); this was not accompanied by thyroid hyperplasia. While there was an increase in uterine adenocarcinomas in rats receiving sertraline at 10-40 mg/kg (0.5-2.0 times the MRHD on a mg/m^2 basis) compared to placebo controls, this effect was not clearly drug related.

Mutagenesis—Sertraline had no genotoxic effects, with or without metabolic activation, based on the following assays: bacterial mutation assay; mouse lymphoma mutation assay; and tests for cytogenetic aberrations *in vivo* in mouse bone marrow and *in vitro* in human lymphocytes.

Impairment of Fertility—A decrease in fertility was seen in one of two rat studies at a dose of 80 mg/kg (4 times the maximum recommended human dose on a mg/m^2 basis).

Pregnancy—Pregnancy Category C—Reproduction studies have been performed in rats and rabbits at doses up to 80 mg/kg/day and 40 mg/kg/day, respectively. These doses correspond to approximately 4 times the maximum recommended human dose (MRHD) on a mg/m^2 basis. There was no evidence of teratogenicity at any dose level. When pregnant rats and rabbits were given sertraline during the period of organogenesis, delayed ossification was observed in fetuses at doses of 10 mg/kg (0.5 times the MRHD on a mg/m^2 basis) in rats and 40 mg/kg (4 times the MRHD on a mg/m^2 basis) in rabbits. When female rats received sertraline during the last third of gestation and throughout lactation, there was an increase in the number of stillborn pups and in the number of pups dying during the first 4 days after birth. Pup body weights were also decreased during the first four days after birth. These effects occurred at a dose of 20 mg/kg (1 times the MRHD on a mg/m^2 basis). The no effect dose for rat pup mortality was 10 mg/kg (0.5 times the MRHD on a mg/m^2 basis). The decrease in pup survival was shown to be due to *in utero* exposure to sertraline. The clinical significance of these effects is unknown. There are no adequate and well-controlled studies in pregnant women. ZOLOFT® (sertraline hydrochloride) should be used during pregnancy only if the potential benefit justifies the potential risk to the fetus.

Labor and Delivery—The effect of ZOLOFT on labor and delivery in humans is unknown.

Nursing Mothers—It is not known whether, and if so in what amount, sertraline or its metabolites are excreted in human milk. Because many drugs are excreted in human milk, caution should be exercised when ZOLOFT is administered to a nursing woman.

Pediatric Use—The efficacy of ZOLOFT for the treatment of obsessive-compulsive disorder was demonstrated in a 12-week, multicenter, placebo-controlled study with 187 outpatients ages 6-17 (see Clinical Trials under CLINICAL PHARMACOLOGY). The efficacy of ZOLOFT in pediatric patients with major depressive disorder, panic disorder, PTSD, PMDD or social anxiety disorder has not been systematically evaluated.

The safety of ZOLOFT use in children and adolescents, ages 6-18, was evaluated in a 12-week, multicenter, placebo-controlled study with 187 outpatients, ages 6-17, and in a flexible dose, 52 week open extension study of 137 patients, ages 6–18, who had completed the initial 12-week, double-blind, placebo-controlled study. ZOLOFT was administered at doses of either 25 mg/day (children, ages 6-12) or 50 mg/day (adolescents, ages 13-18) and then titrated in weekly 25 mg/day or 50 mg/day increments, respectively, to a maximum dose of 200 mg/day based upon clinical response. The mean dose for completers was 157 mg/day. In the acute 12 week pediatric study and in the 52 week study, ZOLOFT had an adverse event profile generally similar to that observed in adults.

Sertraline pharmacokinetics were evaluated in 61 pediatric patients between 6 and 18 years of age with major depressive disorder and/or OCD and revealed similar drug exposures to those of adults when plasma concentration was adjusted for weight (see Pharmacokinetics under CLINICAL PHARMACOLOGY).

More than 250 patients with major depressive disorder and/or OCD between 6 and 18 years of age have received ZOLOFT in clinical trials. The adverse event profile observed in these patients was generally similar to that observed in adult studies with ZOLOFT (see ADVERSE REACTIONS). As with other SSRIs, decreased appetite and weight loss have been observed in association with the use of ZOLOFT. Consequently, regular monitoring of weight and growth is recommended if treatment of a child with an SSRI is to be continued long term. Safety and effectiveness in pediatric patients below the age of 6 have not been established.

The risks, if any, that may be associated with the use of ZOLOFT beyond 1 year in children and adolescents with OCD have not been systematically assessed. The prescriber should be mindful that the evidence relied upon to conclude that sertraline is safe for use in children and adolescents derives from clinical studies that were 12 to 52 weeks in duration and from the extrapolation of experience gained with adult patients. In particular, there are no studies that directly evaluate the effects of long-term sertraline use on the growth, development, and maturation of children and adolescents. Although there is no affirmative finding to suggest that sertraline possesses a capacity to adversely affect growth, development or maturation, the absence of such findings is not compelling evidence of the absence of the potential of sertraline to have adverse effects in chronic use.

Geriatric Use—U.S. geriatric clinical studies of ZOLOFT in major depressive disorder included 663 ZOLOFT-treated subjects $\geq$ 65 years of age, of those, 180 were $\geq$ 75 years of age. No overall differences in the pattern of adverse reactions were observed in the geriatric clinical trial subjects relative to those reported in younger subjects (see ADVERSE REACTIONS), and other reported experience has not identified differences in safety patterns between the elderly and younger subjects. As with all medications, greater sensitivity of some older individuals cannot be ruled out. There were 947 subjects in placebo-controlled geriatric clinical studies of ZOLOFT in major depressive disorder. No overall differences in the pattern of efficacy were observed in the geriatric clinical trial subjects relative to those reported in younger subjects.

Other Adverse Events in Geriatric Patients. In 354 geriatric subjects treated with ZOLOFT in placebo-controlled trials, the overall profile of adverse events was generally similar to that shown in Tables 1 and 2. Urinary tract infection was the only adverse event not appearing in Tables 1 and 2 and reported at an incidence of at least 2% and at a rate greater than placebo in placebo-controlled trials.

As with other SSRIs, ZOLOFT has been associated with cases of clinically significant hyponatremia in elderly patients (see Hyponatremia under PRECAUTIONS).

ADVERSE REACTIONS

During its premarketing assessment, multiple doses of ZOLOFT were administered to over 4000 adult subjects as of February 26, 1998. The conditions and duration of exposure to ZOLOFT varied greatly, and included (in overlapping categories) clinical pharmacology studies, open and double-blind studies, uncontrolled and controlled studies, inpatient and outpatient studies, fixed-dose and titration studies, and studies for multiple indications, including major depressive disorder, OCD, panic disorder, PTSD, PMDD and social anxiety disorder.

Untoward events associated with this exposure were recorded by clinical investigators using terminology of their own choosing. Consequently, it is not possible to provide a meaningful estimate of the proportion of individuals experiencing adverse events without first grouping similar types of untoward events into a smaller number of standardized event categories.

In the tabulations that follow, a World Health Organization dictionary of terminology has been used to classify reported adverse events. The frequencies presented, therefore, represent the proportion of the over 4000 adult individuals exposed to multiple doses of ZOLOFT who experienced a treatment-emergent adverse event of the type cited on at least one occasion while receiving ZOLOFT. An event was considered treatment-emergent if it occurred for the first time or worsened while receiving therapy following baseline evaluation. It is important to emphasize that events reported during therapy were not necessarily caused by it.

The prescriber should be aware that the figures in the tables and tabulations cannot be used to predict the incidence of side effects in the course of usual medical practice where patient characteristics and other factors differ from those that prevailed in the clinical trials. Similarly, the cited frequencies cannot be compared with figures obtained from other clinical investigations involving different treatments, uses, and investigators. The cited figures, however, do provide the prescribing physician with some basis for estimating the relative contribution of drug and nondrug factors to the side effect incidence rate in the population studied.

Incidence in Placebo-Controlled Trials—Table 1 enumerates the most common treatment-emergent adverse events associated with the use of ZOLOFT (incidence of at least 5% for ZOLOFT and at least twice that for placebo within at least one of the indications) for the treatment of adult patients with major depressive disorder/other*, OCD, panic disorder, PTSD, PMDD and social anxiety disorder in placebo-controlled clinical trials. Most patients in major depressive disorder/other*, OCD, panic disorder, PTSD and social anxiety disorder studies received doses of 50 to 200 mg/day. Patients in the PMDD study with daily dosing throughout the menstrual cycle received doses of 50 to 150 mg/day, and in the PMDD study with dosing during the luteal phase of the menstrual cycle received doses of 50 to 100 mg/day. Table 2 enumerates treatment-emergent adverse events that occurred in 2% or more of adult patients treated with ZOLOFT and with incidence greater than placebo who participated in controlled clinical trials comparing ZOLOFT with placebo in the treatment of major depressive disorder/other*, OCD, panic disorder, PTSD, PMDD and social anxiety disorder. Table 2 provides combined data for the pool of studies that are provided separately by indication in Table 1.

[See table 1 on previous page]

TABLE 2
TREATMENT-EMERGENT ADVERSE EVENTS: INCIDENCE IN PLACEBO-CONTROLLED CLINICAL TRIALS
Percentage of Patients Reporting Event
Major Depressive Disorder/Other*, OCD, Panic Disorder, PTSD, PMDD and Social Anxiety Disorder combined

Body System/Adverse Event**	ZOLOFT (N=2799)	Placebo (N=2394)
Autonomic Nervous System Disorders		
Ejaculation Failure[1]	14	1
Mouth Dry	14	8
Sweating Increased	7	2
Centr. & Periph. Nerv. System Disorders		
Somnolence	13	7
Dizziness	12	7
Headache	25	23
Paresthesia	2	1
Tremor	8	2
Disorders of Skin and Appendages		
Rash	3	2
Gastrointestinal Disorders		
Anorexia	6	2
Constipation	6	4
Diarrhea/Loose Stools	20	10
Dyspepsia	8	4
Nausea	25	11
Vomiting	4	2
General		
Fatigue	12	7
Psychiatric Disorders		
Agitation	5	3
Anxiety	4	3
Insomnia	21	11
Libido Decreased	6	2
Nervousness	5	4
Special Senses		
Vision Abnormal	3	2

[1] Primarily ejaculatory delay. Denominator used was for male patients only (N=1118 ZOLOFT; N=926 placebo).
*Major depressive disorder and other premarketing controlled trials.
**Included are events reported by at least 2% of patients taking ZOLOFT except the following events, which had an incidence on placebo greater than or equal to ZOLOFT: abdominal pain, back pain, flatulence, malaise, pain, pharyn-

gitis, respiratory disorder, upper respiratory tract infection.

Associated with Discontinuation in Placebo-Controlled Clinical Trials
Table 3 lists the adverse events associated with discontinuation of ZOLOFT® (sertraline hydrochloride) treatment (incidence at least twice that for placebo and at least 1% for ZOLOFT in clinical trials) in major depressive disorder/other*, OCD, panic disorder, PTSD, PMDD and social anxiety disorder.
[See table 3 at right]

Male and Female Sexual Dysfunction with SSRIs
Although changes in sexual desire, sexual performance and sexual satisfaction often occur as manifestations of a psychiatric disorder, they may also be a consequence of pharmacologic treatment. In particular, some evidence suggests that selective serotonin reuptake inhibitors (SSRIs) can cause such untoward sexual experiences. Reliable estimates of the incidence and severity of untoward experiences involving sexual desire, performance and satisfaction are difficult to obtain, however, in part because patients and physicians may be reluctant to discuss them. Accordingly, estimates of the incidence of untoward sexual experience and performance cited in product labeling, are likely to underestimate their actual incidence.
Table 4 below displays the incidence of sexual side effects reported by at least 2% of patients taking ZOLOFT in placebo-controlled trials.

TABLE 4

Adverse Event	ZOLOFT	Placebo
Ejaculation failure* (primarily delayed ejaculation)	14%	1%
Decreased libido**	6%	1%

*Denominator used was for male patients only (N=1118 ZOLOFT; N=926 placebo)
**Denominator used was for male and female patients (N=2799 ZOLOFT; N=2394 placebo)

There are no adequate and well-controlled studies examining sexual dysfunction with sertraline treatment.
Priapism has been reported with all SSRIs.
While it is difficult to know the precise risk of sexual dysfunction associated with the use of SSRIs, physicians should routinely inquire about such possible side effects.

Other Adverse Events in Pediatric Patients—In approximately N=250 pediatric patients treated with ZOLOFT, the overall profile of adverse events was generally similar to that seen in adult studies, as shown in Tables 1 and 2. However, the following adverse events, not appearing in Tables 1 and 2, were reported at an incidence of at least 2% and occurred at a rate of at least twice the placebo rate in a controlled trial (N=187): hyperkinesia, twitching, fever, malaise, purpura, weight decrease, concentration impaired, manic reaction, emotional lability, thinking abnormal, and epistaxis.

Other Events Observed During the Premarketing Evaluation of ZOLOFT® (sertraline hydrochloride)—Following is a list of treatment-emergent adverse events reported during premarketing assessment of ZOLOFT in clinical trials (over 4000 adult subjects) except those already listed in the previous tables or elsewhere in labeling.
In the tabulations that follow, a World Health Organization dictionary of terminology has been used to classify reported adverse events. The frequencies presented, therefore, represent the proportion of the over 4000 adult individuals exposed to multiple doses of ZOLOFT who experienced an event of the type cited on at least one occasion while receiving ZOLOFT. All events are included except those already listed in the previous tables or elsewhere in labeling and those reported in terms so general as to be uninformative and those for which a causal relationship to ZOLOFT treatment seemed remote. It is important to emphasize that although the events reported occurred during treatment with ZOLOFT, they were not necessarily caused by it. Events are further categorized by body system and listed in order of decreasing frequency according to the following definitions: frequent adverse events are those occurring on one or more occasions in at least 1/100 patients; infrequent adverse events are those occurring in 1/100 to 1/1000 patients; rare events are those occurring in fewer than 1/1000 patients. Events of major clinical importance are also described in the PRECAUTIONS section.

Autonomic Nervous System Disorders—*Frequent:* impotence; *Infrequent:* flushing, increased saliva, cold clammy skin, mydriasis; *Rare:* pallor, glaucoma, priapism, vasodilation.
Body as a Whole—General Disorders—*Rare:* allergic reaction, allergy.
Cardiovascular—*Frequent:* palpitations, chest pain; *Infrequent:* hypertension, tachycardia, postural dizziness, postural hypotension, periorbital edema, peripheral edema, hypotension, peripheral ischemia, syncope, edema, dependent edema; *Rare:* precordial chest pain, substernal chest pain, aggravated hypertension, myocardial infarction, cerebrovascular disorder.
Central and Peripheral Nervous System Disorders—*Frequent:* hypertonia, hypoesthesia; *Infrequent:* twitching, confusion, hyperkinesia, vertigo, ataxia, migraine, abnormal coordination, hyperesthesia, leg cramps, abnormal gait, nystagmus, hypokinesia; *Rare:* dysphonia, coma, dyskinesia, hypotonia, ptosis, choreoathetosis, hyporeflexia.

TABLE 3
MOST COMMON ADVERSE EVENTS ASSOCIATED WITH DISCONTINUATION IN PLACEBO-CONTROLLED CLINICAL TRIALS

Adverse Event	Major Depressive Disorder/Other*, OCD, Panic Disorder, PTSD, PMDD and Social Anxiety Disorder combined (N=2799)	Major Depressive Disorder/Other* (N=861)	OCD (N=533)	Panic Disorder (N=430)	PTSD (N=374)	PMDD Daily Dosing (N=121)	PMDD Luteal Phase Dosing (N=136)	Social Anxiety Disorder (N=344)
Abdominal Pain	–	–	–	–	–	–	–	1%
Agitation	–	1%	–	2%	–	–	–	–
Anxiety	–	–	–	–	–	–	–	2%
Diarrhea/Loose Stools	2%	2%	2%	1%	–	2%	–	–
Dizziness	–	–	1%	–	–	–	–	–
Dry Mouth	–	1%	–	–	–	–	–	–
Dyspepsia	–	–	–	1%	–	–	–	–
Ejaculation Failure[(1)]	1%	1%	1%	2%	–	N/A	N/A	2%
Fatigue	–	–	–	–	–	–	–	2%
Headache	1%	2%	–	–	1%	–	–	2%
Hot Flushes	–	–	–	–	–	–	1%	–
Insomnia	2%	1%	3%	2%	–	–	1%	3%
Nausea	3%	4%	3%	3%	2%	2%	1%	2%
Nervousness	–	–	–	–	–	2%	–	–
Palpitation	–	–	–	–	–	–	1%	–
Somnolence	1%	1%	2%	2%	–	–	–	–
Tremor	–	2%	–	–	–	–	–	–

[(1)]Primarily ejaculatory delay. Denominator used was for male patients only (N=271 major depressive disorder/other*; N=296 OCD; N=216 panic disorder; N=130 PTSD; No male patients in PMDD studies; N=205 social anxiety disorder).
*Major depressive disorder and other premarketing controlled trials.

Disorders of Skin and Appendages—*Infrequent:* pruritus, acne, urticaria, alopecia, dry skin, erythematous rash, photosensitivity reaction, maculopapular rash; *Rare:* follicular rash, eczema, dermatitis, contact dermatitis, bullous eruption, hypertrichosis, skin discoloration, pustular rash.
Endocrine Disorders—*Rare:* exophthalmos, gynecomastia.
Gastrointestinal Disorders—*Frequent:* appetite increased; *Infrequent:* dysphagia, tooth caries aggravated, eructation, esophagitis, gastroenteritis; *Rare:* melena, glossitis, gum hyperplasia, hiccup, stomatitis, tenesmus, colitis, diverticulitis, fecal incontinence, gastritis, rectum hemorrhage, hemorrhagic peptic ulcer, proctitis, ulcerative stomatitis, tongue edema, tongue ulceration.
General—*Frequent:* back pain, asthenia, malaise, weight increase; *Infrequent:* fever, rigors, generalized edema; *Rare:* face edema, aphthous stomatitis.
Hearing and Vestibular Disorders—*Rare:* hyperacusis, labyrinthine disorder.
Hematopoietic and Lymphatic—*Rare:* anemia, anterior chamber eye hemorrhage.
Liver and Biliary System Disorders—*Rare:* abnormal hepatic function.
Metabolic and Nutritional Disorders—*Infrequent:* thirst; *Rare:* hypoglycemia, hypoglycemia reaction.
Musculoskeletal System Disorders—*Frequent:* myalgia; *Infrequent:* arthralgia, dystonia, arthrosis, muscle cramps, muscle weakness.
Psychiatric Disorders—*Frequent:* yawning, other male sexual dysfunction, other female sexual dysfunction; *Infrequent:* depression, amnesia, paroniria, teeth-grinding, emotional lability, apathy, abnormal dreams, euphoria, paranoid reaction, hallucination, aggressive reaction, aggravated depression, delusions; *Rare:* withdrawal syndrome, suicide ideation, libido increased, somnambulism, illusion.
Reproductive—*Infrequent:* menstrual disorder, dysmenorrhea, intermenstrual bleeding, vaginal hemorrhage, amenorrhea, leukorrhea; *Rare:* female breast pain, menorrhagia, balanoposthitis, breast enlargement, atrophic vaginitis, acute female mastitis.
Respiratory System Disorders—*Frequent:* rhinitis; *Infrequent:* coughing, dyspnea, upper respiratory tract infection, epistaxis, bronchospasm, sinusitis; *Rare:* hyperventilation, bradypnea, stridor, apnea, bronchitis, hemoptysis, hypoventilation, laryngismus, laryngitis.
Special Senses—*Frequent:* tinnitus; *Infrequent:* conjunctivitis, earache, eye pain, abnormal accommodation; *Rare:* xerophthalmia, photophobia, diplopia, abnormal lacrimation, scotoma, visual field defect.
Urinary System Disorders—*Infrequent:* micturition frequency, polyuria, urinary retention, dysuria, nocturia, urinary incontinence; *Rare:* cystitis, oliguria, pyelonephritis, hematuria, renal pain, strangury.

Laboratory Tests—In man, asymptomatic elevations in serum transaminases (SGOT [or AST] and SGPT [or ALT]) have been reported infrequently (approximately 0.8%) in association with ZOLOFT® (sertraline hydrochloride) administration. These hepatic enzyme elevations usually occurred within the first 1 to 9 weeks of drug treatment and promptly diminished upon drug discontinuation.
ZOLOFT therapy was associated with small mean increases in total cholesterol (approximately 3%) and triglycerides (approximately 5%), and a small mean decrease in serum uric acid (approximately 7%) of no apparent clinical importance.
The safety profile observed with ZOLOFT treatment in patients with major depressive disorder, OCD, panic disorder, PTSD, PMDD and social anxiety disorder is similar.
Other Events Observed During the Postmarketing Evaluation of ZOLOFT—Reports of adverse events temporally associated with ZOLOFT that have been received since market introduction, that are not listed above and that may have no causal relationship with the drug, include the following: acute renal failure, anaphylactoid reaction, angioedema, blindness, optic neuritis, cataract, increased coagulation times, bradycardia, AV block, atrial arrhythmias, QT-interval prolongation, ventricular tachycardia (including torsade de pointes-type arrhythmias), hypothyroidism, agranulocytosis, aplastic anemia and pancytopenia, leukopenia, thrombocytopenia, lupus-like syndrome, serum sickness, hyperglycemia, galactorrhea, hyperprolactinemia, neuroleptic malignant syndrome-like events, extrapyramidal symptoms, oculogyric crisis, serotonin syndrome, psychosis, pulmonary hypertension, severe skin reactions, which potentially can be fatal, such as Stevens-Johnson syndrome, vasculitis, photosensitivity and other severe cutaneous disorders, rare reports of pancreatitis, and liver events—clinical features (which in the majority of cases appeared to be reversible with discontinuation of ZOLOFT) occurring in one or more patients include: elevated enzymes, increased bilirubin, hepatomegaly, hepatitis, jaundice, abdominal pain, vomiting, liver failure and death.

DRUG ABUSE AND DEPENDENCE
Controlled Substance Class—ZOLOFT® (sertraline hydrochloride) is not a controlled substance.
Physical and Psychological Dependence—In a placebo-controlled, double-blind, randomized study of the comparative abuse liability of ZOLOFT, alprazolam, and d-amphetamine in humans, ZOLOFT did not produce the positive subjective effects indicative of abuse potential, such as euphoria or drug liking, that were observed with the other two drugs. Premarketing clinical experience with ZOLOFT did not reveal any tendency for a withdrawal syndrome or any

Continued on next page

Zoloft—Cont.

drug-seeking behavior. In animal studies ZOLOFT does not demonstrate stimulant or barbiturate-like (depressant) abuse potential. As with any CNS active drug, however, physicians should carefully evaluate patients for history of drug abuse and follow such patients closely, observing them for signs of ZOLOFT misuse or abuse (e.g., development of tolerance, incrementation of dose, drug-seeking behavior).

OVERDOSAGE

Human Experience—Of 1,027 cases of overdose involving sertraline hydrochloride worldwide, alone or with other drugs, there were 72 deaths (circa 1999).

Among 634 overdoses in which sertraline hydrochloride was the only drug ingested, 8 resulted in fatal outcome, 75 completely recovered, and 27 patients experienced sequelae after overdosage to include alopecia, decreased libido, diarrhea, ejaculation disorder, fatigue, insomnia, somnolence and serotonin syndrome. The remaining 524 cases had an unknown outcome. The most common signs and symptoms associated with non-fatal sertraline hydrochloride overdosage were somnolence, vomiting, tachycardia, nausea, dizziness, agitation and tremor.

The largest known ingestion was 13.5 grams in a patient who took sertraline hydrochloride alone and subsequently recovered. However, another patient who took 2.5 grams of sertraline hydrochloride alone experienced a fatal outcome.

Other important adverse events reported with sertraline hydrochloride overdose (single or multiple drugs) include bradycardia, bundle branch block, coma, convulsions, delirium, hallucinations, hypertension, hypotension, manic reaction, pancreatitis, QT-interval prolongation, serotonin syndrome, stupor and syncope.

Overdose Management—Treatment should consist of those general measures employed in the management of overdosage with any antidepressant.

Ensure an adequate airway, oxygenation and ventilation. Monitor cardiac rhythm and vital signs. General supportive and symptomatic measures are also recommended. Induction of emesis is not recommended. Gastric lavage with a large-bore orogastric tube with appropriate airway protection, if needed, may be indicated if performed soon after ingestion, or in symptomatic patients.

Activated charcoal should be administered. Due to large volume of distribution of this drug, forced diuresis, dialysis, hemoperfusion and exchange transfusion are unlikely to be of benefit. No specific antidotes for sertraline are known.

In managing overdosage, consider the possibility of multiple drug involvement. The physician should consider contacting a poison control center on the treatment of any overdose. Telephone numbers for certified poison control centers are listed in the *Physicians' Desk Reference*® (PDR®).

DOSAGE AND ADMINISTRATION

Initial Treatment

Dosage for Adults

Major Depressive Disorder and Obsessive-Compulsive Disorder—ZOLOFT treatment should be administered at a dose of 50 mg once daily.

Panic Disorder, Posttraumatic Stress Disorder and Social Anxiety Disorder—ZOLOFT treatment should be initiated with a dose of 25 mg once daily. After one week, the dose should be increased to 50 mg once daily.

While a relationship between dose and effect has not been established for major depressive disorder, OCD, panic disorder, PTSD or social anxiety disorder, patients were dosed in a range of 50-200 mg/day in the clinical trials demonstrating the effectiveness of ZOLOFT for the treatment of these indications. Consequently, a dose of 50 mg, administered once daily, is recommended as the initial therapeutic dose. Patients not responding to a 50 mg dose may benefit from dose increases up to a maximum of 200 mg/day. Given the 24 hour elimination half-life of ZOLOFT, dose changes should not occur at intervals of less than 1 week.

Premenstrual Dysphoric Disorder—ZOLOFT treatment should be initiated with a dose of 50 mg/day, either daily throughout the menstrual cycle or limited to the luteal phase of the menstrual cycle, depending on physician assessment.

While a relationship between dose and effect has not been established for PMDD, patients were dosed in the range of 50-150 mg/day with dose increases at the onset of each new menstrual cycle (see Clinical Trials under CLINICAL PHARMACOLOGY). Patients not responding to a 50 mg/day dose may benefit from dose increases (at 50 mg increments/menstrual cycle) up to 150 mg/day when dosing daily throughout the menstrual cycle, or 100 mg/day when dosing during the luteal phase of the menstrual cycle. If a 100 mg/day dose has been established with luteal phase dosing, a 50 mg/day titration step for three days should be utilized at the beginning of each luteal phase dosing period.

ZOLOFT should be administered once daily, either in the morning or evening.

Dosage for Pediatric Population (Children and Adolescents)

Obsessive-Compulsive Disorder—ZOLOFT treatment should be initiated with a dose of 25 mg once daily in children (ages 6-12) and at a dose of 50 mg once daily in adolescents (ages 13-17).

While a relationship between dose and effect has not been established for OCD, patients were dosed in a range of 25-200 mg/day in the clinical trials demonstrating the effectiveness of ZOLOFT for pediatric patients (6-17 years) with OCD. Patients not responding to an initial dose of 25 or 50 mg/day may benefit from dose increases up to a maximum of 200 mg/day. For children with OCD, their generally lower body weights compared to adults should be taken into consideration in advancing the dose, in order to avoid excess dosing. Given the 24 hour elimination half-life of ZOLOFT, dose changes should not occur at intervals of less than 1 week.

ZOLOFT should be administered once daily, either in the morning or evening.

Dosage for Hepatically Impaired Patients

The use of sertraline in patients with liver disease should be approached with caution. The effects of sertraline in patients with moderate and severe hepatic impairment have not been studied. If sertraline is administered to patients with liver impairment, a lower or less frequent dose should be used (see CLINICAL PHARMACOLOGY and PRECAUTIONS).

Maintenance/Continuation/Extended Treatment

Major Depressive Disorder—It is generally agreed that acute episodes of major depressive disorder require several months or longer of sustained pharmacologic therapy beyond response to the acute episode. Systematic evaluation of ZOLOFT has demonstrated that its antidepressant efficacy is maintained for periods of up to 44 weeks following 8 weeks of initial treatment at a dose of 50-200 mg/day (mean dose of 70 mg/day) (see Clinical Trials under CLINICAL PHARMACOLOGY). It is not known whether the dose of ZOLOFT needed for maintenance treatment is identical to the dose needed to achieve an initial response. Patients should be periodically reassessed to determine the need for maintenance treatment.

Posttraumatic Stress Disorder—It is generally agreed that PTSD requires several months or longer of sustained pharmacological therapy beyond response to initial treatment. Systematic evaluation of ZOLOFT has demonstrated that its efficacy in PTSD is maintained for periods of up to 28 weeks following 24 weeks of treatment at a dose of 50-200 mg/day (see Clinical Trials under CLINICAL PHARMACOLOGY). It is not known whether the dose of ZOLOFT needed for maintenance treatment is identical to the dose needed to achieve an initial response. Patients should be periodically reassessed to determine the need for maintenance treatment.

Social Anxiety Disorder—Social anxiety disorder is a chronic condition that may require several months or longer of sustained pharmacological therapy beyond response to initial treatment. Systematic evaluation of ZOLOFT has demonstrated that its efficacy in social anxiety disorder is maintained for periods of up to 24 weeks following 20 weeks of treatment at a dose of 50-200 mg/day (see Clinical Trials under CLINICAL PHARMACOLOGY). Dosage adjustments should be made to maintain patients on the lowest effective dose and patients should be periodically reassessed to determine the need for long-term treatment.

Obsessive-Compulsive Disorder and Panic Disorder—It is generally agreed that OCD and Panic Disorder require several months or longer of sustained pharmacological therapy beyond response to initial treatment. Systematic evaluation of continuing ZOLOFT for periods of up to 28 weeks in patients with OCD and Panic Disorder who have responded while taking ZOLOFT during initial treatment phases of 24 to 52 weeks of treatment at a dose range of 50-200 mg/day has demonstrated a benefit of such maintenance treatment (see Clinical Trials under CLINICAL PHARMACOLOGY). It is not known whether the dose of ZOLOFT needed for maintenance treatment is identical to the dose needed to achieve an initial response. Nevertheless, patients should be periodically reassessed to determine the need for maintenance treatment.

Premenstrual Dysphoric Disorder—The effectiveness of ZOLOFT in long-term use, that is, for more than 3 menstrual cycles, has not been systematically evaluated in controlled trials. However, as women commonly report that symptoms worsen with age until relieved by the onset of menopause, it is reasonable to consider continuation of a responding patient. Dosage adjustments, which may include changes between dosage regimens (e.g., daily throughout the menstrual cycle versus during the luteal phase of the menstrual cycle), may be needed to maintain the patient on the lowest effective dosage and patients should be periodically reassessed to determine the need for continued treatment.

Switching Patients to or from a Monoamine Oxidase Inhibitor—At least 14 days should elapse between discontinuation of an MAOI and initiation of therapy with ZOLOFT. In addition, at least 14 days should be allowed after stopping ZOLOFT before starting an MAOI (see CONTRAINDICATIONS and WARNINGS).

ZOLOFT Oral Concentrate

ZOLOFT Oral Concentrate contains 20 mg/mL of sertraline (as the hydrochloride) as the active ingredient and 12% alcohol. ZOLOFT Oral Concentrate must be diluted before use. Just before taking, use the dropper provided to remove the required amount of ZOLOFT Oral Concentrate and mix with 4 oz (1/2 cup) of water, ginger ale, lemon/lime soda, lemonade or orange juice ONLY. Do not mix ZOLOFT Oral Concentrate with anything other than the liquids listed. The dose should be taken immediately after mixing. Do not mix in advance. At times, a slight haze may appear after mixing; this is normal. Note that caution should be exercised for patients with latex sensitivity, as the dropper dispenser contains dry natural rubber.

ZOLOFT Oral Concentrate is contraindicated with ANTABUSE (disulfiram) due to the alcohol content of the concentrate.

HOW SUPPLIED

ZOLOFT® (sertraline hydrochloride) capsular-shaped scored tablets, containing sertraline hydrochloride equivalent to 25, 50 and 100 mg of sertraline, are packaged in bottles.

ZOLOFT® 25 mg Tablets: light green film coated tablets engraved on one side with ZOLOFT and on the other side scored and engraved with 25 mg.

NDC 0049-4960-50	Bottles of 50

ZOLOFT® 50 mg Tablets: light blue film coated tablets engraved on one side with ZOLOFT and on the other side scored and engraved with 50 mg.

NDC 0049-4900-66	Bottles of 100
NDC 0049-4900-73	Bottles of 500
NDC 0049-4900-94	Bottles of 5000
NDC 0049-4900-41	Unit Dose Packages of 100

ZOLOFT® 100 mg Tablets: light yellow film coated tablets engraved on one side with ZOLOFT and on the other side scored and engraved with 100 mg.

NDC 0049-4910-66	Bottles of 100
NDC 0049-4910-73	Bottles of 500
NDC 0049-4910-94	Bottles of 5000
NDC 0049-4910-41	Unit Dose Packages of 100

Store at 25°C (77°F); excursions permitted to 15°-30°C (59°-86°F) [see USP Controlled Room Temperature].

ZOLOFT® Oral Concentrate: ZOLOFT Oral Concentrate is a clear, colorless solution with a menthol scent containing sertraline hydrochloride equivalent to 20 mg of sertraline per mL and 12% alcohol. It is supplied as a 60 mL bottle with an accompanying calibrated dropper.

NDC 0049-4940-23	Bottles of 60 mL

Store at 25°C (77°F); excursions permitted to 15°-30°C (59°-86°F) [see USP Controlled Room Temperature].

Distributed by

Pfizer Roerig

Division of Pfizer Inc, NY, NY 10017

℞ only

69-4721-00-5 Revised February 2003

ZYRTEC® ℞

[*zyür-tĕk*]

(cetirizine hydrochloride)

Tablets and Syrup

For Oral Use

Prescribing information for this product, which appears on pages 2681–2683 of the 2003 PDR, has been completely revised as follows. Please write "See Supplement A" next to the product heading.

DESCRIPTION

Cetirizine hydrochloride, the active component of ZYRTEC® tablets and syrup, is an orally active and selective H_1-receptor antagonist. The chemical name is (±) - [2-[4- [(4- chlorophenyl)phenylmethyl] -1- piperazinyl] ethoxy] acetic acid, dihydrochloride. Cetirizine hydrochloride is a racemic compound with an empirical formula of $C_{21}H_{25}ClN_2O_3 \cdot 2HCl$. The molecular weight is 461.82 and the chemical structure is shown below:

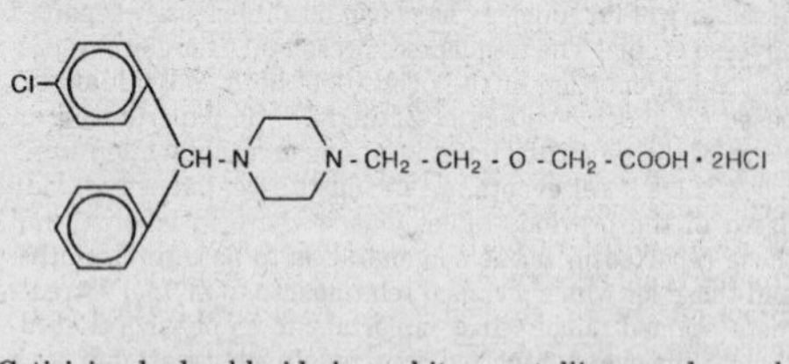

Cetirizine hydrochloride is a white, crystalline powder and is water soluble. ZYRTEC tablets are formulated as white, film-coated, rounded-off rectangular shaped tablets for oral administration and are available in 5 and 10 mg strengths. Inactive ingredients are: lactose; magnesium stearate; povidone; titanium dioxide; hydroxypropyl methylcellulose; polyethylene glycol; and corn starch.

ZYRTEC syrup is a colorless to slightly yellow syrup containing cetirizine hydrochloride at a concentration of 1 mg/mL (5 mg/5 mL) for oral administration. The pH is between 4 and 5. The inactive ingredients of the syrup are: banana flavor; glacial acetic acid; glycerin; grape flavor; methylparaben; propylene glycol; propylparaben; sodium acetate; sugar syrup; and water.

CLINICAL PHARMACOLOGY

Mechanism of Actions: Cetirizine, a human metabolite of hydroxyzine, is an antihistamine; its principal effects are mediated via selective inhibition of peripheral H_1 receptors. The antihistaminic activity of cetirizine has been clearly documented in a variety of animal and human models. *In vivo* and *ex vivo* animal models have shown negligible anticholinergic and antiserotonergic activity. In clinical studies, however, dry mouth was more common with cetirizine than with placebo. *In vitro* receptor binding studies have shown no measurable affinity for other than H_1 receptors. Autoradiographic studies with radiolabeled cetirizine in the rat have shown negligible penetration into the brain. *Ex vivo* experiments in the mouse have shown that systemically administered cetirizine does not significantly occupy cerebral H_1 receptors.

Pharmacokinetics:

Absorption: Cetirizine was rapidly absorbed with a time to maximum concentration (Tmax) of approximately 1 hour following oral administration of tablets or syrup in adults. Comparable bioavailability was found between the tablet and syrup dosage forms. When healthy volunteers were administered multiple doses of cetirizine (10 mg tablets once daily for 10 days), a mean peak plasma concentration (Cmax) of 311 ng/mL was observed. No accumulation was observed. Cetirizine pharmacokinetics were linear for oral doses ranging from 5 to 60 mg. Food had no effect on the extent of cetirizine exposure (AUC) but Tmax was delayed by 1.7 hours and Cmax was decreased by 23% in the presence of food.

Distribution: The mean plasma protein binding of cetirizine is 93%, independent of concentration in the range of 25–1000 ng/mL, which includes the therapeutic plasma levels observed.

Metabolism: A mass balance study in 6 healthy male volunteers indicated that 70% of the administered radioactivity was recovered in the urine and 10% in the feces. Approximately 50% of the radioactivity was identified in the urine as unchanged drug. Most of the rapid increase in peak plasma radioactivity was associated with parent drug, suggesting a low degree of first-pass metabolism. Cetirizine is metabolized to a limited extent by oxidative O-dealkylation to a metabolite with negligible antihistaminic activity. The enzyme or enzymes responsible for this metabolism have not been identified.

Elimination: The mean elimination half-life in 146 healthy volunteers across multiple pharmacokinetic studies was 8.3 hours and the apparent total body clearance for cetirizine was approximately 53 mL/min.

Interaction Studies

Pharmacokinetic interaction studies with cetirizine in adults were conducted with pseudoephedrine, antipyrine, ketoconazole, erythromycin and azithromycin. No interactions were observed. In a multiple dose study of theophylline (400 mg once daily for 3 days) and cetirizine (20 mg once daily for 3 days), a 16% decrease in the clearance of cetirizine was observed. The disposition of theophylline was not altered by concomitant cetirizine administration.

Special Populations

Pediatric Patients: When pediatric patients aged 7 to 12 years received a single, 5-mg oral cetirizine capsule, the mean Cmax was 275 ng/mL. Based on cross-study comparisons, the weight-normalized, apparent total body clearance was 33% greater and the elimination half-life was 33% shorter in this pediatric population than in adults. In pediatric patients aged 2 to 5 years who received 5 mg of cetirizine, the mean Cmax was 660 ng/mL. Based on cross-study comparisons, the weight-normalized apparent total body clearance was 81 to 111% greater and the elimination half-life was 33 to 41% shorter in this pediatric population than in adults. In pediatric patients aged 6 to 23 months who received a single dose of 0.25 mg/kg cetirizine oral solution (mean dose 2.3 mg), the mean Cmax was 390 ng/mL. Based on cross-study comparisons, the weight-normalized, apparent total body clearance was 304% greater and the elimination half-life was 63% shorter in this pediatric population compared to adults. The average AUC(0-t) in children 6 months to <2 years of age receiving the maximum dose of cetirizine solution (2.5 mg twice a day) is expected to be two-fold higher than that observed in adults receiving a dose of 10 mg cetirizine tablets once a day.

Geriatric Patients: Following a single, 10-mg oral dose, the elimination half-life was prolonged by 50% and the apparent total body clearance was 40% lower in 16 geriatric subjects with a mean age of 77 years compared to 14 adult subjects with a mean age of 53 years. The decrease in cetirizine clearance in these elderly volunteers may be related to decreased renal function.

Effect of Gender: The effect of gender on cetirizine pharmacokinetics has not been adequately studied.

Effect of Race: No race-related differences in the kinetics of cetirizine have been observed.

Renal Impairment: The kinetics of cetirizine were studied following multiple, oral, 10-mg daily doses of cetirizine for 7 days in 7 normal volunteers (creatinine clearance 89–128 mL/min), 8 patients with mild renal function impairment (creatinine clearance 42–77 mL/min) and 7 patients with moderate renal function impairment (creatinine clearance 11–31 mL/min). The pharmacokinetics of cetirizine were similar in patients with mild impairment and normal volunteers. Moderately impaired patients had a 3-fold increase in half-life and a 70% decrease in clearance compared to normal volunteers.

Patients on hemodialysis (n=5) given a single, 10-mg dose of cetirizine had a 3-fold increase in half-life and a 70% decrease in clearance compared to normal volunteers. Less than 10% of the administered dose was removed during the single dialysis session.

Dosing adjustment is necessary in patients with moderate or severe renal impairment and in patients on dialysis (see **DOSAGE AND ADMINISTRATION**).

Hepatic Impairment: Sixteen patients with chronic liver diseases (hepatocellular, cholestatic, and biliary cirrhosis), given 10 or 20 mg of cetirizine as a single, oral dose had a 50% increase in half-life along with a corresponding 40% decrease in clearance compared to 16 healthy subjects.

Dosing adjustment may be necessary in patients with hepatic impairment (see **DOSAGE AND ADMINISTRATION**).

Pharmacodynamics: Studies in 69 adult normal volunteers (aged 20 to 61 years) showed that ZYRTEC at doses of 5 and 10 mg strongly inhibited the skin wheal and flare caused by the intradermal injection of histamine. The onset of this activity after a single 10-mg dose occurred within 20 minutes in 50% of subjects and within one hour in 95% of subjects; this activity persisted for at least 24 hours. ZYRTEC at doses of 5 and 10 mg also strongly inhibited the wheal and flare caused by intradermal injection of histamine in 19 pediatric volunteers (aged 5 to 12 years) and the activity persisted for at least 24 hours. In a 35-day study in children aged 5 to 12, no tolerance to the antihistaminic (suppression of wheal and flare response) effects of ZYRTEC was found. In 10 infants 7 to 25 months of age who received 4 to 9 days of cetirizine in an oral solution (0.25 mg/kg bid), there was a 90% inhibition of histamine-induced (10 mg/mL) cutaneous wheal and 87% inhibition of the flare 12 hours after administration of the last dose. The clinical relevance of this suppression of histamine-induced wheal and flare response on skin testing is unknown.

The effects of intradermal injection of various other mediators or histamine releasers were also inhibited by cetirizine, as was response to a cold challenge in patients with cold-induced urticaria. In mildly asthmatic subjects, ZYRTEC at 5 to 20 mg blocked bronchoconstriction due to nebulized histamine, with virtually total blockade after a 20-mg dose. In studies conducted for up to 12 hours following cutaneous antigen challenge, the late phase recruitment of eosinophils, neutrophils and basophils, components of the allergic inflammatory response, was inhibited by ZYRTEC at a dose of 20 mg.

In four clinical studies in healthy adult males, no clinically significant mean increases in QTc were observed in ZYRTEC treated subjects. In the first study, a placebo-controlled crossover trial, ZYRTEC was given at doses up to 60 mg per day, 6 times the maximum clinical dose, for 1 week, and no significant mean QTc prolongation occurred. In the second study, a crossover trial, ZYRTEC 20 mg and erythromycin (500 mg every 8 hours) were given alone and in combination. There was no significant effect on QTc with the combination or with ZYRTEC alone. In the third trial, also a crossover study, ZYRTEC 20 mg and ketoconazole (400 mg per day) were given alone and in combination. ZYRTEC caused a mean increase in QTc of 9.1 msec from baseline after 10 days of therapy. Ketoconazole also increased QTc by 8.3 msec. The combination caused an increase of 17.4 msec, equal to the sum of the individual effects. Thus, there was no significant drug interaction on QTc with the combination of ZYRTEC and ketoconazole. In the fourth study, a placebo-controlled parallel trial, ZYRTEC 20 mg was given alone or in combination with azithromycin (500 mg as a single dose on the first day followed by 250 mg once daily). There was no significant increase in QTc with ZYRTEC 20 mg alone or in combination with azithromycin. In a four-week clinical trial in pediatric patients aged 6 to 11 years, results of randomly obtained ECG measurements before treatment and after 2 weeks of treatment showed that ZYRTEC 5 or 10 mg did not increase QTc versus placebo. In a one week clinical trial (N=86) of ZYRTEC syrup (0.25 mg/kg bid) compared with placebo in pediatric patients 6 to 11 months of age, ECG measurements taken within 3 hours of the last dose did not show any ECG abnormalities or increases in QTc interval in either group compared to baseline assessments. Data from other studies where ZYRTEC was administered to patients 6–23 months of age were consistent with the findings in this study.

The effects of ZYRTEC on the QTc interval at doses higher than 10 mg have not been studied in children less than 12 years of age.

In a six-week, placebo-controlled study of 186 patients (aged 12 to 64 years) with allergic rhinitis and mild to moderate asthma, ZYRTEC 10 mg once daily improved rhinitis symptoms and did not alter pulmonary function. In a two-week, placebo-controlled clinical trial, a subset analysis of 65 pediatric (aged 6 to 11 years) allergic rhinitis patients with asthma showed ZYRTEC did not alter pulmonary function. These studies support the safety of administering ZYRTEC to pediatric and adult allergic rhinitis patients with mild to moderate asthma.

Clinical Studies: Nine multicenter, randomized, double-blind, clinical trials comparing cetirizine 5 to 20 mg to placebo in patients 12 years and older with seasonal or perennial allergic rhinitis were conducted in the United States. Five of these showed significant reductions in symptoms of allergic rhinitis, 3 in seasonal allergic rhinitis (1 to 4 weeks in duration) and 2 in perennial allergic rhinitis for up to 8 weeks in duration. Two 4-week multicenter, randomized, double-blind, clinical trials comparing cetirizine 5 to 20 mg to placebo in patients with chronic idiopathic urticaria were also conducted and showed significant improvement in symptoms of chronic idiopathic urticaria. In general, the 10-mg dose was more effective than the 5-mg dose and the 20-mg dose gave no added effect. Some of these trials included pediatric patients aged 12 to 16 years. In addition, four multicenter, randomized, placebo-controlled, double-blind 2–4 week trials in 534 pediatric patients aged 6 to 11 years with seasonal allergic rhinitis were conducted in the United States at doses up to 10 mg.

INDICATIONS AND USAGE

Seasonal Allergic Rhinitis: ZYRTEC is indicated for the relief of symptoms associated with seasonal allergic rhinitis due to allergens such as ragweed, grass and tree pollens in adults and children 2 years of age and older. Symptoms treated effectively include sneezing, rhinorrhea, nasal pruritus, ocular pruritus, tearing, and redness of the eyes.

Perennial Allergic Rhinitis: ZYRTEC is indicated for the relief of symptoms associated with perennial allergic rhinitis due to allergens such as dust mites, animal dander and molds in adults and children 6 months of age and older. Symptoms treated effectively include sneezing, rhinorrhea, postnasal discharge, nasal pruritus, ocular pruritus, and tearing.

Chronic Urticaria: ZYRTEC is indicated for the treatment of the uncomplicated skin manifestations of chronic idiopathic urticaria in adults and children 6 months of age and older. It significantly reduces the occurrence, severity, and duration of hives and significantly reduces pruritus.

CONTRAINDICATIONS

ZYRTEC is contraindicated in those patients with a known hypersensitivity to it or any of its ingredients or hydroxyzine.

PRECAUTIONS

Activities Requiring Mental Alertness: In clinical trials, the occurrence of somnolence has been reported in some patients taking ZYRTEC; due caution should therefore be exercised when driving a car or operating potentially dangerous machinery. Concurrent use of ZYRTEC with alcohol or other CNS depressants should be avoided because additional reductions in alertness and additional impairment of CNS performance may occur.

Drug-Drug Interactions: No clinically significant drug interactions have been found with theophylline at a low dose, azithromycin, pseudoephedrine, ketoconazole, or erythromycin. There was a small decrease in the clearance of cetirizine caused by a 400-mg dose of theophylline; it is possible that larger theophylline doses could have a greater effect.

Carcinogenesis, Mutagenesis and Impairment of Fertility: In a 2-year carcinogenicity study in rats, cetirizine was not carcinogenic at dietary doses up to 20 mg/kg (approximately 15 times the maximum recommended daily oral dose in adults on a mg/m^2 basis, or approximately 7 times the maximum recommended daily oral dose in infants on a mg/m^2 basis). In a 2-year carcinogenicity study in mice, cetirizine caused an increased incidence of benign liver tumors in males at a dietary dose of 16 mg/kg (approximately 6 times the maximum recommended daily oral dose in adults on a mg/m^2 basis, or approximately 3 times the maximum recommended daily oral dose in infants on a mg/m^2 basis). No increase in the incidence of liver tumors was observed in mice at a dietary dose of 4 mg/kg (approximately 2 times the maximum recommended daily oral dose in adults on a mg/m^2 basis, or approximately equivalent to the maximum recommended daily oral dose in infants on a mg/m^2 basis). The clinical significance of these findings during long-term use of ZYRTEC is not known.

Cetirizine was not mutagenic in the Ames test, and not clastogenic in the human lymphocyte assay, the mouse lymphoma assay, and *in vivo* micronucleus test in rats.

In a fertility and general reproductive performance study in mice, cetirizine did not impair fertility at an oral dose of 64 mg/kg (approximately 25 times the maximum recommended daily oral dose in adults on a mg/m^2 basis).

Pregnancy Category B: In mice, rats, and rabbits, cetirizine was not teratogenic at oral doses up to 96, 225, and 135 mg/kg, respectively (approximately 40, 180 and 220 times the maximum recommended daily oral dose in adults on a mg/m^2 basis). There are no adequate and well-controlled studies in pregnant women. Because animal studies are not always predictive of human response, ZYRTEC should be used in pregnancy only if clearly needed.

Nursing Mothers: In mice, cetirizine caused retarded pup weight gain during lactation at an oral dose in dams of 96 mg/kg (approximately 40 times the maximum recommended daily oral dose in adults on a mg/m^2 basis). Studies in beagle dogs indicated that approximately 3% of the dose was excreted in milk. Cetirizine has been reported to be excreted in human breast milk. Because many drugs are excreted in human milk, use of ZYRTEC in nursing mothers is not recommended.

Geriatric Use: Of the total number of patients in clinical studies of ZYRTEC, 186 patients were 65 years and older, and 39 patients were 75 years and older. No overall differences in safety were observed between these patients and younger patients, but greater sensitivity of some older individuals cannot be ruled out. With regard to efficacy, clinical studies of ZYRTEC for each approved indication did not include sufficient numbers of patients aged 65 years and older to determine whether they respond differently than younger patients.

ZYRTEC is known to be substantially excreted by the kidney, and the risk of toxic reactions to this drug may be greater in patients with impaired renal function. Because elderly patients are more likely to have decreased renal function, care should be taken in dose selection, and it may be useful to monitor renal function. (See Geriatric Patients and Renal Impairment subsections in CLINICAL PHARMACOLOGY.)

Pediatric Use: The safety of ZYRTEC has been demonstrated in pediatric patients aged 6 months to 11 years. The safety of ZYRTEC, at daily doses of 5 or 10 mg, has been demonstrated in 376 pediatric patients aged 6 to 11 years in placebo-controlled trials lasting up to four weeks and in 254 patients in a non-placebo-controlled 12-week trial. The safety of cetirizine has been demonstrated in 168 patients aged 2 to 5 years in placebo-controlled trials of up to 4 weeks duration. On a mg/kg basis, most of the 168 patients

Continued on next page

Zyrtec—Cont.

received between 0.2 and 0.4 mg/kg of cetirizine HCl. The safety of cetirizine in 399 patients aged 12 to 24 months has been demonstrated in a placebo-controlled 18-month trial, in which the average dose was 0.25 mg/kg bid, corresponding to a range of 4 to 11 mg/day. The safety of ZYRTEC syrup has been demonstrated in 42 patients aged 6 to 11 months in a placebo-controlled 7-day trial. The prescribed dose was 0.25 mg/kg bid, which corresponded to a mean of 4.5 mg/day, with a range of 3.4 to 6.2 mg/day.

The effectiveness of ZYRTEC for the treatment of allergic rhinitis and chronic idiopathic urticaria in pediatric patients aged 6 months to 11 years is based on an extrapolation of the demonstrated efficacy of ZYRTEC in adults with these conditions and the likelihood that the disease course, pathophysiology and the drug's effect are substantially similar between these two populations. Efficacy is extrapolated down to 6 months of age for perennial allergic rhinitis and down to 2 years of age for seasonal allergic rhinitis because these diseases are thought to occur down to these ages in children. The recommended doses for the pediatric population are based on cross-study comparisons of the pharmacokinetics and pharmacodynamics of cetirizine in adult and pediatric subjects and on the safety profile of cetirizine in both adult and pediatric patients at doses equal to or higher than the recommended doses. The cetirizine AUC and Cmax in pediatric subjects aged 6 to 23 months who received a mean of 2.3 mg in a single dose, and in subjects aged 2 to 5 years who received a single dose of 5 mg of cetirizine syrup and in pediatric subjects aged 6 to 11 years who received a single dose of 10 mg of cetirizine syrup were estimated to be intermediate between that observed in adults who received a single dose of 10 mg of cetirizine tablets and those who received a single dose of 20 mg of cetirizine tablets.

The safety and effectiveness of cetirizine in pediatric patients under the age of 6 months have not been established.

ADVERSE REACTIONS

Controlled and uncontrolled clinical trials conducted in the United States and Canada included more than 6000 patients aged 12 years and older, with more than 3900 receiving ZYRTEC at doses of 5 to 20 mg per day. The duration of treatment ranged from 1 week to 6 months, with a mean exposure of 30 days.

Most adverse reactions reported during therapy with ZYRTEC were mild or moderate. In placebo-controlled trials, the incidence of discontinuations due to adverse reactions in patients receiving ZYRTEC 5 or 10 mg was not significantly different from placebo (2.9% vs. 2.4%, respectively).

The most common adverse reaction in patients aged 12 years and older that occurred more frequently on ZYRTEC than placebo was somnolence. The incidence of somnolence associated with ZYRTEC was dose related, 6% in placebo, 11% at 5 mg and 14% at 10 mg. Discontinuations due to somnolence for ZYRTEC were uncommon (1.0% on ZYRTEC vs. 0.6% on placebo). Fatigue and dry mouth also appeared to be treatment-related adverse reactions. There were no differences by age, race, gender or by body weight with regard to the incidence of adverse reactions.

Table 1 lists adverse experiences in patients aged 12 years and older which were reported for ZYRTEC 5 and 10 mg in controlled clinical trials in the United States and that were more common with ZYRTEC than placebo.

Table 1.
Adverse Experiences Reported in Patients Aged 12 Years and Older in Placebo-Controlled United States ZYRTEC Trials (Maximum Dose of 10 mg) at Rates of 2% or Greater (Percent Incidence)

Adverse Experience	ZYRTEC (N=2034)	Placebo (N=1612)
Somnolence	13.7	6.3
Fatigue	5.9	2.6
Dry Mouth	5.0	2.3
Pharyngitis	2.0	1.9
Dizziness	2.0	1.2

In addition, headache and nausea occurred in more than 2% of the patients, but were more common in placebo patients.

Pediatric studies were also conducted with ZYRTEC. More than 1300 pediatric patients aged 6 to 11 years with more than 900 treated with ZYRTEC at doses of 1.25 to 10 mg per day were included in controlled and uncontrolled clinical trials conducted in the United States. The duration of treatment ranged from 2 to 12 weeks. Placebo-controlled trials up to 4 weeks duration included 168 pediatric patients aged 2 to 5 years who received cetirizine, the majority of whom received single daily doses of 5 mg. A placebo-controlled trial 18 months in duration included 399 patients aged 12 to 24 months treated with cetirizine (0.25 mg/kg bid), and another placebo-controlled trial of 7 days duration included 42 patients aged 6 to 11 months who were treated with cetirizine (0.25 mg/kg bid).

The majority of adverse reactions reported in pediatric patients aged 2 to 11 years with ZYRTEC were mild or moderate. In placebo-controlled trials, the incidence of discontinuations due to adverse reactions in pediatric patients receiving up to 10 mg of ZYRTEC was uncommon (0.4% on ZYRTEC vs. 1.0% on placebo).

Table 2 lists adverse experiences which were reported for ZYRTEC 5 and 10 mg in pediatric patients aged 6 to 11 years in placebo-controlled clinical trials in the United States and were more common with ZYRTEC than placebo. Of these, abdominal pain was considered treatment-related and somnolence appeared to be dose-related, 1.3% in placebo, 1.9% at 5 mg and 4.2% at 10 mg. The adverse experiences reported in pediatric patients aged 2 to 5 years in placebo-controlled trials were qualitatively similar in nature and generally similar in frequency to those reported in trials with children aged 6 to 11 years.

In the placebo-controlled trials of pediatric patients 6 to 24 months of age, the incidences of adverse experiences, were similar in the cetirizine and placebo treatment groups in each study. Somnolence occurred with essentially the same frequency in patients who received cetirizine and patients who received placebo. In a study of 1 week duration in children 6–11 months of age, patients who received cetirizine exhibited greater irritability/fussiness than patients on placebo. In a study of 18 months duration in patients 12 months and older, insomnia occurred more frequently in patients who received cetirizine compared to patients who received placebo (9.0% v. 5.3%). In those patients who received 5 mg or more per day of cetirizine as compared to patients who received placebo, fatigue (3.6% v. 1.3%) and malaise (3.6% v. 1.8%) occurred more frequently.

Table 2.
Adverse Experiences Reported in Pediatric Patients Aged 6 to 11 Years in Placebo-Controlled United States ZYRTEC Trials (5 or 10 mg Dose) Which Occurred at a Frequency of ≥2% in Either the 5-mg or the 10-mg ZYRTEC Group, and More Frequently Than in the Placebo Group

		ZYRTEC	
Adverse Experiences	Placebo (N=309)	5 mg (N=161)	10 mg (N=215)
Headache	12.3%	11.0%	14.0%
Pharyngitis	2.9%	6.2%	2.8%
Abdominal pain	1.9%	4.4%	5.6%
Coughing	3.9%	4.4%	2.8%
Somnolence	1.3%	1.9%	4.2%
Diarrhea	1.3%	3.1%	1.9%
Epistaxis	2.9%	3.7%	1.9%
Bronchospasm	1.9%	3.1%	1.9%
Nausea	1.9%	1.9%	2.8%
Vomiting	1.0%	2.5%	2.3%

The following events were observed infrequently (less than 2%), in either 3982 adults and children 12 years and older or in 659 pediatric patients aged 6 to 11 years who received ZYRTEC in U.S. trials, including an open adult study of six months duration. A causal relationship of these infrequent events with ZYRTEC administration has not been established.

Autonomic Nervous System: anorexia, flushing, increased salivation, urinary retention.

Cardiovascular: cardiac failure, hypertension, palpitation, tachycardia.

Central and Peripheral Nervous Systems: abnormal coordination, ataxia, confusion, dysphonia, hyperesthesia, hyperkinesia, hypertonia, hypoesthesia, leg cramps, migraine, myelitis, paralysis, paresthesia, ptosis, syncope, tremor, twitching, vertigo, visual field defect.

Gastrointestinal: abnormal hepatic function, aggravated tooth caries, constipation, dyspepsia, eructation, flatulence, gastritis, hemorrhoids, increased appetite, melena, rectal hemorrhage, stomatitis including ulcerative stomatitis, tongue discoloration, tongue edema.

Genitourinary: cystitis, dysuria, hematuria, micturition frequency, polyuria, urinary incontinence, urinary tract infection.

Hearing and Vestibular: deafness, earache, ototoxicity, tinnitus.

Metabolic/Nutritional: dehydration, diabetes mellitus, thirst.

Musculoskeletal: arthralgia, arthritis, arthrosis, muscle weakness, myalgia.

Psychiatric: abnormal thinking, agitation, amnesia, anxiety, decreased libido, depersonalization, depression, emotional lability, euphoria, impaired concentration, insomnia, nervousness, paroniria, sleep disorder.

Respiratory System: bronchitis, dyspnea, hyperventilation, increased sputum, pneumonia, respiratory disorder, rhinitis, sinusitis, upper respiratory tract infection.

Reproductive: dysmenorrhea, female breast pain, intermenstrual bleeding, leukorrhea, menorrhagia, vaginitis.

Reticuloendothelial: lymphadenopathy.

Skin: acne, alopecia, angioedema, bullous eruption, dermatitis, dry skin, eczema, erythematous rash, furunculosis, hyperkeratosis, hypertrichosis, increased sweating, maculopapular rash, photosensitivity reaction, photosensitivity toxic reaction, pruritus, purpura, rash, seborrhea, skin disorder, skin nodule, urticaria.

Special Senses: parosmia, taste loss, taste perversion.

Vision: blindness, conjunctivitis, eye pain, glaucoma, loss of accommodation, ocular hemorrhage, xerophthalmia.

Body as a Whole: accidental injury, asthenia, back pain, chest pain, enlarged abdomen, face edema, fever, generalized edema, hot flashes, increased weight, leg edema, malaise, nasal polyp, pain, pallor, periorbital edema, peripheral edema, rigors.

Occasional instances of transient, reversible hepatic transaminase elevations have occurred during cetirizine therapy. Hepatitis with significant transaminase elevation and elevated bilirubin in association with the use of ZYRTEC has been reported.

In foreign marketing experience the following additional rare, but potentially severe adverse events have been reported: anaphylaxis, cholestasis, glomerulonephritis, hemolytic anemia, hepatitis, orofacial dyskinesia, severe hypotension, stillbirth, and thrombocytopenia.

DRUG ABUSE AND DEPENDENCE

There is no information to indicate that abuse or dependency occurs with ZYRTEC.

OVERDOSAGE

Overdosage has been reported with ZYRTEC. In one adult patient who took 150 mg of ZYRTEC, the patient was somnolent but did not display any other clinical signs or abnormal blood chemistry or hematology results. In an 18 month old pediatric patient who took an overdose of ZYRTEC (approximately 180 mg), restlessness and irritability were observed initially; this was followed by drowsiness. Should overdose occur, treatment should be symptomatic or supportive, taking into account any concomitantly ingested medications. There is no known specific antidote to ZYRTEC. ZYRTEC is not effectively removed by dialysis, and dialysis will be ineffective unless a dialyzable agent has been concomitantly ingested. The acute minimal lethal oral doses were 237 mg/kg in mice (approximately 95 times the maximum recommended daily oral dose in adults on a mg/m^2 basis, or approximately 40 times the maximum recommended daily oral dose in infants on a mg/m^2 basis) and 562 mg/kg in rats (approximately 460 times the maximum recommended daily oral dose in adults on a mg/m^2 basis, or approximately 190 times the maximum recommended daily oral dose in infants on a mg/m^2 basis). In rodents, the target of acute toxicity was the central nervous system, and the target of multiple-dose toxicity was the liver.

DOSAGE AND ADMINISTRATION

Adults and Children 12 Years and Older: The recommended initial dose of ZYRTEC is 5 or 10 mg per day in adults and children 12 years and older, depending on symptom severity. Most patients in clinical trials started at 10 mg. ZYRTEC is given as a single daily dose, with or without food. The time of administration may be varied to suit individual patient needs.

Children 6 to 11 Years: The recommended initial dose of ZYRTEC in children aged 6 to 11 years is 5 or 10 mg (1 or 2 teaspoons) once daily depending on symptom severity. The time of administration may be varied to suit individual patient needs.

Children 2 to 5 Years: The recommended initial dose of ZYRTEC syrup in children aged 2 to 5 years is 2.5 mg (½ teaspoon) once daily. The dosage in this age group can be increased to a maximum dose of 5 mg per day given as 1 teaspoon (5 mg) once daily, or as ½ teaspoon (2.5 mg) given every 12 hours.

Children 6 months to <2 years: The recommended dose of ZYRTEC syrup in children 6 months to 23 months of age is 2.5 mg (½ teaspoon) once daily. The dose in children 12 to 23 months of age can be increased to a maximum dose of 5 mg per day, given as ½ teaspoonful (2.5 mg) every 12 hours.

Dose Adjustment for Renal and Hepatic Impairment: In patients 12 years of age and older with decreased renal function (creatinine clearance 11-31 mL/min), patients on hemodialysis (creatinine clearance less than 7 mL/min), and in hepatically impaired patients, a dose of 5 mg once daily is recommended. Similarly, pediatric patients aged 6 to 11 years with impaired renal or hepatic function should use the lower recommended dose. Because of the difficulty in reliably administering doses of less than 2.5 mg (½ teaspoon) of ZYRTEC syrup and in the absence of pharmacokinetic and safety information for cetirizine in children below the age of 6 years with impaired renal or hepatic function, its use in this impaired patient population is not recommended.

HOW SUPPLIED

ZYRTEC® tablets are white, film-coated, rounded-off rectangular shaped containing 5 mg or 10 mg cetirizine hydrochloride.

5 mg tablets are engraved with "ZYRTEC" on one side and "5" on the other.

Bottles of 100: NDC 0069-5500-66

10 mg tablets are engraved with "ZYRTEC" on one side and "10" on the other.

Bottles of 100: NDC 0069-5510-66

STORAGE: Store at 20°–25°C (68°–77°F) excursions permitted to 15°–30°C (59°–86°F) [see USP Controlled Room Temperature].

ZYRTEC® syrup is colorless to slightly yellow with a banana-grape flavor. Each teaspoonful (5 mL) contains 5 mg cetirizine hydrochloride. ZYRTEC® syrup is supplied as follows:

120 mL amber glass bottles	NDC 0069-5530-47
1 pint amber glass bottles	NDC 0069-5530-93

STORAGE: Store at 20°-25°C (68°-77°F) excursions permitted to 15°-30°C (59°-86°F) [see USP Controlled Room Temperature]; **or Store refrigerated, 2°-8°C (36°-46°F).**

Cetirizine is licensed from UCB Pharma, Inc.

℞ **only**

Manufactured/Marketed by
Pfizer Labs
Division of Pfizer Inc, NY, NY 10017
Marketed by
UCB Pharma, Inc.
Smyrna, GA 30080
70-4573-00-5 Revised October 2002

The Purdue Frederick Company

ONE STAMFORD FORUM
STAMFORD, CT 06901-3431

For Medical Information Contact:
888-726-7535
Adverse Drug Experiences:
888-726-7535
Customer Service:
800-877-5666
FAX 800-877-3210

UNIPHYL® Tablets ℞

[*ū' nī-fĭl*]
theophylline, anhydrous

Prescribing information for this product, which appears on pages 2842–2847 of the 2003 PDR, has been revised as follows. Please write "See Supplement A" next to the product heading.

The following text has been added to the **WARNINGS** *section:*

TABLE II. Clinically significant drug interactions with theophylline

Hypericum perforatum (St. John's Wort) has been moved within the table and now appears alphabetically as St. John's Wort (Hypericum perforatum)

Existing text for **Type of Interaction** has been replaced with:

Decrease in theophylline plasma concentrations.

Under the subhead **Information for Patients,** *after the second sentence:*

Patients should be informed that theophylline interacts with a wide variety of drugs (see Table II). The dietary supplement St. John's Wort (Hypericum perforatum) should not be taken at the same time as theophylline, since it may result in decreased theophylline levels. If patients are already taking St. John's Wort and theophylline together, they should consult their health-care professional before stopping the St. John's Wort, since their theophylline concentrations may rise when this is done, resulting in toxicity.

Under the subhead **Geriatric Use,** *existing text has been replaced with:*

Elderly patients are at a significantly greater risk of experiencing serious toxicity from theophylline than younger patients due to pharmacokinetic and pharmacodynamic changes associated with aging. The clearance of theophylline is decreased by an average of 30% in healthy elderly adults (>60 yrs) compared to healthy young adults. Theophylline clearance may be further reduced by concomitant diseases prevalent in the elderly, which further impair clearance of this drug and have the potential to increase serum levels and potential toxicity. These conditions include impaired renal function, chronic obstructive pulmonary disease, congestive heart failure, hepatic disease and an increased prevalence of use of certain medications (see **PRECAUTIONS: Drug Interactions**) with the potential for pharmacokinetic and pharmacodynamic interaction. Protein binding may be decreased in the elderly resulting in an increased proportion of the total serum theophylline concentration in the pharmacologically active unbound form. Elderly patients also appear to be more sensitive to the toxic effects of theophylline after chronic overdosage than younger patients. Careful attention to dose reduction and frequent monitoring of serum theophylline concentrations are required in elderly patients (see **PRECAUTIONS, Monitoring Serum Theophylline Concentrations,** and **DOSAGE AND ADMINISTRATION**). The maximum daily dose of theophylline in patients greater than 60 years of age ordinarily should not exceed 400 mg/day unless the patient continues to be symptomatic and the peak steady-state serum theophylline concentration is <10 mcg/mL (see **DOSAGE AND ADMINISTRATION**). Theophylline doses greater than 400 mg/d should be prescribed with caution in elderly patients.

Roche Pharmaceuticals

Roche Laboratories Inc.
340 Kingsland Street
Nutley, NJ 07110-1199

For Medical Information:
(Including routine inquiries, adverse drug events and product complaints)
Call: (800) 526-6367
In Emergencies: 24-hour service
For the Medical Needs Program:
Call: (800) 285-4484
Write: Professional Product Information

CELLCEPT® ℞

[*sĕl'sĕpt*]
(mycophenolate mofetil capsules)
(mycophenolate mofetil tablets)
CELLCEPT® ORAL SUSPENSION
(mycophenolate mofetil for oral suspension)
CELLCEPT® INTRAVENOUS
(mycophenolate mofetil hydrochloride for injection)

Prescribing information for this product, which appears on pages 2875–2883 of the 2003 PDR, has been completely revised as follows. Please write "See Supplement A" next to the product heading.

> WARNING
> **Increased susceptibility to infection and the possible development of lymphoma may result from immunosuppression. Only physicians experienced in immunosuppressive therapy and management of renal, cardiac or hepatic transplant patients should use CellCept. Patients receiving the drug should be managed in facilities equipped and staffed with adequate laboratory and supportive medical resources. The physician responsible for maintenance therapy should have complete information requisite for the follow-up of the patient.**

DESCRIPTION

CellCept (mycophenolate mofetil) is the 2-morpholinoethyl ester of mycophenolic acid (MPA), an immunosuppressive agent; inosine monophosphate dehydrogenase (IMPDH) inhibitor.

The chemical name for mycophenolate mofetil (MMF) is 2-morpholinoethyl (E)-6-(1,3-dihydro-4-hydroxy-6-methoxy-7-methyl-3-oxo-5-isobenzofuranyl)-4-methyl-4-hexenoate. It has an empirical formula of $C_{23}H_{31}NO_7$, a molecular weight of 433.50

Mycophenolate mofetil is a white to off-white crystalline powder. It is slightly soluble in water (43 µg/mL at pH 7.4); the solubility increases in acidic medium (4.27 mg/mL at pH 3.6). It is freely soluble in acetone, soluble in methanol, and sparingly soluble in ethanol. The apparent partition coefficient in 1-octanol/water (pH 7.4) buffer solution is 238. The pKa values for mycophenolate mofetil are 5.6 for the morpholino group and 8.5 for the phenolic group.

Mycophenolate mofetil hydrochloride has a solubility of 65.8 mg/mL in 5% Dextrose Injection USP (D5W). The pH of the reconstituted solution is 2.4 to 4.1.

CellCept is available for oral administration as capsules containing 250 mg of mycophenolate mofetil, tablets containing 500 mg of mycophenolate mofetil, and as a powder for oral suspension, which when constituted contains 200 mg/mL mycophenolate mofetil.

Inactive ingredients in CellCept 250 mg capsules include croscarmellose sodium, magnesium stearate, povidone (K-90) and pregelatinized starch. The capsule shells contain black iron oxide, FD&C blue #2, gelatin, red iron oxide, silicon dioxide, sodium lauryl sulfate, titanium dioxide, and yellow iron oxide.

Inactive ingredients in CellCept 500 mg tablets include black iron oxide, croscarmellose sodium, FD&C blue #2 aluminum lake, hydroxypropyl cellulose, hydroxypropyl methylcellulose, magnesium stearate, microcrystalline cellulose, polyethylene glycol 400, povidone (K-90), red iron oxide, talc, and titanium dioxide; may also contain ammonium hydroxide, ethyl alcohol, methyl alcohol, n-butyl alcohol, propylene glycol, and shellac.

Inactive ingredients in CellCept Oral Suspension include aspartame, citric acid anhydrous, colloidal silicon dioxide, methylparaben, mixed fruit flavor, sodium citrate dihydrate, sorbitol, soybean lecithin, and xanthan gum.

CellCept Intravenous is the hydrochloride salt of mycophenolate mofetil. The chemical name for the hydrochloride salt of mycophenolate mofetil is 2-morpholinoethyl (E)-6-(1,3-dihydro-4-hydroxy-6-methoxy-7-methyl-3-oxo-5-isobenzofuranyl)-4-methyl-4-hexenoate hydrochloride. It has an empirical formula of $C_{23}H_{31}NO_7$ HCl and a molecular weight of 469.96.

CellCept Intravenous is available as a sterile white to off-white lyophilized powder in vials containing mycophenolate mofetil hydrochloride for administration by intravenous infusion only. Each vial of CellCept Intravenous contains the equivalent of 500 mg mycophenolate mofetil as the hydrochloride salt. The inactive ingredients are polysorbate 80, 25 mg, and citric acid, 5 mg. Sodium hydroxide may have been used in the manufacture of CellCept Intravenous to adjust the pH. Reconstitution and dilution with 5% Dextrose Injection USP yields a slightly yellow solution of mycophenolate mofetil, 6 mg/mL. (For detailed method of preparation, see DOSAGE AND ADMINISTRATION.)

CLINICAL PHARMACOLOGY

Mechanism of Action: Mycophenolate mofetil has been demonstrated in experimental animal models to prolong the survival of allogeneic transplants (kidney, heart, liver, intestine, limb, small bowel, pancreatic islets, and bone marrow). Mycophenolate mofetil has also been shown to reverse ongoing acute rejection in the canine renal and rat cardiac allograft models. Mycophenolate mofetil also inhibited proliferative arteriopathy in experimental models of aortic and cardiac allografts in rats, as well as in primate cardiac xenografts. Mycophenolate mofetil was used alone or in combination with other immunosuppressive agents in these studies. Mycophenolate mofetil has been demonstrated to inhibit immunologically mediated inflammatory responses in animal models and to inhibit tumor development and prolong survival in murine tumor transplant models.

Mycophenolate mofetil is rapidly absorbed following oral administration and hydrolyzed to form MPA, which is the active metabolite. MPA is a potent, selective, uncompetitive, and reversible inhibitor of inosine monophosphate dehydrogenase (IMPDH), and therefore inhibits the de novo pathway of guanosine nucleotide synthesis without incorporation into DNA. Because T- and B-lymphocytes are critically dependent for their proliferation on de novo synthesis of purines, whereas other cell types can utilize salvage pathways, MPA has potent cytostatic effects on lymphocytes. MPA inhibits proliferative responses of T- and B-lymphocytes to both mitogenic and allospecific stimulation. Addition of guanosine or deoxyguanosine reverses the cytostatic effects of MPA on lymphocytes. MPA also suppresses antibody formation by B-lymphocytes. MPA prevents the glycosylation of lymphocyte and monocyte glycoproteins that are involved in intercellular adhesion to endothelial cells and may inhibit recruitment of leukocytes into sites of inflammation and graft rejection. Mycophenolate mofetil did not inhibit early events in the activation of human peripheral blood mononuclear cells, such as the production of interleukin-1 (IL-1) and interleukin-2 (IL-2), but did block the coupling of these events to DNA synthesis and proliferation.

Pharmacokinetics: Following oral and intravenous administration, mycophenolate mofetil undergoes rapid and complete metabolism to MPA, the active metabolite. Oral absorption of the drug is rapid and essentially complete. MPA is metabolized to form the phenolic glucuronide of MPA (MPAG) which is not pharmacologically active. The parent drug, mycophenolate mofetil, can be measured systemically during the intravenous infusion; however, shortly (about 5 minutes) after the infusion is stopped or after oral administration, MMF concentration is below the limit of quantitation (0.4 µg/mL).

Absorption: In 12 healthy volunteers, the mean absolute bioavailability of oral mycophenolate mofetil relative to intravenous mycophenolate mofetil (based on MPA AUC) was 94%. The area under the plasma-concentration time curve (AUC) for MPA appears to increase in a dose-proportional fashion in renal transplant patients receiving multiple doses of mycophenolate mofetil up to a daily dose of 3 g (see table below on pharmacokinetic parameters).

Food (27 g fat, 650 calories) had no effect on the extent of absorption (MPA AUC) of mycophenolate mofetil when administered at doses of 1.5 g bid to renal transplant patients. However, MPA C_{max} was decreased by 40% in the presence of food (see DOSAGE AND ADMINISTRATION).

Distribution: The mean (±SD) apparent volume of distribution of MPA in 12 healthy volunteers is approximately 3.6 (±1.5) and 4.0 (±1.2) L/kg following intravenous and oral administration, respectively. MPA, at clinically relevant concentrations, is 97% bound to plasma albumin. MPAG is 82% bound to plasma albumin at MPAG concentration ranges that are normally seen in stable renal transplant patients; however, at higher MPAG concentrations (observed in patients with renal impairment or delayed renal graft function), the binding of MPA may be reduced as a result of competition between MPAG and MPA for protein binding. Mean blood to plasma ratio of radioactivity concentrations was approximately 0.6 indicating that MPA and MPAG do not extensively distribute into the cellular fractions of blood.

In vitro studies to evaluate the effect of other agents on the binding of MPA to human serum albumin (HSA) or plasma proteins showed that salicylate (at 25 mg/dL with HSA) and MPAG (at ≥460 µg/mL with plasma proteins) increased the free fraction of MPA. At concentrations that exceeded what is encountered clinically, cyclosporine, digoxin, naproxen, prednisone, propranolol, tacrolimus, theophylline, tolbutamide, and warfarin did not increase the free fraction of MPA. MPA at concentrations as high as 100 µg/mL had little effect on the binding of warfarin, digoxin or propranolol, but decreased the binding of theophylline from 53% to 45% and phenytoin from 90% to 87%.

Metabolism: Following oral and intravenous dosing, mycophenolate mofetil undergoes complete metabolism to MPA, the active metabolite. Metabolism to MPA occurs presystemically after oral dosing. MPA is metabolized principally by glucuronyl transferase to form the phenolic glucuronide of MPA (MPAG) which is not pharmacologically active. In vivo, MPAG is converted to MPA via enterohepatic recirculation. The following metabolites of the 2-hydroxyethyl-morpholino moiety are also recovered in the urine fol-

Continued on next page

Cellcept—Cont.

lowing oral administration of mycophenolate mofetil to healthy subjects: N-(2-carboxymethyl)-morpholine, N-(2-hydroxyethyl)-morpholine, and the N-oxide of N-(2-hydroxyethyl)-morpholine.

Secondary peaks in the plasma MPA concentration-time profile are usually observed 6 to 12 hours postdose. The coadministration of cholestyramine (4 g tid) resulted in approximately a 40% decrease in the MPA AUC (largely as a consequence of lower concentrations in the terminal portion of the profile). These observations suggest that enterohepatic recirculation contributes to MPA plasma concentrations.

Increased plasma concentrations of mycophenolate mofetil metabolites (MPA 50% increase and MPAG about a 3-fold to 6-fold increase) are observed in patients with renal insufficiency (see CLINICAL PHARMACOLOGY: *Special Populations*).

Excretion: Negligible amount of drug is excreted as MPA (<1% of dose) in the urine. Orally administered radiolabeled mycophenolate mofetil resulted in complete recovery of the administered dose, with 93% of the administered dose recovered in the urine and 6% recovered in feces. Most (about 87%) of the administered dose is excreted in the urine as MPAG. At clinically encountered concentrations, MPA and MPAG are usually not removed by hemodialysis. However, at high MPAG plasma concentrations (>100 µg/mL), small amounts of MPAG are removed. Bile acid sequestrants, such as cholestyramine, reduce MPA AUC by interfering with enterohepatic circulation of the drug (see OVERDOSAGE).

Mean (±SD) apparent half-life and plasma clearance of MPA are 17.9 (±6.5) hours and 193 (±48) mL/min following oral administration and 16.6 (±5.8) hours and 177 (±31) mL/min following intravenous administration, respectively.

Pharmacokinetics in Healthy Volunteers, Renal, Cardiac, and Hepatic Transplant Patients: Shown below are the mean (±SD) pharmacokinetic parameters for MPA following the administration of mycophenolate mofetil given as single doses to healthy volunteers and multiple doses to renal, cardiac, and hepatic transplant patients. In the early posttransplant period (<40 days posttransplant), renal, cardiac, and hepatic transplant patients had mean MPA AUCs approximately 20% to 41% lower and mean C_{max} approximately 32% to 44% lower compared to the late transplant period (3 to 6 months posttransplant).

Mean MPA AUC values following administration of 1 g bid intravenous mycophenolate mofetil over 2 hours to renal transplant patients for 5 days were about 24% higher than those observed after oral administration of a similar dose in the immediate posttransplant phase. In hepatic transplant patients, administration of 1 g bid intravenous CellCept followed by 1.5 g bid oral CellCept resulted in mean MPA AUC values similar to those found in renal transplant patients administered 1 g CellCept bid.

[See first table at right]

Two 500 mg tablets have been shown to be bioequivalent to four 250 mg capsules. Five mL of the 200 mg/mL constituted oral suspension have been shown to be bioequivalent to four 250 mg capsules.

Special Populations: Shown below are the mean (±SD) pharmacokinetic parameters for MPA following the administration of oral mycophenolate mofetil given as single doses to non-transplant subjects with renal or hepatic impairment.

[See second table at right]

Renal Insufficiency: In a single-dose study, MMF was administered as capsule or intravenous infusion over 40 minutes. Plasma MPA AUC observed after oral dosing to volunteers with severe chronic renal impairment [glomerular filtration rate (GFR) <25 mL/min/1.73 m^2] was about 75% higher relative to that observed in healthy volunteers (GFR >80 mL/min/1.73 m^2). In addition, the single-dose plasma MPAG AUC was 3-fold to 6-fold higher in volunteers with severe renal impairment than in volunteers with mild renal impairment or healthy volunteers, consistent with the known renal elimination of MPAG. No data are available on the safety of long-term exposure to this level of MPAG.

Plasma MPA AUC observed after single-dose (1 g) intravenous dosing to volunteers (n=4) with severe chronic renal impairment (GFR <25 mL/min/1.73 m^2) was 62.4 µg•h/mL (±19.3). Multiple dosing of mycophenolate mofetil in patients with severe chronic renal impairment has not been studied (see PRECAUTIONS: *General* and DOSAGE AND ADMINISTRATION).

In patients with delayed renal graft function posttransplant, mean MPA AUC(0–12h) was comparable to that seen in posttransplant patients without delayed renal graft function. There is a potential for a transient increase in the free fraction and concentration of plasma MPA in patients with delayed renal graft function. However, dose adjustment does not appear to be necessary in patients with delayed renal graft function. Mean plasma MPAG AUC(0–12h) was 2-fold to 3-fold higher than in posttransplant patients without delayed renal graft function (see PRECAUTIONS: *General* and DOSAGE AND ADMINISTRATION).

In 8 patients with primary graft non-function following renal transplantation, plasma concentrations of MPAG accumulated about 6-fold to 8-fold after multiple dosing for 28 days. Accumulation of MPA was about 1-fold to 2-fold.

The pharmacokinetics of mycophenolate mofetil are not altered by hemodialysis. Hemodialysis usually does not remove MPA or MPAG. At high concentrations of MPAG (>100 µg/mL), hemodialysis removes only small amounts of MPAG.

Hepatic Insufficiency: In a single-dose (1 g oral) study of 18 volunteers with alcoholic cirrhosis and 6 healthy volunteers, hepatic MPA glucuronidation processes appeared to be relatively unaffected by hepatic parenchymal disease when pharmacokinetic parameters of healthy volunteers and alcoholic cirrhosis patients within this study were compared. However, it should be noted that for unexplained reasons, the healthy volunteers in this study had about a 50% lower AUC as compared to healthy volunteers in other studies, thus making comparisons between volunteers with alcoholic cirrhosis and healthy volunteers difficult. Effects of hepatic

Pharmacokinetic Parameters for MPA [mean (±SD)] Following Administration of Mycophenolate Mofetil to Healthy Volunteers (Single Dose), Renal, Cardiac, and Hepatic Transplant Patients (Multiple Doses)

	Dose/Route	T_{max} (h)	C_{max} (µg/mL)	Total AUC (µg•h/mL)
Healthy Volunteers (single dose)	1 g/oral	0.80 (±0.36) (n=129)	24.5 (±9.5) (n=129)	63.9 (±16.2) (n=117)
Renal Transplant Patients (bid dosing) Time After Transplantation	Dose/Route	T_{max} (h)	C_{max} (µg/mL)	Interdosing Interval AUC(0–12h) (µg•h/mL)
5 days	1 g/iv	1.58 (±0.46) (n=31)	12.0 (±3.82) (n=31)	40.8 (±11.4) (n=31)
6 days	1 g/oral	1.33 (±1.05) (n=31)	10.7 (±4.83) (n=31)	32.9 (±15.0) (n=31)
Early (<40 days)	1 g/oral	1.31 (±0.76) (n=25)	8.16 (±4.50) (n=25)	27.3 (±10.9) (n=25)
Early (<40 days)	1.5 g/oral	1.21 (±0.81) (n=27)	13.5 (±8.18) (n=27)	38.4 (±15.4) (n=27)
Late (>3 months)	1.5 g/oral	0.90 (±0.24) (n=23)	24.1 (±12.1) (n=23)	65.3 (±35.4) (n=23)
Cardiac Transplant Patients (bid dosing) Time After Transplantation	Dose/Route	T_{max} (h)	C_{max} (µg/mL)	Interdosing Interval AUC(0–12h) (µg•h/mL)
Early (Day before discharge)	1.5 g/oral	1.8 (±1.3) (n=11)	11.5 (±6.8) (n=11)	43.3 (±20.8) (n=9)
Late (>6 months)	1.5 g/oral	1.1 (±0.7) (n=52)	20.0 (±9.4) (n=52)	54.1* (±20.4) (n=49)
Hepatic Transplant Patients (bid dosing) Time After Transplantation	Dose/Route	T_{max} (h)	C_{max} (µg/mL)	Interdosing Interval AUC(0–12h) (µg•h/mL)
4 to 9 days	1 g/iv	1.50 (±0.517) (n=22)	17.0 (±12.7) (n=22)	34.0 (±17.4) (n=22)
Early (5 to 8 days)	1.5 g/oral	1.15 (±0.432) (n=20)	13.1 (±6.76) (n=20)	29.2 (±11.9) (n=20)
Late (>6 months)	1.5 g/oral	1.54 (±0.51) (n=6)	19.3 (±11.7) (n=6)	49.3 (±14.8) (n=6)

AUC(0–12h) values quoted are extrapolated from data from samples collected over 4 hours.

Pharmacokinetic Parameters for MPA [mean (±SD)] Following Single Doses of Mycophenolate Mofetil Capsules in Chronic Renal and Hepatic Impairment

Renal Impairment (no. of patients)	Dose	T_{max} (h)	C_{max} (µg/mL)	AUC(0–96h) (µg•h/mL)
Healthy Volunteers GFR >80 mL/min/1.73 m^2 (n=6)	1 g	0.75 (±0.27)	25.3 (±7.99)	45.0 (±22.6)
Mild Renal Impairment GFR 50 to 80 mL/min/1.73 m^2 (n=6)	1 g	0.75 (±0.27)	26.0 (±3.82)	59.9 (±12.9)
Moderate Renal Impairment GFR 25 to 49 mL/min/1.73 m^2 (n=6)	1 g	0.75 (±0.27)	19.0 (±13.2)	52.9 (±25.5)
Severe Renal Impairment GFR <25 mL/min/1.73 m^2 (n=7)	1 g	1.00 (±0.41)	16.3 (±10.8)	78.6 (±46.4)
Hepatic Impairment (no. of patients)	Dose	T_{max} (h)	C_{max} (µg/mL)	AUC(0–48h) (µg•h/mL)
Healthy Volunteers (n=6)	1 g	0.63 (±0.14)	24.3 (±5.73)	29.0 (±5.78)
Alcoholic Cirrhosis (n=18)	1 g	0.85 (±0.58)	22.4 (±10.1)	29.8 (±10.7)

disease on this process probably depend on the particular disease. Hepatic disease with other etiologies, such as primary biliary cirrhosis, may show a different effect. In a single-dose (1 g intravenous) study of 6 volunteers with severe hepatic impairment (aminopyrine breath test less than 0.2% of dose) due to alcoholic cirrhosis, MMF was rapidly converted to MPA. MPA AUC was 44.1 µg•h/mL (±15.5).

Pediatrics: The pharmacokinetic parameters of MPA and MPAG have been evaluated in 55 pediatric patients (ranging from 1 year to 18 years of age) receiving CellCept oral suspension at a dose of 600 mg/m^2 bid (up to a maximum of 1 g bid) after allogeneic renal transplantation. The pharmacokinetic data for MPA is provided in the following table:
[See first table at right]

The CellCept oral suspension dose of 600 mg/m^2 bid (up to a maximum of 1 g bid) achieved mean MPA AUC values in pediatric patients similar to those seen in adult renal transplant patients receiving CellCept capsules at a dose of 1 g bid in the early posttransplant period. There was wide variability in the data. As observed in adults, early posttransplant MPA AUC values were approximately 45% to 53% lower than those observed in the later posttransplant period (>3 months). MPA AUC values were similar in the early and late posttransplant period across the 1 year to 18 year age range.

Gender: Data obtained from several studies were pooled to look at any gender-related differences in the pharmacokinetics of MPA (data were adjusted to 1 g oral dose). Mean (±SD) MPA AUC(0–12h) for males (n=79) was 32.0 (±14.5) and for females (n=41) was 36.5 (±18.8) µg•h/mL while mean (±SD) MPA C_{max} was 9.96 (±6.19) in the males and 10.6 (±5.64) µg/mL in the females. These differences are not of clinical significance.

Geriatrics: Pharmacokinetics in the elderly have not been studied.

CLINICAL STUDIES

The safety and efficacy of CellCept in combination with corticosteroids and cyclosporine for the prevention of organ rejection were assessed in randomized, double-blind, multicenter trials in renal (3 trials), in cardiac (1 trial), and in hepatic (1 trial) adult transplant patients.

Renal Transplant: The three renal studies compared two dose levels of oral CellCept (1 g bid and 1.5 g bid) with azathioprine (2 studies) or placebo (1 study) when administered in combination with cyclosporine (Sandimmune®*) and corticosteroids to prevent acute rejection episodes. One study also included antithymocyte globulin (ATGAM®†) induction therapy. These studies are described by geographic location of the investigational sites. One study was conducted in the USA at 14 sites, one study was conducted in Europe at 20 sites, and one study was conducted in Europe, Canada, and Australia at a total of 21 sites.

The primary efficacy endpoint was the proportion of patients in each treatment group who experienced treatment failure within the first 6 months after transplantation (defined as biopsy-proven acute rejection on treatment or the occurrence of death, graft loss or early termination from the study for any reason without prior biopsy-proven rejection). CellCept, when administered with antithymocyte globulin (ATGAM®) induction (one study) and with cyclosporine and corticosteroids (all three studies), was compared to the following three therapeutic regimens: (1) antithymocyte globulin (ATGAM®) induction/azathioprine/cyclosporine/corticosteroids, (2) azathioprine/cyclosporine/corticosteroids, and (3) cyclosporine/corticosteroids.

CellCept, in combination with corticosteroids and cyclosporine reduced (statistically significant at 0.05 level) the incidence of treatment failure within the first 6 months following transplantation. The following tables summarize the results of these studies. These tables show (1) the proportion of patients experiencing treatment failure, (2) the proportion of patients who experienced biopsy-proven acute rejection on treatment, and (3) early termination, for any reason other than graft loss or death, without a prior biopsy-proven acute rejection episode. Patients who prematurely discontinued treatment were followed for the occurrence of death or graft loss, and the cumulative incidence of graft loss and patient death are summarized separately. Patients who prematurely discontinued treatment were not followed for the occurrence of acute rejection after termination. More patients receiving CellCept discontinued without prior biopsy-proven rejection, death or graft loss than discontinued in the control groups, with the highest rate in the CellCept 3 g/day group. Therefore, the acute rejection rates may be underestimates, particularly in the CellCept 3 g/day group.

---
*Sandimmune is a registered trademark of Novartis Pharmaceuticals Corporation.
†ATGAM is a registered trademark of Pharmacia and Upjohn Company.

[See second table at right]

The cumulative incidence of 12-month graft loss or patient death is presented below. No advantage of CellCept with respect to graft loss or patient death was established. Numerically, patients receiving CellCept 2 g/day and 3 g/day experienced a better outcome than controls in all three studies; patients receiving CellCept 2 g/day experienced a better outcome than CellCept 3 g/day in two of the three studies. Patients in all treatment groups who terminated treatment early were found to have a poor outcome with respect to graft loss or patient death at 1 year.
[See first table at top of next page]

Pediatrics: One open-label, safety and pharmacokinetic study of CellCept oral suspension 600 mg/m^2 bid (up to 1 g bid) in combination with cyclosporine and corticosteroids was performed at centers in the US (9), Europe (5) and Australia (1) in 100 pediatric patients (3 months to 18 years of age) for the prevention of renal allograft rejection. CellCept was well tolerated in pediatric patients (see ADVERSE REACTIONS), and the pharmacokinetics profile was similar to that seen in adult patients dosed with 1 g bid CellCept capsules (see CLINICAL PHARMACOLOGY: *Pharmacokinetics*). The rate of biopsy-proven rejection was similar across the age groups (3 months to <6 years, 6 years to <12 years, 12 years to 18 years). The overall biopsy-proven rejection rate at 6 months was comparable to adults. The combined incidence of graft loss (5%) and patient death (2%) at 12 months posttransplant was similar to that observed in adult renal transplant patients.

Cardiac Transplant: A double-blind, randomized, comparative, parallel-group, multicenter study in primary cardiac transplant recipients was performed at 20 centers in the United States, 1 in Canada, 5 in Europe and 2 in Australia. The total number of patients enrolled was 650; 72 never received study drug and 578 received study drug. Patients received CellCept 1.5 g bid (n=289) or azathioprine 1.5 to 3 mg/kg/day (n=289), in combination with cyclosporine (Sandimmune® or Neoral®*) and corticosteroids as maintenance immunosuppressive therapy. The two primary efficacy endpoints were: (1) the proportion of patients who, after transplantation, had at least one endomyocardial biopsy-proven rejection with hemodynamic compromise, or were retransplanted or died, within the first 6 months, and (2) the proportion of patients who died or were retransplanted during the first 12 months following transplantation. Patients who prematurely discontinued treatment were followed for the occurrence of allograft rejection for up to 6 months and for the occurrence of death for 1 year.

(1) Rejection: No difference was established between CellCept and azathioprine (AZA) with respect to biopsy-proven rejection with hemodynamic compromise.

---
*Neoral is a registered trademark of Novartis Pharmaceuticals Corporation.

(2) Survival: CellCept was shown to be at least as effective as AZA in preventing death or retransplantation at 1 year (see table below).
[See second table at top of next page]

Hepatic Transplant: A double-blind, randomized, comparative, parallel-group, multicenter study in primary hepatic transplant recipients was performed at 16 centers in the United States, 2 in Canada, 4 in Europe and 1 in Australia. The total number of patients enrolled was 565. Per protocol, patients received CellCept 1 g bid intravenously for up to 14 days followed by CellCept 1.5 g bid orally or azathioprine 1 to 2 mg/kg/day intravenously followed by azathioprine 1 to 2 mg/kg/day orally, in combination with cyclosporine (Neoral®) and corticosteroids as maintenance immunosuppressive therapy. The actual median oral dose of azathioprine on study was 1.5 mg/kg/day (range of 0.3 to 3.8 mg/

Continued on next page

Mean (±SD) Computed Pharmacokinetic Parameters for MPA by Age and Time After Allogeneic Renal Transplantation

Age Group	(n)	Time	T_{max} (h)		Dose Adjusted[a] C_{max} (µg/mL)		Dose Adjusted[a] AUC_{0-12} (µg·h/mL)	
1 to <2 yr	(6)[d]	Early (Day 7)	3.03	(4.70)	10.3	(5.80)	22.5	(6.66)
1 to <6 yr	(17)		1.63	(2.85)	13.2	(7.16)	27.4	(9.54)
6 to <12 yr	(16)		0.940	(0.546)	13.1	(6.30)	33.2	(12.1)
12 to 18 yr	(21)		1.16	(0.830)	11.7	(10.7)	26.3	(9.14)[b]
1 to <2 yr	(4)[d]	Late (Month 3)	0.725	(0.276)	23.8	(13.4)	47.4	(14.7)
1 to <6 yr	(15)		0.989	(0.511)	22.7	(10.1)	49.7	(18.2)
6 to <12 yr	(14)		1.21	(0.532)	27.8	(14.3)	61.9	(19.6)
12 to 18 yr	(17)		0.978	(0.484)	17.9	(9.57)	53.6	(20.3)[c]
1 to <2 yr	(4)[d]	Late (Month 9)	0.604	(0.208)	25.6	(4.25)	55.8	(11.6)
1 to <6 yr	(12)		0.869	(0.479)	30.4	(9.16)	61.0	(10.7)
6 to <12 yr	(11)		1.12	(0.462)	29.2	(12.6)	66.8	(21.2)
12 to 18 yr	(14)		1.09	(0.518)	18.1	(7.29)	56.7	(14.0)

[a] adjusted to a dose of 600 mg/m^2
[b] n=20
[c] n=16
[d] a subset of 1 to <6 yr

Renal Transplant Studies
Incidence of Treatment Failure
(Biopsy-proven Rejection or Early Termination for Any Reason)

USA Study† (N=499 patients)	CellCept 2 g/day (n=167 patients)	CellCept 3 g/day (n=166 patients)	Azathioprine 1 to 2 mg/kg/day (n=166 patients)
All treatment failures	31.1%	31.3%	47.6%
Early termination without prior acute rejection*	9.6%	12.7%	6.0%
Biopsy-proven rejection episode on treatment	19.8%	17.5%	38.0%
Europe/Canada/ Australia Study‡ (N=503 patients)	**CellCept 2 g/day** (n=173 patients)	**CellCept 3 g/day** (n=164 patients)	**Azathioprine 100 to 150 mg/day** (n=166 patients)
All treatment failures	38.2%	34.8%	50.0%
Early termination without prior acute rejection*	13.9%	15.2%	10.2%
Biopsy-proven rejection episode on treatment	19.7%	15.9%	35.5%
Europe Study§ (N=491 patients)	**CellCept 2 g/day** (n=165 patients)	**CellCept 3 g/day** (n=160 patients)	**Placebo** (n=166 patients)
All treatment failures	30.3%	38.8%	56.0%
Early termination without prior acute rejection*	11.5%	22.5%	7.2%
Biopsy-proven rejection episode on treatment	17.0%	13.8%	46.4%

*Does not include death and graft loss as reason for early termination.
†Antithymocyte globulin induction/MMF or azathioprine/cyclosporine/corticosteroids.
‡MMF or azathioprine/cyclosporine/corticosteroids.
§MMF or placebo/cyclosporine/corticosteroids.

Cellcept—Cont.

kg/day) initially and 1.26 mg/kg/day (range of 0.3 to 3.8 mg/kg/day) at 12 months. The two primary endpoints were: (1) the proportion of patients who experienced, in the first 6 months posttransplantation, one or more episodes of biopsy-proven and treated rejection or death or retransplantation, and (2) the proportion of patients who experienced graft loss (death or retransplantation) during the first 12 months posttransplantation. Patients who prematurely discontinued treatment were followed for the occurrence of allograft rejection and for the occurrence of graft loss (death or retransplantation) for 1 year.

Results: In combination with corticosteroids and cyclosporine, CellCept obtained a lower rate of acute rejection at 6 months and a similar rate of death or retransplantation at 1 year compared to azathioprine.

	Rejection at 6 Months/ Death or Retransplantation at 1 Year	
	AZA N = 287	CellCept N = 278
Biopsy proven, treated rejection at 6 months (includes death or retransplantation)	137 (47.7%)	107 (38.5%)
Death or retransplantation at 1 year	42 (14.6%)	41 (14.7%)

INDICATIONS AND USAGE

Renal, Cardiac, and Hepatic Transplant: CellCept is indicated for the prophylaxis of organ rejection in patients receiving allogeneic renal, cardiac or hepatic transplants. CellCept should be used concomitantly with cyclosporine and corticosteroids.

CellCept Intravenous is an alternative dosage form to CellCept capsules, tablets and oral suspension. CellCept Intravenous should be administered within 24 hours following transplantation. CellCept Intravenous can be administered for up to 14 days; patients should be switched to oral CellCept as soon as they can tolerate oral medication.

CONTRAINDICATIONS

Allergic reactions to CellCept have been observed; therefore, CellCept is contraindicated in patients with a hypersensitivity to mycophenolate mofetil, mycophenolic acid or any component of the drug product. CellCept Intravenous is contraindicated in patients who are allergic to Polysorbate 80 (TWEEN).

WARNINGS (see boxed WARNING)

Patients receiving immunosuppressive regimens involving combinations of drugs, including CellCept, as part of an immunosuppressive regimen are at increased risk of developing lymphomas and other malignancies, particularly of the skin (see ADVERSE REACTIONS). The risk appears to be related to the intensity and duration of immunosuppression rather than to the use of any specific agent. Oversuppression of the immune system can also increase susceptibility to infection, including opportunistic infections, fatal infections, and sepsis.

As usual for patients with increased risk for skin cancer, exposure to sunlight and UV light should be limited by wearing protective clothing and using a sunscreen with a high protection factor.

CellCept has been administered in combination with the following agents in clinical trials: antithymocyte globulin (ATGAM®), OKT3 (Orthoclone OKT® 3*), cyclosporine (Sandimmune®, Neoral®) and corticosteroids. The efficacy and safety of the use of CellCept in combination with other immunosuppressive agents have not been determined.

*Orthoclone OKT is a registered trademark of Ortho Biotech Inc.

Lymphoproliferative disease or lymphoma developed in 0.4% to 1% of patients receiving CellCept (2 g or 3 g) with other immunosuppressive agents in controlled clinical trials of renal, cardiac, and hepatic transplant patients (see ADVERSE REACTIONS).

In pediatric patients, no other malignancies besides lymphoproliferative disorder (2/148 patients) have been observed (see ADVERSE REACTIONS).

Adverse effects on fetal development (including malformations) occurred when pregnant rats and rabbits were dosed during organogenesis. These responses occurred at doses lower than those associated with maternal toxicity, and at doses below the recommended clinical dose for renal, cardiac or hepatic transplantation. There are no adequate and well-controlled studies in pregnant women. However, as CellCept has been shown to have teratogenic effects in animals, it may cause fetal harm when administered to a pregnant woman. Therefore, CellCept should not be used in pregnant women unless the potential benefit justifies the potential risk to the fetus.

Women of childbearing potential should have a negative serum or urine pregnancy test with a sensitivity of at least 50 mIU/mL within 1 week prior to beginning therapy. It is recommended that CellCept therapy should not be initiated by the physician until a report of a negative pregnancy test has been obtained.

Renal Transplant Studies
Cumulative Incidence of Combined Graft Loss or Patient Death at 12 Months

Study	CellCept 2 g/day	CellCept 3 g/day	Control (Azathioprine or Placebo)
USA	8.5%	11.5%	12.2%
Europe/Canada/Australia	11.7%	11.0%	13.6%
Europe	8.5%	10.0%	11.5%

Rejection at 6 Months/Death or Retransplantation at 1 Year

	All Patients		Treated Patients	
	AZA N = 323	CellCept N = 327	AZA N = 289	CellCept N = 289
Biopsy-proven rejection with hemodynamic compromise at 6 months*	121 (38%)	120 (37%)	100 (35%)	92 (32%)
Death or retransplantation at 1 year	49 (15.2%)	42 (12.8%)	33 (11.4%)	18 (6.2%)

* Hemodynamic compromise occurred if any of the following criteria were met: pulmonary capillary wedge pressure ≥20 mm or a 25% increase; cardiac index <2.0 L/min/m^2 or a 25% decrease; ejection fraction ≤30%; pulmonary artery oxygen saturation ≤60% or a 25% decrease; presence of new S_3 gallop; fractional shortening was ≤20% or a 25% decrease; inotropic support required to manage the clinical condition.

Effective contraception must be used before beginning CellCept therapy, during therapy, and for 6 weeks following discontinuation of therapy, even where there has been a history of infertility, unless due to hysterectomy. Two reliable forms of contraception must be used simultaneously unless abstinence is the chosen method (see PRECAUTIONS: *Drug Interactions*). If pregnancy does occur during treatment, the physician and patient should discuss the desirability of continuing the pregnancy (see PRECAUTIONS: *Pregnancy* and *Information for Patients*).

In patients receiving CellCept (2 g or 3 g) in controlled studies for prevention of renal, cardiac or hepatic rejection, fatal infection/sepsis occurred in approximately 2% of renal and cardiac patients and in 5% of hepatic patients (see ADVERSE REACTIONS).

Severe neutropenia [absolute neutrophil count (ANC) <0.5 x 10^3/µL] developed in up to 2.0% of renal, up to 2.8% of cardiac, and up to 3.6% of hepatic transplant patients receiving CellCept 3 g daily (see ADVERSE REACTIONS). Patients receiving CellCept should be monitored for neutropenia (see PRECAUTIONS: *Laboratory Tests*). The development of neutropenia may be related to CellCept itself, concomitant medications, viral infections, or some combination of these causes. If neutropenia develops (ANC <1.3 x 10^3/µL), dosing with CellCept should be interrupted or the dose reduced, appropriate diagnostic tests performed, and the patient managed appropriately (see DOSAGE AND ADMINISTRATION). Neutropenia has been observed most frequently in the period from 31 to 180 days posttransplant in patients treated for prevention of renal, cardiac, and hepatic rejection.

Patients receiving CellCept should be instructed to report immediately any evidence of infection, unexpected bruising, bleeding or any other manifestation of bone marrow depression.

CAUTION: CELLCEPT INTRAVENOUS SOLUTION SHOULD NEVER BE ADMINISTERED BY RAPID OR BOLUS INTRAVENOUS INJECTION.

PRECAUTIONS

General: Gastrointestinal bleeding (requiring hospitalization) has been observed in approximately 3% of renal, in 1.7% of cardiac, and in 5.4% of hepatic transplant patients treated with CellCept 3 g daily. In pediatric renal transplant patients, 5/148 cases of gastrointestinal bleeding (requiring hospitalization) were observed.

Gastrointestinal perforations have rarely been observed. Most patients receiving CellCept were also receiving other drugs known to be associated with these complications. Patients with active peptic ulcer disease were excluded from enrollment in studies with mycophenolate mofetil. Because CellCept has been associated with an increased incidence of digestive system adverse events, including infrequent cases of gastrointestinal tract ulceration, hemorrhage, and perforation, CellCept should be administered with caution in patients with active serious digestive system disease.

Subjects with severe chronic renal impairment (GFR <25 mL/min/1.73 m^2) who have received single doses of CellCept showed higher plasma MPA and MPAG AUCs relative to subjects with lesser degrees of renal impairment or normal healthy volunteers. No data are available on the safety of long-term exposure to these levels of MPAG. Doses of CellCept greater than 1 g administered twice a day to renal transplant patients should be avoided and they should be carefully observed (see CLINICAL PHARMACOLOGY: *Pharmacokinetics* and DOSAGE AND ADMINISTRATION). No data are available for cardiac or hepatic transplant patients with severe chronic renal impairment. CellCept may be used for cardiac or hepatic transplant patients with severe chronic renal impairment if the potential benefits outweigh the potential risks.

In patients with delayed renal graft function posttransplant, mean MPA AUC(0–12h) was comparable, but MPAG AUC(0–12h) was 2-fold to 3-fold higher, compared to that seen in posttransplant patients without delayed renal graft function. In the three controlled studies of prevention of renal rejection, there were 298 of 1483 patients (20%) with delayed graft function. Although patients with delayed graft function have a higher incidence of certain adverse events (anemia, thrombocytopenia, hyperkalemia) than patients without delayed graft function, these events were not more frequent in patients receiving CellCept than azathioprine or placebo. No dose adjustment is recommended for these patients; however, they should be carefully observed (see CLINICAL PHARMACOLOGY: *Pharmacokinetics* and DOSAGE AND ADMINISTRATION).

In cardiac transplant patients, the overall incidence of opportunistic infections was approximately 10% higher in patients treated with CellCept than in those receiving azathioprine therapy, but this difference was not associated with excess mortality due to infection/sepsis among patients treated with CellCept (see ADVERSE REACTIONS).

There were more herpes virus (H. simplex, H. zoster, and cytomegalovirus) infections in cardiac transplant patients treated with CellCept compared to those treated with azathioprine (see ADVERSE REACTIONS).

It is recommended that CellCept not be administered concomitantly with azathioprine because both have the potential to cause bone marrow suppression and such concomitant administration has not been studied clinically.

In view of the significant reduction in the AUC of MPA by cholestyramine, caution should be used in the concomitant administration of CellCept with drugs that interfere with enterohepatic recirculation because of the potential to reduce the efficacy of CellCept (see PRECAUTIONS: *Drug Interactions*).

On theoretical grounds, because CellCept is an IMPDH (inosine monophosphate dehydrogenase) inhibitor, it should be avoided in patients with rare hereditary deficiency of hypoxanthine-guanine phosphoribosyl-transferase (HGPRT) such as Lesch-Nyhan and Kelley-Seegmiller syndrome.

During treatment with CellCept, the use of live attenuated vaccines should be avoided and patients should be advised that vaccinations may be less effective (see PRECAUTIONS: *Drug Interactions: Live Vaccines*).

Phenylketonurics: CellCept Oral Suspension contains aspartame, a source of phenylalanine (0.56 mg phenylalanine/mL suspension). Therefore, care should be taken if CellCept Oral Suspension is administered to patients with phenylketonuria.

Information for Patients: Patients should be informed of the need for repeated appropriate laboratory tests while they are receiving CellCept. Patients should be given complete dosage instructions and informed of the increased risk of lymphoproliferative disease and certain other malignancies. Women of childbearing potential should be instructed of the potential risks during pregnancy, and that they should use effective contraception before beginning CellCept therapy, during therapy, and for 6 weeks after CellCept has been stopped (see WARNINGS and PRECAUTIONS: *Pregnancy*).

Laboratory Tests: Complete blood counts should be performed weekly during the first month, twice monthly for the second and third months of treatment, then monthly through the first year (see WARNINGS, ADVERSE REACTIONS and DOSAGE AND ADMINISTRATION).

Drug Interactions: Drug interaction studies with mycophenolate mofetil have been conducted with acyclovir, antacids, cholestyramine, cyclosporine, ganciclovir, oral contraceptives, and trimethoprim/sulfamethoxazole. Drug interaction studies have not been conducted with other drugs that may be commonly administered to renal, cardiac or hepatic transplant patients. CellCept has not been administered concomitantly with azathioprine.

Acyclovir: Coadministration of mycophenolate mofetil (1 g) and acyclovir (800 mg) to 12 healthy volunteers resulted in no significant change in MPA AUC and C_{max}. However, MPAG and acyclovir plasma AUCs were increased 10.6% and 21.9%, respectively. Because MPAG plasma concentrations are increased in the presence of renal impairment, as are acyclovir concentrations, the potential exists for the two drugs to compete for tubular secretion, further increasing the concentrations of both drugs.

Antacids With Magnesium and Aluminum Hydroxides: Absorption of a single dose of mycophenolate mofetil (2 g) was decreased when administered to ten rheumatoid arthritis patients also taking Maalox®* TC (10 mL qid). The C_{max} and AUC(0–24h) for MPA were 33% and 17% lower, respectively, than when mycophenolate mofetil was administered alone under fasting conditions. CellCept may be administered to patients who are also taking antacids containing magnesium and aluminum hydroxides; however, it is recommended that CellCept and the antacid not be administered simultaneously.

---

*Maalox is a registered trademark of Novartis Consumer Health, Inc.

Cholestyramine: Following single-dose administration of 1.5 g mycophenolate mofetil to 12 healthy volunteers pretreated with 4 g tid of cholestyramine for 4 days, MPA AUC decreased approximately 40%. This decrease is consistent with interruption of enterohepatic recirculation which may be due to binding of recirculating MPAG with cholestyramine in the intestine. Some degree of enterohepatic recirculation is also anticipated following intravenous administration of CellCept. Therefore, CellCept is not recommended to be given with cholestyramine or other agents that may interfere with enterohepatic recirculation.

Cyclosporine: Cyclosporine (Sandimmune®) pharmacokinetics (at doses of 275 to 415 mg/day) were unaffected by single and multiple doses of 1.5 g bid of mycophenolate mofetil in 10 stable renal transplant patients. The mean ($\pm$SD) AUC(0–12h) and C_{max} of cyclosporine after 14 days of multiple doses of mycophenolate mofetil were 3290 ($\pm$822) ng•h/mL and 753 ($\pm$161) ng/mL, respectively, compared to 3245 ($\pm$1088) ng•h/mL and 700 ($\pm$246) ng/mL, respectively, 1 week before administration of mycophenolate mofetil. The effect of cyclosporine on mycophenolate mofetil pharmacokinetics could not be evaluated in this study; however, plasma concentrations of MPA were similar to that for healthy volunteers.

Ganciclovir: Following single-dose administration to 12 stable renal transplant patients, no pharmacokinetic interaction was observed between mycophenolate mofetil (1.5 g) and intravenous ganciclovir (5 mg/kg). Mean ($\pm$SD) ganciclovir AUC and C_{max} (n=10) were 54.3 ($\pm$19.0) µg•h/mL and 11.5 ($\pm$1.8) µg/mL, respectively, after coadministration of the two drugs, compared to 51.0 ($\pm$17.0) µg•h/mL and 10.6 ($\pm$2.0) µg/mL, respectively, after administration of intravenous ganciclovir alone. The mean ($\pm$SD) AUC and C_{max} of MPA (n=12) after coadministration were 80.9 ($\pm$21.6) µg•h/mL and 27.8 ($\pm$13.9) µg/mL, respectively, compared to values of 80.3 ($\pm$16.4) µg•h/mL and 30.9 ($\pm$11.2) µg/mL, respectively, after administration of mycophenolate mofetil alone. Because MPAG plasma concentrations are increased in the presence of renal impairment, as are ganciclovir concentrations, the two drugs will compete for tubular secretion and thus further increases in concentrations of both drugs may occur. In patients with renal impairment in which MMF and ganciclovir are coadministered, patients should be monitored carefully.

Oral Contraceptives: A study of coadministration of CellCept (1 g bid) and combined oral contraceptives containing ethinylestradiol (0.02 mg to 0.04 mg) and levonorgestrel (0.05 mg to 0.20 mg), desogestrel (0.15 mg) or gestodene (0.05 mg to 0.10 mg) was conducted in 18 women with psoriasis over 3 consecutive menstrual cycles. Mean AUC(0–24h) was similar for ethinylestradiol and 3-keto desogestrel; however, mean levonorgestrel AUC(0–24h) significantly decreased by about 15%. There was large interpatient variability (%CV in the range of 60% to 70%) in the data, especially for ethinylestradiol. Mean serum levels of LH, FSH and progesterone were not significantly affected. CellCept may not have any influence on the ovulation-suppressing action of the studied oral contraceptives. However, it is recommended that oral contraceptives are coadministered with CellCept with caution and additional birth control methods be considered (see PRECAUTIONS: *Pregnancy*).

Trimethoprim/sulfamethoxazole: Following single-dose administration of mycophenolate mofetil (1.5 g) to 12 healthy male volunteers on day 8 of a 10 day course of Bactrim™* DS (trimethoprim 160 mg/sulfamethoxazole 800 mg) administered bid, no effect on the bioavailability of MPA was observed. The mean ($\pm$SD) AUC and C_{max} of MPA after concomitant administration were 75.2 ($\pm$19.8) µg•h/mL and 34.0 ($\pm$6.6) µg/mL, respectively, compared to 79.2 ($\pm$27.9) µg•h/mL and 34.2 ($\pm$10.7) µg/mL, respectively, after administration of mycophenolate mofetil alone.

---

*Bactrim is a trademark of Hoffmann-La Roche Inc.

Other Interactions: The measured value for renal clearance of MPAG indicates removal occurs by renal tubular secretion as well as glomerular filtration. Consistent with this, coadministration of probenecid, a known inhibitor of tubular secretion, with mycophenolate mofetil in monkeys results in a 3-fold increase in plasma MPAG AUC and a 2-fold increase in plasma MPA AUC. Thus, other drugs known to undergo renal tubular secretion may compete with MPAG and thereby raise plasma concentrations of MPAG or the other drug undergoing tubular secretion.

Drugs that alter the gastrointestinal flora may interact with mycophenolate mofetil by disrupting enterohepatic recirculation. Interference of MPAG hydrolysis may lead to less MPA available for absorption.

Adverse Events in Controlled Studies in Prevention of Renal, Cardiac or Hepatic Allograft Rejection (Reported in ≥20% of Patients in the CellCept Group)

	Renal Studies			Cardiac Study		Hepatic Study	
	CellCept 2 g/day	CellCept 3 g/day	Azathioprine 1 to 2 mg/kg/day or 100 to 150 mg/day	CellCept 3 g/day	Azathioprine 1.5 to 3 mg/kg/day	CellCept 3 g/day	Azathioprine 1 to 2 mg/kg/day
	(n=336)	(n=330)	(n=326)	(n=289)	(n=289)	(n=277)	(n=287)
	%	%	%	%	%	%	%
Body as a Whole							
Pain	33.0	31.2	32.2	75.8	74.7	74.0	77.7
Abdominal pain	24.7	27.6	23.0	33.9	33.2	62.5	51.2
Fever	21.4	23.3	23.3	47.4	46.4	52.3	56.1
Headache	21.1	16.1	21.2	54.3	51.9	53.8	49.1
Infection	18.2	20.9	19.9	25.6	19.4	27.1	25.1
Sepsis	–	–	–	–	–	27.4	26.5
Asthenia	–	–	–	43.3	36.3	35.4	33.8
Chest pain	–	–	–	26.3	26.0	–	–
Back pain	–	–	–	34.6	28.4	46.6	47.4
Ascites	–	–	–	–	–	24.2	22.6
Hemic and Lymphatic							
Anemia	25.6	25.8	23.6	42.9	43.9	43.0	53.0
Leukopenia	23.2	34.5	24.8	30.4	39.1	45.8	39.0
Thrombocytopenia	–	–	–	23.5	27.0	38.3	42.2
Hypochromic anemia	–	–	–	24.6	23.5	–	–
Leukocytosis	–	–	–	40.5	35.6	22.4	21.3
Urogenital							
Urinary tract infection	37.2	37.0	33.7	–	–	–	–
Kidney function abnormal	–	–	–	21.8	26.3	25.6	28.9
Cardiovascular							
Hypertension	32.4	28.2	32.2	77.5	72.3	62.1	59.6
Hypotension	–	–	–	32.5	36.0	–	–
Cardiovascular disorder	–	–	–	25.6	24.2	–	–
Tachycardia	–	–	–	20.1	18.0	22.0	15.7

(Table continued on next page)

Live Vaccines: During treatment with CellCept, the use of live attenuated vaccines should be avoided and patients should be advised that vaccinations may be less effective (see PRECAUTIONS: *General*). Influenza vaccination may be of value. Prescribers should refer to national guidelines for influenza vaccination.

Carcinogenesis, Mutagenesis, Impairment of Fertility: In a 104-week oral carcinogenicity study in mice, mycophenolate mofetil in daily doses up to 180 mg/kg was not tumorigenic. The highest dose tested was 0.5 times the recommended clinical dose (2 g/day) in renal transplant patients and 0.3 times the recommended clinical dose (3 g/day) in cardiac transplant patients when corrected for differences in body surface area (BSA). In a 104-week oral carcinogenicity study in rats, mycophenolate mofetil in daily doses up to 15 mg/kg was not tumorigenic. The highest dose was 0.08 times the recommended clinical dose in renal transplant patients and 0.05 times the recommended clinical dose in cardiac transplant patients when corrected for BSA. While these animal doses were lower than those given to patients, they were maximal in those species and were considered adequate to evaluate the potential for human risk (see WARNINGS).

The genotoxic potential of mycophenolate mofetil was determined in five assays. Mycophenolate mofetil was genotoxic in the mouse lymphoma/thymidine kinase assay and the in vivo mouse micronucleus assay. Mycophenolate mofetil was not genotoxic in the bacterial mutation assay, the yeast mitotic gene conversion assay or the Chinese hamster ovary cell chromosomal aberration assay.

Mycophenolate mofetil had no effect on fertility of male rats at oral doses up to 20 mg/kg/day. This dose represents 0.1 times the recommended clinical dose in renal transplant patients and 0.07 times the recommended clinical dose in cardiac transplant patients when corrected for BSA. In a female fertility and reproduction study conducted in rats, oral doses of 4.5 mg/kg/day caused malformations (principally of the head and eyes) in the first generation offspring in the absence of maternal toxicity. This dose was 0.02 times the recommended clinical dose in renal transplant patients and 0.01 times the recommended clinical dose in cardiac transplant patients when corrected for BSA. No effects on fertility or reproductive parameters were evident in the dams or in the subsequent generation.

Pregnancy: Category C. In teratology studies in rats and rabbits, fetal resorptions and malformations occurred in rats at 6 mg/kg/day and in rabbits at 90 mg/kg/day, in the absence of maternal toxicity. These levels are equivalent to 0.03 to 0.92 times the recommended clinical dose in renal transplant patients and 0.02 to 0.61 times the recommended clinical dose in cardiac transplant patients on a BSA basis. In a female fertility and reproduction study conducted in rats, oral doses of 4.5 mg/kg/day caused malformations (principally of the head and eyes) in the first generation offspring in the absence of maternal toxicity. This dose was 0.02 times the recommended clinical dose in renal transplant patients and 0.01 times the recommended clinical dose in cardiac transplant patients when corrected for BSA.

There are no adequate and well-controlled studies in pregnant women. CellCept should not be used in pregnant women unless the potential benefit justifies the potential risk to the fetus. Effective contraception must be used before beginning CellCept therapy, during therapy and for 6 weeks after CellCept has been stopped (see WARNINGS and PRECAUTIONS: *Information for Patients*).

Nursing Mothers: Studies in rats treated with mycophenolate mofetil have shown mycophenolic acid to be excreted in milk. It is not known whether this drug is excreted in human milk. Because many drugs are excreted in human milk, and because of the potential for serious adverse reactions in nursing infants from mycophenolate

Continued on next page

Cellcept—Cont.

mofetil, a decision should be made whether to discontinue nursing or to discontinue the drug, taking into account the importance of the drug to the mother.

Pediatric Use: Based on pharmacokinetic and safety data in pediatric patients after renal transplantation, the recommended dose of CellCept oral suspension is 600 mg/m^2 bid (up to a maximum of 1 g bid). Also see CLINICAL PHARMACOLOGY, CLINICAL STUDIES, ADVERSE REACTIONS, and DOSAGE AND ADMINISTRATION.

Safety and effectiveness in pediatric patients receiving allogeneic cardiac or hepatic transplants have not been established.

Geriatric Use: Clinical studies of CellCept did not include sufficient numbers of subjects aged 65 and over to determine whether they respond differently from younger subjects. Other reported clinical experience has not identified differences in responses between the elderly and younger patients. In general dose selection for an elderly patient should be cautious, reflecting the greater frequency of decreased hepatic, renal or cardiac function and of concomitant or other drug therapy. Elderly patients may be at an increased risk of adverse reactions compared with younger individuals (see ADVERSE REACTIONS).

ADVERSE REACTIONS

The principal adverse reactions associated with the administration of CellCept include diarrhea, leukopenia, sepsis, vomiting, and there is evidence of a higher frequency of certain types of infections eg, opportunistic infection (see WARNINGS). The adverse event profile associated with the administration of CellCept Intravenous has been shown to be similar to that observed after administration of oral dosage forms of CellCept.

CellCept Oral: The incidence of adverse events for CellCept was determined in randomized, comparative, double-blind trials in prevention of rejection in renal (2 active, 1 placebo-controlled trials), cardiac (1 active-controlled trial), and hepatic (1 active-controlled trial) transplant patients.

Elderly patients (≥65 years), particularly those who are receiving CellCept as part of a combination immunosuppressive regimen, may be at increased risk of certain infections (including cytomegalovirus [CMV] tissue invasive disease) and possibly gastrointestinal hemorrhage and pulmonary edema, compared to younger individuals (see PRECAUTIONS).

Safety data are summarized below for all active-controlled trials in renal (2 trials), cardiac (1 trial), and hepatic (1 trial) transplantation patients. Approximately 53% of the renal patients, 65% of the cardiac patients, and 48% of the hepatic patients have been treated for more than 1 year. Adverse events reported in ≥20% of patients in the CellCept treatment groups are presented below.

[See table on previous page and below]

The placebo-controlled renal transplant study generally showed fewer adverse events occurring in ≥20% of patients. In addition, those that occurred were not only qualitatively similar to the azathioprine-controlled renal transplant studies, but also occurred at lower rates, particularly for infection, leukopenia, hypertension, diarrhea and respiratory infection.

The above data demonstrate that in three controlled trials for prevention of renal rejection, patients receiving 2 g/day of CellCept had an overall better safety profile than did patients receiving 3 g/day of CellCept.

The above data demonstrate that the types of adverse events observed in multicenter controlled trials in renal, cardiac, and hepatic transplant patients are qualitatively similar except for those that are unique to the specific organ involved.

Sepsis, which was generally CMV viremia, was slightly more common in renal transplant patients treated with CellCept compared to patients treated with azathioprine. The incidence of sepsis was comparable in CellCept and in azathioprine-treated patients in cardiac and hepatic studies.

In the digestive system, diarrhea was increased in renal and cardiac transplant patients receiving CellCept compared to patients receiving azathioprine, but was comparable in hepatic transplant patients treated with CellCept or azathioprine.

Patients receiving CellCept alone or as part of an immunosuppressive regimen are at increased risk of developing lymphomas and other malignancies, particularly of the skin (see WARNINGS). The incidence of malignancies among the 1483 patients treated in controlled trials for the prevention of renal allograft rejection who were followed for ≥1 year was similar to the incidence reported in the literature for renal allograft recipients.

Lymphoproliferative disease or lymphoma developed in 0.4% to 1% of patients receiving CellCept (2 g or 3 g daily) with other immunosuppressive agents in controlled clinical trials of renal, cardiac, and hepatic transplant patients followed for at least 1 year (see WARNINGS). Non-melanoma skin carcinomas occurred in 1.6% to 4.2% of patients, other types of malignancy in 0.7% to 2.1% of patients. Three-year safety data in renal and cardiac transplant patients did not reveal any unexpected changes in incidence of malignancy compared to the 1-year data.

In pediatric patients, no other malignancies besides lymphoproliferative disorder (2/148 patients) have been observed.

Severe neutropenia (ANC <0.5 × 10^3/μL) developed in up to 2.0% of renal transplant patients, up to 2.8% of cardiac transplant patients and up to 3.6% of hepatic transplant patients receiving CellCept 3 g daily (see WARNINGS, PRECAUTIONS: *Laboratory Tests* and DOSAGE AND ADMINISTRATION).

All transplant patients are at increased risk of opportunistic infections. The risk increases with total immunosuppressive load (see WARNINGS). The following table shows the incidence of opportunistic infections that occurred in the renal, cardiac, and hepatic transplant populations in the azathioprine-controlled prevention trials:

[See table at top of next page]

The following other opportunistic infections occurred with an incidence of less than 4% in CellCept patients in the above azathioprine-controlled studies: Herpes zoster, visceral disease; Candida, urinary tract infection, fungemia/disseminated disease, tissue invasive disease; Cryptococcosis; Aspergillus/Mucor; Pneumocystis carinii.

In the placebo-controlled renal transplant study, the same pattern of opportunistic infection was observed compared to the azathioprine-controlled renal studies, with a notably lower incidence of the following: Herpes simplex and CMV tissue-invasive disease.

In patients receiving CellCept (2 g or 3 g) in controlled studies for prevention of renal, cardiac or hepatic rejection, fatal infection/sepsis occurred in approximately 2% of renal and cardiac patients and in 5% of hepatic patients (see WARNINGS).

In cardiac transplant patients, the overall incidence of opportunistic infections was approximately 10% higher in patients treated with CellCept than in those receiving azathioprine, but this difference was not associated with excess mortality due to infection/sepsis among patients treated with CellCept.

Adverse Events in Controlled Studies in Prevention of Renal, Cardiac or Hepatic Allograft Rejection (Reported in ≥20% of Patients in the CellCept Group) *(cont.)*

	Renal Studies			Cardiac Study		Hepatic Study	
	CellCept 2 g/day	CellCept 3 g/day	Azathioprine 1 to 2 mg/kg/day or 100 to 150 mg/day	CellCept 3 g/day	Azathioprine 1.5 to 3 mg/kg/day	CellCept 3 g/day	Azathioprine 1 to 2 mg/kg/day
	(n=336)	(n=330)	(n=326)	(n=289)	(n=289)	(n=277)	(n=287)
	%	%	%	%	%	%	%
Metabolic and Nutritional							
Peripheral edema	28.6	27.0	28.2	64.0	53.3	48.4	47.7
Hypercholesteremia	–	–	–	41.2	38.4	–	–
Edema	–	–	–	26.6	25.6	28.2	28.2
Hypokalemia	–	–	–	31.8	25.6	37.2	41.1
Hyperkalemia	–	–	–	–	–	22.0	23.7
Hyperglycemia	–	–	–	46.7	52.6	43.7	48.8
Creatinine increased	–	–	–	39.4	36.0	–	–
BUN increased	–	–	–	34.6	32.5	–	–
Lactic dehydrogenase increased	–	–	–	23.2	17.0	–	–
Hypomagnesemia	–	–	–	–	–	39.0	37.6
Hypocalcemia	–	–	–	–	–	30.0	30.0
Digestive							
Diarrhea	31.0	36.1	20.9	45.3	34.3	51.3	49.8
Constipation	22.9	18.5	22.4	41.2	37.7	37.9	38.3
Nausea	19.9	23.6	24.5	54.0	54.3	54.5	51.2
Dyspepsia	–	–	–	–	–	22.4	20.9
Vomiting	–	–	–	33.9	28.4	32.9	33.4
Anorexia	–	–	–	–	–	25.3	17.1
Liver function tests abnormal	–	–	–	–	–	24.9	19.2
Respiratory							
Infection	22.0	23.9	19.6	37.0	35.3	–	–
Dyspnea	–	–	–	36.7	36.3	31.0	30.3
Cough increased	–	–	–	31.1	25.6	–	–
Lung disorder	–	–	–	30.1	29.1	22.0	18.8
Sinusitis	–	–	–	26.0	19.0	–	–
Pleural effusion	–	–	–	–	–	34.3	35.9
Skin and Appendages							
Rash	–	–	–	22.1	18.0	–	–
Nervous System							
Tremor	–	–	–	24.2	23.9	33.9	35.5
Insomnia	–	–	–	40.8	37.7	52.3	47.0
Dizziness	–	–	–	28.7	27.7	–	–
Anxiety	–	–	–	28.4	23.9	–	–
Paresthesia	–	–	–	20.8	18.0	–	–

The following adverse events were reported with 3% to <20% incidence in renal, cardiac, and hepatic transplant patients treated with CellCept, in combination with cyclosporine and corticosteroids.

Adverse Events Reported in 3% to <20% of Patients Treated With CellCept in Combination With Cyclosporine and Corticosteroids

Body System	
Body as a Whole	abdomen enlarged, abscess, accidental injury, cellulitis, chills occurring with fever, cyst, face edema, flu syndrome, hemorrhage, hernia, lab test abnormal, malaise, neck pain, pelvic pain, peritonitis
Hemic and Lymphatic	coagulation disorder, ecchymosis, pancytopenia, petechia, polycythemia, prothrombin time increased, thromboplastin time increased
Urogenital	acute kidney failure, albuminuria, dysuria, hydronephrosis, hematuria, impotence, kidney failure, kidney tubular necrosis, nocturia, oliguria, pain, prostatic disorder, pyelonephritis, scrotal edema, urine abnormality, urinary frequency, urinary incontinence, urinary retention, urinary tract disorder
Cardiovascular	angina pectoris, arrhythmia, arterial thrombosis, atrial fibrillation, atrial flutter, bradycardia, cardiovascular disorder, congestive heart failure, extrasystole, heart arrest, heart failure, hypotension, pallor, palpitation, pericardial effusion, peripheral vascular disorder, postural hypotension, pulmonary hypertension, supraventricular tachycardia, supraventricular extrasystoles, syncope, tachycardia, thrombosis, vasodilatation, vasospasm, ventricular extrasystole, ventricular tachycardia, venous pressure increased
Metabolic and Nutritional	abnormal healing, acidosis, alkaline phosphatase increased, alkalosis, bilirubinemia, creatinine increased, dehydration, gamma glutamyl transpeptidase increased, generalized edema, gout, hypercalcemia, hypercholesteremia, hyperlipemia, hyperphosphatemia, hyperuricemia, hypervolemia, hypocalcemia, hypochloremia, hypoglycemia, hyponatremia, hypophosphatemia, hypoproteinemia, hypovolemia, hypoxia, lactic dehydrogenase increased, respiratory acidosis, SGOT increased, SGPT increased, thirst, weight gain, weight loss
Digestive	anorexia, cholangitis, cholestatic jaundice, dysphagia, esophagitis, flatulence, gastritis, gastroenteritis, gastrointestinal disorder, gastrointestinal hemorrhage, gastrointestinal moniliasis, gingivitis, gum hyperplasia, hepatitis, ileus, infection, jaundice, liver damage, liver function tests abnormal, melena, mouth ulceration, nausea and vomiting, oral moniliasis, rectal disorder, stomach ulcer, stomatitis
Respiratory	apnea, asthma, atelectasis, bronchitis, epistaxis, hemoptysis, hiccup, hyperventilation, lung edema, lung disorder, neoplasm, pain, pharyngitis, pleural effusion, pneumonia, pneumothorax, respiratory disorder, respiratory moniliasis, rhinitis, sinusitis, sputum increased, voice alteration
Skin and Appendages	acne, alopecia, fungal dermatitis, hemorrhage, hirsutism, pruritus, rash, skin benign neoplasm, skin carcinoma, skin disorder, skin hypertrophy, skin ulcer, sweating, vesiculobullous rash
Nervous	agitation, anxiety, confusion, convulsion, delirium, depression, dry mouth, emotional lability, hallucinations, hypertonia, hypesthesia, nervousness, neuropathy, paresthesia, psychosis, somnolence, thinking abnormal, vertigo
Endocrine	Cushing's syndrome, diabetes mellitus, hypothyroidism, parathyroid disorder
Musculoskeletal	arthralgia, joint disorder, leg cramps, myalgia, myasthenia, osteoporosis
Special Senses	abnormal vision, amblyopia, cataract (not specified), conjunctivitis, deafness, ear disorder, ear pain, eye hemorrhage, tinnitus, lacrimation disorder

Viral and Fungal Infections in Controlled Studies in Prevention of Renal, Cardiac or Hepatic Transplant Rejection

	Renal Studies			Cardiac Study		Hepatic Study	
	CellCept 2 g/day	CellCept 3 g/day	Azathioprine 1 to 2 mg/kg/day or 100 to 150 mg/day	CellCept 3 g/day	Azathioprine 1.5 to 3 mg/kg/day	CellCept 3 g/day	Azathioprine 1 to 2 mg/kg/day
	(n=336)	(n=330)	(n=326)	(n=289)	(n=289)	(n=277)	(n=287)
	%	%	%	%	%	%	%
Herpes simplex	16.7	20.0	19.0	20.8	14.5	10.1	5.9
CMV							
–Viremia/syndrome	13.4	12.4	13.8	12.1	10.0	14.1	12.2
–Tissue invasive disease	8.3	11.5	6.1	11.4	8.7	5.8	8.0
Herpes zoster	6.0	7.6	5.8	10.7	5.9	4.3	4.9
–Cutaneous disease	6.0	7.3	5.5	10.0	5.5	4.3	4.9
Candida	17.0	17.3	18.1	18.7	17.6	22.4	24.4
–Mucocutaneous	15.5	16.4	15.3	18.0	17.3	18.4	17.4

Pediatrics: The type and frequency of adverse events in a clinical study in 100 pediatric patients 3 months to 18 years of age dosed with CellCept oral suspension 600 mg/m^2 bid (up to 1 g bid) were generally similar to those observed in adult patients dosed with CellCept capsules at a dose of 1 g bid with the exception of abdominal pain, fever, infection, pain, sepsis, diarrhea, vomiting, pharyngitis, respiratory tract infection, hypertension, and anemia, which were observed in a higher proportion in pediatric patients.

CellCept Intravenous: The adverse event profile of CellCept Intravenous was determined from a single, double-blind, controlled comparative study of the safety of 2 g/day of intravenous and oral CellCept in renal transplant patients in the immediate posttransplant period (administered for the first 5 days). The potential venous irritation of CellCept Intravenous was evaluated by comparing the adverse events attributable to peripheral venous infusion of CellCept Intravenous with those observed in the intravenous placebo group; patients in this group received active medication by the oral route.

Adverse events attributable to peripheral venous infusion were phlebitis and thrombosis, both observed at 4% in patients treated with CellCept Intravenous.

In the active controlled study in hepatic transplant patients, 2 g/day of CellCept Intravenous were administered in the immediate posttransplant period (up to 14 days). The safety profile of intravenous CellCept was similar to that of intravenous azathioprine.

Postmarketing Experience

Digestive: colitis (sometimes caused by cytomegalovirus), pancreatitis, isolated cases of intestinal villous atrophy.

Resistance Mechanism Disorders: Serious life-threatening infections such as meningitis and infectious endocarditis have been reported occasionally and there is evidence of a higher frequency of certain types of serious infections such as tuberculosis and atypical mycobacterial infection.

Respiratory: Interstitial lung disorders, including fatal pulmonary fibrosis, have been reported rarely and should be considered in the differential diagnosis of pulmonary symptoms ranging from dyspnea to respiratory failure in posttransplant patients receiving CellCept.

OVERDOSAGE

There has been no reported experience of overdosage of mycophenolate mofetil in humans. The highest dose administered to renal transplant patients in clinical trials has been 4 g/day. In limited experience with cardiac and hepatic transplant patients in clinical trials, the highest doses used were 4 g/day or 5 g/day. At doses of 4 g/day or 5 g/day, there appears to be a higher rate, compared to the use of 3 g/day or less, of gastrointestinal intolerance (nausea, vomiting, and/or diarrhea), and occasional hematologic abnormalities, principally neutropenia, leading to a need to reduce or discontinue dosing.

In acute oral toxicity studies, no deaths occurred in adult mice at doses up to 4000 mg/kg or in adult monkeys at doses up to 1000 mg/kg; these were the highest doses of mycophenolate mofetil tested in these species. These doses represent 11 times the recommended clinical dose in renal transplant patients and approximately 7 times the recommended clinical dose in cardiac transplant patients when corrected for BSA. In adult rats, deaths occurred after single-oral doses of 500 mg/kg of mycophenolate mofetil. The dose represents approximately 3 times the recommended clinical dose in cardiac transplant patients when corrected for BSA.

MPA and MPAG are usually not removed by hemodialysis. However, at high MPAG plasma concentrations (>100 µg/mL), small amounts of MPAG are removed. By increasing excretion of the drug, MPA can be removed by bile acid sequestrants, such as cholestyramine (see CLINICAL PHARMACOLOGY: *Pharmacokinetics*).

DOSAGE AND ADMINISTRATION

RENAL TRANSPLANTATION:

Adults: A dose of 1 g administered orally or intravenously (over NO LESS THAN 2 HOURS) twice a day (daily dose of 2 g) is recommended for use in renal transplant patients. Although a dose of 1.5 g administered twice daily (daily dose of 3 g) was used in clinical trials and was shown to be safe and effective, no efficacy advantage could be established for renal transplant patients. Patients receiving 2 g/day of CellCept demonstrated an overall better safety profile than did patients receiving 3 g/day of CellCept.

Pediatrics: The recommended dose of CellCept oral suspension is 600 mg/m^2 administered twice daily (up to a maximum daily dose of 2 g/10 mL oral suspension). Patients with a body surface area of 1.25 m^2 to 1.5 m^2 may be dosed with CellCept capsules at a dose of 750 mg twice daily (1.5 g daily dose). Patients with a body surface area >1.5 m^2 may be dosed with CellCept capsules or tablets at a dose of 1 g twice daily (2 g daily dose).

CARDIAC TRANSPLANTATION: A dose of 1.5 g bid administered intravenously (over NO LESS THAN 2 HOURS) or 1.5 g bid oral (daily dose of 3 g) is recommended for use in adult cardiac transplant patients.

HEPATIC TRANSPLANTATION: A dose of 1 g bid administered intravenously (over NO LESS THAN 2 HOURS) or 1.5 g bid oral (daily dose of 3 g) is recommended for use in adult hepatic transplant patients.

CellCept Capsules, Tablets, and Oral Suspension: The initial oral dose of CellCept should be given as soon as possible following renal, cardiac or hepatic transplantation. Food had no effect on MPA AUC, but has been shown to decrease MPA C$_{max}$ by 40%. Therefore, it is recommended that CellCept be administered on an empty stomach. However, in stable renal transplant patients, CellCept may be administered with food if necessary.

Note:

If required, CellCept Oral Suspension can be administered via a nasogastric tube with a minimum size of 8 French (minimum 1.7 mm interior diameter).

Patients With Hepatic Impairment: No dose adjustments are recommended for renal patients with severe hepatic parenchymal disease. However, it is not known whether dose adjustments are needed for hepatic disease with other etiologies (see CLINICAL PHARMACOLOGY: *Pharmacokinetics*).

No data are available for cardiac transplant patients with severe hepatic parenchymal disease.

Geriatrics: The recommended oral dose of 1 g bid for renal transplant patients, 1.5 g bid for cardiac transplant patients, and 1 g bid administered intravenously or 1.5 g bid administered orally in hepatic transplant patients is appropriate for elderly patients (see PRECAUTIONS: *Geriatric Use*).

Preparation of Oral Suspension

It is recommended that CellCept Oral Suspension be constituted by the pharmacist prior to dispensing to the patient.

CellCept Oral Suspension should not be mixed with any other medication.

Mycophenolate mofetil has demonstrated teratogenic effects in rats and rabbits. There are no adequate and well-controlled studies in pregnant women. (See WARNINGS, PRECAUTIONS, ADVERSE REACTIONS, and HANDLING AND DISPOSAL.) Care should be taken to avoid inhalation or direct contact with skin or mucous membranes

Continued on next page

Cellcept—Cont.

of the dry powder or the constituted suspension. If such contact occurs, wash thoroughly with soap and water; rinse eyes with water.

1. Tap the closed bottle several times to loosen the powder.
2. Measure 94 mL of water in a graduated cylinder.
3. Add approximately half the total amount of water for constitution to the bottle and shake the closed bottle well for about 1 minute.
4. Add the remainder of water and shake the closed bottle well for about 1 minute.
5. Remove the child-resistant cap and push bottle adapter into neck of bottle.
6. Close bottle with child-resistant cap tightly. This will assure the proper seating of the bottle adapter in the bottle and child-resistant status of the cap.

Dispense with patient instruction sheet and oral dispensers. It is recommended to write the date of expiration of the constituted suspension on the bottle label. (The shelf-life of the constituted suspension is 60 days.)

After constitution the oral suspension contains 200 mg/mL mycophenolate mofetil. Store constituted suspension at 25°C (77°F); excursions permitted to 15° to 30°C (59° to 86°F). Storage in a refrigerator at 2° to 8°C (36° to 46°F) is acceptable. Do not freeze. Discard any unused portion 60 days after constitution.

CellCept Intravenous: CellCept Intravenous is an alternative dosage form to CellCept capsules, tablets and oral suspension recommended for patients unable to take oral CellCept. CellCept Intravenous should be administered within 24 hours following transplantation. CellCept Intravenous can be administered for up to 14 days; patients should be switched to oral CellCept as soon as they can tolerate oral medication.

CellCept Intravenous must be reconstituted and diluted to a concentration of 6 mg/mL using 5% Dextrose Injection USP. CellCept Intravenous is incompatible with other intravenous infusion solutions. Following reconstitution, CellCept Intravenous must be administered by slow intravenous infusion over a period of NO LESS THAN 2 HOURS by either peripheral or central vein.

CAUTION: CELLCEPT INTRAVENOUS SOLUTION SHOULD NEVER BE ADMINISTERED BY RAPID OR BOLUS INTRAVENOUS INJECTION (see WARNINGS).

Preparation of Infusion Solution (6 mg/mL)

Caution should be exercised in the handling and preparation of solutions of CellCept Intravenous. Avoid direct contact of the prepared solution of CellCept Intravenous with skin or mucous membranes. If such contact occurs, wash thoroughly with soap and water; rinse eyes with plain water. (See WARNINGS, PRECAUTIONS, ADVERSE REACTIONS, and HANDLING AND DISPOSAL.)

CellCept Intravenous does not contain an antibacterial preservative; therefore, reconstitution and dilution of the product must be performed under aseptic conditions.

CellCept Intravenous infusion solution must be prepared in two steps: the first step is a reconstitution step with 5% Dextrose Injection USP, and the second step is a dilution step with 5% Dextrose Injection USP. A detailed description of the preparation is given below:

Step 1

a. Two (2) vials of CellCept Intravenous are used for preparing each 1 g dose, whereas three (3) vials are needed for each 1.5 g dose. Reconstitute the contents of each vial by injecting 14 mL of 5% Dextrose Injection USP.
b. Gently shake the vial to dissolve the drug.
c. Inspect the resulting slightly yellow solution for particulate matter and discoloration prior to further dilution. Discard the vials if particulate matter or discoloration is observed.

Step 2

a. To prepare a 1 g dose, further dilute the contents of the two reconstituted vials (approx. 2×15 mL) into 140 mL of 5% Dextrose Injection USP. To prepare a 1.5 g dose, further dilute the contents of the three reconstituted vials (approx. 3×15 mL) into 210 mL of 5% Dextrose Injection USP. The final concentration of both solutions is 6 mg mycophenolate mofetil per mL.
b. Inspect the infusion solution for particulate matter or discoloration. Discard the infusion solution if particulate matter or discoloration is observed.

If the infusion solution is not prepared immediately prior to administration, the commencement of administration of the infusion solution should be within 4 hours from reconstitution and dilution of the drug product. Keep solutions at 25°C (77°F); excursions permitted to 15° to 30°C (59° to 86°F).

CellCept Intravenous should not be mixed or administered concurrently via the same infusion catheter with other intravenous drugs or infusion admixtures.

Dosage Adjustments: In renal transplant patients with severe chronic renal impairment (GFR <25 mL/min/1.73 m^2) outside the immediate posttransplant period, doses of CellCept greater than 1 g administered twice a day should be avoided. These patients should also be carefully observed. No dose adjustments are needed in renal transplant patients experiencing delayed graft function postoperatively (see CLINICAL PHARMACOLOGY: *Pharmacokinetics* and PRECAUTIONS: *General*).

No data are available for cardiac or hepatic transplant patients with severe chronic renal impairment. CellCept may be used for cardiac or hepatic transplant patients with severe chronic renal impairment if the potential benefits outweigh the potential risks.

If neutropenia develops (ANC $<1.3 \times 10^3/\mu L$), dosing with CellCept should be interrupted or the dose reduced, appropriate diagnostic tests performed, and the patient managed appropriately (see WARNINGS, ADVERSE REACTIONS, and PRECAUTIONS: *Laboratory Tests*).

HANDLING AND DISPOSAL: Mycophenolate mofetil has demonstrated teratogenic effects in rats and rabbits (see PRECAUTIONS: Pregnancy). CellCept tablets should not be crushed and CellCept capsules should not be opened or crushed. Avoid inhalation or direct contact with skin or mucous membranes of the powder contained in CellCept capsules and CellCept Oral Suspension (before or after constitution). If such contact occurs, wash thoroughly with soap and water; rinse eyes with plain water. Should a spill occur, wipe up using paper towels wetted with water to remove spilled powder or suspension. Caution should be exercised in the handling and preparation of solutions of CellCept Intravenous. Avoid direct contact of the prepared solution of CellCept Intravenous with skin or mucous membranes. If such contact occurs, wash thoroughly with soap and water; rinse eyes with plain water.

HOW SUPPLIED

CellCept (mycophenolate mofetil capsules)
250 mg

Blue-brown, two-piece hard gelatin capsules, printed in black with "CellCept 250" on the blue cap and "Roche" on the brown body. Supplied in the following presentations:

NDC Number	Size
NDC 0004-0259-01	Bottle of 100
NDC 0004-0259-05	Package containing 12 bottles of 120
NDC 0004-0259-43	Bottle of 500

Storage: Store at 25°C (77°F); excursions permitted to 15° to 30°C (59° to 86°F).

CellCept (mycophenolate mofetil tablets)
500 mg

Lavender-colored, caplet-shaped, film-coated tablets printed in black with "CellCept 500" on one side and "Roche" on the other. Supplied in the following presentations:

NDC Number	Size
NDC 0004-0260-01	Bottle of 100
NDC 0004-0260-43	Bottle of 500

Storage and Dispensing Information: Store at 25°C (77°F); excursions permitted to 15° to 30°C (59° to 86°F). Dispense in light-resistant containers, such as the manufacturer's original containers.

CellCept Oral Suspension (mycophenolate mofetil for oral suspension)

Supplied as a white to off-white powder blend for constitution to a white to off-white mixed-fruit flavor suspension. Supplied in the following presentation:

NDC Number	Size
NDC 0004-0261-29	225 mL bottle with bottle adapter and 2 oral dispensers

Storage: Store dry powder at 25°C (77°F); excursions permitted to 15° to 30°C (59° to 86°F). Store constituted suspension at 25°C (77°F); excursions permitted to 15° to 30°C (59° to 86°F) for up to 60 days. Storage in a refrigerator at 2° to 8°C (36° to 46°F) is acceptable. Do not freeze.

CellCept Intravenous (mycophenolate mofetil hydrochloride for injection)

Supplied in a 20 mL, sterile vial containing the equivalent of 500 mg mycophenolate mofetil as the hydrochloride salt in cartons of 4 vials:

NDC Number
NDC 0004-0298-09

Storage: Store powder and reconstituted/infusion solutions at 25°C (77°F); excursions permitted to 15° to 30°C (59° to 86°F).

Revised: March 2003

HIVID® ℞

[*hī ' vĭd*]
(zalcitabine)
Tablets

Prescribing information for this product, which appears on pages 2898–2902 of the 2003 PDR, has been revised. Please write "See Supplement A" next to the product heading.

Insert the following as the first two paragraphs in the ***PRECAUTIONS: Drug Interactions*** section:

PRECAUTIONS: ***Drug Interactions:*** *Zidovudine:* There is no significant pharmacokinetic interaction between ZDV and zalcitabine which has been confirmed clinically. Zalcitabine also has no significant effect on the intracellular phosphorylation of ZDV, as shown in vitro in peripheral blood mononuclear cells or in two other cell lines (U937 and Molt-4). In the same study it was shown that didanosine and stavudine had no significant effect on the intracellular phosphorylation of zalcitabine in peripheral blood mononuclear cells.

Lamivudine: In vitro studies in peripheral blood mononuclear cells, U937 and Molt-4 cells revealed that lamivudine significantly inhibited zalcitabine phosphorylation in a dose dependent manner. Effects were already seen with doses corresponding to relevant plasma levels in humans, and the intracellular phosphorylation of zalcitabine to its three metabolites (including the active zalcitabine triphosphate metabolite) was significantly inhibited. Zalcitabine inhibited lamivudine phosphorylation at high concentration ratios (10 and 100); however, it is considered to be unlikely that this decrease of phosphorylated lamivudine concentration is of clinical significance, as lamivudine is a more efficient substrate for deoxycytidine kinase than zalcitabine. These in vitro studies suggest that concomitant administration of zalcitabine and lamivudine in humans may result in subtherapeutic concentrations of active phosphorylated zalcitabine, which may lead to a decreased antiretroviral effect of zalcitabine. It is unknown how the effect seen in these in vitro studies translates into clinical consequences. **Concomitant use of zalcitabine and lamivudine is not recommended.**

Revised: September 2002

KLONOPIN® TABLETS Ⓒ ℞

[*klon'o-pin*]
(clonazepam)

KLONOPIN® WAFERS

(clonazepam orally disintegrating tablets)

Prescribing information for this product, which appears on pages 2905–2908 of the 2003 PDR, has been completely revised as follows. Please write "See Supplement A" next to the product heading.

DESCRIPTION

Klonopin, a benzodiazepine, is available as scored tablets with a K-shaped perforation containing 0.5 mg of clonazepam and unscored tablets with a K-shaped perforation containing 1 mg or 2 mg of clonazepam. Each tablet also contains lactose, magnesium stearate, microcrystalline cellulose and corn starch, with the following colorants: 0.5 mg—FD&C Yellow No. 6 Lake; 1 mg—FD&C Blue No. 1 Lake and FD&C Blue No. 2 Lake.

Klonopin is also available as an orally disintegrating tablet containing 0.125 mg, 0.25 mg, 0.5 mg, 1 mg or 2 mg clonazepam. Each orally disintegrating tablet also contains gelatin, mannitol, methylparaben sodium, propylparaben sodium and xanthan gum.

Chemically, clonazepam is 5-(2-chlorophenyl)-1,3-dihydro-7-nitro-2*H*-1,4-benzodiazepin-2-one. It is a light yellow crystalline powder. It has a molecular weight of 315.72.

CLINICAL PHARMACOLOGY

Pharmacodynamics: The precise mechanism by which clonazepam exerts its antiseizure and antipanic effects is unknown, although it is believed to be related to its ability to enhance the activity of gamma aminobutyric acid (GABA), the major inhibitory neurotransmitter in the central nervous system. Convulsions produced in rodents by pentylenetetrazol or, to a lesser extent, electrical stimulation are antagonized, as are convulsions produced by photic stimulation in susceptible baboons. A taming effect in aggressive primates, muscle weakness and hypnosis are also produced. In humans, clonazepam is capable of suppressing the spike and wave discharge in absence seizures (petit mal) and decreasing the frequency, amplitude, duration and spread of discharge in minor motor seizures.

Pharmacokinetics: Clonazepam is rapidly and completely absorbed after oral administration. The absolute bioavailability of clonazepam is about 90%. Maximum plasma concentrations of clonazepam are reached within 1 to 4 hours after oral administration. Clonazepam is approximately 85% bound to plasma proteins. Clonazepam is highly metabolized, with less than 2% unchanged clonazepam being excreted in the urine. Biotransformation occurs mainly by reduction of the 7-nitro group to the 4-amino derivative. This derivative can be acetylated, hydroxylated and glucuronidated. Cytochrome P-450 including CYP3A, may play an important role in clonazepam reduction and oxidation. The elimination half-life of clonazepam is typically 30 to 40 hours. Clonazepam pharmacokinetics are dose-independent throughout the dosing range. There is no evidence that clonazepam induces its own metabolism or that of other drugs in humans.

Pharmacokinetics in Demographic Subpopulations and in Disease States: Controlled studies examining the influence of gender and age on clonazepam pharmacokinetics have not been conducted, nor have the effects of renal or liver disease on clonazepam pharmacokinetics been studied. Because clonazepam undergoes hepatic metabolism, it is possible that liver disease will impair clonazepam elimination. Thus, caution should be exercised when administering clonazepam to these patients.

Clinical Trials: *Panic Disorder:* The effectiveness of Klonopin in the treatment of panic disorder was demonstrated in two double-blind, placebo-controlled studies of adult outpatients who had a primary diagnosis of panic disorder (DSM-IIIR) with or without agoraphobia. In these studies, Klonopin was shown to be significantly more effective than placebo in treating panic disorder on change from baseline in panic attack frequency, the Clinician's Global Impression Severity of Illness Score and the Clinician's Global Impression Improvement Score.

Study 1 was a 9-week, fixed-dose study involving Klonopin doses of 0.5, 1, 2, 3 or 4 mg/day or placebo. This study was conducted in four phases: a 1-week placebo lead-in, a 3-week upward titration, a 6-week fixed dose and a 7-week discontinuance phase. A significant difference from placebo was observed consistently only for the 1 mg/day group. The difference between the 1 mg dose group and placebo in reduction from baseline in the number of full panic attacks was approximately 1 panic attack per week. At endpoint, 74% of patients receiving clonazepam 1 mg/day were free of full panic attacks, compared to 56% of placebo-treated patients.

Study 2 was a 6-week, flexible-dose study involving Klonopin in a dose range of 0.5 to 4 mg/day or placebo. This study was conducted in three phases: a 1-week placebo lead-in, a 6-week optimal-dose and a 6-week discontinuance phase. The mean clonazepam dose during the optimal dosing period was 2.3 mg/day. The difference between Klonopin and placebo in reduction from baseline in the number of full panic attacks was approximately 1 panic attack per week. At endpoint, 62% of patients receiving clonazepam were free of full panic attacks, compared to 37% of placebo-treated patients.

Subgroup analyses did not indicate that there were any differences in treatment outcomes as a function of race or gender.

INDICATIONS AND USAGE

Seizure Disorders: Klonopin is useful alone or as an adjunct in the treatment of the Lennox-Gastaut syndrome (petit mal variant), akinetic and myoclonic seizures. In patients with absence seizures (petit mal) who have failed to respond to succinimides, Klonopin may be useful.

In some studies, up to 30% of patients have shown a loss of anticonvulsant activity, often within 3 months of administration. In some cases, dosage adjustment may reestablish efficacy.

Panic Disorder: Klonopin is indicated for the treatment of panic disorder, with or without agoraphobia, as defined in DSM-IV. Panic disorder is characterized by the occurrence of unexpected panic attacks and associated concern about having additional attacks, worry about the implications or consequences of the attacks, and/or a significant change in behavior related to the attacks.

The efficacy of Klonopin was established in two 6- to 9-week trials in panic disorder patients whose diagnoses corresponded to the DSM-IIIR category of panic disorder (see CLINICAL PHARMACOLOGY: *Clinical Trials*).

Panic disorder (DSM-IV) is characterized by recurrent unexpected panic attacks, ie, a discrete period of intense fear or discomfort in which four (or more) of the following symptoms develop abruptly and reach a peak within 10 minutes: (1) palpitations, pounding heart or accelerated heart rate; (2) sweating; (3) trembling or shaking; (4) sensations of shortness of breath or smothering; (5) feeling of choking; (6) chest pain or discomfort; (7) nausea or abdominal distress; (8) feeling dizzy, unsteady, lightheaded or faint; (9) derealization (feelings of unreality) or depersonalization (being detached from oneself); (10) fear of losing control; (11) fear of dying; (12) paresthesias (numbness or tingling sensations); (13) chills or hot flushes.

The effectiveness of Klonopin in long-term use, that is, for more than 9 weeks, has not been systematically studied in controlled clinical trials. The physician who elects to use Klonopin for extended periods should periodically reevaluate the long-term usefulness of the drug for the individual patient (see DOSAGE AND ADMINISTRATION).

CONTRAINDICATIONS

Klonopin should not be used in patients with a history of sensitivity to benzodiazepines, nor in patients with clinical or biochemical evidence of significant liver disease. It may be used in patients with open angle glaucoma who are receiving appropriate therapy but is contraindicated in acute narrow angle glaucoma.

WARNINGS

Interference With Cognitive and Motor Performance: Since Klonopin produces CNS depression, patients receiving this drug should be cautioned against engaging in hazardous occupations requiring mental alertness, such as operating machinery or driving a motor vehicle. They should also be warned about the concomitant use of alcohol or other CNS-depressant drugs during Klonopin therapy (see PRECAUTIONS: *Drug Interactions* and *Information for Patients*).

Pregnancy Risks: Data from several sources raise concerns about the use of Klonopin during pregnancy.

Animal Findings: In three studies in which Klonopin was administered orally to pregnant rabbits at doses of 0.2, 1, 5 or 10 mg/kg/day (low dose approximately 0.2 times the maximum recommended human dose of 20 mg/day for seizure disorders and equivalent to the maximum dose of 4 mg/day for panic disorder, on a mg/m^2 basis) during the period of organogenesis, a similar pattern of malformations (cleft palate, open eyelid, fused sternebrae and limb defects) was observed in a low, non-dose-related incidence in exposed litters from all dosage groups. Reductions in maternal weight gain occurred at dosages of 5 mg/kg/day or greater and reduction in embryo-fetal growth occurred in one study at a dosage of 10 mg/kg/day. No adverse maternal or embryo-fetal effects were observed in mice and rats following administration during organogenesis of oral doses up to 15 mg/kg/day or 40 mg/kg/day, respectively (4 and 20 times the maximum recommended human dose of 20 mg/day for seizure disorders and 20 and 100 times the maximum dose of 4 mg/day for panic disorder, respectively, on a mg/m^2 basis).

General Concerns and Considerations About Anticonvulsants: Recent reports suggest an association between the use of anticonvulsant drugs by women with epilepsy and an elevated incidence of birth defects in children born to these women. Data are more extensive with respect to diphenylhydantoin and phenobarbital, but these are also the most commonly prescribed anticonvulsants; less systematic or anecdotal reports suggest a possible similar association with the use of all known anticonvulsant drugs.

In children of women treated with drugs for epilepsy, reports suggesting an elevated incidence of birth defects cannot be regarded as adequate to prove a definite cause and effect relationship. There are intrinsic methodologic problems in obtaining adequate data on drug teratogenicity in humans; the possibility also exists that other factors (eg, genetic factors or the epileptic condition itself) may be more important than drug therapy in leading to birth defects. The great majority of mothers on anticonvulsant medication deliver normal infants. It is important to note that anticonvulsant drugs should not be discontinued in patients in whom the drug is administered to prevent seizures because of the strong possibility of precipitating status epilepticus with attendant hypoxia and threat to life. In individual cases where the severity and frequency of the seizure disorder are such that the removal of medication does not pose a serious threat to the patient, discontinuation of the drug may be considered prior to and during pregnancy; however, it cannot be said with any confidence that even mild seizures do not pose some hazards to the developing embryo or fetus.

General Concerns About Benzodiazepines: An increased risk of congenital malformations associated with the use of benzodiazepine drugs has been suggested in several studies. There may also be non-teratogenic risks associated with the use of benzodiazepines during pregnancy. There have been reports of neonatal flaccidity, respiratory and feeding difficulties, and hypothermia in children born to mothers who have been receiving benzodiazepines late in pregnancy. In addition, children born to mothers receiving benzodiazepines late in pregnancy may be at some risk of experiencing withdrawal symptoms during the postnatal period.

Advice Regarding the Use of Klonopin in Women of Childbearing Potential: In general, the use of Klonopin in women of childbearing potential, and more specifically during known pregnancy, should be considered only when the clinical situation warrants the risk to the fetus.

The specific considerations addressed above regarding the use of anticonvulsants for epilepsy in women of childbearing potential should be weighed in treating or counseling these women.

Because of experience with other members of the benzodiazepine class, Klonopin is assumed to be capable of causing an increased risk of congenital abnormalities when administered to a pregnant woman during the first trimester. Because use of these drugs is rarely a matter of urgency in the treatment of panic disorder, their use during the first trimester should almost always be avoided. The possibility that a woman of childbearing potential may be pregnant at the time of institution of therapy should be considered. If this drug is used during pregnancy, or if the patient becomes pregnant while taking this drug, the patient should be apprised of the potential hazard to the fetus. Patients should also be advised that if they become pregnant during therapy or intend to become pregnant, they should communicate with their physician about the desirability of discontinuing the drug.

Withdrawal Symptoms: Withdrawal symptoms of the barbiturate type have occurred after the discontinuation of benzodiazepines (see DRUG ABUSE AND DEPENDENCE).

PRECAUTIONS

General: *Worsening of Seizures:* When used in patients in whom several different types of seizure disorders coexist, Klonopin may increase the incidence or precipitate the onset of generalized tonic-clonic seizures (grand mal). This may require the addition of appropriate anticonvulsants or an increase in their dosages. The concomitant use of valproic acid and Klonopin may produce absence status.

Laboratory Testing During Long-Term Therapy: Periodic blood counts and liver function tests are advisable during long-term therapy with Klonopin.

Risks of Abrupt Withdrawal: The abrupt withdrawal of Klonopin, particularly in those patients on long-term, high-dose therapy, may precipitate status epilepticus. Therefore, when discontinuing Klonopin, gradual withdrawal is essential. While Klonopin is being gradually withdrawn, the simultaneous substitution of another anticonvulsant may be indicated.

Caution in Renally Impaired Patients: Metabolites of Klonopin are excreted by the kidneys; to avoid their excess accumulation, caution should be exercised in the administration of the drug to patients with impaired renal function.

Hypersalivation: Klonopin may produce an increase in salivation. This should be considered before giving the drug to patients who have difficulty handling secretions. Because of this and the possibility of respiratory depression, Klonopin should be used with caution in patients with chronic respiratory diseases.

Information for Patients: Physicians are advised to discuss the following issues with patients for whom they prescribe Klonopin:

Dose Changes: To assure the safe and effective use of benzodiazepines, patients should be informed that, since benzodiazepines may produce psychological and physical dependence, it is advisable that they consult with their physician before either increasing the dose or abruptly discontinuing this drug.

Interference With Cognitive and Motor Performance: Because benzodiazepines have the potential to impair judgment, thinking or motor skills, patients should be cautioned about operating hazardous machinery, including automobiles, until they are reasonably certain that Klonopin therapy does not affect them adversely.

Pregnancy: Patients should be advised to notify their physician if they become pregnant or intend to become pregnant during therapy with Klonopin (see WARNINGS).

Nursing: Patients should be advised not to breastfeed an infant if they are taking Klonopin.

Concomitant Medication: Patients should be advised to inform their physicians if they are taking, or plan to take, any prescription or over-the-counter drugs, since there is a potential for interactions.

Alcohol: Patients should be advised to avoid alcohol while taking Klonopin.

Drug Interactions: *Effect of Clonazepam on the Pharmacokinetics of Other Drugs:* Clonazepam does not appear to alter the pharmacokinetics of phenytoin, carbamazepine or phenobarbital. The effect of clonazepam on the metabolism of other drugs has not been investigated.

Effect of Other Drugs on the Pharmacokinetics of Clonazepam: Literature reports suggest that ranitidine, an agent that decreases stomach acidity, does not greatly alter clonazepam pharmacokinetics.

In a study in which the 2 mg clonazepam orally disintegrating tablet was administered with and without propantheline (an anticholinergic agent with multiple effects on the GI tract) to healthy volunteers, the AUC of clonazepam was 10% lower and the C_{max} of clonazepam was 20% lower when the orally disintegrating tablet was given with propantheline compared to when it was given alone.

Fluoxetine does not affect the pharmacokinetics of clonazepam. Cytochrome P-450 inducers, such as phenytoin, carbamazepine and phenobarbital, induce clonazepam metabolism, causing an approximately 30% decrease in plasma clonazepam levels. Although clinical studies have not been performed, based on the involvement of the cytochrome P-450 3A family in clonazepam metabolism, inhibitors of this enzyme system, notably oral antifungal agents, should be used cautiously in patients receiving clonazepam.

Pharmacodynamic Interactions: The CNS-depressant action of the benzodiazepine class of drugs may be potentiated by alcohol, narcotics, barbiturates, nonbarbiturate hypnotics, antianxiety agents, the phenothiazines, thioxanthene and butyrophenone classes of antipsychotic agents, monoamine oxidase inhibitors and the tricyclic antidepressants, and by other anticonvulsant drugs.

Carcinogenesis, Mutagenesis, Impairment of Fertility: Carcinogenicity studies have not been conducted with clonazepam.

The data currently available are not sufficient to determine the genotoxic potential of clonazepam.

In a two-generation fertility study in which clonazepam was given orally to rats at 10 and 100 mg/kg/day (low dose approximately 5 times and 24 times the maximum recommended human dose of 20 mg/day for seizure disorder and 4 mg/day for panic disorder, respectively, on a mg/m^2 basis), there was a decrease in the number of pregnancies and in the number of offspring surviving until weaning.

Pregnancy: *Teratogenic Effects:* Pregnancy Category D (see WARNINGS).

Labor and Delivery: The effect of Klonopin on labor and delivery in humans has not been specifically studied; however, perinatal complications have been reported in children born to mothers who have been receiving benzodiazepines late in pregnancy, including findings suggestive of either excess benzodiazepine exposure or of withdrawal phenomena (see WARNINGS: *Pregnancy Risks*).

Nursing Mothers: Mothers receiving Klonopin should not breastfeed their infants.

Pediatric Use: Because of the possibility that adverse effects on physical or mental development could become apparent only after many years, a benefit-risk consideration of the long-term use of Klonopin is important in pediatric patients being treated for seizure disorder (see INDICATIONS AND USAGE and DOSAGE AND ADMINISTRATION).

Safety and effectiveness in pediatric patients with panic disorder below the age of 18 have not been established.

Geriatric Use: Clinical studies of Klonopin did not include sufficient numbers of subjects aged 65 and over to determine whether they respond differently from younger subjects. Other reported clinical experience has not identified differences in responses between the elderly and younger patients. In general, dose selection for an elderly patient should be cautious, usually starting at the low end of the dosing range, reflecting the greater frequency of decreased hepatic, renal, or cardiac function, and of concomitant disease or other drug therapy.

Because clonazepam undergoes hepatic metabolism, it is possible that liver disease will impair clonazepam elimination. Metabolites of Klonopin are excreted by the kidneys; to avoid their excess accumulation, caution should be exercised in the administration of the drug to patients with impaired renal function. Because elderly patients are more likely to have decreased hepatic and/or renal function, care should be taken in dose selection, and it may be useful to assess hepatic and/or renal function at the time of dose selection.

Sedating drugs may cause confusion and over-sedation in the elderly; elderly patients generally should be started on low doses of Klonopin and observed closely.

ADVERSE REACTIONS

The adverse experiences for Klonopin are provided separately for patients with seizure disorders and with panic disorder.

Seizure Disorders: The most frequently occurring side effects of Klonopin are referable to CNS depression. Experience in treatment of seizures has shown that drowsiness has occurred in approximately 50% of patients and ataxia in

Continued on next page

Klonopin—Cont.

approximately 30%. In some cases, these may diminish with time; behavior problems have been noted in approximately 25% of patients. Others, listed by system, are:

Neurologic: Abnormal eye movements, aphonia, choreiform movements, coma, diplopia, dysarthria, dysdiadochokinesis, "glassy-eyed" appearance, headache, hemiparesis, hypotonia, nystagmus, respiratory depression, slurred speech, tremor, vertigo

Psychiatric: Confusion, depression, amnesia, hallucinations, hysteria, increased libido, insomnia, psychosis, suicidal attempt (the behavior effects are more likely to occur in patients with a history of psychiatric disturbances). The following paradoxical reactions have been observed: excitability, irritability, aggressive behavior, agitation, nervousness, hostility, anxiety, sleep disturbances, nightmares and vivid dreams

Respiratory: Chest congestion, rhinorrhea, shortness of breath, hypersecretion in upper respiratory passages

Cardiovascular: Palpitations

Dermatologic: Hair loss, hirsutism, skin rash, ankle and facial edema

Gastrointestinal: Anorexia, coated tongue, constipation, diarrhea, dry mouth, encopresis, gastritis, increased appetite, nausea, sore gums

Genitourinary: Dysuria, enuresis, nocturia, urinary retention

Musculoskeletal: Muscle weakness, pains

Miscellaneous: Dehydration, general deterioration, fever, lymphadenopathy, weight loss or gain

Hematopoietic: Anemia, leukopenia, thrombocytopenia, eosinophilia

Hepatic: Hepatomegaly, transient elevations of serum transaminases and alkaline phosphatase

Panic Disorder: Adverse events during exposure to Klonopin were obtained by spontaneous report and recorded by clinical investigators using terminology of their own choosing. Consequently, it is not possible to provide a meaningful estimate of the proportion of individuals experiencing adverse events without first grouping similar types of events into a smaller number of standardized event categories. In the tables and tabulations that follow, CIGY dictionary terminology has been used to classify reported adverse events, except in certain cases in which redundant terms were collapsed into more meaningful terms, as noted below. The stated frequencies of adverse events represent the proportion of individuals who experienced, at least once, a treatment-emergent adverse event of the type listed. An event was considered treatment-emergent if it occurred for the first time or worsened while receiving therapy following baseline evaluation.

Adverse Findings Observed in Short-Term, Placebo-Controlled Trials:

Adverse Events Associated With Discontinuation of Treatment:

Overall, the incidence of discontinuation due to adverse events was 17% in Klonopin compared to 9% for placebo in the combined data of two 6- to 9-week trials. The most common events (≥1%) associated with discontinuation and a dropout rate twice or greater for Klonopin than that of placebo included the following:

Adverse Event	Klonopin (N=574)	Placebo (N=294)
Somnolence	7%	1%
Depression	4%	1%
Dizziness	1%	<1%
Nervousness	1%	0%
Ataxia	1%	0%
Intellectual Ability Reduced	1%	0%

Adverse Events Occurring at an Incidence of 1% or More Among Klonopin-Treated Patients:

Table 1 enumerates the incidence, rounded to the nearest percent, of treatment-emergent adverse events that occurred during acute therapy of panic disorder from a pool of two 6- to 9-week trials. Events reported in 1% or more of patients treated with Klonopin (doses ranging from 0.5 to 4 mg/day) and for which the incidence was greater than that in placebo-treated patients are included.

The prescriber should be aware that the figures in Table 1 cannot be used to predict the incidence of side effects in the course of usual medical practice where patient characteristics and other factors differ from those that prevailed in the clinical trials. Similarly, the cited frequencies cannot be compared with figures obtained from other clinical investigations involving different treatments, uses and investigators. The cited figures, however, do provide the prescribing physician with some basis for estimating the relative contribution of drug and nondrug factors to the side effect incidence in the population studied.

[See table 1 above]

Table 1. Treatment-Emergent Adverse Event Incidence in 6- to 9-Week Placebo-Controlled Clinical Trials*

Adverse Event by Body System	Clonazepam Maximum Daily Dose				All Klonopin Groups N=574 %	Placebo N=294 %
	<1mg n=96 %	1-<2mg n=129 %	2-<3mg n=113 %	≥3mg n=235 %		
Central & Peripheral Nervous System						
Somnolence†	26	35	50	36	37	10
Dizziness	5	5	12	8	8	4
Coordination Abnormal†	1	2	7	9	6	0
Ataxia†	2	1	8	8	5	0
Dysarthria†	0	0	4	3	2	0
Psychiatric						
Depression	7	6	8	8	7	1
Memory Disturbance	2	5	2	5	4	2
Nervousness	1	4	3	4	3	2
Intellectual Ability Reduced	0	2	4	3	2	0
Emotional Lability	0	1	2	2	1	1
Libido Decreased	0	1	3	1	1	0
Confusion	0	2	2	1	1	0
Respiratory System						
Upper Respiratory Tract Infection†	10	10	7	6	8	4
Sinusitis	4	2	8	4	4	3
Rhinitis	3	2	4	2	2	1
Coughing	2	2	4	0	2	0
Pharyngitis	1	1	3	2	2	1
Bronchitis	1	0	2	2	2	1
Gastrointestinal System						
Constipation†	0	1	5	3	2	1
Appetite Decreased	1	1	0	3	1	1
Abdominal Pain†	2	2	2	0	1	1
Body as a Whole						
Fatigue	9	6	7	7	7	4
Allergic Reaction	3	1	4	2	2	1
Musculoskeletal						
Myalgia	2	1	4	0	1	1
Resistance Mechanism Disorders						
Influenza	3	2	5	5	4	3
Urinary System						
Micturition Frequency	1	2	2	1	1	0
Urinary Tract Infection†	0	0	2	2	1	0
Vision Disorders						
Blurred Vision	1	2	3	0	1	1
Reproductive Disorders‡						
Female						
Dysmenorrhea	0	6	5	2	3	2
Colpitis	4	0	2	1	1	1
Male						
Ejaculation Delayed	0	0	2	2	1	0
Impotence	3	0	2	1	1	0

*Events reported by at least 1% of patients treated with Klonopin and for which the incidence was greater than that for placebo.
†Indicates that the p-value for the dose-trend test (Cochran-Mantel-Haenszel) for adverse event incidence was ≤0.10.
‡Denominators for events in gender-specific systems are: n=240 (clonazepam), 102 (placebo) for male, and 334 (clonazepam), 192 (placebo) for female.

Commonly Observed Adverse Events:

Table 2. Incidence of Most Commonly Observed Adverse Events* in Acute Therapy in Pool of 6- to 9-Week Trials

Adverse Event (Roche Preferred Term)	Clonazepam (N=574)	Placebo (N=294)
Somnolence	37%	10%
Depression	7%	1%
Coordination Abnormal	6%	0%
Ataxia	5%	0%

* Treatment-emergent events for which the incidence in the clonazepam patients was ≥5% and at least twice that in the placebo patients.

Treatment-Emergent Depressive Symptoms:

In the pool of two short-term placebo-controlled trials, adverse events classified under the preferred term "depression" were reported in 7% of Klonopin-treated patients compared to 1% of placebo-treated patients, without any clear pattern of dose relatedness. In these same trials, adverse events classified under the preferred term "depression" were reported as leading to discontinuation in 4% of Klonopin-treated patients compared to 1% of placebo-treated patients. While these findings are noteworthy, Hamilton Depression Rating Scale (HAM-D) data collected in these trials revealed a larger decline in HAM-D scores in the clonazepam group than the placebo group suggesting that clonazepam-treated patients were not experiencing a worsening or emergence of clinical depression.

Other Adverse Events Observed During the Premarketing Evaluation of Klonopin in Panic Disorder:

Following is a list of modified CIGY terms that reflect treatment-emergent adverse events reported by patients treated with Klonopin at multiple doses during clinical trials. All reported events are included except those already listed in Table 1 or elsewhere in labeling, those events for which a drug cause was remote, those event terms which were so general as to be uninformative, and events reported only once and which did not have a substantial probability of being acutely life-threatening. It is important to emphasize that, although the events occurred during treatment with Klonopin, they were not necessarily caused by it.

Events are further categorized by body system and listed in order of decreasing frequency. These adverse events were reported infrequently, which is defined as occurring in 1/100 to 1/1000 patients.

Body as a Whole: weight increase, accident, weight decrease, wound, edema, fever, shivering, abrasions, ankle edema, edema foot, edema periorbital, injury, malaise, pain, cellulitis, inflammation localized

Cardiovascular Disorders: chest pain, hypotension postural

Central and Peripheral Nervous System Disorders: migraine, paresthesia, drunkenness, feeling of enuresis, paresis, tremor, burning skin, falling, head fullness, hoarseness, hyperactivity, hypoesthesia, tongue thick, twitching

Gastrointestinal System Disorders: abdominal discomfort, gastrointestinal inflammation, stomach upset, toothache, flatulence, pyrosis, saliva increased, tooth disorder, bowel movements frequent, pain pelvic, dyspepsia, hemorrhoids

Hearing and Vestibular Disorders: vertigo, otitis, earache, motion sickness

Heart Rate and Rhythm Disorders: palpitation
Metabolic and Nutritional Disorders: thirst, gout
Musculoskeletal System Disorders: back pain, fracture traumatic, sprains and strains, pain leg, pain nape, cramps muscle, cramps leg, pain ankle, pain shoulder, tendinitis, arthralgia, hypertonia, lumbago, pain feet, pain jaw, pain knee, swelling knee
Platelet, Bleeding and Clotting Disorders: bleeding dermal
Psychiatric Disorders: insomnia, organic disinhibition, anxiety, depersonalization, dreaming excessive, libido loss, appetite increased, libido increased, reactions decreased, aggressive reaction, apathy, attention lack, excitement, feeling mad, hunger abnormal, illusion, nightmares, sleep disorder, suicide ideation, yawning
Reproductive Disorders, Female: breast pain, menstrual irregularity
Reproductive Disorders, Male: ejaculation decreased
Resistance Mechanism Disorders: infection mycotic, infection viral, infection streptococcal, herpes simplex infection, infectious mononucleosis, moniliasis
Respiratory System Disorders: sneezing excessive, asthmatic attack, dyspnea, nosebleed, pneumonia, pleurisy
Skin and Appendages Disorders: acne flare, alopecia, xeroderma, dermatitis contact, flushing, pruritus, pustular reaction, skin burns, skin disorder
Special Senses Other, Disorders: taste loss
Urinary System Disorders: dysuria, cystitis, polyuria, urinary incontinence, bladder dysfunction, urinary retention, urinary tract bleeding, urine discoloration
Vascular (Extracardiac) Disorders: thrombophlebitis leg
Vision Disorders: eye irritation, visual disturbance, diplopia, eye twitching, styes, visual field defect, xerophthalmia

DRUG ABUSE AND DEPENDENCE

Controlled Substance Class: Clonazepam is a Schedule IV controlled substance.

Physical and Psychological Dependence: Withdrawal symptoms, similar in character to those noted with barbiturates and alcohol (eg, convulsions, psychosis, hallucinations, behavioral disorder, tremor, abdominal and muscle cramps) have occurred following abrupt discontinuance of clonazepam. The more severe withdrawal symptoms have usually been limited to those patients who received excessive doses over an extended period of time. Generally milder withdrawal symptoms (eg, dysphoria and insomnia) have been reported following abrupt discontinuance of benzodiazepines taken continuously at therapeutic levels for several months. Consequently, after extended therapy, abrupt discontinuation should generally be avoided and a gradual dosage tapering schedule followed (see DOSAGE AND ADMINISTRATION). Addiction-prone individuals (such as drug addicts or alcoholics) should be under careful surveillance when receiving clonazepam or other psychotropic agents because of the predisposition of such patients to habituation and dependence.

Following the short-term treatment of patients with panic disorder in Studies 1 and 2 (see CLINICAL PHARMACOLOGY: *Clinical Trials*), patients were gradually withdrawn during a 7-week downward-titration (discontinuance) period. Overall, the discontinuance period was associated with good tolerability and a very modest clinical deterioration, without evidence of a significant rebound phenomenon. However, there are not sufficient data from adequate and well-controlled long-term clonazepam studies in patients with panic disorder to accurately estimate the risks of withdrawal symptoms and dependence that may be associated with such use.

OVERDOSAGE

Human Experience: Symptoms of clonazepam overdosage, like those produced by other CNS depressants, include somnolence, confusion, coma and diminished reflexes.

Overdose Management: Treatment includes monitoring of respiration, pulse and blood pressure, general supportive measures and immediate gastric lavage. Intravenous fluids should be administered and an adequate airway maintained. Hypotension may be combated by the use of levarterenol or metaraminol. Dialysis is of no known value.

Flumazenil, a specific benzodiazepine-receptor antagonist, is indicated for the complete or partial reversal of the sedative effects of benzodiazepines and may be used in situations when an overdose with a benzodiazepine is known or suspected. Prior to the administration of flumazenil, necessary measures should be instituted to secure airway, ventilation and intravenous access. Flumazenil is intended as an adjunct to, not as a substitute for, proper management of benzodiazepine overdose. Patients treated with flumazenil should be monitored for resedation, respiratory depression and other residual benzodiazepine effects for an appropriate period after treatment. **The prescriber should be aware of a risk of seizure in association with flumazenil treatment, particularly in long-term benzodiazepine users and in cyclic antidepressant overdose.** The complete flumazenil package insert, including CONTRAINDICATIONS, WARNINGS and PRECAUTIONS, should be consulted prior to use.

Flumazenil is not indicated in patients with epilepsy who have been treated with benzodiazepines. Antagonism of the benzodiazepine effect in such patients may provoke seizures.

Serious sequelae are rare unless other drugs or alcohol have been taken concomitantly.

DOSAGE AND ADMINISTRATION

Clonazepam is available as a tablet or an orally disintegrating tablet (wafer). The tablets should be administered with water by swallowing the tablet whole. The orally disintegrating tablet should be administered as follows: After opening the pouch, peel back the foil on the blister. Do not push tablet through foil. Immediately upon opening the blister, using dry hands, remove the tablet and place it in the mouth. Tablet disintegration occurs rapidly in saliva so it can be easily swallowed with or without water.

Seizure Disorders: *Adults:* The initial dose for adults with seizure disorders should not exceed 1.5 mg/day divided into three doses. Dosage may be increased in increments of 0.5 to 1 mg every 3 days until seizures are adequately controlled or until side effects preclude any further increase. Maintenance dosage must be individualized for each patient depending upon response. Maximum recommended daily dose is 20 mg.

The use of multiple anticonvulsants may result in an increase of depressant adverse effects. This should be considered before adding Klonopin to an existing anticonvulsant regimen.

Pediatric Patients: Klonopin is administered orally. In order to minimize drowsiness, the initial dose for infants and children (up to 10 years of age or 30 kg of body weight) should be between 0.01 and 0.03 mg/kg/day but not to exceed 0.05 mg/kg/day given in two or three divided doses. Dosage should be increased by no more than 0.25 to 0.5 mg every third day until a daily maintenance dose of 0.1 to 0.2 mg/kg of body weight has been reached, unless seizures are controlled or side effects preclude further increase. Whenever possible, the daily dose should be divided into three equal doses. If doses are not equally divided, the largest dose should be given before retiring.

Geriatric Patients: There is no clinical trial experience with Klonopin in seizure disorder patients 65 years of age and older. In general, elderly patients should be started on low doses of Klonopin and observed closely (see PRECAUTIONS: *Geriatric Use*).

Panic Disorder: *Adults:* The initial dose for adults with panic disorder is 0.25 mg bid. An increase to the target dose for most patients of 1 mg/day may be made after 3 days. The recommended dose of 1 mg/day is based on the results from a fixed dose study in which the optimal effect was seen at 1 mg/day. Higher doses of 2, 3 and 4 mg/day in that study were less effective than the 1 mg/day dose and were associated with more adverse effects. Nevertheless, it is possible that some individual patients may benefit from doses of up to a maximum dose of 4 mg/day, and in those instances, the dose may be increased in increments of 0.125 to 0.25 mg bid every 3 days until panic disorder is controlled or until side effects make further increases undesired. To reduce the inconvenience of somnolence, administration of one dose at bedtime may be desirable.

Treatment should be discontinued gradually, with a decrease of 0.125 mg bid every 3 days, until the drug is completely withdrawn.

There is no body of evidence available to answer the question of how long the patient treated with clonazepam should remain on it. Therefore, the physician who elects to use Klonopin for extended periods should periodically reevaluate the long-term usefulness of the drug for the individual patient.

Pediatric Patients: There is no clinical trial experience with Klonopin in panic disorder patients under 18 years of age.

Geriatric Patients: There is no clinical trial experience with Klonopin in panic disorder patients 65 years of age and older. In general, elderly patients should be started on low doses of Klonopin and observed closely (see PRECAUTIONS: *Geriatric Use*).

HOW SUPPLIED

Klonopin tablets are available as scored tablets with a K-shaped perforation—0.5 mg, orange (NDC 0004-0068-01); and unscored tablets with a K-shaped perforation—1 mg, blue (NDC 0004-0058-01); 2 mg, white (NDC 0004-0098-01)—bottles of 100.

Imprint on tablets:

0.5 mg—1/2 KLONOPIN (front)
ROCHE (scored side)

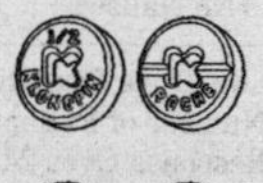

1 mg—1 KLONOPIN (front)
ROCHE (reverse side)

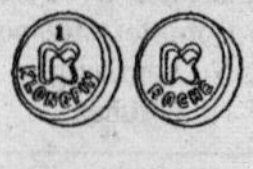

2 mg—2 KLONOPIN (front)
ROCHE (reverse side)

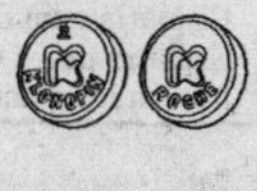

Klonopin Wafers (clonazepam orally disintegrating tablets) are white, round and debossed with the tablet strength expressed as a fraction or whole number (1/8, 1/4, 1/2, 1, or 2). The tablets are available in blister packages of 60 (10 pouches/carton) as follows:

0.125 mg	debossed 1/8, (NDC 0004-0279-22)
0.25 mg	debossed 1/4, (NDC 0004-0280-22)
0.5 mg	debossed 1/2, (NDC 0004-0281-22)
1 mg	debossed 1, (NDC 0004-0282-22)
2 mg	debossed 2, (NDC 0004-0283-22)

Store at 25°C (77°F); excursions permitted to 15° to 30°C (59° to 86°F).

Revised: July 2001

KYTRIL® ℞
(granisetron hydrochloride)
Injection

Prescribing information for this product, which appears on pages 2908–2910 of the 2003 PDR, has been completely revised as follows. Please write "See Supplement A" next to the product heading.

DESCRIPTION

KYTRIL (granisetron hydrochloride) Injection is an antinauseant and antiemetic agent. Chemically it is *endo*-N-(9-methyl-9-azabicyclo [3.3.1] non-3-yl)-1-methyl-1H-indazole-3-carboxamide hydrochloride with a molecular weight of 348.9 (312.4 free base). Its empirical formula is $C_{18}H_{24}N_4O \bullet HCl$.

Granisetron hydrochloride is a white to off-white solid that is readily soluble in water and normal saline at 20°C.

KYTRIL Injection is a clear, colorless, sterile, nonpyrogenic, aqueous solution for intravenous administration.

KYTRIL is available in 1 mL single-dose and 4 mL multi-dose vials.

Single-Dose Vials

Each 1 mL of preservative-free aqueous solution contains 1.12 mg granisetron hydrochloride equivalent to granisetron, 1 mg and sodium chloride, 9 mg. The solution's pH ranges from 4.7 to 7.3.

Multi-Dose Vials

Each 1 mL contains 1.12 mg granisetron hydrochloride equivalent to granisetron, 1 mg; sodium chloride, 9 mg; citric acid, 2 mg; and benzyl alcohol, 10 mg, as a preservative. The solution's pH ranges from 4.0 to 6.0.

CLINICAL PHARMACOLOGY

Granisetron is a selective 5-hydroxytryptamine$_3$ (5-HT$_3$) receptor antagonist with little or no affinity for other serotonin receptors, including 5-HT$_1$; 5-HT$_{1A}$; 5-HT$_{1B/C}$; 5-HT$_2$; for alpha$_1$-, alpha$_2$- or beta-adrenoreceptors; for dopamine-D$_2$; or for histamine-H$_1$; benzodiazepine; picrotoxin or opioid receptors.

Serotonin receptors of the 5-HT$_3$ type are located peripherally on vagal nerve terminals and centrally in the chemoreceptor trigger zone of the area postrema. During chemotherapy-induced vomiting, mucosal enterochromaffin cells release serotonin, which stimulates 5-HT$_3$ receptors. This evokes vagal afferent discharge and may induce vomiting. Animal studies demonstrate that, in binding to 5-HT$_3$ receptors, granisetron blocks serotonin stimulation and subsequent vomiting after emetogenic stimuli such as cisplatin. In the ferret animal model, a single granisetron injection prevented vomiting due to high-dose cisplatin or arrested vomiting within 5 to 30 seconds.

In most human studies, granisetron has had little effect on blood pressure, heart rate or ECG. No evidence of an effect on plasma prolactin or aldosterone concentrations has been found in other studies.

KYTRIL Injection exhibited no effect on oro-cecal transit time in normal volunteers given a single intravenous infusion of 50 mcg/kg or 200 mcg/kg. Single and multiple oral doses slowed colonic transit in normal volunteers.

Pharmacokinetics

Chemotherapy-Induced Nausea and Vomiting

In adult cancer patients undergoing chemotherapy and in volunteers, mean pharmacokinetic data obtained from an infusion of a single 40 mcg/kg dose of KYTRIL Injection are shown in Table 1.

[See table 1 at top of next page]

Distribution

Plasma protein binding is approximately 65% and granisetron distributes freely between plasma and red blood cells.

Metabolism

Granisetron metabolism involves N-demethylation and aromatic ring oxidation followed by conjugation. In vitro liver microsomal studies show that granisetron's major route of metabolism is inhibited by ketoconazole, suggestive of metabolism mediated by the cytochrome P-450 3A subfamily. Animal studies suggest that some of the metabolites may also have 5-HT$_3$ receptor antagonist activity.

Elimination

Clearance is predominantly by hepatic metabolism. In normal volunteers, approximately 12% of the administered dose is eliminated unchanged in the urine in 48 hours. The remainder of the dose is excreted as metabolites, 49% in the urine, and 34% in the feces.

Subpopulations

Gender

There was high inter- and intra-subject variability noted in these studies. No difference in mean AUC was found between males and females, although males had a higher C_{max} generally.

Geriatrics

The ranges of the pharmacokinetic parameters in geriatric volunteers (mean age 71 years), given a single 40 mcg/kg intravenous dose of KYTRIL Injection, were generally similar to those in younger healthy volunteers; mean values were lower for clearance and longer for half-life in the geriatric patients (see Table 1).

Pediatric Patients

A pharmacokinetic study in pediatric cancer patients (2 to 16 years of age), given a single 40 mcg/kg intravenous dose of KYTRIL Injection, showed that volume of distribution and total clearance increased with age. No relationship with age was observed for peak plasma concentration or terminal phase plasma half-life. When volume of distribution and total clearance are adjusted for body weight, the pharmacokinetics of granisetron are similar in pediatric and adult cancer patients.

Continued on next page

Kytril I.V.—Cont.

Renal Failure Patients
Total clearance of granisetron was not affected in patients with severe renal failure who received a single 40 mcg/kg intravenous dose of KYTRIL Injection.

Hepatically Impaired Patients
A pharmacokinetic study in patients with hepatic impairment due to neoplastic liver involvement showed that total clearance was approximately halved compared to patients without hepatic impairment. Given the wide variability in pharmacokinetic parameters noted in patients and the good tolerance of doses well above the recommended 10 mcg/kg dose, dosage adjustment in patients with possible hepatic functional impairment is not necessary.

Postoperative Nausea and Vomiting
In adult patients (age range, 18 to 64 years) recovering from elective surgery and receiving general balanced anesthesia, mean pharmacokinetic data obtained from a single 1 mg dose of KYTRIL Injection administered intravenously over 30 seconds are shown in Table 2.
[See table 2 at right]
The pharmacokinetics of granisetron in patients undergoing surgery were similar to those seen in cancer patients undergoing chemotherapy.

CLINICAL TRIALS

Chemotherapy-Induced Nausea and Vomiting
Single-Day Chemotherapy
Cisplatin-Based Chemotherapy
In a double-blind, placebo-controlled study in 28 cancer patients, KYTRIL Injection, administered as a single intravenous infusion of 40 mcg/kg, was significantly more effective than placebo in preventing nausea and vomiting induced by cisplatin chemotherapy (see Table 3).
[See table 3 at right]
KYTRIL Injection was also evaluated in a randomized dose response study of cancer patients receiving cisplatin ≥75 mg/m². Additional chemotherapeutic agents included: anthracyclines, carboplatin, cytostatic antibiotics, folic acid derivatives, methylhydrazine, nitrogen mustard analogs, podophyllotoxin derivatives, pyrimidine analogs, and vinca alkaloids. KYTRIL Injection doses of 10 and 40 mcg/kg were superior to 2 mcg/kg in preventing cisplatin-induced nausea and vomiting, but 40 mcg/kg was not significantly superior to 10 mcg/kg (see Table 4).
[See table 4 at right]
KYTRIL Injection was also evaluated in a double-blind, randomized dose response study of 353 patients stratified for high (≥80 to 120 mg/m²) or low (50 to 79 mg/m²) cisplatin dose. Response rates of patients for both cisplatin strata are given in Table 5.
[See table 5 at right]
For both the low and high cisplatin strata, the 10, 20, and 40 mcg/kg doses were more effective than the 5 mcg/kg dose in preventing nausea and vomiting within 24 hours of chemotherapy administration. The 10 mcg/kg dose was at least as effective as the higher doses.

Moderately Emetogenic Chemotherapy
KYTRIL Injection, 40 mcg/kg, was compared with the combination of chlorpromazine (50 to 200 mg/24 hours) and dexamethasone (12 mg) in patients treated with moderately emetogenic chemotherapy, including primarily carboplatin >300 mg/m², cisplatin 20 to 50 mg/m² and cyclophosphamide >600 mg/m². KYTRIL Injection was superior to the chlorpromazine regimen in preventing nausea and vomiting (see Table 6).
[See table 6 at top of next page]
In other studies of moderately emetogenic chemotherapy, no significant difference in efficacy was found between KYTRIL doses of 40 mcg/kg and 160 mcg/kg.

Repeat-Cycle Chemotherapy
In an uncontrolled trial, 512 cancer patients received KYTRIL Injection, 40 mcg/kg, prophylactically, for two cycles of chemotherapy, 224 patients received it for at least four cycles, and 108 patients received it for at least six cycles. KYTRIL Injection efficacy remained relatively constant over the first six repeat cycles, with complete response rates (no vomiting and no moderate or severe nausea in 24 hours) of 60% to 69%. No patients were studied for more than 15 cycles.

Pediatric Studies
A randomized double-blind study evaluated the 24-hour response of 80 pediatric cancer patients (age 2 to 16 years) to KYTRIL Injection 10, 20 or 40 mcg/kg. Patients were treated with cisplatin ≥60 mg/m², cytarabine ≥3 g/m², cyclophosphamide ≥1 g/m² or nitrogen mustard ≥6 mg/m² (see Table 7).
[See table 7 at top of next page]
A second pediatric study compared KYTRIL Injection 20 mcg/kg to chlorpromazine plus dexamethasone in 88 patients treated with ifosfamide ≥3 g/m²/day for two or three days. KYTRIL Injection was administered on each day of ifosfamide treatment. At 24 hours, 22% of KYTRIL Injection patients achieved complete response (no vomiting and no moderate or severe nausea in 24 hours) compared with 10% on the chlorpromazine regimen. The median number of vomiting episodes with KYTRIL Injection was 1.5; with chlorpromazine it was 7.0.

Postoperative Nausea and Vomiting
Prevention of Postoperative Nausea and Vomiting
The efficacy of KYTRIL Injection for prevention of postoperative nausea and vomiting was evaluated in 868 patients, of which 833 were women, 35 men, 484 Caucasians, 348 Asians, 18 Blacks, 18 Other, with 61 patients 65 years or older. KYTRIL was evaluated in two randomized, double-blind, placebo-controlled studies in patients who underwent elective gynecological surgery or cholecystectomy and received general anesthesia. Patients received a single intravenous dose of KYTRIL Injection (0.1 mg, 1 mg or 3 mg) or placebo either 5 minutes before induction of anesthesia or immediately before reversal of anesthesia. The primary endpoint was the proportion of patients with no vomiting for 24 hours after surgery. Episodes of nausea and vomiting and use of rescue antiemetic therapy were recorded for 24 hours after surgery. In both studies, KYTRIL Injection (1 mg) was more effective than placebo in preventing postoperative nausea and vomiting (see Table 8). No additional benefit was seen in patients who received the 3 mg dose.
[See table 8 on next page]

Gender/Race
There were too few male and Black patients to adequately assess differences in effect in either population.

Treatment of Postoperative Nausea and Vomiting
The efficacy of KYTRIL Injection for treatment of postoperative nausea and vomiting was evaluated in 844 patients, of which 731 were women, 113 men, 777 Caucasians, 6 Asians, 41 Blacks, 20 Other, with 107 patients 65 years or older. KYTRIL Injection was evaluated in two randomized, double-blind, placebo-controlled studies of adult surgical pa-

Table 1. Pharmacokinetic Parameters in Adult Cancer Patients Undergoing Chemotherapy and in Volunteers, Following a Single Intravenous 40 mcg/kg Dose of KYTRIL Injection

	Peak Plasma Concentration (ng/mL)	Terminal Phase Plasma Half-Life (h)	Total Clearance (L/h/kg)	Volume of Distribution (L/kg)
Cancer Patients				
Mean	63.8*	8.95*	0.38*	3.07*
Range	18.0 to 176	0.90 to 31.1	0.14 to 1.54	0.85 to 10.4
Volunteers				
21 to 42 years				
Mean	64.3†	4.91†	0.79†	3.04†
Range	11.2 to 182	0.88 to 15.2	0.20 to 2.56	1.68 to 6.13
65 to 81 years				
Mean	57.0†	7.69†	0.44†	3.97†
Range	14.6 to 153	2.65 to 17.7	0.17 to 1.06	1.75 to 7.01

*5-minute infusion.
†3-minute infusion.

Table 2. Pharmacokinetic Parameters in 16 Adult Surgical Patients Following a Single Intravenous 1 mg Dose of KYTRIL Injection

	Terminal Phase Plasma Half-Life (h)	Total Clearance (L/h/kg)	Volume of Distribution (L/kg)
Mean	8.63	0.28	2.42
Range	1.77 to 17.73	0.07 to 0.71	0.71 to 4.13

Table 3. Prevention of Chemotherapy-Induced Nausea and Vomiting—Single-Day High-Dose Cisplatin Therapy[1]

	KYTRIL Injection	Placebo	P-Value
Number of Patients	14	14	
Response Over 24 Hours			
Complete Response[2]	93%	7%	<0.001
No Vomiting	93%	14%	<0.001
No More Than Mild Nausea	93%	7%	<0.001

[1] Cisplatin administration began within 10 minutes of KYTRIL Injection infusion and continued for 1.5 to 3.0 hours. Mean cisplatin dose was 86 mg/m² in the KYTRIL Injection group and 80 mg/m² in the placebo group.
[2] No vomiting and no moderate or severe nausea.

Table 4. Prevention of Chemotherapy-Induced Nausea and Vomiting—Single-Day High-Dose Cisplatin Therapy[1]

	KYTRIL Injection (mcg/kg)			P-Value (vs. 2 mcg/kg)	
	2	10	40	10	40
Number of Patients	52	52	53		
Response Over 24 Hours					
Complete Response[2]	31%	62%	68%	<0.002	<0.001
No Vomiting	38%	65%	74%	<0.001	<0.001
No More Than Mild Nausea	58%	75%	79%	NS	0.007

[1] Cisplatin administration began within 10 minutes of KYTRIL Injection infusion and continued for 2.6 hours (mean). Mean cisplatin doses were 96 to 99 mg/m².
[2] No vomiting and no moderate or severe nausea.

Table 5. Prevention of Chemotherapy-Induced Nausea and Vomiting—Single-Day High-Dose and Low-Dose Cisplatin Therapy[1]

	KYTRIL Injection (mcg/kg)				P-Value (vs. 5 mcg/kg)		
	5	10	20	40	10	20	40
High-Dose Cisplatin							
Number of Patients	40	49	48	47			
Response Over 24 Hours							
Complete Response[2]	18%	41%	40%	47%	0.018	0.025	0.004
No Vomiting	28%	47%	44%	53%	NS	NS	0.016
No Nausea	15%	35%	38%	43%	0.036	0.019	0.005
Low-Dose Cisplatin							
Number of Patients	42	41	40	46			
Response Over 24 Hours							
Complete Response[2]	29%	56%	58%	41%	0.012	0.009	NS
No Vomiting	36%	63%	65%	43%	0.012	0.008	NS
No Nausea	29%	56%	38%	33%	0.012	NS	NS

[1] Cisplatin administration began within 10 minutes of KYTRIL Injection infusion and continued for 2 hours (mean). Mean cisplatin doses were 64 and 98 mg/m² for low and high strata.
[2] No vomiting and no use of rescue antiemetic.

Table 6. Prevention of Chemotherapy-Induced Nausea and Vomiting—Single-Day Moderately Emetogenic Chemotherapy

	KYTRIL Injection	Chlorpromazine[1]	P-Value
Number of Patients	133	133	
Response Over 24 Hours			
Complete Response[2]	68%	47%	<0.001
No Vomiting	73%	53%	<0.001
No More Than Mild Nausea	77%	59%	<0.001

[1] Patients also received dexamethasone, 12 mg.
[2] No vomiting and no moderate or severe nausea.

Table 7. Prevention of Chemotherapy-Induced Nausea and Vomiting in Pediatric Patients

	KYTRIL Injection Dose (mcg/kg)		
	10	20	40
Number of Patients	29	26	25
Median Number of Vomiting Episodes	2	3	1
Complete Response Over 24 Hours[1]	21%	31%	32%

[1] No vomiting and no moderate or severe nausea.

Table 8. Prevention of Postoperative Nausea and Vomiting in Adult Patients

Study and Efficacy Endpoint	Placebo	KYTRIL 0.1 mg	KYTRIL 1 mg	KYTRIL 3 mg
Study 1				
Number of Patients	133	132	134	128
No Vomiting				
0 to 24 hours	34%	45%	63%**	62%**
No Nausea				
0 to 24 hours	22%	28%	50%**	42%**
No Nausea or Vomiting				
0 to 24 hours	18%	27%	49%**	42%**
No Use of Rescue Antiemetic Therapy				
0 to 24 hours	60%	67%	75%*	77%*
Study 2				
Number of Patients	117	—	110	114
No Vomiting				
0 to 24 hours	56%	—	77%**	75%*
No Nausea				
0 to 24 hours	37%	—	59%**	56%*

*P<0.05
**P<0.001 versus placebo
Note: No Vomiting = no vomiting and no use of rescue antiemetic therapy; No Nausea = no nausea and no use of rescue antiemetic therapy

Table 9. Treatment of Postoperative Nausea and Vomiting in Adult Patients

Study and Efficacy Endpoint	Placebo	KYTRIL 0.1 mg	KYTRIL 1 mg	KYTRIL 3 mg
Study 3				
Number of Patients	133	128	133	125
No Vomiting				
0 to 6 hours	26%	53%***	58%***	60%***
0 to 24 hours	20%	38%***	46%***	49%***
No Nausea				
0 to 6 hours	17%	40%***	41%***	42%***
0 to 24 hours	13%	27%**	30%**	37%***
No Use of Rescue Antiemetic Therapy				
0 to 6 hours	—	—	—	—
0 to 24 hours	33%	51%**	61%***	61%***
Study 4				
Number of Patients (All Patients)	162	163	—	—
No Vomiting				
0 to 6 hours	20%	32%*	—	—
0 to 24 hours	14%	23%*	—	—
No Nausea				
0 to 6 hours	13%	18%	—	—
0 to 24 hours	9%	14%	—	—
No Nausea to Vomiting				
0 to 6 hours	13%	18%	—	—
0 to 24 hours	9%	14%	—	—
No Use of Rescue Antiemetic Therapy				
0 to 6 hours	—	—	—	—
0 to 24 hours	24%	34%*	—	—
Number of Patients (Treated for Vomiting)[1]	86	103	—	—
No Vomiting				
0 to 6 hours	21%	27%	—	—
0 to 24 hours	14%	20%	—	—

*P<0.05
**P<0.01
***P<0.001 versus placebo
[1]Protocol Specified Analysis: Patients who had vomiting prior to treatment
Note: No vomiting = no vomiting and no use of rescue antiemetic therapy; No nausea = no nausea and no use of rescue antiemetic therapy

tients who received general anesthesia with no prophylactic antiemetic agent, and who experienced nausea or vomiting within 4 hours postoperatively. Patients received a single intravenous dose of KYTRIL Injection (0.1 mg, 1 mg or 3 mg) or placebo after experiencing postoperative nausea or vomiting. Episodes of nausea and vomiting and use of rescue antiemetic therapy were recorded for 24 hours after administration of study medication. KYTRIL Injection was more effective than placebo in treating postoperative nausea and vomiting (see Table 9). No additional benefit was seen in patients who received the 3 mg dose.
[See table above]
Gender/Race
There were too few male and Black patients to adequately assess differences in effect in either population.

INDICATIONS AND USAGE
KYTRIL Injection is indicated for:
- The prevention of nausea and/or vomiting associated with initial and repeat courses of emetogenic cancer therapy, including high-dose cisplatin.
- The prevention and treatment of postoperative nausea and vomiting. As with other antiemetics, routine prophylaxis is not recommended in patients in whom there is little expectation that nausea and/or vomiting will occur postoperatively. In patients where nausea and/or vomiting must be avoided during the postoperative period, KYTRIL Injection is recommended even where the incidence of postoperative nausea and/or vomiting is low.

CONTRAINDICATIONS
KYTRIL Injection is contraindicated in patients with known hypersensitivity to the drug or to any of its components.

WARNINGS
Hypersensitivity reactions may occur in patients who have exhibited hypersensitivity to other selective 5-HT$_3$ receptor antagonists.

PRECAUTIONS
KYTRIL is not a drug that stimulates gastric or intestinal peristalsis. It should not be used instead of nasogastric suction. The use of KYTRIL in patients following abdominal surgery or in patients with chemotherapy-induced nausea and vomiting may mask a progressive ileus and/or gastric distention.

Drug Interactions
Granisetron does not induce or inhibit the cytochrome P-450 drug-metabolizing enzyme system. There have been no definitive drug-drug interaction studies to examine pharmacokinetic or pharmacodynamic interaction with other drugs, but in humans, KYTRIL Injection has been safely administered with drugs representing benzodiazepines, neuroleptics and anti-ulcer medications commonly prescribed with antiemetic treatments. KYTRIL Injection also does not appear to interact with emetogenic cancer chemotherapies. Because granisetron is metabolized by hepatic cytochrome P-450 drug-metabolizing enzymes, inducers or inhibitors of these enzymes may change the clearance and, hence, the half-life of granisetron.

Carcinogenesis, Mutagenesis, Impairment of Fertility
In a 24-month carcinogenicity study, rats were treated orally with granisetron 1, 5 or 50 mg/kg/day (6, 30 or 300 mg/m^2/day). The 50 mg/kg/day dose was reduced to 25 mg/kg/day (150 mg/m^2/day) during week 59 due to toxicity. For a 50 kg person of average height (1.46 m^2 body surface area), these doses represent 16, 81 and 405 times the recommended clinical dose (0.37 mg/m^2, iv) on a body surface area basis. There was a statistically significant increase in the incidence of hepatocellular carcinomas and adenomas in males treated with 5 mg/kg/day (30 mg/m^2/day, 81 times the recommended human dose based on body surface area) and above, and in females treated with 25 mg/kg/day (150 mg/m^2/day, 405 times the recommended human dose based on body surface area). No increase in liver tumors was observed at a dose of 1 mg/kg/day (6 mg/m^2/day, 16 times the recommended human dose based on body surface area) in males and 5 mg/kg/day (30 mg/m^2/day, 81 times the recommended human dose based on body surface area) in females. In a 12-month oral toxicity study, treatment with granisetron 100 mg/kg/day (600 mg/m^2/day, 1622 times the recommended human dose based on body surface area) produced hepatocellular adenomas in male and female rats while no such tumors were found in the control rats. A 24-month mouse carcinogenicity study of granisetron did not show a statistically significant increase in tumor incidence, but the study was not conclusive.
Because of the tumor findings in rat studies, KYTRIL Injection should be prescribed only at the dose and for the indication recommended (see INDICATIONS AND USAGE and DOSAGE AND ADMINISTRATION).
Granisetron was not mutagenic in an in vitro Ames test and mouse lymphoma cell forward mutation assay, and in vivo mouse micronucleus test and in vitro and ex vivo rat hepatocyte UDS assays. It, however, produced a significant increase in UDS in HeLa cells in vitro and a significant increased incidence of cells with polyploidy in an in vitro human lymphocyte chromosomal aberration test.
Granisetron at subcutaneous doses up to 6 mg/kg/day (36 mg/m^2/day, 97 times the recommended human dose based on body surface area) was found to have no effect on fertility and reproductive performance of male and female rats.

Pregnancy
Teratogenic Effects. *Pregnancy Category B.*
Reproduction studies have been performed in pregnant rats at intravenous doses up to 9 mg/kg/day (54 mg/m^2/day, 146 times the recommended human dose based on body surface area) and pregnant rabbits at intravenous doses up to 3 mg/kg/day (35.4 mg/m^2/day, 96 times the recommended human

Continued on next page

Kytril I.V.—Cont.

dose based on body surface area) and have revealed no evidence of impaired fertility or harm to the fetus due to granisetron. There are, however, no adequate and well-controlled studies in pregnant women. Because animal reproduction studies are not always predictive of human response, this drug should be used during pregnancy only if clearly needed.

Nursing Mothers

It is not known whether granisetron is excreted in human milk. Because many drugs are excreted in human milk, caution should be exercised when KYTRIL Injection is administered to a nursing woman.

Pediatric Use

See DOSAGE AND ADMINISTRATION for use in chemotherapy-induced nausea and vomiting in pediatric patients 2 to 16 years of age. Safety and effectiveness in pediatric patients under 2 years of age have not been established. Safety and effectiveness of KYTRIL Injection have not been established in pediatric patients for the prevention or treatment of postoperative nausea or vomiting.

Geriatric Use

During chemotherapy clinical trials, 713 patients 65 years of age or older received KYTRIL Injection. Effectiveness and safety were similar in patients of various ages.

During postoperative nausea and vomiting clinical trials, 168 patients 65 years of age or older, of which 47 were 75 years of age or older, received KYTRIL Injection. Clinical studies of KYTRIL Injection did not include sufficient numbers of subjects aged 65 years and over to determine whether they respond differently from younger subjects. Other reported clinical experience has not identified differences in responses between the elderly and younger patients.

ADVERSE REACTIONS

Chemotherapy-Induced Nausea and Vomiting

The following have been reported during controlled clinical trials or in the routine management of patients. The percentage figures are based on clinical trial experience only. Table 10 gives the comparative frequencies of the five most commonly reported adverse events (≥3%) in patients receiving KYTRIL Injection, in single-day chemotherapy trials. These patients received chemotherapy, primarily cisplatin, and intravenous fluids during the 24-hour period following KYTRIL Injection administration. Events were generally recorded over seven days post-KYTRIL Injection administration. In the absence of a placebo group, there is uncertainty as to how many of these events should be attributed to KYTRIL, except for headache, which was clearly more frequent than in comparison groups.

Table 10. Principal Adverse Events in Clinical Trials—Single-Day Chemotherapy

	Percent of Patients With Event	
	KYTRIL Injection 40 mcg/kg (n=1268)	Comparator[1] (n=422)
Headache	14%	6%
Asthenia	5%	6%
Somnolence	4%	15%
Diarrhea	4%	6%
Constipation	3%	3%

[1] Metoclopramide/dexamethasone and phenothiazines/dexamethasone.

In over 3,000 patients receiving KYTRIL Injection (2 to 160 mcg/kg) in single-day and multiple-day clinical trials with emetogenic cancer therapies, adverse events, other than those in Table 10, were observed; attribution of many of these events to KYTRIL is uncertain.

Hepatic: In comparative trials, mainly with cisplatin regimens, elevations of AST and ALT (>2 times the upper limit of normal) following administration of KYTRIL Injection occurred in 2.8% and 3.3% of patients, respectively. These frequencies were not significantly different from those seen with comparators (AST: 2.1%; ALT: 2.4%).

Cardiovascular: Hypertension (2%); hypotension, arrhythmias such as sinus bradycardia, atrial fibrillation, varying degrees of A-V block, ventricular ectopy including non-sustained tachycardia, and ECG abnormalities have been observed rarely.

Central Nervous System: Agitation, anxiety, CNS stimulation and insomnia were seen in less than 2% of patients. Extrapyramidal syndrome occurred rarely and only in the presence of other drugs associated with this syndrome.

Hypersensitivity: Rare cases of hypersensitivity reactions, sometimes severe (eg, anaphylaxis, shortness of breath, hypotension, urticaria) have been reported.

Other: Fever (3%), taste disorder (2%), skin rashes (1%). In multiple-day comparative studies, fever occurred more frequently with KYTRIL Injection (8.6%) than with comparative drugs (3.4%, $P<0.014$), which usually included dexamethasone.

Postoperative Nausea and Vomiting

The adverse events listed in Table 11 were reported in ≥2% of adults receiving KYTRIL Injection 1 mg during controlled clinical trials.

Table 11. Adverse Events ≥ 2%

	Percent of Patients With Event	
	KYTRIL Injection 1 mg (n=267)	Placebo (n=266)
Pain	10.1	8.3
Constipation	9.4	12.0
Anemia	9.4	10.2
Headache	8.6	7.1
Fever	7.9	4.5
Abdominal Pain	6.0	6.0
Hepatic Enzymes Increased	5.6	4.1
Insomnia	4.9	6.0
Bradycardia	4.5	5.3
Dizziness	4.1	3.4
Leukocytosis	3.7	4.1
Anxiety	3.4	3.8
Hypotension	3.4	3.8
Diarrhea	3.4	1.1
Flatulence	3.0	3.0
Infection	3.0	2.3
Dyspepsia	3.0	1.9
Hypertension	2.6	4.1
Urinary Tract Infection	2.6	3.4
Oliguria	2.2	1.5
Coughing	2.2	1.1

In a clinical study conducted in Japan, the types of adverse events differed notably from those reported above in Table 11. The adverse events in the Japanese study that occurred in ≥2% of patients and were more frequent with KYTRIL 1 mg than with placebo were: fever (56% to 50%), sputum increased (2.7% to 1.7%), and dermatitis (2.7% to 0%).

OVERDOSAGE

There is no specific antidote for KYTRIL Injection overdosage. In case of overdosage, symptomatic treatment should be given. Overdosage of up to 38.5 mg of granisetron hydrochloride injection has been reported without symptoms or only the occurrence of a slight headache.

DOSAGE AND ADMINISTRATION

Prevention of Chemotherapy-Induced Nausea and Vomiting

The recommended dosage for KYTRIL Injection is 10 mcg/kg administered intravenously within 30 minutes before initiation of chemotherapy, and only on the day(s) chemotherapy is given.

Infusion Preparation

KYTRIL Injection may be administered intravenously either undiluted over 30 seconds, or diluted with 0.9% Sodium Chloride or 5% Dextrose and infused over 5 minutes.

Stability

Intravenous infusion of KYTRIL Injection should be prepared at the time of administration. However, KYTRIL Injection has been shown to be stable for at least 24 hours when diluted in 0.9% Sodium Chloride or 5% Dextrose and stored at room temperature under normal lighting conditions.

As a general precaution, KYTRIL Injection should not be mixed in solution with other drugs. Parenteral drug products should be inspected visually for particulate matter and discoloration before administration whenever solution and container permit.

Pediatric Patients

The recommended dose in pediatric patients 2 to 16 years of age is 10 mcg/kg (see CLINICAL TRIALS). Pediatric patients under 2 years of age have not been studied.

Geriatric Patients, Renal Failure Patients or Hepatically Impaired Patients

No dosage adjustment is recommended (see CLINICAL PHARMACOLOGY: Pharmacokinetics).

Prevention and Treatment of Postoperative Nausea and Vomiting

The recommended dosage for prevention of postoperative nausea and vomiting is 1 mg of KYTRIL, undiluted, administered intravenously over 30 seconds, before induction of anesthesia or immediately before reversal of anesthesia.

The recommended dosage for the treatment of nausea and/or vomiting after surgery is 1 mg of KYTRIL, undiluted, administered intravenously over 30 seconds.

Pediatric Patients

Safety and effectiveness of KYTRIL Injection have not been established in pediatric patients for the prevention or treatment of postoperative nausea or vomiting.

Geriatric Patients, Renal Failure Patients or Hepatically Impaired Patients

No dosage adjustment is recommended (see CLINICAL PHARMACOLOGY: Pharmacokinetics).

HOW SUPPLIED

KYTRIL Injection, 1 mg/mL (free base), is supplied in 1 mL Single-Use Vials and 4 mL Multi-Dose Vials.

NDC 0004-0239-09 (package of 1 Single-Dose Vial)

NDC 0004-0240-09 (package of 1 Multi-Dose Vial)

Storage

Store single-dose vials and multi-dose vials at 25°C (77°F); excursions permitted to 15° to 30°C (59° to 86°F). [See USP Controlled Room Temperature]

Once the multi-dose vial is penetrated, its contents should be used within 30 days.

Do not freeze. Protect from light.

Revised: August 2002

LARIAM® ℞

[*lar-ē-um*]

brand of mefloquine hydrochloride TABLETS

Prescribing information for this product, which appears on pages 2912–2914 of the 2003 PDR, has been completely revised as follows. Please write "See Supplement A" next to the product heading.

DESCRIPTION

Lariam (mefloquine hydrochloride) is an antimalarial agent available as 250-mg tablets of mefloquine hydrochloride (equivalent to 228.0 mg of the free base) for oral administration.

Mefloquine hydrochloride is a 4-quinolinemethanol derivative with the specific chemical name of (R*, S*)-(±)-α-2-piperidinyl-2,8-bis (trifluoromethyl)-4-quinolinemethanol hydrochloride. It is a 2-aryl substituted chemical structural analog of quinine. The drug is a white to almost white crystalline compound, slightly soluble in water.

Mefloquine hydrochloride has a calculated molecular weight of 414.78.

The inactive ingredients are ammonium-calcium alginate, corn starch, crospovidone, lactose, magnesium stearate, microcrystalline cellulose, poloxamer #331, and talc.

CLINICAL PHARMACOLOGY

Pharmacokinetics

Absorption

The absolute oral bioavailability of mefloquine has not been determined since an intravenous formulation is not available. The bioavailability of the tablet formation compared with an oral solution was over 85%. The presence of food significantly enhances the rate and extent of absorption, leading to about a 40% increase in bioavailability. In healthy volunteers, plasma concentrations peak 6 to 24 hours (median, about 17 hours) after a single dose of Lariam. In a similar group of volunteers, maximum plasma concentrations in μg/L are roughly equivalent to the dose in milligrams (for example, a single 1000 mg dose produces a maximum concentration of about 1000 μg/L). In healthy volunteers, a dose of 250 mg once weekly, produces maximum steady-state plasma concentrations of 1000 to 2000 μg/L, which are reached after 7 to 10 weeks.

Distribution

In healthy adults, the apparent volume of distribution is approximately 20 L/kg, indicating extensive tissue distribution. Mefloquine may accumulate in parasitized erythrocytes. Experiments conducted in vitro with human blood using concentrations between 50 and 1000 mg/mL showed a relatively constant erythrocyte-to-plasma concentration ratio of about 2 to 1. The equilibrium reached in less than 30 minutes, was found to be reversible. Protein binding is about 98%.

Mefloquine crosses the placenta. Excretion into breast milk appears to be minimal (see **PRECAUTIONS: Nursing Mothers**).

Metabolism

Two metabolites have been identified in humans. The main metabolite, 2,8-*bis*-trifluoromethyl-4-quinoline carboxylic acid, is inactive in *P. falciparum*. In a study in healthy volunteers, the carboxylic acid metabolite appeared in plasma 2 to 4 hours after a single oral dose. Maximum plasma concentrations, which were about 50% higher than those of mefloquine, were reached after 2 weeks. Thereafter, plasma levels of the main metabolite and mefloquine declined at a similar rate. The area under the plasma concentration-time curve (AUC) of the main metabolite was 3 to 5 times larger than that of the parent drug. The other metabolite, an alcohol, was present in minute quantities only.

Elimination

In several studies in healthy adults, the mean elimination half-life of mefloquine varied between 2 and 4 weeks, with an average of about 3 weeks. Total clearance, which is essentially hepatic, is in the order of 30 mL/min. There is evidence that mefloquine is excreted mainly in the bile and feces. In volunteers, urinary excretion of unchanged mefloquine and its main metabolite under steady-state condition accounted for about 9% and 4% of the dose, respectively. Concentrations of other metabolites could not be measured in the urine.

Pharmacokinetics in Special Clinical Situations

Children and the Elderly

No relevant age-related changes have been observed in the pharmacokinetics of mefloquine. Therefore, the dosage for children has been extrapolated from the recommended adult dose.

No pharmacokinetic studies have been performed in patients with renal insufficiency since only a small proportion of the drug is eliminated renally. Mefloquine and its main metabolite are not appreciably removed by hemodialysis. No special chemoprophylactic dosage adjustments are indicated for dialysis patients to achieve concentrations in plasma similar to those in healthy persons.

Although clearance of mefloquine may increase in late pregnancy, in general, pregnancy has no clinically relevant effect on the pharmacokinetics of mefloquine.

The pharmacokinetics of mefloquine may be altered in acute malaria.

Pharmacokinetic differences have been observed between various ethnic populations. In practice, however, these are of minor importance compared with host immune status and sensitivity of the parasite.

During long-term prophylaxis (>2 years), the trough concentrations and the elimination half-life of mefloquine were similar to those obtained in the same population after 6 months of drug use, which is when they reached steady state.

In vitro and in vivo studies showed no hemolysis associated with glucose-6-phosphate dehydrogenase deficiency (see ANIMAL TOXICOLOGY).

Microbiology
Mechanism of Action
Mefloquine is an antimalarial agent which acts as a blood schizonticide. Its exact mechanism of action is not known.
Activity In Vitro and In Vivo
Mefloquine is active against the erythrocytic stages of *Plasmodium* species (see INDICATIONS AND USAGE). However, the drug has no effect against the exoerythrocytic (hepatic) stages of the parasite. Mefloquine is effective against malaria parasites resistant to chloroquine (see INDICATIONS AND USAGE).
Drug Resistance
Strains of *Plasmodium falciparum* with decreased susceptibility to mefloquine can be selected in vitro or in vivo. Resistance of *P. falciparum* to mefloquine has been reported in areas of multi-drug resistance in South East Asia. Increased incidences of resistance have also been reported in other parts of the world.
Cross Resistance
Cross-resistance between mefloquine and halofantrine and cross-resistance between mefloquine and quinine have been observed in some regions.

INDICATIONS AND USAGE
Treatment of Acute Malaria Infections
Lariam is indicated for the treatment of mild to moderate acute malaria caused by mefloquine-susceptible strains of *P. falciparum* (both chloroquine-susceptible and resistant strains) or by *Plasmodium vivax*. There are insufficient clinical data to document the effect of mefloquine in malaria caused by *P. ovale* or *P. malariae*.

Note: Patients with acute *P. vivax* malaria, treated with Lariam, are at high risk of relapse because Lariam does not eliminate exoerythrocytic (hepatic phase) parasites. To avoid relapse, after initial treatment of the acute infection with Lariam, patients should subsequently be treated with an 8-aminoquinoline (eg, primaquine).

Prevention of Malaria
Lariam is indicated for the prophylaxis of *P. falciparum* and *P. vivax* malaria infections, including prophylaxis of chloroquine-resistant strains of *P. falciparum*.

CONTRAINDICATIONS
Use of Lariam is contraindicated in patients with a known hypersensitivity to mefloquine or related compounds (eg, quinine and quinidine) or to any of the excipients contained in the formulation. Lariam should not be prescribed for prophylaxis in patients with active depression, a recent history of depression, generalized anxiety disorder, psychosis, or schizophrenia or other major psychiatric disorders, or with a history of convulsions.

WARNINGS
In case of life-threatening, serious or overwhelming malaria infections due to *P. falciparum*, patients should be treated with an intravenous antimalarial drug. Following completion of intravenous treatment, Lariam may be given to complete the course of therapy.

Data on the use of halofantrine subsequent to administration of Lariam suggest a significant, potentially fatal prolongation of the QTc interval of the ECG. Therefore, halofantrine must not be given simultaneously with or subsequent to Lariam. No data are available on the use of Lariam after halofantrine (see PRECAUTIONS: Drug Interactions).

Mefloquine may cause psychiatric symptoms in a number of patients, ranging from anxiety, paranoia, and depression to hallucinations and psychotic behavior. On occasions, these symptoms have been reported to continue long after mefloquine has been stopped. Rare cases of suicidal ideation and suicide have been reported though no relationship to drug administration has been confirmed. To minimize the chances of these adverse events, mefloquine should not be taken for prophylaxis in patients with active depression or with a recent history of depression, generalized anxiety disorder, psychosis, or schizophrenia or other major psychiatric disorders. Lariam should be used with caution in patients with a previous history of depression.

During prophylactic use, if psychiatric symptoms such as acute anxiety, depression, restlessness or confusion occur, these may be considered prodromal to a more serious event. In these cases, the drug must be discontinued and an alternative medication should be substituted.

Concomitant administration of Lariam and quinine or quinidine may produce electrocardiographic abnormalities.

Concomitant administration of Lariam and quinine or chloroquine may increase the risk of convulsions.

PRECAUTIONS
General
Hypersensitivity reactions ranging from mild cutaneous events to anaphylaxis cannot be predicted.
In patients with epilepsy, Lariam may increase the risk of convulsions. The drug should therefore be prescribed only for curative treatment in such patients and only if there are compelling medical reasons for its use (see PRECAUTIONS: Drug Interactions).

Caution should be exercised with regard to activities requiring alertness and fine motor coordination such as driving, piloting aircraft, operating machinery, and deep-sea diving, as dizziness, a loss of balance, or other disorders of the central or peripheral nervous system have been reported during and following the use of Lariam. These effects may occur after therapy is discontinued due to the long half-life of the drug. Lariam should be used with caution in patients with psychiatric disturbances because mefloquine use has been associated with emotional disturbances (see ADVERSE REACTIONS).

In patients with impaired liver function the elimination of mefloquine may be prolonged, leading to higher plasma levels.

This drug has been administered for longer than 1 year. If the drug is to be administered for a prolonged period, periodic evaluations including liver function tests should be performed. Although retinal abnormalities seen in humans with long-term chloroquine use have not been observed with mefloquine use, long-term feeding of mefloquine to rats resulted in dose-related ocular lesions (retinal degeneration, retinal edema and lenticular opacity at 12.5 mg/kg/day and higher) (see ANIMAL TOXICOLOGY). Therefore, periodic ophthalmic examinations are recommended.

Parenteral studies in animals show that mefloquine, a myocardial depressant, possesses 20% of the antifibrillatory action of quinidine and produces 50% of the increase in the PR interval reported with quinine. The effect of mefloquine on the compromised cardiovascular system has not been evaluated. However, transitory and clinically silent ECG alterations have been reported during the use of mefloquine. Alterations included sinus bradycardia, sinus arrhythmia, first degree AV-block, prolongation of the QTc interval and abnormal T waves (see also cardiovascular effects under PRECAUTIONS: Drug Interactions and ADVERSE REACTIONS). The benefits of Lariam therapy should be weighed against the possibility of adverse effects in patients with cardiac disease.

Laboratory Tests
Periodic evaluation of hepatic function should be performed during prolonged prophylaxis.

Information for Patients
Patients should be advised:
- that malaria can be a life-threatening infection in the traveler;
- that Lariam is being prescribed to help prevent or treat this serious infection;
- that in a small percentage of cases, patients are unable to take this medication because of side effects, and it may be necessary to change medications;
- that when used as prophylaxis, the first dose of Lariam should be taken 1 week prior to arrival in an endemic area;
- that if the patients experience psychiatric symptoms such as acute anxiety, depression, restlessness or confusion, these may be considered prodromal to a more serious event. In these cases, the drug must be discontinued and an alternative medication should be substituted;
- that no chemoprophylactic regimen is 100% effective, and protective clothing, insect repellents, and bednets are important components of malaria prophylaxis;
- to seek medical attention for any febrile illness that occurs after return from a malarious area and to inform their physician that they may have been exposed to malaria.

Drug Interactions
Drug-drug interactions with Lariam have not been explored in detail. There is one report of cardiopulmonary arrest, with full recovery, in a patient who was taking a beta blocker (propranolol) (see PRECAUTIONS: General). The effects of mefloquine on the compromised cardiovascular system have not been evaluated. The benefits of Lariam therapy should be weighed against the possibility of adverse effects in patients with cardiac disease.

Because of the danger of a potentially fatal prolongation of the QTc interval, halofantrine must not be given simultaneously with or subsequent to Lariam (see WARNINGS). Concomitant administration of Lariam and other related compounds (eg, quinine, quinidine and chloroquine) may produce electrocardiographic abnormalities and increase the risk of convulsions (see WARNINGS). If these drugs are to be used in the initial treatment of severe malaria, Lariam administration should be delayed at least 12 hours after the last dose. There is evidence that the use of halofantrine after mefloquine causes a significant lengthening of the QTc interval. Clinically significant QTc prolongation has not been found with mefloquine alone.

This appears to be the only clinically relevant interaction of this kind with Lariam, although theoretically, coadministration of other drugs known to alter cardiac conduction (eg, antiarrhythmic or beta-adrenergic blocking agents, calcium channel blockers, antihistamines or H_1-blocking agents, tricyclic antidepressants and phenothiazines) might also contribute to a prolongation of the QTc interval. There are no data that conclusively establish whether the concomitant administration of mefloquine and the above listed agents has an effect on cardiac function.

In patients taking an anticonvulsant (eg, valproic acid, carbamazepine, phenobarbital or phenytoin), the concomitant use of Lariam may reduce seizure control by lowering the plasma levels of the anticonvulsant. Therefore, patients concurrently taking antiseizure medication and Lariam should have the blood level of their antiseizure medication monitored and the dosage adjusted appropriately (see PRECAUTIONS: General).

When Lariam is taken concurrently with oral live typhoid vaccines, attenuation of immunization cannot be excluded. Vaccinations with attenuated live bacteria should therefore be completed at least 3 days before the first dose of Lariam. No other drug interactions are known. Nevertheless, the effects of Lariam on travelers receiving comedication, particularly diabetics or patients using anticoagulants, should be checked before departure.

In clinical trials, the concomitant administration of sulfadoxine and pyrimethamine did not alter the adverse reaction profile.

Carcinogenesis, Mutagenesis, Impairment of Fertility
Carcinogenesis
The carcinogenic potential of mefloquine was studied in rats and mice in 2-year feeding studies at doses of up to 30 mg/kg/day. No treatment-related increases in tumors of any type were noted.
Mutagenesis
The mutagenic potential of mefloquine was studied in a variety of assay systems including: Ames test, a host-mediated assay in mice, fluctuation tests and a mouse micronucleus assay. Several of these assays were performed with and without prior metabolic activation. In no instance was evidence obtained for the mutagenicity of mefloquine.
Impairment of Fertility
Fertility studies in rats at doses of 5, 20, and 50 mg/kg/day of mefloquine have demonstrated adverse effects on fertility in the male at the high dose of 50 mg/kg/day, and in the female at doses of 20 and 50 mg/kg/day. Histopathological lesions were noted in the epididymides from male rats at doses of 20 and 50 mg/kg/day. Administration of 250 mg/week of mefloquine (base) in adult males for 22-weeks failed to reveal any deleterious effects on human spermatozoa.

Pregnancy
Teratogenic Effects
Pregnancy Category C. Mefloquine has been demonstrated to be teratogenic in rats and mice at a dose of 100 mg/kg/day. In rabbits, a high dose of 160 mg/kg/day was embryotoxic and teratogenic, and a dose of 80 mg/kg/day was teratogenic but not embryotoxic. There are no adequate and well-controlled studies in pregnant women. However, clinical experience with Lariam has not revealed an embryotoxic or teratogenic effect. Mefloquine should be used during pregnancy only if the potential benefit justifies the potential risk to the fetus. Women of childbearing potential who are traveling to areas where malaria is endemic should be warned against becoming pregnant. Women of childbearing potential should also be advised to practice contraception during malaria prophylaxis with Lariam and for up to 3 months thereafter. However, in the case of unplanned pregnancy, malaria chemoprophylaxis with Lariam is not considered an indication for pregnancy termination.

Nursing Mothers
Mefloquine is excreted in human milk in small amounts, the activity of which is unknown. Based on a study in a few subjects, low concentrations (3% to 4%) of mefloquine were excreted in human milk following a dose equivalent to 250 mg of the free base. Because of the potential for serious adverse reactions in nursing infants from mefloquine, a decision should be made whether to discontinue the drug, taking into account the importance of the drug to the mother.

Pediatric Use
Use of Lariam to treat acute, uncomplicated *P. falciparum* malaria in pediatric patients is supported by evidence from adequate and well-controlled studies of Lariam in adults with additional data from published open-label and comparative trials using Lariam to treat malaria caused by *P. falciparum* in patients younger than 16 years of age. The safety and effectiveness of Lariam for the treatment of malaria in pediatric patients below the age of 6 months have not been established.

In several studies, the administration of Lariam for the treatment of malaria was associated with early vomiting in pediatric patients. Early vomiting was cited in some reports as a possible cause of treatment failure. If a second dose is not tolerated, the patient should be monitored closely and alternative malaria treatment considered if improvement is not observed within a reasonable period of time (see DOSAGE AND ADMINISTRATION).

Geriatric Use
Clinical studies of Lariam did not include sufficient numbers of subjects aged 65 and over to determine whether they respond differently from younger subjects. Other reported clinical experience has not identified differences in responses between the elderly and younger patients. Since electrocardiographic abnormalities have been observed in individuals treated with Lariam (see PRECAUTIONS) and underlying cardiac disease is more prevalent in elderly than in younger patients, the benefits of Lariam therapy should be weighed against the possibility of adverse cardiac effects in elderly patients.

ADVERSE REACTIONS
Clinical
At the doses used for treatment of acute malaria infections, the symptoms possibly attributable to drug administration cannot be distinguished from those symptoms usually attributable to the disease itself.

Among subjects who received mefloquine for prophylaxis of malaria, the most frequently observed adverse experience

Continued on next page

Lariam—Cont.

was vomiting (3%). Dizziness, syncope, extrasystoles and other complaints affecting less than 1% were also reported. Among subjects who received mefloquine for treatment, the most frequently observed adverse experiences included: dizziness, myalgia, nausea, fever, headache, vomiting, chills, diarrhea, skin rash, abdominal pain, fatigue, loss of appetite, and tinnitus. Those side effects occurring in less than 1% included bradycardia, hair loss, emotional problems, pruritus, asthenia, transient emotional disturbances and telogen effluvium (loss of resting hair). Seizures have also been reported.

Two serious adverse reactions were cardiopulmonary arrest in one patient shortly after ingesting a single prophylactic dose of mefloquine while concomitantly using propranolol (see **PRECAUTIONS: Drug Interactions**), and encephalopathy of unknown etiology during prophylactic mefloquine administration. The relationship of encephalopathy to drug administration could not be clearly established.

Postmarketing

Postmarketing surveillance indicates that the same kind of adverse experiences are reported during prophylaxis, as well as acute treatment.

The most frequently reported adverse events are nausea, vomiting, loose stools or diarrhea, abdominal pain, dizziness or vertigo, loss of balance, and neuropsychiatric events such as headache, somnolence, and sleep disorders (insomnia, abnormal dreams). These are usually mild and may decrease despite continued use.

Occasionally, more severe neuropsychiatric disorders have been reported such as: sensory and motor neuropathies (including paresthesia, tremor and ataxia), convulsions, agitation or restlessness, anxiety, depression, mood changes, panic attacks, forgetfulness, confusion, hallucinations, aggression, psychotic or paranoid reactions and encephalopathy. Rare cases of suicidal ideation and suicide have been reported though no relationship to drug administration has been confirmed.

Other infrequent adverse events include:

Cardiovascular Disorders: circulatory disturbances (hypotension, hypertension, flushing, syncope), chest pain, tachycardia or palpitation, bradycardia, irregular pulse, extrasystoles, A-V block, and other transient cardiac conduction alterations

Skin Disorders: rash, exanthema, erythema, urticaria, pruritus, edema, hair loss, erythema multiforme, and Stevens-Johnson syndrome

Musculoskeletal Disorders: muscle weakness, muscle cramps, myalgia, and arthralgia

Other Symptoms: visual disturbances, vestibular disorders including tinnitus and hearing impairment, dyspnea, asthenia, malaise, fatigue, fever, sweating, chills, dyspepsia and loss of appetite

Laboratory

The most frequently observed laboratory alterations which could be possibly attributable to drug administration were decreased hematocrit, transient elevation of transaminases, leukopenia and thrombocytopenia. These alterations were observed in patients with acute malaria who received treatment doses of the drug and were attributed to the disease itself.

During prophylactic administration of mefloquine to indigenous populations in malaria-endemic areas, the following occasional alterations in laboratory values were observed: transient elevation of transaminases, leukocytosis or thrombocytopenia.

Because of the long half-life of mefloquine, adverse reactions to Lariam may occur or persist up to several weeks after the last dose.

OVERDOSAGE

In cases of overdosage with Lariam, the symptoms mentioned under **ADVERSE REACTIONS** may be more pronounced. The following procedure is recommended in case of overdosage: Induce vomiting or perform gastric lavage, as appropriate. Monitor cardiac function (if possible by ECG) and neuropsychiatric status for at least 24 hours. Provide symptomatic and intensive supportive treatment as required, particularly for cardiovascular disturbances.

DOSAGE AND ADMINISTRATION (see INDICATIONS AND USAGE)

Adult Patients

Treatment of mild to moderate malaria in adults caused by *P. vivax* or mefloquine-susceptible strains of *P. falciparum*

Five tablets (1250 mg) mefloquine hydrochloride to be given as a single oral dose. The drug should not be taken on an empty stomach and should be administered with at least 8 oz (240 mL) of water.

If a full-treatment course with Lariam does not lead to improvement within 48 to 72 hours, Lariam should not be used for retreatment. An alternative therapy should be used. Similarly, if previous prophylaxis with mefloquine has failed, Lariam should not be used for curative treatment.

Note: Patients with acute *P. vivax* malaria, treated with Lariam, are at high risk of relapse because Lariam does not eliminate exoerythrocytic (hepatic phase) parasites. To avoid relapse after initial treatment of the acute infection with Lariam, patients should subsequently be treated with an 8-aminoquinoline derivative (eg, primaquine).

Malaria Prophylaxis

One 250 mg Lariam tablet once weekly.

Prophylactic drug administration should begin 1 week before arrival in an endemic area. Subsequent weekly doses should be taken regularly, always on the same day of each week, preferably after the main meal. To reduce the risk of malaria after leaving an endemic area, prophylaxis must be continued for 4 additional weeks to ensure suppressive blood levels of the drug when merozoites emerge from the liver. Tablets should not be taken on an empty stomach and should be administered with at least 8 oz (240 mL) of water. In certain cases, eg, when a traveler is taking other medication, it may be desirable to start prophylaxis 2 to 3 weeks prior to departure, in order to ensure that the combination of drugs is well tolerated (see **PRECAUTIONS: Drug Interactions**).

When prophylaxis with Lariam fails, physicians should carefully evaluate which antimalarial to use for therapy.

Pediatric Patients

Treatment of mild to moderate malaria in pediatric patients caused by mefloquine-susceptible strains of *P. falciparum*

Twenty (20) to 25 mg/kg body weight. Splitting the total therapeutic dose into 2 doses taken 6 to 8 hours apart may reduce the occurrence or severity of adverse effects. Experience with Lariam in infants less than 3 months old or weighing less than 5 kg is limited. The drug should not be taken on an empty stomach and should be administered with ample water. The tablets may be crushed and suspended in a small amount of water, milk or other beverage for administration to small children and other persons unable to swallow them whole.

If a full-treatment course with Lariam does not lead to improvement within 48 to 72 hours, Lariam should not be used for retreatment. An alternative therapy should be used. Similarly, if previous prophylaxis with mefloquine has failed, Lariam should not be used for curative treatment.

In pediatric patients, the administration of Lariam for the treatment of malaria has been associated with early vomiting. In some cases, early vomiting has been cited as a possible cause of treatment failure (see **PRECAUTIONS**). If a significant loss of drug product is observed or suspected because of vomiting, a second full dose of Lariam should be administered to patients who vomit less than 30 minutes after receiving the drug. If vomiting occurs 30 to 60 minutes after a dose, an additional half-dose should be given. If vomiting recurs, the patient should be monitored closely and alternative malaria treatment considered if improvement is not observed within a reasonable period of time.

The safety and effectiveness of Lariam to treat malaria in pediatric patients below the age of 6 months have not been established.

Malaria Prophylaxis

The following doses have been extrapolated from the recommended adult dose. Neither the pharmacokinetics, nor the clinical efficacy of these doses have been determined in children owing to the difficulty of acquiring this information in pediatric subjects. The recommended prophylactic dose of Lariam is approximately 5 mg/kg body weight once weekly. One 250 mg Lariam tablet should be taken once weekly in pediatric patients weighing over 45 kg. In pediatric patients weighing less than 45 kg, the weekly dose decreases in proportion to body weight:

30 to 45 kg:	3/4 tablet
20 to 30 kg:	1/2 tablet
10 to 20 kg:	1/4 tablet
5 to 10 kg:	1/8 tablet*

*Approximate tablet fraction based on a dosage of 5 mg/kg body weight. Exact doses for children weighing less than 10 kg may best be prepared and dispensed by pharmacists.

Experience with Lariam in infants less than 3 months old or weighing less than 5 kg is limited.

HOW SUPPLIED

Lariam is available as scored, white, round tablets, containing 250 mg of mefloquine hydrochloride in unit-dose packages of 25 (NDC 0004-0172-02). Imprint on tablets: LARIAM 250 ROCHE

Tablets should be stored at 25°C (77°F); excursions permitted to 15° to 30°C (59° to 86°F).

ANIMAL TOXICOLOGY

Ocular lesions were observed in rats fed mefloquine daily for 2 years. All surviving rats given 30 mg/kg/day had ocular lesions in both eyes characterized by retinal degeneration, opacity of the lens, and retinal edema. Similar but less severe lesions were observed in 80% of female and 22% of male rats fed 12.5 mg/kg/day for 2 years. At doses of 5 mg/kg/day, only corneal lesions were observed. They occurred in 9% of rats studied.

Manufactured by: F. HOFFMANN-LA ROCHE LTD., Basel, Switzerland

Distributed by: Roche Laboratories Inc., Nutley, New Jersey 07110-1199

Revised: January 2003

Schering Corporation

a wholly-owned subsidiary of Schering-Plough Corporation
2000 GALLOPING HILL ROAD
KENILWORTH, NJ 07033

Direct Inquiries to:
(908) 298-4000
CUSTOMER SERVICE:
(800) 222-7579
FAX: (908) 820-6400

For Medical Information Contact:
Schering Laboratories
Drug Information Services
2000 Galloping Hill Road
Kenilworth, NJ 07033
(800) 526-4099
FAX: (908) 298-2188

ELOCON® ℞

[ĕl'ō-cŏn]

brand of mometasone furoate cream, USP
Cream 0.1%
For Dermatologic Use Only
Not for Ophthalmic Use

Prescribing information for this product, which appears on pages 3030–3031 of the 2003 PDR, has been completely revised as follows. Please write "See Supplement A" next to the product heading.

DESCRIPTION

ELOCON® (mometasone furoate cream, USP) Cream 0.1% contains mometasone furoate, USP for dermatologic use. Mometasone furoate is a synthetic corticosteroid with anti-inflammatory activity.

Chemically, mometasone furoate is 9α,21-Dichloro-11β,17-dihydroxy-16α-methylpregna-1,4-diene-3,20-dione 17-(2-furoate), with the empirical formula $C_{27}H_{30}Cl_2O_6$, a molecular weight of 521.4 and the following structural formula:

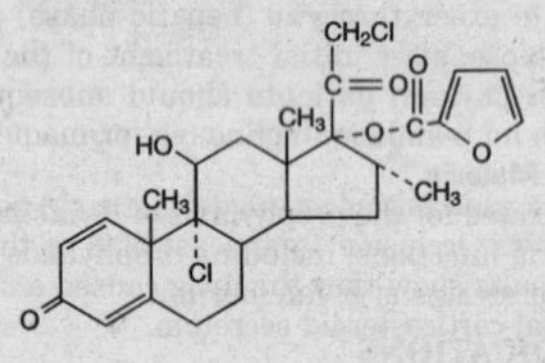

Mometasone furoate is a white to off-white powder practically insoluble in water, slightly soluble in octanol, and moderately soluble in ethyl alcohol.

Each gram of ELOCON Cream 0.1% contains: 1 mg mometasone furoate, USP in a cream base of hexylene glycol, NF; phosphoric acid, NF; propylene glycol stearate (55% monoester); stearyl alcohol and ceteareth-20; titanium dioxide, USP; aluminum starch octenylsuccinate (Gamma Irradiated); white wax, NF; white petrolatum, USP; and purified water, USP.

CLINICAL PHARMACOLOGY

Like other topical corticosteroids, mometasone furoate has anti-inflammatory, antipruritic, and vasoconstrictive properties. The mechanism of the anti-inflammatory activity of the topical steroids, in general, is unclear. However, corticosteroids are thought to act by the induction of phospholipase A_2 inhibitory proteins, collectively called lipocortins. It is postulated that these proteins control the biosynthesis of potent mediators of inflammation such as prostaglandins and leukotrienes by inhibiting the release of their common precursor arachidonic acid. Arachidonic acid is released from membrane phospholipids by phospholipase A_2.

Pharmacokinetics:

The extent of percutaneous absorption of topical corticosteroids is determined by many factors including the vehicle and the integrity of the epidermal barrier. Occlusive dressings with hydrocortisone for up to 24 hours have not been demonstrated to increase penetration; however, occlusion of hydrocortisone for 96 hours markedly enhances penetration. Studies in humans indicate that approximately 0.4% of the applied dose of ELOCON Cream 0.1% enters the circulation after 8 hours of contact on normal skin without occlusion. Inflammation and/or other disease processes in the skin may increase percutaneous absorption.

Studies performed with ELOCON Cream 0.1% indicate that it is in the medium range of potency as compared with other topical corticosteroids.

In a study evaluating the effects of mometasone furoate cream on the hypothalamic-pituitary-adrenal (HPA) axis, 15 grams were applied twice daily for 7 days to six adult patients with psoriasis or atopic dermatitis. The cream was applied without occlusion to at least 30% of the body surface. The results show that the drug caused a slight lowering of adrenal corticosteroid secretion.

In a pediatric trial, 24 atopic dermatitis patients, of which 19 patients were age 2 to 12 years, were treated with ELOCON Cream 0.1% once daily. The majority of patients cleared within 3 weeks.

Ninety-seven pediatric patients ages 6 to 23 months with atopic dermatitis were enrolled in an open-label, hypothalamic-pituitary-adrenal (HPA) axis safety study. ELOCON Cream 0.1% was applied once daily for approximately 3 weeks over a mean body surface area of 41% (range 15% to 94%). In approximately 16% of patients who showed normal adrenal function by Cortrosyn test before starting treatment, adrenal suppression was observed at the end of treatment with ELOCON Cream 0.1%. The criteria for suppression were: basal cortisol level of ≤5 mcg/dL, 30-minute post-stimulation level of ≤18 mcg/dL, or an increase of <7 mcg/dL. Follow-up testing 2 to 4 weeks after stopping treatment, available for 5 of the patients, demonstrated suppressed HPA axis function in one patient, using these same criteria.

INDICATIONS AND USAGE

ELOCON Cream 0.1% is a medium potency corticosteroid indicated for the relief of the inflammatory and pruritic manifestations of corticosteroid-responsive dermatoses. ELOCON (mometasone furoate cream, USP) Cream 0.1% may be used in pediatric patients 2 years of age or older, although the safety and efficacy of drug use for longer than 3 weeks have not been established (see **PRECAUTIONS – Pediatric Use** section). Since safety and efficacy of ELOCON Cream 0.1% have not been established in pediatric patients below 2 years of age, its use in this age group is not recommended.

CONTRAINDICATIONS

ELOCON Cream 0.1% is contraindicated in those patients with a history of hypersensitivity to any of the components in the preparation.

PRECAUTIONS

General:
Systemic absorption of topical corticosteroids can produce reversible hypothalamic-pituitary-adrenal (HPA) axis suppression with the potential for glucocorticosteroid insufficiency after withdrawal of treatment. Manifestations of Cushing's syndrome, hyperglycemia, and glucosuria can also be produced in some patients by systemic absorption of topical corticosteroids while on treatment.
Patients applying a topical steroid to a large surface area or to areas under occlusion should be evaluated periodically for evidence of HPA axis suppression. This may be done by using the ACTH stimulation, A.M. plasma cortisol, and urinary free cortisol tests.
In a study evaluating the effects of mometasone furoate cream on the hypothalamic-pituitary-adrenal (HPA) axis, 15 grams were applied twice daily for 7 days to six adult patients with psoriasis or atopic dermatitis. The cream was applied without occlusion to at least 30% of the body surface. The results show that the drug caused a slight lowering of adrenal corticosteroid secretion.
If HPA axis suppression is noted, an attempt should be made to withdraw the drug, to reduce the frequency of application, or to substitute a less potent corticosteroid. Recovery of HPA axis function is generally prompt upon discontinuation of topical corticosteroids. Infrequently, signs and symptoms of glucocorticosteroid insufficiency may occur requiring supplemental systemic corticosteroids. For information on systemic supplementation, see Prescribing Information for those products.
Pediatric patients may be more susceptible to systemic toxicity from equivalent doses due to their larger skin surface to body mass ratios (see **PRECAUTIONS — Pediatric Use**).
If irritation develops, ELOCON Cream 0.1% should be discontinued and appropriate therapy instituted. Allergic contact dermatitis with corticosteroids is usually diagnosed by observing a failure to heal rather than noting a clinical exacerbation as with most topical products not containing corticosteroids. Such an observation should be corroborated with appropriate diagnostic patch testing.
If concomitant skin infections are present or develop, an appropriate antifungal or antibacterial agent should be used. If a favorable response does not occur promptly, use of ELOCON Cream 0.1% should be discontinued until the infection has been adequately controlled.

Information for Patients:
Patients using topical corticosteroids should receive the following information and instructions:
1. This medication is to be used as directed by the physician. It is for external use only. Avoid contact with the eyes.
2. This medication should not be used for any disorder other than that for which it was prescribed.
3. The treated skin area should not be bandaged or otherwise covered or wrapped so as to be occlusive, unless directed by the physician.
4. Patients should report to their physician any signs of local adverse reactions.
5. Parents of pediatric patients should be advised not to use ELOCON Cream 0.1% in the treatment of diaper dermatitis. ELOCON Cream 0.1% should not be applied in the diaper area as diapers or plastic pants may constitute occlusive dressing (see **DOSAGE AND ADMINISTRATION**).
6. This medication should not be used on the face, underarms, or groin areas unless directed by the physician.
7. As with other corticosteroids, therapy should be discontinued when control is achieved. If no improvement is seen within 2 weeks, contact the physician.
8. Other corticosteroid-containing products should not be used with ELOCON Cream 0.1% without first consulting with the physician.

Laboratory Tests: The following tests may be helpful in evaluating patients for HPA axis suppression:
ACTH stimulation test
A.M. plasma cortisol test
Urinary free cortisol test

Carcinogenesis, Mutagenesis, Impairment of Fertility:
Long-term animal studies have not been performed to evaluate the carcinogenic potential of ELOCON (mometasone furoate cream, USP) Cream 0.1%. Long-term carcinogenicity studies of mometasone furoate were conducted by the inhalation route in rats and mice. In a 2-year carcinogenicity study in Sprague-Dawley rats, mometasone furoate demonstrated no statistically significant increase of tumors at inhalation doses up to 67 mcg/kg (approximately 0.04 times the estimated maximum clinical topical dose from ELOCON Cream 0.1% on a mcg/m^2 basis). In a 19-month carcinogenicity study in Swiss CD-1 mice, mometasone furoate demonstrated no statistically significant increase in the incidence of tumors at inhalation doses up to 160 mcg/kg (approximately 0.05 times the estimated maximum clinical topical dose from ELOCON Cream 0.1% on a mcg/m^2 basis). Mometasone furoate increased chromosomal aberrations in an *in vitro* Chinese hamster ovary cell assay, but did not increase chromosomal aberrations in an *in vitro* Chinese hamster lung cell assay. Mometasone furoate was not mutagenic in the Ames test or mouse lymphoma assay, and was not clastogenic in an *in vivo* mouse micronucleus assay, a rat bone marrow chromosomal aberration assay, or a mouse male germ-cell chromosomal aberration assay. Mometasone furoate also did not induce unscheduled DNA synthesis *in vivo* in rat hepatocytes.
In reproductive studies in rats, impairment of fertility was not produced in male or female rats by subcutaneous doses up to 15 mcg/kg (approximately 0.01 times the estimated maximum clinical topical dose from ELOCON Cream 0.1% on a mcg/m^2 basis).

Pregnancy *Teratogenic Effects: Pregnancy Category C:*
Corticosteroids have been shown to be teratogenic in laboratory animals when administered systemically at relatively low dosage levels. Some corticosteroids have been shown to be teratogenic after dermal application in laboratory animals.
When administered to pregnant rats, rabbits, and mice, mometasone furoate increased fetal malformations. The doses that produced malformations also decreased fetal growth, as measured by lower fetal weights and/or delayed ossification. Mometasone furoate also caused dystocia and related complications when administered to rats during the end of pregnancy.
In mice, mometasone furoate caused cleft palate at subcutaneous doses of 60 mcg/kg and above. Fetal survival was reduced at 180 mcg/kg. No toxicity was observed at 20 mcg/kg. (Doses of 20, 60, and 180 mcg/kg in the mouse are approximately 0.01, 0.02, and 0.05 times the estimated maximum clinical topical dose from ELOCON Cream 0.1% on a mcg/m^2 basis).
In rats, mometasone furoate produced umbilical hernias at topical doses of 600 mcg/kg and above. A dose of 300 mcg/kg produced delays in ossification, but no malformations. (Doses of 300 and 600 mcg/kg in the rat are approximately 0.2 and 0.4 times the estimated maximum clinical topical dose from ELOCON Cream 0.1% on a mcg/m^2 basis).
In rabbits, mometasone furoate caused multiple malformations (eg, flexed front paws, gallbladder agenesis, umbilical hernia, hydrocephaly) at topical doses of 150 mcg/kg and above (approximately 0.2 times the estimated maximum clinical topical dose from ELOCON Cream 0.1% on a mcg/m^2 basis). In an oral study, mometasone furoate increased resorptions and caused cleft palate and/or head malformations (hydrocephaly and domed head) at 700 mcg/kg. At 2800 mcg/kg most litters were aborted or resorbed. No toxicity was observed at 140 mcg/kg. (Doses at 140, 700, and 2800 mcg/kg in the rabbit are approximately 0.2, 0.9, and 3.6 times the estimated maximum clinical topical dose from ELOCON Cream 0.1% on a mcg/m^2 basis).
When rats received subcutaneous doses of mometasone furoate throughout pregnancy or during the later stages of pregnancy, 15 mcg/kg caused prolonged and difficult labor and reduced the number of live births, birth weight, and early pup survival. Similar effects were not observed at 7.5 mcg/kg. (Doses of 7.5 and 15 mcg/kg in the rat are approximately 0.005 and 0.01 times the estimated maximum clinical topical dose from ELOCON Cream 0.1% on a mcg/m^2 basis).
There are no adequate and well-controlled studies of teratogenic effects from topically applied corticosteroids in pregnant women. Therefore, topical corticosteroids should be used during pregnancy only if the potential benefit justifies the potential risk to the fetus.

Nursing Mothers:
Systemically administered corticosteroids appear in human milk and could suppress growth, interfere with endogenous corticosteroid production, or cause other untoward effects. It is not known whether topical administration of corticosteroids could result in sufficient systemic absorption to produce detectable quantities in human milk. Because many drugs are excreted in human milk, caution should be exercised when ELOCON Cream 0.1% is administered to a nursing woman.

Pediatric Use:
ELOCON Cream 0.1% may be used with caution in pediatric patients 2 years of age or older, although the safety and efficacy of drug use for longer than 3 weeks have not been established. Use of ELOCON Cream 0.1% is supported by results from adequate and well-controlled studies in pediatric patients with corticosteroid-responsive dermatoses. Since safety and efficacy of ELOCON Cream 0.1% have not been established in pediatric patients below 2 years of age, its use in this age group is not recommended.
ELOCON Cream 0.1% caused HPA axis suppression in approximately 16% of pediatric patients ages 6 to 23 months, who showed normal adrenal function by Cortrosyn test before starting treatment, and were treated for approximately 3 weeks over a mean body surface area of 41% (range 15% to 94%). The criteria for suppression were: basal cortisol level of ≤5 mcg/dL, 30-minute post-stimulation level of ≤18 mcg/dL, or an increase of <7 mcg/dL. Follow-up testing 2 to 4 weeks after study completion, available for 5 of the patients, demonstrated suppressed HPA axis function in one patient, using these same criteria. Long-term use of topical corticosteroids has not been studied in this population (see **CLINICAL PHARMACOLOGY – Pharmacokinetics** section).
Because of a higher ratio of skin surface area to body mass, pediatric patients are at a greater risk than adults of HPA axis suppression and Cushing's syndrome when they are treated with topical corticosteroids. They are, therefore, also at greater risk of adrenal insufficiency during and/or after withdrawal of treatment. Pediatric patients may be more susceptible than adults to skin atrophy, including striae, when they are treated with topical corticosteroids. Pediatric patients applying topical corticosteroids to greater than 20% of body surface are at higher risk of HPA axis suppression.
HPA axis suppression, Cushing's syndrome, linear growth retardation, delayed weight gain, and intracranial hypertension have been reported in pediatric patients receiving topical corticosteroids. Manifestations of adrenal suppression in children include low plasma cortisol levels, and an absence of response to ACTH stimulation. Manifestations of intracranial hypertension include bulging fontanelles, headaches, and bilateral papilledema.
ELOCON (mometasone furoate cream, USP) Cream 0.1% should not be used in the treatment of diaper dermatitis.

Geriatric Use:
Clinical studies of ELOCON Cream 0.1% included 190 subjects who were 65 years of age and over and 39 subjects who were 75 years of age and over. No overall differences in safety or effectiveness were observed between these subjects and younger subjects, and other reported clinical experience has not identified differences in responses between the elderly and younger patients. However, greater sensitivity of some older individuals cannot be ruled out.

ADVERSE REACTIONS

In controlled clinical studies involving 319 patients, the incidence of adverse reactions associated with the use of ELOCON Cream 0.1% was 1.6%. Reported reactions included burning, pruritus, and skin atrophy. Reports of rosacea associated with the use of ELOCON Cream 0.1% have also been received. In controlled clinical studies (n=74) involving pediatric patients 2 to 12 years of age, the incidence of adverse experiences associated with the use of ELOCON Cream 0.1% was approximately 7%. Reported reactions included stinging, pruritus, and furunculosis.
The following adverse reactions were reported to be possibly or probably related to treatment with ELOCON Cream 0.1% during clinical studies in 4% of 182 pediatric patients 6 months to 2 years of age: decreased glucocorticoid levels, 2; paresthesia, 2; folliculitis,1; moniliasis, 1; bacterial infection, 1; skin depigmentation, 1. The following signs of skin atrophy were also observed among 97 patients treated with ELOCON Cream 0.1% in a clinical study: shininess 4, telangiectasia 1, loss of elasticity 4, loss of normal skin markings 4, thinness 1, and bruising 1. Striae were not observed in this study.
The following additional local adverse reactions have been reported infrequently with topical corticosteroids, but may occur more frequently with the use of occlusive dressings. These reactions are listed in an approximate decreasing order of occurrence: irritation, dryness, folliculitis, hypertrichosis, acneiform eruptions, hypopigmentation, perioral dermatitis, allergic contact dermatitis, secondary infection, striae, and miliaria.

OVERDOSAGE

Topically applied ELOCON Cream 0.1% can be absorbed in sufficient amounts to produce systemic effects (see **PRECAUTIONS** section).

DOSAGE AND ADMINISTRATION

Apply a thin film of ELOCON Cream 0.1% to the affected skin areas once daily. ELOCON Cream 0.1% may be used in pediatric patients 2 years of age or older. Since safety and efficacy of ELOCON Cream 0.1% have not been adequately established in pediatric patients below 2 years of age, its use in this age group is not recommended (see **PRECAUTIONS – Pediatric Use** section).
As with other corticosteroids, therapy should be discontinued when control is achieved. If no improvement is seen within 2 weeks, reassessment of diagnosis may be necessary. Safety and efficacy of ELOCON Cream 0.1% in pediatric patients for more than 3 weeks of use have not been established.
ELOCON Cream 0.1% should not be used with occlusive dressings unless directed by a physician. ELOCON Cream 0.1% should not be applied in the diaper area if the child still requires diapers or plastic pants as these garments may constitute occlusive dressing.

Continued on next page

Elocon-Cream—Cont.

HOW SUPPLIED

ELOCON Cream 0.1% is supplied in 15-g (NDC 0085-0567-01) and 45-g (NDC 0085-0567-02) tubes; boxes of one.

Store ELOCON Cream 0.1% between 2° and 25°C (36° and 77°F).

ELOCON®
brand of mometasone furoate cream, USP
Cream 0.1%
For Dermatologic Use Only
Not for Ophthalmic Use

Schering Corporation
Kenilworth, NJ 07033 USA
Rev. 12/02 17969366
18724332T

ELOCON® ℞

[*ĕl-ō-cŏn*]

brand of mometasone furoate
Lotion 0.1%
For Dermatologic Use Only
Not for Ophthalmic Use

Prescribing information for this product, which appears on page 3031 of the 2003 PDR, has been completely revised as follows. Please write "See Supplement A" next to the product heading.

DESCRIPTION

ELOCON® (mometasone furoate topical solution) Lotion 0.1% contains mometasone furoate, USP for dermatologic use. Mometasone furoate is a synthetic corticosteroid with anti-inflammatory activity.

Chemically, mometasone furoate is 9α,21-dichloro-11β,17-dihydroxy-16α-methylpregna-1,4-diene-3,20-dione 17-(2-furoate), with the empirical formula $C_{27}H_{30}Cl_2O_6$, a molecular weight of 521.4 and the following structural formula:

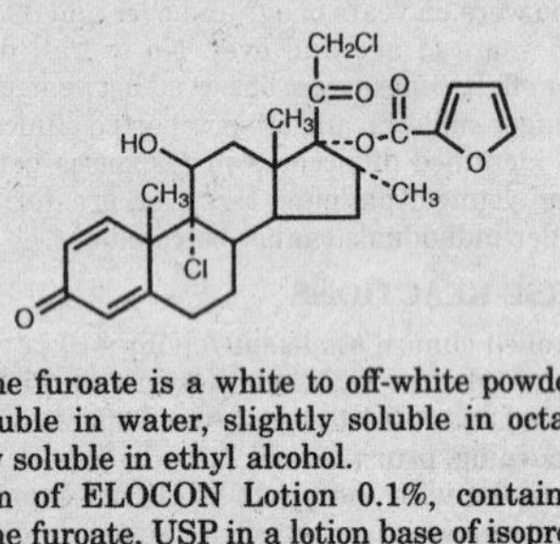

Mometasone furoate is a white to off-white powder practically insoluble in water, slightly soluble in octanol, and moderately soluble in ethyl alcohol.

Each gram of ELOCON Lotion 0.1%, contains: 1 mg mometasone furoate, USP in a lotion base of isopropyl alcohol (40%), propylene glycol, hydroxypropylcellulose, sodium phosphate monobasic monohydrate and water. May also contain phosphoric acid used to adjust the pH to approximately 4.5.

CLINICAL PHARMACOLOGY

Like other topical corticosteroids, mometasone furoate has anti-inflammatory, anti-pruritic, and vasoconstrictive properties. The mechanism of the anti-inflammatory activity of the topical steroids, in general, is unclear. However, corticosteroids are thought to act by the induction of phospholipase A_2 inhibitory proteins, collectively called lipocortins. It is postulated that these proteins control the biosynthesis of potent mediators of inflammation such as prostaglandins and leukotrienes by inhibiting the release of their common precursor arachidonic acid. Arachidonic acid is released from membrane phospholipids by phospholipase A_2.

Pharmacokinetics:

The extent of percutaneous absorption of topical corticosteroids is determined by many factors including the vehicle and the integrity of the epidermal barrier. Occlusive dressings with hydrocortisone for up to 24 hours have not been demonstrated to increase penetration; however, occlusion of hydrocortisone for 96 hours markedly enhances penetration. Studies in humans indicate that approximately 0.7% of the applied dose of ELOCON Ointment 0.1% enters the circulation after 8 hours of contact on normal skin without occlusion. A similar minimal degree of absorption of the corticosteroid from the lotion formulation would be anticipated. Inflammation and/or other disease processes in the skin may increase percutaneous absorption.

Studies performed with ELOCON Lotion 0.1% indicate that it is in the medium range of potency as compared with other topical corticosteroids.

In a study evaluating the effects of mometasone furoate lotion on the hypothalamic-pituitary-adrenal (HPA) axis, 15 mL were applied without occlusion twice daily (30 mL per day) for 7 days to four adult patients with scalp and body psoriasis. At the end of treatment, the plasma cortisol levels for each of the four patients remained within the normal range and changed little from baseline.

Sixty-five pediatric patients ages 6 to 23 months, with atopic dermatitis, were enrolled in an open-label, hypothalamic-pituitary-adrenal (HPA) axis safety study. ELOCON Lotion 0.1% was applied once daily for approximately 3 weeks over a mean body surface area of 40% (range 16% to 90%). In approximately 29% of patients who showed normal adrenal function by Cortrosyn test before starting treatment, adrenal suppression was observed at the end of treatment with ELOCON Lotion 0.1%. The criteria for suppression were: basal cortisol level of ≤5 mcg/dL, 30-minute post-stimulation level of ≤18 mcg/dL, or an increase of <7 mcg/dL. Follow-up testing 2 to 4 weeks after stopping treatment, available for 8 of the patients, demonstrated suppressed HPA axis function in one patient, using these same criteria.

INDICATIONS AND USAGE

ELOCON Lotion, 0.1% is a medium potency corticosteroid indicated for the relief of the inflammatory and pruritic manifestations of corticosteroid-responsive dermatoses. Since safety and efficacy of ELOCON Lotion 0.1% have not been established in pediatric patients below 12 years of age, its use in this age group is not recommended, (see **PRECAUTIONS – Pediatric Use**).

CONTRAINDICATIONS

ELOCON Lotion 0.1% is contraindicated in those patients with a history of hypersensitivity to any of the components in the preparation.

PRECAUTIONS

General:

Systemic absorption of topical corticosteroids can produce reversible hypothalamic-pituitary-adrenal (HPA) axis suppression with the potential for glucocorticosteroid insufficiency after withdrawal of treatment. Manifestations of Cushing's syndrome, hyperglycemia, and glucosuria can also be produced in some patients by systemic absorption of topical corticosteroids while on treatment.

Patients applying a topical steroid to a large surface area or to areas under occlusion should be evaluated periodically for evidence of HPA axis suppression. This may be done by using the ACTH stimulation, A.M. plasma cortisol, and urinary free cortisol tests.

In a study evaluating the effects of mometasone furoate lotion on the hypothalamic-pituitary-adrenal (HPA) axis, 15 mL were applied without occlusion twice daily (30 mL per day) for 7 days to four adult patients with scalp and body psoriasis. At the end of treatment, the plasma cortisol levels for each of the four patients remained within the normal range and changed little from baseline.

If HPA axis suppression is noted, an attempt should be made to withdraw the drug, to reduce the frequency of application, or to substitute a less potent corticosteroid. Recovery of HPA axis function is generally prompt upon discontinuation of topical corticosteroids. Infrequently, signs and symptoms of glucocorticosteroid insufficiency may occur requiring supplemental systemic corticosteroids. For information on systemic supplementation, see Prescribing Information for those products.

Pediatric patients may be more susceptible to systemic toxicity from equivalent doses due to their larger skin surface to body mass ratios (see **PRECAUTIONS—Pediatric Use**).

If irritation develops, ELOCON Lotion 0.1% should be discontinued and appropriate therapy instituted. Allergic contact dermatitis with corticosteroids is usually diagnosed by observing failure to heal rather than noting a clinical exacerbation as with most topical products not containing corticosteroids. Such an observation should be corroborated with appropriate diagnostic patch testing.

If concomitant skin infections are present or develop, an appropriate antifungal or antibacterial agent should be used. If a favorable response does not occur promptly, use of ELOCON Lotion 0.1% should be discontinued until the infection has been adequately controlled.

Information for Patients:

Patients using topical corticosteroids should receive the following information and instructions:

1. This medication is to be used as directed by the physician. It is for external use only. Avoid contact with the eyes.
2. This medication should not be used for any disorder other than that for which it was prescribed.
3. The treated skin area should not be bandaged or otherwise covered or wrapped so as to be occlusive unless directed by the physician.
4. Patients should report to their physician any signs of local adverse reactions.
5. Parents of pediatric patients should be advised not to use ELOCON Lotion 0.1% in the treatment of diaper dermatitis. ELOCON Lotion 0.1% should not be applied in the diaper area, as diapers or plastic pants may constitute occlusive dressing (see **DOSAGE AND ADMINISTRATION**).
6. This medication should not be used on the face, underarms, or groin areas unless directed by the physician.
7. As with other corticosteroids, therapy should be discontinued when control is achieved. If no improvement is seen within 2 weeks, contact the physician.
8. Other corticosteroid-containing products should not be used with ELOCON Lotion 0.1% without first consulting with the physician.

Laboratory Tests:

The following tests may be helpful in evaluating patients for HPA axis suppression:

ACTH stimulation test
A.M. plasma cortisol test
Urinary free cortisol test

Carcinogenesis, Mutagenesis, Impairment of Fertility:

Long-term animal studies have not been performed to evaluate the carcinogenic potential of ELOCON (mometasone furoate lotion) Lotion 0.1%. Long-term carcinogenicity studies of mometasone furoate were conducted by the inhalation route in rats and mice. In a 2-year carcinogenicity study in Sprague-Dawley rats, mometasone furoate demonstrated no statistically significant increase of tumors at inhalation doses up to 67 mcg/kg (approximately 0.04 times the estimated maximum clinical topical dose from ELOCON Lotion 0.1% on a mcg/m² basis). In a 19-month carcinogenicity study in Swiss CD-1 mice, mometasone furoate demonstrated no statistically significant increase in the incidence of tumors at inhalation doses up to 160 mcg/kg (approximately 0.05 times the estimated maximum clinical topical dose from ELOCON Lotion 0.1% on a mcg/m² basis).

Mometasone furoate increased chromosomal aberrations in an *in vitro* Chinese hamster ovary cell assay, but did not increase chromosomal aberrations in an *in vitro* Chinese hamster lung cell assay. Mometasone furoate was not mutagenic in the Ames test or mouse lymphoma assay, and was not clastogenic in an *in vivo* mouse micronucleus assay, a rat bone marrow chromosomal aberration assay, or a mouse male germ-cell chromosomal aberration assay. Mometasone furoate also did not induce unscheduled DNA synthesis *in vivo* in rat hepatocytes.

In reproductive studies in rats, impairment of fertility was not produced in male or female rats by subcutaneous doses up to 15 mcg/kg (approximately 0.01 times the estimated maximum clinical topical dose from ELOCON Lotion 0.1% on a mcg/m² basis).

Pregnancy: ***Teratogenic Effects: Pregnancy Category C:***

Corticosteroids have been shown to be teratogenic in laboratory animals when administered systemically at relatively low dosage levels. Some corticosteroids have been shown to be teratogenic after dermal application in laboratory animals.

When administered to pregnant rats, rabbits, and mice, mometasone furoate increased fetal malformations. The doses that produced malformations also decreased fetal growth, as measured by lower fetal weights and/or delayed ossification. Mometasone furoate also caused dystocia and related complications when administered to rats during the end of pregnancy.

In mice, mometasone furoate caused cleft palate at subcutaneous doses of 60 mcg/kg and above. Fetal survival was reduced at 180 mcg/kg. No toxicity was observed at 20 mcg/kg. (Doses of 20, 60, and 180 mcg/kg in the mouse are approximately 0.01, 0.02, and 0.05 times the estimated maximum clinical topical dose from ELOCON Lotion 0.1% on a mcg/m² basis).

In rats, mometasone furoate produced umbilical hernias at topical doses of 600 mcg/kg and above. A dose of 300 mcg/kg produced delays in ossification, but no malformations. (Doses of 300 and 600 mcg/kg in the rat are approximately 0.2 and 0.4 times the estimated maximum clinical topical dose from ELOCON Lotion 0.1% on a mcg/m² basis).

In rabbits, mometasone furoate caused multiple malformations (e.g., flexed front paws, gallbladder agenesis, umbilical hernia, hydrocephaly) at topical doses of 150 mcg/kg and above (approximately 0.2 times the estimated maximum clinical topical dose from ELOCON Lotion 0.1% on a mcg/m² basis). In an oral study, mometasone furoate increased resorptions and caused cleft palate and/or head malformations (hydrocephaly and domed head) at 700 mcg/kg. At 2800 mcg/kg most litters were aborted or resorbed. No toxicity was observed at 140 mcg/kg. (Doses at 140, 700, and 2800 mcg/kg in the rabbit are approximately 0.2, 0.9, and 3.6 times the estimated maximum clinical topical dose from ELOCON Lotion 0.1% on a mcg/m² basis).

When rats received subcutaneous doses of mometasone furoate throughout pregnancy or during the later stages of pregnancy, 15 mcg/kg caused prolonged and difficult labor and reduced the number of live births, birth weight, and early pup survival. Similar effects were not observed at 7.5 mcg/kg. (Doses of 7.5 and 15 mcg/kg in the rat are approximately 0.005 and 0.01 times the estimated maximum clinical topical dose from ELOCON Lotion 0.1% on a mcg/m² basis).

There are no adequate and well-controlled studies of teratogenic effects from topically applied corticosteroids in pregnant women. Therefore, topical corticosteroids should be used during pregnancy only if the potential benefit justifies the potential risk to the fetus.

Nursing Mothers:

Systemically administered corticosteroids appear in human milk and could suppress growth, interfere with endogenous corticosteroid production, or cause other untoward effects. It is not known whether topical administration of corticosteroids could result in sufficient systemic absorption to produce detectable quantities in human milk. Because many drugs are excreted in human milk, caution should be exercised when ELOCON Lotion 0.1% is administered to a nursing woman.

Pediatric Use:

Since safety and efficacy of ELOCON Lotion 0.1% have not been established in pediatric patients below 12 years of age, its use in this age group is not recommended.

ELOCON Lotion 0.1% caused HPA axis suppression in approximately 29% of pediatric patients ages 6 to 23 months who showed normal adrenal function by Cortrosyn test before starting treatment, and were treated for approximately 3 weeks over a mean body surface area of 40% (range 16% to 90%). The criteria for suppression were: basal cortisol level of ≤5 mcg/dL, 30-minute post-stimulation level of ≤18 mcg/dL, or an increase of <7 mcg/dL. Follow-up testing 2 to 4 weeks after stopping treatment, available for 8 of the patients, demonstrated suppressed HPA axis function in one patient, using these same criteria. Long-term use of topical corticosteroids has not been studied in this population (see **CLINICAL PHARMACOLOGY – Pharmacokinetics**).

Because of a higher ratio of skin surface area to body mass, pediatric patients are at a greater risk than adults of HPA axis suppression and Cushing's syndrome when they are treated with topical corticosteroids. They are, therefore, also at greater risk of adrenal insufficiency during and/or after withdrawal of treatment. Pediatric patients may be more susceptible than adults to skin atrophy, including striae, when they are treated with topical corticosteroids. Pediatric patients applying topical corticosteroids to greater than 20% of body surface are at higher risk of HPA axis suppression.

HPA axis suppression, Cushing's syndrome, linear growth retardation, delayed weight gain, and intracranial hypertension have been reported in pediatric patients receiving topical corticosteroids. Manifestations of adrenal suppression in children include low plasma cortisol levels and absence of response to ACTH stimulation. Manifestations of intracranial hypertension include bulging fontanelles, headaches, and bilateral papilledema.

ELOCON (mometasone furoate lotion) Lotion 0.1% should not be used in the treatment of diaper dermatitis.

Geriatrics Use:

Clinical studies of ELOCON Lotion 0.1% did not include sufficient numbers of subjects aged 65 and over to determine whether they respond differently from younger subjects. Other reported clinical experience has not identified differences in responses between the elderly and younger patients. In general, dose selection for an elderly patient should be cautious.

ADVERSE REACTIONS

In clinical studies involving 209 patients, the incidence of adverse reactions associated with the use of ELOCON Lotion 0.1% was 3%. Reported reactions included acneiform reaction, 2; burning, 4; and itching, 1. In an irritation/sensitization study involving 156 normal subjects, the incidence of folliculitis was 3% (4 subjects).

The following adverse reactions were reported to be possibly or probably related to treatment with ELOCON Lotion 0.1% during a clinical study, in 14% of 65 pediatric patients 6 months to 2 years of age: decreased glucocorticoid levels, 4; paresthesia, 2; dry mouth, 1; an unspecified endocrine disorder, 1; pruritus, 1; and an unspecified skin disorder, 1. The following signs of skin atrophy were also observed among 65 patients treated with ELOCON Lotion 0.1% in a clinical study: shininess 4, telangiectasia 2, loss of elasticity 2, and loss of normal skin markings 3. Striae, thinness and bruising were not observed in this study.

The following additional local adverse reactions have been reported infrequently with topical corticosteroids, but may occur more frequently with the use of occlusive dressings. These reactions are listed in an approximate decreasing order of occurrence: irritation, dryness, hypertrichosis, hypopigmentation, perioral dermatitis, allergic contact dermatitis, secondary infection, skin atrophy, striae, and miliaria.

OVERDOSAGE

Topically applied ELOCON Lotion 0.1% can be absorbed in sufficient amounts to produce systemic effects (see **PRECAUTIONS**).

DOSAGE AND ADMINISTRATION

Apply a few drops of ELOCON Lotion 0.1% to the affected skin areas once daily and massage lightly until it disappears. For the most effective and economical use, hold the nozzle of the bottle very close to the affected areas and gently squeeze. Since safety and efficacy of ELOCON Lotion 0.1% have not been established in pediatric patients below 12 years of age, its use in this age group is not recommended (see **PRECAUTIONS – Pediatric Use**).

As with other corticosteroids, therapy should be discontinued when control is achieved. If no improvement is seen within 2 weeks, reassessment of diagnosis may be necessary.

ELOCON Lotion 0.1% should not be used with occlusive dressings unless directed by a physician. ELOCON Lotion 0.1% should not be applied in the diaper area if the patient still requires diapers or plastic pants as these garments may constitute occlusive dressing.

HOW SUPPLIED

ELOCON Lotion 0.1% is supplied in 30-mL (27.5 g) (NDC 0085-0854-01) and 60-mL (55 g) (NDC 0085-0854-02) bottles; boxes of one.

Store ELOCON Lotion 0.1% between 2° and 30°C (36° and 86°F).

Schering Corporation
Kenilworth, NJ 07033 USA
Rev. 12/02 17980920

Copyright © 1989, 2003, Schering Corporation.
All rights reserved.

ELOCON® ℞

[el'ō-cŏn]

brand of mometasone furoate ointment, USP
Ointment 0.1%
For Dermatologic Use Only
Not for Ophthalmic Use

Prescribing information for this product, which appears on pages 3031–3032 of the 2003 PDR, has been completely revised as follows. Please write "See Supplement A" next to the product heading.

DESCRIPTION

ELOCON® (mometasone furoate ointment, USP) Ointment 0.1% contains mometasone furoate, USP for dermatologic use. Mometasone furoate is a synthetic corticosteroid with anti-inflammatory activity.

Chemically, mometasone furoate is 9α,21-Dichloro-11β,17-dihydroxy-16α-methylpregna-1,4-diene-3,20-dione 17-(2-furoate), with the empirical formula $C_{27}H_{30}Cl_2O_6$, a molecular weight of 521.4 and the following structural formula:

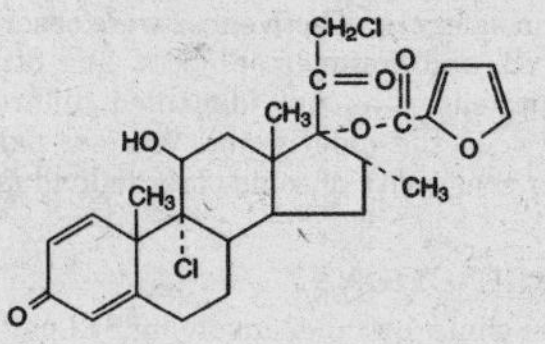

Mometasone furoate is a white to off-white powder practically insoluble in water, slightly soluble in octanol, and moderately soluble in ethyl alcohol.

Each gram contains: 1 mg mometasone furoate, USP in an ointment base of hexylene glycol; phosphoric acid; propylene glycol stearate (55% monoester); white wax; white petrolatum; and purified water.

CLINICAL PHARMACOLOGY

Like other topical corticosteroids, mometasone furoate has anti-inflammatory, anti-pruritic, and vasoconstrictive properties. The mechanism of the anti-inflammatory activity of the topical steroids, in general, is unclear. However, corticosteroids are thought to act by the induction of phospholipase A_2 inhibitory proteins, collectively called lipocortins. It is postulated that these proteins control the biosynthesis of potent mediators of inflammation such as prostaglandins and leukotrienes by inhibiting the release of their common precursor arachidonic acid. Arachidonic acid is released from membrane phospholipids by phospholipase A_2.

Pharmacokinetics The extent of percutaneous absorption of topical corticosteroids is determined by many factors including the vehicle and the integrity of the epidermal barrier. Occlusive dressings with hydrocortisone for up to 24 hours have not been demonstrated to increase penetration; however, occlusion of hydrocortisone for 96 hours markedly enhances penetration. Studies in humans indicate that approximately 0.7% of the applied dose of ELOCON Ointment 0.1% enters the circulation after 8 hours of contact on normal skin without occlusion. Inflammation and/or other disease processes in the skin may increase percutaneous absorption.

Studies performed with ELOCON Ointment 0.1% indicate that it is in the medium range of potency as compared with other topical corticosteroids.

In a study evaluating the effects of mometasone furoate ointment on the hypothalamic-pituitary-adrenal (HPA) axis, 15 grams were applied twice daily for 7 days to six adult patients with psoriasis or atopic dermatitis. The ointment was applied without occlusion to at least 30% of the body surface. The results show that the drug caused a slight lowering of adrenal corticosteroid secretion.

In a pediatric trial, 24 atopic dermatitis patients, of which 19 patients were age 2 to 12 years, were treated with ELOCON Cream 0.1% once daily. The majority of patients cleared within 3 weeks.

Sixty-three pediatric patients ages 6 to 23 months, with atopic dermatitis, were enrolled in an open-label, hypothalamic-pituitary-adrenal (HPA) axis safety study. ELOCON Ointment 0.1% was applied once daily for approximately 3 weeks over a mean body surface area of 39% (range 15% to 99%). In approximately 27% of patients who showed normal adrenal fuction by Cortrosyn test before starting treatment, adrenal suppression was observed at the end of treatment with ELOCON Ointment 0.1%. The criteria for suppression were: basal cortisol level of ≤5 mcg/dL, 30-minute post-stimulation level of ≤18 mcg/dL, or an increase of <7 mcg/dL. Follow-up testing 2 to 4 weeks after stopping treatment, available for 8 of the patients, demonstrated suppressed HPA axis function in 3 patients, using these same criteria.

INDICATIONS AND USAGE

ELOCON Ointment 0.1% is a medium potency corticosteroid indicated for the relief of the inflammatory and pruritic manifestations of corticosteroid-responsive dermatoses.

ELOCON (mometasone furoate ointment, USP) Ointment 0.1% may be used in pediatric patients 2 years of age or older, although the safety and efficacy of drug use for longer than 3 weeks have not been established (see **PRECAUTIONS – Pediatric Use**). Since safety and efficacy of ELOCON Ointment 0.1% have not been adequately established in pediatric patients below 2 years of age, its use in this age group is not recommended.

CONTRAINDICATIONS

ELOCON Ointment 0.1% is contraindicated in those patients with a history of hypersensitivity to any of the components in the preparation.

PRECAUTIONS

General: Systemic absorption of topical corticosteroids can produce reversible hypothalamic-pituitary-adrenal (HPA) axis suppression with the potential for glucocorticosteroid insufficiency after withdrawal of treatment. Manifestations of Cushing's syndrome, hyperglycemia, and glucosuria can also be produced in some patients by systemic absorption of topical corticosteroids while on treatment.

Patients applying a topical steroid to a large surface area or areas under occlusion should be evaluated periodically for evidence of HPA axis suppression. This may be done by using the ACTH stimulation, A.M. plasma cortisol, and urinary free cortisol tests.

In a study evaluating the effects of mometasone furoate ointment on the hypothalamic-pituitary-adrenal (HPA) axis, 15 grams were applied twice daily for 7 days to six adult patients with psoriasis or atopic dermatitis. The ointment was applied without occlusion to at least 30% of the body surface. The results show that the drug caused a slight lowering of adrenal corticosteroid secretion.

If HPA axis suppression is noted, an attempt should be made to withdraw the drug, to reduce the frequency of application, or to substitute a less potent corticosteroid. Recovery of HPA axis function is generally prompt upon discontinuation of topical corticosteroids. Infrequently, signs and symptoms of glucocorticosteroid insufficiency may occur requiring supplemental systemic corticosteroids. For information on systemic supplementation, see Prescribing Information for those products.

Pediatric patients may be more susceptible to systemic toxicity from equivalent doses due to their larger skin surface to body mass ratios (see **PRECAUTIONS – Pediatric Use**).

If irritation develops, ELOCON Ointment 0.1% should be discontinued and appropriate therapy instituted. Allergic contact dermatitis with corticosteroids is usually diagnosed by observing failure to heal rather than noting a clinical exacerbation as with most topical products not containing corticosteroids. Such an observation should be corroborated with appropriate diagnostic patch testing.

If concomitant skin infections are present or develop, an appropriate antifungal or antibacterial agent should be used. If a favorable response does not occur promptly, use of ELOCON Ointment 0.1% should be discontinued until the infection has been adequately controlled.

Information for Patients Patients using topical corticosteroids should receive the following information and instructions:

1. This medication is to be used as directed by the physician. It is for external use only. Avoid contact with the eyes.
2. This medication should not be used for any disorder other than that for which it was prescribed.
3. The treated skin area should not be bandaged or otherwise covered or wrapped so as to be occlusive, unless directed by the physician.
4. Patients should report to their physician any signs of local adverse reactions.
5. Parents of pediatric patients should be advised not to use ELOCON Ointment 0.1% in the treatment of diaper dermatitis. ELOCON Ointment 0.1% should not be applied in the diaper area as diapers or plastic pants may constitute occlusive dressing (see **DOSAGE AND ADMINISTRATION**).
6. This medication should not be used on the face, underarms, or groin areas unless directed by the physician.
7. As with other corticosteroids, therapy should be discontinued when control is achieved. If no improvement is seen within 2 weeks, contact the physician.
8. Other corticosteroid-containing products should not be used with ELOCON Ointment 0.1% without first consulting with the physician.

Laboratory Tests The following tests may be helpful in evaluating patients for HPA axis suppression:

ACTH stimulation test
A.M. plasma cortisol test
Urinary free cortisol test

Carcinogenesis, Mutagenesis, Impairment of Fertility Long-term animal studies have not been performed to evaluate the carcinogenic potential of ELOCON (mometasone furoate ointment, USP) Ointment 0.1%. Long-term carcinogenicity studies of mometasone furoate were conducted by the inhalation route in rats and mice. In a 2-year carcinogenicity study in Sprague-Dawley rats, mometasone furoate demonstrated no statistically significant increase of tumors at inhalation doses up to 67 mcg/kg (approximately 0.04 times the estimated maximum clinical topical dose from ELOCON Ointment 0.1% on a mcg/m^2 basis). In a 19-month carcinogenicity study in Swiss CD-1 mice, mometasone furoate demonstrated no statistically significant increase in the incidence of tumors at inhalation doses up to 160 mcg/kg (approximately 0.05 times the estimated maximum clinical topical dose from ELOCON Ointment 0.1% on a mcg/m^2 basis).

Mometasone furoate increased chromosomal aberrations in an *in vitro* Chinese hamster ovary cell assay, but did not increase chromosomal aberrations in an *in vitro* Chinese hamster lung cell assay. Mometasone furoate was not mutagenic in the Ames test or mouse lymphoma assay, and was not clastogenic in an *in vivo* mouse micronucleus assay, a rat bone marrow chromosomal aberration assay, or a mouse male germ-cell chromosomal aberration assay. Mometasone furoate also did not induce unscheduled DNA synthesis *in vivo* in rat hepatocytes.

In reproductive studies in rats, impairment of fertility was not produced in male or female rats by subcutaneous doses

Continued on next page

Elocon Ointment—Cont.

up to 15 mcg/kg (approximately 0.01 times the estimated maximum clinical topical dose from ELOCON Ointment 0.1% on a mcg/m^2 basis).

Pregnancy *Teratogenic Effects: Pregnancy Category C:* Corticosteroids have been shown to be teratogenic in laboratory animals when administered systemically at relatively low dosage levels. Some corticosteroids have been shown to be teratogenic after dermal application in laboratory animals.

When administered to pregnant rats, rabbits, and mice, mometasone furoate increased fetal malformations. The doses that produced malformations also decreased fetal growth, as measured by lower fetal weights and/or delayed ossification. Mometasone furoate also caused dystocia and related complications when administered to rats during the end of pregnancy.

In mice, mometasone furoate caused cleft palate at subcutaneous doses of 60 mcg/kg and above. Fetal survival was reduced at 180 mcg/kg. No toxicity was observed at 20 mcg/kg. (Doses of 20, 60, and 180 mcg/kg in the mouse are approximately 0.01, 0.02, and 0.05 times the estimated maximum clinical topical dose from ELOCON Ointment 0.1% on a mcg/m^2 basis).

In rats, mometasone furoate produced umbilical hernias at topical doses of 600 mcg/kg and above. A dose of 300 mcg/kg produced delays in ossification, but no malformations. (Doses of 300 and 600 mcg/kg in the rat are approximately 0.2 and 0.4 times the estimated maximum clinical topical dose from ELOCON Ointment 0.1% on a mcg/m^2 basis).

In rabbits, mometasone furoate caused multiple malformations (eg, flexed front paws, gallbladder agenesis, umbilical hernia, hydrocephaly) at topical doses of 150 mcg/kg and above (approximately 0.2 times the estimated maximum clinical topical dose from ELOCON Ointment 0.1% on a mcg/m^2 basis). In an oral study, mometasone furoate increased resorptions and caused cleft palate and/or head malformations (hydrocephaly and domed head) at 700 mcg/kg. At 2800 mcg/kg most litters were aborted or resorbed. No toxicity was observed at 140 mcg/kg. (Doses of 140, 700, and 2800 mcg/kg in the rabbit are approximately 0.2, 0.9, and 3.6 times the estimated maximum clinical topical dose from ELOCON Ointment 0.1% on a mcg/m^2 basis).

When rats received subcutaneous doses of mometasone furoate throughout pregnancy or during the later stages of pregnancy, 15 mcg/kg caused prolonged and difficult labor and reduced the number of live births, birth weight, and early pup survival. Similar effects were not observed at 7.5 mcg/kg. (Doses of 7.5 and 15 mcg/kg in the rat are approximately 0.005 and 0.01 times the estimated maximum clinical topical dose from ELOCON Ointment 0.1% on a mcg/m^2 basis).

There are no adequate and well-controlled studies of teratogenic effects from topically applied corticosteroids in pregnant women. Therefore, topical corticosteroids should be used during pregnancy only if the potential benefit justifies the potential risk to the fetus.

Nursing Mothers Systemically administered corticosteroids appear in human milk and could suppress growth, interfere with endogenous corticosteroid production, or cause other untoward effects. It is not known whether topical administration of corticosteroids could result in sufficient systemic absorption to produce detectable quantities in human milk. Because many drugs are excreted in human milk, caution should be exercised when ELOCON Ointment 0.1% is administered to a nursing woman.

Pediatric Use ELOCON Ointment 0.1% may be used with caution in pediatric patients 2 years of age or older, although the safety and efficacy of drug use for longer than 3 weeks have not been established. Use of ELOCON Ointment 0.1% is supported by results from adequate and well-controlled studies in pediatric patients with corticosteroid-responsive dermatoses. Since safety and efficacy of ELOCON Ointment 0.1% have not been adequately established in pediatric patients below 2 years of age, its use in this age group is not recommended.

ELOCON Ointment 0.1% caused HPA axis suppression in approximately 27% of pediatric patients ages 6 to 23 months, who showed normal adrenal function by Cortrosyn test before starting treatment, and were treated for approximately 3 weeks over a mean body surface area of 39% (range 15% to 99%). The criteria for suppression were: basal cortisol level of ≤5 mcg/dL, 30-minute post-stimulation level of ≤18 mcg/dL, or an increase of <7 mcg/dL. Follow-up testing 2 to 4 weeks after stopping treatment, available for 8 of the patients, demonstrated suppressed HPA axis function in 3 patients, using these same criteria. Long-term use of topical corticosteroids has not been studied in this population (see **CLINICAL PHARMACOLOGY – Pharmacokinetics**).

Because of a higher ratio of skin surface area to body mass, pediatric patients are at a greater risk than adults of HPA axis suppression and Cushing's syndrome when they are treated with topical corticosteroids. They are, therefore, also at greater risk of glucocorticosteroid insufficiency during and/or after withdrawal of treatment. Pediatric patients may be more susceptible than adults to skin atrophy, including striae, when they are treated with topical corticosteroids. Pediatric patients applying topical corticosteroids to greater than 20% of body surface are at higher risk of HPA axis suppression.

HPA axis suppression, Cushing's syndrome, linear growth retardation, delayed weight gain, and intracranial hypertension have been reported in children receiving topical corticosteroids. Manifestations of adrenal suppression in children include low plasma cortisol levels, and absence of response to ACTH stimulation. Manifestations of intracranial hypertension include bulging fontanelles, headaches, and bilateral papilledema.

ELOCON (mometasone furoate ointment, USP) Ointment 0.1% should not be used in the treatment of diaper dermatitis.

Geriatric Use Clinical studies of ELOCON Ointment 0.1% included 310 subjects who were 65 years of age and over and 57 subjects who were 75 years of age and over. No overall differences in safety or effectiveness were observed between these subjects and younger subjects, and other reported clinical experience has not identified differences in responses between the elderly and younger patients. However, greater sensitivity of some older individuals cannot be ruled out.

ADVERSE REACTIONS

In controlled clinical studies involving 812 patients, the incidence of adverse reactions associated with the use of ELOCON Ointment 0.1% was 4.8%. Reported reactions included burning, pruritus, skin atrophy, tingling/stinging, and furunculosis. Reports of rosacea associated with the use of ELOCON Ointment 0.1% have been received. In controlled clinical studies (n=74) involving pediatric patients 2 to 12 years of age, the incidence of adverse experiences associated with the use of ELOCON Cream is approximately 7%. Reported reactions included stinging, pruritus, and furunculosis.

The following adverse reactions were reported to be possibly or probably related to treatment with ELOCON Ointment 0.1% during a clinical study, in 5% of 63 pediatric patients 6 months to 2 years of age: decreased glucocorticoid levels, 1; an unspecified skin disorder, 1; and a bacterial skin infection, 1. The following signs of skin atrophy were also observed among 63 patients treated with ELOCON Ointment 0.1% in a clinical study: shininess 4, telangiectasia 1, loss of elasticity 4, loss of normal skin markings 4, thinness 1. Striae and bruising were not observed in this study.

The following additional local adverse reactions have been reported infrequently with topical corticosteroids, but may occur more frequently with the use of occlusive dressings. These reactions are listed in an approximate decreasing order of occurrence: irritation, dryness, folliculitis, hypertrichosis, acneiform eruptions, hypopigmentation, perioral dermatitis, allergic contact dermatitis, secondary infection, striae, and miliaria.

OVERDOSAGE

Topically applied ELOCON Ointment 0.1% can be absorbed in sufficient amounts to produce systemic effects (see **PRECAUTIONS**).

DOSAGE AND ADMINISTRATION

Apply a thin film of ELOCON Ointment 0.1% to the affected skin areas once daily. ELOCON Ointment 0.1% may be used in pediatric patients 2 years of age or older. Since safety and efficacy of ELOCON Ointment 0.1% have not been adequately established in pediatric patients below 2 years of age, its use in this age group is not recommended (see **PRECAUTIONS – Pediatric Use**).

As with other corticosteroids, therapy should be discontinued when control is achieved. If no improvement is seen within 2 weeks, reassessment of diagnosis may be necessary. Safety and efficacy of ELOCON Ointment 0.1% in pediatric patients for more than 3 weeks have not been established.

ELOCON Ointment 0.1% should not be used with occlusive dressings unless directed by a physician. ELOCON Ointment 0.1% should not be applied in the diaper area if the child still requires diapers or plastic pants as these garments may constitute occlusive dressing.

HOW SUPPLIED

ELOCON Ointment 0.1% is supplied in 15 g (NDC 0085-0370-01) and 45 g (NDC 0085-0370-02) tubes; boxes of one.
Store at 25°C (77°F); excursions permitted to 15–30°C (59–86°F).
[See USP Controlled Room Temperature]
Schering Corporation
Kenilworth, NJ 07033 USA
Rev. 11/02
17969544
18724235T
Copyright © 1987, 2003, Schering Corporation. All rights reserved.

INTRON® A
[in'tr-ŏn]
**Interferon alfa-2b, recombinant
For Injection**

Prescribing information for this product, which appears on pages 3038–3047 of the 2003 PDR, has been completely revised as follows. Please write "Supplement A" next to the product heading.

> **WARNING**
> Alpha interferons, including INTRON® A, cause or aggravate fatal or life-threatening neuropsychiatric, autoimmune, ischemic, and infectious disorders. Patients should be monitored closely with periodic clinical and laboratory evaluations. Patients with persistently severe or worsening signs or symptoms of these conditions should be withdrawn from therapy. In many but not all cases these disorders resolve after stopping INTRON A therapy. See **WARNINGS** and **ADVERSE REACTIONS.**

DESCRIPTION

INTRON A Interferon alfa-2b, recombinant for intramuscular, subcutaneous, intralesional, or intravenous Injection is a purified sterile recombinant interferon product.

Interferon alfa-2b, recombinant for Injection has been classified as an alfa interferon and is a water-soluble protein with a molecular weight of 19,271 daltons produced by recombinant DNA techniques. It is obtained from the bacterial fermentation of a strain of *Escherichia coli* bearing a genetically engineered plasmid containing an interferon alfa-2b gene from human leukocytes. The fermentation is carried out in a defined nutrient medium containing the antibiotic tetracycline hydrochloride at a concentration of 5 to 10 mg/L; the presence of this antibiotic is not detectable in the final product. The specific activity of Interferon alfa-2b, recombinant is approximately 2.6×10^8 IU/mg protein as measured by the HPLC assay.

[See first table at top of next page]

Prior to administration, the INTRON A Powder for Injection is to be reconstituted with the provided Diluent for INTRON A Interferon alfa-2b, recombinant for Injection (bacteriostatic water for injection) containing 0.9% benzyl alcohol as a preservative (see **DOSAGE AND ADMINISTRATION**) INTRON A Powder for Injection is a white to cream-colored powder.

[See second table on next page]
[See third table on next page]

These packages do not require reconstitution prior to administration (see **DOSAGE AND ADMINISTRATION**) INTRON A Solution for Injection is a clear, colorless solution.

CLINICAL PHARMACOLOGY

General The interferons are a family of naturally occurring small proteins and glycoproteins with molecular weights of approximately 15,000 to 27,600 daltons produced and secreted by cells in response to viral infections and to synthetic or biological inducers.

Preclinical Pharmacology Interferons exert their cellular activities by binding to specific membrane receptors on the cell surface. Once bound to the cell membrane, interferons initiate a complex sequence of intracellular events. *In vitro* studies demonstrated that these include the induction of certain enzymes, suppression of cell proliferation, immunomodulating activities such as enhancement of the phagocytic activity of macrophages and augmentation of the specific cytotoxicity of lymphocytes for target cells, and inhibition of virus replication in virus-infected cells.

In a study using human hepatoblastoma cell line, HB 611, the *in vitro* antiviral activity of alfa interferon was demonstrated by its inhibition of hepatitis B virus (HBV) replication.

The correlation between these *in vitro* data and the clinical results is unknown. Any of these activities might contribute to interferon's therapeutic effects.

Pharmacokinetics The pharmacokinetics of INTRON A Interferon alfa-2b, recombinant for Injection were studied in 12 healthy male volunteers following single doses of 5 million IU/m^2 administered intramuscularly, subcutaneously, and as a 30-minute intravenous infusion in a crossover design.

The mean serum INTRON A concentrations following intramuscular and subcutaneous injections were comparable. The maximum serum concentrations obtained via these routes were approximately 18 to 116 IU/mL and occurred 3 to 12 hours after administration. The elimination half-life of INTRON A Interferon alfa-2b, recombinant for Injection following both intramuscular and subcutaneous injections was approximately 2 to 3 hours. Serum concentrations were undetectable by 16 hours after the injections.

After intravenous administration, serum INTRON A concentrations peaked (135 to 273 IU/mL) by the end of the 30-minute infusion, then declined at a slightly more rapid rate than after intramuscular or subcutaneous drug administration, becoming undetectable 4 hours after the infusion. The elimination half-life was approximately 2 hours.

Urine INTRON A concentrations following a single dose (5 million IU/m^2) were not detectable after any of the parenteral routes of administration. This result was expected since preliminary studies with isolated and perfused rabbit kidneys have shown that the kidney may be the main site of interferon catabolism.

There are no pharmacokinetic data available for the intralesional route of administration.

Serum Neutralizing Antibodies In INTRON A treated patients tested for antibody activity in clinical trials, serum anti-interferon neutralizing antibodies were detected in 0% (0/90) of patients with hairy cell leukemia, 0.8% (2/260) of patients treated intralesionally for condylomata acuminata, and 4% (1/24) of patients with AIDS-Related Kaposi's Sarcoma. Serum neutralizing antibodies have been detected in <3% of patients treated with higher INTRON A doses in malignancies other than hairy cell leukemia or AIDS-Related Kaposi's Sarcoma. The clinical significance of the appearance of serum anti-interferon neutralizing activity in these indications is not known.

Serum anti-interferon neutralizing antibodies were detected in 7% (12/168) of patients either during treatment or after completing 12 to 48 weeks of treatment with 3 million IU TIW of INTRON A therapy for chronic hepatitis C and in 13% (6/48) of patients who received INTRON A therapy for chronic hepatitis B at 5 million IU QD for 4 months, and in 3% (1/33) of patients treated at 10 million IU TIW. Serum anti-interferon neutralizing antibodies were detected in 9% (5/53) of pediatric patients who received INTRON A therapy for chronic hepatitis B at 6 million IU/m² TIW. Among all chronic hepatitis B or C patients, pediatric and adults with detectable serum neutralizing antibodies, the titers detected were low (22/24 with titers ≤1:40 and 2/24 with titers ≤ 1:160). The appearance of serum anti-interferon neutralizing activity did not appear to affect safety or efficacy.

Hairy Cell Leukemia In clinical trials in patients with hairy cell leukemia, there was depression of hematopoiesis during the first 1 to 2 months of INTRON A treatment, resulting in reduced numbers of circulating red and white blood cells, and platelets. Subsequently, both splenectomized and non-splenectomized patients achieved substantial and sustained improvements in granulocytes, platelets, and hemoglobin levels in 75% of treated patients and at least some improvement (minor responses) occurred in 90%. INTRON A treatment resulted in a decrease in bone marrow hypercellularity and hairy cell infiltrates. The hairy cell index (HCI), which represents the percent of bone marrow cellularity times the percent of hairy cell infiltrate, was ≥50% at the beginning of the study in 87% of patients. The percentage of patients with such an HCI decreased to 25% after 6 months and to 14% after 1 year. These results indicate that even though hematologic improvement had occurred earlier, prolonged INTRON A treatment may be required to obtain maximal reduction in tumor cell infiltrates in the bone marrow.

The percentage of patients with hairy cell leukemia who required red blood cell or platelet transfusions decreased significantly during treatment and the percentage of patients with confirmed and serious infections declined as granulocyte counts improved. Reversal of splenomegaly and of clinically significant hypersplenism was demonstrated in some patients.

A study was conducted to assess the effects of extended INTRON A treatment on duration of response for patients who responded to initial therapy. In this study, 126 responding patients were randomized to receive additional INTRON A treatment for 6 months or observation for a comparable period, after 12 months of initial INTRON A therapy. During this 6-month period, 3% (2/66) of INTRON A treated patients relapsed compared with 18% (11/60) who were not treated. This represents a significant difference in time to relapse in favor of continued INTRON A treatment (p=0.006/0.01, Log Rank/ Wilcoxon). Since a small proportion of the total population had relapsed, median time to relapse could not be estimated in either group. A similar pattern in relapses was seen when all randomized treatment, including that beyond 6 months, and available follow-up data were assessed. The 15% (10/66) relapses among INTRON A patients occurred over a significantly longer period of time than the 40% (24/60) with observation (p=0.0002/0.0001, Log Rank/Wilcoxon). Median time to relapse was estimated, using the Kaplan-Meier method, to be 6.8 months in the observation group but could not be estimated in the INTRON A group.

Subsequent follow-up with a median time of approximately 40 months demonstrated an overall survival of 87.8%. In a comparable historical control group followed for 24 months, overall median survival was approximately 40%.

Malignant Melanoma The safety and efficacy of INTRON A Interferon alfa-2b, recombinant for Injection was evaluated as adjuvant to surgical treatment in patients with melanoma who were free of disease (postsurgery) but at high risk for systemic recurrence. These included patients with lesions of Breslow thickness >4 mm, or patients with lesions of any Breslow thickness with primary or recurrent nodal involvement. In a randomized, controlled trial in 280 patients, 143 patients received INTRON A therapy at 20 million IU/m² intravenously five times per week for 4 weeks (induction phase) followed by 10 million IU/m² subcutaneously three times per week for 48 weeks (maintenance phase). INTRON A therapy was begun ≤56 days after surgical resection. The remaining 137 patients were observed. INTRON A therapy produced a significant increase in relapse-free and overall survival. Median time to relapse for the INTRON A treated patients vs observation patients was 1.72 years vs 0.98 years (p<0.01, stratified Log Rank). The estimated 5-year relapse-free survival rate, using the Kaplan-Meier method, was 37% for INTRON A treated patients vs 26% for observation patients. Median overall survival time for INTRON A treated patients vs observation patients was 3.82 years vs 2.78 years (p=0.047, stratified Log Rank). The estimated 5-year overall survival rate, using the Kaplan-Meier method, was 46% for INTRON A treated patients vs 37% for observation patients.

In a second study of 642 resected high-risk melanoma patients, subjects were randomized equally to one of three groups: high-dose INTRON A therapy for 1 year (same schedule as above), low-dose INTRON A therapy for 2 years (3 MU/d TIW SC), and observation. Consistent with the earlier trial, high-dose INTRON A therapy demonstrated an improvement in relapse-free survival (3-year estimated RFS 48% vs 41%; median RFS 2.4 vs 1.6 years, p=not significant). Relapse-free survival in the low-dose INTRON A arm was similar to that seen in the observation arm. Neither high-dose nor low-dose INTRON A therapy showed a benefit in overall survival as compared to observation in this study.

Follicular Lymphoma The safety and efficacy of INTRON A in conjunction with CHVP, a combination chemotherapy regimen, was evaluated as initial treatment in patients with clinically aggressive, large tumor burden, Stage III/IV follicular Non-Hodgkin's Lymphoma. Large tumor burden was defined by the presence of any one of the following: a nodal or extranodal tumor mass with a diameter of >7 cm; involvement of at least three nodal sites (each with a diameter of >3 cm); systemic symptoms; splenomegaly; serous effusion, orbital or epidural involvement; ureteral compression; or leukemia.

In a randomized, controlled trial, 130 patients received CHVP therapy and 135 patients received CHVP therapy plus INTRON A therapy at 5 million IU subcutaneously three times weekly for the duration of 18 months. CHVP chemotherapy consisted of cyclophosphamide 600 mg/m², doxorubicin 25 mg/m², and teniposide (VM-26) 60 mg/m², administered intravenously on Day 1 and prednisone at a daily dose of 40 mg/m² given orally on Days 1 to 5. Treatment consisted of six CHVP cycles administered monthly, followed by an additional six cycles administered every 2 months for 1 year. Patients in both treatment groups received a total of 12 CHVP cycles over 18 months.

The group receiving the combination of INTRON A therapy plus CHVP had a significantly longer progression-free survival (2.9 years vs 1.5 years, p=0.0001, Log Rank test). After a median follow-up of 6.1 years, the median survival for patients treated with CHVP alone was 5.5 years while median survival for patients treated with CHVP plus INTRON A therapy had not been reached (p=0.004, Log Rank test). In three additional published, randomized, controlled studies of the addition of interferon alfa to anthracycline-containing combination chemotherapy regimens,[1–3] the addition of interferon alfa was associated with significantly prolonged progression-free survival. Differences in overall survival were not consistently observed.

Condylomata Acuminata Condylomata acuminata (venereal or genital warts) are associated with infections of the human papilloma virus (HPV). The safety and efficacy of INTRON A Interferon alfa-2b, recombinant for Injection in the treatment of condylomata acuminata were evaluated in three controlled double-blind clinical trials. In these studies, INTRON A doses of 1 million IU per lesion were administered intralesionally three times a week (TIW), in ≤5 lesions per patient for 3 weeks. The patients were observed for up to 16 weeks after completion of the full treatment course.

INTRON A treatment of condylomata was significantly more effective than placebo, as measured by disappearance of lesions, decreases in lesion size, and by an overall change in disease status. Of 192 INTRON A treated patients and 206 placebo treated patients who were evaluable for efficacy at the time of best response during the course of the study, 42% of INTRON A patients vs 17% of placebo patients experienced clearing of all treated lesions. Likewise, 24% of INTRON A patients vs 8% of placebo patients experienced marked (≥75% to <100%) reduction in lesion size, 18% vs 9% experienced moderate (≥50% to ≤75%) reduction in lesion size, 10% vs 42% had a slight (<50%) reduction in lesion size, 5% vs 24% had no change in lesion size, and 0% vs 1% experienced exacerbation (p<0.001).

In one of these studies, 43% (54/125) of patients in whom multiple (≤3) lesions were treated, experienced complete clearing of all treated lesions during the course of the study. Of these patients, 81% remained cleared 16 weeks after treatment was initiated.

Patients who did not achieve total clearing of all their treated lesions had these same lesions treated with a second course of therapy. During this second course of treatment, 38% to 67% of patients had clearing of all treated lesions. The overall percentage of patients who had cleared all their treated lesions after two courses of treatment ranged from 57% to 85%.

INTRON A treated lesions showed improvement within 2 to 4 weeks after the start of treatment in the above study; maximal response to INTRON A therapy was noted 4 to 8 weeks after initiation of treatment.

The response to INTRON A therapy was better in patients who had condylomata for shorter durations than in patients with lesions for a longer duration.

Another study involved 97 patients in whom three lesions were treated with either an intralesional injection of 1.5 million IU of INTRON A Interferon alfa-2b, recombinant for Injection per lesion followed by a topical application of 25% podophyllin, or a topical application of 25% podophyllin alone. Treatment was given once a week for 3 weeks. The

Continued on next page

Powder for Injection

Vial Strength	mL Diluent	Final Concentration after Reconstitution million IU/mL*	mg INTRON A† Interferon alfa-2b, recombinant	Route of Administration
5 MIU	1	5	0.019	IM, SC, IV
10 MIU	2	5	0.038	IM, SC, IV, IL††
18 MIU	1	18	0.069	IM, SC, IV
25 MIU	5	5	0.096	IM, SC, IV
50 MIU	1	50	0.192	IM, SC, IV

* Each mL also contains 20 mg glycine, 2.3 mg sodium phosphate dibasic, 0.55 mg sodium phosphate monobasic, and 1.0 mg human albumin.
† Based on the specific activity of approximately 2.6 × 10⁸ IU/mg protein, as measured by HPLC assay.
†† The 10 MIU vial for intralesional use should be reconstituted with 1 mL of the provided diluent.

Solution Vials for Injection

Vial Strength	Final Concentration*	mg INTRON A† Interferon alfa-2b, recombinant	Route of Administration
3 MIU	3 million IU/0.5 mL	0.012	IM, SC
5 MIU	5 million IU/0.5 mL	0.019	IM, SC, IL
10 MIU	10 million IU/1.0 mL	0.038	IM, SC, IL
18‡ MIU multidose	3 million IU/0.5 mL	0.088	IM, SC
25¶ MIU multidose	5 million IU/0.5 mL	0.123	IM, SC, IL

* Each mL contains 7.5 mg sodium chloride, 1.8 mg sodium phosphate dibasic, 1.3 mg sodium phosphate monobasic, 0.1 mg edetate disodium, 0.1 mg polysorbate 80, and 1.5 mg m-cresol as a preservative.
† Based on the specific activity of approximately 2.6 × 10⁸ IU/mg protein as measured by HPLC assay.
‡ This is a multidose vial which contains a total of 22.8 million IU of interferon alfa-2b, recombinant per 3.8 mL in order to provide the delivery of six 0.5-mL doses, each containing 3 million IU of INTRON A Interferon alfa-2b, recombinant for Injection (for a label strength of 18 million IU).
¶ This is a multidose vial which contains a total of 32.0 million IU of interferon alfa-2b, recombinant per 3.2 mL in order to provide the delivery of five 0.5-mL doses, each containing 5 million IU of INTRON A Interferon alfa-2b, recombinant for Injection (for a label strength of 25 million IU).

Solution in Multidose Pens for Injection

Pen Strength	Final Concentration*	INTRON A Dose Delivered (6 doses, 0.2 mL each)	mg INTRON A†	Route of Administration
18 MIU	22.5 MIU/1.5 mL	3 MIU/dose	0.087	SC
30 MIU	37.5 MIU/1.5 mL	5 MIU/dose	0.144	SC
60 MIU	75 MIU/1.5 mL	10 MIU/dose	0.288	SC

* Each mL also contains 7.5 mg sodium chloride, 1.8 mg sodium phosphate dibasic, 1.3 mg sodium phosphate monobasic, 0.1 mg edetate disodium, 0.1 mg polysorbate 80, and 1.5 mg m-cresol as a preservative.
† Based on the specific activity of approximately 2.6 × 10⁸ IU/mg protein as measured by HPLC assay.

Intron A—Cont.

combined treatment of INTRON A Interferon alfa-2b, recombinant for Injection and podophyllin was shown to be significantly more effective than podophyllin alone, as determined by the number of patients whose lesions cleared. This significant difference in response was evident after the second treatment (Week 3) and continued through 8 weeks posttreatment. At the time of the patient's best response, 67% (33/49) of the INTRON A Interferon alfa-2b, recombinant for Injection and podophyllin treated patients had all three treated lesions clear while 42% (20/48) of the podophyllin treated patients had all three clear (p=0.003).

AIDS-Related Kaposi's Sarcoma The safety and efficacy of INTRON A Interferon alfa-2b, recombinant for Injection in the treatment of Kaposi's Sarcoma (KS), a common manifestation of the Acquired Immune Deficiency Syndrome (AIDS), were evaluated in clinical trials in 144 patients.

In one study, INTRON A doses of 30 million IU/m^2 were administered subcutaneously three times per week (TIW), to patients with AIDS-Related KS. Doses were adjusted for patient tolerance. The average weekly dose delivered in the first 4 weeks was 150 million IU; at the end of 12 weeks this averaged 110 million IU/week; and by 24 weeks averaged 75 million IU/week.

Forty-four percent of asymptomatic patients responded vs 7% of symptomatic patients. The median time to response was approximately 2 months and 1 month, respectively, for asymptomatic and symptomatic patients. The median duration of response was approximately 3 months and 1 month, respectively, for the asymptomatic and symptomatic patients. Baseline T4/T8 ratios were 0.46 for responders vs 0.33 for nonresponders.

In another study, INTRON A doses of 35 million IU were administered subcutaneously, daily (QD), for 12 weeks. Maintenance treatment, with every other day dosing (QOD), was continued for up to 1 year in patients achieving antitumor and antiviral responses. The median time to response was 2 months and the median duration of response was 5 months in the asymptomatic patients.

In all studies, the likelihood of response was greatest in patients with relatively intact immune systems as assessed by baseline CD4 counts (interchangeable with T4 counts). Results at doses of 30 million IU/m^2 TIW and 35 million IU/QD were subcutaneously similar and are provided together in TABLE 1. This table demonstrates the relationship of response to baseline CD4 count in both asymptomatic and symptomatic patients in the 30 million IU/m^2 TIW and the 35 million IU/QD treatment groups.

In the 30 million IU study group, 7% (5/72) of patients were complete responders and 22% (16/72) of the patients were partial responders. The 35 million IU study had 13% (3/23 patients) complete responders and 17% (4/23) partial responders.

For patients who received 30 million IU TIW, the median survival time was longer in patients with CD4 >200 (30.7 months) than in patients with CD4 ≤200 (8.9 months). Among responders, the median survival time was 22.6 months vs 9.7 months in nonresponders.

TABLE 1
*RESPONSE BY BASELINE CD4 COUNT**
*IN **AIDS-RELATED KS** PATIENTS*
30 million IU/m^2
TIW, SC and 35 million IU QD, SC

	Asymptomatic		Symptomatic	
CD4<200	4/14	(29%)	0/19	(0%)
200≤CD4≤400	6/12	(50%)	0/5	(0%)
	} 58%			
CD4>400	5/7	(71%)	0/0	(0%)

*Data for CD4, and asymptomatic and symptomatic classification were not available for all patients.

Chronic Hepatitis C The safety and efficacy of INTRON A Interferon alfa-2b, recombinant for Injection in the treatment of chronic hepatitis C was evaluated in 5 randomized clinical studies in which an INTRON A dose of 3 million IU three times a week (TIW) was assessed. The initial three studies were placebo-controlled trials that evaluated a 6-month (24 week) course of therapy. In each of the three studies, INTRON A therapy resulted in a reduction in serum alanine aminotransferase (ALT) in a greater proportion of patients vs control patients at the end of 6 months of dosing. During the 6 months of follow-up, approximately 50% of the patients who responded maintained their ALT response. A combined analysis comparing pretreatment and posttreatment liver biopsies revealed histological improvement in a statistically significantly greater proportion of INTRON A treated patients compared to controls.

Two additional studies have investigated longer treatment durations (up to 24 months).[5,6] Patients in the two studies to evaluate longer duration of treatment had hepatitis with or without cirrhosis in the absence of decompensated liver disease. Complete response to treatment was defined as normalization of the final two serum ALT levels during the treatment period. A sustained response was defined as a complete response at the end of the treatment period with sustained normal ALT values lasting at least 6 months following discontinuation of therapy.

In Study 1, all patients were initially treated with INTRON A 3 million IU TIW subcutaneously for 24 weeks (run-in-period). Patients who completed the initial 24-week treatment period were then randomly assigned to receive no further treatment, or to receive 3 million IU TIW for an additional 48 weeks. In Study 2, patients who met the entry criteria were randomly assigned to receive INTRON A 3 million IU TIW subcutaneously for 24 weeks or to receive INTRON A 3 million IU TIW subcutaneously for 96 weeks. In both studies, patient follow-up was variable and some data collection was retrospective.

TABLE 2
SUSTAINED ALT RESPONSE RATE VS DURATION OF THERAPY
*IN **CHRONIC HEPATITIS C** PATIENTS*
INTRON A 3 Million IU TIW
Treatment Group—Number of Patients (%)*

Study Number	INTRON A 3 million IU 24 weeks of treatment		INTRON A 3 million IU 72 or 96 weeks of treatment†		Difference (Extended– 24 weeks) (95% CI)‡	
ALT response at the end of follow-up						
1	12/101	(12%)	23/104	(22%)	10%	(-3, 24)
2	9/67	(13%)	21/80	(26%)	13%	(-4, 30)
Combined Studies	**21/168**	**(12.5%)**	**44/184**	**(24%)**	**11.4%**	**(2, 21)**
ALT response at the end of treatment						
1	40/101	(40%)	51/104	(49%)	—	
2	32/67	(48%)	35/80	(44%)	—	

*Intent to treat groups.
† Study 1: 72 weeks of treatment; Study 2: 96 weeks of treatment.
‡ Confidence intervals adjusted for multiple comparisons due to 3 treatment arms in the study.

TABLE 3
*VIROLOGIC RESPONSE**
*IN **CHRONIC HEPATITIS B** PATIENTS*
Treatment Group†—Number of Patients (%)

Study Number	INTRON A 5 million IU QD		INTRON A 10 million IU TIW		Untreated Controls		P‡ Value
1[7]	15/38	(39%)	—	—	3/42	(7%)	0.0009
2	—	—	10/24	(42%)	1/22	(5%)	0.005
3[8]	—	—	13/24§	(54%)	2/27	(7%)§	NA§
All Studies	**15/38**	**(39%)**	**23/48**	**(48%)**	**6/91**	**(7%)**	—

*Loss of HBeAg and HBV DNA by 6 months posttherapy.
† Patients pretreated with prednisone not shown.
‡ INTRON A treatment group vs untreated control.
§ Untreated control patients evaluated after 24-week observation period. A subgroup subsequently received INTRON A therapy. A direct comparison is not applicable (NA).

Results show that longer durations of INTRON A therapy improved the sustained response rate (see TABLE 2). In patients with complete responses (CR) to INTRON A therapy after 6 months of treatment (149/352 [42%]), responses were less often sustained if drug was discontinued (21/70 [30%]) than if it was continued for 18 to 24 months (44/79 [56%]). Of all patients randomized, the sustained response rate in the patients receiving 18 or 24 months of therapy was 22% and 26%, respectively, in the two trials. In patients who did not have a CR by 6 months, additional therapy did not result in significantly more responses, since almost all patients who responded to therapy did so within the first 16 weeks of treatment.

A subset (<50%) of patients from the combined extended dosing studies had liver biopsies performed both before and after INTRON A treatment. Improvement in necroinflammatory activity as assessed retrospectively by the Knodell (Study 1) and Scheuer (Study 2) Histology Activity Indices was observed in both studies. A higher number of patients (58%, 45/78) improved with extended therapy than with shorter (6 months) therapy (38%, 34/89) in this subset.

REBETRON® Combination Therapy containing INTRON A and REBETOL® (ribavirin, USP) Capsules has been shown to provide a significant reduction in virologic load and improved histologic response in patients with compensated liver disease who have relapsed following therapy with alfa interferon alone and in patients previously untreated with alfa interferon. See REBETRON Combination Therapy package insert for additional information.

[See table 2 above]

Chronic Hepatitis B ***Adults*** The safety and efficacy of INTRON A Interferon alfa-2b, recombinant for Injection in the treatment of chronic hepatitis B were evaluated in three clinical trials in which INTRON A doses of 30 to 35 million IU per week were administered subcutaneously (SC), as either 5 million IU daily (QD), or 10 million IU three times a week (TIW) for 16 weeks vs no treatment. All patients were 18 years of age or older with compensated liver disease, and had chronic hepatitis B virus (HBV) infection (serum HBsAg positive for at least 6 months) and HBV replication (serum HBeAg positive). Patients were also serum HBV-DNA positive, an additional indicator of HBV replication, as measured by a research assay.[7,8] All patients had elevated serum alanine aminotransferase (ALT) and liver biopsy findings compatible with the diagnosis of chronic hepatitis. Patients with the presence of antibody to human immunodeficiency virus (anti-HIV) or antibody to hepatitis delta virus (anti-HDV) in the serum were excluded from the studies.

Virologic response to treatment was defined in these studies as a loss of serum markers of HBV replication (HBeAg and HBV DNA). Secondary parameters of response included loss of serum HBsAg, decreases in serum ALT, and improvement in liver histology.

In each of two randomized controlled studies, a significantly greater proportion of INTRON A treated patients exhibited a virologic response compared with untreated control patients (see TABLE 3). In a third study without a concurrent control group, a similar response rate to INTRON A therapy was observed. Pretreatment with prednisone, evaluated in two of the studies, did not improve the response rate and provided no additional benefit.

The response to INTRON A therapy was durable. No patient responding to INTRON A therapy at a dose of 5 million IU QD or 10 million IU TIW, relapsed during the follow-up period which ranged from 2 to 6 months after treatment ended. The loss of serum HBeAg and HBV DNA was maintained in 100% of 19 responding patients followed for 3.5 to 36 months after the end of therapy.

In a proportion of responding patients, loss of HBeAg was followed by the loss of HBsAg. HBsAg was lost in 27% (4/15) of patients who responded to INTRON A therapy at a dose of 5 million IU QD, and 35% (8/23) of patients who responded to 10 million IU TIW. No untreated control patient lost HBsAg in these studies.

[See table 3 above]

In an ongoing study to assess the long-term durability of virologic response, 64 patients responding to INTRON A therapy have been followed for 1.1 to 6.6 years after treatment; 95% (61/64) remain serum HBeAg negative and 49% (30/61) have lost serum HBsAg.

INTRON A therapy resulted in normalization of serum ALT in a significantly greater proportion of treated patients compared to untreated patients in each of two controlled studies (see TABLE 4). In a third study without a concurrent control group, normalization of serum ALT was observed in 50% (12/24) of patients receiving INTRON A therapy.

Virologic response was associated with a reduction in serum ALT to normal or near normal (≤1.5 × the upper limit of normal) in 87% (13/15) of patients responding to INTRON A therapy at 5 million IU QD, and 100% (23/23) of patients responding to 10 million IU TIW.

Improvement in liver histology was evaluated in Studies 1 and 3 by comparison of pretreatment and 6-month posttreatment liver biopsies using the semiquantitative Knodell Histology Activity Index.[9] No statistically significant difference in liver histology was observed in treated patients compared to control patients in Study 1. Although statistically significant histological improvement from baseline was observed in treated patients in Study 3 (p≤0.01), there was no control group for comparison. Of those patients exhibiting a virologic response following treatment with 5 million IU QD or 10 million IU TIW, histological improvement was observed in 85% (17/20) compared to 36% (9/25) of patients who were not virologic responders. The histological improvement was due primarily to decreases in severity of necrosis, degeneration, and inflammation in the periportal, lobular, and portal regions of the liver (Knodell Categories I + II + III). Continued histological improvement was observed in four responding patients who lost serum HBsAg and were followed 2 to 4 years after the end of INTRON A therapy.[10]

Pediatrics The safety and efficacy of INTRON A Interferon alfa-2b, recombinant for Injection in the treatment of chronic hepatitis B was evaluated in one randomized controlled trial of 149 patients ranging from 1 year to 17 years of age. Seventy-two patients were treated with 3 million IU/m^2 of INTRON A therapy administered subcutaneously three times a week (TIW) for 1 week; the dose was then escalated to 6 million IU/m^2 TIW for a minimum of 16 weeks up to 24 weeks. The maximum weekly dosage was 10 million IU TIW. Seventy-seven patients were untreated controls. Study entry and response criteria were identical to those described in the adult patient population.

Patients treated with INTRON A therapy had a better response (loss of HBV DNA and HBeAg at 24 weeks of follow up) compared to the untreated controls (24% [17/72] vs 10% [8/77] p=0.05). Sixteen of the 17 responders treated with INTRON A therapy remained HBV DNA and HBeAg negative and had a normal serum ALT 12 to 24 months after completion of treatment. Serum HBsAg became negative in 7 out of 17 patients who responded to INTRON A therapy. None of the control patients who had an HBV DNA and HBeAg response became HBsAg negative. At 24 weeks of follow up, normalization of serum ALT was similar in patients treated with INTRON A therapy (17%, 12/72) and in untreated control patients (16%, 12/77). Patients with a baseline HBV DNA <100 pg/mL were more likely to respond to INTRON A therapy than were patients with a baseline HBV DNA >100 pg/mL (35% vs 9%, respectively). Patients who contracted hepatitis B through maternal vertical transmission had lower response rates than those who contracted the disease by other means (5% vs 31%, respectively). There was no evidence that the effects on HBV DNA and HBeAg were limited to specific subpopulations based on age, gender, or race.

[See table 4 at right]

TABLE 4
*ALT RESPONSES**
*IN **CHRONIC HEPATITIS B** PATIENTS*
Treatment Group—Number of Patients (%)

Study Number	INTRON A 5 million IU QD		INTRON A 10 million IU TIW		Untreated Controls		P† Value
1	16/38	(42%)	—	—	8/42	(19%)	0.03
2	—	—	10/24	(42%)	1/22	(5%)	0.0034
3	—	—	12/24‡	(50%)	2/27	(7%)‡	NA‡
All Studies	**16/38**	**(42%)**	**22/48**	**(46%)**	**11/91**	**(12%)**	**—**

* Reduction in serum ALT to normal by 6 months posttherapy.
† INTRON A treatment group vs untreated control.
‡ Untreated control patients evaluated after 24-week observation period. A subgroup subsequently received INTRON A therapy. A direct comparison is not applicable (NA).

INDICATIONS AND USAGE

Hairy Cell Leukemia INTRON A Interferon alfa-2b, recombinant for Injection is indicated for the treatment of patients 18 years of age or older with hairy cell leukemia.

Malignant Melanoma INTRON A Interferon alfa-2b, recombinant for Injection is indicated as adjuvant to surgical treatment in patients 18 years of age or older with malignant melanoma who are free of disease but at high risk for systemic recurrence, within 56 days of surgery.

Follicular Lymphoma INTRON A Interferon alfa-2b, recombinant for Injection is indicated for the initial treatment of clinically aggressive (see **Clinical Experience**) follicular Non-Hodgkin's Lymphoma in conjunction with anthracycline-containing combination chemotherapy in patients 18 years of age or older. Efficacy of INTRON A therapy in patients with low-grade, low-tumor burden follicular Non-Hodgkin's Lymphoma has not been demonstrated.

Condylomata Acuminata INTRON A Interferon alfa-2b, recombinant for Injection is indicated for intralesional treatment of selected patients 18 years of age or older with condylomata acuminata involving external surfaces of the genital and perianal areas (see **DOSAGE AND ADMINISTRATION**).

The use of this product in adolescents has not been studied.

AIDS-Related Kaposi's Sarcoma INTRON A Interferon alfa-2b, recombinant for Injection is indicated for the treatment of selected patients 18 years of age or older with AIDS-Related Kaposi's Sarcoma. The likelihood of response to INTRON A therapy is greater in patients who are without systemic symptoms, who have limited lymphadenopathy and who have a relatively intact immune system as indicated by total CD4 count.

Chronic Hepatitis C INTRON A Interferon alfa-2b, recombinant for Injection is indicated for the treatment of chronic hepatitis C in patients 18 years of age or older with compensated liver disease who have a history of blood or blood-product exposure and/or are HCV antibody positive. Studies in these patients demonstrated that INTRON A therapy can produce meaningful effects on this disease, manifested by normalization of serum alanine aminotransferase (ALT) and reduction in liver necrosis and degeneration.

A liver biopsy should be performed to establish the diagnosis of chronic hepatitis. Patients should be tested for the presence of antibody to HCV. Patients with other causes of chronic hepatitis, including autoimmune hepatitis, should be excluded. Prior to initiation of INTRON A therapy, the physician should establish that the patient has compensated liver disease. The following patient entrance criteria for compensated liver disease were used in the clinical studies and should be considered before INTRON A treatment of patients with chronic hepatitis C:

- No history of hepatic encephalopathy, variceal bleeding, ascites, or other clinical signs of decompensation
- Bilirubin ≤2 mg/dL
- Albumin Stable and within normal limits
- Prothrombin Time <3 seconds prolonged
- WBC ≥3000/mm³
- Platelets ≥70,000/mm³

Serum creatinine should be normal or near normal.

Prior to initiation of INTRON A therapy, CBC and platelet counts should be evaluated in order to establish baselines for monitoring potential toxicity. These tests should be repeated at weeks 1 and 2 following initiation of INTRON A therapy, and monthly thereafter. Serum ALT should be evaluated at approximately 3-month intervals to assess response to treatment (see **DOSAGE AND ADMINISTRATION**).

Patients with preexisting thyroid abnormalities may be treated if thyroid-stimulating hormone (TSH) levels can be maintained in the normal range by medication. TSH levels must be within normal limits upon initiation of INTRON A treatment and TSH testing should be repeated at 3 and 6 months (see **PRECAUTIONS – Laboratory Tests**).

INTRON A in combination with REBETOL (ribavirin, USP) Capsules is indicated for the treatment of chronic hepatitis C in patients with compensated liver disease previously untreated with alfa interferon therapy or who have relapsed following alfa interferon therapy. See REBETRON Combination Therapy package insert for additional information.

Chronic Hepatitis B INTRON A Interferon alfa-2b, recombinant for Injection is indicated for the treatment of chronic hepatitis B in patients 1 year of age or older with compensated liver disease. Patients who have been serum HBsAg positive for at least 6 months and have evidence of HBV replication (serum HBeAg positive) with elevated serum ALT are candidates for treatment. Studies in these patients demonstrated that INTRON A therapy can produce virologic remission of this disease (loss of serum HBeAg), and normalization of serum aminotransferases. INTRON A therapy resulted in the loss of serum HBsAg in some responding patients.

Prior to initiation of INTRON A therapy, it is recommended that a liver biopsy be performed to establish the presence of chronic hepatitis and the extent of liver damage. The physician should establish that the patient has compensated liver disease. The following patient entrance criteria for compensated liver disease were used in the clinical studies and should be considered before INTRON A treatment of patients with chronic hepatitis B:

- No history of hepatic encephalopathy, variceal bleeding, ascites, or other signs of clinical decompensation
- Bilirubin Normal
- Albumin Stable and within normal limits
- Prothrombin Time *Adults* <3 seconds prolonged; *Pediatrics* ≤2 seconds prolonged
- WBC ≥4000/mm³
- Platelets *Adults* ≥100,000/mm³; *Pediatrics* ≥150,000/mm³

Patients with causes of chronic hepatitis other than chronic hepatitis B or chronic hepatitis C should not be treated with INTRON A Interferon alfa-2b, recombinant for Injection. CBC and platelet counts should be evaluated prior to initiation of INTRON A therapy in order to establish baselines for monitoring potential toxicity. These tests should be repeated at treatment weeks 1, 2, 4, 8, 12, and 16. Liver function tests, including serum ALT, albumin, and bilirubin, should be evaluated at treatment weeks 1, 2, 4, 8, 12, and 16. HBeAg, HBsAg, and ALT should be evaluated at the end of therapy, as well as 3- and 6-months posttherapy, since patients may become virologic responders during the 6-month period following the end of treatment. In clinical studies in adults, 39% (15/38) of responding patients lost HBeAg 1 to 6 months following the end of INTRON A therapy. Of responding patients who lost HBsAg, 58% (7/12) did so 1- to 6-months posttreatment.

A transient increase in ALT ≥2 × baseline value (flare) can occur during INTRON A therapy for chronic hepatitis B. In clinical trials in adults and pediatrics, this flare generally occurred 8 to 12 weeks after initiation of therapy and was more frequent in INTRON A responders (*adults* 63%, 24/38; *pediatrics* 59%, 10/17) than in nonresponders (*adults* 27%, 13/48; *pediatrics* 35%, 19/55). However, in adults and pediatrics, elevations in bilirubin ≥3 mg/dL (≥2 times ULN) occurred infrequently (*adults* 2%, 2/86; *pediatrics* 3%, 2/72) during therapy. When ALT flare occurs, in general, INTRON A therapy should be continued unless signs and symptoms of liver failure are observed. During ALT flare, clinical symptomatology and liver function tests including ALT, prothrombin time, alkaline phosphatase, albumin, and bilirubin, should be monitored at approximately 2-week intervals (see **WARNINGS**).

DOSAGE AND ADMINISTRATION

IMPORTANT: INTRON A Interferon alfa-2b, is packaged as 1) powder for reconstitution/injection; 2) solution for injection; and appropriate dosage form and strength; 3) solution in prefilled, multidose cartridges in a multidose pen device for subcutaneous injection. Not all dosage forms and strengths are appropriate for some indications. It is important that you carefully read the instructions below for the indication you are treating to ensure you are using an appropriate dosage form and strength.

INTRON A SOLUTION FOR INJECTION IS NOT RECOMMENDED FOR INTRAVENOUS ADMINISTRATION.

Hairy Cell Leukemia The recommended dosage of INTRON A Interferon alfa-2b, recombinant for Injection for the treatment of hairy cell leukemia is 2 million IU/m² administered intramuscularly (see **WARNINGS**) or subcutaneously 3 times a week for up to 6 months. Responding patients may benefit from continued treatment. **NOTE: The 50 million IU strength of the INTRON A Powder for Injection is NOT to be used for the treatment of hairy cell leukemia.** Higher doses are not recommended.

If severe adverse reactions develop, the dosage should be modified (50% reduction) or therapy should be temporarily discontinued until the adverse reactions abate. If persistent or recurrent intolerance develops following adequate dosage adjustment, or disease progresses, INTRON A treatment should be discontinued. The minimum effective INTRON A dose has not been established.

Malignant Melanoma The recommended INTRON A treatment regimen includes induction treatment 5 consecutive days per week for 4 weeks as an intravenous (IV) infusion at a dose of 20 million IU/m², followed by maintenance treatment three times per week for 48 weeks as a subcutaneous (SC) injection, at a dose of 10 million IU/m².

In the clinical trial, the median daily INTRON A doses administered to patients were 19.1 million IU/m² during the induction phase and 9.1 million IU/m² during the maintenance phase. **NOTE: INTRON A Solution for Injection is NOT recommended for intravenous administration and should not be used for the induction phase of malignant melanoma.**

Regular laboratory testing should be performed to monitor laboratory abnormalities for the purposes of dose modification (see **PRECAUTIONS – Laboratory Tests**). If adverse reactions develop during INTRON A treatment, particularly if granulocytes decrease to <500/mm³ or SGPT/SGOT rises to >5 × upper limit of normal, treatment should be temporarily discontinued until the adverse reactions abate. INTRON A treatment should be restarted at 50% of the previous dose. If intolerance persists after dose adjustments or if granulocytes decrease to <250/mm³ or SGPT/SGOT rises to >10 × upper limit of normal, INTRON A therapy should be discontinued.

Follicular Lymphoma The recommended dosage of INTRON A Interferon alfa-2b, recombinant for Injection is 5 million IU subcutaneously three times per week for up to 18 months in conjunction with an anthracycline-containing chemotherapy regimen.

In published reports, the doses of myelosuppressive drugs were reduced by 25% from those utilized in a full-dose CHOP regimen, and cycle length increased by 33% (eg, from 21 to 28 days) when an alfa interferon was added to the regimen.[1,4] The dosing regimen should be modified for evidence of serious toxicity. The following dose modification guidelines for hematologic toxicity were used in the clinical trial: the chemotherapy regimen was delayed if either the neutrophil count was <1500/mm³ or the platelet count was <75,000/mm³. Administration of INTRON A therapy was temporarily interrupted for a neutrophil count <1000/mm³, or a platelet count <50,000/mm³, or reduced by 50% to 2.5 MIU TIW for a neutrophil count >1000/mm³ but <1500/mm³.

Reinstitution of the initial INTRON A dose (5 million IU TIW) was tolerated after resolution of hematologic toxicity (≥1500/mm³).

INTRON A therapy should be discontinued if SGOT exceeds >5 × the upper limit of normal or serum creatinine >2.0 mg/dL (see **WARNINGS**).

Condylomata Acuminata The 10 million IU vial of INTRON A Powder for Injection must be reconstituted with 1 mL of Diluent for INTRON A Interferon alfa-2b, recombinant for Injection (bacteriostatic water for injection). Do not reconstitute the 10 million IU vial of INTRON A Powder for Injection with more than 1 mL of diluent since the injection would be subpotent. Do not use the 5 million, 18 million, 25 million, or 50 million IU vials of INTRON A Powder for Injection for the treatment of condylomata acuminata since the resulting reconstituted solution would be either hypertonic or an inappropriate concentration. Do not use the 3 million IU vial or the 18 million IU multidose vial of INTRON A Solution for Injection for the intralesional treatment of condylomata acuminata since the concentrations are inappropriate for such use.

Inject 1.0 million IU of INTRON A Interferon alfa-2b, recombinant for Injection (either 0.1 mL of reconstituted 10 million IU INTRON A Powder for Injection or 0.1 mL of the 5 million IU, 10 million IU, or 25 million IU strengths of INTRON A Solution for Injection, each having a final concentration of 10 million IU/mL) into each lesion three times per week on alternate days, for 3 weeks. The injection should be administered intralesionally using a Tuberculin or similar syringe and a 25- to 30-gauge needle. The needle should be directed at the center of the base of the wart and at an angle almost parallel to the plane of the skin (approximating that in the commonly used PPD test). This will deliver the interferon to the dermal core of the lesion, infiltrating the lesion and causing a small wheal. Care should be taken not to go beneath the lesion too deeply; subcutaneous injection should be avoided, since this area is below the base

Continued on next page

Intron A—Cont.

of the lesion. Do not inject too superficially since this will result in possible leakage, infiltrating only the keratinized layer, and not the dermal core. As many as five lesions can be treated at one time. To reduce side effects, INTRON A injections may be administered in the evening, when possible. Additionally, acetaminophen may be administered at the time of injection to alleviate some of the potential side effects.

The maximum response usually occurs 4 to 8 weeks after initiation of the first treatment course. If results at 12 to 16 weeks after the initial treatment course has concluded are not satisfactory, a second course of treatment using the above dosage schedule may be instituted providing that clinical symptoms and signs, or changes in laboratory parameters (liver function tests, WBC, and platelets) do not preclude such a course of action.

Patients with 6 to 10 condylomata may receive a second (sequential) course of treatment at the above dosage schedule, to treat up to five additional condylomata per course of treatment. Patients with greater than 10 condylomata may receive additional sequences depending on how large a number of condylomata are present.

AIDS-Related Kaposi's Sarcoma The recommended INTRON A dosage is 30 million IU/m^2 three times a week administered subcutaneously or intramuscularly. **NOTE: INTRON A Solution for Injection should NOT be used for AIDS-Related Kaposi's Sarcoma since the concentrations are inappropriate.** The 18 million and 25 million IU multidose strengths of the INTRON A Solution for Injection should not be used for the treatment of AIDS-Related Kaposi's Sarcoma since the concentrations are inappropriate. The selected dosage regimen should be maintained unless the disease progresses rapidly or severe intolerance is manifested. If severe adverse reactions develop, the dosage should be modified (50% reduction) or therapy should be temporarily discontinued until the adverse reactions abate. When patients initiate therapy at 30 million IU/m^2 TIW, the average dose tolerated at the end of 12 weeks of therapy is 110 million IU/week and 75 million IU/week at the end of 24 weeks of therapy.

When disease stabilization or a response to treatment occurs, treatment should continue until there is no further evidence of tumor or until discontinuation is required by evidence of a severe opportunistic infection or adverse effect.

Chronic Hepatitis C The recommended dosage of INTRON A Interferon alfa-2b, recombinant for Injection for the treatment of chronic hepatitis C is 3 million IU three times a week (TIW) administered subcutaneously or intramuscularly. **NOTE: The 10 million IU vial of INTRON A Solution for Injection should NOT be used for chronic hepatitis C.** In patients tolerating therapy with normalization of ALT at 16 weeks of treatment, INTRON A therapy should be extended to 18 to 24 months (72 to 96 weeks) at 3 million IU TIW to improve the sustained response rate (see **CLINICAL PHARMACOLOGY – Chronic Hepatitis C**). Patients who do not normalize their ALTs after 16 weeks of therapy rarely achieve a sustained response with extension of treatment. Consideration should be given to discontinuing these patients from therapy.

If severe adverse reactions develop during INTRON A treatment, the dose should be modified (50% reduction) or therapy should be discontinued as indicated below. If intolerance persists after dose adjustment, INTRON A therapy should be discontinued.

See REBETRON Combination Therapy package insert for dosing when used in combination with REBETOL (ribavirin, USP) Capsules.

Chronic Hepatitis B ***Adults*** The recommended dosage of INTRON A Interferon alfa-2b, recombinant for Injection for the treatment of chronic hepatitis B is 30 to 35 million IU per week, administered subcutaneously or intramuscularly, either as 5 million IU daily (QD) or as 10 million IU three times a week (TIW) for 16 weeks.

Pediatrics The recommended dosage of INTRON A Interferon alfa-2b, recombinant for Injection for the treatment of chronic hepatitis B is 3 million IU/m^2 three times a week (TIW) for the first week of therapy followed by dose escalation to 6 million IU/m^2 TIW (maximum of 10 million IU TIW) administered subcutaneously for a total therapy duration of 16 to 24 weeks. **NOTE: The 3 million IU single-use vial and the 18 million IU multidose vial of INTRON A Solution for Injection should NOT be used for chronic hepatitis B.**

If severe adverse reactions or laboratory abnormalities develop during INTRON A therapy, the dose should be modified (50% reduction), or discontinued if appropriate, until the adverse reactions abate. If intolerance persists after dose adjustment, INTRON A therapy should be discontinued.

For patients with decreases in white blood cell, granulocyte, or platelet counts, the following guidelines for dose modification should be followed:

INTRON A Dose	*White Blood Cell Count*	*Granulocyte Count*	*Platelet Count*
Reduce 50%	$<1.5 \times 10^9$/L	$<0.75 \times 10^9$/L	$<50 \times 10^9$/L
Permanently Discontinue	$<1.0 \times 10^9$/L	$<0.5 \times 10^9$/L	$<25 \times 10^9$/L

INTRON A therapy was resumed at up to 100% of the initial dose when white blood cell, granulocyte, and/or platelet counts returned to normal or baseline values.

INTRON A Interferon alfa-2b, recombinant Powder for Injection

	5 million IU	10 million IU	18 million IU	25 million IU	50 million IU‡
Chronic Hepatitis B	1 mL	1 mL			
Chronic Hepatitis C					
Hairy Cell Leukemia	1 mL	2 mL		5 mL	
AIDS-Related Kaposi's Sarcoma					1 mL
Condylomata Acuminata		1 mL*			
Malignant Melanoma induction phase†	1 mL	1 mL	1 mL	5 mL	1 mL
maintenance phase	1 mL	1 mL	1 mL		1 mL
Follicular Lymphoma	1 mL	1 mL		5 mL	

*IMPORTANT: For patients with condylomata acuminata, reconstitute the 10 million IU vial with only 1 mL of the diluent provided to reach a final concentration of 10 million IU/mL to be administered intralesionally.
† Based on the desired dose, the appropriate vial strengths should be reconstituted and administered intravenously.
‡ This vial strength should be used only for the treatment of patients with AIDS-Related Kaposi's Sarcoma or malignant melanoma since the concentration is inappropriate for all other indications.

INTRON A Interferon alfa-2b, recombinant Solution for Injection

	3 million IU	5 million IU	10 million IU	18 million IU multidose*	25 million IU multidose†
Chronic Hepatitis B		✓	✓		✓§
Chronic Hepatitis C	✓				
Hairy Cell Leukemia	✓	✓	✓	✓	✓
Condylomata Acuminata		✓	✓		✓
Malignant Melanoma	✓‡	✓	✓	✓‡	✓¶
Follicular Lymphoma		✓			

*This is a multidose vial which contains a total of 22.8 million IU of interferon alfa-2b, recombinant per 3.8 mL in order to provide the delivery of six 0.5-mL doses, each containing 3 million IU of INTRON A Interferon alfa-2b, recombinant for Injection (for a label strength of 18 million IU).
† This is a multidose vial which contains a total of 32 million IU of interferon alfa-2b, recombinant per 3.2 mL in order to provide the delivery of five 0.5-mL doses, each containing 5 million IU of INTRON A Interferon alfa-2b, recombinant for Injection (for a label strength of 25 million IU).
‡ Use only for dose reduction.
§ Use only for the 5 MIU daily regimen.
¶ Use only for maintenance treatment.

At the discretion of the physician, the patient may self-administer the medication. (see illustrated **PATIENT INFORMATION SHEET** for instructions).

Preparation and Administration of INTRON A Interferon alfa-2b, recombinant Powder for Injection for Intramuscular, Subcutaneous, or Intralesional Administration

Reconstitution of INTRON A Powder for Injection Inject the amount of Diluent for INTRON A Interferon alfa-2b, recombinant for Injection (bacteriostatic water for injection) stated in the chart below into the INTRON A vial. Swirl gently to hasten complete dissolution of the powder. The appropriate INTRON A dose should then be withdrawn and injected intramuscularly, subcutaneously, or intralesionally (see **PATIENT INFORMATION SHEET** for detailed instructions). After preparation and administration of the INTRON A injection, it is essential to follow the procedure for proper disposal of syringes and needles (see **PATIENT INFORMATION SHEET** for detailed instructions).

INTRON A Powder for Injection is not indicated for use in infants and should not be used in pediatric patients in this age group because when reconstituted with the provided diluent it contains benzyl alcohol (see **WARNINGS Chronic Hepatitis B**).

Preparation and Administration of INTRON A Interferon alfa-2b, recombinant Powder for Injection for Intravenous Infusion

The infusion solution should be prepared immediately prior to use. Based on the desired dose, the appropriate vial strength(s) of INTRON A Interferon alfa-2b, recombinant Powder for Injection should be reconstituted with the diluent provided. The appropriate INTRON A dose should then be withdrawn and injected into a 100-mL bag of 0.9% Sodium Chloride Injection, USP. The final concentration of INTRON A Interferon alfa-2b, recombinant for Injection should be not less than 10 million IU/100 mL. The prepared solution should be infused over a 20-minute period.

[See first table above]

Please refer to the **Patient Information Sheet** for detailed, step-by-step instructions on how to inject the INTRON A dose. After administration of INTRON A, it is essential to follow the procedure for proper disposal of syringes and needles.

Parenteral drug products should be inspected visually for particulate matter and discoloration prior to administration, whenever solution and container permit. INTRON A Interferon alfa-2b, recombinant for Injection may be administered using either sterilized glass or plastic disposable syringes.

Stability INTRON A Interferon alfa-2b, recombinant Powder for Injection provided in vials ranging from 5 to 50 million IU per vial, is stable at 45°C (113°F) for up to 7 days. After reconstitution with Diluent for INTRON A Interferon alfa-2b, recombinant for Injection (bacteriostatic water for injection) the solution is stable for 1 month at 2° to 8°C (36° to 46°F). The reconstituted solution is clear and colorless to light yellow.

Preparation and Administration of INTRON A Interferon alfa-2b, recombinant Solution for Injection

INTRON A Solution for Injection is supplied in single-use vials, multidose vials, and multidose pens. These Solutions for Injection do not require reconstitution prior to administration; the solution is clear and colorless. INTRON A Solution for Injection is not recommended for intravenous infusion.

Solution for Injection in Vials

For INTRON A Solution for Injection vials, the appropriate dose should be withdrawn from the vial and injected intramuscularly, subcutaneously, or intralesionally (5 million IU and 10 million IU single-use vials, and 25 million IU multidose vials only). The single-use 3, 5, and 10 million IU vials are supplied with B-D Safey-Lok* syringes. The Safety-Lok* syringe contains a plastic safety sleeve to be pulled over the needle after use. The syringe locks with an audible click when the green stripe on the safety sleeve covers the red stripe on the needle.

[See second table above]

Solution for Injection in Multidose Pens

The INTRON A Solution for Injection multidose pen contains a prefilled, multidose cartridge for subcutaneous administration. It is designed to deliver individual doses using a simple dial mechanism. The needles provided in the packaging should be used for the INTRON A Solution for Injection multidose pen only. A new needle is to be used each time a dose is delivered using the pen. To avoid the possible transmission of disease, each INTRON A Solution for Injection multidose pen is for single patient use only.

INTRON A Interferon alfa-2b, recombinant Solution in Multidose Pens

	3 million IU/0.2 mL*	5 million IU/0.2 mL**	10 million IU/0.2 mL***
Chronic Hepatitis B		✓	✓
Chronic Hepatitis C	✓		
Hairy Cell Leukemia	✓	✓	
Malignant Melanoma			✓

Follicular Lymphoma			✔

* The 3 million IU multidose pen contains a total of 22.5 million IU of interferon alfa-2b, recombinant per 1.5 mL in order to provide delivery of six 0.2-mL doses each containing 3 million IU of interferon alfa-2b, recombinant Solution for Injection (for a label strength of 18 million IU).

** The 5 million IU multidose pen contains a total of 37.5 million IU of interferon alfa-2b, recombinant per 1.5 mL in order to provide delivery of six 0.2-mL doses each containing 5 million IU of interferon alfa-2b, recombinant Solution for Injection (for a label strength of 30 million IU).

*** The 10 million IU multidose pen contains a total of 75 million IU of interferon alfa-2b, recombinant per 1.5 mL in order to provide delivery of six 0.2-mL doses each containing 10 million IU of interferon alfa-2b, recombinant Solution for Injection (for a label strength of 60 million IU).

Please refer to the **Patient Information Sheet** for detailed, step-by-step instructions on how to inject the INTRON A dose. After administration of INTRON A, it is essential to follow the procedure for proper disposal of syringes and needles.

Parenteral drug products should be inspected visually for particulate matter and discoloration prior to administration, whenever solution and container permit. INTRON A Interferon alfa-2b, recombinant for Injection may be administered using either sterilized glass or plastic disposable syringes.

Stability INTRON A Interferon alfa-2b, recombinant Solution for Injection multidose pens provided in strengths ranging from 18 to 60 million IU per pen is stable at 30°C (86°F) for up to 2 days. INTRON A Interferon alfa-2b, recombinant Solution for Injection provided in vials ranging from 3 to 25 million IU per vial, is stable at 35°C (95°F) for up to 7 days and at 30°C (86°F) for up to 14 days. The solution is clear and colorless.

CONTRAINDICATIONS

INTRON A Interferon alfa-2b, recombinant for Injection is contraindicated in patients with a history of hypersensitivity to interferon alfa or any component of the injection. REBETRON Combination Therapy containing INTRON A and REBETOL (ribavirin, USP) Capsules must not be used by women who are pregnant or by men whose female partners are pregnant. Extreme care must be taken to avoid pregnancy in female patients and in female partners of patients taking combination INTRON A/REBETOL therapy. Patients with autoimmune hepatitis must not be treated with combination INTRON A/REBETOL therapy. See REBETRON Combination Therapy package insert for additional information.

WARNINGS

General Moderate to severe adverse experiences may require modification of the patient's dosage regimen, or in some cases termination of INTRON A therapy. Because of the fever and other "flu-like" symptoms associated with INTRON A administration, it should be used cautiously in patients with debilitating medical conditions, such as those with a history of pulmonary disease (eg, chronic obstructive pulmonary disease), or diabetes mellitus prone to ketoacidosis. Caution should also be observed in patients with coagulation disorders (eg, thrombophlebitis, pulmonary embolism) or severe myelosuppression.

Patients with platelet counts of less than 50,000/mm³ should not be administered INTRON A Interferon alfa-2b, recombinant for Injection intramuscularly, but instead by subcutaneous administration.

INTRON A therapy should be used cautiously in patients with a history of cardiovascular disease. Those patients with a history of myocardial infarction and/or previous or current arrhythmic disorder who require INTRON A therapy should be closely monitored (see **Laboratory Tests**). Cardiovascular adverse experiences, which include hypotension, arrhythmia, or tachycardia of 150 beats per minute or greater, and rarely, cardiomyopathy and myocardial infarction have been observed in some INTRON A treated patients. Some patients with these adverse events had no history of cardiovascular disease. Transient cardiomyopathy was reported in approximately 2% of the AIDS-Related Kaposi's Sarcoma patients treated with INTRON A Interferon alfa-2b, recombinant for Injection. Hypotension may occur during INTRON A administration, or up to 2 days posttherapy, and may require supportive therapy including fluid replacement to maintain intravascular volume.

Supraventricular arrhythmias occurred rarely and appeared to be correlated with preexisting conditions and prior therapy with cardiotoxic agents. These adverse experiences were controlled by modifying the dose or discontinuing treatment, but may require specific additional therapy.
DEPRESSION AND SUICIDAL BEHAVIOR INCLUDING SUICIDAL IDEATION, SUICIDAL ATTEMPTS, AND COMPLETED SUICIDES HAVE BEEN REPORTED IN ASSOCIATION WITH TREATMENT WITH ALFA INTERFERONS, INCLUDING INTRON A THERAPY. Patients with a preexisting psychiatric condition, especially depression, or a history of severe psychiatric disorder should not be treated with INTRON A Interferon alfa-2b, recombinant for Injection.[11] INTRON A therapy should be discontinued for any patient developing severe depression or other psychiatric disorder during treatment. Obtundation and coma have also been observed in some patients, usually elderly, treated at higher doses. While these effects are usually rapidly reversible upon discontinuation of therapy, full resolution of symptoms has taken up to 3 weeks in a few severe episodes. Narcotics, hypnotics, or sedatives may be used concurrently with caution and patients should be closely monitored until the adverse effects have resolved.

Bone marrow toxicity INTRON A therapy suppresses bone marrow function and may result in severe cytopenias including very rare events of aplastic anemia. It is advised that complete blood counts (CBC) be obtained pretreatment and monitored routinely during therapy (see **PRECAUTIONS: Laboratory Tests**). INTRON A therapy should be discontinued in patients who develop severe decreases in neutrophil ($<0.5 \times 10^9$/L) or platelet counts ($<25 \times 10^9$/L) (see **DOSAGE AND ADMINISTRATION**: Guidelines for Dose Modification).

Ophthalmologic Disorders Decrease or loss of vision, retinopathy including macular edema, retinal artery or vein thrombosis, retinal hemorrhages and cotton wool spots; optic neuritis and papilledema may be induced or aggravated by treatment with Interferon alfa-2b or other alpha interferons. All patients should receive an eye examination at baseline. Patients with pre-existing ophthalmologic disorders (eg, diabetic or hypertensive retinopathy) should receive periodic ophthalmologic exams during interferon alpha treatment. Any patient who develops ocular symptoms should receive a prompt and complete eye examination. Interferon alfa-2b treatment should be discontinued in patients who develop new or worsening ophthalmologic disorders.

Infrequently, patients receiving INTRON A therapy developed thyroid abnormalities, either hypothyroid or hyperthyroid. The mechanism by which INTRON A Interferon alfa-2b, recombinant for Injection may alter thyroid status is unknown. Patients with preexisting thyroid abnormalities whose thyroid function cannot be maintained in the normal range by medication should not be treated with INTRON A Interferon alfa-2b, recombinant for Injection. Prior to initiation of INTRON A therapy, serum TSH should be evaluated. Patients developing symptoms consistent with possible thyroid dysfunction during the course of INTRON A therapy should have their thyroid function evaluated and appropriate treatment instituted. Therapy should be discontinued for patients developing thyroid abnormalities during treatment whose thyroid function cannot be normalized by medication. Discontinuation of INTRON A therapy has not always reversed thyroid dysfunction occurring during treatment.

Hepatotoxicity, including fatality, has been observed in interferon alfa treated patients, including those treated with INTRON A Interferon alfa-2b, recombinant for Injection. Any patient developing liver function abnormalities during treatment should be monitored closely and if appropriate, treatment should be discontinued.

Pulmonary infiltrates, pneumonitis and pneumonia, including fatality, have been observed in interferon alfa treated patients, including those treated with INTRON A Interferon alfa-2b, recombinant for Injection. The etiologic explanation for these pulmonary findings has yet to be established. Any patient developing fever, cough, dyspnea, or other respiratory symptoms should have a chest x-ray taken. If the chest x-ray shows pulmonary infiltrates or there is evidence of pulmonary function impairment, the patient should be closely monitored, and, if appropriate, interferon alfa treatment should be discontinued. While this has been reported more often in patients with chronic hepatitis C treated with interferon alfa, it has also been reported in patients with oncologic diseases treated with interferon alfa.

Rare cases of autoimmune diseases including thrombocytopenia, vasculitis, Raynaud's phenomenon, rheumatoid arthritis, lupus erythematosus, and rhabdomyolysis have been observed in patients treated with alfa interferons, including patients treated with INTRON A Interferon alfa-2b, recombinant for Injection. In very rare cases the event resulted in fatality. The mechanism by which these events develop and their relationship to interferon alfa therapy is not clear. Any patient developing an autoimmune disorder during treatment should be closely monitored and, if appropriate, treatment should be discontinued.

Diabetes mellitus and hyperglycemia have been observed rarely in patients treated with INTRON A Interferon alfa-2b, recombinant for Injection. Symptomatic patients should have their blood glucose measured and followed up accordingly. Patients with diabetes mellitus may require adjustment of their antidiabetic regimen.

The 50 million IU strength of the INTRON A Powder for Injection is not to be used for the treatment of hairy cell leukemia, condylomata acuminata, follicular lymphoma, chronic hepatitis C, or chronic hepatitis B. The 5 million, 18 million, and 25 million IU strengths of the INTRON A Powder for Injection are not to be used for the intralesional treatment of condylomata acuminata since the dilution required for the intralesional use would result in a hypertonic solution.

The INTRON A multidose pens, the 3 million IU vial, and the 18 million IU multidose vial of INTRON A Solution for Injection are not to be used for the treatment of condylomata acuminata. The INTRON A multidose pens and the 18 million and 25 million IU multidose vials of INTRON A Solution for Injection are not to be used for the treatment of AIDS-Related Kaposi's Sarcoma. INTRON A Solution for Injection is not recommended for the intravenous treatment of malignant melanoma.

The powder formulations of this product contain albumin, a derivative of human blood. Based on effective donor screening and product manufacturing processes, it carries an extremely remote risk for transmission of viral diseases. A theoretical risk for transmission of Creutzfeldt-Jakob disease (CJD) also is considered extremely remote. No cases of transmission of viral diseases or CJD have ever been identified for albumin.

AIDS-Related Kaposi's Sarcoma INTRON A therapy should not be used for patients with rapidly progressive visceral disease (see **CLINICAL PHARMACOLOGY**). Also of note, there may be synergistic adverse effects between INTRON A Interferon alfa-2b, recombinant for Injection and zidovudine. Patients receiving concomitant zidovudine have had a higher incidence of neutropenia than that expected with zidovudine alone. Careful monitoring of the WBC count is indicated in all patients who are myelosuppressed and in all patients receiving other myelosuppressive medications. The effects of INTRON A Interferon alfa-2b, recombinant for Injection when combined with other drugs used in the treatment of AIDS-Related disease are unknown.

Chronic Hepatitis C and Chronic Hepatitis B Patients with decompensated liver disease, autoimmune hepatitis or a history of autoimmune disease, and patients who are immunosuppressed transplant recipients should not be treated with INTRON A Interferon alfa-2b, recombinant for Injection. There are reports of worsening liver disease, including jaundice, hepatic encephalopathy, hepatic failure, and death following INTRON A therapy in such patients. Therapy should be discontinued for any patient developing signs and symptoms of liver failure.

Chronic hepatitis B patients with evidence of decreasing hepatic synthetic functions, such as decreasing albumin levels or prolongation of prothrombin time, who nevertheless meet the entry criteria to start therapy, may be at increased risk of clinical decompensation if a flare of aminotransferases occurs during INTRON A treatment. In such patients, if increases in ALT occur during INTRON A therapy for chronic hepatitis B, they should be followed carefully including close monitoring of clinical symptomatology and liver function tests, including ALT, prothrombin time, alkaline phosphatase, albumin, and bilirubin. In considering these patients for INTRON A therapy, the potential risks must be evaluated against the potential benefits of treatment.

INTRON A Interferon alfa-2b, recombinant Powder for Injection when reconstituted with the provided Diluent for INTRON A Interferon alfa-2b, recombinant for Injection (bacteriostatic water for injection) contains benzyl alcohol. There have been rare reports of death in infants associated with excessive exposure to benzyl alcohol. The amount of benzyl alcohol at which toxicity or adverse effects may occur in infants is not known. INTRON A **Powder for Injection** is not indicated for use in infants and should not be used in pediatric patients in this age group.

REBETRON Combination Therapy containing INTRON A and REBETOL (ribavirin, USP) Capsules was associated with hemolytic anemia. Hemoglobin <10 g/dL was observed in approximately 10% of patients in clinical trials. Anemia occurred within 1 to 2 weeks of initiation of ribavirin therapy. REBETRON Combination Therapy containing INTRON A and REBETOL is not recommended in patients with severe renal impairment and should be used with caution in patients with moderate renal impairment. See REBETRON Combination Therapy package insert for additional information.

PRECAUTIONS

General Acute serious hypersensitivity reactions (eg, urticaria, angioedema, bronchoconstriction, anaphylaxis) have been observed rarely in INTRON A treated patients; if such an acute reaction develops, the drug should be discontinued immediately and appropriate medical therapy instituted. Transient rashes have occurred in some patients following injection, but have not necessitated treatment interruption. While fever may be related to the flu-like syndrome reported commonly in patients treated with interferon, other causes of persistent fever should be ruled out.

There have been reports of interferon, including INTRON A Interferon alfa-2b, recombinant for Injection, exacerbating preexisting psoriasis and sarcoidosis as well as development of new sarcoidosis. Therefore, INTRON A therapy should be used in these patients only if the potential benefit justifies the potential risk.

Variations in dosage, routes of administration, and adverse reactions exist among different brands of interferon. Therefore, do not use different brands of interferon in any single treatment regimen.

Triglycerides Elevated triglyceride levels have been observed in patients treated with interferons including INTRON A therapy. Elevated triglyceride levels should be managed as clinically appropriate. Hypertriglyceridemia may result in pancreatitis. Discontinuation of INTRON A therapy should be considered for patients with persistently elevated triglycerides (eg, triglycerides > 1000 mg/dL) associated with symptoms of potential pancreatitis, such as abdominal pain, nausea, or vomiting.

Drug Interactions Interactions between INTRON A Interferon alfa-2b, recombinant for Injection and other drugs have not been fully evaluated. Caution should be exercised when administering INTRON A therapy in combination

Continued on next page

Intron A—Cont.

TREATMENT-RELATED ADVERSE EXPERIENCES BY INDICATION
Dosing Regimens
Percentage (%) of Patients*

	Malignant Melanoma 20 MIU/m² Induction (IV) 10 MIU/m² Maintenance (SC)	Follicular Lymphoma 5 MIU TIW/SC	Hairy Cell Leukemia 2 MIU/m² TIW/SC	Condylomata Acuminata 1 MIU lesion	AIDS-Related Kaposi's Sarcoma 30 MIU/m² TIW/SC	35 MIU QD/SC	Chronic Hepatitis C‖ 3 MIU TIW	5 MIU QD	Chronic Hepatitis B Adults 10 MIU/m² TIW	Pediatrics 6 MIU/m² TIW
ADVERSE EXPERIENCE	N=143	N=135	N=145	N=352	N=74	N=29	N=183	N=101	N=78	N=116
Application-Site Disorders										
injection site inflammation	—	1	20	—	—	—	5	3	—	—
other (≤5%)	burning, injection site bleeding, injection site pain, injection site reaction (5% in chronic hepatitis B pediatrics), itching									
Blood Disorders (<5%)	anemia, anemia hypochromic, granulocytopenia, hemolytic anemia, leukopenia, lymphocytosis, neutropenia (9% in chronic hepatitis C, 14% in chronic hepatitis B pediatrics), thrombocytopenia (10% in chronic hepatitis C) (bleeding 8% in malignant melanoma), thrombocytopenic purpura									
Body as a Whole										
facial edema	—	1	—	<1	—	10	<1	3	1	<1
weight decrease	3	13	<1	<1	5	3	10	2	5	3
other (≤5%)	allergic reaction, cachexia, dehydration, earache, hernia, edema, hypercalcemia, hyperglycemia, hypothermia, inflammation nonspecific, lymphadenitis, lymphadenopathy, mastitis, periorbital edema, poor peripheral circulation, peripheral edema (6% in follicular lymphoma), phlebitis superficial, scrotal/penile edema, thirst, weakness, weight increase									
Cardiovascular System Disorders (<5%)	angina, arrhythmia, atrial fibrillation, bradycardia, cardiac failure, cardiomegaly, cardiomyopathy, coronary artery disorder, extrasystoles, heart valve disorder, hematoma, hypertension (9% in chronic hepatitis C), hypotension, palpitations, phlebitis, postural hypotension, pulmonary embolism, Raynaud's disease, tachycardia, thrombosis, varicose vein									
Endocrine System Disorders (<5%)	aggravation of diabetes mellitus, goiter, gynecomastia, hyperglycemia, hyperthyroidism, hypertriglyceridemia, hypothyroidism, virilism									
Flu-like Symptoms										
fever	81	56	68	56	47	55	34	66	86	94
headache	62	21	39	47	36	21	43	61	44	57
chills	54	—	46	45	—	—	—	—	—	—
myalgia	75	16	39	44	34	28	43	59	40	27
fatigue	96	8	61	18	84	48	23	75	69	71
increased sweating	6	13	8	2	4	21	4	1	1	3
asthenia	—	63	7	—	11	—	40	5	15	5
rigors	2	7	—	—	30	14	16	38	42	30
arthralgia	6	8	8	9	—	3	16	19	8	15
dizziness	23	—	12	9	7	24	9	13	10	8
influenza-like symptoms	10	18	37	—	45	79	26	5	—	<1
back pain	—	15	19	6	1	3	—	—	—	—
dry mouth	1	2	19	—	22	28	5	6	5	—
chest pain	2	8	<1	<1	1	28	4	4	—	—
malaise	6	—	—	14	5	—	13	9	6	3
pain (unspecified)	15	9	18	3	3	3	—	—	—	—
other (<5%)	chest pain substernal, hyperthermia, rhinitis, rhinorrhea									
Gastrointestinal System Disorders										
diarrhea	35	19	18	2	18	45	13	19	8	12
anorexia	69	21	19	1	38	41	14	43	53	43
nausea	66	24	21	17	28	21	19	50	33	18
taste alteration	24	2	13	<1	5	7	2	10	—	—
abdominal pain	2	20	<5	1	5	21	16	5	4	23
loose stools	—	1	—	<1	—	10	2	2	—	2
vomiting	†	32	6	2	11	14	8	7	10	27
constipation	1	14	<1	—	1	10	4	5	—	2
gingivitis	2‡	7‡	—	—	—	14	—	1	—	—
dyspepsia	—	2	—	2	4	—	7	3	8	3
other (<5%)	abdominal ascites, abdominal distension, colitis, dysphagia, eructation, esophagitis, flatulence, gallstones, gastric ulcer, gastritis, gastroenteritis, gastrointestinal disorder (7% in follicular lymphoma), gastrointestinal hemorrhage, gastrointestinal mucosal discoloration, gingival bleeding, gum hyperplasia, halitosis, hemorrhoids, increased appetite, increased saliva, intestinal disorder, melena, mouth ulceration, mucositis, oral hemorrhage, oral leukoplakia, rectal bleeding after stool, rectal hemorrhage, stomatitis, stomatitis ulcerative, taste loss, tongue disorder, tooth disorder									
Liver and Biliary System Disorders (<5%)	abnormal hepatic function tests, biliary pain, bilirubinemia, hepatitis, increased lactate dehydrogenase, increased transaminases (SGOT/SGPT) (elevated SGOT 63% in malignant melanoma and 24% in follicular lymphoma), jaundice, right upper quadrant pain (15% in chronic hepatitis C), and very rarely, hepatic encephalopathy, hepatic failure, and death									
Musculoskeletal System Disorders										
musculoskeletal pain	—	18	—	—	—	—	21	9	1	10
other (<5%)	arteritis, arthritis, arthritis aggravated, arthrosis, bone disorder, bone pain, carpal tunnel syndrome, hyporeflexia, leg cramps, muscle atrophy, muscle weakness, polyarteritis nodosa, tendinitis, rheumatoid arthritis, spondylitis									
Nervous System and Psychiatric Disorders										
depression	40	9	6	3	9	28	19	17	6	4
paresthesia	13	13	6	1	3	21	5	6	3	<1
impaired concentration	—	1	—	<1	3	14	3	8	5	3
amnesia	§	1	<5	—	—	14	—	—	—	—
confusion	8	2	<5	4	12	10	1	—	—	2
hypoesthesia	—	1	<5	1	—	10	—	—	—	—
irritability	1	1	—	—	—	—	13	16	12	22
somnolence	1	2	<5	3	3	—	33¶	14	9	5
anxiety	1	9	5	<1	1	3	5	2	—	3
insomnia	5	4	—	<1	3	3	12	11	6	8
nervousness	1	1	—	1	—	3	2	3	—	3
decreased libido	1	1	<5	—	—	—	1	5	1	—
other (<5%)	abnormal coordination, abnormal dreaming, abnormal gait, abnormal thinking, aggravated depression, aggressive reaction, agitation (7% in chronic hepatitis B pediatrics) alcohol intolerance, apathy, aphasia, ataxia, Bell's palsy, CNS dysfunction, coma, convulsions, delirium, dysphonia, emotional lability, extrapyramidal disorder, feeling of ebriety, flushing, hearing disorder, hearing impairment, hot flashes, hyperesthesia, hyperkinesia, hypertonia, hypokinesia, impaired consciousness, labyrinthine disorder, loss of consciousness, manic depression, manic reaction, migraine, neuralgia, neuritis, neuropathy, neurosis, paresis, paroniria, parosmia, personality disorder, polyneuropathy, psychosis, speech disorder, stroke, suicidal ideation, suicide attempt, syncope, tinnitus, tremor, twitching, vertigo (8% in follicular lymphoma)									
Reproduction System Disorders (<5%)	amenorrhea (12% in follicular lymphoma), dysmenorrhea, impotence, leukorrhea, menorrhagia, menstrual irregularity, pelvic pain, penis disorder, sexual dysfunction, uterine bleeding, vaginal dryness									

(Table continued on next page)

TREATMENT-RELATED ADVERSE EXPERIENCES BY INDICATION (cont.)
Dosing Regimens
Percentage (%) of Patients*

	MALIGNANT MELANOMA $20\ MIU/m^2$ Induction (IV) $10\ MIU/m^2$ Maintenance (SC)	FOLLICULAR LYMPHOMA 5 MIU TIW/SC	HAIRY CELL LEUKEMIA $2\ MIU/m^2$ TIW/SC	CONDYLOMATA ACUMINATA 1 MIU lesion	AIDS-RELATED KAPOSI'S SARCOMA $30\ MIU/m^2$ TIW/SC	35 MIU QD/SC	CHRONIC HEPATITIS C[‖] 3 MIU TIW	5 MIU QD	CHRONIC HEPATITIS B Adults 10 MIU TIW	Pediatrics $6\ MIU/m^2$ TIW
ADVERSE EXPERIENCE	N=143	N=135	N=145	N=352	N=74	N=29	N=183	N=101	N=78	N=116
Resistance Mechanism Disorders										
moniliasis	—	1	—	<1	—	17	—	—	—	—
herpes simplex	1	2	—	1	—	3	1	5	—	—
other (<5%)	abscess, conjunctivitis, fungal infection, hemophilus, herpes zoster, infection, infection bacterial, infection nonspecific (7% in follicular lymphoma), infection parasitic, otitis media, sepsis, stye, trichomonas, upper respiratory tract infection, viral infection (7% in chronic hepatitis C)									
Respiratory System Disorders										
dyspnea	15	14	<1	—	1	34	3	5	—	—
coughing	6	13	<1	—	—	31	1	4	—	5
pharyngitis	2	8	<5	1	1	31	3	7	1	7
sinusitis	1	4	—	—	—	21	2	—	—	—
nonproductive coughing	2	7	—	—	—	14	0	1	—	—
nasal congestion	1	7	—	—	—	10	<1	4	—	—
other (≤5%)	asthma, bronchitis (10% in follicular lymphoma), bronchospasm, cyanosis, epistaxis (7% in chronic hepatitis B pediatrics), hemoptysis, hypoventilation, laryngitis, lung fibrosis, pleural effusion, orthopnea, pleural pain, pneumonia, pneumonitis, pneumothorax, rales, respiratory disorder, respiratory insufficiency, sneezing, tonsillitis, tracheitis, wheezing									
Skin and Appendages Disorders										
dermatitis	1	—	8	—	—	—	2	1	—	—
alopecia	29	23	8	—	12	31	28	26	38	17
pruritus	—	10	11	1	7	—	9	6	4	3
rash	19	13	25	—	9	10	5	8	1	5
dry skin	1	3	—	—	9	10	1	—	—	<1
other (<5%)	abnormal hair texture, acne, cellulitis, cyanosis of the hand, cold and clammy skin, dermatitis lichenoides, eczema, epidermal necrolysis, erythema, erythema nodosum, folliculitis, furunculosis, increased hair growth, lacrimal gland disorder, lacrimation, lipoma, maculopapular rash, melanosis, nail disorders, nonherpetic cold sores, pallor, peripheral ischemia, photosensitivity, pruritus genital, psoriasis, psoriasis aggravated, purpura (5% in chronic hepatitis C), rash erythematous, sebaceous cyst, skin depigmentation, skin discoloration, skin nodule, urticaria, vitiligo									
Urinary System Disorders (<5%)	albumin/protein in urine, cystitis, dysuria, hematuria, incontinence, increased BUN, micturition disorder, micturition frequency, nocturia, polyuria (10% in follicular lymphoma), renal insufficiency, urinary tract infection (5% in chronic hepatitis C)									
Vision Disorders (<5%)	abnormal vision, blurred vision, diplopia, dry eyes, eye pain, nystagmus, photophobia									

*Dash (—) indicates not reported
[†] Vomiting was reported with nausea as a single term
[‡] Includes stomatitis/mucositis
[§] Amnesia was reported with confusion as a single term
[‖] Percentages based upon a summary of all adverse events during 18 to 24 months of treatment
[¶] Predominantly lethargy

with other potentially myelosuppressive agents such as zidovudine. Concomitant use of alfa interferon and theophylline decreases theophylline clearance, resulting in a 100% increase in serum theophylline levels.

Information for Patients Patients receiving INTRON A treatment should be directed in its appropriate use, informed of benefits and risks associated with treatment, and referred to the **PATIENT INFORMATION SHEET**. This information is intended to aid in the safe and effective use of this medication. It is not a disclosure of all possible adverse or intended effects.

If home use is prescribed, a puncture-resistant container for the disposal of used syringes and needles should be supplied to the patient. Patients should be thoroughly instructed in the importance of proper disposal and cautioned against any reuse of needles and syringes. The full container should be disposed of according to the directions provided by the physician (see **PATIENT INFORMATION SHEET**).

Patients should be cautioned not to change brands of interferon without medical consultation as a change in dosage may result.

Patients receiving high INTRON A doses should be cautioned against performing tasks that would require complete mental alertness, such as operating machinery or driving a motor vehicle.

The most common adverse experiences occurring with INTRON A therapy are "flu-like" symptoms, such as fever, headache, fatigue, anorexia, nausea, or vomiting (see **ADVERSE REACTIONS**) and appear to decrease in severity as treatment continues. Some of these "flu-like" symptoms may be minimized by bedtime administration. Antipyretics may be used to prevent or partially alleviate the fever and headache. Another common adverse experience is thinning of the hair.

It is advised that patients be well hydrated, especially during the initial stages of treatment.

INTRON A in combination with REBETOL (ribavirin, USP) Capsules therapy must not be used by women who are pregnant or by men whose female partners are pregnant. Extreme care must be taken to avoid pregnancy in female patients and in female partners of patients taking INTRON A/REBETOL therapy. Combination INTRON A/REBETOL therapy should not be initiated until a report of a negative pregnancy test has been obtained immediately prior to initiation of therapy. See REBETRON Combination Therapy package insert for additional information.

Laboratory Tests In addition to those tests normally required for monitoring patients, the following laboratory tests are recommended for all patients on INTRON A therapy, prior to beginning treatment and then periodically thereafter.

- Standard hematologic tests – including hemoglobin, complete and differential white blood cell counts, and platelet count.
- Blood chemistries – electrolytes, liver function tests, and TSH.

Those patients who have preexisting cardiac abnormalities and/or are in advanced stages of cancer should have electrocardiograms taken prior to and during the course of treatment.

Mild-to-moderate leukopenia and elevated serum liver enzyme (SGOT) levels have been reported with intralesional administration of INTRON A Interferon alfa-2b, recombinant for Injection (see **ADVERSE REACTIONS**); therefore, the monitoring of these laboratory parameters should be considered.

Baseline chest x-rays are suggested and should be repeated if clinically indicated.

For malignant melanoma patients, differential WBC count and liver function tests should be monitored weekly during the induction phase of therapy and monthly during the maintenance phase of therapy.

For specific recommendations in chronic hepatitis C and chronic hepatitis B, see **INDICATIONS AND USAGE**.

Carcinogenesis, Mutagenesis, Impairment of Fertility Studies with INTRON A Interferon alfa-2b, recombinant for Injection have not been performed to determine carcinogenicity.

Interferon may impair fertility. In studies of interferon administration in nonhuman primates, menstrual cycle abnormalities have been observed. Decreases in serum estradiol and progesterone concentrations have been reported in women treated with human leukocyte interferon.[12] Therefore, fertile women should not receive INTRON A therapy unless they are using effective contraception during the therapy period. INTRON A therapy should be used with caution in fertile men.

Mutagenicity studies have demonstrated that INTRON A Interferon alfa-2b, recombinant for Injection is not mutagenic.

Studies in mice (0.1, 1.0 million IU/day), rats (4, 20, 100 million IU/kg/day), and cynomolgus monkeys (1.1 million IU/kg/day; 0.25, 0.75, 2.5 million IU/kg/day) injected with INTRON A Interferon alfa-2b, recombinant for Injection for up to 9 days, 3 months, and 1 month, respectively, have revealed no evidence of toxicity. However, in cynomolgus monkeys (4, 20, 100 million IU/kg/day) injected daily for 3 months with INTRON A Interferon alfa-2b, recombinant for Injection toxicity was observed at the mid and high doses and mortality was observed at the high dose.

However, due to the known species-specificity of interferon, the effects in animals are unlikely to be predictive of those in man.

INTRON A in combination with REBETOL (ribavirin, USP) Capsules should be used with caution in fertile men. See the REBETRON Combination Therapy package insert for additional information.

Pregnancy Category C INTRON A Interferon alfa-2b, recombinant for Injection has been shown to have abortifacient effects in *Macaca mulatta* (rhesus monkeys) at 15 and 30 million IU/kg (estimated human equivalent of 5 and 10 million IU/kg, based on body surface area adjustment for a 60 kg adult). There are no adequate and well-controlled studies in pregnant women. INTRON A therapy should be used during pregnancy only if the potential benefit justifies the potential risk to the fetus.

Pregnancy Category X applies to the REBETRON Combination Therapy containing INTRON A and REBETOL (ribavirin, USP) Capsules (see **CONTRAINDICATIONS**). See REBETRON Combination Therapy package insert for additional information.

Nursing Mothers It is not known whether this drug is excreted in human milk. However, studies in mice have shown that mouse interferons are excreted into the milk. Because of the potential for serious adverse reactions from the drug in nursing infants, a decision should be made whether to discontinue nursing or to discontinue INTRON A therapy, taking into account the importance of the drug to the mother.

Pediatric Use *General* Safety and effectiveness in pediatric patients below the age of 18 years have not been established for indications other than chronic hepatitis B.

Chronic Hepatitis B Safety and effectiveness in pediatric patients ranging in age from 1 to 17 years have been established based upon one controlled clinical trial (see **CLINICAL PHARMACOLOGY, INDICATIONS AND USAGE, DOSAGE AND ADMINISTRATION; Chronic Hepatitis B**). Safety and effectiveness in pediatric patients below the age of 1 year have not been established.

INTRON A Interferon alfa-2b, recombinant **Powder for Injection** when reconstituted with the provided Diluent for INTRON A Interferon alfa-2b, recombinant for Injection (bacteriostatic water for injection) contains benzyl alcohol and is not indicated for use in infants. There have been rare reports of death in infants associated with excessive exposure to benzyl alcohol. The amount of benzyl alcohol at which toxicity or adverse effects may occur in infants is not known (see **WARNINGS Chronic Hepatitis B**).

Geriatric Use In all clinical studies of INTRON A (interferon alfa-2b, recombinant), including studies as monotherapy and in combination with REBETOL (ribavirin, USP) Capsules, only a small percentage of the subjects were aged 65 and over. These numbers were too few to de-

Continued on next page

Intron A—Cont.

termine if they respond differently from younger subjects except for the clinical trials of INTRON A in combination with REBETOL, where elderly subjects had a higher frequency of anemia (67%) than did younger patients (28%).

In a database consisting of clinical study and postmarketing reports for various indications, cardiovascular adverse events and confusion were reported more frequently in elderly patients receiving INTRON A therapy compared to younger patients.

In general, INTRON A therapy should be administered to elderly patients cautiously, reflecting the greater frequency of decreased hepatic, renal, bone marrow, and/or cardiac function and concomitant disease or other drug therapy. INTRON A is known to be substantially excreted by the kidney, and the risk of adverse reactions to INTRON A may be greater in patients with impaired renal function. Because elderly patients often have decreased renal function, patients should be carefully monitored during treatment, and dose adjustments made based on symptoms and/or laboratory abnormalities (see **CLINICAL PHARMACOLOGY**, and **DOSAGE AND ADMINISTRATION**).

ADVERSE REACTIONS

General The adverse experiences listed below were reported to be possibly or probably related to INTRON A therapy during clinical trials. Most of these adverse reactions were mild to moderate in severity and were manageable. Some were transient and most diminished with continued therapy.

The most frequently reported adverse reactions were "flu-like" symptoms, particularly fever, headache, chills, myalgia, and fatigue. More severe toxicities are observed generally at higher doses and may be difficult for patients to tolerate. In addition, the following spontaneous adverse experiences have been reported during the marketing surveillance of INTRON A Interferon alfa-2b, recombinant for Injection: nephrotic syndrome, pancreatitis, psychosis, including hallucinations, renal failure, and renal insufficiency. Very rarely, INTRON A used alone or in combination with REBETOL (ribavirin, USP) Capsules may be associated with aplastic anemia. Rarely sarcoidosis or exacerbation of sarcoidosis has been reported.

[See table on pages 298 and 299]

OVERDOSAGE

There is limited experience with overdosage. Postmarketing surveillance includes reports of patients receiving a single dose as great as 10 times the recommended dose. In general, the primary effects of an overdosage are consistent with the effects seen with therapeutic doses of interferon alfa-2b. Hepatic enzyme abnormalities, renal failure, hemorrhage, and myocardial infarction have been reported with single administration overdoses and/or with longer durations of treatment than prescribed (see **ADVERSE REACTIONS**). Toxic effects after ingestion of interferon alfa-2b are not expected because interferons are poorly absorbed orally. Consultation with a poison center is recommended.

Treatment. There is no specific antidote for interferon alfa-2b. Hemodialysis and peritoneal dialysis are not considered effective for treatment of overdose.

HOW SUPPLIED

INTRON A Interferon alfa-2b, recombinant Powder for Injection INTRON A Interferon alfa-2b, recombinant Powder for Injection, 5 million IU per vial and Diluent for INTRON A Interferon alfa-2b, recombinant for Injection (bacteriostatic water for injection) 1 mL per vial; boxes containing 1 INTRON A vial and 1 vial of INTRON A Diluent (NDC 0085-0120-02).

INTRON A Interferon alfa-2b, recombinant Powder for Injection, 10 million IU per vial and Diluent for INTRON A Interferon alfa-2b, recombinant for Injection (bacteriostatic water for injection) 2 mL per vial; boxes containing 1 INTRON A vial and 1 vial of INTRON A Diluent (NDC 0085-0571-02).

INTRON A Interferon alfa-2b, recombinant Powder for Injection, 18 million IU per vial and Diluent for INTRON A Interferon alfa-2b, recombinant for Injection (bacteriostatic water for injection) 1 mL per vial; boxes containing 1 vial of INTRON A and 1 vial of INTRON A Diluent (NDC 0085-1110-01).

INTRON A Interferon alfa-2b, recombinant Powder for Injection, 25 million IU per vial and Diluent for INTRON A Interferon alfa-2b, recombinant for Injection (bacteriostatic water for injection) 5 mL per vial; boxes containing 1 INTRON A vial and 1 vial of INTRON A Diluent (NDC 0085-0285-02).

INTRON A Interferon alfa-2b, recombinant Powder for Injection, 50 million IU per vial and Diluent for INTRON A Interferon alfa-2b, recombinant for Injection (bacteriostatic water for injection) 1 mL per vial; boxes containing 1 INTRON A vial and 1 vial of INTRON A Diluent (NDC 0085-0539-01).

Store INTRON A Interferon alfa-2b, recombinant Powder for Injection both before and after reconstitution between 2° and 8°C (36° and 46°F).

INTRON A Interferon alfa-2b, recombinant Solution for Injection INTRON A Interferon alfa-2b, recombinant Solution for Injection, 6 doses of 3 million IU (18 million IU) multidose pen (22.5 million IU per 1.5 mL per pen); boxes containing 1 INTRON A multidose pen, six disposable needles and alcohol swabs (NDC 0085-1242-01).

INTRON A Interferon alfa-2b, recombinant Solution for Injection, 6 doses of 5 million IU (30 million IU) multidose pen (37.5 million IU per 1.5 mL per pen); boxes containing 1 INTRON A multidose pen, six disposable needles and alcohol swabs (NDC 0085-1235-01).

INTRON A Interferon alfa-2b, recombinant Solution for Injection, 6 doses of 10 million IU (60 million IU) multidose pen (75 million IU per 1.5 mL per pen); boxes containing 1 INTRON A multidose pen, six disposable needles and alcohol swabs (NDC 0085-1254-01).

INTRON A Interferon alfa-2b, recombinant Solution for Injection INTRON A, Pak-3, containing 6 INTRON A vials, 3 million IU per vial; 6 B-D Safety-Lok* syringes with a safety sleeve; and 6 alcohol swabs (NDC 0085-1184-02).

INTRON A Interferon alfa-2b, recombinant Solution for Injection INTRON A, Pak-5, containing 6 INTRON A vials, 5 million IU per vial; 6 B-D Safety-Lok* syringes with a safety sleeve; and 6 alcohol swabs (NDC 0085-1191-02).

INTRON A Interferon alfa-2b, recombinant Solution for Injection INTRON A, Pak-10, containing 6 INTRON A vials, 10 million IU per vial; 6 B-D Safety-Lok* syringes with a safety sleeve; and 6 alcohol swabs (NDC 0085-1179-02).

INTRON A Interferon alfa-2b, recombinant Solution for Injection, 18 million IU multidose vial (22.8 million IU per 3.8 mL per vial); boxes containing 1 vial of INTRON A Solution for Injection (NDC 0085-1168-01).

INTRON A Interferon alfa-2b, recombinant Solution for Injection, 25 million IU multidose vial (32 million IU per 3.2 mL per vial); boxes containing 1 vial of INTRON A Solution for Injection (NDC 0085-1133-01).

Store INTRON A Interferon alfa-2b, recombinant Solution for Injection between 2° and 8°C (36° and 46°F).

Rev. 6/02

Copyright © 1986, 1999, 2002, Schering Corporation. All rights reserved.

*Safety-Lok is a registered trademark of Becton Dickinson and Company.

Schering Corporation
Kenilworth, NJ 07033 USA
B-24937623

REFERENCES

1. Smalley R, et al. *N Engl J Med.* 1992;327:1336-1341.
2. Aviles A, et al. *Leukemia and Lymphoma.* 1996;20:495-499.
3. Unterhalt M, et al. *Blood.* 1996;88 (10Suppl 1):1744A.
4. Schiller J, et al. *J Biol Response Mod.* 1989;8:252-261.
5. Poynard T, et al. *N Engl J Med.* 1995;332:(22)1457-1462.
6. Lin R, et al. *J Hepatol.* 1995;23:487-496.
7. Perrillo R, et al. *N Engl J Med.* 1990;323:295-301.
8. Perez V, et al. *J Hepatol.* 1990;11:S113-S117.
9. Knodell R, et al. *Hepatology.* 1981;1:431-435.
10. Perrillo R, et al. *Ann Intern Med.* 1991;115:113-115.
11. Renault P, et al. *Arch Intern Med.* 1987;147:1577-1580.
12. Kauppila A, et al. *Int J Cancer.* 1982;29:291-294.

NASONEX® ℞

[*nā' zō-nĕks*]

(mometasone furoate monohydrate)
Nasal Spray, 50 mcg*
FOR INTRANASAL USE ONLY

*calculated on the anhydrous basis

Prescribing information for this product, which appears on pages 3052–3055 of the 2003 PDR, has been completely revised as follows. Please write "See Supplement A" next to the product heading.

DESCRIPTION

Mometasone furoate monohydrate, the active component of NASONEX Nasal Spray, 50 mcg, is an anti-inflammatory corticosteroid having the chemical name, 9,21-Dichloro-11β,17-dihydroxy-16α-methylpregna-1,4-diene-3,20-dione 17-(2 furoate) monohydrate, and the following chemical structure:

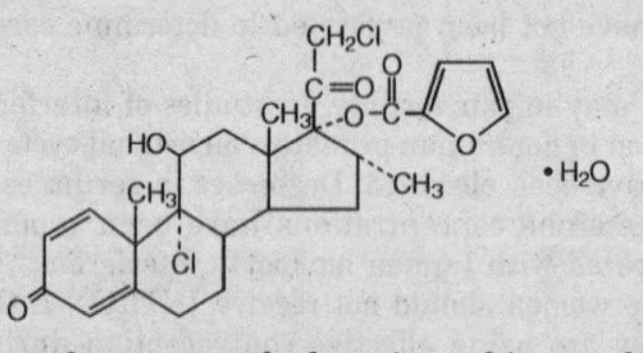

Mometasone furoate monohydrate is a white powder, with an empirical formula of $C_{27}H_{30}Cl_2O_6 \cdot H_2O$, and a molecular weight of 539.45. It is practically insoluble in water; slightly soluble in methanol, ethanol, and isopropanol; soluble in acetone and chloroform; and freely soluble in tetrahydrofuran. Its partition coefficient between octanol and water is greater than 5000.

NASONEX Nasal Spray, 50 mcg is a metered-dose, manual pump spray unit containing an aqueous suspension of mometasone furoate monohydrate equivalent to 0.05% w/w mometasone furoate calculated on the anhydrous basis; in an aqueous medium containing glycerin, microcrystalline cellulose and carboxymethylcellulose sodium, sodium citrate, 0.25% w/w phenylethyl alcohol, citric acid, benzalkonium chloride, and polysorbate 80. The pH is between 4.3 and 4.9.

After initial priming (10 actuations), each actuation of the pump delivers a metered spray containing 100 mg of suspension containing mometasone furoate monohydrate equivalent to 50 mcg of mometasone furoate calculated on the anhydrous basis. Each bottle of NASONEX Nasal Spray, 50 mcg provides 120 sprays.

CLINICAL PHARMACOLOGY

NASONEX Nasal Spray, 50 mcg is a corticosteroid demonstrating anti-inflammatory properties. The precise mechanism of corticosteroid action on allergic rhinitis is not known. Corticosteroids have been shown to have a wide range of effects on multiple cell types (eg, mast cells, eosinophils, neutrophils, macrophages, and lymphocytes) and mediators (eg, histamine, eicosanoids, leukotrienes, and cytokines) involved in inflammation.

In two clinical studies utilizing nasal antigen challenge, NASONEX Nasal Spray, 50 mcg decreased some markers of the early- and late-phase allergic response. These observations included decreases (vs placebo) in histamine and eosinophil cationic protein levels, and reductions (vs baseline) in eosinophils, neutrophils, and epithelial cell adhesion proteins. The clinical significance of these findings is not known.

The effect of NASONEX Nasal Spray, 50 mcg on nasal mucosa following 12 months of treatment was examined in 46 patients with allergic rhinitis. There was no evidence of atrophy and there was a marked reduction in intraepithelial eosinophilia and inflammatory cell infiltration (eg, eosinophils, lymphocytes, monocytes, neutrophils, and plasma cells).

Pharmacokinetics: ***Absorption:*** Mometasone furoate monohydrate administered as a nasal spray is virtually undetectable in plasma from adult and pediatric subjects despite the use of a sensitive assay with a lower quantitation limit (LOQ) of 50 pcg/mL.

Distribution: The *in vitro* protein binding for mometasone furoate was reported to be 98% to 99% in concentration range of 5 to 500 ng/mL.

Metabolism: Studies have shown that any portion of a mometasone furoate dose which is swallowed and absorbed undergoes extensive metabolism to multiple metabolites. There are no major metabolites detectable in plasma. Upon *in vitro* incubation, one of the minor metabolites formed is 6ß-hydroxy-mometasone furoate. In human liver microsomes, the formation of the metabolite is regulated by cytochrome P-450 3A4 (CYP3A4).

Elimination: Following intravenous administration, the effective plasma elimination half-life of mometasone furoate is 5.8 hours. Any absorbed drug is excreted as metabolites mostly via the bile, and to a limited extent, into the urine.

Special Populations: The effects of renal impairment, hepatic impairment, age, or gender on mometasone furoate pharmacokinetics have not been adequately investigated.

Pharmacodynamics: Three clinical pharmacology studies have been conducted in humans to assess the effect of NASONEX Nasal Spray, 50 mcg at various doses on adrenal function. In one study, daily doses of 200 and 400 mcg of NASONEX Nasal Spray, 50 mcg and 10 mg of prednisone were compared to placebo in 64 patients with allergic rhinitis. Adrenal function before and after 36 consecutive days of treatment was assessed by measuring plasma cortisol levels following a 6-hour Cortrosyn (ACTH) infusion and by measuring 24-hour urinary-free cortisol levels. NASONEX Nasal Spray, 50 mcg, at both the 200- and 400-mcg dose, was not associated with a statistically significant decrease in mean plasma cortisol levels post-Cortrosyn infusion or a statistically significant decrease in the 24-hour urinary-free cortisol levels compared to placebo. A statistically significant decrease in the mean plasma cortisol levels post-Cortrosyn infusion and 24-hour urinary-free cortisol levels was detected in the prednisone treatment group compared to placebo.

A second study assessed adrenal response to NASONEX Nasal Spray, 50 mcg (400 and 1600 mcg/day), prednisone (10 mg/day), and placebo, administered for 29 days in 48 male volunteers. The 24-hour plasma cortisol area under the curve (AUC_{0-24}), during and after an 8-hour Cortrosyn infusion and 24-hour urinary-free cortisol levels were determined at baseline and after 29 days of treatment. No statistically significant differences of adrenal function were observed with NASONEX Nasal Spray, 50 mcg compared to placebo.

A third study evaluated single, rising doses of NASONEX Nasal Spray, 50 mcg (1000, 2000, and 4000 mcg/day), orally administered mometasone furoate (2000, 4000, and 8000 mcg/day), orally administered dexamethasone (200, 400, and 800 mcg/day), and placebo (administered at the end of each series of doses) in 24 male volunteers. Dose administrations were separated by at least 72 hours. Determination of serial plasma cortisol levels at 8 AM and for the 24-hour period following each treatment were used to calculate the plasma cortisol area under the curve (AUC_{0-24}). In addition, 24-hour urinary-free cortisol levels were collected prior to initial treatment administration and during the period immediately following each dose. No statistically significant decreases in the plasma cortisol AUC, 8 AM cortisol levels, or 24-hour urinary-free cortisol levels were observed in volunteers treated with either NASONEX Nasal Spray, 50 mcg or oral mometasone, as compared with placebo treatment. Conversely, nearly all volunteers treated with the three doses of dexamethasone demonstrated abnormal 8 AM cortisol levels (defined as a cortisol level <10 mcg/dL), reduced 24-hour plasma AUC values, and decreased 24-hour urinary-free cortisol levels, as compared to placebo treatment.

Three clinical pharmacology studies have been conducted in pediatric patients to assess the effect of mometasone furoate nasal spray, on the adrenal function at daily doses of 50, 100, and 200 mcg vs placebo. In one study, adrenal function before and after 7 consecutive days of treatment was assessed in 48 pediatric patients with allergic rhinitis (ages 6 to 11 years) by measuring morning plasma cortisol and 24-hour urinary-free cortisol levels. Mometasone furoate nasal spray, at all three doses, was not associated with a statistically significant decrease in mean plasma cortisol levels or a statistically significant decrease in the 24-hour urinary-free cortisol levels compared to placebo. In the second study, adrenal function before and after 14 consecutive days of treatment was assessed in 48 pediatric patients (ages 3 to 5 years) with allergic rhinitis by measuring plasma cortisol levels following a 30-minute Cortrosyn infusion. Mometasone furoate nasal spray, 50 mcg, at all three doses (50, 100, and 200 mcg/day), was not associated with a statistically significant decrease in mean plasma cortisol levels post-Cortrosyn infusion compared to placebo. All patients had a normal response to Cortrosyn. In the third study, adrenal function before and after up to 42 consecutive days of once-daily treatment was assessed in 52 patients with allergic rhinitis (ages 2 to 5 years), 28 of whom received mometasone furoate nasal spray, 50 mcg per nostril (total daily dose 100 mcg), by measuring morning plasma cortisol and 24-hour urinary-free cortisol levels. Mometasone furoate nasal spray was not associated with a statistically significant decrease in mean plasma cortisol levels or a statistically significant decrease in the 24-hour urinary-free cortisol levels compared to placebo.

Clinical Studies

The efficacy and safety of NASONEX Nasal Spray, 50 mcg in the prophylaxis and treatment of seasonal allergic rhinitis and the treatment of perennial allergic rhinitis have been evaluated in 18 controlled trials, and one uncontrolled clinical trial, in approximately 3000 adults (ages 17 to 85 years) and adolescents (ages 12 to 16 years). This included 1757 males and 1453 females, including a total of 283 adolescents (182 boys and 101 girls) with seasonal allergic or perennial allergic rhinitis, treated with NASONEX Nasal Spray, 50 mcg at doses ranging from 50 to 800 mcg/day. The majority of patients were treated with 200 mcg/day. These trials evaluated the total nasal symptom scores that included stuffiness, rhinorrhea, itching, and sneezing. Patients treated with NASONEX Nasal Spray, 50 mcg, 200 mcg/day had a significant decrease in total nasal symptom scores compared to placebo-treated patients. No additional benefit was observed for mometasone furoate doses greater than 200 mcg/day. A total of 350 patients have been treated with NASONEX Nasal Spray, 50 mcg for 1 year or longer.

The efficacy and safety of NASONEX Nasal Spray, 50 mcg in the treatment of seasonal allergic and perennial allergic rhinitis in pediatric patients (ages 3 to 11 years) have been evaluated in four controlled trials. This included approximately 990 pediatric patients ages 3 to 11 years (606 males and 384 females) with seasonal allergic or perennial allergic rhinitis treated with mometasone furoate nasal spray at doses ranging from 25 to 200 mcg/day. Pediatric patients treated with NASONEX Nasal Spray, 50 mcg (100 mcg total daily dose, 374 patients) had a significant decrease in total nasal symptom (congestion, rhinorrhea, itching, and sneezing) scores, compared to placebo-treated patients. No additional benefit was observed for the 200-mcg mometasone furoate total daily dose in pediatric patients (ages 3 to 11 years). A total of 163 pediatric patients have been treated for 1 year.

In patients with seasonal allergic rhinitis, NASONEX Nasal Spray, 50 mcg, demonstrated improvement in nasal symptoms (vs placebo) within 11 hours after the first dose based on one single-dose, parallel-group study of patients in an outdoor "park" setting (park study) and one environmental exposure unit (EEU) study, and within 2 days in two randomized, double-blind, placebo-controlled, parallel-group seasonal allergic rhinitis studies. Maximum benefit is usually achieved within 1 to 2 weeks after initiation of dosing.

Prophylaxis of seasonal allergic rhinitis for patients 12 years of age and older with NASONEX Nasal Spray, 50 mcg, given at a dose of 200 mcg/day, was evaluated in two clinical studies in 284 patients. These studies were designed such that patients received 4 weeks of prophylaxis with NASONEX Nasal Spray, 50 mcg prior to the anticipated onset of the pollen season; however, some patients received only 2 to 3 weeks of prophylaxis. Patients receiving 2 to 4 weeks of prophylaxis with NASONEX Nasal Spray, 50 mcg demonstrated a statistically significantly smaller mean increase in total nasal symptom scores with onset of the pollen season as compared to placebo patients.

INDICATIONS AND USAGE

NASONEX Nasal Spray, 50 mcg is indicated for the treatment of the nasal symptoms of seasonal allergic and perennial allergic rhinitis, in adults and pediatric patients 2 years of age and older. NASONEX Nasal Spray, 50 mcg is indicated for the prophylaxis of the nasal symptoms of seasonal allergic rhinitis in adult and adolescent patients 12 years and older. In patients with a known seasonal allergen that precipitates nasal symptoms of seasonal allergic rhinitis, initiation of prophylaxis with NASONEX Nasal Spray, 50 mcg is recommended 2 to 4 weeks prior to the anticipated start of the pollen season. Safety and effectiveness of NASONEX Nasal Spray, 50 mcg in pediatric patients less than 2 years of age have not been established.

CONTRAINDICATIONS

Hypersensitivity to any of the ingredients of this preparation contraindicates its use.

WARNINGS

The replacement of a systemic corticosteroid with a topical corticosteroid can be accompanied by signs of adrenal insufficiency and, in addition, some patients may experience symptoms of withdrawal; ie, joint and/or muscular pain, lassitude, and depression. Careful attention must be given when patients previously treated for prolonged periods with systemic corticosteroids are transferred to topical corticosteroids, with careful monitoring for acute adrenal insufficiency in response to stress. This is particularly important in those patients who have associated asthma or other clinical conditions where too rapid a decrease in systemic corticosteroid dosing may cause a severe exacerbation of their symptoms.

If recommended doses of intranasal corticosteroids are exceeded or if individuals are particularly sensitive or predisposed by virtue of recent systemic steroid therapy, symptoms of hypercorticism may occur, including very rare cases of menstrual irregularities, acneiform lesions, and cushingoid features. If such changes occur, topical corticosteroids should be discontinued slowly, consistent with accepted procedures for discontinuing oral steroid therapy.

Persons who are on drugs which suppress the immune system are more susceptible to infections than healthy individuals. Chickenpox and measles, for example, can have a more serious or even fatal course in nonimmune children or adults on corticosteroids. In such children or adults who have not had these diseases, particular care should be taken to avoid exposure. How the dose, route, and duration of corticosteroid administration affects the risk of developing a disseminated infection is not known. The contribution of the underlying disease and/or prior corticosteroid treatment to the risk is also not known. If exposed to chickenpox, prophylaxis with varicella zoster immune globin (VZIG) may be indicated. If exposed to measles, prophylaxis with pooled intramuscular immunoglobulin (IG) may be indicated. (See the respective package inserts for complete VZIG and IG prescribing information.) If chickenpox develops, treatment with antiviral agents may be considered.

PRECAUTIONS

General:

Intranasal corticosteroids may cause a reduction in growth velocity when administered to pediatric patients (see **PRECAUTIONS, Pediatric Use** section). In clinical studies with NASONEX Nasal Spray, 50 mcg, the development of localized infections of the nose and pharynx with *Candida albicans* has occurred only rarely. When such an infection develops, use of NASONEX Nasal Spray, 50 mcg should be discontinued and appropriate local or systemic therapy instituted, if needed.

Nasal corticosteroids should be used with caution, if at all, in patients with active or quiescent tuberculous infection of the respiratory tract, or in untreated fungal, bacterial, systemic viral infections, or ocular herpes simplex.

Rarely, immediate hypersensitivity reactions may occur after the intranasal administration of mometasone furoate monohydrate. Extreme rare instances of wheezing have been reported.

Rare instances of nasal septum perforation and increased intraocular pressure have also been reported following the intranasal application of aerosolized corticosteroids. As with any long-term topical treatment of the nasal cavity, patients using NASONEX Nasal Spray, 50 mcg over several months or longer should be examined periodically for possible changes in the nasal mucosa.

Because of the inhibitory effect of corticosteroids on wound healing, patients who have experienced recent nasal septum ulcers, nasal surgery, or nasal trauma should not use a nasal corticosteroid until healing has occurred.

Glaucoma and cataract formation was evaluated in one controlled study of 12 weeks' duration and one uncontrolled study of 12 months' duration in patients treated with NASONEX Nasal Spray, 50 mcg at 200 mcg/day, using intraocular pressure measurements and slit lamp examination. No significant change from baseline was noted in the mean intraocular pressure measurements for the 141 NASONEX-treated patients in the 12-week study, as compared with 141 placebo-treated patients. No individual NASONEX-treated patient was noted to have developed a significant elevation in intraocular pressure or cataracts in this 12-week study. Likewise, no significant change from baseline was noted in the mean intraocular pressure measurements for the 139 NASONEX-treated patients in the 12-month study and again, no cataracts were detected in these patients. Nonetheless, nasal and inhaled corticosteroids have been associated with the development of glaucoma and/or cataracts. Therefore, close follow-up is warranted in patients with a change in vision and with a history of glaucoma and/or cataracts.

When nasal corticosteroids are used at excessive doses, systemic corticosteroid effects such as hypercorticism and adrenal suppression may appear. If such changes occur, NASONEX Nasal Spray, 50 mcg should be discontinued slowly, consistent with accepted procedures for discontinuing oral steroid therapy.

Information for Patients:

Patients being treated with NASONEX Nasal Spray, 50 mcg should be given the following information and instructions. This information is intended to aid in the safe and effective use of this medication. It is not a disclosure of all intended or possible adverse effects. Patients should use NASONEX Nasal Spray, 50 mcg at regular intervals (once daily) since its effectiveness depends on regular use. Improvement in nasal symptoms of allergic rhinitis has been shown to occur within 11 hours after the first dose based on one single-dose, parallel-group study of patients in an outdoor "park" setting (park study) and one environmental exposure unit (EEU) study and within 2 days after the first dose in two randomized, double-blind, placebo-controlled, parallel-group seasonal allergic rhinitis studies. Maximum benefit is usually achieved within 1 to 2 weeks after initiation of dosing. Patients should take the medication as directed and should not increase the prescribed dosage by using it more than once a day in an attempt to increase its effectiveness. Patients should contact their physician if symptoms do not improve, or if the condition worsens. To assure proper use of this nasal spray, and to attain maximum benefit, patients should read and follow the accompanying Patient's Instructions for Use carefully. Administration to young children should be aided by an adult.

Patients should be cautioned not to spray NASONEX Nasal Spray, 50 mcg into the eyes or directly onto the nasal septum.

Persons who are on immunosuppressant doses of corticosteroids should be warned to avoid exposure to chickenpox or measles, and patients should also be advised that if they are exposed, medical advice should be sought without delay.

Carcinogenesis, Mutagenesis, Impairment of Fertility:

In a 2-year carcinogenicity study in Sprague Dawley rats, mometasone furoate demonstrated no statistically significant increase in the incidence of tumors at inhalation doses up to 67 mcg/kg (approximately 3 and 2 times the maximum recommended daily intranasal dose in adults and children, respectively, on a mcg/m^2 basis). In a 19-month carcinogenicity study in Swiss CD-1 mice, mometasone furoate demonstrated no statistically significant increase in the incidence of tumors at inhalation doses up to 160 mcg/kg (approximately 3 and 2 times the maximum recommended daily intranasal dose in adults and children, respectively, on a mcg/m^2 basis).

Mometasone furoate increased chromosomal aberrations in an *in vitro* Chinese hamster ovary-cell assay, but did not increase chromosomal aberrations in an *in vitro* Chinese hamster lung cell assay. Mometasone furoate was not mutagenic in the Ames test or mouse-lymphoma assay, and was not clastogenic in an *in vivo* mouse micronucleus assay and a rat bone marrow chromosomal aberration assay or a mouse male germ-cell chromosomal aberration assay. Mometasone furoate also, did not induce unscheduled DNA synthesis *in vivo* in rat hepatocytes.

In reproductive studies in rats, impairment of fertility was not produced by subcutaneous doses up to 15 mcg/kg (less than the maximum recommended daily intranasal dose in adults on a mcg/m^2 basis).

Pregnancy: ***Teratogenic Effects: Pregnancy Category C:***

When administered to pregnant mice, rats and rabbits, mometasone furoate increased fetal malformations. The doses that produced malformations also decreased fetal growth, as measured by lower fetal weights and/or delayed ossification. Mometasone furoate also caused dystocia and related complications when administered to rats during the end of pregnancy.

In mice, mometasone furoate caused cleft palate at subcutaneous doses of 60 mcg/kg and above (approximately equivalent to the maximum recommended daily intranasal dose in adults on a mcg/m^2 basis). Fetal survival was reduced at 180 mcg/kg (approximately 4 times the maximum recommended daily intranasal dose in adults on a mcg/m^2 basis). No toxicity was observed at 20 mcg/kg (less than the maximum recommended daily intranasal dose in adults on a mcg/m^2 basis).

In rats, mometasone furoate produced umbilical hernia at topical dermal doses of 600 mcg/kg and above (approximately 25 times the maximum recommended daily intranasal dose in adults on a mcg/m^2 basis). A dose of 300 mcg/kg (approximately 10 times the maximum recommended daily intranasal dose in adults on a mcg/m^2 basis) produced delays in ossification, but no malformations.

In rabbits, mometasone furoate caused multiple malformations (eg, flexed front paws, gallbladder agenesis, umbilical hernia, hydrocephaly) at topical dermal doses of 150 mcg/kg and above (approximately 10 times the maximum recommended daily intranasal dose in adults on a mcg/m^2 basis). In an oral study, mometasone furoate increased resorptions and caused cleft palate and/or head malformations (hydrocephaly or domed head) at 700 mcg/kg (approximately 55 times the maximum recommended daily intranasal dose in adults on a mcg/m^2 basis). At 2800 mcg/kg (approximately 230 times the maximum recommended daily intranasal dose in adults on a mcg/m^2 basis), most litters were aborted or resorbed. No toxicity was observed at 140 mcg/kg (approximately 10 times the maximum recommended daily intranasal dose in adults on a mcg/m^2 basis).

When rats received subcutaneous doses of mometasone furoate throughout pregnancy or during the later stages of pregnancy, 15 mcg/kg (less than the maximum recommended daily intranasal dose in adults on a mcg/m^2 basis) caused prolonged and difficult labor and reduced the number of live births, birth weight and early pup survival. Similar effects were not observed at 7.5 mcg/kg (less than the maximum recommended daily intranasal dose in adults on a mcg/m^2 basis).

There are no adequate and well-controlled studies in pregnant women. NASONEX Nasal Spray, 50 mcg, like other

Continued on next page

Nasonex—Cont.

corticosteroids, should be used during pregnancy only if the potential benefits justify the potential risk to the fetus. Experience with oral corticosteroids since their introduction in pharmacologic, as opposed to physiologic, doses suggests that rodents are more prone to teratogenic effects from corticosteroids than humans. In addition, because there is a natural increase in corticosteroid production during pregnancy, most women will require a lower exogenous corticosteroid dose and many will not need corticosteroid treatment during pregnancy.

Nonteratogenic Effects:
Hypoadrenalism may occur in infants born to women receiving corticosteroids during pregnancy. Such infants should be carefully monitored.

Nursing Mothers:
It is not known if mometasone furoate is excreted in human milk. Because other corticosteroids are excreted in human milk, caution should be used when NASONEX Nasal Spray, 50 mcg is administered to nursing women.

Pediatric Use:
Controlled clinical studies have shown intranasal corticosteroids may cause a reduction in growth velocity in pediatric patients. This effect has been observed in the absence of laboratory evidence of hypothalamic-pituitary-adrenal (HPA) axis suppression, suggesting that growth velocity is a more sensitive indicator of systemic corticosteroid exposure in pediatric patients than some commonly used tests of HPA axis function. The long-term effects of this reduction in growth velocity associated with intranasal corticosteroids, including the impact on final adult height, are unknown. The potential for "catch up" growth following discontinuation of treatment with intranasal corticosteroids has not been adequately studied. The growth of pediatric patients receiving intranasal corticosteroids, including NASONEX Nasal Spray, 50 mcg should be monitored routinely (eg, via stadiometry). The potential growth effects of prolonged treatment should be weighed against clinical benefits obtained and the availability of safe and effective noncorticosteroid treatment alternatives. To minimize the systemic effects of intranasal corticosteroids, including NASONEX Nasal Spray, 50 mcg, each patient should be titrated to his/her lowest effective dose.

Seven hundred and twenty (720) patients 3 to 11 years of age were treated with mometasone furoate nasal spray, 50 mcg (100 mcg total daily dose) in controlled clinical trials (see **CLINICAL PHARMACOLOGY, Clinical Studies** section). Twenty-eight (28) patients 2 to 5 years of age were treated with mometasone furoate nasal spray, 50 mcg (100 mcg total daily dose) in a controlled trial to evaluate safety (see **CLINICAL PHARMACOLOGY, Pharmacokinetics** section). Safety and effectiveness in children less than 2 years of age have not been established.

A clinical study has been conducted for 1 year in pediatric patients (ages 3 to 9 years) to assess the effect of NASONEX Nasal Spray, 50 mcg (100 mcg total daily dose) on growth velocity. No statistically significant effect on growth velocity was observed for NASONEX Nasal Spray, 50 mcg compared to placebo. No evidence of clinically relevant HPA axis suppression was observed following a 30-minute Cosyntropin infusion.

The potential of NASONEX Nasal Spray, 50 mcg to cause growth suppression in susceptible patients or when given at higher doses cannot be ruled out.

Geriatric Use:
A total of 203 patients above 64 years of age (age range 64 to 85 years) have been treated with NASONEX Nasal Spray, 50 mcg for up to 3 months. The adverse reactions reported in this population were similar in type and incidence to those reported by younger patients.

ADVERSE REACTIONS

In controlled US and International clinical studies, a total of 3210 adult and adolescent patients ages 12 years and older received treatment with NASONEX Nasal Spray, 50 mcg at doses of 50 to 800 mcg/day. The majority of patients (n = 2103) were treated with 200 mcg/day. In controlled US and International studies, a total of 990 pediatric patients (ages 3 to 11 years) received treatment with NASONEX Nasal Spray, 50 mcg, at doses of 25 to 200 mcg/day. The majority of pediatric patients (720) were treated with 100 mcg/day. A total of 513 adult, adolescent, and pediatric patients have been treated for 1 year or longer. The overall incidence of adverse events for patients treated with NASONEX Nasal Spray, 50 mcg was comparable to patients treated with the vehicle placebo. Also, adverse events did not differ significantly based on age, sex, or race. Three percent or less of patients in clinical trials discontinued treatment because of adverse events; this rate was similar for the vehicle and active comparators.

All adverse events (regardless of relationship to treatment) reported by 5% or more of adult and adolescent patients ages 12 years and older who received NASONEX Nasal Spray, 50 mcg, 200 mcg/day and by pediatric patients ages 3 to 11 years who received NASONEX Nasal Spray, 50 mcg, 100 mcg/day in clinical trials vs placebo and that were more common with NASONEX Nasal Spray, 50 mcg than placebo, are displayed in the table below.

[See table below]

Other adverse events which occurred in less than 5% but greater than or equal to 2% of mometasone furoate adult and adolescent patients (ages 12 years and older) treated with 200-mcg doses (regardless of relationship to treatment), and more frequently than in the placebo group included: arthralgia, asthma, bronchitis, chest pain, conjunctivitis, diarrhea, dyspepsia, earache, flu-like symptoms, myalgia, nausea, and rhinitis.

Other adverse events which occurred in less than 5% but greater than or equal to 2% of mometasone furoate pediatric patients ages 3 to 11 years treated with 100-mcg doses vs placebo (regardless of relationship to treatment) and more frequently than in the placebo group included: diarrhea, nasal irritation, otitis media, and wheezing.

The adverse event (regardless of relationship to treatment) reported by 5% of pediatric patients ages 2 to 5 years who received NASONEX Nasal Spray, 50 mcg, 100 mcg/day in a clinical trial vs placebo including 56 subjects (28 each NASONEX Nasal Spray, 50 mcg and placebo) and that was more common with NASONEX Nasal Spray, 50 mcg than placebo, included: upper respiratory tract infection (7% vs 0%, respectively). The other adverse event which occurred in less than 5% but greater than or equal to 2% of mometasone furoate pediatric patients ages 2 to 5 years treated with 100 mcg doses vs placebo (regardless of relationship to treatment) and more frequently than in the placebo group included: skin trauma.

Rare cases of nasal ulcers and nasal and oral candidiasis were also reported in patients treated with NASONEX Nasal Spray, 50 mcg, primarily in patients treated for longer than 4 weeks.

In postmarketing surveillance of this product, cases of nasal burning and irritation, anaphylaxis and angioedema, and rare cases of nasal septal perforation have been reported.

OVERDOSAGE

There are no data available on the effects of acute or chronic overdosage with NASONEX Nasal Spray, 50 mcg. Because of low systemic bioavailability, and an absence of acute drug-related systemic findings in clinical studies, overdose is unlikely to require any therapy other than observation. Intranasal administration of 1600 mcg (8 times the recommended dose of NASONEX Nasal Spray, 50 mcg) daily for 29 days, to healthy human volunteers, was well tolerated with no increased incidence of adverse events. Single intranasal doses up to 4000 mcg have been studied in human volunteers with no adverse effects reported. Single oral doses up to 8000 mcg have been studied in human volunteers with no adverse effects reported. Chronic overdosage with any corticosteroid may result in signs or symptoms of hypercorticism (see **PRECAUTIONS**). Acute overdosage with this dosage form is unlikely since one bottle of NASONEX Nasal Spray, 50 mcg contains approximately 8500 mcg of mometasone furoate.

DOSAGE AND ADMINISTRATION

Adults and Children 12 Years of Age and Older:
The usual recommended dose for prophylaxis and treatment of the nasal symptoms of seasonal allergic rhinitis and treatment of the nasal symptoms of perennial allergic rhinitis is two sprays (50 mcg of mometasone furoate in each spray) in each nostril once daily (total daily dose of 200 mcg).

In patients with a known seasonal allergen that precipitates nasal symptoms of seasonal allergic rhinitis, prophylaxis with NASONEX Nasal Spray, 50 mcg (200 mcg/day) is recommended 2 to 4 weeks prior to the anticipated start of the pollen season.

Children 2 to 11 Years of Age:
The usual recommended dose for treatment of the nasal symptoms of seasonal allergic and perennial allergic rhinitis is one spray (50 mcg of mometasone furoate in each spray) in each nostril once daily (total daily dose of 100 mcg).

Improvement in nasal symptoms of allergic rhinitis has been shown to occur within 11 hours after the first dose based on one single-dose, parallel-group study of patients in an outdoor "park" setting (park study) and one environmental exposure unit (EEU) study and within 2 days after the first dose in two randomized, double-blind, placebo-controlled, parallel-group seasonal allergic rhinitis studies. Maximum benefit is usually achieved within 1 to 2 weeks. Patients should use NASONEX Nasal Spray, 50 mcg only once daily at a regular interval.

Prior to initial use of NASONEX Nasal Spray, 50 mcg, the pump must be primed by actuating ten times or until a fine spray appears. The pump may be stored unused for up to 1 week without repriming. If unused for more than 1 week, reprime by actuating two times, or until a fine spray appears.

Directions for Use:
Illustrated Patient's Instructions for Use accompany each package of NASONEX Nasal Spray, 50 mcg.

HOW SUPPLIED

NASONEX (mometasone furoate monohydrate) Nasal Spray, 50 mcg is supplied in a white, high-density, polyethylene bottle fitted with a white metered-dose, manual spray pump, and teal-green cap. It contains 17 g of product formulation, 120 sprays, each delivering 50 mcg of mometasone furoate per actuation. Supplied with Patient's Instructions for Use (NDC 0085-1197-01).

Store between 2° and 25°C (36° and 77°F). Protect from light.

When NASONEX Nasal Spray, 50 mcg is removed from its cardboard container, prolonged exposure of the product to direct light should be avoided. Brief exposure to light, as with normal use, is acceptable.

SHAKE WELL BEFORE EACH USE.

Schering Corporation
Kenilworth, NJ 07033 USA
Copyright © 1997, 1998, 1999, 2002, Schering Corporation. All rights reserved. Rev. 6/02
26405203T

ADVERSE EVENTS FROM CONTROLLED CLINICAL TRIALS IN SEASONAL ALLERGIC AND PERENNIAL ALLERGIC RHINITIS (PERCENT OF PATIENTS REPORTING)

	Adult and Adolescent Patients 12 years and older		Pediatric Patients Ages 3 to 11 years	
	NASONEX 200 mcg (n = 2103)	VEHICLE PLACEBO (n = 1671)	NASONEX 100 mcg (n = 374)	VEHICLE PLACEBO (n = 376)
Headache	26	22	17	18
Viral Infection	14	11	8	9
Pharyngitis	12	10	10	10
Epistaxis/Blood-Tinged Mucus	11	6	8	9
Coughing	7	6	13	15
Upper Respiratory Tract Infection	6	2	5	4
Dysmenorrhea	5	3	1	0
Musculoskeletal Pain	5	3	1	1
Sinusitis	5	3	4	4
Vomiting	1	1	5	4

NITRO-DUR® ℞

[*nī-trō-dur*]
(nitroglycerin)
Transdermal Infusion System

Prescribing information for this product, which appears on pages 3055–3057 of the 2003 PDR, has been completely revised as follows. Please write "See Supplement A" next to the product heading.

DESCRIPTION

Nitroglycerin is 1,2,3-propanetriol trinitrate, an organic nitrate whose structural formula is:

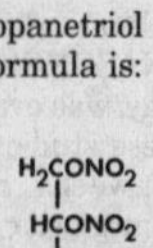
H_2CONO_2
$HCONO_2$
H_2CONO_2

and whose molecular weight is 227.09. The organic nitrates are vasodilators, active on both arteries and veins.

The NITRO-DUR (nitroglycerin) Transdermal Infusion System is a flat unit designed to provide continuous controlled release of nitroglycerin through intact skin. The rate of release of nitroglycerin is linearly dependent upon the area of the applied system; each cm^2 of applied system delivers approximately 0.02 mg of nitroglycerin per hour. Thus, the 5-, 10-, 15-, 20-, 30-, and 40-cm^2 systems deliver approximately 0.1, 0.2, 0.3, 0.4, 0.6, and 0.8 mg of nitroglycerin per hour, respectively.

The remainder of the nitroglycerin in each system serves as a reservoir and is not delivered in normal use. After 12 hours, for example, each system has delivered approximately 6% of its original content of nitroglycerin.

The NITRO-DUR transdermal system contains nitroglycerin in acrylic-based polymer adhesives with a resinous cross-linking agent to provide a continuous source of active ingredient. Each unit is sealed in a paper polyethylene-foil pouch.

Cross section of the system.

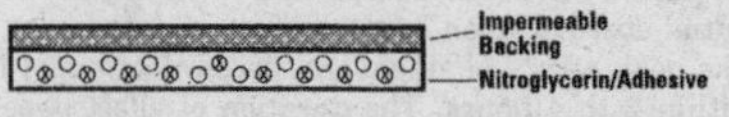

CLINICAL PHARMACOLOGY

The principal pharmacological action of nitroglycerin is relaxation of vascular smooth muscle and consequent dilatation of peripheral arteries and veins, especially the latter. Dilatation of the veins promotes peripheral pooling of blood and decreases venous return to the heart, thereby reducing left ventricular end-diastolic pressure and pulmonary capillary wedge pressure (preload). Arteriolar relaxation reduces systemic vascular resistance, systolic arterial pressure, and mean arterial pressure (afterload). Dilatation of the coronary arteries also occurs. The relative importance of preload reduction, afterload reduction, and coronary dilatation remains undefined.

Dosing regimens for most chronically used drugs are designed to provide plasma concentrations that are continuously greater than a minimally effective concentration. This strategy is inappropriate for organic nitrates. Several well-controlled clinical trials have used exercise testing to assess the antianginal efficacy of continuously delivered nitrates. In the large majority of these trials, active agents were indistinguishable from placebo after 24 hours (or less) of continuous therapy. Attempts to overcome nitrate tolerance by dose escalation, even to doses far in excess of those used acutely, have consistently failed. Only after nitrates have been absent from the body for several hours has their antianginal efficacy been restored.

Pharmacokinetics:

The volume of distribution of nitroglycerin is about 3 L/kg, and nitroglycerin is cleared from this volume at extremely rapid rates, with a resulting serum half-life of about 3 minutes. The observed clearance rates (close to 1 L/kg/min) greatly exceed hepatic blood flow; known sites of extrahepatic metabolism include red blood cells and vascular walls.

The first products in the metabolism of nitroglycerin are inorganic nitrate and the 1,2- and 1,3-dinitroglycerols. The dinitrates are less effective vasodilators than nitroglycerin, but they are longer-lived in the serum, and their net contribution to the overall effect of chronic nitroglycerin regimens is not known. The dinitrates are further metabolized to (nonvasoactive) mononitrates and, ultimately, to glycerol and carbon dioxide.

To avoid development of tolerance to nitroglycerin, drug-free intervals of 10 to 12 hours are known to be sufficient; shorter intervals have not been well studied. In one well-controlled clinical trial, subjects receiving nitroglycerin appeared to exhibit a rebound or withdrawal effect, so that their exercise tolerance at the end of the daily drug-free interval was *less* than that exhibited by the parallel group receiving placebo.

In healthy volunteers, steady-state plasma concentrations of nitroglycerin are reached by about 2 hours after application of a patch and are maintained for the duration of wearing the system (observations have been limited to 24 hours). Upon removal of the patch, the plasma concentration declines with a half-life of about an hour.

Clinical Trials:

Regimens in which nitroglycerin patches were worn for 12 hours daily have been studied in well-controlled trials up to 4 weeks in duration. Starting about 2 hours after application and continuing until 10 to 12 hours after application, patches that deliver at least 0.4 mg of nitroglycerin per hour have consistently demonstrated greater antianginal activity than placebo. Lower-dose patches have not been as well studied, but in one large, well-controlled trial in which higher-dose patches were also studied, patches delivering 0.2 mg/hr had significantly *less* antianginal activity than placebo.

It is reasonable to believe that the rate of nitroglycerin absorption from patches may vary with the site of application, but this relationship has not been adequately studied.

INDICATIONS AND USAGE

Transdermal nitroglycerin is indicated for the prevention of angina pectoris due to coronary artery disease. The onset of action of transdermal nitroglycerin is not sufficiently rapid for this product to be useful in aborting an acute attack.

CONTRAINDICATIONS

Allergic reactions to organic nitrates are extremely rare, but they do occur. Nitroglycerin is contraindicated in patients who are allergic to it. Allergy to the adhesives used in nitroglycerin patches has also been reported, and it similarly constitutes a contraindication to the use of this product.

WARNINGS

Amplification of the vasodilatory effects of the NITRO-DUR patch by sildenafil can result in severe hypotension. The time course and dose dependence of this interaction have not been studied. Appropriate supportive care has not been studied, but it seems reasonable to treat this as a nitrate overdose, with elevation of the extremities and with central volume expansion.

The benefits of transdermal nitroglycerin in patients with acute myocardial infarction or congestive heart failure have not been established. If one elects to use nitroglycerin in these conditions, careful clinical or hemodynamic monitoring must be used to avoid the hazards of hypotension and tachycardia.

A cardioverter/defibrillator should not be discharged through a paddle electrode that overlies a NITRO-DUR patch. The arcing that may be seen in this situation is harmless in itself, but it may be associated with local current concentration that can cause damage to the paddles and burns to the patient.

PRECAUTIONS

General:

Severe hypotension, particularly with upright posture, may occur with even small doses of nitroglycerin, particularly in the elderly. The NITRO-DUR Transdermal Infusion System should therefore be used with caution in elderly patients who may be volume-depleted, are on multiple medications, or who, for whatever reason, are already hypotensive. Hypotension induced by nitroglycerin may be accompanied by paradoxical bradycardia and increased angina pectoris.

Elderly patients may be more susceptible to hypotension and may be at greater risk of falling at the therapeutic doses of nitroglycerin.

Nitrate therapy may aggravate the angina caused by hypertrophic cardiomyopathy, particularly in the elderly.

In industrial workers who have had long-term exposure to unknown (presumably high) doses of organic nitrates, tolerance clearly occurs. Chest pain, acute myocardial infarction, and even sudden death have occurred during temporary withdrawal of nitrates from these workers, demonstrating the existence of true physical dependence.

Several clinical trials in patients with angina pectoris have evaluated nitroglycerin regimens which incorporated a 10- to 12-hour, nitrate-free interval. In some of these trials, an increase in the frequency of anginal attacks during the nitrate-free interval was observed in a small number of patients. In one trial, patients had decreased exercise tolerance at the end of the nitrate-free interval. Hemodynamic rebound has been observed only rarely; on the other hand, few studies were so designed that rebound, if it had occurred, would have been detected. The importance of these observations to the routine, clinical use of transdermal nitroglycerin is unknown.

Information for Patients:

Daily headaches sometimes accompany treatment with nitroglycerin. In patients who get these headaches, the headaches may be a marker of the activity of the drug. Patients should resist the temptation to avoid headaches by altering the schedule of their treatment with nitroglycerin, since loss of headache may be associated with simultaneous loss of antianginal efficacy.

Treatment with nitroglycerin may be associated with lightheadedness on standing, especially just after rising from a recumbent or seated position. This effect may be more frequent in patients who have also consumed alcohol.

After normal use, there is enough residual nitroglycerin in discarded patches that they are a potential hazard to children and pets.

A patient leaflet is supplied with the systems.

Drug Interactions:

The vasodilating effects of nitroglycerin may be additive with those of other vasodilators. Alcohol, in particular, has been found to exhibit additive effects of this variety.

Carcinogenesis, Mutagenesis, Impairment of Fertility:

Animal carcinogenesis studies with topically applied nitroglycerin have not been performed.

Rats receiving up to 434 mg/kg/day of dietary nitroglycerin for 2 years developed dose-related fibrotic and neoplastic changes in liver, including carcinomas, and interstitial cell tumors in testes. At high dose, the incidences of hepatocellular carcinomas in both sexes were 52% vs 0% in controls, and incidences of testicular tumors were 52% vs 8% in controls. Lifetime dietary administration of up to 1058 mg/kg/day of nitroglycerin was not tumorigenic in mice.

Nitroglycerin was weakly mutagenic in Ames tests performed in two different laboratories. Nevertheless, there was no evidence of mutagenicity in an *in vivo* dominant lethal assay with male rats treated with doses up to about 363 mg/kg/day, po, or in *in vitro* cytogenetic tests in rat and dog tissues.

In a three-generation reproduction study, rats received dietary nitroglycerin at doses up to about 434 mg/kg/day for 6 months prior to mating of the F_0 generation with treatment continuing through successive F_1 and F_2 generations. The high dose was associated with decreased feed intake and body weight gain in both sexes at all matings. No specific effect on the fertility of the F_0 generation was seen. Infertility noted in subsequent generations, however, was attributed to increased interstitial cell tissue and aspermatogenesis in the high-dose males. In this three-generation study there was no clear evidence of teratogenicity.

Pregnancy: Pregnancy Category C:

Animal teratology studies have not been conducted with nitroglycerin transdermal systems. Teratology studies in rats and rabbits, however, were conducted with topically applied nitroglycerin ointment at doses up to 80 mg/kg/day and 240 mg/kg/day, respectively.

No toxic effects on dams or fetuses were seen at any dose tested. There are no adequate and well-controlled studies in pregnant women. Nitroglycerin should be given to a pregnant woman only if clearly needed.

Nursing Mothers:

It is not known whether nitroglycerin is excreted in human milk. Because many drugs are excreted in human milk, caution should be exercised when nitroglycerin is administered to a nursing woman.

Pediatric Use:

Safety and effectiveness in pediatric patients have not been established.

Geriatric Use:

Clinical studies of NITRO-DUR Transdermal Infusion System did not include sufficient information to determine whether subjects 65 years and older respond differently from younger subjects. Additional clinical data from the published literature indicate that the elderly demonstrate increased sensitivity to nitrates, which may result in hypotension and increased risk of falling. In general, dose selection for an elderly patient should be cautious, usually starting at the low end of the dosing range, reflecting the greater frequency of the decreased hepatic, renal, or cardiac function, and of concomitant disease or other drug therapy.

ADVERSE REACTIONS

Adverse reactions to nitroglycerin are generally dose related, and almost all of these reactions are the result of nitroglycerin's activity as a vasodilator. Headache, which may be severe, is the most commonly reported side effect. Headache may be recurrent with each daily dose, especially at higher doses. Transient episodes of lightheadedness, occasionally related to blood pressure changes, may also occur. Hypotension occurs infrequently, but in some patients it may be severe enough to warrant discontinuation of therapy. Syncope, crescendo angina, and rebound hypertension have been reported but are uncommon.

Allergic reactions to nitroglycerin are also uncommon, and the great majority of those reported have been cases of contact dermatitis or fixed drug eruptions in patients receiving nitroglycerin in ointments or patches. There have been a few reports of genuine anaphylactoid reactions, and these reactions can probably occur in patients receiving nitroglycerin by any route.

Extremely rarely, ordinary doses of organic nitrates have caused methemoglobinemia in normal-seeming patients. Methemoglobinemia is so infrequent at these doses that further discussion of its diagnosis and treatment is deferred (see **OVERDOSAGE**).

Application-site irritation may occur but is rarely severe.

In two placebo-controlled trials of intermittent therapy with nitroglycerin patches at 0.2 to 0.8 mg/hr, the most frequent adverse reactions among 307 subjects were as follows:

	Placebo	Patch
Headache	18%	63%
Lightheadedness	4%	6%
Hypotension, and/or Syncope	0%	4%
Increased Angina	2%	2%

OVERDOSAGE

Hemodynamic Effects:

Nitroglycerin toxicity is generally mild. The estimated adult oral lethal dose of nitroglycerin is 200 mg to 1,200 mg. Infants may be more susceptible to toxicity from nitroglycerin. Consultation with a poison center should be considered.

Laboratory determinations of serum levels of nitroglycerin and its metabolites are not widely available, and such determinations have, in any event, no established role in the management of nitroglycerin overdose.

No data are available to suggest physiological maneuvers (eg, maneuvers to change the pH of the urine) that might accelerate elimination of nitroglycerin and its active metabolites. Similarly, it is not known which – if any – of these substances can usefully be removed from the body by hemodialysis.

No specific antagonist to the vasodilator effects of nitroglycerin is known, and no intervention has been subject to controlled study as a therapy of nitroglycerin overdose. Because the hypotension associated with nitroglycerin overdose is the result of venodilatation and arterial hypovolemia, prudent therapy in this situation should be directed toward increase in central fluid volume. Passive elevation of the patient's legs may be sufficient, but intravenous infusion of normal saline or similar fluid may also be necessary.

The use of epinephrine or other arterial vasoconstrictors in this setting is likely to do more harm than good.

In patients with renal disease or congestive heart failure, therapy resulting in central volume expansion is not without hazard. Treatment of nitroglycerin overdose in these patients may be subtle and difficult, and invasive monitoring may be required.

Methemoglobinemia:

Nitrate ions liberated during metabolism of nitroglycerin can oxidize hemoglobin into methemoglobin. Even in patients totally without cytochrome b_5 reductase activity, however, and even assuming that the nitrate moieties of nitroglycerin are quantitatively applied to oxidation of hemoglobin, about 1 mg/kg of nitroglycerin should be required before any of these patients manifests clinically significant ($\geq$10%) methemoglobinemia. In patients with normal reductase function, significant production of methemoglobin should require even larger doses of nitroglycerin. In one study in which 36 patients received 2 to 4 weeks of continuous nitroglycerin therapy at 3.1 to 4.4 mg/hr, the average methemoglobin level measured was 0.2%; this was comparable to that observed in parallel patients who received placebo.

Notwithstanding these observations, there are case reports of significant methemoglobinemia in association with moderate overdoses of organic nitrates. None of the affected patients had been thought to be unusually susceptible.

Methemoglobin levels are available from most clinical laboratories. The diagnosis should be suspected in patients who exhibit signs of impaired oxygen delivery despite adequate

Continued on next page

Nitro-Dur—Cont.

cardiac output and adequate arterial PO_2. Classically, methemoglobinemic blood is described as chocolate brown, without color change on exposure to air.
Methemoglobinemia should be treated with methylene blue if the patient develops cardiac or CNS effects of hypoxia. The intial dose is 1 to 2 mg/kg infused intravenously over 5 minutes. Repeat methemoglobin levels should be obtained 30 minutes later and a repeat dose of 0.5 to 1.0 mg/kg may be used if the level remains elevated and the patient is still symptomatic. Relative contraindications for methylene blue include known NADH methemoglobin reductase deficiency or G-6-PD deficiency. Infants under the age of 4 months may not respond to methylene blue due to immature NADH methemoglobin reductase. Exchange transfusion has been used successfully in critically ill patients when methemoglobinemia is refractory to treatment.

DOSAGE AND ADMINISTRATION

The suggested starting dose is between 0.2 mg/hr* and 0.4 mg/hr*. Doses between 0.4 mg/hr* and 0.8 mg/hr* have shown continued effectiveness for 10 to 12 hours daily for at least 1 month (the longest period studied) of intermittent administration. Although the minimum nitrate-free interval has not been defined, data show that a nitrate-free interval of 10 to 12 hours is sufficient (see **CLINICAL PHARMACOLOGY**). Thus, an appropriate dosing schedule for nitroglycerin patches would include a daily patch-on period of 12 to 14 hours and a daily patch-off period of 10 to 12 hours.

* Release rates were formerly described in terms of drug delivered per 24 hours. In these terms, the supplied NITRO-DUR systems would be rated at 2.5 mg/24 hours (0.1 mg/hour), 5 mg/24 hours (0.2 mg/hour), 7.5 mg/24 hours (0.3 mg/hour), 10 mg/24 hours (0.4 mg/hour), and 15 mg/24 hours (0.6 mg/hour).

Although some well-controlled clinical trials using exercise tolerance testing have shown maintenance of effectiveness when patches are worn continuously, the large majority of such controlled trials have shown the development of tolerance (ie, complete loss of effect) within the first 24 hours after therapy was initiated. Dose adjustment, even to levels much higher than generally used, did not restore efficacy.

HOW SUPPLIED

NITRO-DUR

System Rated Release *In Vivo**	Total Nitroglycerin Content	System Size	Package Size
0.1 mg/hr	20 mg	5 cm^2	Unit Dose 30 (NDC 0085-3305-30) Institutional Package 30 (NDC 0085-3305-35)
0.2 mg/hr	40 mg	10 cm^2	Unit Dose 30 (NDC 0085-3310-30) Institutional Package 30 (NDC 0085-3310-35)
0.3 mg/hr	60 mg	15 cm^2	Unit Dose 30 (NDC 0085-3315-30) Institutional Package 30 (NDC 0085-3315-35)
0.4 mg/hr	80 mg	20 cm^2	Unit Dose 30 (NDC 0085-3320-30) Institutional Package 30 (NDC 0085-3320-35)
0.6 mg/hr	120 mg	30 cm^2	Unit Dose 30 (NDC 0085-3330-30) Institutional Package 30 (NDC 0085-3330-35)
0.8 mg/hr	160 mg	40 cm^2	Unit Dose 30 (NDC 0085-0819-30) Institutional Package 30 (NDC 0085-0819-35)

* Release rates were formerly described in terms of drug delivered per 24 hours. In these terms, the supplied NITRO-DUR systems would be rated at 2.5 mg/24 hours (0.1 mg/hour), 5 mg/24 hours (0.2 mg/hour), 7.5 mg/24 hours (0.3 mg/hour), 10 mg/24 hours (0.4 mg/hour), and 15 mg/24 hours (0.6 mg/hour).

Store between 15° and 30°C (59° and 86°F). Do not refrigerate.
Rx only
Key Pharmaceuticals, Inc.
Kenilworth, NJ 07033 USA
Rev. 11/02 18143674
U.S. Patent No. 5,186,938
Copyright © 1987, 2002, Key Pharmaceuticals, Inc.
All rights reserved.

NORMODYNE® ℞

[*nor′mō-dīn*]
brand of labetalol hydrochloride
Tablets, USP

Prescribing information for this product, which appears on pages 3057–3059 of the 2003 PDR, has been completely revised as follows. Please write "See Supplement A" next to the product heading.

DESCRIPTION

NORMODYNE (labetalol HCl) is an adrenergic receptor blocking agent that has both selective alpha$_1$- and nonselective beta-adrenergic receptor blocking actions in a single substance.
Labetalol HCl is a racemate, chemically designated as 5-[1-hydroxy-2-[(1-methyl-3-phenylpropyl) amino] ethyl]salicylamide monohydrochloride, and has the following structure:

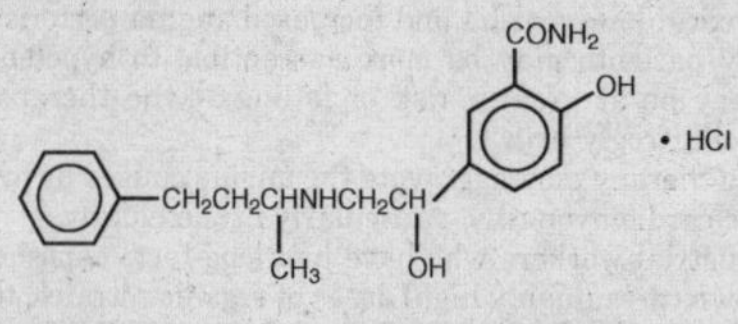

Labetalol HCl has the empirical formula $C_{19}H_{24}N_2O_3 \bullet HCl$ and a molecular weight of 364.9. It has two asymmetric centers and therefore exists as a molecular complex of two diastereoisomeric pairs. Dilevalol, the R,R′ stereoisomer, makes up 25% of racemic labetalol.
Labetalol HCl is a white or off-white crystalline powder, soluble in water.
NORMODYNE Tablets contain 100 mg, 200 mg, or 300 mg labetalol HCl, USP and are taken orally.
The inactive ingredients for NORMODYNE Tablets, 100 mg, include: corn starch, Opaspray Light Brown K-1-2630, hydroxypropyl methylcellulose, lactose, magnesium stearate, methylparaben, PEG, and propylparaben. May also contain: potato starch and wheat starch.
The inactive ingredients for NORMODYNE Tablets, 200 mg, include: corn starch, hydroxypropyl methylcellulose, lactose, magnesium stearate, methylparaben, PEG, propylparaben, and Opaspray White K-1-7000. May also contain: potato starch and wheat starch.
The inactive ingredients for NORMODYNE Tablets, 300 mg, include: corn starch, Opaspray Blue K-1-4212, hydroxypropyl methylcellulose, lactose, magnesium stearate, methylparaben, PEG, and propylparaben. May also contain: potato starch and wheat starch.

CLINICAL PHARMACOLOGY

NORMODYNE (labetalol HCl) combines both selective, competitive alpha$_1$-adrenergic blocking and nonselective, competitive beta-adrenergic blocking activity in a single substance. In man, the ratios of alpha- to beta-blockade have been estimated to be approximately 1:3 and 1:7 following oral and intravenous administration, respectively. Beta$_2$-agonist activity has been demonstrated in animals with minimal beta$_1$-agonist (ISA) activity detected. In animals, at doses greater than those required for alpha- or beta-adrenergic blockade, a membrane-stabilizing effect has been demonstrated.

Pharmacodynamics:
The capacity of labetalol HCl to block alpha receptors in man has been demonstrated by attenuation of the pressor effect of phenylephrine and by a significant reduction of the pressor response caused by immersing the hand in ice-cold water ("cold-pressor test"). Labetalol HCl's beta$_1$-receptor blockade in man was demonstrated by a small decrease in the resting heart rate, attenuation of tachycardia produced by isoproterenol or exercise, and by attenuation of the reflex tachycardia to the hypotension produced by amyl nitrite. Beta$_2$-receptor blockade was demonstrated by inhibition of the isoproterenol-induced fall in diastolic blood pressure. Both the alpha- and beta-blocking actions of orally administered labetalol HCl contribute to a decrease in blood pressure in hypertensive patients. Labetalol HCl consistently, in dose-related fashion, blunted increases in exercise-induced blood pressure and heart rate, and in their double product. The pulmonary circulation during exercise was not affected by labetalol HCl dosing.
Single oral doses of labetalol HCl administered in patients with coronary artery disease had no significant effect on sinus rate, intraventricular conduction, or QRS duration. The AV conduction time was modestly prolonged in 2 of 7 patients. In another study, intravenous labetalol HCl slightly prolonged AV nodal conduction time and atrial effective refractory period with only small changes in heart rate. The effects on AV nodal refractoriness were inconsistent.
Labetalol HCl produces dose-related falls in blood pressure without reflex tachycardia and without significant reduction in heart rate, presumably through a mixture of its alpha-blocking and beta-blocking effects. Hemodynamic effects are variable with small nonsignificant changes in cardiac output seen in some studies but not others, and small decreases in total peripheral resistance. Elevated plasma renins are reduced.
Doses of labetalol HCl that controlled hypertension did not affect renal function in mild to severe hypertensive patients with normal renal function.
Due to the alpha$_1$-receptor blocking activity of labetalol HCl, blood pressure is lowered more in the standing than in the supine position, and symptoms of postural hypotension (2%), including rare instances of syncope, can occur. Following oral administration, when postural hypotension has occurred, it has been transient and is uncommon when the recommended starting dose and titration increments are closely followed (see **DOSAGE AND ADMINISTRATION**). Symptomatic postural hypotension is most likely to occur 2 to 4 hours after a dose, especially following the use of large initial doses or upon large changes in dose.
The peak effects of single oral doses of labetalol HCl occur within 2 to 4 hours. The duration of effect depends upon dose, lasting at least 8 hours following single oral doses of 100 mg and more than 12 hours following single oral doses of 300 mg. The maximum, steady-state blood pressure response upon oral, twice-a-day dosing occurs within 24 to 72 hours.
The antihypertensive effect of labetalol has a linear correlation with the logarithm of labetalol plasma concentration, and there is also a linear correlation between the reduction in exercise-induced tachycardia occurring at 2 hours after oral administration of labetalol HCI and the logarithm of the plasma concentration.
About 70% of the maximum beta-blocking effect is present for 5 hours after the administration of a single oral dose of 400 mg, with suggestion that about 40% remains at 8 hours.
The anti-anginal efficacy of labetalol HCl has not been studied. In 37 patients with hypertension and coronary artery disease, labetalol HCl did not increase the incidence or severity of angina attacks.
Exacerbation of angina and, in some cases, myocardial infarction and ventricular dysrhythmias have been reported after abrupt discontinuation of therapy with beta-adrenergic blocking agents in patients with coronary artery disease. Abrupt withdrawal of these agents in patients without coronary artery disease has resulted in transient symptoms, including tremulousness, sweating, palpitation, headache, and malaise. Several mechanisms have been proposed to explain these phenomena, among them increased sensitivity to catecholamines because of increased numbers of beta receptors.
Although beta-adrenergic receptor blockade is useful in the treatment of angina and hypertension, there are also situations in which sympathetic stimulation is vital. For example, in patients with severely damaged hearts, adequate ventricular function may depend on sympathetic drive. Beta-adrenergic blockade may worsen AV block by preventing the necessary facilitating effects of sympathetic activity on conduction. Beta$_2$-adrenergic blockade results in passive bronchial constriction by interfering with endogenous adrenergic bronchodilator activity in patients subject to bronchospasm and may also interfere with exogenous bronchodilators in such patients.

Pharmacokinetics and Metabolism:
Labetalol HCl is completely absorbed from the gastrointestinal tract with peak plasma levels occurring 1 to 2 hours after oral administration. The relative bioavailability of labetalol HCl tablets compared to an oral solution is 100%. The absolute bioavailability (fraction of drug reaching systemic circulation) of labetalol when compared to an intravenous infusion is 25%; this is due to extensive "first-pass" metabolism. Despite "first-pass" metabolism there is a linear relationship between oral doses of 100 to 3000 mg and peak plasma levels. The absolute bioavailability of labetalol is increased when administered with food.
The plasma half-life of labetalol following oral administration is about 6 to 8 hours. Steady-state plasma levels of labetalol during repetitive dosing are reached by about the third day of dosing. In patients with decreased hepatic or renal function, the elimination half-life of labetalol is not altered; however, the relative bioavailability in hepatically impaired patients is increased due to decreased "first-pass" metabolism.
The metabolism of labetalol is mainly through conjugation to glucuronide metabolites. These metabolites are present in plasma and are excreted in the urine and, via the bile, into the feces. Approximately 55% to 60% of a dose appears in the urine as conjugates or unchanged labetalol within the first 24 hours of dosing.
Labetalol has been shown to cross the placental barrier in humans. Only negligible amounts of the drug crossed the blood-brain barrier in animal studies. Labetalol is approximately 50% protein bound. Neither hemodialysis nor peritoneal dialysis removes a significant amount of labetalol HCl from the general circulation (<1%).

INDICATIONS AND USAGE

NORMODYNE (labetalol HCl) Tablets are indicated in the management of hypertension. NORMODYNE Tablets may be used alone or in combination with other antihypertensive agents, especially thiazide and loop diuretics.

CONTRAINDICATIONS

NORMODYNE (labetalol HCl) Tablets are contraindicated in bronchial asthma, overt cardiac failure, greater than first degree heart block, cardiogenic shock, severe bradycardia, other conditions associated with severe and prolonged hypotension, and in patients with a history of hypersensitivity to any component of the product (see **WARNINGS**). Beta-blockers, even those with apparent cardioselectivity, should not be used in patients with a history of obstructive airway disease, including asthma.

WARNINGS

Hepatic Injury:
Severe hepatocellular injury, confirmed by rechallenge in at least one case, occurs rarely with labetalol therapy. The hepatic injury is usually reversible, but hepatic necrosis and death have been reported. Injury has occurred after both

short- and long-term treatment and may be slowly progressive despite minimal symptomatology. Similar hepatic events have been reported with a related compound, dilevalol HCl, including two deaths. Dilevalol HCl is one of the four isomers of labetalol HCl. Thus, for patients taking labetalol, periodic determination of suitable hepatic laboratory tests would be appropriate. Laboratory testing should also be done at the very first symptom or sign of liver dysfunction (eg, pruritus, dark urine, persistent anorexia, jaundice, right upper quadrant tenderness, or unexplained "flu-like" symptoms). If the patient has jaundice or laboratory evidence of liver injury, labetalol HCl should be stopped and not restarted.

Cardiac Failure:
Sympathetic stimulation is a vital component supporting circulatory function in congestive heart failure. Beta blockade carries a potential hazard of further depressing myocardial contractility and precipitating more severe failure. Although beta-blockers should be avoided in overt congestive heart failure, if necessary, labetalol HCl can be used with caution in patients with a history of heart failure who are well-compensated. Congestive heart failure has been observed in patients receiving labetalol HCl. Labetalol HCl does not abolish the inotropic action of digitalis on heart muscle.

In Patients Without a History of Cardiac Failure:
In patients with latent cardiac insufficiency, continued depression of the myocardium with beta-blocking agents over a period of time can, in some cases, lead to cardiac failure. At the first sign or symptom of impending cardiac failure, patients should be fully digitalized and/or be given a diuretic, and the response observed closely. If cardiac failure continues, despite adequate digitalization and diuretic, NORMODYNE (labetalol HCl) therapy should be withdrawn (gradually if possible).

Exacerbation of Ischemic Heart Disease Following Abrupt Withdrawal: Angina pectoris has not been reported upon labetalol HCl discontinuation. However, hypersensitivity to catecholamines has been observed in patients withdrawn from beta-blocker therapy; exacerbation of angina and, in some cases, myocardial infarction have occurred after *abrupt* discontinuation of such therapy. When discontinuing chronically administered NORMODYNE (labetalol HCl), particularly in patients with ischemic heart disease, the dosage should be gradually reduced over a period of 1 to 2 weeks and the patient should be carefully monitored. If angina markedly worsens or acute coronary insufficiency develops, NORMODYNE (labetalol HCl) administration should be reinstituted promptly, at least temporarily, and other measures appropriate for the management of unstable angina should be taken. Patients should be warned against interruption or discontinuation of therapy without the physician's advice. Because coronary artery disease is common and may be unrecognized, it may be prudent not to discontinue NORMODYNE (labetalol HCl) therapy abruptly even in patients treated only for hypertension.

Nonallergic bronchospasm (eg, chronic bronchitis and emphysema) patients with bronchospastic disease should, in general, not receive beta-blockers. NORMODYNE (labetalol HCl) may be used with caution, however, in patients who do not respond to, or cannot tolerate, other antihypertensive agents. It is prudent, if NORMODYNE (labetalol HCl) is used, to use the smallest effective dose, so that inhibition of endogenous or exogenous beta-agonists is minimized.

Pheochromocytoma:
Labetalol HCl has been shown to be effective in lowering the blood pressure and relieving symptoms in patients with pheochromocytoma. However, paradoxical hypertensive responses have been reported in a few patients with this tumor; therefore, use caution when administering labetalol HCl to patients with pheochromocytoma.

Diabetes Mellitus and Hypoglycemia:
Beta-adrenergic blockade may prevent the appearance of premonitory signs and symptoms (eg, tachycardia) of acute hypoglycemia. This is especially important with labile diabetics. Beta-blockade also reduces the release of insulin in response to hyperglycemia; it may therefore be necessary to adjust the dose of antidiabetic drugs.

Major Surgery:
The necessity or desirability of withdrawing beta-blocking therapy prior to major surgery is controversial. Protracted severe hypotension and difficulty in restarting or maintaining a heartbeat have been reported with beta-blockers. The effect of labetalol HCl's alpha-adrenergic activity has not been evaluated in this setting.

A synergism between labetalol HCl and halothane anesthesia has been shown (see **PRECAUTIONS – Drug Interactions**).

PRECAUTIONS

General:
Impaired Hepatic Function: NORMODYNE (labetalol HCl) Tablets should be used with caution in patients with impaired hepatic function since metabolism of the drug may be diminished.

Jaundice or Hepatic Dysfunction: (See **WARNINGS**.)

Information for Patients:
As with all drugs with beta-blocking activity, certain advice to patients being treated with labetalol HCl is warranted. This information is intended to aid in the safe and effective use of this medication. It is not a disclosure of all possible adverse or intended effects. While no incident of the abrupt withdrawal phenomenon (exacerbation of angina pectoris) has been reported with labetalol HCl, dosing with

	Labetalol HCl (N=227) %	Placebo (N=98) %	Propranolol (N=84) %	Metoprolol (N=49) %
Body as a whole				
fatigue	5	0	12	12
asthenia	1	1	1	0
headache	2	1	1	2
Gastrointestinal				
nausea	6	1	1	2
vomiting	<1	0	0	0
dyspepsia	3	1	1	0
abdominal pain	0	0	1	2
diarrhea	<1	0	2	0
taste distortion	1	0	0	0
Central and Peripheral Nervous Systems				
dizziness	11	3	4	4
paresthesias	<1	0	0	0
drowsiness	<1	2	2	2
Autonomic Nervous System				
nasal stuffiness	3	0	0	0
ejaculation failure	2	0	0	0
impotence	1	0	1	3
increased sweating	<1	0	0	0
Cardiovascular				
edema	1	0	0	0
postural hypotension	1	0	0	0
bradycardia	0	0	5	12
Respiratory				
dyspnea	2	0	1	2
Skin				
rash	1	0	0	0
Special Senses				
vision abnormality	1	0	0	0
vertigo	2	1	0	0

NORMODYNE (labetalol HCl) Tablets should not be interrupted or discontinued without a physician's advice. Patients being treated with NORMODYNE (labetalol HCl) Tablets should consult a physician at any signs or symptoms of impending cardiac failure or hepatic dysfunction (see **WARNINGS**). Also, transient scalp tingling may occur, usually when treatment with NORMODYNE (labetalol HCl) Tablets is initiated (see **ADVERSE REACTIONS**).

Laboratory Tests:
As with any new drug given over prolonged periods, laboratory parameters should be observed over regular intervals. In patients with concomitant illnesses, such as impaired renal function, appropriate tests should be done to monitor these conditions.

Drug Interactions:
In one survey, 2.3% of patients taking labetalol HCl in combination with tricyclic antidepressants experienced tremor as compared to 0.7% reported to occur with labetalol HCl alone. The contribution of each of the treatments to this adverse reaction is unknown but the possibility of a drug interaction cannot be excluded.

Drugs possessing beta-blocking properties can blunt the bronchodilator effect of beta-receptor agonist drugs in patients with bronchospasm; therefore, doses greater than the normal anti-asthmatic dose of beta-agonist bronchodilator drugs may be required.

Cimetidine has been shown to increase the bioavailability of labetalol HCl. Since this could be explained either by enhanced absorption or by an alteration of hepatic metabolism of labetalol HCl, special care should be used in establishing the dose required for blood pressure control in such patients.

Synergism has been shown between halothane anesthesia and intravenously administered labetalol HCl. During controlled hypotensive anesthesia using labetalol HCl in association with halothane, high concentrations (3% or above) of halothane should not be used because the degree of hypotension will be increased and because of the possibility of a large reduction in cardiac output and an increase in central venous pressure. The anesthesiologist should be informed when a patient is receiving labetalol HCl.

Labetalol HCl blunts the reflex tachycardia produced by nitroglycerin without preventing its hypotensive effect. If labetalol HCl is used with nitroglycerin in patients with angina pectoris, additional antihypertensive effects may occur. Care should be taken if labetalol HCl is used concomitantly with calcium antagonists of the verapamil type.

Risk of Anaphylactic Reaction:
While taking beta-blockers, patients with a history of severe anaphylactic reaction to a variety of allergens may be more reactive to repeated challenge, either accidental, diagnostic, or therapeutic. Such patients may be unresponsive to the usual doses of epinephrine used to treat allergic reaction.

Drug/Laboratory Test Interactions:
The presence of labetalol metabolites in the urine may result in falsely elevated levels of urinary catecholamines, metanephrine, normetanephrine, and vanillylmandelic acid (VMA) when measured by fluorimetric or photometric methods. In screening patients suspected of having a pheochromocytoma and being treated with labetalol HCl, a specific method, such as a high performance liquid chromatographic assay with solid phase extraction (eg, *J Chromatogr* 385:241,1987) should be employed in determining levels of catecholamines.

Labetalol HCl has also been reported to produce a false-positive test for amphetamine when screening urine for the presence of drugs using the commercially available assay methods Toxi-Lab A® (thin-layer chromatographic assay) and Emit-d.a.u.® (radioenzymatic assay). When patients being treated with labetalol HCl have a positive urine test for amphetamine using these techniques, confirmation should be made by using more specific methods, such as a gas chromatographic-mass spectrometer technique.

Carcinogenesis, Mutagenesis, Impairment of Fertility:
Long-term oral dosing studies with labetalol HCl for 18 months in mice and for 2 years in rats showed no evidence of carcinogenesis. Studies with labetalol HCl, using dominant lethal assays in rats and mice, and exposing microorganisms according to modified Ames tests, showed no evidence of mutagenesis.

Pregnancy Category C:
Teratogenic studies have been performed with labetalol HCl in rats and rabbits at oral doses up to approximately 6 and 4 times the maximum recommended human dose (MRHD), respectively. No reproducible evidence of fetal malformations was observed. Increased fetal resorptions were seen in both species at doses approximating the MRHD. A teratology study performed with labetalol HCl in rabbits at intravenous doses up to 1.7 times the MRHD revealed no evidence of drug-related harm to the fetus. There are no adequate and well-controlled studies in pregnant women. Labetalol HCl should be used during pregnancy only if the potential benefit justifies the potential risk to the fetus.

Nonteratogenic Effects:
Hypotension, bradycardia, hypoglycemia, and respiratory depression have been reported in infants of mothers who were treated with labetalol HCl for hypertension during pregnancy. Oral administration of labetalol to rats during late gestation through weaning at doses of 2 to 4 times the MRHD caused a decrease in neonatal survival.

Labor and Delivery:
Labetalol HCl given to pregnant women with hypertension did not appear to affect the usual course of labor and delivery.

Nursing Mothers: Small amounts of labetalol (approximately 0.004% of the maternal dose) are excreted in human milk. Caution should be exercised when NORMODYNE (labetalol HCl) Tablets are administered to a nursing woman.

Pediatric Use: Safety and effectiveness in pediatric patients have not been established.

ADVERSE REACTIONS

Most adverse effects are mild, transient and occur early in the course of treatment. In controlled clinical trials of 3 to 4 months duration, discontinuation of NORMODYNE (labetalol HCl) Tablets due to one or more adverse effects was required in 7% of all patients. In these same trials, beta-blocker control agents led to discontinuation in 8% to 10% of patients, and a centrally acting alpha-agonist in 30% of patients.

The incidence rates of adverse reactions listed in the following table were derived from multicenter controlled clinical trials, comparing labetalol HCl, placebo, metoprolol, and propranolol, over treatment periods of 3 and 4 months. Where the frequency of adverse effects for labetalol HCl and placebo is similar, causal relationship is uncertain. The rates are based on adverse reactions considered probably drug related by the investigator. If all reports are considered, the rates are somewhat higher (eg, dizziness 20%, nausea 14%, fatigue 11%), but the overall conclusions are unchanged.

[See table above]

The adverse effects were reported spontaneously and are representative of the incidence of adverse effects that may be observed in a properly selected hypertensive patient pop-

Continued on next page

Normodyne—Cont.

ulation, ie, a group excluding patients with bronchospastic disease, overt congestive heart failure, or other contraindications to beta-blocker therapy.

Clinical trials also included studies utilizing daily doses up to 2400 mg in more severely hypertensive patients. Certain of the side effects increased with increasing dose as shown in the table below which depicts the entire U.S. therapeutic trials data base for adverse reactions that are clearly or possibly drug related.

Labetalol HCl

Daily Dose (mg)	**200**	**300**	**400**	**600**	**800**
Number of patients	522	181	606	608	503
Dizziness (%)	2	3	3	3	5
Fatigue	2	1	4	4	5
Nausea	<1	0	1	2	4
Vomiting	0	0	<1	<1	<1
Dyspepsia	1	0	2	1	1
Paresthesias	2	0	2	2	1
Nasal Stuffiness	1	1	2	2	2
Ejaculation Failure	0	2	1	2	3
Impotence	1	1	1	1	2
Edema	1	0	1	1	1
Daily Dose (mg)	**900**	**1200**	**1600**	**2400**	
Number of Patients	117	411	242	175	
Dizziness (%)	1	9	13	16	
Fatigue	3	7	6	10	
Nausea	0	7	11	19	
Vomiting	0	1	2	3	
Dyspepsia	0	2	2	4	
Paresthesias	1	2	5	5	
Nasal Stuffiness	2	4	5	6	
Ejaculation Failure	0	4	3	5	
Impotence	4	3	4	3	
Edema	0	1	2	2	

In addition, a number of other less common adverse events have been reported:

Body as a Whole: Fever.

Cardiovascular: Hypotension, and rarely, syncope, bradycardia, heart block.

Central and Peripheral Nervous Systems: Paresthesias, most frequently described as scalp tingling. In most cases, it was mild, transient and usually occurred at the beginning of treatment.

Collagen Disorders: Systemic lupus erythematosus; positive antinuclear factor (ANF).

Eyes: Dry eyes.

Immunological System: Antimitochondrial antibodies.

Liver and Biliary System: Hepatic necrosis; hepatitis; cholestatic jaundice; elevated liver function tests.

Musculoskeletal System: Muscle cramps; toxic myopathy.

Respiratory System: Bronchospasm.

Skin and Appendages: Rashes of various types, such as generalized maculopapular; lichenoid; urticarial; bullous lichen planus; psoriaform; facial erythema; Peyronie's disease; reversible alopecia.

Urinary System: Difficulty in micturition, including acute urinary bladder retention.

Hypersensitivity: Rare reports of hypersensitivity (eg, rash, urticaria, pruritus, angioedema, dyspnea) and anaphylactoid reactions.

Following approval for marketing in the United Kingdom, a monitored release survey involving approximately 6,800 patients was conducted for further safety and efficacy evaluation of this product. Results of this survey indicate that the type, severity, and incidence of adverse effects were comparable to those cited above.

Potential Adverse Effects: In addition, other adverse effects not listed above have been reported with other beta-adrenergic blocking agents.

Central Nervous System: Reversible mental depression progressing to catatonia; an acute reversible syndrome characterized by disorientation for time and place, short-term memory loss, emotional lability, slightly clouded sensorium, and decreased performance on neuropsychometrics.

Cardiovascular: Intensification of AV block (see **CONTRAINDICATIONS**).

Allergic: Fever combined with aching and sore throat; laryngospasm; respiratory distress.

Hematologic: Agranulocytosis; thrombocytopenic or nonthrombocytopenic purpura.

Gastrointestinal: Mesenteric artery thrombosis; ischemic colitis.

The oculomucocutaneous syndrome associated with the beta-blocker practolol has not been reported with labetalol HCl.

Clinical Laboratory Tests:

There have been reversible increases of serum transaminases in 4% of patients treated with labetalol HCl and tested, and more rarely, reversible increases in blood urea.

OVERDOSAGE

Overdosage with NORMODYNE (labetalol HCl) Tablets causes excessive hypotension that is posture sensitive, and sometimes, excessive bradycardia. Patients should be placed supine and their legs raised if necessary to improve the blood supply to the brain. If overdosage with labetalol HCl follows oral ingestion, gastric lavage or pharmacologically induced emesis (using syrup of ipecac) may be useful for removal of the drug shortly after ingestion. The following additional measures should be employed if necessary: *Excessive bradycardia* — administer atropine or epinephrine. *Cardiac failure* — administer a digitalis glycoside and a diuretic. Dopamine or dobutamine may also be useful. *Hypotension* — administer vasopressors, eg, norepinephrine. There is pharmacological evidence that norepinephrine may be the drug of choice. *Bronchospasm* — administer epinephrine and/or an aerosolized beta$_2$-agonist. *Seizures* — administer diazepam.

In severe beta-blocker overdose resulting in hypotension and/or bradycardia, glucagon has been shown to be effective when administered in large doses (5 to 10 mg rapidly over 30 seconds, followed by continuous infusion of 5 mg/hr that can be reduced as the patient improves).

Neither hemodialysis nor peritoneal dialysis removes a significant amount of labetalol HCl from the general circulation (<1%).

The oral LD_{50} value of labetalol HCl in the mouse is approximately 600 mg/kg and in the rat is greater than 2 g/kg. The intravenous LD_{50} in these species is 50 to 60 mg/kg.

DOSAGE AND ADMINISTRATION

DOSAGE MUST BE INDIVIDUALIZED. The recommended initial dose is 100 mg twice daily whether used alone or added to a diuretic regimen. After 2 or 3 days, using standing blood pressure as an indicator, dosage may be titrated in increments of 100 mg b.i.d. every 2 or 3 days. The usual maintenance dosage of labetalol HCl is between 200 and 400 mg twice daily.

Since the full antihypertensive effect of labetalol HCl is usually seen within the first 1 to 3 hours of the initial dose or dose increment, the assurance of a lack of an exaggerated hypotensive response can be clinically established in the office setting. The antihypertensive effects of continued dosing can be measured at subsequent visits, approximately 12 hours after a dose, to determine whether further titration is necessary.

Patients with severe hypertension may require from 1200 mg to 2400 mg per day, with or without thiazide diuretics. Should side effects (principally nausea or dizziness) occur with these doses administered b.i.d., the same total daily dose administered t.i.d. may improve tolerability and facilitate further titration. Titration increments should not exceed 200 mg b.i.d.

When a diuretic is added, an additive antihypertensive effect can be expected. In some cases this may necessitate a labetalol HCl dosage adjustment. As with most antihypertensive drugs, optimal dosages of NORMODYNE (labetalol HCl) Tablets are usually lower in patients also receiving a diuretic.

When transferring patients from other antihypertensive drugs, NORMODYNE (labetalol HCl) Tablets should be introduced as recommended and the dosage of the existing therapy progressively decreased.

HOW SUPPLIED

NORMODYNE (labetalol HCl) Tablets, 100 mg, light brown, round, scored, film-coated tablets engraved on one side with Schering and product identification numbers 244, and on the other side the number 100 for the strength and "NORMODYNE"; bottles of 100 (NDC-0085-0244-04), bottles of 500 (NDC-0085-0244-05), and box of 100 for unit-dose dispensing (NDC-0085-0244-08).

NORMODYNE (labetalol HCl) Tablets, 200 mg, white, round, scored,film-coated tablets engraved on one side with Schering and product identification numbers 752, and on the other side the number 200 for the strength and "NORMODYNE"; bottles of 100 (NDC-0085-0752-04), bottles of 500 (NDC-0085-0752-05), and box of 100 for unit-dose dispensing (NDC-0085-0752-08).

NORMODYNE (labetalol HCl) Tablets, 300 mg, blue, round, film-coated tablets engraved on one side with Schering and product identification numbers 438, and on the other side the number 300 for the strength and "NORMODYNE"; bottles of 100 (NDC-0085-0438-03), bottles of 500 (NDC-0085-0438-05), and box of 100 for unit-dose dispensing (NDC-0085-0438-06).

NORMODYNE (labetalol HCl) Tablets should be stored between 2° and 30°C (36° and 86°F).

NORMODYNE (labetalol HCl) Tablets in the unit-dose boxes should be protected from excessive moisture.

Key Pharmaceuticals, Inc.
Kenilworth, NJ 07033 USA
Rev. 5/00 B-16833541
23116715T

Copyright © 1984, 1992, 1994, 1999, Schering Corporation. All rights reserved.

PEG-INTRON® ℞

[*pĕg-ĭntrŏn*]

(Peginterferon alfa-2b)

Powder for Injection

Prescribing information for this product, which appears on pages 3059–3063 of the 2003 PDR, has been completely revised as follows. Please write "See Supplement A" next to the product heading.

Alpha interferons, including PEG-Intron, cause or aggravate fatal or life-threatening neuropsychiatric, autoimmune, ischemic, and infectious disorders. Patients should be monitored closely with periodic clinical and laboratory evaluations. Patients with persistently severe or worsening signs or symptoms of these conditions should be withdrawn from therapy. In many but not all cases these disorders resolve after stopping PEG-Intron therapy. See WARNINGS, ADVERSE REACTIONS.

Use with Ribavirin. Ribavirin may cause birth defects and/or death of the unborn child. Extreme care must be taken to avoid pregnancy in female patients and in female partners of male patients. Ribavirin causes hemolytic anemia. The anemia associated with REBETOL therapy may result in a worsening of cardiac disease. Ribavirin is genotoxic and mutagenic and should be considered a potential carcinogen. (See REBETOL package insert for additional information and other warnings).

DESCRIPTION

PEG-Intron®, peginterferon alfa-2b Powder for Injection, is a covalent conjugate of recombinant alfa-2b interferon with monomethoxypolyethylene glycol (PEG). The average molecular weight of the PEG portion of the molecule is 12,000 daltons. The average molecular weight of the PEG-Intron molecule is approximately 31,000 daltons. The specific activity of peginterferon alfa-2b is approximately 0.7×10^8 IU/mg protein.

Interferon alfa-2b, is a water-soluble protein with a molecular weight of 19,271 daltons produced by recombinant DNA techniques. It is obtained from the bacterial fermentation of a strain of *Escherichia coli* bearing a genetically engineered plasmid containing an interferon gene from human leukocytes.

PEG-Intron is a white to off-white lyophilized powder supplied in 2-mL vials for subcutaneous use. Each vial contains either 74 µg, 118.4 µg, 177.6 µg, or 222 µg of PEG-Intron, and 1.11 mg dibasic sodium phosphate anhydrous, 1.11 mg monobasic sodium phosphate dihydrate, 59.2 mg sucrose and 0.074 mg polysorbate 80. Following reconstitution with 0.7 mL of the supplied diluent (Sterile Water for Injection, USP), each vial contains PEG-Intron at strengths of either 50 µg per 0.5 mL, 80 µg per 0.5 mL, 120 µg per 0.5 mL, or 150 µg per 0.5 mL.

CLINICAL PHARMACOLOGY

General: The biological activity of PEG-Intron is derived from its interferon alfa-2b moiety. Interferons exert their cellular activities by binding to specific membrane receptors on the cell surface and initiate a complex sequence of intracellular events. These include the induction of certain enzymes, suppression of cell proliferation, immunomodulating activities such as enhancement of the phagocytic activity of macrophages and augmentation of the specific cytotoxicity of lymphocytes for target cells, and inhibition of virus replication in virus-infected cells. Interferon alfa upregulates the Th1 T-helper cell subset in *in vitro* studies. The clinical relevance of these findings is not known.

Pharmacodynamics: PEG-Intron raises concentrations of effector proteins such as serum neopterin and 2′5′ oligoadenylate synthetase, raises body temperature, and causes reversible decreases in leukocyte and platelet counts. The correlation between the *in vitro* and *in vivo* pharmacologic and pharmacodynamic and clinical effects is unknown.

Pharmacokinetics: Following a single subcutaneous (SC) dose of PEG-Intron, the mean absorption half-life (t 1/2 k_a) was 4.6 hours. Maximal serum concentrations (C_{max}) occur between 15-44 hours post-dose, and are sustained for up to 48-72 hours. The C_{max} and AUC measurements of PEG-Intron increase in a dose-related manner. After multiple dosing, there is an increase in bioavailability of PEG-Intron. Week 48 mean trough concentrations (320 pg/mL; range 0, 2960) are approximately 3-fold higher than Week 4 mean trough concentrations (94 pg/mL; range 0, 416). The mean PEG-Intron elimination half-life is approximately 40 hours (range 22 to 60 hours) in patients with HCV infection. The apparent clearance of PEG-Intron is estimated to be approximately 22.0 mL/hr•kg. Renal elimination accounts for 30% of the clearance. Single dose peginterferon alfa-2b pharmacokinetics following a subcutaneous 1.0 µg/kg dose suggest the clearance of peginterferon alfa-2b is reduced by approximately half in subjects with impaired renal function (creatinine clearance <50 mL/minute).

Pegylation of interferon alfa-2b produces a product (PEG-Intron) whose clearance is lower than that of non-pegylated interferon alfa-2b. When compared to INTRON A, PEG-Intron (1.0 µg/kg) has approximately a seven-fold lower mean apparent clearance and a five-fold greater mean half-life permitting a reduced dosing frequency. At effective therapeutic doses, PEG-Intron has approximately ten-fold greater C_{max} and 50-fold greater AUC than interferon alfa-2b.

The pharmacokinetics of geriatric subjects (> 65 years of age) treated with a single subcutaneous dose of 1.0 µg/kg of PEG-Intron were similar in C_{max}, AUC, clearance, or elimination half-life as compared to younger subjects (28 to 44 years of age).

During the 48 week treatment period with PEG-Intron, no differences in the pharmacokinetic profiles were observed between male and female patients with chronic hepatitis C infection.

Effect of Food on Absorption of Ribavirin Both AUC_{tf} and C_{max} increased by 70% when REBETOL Capsules were administered with a high-fat meal (841 kcal, 53.8 g fat, 31.6 g protein, and 57.4 g carbohydrate) in a single-dose pharmacokinetic study. (See **DOSAGE AND ADMINISTRATION**).

Drug Interactions: It is not known if PEG-Intron therapy causes clinically significant drug-drug interactions with drugs metabolized by the liver in patients with hepatitis C. In 12 healthy subjects known to be CYP2D6 extensive metabolizers, a single subcutaneous dose of 1 µg/kg PEG-Intron did not inhibit CYP1A2, 2C8/9, 2D6, hepatic 3A4 or N-acetyltransferase; the effects of PEG-Intron on CYP2C19 were not assessed.

CLINICAL STUDIES

PEG-Intron Monotherapy-Study 1

A randomized study compared treatment with PEG-Intron (0.5, 1.0, or 1.5 µg/kg once weekly SC) to treatment with INTRON A, (3 million units three times weekly SC) in 1219 adults with chronic hepatitis from HCV infection. The patients were not previously treated with interferon alfa, had compensated liver disease, detectable HCV RNA, elevated ALT, and liver histopathology consistent with chronic hepatitis. Patients were treated for 48 weeks and were followed for 24 weeks post-treatment. Seventy percent of all patients were infected with HCV genotype 1, and 74 percent of all patients had high baseline levels of HCV RNA (more than 2 million copies per mL of serum), two factors known to predict poor response to treatment.

Response to treatment was defined as undetectable HCV RNA and normalization of ALT at 24 weeks post-treatment. The response rates to the 1.0 and 1.5 µg/kg PEG-Intron doses were similar (approximately 24%) to each other and were both higher than the response rate to INTRON A (12%). (See Table 1)

[See table 1 at right]

TABLE 1. Rates of Response to Treatment-Study 1

	A PEG-Intron 0.5 µg/kg (N=315)	B PEG-Intron 1.0 µg/kg (N=298)	C INTRON A 3 MIU TIW (N=307)	B-C (95% CI) Difference between PEG-Intron 1.0 µg/kg and INTRON A
Treatment Response (Combined Virologic Response and ALT Normalization)	17%	24%	12%	11 (5, 18)
Virologic Response[a]	18%	25%	12%	12 (6, 19)
ALT Normalization	24%	29%	18%	11 (5, 18)

[a]Serum HCV is measured by a research-based quantitative polymerase chain reaction assay by a central laboratory.

Patients with both viral genotype 1 and high serum levels of HCV RNA at baseline were less likely to respond to treatment with PEG-Intron. Among patients with the two unfavorable prognostic variables, 8% (12/157) responded to PEG-Intron treatment and 2% (4/169) responded to INTRON A. Doses of PEG-Intron higher than the recommended dose did not result in higher response rates in these patients.

Patients receiving PEG-Intron with viral genotype 1 had a response rate of 14% (28/199) while patients with other viral genotypes had a 45% (43/96) response rate.

Ninety-six percent of the responders in the PEG-Intron groups and 100% of responders in the INTRON A group first cleared their viral RNA by week-24 of treatment. See **DOSAGE AND ADMINISTRATION**.

The treatment response rates were similar in men and women. Response rates were lower in African American and Hispanic patients and higher in Asians compared to Caucasians. Although African Americans had a higher proportion of poor prognostic factors compared to Caucasians the number of non-Caucasians studied (9% of the total) was insufficient to allow meaningful conclusions about differences in response rates after adjusting for prognostic factors.

Liver biopsies were obtained before and after treatment in 60% of patients. A modest reduction in inflammation compared to baseline that was similar in all four treatment groups was observed.

PEG-Intron/REBETOL Combination Therapy-Study 2

A randomized study compared treatment with two PEG-Intron/REBETOL regimens [PEG-Intron 1.5 µg/kg SC once weekly (QW)/REBETOL 800 mg PO daily (in divided doses); PEG-Intron 1.5 µg/kg SC QW for 4 weeks then 0.5 µg/kg SC QW for 44 weeks/REBETOL 1000/1200 mg PO daily (in divided doses)] with INTRON A (3 MIU SC thrice weekly (TIW)/REBETOL 1000/1200 mg PO daily (in divided doses) in 1530 adults with chronic hepatitis C. Interferon naïve patients were treated for 48 weeks and followed for 24 weeks post-treatment. Eligible patients had compensated liver disease, detectable HCV RNA, elevated ALT, and liver histopathology consistent with chronic hepatitis.

Response to treatment was defined as undetectable HCV RNA at 24 weeks post-treatment. The response rate to the PEG-Intron 1.5 µg/kg plus ribavirin 800 mg dose was higher than the response rate to INTRON A/REBETOL (See **Table 2**). The response rate to PEG-Intron 1.5 → 0.5µg/kg/REBETOL was essentially the same as the response to INTRON A/REBETOL (data not shown).

TABLE 2. Rates of Response to Treatment-Study 2

	PEG-Intron 1.5 µg/kg QW REBETOL 800 mg QD	INTRON A 3 MIU TIW REBETOL 1000/1200 mg QD
Overall[1,2] response	52% (264/511)	46% (231/505)
Genotype 1	41% (141/348)	33% (112/343)
Genotype 2–6	75% (123/163)	73% (119/162)

[1]Serum HCV RNA is measured with a research-based quantitative polymerase chain reaction assay by a central laboratory.

[2]Difference in overall treatment response (PEG-Intron/REBETOL vs. INTRON A/REBETOL) is 6% with 95% confidence interval of (0.18, 11.63) adjusted for viral genotype and presence of cirrhosis at baseline.

Patients with viral genotype 1, regardless of viral load, had a lower response rate to PEG-Intron (1.5 µg/kg)/REBETOL compared to patients with other viral genotypes. Patients with both poor prognostic factors (genotype 1 and high viral load) had a response rate of 30% (78/256) compared to a response rate of 29% (71/247) with INTRON A/REBETOL.

Patients with lower body weight tended to have higher adverse event rates (see **ADVERSE REACTIONS**) and higher response rates than patients with higher body weights. Differences in response rates between treatment arms did not substantially vary with body weight.

Treatment response rates with PEG-Intron/REBETOL were 49% in men and 56% in women. Response rates were lower in African American and Hispanic patients and higher in Asians compared to Caucasians. Although African Americans had a higher proportion of poor prognostic factors compared to Caucasians the number of non-Caucasians studied (11% of the total) was insufficient to allow meaningful conclusions about differences in response rates after adjusting for prognostic factors.

Liver biopsies were obtained before and after treatment in 68% of patients. Compared to baseline approximately 2/3 of patients in all treatment groups were observed to have a modest reduction in inflammation.

INDICATIONS AND USAGE

PEG-Intron, peginterferon alfa-2b, is indicated for use alone or in combination with REBETOL (ribavirin, USP) for the treatment of chronic hepatitis C in patients with compensated liver disease who have not been previously treated with interferon alpha and are at least 18 years of age.

CONTRAINDICATIONS

PEG-Intron is contraindicated in patients with:

- hypersensitivity to PEG-Intron or any other component of the product
- autoimmune hepatitis
- decompensated liver disease

PEG-Intron/REBETOL combination therapy is additionally contraindicated in:

- patients with hypersensitivity to ribavirin or any other component of the product
- women who are pregnant
- men whose female partners are pregnant
- patients with hemoglobinopathies (e.g., thalassemia major, sickle-cell anemia)

WARNINGS

Patients should be monitored for the following serious conditions, some of which may become life threatening. Patients with persistently severe or worsening signs or symptoms should be withdrawn from therapy.

Neuropsychiatric events

Life-threatening or fatal neuropsychiatric events, including suicide, suicidal and homicidal ideation, depression, relapse of drug addiction/overdose, and aggressive behavior have occurred in patients with and without a previous psychiatric disorder during PEG-Intron treatment and follow-up. Psychoses, hallucinations, bipolar disorders, and mania have been observed in patients treated with alpha interferons. PEG-Intron should be used with extreme caution in patients with a history of psychiatric disorders. Patients should be advised to report immediately any symptoms of depression and/or suicidal ideation to their prescribing physicians. Physicians should monitor all patients for evidence of depression and other psychiatric symptoms. In severe cases, PEG-Intron should be stopped immediately and psychiatric intervention instituted. (See **DOSAGE AND ADMINISTRATION: Dose Reduction.**)

Bone marrow toxicity

PEG-Intron suppresses bone marrow function, sometimes resulting in severe cytopenias. PEG-Intron should be discontinued in patients who develop severe decreases in neutrophil or platelet counts. (See **DOSAGE AND ADMINISTRATION: Dose Reduction**). Ribavirin may potentiate the neutropenia induced by interferon alpha. Very rarely alpha interferons may be associated with aplastic anemia.

Endocrine disorders

PEG-Intron causes or aggravates hypothyroidism and hyperthyroidism. Hyperglycemia has been observed in patients treated with PEG-Intron. Diabetes mellitus has been observed in patients treated with alpha interferons. Patients with these conditions who cannot be effectively treated by medication should not begin PEG-Intron therapy. Patients who develop these conditions during treatment and cannot be controlled with medication should not continue PEG-Intron therapy.

Cardiovascular events

Cardiovascular events, which include hypotension, arrhythmia, tachycardia, cardiomyopathy, angina pectoris, and myocardial infarction, have been observed in patients treated with PEG-Intron. PEG-Intron should be used cautiously in patients with cardiovascular disease. Patients with a history of myocardial infarction and arrhythmic disorder who require PEG-Intron therapy should be closely monitored (see **Laboratory Tests**). Patients with a history of significant or unstable cardiac disease should not be treated with PEG-Intron/REBETOL combination therapy. [See **REBETOL package insert**.]

Pulmonary disorders

Dyspnea, pulmonary infiltrates, pneumonia, bronchiolitis obliterans, interstitial pneumonitis and sarcoidosis some resulting in respiratory failure and/or patient deaths, may be induced or aggravated by PEG-Intron or alpha interferon therapy. Recurrence of respiratory failure has been observed with interferon rechallenge. PEG-Intron combination treatment should be suspended in patients who develop pulmonary infiltrates or pulmonary function impairment. Patients who resume interferon treatment should be closely monitored.

Colitis

Fatal and nonfatal ulcerative or hemorrhagic/ischemic colitis have been observed within 12 weeks of the start of alpha interferon treatment. Abdominal pain, bloody diarrhea, and fever are the typical manifestations. PEG-Intron treatment should be discontinued immediately in patients who develop these symptoms and signs. The colitis usually resolves within 1-3 weeks of discontinuation of alpha interferons.

Pancreatitis

Fatal and nonfatal pancreatitis has been observed in patients treated with alpha interferon. PEG-Intron therapy should be suspended in patients with signs and symptoms suggestive of pancreatitis and discontinued in patients diagnosed with pancreatitis.

Autoimmune disorders

Development or exacerbation of autoimmune disorders (e.g. thyroiditis, thrombocytopenia, rheumatoid arthritis, interstitial nephritis, systemic lupus erythematosus, psoriasis) have been observed in patients receiving PEG-Intron. PEG-Intron should be used with caution in patients with autoimmune disorders.

Ophthalmologic disorders

Decrease or loss of vision, retinopathy including macular edema, retinal artery or vein thrombosis, retinal hemorrhages and cotton wool spots, optic neuritis, and papilledema may be induced or aggravated by treatment with peginterferon alfa-2b or other alpha interferons. All patients should receive an eye examination at baseline. Patients with preexisting ophthalmologic disorders (e.g. diabetic or hypertensive retinopathy) should receive periodic ophthalmologic exams during interferon alpha treatment. Any patient who develops ocular symptoms should receive a prompt and complete eye examination. Peginterferon alfa-2b treatment should be discontinued in patients who develop new or worsening ophthalmologic disorders.

Hypersensitivity

Serious, acute hypersensitivity reactions (e.g., urticaria, angioedema, bronchoconstriction, anaphylaxis) have been rarely observed during alpha interferon therapy. If such a reaction develops during treatment with PEG-Intron, discontinue treatment and institute appropriate medical therapy immediately. Transient rashes do not necessitate interruption of treatment.

Use with Ribavirin-(See also **REBETOL Package Insert**)

REBETOL may cause birth defects and/or death of the unborn child. REBETOL therapy should not be started until a report of a negative pregnancy test has been obtained immediately prior to planned initiation of therapy. Patients should use at least two forms of contraception and have monthly pregnancy tests (See BOXED WARNING, CONTRAINDICATIONS and PRECAUTIONS: Information for Patients and REBETOL package insert).

Anemia

Ribavirin caused hemolytic anemia in 10% of PEG-Intron/REBETOL treated patients within 1–4 weeks of initiation of therapy. Complete blood counts should be obtained pretreatment and at week 2 and week 4 of therapy or more frequently if clinically indicated. Anemia associated with REBETOL therapy may result in a worsening of cardiac disease. Decrease in dosage or discontinuation of REBETOL may be necessary. (See **DOSAGE AND ADMINISTRATION: Dose Reduction.**)

PRECAUTIONS

- PEG-Intron alone or in combination with REBETOL has not been studied in patients who have failed other alpha interferon treatments.

Continued on next page

PEG-Intron—Cont.

- The safety and efficacy of PEG-Intron alone or in combination with REBETOL for the treatment of hepatitis C in liver or other organ transplant recipients have not been studied.
- The safety and efficacy of PEG-Intron/REBETOL for the treatment of patients with HCV co-infected with HIV or HBV have not been established.

Patients with renal failure: Patients with impairment of renal function should be closely monitored for signs and symptoms of interferon toxicity and doses of PEG-Intron should be adjusted accordingly. PEG-Intron should be used with caution in patients with creatinine clearance <50 mL/min. See **DOSAGE AND ADMINISTRATION: Dose Modification**.

Immunogenicity: Approximately 2% of patients receiving PEG-Intron (32/1759) or INTRON A (11/728) with or without REBETOL developed low-titer (≤160) neutralizing antibodies to PEG-Intron or INTRON A. The clinical and pathological significance of the appearance of serum neutralizing antibodies is unknown. No apparent correlation of antibody development to clinical response or adverse events was observed. The incidence of post-treatment binding antibody ranged from 8 to 15 percent. The data reflect the percentage of patients whose test results were considered positive for antibodies to PEG-Intron in a Biacore assay that is used to measure binding antibodies, and in an antiviral neutralization assay, which measures serum-neutralizing antibodies. The percentage of patients whose test results were considered positive for antibodies is highly dependent on the sensitivity and specificity of the assays. Additionally the observed incidence of antibody positivity in these assays may be influenced by several factors including sample timing and handling, concomitant medications, and underlying disease. For these reasons, comparison of the incidence of antibodies to PEG-Intron with the incidence of antibodies to other products may be misleading.

Laboratory Tests: PEG-Intron alone or in combination with ribavirin may cause severe decreases in neutrophil and platelet counts, and hematologic, endocrine (e.g.TSH) and hepatic abnormalities. Transient elevations in ALT (2–5 fold above baseline) were observed in 10% of patients treated with PEG-Intron, and was not associated with deterioration of other liver functions.

Patients on PEG-Intron or PEG-Intron/REBETOL combination therapy should have hematology and blood chemistry testing before the start of treatment and then periodically thereafter. In the clinical trial CBC (including hemoglobin, neutrophil and platelet counts) and chemistries (including AST, ALT, bilirubin, and uric acid) were measured during the treatment period at weeks 2, 4, 8, 12, and then at 6-week intervals or more frequently if abnormalities developed. TSH levels were measured every 12 weeks during the treatment period.

HCV RNA should be measured at 6 months of treatment. PEG-Intron or PEG-Intron/REBETOL combination therapy should be discontinued in patients with persistent high viral levels.

Patients who have pre-existing cardiac abnormalities should have electrocardiograms administered before treatment with PEG-Intron/REBETOL.

Information for Patients: Patients receiving PEG-Intron alone or in combination with REBETOL should be directed in its appropriate use, informed of the benefits and risks associated with treatment, and referred to the **MEDICATION GUIDES for PEG-Intron and, if applicable, REBETOL (ribavirin, USP)**.

Patients must be informed that REBETOL may cause birth defects and/or death of the unborn child. Extreme care must be taken to avoid pregnancy in female patients and in female partners of male patients taking combination PEG-Intron/REBETOL therapy. Combination PEG-Intron/REBETOL therapy should not be initiated until a report of a negative pregnancy test has been obtained immediately prior to initiation of therapy. It is recommended that patients undergo monthly pregnancy tests during therapy and for 6 months post-therapy. **(See CONTRAINIDICATIONS and REBETOL package insert)**.

A puncture-resistant container for the disposal of used syringes and needles should be supplied to the patient for at home use. Patients should be thoroughly instructed in the importance of proper disposal and cautioned against any reuse of needles and syringes. The full container should be disposed of according to the directions provided by the physician (see **MEDICATION GUIDE**).

Patients should be informed that there are no data regarding whether PEG-Intron therapy will prevent transmission of HCV infection to others. Also, it is not known if treatment with PEG-Intron will cure hepatitis C or prevent cirrhosis, liver failure, or liver cancer that may be the result of infection with the hepatitis C virus.

Patients should be advised that laboratory evaluations are required before starting therapy and periodically thereafter (see **Laboratory Tests**). It is advised that patients be well-hydrated, especially during the initial stages of treatment. "Flu-like" symptoms associated with administration of PEG-Intron may be minimized by bedtime administration of PEG-Intron or by use of antipyretics.

Carcinogenesis, Mutagenesis, and Impairment of Fertility
Carcinogenesis and Mutagenesis: PEG-Intron has not been tested for its carcinogenic potential. Neither PEG-Intron, nor its components interferon or methoxypolyethylene glycol caused damage to DNA when tested in the standard battery of mutagenesis assays, in the presence and absence of metabolic activation.

Use with Ribavirin: Ribavirin is genotoxic and mutagenic and should be considered a potential carcinogen. See REBETOL package insert for additional warnings relevant to PEG-Intron therapy in combination with ribavirin.

Impairment of Fertility: PEG-Intron may impair human fertility. Irregular menstrual cycles were observed in female cynomolgus monkeys given subcutaneous injections of 4239 µg/m² PEG-Intron alone every other day for one month, (approximately 345 times the recommended weekly human dose based upon body surface area). These effects included transiently decreased serum levels of estradiol and progesterone, suggestive of anovulation. Normal menstrual cycles and serum hormone levels resumed in these animals 2 to 3 months following cessation of PEG-Intron treatment. Every other day dosing with 262 µg/m² (approximately 21 times the weekly human dose) had no effects on cycle duration or reproductive hormone status. The effects of PEG-Intron on male fertility have not been studied.

TABLE 3. Adverse Events Occurring in >5% of Patients

Percentage of Patients Reporting Adverse Events*

Adverse Events	Study 1 PEG-Intron 1.0 µg/kg (n=297)	Study 1 INTRON A 3 MIU (n=303)	Study 2 PEG-Intron 1.5 µg/kg/ REBETOL (n=511)	Study 2 INTRON A/ REBETOL (n=505)
Application Site				
Injection Site Inflammation/Reaction	47	20	75	49
Autonomic Nervous Sys.				
Mouth Dry	6	7	12	8
Sweating Increased	6	7	11	7
Flushing	6	3	4	3
Body as a Whole				
Fatigue/Asthenia	52	54	66	63
Headache	56	52	62	58
Rigors	23	19	48	41
Fever	22	12	46	33
Weight Decrease	11	13	29	20
RUQ pain	8	8	12	6
Chest Pain	6	4	8	7
Malaise	7	6	4	6
Central/Periph. Nerv. Sys.				
Dizziness	12	10	21	17
Endocrine Disorders				
Hypothyroidism	5	3	5	4
Gastrointestinal				
Nausea	26	20	43	33
Anorexia	20	17	32	27
Diarrhea	18	16	22	17
Vomiting	7	6	14	12
Abdominal Pain	15	11	13	13
Dsypepsia	6	7	9	8
Constipation	1	3	5	5
Hemotologic Disorders				
Neutropenia	6	2	26	14
Anemia	0	0	12	17
Leukopenia	<1	0	6	5
Thrombocytopenia	7	<1	5	2
Liver and Biliary System Disorders				
Hepatomegaly	6	5	4	4
Musculoskeletal				
Myalgia	54	53	56	50
Arthralgia	23	27	34	28
Musculoskeletal Pain	28	22	21	19
Psychiatric				
Insomnia	23	23	40	41
Depression	29	25	31	34
Anxiety/Emotional Lability/Irritability	28	34	47	47
Concentration Impaired	10	8	17	21
Agitation	2	2	8	5
Nervousness	4	3	6	6
Reproductive, Female				
Menstrual Disorder	4	3	7	6
Resistance Mechanism				
Infection Viral	11	10	12	12
Infection Fungal	<1	3	6	1
Respiratory System				
Dyspnea	4	2	26	24
Coughing	8	5	23	16
Pharyngitis	10	7	12	13
Rhinitis	2	2	8	6
Sinusitis	7	7	6	5
Skin and Appendages				
Alopecia	22	22	36	32
Pruritus	12	8	29	28
Rash	6	7	24	23
Skin Dry	11	9	24	23
Special Senses Other,				
Taste Perversion	<1	2	9	4
Vision Disorders				
Vision blurred	2	3	5	6
Conjunctivitis	4	2	4	5

* Patients reporting one or more adverse events. A patient may have reported more than one adverse event within a body system/organ class category.

Pregnancy Category C: PEG-Intron monotherapy: Nonpegylated Interferon alfa-2b, has been shown to have abortifacient effects in *Macaca mulatta* (rhesus monkeys) at 15 and 30 million IU/kg (estimated human equivalent of 5 and 10 million IU/kg, based on body surface area adjustment for a 60 kg adult). PEG-Intron should be assumed to also have abortifacient potential. There are no adequate and well-controlled studies in pregnant women. PEG-Intron therapy is to be used during pregnancy only if the potential benefit justifies the potential risk to the fetus. Therefore, PEG-Intron is recommended for use in fertile women only when they are using effective contraception during the treatment period.

Pregnancy Category X : Use with Ribavirin
Significant teratogenic and/or embryocidal effects have been demonstrated in all animal species exposed to ribavirin. REBETOL therapy is contraindicated in women who are pregnant and in the male partners of women who are pregnant. See **CONTRAINDICATIONS** and the **REBETOL Package Insert.**

If pregnancy occurs in a patient or partner of a patient during treatment with PEG-Intron and REBETOL during the 6 months after treatment cessation, physicians should report such cases by calling (800) 727-7064.

Pediatric. Safety and effectiveness in pediatric patients below the age of 18 years have not been established.

Geriatric. In general, younger patients tend to respond better than older patients to interferon-based therapies. Clinical studies of PEG-Intron alone or in combination with REBETOL did not include sufficient numbers of subjects aged 65 and over, however, to determine whether they respond differently than younger subjects. Treatment with alpha interferons, including PEG-Intron, is associated with neuropsychiatric, cardiac, pulmonary, GI and systemic (flu-like) adverse effects. Because these adverse reactions may be more severe in the elderly, caution should be exercised in use of PEG-Intron in this population. This drug is known to be substantially excreted by the kidney. Because elderly patients are more likely to have decreased renal function, the risk of toxic reactions to this drug may be greater in patients with impaired renal function. REBETOL should not be used in patients with creatinine clearance <50 mL/min. When using PEG-Intron/REBETOL therapy, refer also to the REBETOL Medication Guide.

ADVERSE REACTIONS

Nearly all study patients in clinical trials experienced one or more adverse events. In the PEG monotherapy trial the incidence of serious adverse events was similar (about 12%) in all treatment groups. In the PEG-Intron/REBETOL combination trial the incidence of serious adverse events was 17% in the PEG-Intron/REBETOL groups compared to 14% in the INTRON A/REBETOL group.

In many but not all cases, adverse events resolved after dose reduction or discontinuation of therapy. Some patients experienced ongoing or new serious adverse events during the 6-month follow-up period. In the PEG-Intron/REBETOL trial 13 patients experienced life-threatening psychiatric events (suicidal ideation or attempt) and one patient accomplished suicide.

There have been five patient deaths which occurred in clinical trials: one suicide in a patient receiving PEG-Intron monotherapy and one suicide in a patient receiving PEG-Intron/REBETOL combination therapy; two deaths among patients receiving INTRON A monotherapy (1 murder/suicide and 1 sudden death) and one patient death in the INTRON A/REBETOL group (motor vehicle accident).

Overall 10-14% of patients receiving PEG-Intron, alone or in combination with REBETOL, discontinued therapy compared with 6% treated with INTRON A alone and 13% treated with INTRON A in combination with REBETOL. The most common reasons for discontinuation of therapy were related to psychiatric, systemic (e.g. fatigue, headache), or gastrointestinal adverse events.

In the combination therapy trial, dose reductions due to adverse reactions occurred in 42% of patients receiving PEG-Intron (1.5 μg/kg)/REBETOL and in 34% of those receiving INTRON A/REBETOL. The majority of patients (57%) weighing 60 kg or less receiving PEG-Intron (1.5 μg/kg)/REBETOL required dose reduction. Reduction of interferon was dose related (PEG-Intron 1.5 μg/kg > PEG-Intron 0.5 μg/kg or INTRON A), 40%, 27%, 28%, respectively. Dose reduction for REBETOL was similar across all three groups, 33-35%. The most common reasons for dose modifications were neutropenia (18%), or anemia (9%). (see **Laboratory Values**). Other common reasons included depression, fatigue, nausea, and thrombocytopenia.

In the PEG-Intron/REBETOL combination trial the most common adverse events were psychiatric which occurred among 77% of patients and included most commonly depression, irritability, and insomnia, each reported by approximately 30-40% of subjects in all treatment groups. Suicidal behavior (ideation, attempts, and suicides) occurred in 2% of all patients during treatment or during follow-up after treatment cessation (see **WARNINGS**).

PEG-Intron induced fatigue or headache in approximately two-thirds of patients, and induced fever or rigors in approximately half of the patients. The severity of some of these systemic symptoms (e.g. fever and headache) tended to decrease as treatment continues. The incidence tends to be higher with PEG-Intron than with INTRON A therapy alone or in combination with REBETOL.

Application site inflammation and reaction (e.g. bruise, itchiness, irritation) occurred at approximately twice the incidence with PEG-Intron therapies (in up to 75% of patients) compared with INTRON A. However injection site pain was infrequent (2-3%) in all groups.

Other common adverse events in the PEG-Intron/REBETOL group included myalgia (56%), arthralgia (34%), nausea (43%), anorexia (32%), weight loss (29%), alopecia (36%), and pruritus (29%).

In the PEG-Intron monotherapy trial the incidence of severe adverse events was 13% in the INTRON A group and 17% in the PEG-Intron groups. In the PEG-Intron/REBETOL combination therapy trial the incidence of severe adverse events was 23% in the INTRON A/REBETOL group and 31-34% in the PEG-Intron/REBETOL groups. The incidence of life-threatening adverse events was ≤1% across all groups in the monotherapy and combination therapy trials.

Adverse events that occurred in the clinical trial at >5% incidence are provided in **Table 3** by treatment group. Due to potential differences in ascertainment procedures, adverse event rate comparisons across studies should not be made.
[See table 3 at top of previous page]

Many patients continued to experience adverse events several months after discontinuation of therapy. By the end of the 6-month follow-up period the incidence of ongoing adverse events by body class in the PEG-Intron 1.5/REBETOL group was 33% (psychiatric), 20% (musculoskeletal), and 10% (for endocrine and for GI). In approximately 10-15% of patients weight loss, fatigue and headache had not resolved. Individual serious adverse events occurred at a frequency ≤1% and included suicide attempt, suicidal ideation, severe depression; psychosis, aggressive reaction, relapse of drug addiction/overdose; nerve palsy (facial, oculomotor); cardiomyopathy, myocardial infarction, angina, pericardial effusion, retinal ischemia, retinal artery or vein thrombosis, blindness, decreased visual acuity, optic neuritis, transient ischemic attack, supraventricular arrhythmias, loss of consciousness; neutropenia, infection (sepsis, pneumonia, abscess, cellulitis); emphysema, bronchiolitis obliterans, pleural effusion, gastroenteritis, pancreatitis, gout, hyperglycemia, hyperthyroidism and hypothyroidism, autoimmune thrombocytopenia with or without purpura, rheumatoid arthritis, interstitial nephritis, lupus-like syndrome, sarcoidosis, aggravated psoriasis; urticaria, injection-site necrosis, vasculitis, phototoxicity.

The following adverse event has also been reported during the marketing surveillance of PEG-Intron therapy: Seizures.

Laboratory Values

Changes in selected laboratory values during treatment with PEG-Intron alone or in combination with REBETOL treatment are described below. **Decreases in hemoglobin, neutrophils, and platelets may require dose reduction or permanent discontinuation from therapy. (See DOSAGE AND ADMINISTRATION- Dose Reduction)**

Hemoglobin. REBETOL induced a decrease in hemoglobin levels in approximately two thirds of patients. Hemoglobin levels decreased to <11g/dL in about 30% of patients. Severe anemia (<8 g/dL) occurred in <1% of patients. Dose modification was required in 9 and 13% of patients in the PEG-Intron/REBETOL and INTRON A/REBETOL groups. Hemoglobin levels become stable by treatment week 4-6 on average. Hemoglobin levels return to baseline between 4 and 12 weeks posttreatment. In the PEG-Intron monotherapy trial hemoglobin decreases were generally mild and dose modifications were rarely necessary. (See **DOSAGE AND ADMINISTRATION: Dose Modification**).

Neutrophils. Decreases in neutrophil counts were observed in a majority of patients treated with PEG-Intron alone (70%) or as combination therapy with REBETOL (85%) and INTRON A/REBETOL (60%). Severe potentially life-threatening neutropenia (<0.5 × 10^9/L) occurred in 1% of patients treated with PEG-Intron monotherapy, 2% of patients treated with INTRON A/REBETOL and in 4% of patients treated with PEG-Intron/REBETOL. Two percent of patients receiving PEG-Intron monotherapy and 18% of patients receiving PEG-Intron/REBETOL required modification of interferon dosage. Few patients (≤1%) required permanent discontinuation of treatment. Neutrophil counts generally return to pre-treatment levels within 4 weeks of cessation of therapy. (**See DOSAGE AND ADMINISTRATION: Dose Modification**).

Platelets. Platelet counts decrease in approximately 20% of patients treated with PEG-Intron alone or with REBETOL and in 6% of patients treated with INTRON A/REBETOL. Severe decreases in platelet counts (<50,000/mm^3) occur in <1% of patients. Patients may require discontinuation or dose modification as a result of platelet decreases. (See **DOSAGE AND ADMINISTRATION: Dose Modification**). In the PEG-Intron/REBETOL combination therapy trial 1% or 3% of patients required dose modification of INTRON A or PEG-Intron respectively. Platelet counts generally returned to pretreatment levels within 4 weeks of the cessation of therapy.

Thyroid Function. Development of TSH abnormalities, with and without clinical manifestations, are associated with interferon therapies. Clinically apparent thyroid disorders occur among patients treated with either INTRON A or PEG-Intron (with or without REBETOL) at a similar incidence (5% for hypothyroidism and 3% for hyperthyroidism). Subjects developed new onset TSH abnormalities while on treatment and during the follow-up period. At the end of the follow-up period 7% of subjects still had abnormal TSH values.

Bilirubin and uric acid. In the PEG-Intron/REBETOL trial 10-14% of patients developed hyperbilirubinemia and 33-38% developed hyperuricemia in association with hemolysis. Six patients developed mild to moderate gout.

OVERDOSAGE

There is limited experience with overdosage. In the clinical studies, a few patients accidentally received a dose greater than that prescribed. There were no instances in which a participant in the monotherapy or combination therapy trials received more than 10.5 times the intended dose of PEG-Intron. The maximum dose received by any patient was 3.45 μg/kg weekly over a period of approximately 12 weeks. The maximum known overdosage of REBETOL was an intentional ingestion of 10 g (fifty 200 mg capsules). There were no serious reactions attributed to these overdosages. In cases of overdosing, symptomatic treatment and close observation of the patient are recommended.

DOSAGE AND ADMINISTRATION

There are no safety and efficacy data on treatment for longer than one year. A patient should self-inject PEG-Intron only if the physician determines that it is appropriate and the patient agrees to medical follow-up as necessary and training in proper injection technique has been given to him/her. (See illustrated **MEDICATION GUIDE** for instructions.)

It is recommended that patients receiving PEG-Intron, alone or in combination with ribavirin, be discontinued from therapy if HCV viral levels remain high after 6 months of therapy.

PEG-Intron Monotherapy
The recommended dose of PEG-Intron regimen is 1.0 μg/kg/week for one year.
The volume of PEG-Intron to be injected depends on the vial strength used and the patient's weight (see **Table 4 below**).

TABLE 4. Recommended PEG-Intron Monotherapy Dosing

Body weight (kg)	PEG-Intron Vial Strength	Amount of PEG-Intron (μg) to Administer	Volume (mL)* of PEG-Intron to Administer
≤45	50 μg per 0.5 mL	40	0.4
46–56		50	0.5
57–72	80 μg per 0.5 mL	64	0.4
73–88		80	0.5
89–106	120 μg per 0.5 mL	96	0.4
107–136		120	0.5
137–160	150 μg per 0.5 mL	150	0.5

* When reconstituted as directed

PEG-Intron/REBETOL Combination Therapy
When administered in combination with REBETOL, the recommended dose of PEG-Intron is 1.5 micrograms/kg/week. The volume of PEG-Intron to be injected depends on the vial strength of PEG-Intron and patient's body weight. (See **Table 5 below**).

TABLE 5. Recommended PEG-Intron Combination Therapy Dosing

Body weight (kg)	PEG-Intron Vial Strength	Amount of PEG-Intron (μg) to Administer	Volume (mL) of PEG-Intron to Administer
<40	50 μg per 0.5 mL	50	0.5
40–50	80 μg per 0.5 mL	64	0.4
51–60		80	0.5
61–75	120 μg per 0.5 mL	96	0.4
76–85		120	0.5
>85	150 μg per 0.5 mL	150	0.5

The recommended dose of REBETOL is 800 mg/day in 2 divided doses: two capsules (400 mg) with breakfast and two capsules (400 mg) with dinner. REBETOL should not be used in patients with creatinine clearance <50 mL/min.

Dose Reduction
If a serious adverse reaction develops during the course of treatment (See **WARNINGS**) discontinue or modify the dosage of PEG-Intron and/or REBETOL until the adverse event abates or decreases in severity. If persistent or recurrent serious adverse events develop despite adequate dosage adjustment, discontinue treatment. For guidelines for dose modifications and discontinuation based on laboratory parameters, see **Tables 6 and 7**. In the combination therapy trial dose reductions occurred among 42% of patients receiving PEG-Intron 1.5 μg/kg/REBETOL 800 mg daily including 57% of those patients weighing 60 kg or less (see **ADVERSE REACTIONS**).

Continued on next page

PEG-Intron—Cont.

[See table 6 below]
[See table 7 below]

Preparation and Administration

Two Safety-Lok* syringes are provided in the package; one syringe is for the reconstitution steps and one for the patient injection. There is a plastic safety sleeve to be pulled over the needle after use. The syringe locks with an audible click when the green stripe on the safety sleeve covers the red stripe on the needle. Brief instructions for the preparation and administration of PEG-Intron Powder for Injection are provided below. Please refer to the Medication Guide for detailed, step-by-step instructions.

Reconstitute the PEG-Intron lyophilized product with only 0.7 mL of supplied diluent (Sterile Water for Injection, USP). **The diluent vial is for single use only. The remaining diluent should be discarded.** No other medications should be added to solutions containing PEG-Intron, and PEG-Intron should not be reconstituted with other diluents. Swirl gently to hasten complete dissolution of the powder. The reconstituted solution should be clear and colorless. Visually inspect the solution for particulate matter and discoloration prior to administration. The solution should not be used if discolored or cloudy, or if particulates are present (see **MEDICATION GUIDE** for detailed instructions).

The reconstituted solution should be used immediately and cannot be stored for more than 24 hours at 2°–8°C (See **Storage**). The appropriate PEG-Intron dose should be withdrawn and injected subcutaneously. (See **MEDICATION GUIDE** for detailed instructions). The PEG-Intron vial is a single use vial and does not contain a preservative. **DO NOT REENTER VIAL. DISCARD UNUSED PORTION.** Once the dose from a single dose vial has been withdrawn, the sterility of any remaining product can no longer be guaranteed. Pooling of unused portions of some medications has been linked to bacterial contamination and morbidity.

After preparation and administration of the PEG-Intron injection, it is essential to follow the procedure for proper disposal of syringes and needles. A puncture-resistant container should be used for disposal of syringes. Patients should be instructed in the technique and importance of proper syringe disposal and be cautioned against reuse of these items (See **MEDICATION GUIDE** for detailed instructions.)

Storage

PEG-Intron should be stored at 25°C (77°F): excursions permitted to 15°–30°C (59°–86°F)[see USP Controlled Room Temperature]. After reconstitution with supplied Diluent the solution should be used immediately, but may be stored up to 24 hours at 2° to 8°C (36° to 46°F). The reconstituted solution contains no preservative, is clear and colorless. **Do not freeze.**

HOW SUPPLIED

PEG-Intron is a white to off-white lyophilized powder supplied in 2-mL vials. The PEG-Intron Powder for Injection should be reconstituted with 0.7 mL of the supplied Diluent (Sterile Water for Injection, USP) prior to use.

Each PEG-Intron Package Contains:	
A box containing one 50 μg per 0.5 mL vial of PEG-Intron Powder for Injection and one 1 mL vial of Diluent (Sterile Water for Injection, USP), 2 Safety-Lok* syringes with a safety sleeve and 2 alcohol swabs.	(NDC 0085-1368-01)
A box containing one 80 μg per 0.5 mL vial of PEG-Intron Powder for Injection and one 1 mL vial of Diluent (Sterile Water for Injection, USP), 2 Safety-Lok* syringes with a safety sleeve and 2 alcohol swabs.	(NDC 0085-1291-01)
A box containing one 120 μg per 0.5 mL vial of PEG-Intron Powder for Injection and one 1 mL vial of Diluent (Sterile Water for Injection, USP), 2 Safety-Lok* syringes with a safety sleeve and 2 alcohol swabs.	(NDC 0085-1304-01)
A box containing one 150 μg per 0.5 mL vial of PEG-Intron Powder for Injection and one 1 mL vial of Diluent (Sterile Water for Injection, USP), 2 Safety-Lok* syringes with a safety sleeve and 2 alcohol swabs.	(NDC 0085-1279-01)

Schering Corporation
Kenilworth, NJ 07033 USA
Copyright © 2001, Schering Corporation.
All rights reserved.

Rev. 8/02   24564754

*Safety-Lok is a trademark of Becton Dickinson and Company.

REBETOL®   ℞
[rĕ-bĕ-tōl]
(ribavirin, USP)
Capsules

Prescribing information for this product, which appears on pages 3072–3076 of the 2003 PDR, has been completely revised as follows. Please write "See Supplement A" next to the product heading.

- **REBETOL monotherapy is not effective for the treatment of chronic hepatitis C virus infection and should not be used alone for this indication. (See WARNINGS).**
- **The primary toxicity of ribavirin is hemolytic anemia. The anemia associated with REBETOL therapy may result in worsening of cardiac disease that has led to fatal and nonfatal myocardial infarctions. Patients with a history of significant or unstable cardiac disease should not be treated with REBETOL. (See WARNINGS, ADVERSE REACTIONS, and DOSAGE AND ADMINISTRATION).**
- **Significant teratogenic and/or embryocidal effects have been demonstrated in all animal species exposed to ribavirin. In addition, ribavirin has a multiple-dose half-life of 12 days, and so it may persist in nonplasma compartments for as long as 6 months. Therefore, REBETOL therapy is contraindicated in women who are pregnant and in the male partners of women who are pregnant. Extreme care must be taken to avoid pregnancy during therapy and for 6 months after completion of treatment in both female patients and in female partners of male patients who are taking REBETOL therapy. At least two reliable forms of effective contraception must be utilized during treatment and during the 6-month posttreatment follow-up-period. (See CONTRAINDICATIONS, WARNINGS, PRECAUTIONS Information for Patients and Pregnancy Category X).**

DESCRIPTION

REBETOL®

REBETOL is Schering Corporation's brand name for ribavirin, a nucleoside analog. The chemical name of ribavirin is 1-β-D-ribofuranosyl-1H-1,2,4-triazole-3-carboxamide and has the following structural formula:

Ribavirin is a white, crystalline powder. It is freely soluble in water and slightly soluble in anhydrous alcohol. The empirical formula is $C_8H_{12}N_4O_5$ and the molecular weight is 244.21.

REBETOL Capsules consist of a white powder in a white, opaque, gelatin capsule. Each capsule contains 200 mg ribavirin and the inactive ingredients microcrystalline cellulose, lactose monohydrate, croscarmellose sodium, and magnesium stearate. The capsule shell consists of gelatin, sodium lauryl sulfate, silicon dioxide, and titanium dioxide. The capsule is printed with edible blue pharmaceutical ink which is made of shellac, anhydrous ethyl alcohol, isopropyl alcohol, n-butyl alcohol, propylene glycol, ammonium hydroxide, and FD&C Blue #2 aluminum lake.

Mechanism of Action

The mechanism of inhibition of hepatitis C virus (HCV) RNA by combination therapy with interferon products has not been established.

CLINICAL PHARMACOLOGY

Pharmacokinetics

Ribavirin Single- and multiple-dose pharmacokinetic properties in adults with chronic hepatitis C are summarized in **TABLE 1**. Ribavirin was rapidly and extensively absorbed following oral administration. However, due to first-pass metabolism, the absolute bioavailability averaged 64% (44%). There was a linear relationship between dose and AUC_{tf} (AUC from time zero to last measurable concentration) following single doses of 200–1200 mg ribavirin. The relationship between dose and C_{max} was curvilinear, tending to asymptote above single doses of 400–600 mg.

Upon multiple oral dosing, based on $AUC12_{hr}$, a sixfold accumulation of ribavirin was observed in plasma. Following oral dosing with 600 mg BID, steady-state was reached by approximately 4 weeks, with mean steady-state plasma concentrations of 2200 (37%) ng/mL. Upon discontinuation of dosing, the mean half-life was 298 (30%) hours, which probably reflects slow elimination from nonplasma compartments.

Effect of Food on Absorption of Ribavirin Both AUC_{tf} and C_{max} increased by 70% when REBETOL Capsules were administered with a high-fat meal (841 kcal, 53.8 g fat, 31.6 g protein, and 57.4 g carbohydrate) in a single-dose pharma-

---

TABLE 6. Guidelines for Modification or Discontinuation of PEG-Intron or PEG-Intron/REBETOL and for Scheduling Visits for Patients with Depression

Depression Severity[1]	Initial Management (4–8 wks)		Depression		
	Dose modification	Visit schedule	Remains stable	Improves	Worsens
Mild	No change	Evaluate once weekly by visit and/or phone.	Continue weekly visit schedule.	Resume normal visit schedule.	(See moderate or severe depression)
Moderate	Decrease IFN dose 50%	Evaluate once weekly (office visit at least every other week).	Consider psychiatric consultation. Continue reduced dosing.	If symptoms improve and are stable for 4 wks, may resume normal visit schedule. Continue reducing dosing or return to normal dose.	(See severe depression)
Severe	Discontinue IFN/R permanently.	Obtain immediate psychiatric consultation.	Psychiatric therapy necessary		

[1] See DSM-IV for definitions.

TABLE 7. Guidelines for Dose Modification and Discontinuation of PEG-Intron or PEG-Intron/REBETOL for Hematologic Toxicity

Laboratory Values		PEG-Intron	REBETOL
Hgb*	<10.0 g/dL	------------------	Decrease by 200 mg/day
	<8.5 g/dL	Permanently discontinue	Permanently discontinue
WBC	<1.5 × 10⁹/L	Reduce dose by 50%	------------------
	<1.0 × 10⁹/L	Permanently discontinue	Permanently discontinue
Neutrophils	<0.75 × 10⁹/L	Reduce dose by 50%	------------------
	<0.5 × 10⁹/L	Permanently discontinue	Permanently discontinue
Platelets	<80 × 10⁹/L	Reduce dose by 50%	------------------
	<50 × 10⁹/L	Permanently discontinue	Permanently discontinue

*For patients with a history of stable cardiac disease receiving PEG-Intron in combination with ribavirin, the PEG-Intron dose should be reduced by half and the ribavirin dose by 200 mg/day if a >2g/dL decrease in hemoglobin is observed during any 4 week period. Both PEG-Intron and ribavirin should be permanently discontinued if patients have hemoglobin levels <12 g/dL after this ribavirin dose reduction.

cokinetic study. There are insufficient data to address the clinical relevance of these results. Clinical efficacy studies with REBETOL/INTRON A were conducted without instructions with respect to food consumption. During clinical studies with REBETOL/PEG-INTRON, all subjects were instructed to take REBETOL Capsules with food. (See **DOSAGE AND ADMINISTRATION**.)

Effect of Antacid on Absorption of Ribavirin Coadministration with an antacid containing magnesium, aluminum, and simethicone (Mylanta®[1]) resulted in a 14% decrease in mean ribavirin AUC_{tf}. The clinical relevance of results from this single-dose study is unknown.

TABLE 1. Mean (% CV) Pharmacokinetic Parameters for REBETOL When Administered Individually to Adults with Chronic Hepatitis C

Parameter	REBETOL (N=12)	
	Single Dose 600 mg	Multiple Dose 600 mg BID
T_{max} (hr)	1.7 (46)***	3 (60)
C_{max} *	782 (37)	3680 (85)
AUC_{tf} **	13400 (48)	228000 (25)
T½ (hr)	43.6 (47)	298 (30)
Apparent Volume of Distribution (L)	2825 (9)†	
Apparent Clearance (L/hr)	38.2 (40)	
Absolute Bioavailability	64% (44)††	

* ng/mL
** ng.hr/mL
*** N = 11
† data obtained from a single-dose pharmacokinetic study using ^{14}C labeled ribavirin; N = 5
†† N = 6

Ribavirin transport into nonplasma compartments has been most extensively studied in red blood cells, and has been identified to be primarily via an e_s-type equilibrative nucleoside transporter. This type of transporter is present on virtually all cell types and may account for the extensive volume of distribution. Ribavirin does not bind to plasma proteins.

Ribavirin has two pathways of metabolism: (i) a reversible phosphorylation pathway in nucleated cells; and (ii) a degradative pathway involving deribosylation and amide hydrolysis to yield a triazole carboxylic acid metabolite. Ribavirin and its triazole carboxamide and triazole carboxylic acid metabolites are excreted renally. After oral administration of 600 mg of ^{14}C-ribavirin, approximately 61% and 12% of the radioactivity was eliminated in the urine and feces, respectively, in 336 hours. Unchanged ribavirin accounted for 17% of the administered dose.

Results of *in vitro* studies using both human and rat liver microsome preparations indicated little or no cytochrome P450 enzyme-mediated metabolism of ribavirin, with minimal potential for P450 enzyme-based drug interactions.

No pharmacokinetic interactions were noted between INTRON A Injection and REBETOL Capsules in a multiple-dose pharmacokinetic study.

1. Trademark of Johnson & Johnson-Merck Consumer Pharmaceuticals Co.

Special Populations
Renal Dysfunction The pharmacokinetics of ribavirin were assessed after administration of a single oral dose (400 mg) of ribavirin to non HCV-infected subjects with varying degrees of renal dysfunction. The mean AUC_{tf} value was threefold greater in subjects with creatinine clearance values between 10 to 30 mL/min when compared to control subjects (creatinine clearance >90 mL/min). In subjects with creatinine clearance values between 30 to 60 mL/min, AUC_{tf} was twofold greater when compared to control subjects. The increased AUC_{tf} appears to be due to reduction of renal and non-renal clearance in these patients. Phase III efficacy trials included subjects with creatinine clearance values >50 mL/min. The multiple dose pharmacokinetics of ribavirin cannot be accurately predicted in patients with renal dysfunction. Ribavirin is not effectively removed by hemodialysis. Patients with creatinine clearance <50 mL/min should not be treated with REBETOL (See **WARNINGS**).

Hepatic Dysfunction The effect of hepatic dysfunction was assessed after a single oral dose of ribavirin (600 mg). The mean AUC_{tf} values were not significantly different in subjects with mild, moderate, or severe hepatic dysfunction (Child-Pugh Classification A, B, or C) when compared to control subjects. However, the mean C_{max} values increased with severity of hepatic dysfunction and was twofold greater in subjects with severe hepatic dysfunction when compared to control subjects.

Pediatric Patients Pharmacokinetic evaluations in pediatric subjects have not been performed.

Elderly Patients Pharmacokinetic evaluations in elderly subjects have not been performed.

Gender There were no clinically significant pharmacokinetic differences noted in a single-dose study of eighteen male and eighteen female subjects.

In this section of the label, numbers in parenthesis indicate % coefficient of variation.

TABLE 2. Virologic and Histologic Responses: Previously Untreated Patients*

	US Study			
	24 weeks of treatment		48 weeks of treatment	
	INTRON A plus REBETOL (N=228)	INTRON A plus Placebo (N=231)	INTRON A plus REBETOL (N=228)	INTRON A plus Placebo (N=225)
Virologic Response				
-Responder[1]	65 (29)	13 (6)	85 (37)	27 (12)
-Nonresponder	147 (64)	194 (84)	110 (48)	168 (75)
-Missing Data	16 (7)	24 (10)	33 (14)	30 (13)
Histologic Response				
-Improvement[2]	102 (45)	77 (33)	96 (42)	65 (29)
-No improvement	77 (34)	99 (43)	61 (27)	93 (41)
-Missing Data	49 (21)	55 (24)	71 (31)	67 (30)
	International Study			
	24 weeks of treatment		48 weeks of treatment	
		INTRON A plus REBETOL (N=265)	INTRON A plus REBETOL (N=268)	INTRON A plus Placebo (N=266)
Virologic Response				
-Responder[1]		86 (32)	113 (42)	46 (17)
-Nonresponder		158 (60)	120 (45)	196 (74)
-Missing Data		21 (8)	35 (13)	24 (9)
Histologic Response				
-Improvement[2]		103 (39)	102 (38)	69 (26)
-No improvement		85 (32)	58 (22)	111 (41)
-Missing Data		77 (29)	108 (40)	86 (32)

* Number (%) of patients.
1. Defined as HCV RNA below limit of detection using a research based RT-PCR assay at end of treatment and during follow-up period.
2. Defined as posttreatment (end of follow-up) minus pretreatment liver biopsy Knodell HAI score (I+II+III) improvement of ≥2 points.

TABLE 3. Virologic and Histologic Responses: Relapse Patients*

	US Study		International Study	
	INTRON A plus REBETOL (N=77)	INTRON A plus Placebo (N=76)	INTRON A plus REBETOL (N=96)	INTRON A plus Placebo (N=96)
Virologic Responses				
-Responder[1]	33 (43)	3 (4)	46 (48)	5 (5)
-Nonresponder	36 (47)	66 (87)	45 (47)	91 (95)
-Missing Data	8 (10)	7 (9)	5 (5)	0 (0)
Histologic Response				
-Improvement[2]	38 (49)	27 (36)	49 (51)	30 (31)
-No improvement	23 (30)	37 (49)	29 (30)	44 (46)
-Missing Data	16 (21)	12 (16)	18 (19)	22 (23)

* Number (%) of patients.
1. Defined as HCV RNA below limit of detection using a research based RT-PCR assay at end of treatment and during follow-up period.
2. Defined as posttreatment (end of follow-up) minus pretreatment liver biopsy Knodell HAI score (I+II+III) improvement of ≥2 points.

INDICATIONS AND USAGE
REBETOL (ribavirin, USP) Capsules are indicated in combination with INTRON A (interferon alfa-2b, recombinant) Injection for the treatment of chronic hepatitis C in patients with compensated liver disease previously untreated with alpha interferon or who have relapsed following alpha interferon therapy.

REBETOL Capsules are indicated in combination with PEG-INTRON (peg-interferon alfa-2b, recombinant) Injection for the treatment of chronic hepatitis C in patients with compensated liver disease who have not been previously treated with interferon alpha and are at least 18 years of age.

The safety and efficacy of REBETOL Capsules with interferons other than INTRON A or PEG-INTRON products have not been established.

Description of Clinical Studies
REBETOL/INTRON A Combination Therapy
Previously Untreated Patients
Adults with compensated chronic hepatitis C and detectable HCV RNA (assessed by a central laboratory using a research-based RT-PCR assay) who were previously untreated with alpha interferon therapy were enrolled into two multicenter, double-blind trials (US and International) and randomized to receive REBETOL Capsules 1200 mg/day (1000 mg/day for patients weighing ≤75 kg) plus INTRON A Injection 3 MIU TIW or INTRON A Injection plus placebo for 24 or 48 weeks followed by 24 weeks of off-therapy follow-up. The International study did not contain a 24-week INTRON A plus placebo treatment arm. The US study enrolled 912 patients, who, at baseline, were 67% male, 89% Caucasian with a mean Knodell HAI score (I+II+III) of 7.5, and 72% genotype 1. The International study, conducted in Europe, Israel, Canada, and Australia, enrolled 799 patients (65% male, 95% Caucasian, mean Knodell score 6.8, and 58% genotype 1).

Study results are summarized in **TABLE 2**.
[See table 2 above]

Of patients who had not achieved HCV RNA below the limit of detection of the research based assay by week 24 of REBETOL/ INTRON A treatment, less than 5% responded to an additional 24 weeks of combination treatment.

Among patients with HCV Genotype 1 treated with REBETOL/ INTRON A therapy who achieved HCV RNA below the detection limit of the research-based assay by 24 weeks, those randomized to 48 weeks of treatment had higher virologic responses compared to those in the 24 week treatment group. There was no observed increase in response rates for patients with HCV nongenotype 1 randomized to REBETOL/INTRON A therapy for 48 weeks compared to 24 weeks.

Relapse Patients
Patients with compensated chronic hepatitis C and detectable HCV RNA (assessed by a central laboratory using a research-based RT-PCR assay) who had relapsed following one or two courses of interferon therapy (defined as abnormal serum ALT levels) were enrolled into two multi-center, double-blind trials (US and International) and randomized to receive REBETOL 1200 mg/day (1000 mg/day for patients weighing ≤75 kg) plus INTRON A 3 MIU TIW or INTRON A plus placebo for 24 weeks followed by 24 weeks of off-therapy follow-up. The US study enrolled 153 patients who, at baseline, were 67% male, 92% Caucasian with a

Continued on next page

Rebetol—Cont.

mean Knodell HAI score (I+II+III) of 6.8, and 58% genotype 1. The International study, conducted in Europe, Israel, Canada, and Australia, enrolled 192 patients (64% male, 95% Caucasian, mean Knodell score 6.6, and 56% genotype 1).
Study results are summarized in **TABLE 3**.
[See table 3 on previous page]
Virologic and histologic responses were similar among male and female patients in both the previously untreated and relapse studies.

REBETOL/PEG-INTRON Combination Therapy

A randomized study compared treatment with two PEG-INTRON/ REBETOL regimens [PEG-INTRON 1.5 µg/kg SC once weekly (QW)/ REBETOL 800 mg PO daily (in divided doses); PEG-INTRON 1.5 µg/kg SC QW for 4 weeks then 0.5 µg/kg SC QW for 44 weeks/ REBETOL 1000/1200 mg PO daily (in divided doses)] with INTRON A [3 MIU SC thrice weekly (TIW)/REBETOL 1000/1200 mg PO daily (in divided doses)] in 1530 adults with chronic hepatitis C. Interferon naïve patients were treated for 48 weeks and followed for 24 weeks post-treatment. Eligible patients had compensated liver disease, detectable HCV RNA, elevated ALT, and liver histopathology consistent with chronic hepatitis.

Response to treatment was defined as undetectable HCV RNA at 24 weeks posttreatment (See **Table 4**).

TABLE 4. Rates of Response to Combination Treatment

	PEG-INTRON 1.5mg/kg QW REBETOL 800 mg QD	INTRON A 3 MIU TIW REBETOL 1000/1200mg QD
Overall[1,2] response	52% (264/511)	46% (231/505)
Genotype 1	41% (141/348)	33% (112/343)
Genotype 2–6	75% (123/163)	73% (119/162)

1. Serum HCV RNA was measured with a research-based quantitative polymerase chain reaction assay by a central laboratory.
2. Difference in overall treatment response (PEG-INTRON/REBETOL vs. INTRON A/REBETOL) is 6% with 95% confidence interval of (0.18, 11.63) adjusted for viral genotype and presence of cirrhosis at baseline.

The response rate to PEG-INTRON 1.5→0.5µg/kg/REBETOL was essentially the same as the response to INTRON A/REBETOL (data not shown).
Patients with viral genotype 1, regardless of viral load, had a lower response rate to PEG-INTRON (1.5 µg/kg)/REBETOL combination therapy compared to patients with other viral genotypes. Patients with both poor prognostic factors (genotype 1 and high viral load) had a response rate of 30% (78/256) compared to a response rate of 29% (71/247) with INTRON A/REBETOL combination therapy.
Patients with lower body weight tended to have higher adverse event rates (see **ADVERSE REACTIONS**) and higher response rates than patients with higher body weights. Differences in response rates between treatment arms did not substantially vary with body weight.
Treatment response rates with PEG-INTRON/REBETOL combination therapy were 49% in men and 56% in women. Response rates were lower in African American and Hispanic patients and higher in Asians compared to Caucasians. Although African Americans had a higher proportion of poor prognostic factors compared to Caucasians the number of non-Caucasians studied (11% of the total) was insufficient to allow meaningful conclusions about differences in response rates after adjusting for prognostic factors.
Liver biopsies were obtained before and after treatment in 68% of patients. Compared to baseline approximately 2/3 of patients in all treatment groups were observed to have a modest reduction in inflammation.

CONTRAINDICATIONS
Pregnancy
REBETOL Capsules may cause birth defects and/or death of the exposed fetus. REBETOL therapy is contraindicated for use in women who are pregnant or in men whose female partners are pregnant. (See **WARNINGS, PRECAUTIONS**-Information for Patients and Pregnancy Category X).
REBETOL Capsules are contraindicated in patients with a history of hypersensitivity to ribavirin or any component of the capsule.
Patients with autoimmune hepatitis must not be treated with combination REBETOL/INTRON A therapy because using these medicines can make the hepatitis worse.
Patients with hemoglobinopathies (eg, thalassemia major, sickle-cell anemia) should not be treated with REBETOL Capsules.

WARNINGS
Based on results of clinical trials ribavirin monotherapy is not effective for the treatment of chronic hepatitis C virus infection; therefore, REBETOL Capsules must not be used alone. The safety and efficacy of REBETOL Capsules have only been established when used together with INTRON A (interferon alfa-2b, recombinant) as REBETRON Combination Therapy or with PEG-INTRON Injection.
There are significant adverse events caused by REBETOL/INTRON A or PEG-INTRON therapy, including severe depression and suicidal ideation, hemolytic anemia, suppression of bone marrow function, autoimmune and infectious disorders, pulmonary dysfunction, pancreatitis, and diabetes. The REBETRON Combination Therapy and PEG-INTRON package inserts should be reviewed in their entirety prior to initiation of combination treatment for additional safety information.

Pregnancy
REBETOL Capsules may cause birth defects and/or death of the exposed fetus. Extreme care must be taken to avoid pregnancy in female patients and in female partners of male patients. REBETOL has demonstrated significant teratogenic and/or embryocidal effects in all animal species in which adequate studies have been conducted. These effects occurred at doses as low as one twentieth of the recommended human dose of ribavirin. REBETOL THERAPY SHOULD NOT BE STARTED UNTIL A REPORT OF A NEGATIVE PREGNANCY TEST HAS BEEN OBTAINED IMMEDIATELY PRIOR TO PLANNED INITIATION OF THERAPY. Patients should be instructed to use at least two forms of effective contraception during treatment and during the six month period after treatment has been stopped based on multiple dose half-life of ribavirin of 12 days. Pregnancy testing should occur monthly during REBETOL therapy and for six months after therapy has stopped (see **CONTRAINDICATIONS and PRECAUTIONS**: Information for Patients and Pregnancy Category X).

Anemia
The primary toxicity of ribavirin is hemolytic anemia, which was observed in approximately 10% of REBETOL/INTRON A-treated patients in clinical trials (See **ADVERSE REACTIONS**: Laboratory Values—*Hemoglobin*). The anemia associated with REBETOL capsules occurs within 1–2 weeks of initiation of therapy. BECAUSE THE INITIAL DROP IN HEMOGLOBIN MAY BE SIGNIFICANT, IT IS ADVISED THAT HEMOGLOBIN OR HEMATOCRIT BE OBTAINED PRETREATMENT AND AT WEEK 2 AND WEEK 4 OF THERAPY, OR MORE FREQUENTLY IF CLINICALLY INDICATED. Patients should then be followed as clinically appropriate.

Fatal and nonfatal myocardial infarctions have been reported in patients with anemia caused by REBETOL. Patients should be assessed for underlying cardiac disease before initiation of ribavirin therapy. Patients with pre-existing cardiac disease should have electrocardiograms administered before treatment, and should be appropriately monitored during therapy. If there is any deterioration of cardiovascular status, therapy should be suspended or discontinued. (See **DOSAGE AND ADMINISTRATION**: Guidelines for Dose Modification.) Because cardiac disease may be worsened by drug induced anemia, patients with a history of significant or unstable cardiac disease should not use REBETOL. (See **ADVERSE REACTIONS**.)

REBETOL and INTRON A or PEG-INTRON therapy should be suspended in patients with signs and symptoms of pancreatitis and discontinued in patients with confirmed pancreatitis.
REBETOL should not be used in patients with creatinine clearance <50 mL/min. (See **Clinical Pharmacology**, Special populations.)

Pulmonary symptoms, including dyspnea, pulmonary infiltrates, pneumonitis and pneumonia, have been reported during therapy with REBETOL/INTRON A; occasional cases of fatal pneumonia have occurred. In addition, sarcoidosis or the exacerbation of sarcoidosis has been reported. If there is evidence of pulmonary infiltrates or pulmonary function impairment, the patient should be closely monitored, and if appropriate, combination REBETOL/INTRON A treatment should be discontinued.

PRECAUTIONS
The safety and efficacy of REBETOL/INTRON A and PEG-INTRON therapy for the treatment of HIV infection, adenovirus, RSV, parainfluenza, or influenza infections have not been established. REBETOL Capsules should not be used for these indications. Ribavirin for inhalation has a separate package insert, which should be consulted if ribavirin inhalation therapy is being considered.
The safety and efficacy of REBETOL/INTRON A therapy has not been established in liver or other organ transplant patients, patients with decompensated liver disease due to hepatitis C infection, patients who are nonresponders to interferon therapy, or patients coinfected with HBV or HIV.

Information for Patients
Patients must be informed that REBETOL Capsules may cause birth defects and/or death of the exposed fetus. REBETOL must not be used by women who are pregnant or by men whose female partners are pregnant. Extreme care must be taken to avoid pregnancy in female patients and in female partners of male patients taking REBETOL. REBETOL should not be initiated until a report of a negative pregnancy test has been obtained immediately prior to initiation of therapy. Patients must perform a pregnancy test monthly during therapy and for 6 months posttherapy. Women of childbearing potential must be counseled about use of effective contraception (two reliable forms) prior to initiating therapy. Patients (male and female) must be advised of the teratogenic/embryocidal risks and must be instructed to practice effective contraception during REBETOL and for 6 months posttherapy. Patients (male and female) should be advised to notify the physician immediately in the event of a pregnancy. (See **CONTRAINDICATIONS and WARNINGS**.)

If pregnancy does occur during treatment or during 6 months posttherapy, the patient must be advised of the teratogenic risk of REBETOL therapy to the fetus. Patients, or partners of patients, should immediately report any pregnancy that occurs during treatment or within 6 months after treatment cessation to their physician. Physicians should report such cases by calling 1-800-727-7064.

Patients receiving REBETOL Capsules should be informed of the benefits and risks associated with treatment, directed in its appropriate use, and referred to the patient **MEDICATION GUIDE**. Patients should be informed that the effect of treatment of hepatitis C infection on transmission is not known, and that appropriate precautions to prevent transmission of the hepatitis C virus should be taken.

The most common adverse experience occurring with REBETOL Capsules is anemia, which may be severe. (See **ADVERSE REACTIONS**.) Patients should be advised that laboratory evaluations are required prior to starting therapy and periodically thereafter. (See **Laboratory Tests**.) It is advised that patients be well hydrated, especially during the initial stages of treatment.

Laboratory Tests The following laboratory tests are recommended for all patients treated with REBETOL Capsules, prior to beginning treatment and then periodically thereafter.
- Standard hematologic tests - including hemoglobin (pretreatment, week 2 and week 4 of therapy, and as clinically appropriate [see **WARNINGS**]), complete and differential white blood cell counts, and platelet count.
- Blood chemistries - liver function tests and TSH.
- Pregnancy - including monthly monitoring for women of child-bearing potential.
- ECG (See **WARNINGS**)

Carcinogenesis and Mutagenesis Adequate studies to assess the carcinogenic potential of ribavirin in animals have not been conducted. However, ribavirin is a nucleoside analogue that has produced positive findings in multiple *in vitro* and animal *in vivo* genotoxicity assays, and should be considered a potential carcinogen. Further studies to assess the carcinogenic potential of ribavirin in animals are ongoing.

Ribavirin demonstrated increased incidences of mutation and cell transformation in multiple genotoxicity assays. Ribavirin was active in the Balb/3T3 *In Vitro* Cell Transformation Assay. Mutagenic activity was observed in the mouse lymphoma assay, and at doses of 20–200 mg/kg (estimated human equivalent of 1.67–16.7 mg/kg, based on body surface area adjustment for a 60 kg adult; 0.1–1 X the maximum recommended human 24-hour dose of ribavirin) in a mouse micronucleus assay. A dominant lethal assay in rats was negative, indicating that if mutations occurred in rats they were not transmitted through male gametes.

Impairment of Fertility Ribavirin demonstrated significant embryocidal and/or teratogenic effects at doses well below the recommended human dose in all animal species in which adequate studies have been conducted.

Fertile women and partners of fertile women should not receive REBETOL unless the patient and his/her partner are using effective contraception (two reliable forms). Based on a multiple dose half-life (t½) of ribavirin of 12 days, effective contraception must be utilized for 6 months posttherapy (eg, 15 half-lives of clearance for ribavirin).

REBETOL should be used with caution in fertile men. In studies in mice to evaluate the time course and reversibility of ribavirin-induced testicular degeneration at doses of 15 to 150 mg/kg/day (estimated human equivalent of 1.25–12.5 mg/kg/day, based on body surface area adjustment for a 60 kg adult; 0.1–0.8 X the maximum human 24-hour dose of ribavirin) administered for 3 or 6 months, abnormalities in sperm occurred. Upon cessation of treatment, essentially total recovery from ribavirin-induced testicular toxicity was apparent within 1 or 2 spermatogenesis cycles.

Animal Toxicology Long-term studies in the mouse and rat (18–24 months; doses of 20–75 and 10–40 mg/kg/day, respectively [estimated human equivalent doses of 1.67–6.25 and 1.43–5.71 mg/kg/day, respectively, based on body surface area adjustment for a 60 kg adult; approximately 0.1–0.4 X the maximum human 24-hour dose of ribavirin]) have demonstrated a relationship between chronic ribavirin exposure and increased incidences of vascular lesions (microscopic hemorrhages) in mice. In rats, retinal degeneration occurred in controls, but the incidence was increased in ribavirin-treated rats.

Pregnancy Category X (see **CONTRAINDICATIONS**)
Ribavirin produced significant embryocidal and/or teratogenic effects in all animal species in which adequate studies have been conducted. Malformations of the skull, palate, eye, jaw, limbs, skeleton, and gastrointestinal tract were noted. The incidence and severity of teratogenic effects increased with escalation of the drug dose. Survival of fetuses and offspring was reduced. In conventional embryotoxicity/teratogenicity studies in rats and rabbits, observed no effect dose levels were well below those for proposed clinical use (0.3 mg/kg/day for both the rat and rabbit; approximately 0.06 X the recommended human 24-hour dose of ribavirin). No maternal toxicity or effects on offspring were observed in a peri/postnatal toxicity study in rats dosed orally at up to 1 mg/kg/day (estimated human equivalent dose of 0.17 mg/kg based on body surface area adjustment for a 60 kg adult; approximately 0.01 X the maximum recommended human 24-hour dose of ribavirin).

TABLE 5. Selected Treatment-Emergent Adverse Events:
Previously Untreated and Relapse Patients

Percentage of Patients

	US Previously Untreated Study				US Relapse Study	
	24 weeks of treatment		48 weeks of treatment		24 weeks of treatment	
Patients Reporting Adverse Events*	INTRON A plus REBETOL (N=228)	INTRON A plus Placebo (N=231)	INTRON A plus REBETOL (N=228)	INTRON A plus Placebo (N=225)	INTRON A plus REBETOL (N=77)	INTRON A plus Placebo (N=76)
Application Site Disorders						
injection site inflammation	13	10	12	14	6	8
injection site reaction	7	9	8	9	5	3
Body as a Whole – General Disorders						
Headache	63	63	66	67	66	68
Fatigue	68	62	70	72	60	53
Rigors	40	32	42	39	43	37
Fever	37	35	41	40	32	36
influenza-like symptoms	14	18	18	20	13	13
Asthenia	9	4	9	9	10	4
chest pain	5	4	9	8	6	7
Central & Peripheral Nervous System Disorders						
Dizziness	17	15	23	19	26	21
Gastrointestinal System Disorders						
Nausea	38	35	46	33	47	33
Anorexia	27	16	25	19	21	14
Dyspepsia	14	6	16	9	16	9
Vomiting	11	10	9	13	12	8
Musculoskeletal System Disorders						
Myalgia	61	57	64	63	61	58
Arthralgia	30	27	33	36	29	29
musculoskeletal pain	20	26	28	32	22	28
Psychiatric Disorders						
Insomnia	39	27	39	30	26	25
Irritability	23	19	32	27	25	20
Depression	32	25	36	37	23	14
emotional lability	7	6	11	8	12	8
concentration impaired	11	14	14	14	10	12
nervousness	4	2	4	4	5	4
Respiratory System Disorders						
Dyspnea	19	9	18	10	17	12
Sinusitis	9	7	10	14	12	7
Skin and Appendages Disorders						
Alopecia	28	27	32	28	27	26
Rash	20	9	28	8	21	5
Pruritus	21	9	19	8	13	4
Special Senses, Other Disorders						
taste perversion	7	4	8	4	6	5

* Patients reporting one or more adverse events. A patient may have reported more than one adverse event within a body system/organ class category.

Treatment and Posttreatment: Potential Risk to the Fetus
Ribavirin is known to accumulate in intracellular components from where it is cleared very slowly. It is not known whether ribavirin contained in sperm will exert a potential teratogenic effect upon fertilization of the ova. In a study in rats, it was concluded that dominant lethality was not induced by ribavirin at doses up to 200 mg/kg for 5 days (estimated human equivalent doses of 7.14–28.6 mg/kg, based on body surface area adjustment for a 60 kg adult; up to 1.7 X the maximum recommended human dose of ribavirin). However, because of the potential human teratogenic effects of ribavirin, male patients should be advised to take every precaution to avoid risk of pregnancy for their female partners.

Women of childbearing potential should not receive REBETOL unless they are using effective contraception (two reliable forms) during the therapy period. In addition, effective contraception should be utilized for 6 months posttherapy based on a multiple-dose half-life (t½) of ribavirin of 12 days. Male patients and their female partners must practice effective contraception (two reliable forms) during treatment with REBETOL and for the 6-month posttherapy period (eg, 15 half-lives for ribavirin clearance from the body).

If pregnancy occurs in a patient or partner of a patient during treatment or during the 6 months after treatment cessation, physicians should report such cases by calling 1-800-727-7064.

Nursing Mothers It is not known whether the REBETOL product is excreted in human milk. Because of the potential for serious adverse reactions from the drug in nursing infants, a decision should be made whether to discontinue nursing or to delay or discontinue REBETOL.

Geriatric Use Clinical studies of REBETOL/INTRON A or PEG-INTRON therapy did not include sufficient numbers of subjects aged 65 and over to determine if they respond differently from younger subjects.

REBETOL is known to be substantially excreted by the kidney, and the risk of toxic reactions to this drug may be greater in patients with impaired renal function. Because elderly patients often have decreased renal function, care should be taken in dose selection. Renal function should be monitored and dosage adjustments should be made accordingly. REBETOL should not be used in patients with creatinine clearance <50 mL/min. (See **WARNINGS**.)

In general, REBETOL Capsules should be administered to elderly patients cautiously, starting at the lower end of the dosing range, reflecting the greater frequency of decreased hepatic and/or cardiac function, and of concomitant disease or other drug therapy. In clinical trials, elderly subjects had a higher frequency of anemia (67%) than did younger patients (28%). (See **WARNINGS**.)

Pediatric Use Safety and effectiveness in pediatric patients have not been established.

ADVERSE REACTIONS

The primary toxicity of ribavirin is hemolytic anemia. Reductions in hemoglobin levels occurred within the first 1–2 weeks of oral therapy. (See WARNINGS.) Cardiac and pulmonary events associated with anemia occurred in approximately 10% of patients. (See WARNINGS.)

REBETOL/INTRON A Combination Therapy
In clinical trials, 19% and 6% of previously untreated and relapse patients, respectively, discontinued therapy due to adverse events in the combination arms compared to 13% and 3% in the interferon arms. Selected treatment-emergent adverse events that occurred in the US studies with ≥5% incidence are provided in **TABLE 5** by treatment group. In general, the selected treatment-emergent adverse events reported with lower incidence in the international studies as compared to the US studies with the exception of asthenia, influenza-like symptoms, nervousness, and pruritus.
[See table 5 above]

In addition, the following spontaneous adverse events have been reported during the marketing surveillance of REBETOL/INTRON A therapy: hearing disorder and vertigo.

REBETOL/PEG-INTRON Combination Therapy
Overall, in clinical trials, 14% of patients receiving REBETOL in combination with PEG-INTRON, discontinued therapy compared with 13% treated with REBETOL in combination with INTRON A. The most common reasons for discontinuation of therapy were related to psychiatric, systemic (e.g. fatigue, headache), or gastrointestinal adverse events. Adverse events that occurred in clinical trial at >5% incidence are provided in **Table 6** by treatment group.

TABLE 6. Adverse Events Occurring in > 5% of Patients

	Percentage of Patients Reporting Adverse Events*	
Adverse Events	PEG-INTRON 1.5 µg.kg/ REBETOL (N=511)	INTRON A/ REBETOL (N=505)
Application Site		
Injection Site Inflammation	25	18
Injection Site Reaction	58	36
Autonomic Nervous System		
Mouth Dry	12	8
Sweating Increased	11	7
Flushing	4	3
Body as a Whole		
Fatigue/Asthenia	66	63
Headache	62	58
Rigors	48	41
Fever	46	33
Weight Decrease	29	20
RUQ Pain	12	6
Chest Pain	8	7
Malaise	4	6
Central & Peripheral Nervous System		
Dizziness	21	17
Endocrine		
Hypothyroidism	5	4
Gastrointestinal		
Nausea	43	33
Anorexia	32	27
Diarrhea	22	17
Vomiting	14	12
Abdominal Pain	13	13
Dyspepsia	9	8
Constipation	5	5
Hematologic Disorders		
Neutropenia	26	14
Anemia	12	17
Leukopenia	6	5
Thrombocytopenia	5	2
Liver and Biliary System		
Hepatomegaly	4	4
Musculoskeletal		
Myalgia	56	50
Arthralgia	34	28
Musculoskeletal Pain	21	19
Psychiatric		
Insomnia	40	41
Depression	31	34
Anxiety/Emotional Lability/Irritability	47	47
Concentration Impaired	17	21
Agitation	8	5
Nervousness	6	6
Reproductive, Female		
Menstrual Disorder	7	6
Resistance Mechanism		
Infection Viral	12	12
Infection Fungal	6	1
Respiratory System		
Dyspnea	26	24
Coughing	23	16
Pharyngitis	12	13
Rhinitis	8	6
Sinusitis	6	5
Skin and Appendages		
Alopecia	36	32
Pruritus	29	28
Rash	24	23

Continued on next page

Rebetol—Cont.

Skin Dry	24	23
Special Senses, Other		
Taste Perversion	9	4
Vision Disorders		
Vision Blurred	5	6
Conjunctivitis	4	5

*Patients reporting one or more adverse events. A patient may have reported more than one adverse event within a body system/organ class category.

Laboratory Values
REBETOL/INTRON A Combination Therapy
Changes in selected hematologic values (hemoglobin, white blood cells, neutrophils, and platelets) during therapy are described below. (See **TABLE 7**.)

Hemoglobin Hemoglobin decreases among patients receiving REBETOL therapy began at Week 1, with stabilization by Week 4. In previously untreated patients treated for 48 weeks the mean maximum decrease from baseline was 3.1 g/dL in the US study and 2.9 g/dL in the International study. In relapse patients the mean maximum decrease from baseline was 2.8 g/dL in the US study and 2.6 g/dL in the International study. Hemoglobin values returned to pretreatment levels within 4–8 weeks of cessation of therapy in most patients.

Bilirubin and Uric Acid Increases in both bilirubin and uric acid, associated with hemolysis, were noted in clinical trials. Most were moderate biochemical changes and were reversed within 4 weeks after treatment discontinuation. This observation occurs most frequently in patients with a previous diagnosis of Gilbert's syndrome. This has not been associated with hepatic dysfunction or clinical morbidity.
[See table 7 below]

REBETOL/PEG-INTRON Combination Therapy
Changes in selected hematologic values (hemoglobin, white blood cells, neutrophils, and platelets) during therapy are described below. (See **TABLE 8**.)

Hemoglobin
REBETOL induced a decrease in hemoglobin levels in approximately two thirds of patients. Hemoglobin levels decreased to <11g/dL in about 30% of patients. Severe anemia (<8 g/dl) occurred in <1% of patients. Dose modification was required in 9 and 13% of patients in the PEG-INTRON/REBETOL and INTRON A/REBETOL groups.

Bilirubin and Uric
In the REBETOL/PEG-INTRON combination trial 10–14% of patients developed hyperbilirubinemia and 33–38% developed hyperuricemia in association with hemolysis. Six patients developed mild to moderate gout.

TABLE 8. Selected Hematologic Values During Treatment with REBETOL plus PEG-INTRON

	Number (%) of Subjects	
	PEG-INTRON plus REBETOL (N=511)	INTRON A plus Placebo (N=505)
Hemoglobin (g/dL)		
9.5-10.9	26	27
8.0-9.4	3	3
6.5-7.9	0.2	0.2
<6.5	0	0
Leukocytes (×10⁹/L)		
2.0-2.9	46	41
1.5-1.9	24	8
1.0-1.4	5	1
<1.0	0	0
Neutrophils (×10⁹/L)		
1.0-1.49	33	37
0.75-0.99	25	13
0.5-0.74	18	7
<0.5	4	2
Platelets (×10⁹/L)		
70-99	15	5
50-69	3	0.8
30-49	0.2	0.2
<30	0	0
Total Bilirubin (mg/dL)		
1.5-3.0	10	13
3.1-6.0	0.6	0.2
6.1-12.0	0	0.2
>12.0	0	0
ALT (SGPT)		
2 × Baseline	0.6	0.2
2.1-5 × Baseline	3	1
5.1-10 × Baseline	0	0
>10 × Baseline	0	0

OVERDOSAGE
There is limited experience with overdosage. Acute ingestion of up to 20 grams of REBETOL Capsules, INTRON A ingestion of up to 120 million units, and subcutaneous doses of INTRON A up to 10 times the recommended doses have been reported. Primary effects that have been observed are increased incidence and severity of the adverse events related to the therapeutic use of INTRON A and REBETOL products. However, hepatic enzyme abnormalities, renal failure, hemorrhage, and myocardial infarction have been reported with administration of single subcutaneous doses of INTRON A that exceed dosing recommendations.

There is no specific antidote for INTRON A or REBETOL overdose, and hemodialysis and peritoneal dialysis are not effective for treatment of overdose of either agent.

DOSAGE AND ADMINISTRATION (see CLINICAL PHARMACOLOGY, Special Populations; see WARNINGS)
REBETOL/INTRON A Combination Therapy
The recommended dose of REBETOL Capsules depends on the patient's body weight. The recommended dose of REBETOL is provided in **TABLE 9**.
The recommended duration of treatment for patients previously untreated with interferon is 24 to 48 weeks. The duration of treatment should be individualized to the patient depending on baseline disease characteristics, response to therapy, and tolerability of the regimen. (See **Description of Clinical Studies** and **ADVERSE REACTIONS**.) After 24 weeks of treatment virologic response should be assessed. Treatment discontinuation should be considered in any patient who has not achieved an HCV RNA below the limit of detection of the assay by 24 weeks. There are no safety and efficacy data on treatment for longer than 48 weeks in the previously untreated patient population.
In patients who relapse following interferon therapy, the recommended duration of treatment is 24 weeks. There are no safety and efficacy data on treatment for longer than 24 weeks in the relapse patient population.

TABLE 9. Recommended Dosing

Body weight	REBETOL Capsules
≤ 75 kg	2 × 200-mg capsules AM, 3 × 200-mg capsules PM daily p.o.
> 75 kg	3 × 200 mg capsules AM, 3 × 200 mg capsules PM daily p.o.

REBETOL may be administered without regard to food, but should be administered in a consistent manner with respect to food intake. (See **CLINICAL PHARMACOLOGY**.)
REBETOL/PEG-INTRON Combination Therapy
The recommended dose of REBETOL Capsules is 800 mg/day in 2 divided doses: two capsules (400 mg) in the morning with food and two capsules (400 mg) in the evening with food.

Dose Modifications (TABLE 10)
If severe adverse reactions or laboratory abnormalities develop during combination REBETOL/INTRON A therapy the dose should be modified, or discontinued if appropriate, until the adverse reactions abate. If intolerance persists after dose adjustment, REBETOL/INTRON A therapy should be discontinued.
REBETOL should not be used in patients with creatinine clearance <50 mL/min. (See **WARNINGS** and **CLINICAL PHARMACOLOGY, Special Populations**.)
REBETOL should be administered with caution to patients with pre-existing cardiac disease. Patients should be assessed before commencement of therapy and should be appropriately monitored during therapy. If there is any deterioration of cardiovascular status, therapy should be stopped. (See **WARNINGS**.)
For patients with a history of stable cardiovascular disease, a permanent dose reduction is required if the hemoglobin decreases by ≥2 g/dL during any 4-week period. In addition, for these cardiac history patients, if the hemoglobin remains <12 g/dL after 4 weeks on a reduced dose, the patient should discontinue combination REBETOL/INTRON A therapy.
It is recommended that a patient whose hemoglobin level falls below 10 g/dL have his/her REBETOL dose reduced to 600 mg daily (1 × 200-mg capsule AM, 2 × 200 mg capsules PM). A patient whose hemoglobin level falls below 8.5 g/dL should be permanently discontinued from REBETOL therapy. (See **WARNINGS**.)

TABLE 10. Guidelines for Dose Modifications and Discontinuation for Anemia

Hemoglobin	Dose Reduction* REBETOL- 600 mg daily	Permanent Discontinuation of REBETOL Treatment
No Cardiac History	<10 g/dL	<8.5 g/dL
Cardiac History Patients	≥2 g/dL decrease during any 4-week period during treatment	<12 g/dL after 4 weeks of dose reduction

HOW SUPPLIED
REBETOL 200-mg Capsules are white, opaque capsules with REBETOL, 200 mg, and the Schering Corporation logo imprinted on the capsule shell; the capsules are packaged in a bottle containing 42 capsules (NDC-0085-1327-04), 56 capsules (NDC 0085-1351-05), 70 capsules (NDC 0085-1385-07), and 84 capsules (NDC 0085-1194-03).
Storage Conditions
The bottle of REBETOL Capsules should be stored at 25°C (77°F); excursions are permitted between 15° and 30°C (59° and 86°F).
Schering Corporation
Kenilworth, NJ 07033 USA

TABLE 7. Selected Hematologic Values During Treatment with REBETOL plus INTRON A: Previously Untreated and Relapse Patients

	Percentage of Patients					
	US Previously Untreated Study				US Relapse Study	
	24 weeks of treatment		48 weeks of treatment		24 weeks of treatment	
	INTRON A plus REBETOL (N=228)	INTRON A plus Placebo (N=231)	INTRON A plus REBETOL (N=228)	INTRON A plus Placebo (N=225)	INTRON A plus REBETOL (N=77)	INTRON A plus Placebo (N=76)
Hemoglobin (g/dL)						
9.5-10.9	24	1	32	1	21	3
8.0-9.4	5	0	4	0	4	0
6.5-7.9	0	0	0	0.4	0	0
<6.5	0	0	0	0	0	0
Leukocytes (×10⁹/L)						
2.0-2.9	40	20	38	23	45	26
1.5-1.9	4	1	9	2	5	3
1.0-1.4	0.9	0	2	0	0	0
<1.0	0	0	0	0	0	0
Neutrophils (×10⁹/L)						
1.0-1.49	30	32	31	44	42	34
0.75-0.99	14	15	14	11	16	18
0.5-0.74	9	9	14	7	8	4
<0.5	11	8	11	5	5	8
Platelets (×10⁹/L)						
70-99	9	11	11	14	6	12
50-69	2	3	2	3	0	5
30-49	0	0.4	0	0.4	0	0
<30	0.9	0	1	0.9	0	0
Total Bilirubin (mg/dL)						
1.5-3.0	27	13	32	13	21	7
3.1-6.0	0.9	0.4	2	0	3	0
6.1-12.0	0	0	0.4	0	0	0
>12.0	0	0	0	0	0	0

B-24819639 Rev. 9/02

REBETRON® ℞
[*rĕb-ē-trŏn*]
Combination Therapy *containing*
REBETOL® (ribavirin, USP) Capsules *and*
INTRON® A (interferon alfa-2b, recombinant) Injection

Prescribing information for this product, which appears on pages 3076–3081 of the 2003 PDR, has been completely revised as follows. Please write "See Supplement A" next to the product heading.

CONTRAINDICATIONS AND WARNINGS

Combination REBETOL/INTRON A therapy is contraindicated in females who are pregnant and in the male partners of females who are pregnant. Extreme care must be taken to avoid pregnancy during therapy and for 6 months after completion of treatment in female patients, and in female partners of male patients who are taking combination REBETOL/INTRON A therapy. Females of childbearing potential and males must use two reliable forms of effective contraception during treatment and during the 6-month posttreatment follow-up period. Significant teratogenic and/or embryocidal effects have been demonstrated for ribavirin in all animal species studied. See CONTRAINDICATIONS and WARNINGS. REBETOL monotherapy is not effective for the treatment of chronic hepatitis C and should not be used for this indication. See WARNINGS.

Alpha interferons, including INTRON® A, cause or aggravate fatal or life-threatening neuropsychiatric, autoimmune, ischemic, and infectious disorders. Patients should be monitored closely with periodic clinical and laboratory evaluations. Patients with persistently severe or worsening signs or symptoms of these conditions should be withdrawn from therapy. In many but not all cases these disorders resolve after stopping INTRON A therapy. See **WARNINGS**, and **ADVERSE REACTIONS**.

DESCRIPTION

REBETOL®

REBETOL is Schering Corporation's brand name for ribavirin, a nucleoside analog with antiviral activity. The chemical name of ribavirin is 1-β-D-ribofuranosyl-1*H*-1,2,4-triazole-3-carboxamide and has the following structural formula:

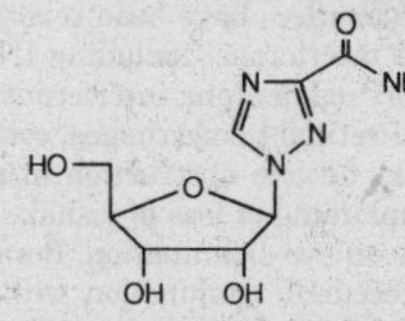

Ribavirin is a white, crystalline powder. It is freely soluble in water and slightly soluble in anhydrous alcohol. The empirical formula is $C_8H_{12}N_4O_5$ and the molecular weight is 244.21.

REBETOL Capsules consist of a white powder in a white, opaque, gelatin capsule. Each capsule contains 200 mg ribavirin and the inactive ingredients microcrystalline cellulose, lactose monohydrate, croscarmellose sodium, and magnesium stearate. The capsule shell consists of gelatin and titanium dioxide. The capsule is printed with edible blue pharmaceutical ink which is made of shellac, anhydrous ethyl alcohol, isopropyl alcohol, n-butyl alcohol, propylene glycol, ammonium hydroxide, and FD&C Blue #2 aluminum lake.

INTRON® A

INTRON A is Schering Corporation's brand name for interferon alfa-2b, recombinant, a purified, sterile, recombinant interferon product.

Interferon alfa-2b, recombinant has been classified as an alpha interferon and is a water-soluble protein composed of 165 amino acids with a molecular weight of 19,271 daltons produced by recombinant DNA techniques. It is obtained from the bacterial fermentation of a strain of *Escherichia coli* bearing a genetically engineered plasmid containing an interferon alfa-2b gene from human leukocytes. The fermentation is carried out in a defined nutrient medium containing the antibiotic tetracycline hydrochloride at a concentration of 5 to 10 mg/L; the presence of this antibiotic is not detectable in the final product.

INTRON A Injection is a clear, colorless solution. The 3 million IU vial of INTRON A Injection contains 3 million IU of interferon alfa-2b, recombinant per 0.5 mL. The 18 million IU multidose vial of INTRON A Injection contains a total of 22.8 million IU of interferon alfa-2b, recombinant per 3.8 mL (3 million IU/0.5 mL) in order to provide the delivery of six 0.5-mL doses, each containing 3 million IU of INTRON A (for a label strength of 18 million IU). The 18 million IU INTRON A Injection multidose pen contains a total of 22.5 million IU of interferon alfa-2b, recombinant per 1.5 mL (3 million IU/0.2 mL) in order to provide the delivery of six 0.2-mL doses, each containing 3 million IU of INTRON A (for a label strength of 18 million IU). Each mL also contains 7.5 mg sodium chloride, 1.8 mg sodium phosphate dibasic, 1.3 mg sodium phosphate monobasic, 0.1 mg edetate disodium, 0.1 mg polysorbate 80, and 1.5 mg m-cresol as a preservative.

Based on the specific activity of approximately 2.6 × 10^8 IU/mg protein as measured by HPLC assay, the corresponding quantities of interferon alfa-2b, recombinant in the vials and pen described above are approximately 0.012 mg, 0.088 mg, and 0.087 mg protein, respectively.

Mechanism of Action

Ribavirin/Interferon alfa-2b, recombinant The mechanism of inhibition of hepatitis C virus (HCV) RNA by combination therapy with REBETOL and INTRON A has not been established.

CLINICAL PHARMACOLOGY

Pharmacokinetics

Interferon alfa-2b, recombinant Single- and multiple-dose pharmacokinetic properties of INTRON A (interferon alfa-2b, recombinant) are summarized in **TABLE 1**. Following a single 3 million IU (MIU) subcutaneous dose in 12 patients with chronic hepatitis C, mean (% CV*) serum concentrations peaked at 7 (44%) hours. Following 4 weeks of subcutaneous dosing with 3 MIU three times a week (TIW), interferon serum concentrations were undetectable predose. However, a twofold increase in bioavailability was noted upon multiple dosing of interferon; the reason for this is unknown. Mean half-life values following single- and multiple-dose administrations were 6.8 (24%) hours and 6.5 (29%) hours, respectively.

Ribavirin Single- and multiple-dose pharmacokinetic properties in adults with chronic hepatitis C are summarized in **TABLE 1**. Ribavirin was rapidly and extensively absorbed following oral administration. However, due to first-pass metabolism, the absolute bioavailability averaged 64% (44%). There was a linear relationship between dose and AUC_{tf} (AUC from time zero to last measurable concentration) following single doses of 200-1200 mg ribavirin. The relationship between dose and C_{max} was curvilinear, tending to asymptote above single doses of 400-600 mg.

Upon multiple oral dosing, based on $AUC12_{hr}$, a sixfold accumulation of ribavirin was observed in plasma. Following oral dosing with 600 mg BID, steady-state was reached by approximately 4 weeks, with mean steady-state plasma concentrations of 2200 (37%) ng/mL. Upon discontinuation of dosing, the mean half-life was 298 (30%) hours, which probably reflects slow elimination from nonplasma compartments.

Effect of Food on Absorption of Ribavirin Both AUC_{tf} and C_{max} increased by 70% when REBETOL Capsules were administered with a high-fat meal (841 kcal, 53.8 g fat, 31.6 g protein, and 57.4 g carbohydrate) in a single-dose pharmacokinetic study. There are insufficient data to address the clinical relevance of these results. Clinical efficacy studies were conducted without instructions with respect to food consumption. (See **DOSAGE AND ADMINISTRATION**.)

Effect of Antacid on Absorption of Ribavirin Coadministration with an antacid containing magnesium, aluminum, and simethicone (Mylanta®) resulted in a 14% decrease in mean ribavirin AUC_{tf}. The clinical relevance of results from this single-dose study is unknown.

[See table 1 above]

TABLE 1. Mean (% CV) Pharmacokinetic Parameters for INTRON A and REBETOL When Administered Individually to Adults with Chronic Hepatitis C

Parameter	INTRON A (N=12)		REBETOL (N=12)	
	Single Dose 3 MIU	Multiple Dose 3 MIU TIW	Single Dose 600 mg	Multiple Dose 600 mg BID
T_{max} (hr)	7 (44)	5 (37)	1.7 (46)***	3 (60)
C_{max}*	13.9 (32)	29.7 (33)	782 (37)	3680 (85)
AUC_{tf}**	142 (43)	333 (39)	13400 (48)	228000 (25)
$T_{1/2}$ (hr)	6.8 (24)	6.5 (29)	43.6 (47)	298 (30)
Apparent Volume of Distribution (L)			2825 (9)†	
Apparent Clearance (L/hr)	14.3 (17)		38.2 (40)	
Absolute Bioavailability			64% (44)††	

* IU/mL for INTRON A and ng/mL for REBETOL
** IU.hr/mL for INTRON A and ng.hr/mL for REBETOL
† Data obtained from a single-dose pharmacokinetic study using ^{14}C labeled ribavirin; N=5
†† N=6
*** N=11

Ribavirin transport into nonplasma compartments has been most extensively studied in red blood cells, and has been identified to be primarily via an e_s-type equilibrative nucleoside transporter. This type of transporter is present on virtually all cell types and may account for the extensive volume of distribution. Ribavirin does not bind to plasma proteins.

Ribavirin has two pathways of metabolism: (i) a reversible phosphorylation pathway in nucleated cells; and (ii) a degradative pathway involving deribosylation and amide hydrolysis to yield a triazole carboxylic acid metabolite. Ribavirin and its triazole carboxamide and triazole carboxylic acid metabolites are excreted renally. After oral administration of 600 mg of ^{14}C-ribavirin, approximately 61% and 12% of the radioactivity was eliminated in the urine and feces, respectively, in 336 hours. Unchanged ribavirin accounted for 17% of the administered dose.

Results of *in vitro* studies using both human and rat liver microsome preparations indicated little or no cytochrome P450 enzyme-mediated metabolism of ribavirin, with minimal potential for P450 enzyme-based drug interactions.

No pharmacokinetic interactions were noted between INTRON A Injection and REBETOL Capsules in a multiple-dose pharmacokinetic study.

Special Populations

Renal Dysfunction The pharmacokinetics of ribavirin were assessed after administration of a single oral dose (400 mg) of ribavirin to subjects with varying degrees of renal dysfunction. The mean AUC_{tf} value was threefold greater in subjects with creatinine clearance values between 10 to 30 mL/min when compared to control subjects (creatinine clearance >90 mL/min). This appears to be due to reduction of apparent clearance in these patients. Ribavirin was not removed by hemodialysis. Patients with creatinine clearance <50 mL/min should not be treated with REBETOL (see **WARNINGS**).

Hepatic Dysfunction The effect of hepatic dysfunction was assessed after a single oral dose of ribavirin (600 mg). The mean AUC_{tf} values were not significantly different in subjects with mild, moderate, or severe hepatic dysfunction (Child-Pugh Classification A, B, or C) when compared to control subjects. However, the mean C_{max} values increased with severity of hepatic dysfunction and was twofold greater in subjects with severe hepatic dysfunction when compared to control subjects.

Pediatric Patients Multiple-dose pharmacokinetic properties for ribavirin in pediatric patients with chronic hepatitis C between 5 and 16 years of age are summarized in **TABLE 2**.

TABLE 2. Mean (% CV) Pharmacokinetic Parameters for REBETOL When Administered to Pediatric Patients with Chronic Hepatitis C

Parameter	12 mg/kg/day as 2 divided doses (n=19)	15 mg/kg/day as 2 divided doses (n=19)
T_{max} (hr)	1.4 (60)	1.9 (81)
C_{max} (ng/mL)	2705 (17)	3243 (24)
AUC_{12} (ng*hr/mL)	25049 (16)	29620 (25)
Apparent Clearance (L/hr/kg)	0.25 (16)	0.27 (25)

Elderly Patients Pharmacokinetic evaluations for elderly subjects have not been performed.

Gender There were no clinically significant pharmacokinetic differences noted in a single-dose study of eighteen male and eighteen female subjects.

****In this section of the label, numbers in parenthesis indicate % coefficient of variation.***

INDICATIONS AND USAGE

REBETOL (ribavirin, USP) Capsules is indicated in combination with INTRON A (interferon alfa-2b, recombinant) Injection for the treatment of chronic hepatitis C in patients with compensated liver disease previously untreated with alpha interferon or who have relapsed following alpha interferon therapy.

Description of Clinical Studies

Previously Untreated Patients Adults with compensated chronic hepatitis C and detectable HCV RNA (assessed by a central laboratory using a research-based RT-PCR assay) who were previously untreated with alpha interferon therapy were enrolled into two multicenter, double-blind trials (US and International) and randomized to receive REBETOL Capsules 1200 mg/day (1000 mg/day for patients weighing ≤75 kg) plus INTRON A Injection 3 MIU TIW or INTRON A Injection plus placebo for 24 or 48 weeks followed by 24 weeks of off-therapy follow-up. The International study did not contain a 24-week INTRON A plus placebo treatment arm. The US study enrolled 912 patients who, at baseline, were 67% male, 89% caucasian with a mean Knodell HAI score (I+II+III) of 7.5, and 72% genotype 1. The International study, conducted in Europe, Israel, Canada, and Australia, enrolled 799 patients (65%

Continued on next page

Rebetron—Cont.

male, 95% caucasian, mean Knodell score 6.8, and 58% genotype 1).
Study results are summarized in **TABLE 3**.
[See table 3 at right]
Of patients who had not achieved HCV RNA below the limit of detection of the research-based assay by week 24 of REBETOL/INTRON A treatment, less than 5% responded to an additional 24 weeks of combination treatment.
Among patients with HCV genotype 1 treated with REBETOL/INTRON A therapy who achieved HCV RNA below the detection limit of the research-based assay by 24 weeks, those randomized to 48 weeks of treatment had higher virologic responses compared to those in the 24-week treatment group. There was no observed increase in response rates for patients with HCV nongenotype 1 randomized to REBETOL/INTRON A therapy for 48 weeks compared to 24 weeks.
Relapse Patients Patients with compensated chronic hepatitis C and detectable HCV RNA (assessed by a central laboratory using a research-based RT-PCR assay) who had relapsed following one or two courses of interferon therapy (defined as abnormal serum ALT levels) were enrolled into two multicenter, double-blind trials (US and International) and randomized to receive REBETOL 1200 mg/day (1000 mg/day for patients weighing ≤75 kg) plus INTRON A 3 MIU TIW or INTRON A plus placebo for 24 weeks followed by 24 weeks of off-therapy follow-up. The US study enrolled 153 patients who, at baseline, were 67% male, 92% caucasian with a mean Knodell HAI score (I+II+III) of 6.8, and 58% genotype 1. The International study, conducted in Europe, Israel, Canada, and Australia, enrolled 192 patients (64% male, 95% caucasian, mean Knodell score 6.6, and 56% genotype 1).
Study results are summarized in **TABLE 4**.
[See table 4 at right]
Virologic and histologic responses were similar among male and female patients in both the previously untreated and relapse studies.

CONTRAINDICATIONS
Combination REBETOL/INTRON A therapy must not be used by females who are pregnant or by males whose female partners are pregnant. Extreme care must be taken to avoid pregnancy in female patients and in female partners of male patients taking combination REBETOL/INTRON A therapy. Combination REBETOL/INTRON A therapy should not be initiated until a report of a negative pregnancy test has been obtained immediately prior to initiation of therapy. Females of childbearing potential and males must use two forms of effective contraception during treatment and during the 6 months after treatment has been concluded. Significant teratogenic and/or embryocidal effects have been demonstrated for ribavirin in all animal species in which adequate studies have been conducted. These effects occurred at doses as low as one twentieth of the recommended human dose of REBETOL Capsules. If pregnancy occurs in a patient or partner of a patient during treatment or during the 6 months after treatment stops, physicians are encouraged to report such cases by calling (800) 727-7064. See boxed **CONTRAINDICATIONS AND WARNINGS**. See **WARNINGS**.
REBETOL Capsules in combination with INTRON A Injection is contraindicated in patients with a history of hypersensitivity to ribavirin and/or alpha interferon or any component of the capsule and/or injection.
Patients with autoimmune hepatitis must not be treated with combination REBETOL/INTRON A therapy.

WARNINGS
Pregnancy
Category X, may cause birth defects. See boxed CONTRAINDICATIONS AND WARNINGS. See CONTRAINDICATIONS.
Anemia
HEMOLYTIC ANEMIA (HEMOGLOBIN <10 G/DL) WAS OBSERVED IN APPROXIMATELY 10% OF REBETOL/INTRON A-TREATED PATIENTS IN CLINICAL TRIALS (SEE ADVERSE REACTIONS LABORATORY VALUES - *HEMOGLOBIN*). ANEMIA OCCURRED WITHIN 1-2 WEEKS OF INITIATION OF RIBAVIRIN THERAPY. BECAUSE OF THIS INITIAL ACUTE DROP IN HEMOGLOBIN, IT IS ADVISED THAT COMPLETE BLOOD COUNTS (CBC) SHOULD BE OBTAINED PRETREATMENT AND AT WEEK 2 AND WEEK 4 OF THERAPY OR MORE FREQUENTLY IF CLINICALLY INDICATED. PATIENTS SHOULD THEN BE FOLLOWED AS CLINICALLY APPROPRIATE.

The anemia associated with REBETOL/INTRON A therapy may result in deterioration of cardiac function and/or exacerbation of the symptoms of coronary disease. Patients should be assessed before initiation of therapy and should be appropriately monitored during therapy. If there is any deterioration of cardiovascular status, therapy should be suspended or discontinued. (See **DOSAGE AND ADMINISTRATION**.) Because cardiac disease may be worsened by drug induced anemia, patients with a history of significant or unstable cardiac disease should not use combination REBETOL/INTRON A therapy. (See **ADVERSE REACTIONS**.)
Similarly, patients with hemoglobinopathies (eg, thalassemia, sickle-cell anemia) should not be treated with combination REBETOL/INTRON A therapy.

TABLE 3. Virologic and Histologic Responses: Previously Untreated Patients*

	US Study				International Study		
	24 weeks of treatment		48 weeks of treatment		24 weeks of treatment	48 weeks of treatment	
	INTRON A plus REBETOL (N=228)	INTRON A plus Placebo (N=231)	INTRON A plus REBETOL (N=228)	INTRON A plus Placebo (N=225)	INTRON A plus REBETOL (N=265)	INTRON A plus REBETOL (N=268)	INTRON A plus Placebo (N=266)
Virologic Response							
–Responder[1]	65 (29)	13 (6)	85 (37)	27 (12)	86 (32)	113 (42)	46 (17)
–Nonresponder	147 (64)	194 (84)	110 (48)	168 (75)	158 (60)	120 (45)	196 (74)
–Missing data	16 (7)	24 (10)	33 (14)	30 (13)	21 (8)	35 (13)	24 (9)
Histologic Response							
–Improvement[2]	102 (45)	77 (33)	96 (42)	65 (29)	103 (39)	102 (38)	69 (26)
–No improvement	77 (34)	99 (43)	61 (27)	93 (41)	85 (32)	58 (22)	111 (41)
–Missing data	49 (21)	55 (24)	71 (31)	67 (30)	77 (29)	108 (40)	86 (32)

* Number (%) of patients
[1] Defined as HCV RNA below limit of detection using a research-based RT-PCR assay at end of treatment and during follow-up period.
[2] Defined as posttreatment (end of follow-up) minus pretreatment liver biopsy Knodell HAI score (I+II+III) improvement of ≥2 points.

TABLE 4. Virologic and Histologic Responses: Relapse Patients*

	US Study		International Study	
	INTRON A plus REBETOL (N=77)	INTRON A plus Placebo (N=76)	INTRON A plus REBETOL (N=96)	INTRON A plus Placebo (N=96)
Virologic Response				
–Responder[1]	33 (43)	3 (4)	46 (48)	5 (5)
–Nonresponder	36 (47)	66 (87)	45 (47)	91 (95)
–Missing data	8 (10)	7 (9)	5 (5)	0 (0)
Histologic Response				
–Improvement[2]	38 (49)	27 (36)	49 (51)	30 (31)
–No improvement	23 (30)	37 (49)	29 (30)	44 (46)
–Missing data	16 (21)	12 (16)	18 (19)	22 (23)

* Number (%) of patients
[1] Defined as HCV RNA below limit of detection using a research-based RT-PCR assay at end of treatment and during follow-up period.
[2] Defined as posttreatment (end of follow-up) minus pretreatment liver biopsy Knodell HAI score (I+II+III) improvement of ≥2 points.

Psychiatric
Severe psychiatric adverse events, including depression, psychoses, aggressive behavior, hallucinations, violent behavior (suicidal ideation, suicidal attempts, suicides), and rare instances of homicidal ideation have occurred during combination REBETOL/INTRON A therapy, both in patients with and without a previous psychiatric disorder. REBETOL/INTRON A therapy should be used with extreme caution in patients with a history of pre-existing psychiatric disorders, and all patients should be carefully monitored for evidence of depression and other psychiatric symptoms. Suspension of REBETOL/INTRON A therapy should be considered if psychiatric intervention and/or dose reduction is unsuccessful in controlling psychiatric symptoms. In severe cases, therapy should be stopped immediately and psychiatric intervention sought. (See ADVERSE REACTIONS.)
Bone Marrow Toxicity
INTRON A therapy suppresses bone marrow function and may result in severe cytopenias including very rare events of aplastic anemia. It is advised that complete blood counts (CBC) be obtained pre-treatment and monitored routinely during therapy (see **PRECAUTIONS: Laboratory Tests**). INTRON A therapy should be discontinued in patients who develop severe decreases in neutrophil ($<0.5 \times 10^9/L$) or platelet counts ($<25 \times 10^9/L$) (See **DOSAGE AND ADMINISTRATION: Guidelines for Dose Modifications**).
Pulmonary
Pulmonary symptoms, including dyspnea, pulmonary infiltrates, pneumonitis and pneumonia, have been reported during therapy with REBETOL/INTRON A; occasional cases of fatal pneumonia have occurred. In addition, sarcoidosis or the exacerbation of sarcoidosis has been reported. If there is evidence of pulmonary infiltrates or pulmonary function impairment, the patient should be closely monitored, and if appropriate, combination REBETOL/INTRON A treatment should be discontinued.
Other
- REBETOL Capsule monotherapy is not effective for the treatment of chronic hepatitis C and should not be used for this indication.
- Fatal and nonfatal pancreatitis has been observed in patients treated with REBETOL/INTRON A therapy. REBETOL/INTRON A therapy should be suspended in patients with signs and symptoms of pancreatitis and discontinued in patients with confirmed pancreatitis.
- Combination REBETOL/INTRON A therapy should not be used in patients with creatinine clearance <50 mL/min.
- Diabetes mellitus and hyperglycemia have been observed in patients treated with INTRON A.
- Ophthalmologic disorders have been reported with treatment with alpha interferons (including INTRON A therapy). Investigators using alpha interferons have reported the occurrence of retinal hemorrhages, cotton wool spots, and retinal artery or vein obstruction in rare instances. Any patient complaining of loss of visual acuity or visual field should have an eye examination. Because these ocular events may occur in conjunction with other disease states, a visual exam prior to initiation of combination REBETOL/INTRON A therapy is recommended in patients with diabetes mellitus or hypertension.
- Acute serious hypersensitivity reactions (eg, urticaria, angioedema, bronchoconstriction, anaphylaxis) have been observed in INTRON A-treated patients; if such an acute reaction develops, combination REBETOL/INTRON A therapy should be discontinued immediately and appropriate medical therapy instituted.
- Combination REBETOL/INTRON A therapy should be discontinued for patients developing thyroid abnormalities during treatment whose thyroid function cannot be controlled by medication.

PRECAUTIONS
Exacerbation of autoimmune disease has been reported in patients receiving alpha interferon therapy (including INTRON A therapy). REBETOL/INTRON A therapy should be used with caution in patients with other autoimmune disorders.
There have been reports of interferon, including INTRON A (interferon alfa-2b, recombinant) exacerbating pre-existing psoriasis; therefore, combination REBETOL/INTRON A therapy should be used in these patients only if the potential benefit justifies the potential risk.
The safety and efficacy of REBETOL/INTRON A therapy has not been established in liver or other organ transplant patients, decompensated hepatitis C patients, patients who are nonresponders to interferon therapy, or patients coinfected with HBV or HIV.
The safety and efficacy of REBETOL Capsule monotherapy for the treatment of HIV infection, adenovirus, early RSV infection, parainfluenza, or influenza have not been established and REBETOL Capsules should not be used for these indications.
There is no information regarding the use of REBETOL Capsules with other interferons.
Triglycerides Elevated triglyceride levels have been observed in patients treated with interferon including REBETOL/INTRON A therapy. Elevated triglyceride levels should be managed as clinically appropriate. Severe hypertriglyceridemia (triglycerides >1000 mg/dL) may result in

pancreatitis. Discontinuation of REBETOL/INTRON A therapy should be considered for patients with persistently elevated triglycerides (triglycerides >1000 mg/dL) associated with symptoms of potential pancreatitis, such as abdominal pain, nausea, or vomiting (see **WARNINGS - Other**).

Drug Interactions Nucleoside Analogues: Administration of nucleoside analogues has resulted in fatal and nonfatal lactic acidosis. Coadministration of ribavirin and nucleoside analogues should be undertaken with caution and only if the potential benefit outweighs the potential risks.

Information for Patients Combination REBETOL/INTRON A therapy must not be used by females who are pregnant or by males whose female partners are pregnant. Extreme care must be taken to avoid pregnancy in female patients and in female partners of male patients taking combination REBETOL/INTRON A therapy. Combination REBETOL/INTRON A therapy should not be initiated until a report of a negative pregnancy test has been obtained immediately prior to initiation of therapy. Patients must perform a pregnancy test monthly during therapy and for 6 months posttherapy. Females of childbearing potential must be counseled about use of effective contraception (two reliable forms) prior to initiating therapy. Patients (male and female) must be advised of the teratogenic/embryocidal risks and must be instructed to practice effective contraception during combination REBETOL/INTRON A therapy and for 6 months posttherapy. Patients (male and female) should be advised to notify the physician immediately in the event of a pregnancy. (See **CONTRAINDICATIONS.**)

If pregnancy does occur during treatment or during 6 months posttherapy, the patient must be advised of the significant teratogenic risk of REBETOL therapy to the fetus. Patients, or partners of patients, should immediately report any pregnancy that occurs during treatment or within 6 months after treatment cessation to their physician. Physicians are encouraged to report such cases by calling (800) 727-7064.

Patients receiving combination REBETOL/INTRON A treatment should be directed in its appropriate use, informed of the benefits and risks associated with treatment, and referred to the patient **MEDICATION GUIDE**. There are no data evaluating whether REBETOL/INTRON A therapy will prevent transmission of infection to others. Also, it is not known if treatment with REBETOL/INTRON A therapy will cure hepatitis C or prevent cirrhosis, liver failure, or liver cancer that may be the result of infection with the hepatitis C virus.

If home use is prescribed, a puncture-resistant container for the disposal of used syringes and needles should be supplied to the patient. Patients should be thoroughly instructed in the importance of proper disposal and cautioned against any reuse of needles and syringes. The full container should be disposed of according to the directions provided by the physician (see **MEDICATION GUIDE**). To avoid possible transmission of disease, do not share your multidose pen with anyone; it is for you and you alone.

The most common adverse experiences occurring with combination REBETOL/INTRON A therapy are "flu-like" symptoms, such as headache, fatigue, myalgia, and fever (see **ADVERSE REACTIONS**) and appear to decrease in severity as treatment continues. Some of these "flu-like" symptoms may be minimized by bedtime administration of INTRON A therapy. Antipyretics should be considered to prevent or partially alleviate the fever and headache. Another common adverse experience associated with INTRON A therapy is thinning of the hair.

Patients should be advised that laboratory evaluations are required prior to starting therapy and periodically thereafter (see **Laboratory Tests**). It is advised that patients be well hydrated, especially during the initial stages of treatment.

Laboratory Tests The following laboratory tests are recommended for all patients on combination REBETOL/INTRON A therapy, prior to beginning treatment and then periodically thereafter.

- Standard hematologic tests – including hemoglobin (pretreatment, week 2 and week 4 of therapy, and as clinically appropriate [see **WARNINGS**]), complete and differential white blood cell counts, and platelet count.
- Blood chemistries – liver function tests and TSH.
- Pregnancy – including monthly monitoring for females of childbearing potential.

Carcinogenesis and Mutagenesis Carcinogenicity studies with interferon alfa-2b, recombinant have not been performed because neutralizing activity appears in the serum after multiple dosing in all of the animal species tested.

Adequate studies to assess the carcinogenic potential of ribavirin in animals have not been conducted. However, ribavirin is a nucleoside analog that has produced positive findings in multiple *in vitro* and animal *in vivo* genotoxicity assays, and should be considered a potential carcinogen. Further studies to assess the carcinogenic potential of ribavirin in animals are ongoing.

Mutagenicity studies have demonstrated that interferon alfa-2b, recombinant is not mutagenic. Ribavirin demonstrated increased incidences of mutation and cell transformation in multiple genotoxicity assays. Ribavirin was active in the Balb/3T3 *In Vitro* Cell Transformation Assay. Mutagenic activity was observed in the mouse lymphoma assay, and at doses of 20-200 mg/kg (estimated human equivalent of 1.67-16.7 mg/kg, based on body surface area adjustment for a 60 kg adult; 0.1-1 × the maximum recommended human 24-hour dose of ribavirin) in a mouse micronucleus assay. A dominant lethal assay in rats was negative, indicating that if mutations occurred in rats they were not transmitted through male gametes.

TABLE 5. Selected Treatment-Emergent Adverse Events: Previously Untreated and Relapse Patients

	Percentage of Patients					
	US Previously Untreated Study				US Relapse Study	
	24 weeks of treatment		48 weeks of treatment		24 weeks of treatment	
Patients Reporting Adverse Events*	**INTRON A plus REBETOL (N=228)**	**INTRON A plus Placebo (N=231)**	**INTRON A plus REBETOL (N=228)**	**INTRON A plus Placebo (N=225)**	**INTRON A plus REBETOL (N=77)**	**INTRON A plus Placebo (N=76)**
Application Site Disorders						
injection site inflammation	13	10	12	14	6	8
injection site reaction	7	9	8	9	5	3
Body as a Whole - General Disorders						
headache	63	63	66	67	66	68
fatigue	68	62	70	72	60	53
rigors	40	32	42	39	43	37
fever	37	35	41	40	32	36
influenza-like symptoms	14	18	18	20	13	13
asthenia	9	4	9	9	10	4
chest pain	5	4	9	8	6	7
Central & Peripheral Nervous System Disorders						
dizziness	17	15	23	19	26	21
Gastrointestinal System Disorders						
nausea	38	35	46	33	47	33
anorexia	27	16	25	19	21	14
dyspepsia	14	6	16	9	16	9
vomiting	11	10	9	13	12	8
Musculoskeletal System Disorders						
myalgia	61	57	64	63	61	58
arthralgia	30	27	33	36	29	29
musculoskeletal pain	20	26	28	32	22	28
Psychiatric Disorders						
insomnia	39	27	39	30	26	25
irritability	23	19	32	27	25	20
depression	32	25	36	37	23	14
emotional lability	7	6	11	8	12	8
concentration impaired	11	14	14	14	10	12
nervousness	4	2	4	4	5	4
Respiratory System Disorders						
dyspnea	19	9	18	10	17	12
sinusitis	9	7	10	14	12	7
Skin and Appendages Disorders						
alopecia	28	27	32	28	27	26
rash	20	9	28	8	21	5
pruritus	21	9	19	8	13	4
Special Senses, Other Disorders						
taste perversion	7	4	8	4	6	5

* Patients reporting one or more adverse events. A patient may have reported more than one adverse event within a body system/organ class category.

Impairment of Fertility No reproductive toxicology studies have been performed using interferon alfa-2b, recombinant in combination with ribavirin. However, evidence provided below for interferon alfa-2b, recombinant and ribavirin when administered alone indicate that both agents have adverse effects on reproduction. It should be assumed that the effects produced by either agent alone will also be caused by the combination of the two agents. Interferons may impair human fertility. In studies of interferon alfa-2b, recombinant administration in nonhuman primates, menstrual cycle abnormalities have been observed. Decreases in serum estradiol and progesterone concentrations have been reported in females treated with human leukocyte interferon. In addition, ribavirin demonstrated significant embryocidal and/or teratogenic effects at doses well below the recommended human dose in all animal species in which adequate studies have been conducted.

Fertile females and partners of fertile females should not receive combination REBETOL/INTRON A therapy unless the patient and his/her partner are using effective contraception (two reliable forms). Based on a multiple dose half-life ($t_{1/2}$) of ribavirin of 12 days, effective contraception must be utilized for 6 months posttherapy (eg, 15 half-lives of clearance for ribavirin).

Combination REBETOL/INTRON A therapy should be used with caution in fertile males. In studies in mice to evaluate the time course and reversibility of ribavirin-induced testicular degeneration at doses of 15 to 150 mg/kg/day (estimated human equivalent of 1.25-12.5 mg/kg/day, based on body surface area adjustment for a 60 kg adult; 0.1-0.8 × the maximum human 24-hour dose of ribavirin) administered for 3 or 6 months, abnormalities in sperm occurred. Upon cessation of treatment, essentially total recovery from ribavirin-induced testicular toxicity was apparent within 1 or 2 spermatogenesis cycles.

Animal Toxicology Long-term studies in the mouse and rat (18-24 months; doses of 20-75 and 10-40 mg/kg/day, respectively [estimated human equivalent doses of 1.67-6.25 and 1.43-5.71 mg/kg/day, respectively, based on body surface area adjustment for a 60 kg adult; approximately 0.1-0.4 × the maximum human 24-hour dose of ribavirin]) have demonstrated a relationship between chronic ribavirin exposure and increased incidences of vascular lesions (microscopic hemorrhages) in mice. In rats, retinal degeneration occurred in controls, but the incidence was increased in ribavirin-treated rats.

Pregnancy Category X (see **CONTRAINDICATIONS**)

Interferon alfa-2b, recombinant has been shown to have abortifacient effects in *Macaca mulatta* (rhesus monkeys) at 15 and 30 million IU/kg (estimated human equivalent of 5 and 10 million IU/kg, based on body surface area adjustment for a 60 kg adult). There are no adequate and well-controlled studies in pregnant females.

Ribavirin produced significant embryocidal and/or teratogenic effects in all animal species in which adequate studies have been conducted. Malformations of the skull, palate, eye, jaw, limbs, skeleton, and gastrointestinal tract were noted. The incidence and severity of teratogenic effects increased with escalation of the drug dose. Survival of fetuses and offspring was reduced. In conventional embryotoxicity/teratogenicity studies in rats and rabbits, observed no effect dose levels were well below those for proposed clinical use (0.3 mg/kg/day for both the rat and rabbit; approximately 0.06 × the recommended human 24-hour dose of ribavirin). No maternal toxicity or effects on offspring were observed in a peri/postnatal toxicity study in rats dosed orally at up to 1 mg/kg/day (estimated human equivalent dose of 0.17 mg/kg based on body surface area adjustment for a 60 kg adult; approximately 0.01 × the maximum recommended human 24-hour dose of ribavirin).

Treatment and Posttreatment: Potential Risk to the Fetus

Ribavirin is known to accumulate in intracellular components from where it is cleared very slowly. It is not known whether ribavirin contained in sperm will exert a potential teratogenic effect upon fertilization of the ova. In a study in rats, it was concluded that dominant lethality was not induced by ribavirin at doses up to 200 mg/kg for 5 days (estimated human equivalent doses of 7.14–28.6 mg/kg, based on body surface area adjustment for a 60 kg adult; up to 1.7

Continued on next page

Rebetron—Cont.

× the maximum recommended human dose of ribavirin). However, because of the potential human teratogenic effects of ribavirin, male patients should be advised to take every precaution to avoid risk of pregnancy for their female partners.

Females of childbearing potential should not receive combination REBETOL/INTRON A therapy unless they are using effective contraception (two reliable forms) during the therapy period. In addition, effective contraception should be utilized for 6 months posttherapy based on a multiple dose half-life ($t_{1/2}$) of ribavirin of 12 days.

Male patients and their female partners must practice effective contraception (two reliable forms) during treatment with combination REBETOL/INTRON A therapy and for the 6-month posttherapy period (eg, 15 half-lives for ribavirin clearance from the body).

If pregnancy occurs in a patient or partner of a patient during treatment or during the 6 months after treatment cessation, physicians are encouraged to report such cases by calling (800) 727-7064.

Nursing Mothers It is not known whether REBETOL and INTRON A are excreted in human milk. However, studies in mice have shown that mouse interferons are excreted into the milk. Because of the potential for serious adverse reactions from the drugs in nursing infants, a decision should be made whether to discontinue nursing or to discontinue combination REBETOL/INTRON A therapy, taking into account the importance of the therapy to the mother.

Pediatric Use One hundred twenty-five pediatric patients between three and sixteen years of age with chronic hepatitis C virus infection (median duration 10.7 years) received REBETOL Capsules with INTRON A for up to 48 weeks. The overall sustained response rate cannot be calculated since all patients have not yet completed 24-weeks of off-therapy follow-up.

Suicidal ideation or attempts occurred more frequently among pediatric patients compared to adult patients (2.4% versus 1%) during treatment and off-therapy follow-up (see WARNINGS). As in adult patients, pediatric patients experienced other psychiatric adverse events (eg, depression, emotional lability, somnolence), anemia, and neutropenia (see **WARNINGS**). During a 48-week course of therapy there was a decrease in the rate of linear growth (mean percentile assignment decrease of 7%) and a decrease in the rate of weight gain (mean percentile assignment decrease of 9%). A general reversal of these trends was noted during the 24-week posttreatment period.

Injection site disorders, fever, anorexia, vomiting, and emotional lability occurred more frequently in pediatric patients compared to adult patients. Conversely, pediatric patients experienced less fatigue, dyspepsia, arthralgia, insomnia, irritability, impaired concentration, dyspnea, and pruritus compared to adult patients.

Geriatric Use Clinical studies of REBETRON Combination Therapy did not include sufficient numbers of subjects aged 65 and over to determine if they respond differently from younger subjects. In clinical trials, elderly subjects had a higher frequency of anemia (67%) than did younger patients (28%) (see **WARNINGS**).

In general, REBETOL (ribavirin) should be administered to elderly patients cautiously, starting at the lower end of the dosing range, reflecting the greater frequency of decreased renal, hepatic and/or cardiac function, and of concomitant disease or other drug therapy.

REBETOL (ribavirin) is known to be substantially excreted by the kidney, and the risk of adverse reactions to ribavirin may be greater in patients with impaired renal function. Because elderly patients often have decreased renal function, care should be taken in dose selection. Renal function should be monitored and dosage adjustments of ribavirin should be made accordingly (see **DOSAGE AND ADMINISTRATION: Guidelines for Dose Modifications**). REBETOL should not be used in elderly patients with creatinine clearance <50mL/min (see **WARNINGS**).

REBETRON Combination Therapy should be used very cautiously in elderly patients with a history of psychiatric disorders (see **WARNINGS**).

ADVERSE REACTIONS

The safety of combination REBETOL/INTRON A therapy was evaluated in controlled trials of 1010 HCV-infected adults who were previously untreated with interferon therapy and were subsequently treated for 24 or 48 weeks with combination REBETOL/INTRON A therapy and in 173 HCV-infected patients who had relapsed after interferon therapy and were subsequently treated for 24 weeks with combination REBETOL/INTRON A therapy. (See **Description of Clinical Studies**.) Overall, 19% and 6% of previously untreated and relapse patients, respectively, discontinued therapy due to adverse events in the combination arms compared to 13% and 3% in the interferon arms.

The primary toxicity of ribavirin is hemolytic anemia. Reductions in hemoglobin levels occurred within the first 1–2 weeks of therapy (see WARNINGS). Cardiac and pulmonary events associated with anemia occurred in approximately 10% of patients treated with REBETOL/INTRON A therapy. (See WARNINGS.)

The most common psychiatric events occurring in US studies of previously untreated and relapse patients treated with REBETOL/INTRON A therapy, respectively, were insomnia (39%, 26%), depression (34%, 23%), and irritability (27%, 25%). Suicidal behavior (ideation, attempts, and suicides) occurred in 1% of patients. (See **WARNINGS**.) In addition, hearing disorders (tinnitus and hearing loss) and vertigo have occurred in patients treated with combination REBETOL/INTRON A therapy.

Selected treatment-emergent adverse events that occurred in the US studies with ≥5% incidence are provided in **TABLE 5** by treatment group. In general, the selected treatment-emergent adverse events reported with lower incidence in the international studies as compared to the US studies with the exception of asthenia, influenza-like symptoms, nervousness, and pruritus.

[See table 5 at top of previous page]

Laboratory Values

Changes in selected hematologic values (hemoglobin, white blood cells, neutrophils, and platelets) during combination REBETOL/INTRON A treatment are described below (see **TABLE 6**).

Hemoglobin Hemoglobin decreases among patients on combination therapy began at Week 1, with stabilization by Week 4. In previously untreated patients treated for 48 weeks, the mean maximum decrease from baseline was 3.1 g/dL in the US study and 2.9 g/dL in the International study. In relapse patients, the mean maximum decrease from baseline was 2.8 g/dL in the US study and 2.6 g/dL in the International study. Hemoglobin values returned to pretreatment levels within 4 to 8 weeks of cessation of therapy in most patients.

Neutrophils There were decreases in neutrophil counts in both the combination REBETOL/INTRON A and INTRON A plus placebo dose groups. In previously untreated patients treated for 48 weeks, the mean maximum decrease in neutrophil count in the US study was 1.3×10^9/L and in the International study was 1.5×10^9/L. In relapse patients the mean maximum decrease in neutrophil count in the US study was 1.3×10^9/L and in the International study was 1.6×10^9/L. Neutrophil counts returned to pretreatment levels within 4 weeks of cessation of therapy in most patients.

Platelets In both previously untreated and relapse patients mean platelet counts generally remained in the normal range in all treatment groups; however, mean platelet counts were 10% to 15% lower in the INTRON A plus placebo group than the REBETOL/INTRON A group. Mean platelet counts returned to baseline levels within 4 weeks after treatment discontinuation.

Thyroid Function Of patients who entered the previously untreated (24 and 48 week treatments) and relapse (24 week treatment) studies without thyroid abnormalities, approximately 3% to 6% and 1% to 2%, respectively, developed thyroid abnormalities requiring clinical intervention.

Bilirubin and Uric Acid Increases in both bilirubin and uric acid, associated with hemolysis, were noted in clinical trials. Most were moderate biochemical changes and were reversed within 4 weeks after treatment discontinuation. This observation occurs most frequently in patients with a previous diagnosis of Gilbert's syndrome. This has not been associated with hepatic dysfunction or clinical morbidity.

[See table 6 above]

OVERDOSAGE

There is limited experience with overdosage. Acute ingestion of up to 20 grams of REBETOL Capsules, INTRON A ingestion of up to 120 million units, and subcutaneous doses of INTRON A up to 10 times the recommended doses have been reported. Primary effects that have been observed are increased incidence and severity of the adverse events related to the therapeutic use of INTRON A and REBETOL. However, hepatic enzyme abnormalities, renal failure, hem-

TABLE 6. Selected Hematologic Values During Treatment with REBETOL plus INTRON A: Previously Untreated and Relapse Patients

	Percentage of Patients					
	US Previously Untreated Study				US Relapse Study	
	24 weeks of treatment		48 weeks of treatment		24 weeks of treatment	
	INTRON A plus REBETOL (N=228)	INTRON A plus Placebo (N=231)	INTRON A plus REBETOL (N=228)	INTRON A plus Placebo (N=225)	INTRON A plus REBETOL (N=77)	INTRON A plus Placebo (N=76)
Hemoglobin (g/dL)						
9.5-10.9	24	1	32	1	21	3
8.0-9.4	5	0	4	0	4	0
6.5-7.9	0	0	0	0.4	0	0
<6.5	0	0	0	0	0	0
Leukocytes ($\times 10^9$/L)						
2.0-2.9	40	20	38	23	45	26
1.5-1.9	4	1	9	2	5	3
1.0-1.4	0.9	0	2	0	0	0
<1.0	0	0	0	0	0	0
Neutrophils ($\times 10^9$/L)						
1.0-1.49	30	32	31	44	42	34
0.75-0.99	14	15	14	11	16	18
0.5-0.74	9	9	14	7	8	4
<0.5	11	8	11	5	5	8
Platelets ($\times 10^9$/L)						
70-99	9	11	11	14	6	12
50-69	2	3	2	3	0	5
30-49	0	0.4	0	0.4	0	0
<30	0.9	0	1	0.9	0	0
Total Bilirubin (mg/dL)						
1.5-3.0	27	13	32	13	21	7
3.1-6.0	0.9	0.4	2	0	3	0
6.1-12.0	0	0	0.4	0	0	0
>12.0	0	0	0	0	0	0

TABLE 7. Recommended Adult Dosing

Body weight	REBETOL Capsules	INTRON A Injection
≤75 kg	2 × 200-mg capsules AM, 3 × 200-mg capsules PM daily p.o.	3 million IU 3 times weekly s.c.
>75 kg	3 × 200-mg capsules AM, 3 × 200-mg capsules PM daily p.o.	3 million IU 3 times weekly s.c.

Table 8. Pediatric Dosing

Body weight	REBETOL Capsules	INTRON A Injection
25-36 kg	1 × 200-mg capsule AM 1 × 200-mg capsule PM daily p.o.	3 million IU/m² 3 times weekly s.c.
37-49 kg	1 × 200-mg capsule AM 2 × 200-mg capsule PM daily p.o.	3 million IU/m² 3 times weekly s.c.
50-61 kg	2 × 200-mg capsules AM 2 × 200-mg capsules PM daily p.o.	3 million IU/m² 3 times weekly s.c.
>61 kg	Refer to adult dosing table	Refer to adult dosing table

orrhage, and myocardial infarction have been reported with administration of single subcutaneous doses of INTRON A that exceed dosing recommendations.
There is no specific antidote for INTRON A or REBETOL, and hemodialysis and peritoneal dialysis are not effective for treatment of overdose of either agent.

DOSAGE AND ADMINISTRATION

INTRON A Injection should be administered subcutaneously and REBETOL Capsules should be administered orally. REBETOL may be administered without regard to food, but should be administered in a consistent manner. (See **CLINICAL PHARMACOLOGY**.)

Adults
The recommended dose of REBETOL Capsules depends on the patient's body weight. The recommended doses of REBETOL and INTRON A are given in **TABLE 7**.
The recommended duration of treatment for patients previously untreated with interferon is 24 to 48 weeks. The duration of treatment should be individualized to the patient depending on baseline disease characteristics, response to therapy, and tolerability of the regimen (see **Description of Clinical Studies** and **ADVERSE REACTIONS**). After 24 weeks of treatment virologic response should be assessed. Treatment discontinuation should be considered in any patient who has not achieved an HCV RNA below the limit of detection of the assay by 24 weeks. There are no safety and efficacy data on treatment for longer than 48 weeks in the previously untreated patient population.
In patients who relapse following interferon therapy, the recommended duration of treatment is 24 weeks. There are no safety and efficacy data on treatment for longer than 24 weeks in the relapse patient population.
[See table 7 on previous page]

Pediatrics
Efficacy of REBETOL and INTRON A for pediatric patients has not been established. Based on pharmacokinetic data, the following doses of REBETOL and INTRON A provide similar exposures in pediatric patients as observed in adult patients treated with the approved doses of REBETOL and INTRON A (see **TABLE 8**).
[See table 8 on previous page]
Under no circumstances should REBETOL Capsules be opened, crushed, or broken (See **CONTRAINDICATIONS** and **WARNINGS**).

Dose Modifications (**TABLE 9**)
In clinical trials, approximately 26% of patients required modification of their dose of REBETOL Capsules, INTRON A Injection, or both agents. If severe adverse reactions or laboratory abnormalities develop during combination REBETOL/INTRON A therapy, the dose should be modified, or discontinued if appropriate, until the adverse reactions abate. If intolerance persists after dose adjustment, REBETOL/INTRON A therapy should be discontinued.
REBETOL/INTRON A therapy should be administered with caution to patients with pre-existing cardiac disease. Patients should be assessed before commencement of therapy and should be appropriately monitored during therapy. If there is any deterioration of cardiovascular status, therapy should be stopped. (See **WARNINGS**.)
For patients with a history of stable cardiovascular disease, a permanent dose reduction is required if the hemoglobin decreases by ≥2 g/dL during any 4-week period. In addition, for these cardiac history patients, if the hemoglobin remains <12 g/dL after 4 weeks on a reduced dose, the patient should discontinue combination REBETOL/INTRON A therapy.
It is recommended that a patient whose hemoglobin level falls below 10 g/dL have his/her REBETOL dose reduced to 600 mg daily (1 × 200-mg capsule AM, 2 × 200-mg capsules PM). A patient whose hemoglobin level falls below 8.5 g/dL should be permanently discontinued from REBETOL/INTRON A therapy. (See **WARNINGS**.)
It is recommended that a patient who experiences moderate depression (persistent low mood, loss of interest, poor self image, and/or hopelessness) have his/her INTRON A dose temporarily reduced and/or be considered for medical therapy. A patient experiencing severe depression or suicidal ideation/attempt should be discontinued from REBETOL/INTRON A therapy and followed closely with appropriate medical management. (See **WARNINGS**.)
[See table 9 above]

Administration of INTRON A Injection
At the discretion of the physician, the patient may self-administer the INTRON A. (See illustrated **MEDICATION GUIDE** for instructions.)
The INTRON A Injection is supplied as a clear and colorless solution. The appropriate INTRON A dose should be withdrawn from the vial or set on the multidose pen and injected subcutaneously. The INTRON A Injection supplied with the B-D Safety Lok™ syringes contain a plastic sleeve to be pulled over the needle after use. The syringe locks with an audible click when the green stripe on the safety sleeve covers the red stripe on the needle. After administration of INTRON A Injection, it is essential to follow the procedure for proper disposal of syringes and needles. (See **MEDICATION GUIDE** for detailed instructions.)
[See second table above]
Parenteral drug products should be inspected visually for particulate matter and discoloration prior to administration, whenever solution and container permit. INTRON A Injection may be administered using either sterilized glass or plastic disposable syringes.

TABLE 9. Guidelines for Dose Modifications

	Dose Reduction* REBETOL - Adults: 600 mg daily Pediatrics: half the dose INTRON A - Adults: 1.5 million IU TIW Pediatrics: 1.5 million IU/m² TIW	Permanent Discontinuation of Treatment REBETOL and INTRON A
Hemoglobin	<10 g/dL (REBETOL) Cardiac History Patients Only. ≥2 g/dL decrease during any 4-week period during treatment (REBETOL/INTRON A)	<8.5 g/dL Cardiac History Patients Only. <12 g/dL after 4 weeks of dose reduction
White blood count	<1.5 × 10⁹/L (INTRON A)	<1.0 × 10⁹/L
Neutrophil count	<0.75 × 10⁹/L (INTRON A)	<0.5 × 10⁹/L
Platelet count	Adults: <50 × 10⁹/L (INTRON A) Pediatrics: <80 × 10⁹/L (INTRON A)	Adults: <25 × 10⁹/L Pediatrics: <50 × 10⁹/L

*Study medication to be dose reduced is shown in parenthesis.

Vial/Pen Label Strength	Fill Volume	Concentration
3 million IU vial	0.5 mL	3 million IU/0.5 mL
18 million IU multidose vial†	3.8 mL	3 million IU/0.5 mL
18 million IU multidose pen††	1.5 mL	3 million IU/0.2 mL

† This is a multidose vial which contains a total of 22.8 million IU of interferon alfa-2b, recombinant per 3.8 mL in order to provide the delivery of six 0.5-mL doses, each containing 3 million IU of interferon alfa-2b, recombinant (for a label strength of 18 million IU).

†† This is a multidose pen which contains a total of 22.5 million IU of interferon alfa-2b, recombinant per 1.5 mL in order to provide the delivery of six 0.2-mL doses, each containing 3 million IU of interferon alfa-2b, recombinant (for a label strength of 18 million IU).

	Each REBETRON Combination Package Consists of:	
For Patients ≤75 kg	A box containing 6 vials of INTRON A Injection (3 million IU in 0.5 mL per vial), 6 B-D Safety-Lok™ syringes with a safety sleeve, alcohol swabs, and one bottle containing 70 REBETOL Capsules.	(NDC 0085-1241-02)
	One 18 million IU multidose vial of INTRON A Injection (22.8 million IU per 3.8 mL; 3 million IU/0.5 mL), 6 B-D Safety Lok™ syringes with a safety sleeve, alcohol swabs, and one bottle containing 70 REBETOL Capsules.	(NDC 0085-1236-02)
	One 18 million IU INTRON A Injection multidose pen (22.5 million IU per 1.5 mL; 3 million IU/0.2 mL), 6 disposable needles, alcohol swabs, and one bottle containing 70 REBETOL Capsules.	(NDC 0085-1258-02)
For Patients >75 kg	A box containing 6 vials of INTRON A Injection (3 million IU in 0.5 mL per vial), 6 B-D Safety-Lok™ syringes with a safety sleeve, alcohol swabs, and one bottle containing 84 REBETOL Capsules.	(NDC 0085-1241-01)
	One 18 million IU multidose vial of INTRON A Injection (22.8 million IU per 3.8 mL; 3 million IU/0.5 mL), 6 B-D Safety Lok™ syringes with a safety sleeve, alcohol swabs, and one bottle containing 84 REBETOL Capsules.	(NDC 0085-1236-01)
	One 18 million IU INTRON A Injection multidose pen (22.5 million IU per 1.5 mL; 3 million IU/0.2 mL), 6 disposable needles, alcohol swabs, and one bottle containing 84 REBETOL Capsules.	(NDC 0085-1258-01)
For REBETOL Dose Reduction	A box containing 6 vials of INTRON A Injection (3 million IU in 0.5 mL per vial), 6 B-D Safety-Lok™ syringes with a safety sleeve, alcohol swabs, and one bottle containing 42 REBETOL Capsules.	(NDC 0085-1241-03)
	One 18 million IU multidose vial of INTRON A Injection (22.8 million IU per 3.8 mL; 3 million IU/0.5 mL), 6 B-D Safety Lok™ syringes with a safety sleeve, alcohol swabs, and one bottle containing 42 REBETOL Capsules.	(NDC 0085-1236-03)
	One 18 million IU INTRON A Injection multidose pen (22.5 million IU per 1.5 mL; 3 million IU/0.2 mL), 6 disposable needles, alcohol swabs, and one bottle containing 42 REBETOL Capsules.	(NDC 0085-1258-03)

Stability INTRON A Injection provided in vials is stable at 35°C (95°F) for up to 7 days and at 30°C (86°F) for up to 14 days. INTRON A Injection provided in a multidose pen is stable at 30°C (86°F) for up to 2 days. The solution is clear and colorless.

HOW SUPPLIED
REBETOL 200-mg Capsules are white, opaque capsules with REBETOL, 200 mg, and the Schering Corporation logo imprinted on the capsule shell; the capsules are packaged in a bottle.
INTRON A Injection is a clear, colorless solution packaged in single-dose and multidose vials, and a multidose pen.
INTRON A Injection and REBETOL Capsules are available in the following combination package presentations:
[See third table above]

STORAGE CONDITIONS
Store the REBETOL Capsules plus INTRON A Injection combination package refrigerated between 2° and 8°C (36° and 46°F).
When separated, the individual bottle of REBETOL Capsules should be stored refrigerated between 2° and 8°C (36° and 46°F) or at 25°C (77°F); excursions are permitted between 15° and 30°C (59° and 86°F).
When separated, the individual vials of INTRON A Injection and INTRON A multidose pen should be stored refrigerated between 2° and 8°C (36° and 46°F).

Schering Corporation
Kenilworth, NJ 07033 USA
Copyright © 1998, 2002, Schering Corporation.
All rights reserved.

B-25930614 Rev. 9/02
25272927T

To keep your **PDR** up to date throughout the year, note these revisions on the corresponding pages of the annual volume. Simply write "See Supplement A" next to the product heading.

Solvay Pharmaceuticals, Inc.
901 SAWYER ROAD
MARIETTA, GA 30062

www.solvaypharmaceuticals-us.com
For Medical Information Contact:
Generally:
Medical Information Department
(888) 410-2806

Sales and Ordering:
Orders may be placed by calling this toll free number:
(800) 241-1643
Fax # 770 578-5901
Mail orders should be sent to:
Solvay Pharmaceuticals
Order Entry Department
901 Sawyer Road
Marietta, GA 30062

LITHOBID® ℞
[lĭth-ō-bĭd]
(Lithium Carbonate, USP)
Slow-Release Tablets 300 mg
℞ only

Prescribing information for this product, which appears on pages 3165–3166 of the 2003 PDR, has been completely revised as follows. Please write "See Supplement A" next to the product heading.

> **WARNING**
> Lithium toxicity is closely related to serum lithium levels, and can occur at doses close to therapeutic levels. Facilities for prompt and accurate serum lithium determinations should be available before initiating therapy (see **DOSAGE AND ADMINISTRATION**).

DESCRIPTION
LITHOBID® Tablets contain lithium carbonate, a white, odorless alkaline powder with molecular formula Li_2CO_3 and molecular weight 73.89. Lithium is an element of the alkali-metal group with atomic number 3, atomic weight 6.94 and an emission line at 671 nm on the flame photometer.

Each peach-colored, film-coated, slow-release tablet contains 300 mg of lithium carbonate. This slowly dissolving, film-coated tablet is designed to give lower serum lithium peak concentrations than obtained with conventional oral lithium dosage forms. Inactive ingredients consist of calcium stearate, carnauba wax, cellulose compounds, FD&C Blue No. 2 Aluminum Lake, FD&C Red No. 40 Aluminum Lake, FD&C Yellow No. 6 Aluminum Lake, povidone, propylene glycol, sodium chloride, sodium lauryl sulfate, sodium starch glycolate, sorbitol and titanium dioxide. Product meets USP Drug Release Test 1.

ACTIONS
Preclinical studies have shown that lithium alters sodium transport in nerve and muscle cells and effects a shift toward intraneuronal metabolism of catecholamines, but the specific biochemical mechanism of lithium action in mania is unknown.

INDICATIONS
Lithium is indicated in the treatment of manic episodes of manic-depressive illness. Maintenance therapy prevents or diminishes the intensity of subsequent episodes in those manic-depressive patients with a history of mania.
Typical symptoms: of mania include pressure of speech, motor hyperactivity, reduced need for sleep, flight of ideas, grandiosity, elation, poor judgment, aggressiveness, and possibly hostility. When given to a patient experiencing a manic episode, lithium may produce a normalization of symptomatology within 1 to 3 weeks.

WARNINGS
Lithium should generally not be given to patients with significant renal or cardiovascular disease, severe debilitation, dehydration, sodium depletion, and to patients receiving diuretics, or angiotensin converting enzyme (ACE) inhibitors, since the risk of lithium toxicity is very high in such patients. If the psychiatric indication is life threatening, and if such a patient fails to respond to other measures, lithium treatment may be undertaken with extreme caution, including daily serum lithium determinations and adjustment to the usually low doses ordinarily tolerated by these individuals. In such instances, hospitalization is a necessity.

Chronic lithium therapy may be associated with diminution of renal concentrating ability, occasionally presenting as nephrogenic diabetes insipidus, with polyuria and polydipsia. Such patients should be carefully managed to avoid dehydration with resulting lithium retention and toxicity. This condition is usually reversible when lithium is discontinued. Morphologic changes with glomerular and interstitial fibrosis and nephron atrophy have been reported in patients on chronic lithium therapy. Morphologic changes have also been seen in manic-depressive patients never exposed to lithium. The relationship between renal function and morphologic changes and their association with lithium therapy have not been established.

Kidney function should be assessed prior to and during lithium therapy. Routine urinalysis and other tests may be used to evaluate tubular function (e.g., urine specific gravity or osmolality following a period of water deprivation, or 24-hour urine volume) and glomerular function (e.g., serum creatinine or creatinine clearance). During lithium therapy, progressive or sudden changes in renal function, even within the normal range, indicate the need for re-evaluation of treatment.

An encephalopathic syndrome (characterized by weakness, lethargy, fever, tremulousness and confusion, extrapyramidal symptoms, leukocytosis, elevated serum enzymes, BUN and FBS) has occurred in a few patients treated with lithium plus a neuroleptic, most notably haloperidol. In some instances, the syndrome was followed by irreversible brain damage. Because of possible causal relationship between these events and the concomitant administration of lithium and neuroleptic drugs, patients receiving such combined therapy or patients with organic brain syndrome or other CNS impairment should be monitored closely for early evidence of neurologic toxicity and treatment discontinued promptly if such signs appear. This encephalopathic syndrome may be similar to or the same as Neuroleptic Malignant Syndrome (NMS).

Lithium toxicity is closely related to serum lithium concentrations and can occur at doses close to the therapeutic concentrations (see **DOSAGE AND ADMINISTRATION**).

Outpatients and their families should be warned that the patient must discontinue lithium therapy and contact his physician if such clinical signs of lithium toxicity as diarrhea, vomiting, tremor, mild ataxia, drowsiness, or muscular weakness occur.

Lithium may prolong the effects of neuromuscular blocking agents. Therefore, neuromuscular blocking agents should be given with caution to patients receiving lithium.

Usage in Pregnancy
Adverse effects on nidation in rats, embryo viability in mice, and metabolism in vitro of rat testis and human spermatozoa have been attributed to lithium, as have teratogenicity in submammalian species and cleft palate in mice.

In humans, lithium may cause fetal harm when administered to a pregnant woman. Data from lithium birth registries suggest an increase in cardiac and other anomalies especially Ebstein's anomaly. If this drug is used in women of childbearing potential, or during pregnancy, or if a patient becomes pregnant while taking this drug, the patient should be apprised by their physician of the potential hazard to the fetus.

Usage in Nursing Mothers
Lithium is excreted in human milk. Nursing should not be undertaken during lithium therapy except in rare and unusual circumstances where, in the view of the physician, the potential benefits to the mother outweigh possible hazard to the infant or neonate. Signs and symptoms of lithium toxicity such as hypertonia, hypothermia, cyanosis and ECG changes have been reported in some infants and neonates.

Pediatric Use
Safety and effectiveness in pediatric patients under 12 years of age have not been determined; its use in these patients is not recommended.

There has been a report of transient syndrome of acute dystonia and hyperreflexia occurring in a 15 kg pediatric patient who ingested 300 mg of lithium carbonate.

PRECAUTIONS
The ability to tolerate lithium is greater during the acute manic phase and decreases when manic symptoms subside (see **DOSAGE AND ADMINISTRATION**).

The distribution space of lithium approximates that of total body water. Lithium is primarily excreted in urine with insignificant excretion in feces. Renal excretion of lithium is proportional to its plasma concentration. The elimination half-life of lithium is approximately 24 hours. Lithium decreases sodium reabsorption by the renal tubules which could lead to sodium depletion. Therefore, it is essential for the patient to maintain a normal diet, including salt, and an adequate fluid intake (2500-3500 mL) at least during the initial stabilization period. Decreased tolerance to lithium has been reported to ensue from protracted sweating or diarrhea and, if such occur, supplemental fluid and salt should be administered under careful medical supervision and lithium intake reduced or suspended until the condition is resolved.

In addition to sweating and diarrhea, concomitant infection with elevated temperatures may also necessitate a temporary reduction or cessation of medication.

Previously existing thyroid disorders do not necessarily constitute a contraindication to lithium treatment. Where hypothyroidism preexists, careful monitoring of thyroid function during lithium stabilization and maintenance allows for correction of changing thyroid parameters and/or adjustment of lithium doses, if any. If hypothyroidism occurs during lithium stabilization and maintenance, supplemental thyroid treatment may be used.

In general, the concomitant use of diuretics or angiotensin converting enzyme (ACE) inhibitors with lithium carbonate should be avoided. In those cases where concomitant use is necessary, extreme caution is advised since sodium loss from these drugs may reduce the renal clearance of lithium resulting in increased serum lithium concentrations with the risk of lithium toxicity. When such combinations are used, the lithium dosage may need to be decreased, and more frequent monitoring of lithium serum concentrations is recommended. See **WARNINGS** for additional caution information.

Concomitant administration of carbamazepine and lithium may increase the risk of neurotoxic side effects.

The following drugs can lower serum lithium concentrations by increasing urinary lithium excretion: acetazolamide, urea, xanthine preparations and alkalinizing agents such as sodium bicarbonate.

Concomitant extended use of iodide preparations, especially potassium iodide, with lithium may produce hypothyroidism.

Concurrent use of calcium channel blocking agents with lithium may increase the risk of neurotoxicity in the form of ataxia, tremors, nausea, vomiting, diarrhea and/or tinnitus. Concurrent use of metronidazole with lithium may provoke lithium toxicity due to reduced renal clearance. Patients receiving such combined therapy should be monitored closely. Concurrent use of fluoxetine with lithium has resulted in both increased and decreased serum lithium concentrations. Patients receiving such combined therapy should be monitored closely.

Nonsteroidal anti-inflammatory drugs (NSAIDS): Lithium levels should be closely monitored when patients initiate or discontinue NSAID use. In some cases, lithium toxicity has resulted from interactions between an NSAID and lithium. Indomethacin and piroxicam have been reported to increase significantly steady-state plasma lithium concentrations. There is also evidence that other nonsteroidal anti-inflammatory agents, including the selective cyclooxygenase-2 (COX-2) inhibitors, have the same effect. In a study conducted in healthy subjects, mean steady-state lithium plasma levels increased approximately 17% in subjects receiving lithium 450 mg BID with celecoxib 200 mg BID as compared to subjects receiving lithium alone.

Lithium may impair mental and/or physical abilities. Patients should be cautioned about activities requiring alertness (e.g., operating vehicles or machinery).

Usage in Pregnancy
Pregnancy Category D. (see **WARNINGS**).

Usage in Nursing Mothers
Because of the potential for serious adverse reactions in nursing infants and neonates from lithium, a decision should be made whether to discontinue nursing or to discontinue the drug, taking into account the importance of the drug to the mother (see **WARNINGS**).

Pediatric Use
Safety and effectiveness in pediatric patients below the age of 12 have not been established (see **WARNINGS**).

Geriatric Use
Clinical studies of LITHOBID® Tablets did not include sufficient numbers of subjects aged 65 and over to determine whether they respond differently from younger subjects. Other reported clinical experience has not identified differences in responses between the elderly and younger patients. In general, dose selection for an elderly patient should be cautious, usually starting at the low end of the dosing range, reflecting the greater frequency of decreased hepatic, renal, or cardiac function, and of concomitant disease or other therapy.

This drug is known to be substantially excreted by the kidney, and the risk of toxic reactions to this drug may be greater in patients with impaired renal function. Because elderly patients are more likely to have decreased renal function, care should be taken in dose selection, and it may be useful to monitor renal function.

ADVERSE REACTIONS
The occurrence and severity of adverse reactions are generally directly related to serum lithium concentrations and to individual patient sensitivity to lithium. They generally occur more frequently and with greater severity at higher concentrations.

Adverse reactions may be encountered at serum lithium concentrations below 1.5 mEq/L. Mild to moderate adverse reactions may occur at concentrations from 1.5-2.5 mEq/L, and moderate to severe reactions may be seen at concentrations from 2.0 mEq/L and above.

Fine hand tremor, polyuria and mild thirst may occur during initial therapy for the acute manic phase and may persist throughout treatment. Transient and mild nausea and general discomfort may also appear during the first few days of lithium administration.

These side effects usually subside with continued treatment or with a temporary reduction or cessation of dosage. If persistent, a cessation of lithium therapy may be required. Diarrhea, vomiting, drowsiness, muscular weakness and lack of coordination may be early signs of lithium intoxication, and can occur at lithium concentrations below 2.0 mEq/L. At higher concentrations, giddiness, ataxia, blurred vision, tinnitus and a large output of dilute urine may be seen. Serum lithium concentrations above 3.0 mEq/L may produce a complex clinical picture involving multiple organs and organ systems. Serum lithium concentrations should not be permitted to exceed 2.0 mEq/L during the acute treatment phase.

The following reactions have been reported and appear to be related to serum lithium concentrations, including concentrations within the therapeutic range:

Central Nervous System: tremor, muscle hyperirritability (fasciculations, twitching, clonic movements of whole limbs), hypertonicity, ataxia, choreoathetotic movements, hyperactive deep tendon reflex, extrapyramidal symptoms including acute dystonia, cogwheel rigidity, blackout spells, epileptiform seizures, slurred speech, dizziness, vertigo, downbeat nystagmus, incontinence of urine or feces, somnolence, psychomotor retardation, restlessness, confusion, stupor, coma, tongue movements, tics, tinnitus, hallucinations, poor memory, slowed intellectual functioning, startled response, worsening of organic brain syndromes. Cases of Pseudotumor Cerebri (increased intracranial pressure and papilledema) have been reported with lithium use. If undetected, this condition may result in enlargement of the blind spot, constriction of visual fields and eventual blindness due to optic atrophy. Lithium should be discontinued, if clinically possible, if this syndrome occurs. **Cardiovascular:** cardiac arrhythmia, hypotension, peripheral circulatory collapse, bradycardia, sinus node dysfunction with severe bradycardia (which may result in syncope); **Gastrointestinal:** anorexia, nausea, vomiting, diarrhea, gastritis, salivary gland swelling, abdominal pain, excessive salivation, flatulence, indigestion; **Genitourinary:** glycosuria, decreased creatinine clearance, albuminuria, oliguria, and symptoms of nephrogenic diabetes insipidus including polyuria, thirst and polydipsia; **Dermatologic:** drying and thinning of hair, alopecia, anesthesia of skin, acne, chronic folliculitis, xerosis cutis, psoriasis or its exacerbation, generalized pruritus with or without rash, cutaneous ulcers, angioedema; **Autonomic Nervous System:** blurred vision, dry mouth, impotence/sexual dysfunction; **Thyroid Abnormalities:** euthyroid goiter and/or hypothyroidism (including myxedema) accompanied by lower T_3 and T_4. ^{131}Iodine uptake may be elevated (see **PRECAUTIONS**). Paradoxically, rare cases of hyperthyroidism have been reported. **EEG Changes:** diffuse slowing, widening of frequency spectrum, potentiation and disorganization of background rhythm. **EKG Changes:** reversible flattening, isoelectricity or inversion of T-waves. **Miscellaneous:** Fatigue, lethargy, transient scotomata, exophthalmos, dehydration, weight loss, leucocytosis, headache, transient hyperglycemia, hypercalcemia, hyperparathyroidism, albuminuria, excessive weight gain, edematous swelling of ankles or wrists, metallic taste, dysgeusia/taste distortion, salty taste, thirst, swollen lips, tightness in chest, swollen and/or painful joints, fever, polyarthralgia, and dental caries.

Some reports of nephrogenic diabetes insipidus, hyperparathyroidism and hypothyroidism which persist after lithium discontinuation have been received.

A few reports have been received of the development of painful discoloration of fingers and toes and coldness of the extremities within one day of starting lithium treatment. The mechanism through which these symptoms (resembling Raynaud's Syndrome) developed is not known. Recovery followed discontinuance.

DOSAGE AND ADMINISTRATION

Acute Mania

Optimal patient response can usually be established with 1800 mg/day in the following dosages:

ACUTE MANIA

	Morning	Afternoon	Nighttime
LITHOBID® Slow-Release Tablets[1]	3 tabs (900 mg)		3 tabs (900 mg)

[1] Can also be administered on 600 mg t.i.d. recommended dosing interval.

Such doses will normally produce an effective serum lithium concentration ranging between 1.0 and 1.5 mEq/L. Dosage must be individualized according to serum concentrations and clinical response. Regular monitoring of the patient's clinical state and of serum lithium concentrations is necessary. Serum concentrations should be determined twice per week during the acute phase, and until the serum concentrations and clinical condition of the patient have been stabilized.

Long-Term Control

Desirable serum lithium concentrations are 0.6 to 1.2 mEq/L which can usually be achieved with 900-1200 mg/day. Dosage will vary from one individual to another, but generally the following dosages will maintain this concentration.

LONG-TERM CONTROL

	Morning	Afternoon	Nighttime
LITHOBID® Slow-Release Tablets[1]	2 tabs (600 mg)		2 tabs (600 mg)

[1] Can be administered on t.i.d. recommended dosing interval up to 1200 mg/day.

Serum lithium concentrations in uncomplicated cases receiving maintenance therapy during remission should be monitored at least every two months. Patients abnormally sensitive to lithium may exhibit toxic signs at serum concentrations of 1.0 to 1.5 mEq/L. Geriatric patients often respond to reduced dosage, and may exhibit signs of toxicity at serum concentrations ordinarily tolerated by other patients. In general, dose selection for an elderly patient should be cautious, usually starting at the low end of the dosing range, reflecting the greater frequency of decreased hepatic, renal, or cardiac function, and of concomitant disease or other drug therapy.

Important Considerations

- Blood samples for serum lithium determinations should be drawn immediately prior to the next dose when lithium concentrations are relatively stable (i.e., 8-12 hours after previous dose). Total reliance must not be placed on serum concentrations alone. Accurate patient evaluation requires both clinical and laboratory analysis.
- LITHOBID® Slow-Release Tablets must be swallowed whole and never chewed or crushed.

OVERDOSAGE

The toxic concentrations for lithium (≥1.5 mEq/L) are close to the therapeutic concentrations (0.6-1.2 mEq/L). It is therefore important that patients and their families be cautioned to watch for early toxic symptoms and to discontinue the drug and inform the physician should they occur. (Toxic symptoms are listed in detail under **ADVERSE REACTIONS**.)

Treatment

No specific antidote for lithium poisoning is known. Treatment is supportive. Early symptoms of lithium toxicity can usually be treated by reduction or cessation of dosage of the drug and resumption of the treatment at a lower dose after 24 to 48 hours. In severe cases of lithium poisoning, the first and foremost goal of treatment consists of elimination of this ion from the patient.

Treatment is essentially the same as that used in barbiturate poisoning: 1) gastric lavage, 2) correction of fluid and electrolyte imbalance and, 3) regulation of kidney functioning. Urea, mannitol, and aminophylline all produce significant increases in lithium excretion. Hemodialysis is an effective and rapid means of removing the ion from the severely toxic patient. However, patient recovery may be slow.

Infection prophylaxis, regular chest X-rays, and preservation of adequate respiration are essential.

HOW SUPPLIED

LITHOBID® (Lithium Carbonate, USP) Slow-Release Tablets, 300 mg, peach-colored imprinted "SOLVAY 4492"
NDC 0032-4492-01 (Bottle of 100)
NDC 0032-4492-10 (Bottle of 1000)

Storage Conditions

Store between 59°-86°F (15°-30°C). Protect from moisture. Dispense in tight, child-resistant container (USP).

Solvay
Pharmaceuticals, Inc.
Marietta, GA 30062
0990
10E Rev 12/2002

Wyeth Pharmaceuticals

Division of Wyeth
P.O. BOX 8299
PHILADELPHIA, PA 19101

For Product Information Contact:
(800) 934-5556
For Product Quality Contact:
(800) 999-9384
For Professional Services Contact:
(800) 395-9938
For Customer Service and Ordering Information Contact:
Pharmaceuticals: (800) 666-7248
Vaccines: (800) 572-8221
For Patient Assistance Program Contact:
(800) 568-9938
For All Other Inquiries:
(610) 688-4400
www.wyeth.com

Information on these Wyeth Pharmaceuticals products is based on labeling in effect as of May 2003. Since the publication of this reference book, there may have been revisions to the labeling of these products.

For further product information and current package inserts please visit www.wyeth.com or call our Global Medical Communications Department toll-free at 1-800-934-5556.

CORDARONE® ℞

[*kōr' dă-rōn*]
(amiodarone HCl)
TABLETS

Prescribing information for this product, which appears on pages 3384–3387 of the 2003 PDR, has been completely revised as follows. Please write "See Supplement A" next to the product heading.

DESCRIPTION

Cordarone is a member of a new class of antiarrhythmic drugs with predominantly Class III (Vaughan Williams' classification) effects, available for oral administration as pink, scored tablets containing 200 mg of amiodarone hydrochloride. The inactive ingredients present are colloidal silicon dioxide, lactose, magnesium stearate, povidone, starch, and FD&C Red 40. Cordarone is a benzofuran derivative: 2-butyl-3-benzo-furanyl 4-[2-(diethylamino)-ethoxy]-3,5-diiodophenyl ketone hydrochloride. It is not chemically related to any other available antiarrhythmic drug.

The structural formula is as follows:

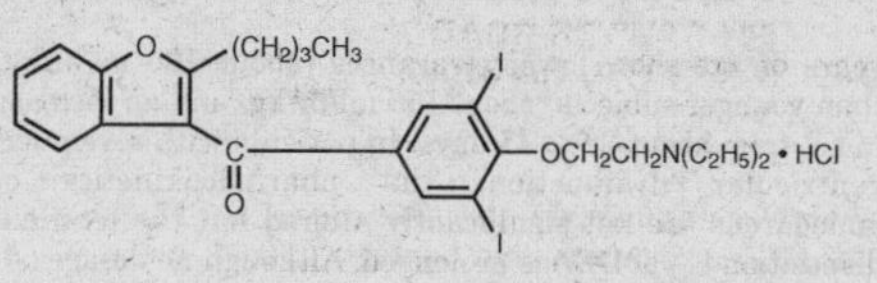

$C_{25}H_{29}I_2NO_3$•HCl Molecular Weight: 681.8

Amiodarone HCl is a white to cream-colored crystalline powder. It is slightly soluble in water, soluble in alcohol, and freely soluble in chloroform. It contains 37.3% iodine by weight.

CLINICAL PHARMACOLOGY

Electrophysiology/Mechanisms of Action

In animals, Cordarone is effective in the prevention or suppression of experimentally-induced arrhythmias. The antiarrhythmic effect of Cordarone may be due to at least two major properties: 1) a prolongation of the myocardial cell-action potential duration and refractory period and 2) noncompetitive α- and β-adrenergic inhibition.

Cordarone prolongs the duration of the action potential of all cardiac fibers while causing minimal reduction of dV/dt (maximal upstroke velocity of the action potential). The refractory period is prolonged in all cardiac tissues. Cordarone increases the cardiac refractory period without influencing resting membrane potential, except in automatic cells where the slope of the prepotential is reduced, generally reducing automaticity. These electrophysiologic effects are reflected in a decreased sinus rate of 15 to 20%, increased PR and QT intervals of about 10%, the development of U-waves, and changes in T-wave contour. These changes should not require discontinuation of Cordarone as they are evidence of its pharmacological action, although Cordarone can cause marked sinus bradycardia or sinus arrest and heart block. On rare occasions, QT prolongation has been associated with worsening of arrhythmia (see "**WARNINGS**").

Hemodynamics

In animal studies and after intravenous administration in man, Cordarone relaxes vascular smooth muscle, reduces peripheral vascular resistance (afterload), and slightly increases cardiac index. After oral dosing, however, Cordarone produces no significant change in left ventricular ejection fraction (LVEF), even in patients with depressed LVEF. After acute intravenous dosing in man, Cordarone may have a mild negative inotropic effect.

Pharmacokinetics

Following oral administration in man, Cordarone is slowly and variably absorbed. The bioavailability of Cordarone is approximately 50%, but has varied between 35 and 65% in various studies. Maximum plasma concentrations are attained 3 to 7 hours after a single dose. Despite this, the onset of action may occur in 2 to 3 days, but more commonly takes 1 to 3 weeks, even with loading doses. Plasma concentrations with chronic dosing at 100 to 600 mg/day are approximately dose proportional, with a mean 0.5 mg/L increase for each 100 mg/day. These means, however, include considerable individual variability. Food increases the rate and extent of absorption of Cordarone. The effects of food upon the bioavailability of Cordarone have been studied in 30 healthy subjects who received a single 600-mg dose immediately after consuming a high fat meal and following an overnight fast. The area under the plasma concentration-time curve (AUC) and the peak plasma concentration (C_{max}) of amiodarone increased by 2.3 (range 1.7 to 3.6) and 3.8 (range 2.7 to 4.4) times, respectively, in the presence of food. Food also increased the rate of absorption of amiodarone, decreasing the time to peak plasma concentration (T_{max}) by 37%. The mean AUC and mean C_{max} of desethylamiodarone increased by 55% (range 58 to 101%) and 32% (range 4 to 84%), respectively, but there was no change in the T_{max} in the presence of food.

Cordarone has a very large but variable volume of distribution, averaging about 60 L/kg, because of extensive accumulation in various sites, especially adipose tissue and highly perfused organs, such as the liver, lung, and spleen. One major metabolite of Cordarone, desethylamiodarone (DEA), has been identified in man; it accumulates to an even greater extent in almost all tissues. No data are available on the activity of DEA in humans, but in animals, it has significant electrophysiologic and antiarrhythmic effects generally similar to amiodarone itself. DEA's precise role and contribution to the antiarrhythmic activity of oral amiodarone are not certain. The development of maximal ventricular class III effects after oral Cordarone administration in humans correlates more closely with DEA accumulation over time than with amiodarone accumulation.

Amiodarone is eliminated primarily by hepatic metabolism and biliary excretion and there is negligible excretion of amiodarone or DEA in urine. Neither amiodarone nor DEA is dialyzable.

In clinical studies of 2 to 7 days, clearance of amiodarone after intravenous administration in patients with VT and VF ranged between 220 and 440 ml/hr/kg. Age, sex, renal disease, and hepatic disease (cirrhosis) do not have marked effects on the disposition of amiodarone or DEA. Renal impairment does not influence the pharmacokinetics of amiodarone. After a single dose of intravenous amiodarone in cirrhotic patients, significantly lower C_{max} and average concentration values are seen for DEA, but mean amiodarone levels are unchanged. Normal subjects over 65

Continued on next page

Cordarone Tablets—Cont.

years of age show lower clearances (about 100 ml/hr/kg) than younger subjects (about 150 ml/hr/kg) and an increase in $t_{1/2}$ from about 20 to 47 days. In patients with severe left ventricular dysfunction, the pharmacokinetics of amiodarone are not significantly altered but the terminal disposition $t_{1/2}$ of DEA is prolonged. Although no dosage adjustment for patients with renal, hepatic, or cardiac abnormalities has been defined during chronic treatment with Cordarone, close clinical monitoring is prudent for elderly patients and those with severe left ventricular dysfunction.

Following single dose administration in 12 healthy subjects, Cordarone exhibited multicompartmental pharmacokinetics with a mean apparent plasma terminal elimination half-life of 58 days (range 15 to 142 days) for amiodarone and 36 days (range 14 to 75 days) for the active metabolite (DEA). In patients, following discontinuation of chronic oral therapy, Cordarone has been shown to have a biphasic elimination with an initial one-half reduction of plasma levels after 2.5 to 10 days. A much slower terminal plasma-elimination phase shows a half-life of the parent compound ranging from 26 to 107 days, with a mean of approximately 53 days and most patients in the 40- to 55-day range. In the absence of a loading-dose period, steady-state plasma concentrations, at constant oral dosing, would therefore be reached between 130 and 535 days, with an average of 265 days. For the metabolite, the mean plasma-elimination half-life was approximately 61 days. These data probably reflect an initial elimination of drug from well-perfused tissue (the 2.5- to 10-day half-life phase), followed by a terminal phase representing extremely slow elimination from poorly perfused tissue compartments such as fat.

The considerable intersubject variation in both phases of elimination, as well as uncertainty as to what compartment is critical to drug effect, requires attention to individual responses once arrhythmia control is achieved with loading doses because the correct maintenance dose is determined, in part, by the elimination rates. Daily maintenance doses of Cordarone should be based on individual patient requirements (see **"DOSAGE AND ADMINISTRATION"**).

Cordarone and its metabolite have a limited transplacental transfer of approximately 10 to 50%. The parent drug and its metabolite have been detected in breast milk.

Cordarone is highly protein-bound (approximately 96%).

Although electrophysiologic effects, such as prolongation of QTc, can be seen within hours after a parenteral dose of Cordarone, effects on abnormal rhythms are not seen before 2 to 3 days and usually require 1 to 3 weeks, even when a loading dose is used. There may be a continued increase in effect for longer periods still. There is evidence that the time to effect is shorter when a loading-dose regimen is used.

Consistent with the slow rate of elimination, antiarrhythmic effects persist for weeks or months after Cordarone is discontinued, but the time of recurrence is variable and unpredictable. In general, when the drug is resumed after recurrence of the arrhythmia, control is established relatively rapidly compared to the initial response, presumably because tissue stores were not wholly depleted at the time of recurrence.

Pharmacodynamics

There is no well-established relationship of plasma concentration to effectiveness, but it does appear that concentrations much below 1 mg/L are often ineffective and that levels above 2.5 mg/L are generally not needed. Within individuals dose reductions and ensuing decreased plasma concentrations can result in loss of arrhythmia control. Plasma-concentration measurements can be used to identify patients whose levels are unusually low, and who might benefit from a dose increase, or unusually high, and who might have dosage reduction in the hope of minimizing side effects. Some observations have suggested a plasma concentration, dose, or dose/duration relationship for side effects such as pulmonary fibrosis, liver-enzyme elevations, corneal deposits and facial pigmentation, peripheral neuropathy, gastrointestinal and central nervous system effects.

Monitoring Effectiveness

Predicting the effectiveness of any antiarrhythmic agent in long-term prevention of recurrent ventricular tachycardia and ventricular fibrillation is difficult and controversial, with highly qualified investigators recommending use of ambulatory monitoring, programmed electrical stimulation with various stimulation regimens, or a combination of these, to assess response. There is no present consensus on many aspects of how best to assess effectiveness, but there is a reasonable consensus on some aspects:

1. If a patient with a history of cardiac arrest does not manifest a hemodynamically unstable arrhythmia during electrocardiographic monitoring prior to treatment, assessment of the effectiveness of Cordarone requires some provocative approach, either exercise or programmed electrical stimulation (PES).
2. Whether provocation is also needed in patients who do manifest their life-threatening arrhythmia spontaneously is not settled, but there are reasons to consider PES or other provocation in such patients. In the fraction of patients whose PES-inducible arrhythmia can be made noninducible by Cordarone (a fraction that has varied widely in various series from less than 10% to almost 40%, perhaps due to different stimulation criteria), the prognosis has been almost uniformly excellent, with very low recurrence (ventricular tachycardia or sudden death) rates. More controversial is the meaning of continued inducibility. There has been an impression that continued inducibility in Cordarone patients may not foretell a poor prognosis but, in fact, many observers have found greater recurrence rates in patients who remain inducible than in those who do not. A number of criteria have been proposed, however, for identifying patients who remain inducible but who seem likely nonetheless to do well on Cordarone. These criteria include increased difficulty of induction (more stimuli or more rapid stimuli), which has been reported to predict a lower rate of recurrence, and ability to tolerate the induced ventricular tachycardia without severe symptoms, a finding that has been reported to correlate with better survival but not with lower recurrence rates. While these criteria require confirmation and further study in general, *easier* inducibility or *poorer* tolerance of the induced arrhythmia should suggest consideration of a need to revise treatment.

Several predictors of success not based on PES have also been suggested, including complete elimination of all nonsustained ventricular tachycardia on ambulatory monitoring and very low premature ventricular-beat rates (less than 1 VPB/1,000 normal beats).

While these issues remain unsettled for Cordarone, as for other agents, the prescriber of Cordarone should have access to (direct or through referral), and familiarity with, the full range of evaluatory procedures used in the care of patients with life-threatening arrhythmias.

It is difficult to describe the effectiveness rates of Cordarone, as these depend on the specific arrhythmia treated, the success criteria used, the underlying cardiac disease of the patient, the number of drugs tried before resorting to Cordarone, the duration of follow-up, the dose of Cordarone, the use of additional antiarrhythmic agents, and many other factors. As Cordarone has been studied principally in patients with refractory life-threatening ventricular arrhythmias, in whom drug therapy must be selected on the basis of response and cannot be assigned arbitrarily, randomized comparisons with other agents or placebo have not been possible. Reports of series of treated patients with a history of cardiac arrest and mean follow-up of one year or more have given mortality (due to arrhythmia) rates that were highly variable, ranging from less than 5% to over 30%, with most series in the range of 10 to 15%. Overall arrhythmia-recurrence rates (fatal and nonfatal) also were highly variable (and, as noted above, depended on response to PES and other measures), and depend on whether patients who do not seem to respond initially are included. In most cases, considering only patients who seemed to respond well enough to be placed on long-term treatment, recurrence rates have ranged from 20 to 40% in series with a mean follow-up of a year or more.

INDICATIONS AND USAGE

Because of its life-threatening side effects and the substantial management difficulties associated with its use (see **"WARNINGS"** below), Cordarone is indicated only for the treatment of the following documented, life-threatening recurrent ventricular arrhythmias when these have not responded to documented adequate doses of other available antiarrhthymics or when alternative agents could not be tolerated.

1. Recurrent ventricular fibrillation.
2. Recurrent hemodynamically unstable ventricular tachycardia.

As is the case for other antiarrhythmic agents, there is no evidence from controlled trials that the use of Cordarone (amiodarone HCl) Tablets favorably affects survival.

Cordarone should be used only by physicians familiar with and with access to (directly or through referral) the use of all available modalities for treating recurrent life-threatening ventricular arrhythmias, and who have access to appropriate monitoring facilities, including in-hospital and ambulatory continuous electrocardiographic monitoring and electrophysiologic techniques. Because of the life-threatening nature of the arrhythmias treated, potential interactions with prior therapy, and potential exacerbation of the arrhythmia, initiation of therapy with Cordarone should be carried out in the hospital.

CONTRAINDICATIONS

Cordarone is contraindicated in severe sinus-node dysfunction, causing marked sinus bradycardia; second- and third-degree atrioventricular block; and when episodes of bradycardia have caused syncope (except when used in conjunction with a pacemaker).

Cordarone is contraindicated in patients with a known hypersensitivity to the drug.

WARNINGS

Cordarone is intended for use only in patients with the indicated life-threatening arrhythmias because its use is accompanied by substantial toxicity.

Cordarone has several potentially fatal toxicities, the most important of which is pulmonary toxicity (hypersensitivity pneumonitis or interstitial/alveolar pneumonitis) that has resulted in clinically manifest disease at rates as high as 10 to 17% in some series of patients with ventricular arrhythmias given doses around 400 mg/day, and as abnormal diffusion capacity without symptoms in a much higher percentage of patients. Pulmonary toxicity has been fatal about 10% of the time. Liver injury is common with Cordarone, but is usually mild and evidenced only by abnormal liver enzymes. Overt liver disease can occur, however, and has been fatal in a few cases. Like other antiarrhythmics, Cordarone can exacerbate the arrhythmia, e.g., by making the arrhythmia less well tolerated or more difficult to reverse. This has occurred in 2 to 5% of patients in various series, and significant heart block or sinus bradycardia has been seen in 2 to 5%. All of these events should be manageable in the proper clinical setting in most cases. Although the frequency of such proarrhythmic events does not appear greater with Cordarone than with many other agents used in this population, the effects are prolonged when they occur. Even in patients at high risk of arrhythmic death, in whom the toxicity of Cordarone is an acceptable risk, Cordarone poses major management problems that could be life-threatening in a population at risk of sudden death, so that every effort should be made to utilize alternative agents first.

The difficulty of using Cordarone effectively and safely itself poses a significant risk to patients. Patients with the indicated arrhythmias must be hospitalized while the loading dose of Cordarone is given, and a response generally requires at least one week, usually two or more. Because absorption and elimination are variable, maintenance-dose selection is difficult, and it is not unusual to require dosage decrease or discontinuation of treatment. In a retrospective survey of 192 patients with ventricular tachyarrhythmias, 84 required dose reduction and 18 required at least temporary discontinuation because of adverse effects, and several series have reported 15 to 20% overall frequencies of discontinuation due to adverse reactions. The time at which a previously controlled life-threatening arrhythmia will recur after discontinuation or dose adjustment is unpredictable, ranging from weeks to months. The patient is obviously at great risk during this time and may need prolonged hospitalization. Attempts to substitute other antiarrhythmic agents when Cordarone must be stopped will be made difficult by the gradually, but unpredictably, changing amiodarone body burden. A similar problem exists when Cordarone is not effective; it still poses the risk of an interaction with whatever subsequent treatment is tried.

Mortality

In the National Heart, Lung and Blood Institute's Cardiac Arrhythmia Suppression Trial (CAST), a long-term, multicentered, randomized, double-blind study in patients with asymptomatic non-life-threatening ventricular arrhythmias who had had myocardial infarctions more than six days but less than two years previously, an excessive mortality or non-fatal cardiac arrest rate was seen in patients treated with encainide or flecainide (56/730) compared with that seen in patients assigned to matched placebo-treated groups (22/725). The average duration of treatment with encainide or flecainide in this study was ten months.

Cordarone therapy was evaluated in two multi-centered, randomized, double-blind, placebo-controlled trials involving 1202 (Canadian Amiodarone Myocardial Infarction Arrhythmia Trial; CAMIAT) and 1486 (European Myocardial Infarction Amiodarone Trial; EMIAT) post-MI patients followed for up to 2 years. Patients in CAMIAT qualified with ventricular arrhythmias, and those randomized to amiodarone received weight- and response-adjusted doses of 200 to 400 mg/day. Patients in EMIAT qualified with ejection fraction <40%, and those randomized to amiodarone received fixed doses of 200 mg/day. Both studies had weeks-long loading dose schedules. Intent-to-treat all-cause mortality results were as follows:

[See table below]

These data are consistent with the results of a pooled analysis of smaller, controlled studies involving patients with structural heart disease (including myocardial infarction).

Pulmonary Toxicity

Cordarone (amiodarone HCl) Tablets may cause a clinical syndrome of cough and progressive dyspnea accompanied by functional, radiographic, gallium-scan, and pathological data consistent with pulmonary toxicity, the frequency of which varies from 2 to 7% in most published reports, but is as high as 10 to 17% in some reports. Therefore, when Cordarone therapy is initiated, a baseline chest X-ray and pulmonary-function tests, including diffusion capacity, should be performed. The patient should return for a history, physical exam, and chest X-ray every 3 to 6 months.

Preexisting pulmonary disease does not appear to increase the risk of developing pulmonary toxicity; however, these patients have a poorer prognosis if pulmonary toxicity does develop.

	Placebo		Amiodarone		Relative Risk	
	N	Deaths	N	Deaths		95% CI
EMIAT	743	102	743	103	0.99	0.76-1.31
CAMIAT	596	68	606	57	0.88	0.58-1.16

Pulmonary toxicity secondary to Cordarone seems to result from either indirect or direct toxicity as represented by hypersensitivity pneumonitis or interstitial/alveolar pneumonitis, respectively.

Hypersensitivity pneumonitis usually appears earlier in the course of therapy, and rechallenging these patients with Cordarone results in a more rapid recurrence of greater severity. Bronchoalveolar lavage is the procedure of choice to confirm this diagnosis, which can be made when a T suppressor/cytotoxic (CD8-positive) lymphocytosis is noted. Steroid therapy should be instituted and Cordarone therapy discontinued in these patients.

Interstitial/alveolar pneumonitis may result from the release of oxygen radicals and/or phospholipidosis and is characterized by findings of diffuse alveolar damage, interstitial pneumonitis or fibrosis in lung biopsy specimens. Phospholipidosis (foamy cells, foamy macrophages), due to inhibition of phospholipase, will be present in most cases of Cordarone-induced pulmonary toxicity; however, these changes also are present in approximately 50% of all patients on Cordarone therapy. These cells should be used as markers of therapy, but not as evidence of toxicity. A diagnosis of Cordarone-induced interstitial/alveolar pneumonitis should lead, at a minimum, to dose reduction or, preferably, to withdrawal of the Cordarone to establish reversibility, especially if other acceptable antiarrhythmic therapies are available. Where these measures have been instituted, a reduction in symptoms of amiodarone-induced pulmonary toxicity was usually noted within the first week, and a clinical improvement was greatest in the first two to three weeks. Chest X-ray changes usually resolve within two to four months. According to some experts, steroids may prove beneficial. Prednisone in doses of 40 to 60 mg/day or equivalent doses of other steroids have been given and tapered over the course of several weeks depending upon the condition of the patient. In some cases rechallenge with Cordarone at a lower dose has not resulted in return of toxicity. Recent reports suggest that the use of lower loading and maintenance doses of Cordarone are associated with a decreased incidence of Cordarone-induced pulmonary toxicity.

In a patient receiving Cordarone, any new respiratory symptoms should suggest the possibility of pulmonary toxicity, and the history, physical exam, chest X-ray, and pulmonary-function tests (with diffusion capacity) should be repeated and evaluated. A 15% decrease in diffusion capacity has a high sensitivity but only a moderate specificity for pulmonary toxicity; as the decrease in diffusion capacity approaches 30%, the sensitivity decreases but the specificity increases. A gallium-scan also may be performed as part of the diagnostic workup.

Fatalities, secondary to pulmonary toxicity, have occurred in approximately 10% of cases. However, in patients with life-threatening arrhythmias, discontinuation of Cordarone therapy due to suspected drug-induced pulmonary toxicity should be undertaken with caution, as the most common cause of death in these patients is sudden cardiac death. Therefore, every effort should be made to rule out other causes of respiratory impairment (i.e., congestive heart failure with Swan-Ganz catheterization if necessary, respiratory infection, pulmonary embolism, malignancy, etc.) before discontinuing Cordarone in these patients. In addition, bronchoalveolar lavage, transbronchial lung biopsy and/or open lung biopsy may be necessary to confirm the diagnosis, especially in those cases where no acceptable alternative therapy is available.

If a diagnosis of Cordarone-induced hypersensitivity pneumonitis is made, Cordarone should be discontinued, and treatment with steroids should be instituted. If a diagnosis of Cordarone-induced interstitial/alveolar pneumonitis is made, steroid therapy should be instituted and, preferably, Cordarone discontinued or, at a minimum, reduced in dosage. Some cases of Cordarone-induced interstitial/alveolar pneumonitis may resolve following a reduction in Cordarone dosage in conjunction with the administration of steroids. In some patients, rechallenge at a lower dose has not resulted in return of interstitial/alveolar pneumonitis; however, in some patients (perhaps because of severe alveolar damage) the pulmonary lesions have not been reversible.

Worsened Arrhythmia

Cordarone, like other antiarrhythmics, can cause serious exacerbation of the presenting arrhythmia, a risk that may be enhanced by the presence of concomitant antiarrhythmics. Exacerbation has been reported in about 2 to 5% in most series, and has included new ventricular fibrillation, incessant ventricular tachycardia, increased resistance to cardioversion, and polymorphic ventricular tachycardia associated with QTc prolongation (Torsade de Pointes). In addition, Cordarone has caused symptomatic bradycardia or sinus arrest with suppression of escape foci in 2 to 4% of patients.

The need to co-administer amiodarone with any other drug known to prolong the QTc interval must be based on a careful assessment of the potential risks and benefits of doing so for each patient. A careful assessment of the potential risks and benefits of administering Cordarone must be made in patients with thyroid dysfunction due to the possibility of arrhythmia breakthrough or exacerbation of arrhythmia in these patients.

Liver Injury

Elevations of hepatic enzyme levels are seen frequently in patients exposed to Cordarone and in most cases are asymptomatic. If the increase exceeds three times normal, or doubles in a patient with an elevated baseline, discontinuation of Cordarone or dosage reduction should be considered. In a few cases in which biopsy has been done, the histology has resembled that of alcoholic hepatitis or cirrhosis. Hepatic failure has been a rare cause of death in patients treated with Cordarone.

Loss of Vision

Cases of optic neuropathy and/or optic neuritis, usually resulting in visual impairment, have been reported in patients treated with amiodarone. In some cases, visual impairment has progressed to permanent blindness. Optic neuropathy and/or neuritis may occur at any time following initiation of therapy. A causal relationship to the drug has not been clearly established. If symptoms of visual impairment appear, such as changes in visual acuity and decreases in peripheral vision, prompt ophthalmic examination is recommended. Appearance of optic neuropathy and/or neuritis calls for re-evaluation of Cordarone therapy. The risks and complications of antiarrhythmic therapy with Cordarone must be weighed against its benefits in patients whose lives are threatened by cardiac arrhythmias. Regular ophthalmic examination, including fundoscopy and slit-lamp examination, is recommended during administration of Cordarone. (See "**ADVERSE REACTIONS**").

Neonatal Hypo- or Hyperthyroidism

Cordarone can cause fetal harm when administered to a pregnant woman. Although Cordarone use during pregnancy is uncommon, there have been a small number of published reports of congenital goiter/hypothyroidism and hyperthyroidism. If Cordarone is used during pregnancy, or if the patient becomes pregnant while taking Cordarone, the patient should be apprised of the potential hazard to the fetus.

In general, Cordarone (amiodarone HCl) Tablets should be used during pregnancy only if the potential benefit to the mother justifies the unknown risk to the fetus.

In pregnant rats and rabbits, amiodarone HCl in doses of 25 mg/kg/day (approximately 0.4 and 0.9 times, respectively, the maximum recommended human maintenance dose*) had no adverse effects on the fetus. In the rabbit, 75 mg/kg/day (approximately 2.7 times the maximum recommended human maintenance dose*) caused abortions in greater than 90% of the animals. In the rat, doses of 50 mg/kg/day or more were associated with slight displacement of the testes and an increased incidence of incomplete ossification of some skull and digital bones; at 100 mg/kg/day or more, fetal body weights were reduced; at 200 mg/kg/day, there was an increased incidence of fetal resorption. (These doses in the rat are approximately 0.8, 1.6 and 3.2 times the maximum recommended human maintenance dose.*) Adverse effects on fetal growth and survival also were noted in one of two strains of mice at a dose of 5 mg/kg/day (approximately 0.04 times the maximum recommended human maintenance dose*).

*600 mg in a 50 kg patient (doses compared on a body surface area basis)

PRECAUTIONS

Impairment of Vision

Optic Neuropathy and/or Neuritis

Cases of optic neuropathy and optic neuritis have been reported (see "**WARNINGS**").

Corneal Microdeposits

Corneal microdeposits appear in the majority of adults treated with Cordarone. They are usually discernible only by slit-lamp examination, but give rise to symptoms such as visual halos or blurred vision in as many as 10% of patients. Corneal microdeposits are reversible upon reduction of dose or termination of treatment. Asymptomatic microdeposits alone are not a reason to reduce dose or discontinue treatment (see "**ADVERSE REACTIONS**").

Neurologic

Chronic administration of oral amiodarone in rare instances may lead to the development of peripheral neuropathy that may resolve when amiodarone is discontinued, but this resolution has been slow and incomplete.

Photosensitivity

Cordarone has induced photosensitization in about 10% of patients; some protection may be afforded by the use of sun-barrier creams or protective clothing. During long-term treatment, a blue-gray discoloration of the exposed skin may occur. The risk may be increased in patients of fair complexion or those with excessive sun exposure, and may be related to cumulative dose and duration of therapy.

Thyroid Abnormalities

Cordarone inhibits peripheral conversion of thyroxine (T_4) to triiodothyronine (T_3) and may cause increased thyroxine levels, decreased T_3 levels, and increased levels of inactive reverse T_3 (rT_3) in clinically euthyroid patients. It is also a potential source of large amounts of inorganic iodine. Because of its release of inorganic iodine, or perhaps for other reasons, Cordarone can cause either hypothyroidism or hyperthyroidism. Thyroid function should be monitored prior to treatment and periodically thereafter, particularly in elderly patients, and in any patient with a history of thyroid nodules, goiter, or other thyroid dysfunction. Because of the slow elimination of Cordarone and its metabolites, high plasma iodide levels, altered thyroid function, and abnormal thyroid-function tests may persist for several weeks or even months following Cordarone withdrawal. Hypothyroidism has been reported in 2 to 4% of patients in most series, but in 8 to 10% in some series. This condition may be identified by relevant clinical symptoms and particularly by elevated serum TSH levels. In some clinically hypothyroid amiodarone-treated patients, free thyroxine index values may be normal. Hypothyroidism is best managed by Cordarone dose reduction and/or thyroid hormone supplement. However, therapy must be individualized, and it may be necessary to discontinue Cordarone® (amiodarone HCl) Tablets in some patients. Hyperthyroidism occurs in about 2% of patients receiving Cordarone, but the incidence may be higher among patients with prior inadequate dietary iodine intake. Cordarone-induced hyperthyroidism usually poses a greater hazard to the patient than hypothyroidism because of the possibility of arrhythmia breakthrough or aggravation, which may result in death. In fact, IF ANY NEW SIGNS OF ARRHYTHMIA APPEAR, THE POSSIBILITY OF HYPERTHYROIDISM SHOULD BE CONSIDERED. Hyperthyroidism is best identified by relevant clinical symptoms and signs, accompanied usually by abnormally elevated levels of serum T_3 RIA, and further elevations of serum T_4, and a subnormal serum TSH level (using a sufficiently sensitive TSH assay). The finding of a flat TSH response to TRH is confirmatory of hyperthyroidism and may be sought in equivocal cases. Since arrhythmia breakthroughs may accompany Cordarone-induced hyperthyroidism, aggressive medical treatment is indicated, including, if possible, dose reduction or withdrawal of Cordarone. The institution of antithyroid drugs, β-adrenergic blockers and/or temporary corticosteroid therapy may be necessary. The action of antithyroid drugs may be especially delayed in amiodarone-induced thyrotoxicosis because of substantial quantities of preformed thyroid hormones stored in the gland. Radioactive iodine therapy is contraindicated because of the low radioiodine uptake associated with amiodarone-induced hyperthyroidism. Experience with thyroid surgery in this setting is extremely limited, and this form of therapy runs the theoretical risk of inducing thyroid storm. Cordarone-induced hyperthyroidism may be followed by a transient period of hypothyroidism.

Surgery

Volatile Anesthetic Agents: Close perioperative monitoring is recommended in patients undergoing general anesthesia who are on amiodarone therapy as they may be more sensitive to the myocardial depressant and conduction effects of halogenated inhalational anesthetics.

Hypotension Postbypass: Rare occurrences of hypotension upon discontinuation of cardiopulmonary bypass during open-heart surgery in patients receiving Cordarone have been reported. The relationship of this event to Cordarone therapy is unknown.

Adult Respiratory Distress Syndrome (ARDS): Postoperatively, occurrences of ARDS have been reported in patients receiving Cordarone therapy who have undergone either cardiac or noncardiac surgery. Although patients usually respond well to vigorous respiratory therapy, in rare instances the outcome has been fatal. Until further studies have been performed, it is recommended that FiO_2 and the determinants of oxygen delivery to the tissues (e.g., SaO_2, PaO_2) be closely monitored in patients on Cordarone.

Laboratory Tests

Elevations in liver enzymes (SGOT and SGPT) can occur. Liver enzymes in patients on relatively high maintenance doses should be monitored on a regular basis. Persistent significant elevations in the liver enzymes or hepatomegaly should alert the physician to consider reducing the maintenance dose of Cordarone or discontinuing therapy.

Cordarone alters the results of thyroid-function tests, causing an increase in serum T_4 and serum reverse T_3, and a decline in serum T_3 levels. Despite these biochemical changes, most patients remain clinically euthyroid.

Drug Interactions

Amiodarone is metabolized to desethylamiodarone by the cytochrome P450 (CYP450) enzyme group, specifically cytochrome P450 3A4 (CYP3A4). This isoenzyme is present in both the liver and intestines (see "**CLINICAL PHARMACOLOGY, Pharmacokinetics and Metabolism**"). Amiodarone is also known to be an inhibitor of CYP3A4. Therefore, amiodarone has the **potential** for interactions with drugs or substances that may be substrates, inhibitors or inducers of CYP3A4. While only a limited number of *in vivo* drug-drug interactions with amiodarone have been reported, the potential for other interactions should be anticipated. This is especially important for drugs associated with serious toxicity, such as other antiarrhythmics. If such drugs are needed, their dose should be reassessed and, where appropriate, plasma concentration measured.

In view of the long and variable half-life of amiodarone, potential for drug interactions exists not only with concomitant medication but also with drugs administered after discontinuation of amiodarone.

Since amiodarone is a substrate for CYP3A4, drugs/substances that inhibit CYP3A4 may decrease the metabolism and increase serum concentrations of amiodarone, with the potential for toxic effects. Reported examples of this interaction include the following:

Protease Inhibitors:

Protease inhibitors are known to inhibit CYP3A4 to varying degrees. Inhibition of CYP3A4 by **indinavir** has been reported to result in increased serum concentrations of amiodarone. Monitoring for amiodarone toxicity and serial measurement of amiodarone serum concentration during concomitant protease inhibitor therapy should be considered.

Histamine H_2 antagonists:

Cimetidine inhibits CYP3A4 and can increase serum amiodarone levels.

Continued on next page

Cordarone Tablets—Cont.

Other substances:
Grapefruit juice inhibits CYP3A4-mediated metabolism of oral amiodarone in the intestinal mucosa, resulting in increased plasma levels of amiodarone; therefore, grapefruit juice should not be taken during treatment with oral amiodarone (see "**DOSAGE AND ADMINISTRATION**").
Amiodarone may suppress certain CYP450 enzymes (enzyme inhibition). This can result in unexpectedly high plasma levels of other drugs which are metabolized by those CYP450 enzymes and may lead to toxic effects. Reported examples of this interaction include the following:
Immunosuppressives:
Cyclosporine (CYP3A4 substrate) administered in combination with oral amiodarone has been reported to produce persistently elevated plasma concentrations of cyclosporine resulting in elevated creatinine, despite reduction in dose of cyclosporine.
HMG-CoA Reductase Inhibitors:
Simvastatin (CYP3A4 substrate) in combination with amiodarone has been associated with reports of myopathy/rhabdomyolysis.
Cardiovasculars:
Cardiac glycosides: In patients receiving **digoxin** therapy, administration of oral amiodarone regularly results in an increase in the serum digoxin concentration that may reach toxic levels with resultant clinical toxicity. Amiodarone taken concomitantly with digoxin increases the serum digoxin concentration by 70% after one day. **On initiation of oral amiodarone, the need for digitalis therapy should be reviewed and the dose reduced by approximately 50% or discontinued.** If digitalis treatment is continued, serum levels should be closely monitored and patients observed for clinical evidence of toxicity. These precautions probably should apply to digitoxin administration as well.
Antiarrhythmics:
Other antiarrhythmic drugs, such as **quinidine, procainamide, disopyramide,** and **phenytoin,** have been used concurrently with oral amiodarone.
There have been case reports of increased steady-state levels of quinidine, procainamide, and phenytoin during concomitant therapy with amiodarone. Phenytoin decreases serum amiodarone levels. Amiodarone taken concomitantly with quinidine increases quinidine serum concentration by 33% after two days. Amiodarone taken concomitantly with procainamide for less than seven days increases plasma concentrations of procainamide and n-acetyl procainamide by 55% and 33%, respectively. Quinidine and procainamide doses should be reduced by one-third when either is administered with amiodarone. Plasma levels of **flecainide** have been reported to increase in the presence of oral amiodarone; because of this, the dosage of flecainide should be adjusted when these drugs are administered concomitantly. In general, any added antiarrhythmic drug should be initiated at a lower than usual dose with careful monitoring. Combination of amiodarone with other antiarrhythmic therapy should be reserved for patients with life-threatening ventricular arrhythmias who are incompletely responsive to a single agent or incompletely responsive to amiodarone. During transfer to amiodarone the dose levels of previously administered agents should be reduced by 30 to 50% several days after the addition of amiodarone, when arrhythmia suppression should be beginning. The continued need for the other antiarrhythmic agent should be reviewed after the effects of amiodarone have been established, and discontinuation ordinarily should be attempted. If the treatment is continued, these patients should be particularly carefully monitored for adverse effects, especially conduction disturbances and exacerbation of tachyarrhythmias, as amiodarone is continued. In amiodarone-treated patients who require additional antiarrhythmic therapy, the initial dose of such agents should be approximately half of the usual recommended dose.
Antihypertensives:
Amiodarone should be used with caution in patients receiving **β-receptor blocking agents** (e.g., propanolol, a CYP3A4 inhibitor) or **calcium channel antagonists** (e.g., verapamil, a CYP3A4 substrate, and diltiazem, a CYP3A4 inhibitor) because of the possible potentiation of bradycardia, sinus arrest, and AV block; if necessary, amiodarone can continue to be used after insertion of a pacemaker in patients with severe bradycardia or sinus arrest.
Anticoagulants:
Potentiation of **warfarin**-type (CYP2C9 and CYP3A4 substrate) anticoagulant response is almost always seen in patients receiving amiodarone and can result in serious or fatal bleeding. Since the concomitant administration of warfarin with amiodarone increases the prothrombin time by 100% after 3 to 4 days, **the dose of the anticoagulant should be reduced by one-third to one-half, and prothrombin times should be monitored closely.**
Some drugs/substances are known to accelerate the metabolism of amiodarone by stimulating the synthesis of CYP3A4 (enzyme induction). This may lead to low amiodarone serum levels and potential decrease in efficacy. Reported examples of this interaction include the following:
Antibiotics:
Rifampin is a potent inducer of CYP3A4. Administration of rifampin concomitantly with oral amiodarone has been shown to result in decreases in serum concentrations of amiodarone and desethylamiodarone.

Other substances, including herbal preparations:
St. John's Wort (Hypericum perforatum) induces CYP3A4. Since amiodarone is a substrate for CYP3A4, there is the potential that the use of St. John's Wort in patients receiving amiodarone could result in reduced amiodarone levels.
Other reported interactions with amiodarone:
Fetanyl (CYP3A4 substrate) in combination with amiodarone may cause hypotension, bradycardia, decreased cardiac output.
Sinus bradycardia has been reported with oral amiodarone in combination with **lidocaine** (CYP3A4 substrate) given for local anesthesia. Seizure, associated with increased lidocaine concentrations, has been reported with concomitant administration of intravenous amiodarone.
Dextromethorphan is a substrate for both CYP2D6 and CYP3A4. Amiodarone inhibits CYP2D6.
Cholestyramine increases enterohepatic elimination of amiodarone and may reduce serum levels and $t_{1/2}$.
Disopyramide increases QT prolongation which could cause arrhythmia.
Hemodynamic and electrophysiologic interactions have also been observed after concomitant administration with **propranolol, diltiazem,** and **verapamil**.
Volatile Anesthetic Agents (See "**PRECAUTIONS,** Surgery, *Volatile Anesthetic Agents.*")
In addition to the interactions noted above, chronic (> 2 weeks) *oral* Cordarone administration impairs metabolism of phenytoin, dextromethorphan, and methotrexate.
Electrolyte Disturbances
Since antiarrhythmic drugs may be ineffective or may be arrhythmogenic in patients with hypokalemia, any potassium or magnesium deficiency should be corrected before instituting and during Cordarone therapy. Use caution when coadministering Cordarone with drugs which may induce hypokalemia and/or hypomagnesemia.
Carcinogenesis, Mutagenesis, Impairment of Fertility
Amiodarone HCl was associated with a statistically significant, dose-related increase in the incidence of thyroid tumors (follicular adenoma and/or carcinoma) in rats. The incidence of thyroid tumors was greater than control even at the lowest dose level tested, i.e., 5 mg/kg/day (approximately 0.08 times the maximum recommended human maintenance dose*).
Mutagenicity studies (Ames, micronucleus, and lysogenic tests) with Cordarone were negative.
In a study in which amiodarone HCl was administered to male and female rats, beginning 9 weeks prior to mating, reduced fertility was observed at a dose level of 90 mg/kg/day (approximately 1.4 times the maximum recommended human maintenance dose*).

___
*600 mg in a 50 kg patient (dose compared on a body surface area basis)
Pregnancy: Pregnancy Category D
See "**WARNINGS**, Neonatal Hypo- or Hyperthyroidism."
Labor and Delivery
It is not known whether the use of Cordarone during labor or delivery has any immediate or delayed adverse effects. Preclinical studies in rodents have not shown any effect of Cordarone on the duration of gestation or on parturition.
Nursing Mothers
Cordarone is excreted in human milk, suggesting that breast-feeding could expose the nursing infant to a significant dose of the drug. Nursing offspring of lactating rats administered Cordarone have been shown to be less viable and have reduced body-weight gains. Therefore, when Cordarone therapy is indicated, the mother should be advised to discontinue nursing.
Pediatric Use
The safety and effectiveness of Cordarone (amiodarone HCl) Tablets in pediatric patients have not been established.
Geriatric Use
Clinical studies of Cordarone Tablets did not include sufficient numbers of subjects aged 65 and over to determine whether they respond differently from younger subjects. Other reported clinical experience has not identified differences in responses between the elderly and younger patients. In general, dose selection for an elderly patient should be cautious, usually starting at the low end of the dosing range, reflecting the greater frequency of decreased hepatic, renal, or cardiac function, and of concomitant disease or other drug therapy.

ADVERSE REACTIONS
Adverse reactions have been very common in virtually all series of patients treated with Cordarone for ventricular arrhythmias with relatively large doses of drug (400 mg/day and above), occurring in about three-fourths of all patients and causing discontinuation in 7 to 18%. The most serious reactions are pulmonary toxicity, exacerbation of arrhythmia, and rare serious liver injury (see "**WARNINGS**"), but other adverse effects constitute important problems. They are often reversible with dose reduction or cessation of Cordarone treatment. Most of the adverse effects appear to become more frequent with continued treatment beyond six months, although rates appear to remain relatively constant beyond one year. The time and dose relationships of adverse effects are under continued study.
Neurologic problems are extremely common, occurring in 20 to 40% of patients and including malaise and fatigue, tremor and involuntary movements, poor coordination and gait, and peripheral neuropathy; they are rarely a reason to stop therapy and may respond to dose reductions or discontinuation (see "**PRECAUTIONS**").

Gastrointestinal complaints, most commonly nausea, vomiting, constipation, and anorexia, occur in about 25% of patients but rarely require discontinuation of drug. These commonly occur during high-dose administration (i.e., loading dose) and usually respond to dose reduction or divided doses.
Ophthalmic abnormalities including optic neuropathy and/or optic neuritis, in some cases progressing to permanent blindness, papilledema, corneal degeneration, photosensitivity, eye discomfort, scotoma, lens opacities, and macular degeneration have been reported. (See "**WARNINGS**.") Asymptomatic corneal microdeposits are present in virtually all adult patients who have been on drug for more than 6 months. Some patients develop eye symptoms of halos, photophobia, and dry eyes. Vision is rarely affected and drug discontinuation is rarely needed.
Dermatological adverse reactions occur in about 15% of patients, with photosensitivity being most common (about 10%). Sunscreen and protection from sun exposure may be helpful, and drug discontinuation is not usually necessary. Prolonged exposure to Cordarone occasionally results in a blue-gray pigmentation. This is slowly and occasionally incompletely reversible on discontinuation of drug but is of cosmetic importance only.
Cardiovascular adverse reactions, other than exacerbation of the arrhythmias, include the uncommon occurrence of congestive heart failure (3%) and bradycardia. Bradycardia usually responds to dosage reduction but may require a pacemaker for control. CHF rarely requires drug discontinuation. Cardiac conduction abnormalities occur infrequently and are reversible on discontinuation of drug.
The following side-effect rates are based on a retrospective study of 241 patients treated for 2 to 1,515 days (mean 441.3 days).
The following side effects were each reported in 10 to 33% of patients:
Gastrointestinal: Nausea and vomiting.
The following side effects were each reported in 4 to 9% of patients:
Dermatologic: Solar dermatitis/photosensitivity.
Neurologic: Malaise and fatigue, tremor/abnormal involuntary movements, lack of coordination, abnormal gait/ataxia, dizziness, paresthesias.
Gastrointestinal: Constipation, anorexia.
Ophthalmologic: Visual disturbances.
Hepatic: Abnormal liver-function tests.
Respiratory: Pulmonary inflammation or fibrosis.
The following side effects were each reported in 1 to 3% of patients:
Thyroid: Hypothyroidism, hyperthyroidism.
Neurologic: Decreased libido, insomnia, headache, sleep disturbances.
Cardiovascular: Congestive heart failure, cardiac arrhythmias, SA node dysfunction.
Gastrointestinal: Abdominal pain.
Hepatic: Nonspecific hepatic disorders.
Other: Flushing, abnormal taste and smell, edema, abnormal salivation, coagulation abnormalities.
The following side effects were each reported in less than 1% of patients:
Blue skin discoloration, rash, spontaneous ecchymosis, alopecia, hypotension, and cardiac conduction abnormalities.
In surveys of almost 5,000 patients treated in open U.S. studies and in published reports of treatment with Cordarone, the adverse reactions most frequently requiring discontinuation of Cordarone included pulmonary infiltrates or fibrosis, paroxysmal ventricular tachycardia, congestive heart failure, and elevation of liver enzymes. Other symptoms causing discontinuations less often included visual disturbances, solar dermatitis, blue skin discoloration, hyperthyroidism, and hypothyroidism.
Postmarketing Reports
In postmarketing surveillance, sinus arrest, hepatitis, cholestatic hepatitis, cirrhosis, epididymitis, impotence, vasculitis, pseudotumor cerebri, thrombocytopenia, angioedema, bronchiolitis obliterans organizing pneumonia (possibly fatal), bronchospasm, pleuritis, pancreatitis, toxic epidermal necrolysis, myopathy, rhabdomyolysis, hemolytic anemia, aplastic anemia, pancytopenia, neutropenia, erythema multiforme, Stevens-Johnson syndrome, and exfoliative dermatitis, also have been reported in patients receiving Cordarone.

OVERDOSAGE
There have been cases, some fatal, of Cordarone overdose. In addition to general supportive measures, the patient's cardiac rhythm and blood pressure should be monitored, and if bradycardia ensues, a β-adrenergic agonist or a pacemaker may be used. Hypotension with inadequate tissue perfusion should be treated with positive inotropic and/or vasopressor agents. Neither Cordarone nor its metabolite is dialyzable.
The acute oral LD_{50} of amiodarone HCl in mice and rats is greater than 3,000 mg/kg.

DOSAGE AND ADMINISTRATION
BECAUSE OF THE UNIQUE PHARMACOKINETIC PROPERTIES, DIFFICULT DOSING SCHEDULE, AND SEVERITY OF THE SIDE EFFECTS IF PATIENTS ARE IMPROPERLY MONITORED, CORDARONE SHOULD BE ADMINISTERED ONLY BY PHYSICIANS WHO ARE EXPERIENCED IN THE TREATMENT OF LIFE-THREATENING ARRHYTHMIAS WHO ARE THOROUGHLY FAMILIAR WITH THE RISKS AND BENEFITS OF CORDARONE THERAPY, AND WHO HAVE ACCESS

TO LABORATORY FACILITIES CAPABLE OF ADEQUATELY MONITORING THE EFFECTIVENESS AND SIDE EFFECTS OF TREATMENT.

In order to insure that an antiarrhythmic effect will be observed without waiting several months, loading doses are required. A uniform, optimal dosage schedule for administration of Cordarone has not been determined. Because of the food effect on absorption, Cordarone should be administered consistently with regard to meals (see **"CLINICAL PHARMACOLOGY"**). Individual patient titration is suggested according to the following guidelines.

For life-threatening ventricular arrhythmias, such as ventricular fibrillation or hemodynamically unstable ventricular tachycardia: Close monitoring of the patients is indicated during the loading phase, particularly until risk of recurrent ventricular tachycardia or fibrillation has abated. Because of the serious nature of the arrhythmia and the lack of predictable time course of effect, loading should be performed in a hospital setting. Loading doses of 800 to 1,600 mg/day are required for 1 to 3 weeks (occasionally longer) until initial therapeutic response occurs. (Administration of Cordarone in divided doses with meals is suggested for total daily doses of 1,000 mg or higher, or when gastrointestinal intolerance occurs.) If side effects become excessive, the dose should be reduced. Elimination of recurrence of ventricular fibrillation and tachycardia usually occurs within 1 to 3 weeks, along with reduction in complex and total ventricular ectopic beats.

Since grapefruit juice is known to inhibit CYP3A4-mediated metabolism of oral amiodarone in the intestinal mucosa, resulting in increased plasma levels of amiodarone; grapefruit juice should not be taken during treatment with oral amiodarone (see **"PRECAUTIONS, Drug Interactions"**).

Upon starting Cordarone therapy, an attempt should be made to gradually discontinue prior antiarrhythmic drugs (see section on **"Drug Interactions"**). When adequate arrhythmia control is achieved, or if side effects become prominent, Cordarone dose should be reduced to 600 to 800 mg/day for one month and then to the maintenance dose, usually 400 mg/day (see **"CLINICAL PHARMACOLOGY–Monitoring Effectiveness"**). Some patients may require larger maintenance doses, up to 600 mg/day, and some can be controlled on lower doses. Cordarone may be administered as a single daily dose, or in patients with severe gastrointestinal intolerance, as a b.i.d. dose. In each patient, the chronic maintenance dose should be determined according to antiarrhythmic effect as assessed by symptoms, Holter recordings, and/or programmed electrical stimulation and by patient tolerance. Plasma concentrations may be helpful in evaluating nonresponsiveness or unexpectedly severe toxicity (see **"CLINICAL PHARMACOLOGY"**).

The lowest effective dose should be used to prevent the occurrence of side effects. In all instances, the physician must be guided by the severity of the individual patient's arrhythmia and response to therapy.

When dosage adjustments are necessary, the patient should be closely monitored for an extended period of time because of the long and variable half-life of Cordarone and the difficulty in predicting the time required to attain a new steady-state level of drug. Dosage suggestions are summarized below:

	Loading Dose (Daily)	Adjustment and Maintenance Dose (Daily)	
Ventricular Arrhythmias	1 to 3 weeks	~1 month	usual maintenance
	800 to 1,600 mg	600 to 800 mg	400 mg

HOW SUPPLIED

Cordarone® (amiodarone HCl) Tablets are available in bottles of 60 tablets and in Redipak® cartons containing 100 tablets (10 blister strips of 10) as follows:

200 mg, NDC 0008-4188, round, convex-faced, pink tablets with a raised "C" and marked "200" on one side, with reverse side scored and marked "WYETH" and "4188."

Keep tightly closed.

Store at room temperature, approximately 25°C (77°F).

Protect from light.

Dispense in a light-resistant, tight container.

Use carton to protect contents from light.

℞ only

Manufactured for
Wyeth Laboratories
A Wyeth-Ayerst Company
Philadelphia, PA 19101
by Sanofi Winthrop Industrie
1, rue de la Vierge
33440 Ambares, France

CI 6036-4 Revised August 30, 2002

CORDARONE® INTRAVENOUS ℞

[*kōr'dă-rōn*]

(amiodarone hydrochloride)

℞ only

Prescribing information for this product, which appears on pages 3387–3390 of the 2003 PDR, has been completely revised as follows. Please write "See Supplement A" next to the product heading.

DESCRIPTION

Cordarone Intravenous (Cordarone I.V.) contains amiodarone HCl ($C_{25}H_{29}I_2NO_3 \cdot HCl$), a class III antiarrhythmic drug. Amiodarone HCl is (2-butyl-3-benzofuranyl)[4-[2-(diethylamino)ethoxy]-3,5-diiodophenyl]methanone hydrochloride. Amiodarone HCl has the following structural formula:

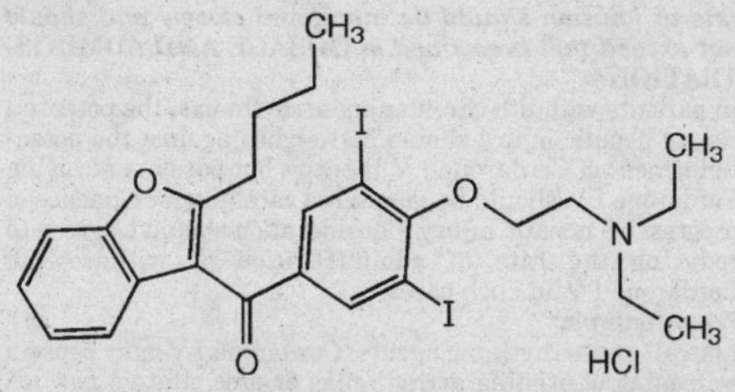

Amiodarone HCl is a white to slightly yellow crystalline powder, and is very slightly soluble in water. It has a molecular weight of 681.78 and contains 37.3% iodine by weight. Cordarone I.V. is a sterile clear, pale-yellow solution visually free from particulates. Each milliliter of the Cordarone I.V. formulation contains 50 mg of amiodarone HCl, 20.2 mg of benzyl alcohol, 100 mg of polysorbate 80, and water for injection.

CLINICAL PHARMACOLOGY

Mechanisms of Action

Amiodarone is generally considered a class III antiarrhythmic drug, but it possesses electrophysiologic characteristics of all four Vaughan Williams classes. Like class I drugs, amiodarone blocks sodium channels at rapid pacing frequencies, and like class II drugs, it exerts a noncompetitive antisympathetic action. One of its main effects, with prolonged administration, is to lengthen the cardiac action potential, a class III effect. The negative chronotropic effect of amiodarone in nodal tissues is similar to the effect of class IV drugs. In addition to blocking sodium channels, amiodarone blocks myocardial potassium channels, which contributes to slowing of conduction and prolongation of refractoriness. The antisympathetic action and the block of calcium and potassium channels are responsible for the negative dromotropic effects on the sinus node and for the slowing of conduction and prolongation of refractoriness in the atrioventricular (AV) node. Its vasodilatory action can decrease cardiac workload and consequently myocardial oxygen consumption.

Cordarone I.V. administration prolongs intranodal conduction (Atrial-His, AH) and refractoriness of the atrioventricular node (ERP AVN), but has little or no effect on sinus cycle length (SCL), refractoriness of the right atrium and right ventricle (ERP RA and ERP RV), repolarization (QTc), intraventricular conduction (QRS), and infranodal conduction (His-ventricular, HV). A comparison of the electrophysiologic effects of Cordarone I.V. and oral Cordarone is shown in the table below.

EFFECTS OF INTRAVENOUS AND ORAL CORDARONE ON ELECTROPHYSIOLOGIC PARAMETERS

Formulation	SCL	QRS	QTc	AH	HV	ERP RA	ERP RV	ERP AVN
I.V.	↔	↔	↔	↑	↔	↔	↔	↑
Oral	↑	↔	↑	↑	↔	↑	↑	↑

↔ No change

At higher doses (>10 mg/kg) of Cordarone I.V., prolongation of the ERP RV and modest prolongation of the QRS have been seen. These differences between oral and intravenous administration suggest that the initial acute effects of Cordarone I.V. may be predominantly focused on the AV node, causing an intranodal conduction delay and increased nodal refractoriness due to slow channel blockade (class IV activity) and noncompetitive adrenergic antagonism (class II activity).

Pharmacokinetics and Metabolism

Amiodarone exhibits complex disposition characteristics after intravenous administration. Peak serum concentrations after single 5 mg/kg 15-minute intravenous infusions in healthy subjects range between 5 and 41 mg/L. Peak concentrations after 10-minute infusions of 150 mg Cordarone I.V. in patients with ventricular fibrillation (VF) or hemodynamically unstable ventricular tachycardia (VT) range between 7 and 26 mg/L. Due to rapid distribution, serum concentrations decline to 10% of peak values within 30 to 45 minutes after the end of the infusion. In clinical trials, after 48 hours of continued infusions (125, 500, or 1000 mg/day) plus supplemental (150 mg) infusions (for recurrent arrhythmias), amiodarone mean serum concentrations between 0.7 to 1.4 mg/L were observed (n = 260).

N-desethylamiodarone (DEA) is the major active metabolite of amiodarone in humans. DEA serum concentrations above 0.05 mg/L are not usually seen until after several days of continuous infusion but with prolonged therapy reach approximately the same concentration as amiodarone. The enzymes responsible for the N-deethylation are believed to be the cytochrome P-450 3A (CYP3A) subfamily, principally CYP3A4. This isozyme is present in both the liver and intestines. The highly variable systemic availability of oral amiodarone may be attributed potentially to large interindividual variability in CYP3A4 activity.

Amiodarone is eliminated primarily by hepatic metabolism and biliary excretion and there is negligible excretion of amiodarone or DEA in urine. Neither amiodarone nor DEA is dialyzable. Amiodarone and DEA cross the placenta and both appear in breast milk.

No data are available on the activity of DEA in humans, but in animals, it has significant electrophysiologic and antiarrhythmic effects generally similar to amiodarone itself. DEA's precise role and contribution to the antiarrhythmic activity of oral amiodarone are not certain. The development of maximal ventricular class III effects after oral Cordarone administration in humans correlates more closely with DEA accumulation over time than with amiodarone accumulation. On the other hand (see **Clinical Trials**), after Cordarone I.V. administration, there is evidence of activity well before significant concentrations of DEA are attained.

The following table summarizes the mean ranges of pharmacokinetic parameters of amiodarone reported in single dose i.v. (5 mg/kg over 15 min) studies of healthy subjects.

PHARMACOKINETIC PROFILE AFTER I.V. AMIODARONE ADMINISTRATION

Drug	Clearance (mL/h/kg)	V_c (L/kg)	V_{ss} (L/kg)	$t_{1/2}$ (days)
Amiodarone	90-158	0.2	40-84	20-47
Desethylamiodarone	197-290	—	68-168	≥AMI $t_{1/2}$

Notes: V_c and V_{ss} denote the central and steady-state volumes of distribution from i.v. studies.
"—" denotes not available.

Desethylamiodarone clearance and volume involve an unknown biotransformation factor. The systemic availability of ***oral*** amiodarone in healthy subjects ranges between 33% and 65%. From *in vitro* studies, the protein binding of amiodarone is >96%.

In clinical studies of 2 to 7 days, clearance of amiodarone after intravenous administration in patients with VT and VF ranged between 220 and 440 mL/h/kg. Age, sex, renal disease, and hepatic disease (cirrhosis) do not have marked effects on the disposition of amiodarone or DEA. Renal impairment does not influence the pharmacokinetics of amiodarone. After a single dose of Cordarone I.V. in cirrhotic patients, significantly lower C_{max} and average concentration values are seen for DEA, but mean amiodarone levels are unchanged. Normal subjects over 65 years of age show lower clearances (about 100 mL/hr/kg) than younger subjects (about 150 mL/hr/kg) and an increase in $t_{1/2}$ from about 20 to 47 days. In patients with severe left ventricular dysfunction, the pharmacokinetics of amiodarone are not significantly altered but the terminal disposition $t_{1/2}$ of DEA is prolonged. Although no dosage adjustment for patients with renal, hepatic, or cardiac abnormalities has been defined during chronic treatment with ***oral*** Cordarone, close clinical monitoring is prudent for elderly patients and those with severe left ventricular dysfunction.

There is no established relationship between drug concentration and therapeutic response for short-term intravenous use. Steady-state amiodarone concentrations of 1 to 2.5 mg/L have been associated with antiarrhythmic effects and acceptable toxicity following chronic ***oral*** Cordarone therapy.

Pharmacodynamics

Cordarone I.V. has been reported to produce negative inotropic and vasodilatory effects in animals and humans. In clinical studies of patients with refractory VF or hemodynamically unstable VT, treatment-emergent, drug-related hypotension occurred in 288 of 1836 patients (16%) treated with Cordarone I.V. No correlations were seen between the baseline ejection fraction and the occurrence of clinically significant hypotension during infusion of Cordarone I.V.

Clinical Trials

Apart from studies in patients with VT or VF, described below, there are two other studies of amiodarone showing an antiarrhythmic effect before significant levels of DEA could have accumulated. A placebo-controlled study of i.v. amiodarone (300 mg over 2 hours followed by 1200 mg/day) in post-coronary artery bypass graft patients with supraventricular and 2- to 3-consecutive-beat ventricular arrhythmias showed a reduction in arrhythmias from 12 hours on. A baseline-controlled study using a similar i.v. regimen in patients with recurrent, refractory VT/VF also showed rapid onset of antiarrhythmic activity; amiodarone therapy reduced episodes of VT by 85% compared to baseline.

The acute effectiveness of Cordarone I.V. in suppressing recurrent VF or hemodynamically unstable VT is supported by two randomized, parallel, dose-response studies of approximately 300 patients each. In these studies, patients with at least two episodes of VF or hemodynamically unstable VT in the preceding 24 hours were randomly assigned to receive doses of approximately 125 or 1000 mg over the first 24 hours, an 8-fold difference. In one study, a middle dose of approximately 500 mg was evaluated. The dose regimen consisted of an initial rapid loading infusion, followed by a slower 6-hour loading infusion, and then an 18-hour maintenance infusion. The maintenance infusion was continued up to hour 48. Additional 10-minute infusions of 150 mg Cordarone I.V. were given for "breakthrough" VT/VF more frequently to the 125-mg dose group, thereby considerably reducing the planned 8-fold differences in total dose to 1.8- and 2.6- fold, respectively, in the two studies.

The prospectively defined primary efficacy end point was the rate of VT/VF episodes per hour. For both studies, the median rate was 0.02 episodes per hour in patients receiv-

Continued on next page

Cordarone IV—Cont.

ing the high dose and 0.07 episodes per hour in patients receiving the low dose, or approximately 0.5 versus 1.7 episodes per day (p = 0.07, 2-sided, in both studies). In one study, the time to first episode of VT/VF was significantly prolonged (approximately 10 hours in patients receiving the low dose and 14 hours in patients receiving the high dose). In both studies, significantly fewer supplemental infusions were given to patients in the high-dose group. Mortality was not affected in these studies; at the end of double-blind therapy or after 48 hours, all patients were given open access to whatever treatment (including Cordarone I.V.) was deemed necessary.

INDICATIONS AND USAGE
Cordarone I.V. is indicated for initiation of treatment and prophylaxis of frequently recurring ventricular fibrillation and hemodynamically unstable ventricular tachycardia in patients refractory to other therapy. Cordarone I.V. also can be used to treat patients with VT/VF for whom oral Cordarone is indicated, but who are unable to take oral medication. During or after treatment with Cordarone I.V., patients may be transferred to oral Cordarone therapy (see **DOSAGE AND ADMINISTRATION**).

Cordarone I.V. should be used for acute treatment until the patient's ventricular arrhythmias are stabilized. Most patients will require this therapy for 48 to 96 hours, but Cordarone I.V. may be safely administered for longer periods if necessary.

CONTRAINDICATIONS
Cordarone I.V. is contraindicated in patients with known hypersensitivity to any of the components of Cordarone I.V., or in patients with cardiogenic shock, marked sinus bradycardia, and second- or third-degree AV block unless a functioning pacemaker is available.

WARNINGS
Hypotension
Hypotension is the most common adverse effect seen with Cordarone I.V. In clinical trials, treatment-emergent, drug-related hypotension was reported as an adverse effect in 288 (16%) of 1836 patients treated with Cordarone I.V. Clinically significant hypotension during infusions was seen most often in the first several hours of treatment and was not dose related, but appeared to be related to the rate of infusion. Hypotension necessitating alterations in Cordarone I.V. therapy was reported in 3% of patients, with permanent discontinuation required in less than 2% of patients.

Hypotension should be treated initially by slowing the infusion; additional standard therapy may be needed, including the following: vasopressor drugs, positive inotropic agents, and volume expansion.

The initial rate of infusion should be monitored closely and should not exceed that prescribed in **DOSAGE AND ADMINISTRATION.**

In some cases, hypotension may be refractory resulting in fatal outcome (see **ADVERSE REACTIONS, Postmarketing Reports**).

Bradycardia and AV Block
Drug-related bradycardia occurred in 90 (4.9%) of 1836 patients in clinical trials while they were receiving Cordarone I.V. for life-threatening VT/VF; it was not dose-related. Bradycardia should be treated by slowing the infusion rate or discontinuing Cordarone I.V. In some patients, inserting a pacemaker is required. Despite such measures, bradycardia was progressive and terminal in 1 patient during the controlled trials. Patients with a known predisposition to bradycardia or AV block should be treated with Cordarone I.V. in a setting where a temporary pacemaker is available.

Long-Term Use
See labeling for oral Cordarone. There has been limited experience in patients receiving Cordarone I.V. for longer than 3 weeks.

Neonatal Hypo- or Hyperthyroidism
Although Cordarone use during pregnancy is uncommon, there have been a small number of published reports of congenital goiter/hypothyroidism and hyperthyroidism associated with its oral administration. If Cordarone I.V. is administered during pregnancy, the patient should be apprised of the potential hazard to the fetus.

PRECAUTIONS
Cordarone I.V. should be administered only by physicians who are experienced in the treatment of life-threatening arrhythmias, who are thoroughly familiar with the risks and benefits of Cordarone therapy, and who have access to facilities adequate for monitoring the effectiveness and side effects of treatment.

Liver Enzyme Elevations
Elevations of blood hepatic enzyme values—alanine aminotransferase (ALT), aspartate aminotransferase (AST), and gamma-glutamyl transferase (GGT)—are seen commonly in patients with immediately life-threatening VT/VF. Interpreting elevated AST activity can be difficult because the values may be elevated in patients who have had recent myocardial infarction, congestive heart failure, or multiple electrical defibrillations. Approximately 54% of patients receiving Cordarone I.V. in clinical studies had baseline liver enzyme elevations, and 13% had clinically significant elevations. In 81% of patients with both baseline and on-therapy data available, the liver enzyme elevations either improved during therapy or remained at baseline levels. Baseline abnormalities in hepatic enzymes are not a contraindication to treatment.

Rare cases of fatal hepatocellular necrosis after treatment with Cordarone I.V. have been reported. Two patients, one 28 years of age and the other 60 years of age, were treated for atrial arrhythmias with an initial infusion of 1500 mg over 5 hours, a rate much higher than recommended. Both patients developed hepatic and renal failure within 24 hours after the start of Cordarone I.V. treatment and died on day 14 and day 4, respectively. Because these episodes of hepatic necrosis may have been due to the rapid rate of infusion with possible rate-related hypotension, *the initial rate of infusion should be monitored closely and should not exceed that prescribed in* DOSAGE AND ADMINISTRATION.

In patients with life-threatening arrhythmias, the potential risk of hepatic injury should be weighed against the potential benefit of Cordarone I.V. therapy, but patients receiving Cordarone I.V. should be monitored carefully for evidence of progressive hepatic injury. Consideration should be given to reducing the rate of administration or withdrawing Cordarone I.V. in such cases.

Proarrhythmia
Like all antiarrhythmic agents, Cordarone I.V. may cause a worsening of existing arrhythmias or precipitate a new arrhythmia. Proarrhythmia, primarily torsades de pointes, has been associated with prolongation by Cordarone I.V. of the QTc interval to 500 ms or greater. Although QTc prolongation occurred frequently in patients receiving Cordarone I.V., torsades de pointes or new-onset VF occurred infrequently (less than 2%). Patients should be monitored for QTc prolongation during infusion with Cordarone I.V. Combination of amiodarone with other antiarrhythmic therapy that prolongs the QTc should be reserved for patients with life-threatening ventricular arrhythmias who are incompletely responsive to a single agent.

The need to co-administer amiodarone with any other drug known to prolong the QTc interval must be based on a careful assessment of the potential risks and benefits of doing so for each patient.

A careful assessment of the potential risks and benefits of administering Cordarone I.V. must be made in patients with thyroid dysfunction due to the possibility of arrhythmia breakthrough or exacerbation of arrhythmia, which may result in death, in these patients.

Pulmonary Disorders
ARDS
Two percent (2%) of patients were reported to have adult respiratory distress syndrome (ARDS) during clinical studies. ARDS is a disorder characterized by bilateral, diffuse pulmonary infiltrates with pulmonary edema and varying degrees of respiratory insufficiency. The clinical and radiographic picture can arise after a variety of lung injuries, such as those resulting from trauma, shock, prolonged cardiopulmonary resuscitation, and aspiration pneumonia, conditions present in many of the patients enrolled in the clinical studies. It is not possible to determine what role, if any, Cordarone I.V. played in causing or exacerbating the pulmonary disorder in those patients.

Postoperatively, occurrences of ARDS have been reported in patients receiving *oral* Cordarone therapy who have undergone either cardiac or noncardiac surgery. Although patients usually respond well to vigorous respiratory therapy, in rare instances the outcome has been fatal. Until further studies have been performed, it is recommended that FiO_2 and the determinants of oxygen delivery to the tissues (e.g., SaO_2, PaO_2) be closely monitored in patients on Cordarone.

Pulmonary fibrosis
Only 1 of more than 1000 patients treated with Cordarone I.V. in clinical studies developed pulmonary fibrosis. In that patient, the condition was diagnosed 3 months after treatment with Cordarone I.V., during which time she received *oral* Cordarone. Pulmonary toxicity is a well-recognized complication of long-term Cordarone use (see labeling for oral Cordarone).

Surgery
Close perioperative monitoring is recommended in patients undergoing general anesthesia who are on amiodarone therapy as they may be more sensitive to the myocardial depressant and conduction defects of halogenated inhalational anesthetics.

Drug Interactions
Amiodarone is metabolized to desethylamiodarone by the cytochrome P450 (CYP450) enzyme group, specifically cytochrome P450 3A4 (CYP3A4). This isoenzyme is present in both the liver and intestines (see **CLINICAL PHARMACOLOGY, Pharmacokinetics and Metabolism**). Amiodarone is also known to be an inhibitor of CYP3A4. Therefore, amiodarone has the **potential** for interactions with drugs or substances that may be substrates, inhibitors or inducers of CYP3A4. While only a limited number of *in vivo* drug-drug interactions with amiodarone have been reported, chiefly with the oral formulation, the potential for other interactions should be anticipated. This is especially important for drugs associated with serious toxicity, such as other antiarrhythmics. If such drugs are needed, their dose should be reassessed and, where appropriate, plasma concentration measured. In view of the long and variable half-life of amiodarone, potential for drug interactions exists not only with concomitant medication but also with drugs administered after discontinuation of amiodarone.

Since amiodarone is a substrate for CYP3A4, drugs/substances that inhibit CYP3A4 may decrease the metabolism and increase serum concentrations of amiodarone, with the potential for toxic effects. Reported examples of this interaction include the following:
Protease Inhibitors:
Protease inhibitors are known to inhibit CYP3A4 to varying degrees. Inhibition of CYP3A4 by **indinavir** has been reported to result in increased serum concentrations of amiodarone. Monitoring for amiodarone toxicity and serial measurement of amiodarone serum concentration during concomitant protease inhibitor therapy should be considered.
Histamine H_2 antagonists:
Cimetidine inhibits CYP3A4 and can increase serum amiodarone levels.
Other substances:
Grapefruit juice inhibits CYP3A4-mediated metabolism of oral amiodarone in the intestinal mucosa, resulting in increased plasma levels of amiodarone; therefore, grapefruit juice should not be taken during treatment with oral amiodarone. This information should be considered when changing from intravenous amiodarone to oral amiodarone (see **DOSAGE AND ADMINISTRATION, Intravenous to Oral Transition**).

Amiodarone may suppress certain CYP450 enzymes (enzyme inhibition). This can result in unexpectedly high plasma levels of other drugs which are metabolized by those CYP450 enzymes and may lead to toxic effects. Reported examples of this interaction include the following:
Immunosuppressives:
Cyclosporine (CYP3A4 substrate) administered in combination with oral amiodarone has been reported to produce persistently elevated plasma concentrations of cyclosporine resulting in elevated creatinine, despite reduction in dose of cyclosporine.
HMG-CoA Reductase Inhibitors:
Simvastatin (CYP3A4 substrate) in combination with amiodarone has been associated with reports of myopathy/rhabdomyolysis.
Cardiovasculars:
Cardiac glycosides: In patients receiving **digoxin** therapy, administration of oral amiodarone regularly results in an increase in serum digoxin concentration that may reach toxic levels with resultant clinical toxicity. Amiodarone taken concomitantly with digoxin increases the serum digoxin concentration by 70% after one day. **On administration of oral amiodarone, the need for digitalis therapy should be reviewed and the dose reduced by approximately 50% or discontinued.** If digitalis treatment is continued, serum levels should be closely monitored and patients observed for clinical evidence of toxicity. These precautions probably should apply to digitoxin administration as well.

Antiarrhythmics: Other antiarrhythmic drugs, such as **quinidine, procainamide, disopyramide**, and **phenytoin**, have been used concurrently with amiodarone. There have been case reports of increased steady-state levels of quinidine, procainamide, and phenytoin during concomitant therapy with amiodarone. Phenytoin decreases serum amiodarone levels. Amiodarone taken concomitantly with quinidine increases quinidine serum concentration by 33% after two days. Amiodarone taken concomitantly with procainamide for less than seven days increases plasma concentrations of procainamide and n-acetyl procainamide by 55% and 33%, respectively. Quinidine and procainamide doses should be reduced by one-third when either is administered with amiodarone. Plasma levels of **flecainide** have been reported to increase in the presence of oral amiodarone; because of this, the dosage of flecainide should be adjusted when these drugs are administered concomitantly. In general, any added antiarrhythmic drug should be initiated at a lower than usual dose with careful monitoring. Combination of amiodarone with other antiarrhythmic therapy should be reserved for patients with life-threatening ventricular arrhythmias who are incompletely responsive to a single agent or incompletely responsive to amiodarone. During transfer to oral amiodarone, the dose levels of previously administered agents should be reduced by 30 to 50% several days after the addition of oral amiodarone (see **DOSAGE AND ADMINISTRATION, Intravenous to Oral Transition**). The continued need for the other antiarrhythmic agent should be reviewed after the effects of amiodarone have been established, and discontinuation ordinarily should be attempted. If the treatment is continued, these patients should be particularly carefully monitored for adverse effects, especially conduction disturbances and exacerbation of tachyarrhythmias, as amiodarone is continued. In amiodarone-treated patients who require additional antiarrhythmic therapy, the initial dose of such agents should be approximately half of the usual recommended dose.

Antihypertensives: Amiodarone should be used with caution in patients receiving β-receptor blocking agents (e.g., propanolol, a CYP3A4 inhibitor) or **calcium channel antagonists** (e.g., verapamil, a CYP3A4 substrate, and diltiazem, a CYP3A4 inhibitor) because of the possible potentiation of bradycardia, sinus arrest, and AV block; if necessary, amiodarone can continue to be used after insertion of a pacemaker in patients with severe bradycardia or sinus arrest.

Anticoagulants: Potentiation of **warfarin**-type (CYP2C9 and CYP3A4 substrate) anticoagulant response is almost always seen in patients receiving amiodarone and can result in serious or fatal bleeding. Since the concomitant administration of warfarin with amiodarone increases the prothrombin time by 100% after 3 to 4 days, **the dose of the anticoagulant should be reduced by one-third to one-half, and prothrombin times should be monitored closely.**

Some drugs/substances are known to accelerate the metabolism of amiodarone by stimulating the synthesis of CYP3A4 (enzyme induction). This may lead to low amiodarone serum levels and potential decrease in efficacy. Reported examples of this interaction include the following:
Antibiotics:
Rifampin is a potent inducer of CYP3A4. Administration of rifampin concomitantly with oral amiodarone has been shown to result in decreases in serum concentrations of amiodarone and desethylamiodarone.

Other substances, including herbal preparations:
St. John's Wort (Hypericum perforatum) induces CYP3A4. Since amiodarone is a substrate for CYP3A4, there is the potential that the use of St. John's Wort in patients receiving amiodarone could result in reduced amiodarone levels.
Other reported interactions with amiodarone:
Fentanyl (CYP3A4 substrate) in combination with amiodarone may cause hypotension, bradycardia, decreased cardiac output.
Sinus bradycardia has been reported with oral amiodarone in combination with **lidocaine** (CYP3A4 substrate) given for local anesthesia. Seizure, associated with increased lidocaine concentrations, has been reported with concomitant administration of intravenous amiodarone.
Dextromethorphan is a substrate for both CYP2D6 and CYP3A4. Amiodarone inhibits CYP2D6.
Cholestyramine increases enterohepatic elimination of amiodarone and may reduce serum levels and $t_{1/2}$.
Disopyramide increases QT prolongation which could cause arrhythmia.
Hemodynamic and electrophysiologic interactions have also been observed after concomitant administration with **propranolol, diltiazem**, and **verapamil**.
Volatile Anesthetic Agents: (see **PRECAUTIONS, Surgery**).
In addition to the interactions noted above, chronic (> 2 weeks) ***oral*** Cordarone administration impairs metabolism of phenytoin, dextromethorphan, and methotrexate.

Electrolyte Disturbances
Patients with hypokalemia or hypomagnesemia should have the condition corrected whenever possible before being treated with Cordarone I.V., as these disorders can exaggerate the degree of QTc prolongation and increase the potential for torsades de pointes. Special attention should be given to electrolyte and acid-base balance in patients experiencing severe or prolonged diarrhea or in patients receiving concomitant diuretics.

Carcinogenesis, Mutagenesis, Impairment of Fertility
No carcinogenicity studies were conducted with Cordarone I.V. However, **oral** Cordarone caused a statistically significant, dose-related increase in the incidence of thyroid tumors (follicular adenoma and/or carcinoma) in rats. The incidence of thyroid tumors in rats was greater than the incidence in controls even at the lowest dose level tested, i.e., 5 mg/kg/day (approximately 0.08 times the maximum recommended human maintenance dose*).
Mutagenicity studies conducted with amiodarone HCl (Ames, micronucleus, and lysogenic induction tests) were negative.
No fertility studies were conducted with Cordarone I.V. However, in a study in which amiodarone HCl was orally administered to male and female rats, beginning 9 weeks prior to mating, reduced fertility was observed at a dose level of 90 mg/kg/day (approximately 1.4 times the maximum recommended human maintenance dose*).

*600 mg in a 50 kg patient (dose compared on a body surface area basis)

Pregnancy
Category D. See **WARNINGS, Neonatal Hypo- or Hyperthyroidism**. In addition to causing infrequent congenital goiter/hypothyroidism and hyperthyroidism, amiodarone has caused a variety of adverse effects in animals.
In a reproductive study in which amiodarone was given intravenously to rabbits at dosages of 5, 10, or 25 mg/kg per day (about 0.1, 0.3, and 0.7 times the maximum recommended human dose [MRHD] on a body surface area basis), maternal deaths occurred in all groups, including controls. Embryotoxicity (as manifested by fewer full-term fetuses and increased resorptions with concomitantly lower litter weights) occurred at dosages of 10 mg/kg and above. No evidence of embryotoxicity was observed at 5 mg/kg and no teratogenicity was observed at any dosages.
In a teratology study in which amiodarone was administered by continuous i.v. infusion to rats at dosages of 25, 50, or 100 mg/kg per day (about 0.4, 0.7, and 1.4 times the MRHD when compared on a body surface area basis), maternal toxicity (as evidenced by reduced weight gain and food consumption) and embryotoxicity (as evidenced by increased resorptions, decreased live litter size, reduced body weights, and retarded sternum and metacarpal ossification) were observed in the 100 mg/kg group.
Cordarone® I.V. (amiodarone HCl) should be used during pregnancy only if the potential benefit to the mother justifies the risk to the fetus.

Nursing Mothers
Amiodarone is excreted in human milk, suggesting that breast-feeding could expose the nursing infant to a significant dose of the drug. Nursing offspring of lactating rats administered amiodarone have demonstrated reduced viability and reduced body weight gains. The risk of exposing the infant to amiodarone should be weighed against the potential benefit of arrhythmia suppression in the mother. The mother should be advised to discontinue nursing.

Labor and Delivery
It is not known whether the use of Cordarone during labor or delivery has any immediate or delayed adverse effects. Preclinical studies in rodents have not shown any effect on the duration of gestation or on parturition.

Pediatric Use
The safety and efficacy of Cordarone in the pediatric population have not been established; therefore, its use in pediatric patients is not recommended.
Cordarone I.V. contains the preservative benzyl alcohol (see **DESCRIPTION**). There have been reports of fatal "gasping syndrome" in neonates (children less than one month of age) following the administration of intravenous solutions containing the preservative benzyl alcohol. Symptoms include a striking onset of gasping respiration, hypotension, bradycardia, and cardiovascular collapse.

SUMMARY TABULATION OF TREATMENT-EMERGENT DRUG-RELATED STUDY EVENTS IN PATIENTS RECEIVING CORDARONE I.V. IN CONTROLLED AND OPEN-LABEL STUDIES (≥2% INCIDENCE)

Study Event	Controlled Studies (n=814)	Open-Label Studies (n=1022)	Total (n=1836)
Body as a Whole			
Fever	24 (2.9%)	13 (1.2%)	37 (2.0%)
Cardiovascular System			
Bradycardia	49 (6.0%)	41 (4.0%)	90 (4.9%)
Congestive heart failure	18 (2.2%)	21 (2.0%)	39 (2.1%)
Heart arrest	29 (3.5%)	26 (2.5%)	55 (2.9%)
Hypotension	165 (20.2%)	123 (12.0%)	288 (15.6%)
Ventricular tachycardia	15 (1.8%)	30 (2.9%)	45 (2.4%)
Digestive System			
Liver function tests abnormal	35 (4.2%)	29 (2.8%)	64 (3.4%)
Nausea	29 (3.5%)	43 (4.2%)	72 (3.9%)

AMIODARONE HCl SOLUTION STABILITY

Solution	Concentration (mg/mL)	Container	Comments
5% Dextrose in Water (D_5W)	1.0 - 6.0	PVC	Physically compatible, with amiodarone loss <10% at 2 hours.
5% Dextrose in Water (D_5W)	1.0 - 6.0	Polyolefin, Glass	Physically compatible, with no amiodarone loss at 24 hours.

Y-SITE INJECTION INCOMPATIBILITY

Drug	Vehicle	Amiodarone Concentration	Comments
Aminophylline	D_5W	4 mg/mL	Precipitate
Cefamandole Nafate	D_5W	4 mg/mL	Precipitate
Cefazolin Sodium	D_5W	4 mg/mL	Precipitate
Mezlocillin Sodium	D_5W	4 mg/mL	Precipitate
Heparin Sodium	D_5W	—	Precipitate
Sodium Bicarbonate	D_5W	3 mg/mL	Precipitate

Geriatric Use
Clinical studies of Cordarone I.V. did not include sufficient numbers of subjects aged 65 and over to determine whether they respond differently from younger subjects. Other reported clinical experience has not identified differences in responses between the elderly and younger patients. In general, dose selection for an elderly patient should be cautious, usually starting at the low end of the dosing range, reflecting the greater frequency of decreased hepatic, renal, or cardiac function, and of concomitant disease or other drug therapy.

ADVERSE REACTIONS
In a total of 1836 patients in controlled and uncontrolled clinical trials, 14% of patients received Cordarone I.V. for at least 1 week, 5% received it for at least 2 weeks, 2% received it for at least 3 weeks, and 1% received it for more than 3 weeks, without an increased incidence of severe adverse reactions. The mean duration of therapy in these studies was 5.6 days; median exposure was 3.7 days.
The most important treatment-emergent adverse effects were hypotension, asystole/cardiac arrest/electromechanical dissociation (EMD), cardiogenic shock, congestive heart failure, bradycardia, liver function test abnormalities, VT, and AV block. Overall, treatment was discontinued for about 9% of the patients because of adverse effects. The most common adverse effects leading to discontinuation of Cordarone I.V. therapy were hypotension (1.6%), asystole/cardiac arrest/EMD (1.2%), VT (1.1%), and cardiogenic shock (1%).
The following table lists the most common (incidence ≥ 2%) treatment-emergent adverse events during Cordarone I.V. therapy considered at least possibly drug-related. These data were collected from the Wyeth-Ayerst clinical trials involving 1836 patients with life-threatening VT/VF. Data from all assigned treatment groups are pooled because none of the adverse events appeared to be dose-related.
[See first table above]
Other treatment-emergent possibly drug-related adverse events reported in less than 2% of patients receiving Cordarone I.V. in Wyeth-Ayerst controlled and uncontrolled studies included the following: abnormal kidney function, atrial fibrillation, diarrhea, increased ALT, increased AST, lung edema, nodal arrhythmia, prolonged QT interval, respiratory disorder, shock, sinus bradycardia, Stevens-Johnson syndrome, thrombocytopenia, VF, and vomiting.

Postmarketing Reports
In postmarketing surveillance, hypotension (sometimes fatal), sinus arrest, pseudotumor cerebri, toxic epidermal necrolysis, exfoliative dermatitis, pancytopenia, neutropenia, erythema multiforme, angioedema, bronchospasm, and anaphylactic shock also have been reported with amiodarone therapy.
Also, in patients receiving recommended dosages, there have been postmarketing reports of the following injection site reactions: pain, erythema, edema, pigment changes, venous thrombosis, phlebitis, thrombophlebitis, cellulitis, necrosis, and skin sloughing (see **DOSAGE AND ADMINISTRATION**).

OVERDOSAGE
There have been cases, some fatal, of amiodarone overdose. Effects of an inadvertent overdose of Cordarone I.V. include hypotension, cardiogenic shock, bradycardia, AV block, and hepatotoxicity. Hypotension and cardiogenic shock should be treated by slowing the infusion rate or with standard therapy: vasopressor drugs, positive inotropic agents, and volume expansion. Bradycardia and AV block may require temporary pacing. Hepatic enzyme concentrations should be monitored closely. Amiodarone is not dialyzable.

DOSAGE AND ADMINISTRATION
Amiodarone shows considerable interindividual variation in response. Thus, although a starting dose adequate to suppress life-threatening arrhythmias is needed, close monitoring with adjustment of dose as needed is essential. The recommended starting dose of Cordarone I.V. is about 1000 mg over the first 24 hours of therapy, delivered by the following infusion regimen:

CORDARONE I.V. DOSE RECOMMENDATIONS — FIRST 24 HOURS —

Loading infusions	
***First* Rapid:**	**150 mg over the FIRST 10 minutes (15 mg/min).** Add 3 mL of Cordarone I.V. (150 mg) to 100 mL D_5W (concentration = 1.5 mg/mL). Infuse 100 mL over 10 minutes.
***Followed by* Slow:**	**360 mg over the NEXT 6 hours (1 mg/min).** Add 18 mL of Cordarone I.V. (900 mg) to 500 mL D_5W (concentration = 1.8 mg/mL).
Maintenance infusion	**540 mg over the REMAINING 18 hours (0.5 mg/min).** Decrease the rate of the slow loading infusion to 0.5 mg/min.

After the first 24 hours, the maintenance infusion rate of 0.5 mg/min (720 mg/24 hours) should be continued utilizing a concentration of 1 to 6 mg/mL (Cordarone I.V. concentrations greater than 2 mg/mL should be administered via a central venous catheter). In the event of breakthrough episodes of VF or hemodynamically unstable VT, 150-mg supplemental infusions of Cordarone I.V. mixed in 100 mL of D_5W may be administered. Such infusions should be administered over 10 minutes to minimize the potential for hypotension. The rate of the maintenance infusion may be increased to achieve effective arrhythmia suppression.
The first 24-hour dose may be individualized for each patient; however, in controlled clinical trials, mean daily doses above 2100 mg were associated with an increased risk of hypotension. The initial infusion rate should not exceed 30 mg/min.
Based on the experience from clinical studies of Cordarone I.V., a maintenance infusion of up to 0.5 mg/min can be cautiously continued for 2 to 3 weeks regardless of the patient's

Continued on next page

Cordarone IV—Cont.

age, renal function, or left ventricular function. There has been limited experience in patients receiving Cordarone I.V. for longer than 3 weeks.

The surface properties of solutions containing injectable amiodarone are altered such that the drop size may be reduced. This reduction may lead to underdosage of the patient by up to 30% if drop counter infusion sets are used. Cordarone I.V. must be delivered by a volumetric infusion pump.

Cordarone I.V. should, whenever possible, be administered through a central venous catheter dedicated to that purpose. An in-line filter should be used during administration. Cordarone I.V. concentrations greater than 3 mg/mL in D_5W have been associated with a high incidence of peripheral vein phlebitis; however, concentrations of 2.5 mg/mL or less appear to be less irritating. Therefore, for infusions longer than 1 hour, Cordarone I.V. concentrations should not exceed 2 mg/mL unless a central venous catheter is used (see **ADVERSE REACTIONS, Postmarketing Reports**).

Cordarone I.V. infusions exceeding 2 hours must be administered in glass or polyolefin bottles containing D_5W. Use of **evacuated glass containers** for admixing Cordarone I.V. is not recommended as incompatibility with a buffer in the container may cause precipitation.

It is well known that amiodarone adsorbs to polyvinyl chloride (PVC) tubing and the clinical trial dose administration schedule was designed to account for this adsorption. All of the clinical trials were conducted using PVC tubing and its use is therefore recommended. The concentrations and rates of infusion provided in **DOSAGE AND ADMINISTRATION** reflect doses identified in these studies. It is important that the recommended infusion regimen be followed closely.

Cordarone I.V. has been found to leach out plasticizers, including DEHP [di-(2-ethylhexyl)phthalate] from intravenous tubing (including PVC tubing). The degree of leaching increases when infusing Cordarone I.V. at higher concentrations and lower flow rates than provided in **DOSAGE AND ADMINISTRATION**.

Cordarone I.V. does not need to be protected from light during administration.

[See second table at top of previous page]

Admixture Incompatibility

Cordarone I.V. in D_5W is incompatible with the drugs shown below.

[See third table at top of previous page]

Intravenous to Oral Transition

Patients whose arrhythmias have been suppressed by Cordarone I.V. may be switched to oral Cordarone. The optimal dose for changing from intravenous to oral administration of Cordarone will depend on the dose of Cordarone I.V. already administered, as well as the bioavailability of oral Cordarone. When changing to oral Cordarone therapy, clinical monitoring is recommended, particularly for elderly patients.

Since there are some differences between the safety and efficacy profiles of the intravenous and oral formulations, the prescriber is advised to review the package insert for oral amiodarone when switching from intravenous to oral amiodarone therapy.

Since grapefruit juice is known to inhibit CYP3A4-mediated metabolism of oral amiodarone in the intestinal mucosa, resulting in increased plasma levels of amiodarone; grapefruit juice should not be taken during treatment with oral amiodarone (see **PRECAUTIONS, Drug Interactions**).

The following table provides suggested doses of oral Cordarone to be initiated after varying durations of Cordarone I.V. administration. These recommendations are made on the basis of a comparable total body amount of amiodarone delivered by the intravenous and oral routes, based on 50% bioavailability of oral amiodarone.

RECOMMENDATIONS FOR ORAL DOSAGE AFTER I.V. INFUSION

Duration of Cordarone I.V. Infusion#	Initial Daily Dose of Oral Cordarone
<1 week	800-1600 mg
1-3 weeks	600-800 mg
>3 weeks*	400 mg

Assuming a 720 mg/day infusion (0.5 mg/min).
* Cordarone I.V is not intended for maintenance treatment.

HOW SUPPLIED

Cordarone® I.V. (amiodarone HCl) is available in packages of 10 ampuls (2 cartons each containing 5 ampuls), 3 mL each, as follows:
50 mg per mL, NDC 0008-0814-01.
Store at room temperature, 15° to 25°C (59° to 77°F).
Protect from light and excessive heat.
Use carton to protect contents from light until used.

Wyeth Laboratories
A Wyeth-Ayerst Company
Philadelphia, PA 19101
by arrangement with Sanofi S.A.
CI 5032-7 Revised October 2, 2002

EFFEXOR® ℞

[ĕf-fĕks'ŏr]
(venlafaxine hydrochloride)
Tablets
℞ only

Prescribing information for this product, which appears on pages 3392–3396 of the 2003 PDR, has been revised as follows. Please write "See Supplement A" next to the product heading.

In the **CLINICAL TRIALS** *section, the first sentence of the fourth paragraph has been revised as follows:*

In a second longer-term trial, outpatients meeting DSM-III-R criteria for major depressive disorder, recurrent type, who had responded (HAM-D-21 total score ≤12 at the day 56 evaluation) and continued to be improved [defined as the following criteria being met for days 56 through 180: (1) no HAM-D-21 total score ≥20; (2) no more than 2 HAM-D-21 total scores >10; and (3) no single CGI Severity of Illness item score ≥4 (moderately ill)] during an initial 26 weeks of treatment on Effexor (100 to 200 mg/day, on a b.i.d. schedule) were randomized to continuation of their same Effexor dose or to placebo.

In the **PRECAUTIONS** *section, the "Abnormal Bleeding" section has been revised as follows:*

Abnormal Bleeding

There have been reports of abnormal bleeding (most commonly ecchymosis) associated with venlafaxine treatment. While a causal relationship to venlafaxine is unclear, impaired platelet aggregation may result from platelet serotonin depletion and contribute to such occurrences.

In the **PRECAUTIONS** *section, the following has been added after the "Abnormal Bleeding" section:*

Serum Cholesterol Elevation

Clinically relevant increases in serum cholesterol were recorded in 5.3% of venlafaxine-treated patients and 0.0% of placebo-treated patients treated for at least 3 months in placebo-controlled trials (see **ADVERSE REACTIONS–Laboratory Changes**). Measurement of serum cholesterol levels should be considered during long-term treatment.

In the **ADVERSE REACTIONS** *section, the "Laboratory Changes" subsection has been revised as follows:*

Laboratory Changes

Of the serum chemistry and hematology parameters monitored during clinical trials with Effexor, a statistically significant difference with placebo was seen only for serum cholesterol. In premarketing trials, treatment with Effexor tablets was associated with a mean final on-therapy increase in total cholesterol of 3 mg/dL.

Patients treated with Effexor tablets for at least 3 months in placebo-controlled 12-month extension trials had a mean final on-therapy increase in total cholesterol of 9.1 mg/dL compared with a decrease of 7.1 mg/dL among placebo-treated patients. This increase was duration dependent over the study period and tended to be greater with higher doses. Clinically relevant increases in serum cholesterol, defined as 1) a final on-therapy increase in serum cholesterol ≥50 mg/dL from baseline and to a value ≥261 mg/dL or 2) an average on-therapy increase in serum cholesterol ≥50 mg/dL from baseline and to a value ≥261 mg/dL, were recorded in 5.3% of venlafaxine-treated patients and 0.0% of placebo-treated patients (see **PRECAUTIONS-General-***Serum Cholesterol Elevation*).

In the **DOSAGE AND ADMINISTRATION** *section, the* **Maintenance/Continuation/Extended Treatment** *section has been revised as follows:*

Maintenance Treatment

It is generally agreed that acute episodes of depression require several months or longer of sustained pharmacological therapy beyond response to the acute episode. In one study, in which patients responding during 8 weeks of acute treatment with Effexor XR were assigned randomly to placebo or to the same dose of Effexor XR (75, 150, or 225 mg/day, qAM) during 26 weeks of maintenance treatment as they had received during the acute stabilization phase, longer-term efficacy was demonstrated. A second longer-term study has demonstrated the efficacy of Effexor in maintaining an antidepressant response in patients with recurrent depression who had responded and continued to be improved during an initial 26 weeks of treatment and were then randomly assigned to placebo or Effexor for periods of up to 52 weeks on the same dose (100 to 200 mg/day, on a b.i.d. schedule) (see **CLINICAL TRIALS**). Based on these limited data, it is not known whether or not the dose of Effexor/Effexor XR needed for maintenance treatment is identical to the dose needed to achieve an initial response. Patients should be periodically reassessed to determine the need for maintenance treatment and the appropriate dose for such treatment.

Wyeth Laboratories W10402C002
A Wyeth-Ayerst Company CI 6027-9
Philadelphia, PA 19101 Rev 09/02

EFFEXOR® XR ℞

[ĕf-feks' ŏr xr]
(venlafaxine hydrochloride)
Extended-Release Capsules
℞ only

Prescribing information for this product, which appears on pages 3397–3402 of the 2003 PDR, has been completely revised as follows. Please write "See Supplement A" next to the product heading.

DESCRIPTION

Effexor XR is an extended-release capsule for oral administration that contains venlafaxine hydrochloride, a structurally novel antidepressant. It is designated (R/S)-1-[2-(dimethylamino)-1-(4-methoxyphenyl)ethyl] cyclohexanol hydrochloride or (±)-1-[α-[(dimethylamino)methyl]-p-methoxybenzyl] cyclohexanol hydrochloride and has the empirical formula of $C_{17}H_{27}NO_2$ hydrochloride. Its molecular weight is 313.87. The structural formula is shown below.

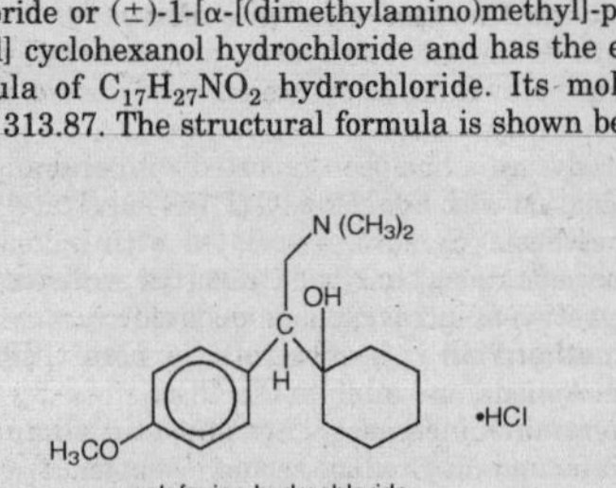

venlafaxine hydrochloride

Venlafaxine hydrochloride is a white to off-white crystalline solid with a solubility of 572 mg/mL in water (adjusted to ionic strength of 0.2 M with sodium chloride). Its octanol: water (0.2 M sodium chloride) partition coefficient is 0.43.

Effexor XR is formulated as an extended-release capsule for once-a-day oral administration. Drug release is controlled by diffusion through the coating membrane on the spheroids and is not pH dependent. Capsules contain venlafaxine hydrochloride equivalent to 37.5 mg, 75 mg, or 150 mg venlafaxine. Inactive ingredients consist of cellulose, ethylcellulose, gelatin, hypromellose, iron oxide, and titanium dioxide. The 37.5 mg capsule also contains D&C Red #28, D&C Yellow #10, and FD&C Blue #1.

CLINICAL PHARMACOLOGY

Pharmacodynamics

The mechanism of the antidepressant action of venlafaxine in humans is believed to be associated with its potentiation of neurotransmitter activity in the CNS. Preclinical studies have shown that venlafaxine and its active metabolite, O-desmethylvenlafaxine (ODV), are potent inhibitors of neuronal serotonin and norepinephrine reuptake and weak inhibitors of dopamine reuptake. Venlafaxine and ODV have no significant affinity for muscarinic cholinergic, H_1-histaminergic, or α_1-adrenergic receptors in vitro. Pharmacologic activity at these receptors is hypothesized to be associated with the various anticholinergic, sedative, and cardiovascular effects seen with other psychotropic drugs. Venlafaxine and ODV do not possess monoamine oxidase (MAO) inhibitory activity.

Pharmacokinetics

Steady-state concentrations of venlafaxine and ODV in plasma are attained within 3 days of oral multiple dose therapy. Venlafaxine and ODV exhibited linear kinetics over the dose range of 75 to 450 mg/day. Mean±SD steady-state plasma clearance of venlafaxine and ODV is 1.3±0.6 and 0.4±0.2 L/h/kg, respectively; apparent elimination half-life is 5±2 and 11±2 hours, respectively; and apparent (steady-state) volume of distribution is 7.5±3.7 and 5.7±1.8 L/kg, respectively. Venlafaxine and ODV are minimally bound at therapeutic concentrations to plasma proteins (27% and 30%, respectively).

Absorption

Venlafaxine is well absorbed and extensively metabolized in the liver. O-desmethylvenlafaxine (ODV) is the only major active metabolite. On the basis of mass balance studies, at least 92% of a single oral dose of venlafaxine is absorbed. The absolute bioavailability of venlafaxine is about 45%.

Administration of Effexor XR (150 mg q24 hours) generally resulted in lower C_{max} (150 ng/mL for venlafaxine and 260 ng/mL for ODV) and later T_{max} (5.5 hours for venlafaxine and 9 hours for ODV) than for immediate release venlafaxine tablets (C_{max}'s for immediate release 75 mg q12 hours were 225 ng/mL for venlafaxine and 290 ng/mL for ODV; T_{max}'s were 2 hours for venlafaxine and 3 hours for ODV). When equal daily doses of venlafaxine were administered as either an immediate release tablet or the extended-release capsule, the exposure to both venlafaxine and ODV was similar for the two treatments, and the fluctuation in plasma concentrations was slightly lower with the Effexor XR capsule. Effexor XR, therefore, provides a slower rate of absorption, but the same extent of absorption compared with the immediate release tablet.

Food did not affect the bioavailability of venlafaxine or its active metabolite, ODV. Time of administration (AM vs PM) did not affect the pharmacokinetics of venlafaxine and ODV from the 75 mg Effexor XR capsule.

Metabolism and Excretion

Following absorption, venlafaxine undergoes extensive presystemic metabolism in the liver, primarily to ODV, but also to N-desmethylvenlafaxine, N,O-didesmethylvenlafaxine, and other minor metabolites. In vitro studies indicate that the formation of ODV is catalyzed by CYP2D6; this has been confirmed in a clinical study showing that patients with low CYP2D6 levels ("poor metabolizers") had increased levels of venlafaxine and reduced levels of ODV compared to people with normal CYP2D6 ("extensive metabolizers"). The differences between the CYP2D6 poor and extensive metabolizers, however, are not expected to be clinically important because the sum of venlafaxine and ODV is similar in the two groups and venlafaxine and ODV are pharmacologically approximately equiactive and equipotent.

Approximately 87% of a venlafaxine dose is recovered in the urine within 48 hours as unchanged venlafaxine (5%), unconjugated ODV (29%), conjugated ODV (26%), or other minor inactive metabolites (27%). Renal elimination of venlafaxine and its metabolites is thus the primary route of excretion.

Special Populations

Age and Gender: A population pharmacokinetic analysis of 404 venlafaxine-treated patients from two studies involving both b.i.d. and t.i.d. regimens showed that dose-normalized trough plasma levels of either venlafaxine or ODV were unaltered by age or gender differences. Dosage adjustment based on the age or gender of a patient is generally not necessary (see DOSAGE AND ADMINISTRATION).

Extensive/Poor Metabolizers: Plasma concentrations of venlafaxine were higher in CYP2D6 poor metabolizers than extensive metabolizers. Because the total exposure (AUC) of venlafaxine and ODV was similar in poor and extensive metabolizer groups, however, there is no need for different venlafaxine dosing regimens for these two groups.

Liver Disease: In 9 patients with hepatic cirrhosis, the pharmacokinetic disposition of both venlafaxine and ODV was significantly altered after oral administration of venlafaxine. Venlafaxine elimination half-life was prolonged by about 30%, and clearance decreased by about 50% in cirrhotic patients compared to normal subjects. ODV elimination half-life was prolonged by about 60%, and clearance decreased by about 30% in cirrhotic patients compared to normal subjects. A large degree of intersubject variability was noted. Three patients with more severe cirrhosis had a more substantial decrease in venlafaxine clearance (about 90%) compared to normal subjects. Dosage adjustment is necessary in these patients (see DOSAGE AND ADMINISTRATION).

Renal Disease: In a renal impairment study, venlafaxine elimination half-life after oral administration was prolonged by about 50% and clearance was reduced by about 24% in renally impaired patients (GFR=10 to 70 mL/min), compared to normal subjects. In dialysis patients, venlafaxine elimination half-life was prolonged by about 180% and clearance was reduced by about 57% compared to normal subjects. Similarly, ODV elimination half-life was prolonged by about 40% although clearance was unchanged in patients with renal impairment (GFR=10 to 70 mL/min) compared to normal subjects. In dialysis patients, ODV elimination half-life was prolonged by about 142% and clearance was reduced by about 56% compared to normal subjects. A large degree of intersubject variability was noted. Dosage adjustment is necessary in these patients (see DOSAGE AND ADMINISTRATION).

Clinical Trials

Major Depressive Disorder

The efficacy of Effexor XR (venlafaxine hydrochloride) extended-release capsules as a treatment for major depressive disorder was established in two placebo-controlled, short-term, flexible-dose studies in adult outpatients meeting DSM-III-R or DSM-IV criteria for major depressive disorder.

A 12-week study utilizing Effexor XR doses in a range 75 to 150 mg/day (mean dose for completers was 136 mg/day) and an 8-week study utilizing Effexor XR doses in a range 75 to 225 mg/day (mean dose for completers was 177 mg/day) both demonstrated superiority of Effexor XR over placebo on the HAM-D total score, HAM-D Depressed Mood Item, the MADRS total score, the Clinical Global Impressions (CGI) Severity of Illness item, and the CGI Global Improvement item. In both studies, Effexor XR was also significantly better than placebo for certain factors of the HAM-D, including the anxiety/somatization factor, the cognitive disturbance factor, and the retardation factor, as well as for the psychic anxiety score.

A 4-week study of inpatients meeting DSM-III-R criteria for major depressive disorder with melancholia utilizing Effexor (the immediate release form of venlafaxine) in a range of 150 to 375 mg/day (t.i.d. schedule) demonstrated superiority of Effexor over placebo. The mean dose in completers was 350 mg/day.

Examination of gender subsets of the population studied did not reveal any differential responsiveness on the basis of gender.

In one longer-term study, outpatients meeting DSM-IV criteria for major depressive disorder who had responded during an 8-week open trial on Effexor XR (75, 150, or 225 mg, qAM) were randomized to continuation of their same Effexor XR dose or to placebo, for up to 26 weeks of observation for relapse. Response during the open phase was defined as a CGI Severity of Illness item score of ≤3 and a HAM-D-21 total score of ≤10 at the day 56 evaluation. Relapse during the double-blind phase was defined as follows: (1) a reappearance of major depressive disorder as defined by DSM-IV criteria and a CGI Severity of Illness item score of ≥4 (moderately ill), (2) 2 consecutive CGI Severity of Illness item scores of ≥4, or (3) a final CGI Severity of Illness item score of ≥4 for any patient who withdrew from the study for any reason. Patients receiving continued Effexor XR treatment experienced significantly lower relapse rates over the subsequent 26 weeks compared with those receiving placebo.

In a second longer-term trial, outpatients meeting DSM-III-R criteria for major depressive disorder, recurrent type, who had responded (HAM-D-21 total score ≤12 at the day 56 evaluation) and continued to be improved [defined as the following criteria being met for days 56 through 180: (1) no HAM-D-21 total score ≥20; (2) no more than 2 HAM-D-21 total scores >10, and (3) no single CGI Severity of Illness item score ≥4 (moderately ill)] during an initial 26 weeks of treatment on Effexor (100 to 200 mg/day, on a b.i.d. schedule) were randomized to continuation of their same Effexor dose or to placebo. The follow-up period to observe patients for relapse, defined as a CGI Severity of Illness item score ≥4, was for up to 52 weeks. Patients receiving continued Effexor treatment experienced significantly lower relapse rates over the subsequent 52 weeks compared with those receiving placebo.

Generalized Anxiety Disorder

The efficacy of Effexor XR capsules as a treatment for Generalized Anxiety Disorder (GAD) was established in two 8-week, placebo-controlled, fixed-dose studies, one 6-month, placebo-controlled, fixed-dose study, and one 6-month, placebo-controlled, flexible-dose study in outpatients meeting DSM-IV criteria for GAD.

One 8-week study evaluating Effexor XR doses of 75, 150, and 225 mg/day, and placebo showed that the 225 mg/day dose was more effective than placebo on the Hamilton Rating Scale for Anxiety (HAM-A) total score, both the HAM-A anxiety and tension items, and the Clinical Global Impressions (CGI) scale. While there was also evidence for superiority over placebo for the 75 and 150 mg/day doses, these doses were not as consistently effective as the highest dose. A second 8-week study evaluating Effexor XR doses of 75 and 150 mg/day and placebo showed that both doses were more effective than placebo on some of these same outcomes; however, the 75 mg/day dose was more consistently effective than the 150 mg/day dose. A dose-response relationship for effectiveness in GAD was not clearly established in the 75 to 225 mg/day dose range utilized in these two studies.

Two 6-month studies, one evaluating Effexor XR doses of 37.5, 75, and 150 mg/day and the other evaluating Effexor XR doses of 75 to 225 mg/day, showed that daily doses of 75 mg or higher were more effective than placebo on the HAM-A total, both the HAM-A anxiety and tension items, and the CGI scale during 6 months of treatment. While there was also evidence for superiority over placebo for the 37.5 mg/day dose, this dose was not as consistently effective as the higher doses.

Examination of gender subsets of the population studied did not reveal any differential responsiveness on the basis of gender.

Social Anxiety Disorder (Social Phobia)

The efficacy of Effexor XR capsules as a treatment for Social Anxiety Disorder (also known as Social Phobia) was established in two double-blind, parallel group, 12-week, multicenter, placebo-controlled, flexible-dose studies in adult outpatients meeting DSM-IV criteria for Social Anxiety Disorder. Patients received doses in a range of 75 to 225 mg/day. Efficacy was assessed with the Liebowitz Social Anxiety Scale (LSAS). In these two trials, Effexor XR was significantly more effective than placebo on change from baseline to endpoint on the LSAS total score.

Examination of subsets of the population studied did not reveal any differential responsiveness on the basis of gender. There was insufficient information to determine the effect of age or race on outcome in these studies.

INDICATIONS AND USAGE

Major Depressive Disorder

Effexor XR (venlafaxine hydrochloride) extended-release capsules is indicated for the treatment of major depressive disorder.

The efficacy of Effexor XR in the treatment of major depressive disorder was established in 8- and 12-week controlled trials of outpatients whose diagnoses corresponded most closely to the DSM-III-R or DSM-IV category of major depressive disorder (see Clinical Trials).

A major depressive episode (DSM-IV) implies a prominent and relatively persistent (nearly every day for at least 2 weeks) depressed mood or the loss of interest or pleasure in nearly all activities, representing a change from previous functioning, and includes the presence of at least five of the following nine symptoms during the same two-week period: depressed mood, markedly diminished interest or pleasure in usual activities, significant change in weight and/or appetite, insomnia or hypersomnia, psychomotor agitation or retardation, increased fatigue, feelings of guilt or worthlessness, slowed thinking or impaired concentration, a suicide attempt or suicidal ideation.

The efficacy of Effexor (the immediate release form of venlafaxine) in the treatment of major depressive disorder in inpatients meeting diagnostic criteria for major depressive disorder with melancholia was established in a 4-week controlled trial (see Clinical Trials). The safety and efficacy of Effexor XR in hospitalized depressed patients have not been adequately studied.

The efficacy of Effexor XR in maintaining a response in major depressive disorder for up to 26 weeks following 8 weeks of acute treatment was demonstrated in a placebo-controlled trial. The efficacy of Effexor in maintaining a response in patients with recurrent major depressive disorder who had responded and continued to be improved during an initial 26 weeks of treatment and were then followed for a period of up to 52 weeks was demonstrated in a second placebo-controlled trial (see Clinical Trials). Nevertheless, the physician who elects to use Effexor/Effexor XR for extended periods should periodically re-evaluate the long-term usefulness of the drug for the individual patient (see DOSAGE AND ADMINISTRATION).

Generalized Anxiety Disorder

Effexor XR is indicated for the treatment of Generalized Anxiety Disorder (GAD) as defined in DSM-IV. Anxiety or tension associated with the stress of everyday life usually does not require treatment with an anxiolytic.

The efficacy of Effexor XR in the treatment of GAD was established in 8-week and 6-month placebo-controlled trials in outpatients diagnosed with GAD according to DSM-IV criteria (see Clinical Trials).

Generalized Anxiety Disorder (DSM-IV) is characterized by excessive anxiety and worry (apprehensive expectation) that is persistent for at least 6 months and which the person finds difficult to control. It must be associated with at least 3 of the following 6 symptoms: restlessness or feeling keyed up or on edge, being easily fatigued, difficulty concentrating or mind going blank, irritability, muscle tension, sleep disturbance.

Although the effectiveness of Effexor XR has been demonstrated in 6-month clinical trials in patients with GAD, the physician who elects to use Effexor XR for extended periods should periodically re-evaluate the long-term usefulness of the drug for the individual patient (see DOSAGE AND ADMINISTRATION).

Social Anxiety Disorder

Effexor XR is indicated for the treatment of Social Anxiety Disorder, also known as Social Phobia, as defined in DSM-IV (300.23).

Social Anxiety Disorder (DSM-IV) is characterized by a marked and persistent fear of 1 or more social or performance situations in which the person is exposed to unfamiliar people or to possible scrutiny by others. Exposure to the feared situation almost invariably provokes anxiety, which may approach the intensity of a panic attack. The feared situations are avoided or endured with intense anxiety or distress. The avoidance, anxious anticipation, or distress in the feared situation(s) interferes significantly with the person's normal routine, occupational or academic functioning, or social activities or relationships, or there is a marked distress about having the phobias. Lesser degrees of performance anxiety or shyness generally do not require psychopharmacological treatment.

The efficacy of Effexor XR in the treatment of Social Anxiety Disorder was established in two 12-week placebo-controlled trials in adult outpatients with Social Anxiety Disorder (DSM-IV). Effexor XR has not been studied in children or adolescents with Social Anxiety Disorder (see Clinical Trials).

The effectiveness of Effexor XR in the long-term treatment of Social Anxiety Disorder, ie, for more than 12 weeks, has not been systematically evaluated in adequate and well-controlled trials. Therefore, the physician who elects to use Effexor XR for extended periods should periodically re-evaluate the long-term usefulness of the drug for the individual patient (see DOSAGE AND ADMINISTRATION).

CONTRAINDICATIONS

Hypersensitivity to venlafaxine hydrochloride or to any excipients in the formulation.

Concomitant use in patients taking monoamine oxidase inhibitors (MAOIs) is contraindicated (see WARNINGS).

WARNINGS

Potential for Interaction with Monoamine Oxidase Inhibitors

Adverse reactions, some of which were serious, have been reported in patients who have recently been discontinued from a monoamine oxidase inhibitor (MAOI) and started on venlafaxine, or who have recently had venlafaxine therapy discontinued prior to initiation of an MAOI. These reactions have included tremor, myoclonus, diaphoresis, nausea, vomiting, flushing, dizziness, hyperthermia with features resembling neuroleptic malignant syndrome, seizures, and death. In patients receiving antidepressants with pharmacological properties similar to venlafaxine in combination with an MAOI, there have also been reports of serious, sometimes fatal, reactions. For a selective serotonin reuptake inhibitor, these reactions have included hyperthermia, rigidity, myoclonus, autonomic instability with possible rapid fluctuations of vital signs, and mental status changes that include extreme agitation progressing to delirium and coma. Some cases presented with features resembling neuroleptic malignant syndrome. Severe hyperthermia and seizures, sometimes fatal, have been reported in association with the combined use of tricyclic antidepressants and MAOIs. These reactions have also been reported in patients who have recently discontinued these drugs and have been started on an MAOI. The effects of combined use of venlafaxine and MAOIs have not been evaluated in humans or animals. Therefore, because venlafaxine is an inhibitor of both norepinephrine and serotonin reuptake, it is recommended that Effexor XR (venlafaxine hydrochloride) extended-release capsules not be used in combination with an MAOI, or within at least 14 days of discontinuing treatment with an MAOI. Based on the half-life of venlafaxine, at least 7 days should be allowed after stopping venlafaxine before starting an MAOI.

Sustained Hypertension

Venlafaxine treatment is associated with sustained increases in blood pressure in some patients. Among patients treated with 75 to 375 mg/day of Effexor XR in premarketing studies in patients with major depressive disorder, 3% (19/705) experienced sustained hypertension [defined as treatment-emergent supine diastolic blood pressure (SDBP) ≥ 90 mm Hg and ≥ 10 mm Hg above baseline for 3 consecutive on-therapy visits]. Among patients treated with 37.5 to 225 mg/day of Effexor XR in premarketing GAD studies, 0.5% (5/1011) experienced sustained hypertension. Among patients treated with 75 to 225 mg/day of Effexor XR in premarketing Social Anxiety Disorder studies, 1.4% (4/277)

Continued on next page

Effexor XR—Cont.

experienced sustained hypertension. Experience with the immediate-release venlafaxine showed that sustained hypertension was dose-related, increasing from 3% to 7% at 100 to 300 mg/day to 13% at doses above 300 mg/day. An insufficient number of patients received mean doses of Effexor XR over 300 mg/day to fully evaluate the incidence of sustained increases in blood pressure at these higher doses.

In placebo-controlled premarketing studies in patients with major depressive disorder with Effexor XR 75 to 225 mg/day, a final on-drug mean increase in supine diastolic blood pressure (SDBP) of 1.2 mm Hg was observed for Effexor XR-treated patients compared with a mean decrease of 0.2 mm Hg for placebo-treated patients. In placebo-controlled premarketing GAD studies with Effexor XR 37.5 to 225 mg/day, up to 8 weeks or up to 6 months, a final on-drug mean increase in SDBP of 0.3 mm Hg was observed for Effexor XR-treated patients compared with a mean decrease of 0.9 and 0.8 mm Hg, respectively, for placebo-treated patients.

In placebo-controlled premarketing Social Anxiety Disorder studies with Effexor XR 75 to 225 mg/day up to 12 weeks, a final on-drug mean increase in SDBP of 1.6 mm Hg was observed for Effexor XR-treated patients compared with a mean decrease of 1.1 mm Hg for placebo-treated patients.

In premarketing major depressive disorder studies, 0.7% (5/705) of the Effexor XR-treated patients discontinued treatment because of elevated blood pressure. Among these patients, most of the blood pressure increases were in a modest range (12 to 16 mm Hg, SDBP). In premarketing GAD studies up to 8 weeks and up to 6 months, 0.7% (10/1381) and 1.3% (7/535) of the Effexor XR-treated patients, respectively, discontinued treatment because of elevated blood pressure. Among these patients, most of the blood pressure increases were in a modest range (12 to 25 mm Hg, SDBP up to 8 weeks; 8 to 28 mm Hg up to 6 months). In premarketing Social Anxiety Disorder studies up to 12 weeks, 0.4% (1/277) of the Effexor XR-treated patients discontinued treatment because of elevated blood pressure. In this patient, the blood pressure increase was modest (13 mm Hg, SDBP).

Sustained increases of SDBP could have adverse consequences. Therefore, it is recommended that patients receiving Effexor XR have regular monitoring of blood pressure. For patients who experience a sustained increase in blood pressure while receiving venlafaxine, either dose reduction or discontinuation should be considered.

PRECAUTIONS

General

Insomnia and Nervousness

Treatment-emergent insomnia and nervousness were more commonly reported for patients treated with Effexor XR (venlafaxine hydrochloride) extended-release capsules than with placebo in pooled analyses of short-term major depressive disorder, GAD, and Social Anxiety Disorder studies, as shown in Table 1.

[See table 1 below]

Insomnia and nervousness each led to drug discontinuation in 0.9% of the patients treated with Effexor XR in major depressive disorder studies.

In GAD trials, insomnia and nervousness led to drug discontinuation in 3% and 2%, respectively, of the patients treated with Effexor XR up to 8 weeks and 2% and 0.7%, respectively, of the patients treated with Effexor XR up to 6 months.

In Social Anxiety Disorder trials, insomnia and nervousness led to drug discontinuation in 3% and 0%, respectively, of the patients treated with Effexor XR up to 12 weeks.

Changes in Appetite and Weight

Treatment-emergent anorexia was more commonly reported for Effexor XR-treated (8%) than placebo-treated patients (4%) in the pool of short-term studies in major depressive disorder. Significant weight loss, especially in underweight depressed patients, may be an undesirable result of Effexor XR treatment. A loss of 5% or more of body weight occurred in 7% of Effexor XR-treated and 2% of placebo-treated patients in placebo-controlled major depressive disorder trials. Discontinuation rates for anorexia and weight loss associated with Effexor XR were low (1.0% and 0.1%, respectively, of Effexor XR-treated patients in major depressive disorder studies).

In the pool of GAD studies, treatment-emergent anorexia was reported in 8% and 2% of patients receiving Effexor XR and placebo up to 8 weeks, respectively. A loss of 7% or more of body weight occurred in 3% of the Effexor XR-treated and 1% of the placebo-treated patients up to 6 months in these trials. Discontinuation rates for anorexia and weight loss were low for patients receiving Effexor XR up to 8 weeks (0.9% and 0.3%, respectively).

In the pool of Social Anxiety Disorder studies, treatment-emergent anorexia was reported in 20% and 2% of patients receiving Effexor XR and placebo up to 12 weeks, respectively. A loss of 7% or more of body weight occurred in none of the Effexor XR-treated or the placebo-treated patients up to 12 weeks in these trials. Discontinuation rates for anorexia and weight loss were low for patients receiving Effexor XR up to 12 weeks (0.4% and 0.0%, respectively).

The safety and efficacy of venlafaxine therapy in combination with weight loss agents, including phentermine, have not been established. Co-administration of Effexor XR and weight loss agents is not recommended. Effexor XR is not indicated for weight loss alone or in combination with other products.

Activation of Mania/Hypomania

During premarketing major depressive disorder studies, mania or hypomania occurred in 0.3% of Effexor XR-treated patients and 0.0% placebo patients. In premarketing GAD studies, 0.0% of Effexor XR-treated patients and 0.2% of placebo-treated patients experienced mania or hypomania. In premarketing Social Anxiety Disorder studies, no Effexor XR-treated patients and no placebo-treated patients experienced mania or hypomania. In all premarketing major depressive disorder trials with Effexor, mania or hypomania occurred in 0.5% of venlafaxine-treated patients compared with 0% of placebo patients. Mania/hypomania has also been reported in a small proportion of patients with mood disorders who were treated with other marketed drugs to treat major depressive disorder. As with all drugs effective in the treatment of major depressive disorder, Effexor XR should be used cautiously in patients with a history of mania.

Hyponatremia

Hyponatremia and/or the syndrome of inappropriate antidiuretic hormone secretion (SIADH) may occur with venlafaxine. This should be taken into consideration in patients who are, for example, volume-depleted, elderly, or taking diuretics.

Mydriasis

Mydriasis has been reported in association with venlafaxine; therefore patients with raised intraocular pressure or those at risk of acute narrow-angle glaucoma should be monitored.

Seizures

During premarketing experience, no seizures occurred among 705 Effexor XR-treated patients in the major depressive disorder studies, among 1381 Effexor XR-treated patients in GAD studies, or among 277 Effexor XR-treated patients in Social Anxiety Disorder studies. In all premarketing major depressive disorder trials with Effexor, seizures were reported at various doses in 0.3% (8/3082) of venlafaxine-treated patients. Effexor XR, like many antidepressants, should be used cautiously in patients with a history of seizures and should be discontinued in any patient who develops seizures.

Abnormal Bleeding

There have been reports of abnormal bleeding (most commonly ecchymosis) associated with venlafaxine treatment. While a causal relationship to venlafaxine is unclear, impaired platelet aggregation may result from platelet serotonin depletion and contribute to such occurrences.

Serum Cholesterol Elevation

Clinically relevant increases in serum cholesterol were recorded in 5.3% of venlafaxine-treated patients and 0.0% of placebo-treated patients treated for at least 3 months in placebo-controlled trials (see **ADVERSE REACTIONS-Laboratory Changes**). Measurement of serum cholesterol levels should be considered during long-term treatment.

Suicide

The possibility of a suicide attempt is inherent in major depressive disorder and may persist until significant remission occurs. Close supervision of high-risk patients should accompany initial drug therapy. Prescriptions for Effexor XR should be written for the smallest quantity of capsules consistent with good patient management in order to reduce the risk of overdose.

The same precautions observed when treating patients with major depressive disorder should be observed when treating patients with GAD or Social Anxiety Disorder.

Use in Patients With Concomitant Illness

Premarketing experience with venlafaxine in patients with concomitant systemic illness is limited. Caution is advised in administering Effexor XR to patients with diseases or conditions that could affect hemodynamic responses or metabolism.

Venlafaxine has not been evaluated or used to any appreciable extent in patients with a recent history of myocardial infarction or unstable heart disease. Patients with these diagnoses were systematically excluded from many clinical studies during venlafaxine's premarketing testing. The electrocardiograms were analyzed for 275 patients who received Effexor XR and 220 patients who received placebo in 8- to 12-week double-blind, placebo-controlled trials in major depressive disorder, for 610 patients who received Effexor XR and 298 patients who received placebo in 8-week double-blind, placebo-controlled trials in GAD, and for 195 patients who received Effexor XR and 228 patients who received placebo in 12-week double-blind, placebo-controlled trials in Social Anxiety Disorder. The mean change from baseline in corrected QT interval (QTc) for Effexor XR-treated patients in major depressive disorder studies was increased relative to that for placebo-treated patients (increase of 4.7 msec for Effexor XR and decrease of 1.9 msec for placebo). The mean change from baseline in corrected QT interval (QTc) for Effexor XR-treated patients in the GAD studies did not differ significantly from that with placebo. The mean change from baseline in QTc for Effexor XR-treated patients in the Social Anxiety Disorder studies was increased relative to that for placebo-treated patients (increase of 2.8 msec for Effexor XR and decrease of 2.0 msec for placebo).

In these same trials, the mean change from baseline in heart rate for Effexor XR-treated patients in the major depressive disorder studies was significantly higher than that for placebo (a mean increase of 4 beats per minute for Effexor XR and 1 beat per minute for placebo). The mean change from baseline in heart rate for Effexor XR-treated patients in the GAD studies was significantly higher than that for placebo (a mean increase of 3 beats per minute for Effexor XR and no change for placebo). The mean change from baseline in heart rate for Effexor XR-treated patients in the Social Anxiety Disorder studies was significantly higher than that for placebo (a mean increase of 5 beats per minute for Effexor XR and no change for placebo).

In a flexible-dose study, with Effexor doses in the range of 200 to 375 mg/day and mean dose greater than 300 mg/day, Effexor-treated patients had a mean increase in heart rate of 8.5 beats per minute compared with 1.7 beats per minute in the placebo group.

As increases in heart rate were observed, caution should be exercised in patients whose underlying medical conditions might be compromised by increases in heart rate (eg, patients with hyperthyroidism, heart failure, or recent myocardial infarction), particularly when using doses of Effexor above 200 mg/day.

Evaluation of the electrocardiograms for 769 patients who received immediate release Effexor in 4- to 6-week double-blind, placebo-controlled trials showed that the incidence of trial-emergent conduction abnormalities did not differ from that with placebo.

In patients with renal impairment (GFR = 10 to 70 mL/min) or cirrhosis of the liver, the clearances of venlafaxine and its active metabolites were decreased, thus prolonging the elimination half-lives of these substances. A lower dose may be necessary (see **DOSAGE AND ADMINISTRATION**).

Effexor XR, like all drugs effective in the treatment of major depressive disorder, should be used with caution in such patients.

Information for Patients

Physicians are advised to discuss the following issues with patients for whom they prescribe Effexor XR (venlafaxine hydrochloride) extended-release capsules:

Interference with Cognitive and Motor Performance

Clinical studies were performed to examine the effects of venlafaxine on behavioral performance of healthy individuals. The results revealed no clinically significant impairment of psychomotor, cognitive, or complex behavior performance. However, since any psychoactive drug may impair judgment, thinking, or motor skills, patients should be cautioned about operating hazardous machinery, including automobiles, until they are reasonably certain that venlafaxine therapy does not adversely affect their ability to engage in such activities.

Concomitant Medication

Patients should be advised to inform their physicians if they are taking, or plan to take, any prescription or over-the-counter drugs, including herbal preparations, since there is a potential for interactions.

Alcohol

Although venlafaxine has not been shown to increase the impairment of mental and motor skills caused by alcohol, patients should be advised to avoid alcohol while taking venlafaxine.

Allergic Reactions

Patients should be advised to notify their physician if they develop a rash, hives, or a related allergic phenomenon.

Pregnancy

Patients should be advised to notify their physician if they become pregnant or intend to become pregnant during therapy.

Nursing

Patients should be advised to notify their physician if they are breast-feeding an infant.

Laboratory Tests

There are no specific laboratory tests recommended.

Drug Interactions

As with all drugs, the potential for interaction by a variety of mechanisms is a possibility.

Alcohol

A single dose of ethanol (0.5 g/kg) had no effect on the pharmacokinetics of venlafaxine or O-desmethylvenlafaxine (ODV) when venlafaxine was administered at 150 mg/day in 15 healthy male subjects. Additionally, administration of venlafaxine in a stable regimen did not exaggerate the psychomotor and psychometric effects induced by ethanol in these same subjects when they were not receiving venlafaxine.

Table 1
Incidence of Insomnia and Nervousness in Placebo-Controlled Major Depressive Disorder, GAD, and Social Anxiety Disorder Trials

	Major Depressive Disorder		GAD		Social Anxiety Disorder	
Symptom	Effexor XR n = 357	Placebo n = 285	Effexor XR n = 1381	Placebo n = 555	Effexor XR n = 277	Placebo n = 274
Insomnia	17%	11%	15%	10%	23%	7%
Nervousness	10%	5%	6%	4%	11%	3%

Cimetidine
Concomitant administration of cimetidine and venlafaxine in a steady-state study for both drugs resulted in inhibition of first-pass metabolism of venlafaxine in 18 healthy subjects. The oral clearance of venlafaxine was reduced by about 43%, and the exposure (AUC) and maximum concentration (C_{max}) of the drug were increased by about 60%. However, coadministration of cimetidine had no apparent effect on the pharmacokinetics of ODV, which is present in much greater quantity in the circulation than venlafaxine. The overall pharmacological activity of venlafaxine plus ODV is expected to increase only slightly, and no dosage adjustment should be necessary for most normal adults. However, for patients with pre-existing hypertension, and for elderly patients or patients with hepatic dysfunction, the interaction associated with the concomitant use of venlafaxine and cimetidine is not known and potentially could be more pronounced. Therefore, caution is advised with such patients.

Diazepam
Under steady-state conditions for venlafaxine administered at 150 mg/day, a single 10 mg dose of diazepam did not appear to affect the pharmacokinetics of either venlafaxine or ODV in 18 healthy male subjects. Venlafaxine also did not have any effect on the pharmacokinetics of diazepam or its active metabolite, desmethyldiazepam, or affect the psychomotor and psychometric effects induced by diazepam.

Haloperidol
Venlafaxine administered under steady-state conditions at 150 mg/day in 24 healthy subjects decreased total oral-dose clearance (Cl/F) of a single 2 mg dose of haloperidol by 42%, which resulted in a 70% increase in haloperidol AUC. In addition, the haloperidol C_{max} increased 88% when coadministered with venlafaxine, but the haloperidol elimination half-life ($t_{1/2}$) was unchanged. The mechanism explaining this finding is unknown.

Lithium
The steady-state pharmacokinetics of venlafaxine administered at 150 mg/day were not affected when a single 600 mg oral dose of lithium was administered to 12 healthy male subjects. ODV also was unaffected. Venlafaxine had no effect on the pharmacokinetics of lithium.

Drugs Highly Bound to Plasma Proteins
Venlafaxine is not highly bound to plasma proteins; therefore, administration of Effexor XR to a patient taking another drug that is highly protein bound should not cause increased free concentrations of the other drug.

Drugs that Inhibit Cytochrome P450 Isoenzymes
CYP2D6 Inhibitors: In vitro and in vivo studies indicate that venlafaxine is metabolized to its active metabolite, ODV, by CYP2D6, the isoenzyme that is responsible for the genetic polymorphism seen in the metabolism of many antidepressants. Therefore, the potential exists for a drug interaction between drugs that inhibit CYP2D6-mediated metabolism of venlafaxine, reducing the metabolism of venlafaxine to ODV, resulting in increased plasma concentrations of venlafaxine and decreased concentrations of the active metabolite. CYP2D6 inhibitors such as quinidine would be expected to do this, but the effect would be similar to what is seen in patients who are genetically CYP2D6 poor metabolizers (see *Metabolism and Excretion* under **CLINICAL PHARMACOLOGY**). Therefore, no dosage adjustment is required when venlafaxine is coadministered with a CYP2D6 inhibitor.
The concomitant use of venlafaxine with drug treatment(s) that potentially inhibits both CYP2D6 and CYP3A4, the primary metabolizing enzymes for venlafaxine, has not been studied.
Therefore, caution is advised should a patient's therapy include venlafaxine and any agent(s) that produce simultaneous inhibition of these two enzyme systems.

Drugs Metabolized by Cytochrome P450 Isoenzymes
CYP2D6: In vitro studies indicate that venlafaxine is a relatively weak inhibitor of CYP2D6. These findings have been confirmed in a clinical drug interaction study comparing the effect of venlafaxine with that of fluoxetine on the CYP2D6-mediated metabolism of dextromethorphan to dextrorphan.
Imipramine - Venlafaxine did not affect the pharmacokinetics of imipramine and 2-OH-imipramine. However, desipramine AUC, C_{max}, and C_{min} increased by about 35% in the presence of venlafaxine. The 2-OH-desipramine AUC's increased by at least 2.5 fold (with venlafaxine 37.5 mg q12h) and by 4.5 fold (with venlafaxine 75 mg q12h). Imipramine did not affect the pharmacokinetics of venlafaxine and ODV. The clinical significance of elevated 2-OH-desipramine levels is unknown.
Risperidone - Venlafaxine administered under steady-state conditions at 150 mg/day slightly inhibited the CYP2D6-mediated metabolism of risperidone (administered as a single 1 mg oral dose) to its active metabolite, 9-hydroxyrisperidone, resulting in an approximate 32% increase in risperidone AUC. However, venlafaxine coadministration did not significantly alter the pharmacokinetic profile of the total active moiety (risperidone plus 9-hydroxyrisperidone).
CYP3A4: Venlafaxine did not inhibit CYP3A4 in vitro. This finding was confirmed in vivo by clinical drug interaction studies in which venlafaxine did not inhibit the metabolism of several CYP3A4 substrates, including alprazolam, diazepam, and terfenadine.
Indinavir - In a study of 9 healthy volunteers, venlafaxine administered under steady-state conditions at 150 mg/day resulted in a 28% decrease in the AUC of a single 800 mg oral dose of indinavir and a 36% decrease in indinavir C_{max}.

Table 2
Common Adverse Events Leading to Discontinuation of Treatment in Placebo-Controlled Trials[1]

Adverse Event	Percentage of Patients Discontinuing Due to Adverse Event: Major Depressive Disorder Indication[2]		GAD Indication[3,4]		Social Anxiety Disorder Indication	
	Effexor XR n=357	Placebo n=285	Effexor XR n=1381	Placebo n=555	Effexor XR n=277	Placebo n=274
Body as a Whole						
Asthenia	—	—	3%	<1%	1%	<1%
Headache	—	—	—	—	2%	<1%
Digestive System						
Nausea	4%	<1%	8%	<1%	4%	0%
Anorexia	1%	<1%	—	—	—	—
Dry Mouth	1%	0%	2%	<1%	—	—
Vomiting	—	—	1%	<1%	—	—
Nervous System						
Dizziness	2%	1%	—	—	2%	0%
Insomnia	1%	<1%	3%	<1%	3%	<1%
Somnolence	2%	<1%	3%	<1%	2%	<1%
Nervousness	—	—	2%	<1%	—	—
Tremor	—	—	1%	0%	—	—
Anxiety	—	—	—	—	1%	<1%
Skin						
Sweating	—	—	2%	<1%	1%	0%
Urogenital System						
Impotence[5]	—	—	—	—	3%	0%

[1] Two of the major depressive disorder studies were flexible dose and one was fixed dose. Four of the GAD studies were fixed dose and one was flexible dose. Both of the Social Anxiety Disorder studies were flexible dose.
[2] In U.S. placebo-controlled trials for major depressive disorder, the following were also common events leading to discontinuation and were considered to be drug-related for Effexor XR-treated patients (% Effexor XR [n = 192], % Placebo [n = 202]): hypertension (1%, <1%); diarrhea (1%, 0%); paresthesia (1%, 0%); tremor (1%, 0%); abnormal vision, mostly blurred vision (1%, 0%); and abnormal, mostly delayed, ejaculation (1%, 0%).
[3] In two short-term U.S. placebo-controlled trials for GAD, the following were also common events leading to discontinuation and were considered to be drug-related for Effexor XR-treated patients (% Effexor XR [n = 476]), % Placebo [n = 201]): headache (4%, <1%); vasodilatation (1%, 0%); anorexia (2%, <1%); dizziness (4%, 1%); thinking abnormal (1%, 0%); and abnormal vision (1%, 0%).
[4] In long-term placebo-controlled trials for GAD, the following was also a common event leading to discontinuation and was considered to be drug-related for Effexor XR-treated patients (% Effexor XR [n = 535], % Placebo [n = 257]): decreased libido (1%, 0%).
[5]Incidence is based on the number of men (Effexor XR = 158, placebo = 153).

Indinavir did not affect the pharmacokinetics of venlafaxine and ODV. The clinical significance of this finding is unknown.
CYP1A2: Venlafaxine did not inhibit CYP1A2 in vitro. This finding was confirmed in vivo by a clinical drug interaction study in which venlafaxine did not inhibit the metabolism of caffeine, a CYP1A2 substrate.
CYP2C9: Venlafaxine did not inhibit CYP2C9 in vitro. The clinical significance of this finding is unknown.
CYP2C19: Venlafaxine did not inhibit the metabolism of diazepam, which is partially metabolized by CYP2C19 (see *Diazepam* above).

Monoamine Oxidase Inhibitors
See **CONTRAINDICATIONS** and **WARNINGS**.

CNS-Active Drugs
The risk of using venlafaxine in combination with other CNS-active drugs has not been systematically evaluated (except in the case of those CNS-active drugs noted above). Consequently, caution is advised if the concomitant administration of venlafaxine and such drugs is required.

Electroconvulsive Therapy
There are no clinical data establishing the benefit of electroconvulsive therapy combined with Effexor XR (venlafaxine hydrochloride) extended-release capsules treatment.

Postmarketing Spontaneous Drug Interaction Reports
See **ADVERSE REACTIONS, Postmarketing Reports.**

Carcinogenesis, Mutagenesis, Impairment of Fertility

Carcinogenesis
Venlafaxine was given by oral gavage to mice for 18 months at doses up to 120 mg/kg per day, which was 1.7 times the maximum recommended human dose on a mg/m^2 basis. Venlafaxine was also given to rats by oral gavage for 24 months at doses up to 120 mg/kg per day. In rats receiving the 120 mg/kg dose, plasma concentrations of venlafaxine at necropsy were 1 times (male rats) and 6 times (female rats) the plasma concentrations of patients receiving the maximum recommended human dose. Plasma levels of the O-desmethyl metabolite were lower in rats than in patients receiving the maximum recommended dose. Tumors were not increased by venlafaxine treatment in mice or rats.

Mutagenesis
Venlafaxine and the major human metabolite, O-desmethylvenlafaxine (ODV), were not mutagenic in the Ames reverse mutation assay in Salmonella bacteria or the Chinese hamster ovary/HGPRT mammalian cell forward gene mutation assay. Venlafaxine was also not mutagenic or clastogenic in the in vitro BALB/c-3T3 mouse cell transformation assay, the sister chromatid exchange assay in cultured Chinese hamster ovary cells, or in the in vivo chromosomal aberration assay in rat bone marrow. ODV was not clastogenic in the in vitro Chinese hamster ovary cell chromosomal aberration assay, but elicited a clastogenic response in the in vivo chromosomal aberration assay in rat bone marrow.

Impairment of Fertility
Reproduction and fertility studies in rats showed no effects on male or female fertility at oral doses of up to 2 times the maximum recommended human dose on a mg/m^2 basis.

Pregnancy

Teratogenic Effects - Pregnancy Category C
Venlafaxine did not cause malformations in offspring of rats or rabbits given doses up to 2.5 times (rat) or 4 times (rabbit) the maximum recommended human daily dose on a mg/m^2 basis. However, in rats, there was a decrease in pup weight, an increase in stillborn pups, and an increase in pup deaths during the first 5 days of lactation, when dosing began during pregnancy and continued until weaning. The cause of these deaths is not known. These effects occurred at 2.5 times (mg/m^2) the maximum human daily dose. The no effect dose for rat pup mortality was 0.25 times the human dose on a mg/m^2 basis. There are no adequate and well-controlled studies in pregnant women. Because animal reproduction studies are not always predictive of human response, this drug should be used during pregnancy only if clearly needed.

Non-teratogenic Effects
If venlafaxine is used until or shortly before birth, discontinuation effects in the newborn should be considered.

Labor and Delivery
The effect of venlafaxine on labor and delivery in humans is unknown.

Nursing Mothers
Venlafaxine and ODV have been reported to be excreted in human milk. Because of the potential for serious adverse reactions in nursing infants from Effexor XR, a decision should be made whether to discontinue nursing or to discontinue the drug, taking into account the importance of the drug to the mother.

Pediatric Use
Safety and effectiveness in pediatric patients have not been established.

Geriatric Use
Approximately 4% (14/357), 6% (77/1381), and 2% (6/277) of Effexor XR-treated patients in placebo-controlled premarketing major depressive disorder, GAD, and Social Anxiety Disorder trials, respectively, were 65 years of age or over. Of 2,897 Effexor-treated patients in premarketing phase major depressive disorder studies, 12% (357) were 65 years of age or over. No overall differences in effectiveness or safety were observed between geriatric patients and younger patients, and other reported clinical experience generally has not identified differences in response between the elderly and younger patients. However, greater sensitivity of some older individuals cannot be ruled out. As with other antidepressants, several cases of hyponatremia and syndrome of inappropriate antidiuretic hormone secretion (SIADH) have been reported, usually in the elderly.
The pharmacokinetics of venlafaxine and ODV are not substantially altered in the elderly (see **CLINICAL PHARMACOLOGY**). No dose adjustment is recommended for the elderly on the basis of age alone, although other clinical circumstances, some of which may be more common in the elderly, such as renal or hepatic impairment, may warrant a dose reduction (see **DOSAGE AND ADMINISTRATION**).

ADVERSE REACTIONS

The information included in the **Adverse Findings Observed in Short-Term, Placebo-Controlled Studies with Effexor XR**

Continued on next page

Effexor XR—Cont.

subsection is based on data from a pool of three 8- and 12-week controlled clinical trials in major depressive disorder (includes two U.S. trials and one European trial) and on data up to 8 weeks from a pool of five controlled clinical trials in GAD with Effexor XR®, and on data up to 12 weeks from a pool of two controlled clinical trials in Social Anxiety Disorder. Information on additional adverse events associated with Effexor XR in the entire development program for the formulation and with Effexor (the immediate release formulation of venlafaxine) is included in the **Other Adverse Events Observed During the Premarketing Evaluation of Effexor and Effexor XR** subsection (see also **WARNINGS** and **PRECAUTIONS**).

Adverse Findings Observed in Short-Term, Placebo-Controlled Studies with Effexor XR

Adverse Events Associated with Discontinuation of Treatment

Approximately 11% of the 357 patients who received Effexor® XR (venlafaxine hydrochloride) extended-release capsules in placebo-controlled clinical trials for major depressive disorder discontinued treatment due to an adverse experience, compared with 6% of the 285 placebo-treated patients in those studies. Approximately 18% of the 1381 patients who received Effexor XR capsules in placebo-controlled clinical trials for GAD discontinued treatment due to an adverse experience, compared with 12% of the 555 placebo-treated patients in those studies. Approximately 17% of the 277 patients who received Effexor XR capsules in placebo-controlled clinical trials for Social Anxiety Disorder discontinued treatment due to an adverse experience, compared with 5% of the 274 placebo-treated patients in those studies. The most common events leading to discontinuation and considered to be drug-related (ie, leading to discontinuation in at least 1% of the Effexor XR-treated patients at a rate at least twice that of placebo for either indication) are shown in Table 2.

[See table 2 at top of previous page]

Adverse Events Occurring at an Incidence of 2% or More Among Effexor XR-Treated Patients

Tables 3, 4, and 5 enumerate the incidence, rounded to the nearest percent, of treatment-emergent adverse events that occurred during acute therapy of major depressive disorder (up to 12 weeks; dose range of 75 to 225 mg/day), of GAD (up to 8 weeks; dose range of 37.5 to 225 mg/day), and of Social Anxiety Disorder (up to 12 weeks; dose range of 75 to 225 mg/day, respectively, in 2% or more of patients treated with Effexor XR® (venlafaxine hydrochloride) where the incidence in patients treated with Effexor XR was greater than the incidence for the respective placebo-treated patients. The table shows the percentage of patients in each group who had at least one episode of an event at some time during their treatment. Reported adverse events were classified using a standard COSTART-based Dictionary terminology.

The prescriber should be aware that these figures cannot be used to predict the incidence of side effects in the course of usual medical practice where patient characteristics and other factors differ from those which prevailed in the clinical trials. Similarly, the cited frequencies cannot be compared with figures obtained from other clinical investigations involving different treatments, uses and investigators. The cited figures, however, do provide the prescribing physician with some basis for estimating the relative contribution of drug and nondrug factors to the side effect incidence rate in the population studied.

Commonly Observed Adverse Events from Tables 3, 4, and 5:

Major Depressive Disorder

Note in particular the following adverse events that occurred in at least 5% of the Effexor XR patients and at a rate at least twice that of the placebo group for all placebo-controlled trials for the major depressive disorder (Table 3): Abnormal ejaculation, gastrointestinal complaints (nausea, dry mouth, and anorexia), CNS complaints (dizziness, somnolence, and abnormal dreams), and sweating. In the two U.S. placebo-controlled trials, the following additional events occurred in at least 5% of Effexor XR-treated patients (n = 192) and at a rate at least twice that of the placebo group: Abnormalities of sexual function (impotence in men, anorgasmia in women, and libido decreased), gastrointestinal complaints (constipation and flatulence), CNS complaints (insomnia, nervousness, and tremor), problems of special senses (abnormal vision), cardiovascular effects (hypertension and vasodilatation), and yawning.

Generalized Anxiety Disorder

Note in particular the following adverse events that occurred in at least 5% of the Effexor XR patients and at a rate at least twice that of the placebo group for all placebo-controlled trials for the GAD indication (Table 4): Abnormalities of sexual function (abnormal ejaculation and impotence), gastrointestinal complaints (nausea, dry mouth, anorexia, and constipation), problems of special senses (abnormal vision), and sweating.

Social Anxiety Disorder

Note in particular the following adverse events that occurred in at least 5% of the Effexor XR patients and at a rate at least twice that of the placebo group for the 2 placebo-controlled trials for the Social Anxiety Disorder indication (Table 5):

Asthenia, gastrointestinal complaints (anorexia, dry mouth, nausea), CNS complaints (anxiety, insomnia, libido decreased, nervousness, somnolence, dizziness), abnormalities of sexual function (abnormal ejaculation, orgasmic dysfunction, impotence), yawn, sweating, and abnormal vision.

Table 3
Treatment-Emergent Adverse Event Incidence in Short-Term Placebo-Controlled Effexor XR Clinical Trials in Patients with Major Depressive Disorder[1,2]

Body System Preferred Term	% Reporting Event Effexor XR (n=357)	 Placebo (n=285)
Body as a Whole		
Asthenia	8%	7%
Cardiovascular System		
Vasodilatation[3]	4%	2%
Hypertension	4%	1%
Digestive System		
Nausea	31%	12%
Constipation	8%	5%
Anorexia	8%	4%
Vomiting	4%	2%
Flatulence	4%	3%
Metabolic/Nutritional		
Weight Loss	3%	0%
Nervous System		
Dizziness	20%	9%
Somnolence	17%	8%
Insomnia	17%	11%
Dry Mouth	12%	6%
Nervousness	10%	5%
Abnormal Dreams[4]	7%	2%
Tremor	5%	2%
Depression	3%	<1%
Paresthesia	3%	1%
Libido Decreased	3%	<1%
Agitation	3%	1%
Respiratory System		
Pharyngitis	7%	6%
Yawn	3%	0%
Skin		
Sweating	14%	3%
Special Senses		
Abnormal Vision[5]	4%	<1%
Urogenital System		
Abnormal Ejaculation (male)[6,7]	16%	<1%
Impotence[7]	4%	<1%
Anorgasmia (female)[8,9]	3%	<1%

[1] Incidence, rounded to the nearest %, for events reported by at least 2% of patients treated with Effexor XR, except the following events which had an incidence equal to or less than placebo: abdominal pain, accidental injury, anxiety, back pain, bronchitis, diarrhea, dysmenorrhea, dyspepsia, flu syndrome, headache, infection, pain, palpitation, rhinitis, and sinusitis.
[2] <1% indicates an incidence greater than zero but less than 1%.
[3] Mostly "hot flashes."
[4] Mostly "vivid dreams," "nightmares," and "increased dreaming."
[5] Mostly "blurred vision" and "difficulty focusing eyes."
[6] Mostly "delayed ejaculation."
[7] Incidence is based on the number of male patients.
[8] Mostly "delayed orgasm" or "anorgasmia."
[9] Incidence is based on the number of female patients.

Table 4
Treatment-Emergent Adverse Event Incidence in Short-Term Placebo-Controlled Effexor XR Clinical Trials in GAD Patients[1,2]

Body System Preferred Term	% Reporting Event Effexor XR (n=1381)	 Placebo (n=555)
Body as a Whole		
Asthenia	12%	8%
Cardiovascular System		
Vasodilatation[3]	4%	2%
Digestive System		
Nausea	35%	12%
Constipation	10%	4%
Anorexia	8%	2%
Vomiting	5%	3%
Nervous System		
Dizziness	16%	11%
Dry Mouth	16%	6%
Insomnia	15%	10%
Somnolence	14%	8%
Nervousness	6%	4%
Libido Decreased	4%	2%
Tremor	4%	<1%
Abnormal Dreams[4]	3%	2%
Hypertonia	3%	2%
Paresthesia	2%	1%
Respiratory System		
Yawn	3%	<1%
Skin		
Sweating	10%	3%
Special Senses		
Abnormal Vision[5]	5%	<1%
Urogenital System		
Abnormal Ejaculation[6,7]	11%	<1%
Impotence[7]	5%	<1%
Orgasmic Dysfunction (female)[8,9]	2%	0%

[1] Adverse events for which the Effexor XR reporting rate was less than or equal to the placebo rate are not included. These events are: abdominal pain, accidental injury, anxiety, back pain, diarrhea, dysmenorrhea, dyspepsia, flu syndrome, headache, infection, myalgia, pain, palpitation, pharyngitis, rhinitis, tinnitus, and urinary frequency.
[2] <1% means greater than zero but less than 1%.
[3] Mostly "hot flashes."
[4] Mostly "vivid dreams," "nightmares," and "increased dreaming."
[5] Mostly "blurred vision" and "difficulty focusing eyes."
[6] Includes "delayed ejaculation," and "anorgasmia."
[7] Percentage based on the number of males (Effexor XR= 525, placebo=220).
[8] Includes "delayed orgasm," "abnormal orgasm," and "anorgasmia."
[9] Percentage based on the number of females (Effexor XR= 856, placebo=335).

Table 5
Treatment-Emergent Adverse Event Incidence in Short-Term Placebo-Controlled Effexor XR Clinical Trials in Social Anxiety Disorder Patients[1,2]

Body System Preferred Term	% Reporting Event Effexor XR (n=277)	 Placebo (n=274)
Body as a Whole		
Headache	34%	33%
Asthenia	17%	8%
Flu Syndrome	6%	5%
Accidental Injury	5%	3%
Abdominal Pain	4%	3%
Cardiovascular System		
Hypertension	5%	4%
Vasodilatation[3]	3%	1%
Palpitation	3%	1%
Digestive System		
Nausea	29%	9%
Anorexia[4]	20%	1%
Constipation	8%	4%
Diarrhea	6%	5%
Vomiting	3%	2%
Eructation	2%	0%
Metabolic/Nutritional		
Weight Loss	4%	0%
Nervous System		
Insomnia	23%	7%
Dry Mouth	17%	4%
Dizziness	16%	8%
Somnolence	16%	8%
Nervousness	11%	3%
Libido Decreased	9%	<1%
Anxiety	5%	3%
Agitation	4%	1%
Tremor	4%	<1%
Abnormal Dreams[5]	4%	<1%
Paresthesia	3%	<1%
Twitching	2%	0%
Respiratory System		
Yawn	5%	<1%
Sinusitis	2%	1%
Skin		
Sweating	13%	2%
Special Senses		
Abnormal Vision[6]	6%	3%
Urogenital System		
Abnormal Ejaculation[7,8]	16%	1%
Impotence[8]	10%	1%
Orgasmic Dysfunction[9,10]	8%	0%

[1] Adverse events for which the Effexor XR reporting rate was less than or equal to the placebo rate are not included. These events are: back pain, depression, dysmenorrhea, dyspepsia, infection, myalgia, pain, pharyngitis, rash, rhinitis, and upper respiratory infection.
[2] <1% means greater than zero but less than 1%.
[3] Mostly "hot flashes."
[4] Mostly "decreased appetite" and "loss of appetite."
[5] Mostly "vivid dreams," "nightmares," and "increased dreaming."
[6] Mostly "blurred vision."
[7] Includes "delayed ejaculation" and "anorgasmia."
[8] Percentage based on the number of males (Effexor XR = 158, placebo = 153).
[9] Includes "abnormal orgasm" and "anorgasmia."
[10] Percentage based on the number of females (Effexor XR = 119, placebo = 121).

Vital Sign Changes

Effexor XR (venlafaxine hydrochloride) extended-release capsules treatment for up to 12 weeks in premarketing placebo-controlled major depressive disorder trials was associated with a mean final on-therapy increase in pulse rate of approximately 2 beats per minute, compared with 1 beat per minute for placebo. Effexor XR treatment for up to 8 weeks in premarketing placebo-controlled GAD trials was associated with a mean final on-therapy increase in pulse rate of approximately 2 beats per minute, compared with less than 1 beat per minute for placebo. Effexor XR treatment for up to 12 weeks in premarketing placebo-controlled Social Anxiety Disorder trials was associated with mean final on-therapy increase in pulse rate of approximately 4 beats per minute, compared with no change for placebo. (See the **Sustained Hypertension** section of **WARNINGS** for effects on blood pressure.)

In a flexible-dose study, with Effexor doses in the range of 200 to 375 mg/day and mean dose greater than 300 mg/day, the mean pulse was increased by about 2 beats per minute compared with a decrease of about 1 beat per minute for placebo.

Laboratory Changes

Effexor XR (venlafaxine hydrochloride) extended-release capsules treatment for up to 12 weeks in premarketing placebo-controlled trials for major depressive disorder was associated with a mean final on-therapy increase in serum cholesterol concentration of approximately 1.5 mg/dL compared with a mean final decrease of 7.4 mg/dL for placebo. Effexor XR treatment for up to 8 weeks and up to 6 months in premarketing placebo-controlled GAD trials was associated with mean final on-therapy increases in serum cholesterol concentration of approximately 1.0 mg/dL and 2.3 mg/dL, respectively while placebo subjects experienced mean final decreases of 4.9 mg/dL and 7.7 mg/dL, respectively. Effexor XR treatment for up to 12 weeks in premarketing placebo-controlled Social Anxiety Disorder trials was associated with mean final on-therapy increases in serum cholesterol concentration of approximately 11.4 mg/dL compared with a mean final decrease of 2.2 mg/dL for placebo. Patients treated with Effexor tablets (the immediate-release form of venlafaxine) for at least 3 months in placebo-controlled 12-month extension trials had a mean final on-therapy increase in total cholesterol of 9.1 mg/dL compared with a decrease of 7.1 mg/dL among placebo-treated patients. This increase was duration dependent over the study period and tended to be greater with higher doses. Clinically relevant increases in serum cholesterol, defined as 1) a final on-therapy increase in serum cholesterol ≥50 mg/dL from baseline and to a value ≥261 mg/dL, or 2) an average on-therapy increase in serum cholesterol ≥50 mg/dL from baseline and to a value ≥261 mg/dL, were recorded in 5.3% of venlafaxine-treated patients and 0.0% of placebo-treated patients (see **PRECAUTIONS-General**-*Serum Cholesterol Elevation*).

ECG Changes

In a flexible-dose study, with Effexor doses in the range of 200 to 375 mg/day and mean dose greater than 300 mg/day, the mean change in heart rate was 8.5 beats per minute compared with 1.7 beats per minute for placebo.

(See the *Use in Patients with Concomitant Illness* section of **PRECAUTIONS**).

Other Adverse Events Observed During the Premarketing Evaluation of Effexor and Effexor XR

During its premarketing assessment, multiple doses of Effexor XR were administered to 705 patients in Phase 3 major depressive disorder studies and Effexor was administered to 96 patients. During its premarketing assessment, multiple doses of Effexor XR were also administered to 1381 patients in Phase 3 GAD studies and 277 patients in Phase 3 Social Anxiety Disorder studies. In addition, in premarketing assessment of Effexor, multiple doses were administered to 2897 patients in Phase 2 to Phase 3 studies for major depressive disorder. The conditions and duration of exposure to venlafaxine in both development programs varied greatly, and included (in overlapping categories) open and double-blind studies, uncontrolled and controlled studies, inpatient (Effexor only) and outpatient studies, fixed-dose, and titration studies. Untoward events associated with this exposure were recorded by clinical investigators using terminology of their own choosing. Consequently, it is not possible to provide a meaningful estimate of the proportion of individuals experiencing adverse events without first grouping similar types of untoward events into a smaller number of standardized event categories.

In the tabulations that follow, reported adverse events were classified using a standard COSTART-based Dictionary terminology. The frequencies presented, therefore, represent the proportion of the 5356 patients exposed to multiple doses of either formulation of venlafaxine who experienced an event of the type cited on at least one occasion while receiving venlafaxine. All reported events are included except those already listed in Tables 3, 4, and 5 and those events for which a drug cause was remote. If the COSTART term for an event was so general as to be uninformative, it was replaced with a more informative term. It is important to emphasize that, although the events reported occurred during treatment with venlafaxine, they were not necessarily caused by it.

Events are further categorized by body system and listed in order of decreasing frequency using the following definitions: **frequent** adverse events are defined as those occurring on one or more occasions in at least 1/100 patients; **infrequent** adverse events are those occurring in 1/100 to 1/1000 patients; **rare** events are those occurring in fewer than 1/1000 patients.

Body as a whole - **Frequent**: chest pain substernal, chills, fever, neck pain; **Infrequent**: face edema, intentional injury, malaise, moniliasis, neck rigidity, pelvic pain, photosensitivity reaction, suicide attempt, withdrawal syndrome; **Rare**: appendicitis, bacteremia, carcinoma, cellulitis.

Cardiovascular system - **Frequent**: migraine, postural hypotension, tachycardia; **Infrequent**: angina pectoris, arrhythmia, extrasystoles, hypotension, peripheral vascular disorder (mainly cold feet and/or cold hands), syncope, thrombophlebitis; **Rare**: aortic aneurysm, arteritis, first-degree atrioventricular block, bigeminy, bradycardia, bundle branch block, capillary fragility, cerebral ischemia, coronary artery disease, congestive heart failure, heart arrest, cardiovascular disorder (mitral valve and circulatory disturbance), mucocutaneous hemorrhage, myocardial infarct, pallor.

Digestive system - **Frequent**: increased appetite; **Infrequent**: bruxism, colitis, dysphagia, tongue edema, esophagitis, gastritis, gastroenteritis, gastrointestinal ulcer, gingivitis, glossitis, rectal hemorrhage, hemorrhoids, melena, oral moniliasis, stomatitis, mouth ulceration; **Rare**: cheilitis, cholecystitis, cholelithiasis, esophageal spasms, duodenitis, hematemesis, gastrointestinal hemorrhage, gum hemorrhage, hepatitis, ileitis, jaundice, intestinal obstruction, parotitis, periodontitis, proctitis, increased salivation, soft stools, tongue discoloration.

Endocrine system - **Rare**: goiter, hyperthyroidism, hypothyroidism, thyroid nodule, thyroiditis.

Hemic and lymphatic system - **Frequent**: ecchymosis; **Infrequent**: anemia, leukocytosis, leukopenia, lymphadenopathy, thrombocythemia, thrombocytopenia; **Rare**: basophilia, bleeding time increased, cyanosis, eosinophilia, lymphocytosis, multiple myeloma, purpura.

Metabolic and nutritional - **Frequent**: edema, weight gain; **Infrequent**: alkaline phosphatase increased, dehydration, hypercholesteremia, hyperglycemia, hyperlipemia, hypokalemia, SGOT increased, SGPT increased, thirst; **Rare**: alcohol intolerance, bilirubinemia, BUN increased, creatinine increased, diabetes mellitus, glycosuria, gout, healing abnormal, hemochromatosis, hypercalcinuria, hyperkalemia, hyperphosphatemia, hyperuricemia, hypocholesteremia, hypoglycemia, hyponatremia, hypophosphatemia, hypoproteinemia, uremia.

Musculoskeletal system - **Frequent**: arthralgia; **Infrequent**: arthritis, arthrosis, bone pain, bone spurs, bursitis, leg cramps, myasthenia, tenosynovitis; **Rare**: pathological fracture, myopathy, osteoporosis, osteosclerosis, plantar fasciitis, rheumatoid arthritis, tendon rupture.

Nervous system - **Frequent**: amnesia, confusion, depersonalization, hypesthesia, thinking abnormal, trismus, vertigo; **Infrequent**: akathisia, apathy, ataxia, circumoral paresthesia, CNS stimulation, emotional lability, euphoria, hallucinations, hostility, hyperesthesia, hyperkinesia, hypotonia, incoordination, libido increased, manic reaction, myoclonus, neuralgia, neuropathy, psychosis, seizure, abnormal speech, stupor; **Rare**: akinesia, alcohol abuse, aphasia, bradykinesia, buccoglossal syndrome, cerebrovascular accident, feeling drunk, loss of consciousness, delusions, dementia, dystonia, facial paralysis, abnormal gait, Guillain-Barre Syndrome, hyperchlorhydria, hypokinesia, impulse control difficulties, neuritis, nystagmus, paranoid reaction, paresis, psychotic depression, reflexes decreased, reflexes increased, suicidal ideation, torticollis.

Respiratory system - **Frequent**: cough increased, dyspnea; **Infrequent**: asthma, chest congestion, epistaxis, hyperventilation, laryngismus, laryngitis, pneumonia, voice alteration; **Rare**: atelectasis, hemoptysis, hypoventilation, hypoxia, larynx edema, pleurisy, pulmonary embolus, sleep apnea.

Skin and appendages - **Frequent**: pruritus; **Infrequent**: acne, alopecia, brittle nails, contact dermatitis, dry skin, eczema, skin hypertrophy, maculopapular rash, psoriasis, urticaria; **Rare**: erythema nodosum, exfoliative dermatitis, lichenoid dermatitis, hair discoloration, skin discoloration, furunculosis, hirsutism, leukoderma, petechial rash, pustular rash, vesiculobullous rash, seborrhea, skin atrophy, skin striae.

Special senses - **Frequent**: abnormality of accommodation, mydriasis, taste perversion; **Infrequent**: cataract, conjunctivitis, corneal lesion, diplopia, dry eyes, eye pain, hyperacusis, otitis media, parosmia, photophobia, taste loss, visual field defect; **Rare**: blepharitis, chromatopsia, conjunctival edema, deafness, exophthalmos, glaucoma, retinal hemorrhage, subconjunctival hemorrhage, keratitis, labyrinthitis, miosis, papilledema, decreased pupillary reflex, otitis externa, scleritis, uveitis.

Urogenital system - **Frequent**: metrorrhagia,* prostatic disorder (prostatitis and enlarged prostate),* urination impaired, vaginitis*; **Infrequent**: albuminuria, amenorrhea,* cystitis, dysuria, hematuria, leukorrhea,* menorrhagia,* nocturia, bladder pain, breast pain, polyuria, pyuria, urinary incontinence, urinary retention, urinary urgency, vaginal hemorrhage*; **Rare**: abortion,* anuria, breast discharge, breast engorgement, balanitis,* breast enlargement, endometriosis,* female lactation,* fibrocystic breast, calcium crystalluria, cervicitis,* orchitis,* ovarian cyst,* prolonged erection,* gynecomastia (male),* hypomenorrhea,* kidney calculus, kidney pain, kidney function abnormal, mastitis, menopause,* pyelonephritis, oliguria, salpingitis,* urolithiasis, uterine hemorrhage,* uterine spasm,* vaginal dryness.*

---

*Based on the number of men and women as appropriate.

Postmarketing Reports

Voluntary reports of other adverse events temporally associated with the use of venlafaxine that have been received since market introduction and that may have no causal relationship with the use of venlafaxine include the following: agranulocytosis, anaphylaxis, aplastic anemia, catatonia, congenital anomalies, CPK increased, deep vein thrombophlebitis, delirium, EKG abnormalities such as QT prolongation; cardiac arrhythmias including atrial fibrillation, supraventricular tachycardia, ventricular extrasystoles, and rare reports of ventricular fibrillation and ventricular tachycardia, including torsade de pointes; epidermal necrosis/Stevens-Johnson Syndrome, erythema multiforme, extrapyramidal symptoms (including tardive dyskinesia), hemorrhage (including eye and gastrointestinal bleeding), hepatic events (including GGT elevation; abnormalities of unspecified liver function tests; liver damage, necrosis, or failure; and fatty liver), involuntary movements, LDH increased, neuroleptic malignant syndrome-like events (including a case of a 10-year-old who may have been taking methylphenidate, was treated and recovered), neutropenia, night sweats, pancreatitis, pancytopenia, panic, prolactin increased, pulmonary eosinophilia, renal failure, serotonin syndrome, shock-like electrical sensations (in some cases, subsequent to the discontinuation of venlafaxine or tapering of dose), and syndrome of inappropriate antidiuretic hormone secretion (usually in the elderly).

There have been reports of elevated clozapine levels that were temporally associated with adverse events, including seizures, following the addition of venlafaxine. There have been reports of increases in prothrombin time, partial thromboplastin time, or INR when venlafaxine was given to patients receiving warfarin therapy.

DRUG ABUSE AND DEPENDENCE

Controlled Substance Class

Effexor XR (venlafaxine hydrochloride) extended-release capsules is not a controlled substance.

Physical and Psychological Dependence

In vitro studies revealed that venlafaxine has virtually no affinity for opiate, benzodiazepine, phencyclidine (PCP), or N-methyl-D-aspartic acid (NMDA) receptors.

Venlafaxine was not found to have any significant CNS stimulant activity in rodents. In primate drug discrimination studies, venlafaxine showed no significant stimulant or depressant abuse liability.

Discontinuation effects have been reported in patients receiving venlafaxine (see **DOSAGE AND ADMINISTRATION**).

While venlafaxine has not been systematically studied in clinical trials for its potential for abuse, there was no indication of drug-seeking behavior in the clinical trials. However, it is not possible to predict on the basis of premarketing experience the extent to which a CNS active drug will be misused, diverted, and/or abused once marketed. Consequently, physicians should carefully evaluate patients for history of drug abuse and follow such patients closely, observing them for signs of misuse or abuse of venlafaxine (eg, development of tolerance, incrementation of dose, drug-seeking behavior).

OVERDOSAGE

Human Experience

Among the patients included in the premarketing evaluation of Effexor XR, there were 2 reports of acute overdosage with Effexor XR in major depressive disorder trials, either alone or in combination with other drugs. One patient took a combination of 6 g of Effexor XR and 2.5 mg of lorazepam. This patient was hospitalized, treated symptomatically, and recovered without any untoward effects. The other patient took 2.85 g of Effexor XR. This patient reported paresthesia of all four limbs but recovered without sequelae.

There were 2 reports of acute overdose with Effexor XR in GAD trials. One patient took a combination of 0.75 g of Effexor XR and 200 mg of paroxetine and 50 mg of zolpidem. This patient was described as being alert, able to communicate, and a little sleepy. This patient was hospitalized, treated with activated charcoal, and recovered without any untoward effects. The other patient took 1.2 g of Effexor XR. This patient recovered and no other specific problems were found. The patient had moderate dizziness, nausea, numb hands and feet, and hot-cold spells 5 days after the overdose. These symptoms resolved over the next week.

There were no reports of acute overdose with Effexor XR in Social Anxiety Disorder trials.

Among the patients included in the premarketing evaluation with Effexor, there were 14 reports of acute overdose with venlafaxine, either alone or in combination with other drugs and/or alcohol. The majority of the reports involved ingestion in which the total dose of venlafaxine taken was estimated to be no more than several-fold higher than the usual therapeutic dose. The 3 patients who took the highest doses were estimated to have ingested approximately 6.75 g, 2.75 g, and 2.5 g. The resultant peak plasma levels of venlafaxine for the latter 2 patients were 6.24 and 2.35 μg/mL, respectively, and the peak plasma levels of O-desmethylvenlafaxine were 3.37 and 1.30 μg/mL, respectively. Plasma venlafaxine levels were not obtained for the patient who ingested 6.75 g of venlafaxine. All 14 patients recovered without sequelae. Most patients reported no symptoms. Among the remaining patients, somnolence was the most commonly reported symptom. The patient who ingested 2.75 g of venlafaxine was observed to have 2 generalized convulsions and a prolongation of QTc to 500 msec, compared with 405 msec at baseline. Mild sinus tachycardia was reported in 2 of the other patients.

In postmarketing experience, overdose with venlafaxine has occurred predominantly in combination with alcohol and/or other drugs. Electrocardiogram changes (eg, prolongation of QT interval, bundle branch block, QRS prolongation), sinus and ventricular tachycardia, bradycardia, hypotension, altered level of consciousness (ranging from somnolence to coma), seizures, vertigo, and death have been reported.

Continued on next page

Effexor XR—Cont.

Management of Overdosage
Treatment should consist of those general measures employed in the management of overdosage with any antidepressant. Ensure an adequate airway, oxygenation, and ventilation. Monitor cardiac rhythm and vital signs. General supportive and symptomatic measures are also recommended. Induction of emesis is not recommended. Gastric lavage with a large bore orogastric tube with appropriate airway protection, if needed, may be indicated if performed soon after ingestion or in symptomatic patients.
Activated charcoal should be administered. Due to the large volume of distribution of this drug, forced diuresis, dialysis, hemoperfusion, and exchange transfusion are unlikely to be of benefit. No specific antidotes for venlafaxine are known.
In managing overdosage, consider the possibility of multiple drug involvement. The physician should consider contacting a poison control center for additional information on the treatment of any overdose. Telephone numbers for certified poison control centers are listed in the *Physicians' Desk Reference® (PDR).*

DOSAGE AND ADMINISTRATION

Effexor XR should be administered in a single dose with food either in the morning or in the evening at approximately the same time each day. Each capsule should be swallowed whole with fluid and not divided, crushed, chewed, or placed in water, or it may be administered by carefully opening the capsule and sprinkling the entire contents on a spoonful of applesauce. This drug/food mixture should be swallowed immediately without chewing and followed with a glass of water to ensure complete swallowing of the pellets.

Initial Treatment
Major Depressive Disorder
For most patients, the recommended starting dose for Effexor XR is 75 mg/day, administered in a single dose. In the clinical trials establishing the efficacy of Effexor XR in moderately depressed outpatients, the initial dose of venlafaxine was 75 mg/day. For some patients, it may be desirable to start at 37.5 mg/day for 4 to 7 days, to allow new patients to adjust to the medication before increasing to 75 mg/day. While the relationship between dose and antidepressant response for Effexor XR has not been adequately explored, patients not responding to the initial 75 mg/day dose may benefit from dose increases to a maximum of approximately 225 mg/day. Dose increases should be in increments of up to 75 mg/day, as needed, and should be made at intervals of not less than 4 days, since steady state plasma levels of venlafaxine and its major metabolites are achieved in most patients by day 4. In the clinical trials establishing efficacy, upward titration was permitted at intervals of 2 weeks or more; the average doses were about 140 to 180 mg/day (see **Clinical Trials** under **CLINICAL PHARMACOLOGY**).
It should be noted that, while the maximum recommended dose for moderately depressed outpatients is also 225 mg/day for Effexor (the immediate release form of venlafaxine), more severely depressed inpatients in one study of the development program for that product responded to a mean dose of 350 mg/day (range of 150 to 375 mg/day). Whether or not higher doses of Effexor XR are needed for more severely depressed patients is unknown; however, the experience with Effexor XR doses higher than 225 mg/day is very limited. (See **PRECAUTIONS-General**-*Use in Patients with Concomitant Illness.*)
Generalized Anxiety Disorder
For most patients, the recommended starting dose for Effexor XR is 75 mg/day, administered in a single dose. In clinical trials establishing the efficacy of Effexor XR in outpatients with Generalized Anxiety Disorder (GAD), the initial dose of venlafaxine was 75 mg/day. For some patients, it may be desirable to start at 37.5 mg/day for 4 to 7 days, to allow new patients to adjust to the medication before increasing to 75 mg/day. Although a dose-response relationship for effectiveness in GAD was not clearly established in fixed-dose studies, certain patients not responding to the initial 75 mg/day dose may benefit from dose increases to a maximum of approximately 225 mg/day. Dose increases should be in increments of up to 75 mg/day, as needed, and should be made at intervals of not less than 4 days. (See the *Use in Patients with Concomitant Illness* section of **PRECAUTIONS**.)
Social Anxiety Disorder (Social Phobia)
For most patients, the recommended starting dose for Effexor XR is 75 mg/day, administered in a single dose. In clinical trials establishing the efficacy of Effexor XR in outpatients with Social Anxiety Disorder, the initial dose of Effexor XR was 75 mg/day and the maximum dose was 225 mg/day. For some patients, it may be desirable to start at 37.5 mg/day for 4 to 7 days, to allow new patients to adjust to the medication before increasing to 75 mg/day. Although a dose-response relationship for effectiveness in patients with Social Anxiety Disorder was not clearly established in fixed-dose studies, certain patients not responding to the initial 75 mg/day dose may benefit from dose increases to a maximum of approximately 225 mg/day. Dose increases should be in increments of up to 75 mg/day, as needed, and should be made at intervals of not less than 4 days. (See the *Use in Patients with Concomitant Illness* section of **PRECAUTIONS**).

Switching Patients from Effexor Tablets
Depressed patients who are currently being treated at a therapeutic dose with Effexor may be switched to Effexor XR at the nearest equivalent dose (mg/day), eg, 37.5 mg venlafaxine two-times-a-day to 75 mg Effexor XR once daily. However, individual dosage adjustments may be necessary.

Patients with Hepatic Impairment
Given the decrease in clearance and increase in elimination half-life for both venlafaxine and ODV that is observed in patients with hepatic cirrhosis compared with normal subjects (see **CLINICAL PHARMACOLOGY**), it is recommended that the starting dose be reduced by 50% in patients with moderate hepatic impairment. Because there was much individual variability in clearance between patients with cirrhosis, individualization of dosage may be desirable in some patients.

Patients with Renal Impairment
Given the decrease in clearance for venlafaxine and the increase in elimination half-life for both venlafaxine and ODV that is observed in patients with renal impairment (GFR = 10 to 70 mL/min) compared with normal subjects (see **CLINICAL PHARMACOLOGY**), it is recommended that the total daily dose be reduced by 25% to 50%. In patients undergoing hemodialysis, it is recommended that the total daily dose be reduced by 50% and that the dose be withheld until the dialysis treatment is completed (4 hrs). Because there was much individual variability in clearance between patients with renal impairment, individualization of dosage may be desirable in some patients.

Elderly Patients
No dose adjustment is recommended for elderly patients solely on the basis of age. As with any drug for the treatment of major depressive disorder, Generalized Anxiety Disorder, or Social Anxiety Disorder, however, caution should be exercised in treating the elderly. When individualizing the dosage, extra care should be taken when increasing the dose.

Maintenance Treatment
There is no body of evidence available from controlled trials to indicate how long patients with major depressive disorder, Generalized Anxiety Disorder, or Social Anxiety Disorder should be treated with Effexor XR.
It is generally agreed that acute episodes of major depressive disorder require several months or longer of sustained pharmacological therapy beyond response to the acute episode. In one study, in which patients responding during 8 weeks of acute treatment with Effexor XR were assigned randomly to placebo or to the same dose of Effexor XR (75, 150, or 225 mg/day, qAM) during 26 weeks of maintenance treatment as they had received during the acute stabilization phase, longer-term efficacy was demonstrated. A second longer-term study has demonstrated the efficacy of Effexor in maintaining a response in patients with recurrent major depressive disorder who had responded and continued to be improved during an initial 26 weeks of treatment and were then randomly assigned to placebo or Effexor for periods of up to 52 weeks on the same dose (100 to 200 mg/day, on a b.i.d. schedule) (see **Clinical Trials** under **CLINICAL PHARMACOLOGY**). Based on these limited data, it is not known whether or not the dose of Effexor/Effexor XR needed for maintenance treatment is identical to the dose needed to achieve an initial response. Patients should be periodically reassessed to determine the need for maintenance treatment and the appropriate dose for such treatment.
In patients with Generalized Anxiety Disorder, Effexor XR has been shown to be effective in 6-month clinical trials. The need for continuing medication in patients with GAD who improve with Effexor XR treatment should be periodically reassessed.
In patients with Social Anxiety Disorder, there are no efficacy data beyond 12 weeks of treatment with Effexor XR. The need for continuing medication in patients with Social Anxiety Disorder who improve with Effexor XR treatment should be periodically reassessed.

Discontinuing Effexor XR
When discontinuing Effexor XR after more than 1 week of therapy, it is generally recommended that the dose be tapered to minimize the risk of discontinuation symptoms. Patients who have received Effexor XR for 6 weeks or more should have their dose tapered over at least a 2-week period. In clinical trials with Effexor XR, tapering was achieved by reducing the daily dose by 75 mg at 1 week intervals. Individualization of tapering may be necessary.
Discontinuation symptoms have been systematically evaluated in patients taking venlafaxine, to include prospective analyses of clinical trials in Generalized Anxiety Disorder and retrospective surveys of trials of major depressive disorder. Abrupt discontinuation or dose reduction of venlafaxine at various doses has been found to be associated with the appearance of new symptoms, the frequency of which increased with increased dose level and with longer duration of treatment. Reported symptoms include agitation, anorexia, anxiety, confusion, coordination impaired, diarrhea, dizziness, dry mouth, dysphoric mood, fasciculation, fatigue, headaches, hypomania, insomnia, nausea, nervousness, nightmares, sensory disturbances (including shock-like electrical sensations), somnolence, sweating, tremor, vertigo, and vomiting. It is therefore recommended that the dosage of Effexor XR be tapered gradually and the patient monitored. The period required for tapering may depend on the dose, duration of therapy and the individual patient. Discontinuation effects are well known to occur with antidepressants.

Switching Patients To or From a Monoamine Oxidase Inhibitor
At least 14 days should elapse between discontinuation of an MAOI and initiation of therapy with Effexor XR. In addition, at least 7 days should be allowed after stopping Effexor XR before starting an MAOI (see **CONTRAINDICATIONS** and **WARNINGS**).

HOW SUPPLIED

Effexor® XR (venlafaxine hydrochloride) extended-release capsules are available as follows:
37.5 mg, grey cap/peach body with W and "Effexor XR" on the cap and "37.5" on the body.
NDC 0008-0837-01, bottle of 100 capsules.
NDC 0008-0837-03, carton of 10 Redipak® blister strips of 10 capsules each.
Store at controlled room temperature, 20°C to 25°C (68°F to 77°F).
Bottles: Protect from light. Dispense in light-resistant container.
Blisters: Protect from light. Use blister carton to protect contents from light.
75 mg, peach cap and body with W and "Effexor XR" on the cap and "75" on the body.
NDC 0008-0833-01, bottle of 100 capsules.
NDC 0008-0833-03, carton of 10 Redipak® blister strips of 10 capsules each.
Store at controlled room temperature, 20°C to 25°C (68°F to 77°F).
150 mg, dark orange cap and body with W and "Effexor XR" on the cap and "150" on the body.
NDC 0008-0836-01, bottle of 100 capsules.
NDC 0008-0836-03, carton of 10 Redipak® blister strips of 10 capsules each.
Store at controlled room temperature, 20°C to 25°C (68°F to 77°F).
The appearance of these capsules is a trademark of Wyeth-Ayerst Laboratories.
Wyeth Laboratories
A Wyeth-Ayerst Company
Philadelphia, PA 19101 W10404C002
CI 7845-1 Rev 02/03

INDERAL® LA ℞
[ĭn'dûr-ăl]
(propranolol hydrochloride)
Long-Acting Capsules
℞ only

Prescribing information for this product, which appears on pages 3404–3406 of the 2003 PDR, has been revised as follows. Please write "See Supplement A" next to the product heading.
In the **DESCRIPTION** *section, the fourth paragraph has been revised as follows:*
Inderal LA capsules contain the following inactive ingredients: cellulose, ethylcellulose, gelatin capsules, hypromellose, and titanium dioxide. In addition, Inderal LA 60 mg, 80 mg, and 120 mg capsules contain D&C Red No. 28 and FD&C Blue No. 1; Inderal LA 160 mg capsules contain FD&C Blue No. 1.
In the **WARNINGS** *section, the subheading* **"Diabetes and Hypoglycemia"** *has been revised as follows:*
Diabetes and Hypoglycemia: Beta-adrenergic blockade may prevent the appearance of certain premonitory signs and symptoms (pulse rate and pressure changes) of acute hypoglycemia in labile insulin-dependent diabetes. In these patients, it may be more difficult to adjust the dosage of insulin. Hypoglycemic attacks may be accompanied by a precipitous elevation of blood pressure in patients on propranolol.
Propranolol therapy, particularly in infants and children, diabetic or not, has been associated with hypoglycemia especially during fasting as in preparation for surgery. Hypoglycemia also has been found after this type of drug therapy and prolonged physical exertion and has occurred in renal insufficiency, both during dialysis and sporadically, in patients on propranolol.
Acute increases in blood pressure have occurred after insulin-induced hypoglycemia in patients on propranolol.
Ayerst Laboratories
A Wyeth-Ayerst Company
Philadelphia, PA 19101
CI 4628-6 Revised June 10, 2002

METHOTREXATE SODIUM FOR INJECTION, ℞ METHOTREXATE LPF® SODIUM (METHOTREXATE SODIUM INJECTION) AND METHOTREXATE SODIUM INJECTION

Prescribing information for this product, which appears on pages 3415–3420 of the 2003 PDR, has been revised as follows. Please write "See Supplement A" next to the product heading.
Xanodyne Pharmacal, Inc. has distribution rights to the Methotrexate Injectable product. As a courtesy to PDR readers by Wyeth Pharmaceuticals, the current package insert for the product may be found on www.wyeth.com.

MYLOTARG® ℞
[*mī'lō-tärg*]
(gemtuzumab ozogamicin for Injection)
FOR INTRAVENOUS USE ONLY
℞ **only**

Prescribing information for this product, which appears on pages 3424–3427 of the 2003 PDR, has been revised as follows. Please write "See Supplement A" next to the product heading.

In the **DOSAGE AND ADMINISTRATION** *section, the* **"Stability and Storage"** *subsection has been revised as follows:*

Stability and Storage: Mylotarg should be stored refrigerated 2° to 8° C (36° to 46° F) and protected from light.

Wyeth Laboratories
Division of Wyeth-Ayerst Pharmaceuticals Inc.
Philadelphia, PA 19101
CI 7407-4
Revised May 28, 2002

NEUMEGA® ℞
[*nu-meg<a*]
(oprelvekin)
Rx ONLY

Prescribing information for this product, which appears on pages 3427–3429 of the 2003 PDR, has been completely revised as follows. Please write "See Supplement A" next to the product heading.

BOXED WARNING

Allergic Reactions Including Anaphylaxis
Neumega has caused allergic or hypersensitivity reactions, including anaphylaxis. Administration of Neumega should be permanently discontinued in any patient who develops an allergic or hypersensitivity reaction (see **WARNINGS, CONTRAINDICATIONS, ADVERSE REACTIONS** and **ADVERSE REACTIONS, Immunogenicity**).

DESCRIPTION

Interleukin eleven (IL-11) is a thrombopoietic growth factor that directly stimulates the proliferation of hematopoietic stem cells and megakaryocyte progenitor cells and induces megakaryocyte maturation resulting in increased platelet production. IL-11 is a member of a family of human growth factors which includes human growth hormone, granulocyte colony-stimulating factor (G-CSF), and other growth factors.

Oprelvekin, the active ingredient in Neumega, is produced in *Escherichia coli (E. coli)* by recombinant DNA technology. The protein has a molecular mass of approximately 19,000 daltons, and is non-glycosylated. The polypeptide is 177 amino acids in length and differs from the 178 amino acid length of native IL-11 only in lacking the amino-terminal proline residue. This alteration has not resulted in measurable differences in bioactivity either *in vitro* or *in vivo*.

Neumega is formulated in single-use vials containing 5 mg of oprelvekin (specific activity approximately 8×10^6 Units/mg) as a sterile, lyophilized powder with 23 mg Glycine, USP, 1.6 mg Dibasic Sodium Phosphate Heptahydrate, USP, and 0.55 mg Monobasic Sodium Phosphate Monohydrate, USP. When reconstituted with 1 mL of Sterile Water for Injection, USP, the resulting solution has a pH of 7.0 and a concentration of 5 mg/mL.

CLINICAL PHARMACOLOGY

The primary hematopoietic activity of Neumega is stimulation of megakaryocytopoiesis and thrombopoiesis. Neumega has shown potent thrombopoietic activity in animal models of compromised hematopoiesis, including moderately to severely myelosuppressed mice and nonhuman primates. In these models, Neumega improved platelet nadirs and accelerated platelet recoveries compared to controls.

Preclinical trials have shown that mature megakaryocytes which develop during *in vivo* treatment with Neumega are ultrastructurally normal. Platelets produced in response to Neumega were morphologically and functionally normal and possessed a normal life span.

IL-11 has also been shown to have non-hematopoietic activities in animals including the regulation of intestinal epithelium growth (enhanced healing of gastrointestinal lesions), the inhibition of adipogenesis, the induction of acute phase protein synthesis, inhibition of pro-inflammatory cytokine production by macrophages, and the stimulation of osteoclastogenesis and neurogenesis. Non-hematopoietic pathologic changes observed in animals include fibrosis of tendons and joint capsules, periosteal thickening, papilledema, and embryotoxicity (see **PRECAUTIONS, Pediatric Use** and **PRECAUTIONS, Pregnancy Category C**).

IL-11 is produced by bone marrow stromal cells and is part of the cytokine family that shares the gp130 signal transducer. Primary osteoblasts and mature osteoclasts express mRNAs for both IL-11 receptor (IL-11R alpha) and gp130. Both bone-forming and bone-resorbing cells are potential targets of IL-11. (1)

Pharmacokinetics

The pharmacokinetics of Neumega have been evaluated in studies of healthy, adult subjects and cancer patients receiving chemotherapy. In a study in which a single 50 µg/kg subcutaneous dose was administered to eighteen healthy men, the peak serum concentration (C_{max}) of 17.4 ± 5.4 ng/mL (mean ± S.D.) was reached at 3.2 ± 2.4 hrs (T_{max}) following dosing. The terminal half-life was 6.9 ± 1.7 hrs. In a second study in which single 75 µg/kg subcutaneous and intravenous doses were administered to twenty-four healthy subjects, the pharmacokinetic profiles were similar between men and women. The absolute bioavailability of Neumega was >80%. In a study in which multiple, subcutaneous doses of both 25 and 50 µg/kg were administered to cancer patients receiving chemotherapy, Neumega did not accumulate and clearance of Neumega was not impaired following multiple doses.

In a dose escalation Phase 1 study, Neumega was also administered to 43 pediatric (ages 8 months to 18 years) and 1 adult patient receiving ICE (ifosfamide, carboplatin, etoposide) chemotherapy. Administered doses ranged from 25 to 125 µg/kg. Analysis of data from 40 pediatric patients showed that C_{max}, T_{max}, and terminal half-life were comparable to that in adults. The mean area under the concentration-time curve (AUC) for pediatric patients (8 months to 18 years), receiving 50 µg/kg was approximately half that achieved in healthy adults receiving 50 µg/kg. Available data suggest that clearance of IL-11 decreases with increasing age.

In preclinical trials in rats, radiolabeled Neumega was rapidly cleared from the serum and distributed to highly perfused organs. The kidney was the primary route of elimination. The amount of intact Neumega in urine was low, indicating that the molecule was metabolized before excretion. In a clinical study, a single dose of Neumega was administered to subjects with severely impaired renal function (creatinine clearance <15 mL/min). The mean ± S.D. values for C_{max} and AUC were 30.8 ± 8.6 ng/mL and 373 ± 106 ng*hr/mL, respectively. When compared with control subjects in this study with normal renal function, the mean C_{max} was 2.2 fold higher and the mean AUC was 2.6 fold (95% confidence interval, 1.7%-3.8%) higher in the subjects with severe renal impairment. In the subjects with severe renal impairment, clearance was approximately 40% of the value seen in subjects with normal renal function. The average terminal half-life was similar in subjects with severe renal impairment and those with normal renal function.

Pharmacodynamics

In a study in which Neumega was administered to non-myelosuppressed cancer patients, daily subcutaneous dosing for 14 days with Neumega increased the platelet count in a dose-dependent manner. Platelet counts began to increase relative to baseline between 5 and 9 days after the start of dosing with Neumega. After cessation of treatment, platelet counts continued to increase for up to 7 days then returned toward baseline within 14 days. No change in platelet reactivity as measured by platelet activation in response to ADP, and platelet aggregation in response to ADP, epinephrine, collagen, ristocetin and arachidonic acid has been observed in association with Neumega treatment.

In a randomized, double-blind, placebo-controlled study in normal volunteers, subjects receiving Neumega had a mean increase in plasma volume of >20%, and all subjects receiving Neumega had at least a 10% increase in plasma volume. Red blood cell volume decreased similarly (due to repeated phlebotomy) in the Neumega and placebo groups. As a result, whole blood volume increased approximately 10% and hemoglobin concentration decreased approximately 10% in subjects receiving Neumega compared with subjects receiving placebo. Mean 24 hour sodium excretion decreased, and potassium excretion did not increase, in subjects receiving Neumega compared with subjects receiving placebo.

CLINICAL STUDIES

Two randomized, double-blind, placebo-controlled trials in adults studied Neumega for the prevention of severe thrombocytopenia following single or repeated sequential cycles of various myelosuppressive chemotherapy regimens.

One study evaluated the effectiveness of Neumega in eliminating the need for platelet transfusions in patients who had recovered from an episode of severe chemotherapy-induced thrombocytopenia (defined as a platelet count ≤20,000/µL), and were to receive one additional cycle of the same chemotherapy without dose reduction. Patients had various underlying non-myeloid malignancies, and were undergoing dose-intensive chemotherapy with a variety of regimens. Patients were randomized to receive Neumega at a dose of 25 µg/kg or 50 µg/kg, or placebo.

The primary endpoint was whether the patient required one or more platelet transfusions in the subsequent chemotherapy cycle. Ninety-three patients were randomized. Five patients withdrew from the study prior to receiving study drug. As a result, eighty-eight patients were included in a modified intent-to-treat analysis. The results for the Neumega 50 µg/kg and placebo groups are summarized in Table 1. The placebo group includes one patient who underwent chemotherapy dose reduction and who avoided platelet transfusions.

TABLE 1
STUDY RESULTS

	Placebo n=30	Neumega 50 µg/kg n=29
Number (%) of patients avoiding platelet transfusion	2 (7%)	8 (28%)
Number (%) of patients requiring platelet transfusion	28 (93%)	21 (72%)
Median (mean) number of platelet transfusion events	2.5 (3.3)	1 (2.2)

In the primary efficacy analysis, more patients avoided platelet transfusion in the Neumega 50 µg/kg arm than in the placebo arm (p = 0.04, Fisher's Exact test, 2-tailed). The difference in the proportion of patients avoiding platelet transfusions in the Neumega 50 µg/kg and placebo groups was 21% (95% confidence interval, 2%-40%). The results observed in patients receiving 25 µg/kg of Neumega were intermediate between those of the placebo and the 50 µg/kg groups.

A second study evaluated the effectiveness of Neumega in eliminating platelet transfusions over two dose-intensive chemotherapy cycles in breast cancer patients who had not previously experienced severe chemotherapy-induced thrombocytopenia. All patients received the same chemotherapy regimen (cyclophosphamide 3,200 mg/m² and doxorubicin 75 mg/m²). All patients received concomitant filgrastim (G-CSF) in all cycles. The patients were stratified by whether or not they had received prior chemotherapy, and randomized to receive Neumega 50 µg/kg or placebo. The primary endpoint was whether or not a patient required one or more platelet transfusions in the two study cycles. Seventy-seven patients were randomized. Thirteen patients failed to complete both study cycles—eight of these had insufficient data to be evaluated for the primary endpoint. The results of this trial are summarized in Table 2.

TABLE 2
STUDY RESULTS

	Overall n=77		No Prior Chemotherapy n=54		Prior Chemotherapy n=23	
	Placebo n=37	Neumega n=40	Placebo n=27	Neumega n=27	Placebo n=10	Neumega n=13
Number (%) of patients avoiding platelet transfusion	15 (41%)	26 (65%)	14 (52%)	19 (70%)	1 (10%)	7 (54%)
Number (%) of patients requiring platelet transfusion	16 (43%)	12 (30%)	9 (33%)	7 (26%)	7 (70%)	5 (38%)
Number (%) of patients not evaluable	6 (16%)	2 (5%)	4 (15%)	1 (4%)	2 (20%)	1 (8%)

This study showed a trend in favor of Neumega, particularly in the subgroup of patients with prior chemotherapy. Open-label treatment with Neumega has been continued for up to four consecutive chemotherapy cycles without evidence of any adverse effect on the rate of neutrophil recovery or red blood cell transfusion requirements. Some patients continued to maintain platelet nadirs >20,000/µL for at least four sequential cycles of chemotherapy without the need for transfusions, chemotherapy dose reduction, or changes in treatment schedules.

Platelet activation studies done on a limited number of patients showed no evidence of abnormal spontaneous platelet activation, or an abnormal response to ADP. In an unblinded, retrospective analysis of the two placebo-controlled studies, 19 of 69 patients (28%) receiving Neumega 50 µg/kg and 34 of 67 patients (51%) receiving placebo reported at least one hemorrhagic adverse event which involved bleeding.

In a randomized, double-blind, placebo-controlled, Phase 2 study conducted in patients who received autologous bone marrow transplantation following myeloablative chemotherapy, the incidence of platelet transfusions and time to neutrophil and platelet engraftment were similar in the Neumega and placebo-treated arms.

[See table 2 above]

In long term follow-up of patients, the distribution of survival and progression-free survival times was similar between patients randomized to Neumega therapy and those randomized to receive placebo.

INDICATIONS AND USAGE

Neumega is indicated for the prevention of severe thrombocytopenia and the reduction of the need for platelet transfusions following myelosuppressive chemotherapy in adult patients with nonmyeloid malignancies who are at high risk of severe thrombocytopenia. Efficacy was demonstrated in patients who had experienced severe thrombocytopenia following the previous chemotherapy cycle. Neumega is not in-

Continued on next page

Neumega—Cont.

dicated following myeloablative chemotherapy. The safety and effectiveness of Neumega have not been established in pediatric patients.

CONTRAINDICATIONS
Neumega is contraindicated in patients with a history of hypersensitivity to Neumega or any component of the product (see WARNINGS, Allergic Reactions Including Anaphylaxis).

WARNINGS
Allergic Reactions Including Anaphylaxis
In the post-marketing setting, Neumega has caused allergic or hypersensitivity reactions, including anaphylaxis. The administration of Neumega should be attended by appropriate precautions in case allergic reactions occur. In addition, patients should be counseled about the symptoms for which they should seek medical attention (see PRECAUTIONS, Information for Patients). Signs and symptoms reported included edema of the face, tongue, or larynx; shortness of breath; wheezing; chest pain; hypotension (including shock); dysarthria; loss of consciousness; mental status changes; rash; urticaria; flushing and fever. Reactions occurred after the first dose or subsequent doses of Neumega. Administration of Neumega should be permanently discontinued in any patient who develops an allergic or hypersensitivity reaction (see BOXED WARNING, CONTRAINDICATIONS, ADVERSE REACTIONS, and ADVERSE REACTIONS, Immunogenicity).

Fluid Retention
Neumega is known to cause serious fluid retention that can result in peripheral edema, dyspnea on exertion, pulmonary edema, capillary leak syndrome, atrial arrhythmias, and exacerbation of pre-existing pleural effusions. (see CLINICAL PHARMACOLOGY, Pharmacodynamics; WARNINGS, Cardiovascular Events; and WARNINGS, Dilutional Anemia). It should be used with caution in patients with clinically evident congestive heart failure, patients who may be susceptible to developing congestive heart failure, patients receiving aggressive hydration, patients with a history of heart failure who are well-compensated and receiving appropriate medical therapy, and patients who may develop fluid retention as a result of associated medical conditions or whose medical condition may be exacerbated by fluid retention.

Fluid retention is reversible within several days following discontinuation of Neumega. During dosing with Neumega, fluid balance should be monitored and appropriate medical management is advised.

Close monitoring of fluid and electrolyte status should be performed in patients receiving chronic diuretic therapy. Sudden deaths have occurred in oprelvekin-treated patients receiving chronic diuretic therapy and ifosfamide who developed severe hypokalemia (see ADVERSE REACTIONS).

Pre-existing fluid collections, including pericardial effusions or ascites, should be monitored. Drainage should be considered if medically indicated.

Dilutional Anemia
Moderate decreases in hemoglobin concentration, hematocrit, and red blood cell count (~10% to 15%) without a decrease in red blood cell mass have been observed. These changes are predominantly due to an increase in plasma volume (dilutional anemia) that is primarily related to renal sodium and water retention. The decrease in hemoglobin concentration typically begins within 3 to 5 days of the initiation of Neumega, and is reversible over approximately a week following discontinuation of Neumega (see WARNINGS, Fluid Retention).

Cardiovascular Events
Neumega use is associated with cardiovascular events including arrhythmias and pulmonary edema. Cardiac arrest has been reported, but the causal relationship to Neumega is uncertain. Use with caution in patients with a history of atrial arrhythmias, and only after consideration of the potential risks in relation to anticipated benefit. In clinical trials, cardiac events including atrial arrhythmias (atrial fibrillation or atrial flutter) occurred in 15% (23/157) of patients treated with Neumega at doses of 50 µg/kg. Arrhythmias were usually brief in duration; conversion to sinus rhythm typically occurred spontaneously or after rate-control drug therapy. Approximately one-half (11/24) of the patients who were rechallenged had recurrent atrial arrhythmias. Clinical sequelae, including stroke, have been reported in patients who experienced atrial arrhythmias while receiving Neumega.

The mechanism for induction of arrhythmias is not known. Neumega was not directly arrhythmogenic in animal models. In some patients, development of atrial arrhythmias may be due to increased plasma volume associated with fluid retention (see WARNINGS, Fluid Retention).

Nervous System Events
Stroke has been reported in the setting of patients who develop atrial fibrillation/flutter while receiving Neumega (see WARNINGS, Cardiovascular Events). Patients with a history of stroke or transient ischemic attack may also be at increased risk for these events.

Papilledema
Papilledema has been reported in 2% (10/405) of patients receiving Neumega in clinical trials following repeated cycles of exposure. The incidence was higher, 16% (7/43) in children than in adults, 1% (3/362). Nonhuman primates treated with Neumega at a dose of 1,000 µg/kg SC once daily for 4 to 13 weeks developed papilledema that was not associated with inflammation or any other histologic abnormality and was reversible after dosing was discontinued. Neumega should be used with caution in patients with pre-existing papilledema, or with tumors involving the central nervous system since it is possible that papilledema could worsen or develop during treatment (see ADVERSE REACTIONS).

PRECAUTIONS
General
Dosing with Neumega should begin 6 to 24 hours following the completion of chemotherapy dosing. The safety and efficacy of Neumega given immediately prior to or concurrently with cytotoxic chemotherapy or initiated at the time of expected nadir have not been established (see DOSAGE AND ADMINISTRATION).

The effectiveness of Neumega has not been evaluated in patients receiving chemotherapy regimens of greater than 5 days duration or regimens associated with delayed myelosuppression (eg, nitrosoureas, mitomycin-C).

Chronic Administration
Neumega has been administered safely using the recommended dosage schedule (see DOSAGE AND ADMINISTRATION) for up to 6 cycles following chemotherapy. The safety and efficacy of chronic administration of Neumega have not been established. Continuous dosage (2 to 13 weeks) in nonhuman primates produced joint capsule and tendon fibrosis and periosteal hyperostosis (see PRECAUTIONS, Pediatric Use). The relevance of these findings to humans is unclear.

Information for Patients
Neumega should be used under the guidance and supervision of a health care professional. However, when the physician determines that Neumega may be used outside of the hospital or office setting, persons who will be administering Neumega should be instructed as to the proper dose, and the method for reconstituting and administering Neumega (see DOSAGE AND ADMINISTRATION). If home use is prescribed, patients should be instructed in the importance of proper disposal and cautioned against the reuse of needles, syringes, drug product, and diluent. A puncture resistant container should be used by the patient for the disposal of used needles.

Patients should be informed of the serious and most common adverse reactions associated with Neumega administration, including those symptoms related to allergic or hypersensitivity reactions (see BOXED WARNING). Patients should be advised to immediately seek medical attention if any of the following signs or symptoms develop: swelling of the face, tongue, or throat; difficulty breathing, swallowing or talking; shortness of breath; wheezing; chest pain; throat tightness; lightheadedness; loss of consciousness; confusion; drowsiness; rash; itching; hives; flushing and/or fever. Mild to moderate peripheral edema and shortness of breath on exertion can occur within the first week of treatment and may continue for the duration of administration of Neumega. Patients who have preexisting pleural or other effusions or a history of congestive heart failure should be advised to contact their physician for worsening of dyspnea (see ADVERSE REACTIONS and WARNINGS, Fluid Retention). Most patients who receive Neumega develop anemia. Patients should be advised to contact their physician if symptoms attributable to atrial arrhythmia develop. Female patients of childbearing potential should be advised of the possible risks to the fetus of Neumega (see PRECAUTIONS, Pregnancy Category C).

Laboratory Monitoring
A complete blood count should be obtained prior to chemotherapy and at regular intervals during Neumega therapy (see DOSAGE AND ADMINISTRATION). Platelet counts should be monitored during the time of the expected nadir and until adequate recovery has occurred (post-nadir counts ≥50,000/µL).

Drug Interactions
Most patients in trials evaluating Neumega were treated concomitantly with filgrastim (G-CSF) with no adverse effect of Neumega on the activity of G-CSF. No information is available on the clinical use of sargramostim (GM-CSF) with Neumega in human subjects. However, in a study in nonhuman primates in which Neumega and GM-CSF were coadministered, there were no adverse interactions between Neumega and GM-CSF and no apparent difference in the pharmacokinetic profile of Neumega.

Drug interactions between Neumega and other drugs have not been fully evaluated. Based on in vitro and nonclinical in vivo evaluations of Neumega, drug-drug interactions with known substrates of P450 enzymes would not be predicted.

Carcinogenesis, Mutagenesis, Impairment of Fertility
No studies have been performed to assess the carcinogenic potential of Neumega. In vitro, Neumega did not stimulate the growth of tumor colony-forming cells harvested from patients with a variety of human malignancies. Neumega has been shown to be non-genotoxic in in vitro studies. These data suggest that Neumega is not mutagenic. Although prolonged estrus cycles have been noted at 2 to 20 times the human dose, no effects on fertility have been observed in rats treated with Neumega at doses up to 1000 µg/kg/day.

Pregnancy Category C
Neumega has been shown to have embryocidal effects in pregnant rats and rabbits when given in doses of 0.2 to 20 times the human dose. There are no adequate and well-controlled studies of Neumega in pregnant women. Neumega should be used during pregnancy only if the potential benefit justifies the potential risk to the fetus.

Neumega has been tested in studies of fertility, early embryonic development, and pre and postnatal development in rats and in studies of organogenesis (teratogenicity) in rats and rabbits. Parental toxicity has been observed when Neumega is given at doses of 2 to 20 times the human dose (≥100 µg/kg/day) in the rat and at 0.02 to 2.0 times the human dose (≥1 µg/kg/day) in the rabbit. Findings in pregnant rats consisted of transient hypoactivity and dyspnea after administration (maternal toxicity), as well as prolonged estrus cycle, increased early embryonic deaths and decreased numbers of live fetuses. In addition, low fetal body weights and a reduced number of ossified sacral and caudal vertebrae (ie, retarded fetal development) occurred in rats at 20 times the human dose. Findings in pregnant rabbits consisted of decreased fecal/urine eliminations (the only toxicity noted at 1 µg/kg/day in dams) as well as decreased food consumption, body weight loss, abortion, increased embryonic and fetal deaths, and decreased numbers of live fetuses. No teratogenic effects of Neumega were observed in rabbits at doses up to 0.6 times the human dose (30 µg/kg/day).

Adverse effects in the first generation offspring of rats given Neumega at maternally toxic doses ≥2 times the human dose (≥100 µg/kg/day) during both gestation and lactation included increased newborn mortality, decreased viability index on day 4 of lactation, and decreased body weights during lactation. In rats given 20 times the human dose (1000 µg/kg/day) during both gestation and lactation, maternal toxicity and growth retardation of the first generation offspring resulted in an increased rate of fetal death of the second generation offspring.

Nursing Mothers
It is not known if Neumega is excreted in human milk. Because many drugs are excreted in human milk and because of the potential for serious adverse reactions in nursing infants from Neumega, a decision should be made whether to discontinue nursing or to discontinue Neumega, taking into account the importance of the drug to the mother.

Pediatric Use
A safe and effective dose of Neumega has not been established in children. In a Phase 1, single arm, dose-escalation study, 43 pediatric patients were treated with Neumega at doses ranging from 25 to 125 µg/kg/day following ICE chemotherapy. All patients required platelet transfusions and the lack of a comparator arm made the study design inadequate to assess efficacy. The projected effective dose (based on comparable AUC observed for the effective dose in healthy adults) in children appears to exceed the maximum tolerated pediatric dose of 50 µg/kg/day (see CLINICAL PHARMACOLOGY, Pharmacokinetics). Papilledema was dose-limiting and occurred in 16% of children (see WARNINGS, Papilledema).

The most common adverse events seen in pediatric studies included tachycardia (84%), conjunctival injection (58%), radiographic and echocardiographic evidence of cardiomegaly (21%) and periosteal changes (11%). These events occurred at a higher frequency in children than adults. The incidence of other adverse events were generally similar to those observed using Neumega at a dose of 50 µg/kg in the randomized studies in adults receiving chemotherapy (see ADVERSE REACTIONS).

Studies in animals were predictive of the effect of Neumega on developing bone in children. In growing rodents treated with 100, 300, or 1000 µg/kg/day for a minimum of 28 days, thickening of femoral and tibial growth plates was noted, which did not completely resolve after a 28-day non-treatment period. In a nonhuman primate toxicology study of Neumega, animals treated for 2 to 13 weeks at doses of 10 to 1000 µg/kg showed partially reversible joint capsule and tendon fibrosis and periosteal hyperostosis. An asymptomatic, laminated periosteal reaction in the diaphyses of the femur, tibia, and fibula has been observed in one patient during pediatric studies involving multiple courses of Neumega treatment. The relationship of these findings to treatment with Neumega is unclear. No studies have been performed to assess the long-term effects of Neumega on growth and development.

Use in Patients with Renal Impairment
Neumega is eliminated primarily by the kidneys. The pharmacokinetics of Neumega have not been studied in patients with mild or moderate renal impairment (creatinine clearance ≥15 mL/min). Fluid retention associated with Neumega treatment has not been studied in patients with renal impairment, but fluid balance should be carefully monitored in these patients (see WARNINGS, Fluid Retention).

ADVERSE REACTIONS
Because clinical trials are conducted under widely varying conditions, adverse reaction rates observed in the clinical studies of a drug cannot be directly compared to rates in the clinical studies of another drug and may not reflect the rates observed in practice. The adverse reaction information from clinical trials does, however, provide a basis for identifying the adverse events that appear to be related to drug use and for approximating rates.

Three hundred twenty-four subjects, with ages ranging from 8 months to 75 years, have been exposed to Neumega treatment in clinical studies. Subjects have received up to six (eight in pediatric patients) sequential courses of Neumega treatment, with each course lasting from 1 to 28 days. Apart from the sequelae of the underlying malignancy or cytotoxic chemotherapy, most adverse events were mild or moderate in severity and reversible after discontinuation of Neumega dosing.

In general, the incidence and type of adverse events were similar between Neumega 50 µg/kg and placebo groups. The most frequently reported serious adverse events were neutropenic fever, syncope, atrial fibrillation, fever and pneumonia. The most commonly reported adverse events were edema, dyspnea, tachycardia, conjunctival injection, palpitations, atrial arrhythmias, and pleural effusions. The most frequently reported adverse reactions resulting in clinical intervention (eg, discontinuation of Neumega, adjustment in dosage, or the need for concomitant medication to treat an adverse reaction symptom) were atrial arrhythmias, syncope, dyspnea, congestive heart failure, and pulmonary edema (see **WARNINGS**). Selected adverse events that occurred in ≥10% of Neumega-treated patients are listed in Table 3.
The following adverse events also occurred more frequently in cancer patients receiving Neumega than in those receiving placebo: amblyopia, paresthesia, dehydration, skin discoloration, exfoliative dermatitis, and eye hemorrhage; a statistically significant association of Neumega to these events has not been established. Other than a higher incidence of severe asthenia in Neumega treated patients (10 [14%] in Neumega patients versus 2 [3%] in placebo patients), the incidence of severe or life-threatening adverse events was comparable in the Neumega and placebo treatment groups.
Two patients with cancer treated with Neumega experienced sudden death which the investigator considered possibly or probably related to Neumega. Both deaths occurred in patients with severe hypokalemia (<3.0 mEq/L) who had received high doses of ifosfamide and were receiving daily doses of a diuretic (see **WARNINGS, Cardiovascular Events**).
Other serious events associated with Neumega were cardiovascular events including atrial arrhythmias, stroke and papilledema. In addition, cardiomegaly was reported in children.
The following adverse events, occurring in ≥10% of patients, were observed at equal or greater frequency in placebo-treated patients: asthenia, pain, chills, abdominal pain, infection, anorexia, constipation, dyspepsia, ecchymosis, myalgia, bone pain, nervousness, and alopecia. The incidence of fever, neutropenic fever, flu-like symptoms, thrombocytosis, thrombotic events, the average number of units of red blood cells transfused per patient, and the duration of neutropenia <500 cells/µL were similar in the Neumega 50 µg/kg and placebo groups.

Immunogenicity
In clinical studies that evaluated the immunogenicity of Neumega, two of 181 patients (1%) developed antibodies to Neumega. In one of these two patients, neutralizing antibodies to Neumega were detected in an unvalidated assay. The clinical relevance of the presence of these antibodies is unknown. In the post-marketing setting, cases of allergic reactions, including anaphylaxis have been reported (see **WARNINGS, Allergic Reactions Including Anaphylaxis**). The presence of antibodies to Neumega was not assessed in these patients.

TABLE 3
SELECTED ADVERSE EVENTS

Body System Adverse Event	Placebo n=67 (%)	50 µg/kg n=69 (%)
Body as a Whole		
Edema*	10 (15)	41 (59)
Neutropenic fever	28 (42)	33 (48)
Headache	24 (36)	28 (41)
Fever	19 (28)	25 (36)
Cardiovascular System		
Tachycardia*	2 (3)	14 (20)
Vasodilatation	6 (9)	13 (19)
Palpitations*	2 (3)	10 (14)
Syncope	4 (6)	9 (13)
Atrial fibrillation/ flutter*	1 (1)	8 (12)
Digestive System		
Nausea/vomiting	47 (70)	53 (77)
Mucositis	25 (37)	30 (43)
Diarrhea	22 (33)	30 (43)
Oral moniliasis*	1 (1)	10 (14)
Nervous System		
Dizziness	19 (28)	26 (38)
Insomnia	18 (27)	23 (33)
Respiratory System		
Dyspnea*	15 (22)	33 (48)
Rhinitis	21 (31)	29 (42)
Cough increased	15 (22)	20 (29)
Pharyngitis	11 (16)	17 (25)
Pleural effusions	0 (0)	7 (10)
Skin and Appendages		
Rash	11 (16)	17 (25)
Special Senses		
Conjunctival injection	2 (3)	13 (19)

*Occurred in significantly more Neumega-treated patients than in placebo-treated patients.

The data reflect the percentage of patients whose test results were considered positive for antibodies to Neumega and are highly dependent on the sensitivity and specificity of the assay. Additionally the observed incidence of antibody positivity in an assay may be influenced by several factors including sample handling, concomitant medications, and underlying disease. For these reasons, comparisons of the incidence of antibodies to Neumega with incidence of antibodies to other products may be misleading.

Abnormal Laboratory Values
The most common laboratory abnormality reported in patients in clinical trials was a decrease in hemoglobin concentration predominantly as a result of expansion of the plasma volume (see **WARNINGS, Fluid Retention**). The increase in plasma volume is also associated with a decrease in the serum concentration of albumin and several other proteins (eg, transferrin and gamma globulins). A parallel decrease in calcium without clinical effects has been documented.
After daily SC injections, treatment with Neumega resulted in a two-fold increase in plasma fibrinogen. Other acute-phase proteins also increased. These protein levels returned to normal after dosing with Neumega was discontinued. Von Willebrand factor (vWF) concentrations increased with a normal multimer pattern in healthy subjects receiving Neumega.

Postmarketing Reports
The following adverse reactions have been reported during the post-approval use of Neumega: allergic reactions, anaphylaxis (see **BOXED WARNING, WARNINGS, Allergic Reactions Including Anaphylaxis** and **CONTRAINDICATIONS**).
Because these reactions are reported voluntarily from a population of uncertain size, it is not always possible to reliably estimate their frequency or establish a causal relationship to drug exposure. Decisions to include these reactions in labeling are typically based on one or more of the following factors: (1) seriousness of the reactions, (2) frequency of reporting, or (3) strength of causal connection to Neumega.

OVERDOSAGE
Doses of Neumega above 125 µg/kg have not been administered to humans. While clinical experience is limited, doses of Neumega greater than 50 µg/kg may be associated with an increased incidence of cardiovascular events in adult patients (see **WARNINGS, Fluid Retention** and **Cardiovascular Events**). If an overdose of Neumega is administered, Neumega should be discontinued, and the patient should be closely observed for signs of toxicity (see **WARNINGS** and **ADVERSE REACTIONS**). Reinstitution of Neumega therapy should be based upon individual patient factors (eg, evidence of toxicity, continued need for therapy).

DOSAGE AND ADMINISTRATION
The recommended dose of Neumega in adults is 50 µg/kg given once daily. Neumega should be administered subcutaneously as a single injection in either the abdomen, thigh, or hip (or upper arm if not self-injecting). A safe and effective dose has not been established in children (see **PRECAUTIONS, Pediatric Use**).
Dosing should be initiated 6 to 24 hours after the completion of chemotherapy. Platelet counts should be monitored periodically to assess the optimal duration of therapy. Dosing should be continued until the post-nadir platelet count is ≥50,000/µL. In controlled clinical trials, doses were administered in courses of 10 to 21 days. Dosing beyond 21 days per treatment course is not recommended.
Treatment with Neumega should be discontinued at least 2 days before starting the next planned cycle of chemotherapy.

Preparation of Neumega
1. Neumega is a sterile, white, preservative-free, lyophilized powder for subcutaneous injection upon reconstitution. Neumega (5 mg vials) should be reconstituted aseptically with 1.0 mL of Sterile Water for Injection, USP (without preservative). The reconstituted Neumega solution is clear, colorless, isotonic, with a pH of 7.0, and contains 5 mg/mL of Neumega. The single-use vial should not be re-entered or reused. Any unused portion of either reconstituted Neumega solution or Sterile Water for Injection, USP should be discarded.
2. During reconstitution, the Sterile Water for Injection, USP should be directed at the side of the vial and the contents gently swirled. EXCESSIVE OR VIGOROUS AGITATION SHOULD BE AVOIDED.
3. Parenteral drug products should be inspected visually for particulate matter and discoloration prior to administration, whenever solution and container permit. If particulate matter is present or the solution is discolored, the vial should not be used.
4. Because neither Neumega powder for injection nor its accompanying diluent, Sterile Water for Injection, USP contains a preservative, Neumega should be used within 3 hours following reconstitution. Reconstituted Neumega may be refrigerated [2°C to 8°C (36°F to 46°F)] or at room temperature [up to 25°C (77°F)]. DO NOT FREEZE OR SHAKE THE RECONSTITUTED SOLUTION.

HOW SUPPLIED
Neumega is supplied as a sterile, white, preservative-free, lyophilized powder in vials containing 5 mg oprelvekin. Neumega is available in boxes containing one single-dose Neumega vial and one 1-mL vial of diluent for Neumega (Sterile Water for Injection, USP) - NDC 58394-004-01, and boxes containing seven single-dose Neumega vials and seven 1-mL vials of diluent for Neumega (Sterile Water for Injection, USP) - NDC 58394-004-02.

Storage
Lyophilized Neumega and diluent should be stored in a refrigerator at 2°C to 8°C (36°F to 46°F). Protect from light. DO NOT FREEZE. Reconstituted Neumega must be used within 3 hours of reconstitution and can be stored in the vial either at 2°C to 8°C (36°F to 46°F) or at room temperature up to 25°C (77°F).

REFERENCES
(1) Du, X. and Williams, D., Interleukin 11: review of molecular, cell biology and clinical use. *Blood.* 1997;89(11):3897-3908.
Genetics Institute, Inc.
Cambridge, MA 02140-2387, USA
US License Number 1163
Telephone: 1-800-934-5556
Rev. 9/02
4004G110

OVRETTE® Tablets ℞
[*oh-vrĕt'*]
(norgestrel tablets)
℞ only

Prescribing information for this product, which appears on pages 3431–3432 of the 2003 PDR, has been revised as follows. Please write "See Supplement A" next to the product heading.
The **HOW SUPPLIED** *section was revised as follows:*
HOW SUPPLIED
OVRETTE® tablets (0.075 mg norgestrel) are available in packages of 6 PILPAK® dispensers with 28 tablets each as follows: NDC 0008-0062-01, yellow, round tablet marked "WYETH" on one side and "62" on reverse side.
Wyeth Laboratories
A Wyeth-Ayerst Company
Philadelphia, PA 19101 CI 7782-1 Issued October 16, 2002

PIPRACIL® ℞
[*pĭp'rā-sĭl*]
(piperacillin for injection)
For intravenous and Intramuscular Use
℞ only

Prescribing infomation for this product, which appears on pages 3434–3437 of the 2003 PDR, has been revised as follows. Please write "See Supplement A" next to the product heading.
The **DESCRIPTION** *section has been revised as follows:*
DESCRIPTION
PIPRACIL® (piperacillin for injection) is a semisynthetic broad-spectrum penicillin for parenteral use derived from D(-)-α-aminobenzylpenicillin. The chemical name of piperacillin sodium is 4-Thia-1-azabicyclo[3.2.0]heptane-2-carboxylic acid, 6-[[[[(4-ethyl-2,3-dioxo-1-piperazinyl)carbonyl]amino]phenylacetyl] amino]-3,3-dimethyl-7-oxo-, monosodium salt, [2*S*-[2α,5α,6β(*S**)]]. The chemical formula is $C_{23}H_{26}N_5NaO_7S$ and the molecular weight is 539.54. Its structural formula is:

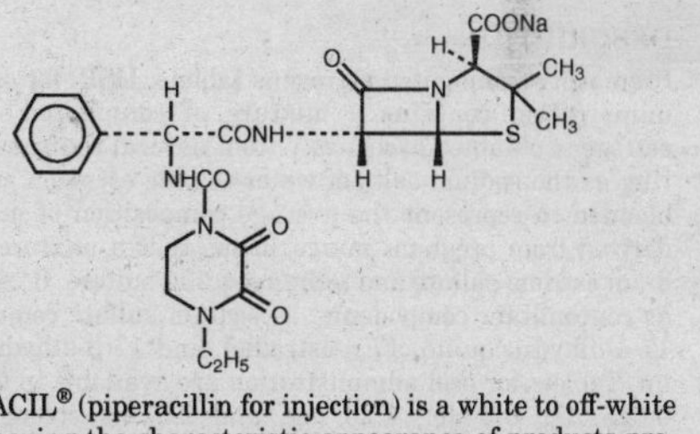

PIPRACIL® (piperacillin for injection) is a white to off-white solid having the characteristic appearance of products prepared by freeze-drying. Freely soluble in water and in alcohol. The pH of the aqueous solution is 5.5 to 7.5. One g contains 1.85 mEq (42.5 mg) of sodium (Na^+).
In the **DOSAGE AND ADMINISTRATION** *section, the subheading* **"Intravenous Administration"** *has been revised as follows:*
Intravenous Administration
Reconstitution Directions for Conventional Vials: Reconstitute each gram of PIPRACIL with at least 5 mL of a suitable diluent (except Lidocaine HCl 0.5%-1% without epinephrine) listed above. Shake well until dissolved. Reconstituted solution may be further diluted to the desired volume (eg, 50 or 100 mL) in the above listed intravenous solutions and admixtures.
Reconstitution Directions for ADD-Vantage Vials: See Instruction Sheet provided in box.
DIRECTIONS FOR ADMINISTRATION
Intermittent IV Infusion
Infuse diluted solution over period of about 30 minutes. During infusion it is desirable to discontinue the primary intravenous solution.
Intravenous Injection (Bolus)
Reconstituted solution should be injected slowly over a 3- to 5-minute period to help avoid vein irritation.
The **HOW SUPPLIED** *section has been revised as follows:*
HOW SUPPLIED
PIPRACIL® (piperacillin for injection) is available in vials containing freeze-dried piperacillin sodium powder equivalent to two, three, and four g of piperacillin. One g of piperacillin (as a monosodium salt) contains 1.85 mEq (42.5 mg) of sodium.

Continued on next page

Pipracil—Cont.

Product Numbers
2 gram/Vial - 10 per box - NDC 0206-3879-16
3 gram/Vial - 10 per box - NDC 0206-3882-55
4 gram/Vial - 10 per box - NDC 0206-3880-25
3 gram ADD-Vantage Vial - 10 per box - NDC 0206-3882-28
4 gram ADD-Vantage Vial - 10 per box - NDC 0206-3880-29

Store at controlled room temperature 20° to 25°C (68° to 77°F).
LEDERLE
PIPERACILLIN, INC.
Carolina, Puerto Rico 00987
CI 4579-4   Revised 10/2002

PREMARIN® ℞
[prĕm'ărĭn]
(conjugated estrogens tablets, USP)
℞ only

Prescribing information for this product, which appears on pages 3444–3447 of the 2003 PDR, has been completely revised as follows. Please write "See Supplement A" next to the product heading.

ESTROGENS INCREASE THE RISK OF ENDOMETRIAL CANCER

Close clinical surveillance of all women taking estrogens is important. Adequate diagnostic measures, including endometrial sampling when indicated, should be undertaken to rule out malignancy in all cases of undiagnosed persistent or recurring abnormal vaginal bleeding. There is no evidence that the use of "natural" estrogens results in a different endometrial risk profile than synthetic estrogens of equivalent estrogen dose.

CARDIOVASCULAR AND OTHER RISKS

Estrogens with or without progestins should not be used for the prevention of cardiovascular disease.
The Women's Health Initiative (WHI) reported increased risks of myocardial infarction, stroke, invasive breast cancer, pulmonary emboli, and deep vein thrombosis in postmenopausal women during 5 years of treatment with conjugated equine estrogens (0.625 mg) combined with medroxyprogesterone acetate (2.5 mg) relative to placebo (see **CLINICAL PHARMACOLOGY, Clinical Studies**). Other doses of conjugated estrogens and medroxyprogesterone acetate, and other combinations of estrogens and progestins were not studied in the WHI and, in the absence of comparable data, these risks should be assumed to be similar. Because of these risks, estrogens with or without progestins should be prescribed at the lowest effective doses and for the shortest duration consistent with treatment goals and risks for the individual woman.

DESCRIPTION

Premarin® (conjugated estrogens tablets, USP) for oral administration contains a mixture of conjugated equine estrogens obtained exclusively from natural sources, occurring as the sodium salts of water-soluble estrogen sulfates blended to represent the average composition of material derived from pregnant mares' urine. It is a mixture of sodium estrone sulfate and sodium equilin sulfate. It contains as concomitant components, as sodium sulfate conjugates, 17 α-dihydroequilin, 17 α-estradiol, and 17 β-dihydroequilin. Tablets for oral administration are available in 0.3 mg, 0.625 mg, 0.9 mg, 1.25 mg, and 2.5 mg strengths of conjugated estrogens.

Premarin Tablets contain the following inactive ingredients: calcium phosphate tribasic, calcium sulfate, carnauba wax, cellulose, glyceryl monooleate, lactose, magnesium stearate, methylcellulose, pharmaceutical glaze, polyethylene glycol, stearic acid, sucrose, titanium dioxide.

— 0.3 mg tablets also contain: D&C Yellow No. 10, FD&C Blue No. 1, FD&C Blue No. 2, FD&C Yellow No. 6; these tablets comply with USP Drug Release Test 1.
— 0.625 mg tablets also contain: FD&C Blue No. 2, D&C Red No. 27, FD&C Red No. 40; these tablets comply with USP Drug Release Test 1.
— 0.9 mg tablets also contain: D&C Red No. 6, D&C Red No. 7; these tablets comply with USP Drug Release Test 2.
— 1.25 mg tablets also contain: black iron oxide, D&C Yellow No. 10, FD&C Yellow No. 6; these tablets comply with USP Drug Release Test 3.
— 2.5 mg tablets also contain: FD&C Blue No. 2, D&C Red No. 7; these tablets comply with USP Drug Release Test 3.

CLINICAL PHARMACOLOGY

Endogenous estrogens are largely responsible for the development and maintenance of the female reproductive system and secondary sexual characteristics. Although circulating estrogens exist in a dynamic equilibrium of metabolic interconversions, estradiol is the principal intracellular human estrogen and is substantially more potent than its metabolites, estrone and estriol, at the receptor level.

The primary source of estrogen in normally cycling adult women is the ovarian follicle, which secretes 70 to 500 mcg of estradiol daily, depending on the phase of the menstrual cycle. After menopause, most endogenous estrogen is produced by conversion of androstenedione, secreted by the adrenal cortex, to estrone by peripheral tissues. Thus, estrone and the sulfate-conjugated form, estrone sulfate, are the most abundant circulating estrogens in postmenopausal women.

Estrogens act through binding to nuclear receptors in estrogen-responsive tissues. To date, two estrogen receptors have been identified. These vary in proportion from tissue to tissue.

Circulating estrogens modulate the pituitary secretion of the gonadotropins, luteinizing hormone (LH) and follicle stimulating hormone (FSH) through a negative feedback mechanism. Estrogens act to reduce the elevated levels of these gonadotropins seen in postmenopausal women.

Pharmacokinetics

Absorption
Conjugated estrogens are soluble in water and are well absorbed from the gastrointestinal tract after release from the drug formulation. The Premarin tablet releases conjugated estrogens slowly over several hours. The pharmacokinetic profile of unconjugated and conjugated estrogens following a dose of 2 × 0.625 mg is provided in Table 1.

Distribution
The distribution of exogenous estrogens is similar to that of endogenous estrogens. Estrogens are widely distributed in the body and are generally found in higher concentrations in the sex hormone target organs. Estrogens circulate in the blood largely bound to sex hormone binding globulin (SHBG) and albumin.

Metabolism
Exogenous estrogens are metabolized in the same manner as endogenous estrogens. Circulating estrogens exist in a dynamic equilibrium of metabolic interconversions. These transformations take place mainly in the liver. Estradiol is converted reversibly to estrone, and both can be converted to estriol, which is the major urinary metabolite. Estrogens also undergo enterohepatic recirculation via sulfate and glucuronide conjugation in the liver, biliary secretion of conjugates into the intestine, and hydrolysis in the gut followed by reabsorption. In postmenopausal women a significant proportion of the circulating estrogens exists as sulfate conjugates, especially estrone sulfate, which serves as a circulating reservoir for the formation of more active estrogens.

Excretion
Estradiol, estrone, and estriol are excreted in the urine along with glucuronide and sulfate conjugates.
[See table 1 above]

Special Populations
No pharmacokinetic studies were conducted in special populations, including patients with renal or hepatic impairment.

Table 1. PHARMACOKINETIC PARAMETERS FOR PREMARIN

Pharmacokinetic Profile of Unconjugated Estrogens Following a Dose of 2 × 0.625 mg*

Drug	C_{max} (pg/mL)	t_{max} (h)	$t_{1/2}$** (h)	AUC (pg•h/mL)
estrone	139 (37)	8.8 (20)	28.0 (13)	5016 (34)
baseline-adjusted estrone	120 (42)	8.8 (20)	17.4 (37)	2956 (39)
equilin	66 (42)	7.9 (19)	13.6 (52)	1210 (37)

*Mean (Coefficient of Variation, %)
**$t_{1/2}$ = terminal-phase disposition half-life $(0.693/\gamma_2)$

Pharmacokinetic Profile of Conjugated Estrogens Following a Dose of 2 × 0.625 mg*

Drug	C_{max} (ng/mL)	t_{max} (h)	$t_{1/2}$** (h)	AUC (ng•h/mL)
total estrone	7.3 (41)	7.3 (51)	15.0 (25)	134 (42)
baseline-adjusted total estrone	7.1 (41)	7.3 (25)	13.6 (27)	122 (39)
total equilin	5.0 (42)	6.2 (26)	10.1 (27)	65 (45)

*Mean (Coefficient of Variation, %)
**$t_{1/2}$ = terminal-phase disposition half-life $(0.693/\gamma_2)$

Table 2. MEAN PERCENTAGE CHANGE FROM BASELINE IN BMD AT 36 MONTHS IN INTENT-TO-TREAT SUBJECTS**

	Spine			Hip		
Regimen	n	Mean % Change	95% CI	n	Mean % Change	95% CI
Premarin 0.625 mg	175	+3.46%*†	2.78, 4.14	175	+1.31%*†	0.76, 1.86
Premarin 0.625 mg/ MPA 2.5 mg	174	+4.87%*†	4.21, 5.52	174	+1.94%*†	1.50, 2.39
Placebo	174	-1.81%*	-2.51, -1.12	173	-1.62%*	-2.16, -1.08

* denotes a statistically significant mean change from baseline at the 0.001 level.
† denotes mean percentage change from baseline is significantly different from placebo at the 0.001 level.
** includes all 523 women who were randomized to either Premarin, Premarin/MPA or placebo whether or not they completed the study. If BMD was not available at 36 months, then the 12 months value was carried forward and analyzed. Baseline values were carried forward if 12 months and 36 months data were unavailable. Most patients who discontinued study medication were followed through month 36 and could have been off therapy for an extended period prior to their month 36 evaluation.

Table 3. MEAN PERCENTAGE CHANGE FROM BASELINE IN BMD AT 36 MONTHS IN ADHERENT SUBJECTS**

	Spine			Hip		
Regimen	n	Mean % Change	95% CI	n	Mean % Change	95% CI
Premarin 0.625 mg	95	+5.16%*†	4.32, 6.00	95	+2.60%*†	1.97, 3.23
Premarin 0.625 mg/ MPA 2.5 mg	144	+5.49%*†	4.79, 6.18	144	+2.23%*†	1.75, 2.71
Placebo	124	-2.82%*	-3.54, -2.10	123	-2.17%*	-2.78, -1.56

* denotes a statistically significant mean change from baseline at the 0.001 level.
† denotes mean percentage change from baseline is significantly different from placebo at the 0.001 level.
** women who completed the study had BMD reported at month 36, and took 80% or more of their prescribed medication.

Table 4. MEAN PERCENTAGE CHANGE FROM BASELINE IN BMD FOR WOMEN 45 TO 54 YEARS OF AGE

	Intent-To-Treat Subjects				Adherent Subjects			
Regimen	n	Mean % Change at the Spine	n	Mean % Change at the Hip	n	Mean % Change at the Spine	n	Mean % Change at the Hip
Premarin 0.625 mg	74	+2.45%†**	74	+1.37%†**	43	+3.73%†**	43	+2.20%†**
Premarin 0.625 mg/ MPA 2.5 mg	69	+3.53%†**	69	+1.26%†**	58	+3.97%†**	58	+1.48%†**
Placebo	78	-2.82%**	78	-2.23%**	50	-4.02%**	50	-3.04%**

** denotes a statistically significant mean change from baseline at the 0.001 level.
† denotes mean percentage change from baseline is significantly different from placebo at the 0.001 level.

Drug Interactions

Data from a single-dose drug-drug interaction study involving conjugated estrogens and medroxyprogesterone acetate indicate that the pharmacokinetic dispositions of both drugs are not significantly altered. No other clinical drug-drug interaction studies have been conducted with conjugated estrogens.

In vitro and in vivo studies have shown that estrogens are metabolized partially by cytochrome P450 3A4 (CYP3A4). Therefore, inducers or inhibitors of CYP3A4 may affect estrogen drug metabolism. Inducers of CYP3A4 such as St. John's Wort preparations (Hypericum perforatum), phenobarbital, carbamazepine, and rifampin may reduce plasma concentrations of estrogens, possibly resulting in a decrease in therapeutic effects and/or changes in the uterine bleeding profile. Inhibitors of CYP3A4 such as erythromycin, clarithromycin, ketoconazole, itraconazole, ritonavir and grapefruit juice may increase plasma concentrations of estrogens and may result in side effects.

Clinical Studies

Effects on bone mineral density.

In the 3-year, randomized, double-blind, placebo-controlled Postmenopausal Estrogen/Progestin Interventions (PEPI) trial, the effect of Premarin 0.625 mg (conjugated estrogens tablets, USP), given alone or in combination with medroxyprogesterone acetate (MPA), on bone mineral density (BMD) was evaluated in postmenopausal women. One of the regimens evaluated was continuous combined Premarin 0.625 mg/MPA 2.5 mg, a regimen similar to Prempro™.

Intent-to-treat subjects

In the intent-to-treat subjects, BMD increased significantly (p<0.001) compared to baseline or placebo at both the hip and the spine in women assigned to Premarin or the continuous Premarin/MPA regimen. Spinal BMD increased 3.46% among women assigned to Premarin, increased 4.87% in women assigned to the Premarin/MPA regimen and decreased 1.81% in women assigned to placebo. At the hip, women assigned to Premarin gained 1.31%, women assigned to Premarin/MPA gained 1.94%, while women assigned to placebo lost 1.62%.

Adherent subjects

In the adherent subjects, BMD also increased significantly (p<0.001) compared to baseline or placebo at both the hip and the spine in women assigned to Premarin or continuous Premarin/MPA. Spinal BMD increased 5.16% among women assigned to Premarin, increased 5.49% in women assigned to Premarin/MPA and decreased 2.82% in women assigned to placebo. At the hip, women assigned to Premarin gained 2.60%, women assigned to Premarin/MPA gained 2.23%, while women assigned to placebo lost 2.17%.

These results are summarized in Tables 2 and 3 below.

[See table 2 on previous page]
[See table 3 on previous page]

In general, older women (55-64 years of age) taking placebo in the PEPI study lost bone at a lower rate than younger women (45-54 years of age). Conversely, older women receiving Premarin or Premarin 0.625 mg/MPA 2.5 mg had greater increases in BMD than younger women. Tables 4 and 5 present data for women 45 to 54 years of age and women 55 to 64 years of age.

[See table 4 on previous page]
[See table 5 above]

Women's Health Initiative Studies.

The Women's Health Initiative (WHI) enrolled a total of 27,000 predominantly healthy postmenopausal women to assess the risks and benefits of either the use of Premarin (0.625 mg conjugated equine estrogens per day) alone or the use of Prempro (0.625 mg conjugated equine estrogens plus 2.5 mg medroxyprogesterone acetate per day) compared to placebo in the prevention of certain chronic diseases. The primary endpoint was the incidence of coronary heart disease (CHD) (nonfatal myocardial infarction and CHD death), with invasive breast cancer as the primary adverse outcome studied. A "global index" included the earliest occurrence of CHD, invasive breast cancer, stroke, pulmonary embolism (PE), endometrial cancer, colorectal cancer, hip fracture, or death due to other cause. The study did not evaluate the effects of Premarin or Prempro on menopausal symptoms.

The Premarin-only substudy is continuing and results have not been reported. The Prempro substudy was stopped early because, according to the predefined stopping rule, the increased risk of breast cancer and cardiovascular events exceeded the specified benefits included in the "global index." Results of the Prempro substudy, which included 16,608 women (average age of 63 years, range 50 to 79; 83.9% White, 6.5% Black, 5.5% Hispanic), after an average follow-up of 5.2 years are presented in Table 6 below:

[See table 6 above]

For those outcomes included in the "global index", absolute excess risks per 10,000 person-years in the group treated with Prempro were 7 more CHD events, 8 more strokes, 8 more PEs, and 8 more invasive breast cancers, while absolute risk reductions per 10,000 person-years were 6 fewer colorectal cancers and 5 fewer hip fractures. The absolute excess risk of events included in the "global index" was 19 per 10,000 person-years. There was no difference between the groups in terms of all-cause mortality. (See **BOXED WARNINGS, WARNINGS,** and **PRECAUTIONS.**)

INDICATIONS AND USAGE

Premarin therapy is indicated in the:
1. Treatment of moderate to severe vasomotor symptoms associated with the menopause.
2. Treatment of moderate to severe symptoms of vulvar and vaginal atrophy associated with the menopause. When prescribing solely for the treatment of symptoms of vulvar and vaginal atrophy, topical vaginal products should be considered.
3. Treatment of hypoestrogenism due to hypogonadism, castration or primary ovarian failure.
4. Treatment of breast cancer (for palliation only) in appropriately selected women and men with metastatic disease.
5. Treatment of advanced androgen-dependent carcinoma of the prostate (for palliation only).
6. Prevention of postmenopausal osteoporosis. When prescribing solely for the prevention of postmenopausal osteoporosis, therapy should only be considered for women at significant risk of osteoporosis and non-estrogen medications should be carefully considered.

The mainstays for decreasing the risk of postmenopausal osteoporosis are weight-bearing exercise, adequate calcium and vitamin D intake, and when indicated, pharmacologic therapy. Postmenopausal women require an average of 1500 mg/day of elemental calcium. Therefore, when not contraindicated, calcium supplementation may be helpful for women with suboptimal dietary intake. Vitamin D supplementation of 400-800 IU/day may also be required to ensure adequate daily intake in postmenopausal women.

CONTRAINDICATIONS

Estrogens should not be used in individuals with any of the following conditions:
1. Undiagnosed abnormal genital bleeding.
2. Known, suspected, or history of cancer of the breast except in appropriately selected patients being treated for metastatic disease.
3. Known or suspected estrogen-dependent neoplasia.
4. Active deep vein thrombosis, pulmonary embolism or a history of these conditions.
5. Active or recent (e.g., within past year) arterial thromboembolic disease (e.g., stroke, myocardial infarction).
6. Liver dysfunction or disease.
7. Premarin Tablets should not be used in patients with known hypersensitivity to their ingredients.
8. Known or suspected pregnancy. There is no indication for Premarin in pregnancy. There appears to be little or no increased risk of birth defects in women who have used estrogen and progestins from oral contraceptives inadvertently during pregnancy. (See **PRECAUTIONS.**)

WARNINGS

See **BOXED WARNINGS.**

The use of unopposed estrogens in women who have a uterus is associated with an increased risk of endometrial cancer.

1. **Cardiovascular disorders.**

Estrogen and estrogen/progestin therapy have been associated with an increased risk of cardiovascular events such as myocardial infarction and stroke, as well as venous thrombosis and pulmonary embolism (venous thromboembolism or VTE). Should any of these occur or be suspected, estrogens should be discontinued immediately.

Risk factors for cardiovascular disease (e.g., hypertension, diabetes mellitus, tobacco use, hypercholesterolemia, and obesity) should be managed appropriately.

a. Coronary heart disease and stroke. In the Premarin substudy of the Women's Health Initiative (WHI), an increase in the number of myocardial infarctions and strokes has been observed in women receiving Premarin compared to placebo. These observations are preliminary, and the study is continuing. (See **CLINICAL PHARMACOLOGY, Clinical Studies.**)

In the Prempro substudy of WHI, an increased risk of coronary heart disease (CHD) events (defined as non-fatal myocardial infarction and CHD death) was observed in women receiving Prempro compared to women receiving placebo (37 vs 30 per 10,000 person-years). The increase in risk was observed in year one and persisted.

In the same substudy of WHI, an increased risk of stroke was observed in women receiving Prempro compared to women receiving placebo (29 vs 21 per 10,000 person-years). The increase in risk was observed after the first year and persisted.

In postmenopausal women with documented heart disease (n = 2,763, average age 66.7 years) a controlled clinical trial

Continued on next page

Table 5. MEAN PERCENTAGE CHANGE FROM BASELINE IN BMD FOR WOMEN 55 TO 64 YEARS OF AGE

Regimen	Intent-To-Treat Subjects				Adherent Subjects			
	n	Mean % Change at the Spine	n	Mean % Change at the Hip	n	Mean % Change at the Spine	n	Mean % Change at the Hip
Premarin 0.625 mg	101	+4.21%†‡**	101	+1.27%†**	52	+6.34%†‡**	52	+2.93%†**
Premarin 0.625 mg/ MPA 2.5 mg	105	+5.75%†‡**	105	+2.39%†**	86	+6.51%†‡**	86	+2.73%†**
Placebo	95	-1.01%*	94	-1.14%*	73	-2.04%‡**	72	-1.60%**

* denotes a statistically significant mean change from baseline at the 0.05 level.
** denotes a statistically significant mean change from baseline at the 0.001 level.
† denotes mean percentage change from baseline is significantly different from placebo at the 0.001 level.
‡ denotes mean percentage change from baseline in the older age group is significantly different from the mean percentage change in the younger age group at the 0.05 level.

Table 6. RELATIVE AND ABSOLUTE RISK SEEN IN THE PREMPRO SUBSTUDY OF WHI[a]

Event[c]	Relative Risk Prempro vs Placebo at 5.2 Years (95% CI*)	Placebo n = 8102	Prempro n = 8506
		Absolute Risk per 10,000 Person-years	
CHD events	1.29 (1.02-1.63)	30	37
Non-fatal MI	*1.32 (1.02-1.72)*	*23*	*30*
CHD death	*1.18 (0.70-1.97)*	*6*	*7*
Invasive breast cancer[b]	1.26 (1.00-1.59)	30	38
Stroke	1.41 (1.07-1.85)	21	29
Pulmonary embolism	2.13 (1.39-3.25)	8	16
Colorectal cancer	0.63 (0.43-0.92)	16	10
Endometrial cancer	0.83 (0.47-1.47)	6	5
Hip fracture	0.66 (0.45-0.98)	15	10
Death due to causes other than the events above	0.92 (0.74-1.14)	40	37
Global Index[c]	1.15 (1.03-1.28)	151	170
Deep vein thrombosis[d]	2.07 (1.49-2.87)	13	26
Vertebral fractures[d]	0.66 (0.44-0.98)	15	9
Other osteoporotic fractures[d]	0.77 (0.69-0.86)	170	131

[a] adapted from JAMA, 2002; 288:321-333
[b] includes metastatic and non-metastatic breast cancer with the exception of in situ breast cancer
[c] a subset of the events was combined in a "global index", defined as the earliest occurrence of CHD events, invasive breast cancer, stroke, pulmonary embolism, endometrial cancer, colorectal cancer, hip fracture, or death due to other causes
[d] not included in Global Index
*nominal confidence intervals unadjusted for multiple looks and multiple comparisons

Premarin—Cont.

of secondary prevention of cardiovascular disease (Heart and Estrogen/progestin Replacement Study; HERS) treatment with Prempro (0.625 mg conjugated equine estrogen plus 2.5 mg medroxyprogesterone acetate per day) demonstrated no cardiovascular benefit. During an average follow-up of 4.1 years, treatment with Prempro did not reduce the overall rate of CHD events in postmenopausal women with established coronary heart disease. There were more CHD events in the Prempro-treated group than in the placebo group in year 1, but not during the subsequent years. Two thousand three hundred and twenty one women from the original HERS trial agreed to participate in an open label extension of HERS, HERS II. Average follow-up in HERS II was an additional 2.7 years, for a total of 6.8 years overall. Rates of CHD events were comparable among women in the Prempro group and the placebo group in HERS, HERS II, and overall.

Large doses of estrogen (5 mg conjugated estrogens per day), comparable to those used to treat cancer of the prostate and breast, have been shown in a large prospective clinical trial in men to increase the risks of nonfatal myocardial infarction, pulmonary embolism, and thrombophlebitis.

b. Venous thromboembolism (VTE). In the Premarin substudy of the Women's Health Initiative (WHI), an increase in VTE has been observed in women receiving Premarin compared to placebo. These observations are preliminary, and the study is continuing. (See **CLINICAL PHARMACOLOGY, Clinical Studies**.)

In the Prempro substudy of WHI, a 2-fold greater rate of VTE, including deep venous thrombosis and pulmonary embolism, was observed in women receiving Prempro compared to women receiving placebo. The rate of VTE was 34 per 10,000 woman-years in the Prempro group compared to 16 per 10,000 woman-years in the placebo group. The increase in VTE risk was observed during the first year and persisted.

If feasible, estrogens should be discontinued at least 4 to 6 weeks before surgery of the type associated with an increased risk of thromboembolism, or during periods of prolonged immobilization.

Recognized risk factors for VTE include, but are not limited to, a personal history or family history of VTE, obesity, and systemic lupus erythematosus.

2. Malignant neoplasms.

a. Endometrial cancer. The use of unopposed estrogens in women with intact uteri has been associated with an increased risk of endometrial cancer. The reported endometrial cancer risk among unopposed estrogen users is about 2- to 12-fold greater than in non-users, and appears dependent on duration of treatment and on estrogen dose. Most studies show no significant increased risk associated with the use of estrogens for less than one year. The greatest risk appears associated with prolonged use, with increased risks of 15- to 24-fold for five to ten years or more and this risk has been shown to persist for at least 8 to 15 years after estrogen therapy is discontinued.

Clinical surveillance of all women taking estrogen/progestin combinations is important. Adequate diagnostic measures, including endometrial sampling when indicated, should be undertaken to rule out malignancy in all cases of undiagnosed persistent or recurring abnormal vaginal bleeding. There is no evidence that the use of natural estrogens results in a different endometrial risk profile than synthetic estrogens of equivalent estrogen dose. Adding a progestin to postmenopausal estrogen therapy has been shown to reduce the risk of endometrial hyperplasia, which may be a precursor to endometrial cancer.

b. Breast cancer. Estrogen and estrogen/progestin therapy in postmenopausal women have been associated with an increased risk of breast cancer. In the Prempro substudy of the Women's Health Initiative study (WHI), a 26% increase of invasive breast cancer (38 vs 30 per 10,000 woman-years) after an average of 5.2 years of treatment was observed in women receiving Prempro compared to women receiving placebo. The increased risk of breast cancer became apparent after 4 years on Prempro. The women reporting prior postmenopausal use of estrogen and/or estrogen with progestin had a higher relative risk for breast cancer associated with Prempro than those who had never used these hormones. (See **CLINICAL PHARMACOLOGY, Clinical Studies**.)

In the Premarin substudy of WHI, no increased risk of breast cancer in estrogen-treated women compared to placebo was reported after an average of 5.2 years of therapy. These data are preliminary and that substudy of WHI is continuing.

Epidemiologic studies have reported an increased risk of breast cancer in association with increasing duration of postmenopausal treatment with estrogens, with or without progestin. This association was reanalyzed in original data from 51 studies that involved treatment with various doses and types of estrogens, with and without progestin. In the reanalysis, an increased risk of having breast cancer diagnosed became apparent after about 5 years of continued treatment, and subsided after treatment had been discontinued for about 5 years. Some later studies have suggested that treatment with estrogen and progestin increases the risk of breast cancer more than treatment with estrogen alone.

A postmenopausal woman without a uterus who requires estrogen should receive estrogen-alone therapy, and should not be exposed unnecessarily to progestins. All postmenopausal women should receive yearly breast exams by a healthcare provider and perform monthly breast self-examinations. In addition, mammography examinations should be scheduled based on patient age and risk factors.

3. Gallbladder disease.
A 2- to 4-fold increase in the risk of gallbladder disease requiring surgery in postmenopausal women receiving postmenopausal estrogens has been reported.

4. Hypercalcemia.
Estrogen administration may lead to severe hypercalcemia in patients with breast cancer and bone metastases. If hypercalcemia occurs, use of the drug should be stopped and appropriate measures taken to reduce the serum calcium level.

5. Visual abnormalities. Retinal vascular thrombosis has been reported in patients receiving estrogens. Discontinue medication pending examination if there is sudden partial or complete loss of vision, or a sudden onset of proptosis, diplopia, or migraine. If examination reveals papilledema or retinal vascular lesions, estrogens should be discontinued.

PRECAUTIONS

A. General

1. Addition of a progestin when a woman has not had a hysterectomy.
Studies of the addition of a progestin for 10 or more days of a cycle of estrogen administration or daily with estrogen in a continuous regimen, have reported a lowered incidence of endometrial hyperplasia than would be induced by estrogen treatment alone. Endometrial hyperplasia may be a precursor to endometrial cancer.

There are, however, possible risks that may be associated with the use of progestins with estrogens compared to estrogen-alone regimens. These include a possible increased risk of breast cancer, adverse effects on lipoprotein metabolism (e.g., lowering HDL, raising LDL) and impairment of glucose tolerance.

2. Elevated blood pressure.
In a small number of case reports, substantial increases in blood pressure have been attributed to idiosyncratic reactions to estrogens. In a large, randomized, placebo-controlled clinical trial, a generalized effect of estrogen therapy on blood pressure was not seen. Blood pressure should be monitored at regular intervals with estrogen use.

3. Hypertriglyceridemia.
In patients with pre-existing hypertriglyceridemia, estrogen therapy may be associated with elevations of plasma triglycerides leading to pancreatitis and other complications.

4. Impaired liver function and past history of cholestatic jaundice.
Estrogens may be poorly metabolized in patients with impaired liver function. For patients with a history of cholestatic jaundice associated with past estrogen use or with pregnancy, caution should be exercised and in the case of recurrence, medication should be discontinued.

5. Hypothyroidism.
Estrogen administration leads to increased thyroid-binding globulin (TBG) levels. Patients with normal thyroid function can compensate for the increased TBG by making more thyroid hormone, thus maintaining free T_4 and T_3 serum concentrations in the normal range. Patients dependent on thyroid hormone replacement therapy who are also receiving estrogens may require increased doses of their thyroid replacement therapy. These patients should have their thyroid function monitored in order to maintain their free thyroid hormone levels in an acceptable range.

6. Fluid retention.
Because estrogens may cause some degree of fluid retention, patients with conditions that might be influenced by this factor, such as a cardiac or renal dysfunction, warrant careful observation when estrogens are prescribed.

7. Hypocalcemia.
Estrogens should be used with caution in individuals with severe hypocalcemia.

8. Ovarian cancer
Use of estrogen-only products, in particular for ten or more years, has been associated with an increased risk of ovarian cancer in some epidemiological studies. Other studies did not show a significant association. Data are insufficient to determine whether there is an increased risk with combined estrogen/progestin therapy in postmenopausal women.

9. Exacerbation of endometriosis.
Endometriosis may be exacerbated with administration of estrogens.
The addition of a progestin should be considered in women who have undergone hysterectomy but are known to have residual endometriosis, since a few cases of malignant transformation after estrogen-only therapy have been reported.

10. Exacerbation of other conditions.
Estrogens may cause an exacerbation of asthma, diabetes mellitus, epilepsy, migraine, porphyria, systemic lupus erythematosus, and hepatic hemangiomas and should be used with caution in patients with these conditions.

B. Patient Information
Physicians are advised to discuss the contents of the PATIENT INFORMATION leaflet with patients for whom they prescribe Premarin.

C. Laboratory Tests
Estrogen administration should be initiated at the lowest dose for the treatment of postmenopausal moderate to severe vasomotor symptoms and moderate to severe symptoms of postmenopausal vulvar and vaginal atrophy and then guided by clinical response rather than by serum hormone levels (e.g., estradiol, FSH). Laboratory parameters may be useful in guiding dosage for the treatment of hypoestrogenism due to hypogonadism, castration and primary ovarian failure.

D. Drug/Laboratory Test Interactions

1. Accelerated prothrombin time, partial thromboplastin time, and platelet aggregation time; increased platelet count; increased factors II, VII antigen, VIII antigen, VIII coagulant activity, IX, X, XII, VII-X complex, II-VII-X complex, and beta-thromboglobulin; decreased levels of anti-factor Xa and antithrombin III, decreased antithrombin III activity; increased levels of fibrinogen and fibrinogen activity; increased plasminogen antigen and activity.

2. Increased thyroid binding globulin (TBG) levels leading to increased circulating total thyroid hormone levels as measured by protein-bound iodine (PBI), T_4 levels (by column or by radioimmunoassay), or T_3 levels by radioimmunoassay. T_3 resin uptake is decreased, reflecting the elevated TBG. Free T_4 and free T_3 concentrations are unaltered. Patients on thyroid replacement therapy may require higher doses of thyroid hormone.

3. Other binding proteins may be elevated in serum, i.e., corticosteroid binding globulin (CBG), sex hormone binding globulin (SHBG), leading to increased circulating corticosteroids and sex steroids, respectively. Free or biologically active hormone concentrations are unchanged. Other plasma proteins may be increased (angiotensinogen/renin substrate, alpha-1-antitrypsin, ceruloplasmin).

4. Increased plasma HDL and HDL_2 cholesterol subfraction concentrations, reduced LDL cholesterol concentration, increased triglyceride levels.

5. Impaired glucose tolerance.

6. Reduced response to metyrapone test.

E. Carcinogenesis, Mutagenesis, Impairment of Fertility
Long-term continuous administration of natural and synthetic estrogens in certain animal species increases the frequency of carcinomas of the breast, uterus, cervix, vagina, testis, and liver. (See **BOXED WARNINGS, CONTRAINDICATIONS, and WARNINGS**.)

F. Pregnancy
Premarin should not be used during pregnancy. (See **CONTRAINDICATIONS**.)

G. Nursing Mothers
Estrogen administration to nursing mothers has been shown to decrease the quantity and quality of the milk. Detectable amounts of estrogens have been identified in the milk of mothers receiving this drug. Caution should be exercised when Premarin is administered to a nursing woman.

H. Pediatric Use
Estrogen therapy has been used for the induction of puberty in adolescents with some forms of pubertal delay. Safety and effectiveness in pediatric patients have not otherwise been established.

Large and repeated doses of estrogen over an extended time period have been shown to accelerate epiphyseal closure, which could result in short adult stature if treatment is initiated before the completion of physiologic puberty in normally developing children. If estrogen is administered to patients whose bone growth is not complete, periodic monitoring of bone maturation and effects on epiphyseal centers is recommended during estrogen administration.

Estrogen treatment of prepubertal girls also induces premature breast development and vaginal cornification, and may induce vaginal bleeding. In boys, estrogen treatment may modify the normal pubertal process and induce gynecomastia. See **INDICATIONS** and **DOSAGE AND ADMINISTRATION** sections.

I. Geriatric Use
Of the total number of subjects in the Prempro substudy of the Women's Health Initiative study, 44% (n=7320) were 65 years and over, while 6.6% (n=1,095) were 75 and over (see **CLINICAL PHARMACOLOGY, Clinical Studies**). No significant differences in safety were observed between subjects 65 years and over compared to younger subjects. There was a higher incidence of stroke and invasive breast cancer in women 75 and over compared to younger subjects.

With respect to efficacy in the approved indications, there have not been sufficient numbers of geriatric patients involved in studies utilizing Premarin to determine whether those over 65 years of age differ from younger subjects in their response to Premarin.

ADVERSE REACTIONS

See **BOXED WARNINGS, WARNINGS**, and **PRECAUTIONS**.
The following additional adverse reactions have been reported with estrogen therapy and/or progestin therapy:

1. *Genitourinary system*
Changes in vaginal bleeding pattern and abnormal withdrawal bleeding or flow; breakthrough bleeding, spotting, dysmenorrhea.
Increase in size of uterine leiomyomata.
Vaginitis, including vaginal candidiasis.
Change in amount of cervical secretion.
Change in cervical ectropion.
Ovarian cancer.
Endometrial hyperplasia.
Endometrial cancer.

2. *Breasts*
Tenderness, enlargement, pain, discharge, galactorrhea.
Fibrocystic breast changes.
Breast cancer.

3. *Cardiovascular*
Deep and superficial venous thrombosis.
Pulmonary embolism.
Thrombophlebitis.
Myocardial infarction.
Stroke.
Increase in blood pressure.

4. *Gastrointestinal*
Nausea, vomiting.
Abdominal cramps, bloating.
Cholestatic jaundice.
Increased incidence of gallbladder disease.
Pancreatitis.
Enlargement of hepatic hemangiomas.

5. *Skin*
Chloasma or melasma that may persist when drug is discontinued.
Erythema multiforme.
Erythema nodosum.
Hemorrhagic eruption.
Loss of scalp hair.
Hirsutism.
Pruritus, rash.

6. *Eyes*
Retinal vascular thrombosis.
Steepening of corneal curvature.
Intolerance to contact lenses.

7. *Central Nervous System*
Headache.
Migraine.
Dizziness.
Mental depression.
Chorea.
Nervousness.
Mood disturbances.
Irritability.
Exacerbation of epilepsy.

8. *Miscellaneous*
Increase or decrease in weight.
Reduced carbohydrate tolerance.
Aggravation of porphyria.
Edema.
Arthralgias.
Leg cramps.
Changes in libido.
Urticaria, angioedema, anaphylactoid/anaphylactic reactions.
Hypocalcemia.
Exacerbation of asthma.
Increased triglycerides.

OVERDOSAGE

Serious ill effects have not been reported following acute ingestion of large doses of estrogen-containing oral contraceptives by young children. Overdosage of estrogen may cause nausea and vomiting, and withdrawal bleeding may occur in females.

DOSAGE AND ADMINISTRATION

When estrogen is prescribed for a postmenopausal woman with a uterus, progestin should also be initiated to reduce the risk of endometrial cancer. A woman without a uterus does not need progestin. Use of estrogen, alone or in combination with a progestin, should be limited to the shortest duration consistent with treatment goals and risks for the individual woman. Patients should be re-evaluated periodically as clinically appropriate (e.g., at 3-month to 6-month intervals) to determine if treatment is still necessary (see **BOXED WARNINGS** and **WARNINGS**). For women who have a uterus, adequate diagnostic measures, such as endometrial sampling, when indicated, should be undertaken to rule out malignancy in cases of undiagnosed persistent or recurring abnormal vaginal bleeding.

1. For treatment of moderate to severe vasomotor symptoms and/or moderate to severe symptoms of vulvar and vaginal atrophy associated with the menopause:
Patients should be started at the lowest dose.
Premarin therapy may be given continuously with no interruption in therapy, or in cyclical regimens (regimens such as 25 days on drug followed by five days off drug) as is medically appropriate on an individualized basis.

2. For prevention of postmenopausal osteoporosis.
0.625 mg daily.
Premarin therapy may be given continuously with no interruption in therapy, or in cyclical regimens (regimens such as 25 days on drug followed by five days off drug) as is medically appropriate on an individualized basis. When using Premarin solely for the prevention of postmenopausal osteoporosis, alternative non-estrogen treatments should be carefully considered.

3. For treatment of female hypoestrogenism due to hypogonadism, castration, or primary ovarian failure:
Female hypogonadism—0.3 mg to 0.625 mg daily, administered cyclically (e.g., three weeks on and one week off). Doses are adjusted depending on the severity of symptoms and responsiveness of the endometrium.
In clinical studies of delayed puberty due to female hypogonadism, breast development was induced by doses as low as 0.15 mg. The dosage may be gradually titrated upward at 6 to 12 month intervals as needed to achieve appropriate bone age advancement and eventual epiphyseal closure. Clinical studies suggest that doses of 0.15 mg, 0.3 mg, and 0.6 mg are associated with mean ratios of bone age advancement to chronological age progression ($\Delta BA/\Delta CA$) of 1.1, 1.5, and 2.1, respectively. (Premarin in the dose strength of 0.15 mg is not available commercially). Available data suggest that chronic dosing with 0.625 mg is sufficient to induce artificial cyclic menses with sequential progestin treatment and to maintain bone mineral density after skeletal maturity is achieved. Female castration or primary ovarian failure—1.25 mg daily, cyclically. Adjust dosage, upward or downward, according to severity of symptoms and response of the patient. For maintenance, adjust dosage to lowest level that will provide effective control.

4. For treatment of breast cancer, for palliation only, in appropriately selected women and men with metastatic disease:
Suggested dosage is 10 mg three times daily for a period of at least three months.

5. For treatment of advanced androgen-dependent carcinoma of the prostate, for palliation only:
1.25 mg to 2.5 mg three times daily. The effectiveness of therapy can be judged by phosphatase determinations as well as by symptomatic improvement of the patient.

HOW SUPPLIED

Premarin® (conjugated estrogens tablets, USP)
— Each oval purple tablet contains 2.5 mg, in bottles of 100 (NDC 0046-0865-81) and 1,000 (NDC 0046-0865-91).
— Each oval yellow tablet contains 1.25 mg, in bottles of 100 (NDC 0046-0866-81); 1,000 (NDC 0046-0866-91); and Unit-Dose Packages of 100 (NDC 0046-0866-99).
— Each oval white tablet contains 0.9 mg, in bottles of 100 (NDC 0046-0864-81).
— Each oval maroon tablet contains 0.625 mg, in bottles of 100 (NDC 0046-0867-81); 1,000 (NDC 0046-0867-91); and Unit-Dose Packages of 100 (NDC 0046-0867-99).
— Each oval green tablet contains 0.3 mg, in bottles of 100 (NDC 0046-0868-81) and 1,000 (NDC 0046-0868-91).
The appearance of these tablets is a trademark of Wyeth Pharmaceuticals.
Store at room temperature (approximately 25°C).
Dispense in a well-closed container as defined in the USP.

PATIENT INFORMATION
(Updated January 23, 2003)
Premarin®
(conjugated estrogens tablets, USP)

Read this PATIENT INFORMATION before you start taking Premarin and read what you get each time you refill Premarin. There may be new information. This information does not take the place of talking to your healthcare provider about your medical condition or your treatment.

What is the most important information I should know about Premarin (an estrogen mixture)?

- Estrogens increase the chances of getting cancer of the uterus.
Report any unusual vaginal bleeding right away while you are taking Premarin. Vaginal bleeding after menopause may be a warning sign of cancer of the uterus (womb). Your healthcare provider should check any unusual vaginal bleeding to find out the cause.
- Do not use estrogens with or without progestins to prevent heart disease, heart attacks, or strokes.
Using estrogens with or without progestins may increase your chances of getting heart attacks, strokes, breast cancer, and blood clots. You and your healthcare provider should talk regularly about whether you still need treatment with estrogens.

What is Premarin?
Premarin is a medicine that contains a mixture of estrogen hormones.

Premarin is used after menopause to:
- **reduce moderate to severe hot flashes.** Estrogens are hormones made by a woman's ovaries. The ovaries normally stop making estrogens when a woman is between 45 and 55 years old. This drop in body estrogen levels causes the "change of life" or menopause (the end of monthly menstrual periods). Sometimes both ovaries are removed during an operation before natural menopause takes place. The sudden drop in estrogen levels causes "surgical menopause."
When the estrogen levels begin dropping, some women develop very uncomfortable symptoms, such as feelings of warmth in the face, neck, and chest, or sudden strong feelings of heat and sweating ("hot flashes" or "hot flushes"). In some women the symptoms are mild, and they will not need to take estrogens. In other women, symptoms can be more severe. You and your healthcare provider should talk regularly about whether you still need treatment with Premarin.
- **treat moderate to severe dryness, itching, and burning, in and around the vagina.** You and your healthcare provider should talk regularly about whether you still need treatment with Premarin to control these problems.
- **help reduce your chances of getting osteoporosis (thin weak bones).** Osteoporosis from menopause is a thinning of the bones that makes them weaker and easier to break. If you use Premarin only to prevent osteoporosis from menopause, talk with your healthcare provider about whether a different treatment or medicine without estrogens might be better for you. You and your healthcare provider should talk regularly about whether you should continue with Premarin.
Weight-bearing exercise, like walking or running, and taking calcium and vitamin D supplements may also lower your chances for getting postmenopausal osteoporosis. It is important to talk about exercise and supplements with your healthcare provider before starting them.

Premarin is also used to:
- **treat certain conditions in women before menopause if their ovaries do not make enough estrogen.**
- **ease symptoms of certain cancers that have spread through the body, in men and women.**

Who should not take Premarin?
Do not start taking Premarin if you:
- **have unusual vaginal bleeding.**
- **currently have or have had certain cancers.** Estrogens may increase the chances of getting certain types of cancers, including cancer of the breast or uterus. If you have or have had cancer, talk with your healthcare provider about whether you should take Premarin.
- **had a stroke or heart attack in the past year.**
- **currently have or have had blood clots.**
- **are allergic to Premarin tablets or any of its ingredients.** See the end of this leaflet for a list of all the ingredients in Premarin.
- **think you may be pregnant.**

Tell your healthcare provider:
- **if you are breast feeding.** The hormones in Premarin can pass into your milk.
- **about all of your medical problems.** Your healthcare provider may need to check you more carefully if you have certain conditions, such as asthma (wheezing), epilepsy (seizures), migraine, endometriosis, lupus, problems with your heart, liver, thyroid, kidneys, or have high calcium levels in your blood.
- **about all the medicines you take,** including prescription and nonprescription medicines, vitamins, and herbal supplements. Some medicines may affect how Premarin works. Premarin may also affect how your other medicines work.
- **if you are going to have surgery or will be on bedrest.** You may need to stop taking estrogens.

How should I take Premarin?
- Take one Premarin tablet at the same time each day.
- If you miss a dose, take it as soon as possible. If it is almost time for your next dose, skip the missed dose and go back to your normal schedule. Do not take 2 doses at the same time.
- Estrogens should be used only as long as needed. You and your healthcare provider should talk regularly (for example, every 3 to 6 months) about whether you still need treatment with Premarin.

What are the possible side effects of Premarin?
Less common but serious side effects include:
- Breast cancer
- Cancer of the uterus
- Stroke
- Heart attack
- Blood clots
- Gallbladder disease
- Ovarian cancer

These are some of the warning signs of serious side effects:
- Breast lumps
- Unusual vaginal bleeding
- Dizziness and faintness
- Changes in speech
- Severe headaches
- Chest pain
- Shortness of breath
- Pains in your legs
- Changes in vision
- Vomiting

Call your healthcare provider right away if you get any of these warning signs, or any other unusual symptom that concerns you.

Common side effects include:
- Headache
- Breast pain
- Irregular vaginal bleeding or spotting
- Stomach/abdominal cramps, bloating
- Nausea and vomiting
- Hair loss

Other side effects include:
- High blood pressure
- Liver problems
- High blood sugar
- Fluid retention
- Enlargement of benign tumors of the uterus ("fibroids")
- Vaginal yeast infections

These are not all the possible side effects of Premarin. For more information, ask your healthcare provider or pharmacist.

What can I do to lower my chances of getting a serious side effect with Premarin?
- Talk with your healthcare provider regularly about whether you should continue taking Premarin.
- See your healthcare provider right away if you get vaginal bleeding while taking Premarin.
- Have a breast exam and mammogram (breast X-ray) every year unless your healthcare provider tells you something else. If members of your family have had breast cancer or if you have ever had breast lumps or an abnormal mammogram, you may need to have breast exams more often.
- If you have high blood pressure, high cholesterol (fat in the blood), diabetes, are overweight, or if you use tobacco,

Continued on next page

Premarin—Cont.

you may have higher chances for getting heart disease. Ask your healthcare provider for ways to lower your chances for getting heart disease.

General information about the safe and effective use of Premarin

Medicines are sometimes prescribed for conditions that are not mentioned in patient information leaflets. Do not take Premarin for conditions for which it was not prescribed. Do not give Premarin to other people, even if they have the same symptoms you have. It may harm them.

Keep Premarin out of the reach of children.

This leaflet provides a summary of the most important information about Premarin. If you would like more information, talk with your healthcare provider or pharmacist. You can ask for information about Premarin that is written for health professionals. You can get more information by calling the toll free number 800-934-5556.

What are the ingredients in Premarin?

Premarin contains a mixture of conjugated equine estrogens, which are a mixture of sodium estrone sulfate and sodium equilin sulfate and other components including sodium sulfate conjugates, 17 α-dihydroequilin, 17 α-estradiol, and 17 β-dihydroequilin. Premarin also contains calcium phosphate tribasic, calcium sulfate, carnauba wax, cellulose, glyceryl monooleate, lactose, magnesium stearate, methylcellulose, pharmaceutical glaze, polyethylene glycol, stearic acid, sucrose, and titanium dioxide. The tablets come in different strengths and each strength tablet is a different color. The color ingredients are:

- 0.3 mg tablet (green color): D&C Yellow No. 10, FD&C Blue No. 1, FD&C Blue No. 2, and FD&C Yellow No. 6.
- 0.625 mg tablet (maroon color): FD&C Blue No. 2, D&C Red No. 27, and FD&C Red No. 40.
- 0.9 mg tablet (white color): D&C Red No. 6 and D&C Red No. 7.
- 1.25 mg tablet (yellow color): black iron oxide, D&C Yellow No. 10, and FD&C Yellow No. 6.
- 2.5 mg tablet (purple color): FD&C Blue No. 2 and D&C Red No. 7.

Ayerst Laboratories
A Wyeth-Ayerst Company
Philadelphia, PA 19101
CI 7755-6
W10405C004
Revised January 23, 2003

PREMPRO™ ℞

[*prĕm'prō*]

(conjugated estrogens/medroxyprogesterone acetate tablets)

PREMPHASE®

[*prĕm'fāz*]

(conjugated estrogens/medroxyprogesterone acetate tablets)

℞ only

Prescribing information for this product, which appears on pages 3450–3455 of the 2003 PDR, has been completely revised as follows. Please write "See Supplement A" next to the product heading.

WARNING

Estrogens and progestins should not be used for the prevention of cardiovascular disease.

The Women's Health Initiative (WHI) reported increased risks of myocardial infarction, stroke, invasive breast cancer, pulmonary emboli, and deep vein thrombosis in postmenopausal women during 5 years of treatment with conjugated equine estrogens (0.625 mg) combined with medroxyprogesterone acetate (2.5 mg) relative to placebo (see **CLINICAL PHARMACOLOGY, Clinical Studies**). Other doses of conjugated estrogens and medroxyprogesterone acetate, and other combinations of estrogens and progestins were not studied in the WHI and, in the absence of comparable data, these risks should be assumed to be similar. Because of these risks, estrogens and progestins should be prescribed at the lowest effective doses and for the shortest duration consistent with treatment goals and risks for the individual woman.

DESCRIPTION

PREMPRO™ therapy consists of a single tablet containing 0.625 mg of the conjugated estrogens found in Premarin® tablets and 2.5 mg or 5 mg of medroxyprogesterone acetate (MPA) for oral administration.

PREMPHASE® therapy consists of two separate tablets, a maroon Premarin tablet containing 0.625 mg of conjugated estrogens that is taken orally on days 1 through 14 and a light-blue tablet containing 0.625 mg of the conjugated estrogens found in Premarin tablets and 5 mg of medroxyprogesterone acetate (MPA) that is taken orally on days 15 through 28.

The conjugated equine estrogens found in Premarin tablets are a mixture of sodium estrone sulfate and sodium equilin sulfate. They contain as concomitant components, as sodium sulfate conjugates, 17 α-dihydroequilin, 17 α-estradiol and 17 β-dihydroequilin.

Medroxyprogesterone acetate is a derivative of progesterone. It is a white to off-white, odorless, crystalline powder, stable in air, melting between 200°C and 210°C. It is freely soluble in chloroform, soluble in acetone and in dioxane, sparingly soluble in alcohol and in methanol, slightly soluble in ether, and insoluble in water. The chemical name for MPA is pregn-4-ene-3, 20-dione, 17-(acetyloxy)-6-methyl-, (6α)-. Its molecular formula is $C_{24}H_{34}O_4$, with a molecular weight of 386.53. Its structural formula is:

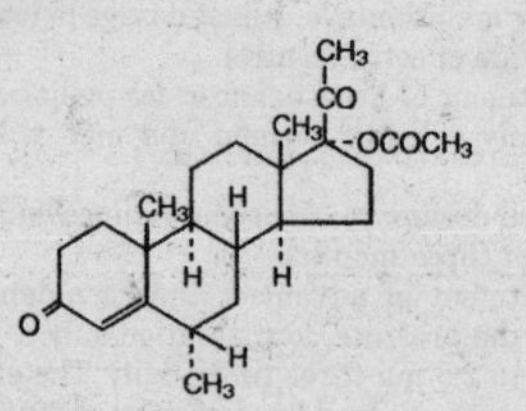

<u>PREMPRO 2.5 mg</u>

Each peach tablet for oral administration contains 0.625 mg conjugated estrogens, 2.5 mg of medroxyprogesterone acetate and the following inactive ingredients: calcium phosphate tribasic, calcium sulfate, carnauba wax, cellulose, glyceryl monooleate, lactose, magnesium stearate, methylcellulose, pharmaceutical glaze, polyethylene glycol, sucrose, povidone, titanium dioxide, red ferric oxide.

<u>PREMPRO 5 mg</u>

Each light-blue tablet for oral administration contains 0.625 mg conjugated estrogens, 5 mg of medroxyprogesterone acetate and the following inactive ingredients: calcium phosphate tribasic, calcium sulfate, carnauba wax, cellulose, glyceryl monooleate, lactose, magnesium stearate, methylcellulose, pharmaceutical glaze, polyethylene glycol, sucrose, povidone, titanium dioxide, FD&C Blue No. 2.

<u>PREMPHASE</u>

Each maroon Premarin tablet for oral administration contains 0.625 mg of conjugated estrogens and the following inactive ingredients: calcium phosphate tribasic, calcium sulfate, carnauba wax, cellulose, glyceryl monooleate, lactose, magnesium stearate, methylcellulose, pharmaceutical glaze, polyethylene glycol, stearic acid, sucrose, titanium dioxide, FD&C Blue No. 2, D&C Red No. 27, FD&C Red No. 40. These tablets comply with USP Drug Release Test 1.

Each light-blue tablet for oral administration contains 0.625 mg of conjugated estrogens and 5 mg of medroxyprogesterone acetate and the following inactive ingredients: calcium phosphate tribasic, calcium sulfate, carnauba wax, cellulose, glyceryl monooleate, lactose, magnesium stearate, methylcellulose, pharmaceutical glaze, polyethylene glycol, sucrose, povidone, titanium dioxide, FD&C Blue No. 2.

CLINICAL PHARMACOLOGY

Endogenous estrogens are largely responsible for the development and maintenance of the female reproductive system and secondary sexual characteristics. Although circulating estrogens exist in a dynamic equilibrium of metabolic interconversions, estradiol is the principal intracellular human estrogen and is substantially more potent than its metabolites, estrone and estriol, at the receptor level.

The primary source of estrogen in normally cycling adult women is the ovarian follicle, which secretes 70 to 500 mcg of estradiol daily, depending on the phase of the menstrual cycle. After menopause, most endogenous estrogen is produced by conversion of androstenedione, secreted by the adrenal cortex, to estrone by peripheral tissues. Thus, estrone and the sulfate-conjugated form, estrone sulfate, are the most abundant circulating estrogens in postmenopausal women.

Estrogens act through binding to nuclear receptors in estrogen-responsive tissues. To date, two estrogen receptors have been identified. These vary in proportion from tissue to tissue.

Circulating estrogens modulate the pituitary secretion of the gonadotropins, luteinizing hormone (LH) and follicle stimulating hormone (FSH), through a negative feedback mechanism. Estrogens act to reduce the elevated levels of these gonadotropins seen in postmenopausal women.

Parenterally administered medroxyprogesterone acetate (MPA) inhibits gonadotropin production, which in turn prevents follicular maturation and ovulation, although available data indicate that this does not occur when the usually recommended oral dosage is given as single daily doses. MPA may achieve its beneficial effect on the endometrium in part by decreasing nuclear estrogen receptors and suppression of epithelial DNA synthesis in endometrial tissue. Androgenic and anabolic effects of MPA have been noted, but the drug is apparently devoid of significant estrogenic activity.

Pharmacokinetics

Absorption

Conjugated estrogens are soluble in water and are well absorbed from the gastrointestinal tract after release from the drug formulation. However, PREMPRO and PREMPHASE contain a formulation of medroxyprogesterone acetate (MPA) that is immediately released and conjugated estrogens that are slowly released over several hours. MPA is well absorbed from the gastrointestinal tract. Table 1 summarizes the mean pharmacokinetic parameters for unconjugated and conjugated estrogens, and medroxyprogesterone acetate following administration of 0.625 mg/2.5 mg and 0.625 mg/5 mg tablets to healthy postmenopausal women.

Food-Effect: Single dose studies in healthy, postmenopausal women were conducted to investigate any potential drug interaction when PREMPRO or PREMPHASE is administered with a high fat breakfast. Administration with food decreased the C_{max} of total estrone by 18 to 34% and increased total equilin C_{max} by 38% compared to the fasting state, with no other effect on the rate or extent of absorption of other conjugated or unconjugated estrogens. Administration with food approximately doubles MPA C_{max} and increases MPA AUC by approximately 20 to 30%.

Dose Proportionality: The C_{max} and AUC values for MPA observed in two separate pharmacokinetic studies conducted with PREMPRO or PREMPHASE 2 × 0.625 mg/2.5 mg and 2 × 0.625 mg/5 mg tablets exhibited nonlinear dose proportionality; doubling the MPA dose from 2 × 2.5 to 2 × 5.0 mg increased the mean C_{max} and AUC by 3.2 and 2.8 folds, respectively. The apparent clearance (Cl/F) of MPA obtained with 2 × 0.625 mg/5 mg tablets was lower than that observed with 2 × 0.625 mg/2.5 mg tablets.

[See table below]

Distribution

The distribution of exogenous estrogens is similar to that of endogenous estrogens. Estrogens are widely distributed in the body and are generally found in higher concentrations in the sex hormone target organs. Estrogens circulate in the blood largely bound to sex hormone binding globulin (SHBG) and albumin. MPA is approximately 90% bound to plasma proteins but does not bind to SHBG.

Metabolism

Exogenous estrogens are metabolized in the same manner as endogenous estrogens. Circulating estrogens exist in a dynamic equilibrium of metabolic interconversions. These transformations take place mainly in the liver. Estradiol is converted reversibly to estrone, and both can be converted to estriol, which is the major urinary metabolite. Estrogens also undergo enterohepatic recirculation via sulfate and glucuronide conjugation in the liver, biliary secretion of conjugates into the intestine, and hydrolysis in the gut followed

Table 1. PHARMACOKINETIC PARAMETERS FOR UNCONJUGATED AND CONJUGATED ESTROGENS (CE), AND MEDROXYPROGESTERONE ACETATE (MPA)

DRUG	2 × 0.625 mg CE/2.5 mg MPA Combination Tablets (n=54)				2 × 0.625 mg CE/5 mg MPA Combination Tablets (n=51)			
PK Parameter Geometric Mean (SD)	C_{max} (pg/mL)	t_{max} (h)	$t_{1/2}$ (h)	AUC (pg•h/mL)	C_{max} (pg/mL)	t_{max} (h)	$t_{1/2}$ (h)	AUC (pg•h/mL)
Unconjugated Estrogens								
Estrone	175 (41)	7.6 (1.8)	31.6 (7.4)	5358 (1840)	124 (53)	10 (3.5)	62.2 (85.2)	6303 (2542)
BA*-Estrone	159 (41)	7.6 (1.8)	16.9 (5.8)	3313 (1310)	104 (51)	10 (3.5)	26.0 (25.9)	3136 (1598)
Equilin	71 (22)	5.8 (2.0)	9.9 (3.5)	951 (413)	54 (23)	8.9 (3.0)	15.5 (8.2)	1179 (540)
PK Parameter Geometric Mean (SD)	C_{max} (ng/mL)	t_{max} (h)	$t_{1/2}$ (h)	AUC (ng•h/mL)	C_{max} (ng/mL)	t_{max} (h)	$t_{1/2}$ (h)	AUC (ng•h/mL)
Conjugated Estrogens								
Total Estrone	6.6 (2.5)	6.1 (1.7)	20.7 (7.0)	116 (68)	6.3 (3.0)	9.1 (2.6)	23.6 (8.4)	151 (63)
BA*-Total Estrone	6.4 (2.5)	6.1 (1.7)	15.4 (5.2)	100 (57)	6.2 (3.0)	9.1 (2.6)	20.6 (7.3)	139 (56)
Total Equilin	5.1 (2.3)	4.6 (1.6)	11.4 (2.9)	50 (35)	4.2 (2.2)	7.0 (2.5)	17.2 (22.6)	72 (36)
Medroxyprogesterone Acetate	C_{max} (ng/mL)	t_{max} (h)	$t_{1/2}$ (h)	Cl/F (L/h/kg)	C_{max} (ng/mL)	t_{max} (h)	$t_{1/2}$ (h)	Cl/F (L/h/kg)
MPA	1.5 (0.6)	2.8 (1.5)	37.6 (11.2)	2.3 (0.7)	4.8 (1.5)	2.4 (1.2)	46.3 (18.0)	1.6 (0.5)

BA* = Baseline Adjusted
C_{max} = peak plasma concentration
t_{max} = time peak concentration occurs
$t_{1/2}$ = terminal-phase disposition half-life (0.693/λz)
AUC = total area under the curve
Cl/F = apparent oral clearance

by reabsorption. In postmenopausal women a significant proportion of the circulating estrogens exists as sulfate conjugates, especially estrone sulfate, which serves as a circulating reservoir for the formation of more active estrogens. Metabolism and elimination of MPA occurs primarily in the liver via hydroxylation, with subsequent conjugation and elimination in the urine.

Excretion
Estradiol, estrone, and estriol are excreted in the urine along with glucuronide and sulfate conjugates. Most metabolites of MPA are excreted as glucuronide conjugates with only minor amounts excreted as sulfates.

Special Populations
No pharmacokinetic studies were conducted in special populations, including patients with renal or hepatic impairment.

Drug Interactions
Data from a single-dose drug-drug interaction study involving conjugated estrogens and medroxyprogesterone acetate indicate that the pharmacokinetic disposition of both drugs is not altered when the drugs are coadministered. No other clinical drug-drug interaction studies have been conducted with conjugated estrogens.

In vitro and in vivo studies have shown that estrogens are metabolized partially by cytochrome P450 3A4 (CYP3A4). Therefore, inducers or inhibitors of CYP3A4 may affect estrogen drug metabolism. Inducers of CYP3A4 such as St. John's Wort preparations (Hypericum perforatum), phenobarbital, carbamazepine, and rifampicin may reduce plasma concentrations of estrogens, possibly resulting in a decrease in therapeutic effects and/or changes in the uterine bleeding profile. Inhibitors of CYP3A4 such as erythromycin, clarithromycin, ketoconazole, itraconazole, ritonavir and grapefruit juice may increase plasma concentrations of estrogens and may result in side effects.

Clinical Studies
Effects on the endometrium.
In a 1-year clinical trial of 1376 women (average age 54.0 ± 4.6 years) randomized to PREMPRO 0.625 mg/2.5 mg (Group A, n=340), PREMPRO 0.625 mg/5 mg (Group B, n=338), PREMPHASE 0.625 mg/5 mg (Group C, n=351), or Premarin 0.625 mg alone (n=347), results of evaluable biopsies at 12 months (n=279 for Group A, 274 for Group B, 277 for Group C, and 283 for Premarin alone) showed a reduced risk of endometrial hyperplasia in the two PREMPRO treatment groups (less than 1%) and in the PREMPHASE treatment group (less than 1%; 1% when focal hyperplasia was included) compared to the Premarin group (8%; 20% when focal hyperplasia was included). See Table 2.
[See table 2 at right]

Effects on uterine bleeding or spotting.
The effects of PREMPRO on uterine bleeding or spotting, as recorded on daily diary cards, were evaluated in this same clinical trial. Results are shown in Figures 1 and 2.

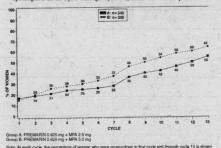

Figure 1. Patients with Cumulative Amenorrhea Over Time
(Percentage of Women With No Bleeding or Spotting at a Given Cycle Through Cycle 13), Intent-To-Treat Population

Group A: PREMARIN 0.625 mg + MPA 2.5 mg
Group B: PREMARIN 0.625 mg + MPA 5.0 mg
Note: At each cycle, the percentage of women who were amenorrheic in that cycle and through cycle 13 is shown

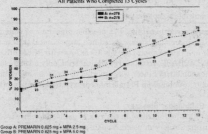

Figure 2. Patients with Cumulative Amenorrhea Over Time
(Percentage of Women With No Bleeding or Spotting at a Given Cycle Through Cycle 13)
All Patients Who Completed 13 Cycles

Group A: PREMARIN 0.625 mg + MPA 2.5 mg
Group B: PREMARIN 0.625 mg + MPA 5.0 mg
Note: At each cycle, the percentage of women who were amenorrheic in that cycle and through cycle 13 is shown

Effects on bone mineral density.
In the 3-year, randomized, double-blind, placebo-controlled Postmenopausal Estrogen/Progestin Interventions (PEPI) trial, the effect of Premarin 0.625 mg (conjugated estrogens tablets, USP), given alone or in combination with medroxyprogesterone acetate (MPA), on bone mineral density (BMD) was evaluated in postmenopausal women. One of the regimens evaluated was continuous combined Premarin 0.625 mg/MPA 2.5 mg.

Intent-to-treat subjects
In the intent-to-treat subjects, BMD increased significantly (p<0.001) compared to baseline or placebo at both the hip and the spine in women assigned to Premarin or the continuous Premarin/MPA regimen. Spinal BMD increased 3.46% among women assigned to Premarin, increased 4.87% in women assigned to the Premarin/MPA regimen, and decreased 1.81% in women assigned to placebo. At the hip, women assigned to Premarin gained 1.31%, women assigned to Premarin/MPA gained 1.94%, while women assigned to placebo lost 1.62%.

Adherent subjects
In the adherent subjects, BMD also increased significantly (p<0.001) compared to baseline or placebo at both the hip and the spine in women assigned to Premarin or continuous Premarin/MPA. Spinal BMD increased 5.16% among women assigned to Premarin, increased 5.49% in women assigned to Premarin/MPA and decreased 2.82% in women assigned to placebo. At the hip, women assigned to Premarin gained 2.60%, women assigned to Premarin/MPA gained 2.23%, while women assigned to placebo lost 2.17%.

These results are summarized in Tables 3 and 4 below.
[See table 3 above]
[See table 4 above]

In general, older women (55-64 years of age) taking placebo in the PEPI study lost bone at a lower rate than younger women (45-54 years of age). Conversely, older women receiving Premarin or Premarin 0.625 mg/MPA 2.5 mg had greater increases in BMD than younger women. Tables 5 and 6 present data for women 45 to 54 years of age and women 55 to 64 years of age.
[See table 5 at top of next page]
[See table 6 at top of next page]

Women's Health Initiative Studies.
A substudy of the Women's Health Initiative (WHI) enrolled 16,608 predominantly healthy postmenopausal women (average age of 63 years, range 50 to 79; 83.9% White, 6.5% Black, 5.5% Hispanic) to assess the risks and benefits of the use of PREMPRO (0.625 mg conjugated equine estrogens plus 2.5 mg medroxyprogesterone acetate per day) compared to placebo in the prevention of certain chronic diseases. The primary endpoint was the incidence of coronary heart disease (CHD) (nonfatal myocardial infarction and CHD death), with invasive breast cancer as the primary adverse outcome studied. A "global index" included the earliest occurrence of CHD, invasive breast cancer, stroke, pulmonary embolism (PE), endometrial cancer, colorectal cancer, hip fracture, or death due to other cause. The study did not evaluate the effects of PREMPRO on menopausal symptoms. The PREMPRO substudy was stopped early because, according to the predefined stopping rule, the increased risk of breast cancer and cardiovascular events exceeded the specified benefits included in the "global index." Results are presented in Table 7 below:
[See table 7 at top of next page]

For those outcomes included in the "global index", absolute excess risks per 10,000 person-years in the group treated with PREMPRO were 7 more CHD events, 8 more strokes, 8 more PEs, and 8 more invasive breast cancers, while absolute risk reductions per 10,000 person-years were 6 fewer colorectal cancers and 5 fewer hip fractures. The absolute excess risk of events included in the "global index" was 19 per 10,000 person-years. There was no difference between the groups in terms of all-cause mortality. (See **BOXED WARNING, WARNINGS,** and **PRECAUTIONS.**)

INDICATIONS AND USAGE

PREMPRO or PREMPHASE therapy is indicated in women who have a uterus for the:
1. Treatment of moderate to severe vasomotor symptoms associated with the menopause.
2. Treatment of moderate to severe symptoms of vulvar and vaginal atrophy associated with the menopause. When prescribing solely for the treatment of symptoms of vulvar and vaginal atrophy, topical vaginal products should be considered.
3. Prevention of postmenopausal osteoporosis. When prescribing solely for the prevention of postmenopausal osteoporosis, therapy should only be considered for women at significant risk of osteoporosis and non-estrogen medications should be carefully considered.

The mainstays for decreasing the risk of postmenopausal osteoporosis are weight-bearing exercise, adequate calcium and vitamin D intake, and when indicated, pharmacologic therapy. Postmenopausal women require an average of 1500 mg/day of elemental calcium. Therefore, when not contraindicated, calcium supplementation may be helpful for women with suboptimal dietary intake. Vitamin D supplementation of 400-800 IU/day may also be required to ensure adequate daily intake in postmenopausal women.

CONTRAINDICATIONS

Estrogens/progestins combined should not be used in women with any of the following conditions:
1. Undiagnosed abnormal genital bleeding.
2. Known, suspected, or history of cancer of the breast.
3. Known or suspected estrogen-dependent neoplasia.
4. Active deep vein thrombosis, pulmonary embolism or a history of these conditions.
5. Active or recent (e.g., within past year) arterial thromboembolic disease (e.g., stroke, myocardial infarction).
6. Liver dysfunction or disease.

Continued on next page

Table 2. INCIDENCE OF ENDOMETRIAL HYPERPLASIA AFTER ONE YEAR OF TREATMENT

	Groups			
Patient	PREMPRO 0.625 mg/2.5 mg	PREMPRO 0.625 mg/5 mg	PREMPHASE 0.625 mg/5 mg	Premarin 0.625 mg
Total number of patients	340	338	351	347
Number of patients with evaluable biopsies	279	274	277	283
No. (%) of patients with biopsies				
• all focal and non-focal hyperplasia	2 (<1)*	0 (0)*	3 (1)*	57 (20)
• excluding focal cystic hyperplasia	2 (<1)*	0 (0)*	1 (<1)*	25 (8)

*Significant (p < 0.001) in comparison with Premarin (0.625 mg) alone.

Table 3. MEAN PERCENTAGE CHANGE FROM BASELINE IN BMD AT 36 MONTHS IN INTENT-TO-TREAT SUBJECTS**

	Spine			Hip		
Regimen	n	Mean % Change	95% CI	n	Mean % Change	95% CI
Premarin 0.625 mg	175	+3.46%*†	2.78, 4.14	175	+1.31%*†	0.76, 1.86
Premarin 0.625 mg/ MPA 2.5 mg	174	+4.87%*†	4.21, 5.52	174	+1.94%*†	1.50, 2.39
Placebo	174	-1.81%*	-2.51, -1.12	173	-1.62%*	-2.16, -1.08

* denotes a statistically significant mean change from baseline at the 0.001 level.
† denotes mean percentage change from baseline is significantly different from placebo at the 0.001 level.
**includes all 523 women who were randomized to either Premarin, Premarin/MPA or placebo whether or not they completed the study. If BMD was not available at 36 months, then the 12 months value was carried forward and analyzed. Baseline values were carried forward if 12 months and 36 months data were unavailable. Most patients who discontinued study medication were followed through month 36 and could have been off therapy for an extended period prior to their month 36 evaluation.

Table 4. MEAN PERCENTAGE CHANGE FROM BASELINE IN BMD AT 36 MONTHS IN ADHERENT SUBJECTS**

	Spine			Hip		
Regimen	n	Mean % Change	95% CI	n	Mean % Change	95% CI
Premarin 0.625 mg	95	+5.16%*†	4.32, 6.00	95	+2.60%*†	1.97, 3.23
Premarin 0.625 mg/ MPA 2.5 mg	144	+5.49%*†	4.79, 6.18	144	+2.23%*†	1.75, 2.71
Placebo	124	-2.82%*	-3.54, -2.10	123	-2.17%*	-2.78, -1.56

* denotes a statistically significant mean change from baseline at the 0.001 level.
† denotes mean percentage change from baseline is significantly different from placebo at the 0.001 level.
**women who completed the study had BMD reported at month 36, and took 80% or more of their prescribed study medication.

Prempro—Cont.

7. PREMPRO or PREMPHASE therapy should not be used in patients with known hypersensitivity to their ingredients.
8. Known or suspected pregnancy. There is no indication for PREMPRO or PREMPHASE in pregnancy. There appears to be little or no increased risk of birth defects in women who have used estrogen and progestins from oral contraceptives inadvertently during pregnancy. (See **PRECAUTIONS**.)

WARNINGS
See **BOXED WARNING**.

1. Cardiovascular disorders.
Estrogen/progestin therapy has been associated with an increased risk of cardiovascular events such as myocardial infarction and stroke, as well as venous thrombosis and pulmonary embolism (venous thromboembolism or VTE). Should any of these occur or be suspected, estrogen/progestin therapy should be discontinued immediately.
Risk factors for cardiovascular disease (e.g., hypertension, diabetes mellitus, tobacco use, hypercholesterolemia, and obesity) should be managed appropriately.

a. Coronary heart disease and stroke. In the PREMPRO substudy of the Women's Health Initiative study (WHI), an increased risk of coronary heart disease (CHD) events (defined as non-fatal myocardial infarction and CHD death) was observed in women receiving PREMPRO compared to women receiving placebo (37 vs 30 per 10,000 person-years). The increase in risk was observed in year one and persisted. (See **CLINICAL PHARMACOLOGY, Clinical Studies**.)
In the same substudy of WHI, an increased risk of stroke was observed in women receiving PREMPRO compared to women receiving placebo (29 vs 21 per 10,000 person-years). The increase in risk was observed after the first year and persisted.
In postmenopausal women with documented heart disease (n = 2,763, average age 66.7 years) a controlled clinical trial of secondary prevention of cardiovascular disease (Heart and Estrogen/progestin Replacement Study; HERS) treatment with PREMPRO (0.625 mg conjugated equine estrogens plus 2.5 mg medroxyprogesterone acetate per day) demonstrated no cardiovascular benefit. During an average follow-up of 4.1 years, treatment with PREMPRO did not reduce the overall rate of CHD events in postmenopausal women with established coronary heart disease. There were more CHD events in the PREMPRO-treated group than in the placebo group in year 1, but not during the subsequent years. Two thousand three hundred and twenty one women from the original HERS trial agreed to participate in an open label extension of HERS, HERS II. Average follow-up in HERS II was an additional 2.7 years, for a total of 6.8 years overall. Rates of CHD events were comparable among women in the PREMPRO group and the placebo group in HERS, HERS II, and overall.
Large doses of estrogen (5 mg conjugated estrogens per day), comparable to those used to treat cancer of the prostate and breast, have been shown in a large prospective clinical trial in men to increase the risk of nonfatal myocardial infarction, pulmonary embolism, and thrombophlebitis.

b. Venous thromboembolism (VTE). In the PREMPRO substudy of WHI, a 2-fold greater rate of VTE, including deep venous thrombosis and pulmonary embolism, was observed in women receiving PREMPRO compared to women receiving placebo. The rate of VTE was 34 per 10,000 woman-years in the PREMPRO group compared to 16 per 10,000 woman-years in the placebo group. The increase in VTE risk was observed during the first year and persisted. (See **CLINICAL PHARMACOLOGY, Clinical Studies**.)
If feasible, estrogens should be discontinued at least 4 to 6 weeks before surgery of the type associated with an increased risk of thromboembolism, or during periods of prolonged immobilization.
Recognized risk factors for VTE include, but are not limited to, a personal history or family history of VTE, obesity, and systemic lupus erythematosus.

2. Malignant neoplasms.
a. Breast cancer. Estrogen/progestin therapy in postmenopausal women has been associated with an increased risk of breast cancer. In the PREMPRO substudy of the Women's Health Initiative study, a 26% increase of invasive breast cancer (38 vs 30 per 10,000 woman-years) after an average of 5.2 years of treatment was observed in women receiving PREMPRO compared to women receiving placebo. The increased risk of breast cancer became apparent after 4 years on PREMPRO. The women reporting prior postmenopausal use of estrogen and/or estrogen with progestin had a higher relative risk for breast cancer associated with PREMPRO than those who had never used these hormones. (See **CLINICAL PHARMACOLOGY, Clinical Studies**.)
Epidemiologic studies have reported an increased risk of breast cancer in association with increasing duration of postmenopausal treatment with estrogens, with or without progestin. This association was reanalyzed in original data from 51 studies that involved treatment with various doses and types of estrogens, with and without progestin. In the reanalysis, an increased risk of having breast cancer diagnosed became apparent after about 5 years of continued treatment, and subsided after treatment had been discontinued for about 5 years. Some later studies have suggested that treatment with estrogen and progestin increases the risk of breast cancer more than treatment with estrogen alone.

Table 5. MEAN PERCENTAGE CHANGE FROM BASELINE IN BMD FOR WOMEN 45 TO 54 YEARS OF AGE

Regimen	Intent-To-Treat Subjects				Adherent Subjects			
	n	Mean % Change at the Spine	n	Mean % Change at the Hip	n	Mean % Change at the Spine	n	Mean % Change at the Hip
Premarin 0.625 mg	74	+2.45%†**	74	+1.37%†**	43	+3.73%†**	43	+2.20%†**
Premarin 0.625 mg/ MPA 2.5 mg	69	+3.53%†**	69	+1.26%†**	58	+3.97%†**	58	+1.48%†**
Placebo	78	-2.82%**	78	-2.23%**	50	-4.02%**	50	-3.04%**

**denotes a statistically significant mean change from baseline at the 0.001 level.
† denotes mean percentage change from baseline is significantly different from placebo at the 0.001 level.

Table 6. MEAN PERCENTAGE CHANGE FROM BASELINE IN BMD FOR WOMEN 55 TO 64 YEARS OF AGE

Regimen	Intent-To-Treat Subjects				Adherent Subjects			
	n	Mean % Change at the Spine	n	Mean % Change at the Hip	n	Mean % Change at the Spine	n	Mean % Change at the Hip
Premarin 0.625 mg	101	+4.21%†‡**	101	+1.27%†**	52	+6.34%†‡**	52	+2.93%†**
Premarin 0.625 mg/ MPA 2.5 mg	105	+5.75%†‡**	105	+2.39%†**	86	+6.51%†‡**	86	+2.73%†**
Placebo	95	-1.01%*	94	-1.14%*	73	-2.04%‡**	72	-1.60%**

* denotes a statistically significant mean change from baseline at the 0.05 level.
** denotes a statistically significant mean change from baseline at the 0.001 level.
† denotes mean percentage change from baseline is significantly different from placebo at the 0.001 level.
‡ denotes mean percentage change from baseline in the older age group is significantly different from the mean percentage change in the younger age group at the 0.05 level.

Table 7. RELATIVE AND ABSOLUTE RISK SEEN IN THE PREMPRO SUBSTUDY OF WHI[a]

Event[c]	Relative Risk PREMPRO vs Placebo at 5.2 Years (95% CI*)	Placebo n = 8102	PREMPRO n = 8506
		Absolute Risk per 10,000 Person-years	
CHD events	1.29 (1.02-1.63)	30	37
Non-fatal MI	*1.32 (1.02-1.72)*	*23*	*30*
CHD death	*1.18 (0.70-1.97)*	*6*	*7*
Invasive breast cancer[b]	1.26 (1.00-1.59)	30	38
Stroke	1.41 (1.07-1.85)	21	29
Pulmonary embolism	2.13 (1.39-3.25)	8	16
Colorectal cancer	0.63 (0.43-0.92)	16	10
Endometrial cancer	0.83 (0.47-1.47)	6	5
Hip fracture	0.66 (0.45-0.98)	15	10
Death due to causes other than the events above	0.92 (0.74-1.14)	40	37
Global Index[c]	1.15 (1.03-1.28)	151	170
Deep vein thrombosis[d]	2.07 (1.49-2.87)	13	26
Vertebral fractures[d]	0.66 (0.44-0.98)	15	9
Other osteoporotic fractures[d]	0.77 (0.69-0.86)	170	131

[a] adapted from JAMA, 2002; 288:321-333
[b] includes metastatic and non-metastatic breast cancer with the exception of in situ breast cancer
[c] a subset of the events was combined in a "global index", defined as the earliest occurrence of CHD events, invasive breast cancer, stroke, pulmonary embolism, endometrial cancer, colorectal cancer, hip fracture, or death due to other causes
[d] not included in Global Index
* nominal confidence intervals unadjusted for multiple looks and multiple comparisons.

A postmenopausal woman without a uterus who requires estrogen should receive estrogen-alone therapy, and should not be exposed unnecessarily to progestins. All postmenopausal women should receive yearly breast exams by a healthcare provider and perform monthly breast self-examinations. In addition, mammography examinations should be scheduled based on patient age and risk factors.

b. Endometrial cancer. The reported endometrial cancer risk among unopposed estrogen users is about 2- to 12-fold greater than in non-users, and appears dependent on duration of treatment and on estrogen dose. Most studies show no significant increased risk associated with the use of estrogens for less than one year. The greatest risk appears associated with prolonged use, with increased risks of 15- to 24-fold for five to ten years or more and this risk has been shown to persist for at least 8 to 15 years after estrogen therapy is discontinued.
Clinical surveillance of all women taking estrogen/progestin combinations is important. Adequate diagnostic measures, including endometrial sampling when indicated, should be undertaken to rule out malignancy in all cases of undiagnosed persistent or recurring abnormal vaginal bleeding. There is no evidence that the use of natural estrogens results in a different endometrial risk profile than synthetic estrogens of equivalent estrogen dose.

Endometrial hyperplasia (a possible precursor of endometrial cancer) has been reported in a large clinical trial to occur at a rate of approximately 1% or less with PREMPRO or PREMPHASE. In this large clinical trial, only a single case of endometrial cancer was reported to occur among women taking combination Premarin/medroxyprogesterone acetate therapy.

3. Gallbladder disease.
A 2- to 4-fold increase in the risk of gallbladder disease requiring surgery in postmenopausal women receiving estrogens has been reported.

4. Hypercalcemia.
Estrogen administration may lead to severe hypercalcemia in patients with breast cancer and bone metastases. If hypercalcemia occurs, use of the drug should be stopped and appropriate measures taken to reduce the serum calcium level.

5. Visual abnormalities.
Retinal vascular thrombosis has been reported in patients receiving estrogens. Discontinue medication pending examination if there is sudden partial or complete loss of vision, or a sudden onset of proptosis, diplopia, or migraine. If examination reveals papilledema or retinal vascular lesions, estrogens should be discontinued.

PRECAUTIONS

A. General

1. Addition of a progestin when a woman has not had a hysterectomy.
Studies of the addition of a progestin for 10 or more days of a cycle of estrogen administration, or daily with estrogen in a continuous regimen, have reported a lowered incidence of endometrial hyperplasia than would be induced by estrogen treatment alone. Endometrial hyperplasia may be a precursor to endometrial cancer.
There are, however, possible risks that may be associated with the use of progestins with estrogens compared to estrogen-alone regimens. These include a possible increased risk of breast cancer, adverse effects on lipoprotein metabolism (e.g., lowering HDL, raising LDL) and impairment of glucose tolerance.

2. Elevated blood pressure.
In a small number of case reports, substantial increases in blood pressure have been attributed to idiosyncratic reactions to estrogens. In a large, randomized, placebo-controlled clinical trial, a generalized effect of estrogen therapy on blood pressure was not seen. Blood pressure should be monitored at regular intervals with estrogen use.

3. Hypertriglyceridemia.
In patients with pre-existing hypertriglyceridemia, estrogen therapy may be associated with elevations of plasma triglycerides leading to pancreatitis and other complications.

4. Impaired liver function and past history of cholestatic jaundice.
Estrogens may be poorly metabolized in patients with impaired liver function. For patients with a history of cholestatic jaundice associated with past estrogen use or with pregnancy, caution should be exercised and in the case of recurrence, medication should be discontinued.

5. Hypothyroidism.
Estrogen administration leads to increased thyroid-binding globulin (TBG) levels. Patients with normal thyroid function can compensate for the increased TBG by making more thyroid hormone, thus maintaining free T_4 and T_3 serum concentrations in the normal range. Patients dependent on thyroid hormone replacement therapy who are also receiving estrogens may require increased doses of their thyroid replacement therapy. These patients should have their thyroid function monitored in order to maintain their free thyroid hormone levels in an acceptable range.

6. Fluid retention.
Because estrogens/progestins may cause some degree of fluid retention, patients with conditions that might be influenced by this factor, such as cardiac or renal dysfunction, warrant careful observation when estrogens are prescribed.

7. Hypocalcemia.
Estrogens should be used with caution in individuals with severe hypocalcemia.

8. Ovarian cancer.
Use of estrogen-only products, in particular for ten or more years, has been associated with an increased risk of ovarian cancer in some epidemiological studies. Other studies did not show a significant association. Data are insufficient to determine whether there is an increased risk with combined estrogen/progestin therapy in postmenopausal women.

9. Exacerbation of endometriosis.
Endometriosis may be exacerbated with administration of estrogens.

10. Exacerbation of other conditions.
Estrogens may cause an exacerbation of asthma, diabetes mellitus, epilepsy, migraine, porphyria, systemic lupus erythematosus, and hepatic hemangiomas and should be used with caution in women with these conditions.

B. Patient Information
Physicians are advised to discuss the contents of the PATIENT INFORMATION leaflet with patients for whom they prescribe PREMPRO or PREMPHASE.

C. Laboratory Tests
Estrogen administration should be initiated at the lowest dose approved for the indication and then guided by clinical response rather than by serum hormone levels (e.g., estradiol, FSH).

D. Drug/Laboratory Test Interactions
1. Accelerated prothrombin time, partial thromboplastin time, and platelet aggregation time; increased platelet count; increased factors II, VII antigen, VIII coagulant activity, IX, X, XII, VII-X complex, II-VII-X complex, and beta-thromboglobulin; decreased levels of anti-factor Xa and antithrombin III, decreased antithrombin III activity; increased levels of fibrinogen and fibrinogen activity; increased plasminogen antigen and activity.
2. Increased thyroid binding globulin (TBG) levels leading to increased circulating total thyroid hormone levels as measured by protein-bound iodine (PBI), T_4 levels (by column or by radioimmunoassay), or T_3 levels by radioimmunoassay. T_3 resin uptake is decreased, reflecting the elevated TBG. Free T_4 and free T_3 concentrations are unaltered. Patients on thyroid replacement therapy may require higher doses of thyroid hormone.
3. Other binding proteins may be elevated in serum, i.e., corticosteroid binding globulin (CBG), sex hormone binding globulin (SHBG), leading to increased circulating corticosteroids and sex steroids, respectively. Free or biologically active hormone concentrations are unchanged. Other plasma proteins may be increased (angiotensinogen/renin substrate, alpha-1-antitrypsin, ceruloplasmin).
4. Increased plasma HDL and HDL_2 cholesterol subfraction concentrations, reduced LDL cholesterol concentration, increased triglyceride levels.
5. Impaired glucose tolerance.
6. Reduced response to metyrapone test.
7. Aminoglutethimide administered concomitantly with medroxyprogesterone acetate (MPA) may significantly depress the bioavailability of MPA.

E. Carcinogenesis, Mutagenesis, Impairment of Fertility
Long-term continuous administration of natural and synthetic estrogens in certain animal species increases the frequency of carcinomas of the breasts, uterus, cervix, vagina, testis, and liver. (See **BOXED WARNING, CONTRAINDICATIONS, and WARNINGS**.)
In a two-year oral study of medroxyprogesterone acetate (MPA) in which female rats were exposed to dosages of up to 5000 mcg/kg/day in their diets (50 times higher – based on AUC values – than the level observed experimentally in women taking 10 mg of MPA), a dose-related increase in pancreatic islet cell tumors (adenomas and carcinomas) occurred. Pancreatic tumor incidence was increased at 1000 and 5000 mcg/kg/day, but not at 200 mcg/kg/day.
A decreased incidence of spontaneous mammary gland tumors was observed in all three MPA-treated groups, compared to controls, in the two-year rat study. The mechanism for the decreased incidence of mammary gland tumors observed in the MPA-treated rats may be linked to the significant decrease in serum prolactin concentration observed in rats.
Beagle dogs treated with MPA developed mammary nodules, some of which were malignant. Although nodules occasionally appeared in control animals, they were intermittent in nature, whereas the nodules in the drug-treated animals were larger, more numerous, persistent, and there were some breast malignancies with metastases. It is known that progestogens stimulate synthesis and release of growth hormone in dogs. The growth hormone, along with the progestogen, stimulates mammary growth and function. In contrast, growth hormone in humans is not increased, nor does growth hormone have any significant mammotrophic role. No pancreatic tumors occurred in dogs.

F. Pregnancy
PREMPRO and PREMPHASE should not be used during pregnancy. (See **CONTRAINDICATIONS**.)

G. Nursing Mothers
Estrogen administration to nursing mothers has been shown to decrease the quantity and quality of the milk. Detectable amounts of estrogen and progestin have been identified in the milk of mothers receiving these drugs. Caution should be exercised when PREMPRO or PREMPHASE are administered to a nursing woman.

H. Pediatric Use
PREMPRO and PREMPHASE are not indicated in children.

I. Geriatric Use
Of the total number of subjects in the PREMPRO substudy of the Women's Health Initiative study, 44% (n=7320) were 65 years and over, while 6.6% (n=1,095) were 75 and over (see **CLINICAL PHARMACOLOGY, Clinical Studies**). No significant differences in safety were observed between subjects 65 years and over compared to younger subjects. There was a higher incidence of stroke and invasive breast cancer in women 75 and over compared to younger subjects.
With respect to efficacy in the approved indications, there have not been sufficient numbers of geriatric patients involved in studies utilizing Premarin and medroxyprogesterone acetate to determine whether those over 65 years of age differ from younger subjects in their response to PREMPRO or PREMPHASE.

ADVERSE REACTIONS

See **BOXED WARNING, WARNINGS, and PRECAUTIONS**.
Because clinical trials are conducted under widely varying conditions, adverse reaction rates observed in the clinical trials of a drug cannot be directly compared to rates in the clinical trials of another drug and may not reflect the rates observed in practice. The adverse reaction information from clinical trials does, however, provide a basis for identifying the adverse events that appear to be related to drug use and for approximating rates.
In a one-year clinical trial that included 678 women treated with PREMPRO, 351 women treated with PREMPHASE, and 347 women treated with Premarin, the following adverse events occurred at a rate ≥5% (see Table 8):
[See table 8 above]
The following additional adverse reactions have been reported with estrogen and/or progestin therapy:

1. Genitourinary system
Changes in vaginal bleeding pattern and abnormal withdrawal bleeding or flow, breakthrough bleeding, spotting, change in amount of cervical secretion, premenstrual-like syndrome, cystitis-like syndrome, increase in size of uterine leiomyomata, vaginal candidiasis, amenorrhea, changes in cervical erosion, ovarian cancer, endometrial hyperplasia, endometrial cancer.

2. Breasts
Tenderness, enlargement, galactorrhea, discharge, fibrocystic breast changes, breast cancer.

3. Cardiovascular
Deep and superficial venous thrombosis, pulmonary embolism, thrombophlebitis, myocardial infarction, stroke, increase in blood pressure.

4. Gastrointestinal
Nausea, cholestatic jaundice, changes in appetite, vomiting, abdominal cramps, bloating, increased incidence of gallbladder disease, pancreatitis, enlargement of hepatic hemangiomas.

Continued on next page

Table 8. ALL TREATMENT EMERGENT STUDY EVENTS REGARDLESS OF DRUG RELATIONSHIP REPORTED AT A FREQUENCY ≥ 5%

	PREMPRO 0.625 mg/2.5 mg continuous (n=340)	PREMPRO 0.625 mg/5.0 mg continuous (n=338)	PREMPHASE 0.625 mg/5.0 mg sequential (n=351)	PREMARIN 0.625 mg daily (n=347)
Body as a whole				
abdominal pain	16%	21%	23%	17%
accidental injury	5%	4%	5%	5%
asthenia	6%	8%	10%	8%
back pain	14%	13%	16%	14%
flu syndrome	10%	13%	12%	14%
headache	36%	28%	37%	38%
infection	16%	16%	18%	14%
pain	11%	13%	12%	13%
pelvic pain	4%	5%	5%	5%
Digestive system				
diarrhea	6%	6%	5%	10%
dyspepsia	6%	6%	5%	5%
flatulence	8%	9%	8%	5%
nausea	11%	9%	11%	11%
Metabolic and Nutritional				
peripheral edema	4%	4%	3%	5%
Musculoskeletal system				
arthralgia	9%	7%	9%	7%
leg cramps	3%	4%	5%	4%
Nervous system				
depression	6%	11%	11%	10%
dizziness	5%	3%	4%	6%
hypertonia	4%	3%	3%	7%
Respiratory system				
pharyngitis	11%	11%	13%	12%
rhinitis	8%	6%	8%	7%
sinusitis	8%	7%	7%	5%
Skin and appendages				
pruritus	10%	8%	5%	4%
rash	4%	6%	4%	3%
Urogenital system				
breast pain	33%	38%	32%	12%
cervix disorder	4%	4%	5%	5%
dysmenorrhea	8%	5%	13%	5%
leukorrhea	6%	5%	9%	8%
vaginal hemorrhage	2%	1%	3%	6%
vaginitis	7%	7%	5%	3%

Prempro—Cont.

5. *Skin*
Chloasma or melasma that may persist when drug is discontinued, erythema multiforme, erythema nodosum, hemorrhagic eruption, loss of scalp hair, hirsutism, itching, urticaria, pruritus, generalized rash, rash (allergic) with and without pruritus, acne.

6. *Eyes*
Neuro-ocular lesions, e.g., retinal vascular thrombosis and optic neuritis, steepening of corneal curvature, intolerance of contact lenses.

7. *CNS*
Headache, dizziness, mental depression, mood disturbances, anxiety, irritability, nervousness, migraine, chorea, insomnia, somnolence, exacerbation of epilepsy.

8. *Miscellaneous*
Increase or decrease in weight, edema, changes in libido, fatigue, backache, reduced carbohydrate tolerance, aggravation of porphyria, pyrexia, urticaria, angioedema, anaphylactoid/anaphylactic reactions, hypocalcemia, exacerbation of asthma, increased triglycerides.

OVERDOSAGE
Serious ill effects have not been reported following acute ingestion of large doses of estrogen/progestin-containing oral contraceptives by young children. Overdosage of estrogen/progestin may cause nausea and vomiting, and withdrawal bleeding may occur in females.

DOSAGE AND ADMINISTRATION
Use of estrogen, alone or in combination with a progestin, should be limited to the shortest duration consistent with treatment goals and risks for the individual woman. Patients should be re-evaluated periodically as clinically appropriate (e.g., at 3-month to 6-month intervals) to determine if treatment is still necessary (see **BOXED WARNING** and **WARNINGS**). For women who have a uterus, adequate diagnostic measures, such as endometrial sampling, when indicated, should be undertaken to rule out malignancy in cases of undiagnosed persistent or recurring abnormal vaginal bleeding.
PREMPRO therapy consists of a single tablet to be taken once daily. Patients should be started at the lowest available dose.
In patients where bleeding or spotting remains a problem, after appropriate evaluation, consideration should be given to increasing the medroxyprogesterone acetate (MPA) dose to PREMPRO 0.625 mg/ 5 mg daily. This dose should be periodically reassessed by the healthcare provider.
PREMPHASE therapy consists of two separate tablets; one maroon 0.625 mg Premarin tablet taken daily on days 1 through 14 and one light-blue tablet, containing 0.625 mg conjugated estrogens and 5 mg of medroxyprogesterone acetate, taken on days 15 through 28.

HOW SUPPLIED
PREMPRO™ therapy consists of a single tablet to be taken once daily.
PREMPRO 0.625 mg/2.5 mg
Each carton includes 3 EZ DIAL™ dispensers containing 28 tablets. One EZ DIAL dispenser contains 28 oval, peach tablets containing 0.625 mg of the conjugated estrogens found in Premarin® tablets and 2.5 mg of medroxyprogesterone acetate for oral administration.
PREMPRO 0.625 mg/5 mg
Each carton includes 3 EZ DIAL dispensers containing 28 tablets. One EZ DIAL dispenser contains 28 oval, light-blue tablets containing 0.625 mg of the conjugated estrogens found in Premarin tablets and 5 mg of medroxyprogesterone acetate for oral administration.
PREMPHASE® therapy consists of two separate tablets; one maroon Premarin tablet taken daily on days 1 through 14 and one light-blue tablet taken on days 15 through 28.
Each carton includes 3 EZ DIAL dispensers containing 28 tablets. One EZ DIAL dispenser contains 14 oval, maroon Premarin® tablets containing 0.625 mg of conjugated estrogens and 14 oval, light-blue tablets that contain 0.625 mg of the conjugated estrogens found in Premarin tablets and 5 mg of medroxyprogesterone acetate for oral administration.
The appearance of PREMPRO tablets is a trademark of Wyeth Pharmaceuticals.
The appearance of Premarin tablets is a trademark of Wyeth Pharmaceuticals. The appearance of the conjugated estrogens/medroxyprogesterone acetate combination tablets is a registered trademark.
Store at controlled room temperature 20° to 25°C (68° to 77°F).

PATIENT INFORMATION
(Updated January 23, 2003)
PREMPRO™
(conjugated estrogens/medroxyprogesterone acetate tablets)
PREMPHASE®
(conjugated estrogens/medroxyprogesterone acetate tablets)
Read this PATIENT INFORMATION before you start taking PREMPRO or PREMPHASE and read what you get each time you refill PREMPRO or PREMPHASE. There may be new information. This information does not take the place of talking to your healthcare provider about your medical condition or your treatment.

What is the most important information I should know about PREMPRO and PREMPHASE (combinations of estrogens and a progestin)?
Do not use estrogens and progestins to prevent heart disease, heart attacks, or strokes.
Using estrogens and progestins may increase your chances of getting heart attacks, strokes, breast cancer, or blood clots. You and your healthcare provider should talk regularly about whether you still need treatment with PREMPRO or PREMPHASE.

What is PREMPRO or PREMPHASE?
PREMPRO or PREMPHASE are medicines that contain two kinds of hormones, estrogens and a progestin.
PREMPRO or PREMPHASE is used after menopause to:
- **reduce moderate to severe hot flashes.** Estrogens are hormones made by a woman's ovaries. The ovaries normally stop making estrogens when a woman is between 45 and 55 years old. This drop in body estrogen levels causes the "change of life" or menopause (the end of monthly menstrual periods). Sometimes, both ovaries are removed during an operation before natural menopause takes place. The sudden drop in estrogen levels causes "surgical menopause."
When the estrogen levels begin dropping, some women develop very uncomfortable symptoms, such as feelings of warmth in the face, neck, and chest, or sudden strong feelings of heat and sweating ("hot flashes" or "hot flushes"). In some women the symptoms are mild, and they will not need to take estrogens. In other women, symptoms can be more severe. You and your healthcare provider should talk regularly about whether you still need treatment with PREMPRO or PREMPHASE.
- **treat moderate to severe dryness, itching, and burning, in and around the vagina.** You and your healthcare provider should talk regularly about whether you still need treatment with PREMPRO or PREMPHASE to control these problems.
- **help reduce your chances of getting osteoporosis (thin weak bones).** Osteoporosis from menopause is a thinning of the bones that makes them weaker and easier to break. If you use PREMPRO or PREMPHASE only to prevent osteoporosis from menopause, talk with your healthcare provider about whether a different treatment or medicine without estrogens might be better for you. You and your healthcare provider should talk regularly about whether you should continue with PREMPRO or PREMPHASE. Weight-bearing exercise, like walking or running, and taking calcium and vitamin D supplements may also lower your chances for getting postmenopausal osteoporosis. It is important to talk about exercise and supplements with your healthcare provider before starting them.

Who should not take PREMPRO or PREMPHASE?
Do not take PREMPRO or PREMPHASE if you have had your uterus removed (hysterectomy).
PREMPRO and PREMPHASE contain a progestin to decrease the chances of getting cancer of the uterus. If you do not have a uterus, you do not need a progestin and you should not take PREMPRO or PREMPHASE.
Do not start taking PREMPRO or PREMPHASE if you:
- **have unusual vaginal bleeding.**
- **currently have or have had certain cancers.** Estrogens may increase the chances of getting certain types of cancers, including cancer of the breast or uterus. If you have or had cancer, talk with your healthcare provider about whether you should take PREMPRO or PREMPHASE.
- **had a stroke or heart attack in the past year.**
- **currently have or have had clots.**
- **have liver problems.**
- **are allergic to PREMPRO or PREMPHASE or any of their ingredients.** See the end of this leaflet for a list of all the ingredients in PREMPRO and PREMPHASE.
- **think you may be pregnant.**

Tell your healthcare provider:
- **if you are breastfeeding.** The hormones in PREMPRO and PREMPHASE can pass into your milk.
- **about all of your medical problems.** Your healthcare provider may need to check you more carefully if you have certain conditions, such as asthma (wheezing), epilepsy (seizures), migraine, endometriosis, lupus, problems with your heart, liver, thyroid, kidneys, or have high calcium levels in your blood.
- **about all the medicines you take,** including prescription and nonprescription medicines, vitamins, and herbal supplements. Some medicines may affect how PREMPRO or PREMPHASE works. PREMPRO or PREMPHASE may also affect how your other medicines work.
- **if you are going to have surgery or will be on bedrest.** You may need to stop taking estrogens and progestins.

How should I take PREMPRO or PREMPHASE?
- Take one PREMPRO or PREMPHASE tablet at the same time each day.
- If you miss a dose, take it as soon as possible. If it is almost time for your next dose, skip the missed dose and go back to your normal schedule. Do not take 2 doses at the same time.
- Estrogens should be used only as long as needed. You and your healthcare provider should talk regularly (for example, every 3 to 6 months) about whether you still need treatment with PREMPRO or PREMPHASE.

What are the possible side effects of PREMPRO or PREMPHASE?
Less common but serious side effects include:
- Breast cancer
- Cancer of the uterus
- Stroke
- Heart attack
- Blood clots
- Gallbladder disease
- Ovarian cancer

These are some of the warning signs of serious side effects:
- Breast lumps
- Unusual vaginal bleeding
- Dizziness and faintness
- Changes in speech
- Severe headaches
- Chest pain
- Shortness of breath
- Pains in your legs
- Changes in vision
- Vomiting

Call your healthcare provider right away if you get any of these warning signs, or any other unusual symptom that concerns you.

Common side effects include:
- Headache
- Breast pain
- Irregular vaginal bleeding or spotting
- Stomach/abdominal cramps, bloating
- Nausea and vomiting
- Hair loss

Other side effects include:
- High blood pressure
- Liver problems
- High blood sugar
- Fluid retention
- Enlargement of benign tumors of the uterus ("fibroids")
- Vaginal yeast infections
- Mental depression

These are not all the possible side effects of PREMPRO or PREMPHASE. For more information, ask your healthcare provider or pharmacist.

What can I do to lower my chances of getting a serious side effect with PREMPRO or PREMPHASE?
- Talk with your healthcare provider regularly about whether you should continue taking PREMPRO or PREMPHASE.
- See your healthcare provider right away if you get vaginal bleeding while taking PREMPRO or PREMPHASE.
- Have a breast exam and mammogram (breast X-ray) every year unless your healthcare provider tells you something else. If members of your family have had breast cancer or if you have ever had breast lumps or an abnormal mammogram, you may need to have breast exams more often.
- If you have high blood pressure, high cholesterol (fat in the blood), diabetes, are overweight, or if you use tobacco, you may have higher chances for getting heart disease. Ask your healthcare provider for ways to lower your chances for getting heart disease.

General information about the safe and effective use of PREMPRO and PREMPHASE
Medicines are sometimes prescribed for conditions that are not mentioned in patient information leaflets. Do not take PREMPRO or PREMPHASE for conditions for which they were not prescribed. Do not give PREMPRO or PREMPHASE to other people, even if they have the same symptoms you have. It may harm them. **Keep PREMPRO and PREMPHASE out of the reach of children.**
This leaflet provides a summary of the most important information about PREMPRO and PREMPHASE. If you would like more information, talk with your healthcare provider or pharmacist. You can ask for information about PREMPRO and PREMPHASE that is written for health professionals. You can get more information by calling the toll free number 800-934-5556.

What are the ingredients in PREMPRO and PREMPHASE?
PREMPRO contains 0.625 mg of the same conjugated estrogens found in Premarin® which are a mixture of sodium estrone sulfate and sodium equilin sulfate and other components including sodium sulfate conjugates, 17 α-dihydroequilin, 17 α-estradiol and 17 β-dihydroequilin. PREMPRO also contains either 2.5 or 5 mg of medroxyprogesterone acetate. PREMPRO also contains calcium phosphate tribasic, calcium sulfate, carnauba wax, cellulose, glyceryl monooleate, lactose, magnesium stearate, methylcellulose, pharmaceutical glaze, polyethylene glycol, sucrose, povidone, titanium dioxide, and red ferric oxide or FD&C Blue No. 2.
PREMPHASE is two separate tablets. One tablet (maroon color) is 0.625 mg of Premarin® which is a mixture of sodium estrone sulfate and sodium equilin sulfate and other components including sodium sulfate conjugates, 17 α-dihydroequilin, 17 α-estradiol and 17 β-dihydroequilin. The maroon tablet also contains calcium phosphate tribasic, calcium sulfate, carnauba wax, cellulose, glyceryl monooleate, lactose, magnesium stearate, methylcellulose, pharmaceutical glaze, polyethylene glycol, stearic acid, sucrose, titanium dioxide, FD&C Blue No. 2, D&C Red No. 27, FD&C Red No. 40. The second tablet (light blue color) contains 0.625 mg of the same ingredients as the maroon color tablet plus 5 mg of medroxyprogesterone acetate. The light blue tablet also contains calcium phosphate tribasic, calcium sulfate, carnauba wax, cellulose, glyceryl monooleate, lactose, magnesium

stearate, methylcellulose, pharmaceutical glaze, polyethylene glycol, sucrose, povidone, titanium dioxide, and FD&C Blue No. 2.

PREMPRO™ therapy consists of a single tablet to be taken once daily.

PREMPRO 0.625 mg/2.5 mg

Each carton includes 3 EZ DIAL™ dispensers containing 28 tablets. One EZ DIAL dispenser contains 28 oval, peach tablets containing 0.625 mg of the conjugated estrogens found in Premarin® tablets and 2.5 mg of medroxyprogesterone acetate for oral administration.

PREMPRO 0.625 mg/5 mg

Each carton includes 3 EZ DIAL dispensers containing 28 tablets. One EZ DIAL dispenser contains 28 oval, light-blue tablets containing 0.625 mg of the conjugated estrogens found in Premarin tablets and 5 mg of medroxyprogesterone acetate for oral administration.

PREMPHASE® therapy consists of two separate tablets; one maroon Premarin tablet taken daily on days 1 through 14 and one light-blue tablet taken on days 15 through 28. Each carton includes 3 EZ DIAL dispensers containing 28 tablets. One EZ DIAL dispenser contains 14 oval, maroon Premarin® tablets containing 0.625 mg of conjugated estrogens and 14 oval, light-blue tablets that contain 0.625 mg of the conjugated estrogens found in Premarin tablets and 5 mg of medroxyprogesterone acetate for oral administration.

The appearance of PREMPRO tablets is a trademark of Wyeth Pharmaceuticals.

The appearance of Premarin tablets is a trademark of Wyeth Pharmaceuticals. The appearance of the conjugated estrogens/medroxyprogesterone acetate combination tablets is a registered trademark.

Store at controlled room temperature 20° to 25°C (68° to 77°F).

Ayerst Laboratories
A Wyeth-Ayerst Company CI7754-6
Philadelphia, PA 19101 W10407C004
Revised January 23, 2003

PREVNAR® ℞

[prĕv' năr]

Pneumococcal 7-valent Conjugate Vaccine (Diphtheria CRM_{197} Protein)

℞ only

For Intramuscular Injection Only

Prescribing information for this product, which appears on pages 3455–3461 of the 2003 PDR, has been completely revised as follows. Please write "See Supplement A" next to the product heading.

DESCRIPTION

Pneumococcal 7-valent Conjugate Vaccine (Diphtheria CRM_{197} Protein), Prevnar®, is a sterile solution of saccharides of the capsular antigens of *Streptococcus pneumoniae* serotypes 4, 6B, 9V, 14, 18C, 19F, and 23F individually conjugated to diphtheria CRM_{197} protein. Each serotype is grown in soy peptone broth. The individual polysaccharides are purified through centrifugation, precipitation, ultrafiltration, and column chromatography. The polysaccharides are chemically activated to make saccharides which are directly conjugated to the protein carrier CRM_{197} to form the glycoconjugate. This is effected by reductive amination. CRM_{197} is a nontoxic variant of diphtheria toxin isolated from cultures of *Corynebacterium diphtheriae* strain C7 (β197) grown in a casamino acids and yeast extract-based medium. CRM_{197} is purified through ultrafiltration, ammonium sulfate precipitation, and ion-exchange chromatography. The individual glycoconjugates are purified by ultrafiltration and column chromatography and are analyzed for saccharide to protein ratios, molecular size, free saccharide, and free protein.

The individual glycoconjugates are compounded to formulate the vaccine, Prevnar®. Potency of the formulated vaccine is determined by quantification of each of the saccharide antigens, and by the saccharide to protein ratios in the individual glycoconjugates.

Prevnar® is manufactured as a liquid preparation. Each 0.5 mL dose is formulated to contain: 2 µg of each saccharide for serotypes 4, 9V, 14, 18C, 19F, and 23F, and 4 µg of serotype 6B per dose (16 µg total saccharide); approximately 20 µg of CRM_{197} carrier protein; and 0.125 mg of aluminum per 0.5 mL dose as aluminum phosphate adjuvant. After shaking, the vaccine is a homogeneous, white suspension.

CLINICAL PHARMACOLOGY

S. pneumoniae is an important cause of morbidity and mortality in persons of all ages worldwide. The organism causes invasive infections, such as bacteremia and meningitis, as well as pneumonia and upper respiratory tract infections including otitis media and sinusitis. In children older than 1 month, *S. pneumoniae* is the most common cause of invasive disease.[1] Data from community-based studies performed between 1986 and 1995, indicate that the overall annual incidence of invasive pneumococcal disease in the United States (US) is an estimated 10 to 30 cases per 100,000 persons, with the highest risk in children aged less than or equal to 2 years of age (140 to 160 cases per 100,000 persons).[2,3,4,5,6] Children in group child care have an increased risk for invasive pneumococcal disease.[7,8] Immunocompromised individuals with neutropenia, asplenia, sickle cell disease, disorders of complement and humoral immunity, human immunodeficiency virus (HIV) infections or chronic underlying disease are also at increased risk for invasive pneumococcal disease.[8] *S. pneumoniae* is the most common cause of bacterial meningitis in the US.[1] The annual incidence of pneumococcal meningitis in children between 1 to 23 months of age is approximately 7 cases per 100,000 persons.[1] Pneumococcal meningitis in childhood has been associated with 8% mortality and may result in neurological sequelae (25%) and hearing loss (32%) in survivors.[9]

Acute otitis media (AOM) is a common childhood disease, with more than 60% of children experiencing an episode by one year of age, and more than 90% of children experiencing an episode by age 5. Prior to the US introduction of Prevnar® in the year 2000, approximately 24.5 million ambulatory care visits and 490,000 procedures for myringotomy with tube placement were attributed to otitis media annually.[10,11] The peak incidence of AOM is 6 to 18 months of age.[12] Otitis media is less common, but occurs, in older children. In a 1990 surveillance by the Centers for Disease Control and Prevention (CDC), otitis media was the most common principal illness diagnosis in children 2-10 years of age.[13] Complications of AOM include persistent middle ear effusion, chronic otitis media, transient hearing loss, or speech delays and, if left untreated, may lead to more serious diseases such as mastoiditis and meningitis. *S. pneumoniae* is an important cause of AOM. It is the bacterial pathogen most commonly isolated from middle ear fluid, identified in 20% to 40% of middle ear fluid cultures in AOM.[14,15] Pneumococcal otitis media is associated with higher rates of fever, and is less likely to resolve spontaneously than AOM due to either nontypeable *H. influenzae* or *M. catarrhalis*.[16,17] Prior to the introduction of Prevnar®, the seven serotypes contained in the vaccine accounted for approximately 60% of AOM due to *S. pneumoniae* (12%-24% of all AOM).[18]

The exact contribution of *S. pneumoniae* to childhood pneumonia is unknown, as it is often not possible to identify the causative organisms. In studies of children less than 5 years of age with community-acquired pneumonia, where diagnosis was attempted using serological methods, antigen testing, or culture data, 30% of cases were classified as bacterial pneumonia, and 70% of these (21% of total community-acquired pneumonia) were found to be due to *S. pneumoniae*.[19,20]

In the past decade the proportion of *S. pneumoniae* isolates resistant to antibiotics has been on the rise in the US and worldwide. In a multi-center US surveillance study, the prevalence of penicillin and cephalosporin-nonsusceptible (intermediate or high level resistance) invasive disease isolates from children was 21% (range <5% to 38% among centers), and 9.3% (range 0%-18%), respectively. Over the 3-year surveillance period (1993-1996), there was a 50% increase in penicillin-nonsusceptible *S. pneumoniae* (PNSP) strains and a three-fold rise in cephalosporin-nonsusceptible strains.[8] Although generally less common than PNSP, pneumococci resistant to macrolides and trimethoprim-sulfamethoxazole have also been observed.[4] Day care attendance, a history of ear infection, and a recent history of antibiotic exposure, have also been associated with invasive infections with PNSP in children 2 months to 59 months of age.[7,8] There has been no difference in mortality associated with PNSP strains.[8,9] However, the American Academy of Pediatrics (AAP) revised the antibiotic treatment guidelines in 1997 in response to the increased prevalence of antibiotic-resistant pneumococci.[21]

Approximately 90 serotypes of *S. pneumoniae* have been identified based on antigenic differences in their capsular polysaccharides. The distribution of serotypes responsible for disease differ with age and geographic location.[22]

Serotypes 4, 6B, 9V, 14, 18C, 19F, and 23F have been responsible for approximately 80% of invasive pneumococcal disease in children <6 years of age in the US.[18] These 7 serotypes also accounted for 74% of PNSP and 100% of pneumococci with high level penicillin resistance isolated from children <6 years with invasive disease during a 1993-1994 surveillance by the CDC.[23]

Results of Clinical Evaluations

Efficacy Against Invasive Disease

Efficacy was assessed in a randomized, double-blinded clinical trial in a multiethnic population at Northern California Kaiser Permanente (NCKP) from October 1995 through August 20, 1998, in which 37,816 infants were randomized to receive either Prevnar® or a control vaccine (an investigational meningococcal group C conjugate vaccine [MnCC]) at 2, 4, 6, and 12-15 months of age. Prevnar® was administered to 18,906 children and the control vaccine to 18,910 children. Routinely recommended vaccines were also administered which changed during the trial to reflect changing AAP and Advisory Committee on Immunization Practices (ACIP) recommendations. A planned interim analysis was performed upon accrual of 17 cases of invasive disease due to vaccine-type *S. pneumoniae* (August 1998). Ancillary endpoints for evaluation of efficacy against pneumococcal disease were also assessed in this trial.

Invasive disease was defined as isolation and identification of *S. pneumoniae* from normally sterile body sites in children presenting with an acute illness consistent with pneumococcal disease. Weekly surveillance of listings of cultures from the NCKP Regional Microbiology database was conducted to assure ascertainment of all cases. The primary endpoint was efficacy against invasive pneumococcal disease due to vaccine serotypes. The per protocol analysis of the primary endpoint included cases which occurred ≥14 days after the third dose. The intent-to-treat (ITT) analysis included all cases of invasive pneumococcal disease due to vaccine serotypes in children who received at least one dose of vaccine. Secondary analyses of efficacy against all invasive pneumococcal disease, regardless of serotype, were also performed according to these same per protocol and ITT definitions. Results of these analyses are presented in Table 1.

[See table 1 above]

All 22 cases of invasive disease due to vaccine serotype strains in the ITT population were bacteremic. In addition, the following diagnoses were also reported: meningitis (2), pneumonia (2), and cellulitis (1).

TABLE 1
Efficacy of Prevnar® Against Invasive Disease Due to *S. pneumoniae* in Cases Accrued From October 15, 1995 Through August 20, 1998[24,25]

	Prevnar® Number of Cases	Control* Number of Cases	Efficacy	95% CI
Vaccine serotypes				
Per protocol	0	17	100%	75.4, 100
Intent-to-treat	0	22	100%	81.7, 100
All pneumococcal serotypes				
Per protocol	2	20	90.0%	58.3, 98.9
Intent-to-treat	3	27†	88.9%	63.8, 97.9

* Investigational meningococcal group C conjugate vaccine (MnCC).
† Includes one case in an immunocompromised subject.

TABLE 2
Efficacy of Prevnar® Against Otitis Media in the Finnish and NCKP Trials[24,25,26,27]

	Per Protocol		Intent-to-Treat	
	Vaccine Efficacy Estimate*	95% Confidence Interval	Vaccine Efficacy Estimate*	95% Confidence Interval
Finnish Trial	N=1632		N=1662	
AOM due to Vaccine Serotypes	57%	44, 67	54%	41, 64
All culture-confirmed pneumococcal AOM regardless of serotype	34%	21, 45	32%	19, 42
NCKP Trial	N=23,746		N=34,146	
All Otitis Media Episodes regardless of etiology†	7%	4, 10	6%	4, 9

* All vaccine efficacy estimates in the table are statistically significant.
† The vaccine efficacy against all AOM episodes in the Finnish trial, while not reaching statistical significance, was 6% (95% CI: -4, 16) in the per protocol population and 4% (95% CI: -7, 14) in the intent-to-treat population.

Continued on next page

Prevnar—Cont.

Data accumulated through an extended follow-up period to April 20, 1999, resulted in a similar efficacy estimate (Per protocol: 1 case in Pneumococcal 7-valent Conjugate Vaccine (Diphtheria CRM_{197} Protein), Prevnar® group, 39 cases in control group; ITT: 3 cases in Prevnar® group, 49 cases in the control group).[25]

Efficacy Against Otitis Media

The efficacy of Prevnar® against otitis media was assessed in two clinical trials: a trial in Finnish infants at the National Public Health Institute and the invasive disease efficacy trial in US infants at Northern California Kaiser Permanente (NCKP).

The trial in Finland was a randomized, double-blind trial in which 1,662 infants were equally randomized to receive either Prevnar® or a control vaccine (Hepatitis B vaccine [Hep B]) at 2, 4, 6, and 12-15 months of age. All infants received a DTP-Hib combination vaccine concurrently at 2, 4, and 6 months of age, and Inactivated Poliovirus Vaccine (IPV) concurrently at 12 months of age. Parents of study participants were asked to bring their children to the study clinics if the child had respiratory infections or symptoms suggesting acute otitis media (AOM). If AOM was diagnosed, tympanocentesis was performed, and the middle ear fluid was cultured. If S. pneumoniae was isolated, serotyping was performed.

AOM was defined as a visually abnormal tympanic membrane suggesting effusion in the middle ear cavity, concomitantly with at least one of the following symptoms of acute infection: fever, ear ache, irritability, diarrhea, vomiting, acute otorrhea not caused by external otitis, or other symptoms of respiratory infection. A new visit or "episode" was defined as a visit with a study physician at which time a diagnosis of AOM was made and at least 30 days had elapsed since any previous visit for otitis media. The primary endpoint was efficacy against AOM episodes caused by vaccine serotypes in the per protocol population.

In the NCKP invasive disease efficacy trial, the effectiveness of Prevnar® in reducing the incidence of otitis media was assessed from the beginning of the trial in October 1995 through April 1998. During this time, 34,146 infants were randomized to receive either Prevnar® (N=17,070), or the control, an investigational meningococcal group C conjugate vaccine (N=17,076), at 2, 4, 6, and 12-15 months of age. Physician visits for otitis media were identified by physician coding of outpatient encounter forms. Because visits may have included both acute and follow-up care, a new visit or "episode" was defined as a visit that was at least 21 days following a previous visit for otitis media (at least 42 days, if the visit appointment was made > 3 days in advance). Data on placement of ear tubes were collected from automated databases. No routine tympanocentesis was performed, and no standard definition of otitis media was used by study physicians. The primary otitis media endpoint was efficacy against all otitis media episodes in the per protocol population.

Table 2 presents the per protocol and intent-to-treat results of key otitis media analyses for both studies. The per protocol analyses include otitis media episodes that occurred ≥14 days after the third dose. The intent-to-treat analyses include all otitis media episodes in children who received at least one dose of vaccine.[25]

[See table 2 at top of previous page]

The vaccine efficacy against AOM episodes due to vaccine-related serotypes (6A, 9N, 18B, 19A, 23A), also assessed in the Finnish trial, was 51% (95% CI: 27, 67) in the per protocol population and 44% (95% CI: 20, 62) in the intent-to-treat population. The vaccine efficacy against AOM episodes caused by serotypes unrelated to the vaccine was -33% (95% CI: -80, 1) in the per protocol population and -39% (95% CI: -86, -3) in the intent-to-treat population, indicating that children who received Prevnar® appear to be at increased risk of otitis media due to pneumococcal serotypes not represented in the vaccine, compared to children who received the control vaccine. However, vaccination with Prevnar® reduced pneumococcal otitis media episodes overall.

Several other otitis media endpoints were also assessed in the two trials. Recurrent AOM, defined as 3 episodes in 6 months or 4 episodes in 12 months, was reduced by 9% in both the per protocol and intent-to-treat populations (95% CI: 3, 15 in per protocol and 95% CI: 4, 14 in intent-to-treat) in the NCKP trial. This observation was supported by a similar trend, although not statistically significant, seen in the Finnish trial. The NCKP trial also demonstrated a 20% reduction (95% CI: 2, 35) in the placement of tympanostomy tubes in the per protocol population and a 21% reduction (95% CI: 4, 34) in the intent-to-treat population.

Data from the NCKP trial accumulated through an extended follow-up period to April 20, 1999, in which a total of 37,866 children were included (18,925 in Prevnar® group and 18,941 in MnCC control group), resulted in similar otitis media efficacy estimates for all endpoints.[28]

Immunogenicity

Routine Schedule

Subjects from a subset of selected study sites in the NCKP efficacy study were approached for participation in the immunogenicity portion of the study on a volunteer basis. Immune responses following three or four doses of Prevnar® or the control vaccine were evaluated in children who received either concurrent Diphtheria and Tetanus Toxoids and Pertussis Vaccine Adsorbed and Haemophilus b Conjugate Vaccine (Diphtheria CRM_{197} Protein Conjugate), (DTP-HbOC), or Diphtheria and Tetanus Toxoids and Acellular Pertussis Vaccine Adsorbed (DTaP), and Haemophilus b Conjugate Vaccine (Diphtheria CRM_{197} Protein Conjugate), (HbOC) vaccines at 2, 4, and 6 months of age. The use of Hepatitis B (Hep B), Oral Polio Vaccine (OPV), Inactivated Polio Vaccine (IPV), Measles-Mumps-Rubella (MMR), and Varicella vaccines were permitted according to the AAP and ACIP recommendations.

Table 3 presents the geometric mean concentrations (GMC) of pneumococcal antibodies following the third and fourth doses of Prevnar® or the control vaccine when administered concurrently with DTP-HbOC vaccine in the efficacy study.

[See table 3 above]

In another randomized study (Manufacturing Bridging Study, 118-16), immune responses were evaluated following three doses of Pneumococcal 7-valent Conjugate Vaccine (Diphtheria CRM_{197} Protein), Prevnar® administered concomitantly with DTaP and HbOC vaccines at 2, 4, and 6 months of age, IPV at 2 and 4 months of age, and Hep B at 2 and 6 months of age. The control group received concomitant vaccines only. Table 4 presents the immune responses to pneumococcal polysaccharides observed in both this study and in the subset of subjects from the efficacy study that received concomitant DTaP and HbOC vaccines.

[See table 4 above]

In all studies in which the immune responses to Prevnar® were contrasted to control, a significant antibody response was seen to all vaccine serotypes following three or four doses, although geometric mean concentrations of antibody varied among serotypes.[24,25,27,29,30,31,32,33,34] The minimum serum antibody concentration necessary for protection against invasive pneumococcal disease or against pneumococcal otitis media has not been determined for any serotype. Prevnar® induces functional antibodies to all vaccine serotypes, as measured by opsonophagocytosis following three doses.[34]

Previously Unvaccinated Older Infants and Children

To determine an appropriate schedule for children 7 months of age or older at the time of the first immunization with Prevnar®, 483 children in 4 ancillary studies received Prevnar® at various schedules and were evaluated for immunogenicity. GMCs attained using the various schedules

TABLE 3
Geometric Mean Concentrations (μg/mL) of Pneumococcal Antibodies Following the Third and Fourth Doses of Prevnar® or Control* When Administered Concurrently With DTP-HbOC in the Efficacy Study[24,25]

Serotype	Post dose 3 GMC† (95% CI for Prevnar®)		Post dose 4 GMC‡ (95% CI for Prevnar®)	
	Prevnar®§	Control*	Prevnar®§	Control*
	N=88	N=92	N=68	N=61
4	1.46 (1.19, 1.78)	0.03	2.38 (1.88, 3.03)	0.04
6B	4.70 (3.59, 6.14)	0.08	14.45 (11.17, 18.69)	0.17
9V	1.99 (1.64, 2.42)	0.05	3.51 (2.75, 4.48)	0.06
14	4.60 (3.70, 5.74)	0.05	6.52 (5.18, 8.21)	0.06
18C	2.16 (1.73, 2.69)	0.04	3.43 (2.70, 4.37)	0.07
19F	1.39 (1.16, 1.68)	0.09	2.07 (1.66, 2.57)	0.18
23F	1.85 (1.46, 2.34)	0.05	3.82 (2.85, 5.11)	0.09

* Control was investigational meningococcal group C conjugate vaccine (MnCC).
† Mean age of Prevnar® group was 7.8 months and of control group was 7.7 months. N is slightly less for some serotypes in each group.
‡ Mean age of Prevnar® group was 14.2 months and of control group was 14.4 months. N is slightly less for some serotypes in each group.
§ $p<0.001$ when Prevnar® compared to control for each serotype using a Wilcoxon's test.

TABLE 4
Geometric Mean Concentrations (μg/mL) of Pneumococcal Antibodies Following the Third Dose of Prevnar® or Control* When Administered Concurrently With DTaP and HbOC in the Efficacy Study† and Manufacturing Bridging Study[24,25,29]

	Efficacy Study		Manufacturing Bridging Study	
Serotype	Post dose 3 GMC‡ (95% CI for Prevnar®)		Post dose 3 GMC§ (95% CI for Prevnar®)	
	Prevnar® ‖	Control*	Prevnar® ‖	Control*
	N=32	N=32	N=159	N=83
4	1.47 (1.08, 2.02)	0.02	2.03 (1.75, 2.37)	0.02
6B	2.18 (1.20, 3.96)	0.06	2.97 (2.43, 3.65)	0.07
9V	1.52 (1.04, 2.22)	0.04	1.18 (1.01, 1.39)	0.04
14	5.05 (3.32, 7.70)	0.04	4.64 (3.80, 5.66)	0.04
18C	2.24 (1.65, 3.02)	0.04	1.96 (1.66, 2.30)	0.04
19F	1.54 (1.09, 2.17)	0.10	1.91 (1.63, 2.25)	0.08
23F	1.48 (0.97, 2.25)	0.05	1.71 (1.44, 2.05)	0.05

* Control in efficacy was investigational meningococcal group C conjugate vaccine (MnCC) and in Manufacturing Bridging Study was concomitant vaccines only.
† Sufficient data are not available to reliably assess GMCs following 4 doses of Prevnar® when administered with DTaP in the NCKP efficacy study.
‡ Mean age of the Prevnar® group was 7.4 months and of the control group was 7.6 months. N is slightly less for some serotypes in each group.
§ Mean age of the Prevnar® group and the control group was 7.2 months.
‖ $p<0.001$ when Prevnar® compared to control for each serotype using a Wilcoxon's test in the efficacy study and two-sample t-test in the Manufacturing Bridging Study.

among older infants and children were comparable to immune responses of children, who received concomitant DTaP, in the NCKP efficacy study (118-8) after 3 doses for most serotypes, as shown in Table 5. These data support the schedule for previously unvaccinated older infants and children who are beyond the age of the infant schedule. For usage in older infants and children, see **DOSAGE AND ADMINISTRATION**.
[See table 5 at right]

INDICATIONS AND USAGE
Prevnar® is indicated for active immunization of infants and toddlers against invasive disease caused by *S. pneumoniae* due to capsular serotypes included in the vaccine (4, 6B, 9V, 14, 18C, 19F, and 23F). The routine schedule is 2, 4, 6, and 12-15 months of age.
The decision to administer Pneumococcal 7-valent Conjugate Vaccine (Diphtheria CRM_{197} Protein), Prevnar® should be based primarily on its efficacy in preventing invasive pneumococcal disease. As with any vaccine, Prevnar® may not protect all individuals receiving the vaccine from invasive pneumococcal disease.
Prevnar® is also indicated for active immunization of infants and toddlers against otitis media caused by serotypes included in the vaccine. However, for vaccine serotypes, protection against otitis media is expected to be substantially lower than protection against invasive disease. Additionally, because otitis media is caused by many organisms other than serotypes of *S. pneumoniae* represented in the vaccine, protection against all causes of otitis media is expected to be low.
(See **CLINICAL PHARMACOLOGY** for estimates of efficacy against invasive disease and otitis media).
For additional information on usage, see **DOSAGE AND ADMINISTRATION**.
This vaccine is not intended to be used for treatment of active infection.

CONTRAINDICATIONS
Hypersensitivity to any component of the vaccine, including diphtheria toxoid, is a contraindication to use of this vaccine.
The decision to administer or delay vaccination because of a current or recent febrile illness depends largely on the severity of the symptoms and their etiology. Although a severe or even a moderate febrile illness is sufficient reason to postpone vaccinations, minor illnesses, such as a mild upper respiratory infection with or without low-grade fever, are not generally contraindications.[36,37]

WARNINGS
THIS VACCINE WILL NOT PROTECT AGAINST *S. PNEUMONIAE* DISEASE CAUSED BY SEROTYPES UNRELATED TO THOSE IN THE VACCINE, NOR WILL IT PROTECT AGAINST OTHER MICROORGANISMS THAT CAUSE INVASIVE INFECTIONS SUCH AS BACTEREMIA AND MENINGITIS OR NON-INVASIVE INFECTIONS SUCH AS OTITIS MEDIA.
This vaccine should not be given to infants or children with thrombocytopenia or any coagulation disorder that would contraindicate intramuscular injection unless the potential benefit clearly outweighs the risk of administration. If the decision is made to administer this vaccine to children with coagulation disorders, it should be given with caution. (See **DRUG INTERACTIONS**.)
Immunization with Prevnar® does not substitute for routine diphtheria immunization.
Healthcare professionals should prescribe and/or administer this product with caution to patients with a possible history of latex sensitivity since the packaging contains dry natural rubber.

PRECAUTIONS
Prevnar® is for intramuscular use only. Prevnar® SHOULD UNDER NO CIRCUMSTANCES BE ADMINISTERED INTRAVENOUSLY. The safety and immunogenicity for other routes of administration (eg, subcutaneous) have not been evaluated.
Fever, and rarely febrile seizure, have been reported in children receiving Prevnar®. For children at higher risk of seizures than the general population, acetaminophen or other appropriate antipyretics (dosed according to respective prescribing information) may be administered around the time of vaccination, to reduce the possibility of post-vaccination fever.

General
CARE IS TO BE TAKEN BY THE HEALTHCARE PROFESSIONAL FOR THE SAFE AND EFFECTIVE USE OF THIS PRODUCT.
1. PRIOR TO ADMINISTRATION OF ANY DOSE OF THIS VACCINE, THE PARENT OR GUARDIAN SHOULD BE ASKED ABOUT THE PERSONAL HISTORY, FAMILY HISTORY, AND RECENT HEALTH STATUS OF THE VACCINE RECIPIENT. THE HEALTHCARE PROFESSIONAL SHOULD ASCERTAIN PREVIOUS IMMUNIZATION HISTORY, CURRENT HEALTH STATUS, AND OCCURRENCE OF ANY SYMPTOMS AND/OR SIGNS OF AN ADVERSE EVENT AFTER PREVIOUS IMMUNIZATIONS IN THE CHILD TO BE IMMUNIZED, IN ORDER TO DETERMINE THE EXISTENCE OF ANY CONTRAINDICATION TO IMMUNIZATION WITH THIS VACCINE AND TO ALLOW AN ASSESSMENT OF RISKS AND BENEFITS.
2. BEFORE THE ADMINISTRATION OF ANY BIOLOGICAL, THE HEALTHCARE PROFESSIONAL SHOULD TAKE ALL PRECAUTIONS KNOWN FOR THE PREVENTION OF ALLERGIC OR ANY OTHER ADVERSE REACTIONS. This should include a review of the patient's history regarding possible sensitivity; the ready availability of epinephrine 1:1000 and other appropriate agents used for control of immediate allergic reactions; and a knowledge of the recent literature pertaining to use of the biological concerned, including the nature of side effects and adverse reactions that may follow its use.
3. Children with impaired immune responsiveness, whether due to the use of immunosuppressive therapy (including irradiation, corticosteroids, antimetabolites, alkylating agents, and cytotoxic agents), a genetic defect, HIV infection, or other causes, may have reduced antibody response to active immunization.[36,37,38] (See **DRUG INTERACTIONS**.)
4. The use of pneumococcal conjugate vaccine does not replace the use of 23-valent pneumococcal polysaccharide vaccine in children ≥ 24 months of age with sickle cell disease, asplenia, HIV infection, chronic illness or who are immunocompromised. Data on sequential vaccination with Prevnar® followed by 23-valent pneumococcal polysaccharide vaccine are limited. In a randomized study, 23

Continued on next page

TABLE 5
Geometric Mean Concentrations (µg/mL) of Pneumococcal Antibodies Following Immunization of Children From 7 Months Through 9 Years of Age With Prevnar®[35]

Age group, Vaccinations	Study	Sample Size(s)	4	6B	9V	14	18C	19F	23F
7-11 mo. 3 doses	118-12	22	2.34	3.66	2.11	**9.33**	2.31	1.60	**2.50**
	118-16	39	**3.60**	**4.63**	**2.04**	**5.48**	1.98	**2.15**	**1.93**
12-17 mo. 2 doses	118-15*	82-84†	**3.91**	**4.67**	**1.94**	**6.92**	**2.25**	**3.78**	**3.29**
	118-18	33	**7.02**	**4.25**	**3.26**	**6.31**	**3.60**	**3.29**	**2.92**
18-23 mo. 2 doses	118-15*	52-54†	**3.36**	**4.92**	**1.80**	**6.69**	**2.65**	**3.17**	**2.71**
	118-18	45	**6.85**	**3.71**	**3.86**	**6.48**	**3.42**	**3.86**	**2.75**
24-35 mo. 1 dose	118-18	53	**5.34**	**2.90**	**3.43**	1.88	**3.03**	**4.07**	1.56
36-59 mo. 1 dose	118-18	52	**6.27**	**6.40**	**4.62**	**5.95**	**4.08**	**6.37**	**2.95**
5-9 yrs. 1 dose	118-18	101	**6.92**	**20.84**	**7.49**	**19.32**	**6.72**	**12.51**	**11.57**
118-8, DTaP	Post dose 3	31-32†	1.47	2.18	1.52	5.05	2.24	1.54	1.48

Bold = GMC not inferior to 118-8, DTaP post dose 3 (one-sided lower limit of the 95% CI of GMC ratio ≥0.50).
*Study in Navajo and Apache populations.
† Numbers vary with serotype.

TABLE 6
Concurrent Administration of Prevnar® With Other Vaccines to Infants in Non-Efficacy Studies[29,32]

Antigen*	GMC*		% Responders†		Study	Vaccine Schedule‡	N	
	Prevnar®	Control§	Prevnar®	Control§		(mo.)	Prevnar®	Control§
Hib	6.2	4.4	99.5, 88.3	97.0, 88.1	118-12	2, 4, 6	214	67
Diphtheria	0.9	0.8	100	97.0				
Tetanus	3.5	4.1‖	100	100				
PT	19.1	17.8	74.0	69.7				
FHA	43.8	46.7	66.4	69.7				
Pertactin	40.1	50.9	65.6	77.3				
Fimbriae 2	3.3	4.2	44.7	62.5‖				
Hib	11.9	7.8‖	100, 96.9	98.8, 92.8	118-16	2, 4, 6	159	83
Hep B	—	—	99.4	96.2	118-16	0, 2, 6	156	80
IPV Type 1	—	—	89.0	93.6¶	118-16	2, 4	156	80
Type 2	—	—	94.2	93.6				
Type 3	—	—	83.8	80.8				

* Hib vaccine was HibTITER®, DTaP vaccine was Acel-Imune®. Hib (µg/mL) Dip, Tet (IU/mL); Pertussis Antigens (PT, FHA, Ptn, Fim) (units/mL).
† Responders = Hib (≥0.15 µg/mL, ≥1.0 µg/mL); Dip, Tet (≥0.1 IU/mL); Pertussis Antigens (PT, FHA, Ptn, Fim) [4-fold rise]; IPV (≥1:10); Hep B (≥10 mIU/mL).
‡ Schedule for concurrently administered vaccines; Pneumococcal 7-valent Conjugate Vaccine (Diphtheria CRM_{197} Protein), Prevnar® administered at 2, 4, 6 mos.; blood for antibody assessment attained 1 month after third dose, except for IPV (3 months post-immunization).
§ Concurrent vaccines only.
‖ $p<0.05$ when Prevnar® compared to control group using the following tests: ANCOVA for GMCs in 118-12; ANOVA for GMCs in 118-16; and Fisher's Exact test for % Responders in 118-12.
¶ Lower bound of 90% CI of difference >10%.

TABLE 7
Concurrent Administration of Prevnar® With Other Vaccines to Toddlers in a Non-Efficacy Study[31]

Antigen*	GMC*		% Responders†		Study‡	Vaccine Schedule§	N	
	Prevnar®	Control‖	Prevnar®	Control‖		(mo.)	Prevnar®	Control‖
Hib	22.7	47.9¶	100, 97.9	100, 100	118-7	12-15	47	26
Diphtheria	2.0	3.2¶	100	100				
Tetanus	14.4	18.8	100	100				
PT	68.6	121.2¶	68.1	73.1				
FHA	29.0	48.2¶	68.1	84.6				
Pertactin	84.4	83.0	83.0	96.2				
Fimbriae 2	5.2	3.8	63.8	50.0				

* Hib vaccine was HibTITER®, DTaP vaccine was Acel-Imune®. Hib (µg/mL); Dip, Tet (IU/mL); Pertussis Antigens (PT, FHA, Ptn, Fim) (units/mL).
† Responders = Hib (≥0.15 µg/mL, ≥1.0 µg/mL); Dip, Tet (≥0.1 IU/mL); Pertussis Antigens (PT, FHA, Ptn, Fim) [4-fold rise].
‡ Children received a primary series of DTP-HbOC (Tetramune®).
§ Blood for antibody assessment obtained 1 month after dose.
‖ Concurrent vaccines only.
¶ $p<0.05$ when Prevnar® compared to control group using a two-sample t-test.

Prevnar—Cont.

children ≥ 2 years of age with sickle cell disease were administered either 2 doses of Prevnar® followed by a dose of polysaccharide vaccine or a single dose of polysaccharide vaccine alone. In this small study, safety and immune responses with the combined schedule were similar to polysaccharide vaccine alone.[39]

5. Since this product is a suspension containing an aluminum adjuvant, shake vigorously immediately prior to use to obtain a uniform suspension prior to withdrawing the dose.
6. A separate sterile syringe and needle or a sterile disposable unit should be used for each individual to prevent transmission of hepatitis or other infectious agents from one person to another. Needles should be disposed of properly and should not be recapped.
7. The vaccine is to be administered immediately after being drawn up into a syringe.
8. Special care should be taken to prevent injection into or near a blood vessel or nerve.
9. Healthcare professionals should prescribe and/or administer this product with caution to patients with a possible history of latex sensitivity since the packaging contains dry natural rubber.

Information for Parents or Guardians
Prior to administration of this vaccine, the healthcare professional should inform the parent, guardian, or other responsible adult of the potential benefits and risks to the patient (see **ADVERSE REACTIONS** and **WARNINGS** sections), and the importance of completing the immunization series unless contraindicated. Parents or guardians should be instructed to report any suspected adverse reactions to their healthcare professional. The healthcare professional should provide vaccine information statements prior to each vaccination.

DRUG INTERACTIONS
Children receiving therapy with immunosuppressive agents (large amounts of corticosteroids, antimetabolites, alkylating agents, cytotoxic agents) may not respond optimally to active immunization.[37,38,40,41] (See **PRECAUTIONS, General**.)
As with other intramuscular injections, Prevnar® should be given with caution to children on anticoagulant therapy.

Simultaneous Administration with Other Vaccines
During clinical studies, Prevnar® was administered simultaneously with DTP-HbOC or DTaP and HbOC, OPV or IPV, Hep B vaccines, MMR, and Varicella vaccine. Thus, the safety experience with Prevnar® reflects the use of this product as part of the routine immunization schedule.[24,25,29,31,32,34]
The immune response to routine vaccines when administered with Prevnar® (at separate sites) was assessed in 3 clinical studies in which there was a control group for comparison. Results for the concurrent immunizations in infants are shown in Table 6 and for toddlers in Table 7. Enhancement of antibody response to HbOC in the infant series was observed. Some suppression of *Haemophilus influenzae* type b (Hib) response was seen at the 4th dose, but over 97% of children achieved titers ≥1 µg/mL. Although some inconsistent differences in response to pertussis antigens were observed, the clinical relevance is unknown. The response to 2 doses of IPV given concomitantly with Prevnar®, assessed 3 months after the second dose, was equivalent to controls for poliovirus Types 2 and 3, but lower for Type 1. MMR and Varicella immunogenicity data from controlled clinical trials with concurrent administration of Prevnar® are not available.
[See table 6 on previous page]
[See table 7 on previous page]

CARCINOGENESIS, MUTAGENESIS, IMPAIRMENT OF FERTILITY
Prevnar® has not been evaluated for any carcinogenic or mutagenic potential, or impairment of fertility.

PREGNANCY
Pregnancy Category C
Animal reproductive studies have not been conducted with this product. It is not known whether Prevnar® can cause fetal harm when administered to a pregnant woman or whether it can affect reproductive capacity. This vaccine is not recommended for use in pregnant women.

Nursing Mothers
It is not known whether vaccine antigens or antibodies are excreted in human milk. This vaccine is not recommended for use in a nursing mother.

PEDIATRIC USE
Prevnar® has been shown to be usually well-tolerated and immunogenic in infants. The safety and effectiveness of Prevnar® in children below the age of 6 weeks or on or after the 10th birthday have not been established. Immune responses elicited by Prevnar® among infants born prematurely have not been studied. See **DOSAGE AND ADMINISTRATION** for the recommended pediatric dosage.

GERIATRIC USE
This vaccine is NOT recommended for use in adult populations. It is not to be used as a substitute for the pneumococcal polysaccharide vaccine in geriatric populations.

ADVERSE REACTIONS
Pre-Licensure Clinical Trial Experience
The majority of the safety experience with Prevnar® comes from the NCKP Efficacy Trial in which 17,066 infants received 55,352 doses of Prevnar®, along with other routine childhood vaccines through April 1998 (see **CLINICAL PHARMACOLOGY** section). The number of Prevnar® recipients in the safety analysis differs from the number included in the efficacy analysis due to the different lengths of follow-up for these study endpoints. Safety was monitored in this study using several modalities. Local reactions and systemic events occurring within 48 hours of each dose of vaccine were ascertained by scripted telephone interview on a randomly selected subset of approximately 3,000 children in each vaccine group. The rate of relatively rare events requiring medical attention was evaluated across all doses in all study participants using automated databases. Specifically, rates of hospitalizations within 3, 14, 30, and 60 days of immunization, and of emergency room visits within 3, 14, and 30 days of immunization were assessed and compared between vaccine groups for each diagnosis. Seizures within 3 and 30 days of immunization were ascertained across multiple settings (hospitalizations, emergency room or clinic visits, telephone interviews). Deaths and SIDS were ascertained through April 1999. Hospitalizations due to diabetes, autoimmune disorders, and blood disorders were ascertained through August 1999.
In Tables 8 and 9 the rate of local reactions at the Prevnar® injection site is compared at each dose to the DTP or DTaP injection site in the same children.
[See table 8 above]
[See table 9 above]
Table 10 presents the rates of local reactions in previously unvaccinated older infants and children.
[See table 10 at bottom of next page]
Tables 11 and 12 present the rates of systemic events observed in the efficacy study when Prevnar® was administered concomitantly with DTP or DTaP.
[See table 11 at bottom of next page]
[See table 12 at top of page 352]

Table 13 presents results from a second study (Manufacturing Bridging Study) conducted at Northern California and Denver Kaiser sites, in which children were randomized to receive one of three lots of Pneumococcal 7-valent Conjugate Vaccine (Diphtheria CRM$_{197}$ Protein), Prevnar®, with concomitant vaccines including DTaP, or the same concomitant vaccines alone. Information was ascertained by scripted telephone interview, as described above.
[See table 13 on page 352]
Fever (≥38.0°C) within 48 hours of a vaccine dose was reported by a greater proportion of subjects who received Prevnar®, compared to control (investigational meningococcal group C conjugate vaccine [MnCC]), after each dose when administered concurrently with DTP-HbOC or DTaP in the efficacy study. In the Manufacturing Bridging Study, fever within 48-72 hours was also reported more commonly after each dose compared to infants in the control group who received only recommended vaccines. When administered concurrently with DTaP in either study, fever rates among Prevnar® recipients ranged from 15% to 34%, and were greatest after the 2nd dose.
Table 14 presents the frequencies of systemic reactions in previously unvaccinated older infants and children.
[See table 14 at bottom of page 352]
Of the 17,066 subjects who received at least one dose of Prevnar® in the efficacy trial, there were 24 hospitalizations (for 29 diagnoses) within 3 days of a dose from October 1995 through April 1998. Diagnoses were as follows: bronchiolitis (5); congenital anomaly (4); elective procedure, UTI (3 each); acute gastroenteritis, asthma, pneumonia (2 each); aspiration, breath holding, influenza, inguinal hernia repair, otitis media, febrile seizure, viral syndrome, well child/reassurance (1 each). There were 162 visits to the emergency room

TABLE 8
Percentage of Subjects Reporting Local Reactions Within 2 Days Following Immunization With Prevnar® and DTP-HbOC* Vaccines at 2, 4, 6, and 12–15 Months of Age[24,25]

Reaction	Dose 1		Dose 2		Dose 3		Dose 4	
	Prevnar® Site	DTP-HbOC Site†	Prevnar® Site	DTP-HbOC Site†	Prevnar® Site	DTP-HbOC Site†	Prevnar® Site	DTP-HbOC Site†
	N=2890	N=2890	N=2725	N=2725	N=2538	N=2538	N=599	N=599
Erythema								
Any	12.4	21.9	14.3	25.1	15.2	26.5	12.7	23.4
>2.4 cm	1.2	4.6	1.0	2.9	2.0	4.4	1.7	6.4
Induration								
Any	10.9	22.4	12.3	23.0	12.8	23.3	11.4	20.5
>2.4 cm	2.6	7.2	2.4	5.6	2.9	6.7	2.8	7.2
Tenderness								
Any	28.0	36.4	25.2	30.5	25.6	32.8	36.5	45.1
Interfered with limb movement	7.9	10.7	7.4	8.4	7.8	10.0	18.5	22.2

*If Hep B vaccine was administered simultaneously, it was administered into the same limb as the DTP-HbOC vaccine. If reactions occurred at either or both sites on that limb, the more severe reaction was recorded.
† p<0.05 when Prevnar® site compared to the DTP-HbOC site using the sign test.

TABLE 9
Percentage of Subjects Reporting Local Reactions Within 2 Days Following Immunization With Prevnar®* and DTaP Vaccines† at 2, 4, 6, and 12-15 Months of Age[24,25]

Reaction	Dose 1		Dose 2		Dose 3		Dose 4	
	Prevnar® Site	DTaP Site	Prevnar® Site	DTaP Site	Prevnar® Site	DTaP Site	Prevnar® Site	DTPaP Site‡
	N=693	N=693	N=526	N=526	N=422	N=422	N=165	N=165
Erythema								
Any	10.0	6.7§	11.6	10.5	13.8	11.4	10.9	3.6§
>2.4 cm	1.3	0.4§	0.6	0.6	1.4	1.0	3.6	0.6
Induration								
Any	9.8	6.6§	12.0	10.5	10.4	10.4	12.1	5.5§
>2.4 cm	1.6	0.9	1.3	1.7	2.4	1.9	5.5	1.8
Tenderness								
Any	17.9	16.0	19.4	17.3	14.7	13.1	23.3	18.4
Interfered with limb movement	3.1	1.8§	4.1	3.3	2.9	1.9	9.2	8.0

*HbOC was administered in the same limb as Pneumococcal 7-valent Conjugate Vaccine (Diphtheria CRM$_{197}$ Protein), Prevnar®. If reactions occurred at either or both sites on that limb, the more severe reaction was recorded.
† If Hep B vaccine was administered simultaneously, it was administered into the same limb as DTaP. If reactions occurred at either or both sites on that limb, the more severe reaction was recorded.
‡ Subjects may have received DTP or a mixed DTP/DTaP regimen for the primary series. Thus, this is the 4th dose of a pertussis vaccine, but not a 4th dose of DTaP.
§ p<0.05 when Prevnar® site compared to DTaP site using the sign test.

(for 182 diagnoses) within 3 days of a dose from October 1995 through April 1998. Diagnoses were as follows: febrile illness (20); acute gastroenteritis (19); trauma, URI (16 each); otitis media (15); well child (13); irritable child, viral syndrome (10 each); rash (8); croup, pneumonia (6 each); poisoning/ingestion (5); asthma, bronchiolitis (4 each); febrile seizure, UTI (3 each); thrush, wheezing, breath holding, choking, conjunctivitis, inguinal hernia repair, pharyngitis (2 each); colic, colitis, congestive heart failure, elective procedure, hives, influenza, ingrown toenail, local swelling, roseola, sepsis (1 each).[24,25]

In the large-scale efficacy study, urticaria-like rash was reported in 0.4%-1.4% of children within 48 hours following immunization with Prevnar® administered concurrently with other routine childhood vaccines. Urticaria-like rash was reported in 1.3%-6% of children in the period from 3 to 14 days following immunization, and was most often reported following the fourth dose when it was administered concurrently with MMR vaccine. Based on limited data, it appears that children with urticaria-like rash after a dose of Prevnar® may be more likely to report urticaria-like rash following a subsequent dose of Prevnar®.

One case of a hypotonic-hyporesponsive episode (HHE) was reported in the efficacy study following Prevnar® and concurrent DTP vaccines in the study period from October 1995 through April 1998. Two additional cases of HHE were reported in four other studies and these also occurred in children who received Prevnar® concurrently with DTP vaccine.[31,34]

In the Kaiser efficacy study in which 17,066 children received a total of 55,352 doses of Prevnar® and 17,080 children received a total of 55,387 doses of the control vaccine (investigational meningococcal group C conjugate vaccine [MnCC]), seizures were reported in 8 Prevnar® recipients and 4 control vaccine recipients within 3 days of immunization from October 1995 through April 1998. Of the 8 Prevnar® recipients, 7 received concomitant DTP-containing vaccines and one received DTaP. Of the 4 control vaccine recipients, 3 received concomitant DTP-containing vaccines and one received DTaP.[24,25] In the other 4 studies combined, in which 1,102 children were immunized with 3,347 doses of Prevnar® and 408 children were immunized with 1,310 doses of control vaccine (either investigational meningococcal group C conjugate vaccine [MnCC] or concurrent vaccines), there was one seizure event reported within 3 days of immunization.[32] This subject received Prevnar® concurrent with DTaP vaccine.

Twelve deaths (5 SIDS and 7 with clear alternative cause) occurred among subjects receiving Prevnar®, of which 11 (4 SIDS and 7 with clear alternative cause) occurred in the Kaiser efficacy study from October 1995 until April 20, 1999. In comparison, 21 deaths (8 SIDS, 12 with clear alternative cause and one SIDS-like death in an older child), occurred in the control vaccine group during the same time period in the efficacy study.[24,25,29] The number of SIDS deaths in the efficacy study from October 1995 until April 20, 1999 was similar to or lower than the age and season-adjusted expected rate from the California State data from 1995-1997 and are presented in Table 15.

[See table 15 on page 353]

In a review of all hospitalizations that occurred between October 1995 and August 1999 in the efficacy study for the specific diagnoses of aplastic anemia, autoimmune disease, autoimmune hemolytic anemia, diabetes mellitus, neutropenia, and thrombocytopenia, the numbers of such cases were equal to or less than the expected numbers based on the 1995 Kaiser Vaccine Safety Data Link (VSD) data set. Overall, the safety of Prevnar® was evaluated in a total of five clinical studies in the US in which 18,168 infants and children received a total of 58,699 doses of vaccine at 2, 4, 6, and 12-15 months of age. In addition, the safety of Prevnar® was evaluated in 831 Finnish infants using the same schedule, and the overall safety profile was similar to that in US infants. The safety of Prevnar® was also evaluated in 560 children from 4 ancillary studies in the US who started immunization at 7 months to 9 years of age. Tables 16 and 17 summarize systemic reactogenicity data within 2 or 3 days across 4,748 subjects in US studies (13,039 infant doses and 1,706 toddler doses) for whom these data were collected and according to the pertussis vaccine administered concurrently.

[See table 16 on page 353]
[See table 17 at bottom of page 353]

With vaccines in general, including Pneumococcal 7-valent Conjugate Vaccine (Diphtheria CRM_{197} Protein), Prevnar®, it is not uncommon for patients to note within 48 to 72 hours at or around the injection site the following minor reactions: edema; pain or tenderness; redness, inflammation or skin discoloration; mass; or local hypersensitivity reaction. Such local reactions are usually self-limited and require no therapy.

As with other aluminum-containing vaccines, a nodule may occasionally be palpable at the injection site for several weeks.[42]

Postmarketing Experience

Additional adverse reactions identified from postmarketing experience are listed below:

Administration site conditions: injection site dermatitis, injection site urticaria, injection site pruritus

Blood and lymphatic system disorders: lymphadenopathy localized to the region of the injection site

Immune system disorders: hypersensitivity reaction including face edema, dyspnea, bronchospasm; anaphylactic/anaphylactoid reaction including shock

Skin and subcutaneous tissue disorders: angioneurotic edema, erythema multiforme

ADVERSE EVENT REPORTING

Any suspected adverse events following immunization should be reported by the healthcare professional to the US Department of Health and Human Services (DHHS). The National Vaccine Injury Compensation Program requires that the manufacturer and lot number of the vaccine administered be recorded by the healthcare professional in the vaccine recipient's permanent medical record (or in a permanent office log or file), along with the date of administration of the vaccine and the name, address, and title of the person administering the vaccine.

The US DHHS has established the Vaccine Adverse Event Reporting System (VAERS) to accept all reports of suspected adverse events after the administration of any vaccine including, but not limited to, the reporting of events required by the National Childhood Vaccine Injury Act of 1986. The FDA web site is: http://www.fda.gov/cber/vaers/vaers.htm.

The VAERS toll-free number for VAERS forms and information is 800-822-7967.[43]

OVERDOSAGE

There have been reports of overdose with Prevnar®, including cases of administration of a higher than recommended dose and cases of subsequent doses administered closer than recommended to the previous dose. Most individuals were asymptomatic. In general, adverse events reported with overdose have also been reported with recommended single doses of Prevnar®.

DOSAGE AND ADMINISTRATION

For intramuscular injection only. *Do not inject intravenously.*

The dose is 0.5 mL to be given intramuscularly.

Since this product is a suspension containing an adjuvant, shake vigorously immediately prior to use to obtain a uniform suspension in the vaccine container. The vaccine should not be used if it cannot be resuspended.

After shaking, the vaccine is a homogeneous, white suspension.

Parenteral drug products should be inspected visually for particulate matter and discoloration prior to administration (see **DESCRIPTION**). This product should not be used if particulate matter or discoloration is found.

The vaccine should be injected intramuscularly. The preferred sites are the anterolateral aspect of the thigh in infants or the deltoid muscle of the upper arm in toddlers and young children. The vaccine should not be injected in the gluteal area or areas where there may be a major nerve trunk and/or blood vessel. Before injection, the skin at the injection site should be cleansed and prepared with a suitable germicide. After insertion of the needle, aspirate and wait to see if any blood appears in the syringe, which will help avoid inadvertent injection into a blood vessel. If blood appears, withdraw the needle and prepare for a new injection at another site.

Vaccine Schedule

For infants, the immunization series of Prevnar® consists of three doses of 0.5 mL each, at approximately 2-month intervals, followed by a fourth dose of 0.5 mL at 12-15 months of age. The customary age for the first dose is 2 months of age,

Continued on next page

TABLE 10
Percentage of Subjects Reporting Local Reactions Within 3 Days of Immunization with Prevnar® in Infants and Children from 7 Months Through 9 Years of Age[35]

Age at 1st Vaccination	7 - 11 Mos.						12 - 23 Mos.			24 - 35 Mos.	36 - 59 Mos.	5 - 9 Yrs.
Study No.	118-12			118-16			118-9*	118-18		118-18	118-18	118-18
Dose Number	1	2	3†	1	2	3†	1	1	1	1	1	1
Number of Subjects	54	51	24	81	76	50	60	114	117	46	48	49
Reaction												
Erythema												
Any	16.7	11.8	20.8	7.4	7.9	14.0	48.3	10.5	9.4	6.5	29.2	24.2
>2.4 cm‡	1.9	0.0	0.0	0.0	0.0	0.0	6.7	1.8	1.7	0.0	8.3	7.1
Induration												
Any	16.7	11.8	8.3	7.4	3.9	10.0	48.3	8.8	6.0	10.9	22.9	25.5
>2.4 cm‡	3.7	0.0	0.0	0.0	0.0	0.0	3.3	0.9	0.9	2.2	6.3	9.3
Tenderness												
Any	13.0	11.8	12.5	8.6	10.5	12.0	46.7	25.7	26.5	41.3	58.3	82.8
Interfered with limb movement§	1.9	2.0	4.2	1.2	1.3	0.0	3.3	6.2	8.5	13.0	20.8	39.4

* For 118-9, 2 of 60 subjects were ≥24 months of age.
† For 118-12, dose 3 was administered at 15 - 18 mos. of age, For 118-16, dose 3 was administered at 12 - 15 mos. of age.
‡ For 118-16 and 118-18, ≥2 cm.
§ Tenderness interfering with limb movement.

TABLE 11
Percentage of Subjects* Reporting Systemic Events Within 2 Days Following Immunization With Prevnar® or Control† Vaccine Concurrently With DTP-HbOC Vaccine at 2, 4, 6, and 12-15 Months of Age[24,25]

Reaction	Dose 1		Dose 2		Dose 3		Dose 4	
	Prevnar®	Control†	Prevnar®	Control†	Prevnar®	Control†	Prevnar®	Control†
	N=2998	N=2982	N=2788	N=2761	N=2596	N=2591	N=709	N=733
Fever								
≥38.0°C	33.4	28.7‡	34.7	27.4‡	40.6	32.4‡	41.9	36.9
>39.0°C	1.3	1.3	3.0	1.6‡	5.3	3.4‡	4.5	4.5
Irritability	71.3	67.9‡	69.4	63.8‡	68.9	61.6‡	72.8	65.8‡
Drowsiness	49.2	50.6	32.5	33.6	25.9	23.4‡	21.3	22.7
Restless Sleep	18.1	17.9	27.3	24.3‡	33.3	30.1‡	29.9	28.0
Decreased Appetite	24.7	23.6	22.8	20.3‡	27.7	25.6	33.0	27.4‡
Vomiting	17.9	14.9‡	16.2	14.4	15.5	12.7‡	9.6	6.8
Diarrhea	12.0	10.7	10.9	9.9	11.5	10.4	12.1	11.2
Urticaria-like Rash	0.7	0.6	0.8	0.8	1.4	1.1	1.4	0.8

* Approximately 90% of subjects received prophylactic or therapeutic antipyretics within 48 hours of each dose.
† Investigational meningococcal group C conjugate vaccine (MnCC).
‡ p<0.05 when Prevnar® compared to control group using a Chi-Square test.

Prevnar—Cont.

but it can be given as young as 6 weeks of age. The recommended dosing interval is 4 to 8 weeks. The fourth dose should be administered at least 2 months after the third dose.

Previously Unvaccinated Older Infants and Children
For previously unvaccinated older infants and children, who are beyond the age of the routine infant schedule, the following schedule applies:[35]

Age at First Dose	Total Number of 0.5 mL Doses
7-11 months of age	3*
12-23 months of age	2†
≥24 months through 9 years of age	1

*2 doses at least 4 weeks apart; third dose after the one-year birthday, separated from the second dose by at least 2 months.
† 2 doses at least 2 months apart.

(See **CLINICAL PHARMACOLOGY** section for the limited available immunogenicity data and **ADVERSE EVENTS** section for limited safety data corresponding to the previously noted vaccination schedule for older children).

Safety and immunogenicity data are either limited or not available for children in specific high risk groups for invasive pneumococcal disease (eg, persons with sickle cell disease, asplenia, HIV-infected).

HOW SUPPLIED
Vial, 1 Dose (5 per package) - NDC 0005-1970-67
CPT Code 90669

STORAGE
DO NOT FREEZE. STORE REFRIGERATED, AWAY FROM FREEZER COMPARTMENT, AT 2°C TO 8°C (36°F TO 46°F).

REFERENCES
1. Schuchat A, Robinson K, Wenger JD, et al. Bacterial meningitis in the United States in 1995. N Engl J Med. 1997; 337:970-6.
2. Zangwill KM, Vadheim CM, Vannier AM, et al. Epidemiology of invasive pneumococcal disease in Southern California: implications for the design and conduct of a pneumococcal conjugate vaccine efficacy trial. J Infect Dis. 1996; 174:752-9.
3. Pastor P, Medley F, Murphy T. Invasive pneumococcal disease in Dallas County, Texas: results from population-based surveillance in 1995. Clin Infect Dis. 1998; 26:590-5.
4. Hofmann J, Cetron MS, Farley MM, et al. The prevalence of drug-resistant Streptococcus pneumoniae in Atlanta. N Engl J Med. 1995; 333:481-515.
5. Breiman R, Spika J, Navarro V, et al. Pneumococcal bacteremia in Charleston County, South Carolina. Arch Intern Med. 1990; 150:1401-5.
6. Plouffe J, Breiman R, Facklam R. Franklin County Study Group. Bacteremia with Streptococcus pneumoniae in adults-implications for therapy and prevention. JAMA. 1996; 275:194-8.
7. Levine O, Farley M, Harrison LH, et al. Risk factors for invasive pneumococcal disease in children: a population-based case-control study in North America. Pediatrics. 1999; 103:1-5.
8. Kaplan SL, Mason EO, Barson WJ, et al. Three-year multicenter surveillance of systemic pneumococcal infections in children. Pediatrics. 1998; 102:538-44.
9. Arditi M, Mason E, Bradley J, et al. Three-year multicenter surveillance of pneumococcal meningitis in children: clinical characteristics and outcome related to penicillin susceptibility and dexamethasone use. Pediatrics. 1998; 102:1087-97.
10. Shappert SM. Ambulatory care visits to physician offices, hospital outpatient departments, and emergency departments: United States, 1997. National Center for Health Statistics. Vital Health Sat. 1999; 13(143):1-41.
11. Hall MJ, Lawrence L. Ambulatory surgery in the United States, 1996. Adv Data Vital Health Stat. 1998; 300:1-16.
12. Teele DW, Klein JO, Rosner B, et al. Epidemiology of otitis media during the first seven years of life in children in greater Boston: a prospective, cohort study. J Infect Dis. 1989; 160:83-94.
13. Shappert, SM. Office visits for otitis media: United States, 1975-1990. Adv Data Vital Health Stat. 1992; 214:1-20.
14. Bluestone CD, Stephenson BS, Martin LM. Ten-year review of otitis media pathogens. Pediatr Infect Dis J. 1992; 11:S7-S11.
15. Giebink GS. The microbiology of otitis media. Pediatr Infect Dis J. 1989; 8:S18-S20.
16. Rodriguez WJ, Schwartz RH. Streptococcus pneumoniae causes otitis media with higher fever and more redness of tympanic membrane than Haemophilus influenzae or Moraxella catarrhalis. Pediatr Infect Dis J. 1999; 18:942-4.
17. Barnett ED, Klein JO. The problem of resistant bacteria for the management of acute otitis media. Ped Clin North Am. 1995; 42:509-17.
18. Butler JC, Breiman RF, Lipman HB, et al. Serotype distribution of Streptococcus pneumoniae infections among pre-school children in the United States, 1978-1994: implications for development of a conjugate vaccine. J Infect Dis. 1995; 171:885-9.
19. Paisley JW, Lauer BA, McIntosh K, et al. Pathogens associated with acute lower respiratory tract infection in young children. Pediatr Infect Dis J. 1984; 3:14-9.
20. Heiskanen-Kosma T, Korppi M, Jokinen C, et al. Etiology of childhood pneumonia: serologic results of a prospective, population-based study. Pediatr Infect Dis J. 1998; 17:986-91.
21. American Academy of Pediatrics Committee on Infectious Diseases. Therapy for children with invasive pneumococcal infections. Pediatrics. 1997; 99:289-300.
22. Hausdorff WP, Bryant J, Paradiso PR, Siber GR. Which pneumococcal serogroups cause the most invasive disease: implications for conjugate vaccine formulation and use, part I. Clin Infect Dis. 2000; 30:100-21.
23. Butler JC, Hoffman J, Cetron MS, et al. The continued emergence of drug-resistant Streptococcus pneumoniae in the United States. An Update from the Centers for Disease Control and Prevention's Pneumococcal Sentinel Surveillance System. J Infect Dis. 1996; 174:986-93.

TABLE 12
Percentage of Subjects* Reporting Systemic Events Within 2 Days Following Immunization With Prevnar® or Control† Vaccine Concurrently With DTaP Vaccine at 2, 4, 6, and 12-15 Months of Age[24,25]

Reaction	Dose 1		Dose 2		Dose 3		Dose 4‡	
	Prevnar®	Control†	Prevnar®	Control†	Prevnar®	Control†	Prevnar®	Control†
	N=710	N=711	N=559	N=508	N=461	N=414	N=224	N=230
Fever								
≥38.0°C	15.1	9.4§	23.9	10.8§	19.1	11.8§	21.0	17.0
>39.0°C	0.9	0.3	2.5	0.8§	1.7	0.7	1.3	1.7
Irritability	48.0	48.2	58.7	45.3§	51.2	44.8	44.2	42.6
Drowsiness	40.7	42.0	25.6	22.8	19.5	21.9	17.0	16.5
Restless Sleep	15.3	15.1	20.2	19.3	25.2	19.0§	20.2	19.1
Decreased Appetite	17.0	13.5	17.4	13.4	20.7	13.8§	20.5	23.1
Vomiting	14.6	14.5	16.8	14.4	10.4	11.6	4.9	4.8
Diarrhea	11.9	8.4§	10.2	9.3	8.3	9.4	11.6	9.2
Urticaria-like Rash	1.4	0.3§	1.3	1.4	0.4	0.5	0.5	1.7

*Approximately 75% of subjects received prophylactic or therapeutic antipyretics within 48 hours of each dose.
† Investigational meningococcal group C conjugate vaccine (MnCC).
‡ Most of these children had received DTP for the primary series. Thus, this is a 4th dose of a pertussis vaccine, but not of DTaP.
§ $p<0.05$ when Prevnar® compared to control group using a Chi-Square test.

TABLE 13
Percentage of Subjects* Reporting Systemic Reactions Within 3 Days Following Immunization With Prevnar®, DTaP, HbOC, Hep B, and IPV vs. Control† in Manufacturing Bridging Study[29]

Reaction	Dose 1		Dose 2		Dose 3	
	Prevnar®	Control†	Prevnar®	Control†	Prevnar®	Control†
	N=498	N=108	N=452	N=99	N=445	N=89
Fever						
≥38.0°C	21.9	10.2‡	33.6	17.2‡	28.1	23.6
>39.0°C	0.8	0.9	3.8	0.0	2.2	0.0
Irritability	59.7	60.2	65.3	52.5‡	54.2	50.6
Drowsiness	50.8	38.9‡	30.3	31.3	21.2	20.2
Decreased Appetite	19.1	15.7	20.6	11.1‡	20.4	9.0‡

*Approximately 72% of subjects received prophylactic or therapeutic antipyretics within 48 hours of each dose.
† Control group received concomitant vaccines only in the same schedule as the Prevnar® group (DTaP, HbOC at dose 1, 2, 3; IPV at doses 1 and 2; Hep B at doses 1 and 3).
‡ $p<0.05$ when Prevnar® compared to control group using Fisher's Exact test.

TABLE 14
Percentage of Subjects Reporting Systemic Reactions Within 3 Days of Immunization With Prevnar® in Infants and Children from 7 Months Through 9 Years of Age[35]

Age at 1st Vaccination	7 - 11 Mos.			12 - 23 Mos.				24 - 35 Mos.	36 - 59 Mos.	5 - 9 Yrs.
Study No.	118-12			118-16			118-9*	118-18	118-18	118-18	118-18
Dose Number	1	2	3†	1	2	3†	1	1	2	1	1	1
Number of Subjects	54	51	24	85	80	50	60	120	117	47	52	100
Reaction												
Fever												
≥38.0°C	20.8	21.6	25.0	17.6	18.8	22.0	36.7	11.7	6.8	14.9	11.5	7.0
>39.0°C	1.9	5.9	0.0	1.6	3.9	2.6	0.0	4.4	0.0	4.2	2.3	1.2
Fussiness	29.6	39.2	16.7	54.1	41.3	38.0	40.0	37.5	36.8	46.8	34.6	29.3
Drowsiness	11.1	17.6	16.7	24.7	16.3	14.0	13.3	18.3	11.1	12.8	17.3	11.0
Decreased Appetite	9.3	15.7	0.0	15.3	15.0	30.0	25.0	20.8	16.2	23.4	11.5	9.0

*For 118-9, 2 of 60 subjects were ≥24 months of age.
† For 118-12, dose 3 was administered at 15 - 18 mos. of age. For 118-16, dose 3 was administered at 12 - 15 mos. of age.

24. Lederle Laboratories, Data on File: D118-P8.
25. Black S, Shinefield H, Ray P, et al. Efficacy, safety and immunogenicity of heptavalent pneumococcal conjugate vaccine in children. Pediatr Infect Dis J. 2000; 19:187-195.
26. Lederle Laboratories, Data on File: D118-P809.
27. Eskola J, Kilpi T, Palma A, et al. Efficacy of a pneumococcal conjugate vaccine against acute otitis media. N Engl J Med. 2001; 344:403-409.
28. Fireman B, Black S, Shinefield H, et al. The impact of the pneumococcal conjugate vaccine on otitis media. Pediatr Infect Dis J. In press.
29. Lederle Laboratories, Data on File: D118-P16.
30. Lederle Laboratories, Data on File: D118-P8 Addendum DTaP Immunogenicity.
31. Shinefield HR, Black S, Ray P. Safety and immunogenicity of heptavalent pneumococcal CRM_{197} conjugate vaccine in infants and toddlers. Pediatr Infect Dis J. 1999; 18:757-63.
32. Lederle Laboratories, Data on File: D118-P12.
33. Rennels MD, Edwards KM, Keyserling HL, et al. Safety and immunogenicity of heptavalent pneumococcal vaccine conjugated to CRM_{197} in United States infants. Pediatrics. 1998; 101(4):604-11.
34. Lederle Laboratories, Data on File: D118-P3.
35. Lederle Laboratories, Data on File: Integrated Summary on Catch-Up.
36. Report of the Committee on Infectious Diseases 24th Edition. Elk Grove Village, IL: American Academy of Pediatrics. 1997; 31-3.
37. Update: Vaccine Side Effects, Adverse Reactions, Contraindications, and Precautions. MMWR. 1996; 45(RR-12):1-35.
38. Recommendations of the Advisory Committee on Immunization Practices (ACIP): use of vaccines and immunoglobulins in persons with altered immunocompetence. MMWR. 1993; 43(RR-4):1-18.
39. Vernacchio L, Neufeld EJ, MacDonald K, et al. Combined schedule of 7-valent pneumococcal conjugate vaccine followed by 23-valent pneumococcal vaccine in children and young adults with sickle cell disease. J Pediatr. 1998; 103:275-8.
40. Immunization of children infected with human immunodeficiency virus – supplementary ACIP statement. MMWR. 1988; 37(12):181-83.
41. Centers for Disease Control and Prevention. General recommendations on immunization. Recommendations of the Advisory Committee on Immunization Practices (ACIP) and the American Academy of Family Physicians (AAFP). MMWR. 2002; 51(RR-2):1-36.
42. Fawcett HA, Smith NP. Injection-site granuloma due to aluminum. Archives Dermatology. 1984; 120:1318-22.
43. Vaccines Adverse Event Reporting System – United States. MMWR. 1990; 39:730-3.

Manufactured by:
LEDERLE LABORATORIES
Division American Cyanamid Company
Pearl River, NY 10965 USA
US GOVERNMENT LICENSE NO. 17
Marketed by:
WYETH LEDERLE
VACCINES
Wyeth-Ayerst Laboratories
Philadelphia, PA 19101
CI 6188-2   Revised January 13, 2003

TABLE 15
Age and Season-Adjusted Comparison of SIDS Rates in the NCKP Efficacy Trial With the Expected Rate from the California State Data for 1995-1997[24,25]

Vaccine	<One Week After Immunization		≤Two Weeks After Immunization		≤One Month After Immunization		≤One Year After Immunization	
	Exp	Obs	Exp	Obs	Exp	Obs	Exp	Obs
Prevnar®	1.06	1	2.09	2	4.28	2	8.08	4
Control*	1.06	2	2.09	3[†]	4.28	3[†]	8.08	8[†]

* Investigational meningococcal group C conjugate vaccine (MnCC).
[†] Does not include one additional case of SIDS-like death in a child older than the usual SIDS age (448 days).

TABLE 16
Overall Percentage of Doses Associated With Systemic Events Within 2 or 3 Days For The US Efficacy Study and All US Ancillary Studies When Prevnar® Administered To Infants As a Primary Series at 2, 4, and 6 Months of Age[24,25,29,31,32,33]

Systemic Event	Prevnar® Concurrently With DTP-HbOC (9,191 Doses)*	Prevnar® Concurrently With DTaP and HbOC (3,848 Doses)[†]	DTaP and HbOC Control (538 Doses)[‡]
Fever			
≥38.0°C	35.6	21.1	14.2
>39.0°C	3.1	1.8	0.4
Irritability	69.1	52.5	45.2
Drowsiness	36.9	32.9	27.7
Restless Sleep	25.8	20.6	22.3
Decreased Appetite	24.7	18.1	13.6
Vomiting	16.2	13.4	9.8
Diarrhea	11.4	9.8	4.4
Urticaria-like Rash	0.9	0.6	0.3

* Total from which reaction data are available varies between reactions from 8,874-9,191 doses. Data from studies 118-3, 118-7, 118-8.
[†] Total from which reaction data are available varies between reactions from 3,121-3,848 doses. Data from studies 118-8, 118-12, 118-16.
[‡] Total from which reaction data are available varies between reactions from 295-538 doses. Data from studies 118-12 and 118-16.

TABLE 17
Overall Percentage of Doses Associated With Systemic Events Within 2 or 3 Days For The US Efficacy Study and All US Ancillary Studies When Prevnar® Administered To Toddlers as a Fourth Dose At 12 to 15 Months of Age[24,25,31]

Systemic Event	Prevnar® Concurrently With DTP-HbOC (709 Doses)*	Prevnar® Concurrently With DTaP and HbOC (270 Doses)[†]	Prevnar® Only No Concurrent Vaccines (727 Doses)[‡]
Fever			
≥38.0°C	41.9	19.6	13.4
>39.0°C	4.5	1.5	1.2
Irritability	72.8	45.9	45.8
Drowsiness	21.3	17.5	15.9
Restless Sleep	29.9	21.2	21.2
Decreased Appetite	33.0	21.1	18.3
Vomiting	9.6	5.6	6.3
Diarrhea	12.1	13.7	12.8
Urticaria-like Rash	1.4	0.7	1.2

* Total from which reaction data are available varies between reactions from 706-709 doses. Data from study 118-8.
[†] Total from which reaction data are available varies between reactions from 269-270 doses. Data from studies 118-7 and 118-8.
[‡] Total from which reaction data are available varies between reactions from 725-727 doses. Data from studies 118-7 and 118-8.

RAPAMUNE®   ℞
[răp' ă-mūn]
(sirolimus)
Oral Solution and Tablets

Prescribing information for this product, which appears on pages 3469–3474 of the 2003 PDR, has been completely revised as follows. Please write "See Supplement A" next to the product heading.

> **WARNING:**
> Increased susceptibility to infection and the possible development of lymphoma may result from immunosuppression. Only physicians experienced in immunosuppressive therapy and management of renal transplant patients should use Rapamune®. Patients receiving the drug should be managed in facilities equipped and staffed with adequate laboratory and supportive medical resources. The physician responsible for maintenance therapy should have complete information requisite for the follow-up of the patient.

DESCRIPTION
Rapamune® (sirolimus) is an immunosuppressive agent. Sirolimus is a macrocyclic lactone produced by *Streptomyces hygroscopicus*. The chemical name of sirolimus (also known as rapamycin) is (3S,6R,7E,9R,10R,12R,14S,15E,17E, 19E,21S,23S,26R,27R,34aS)-9,10,12,13,14,21,22,23,24,25, 26,27,32,33,34, 34a-hexadecahydro-9,27-dihydroxy-3-[(1R)-2-[(1S,3R,4R)-4-hydroxy-3-methoxycyclohexyl]-1-methylethyl]-10,21-dimethoxy-6,8,12,14,20,26-hexamethyl-23,27-epoxy-3H-pyrido[2,1-c][1,4] oxaazacyclohentriacontine-1,5,11,28,29 (4H,6H,31H)-pentone. Its molecular formula is $C_{51}H_{79}NO_{13}$ and its molecular weight is 914.2. The structural formula of sirolimus is shown below.

Sirolimus is a white to off-white powder and is insoluble in water, but freely soluble in benzyl alcohol, chloroform, acetone, and acetonitrile.

Continued on next page

Rapamune—Cont.

Rapamune® is available for administration as an oral solution containing 1 mg/mL sirolimus. Rapamune is also available as a white, triangular-shaped tablet containing 1 mg sirolimus, and as a yellow to beige triangular-shaped tablet containing 2 mg sirolimus.

The inactive ingredients in Rapamune® Oral Solution are Phosal 50 PG® (phosphatidylcholine, propylene glycol, mono- and di-glycerides, ethanol, soy fatty acids, and ascorbyl palmitate) and polysorbate 80. Rapamune Oral Solution contains 1.5%–2.5% ethanol.

The inactive ingredients in Rapamune® Tablets include sucrose, lactose, polyethylene glycol 8000, calcium sulfate, microcrystalline cellulose, pharmaceutical glaze, talc, titanium dioxide, magnesium stearate, povidone, poloxamer 188, polyethylene glycol 20,000, glyceryl monooleate, carnauba wax, and other ingredients. The 2 mg dosage strength also contains iron oxide yellow 10 and iron oxide brown 70.

CLINICAL PHARMACOLOGY

Mechanism of Action

Sirolimus inhibits T lymphocyte activation and proliferation that occurs in response to antigenic and cytokine (Interleukin [IL]-2, IL-4, and IL-15) stimulation by a mechanism that is distinct from that of other immunosuppressants. Sirolimus also inhibits antibody production. In cells, sirolimus binds to the immunophilin, FK Binding Protein-12 (FKBP-12), to generate an immunosuppressive complex. The sirolimus:FKBP-12 complex has no effect on calcineurin activity. This complex binds to and inhibits the activation of the mammalian Target Of Rapamycin (mTOR), a key regulatory kinase. This inhibition suppresses cytokine-driven T-cell proliferation, inhibiting the progression from the G_1 to the S phase of the cell cycle.

Studies in experimental models show that sirolimus prolongs allograft (kidney, heart, skin, islet, small bowel, pancreatico-duodenal, and bone marrow) survival in mice, rats, pigs, and/or primates. Sirolimus reverses acute rejection of heart and kidney allografts in rats and prolonged the graft survival in presensitized rats. In some studies, the immunosuppressive effect of sirolimus lasted up to 6 months after discontinuation of therapy. This tolerization effect is alloantigen specific.

In rodent models of autoimmune disease, sirolimus suppresses immune-mediated events associated with systemic lupus erythematosus, collagen-induced arthritis, autoimmune type I diabetes, autoimmune myocarditis, experimental allergic encephalomyelitis, graft-versus-host disease, and autoimmune uveoretinitis.

Pharmacokinetics

Sirolimus pharmacokinetic activity has been determined following oral administration in healthy subjects, pediatric dialysis patients, hepatically-impaired patients, and renal transplant patients.

Absorption

Following administration of Rapamune® (sirolimus) Oral Solution, sirolimus is rapidly absorbed, with a mean time-to-peak concentration (t_{max}) of approximately 1 hour after a single dose in healthy subjects and approximately 2 hours after multiple oral doses in renal transplant recipients. The systemic availability of sirolimus was estimated to be approximately 14% after the administration of Rapamune Oral Solution. The mean bioavailability of sirolimus after administration of the tablet is about 27% higher relative to the oral solution. Sirolimus oral tablets are not bioequivalent to the oral solution; however, clinical equivalence has been demonstrated at the 2-mg dose level. (See **CLINICAL STUDIES** and **DOSAGE AND ADMINISTRATION**). Sirolimus concentrations, following the administration of Rapamune Oral Solution to stable renal transplant patients, are dose proportional between 3 and 12 mg/m^2.

Food effects: In 22 healthy volunteers receiving Rapamune Oral Solution, a high-fat meal (861.8 kcal, 54.9% kcal from fat) altered the bioavailability characteristics of sirolimus. Compared to fasting, a 34% decrease in the peak blood sirolimus concentration (C_{max}), a 3.5-fold increase in the time-to-peak concentration (t_{max}), and a 35% increase in total exposure (AUC) was observed. After administration of Rapamune Tablets and a high-fat meal in 24 healthy volunteers, C_{max}, t_{max}, and AUC showed increases of 65%, 32%, and 23%, respectively. To minimize variability, both Rapamune Oral Solution and Tablets should be taken consistently with or without food (See **DOSAGE AND ADMINISTRATION**).

Distribution

The mean (± SD) blood-to-plasma ratio of sirolimus was 36 (± 17.9) in stable renal allograft recipients, indicating that sirolimus is extensively partitioned into formed blood elements. The mean volume of distribution (V_{ss}/F) of sirolimus is 12 ± 7.52 L/kg. Sirolimus is extensively bound (approximately 92%) to human plasma proteins. In man, the binding of sirolimus was shown mainly to be associated with serum albumin (97%), α_1-acid glycoprotein, and lipoproteins.

Metabolism

Sirolimus is a substrate for both cytochrome P450 IIIA4 (CYP3A4) and P-glycoprotein. Sirolimus is extensively metabolized by O-demethylation and/or hydroxylation. Seven (7) major metabolites, including hydroxy, demethyl, and hydroxydemethyl, are identifiable in whole blood. Some of these metabolites are also detectable in plasma, fecal, and urine samples. Glucuronide and sulfate conjugates are not

SIROLIMUS PHARMACOKINETIC PARAMETERS (MEAN ± SD) IN RENAL TRANSPLANT PATIENTS (MULTIPLE DOSE ORAL SOLUTION)[a,b]

n	Dose	$C_{max,ss}$[c] (ng/mL)	$t_{max,ss}$ (h)	$AUC_{\tau,ss}$[c] (ng•h/mL)	CL/F/WT[d] (mL/h/kg)
19	2 mg	12.2 ± 6.2	3.01 ± 2.40	158 ± 70	182 ± 72
23	5 mg	37.4 ± 21	1.84 ± 1.30	396 ± 193	221 ± 143

a: Sirolimus administered four hours after cyclosporine oral solution (MODIFIED) (e.g., Neoral® Oral Solution) and/or cyclosporine capsules (MODIFIED) (e.g., Neoral® Soft Gelatin Capsules).
b: As measured by the Liquid Chromatographic/Tandem Mass Spectrometric Method (LC/MS/MS).
c: These parameters were dose normalized prior to the statistical comparison.
d: CL/F/WT = oral dose clearance.

SIROLIMUS PHARMACOKINETIC PARAMETERS (MEAN ± SD) IN RENAL TRANSPLANT PATIENTS (MULTIPLE DOSE TABLETS)[a,b]

n	Dose (2 mg/day)	$C_{max,ss}$[c] (ng/mL)	$t_{max,ss}$ (h)	$AUC_{\tau,ss}$[c] (ng•h/mL)	CL/F/WT[d] (mL/h/kg)
17	Oral solution	14.4 ± 5.3	2.12 ± 0.84	194 ± 78	173 ± 50
13	Tablets	15.0 ± 4.9	3.46 ± 2.40	230 ± 67	139 ± 63

a: Sirolimus administered four hours after cyclosporine oral solution (MODIFIED) (e.g., Neoral® Oral Solution) and/or cyclosporine capsules (MODIFIED) (e.g., Neoral® Soft Gelatin Capsules).
b: As measured by the Liquid Chromatographic/Tandem Mass Spectrometric Method (LC/MS/MS).
c: These parameters were dose normalized prior to the statistical comparison.
d: CL/F/WT = oral dose clearance.

SIROLIMUS PHARMACOKINETIC PARAMETERS (MEAN ± SD) IN 18 HEALTHY SUBJECTS AND 18 PATIENTS WITH HEPATIC IMPAIRMENT (15 MG SINGLE DOSE – ORAL SOLUTION)

Population	$C_{max,ss}$[a] (ng/mL)	t_{max} (h)	$AUC_{0-\infty}$ (ng•h/mL)	CL/F/WT (mL/h/kg)
Healthy subjects	78.2 ± 18.3	0.82 ± 0.17	970 ± 272	215 ± 76
Hepatic impairment	77.9 ± 23.1	0.84 ± 0.17	1567 ± 616	144 ± 62

a: As measured by (LC/MS/MS)

SIROLIMUS PHARMACOKINETIC PARAMETERS (MEAN ± SD) IN PEDIATRIC PATIENTS WITH STABLE CHRONIC RENAL FAILURE MAINTAINED ON HEMODIALYSIS OR PERITONEAL DIALYSIS (1, 3, 9, 15 MG/M^2 SINGLE DOSE)

Age Group (y)	n	t_{max} (h)	$t_{1/2}$ (h)	CL/F/WT (mL/h/kg)
5–11	9	1.1 ± 0.5	71 ± 40	580 ± 450
12–18	11	0.79 ± 0.17	55 ± 18	450 ± 232

present in any of the biologic matrices. Sirolimus is the major component in human whole blood and contributes to more than 90% of the immunosuppressive activity.

Excretion

After a single dose of [^{14}C]sirolimus in healthy volunteers, the majority (91%) of radioactivity was recovered from the feces, and only a minor amount (2.2%) was excreted in urine.

Pharmacokinetics in renal transplant patients

Rapamune Oral Solution: Pharmacokinetic parameters for sirolimus oral solution given daily in combination with cyclosporine and corticosteroids in renal transplant patients are summarized below based on data collected at months 1, 3, and 6 after transplantation. There were no significant differences in any of these parameters with respect to treatment group or month.

[See first table above]

Whole blood sirolimus trough concentrations (mean ± SD), as measured by immunoassay, for the 2 mg/day and 5 mg/day dose groups were 8.59 ± 4.01 ng/mL (n = 226) and 17.3 ± 7.4 ng/mL (n = 219), respectively. Whole blood trough sirolimus concentrations, as measured by LC/MS/MS, were significantly correlated (r^2 = 0.96) with $AUC_{\tau,ss}$. Upon repeated twice daily administration without an initial loading dose in a multiple-dose study, the average trough concentration of sirolimus increases approximately 2 to 3-fold over the initial 6 days of therapy at which time steady state is reached. A loading dose of 3 times the maintenance dose will provide near steady-state concentrations within 1 day in most patients. The mean ± SD terminal elimination half life ($t_{1/2}$) of sirolimus after multiple dosing in stable renal transplant patients was estimated to be about 62 ± 16 hours.

Rapamune Tablets: Pharmacokinetic parameters for sirolimus tablets administered daily in combination with cyclosporine and corticosteroids in renal transplant patients are summarized below based on data collected at months 1 and 3 after transplantation.

[See second table above]

Whole blood sirolimus trough concentrations (mean ± SD), as measured by immunoassay, for the 2 mg oral solution and 2 mg tablets over 6 months, were 8.94 ± 4.36 ng/mL (n = 172) and 9.48 ± 3.85 ng/mL (n = 179), respectively. Whole blood trough sirolimus concentrations, as measured by LC/MS/MS, were significantly correlated (r^2 = 0.85) with $AUC_{\tau,ss}$. Mean whole blood sirolimus trough concentrations in patients receiving either Rapamune Oral Solution or Rapamune Tablets with a loading dose of three times the maintenance dose achieved steady-state concentrations within 24 hours after the start of dose administration.

Special Populations

Hepatic impairment: Sirolimus (15 mg) was administered as a single oral dose to 18 subjects with normal hepatic function and to 18 patients with Child-Pugh classification A or B hepatic impairment, in which hepatic impairment was primary and not related to an underlying systemic disease. Shown below are the mean ± SD pharmacokinetic parameters following the administration of sirolimus oral solution.

[See third table above]

Compared with the values in the normal hepatic group, the hepatic impairment group had higher mean values for sirolimus AUC (61%) and $t_{1/2}$ (43%) and had lower mean values for sirolimus CL/F/WT (33%). The mean $t_{1/2}$ increased from 79 ± 12 hours in subjects with normal hepatic function to 113 ± 41 hours in patients with impaired hepatic function. The rate of absorption of sirolimus was not altered by hepatic disease, as evidenced by C_{max} and t_{max} values. However, hepatic diseases with varying etiologies may show different effects and the pharmacokinetics of sirolimus in patients with severe hepatic dysfunction is unknown. Dosage adjustment is recommended for patients with mild to moderate hepatic impairment (see **DOSAGE AND ADMINISTRATION**).

Renal impairment: The effect of renal impairment on the pharmacokinetics of sirolimus is not known. However, there is minimal (2.2%) renal excretion of the drug or its metabolites.

Pediatric: Limited pharmacokinetic data are available in pediatric patients. The table below summarizes pharmacokinetic data obtained in pediatric dialysis patients with chronically impaired renal function.

[See fourth table above]

Geriatric: Clinical studies of Rapamune did not include a sufficient number of patients >65 years of age to determine whether they will respond differently than younger patients. After the administration of Rapamune Oral Solution, sirolimus trough concentration data in 35 renal transplant patients >65 years of age were similar to those in the adult population (n = 822) 18 to 65 years of age. Similar results were obtained after the administration of Rapamune Tablets to 12 renal transplant patients >65 years of age compared with adults (n = 167) 18 to 65 years of age.

Gender: After the administration of Rapamune Oral Solution, sirolimus oral dose clearance in males was 12% lower than that in females; male subjects had a significantly longer $t_{1/2}$ than did female subjects (72.3 hours versus 61.3 hours). A similar trend in the effect of gender on sirolimus oral dose clearance and $t_{1/2}$ was observed after the administration of Rapamune Tablets. Dose adjustments based on gender are not recommended.

Race: In large phase III trials using Rapamune Oral Solution and cyclosporine oral solution (MODIFIED) (e.g., Neoral® Oral Solution) and/or cyclosporine capsules (MODIFIED) (e.g., Neoral® Soft Gelatin Capsules), there were no significant differences in mean trough sirolimus concentrations over time between black (n = 139) and non-black (n = 724) patients during the first 6 months after transplantation at sirolimus doses of 2 mg/day and 5 mg/day. Similarly, after administration of Rapamune Tablets (2 mg/day) in a phase III trial, mean sirolimus trough concentrations over 6 months were not significantly different among black (n = 51) and non-black (n = 128) patients.

CLINICAL STUDIES

Rapamune® (sirolimus) Oral Solution: The safety and efficacy of Rapamune® Oral Solution for the prevention of organ rejection following renal transplantation were assessed in two randomized, double-blind, multicenter, controlled trials. These studies compared two dose levels of Rapamune Oral Solution (2 mg and 5 mg, once daily) with azathioprine (Study 1) or placebo (Study 2) when administered in combination with cyclosporine and corticosteroids. Study 1 was conducted in the United States at 38 sites. Seven hundred nineteen (719) patients were enrolled in this trial and randomized following transplantation; 284 were randomized to receive Rapamune Oral Solution 2 mg/day, 274 were randomized to receive Rapamune Oral Solution 5 mg/day, and 161 to receive azathioprine 2–3 mg/kg/day. Study 2 was conducted in Australia, Canada, Europe, and the United States, at a total of 34 sites. Five hundred seventy-six (576) patients were enrolled in this trial and randomized before transplantation; 227 were randomized to receive Rapamune Oral Solution 2 mg/day, 219 were randomized to receive Rapamune Oral Solution 5 mg/day, and 130 to receive placebo. In both studies, the use of antilymphocyte antibody induction therapy was prohibited. In both studies, the primary efficacy endpoint was the rate of efficacy failure in the first 6 months after transplantation. Efficacy failure was defined as the first occurrence of an acute rejection episode (confirmed by biopsy), graft loss, or death.

The tables below summarize the results of the primary efficacy analyses from these trials. Rapamune Oral Solution, at doses of 2 mg/day and 5 mg/day, significantly reduced the incidence of efficacy failure (statistically significant at the <0.025 level; nominal significance level adjusted for multiple [2] dose comparisons) at 6 months following transplantation compared to both azathioprine and placebo.
[See first table at right]
[See second table at right]
Patient and graft survival at 1 year were co-primary endpoints. The table below shows graft and patient survival at 1 year in Study 1 and Study 2. The graft and patient survival rates at 1 year were similar in patients treated with Rapamune and comparator-treated patients.
[See third table at right]
The reduction in the incidence of first biopsy-confirmed acute rejection episodes in patients treated with Rapamune compared to the control groups included a reduction in all grades of rejection.
[See fourth table at right]
In Study 1, which was prospectively stratified by race within center, efficacy failure was similar for Rapamune Oral Solution 2 mg/day and lower for Rapamune Oral Solution 5 mg/day compared to azathioprine in black patients. In Study 2, which was not prospectively stratified by race, efficacy failure was similar for both Rapamune Oral Solution doses compared to placebo in black patients. The decision to use the higher dose of Rapamune Oral Solution in black patients must be weighed against the increased risk of dose-dependent adverse events that were observed with the Rapamune Oral Solution 5 mg dose (see **ADVERSE REACTIONS**).
[See first table at top of next page]
Mean glomerular filtration rates (GFR) at one year post transplant were calculated by using the Nankivell equation for all subjects in Studies 1 and 2 who had serum creatinine measured at 12 months. In Studies 1 and 2 mean GFR, at 12 months, were lower in patients treated with cyclosporine and Rapamune Oral Solution compared to those treated with cyclosporine and the respective azathioprine or placebo control.

Within each treatment group in Studies 1 and 2, mean GFR at one year post transplant was lower in patients who experienced at least 1 episode of biopsy-proven acute rejection, compared to those who did not.

Renal function should be monitored and appropriate adjustment of the immunosuppression regimen should be considered in patients with elevated serum creatinine levels (see **PRECAUTIONS**).

Rapamune® Tablets: The safety and efficacy of Rapamune Oral Solution and Rapamune Tablets for the prevention of organ rejection following renal transplantation were compared in a randomized multicenter controlled trial (Study 3). This study compared a single dose level (2 mg, once daily) of Rapamune Oral Solution and Rapamune Tablets when administered in combination with cyclosporine and corticosteroids. The study was conducted at 30 centers in Australia, Canada, and the United States. Four hundred seventy-seven (477) patients were enrolled in this study and randomized before transplantation; 238 patients were randomized to receive Rapamune Oral Solution 2 mg/day and 239 patients were randomized to receive Rapamune Tablets 2 mg/day. In this study, the use of antilymphocyte antibody induction therapy was prohibited. The primary efficacy endpoint was the rate of efficacy failure in the first 3 months after transplantation. Efficacy failure was defined as the first occurrence of an acute rejection episode (confirmed by biopsy), graft loss, or death.

The table below summarizes the result of the primary efficacy analysis at 3 months from this trial. The overall rate of efficacy failure in the tablet treatment group was equivalent to the rate in the oral solution treatment group.
[See second table at top of next page]
The table below summarizes the results of the primary efficacy analysis at 6 months after transplantation.
[See third table at top of next page]
Graft and patient survival at 12 months were co-primary efficacy endpoints. There was no significant difference between the oral solution and tablet formulations for both graft and patient survival. Graft survival was 92.0% and 88.7% for the oral solution and tablet treatment groups, respectively. The patient survival rates in the oral solution and tablet treatment groups were 95.8% and 96.2%, respectively.

The mean GFR at 12 months, calculated by the Nankivell equation, were not significantly different for the oral solution group and for the tablet group.

The table below summarizes the mean GFR at one-year post-transplantation for all subjects in Study 3 who had serum creatinine measured at 12 months.

OVERALL CALCULATED GLOMERULAR FILTRATION RATES (CC/MIN) BY NANKIVELL EQUATION AT 12 MONTHS POST TRANSPLANT: STUDY 3

	Rapamune® Oral Solution	Rapamune® Tablets
Mean (SE)	58.3 (1.64)	58.5 (1.44)
	n = 166	n = 162

INDICATIONS AND USAGE

Rapamune® (sirolimus) is indicated for the prophylaxis of organ rejection in patients receiving renal transplants. It is recommended that Rapamune be used in a regimen with cyclosporine and corticosteroids.

CONTRAINDICATIONS

Rapamune is contraindicated in patients with a hypersensitivity to sirolimus or its derivatives or any component of the drug product.

INCIDENCE (%) OF THE PRIMARY ENDPOINT AT 6 MONTHS: STUDY 1[a]

Parameter	Rapamune® Oral Solution 2 mg/day (n = 284)	Rapamune® Oral Solution 5 mg/day (n = 274)	Azathioprine 2–3 mg/kg/day (n = 161)
Efficacy failure at 6 months	18.7	16.8	32.3
Components of efficacy failure			
Biopsy-proven acute rejection	16.5	11.3	29.2
Graft loss	1.1	2.9	2.5
Death	0.7	1.8	0
Lost to follow-up	0.4	0.7	0.6

a: Patients received cyclosporine and corticosteroids.

INCIDENCE (%) OF THE PRIMARY ENDPOINT AT 6 MONTHS: STUDY 2[a]

Parameter	Rapamune® Oral Solution 2 mg/day (n = 227)	Rapamune® Oral Solution 5 mg/day (n = 219)	Placebo (n = 130)
Efficacy failure at 6 months	30.0	25.6	47.7
Components of efficacy failure			
Biopsy-proven acute rejection	24.7	19.2	41.5
Graft loss	3.1	3.7	3.9
Death	2.2	2.7	2.3
Lost to follow-up	0	0	0

a: Patients received cyclosporine and corticosteroids.

1 YEAR GRAFT AND PATIENT SURVIVAL (%)[a]

Parameter	Rapamune® Oral Solution 2 mg/day	Rapamune® Oral Solution 5 mg/day	Azathioprine 2–3 mg/kg/day	Placebo
Study 1	(n = 284)	(n = 274)	(n = 161)	
Graft survival	94.7	92.7	93.8	
Patient survival	97.2	96.0	98.1	
Study 2	(n = 227)	(n = 219)		(n = 130)
Graft survival	89.9	90.9		87.7
Patient survival	96.5	95.0		94.6

a: Patients received cyclosporine and corticosteroids.

PERCENTAGE OF EFFICACY FAILURE BY RACE AT 6 MONTHS

Parameter	Rapamune® Oral Solution 2 mg/day	Rapamune® Oral Solution 5 mg/day	Azathioprine 2–3 mg/kg/day	Placebo
Study 1				
Black (n = 166)	34.9 (n = 63)	18.0 (n = 61)	33.3 (n = 42)	
Non-black (n = 553)	14.0 (n = 221)	16.4 (n = 213)	31.9 (n = 119)	
Study 2				
Black (n = 66)	30.8 (n = 26)	33.7 (n = 27)		38.5 (n = 13)
Non-black (n = 510)	29.9 (n = 201)	24.5 (n = 192)		48.7 (n = 117)

WARNINGS

Increased susceptibility to infection and the possible development of lymphoma and other malignancies, particularly of the skin, may result from immunosuppression (see **ADVERSE REACTIONS**). Oversuppression of the immune system can also increase susceptibility to infection including opportunistic infections, fatal infections, and sepsis. Only physicians experienced in immunosuppressive therapy and management of organ transplant patients should use Rapamune. Patients receiving the drug should be managed in facilities equipped and staffed with adequate laboratory and supportive medical resources. The physician responsible for maintenance therapy should have complete information requisite for the follow-up of the patient.

As usual for patients with increased risk for skin cancer, exposure to sunlight and UV light should be limited by wearing protective clothing and using a sunscreen with a high protection factor.

Increased serum cholesterol and triglycerides, that may require treatment, occurred more frequently in patients treated with Rapamune compared to azathioprine or placebo controls (see **PRECAUTIONS**).

In phase III studies, mean serum creatinine was increased and mean glomerular filtration rate was decreased in patients treated with Rapamune and cyclosporine compared to those treated with cyclosporine and placebo or azathioprine controls (see **CLINICAL STUDIES**). Renal function should be monitored during the administration of maintenance immunosuppression regimens including Rapamune in combination with cyclosporine, and appropriate adjustment of the immunosuppression regimen should be considered in patients with elevated serum creatinine levels. Caution should be exercised when using agents which are known to impair renal function (see **PRECAUTIONS**).

In clinical trials, Rapamune has been administered concurrently with corticosteroids and with the following formulations of cyclosporine:

Sandimmune® Injection (cyclosporine injection)
Sandimmune® Oral Solution (cyclosporine oral solution)

Continued on next page

Rapamune—Cont.

Sandimmune® Soft Gelatin Capsules (cyclosporine capsules)
Neoral® Soft Gelatin Capsules (cyclosporine capsules [MODIFIED])
Neoral® Oral Solution (cyclosporine oral solution [MODIFIED])

The efficacy and safety of the use of Rapamune in combination with other immunosuppressive agents has not been determined.

Liver Transplantation – Excess Mortality, Graft Loss, and Hepatic Artery Thrombosis (HAT): The use of sirolimus in combination with tacrolimus was associated with excess mortality and graft loss in a study in de novo liver transplant recipients. Many of these patients had evidence of infection at or near the time of death.

In this and another study in de novo liver transplant recipients, the use of sirolimus in combination with cyclosporine or tacrolimus was associated with an increase in HAT; most cases of HAT occurred within 30 days post-transplantation and most led to graft loss or death.

Lung Transplantation – Bronchial Anastomotic Dehiscence:
Cases of bronchial anastomotic dehiscence, most fatal, have been reported in de novo lung transplant patients when sirolimus has been used as part of an immunosuppressive regimen.

The safety and efficacy of Rapamune® (sirolimus) as immunosuppressive therapy have not been established in liver or lung transplant patients, and therefore, such use is not recommended.

PRECAUTIONS

General

Rapamune is intended for oral administration only.

Lymphocele, a known surgical complication of renal transplantation, occurred significantly more often in a dose-related fashion in patients treated with Rapamune. Appropriate post-operative measures should be considered to minimize this complication.

Lipids

The use of Rapamune® (sirolimus) in renal transplant patients was associated with increased serum cholesterol and triglycerides that may require treatment.

In phase III clinical trials, in *de novo* renal transplant recipients who began the study with normal, fasting, total serum cholesterol (fasting serum cholesterol <200 mg/dL), there was an increased incidence of hypercholesterolemia (fasting serum cholesterol >240 mg/dL) in patients receiving both Rapamune® 2 mg and Rapamune® 5 mg compared to azathioprine and placebo controls.

In phase III clinical trials, in *de novo* renal transplant recipients who began the study with normal, fasting, total serum triglycerides (fasting serum triglycerides <200 mg/dL), there was an increased incidence of hypertriglyceridemia (fasting serum triglycerides >500 mg/dL) in patients receiving Rapamune® 2 mg and Rapamune® 5 mg compared to azathioprine and placebo controls.

Treatment of new-onset hypercholesterolemia with lipid-lowering agents was required in 42–52% of patients enrolled in the Rapamune arms of the study compared to 16% of patients in the placebo arm and 22% of patients in the azathioprine arm.

Renal transplant patients have a higher prevalence of clinically significant hyperlipidemia. Accordingly, the risk/benefit should be carefully considered in patients with established hyperlipidemia before initiating an immunosuppressive regimen including Rapamune.

Any patient who is administered Rapamune should be monitored for hyperlipidemia using laboratory tests and if hyperlipidemia is detected, subsequent interventions such as diet, exercise, and lipid-lowering agents, as outlined by the National Cholesterol Education Program guidelines, should be initiated.

In clinical trials, the concomitant administration of Rapamune and HMG-CoA reductase inhibitors and/or fibrates appeared to be well tolerated.

During Rapamune therapy with cyclosporine, patients administered an HMG-CoA reductase inhibitor and/or fibrate should be monitored for the possible development of rhabdomyolysis and other adverse effects as described in the respective labeling for these agents.

Renal Function

Patients treated with cyclosporine and Rapamune were noted to have higher serum creatinine levels and lower glomerular filtration rates compared with patients treated with cyclosporine and placebo or azathioprine controls. Renal function should be monitored during the administration of maintenance immunosuppression regimens including Rapamune in combination with cyclosporine, and appropriate adjustment of the immunosuppression regimen should be considered in patients with elevated serum creatinine levels. Caution should be exercised when using agents (e.g., aminoglycosides, and amphotericin B) that are known to have a deleterious effect on renal function.

Antimicrobial Prophylaxis

Cases of *Pneumocystis carinii* pneumonia have been reported in patients not receiving antimicrobial prophylaxis. Therefore, antimicrobial prophylaxis for *Pneumocystis carinii* pneumonia should be administered for 1 year following transplantation.

OVERALL CALCULATED GLOMERULAR FILTRATION RATES (CC/MIN) BY NANKIVELL EQUATION AT 12 MONTHS POST TRANSPLANT

Parameter	Rapamune® Oral Solution 2 mg/day	Rapamune® Oral Solution 5 mg/day	Azathioprine 2–3 mg/kg/day	Placebo
Study 1	(n = 233)	(n = 226)	(n = 127)	
Mean (SE)	57.4 (1.28)	55.1 (1.28)	65.9 (1.69)	
Study 2	(n = 190)	(n = 175)		(n = 101)
Mean (SE)	54.9 (1.26)	52.9 (1.46)		61.7 (1.81)

INCIDENCE (%) OF THE PRIMARY ENDPOINT AT 3 MONTHS: STUDY 3[a]

	Rapamune® Oral Solution (n = 238)	Rapamune® Tablets (n = 239)
Efficacy Failure at 3 months	23.5	24.7
Components of efficacy failure		
Biopsy-proven acute rejection	18.9	17.6
Graft loss	3.4	6.3
Death	1.3	0.8

a: Patients received cyclosporine and corticosteroids.

INCIDENCE (%) OF THE PRIMARY ENDPOINT AT 6 MONTHS: STUDY 3[a]

	Rapamune® Oral Solution (n = 238)	Rapamune® Tablets (n = 239)
Efficacy Failure at 6 months	26.1	27.2
Components of efficacy failure		
Biopsy-proven acute rejection	21.0	19.2
Graft loss	3.4	6.3
Death	1.7	1.7

a: Patients received cyclosporine and corticosteroids.

Cytomegalovirus (CMV) prophylaxis is recommended for 3 months after transplantation, particularly for patients at increased risk for CMV disease.

Interstitial Lung Disease

Cases of interstitial lung disease (including pneumonitis, and infrequently bronchiolitis obliterans organizing pneumonia [BOOP] and pulmonary fibrosis), some fatal, with no identified infectious etiology have occurred in patients receiving immunosuppressive regimens including Rapamune. In some cases, the interstitial lung disease has resolved upon discontinuation or dose reduction of Rapamune. The risk may be increased as the trough Rapamune level increases (see **ADVERSE REACTIONS**).

Information for Patients

Patients should be given complete dosage instructions (see **Patient Instructions**). Women of childbearing potential should be informed of the potential risks during pregnancy and that they should use effective contraception prior to initiation of Rapamune therapy, during Rapamune therapy and for 12 weeks after Rapamune therapy has been stopped (see **PRECAUTIONS: Pregnancy**).

Patients should be told that exposure to sunlight and UV light should be limited by wearing protective clothing and using a sunscreen with a high protection factor because of the increased risk for skin cancer (see **WARNINGS**).

Laboratory Tests

It is prudent to monitor blood sirolimus levels in patients likely to have altered drug metabolism, in patients ≥13 years who weigh less than 40 kg, in patients with hepatic impairment, and during concurrent administration of potent CYP3A4 inducers and inhibitors (see **PRECAUTIONS: Drug Interactions**).

Drug Interactions

Sirolimus is known to be a substrate for both cytochrome CYP3A4 and P-glycoprotein. The pharmacokinetic interaction between sirolimus and concomitantly administered drugs is discussed below. Drug interaction studies have not been conducted with drugs other than those described below.

Cyclosporine capsules MODIFIED:

Rapamune Oral Solution: In a single dose drug-drug interaction study, 24 healthy volunteers were administered 10 mg sirolimus either simultaneously or 4 hours after a 300 mg dose of Neoral® Soft Gelatin Capsules (cyclosporine capsules [MODIFIED]). For simultaneous administration, the mean C_{max} and AUC of sirolimus were increased by 116% and 230%, respectively, relative to administration of sirolimus alone. However, when given 4 hours after Neoral® Soft Gelatin Capsules (cyclosporine capsules [MODIFIED]) administration, sirolimus C_{max} and AUC were increased by 37% and 80%, respectively, compared to administration of sirolimus alone.

Mean cyclosporine C_{max} and AUC were not significantly affected when sirolimus was given simultaneously or when administered 4 hours after Neoral® Soft Gelatin Capsules (cyclosporine capsules [MODIFIED]). However, after multiple-dose administration of sirolimus given 4 hours after Neoral® in renal post-transplant patients over 6 months, cyclosporine oral-dose clearance was reduced, and lower doses of Neoral® Soft Gelatin Capsules (cyclosporine capsules [MODIFIED]) were needed to maintain target cyclosporine concentration.

Rapamune (sirolimus) Tablets: In a single-dose drug-drug interaction study, 24 healthy volunteers were administered 10 mg sirolimus (Rapamune Tablets) either simultaneously or 4 hours after a 300-mg dose of Neoral® Soft Gelatin Capsules (cyclosporine capsules [MODIFIED]). For simultaneous administration, mean C_{max} and AUC were increased by 512% and 148%, respectively, relative to administration of sirolimus alone. However, when given 4 hours after cyclosporine administration, sirolimus C_{max} and AUC were both increased by only 33% compared with administration of sirolimus alone.

Because of the effect of cyclosporine capsules (MODIFIED), it is recommended that sirolimus should be taken 4 hours after administration of cyclosporine oral solution (MODIFIED) and/or cyclosporine capsules (MODIFIED), (see DOSAGE AND ADMINISTRATION).

Cyclosporine oral solution: In a multiple-dose study in 150 psoriasis patients, sirolimus 0.5, 1.5, and 3 mg/m²/day was administered simultaneously with Sandimmune® Oral Solution (cyclosporine Oral Solution) 1.25 mg/kg/day. The increase in average sirolimus trough concentrations ranged between 67% to 86% relative to when sirolimus was administered without cyclosporine. The intersubject variability (%CV) for sirolimus trough concentrations ranged from 39.7% to 68.7%. There was no significant effect of multiple-dose sirolimus on cyclosporine trough concentrations following Sandimmune® Oral Solution (cyclosporine oral solution) administration. However, the %CV was higher (range 85.9%–165%) than those from previous studies.

Sandimmune® Oral Solution (cyclosporine oral solution) is not bioequivalent to Neoral® Oral Solution (cyclosporine oral solution MODIFIED), and should not be used interchangeably. Although there is no published data comparing Sandimmune® Oral Solution (cyclosporine oral solution) to SangCya® Oral Solution (cyclosporine oral solution [MODIFIED]), they should not be used interchangeably. Likewise, Sandimmune® Soft Gelatin Capsules (cyclosporine capsules) are not bioequivalent to Neoral® Soft Gelatin Capsules (cyclosporine capsules [MODIFIED]) and should not be used interchangeably.

Diltiazem: The simultaneous oral administration of 10 mg of sirolimus oral solution and 120 mg of diltiazem to 18 healthy volunteers significantly affected the bioavailability of sirolimus. Sirolimus C_{max}, t_{max}, and AUC were increased 1.4-, 1.3-, and 1.6-fold, respectively. Sirolimus did not affect the pharmacokinetics of either diltiazem or its metabolites desacetyldiltiazem and desmethyldiltiazem. If diltiazem is administered, sirolimus should be monitored and a dose adjustment may be necessary.

Ketoconazole: Multiple-dose ketoconazole administration significantly affected the rate and extent of absorption and sirolimus exposure after administration of Rapamune® (sirolimus) Oral Solution, as reflected by increases in sirolimus C_{max}, t_{max}, and AUC of 4.3-fold, 38%, and 10.9-fold, respectively. However, the terminal $t_{1/2}$ of sirolimus was not changed. Single-dose sirolimus did not affect steady-state 12-hour plasma ketoconazole concentrations. It is recommended that sirolimus oral solution and oral tablets should not be administered with ketoconazole.

Rifampin: Pretreatment of 14 healthy volunteers with multiple doses of rifampin, 600 mg daily for 14 days, followed by a single 20-mg dose of sirolimus, greatly increased sirolimus oral-dose clearance by 5.5-fold (range = 2.8 to 10), which represents mean decreases in AUC and C_{max} of about 82% and 71%, respectively. In patients where rifampin is indicated, alternative therapeutic agents with less enzyme induction potential should be considered.

Drugs which may be coadministered without dose adjustment

Clinically significant pharmacokinetic drug-drug interactions were not observed in studies of drugs listed below. A synopsis of the type of study performed for each drug is provided. Sirolimus and these drugs may be coadministered without dose adjustments.

Acyclovir: Acyclovir, 200 mg, was administered once daily for 3 days followed by a single 10-mg dose of sirolimus oral solution on day 3 in 20 adult healthy volunteers.

Digoxin: Digoxin, 0.25 mg, was administered daily for 8 days and a single 10-mg dose of sirolimus oral solution was given on day 8 to 24 healthy volunteers.

Glyburide: A single 5-mg dose of glyburide and a single 10-mg dose of sirolimus oral solution were administered to 24 healthy volunteers. Sirolimus did not affect the hypoglycemic action of glyburide.

Nifedipine: A single 60-mg dose of nifedipine and a single 10-mg dose of sirolimus oral solution were administered to 24 healthy volunteers.

Norgestrel/ethinyl estradiol (Lo/Ovral®): Sirolimus oral solution, 2 mg, was given daily for 7 days to 21 healthy female volunteers on norgestrel/ethinyl estradiol.

Prednisolone: Pharmacokinetic information was obtained from 42 stable renal transplant patients receiving daily doses of prednisone (5–20 mg/day) and either single or multiple doses of sirolimus oral solution (0.5–5 mg/m^2 q 12h).

Sulfamethoxazole/trimethoprim (Bactrim®): A single oral dose of sulfamethoxazole (400 mg)/trimethoprim (80 mg) was given to 15 renal transplant patients receiving daily oral doses of sirolimus (8 to 25 mg/m^2).

Other drug interactions

Sirolimus is extensively metabolized by the CYP3A4 isoenzyme in the gut wall and liver. Therefore, absorption and the subsequent elimination of systemically absorbed sirolimus may be influenced by drugs that affect this isoenzyme. Inhibitors of CYP3A4 may decrease the metabolism of sirolimus and increase sirolimus levels, while inducers of CYP3A4 may increase the metabolism of sirolimus and decrease sirolimus levels.

Drugs that may increase sirolimus blood concentrations include:

- Calcium channel blockers: nicardipine, verapamil.
- Antifungal agents: clotrimazole, fluconazole, itraconazole.
- Macrolide antibiotics: clarithromycin, erythromycin, troleandomycin.
- Gastrointestinal prokinetic agents: cisapride, metoclopramide.
- Other drugs: bromocriptine, cimetidine, danazol, HIV-protease inhibitors (e.g., ritonavir, indinavir).

Drugs that may decrease sirolimus levels include:

- Anticonvulsants: carbamazepine, phenobarbital, phenytoin.
- Antibiotics: rifabutin, rifapentine.

This list is not all inclusive.

Care should be exercised when drugs or other substances that are metabolized by CYP3A4 are administered concomitantly with Rapamune. Grapefruit juice reduces CYP3A4-mediated metabolism of Rapamune and must not be used for dilution (see **DOSAGE AND ADMINISTRATION**).

Herbal Preparations

St. John's Wort (*hypericum perforatum*) induces CYP3A4 and P-glycoprotein. Since sirolimus is a substrate for both cytochrome CYP3A4 and P-glycoprotein, there is the potential that the use of St. John's Wort in patients receiving Rapamune could result in reduced sirolimus levels.

Vaccination

Immunosuppressants may affect response to vaccination. Therefore, during treatment with Rapamune, vaccination may be less effective. The use of live vaccines should be avoided; live vaccines may include, but are not limited to measles, mumps, rubella, oral polio, BCG, yellow fever, varicella, and TY21a typhoid.

Drug-Laboratory Test Interactions

There are no studies on the interactions of sirolimus in commonly employed clinical laboratory tests.

Carcinogenesis, Mutagenesis, and Impairment of Fertility

Sirolimus was not genotoxic in the in vitro bacterial reverse mutation assay, the Chinese hamster ovary cell chromosomal aberration assay, the mouse lymphoma cell forward mutation assay, or the in vivo mouse micronucleus assay.

Carcinogenicity studies were conducted in mice and rats. In an 86-week female mouse study at dosages of 0, 12.5, 25 and 50/6 (dosage lowered from 50 to 6 mg/kg/day at week 31 due to infection secondary to immunosuppression) there was a statistically significant increase in malignant lymphoma at all dose levels (approximately 16 to 135 times the clinical doses adjusted for body surface area) compared to controls. In a second mouse study at dosages of 0, 1, 3 and 6 mg/kg (approximately 3 to 16 times the clinical dose adjusted for body surface area), hepatocellular adenoma and carcinoma (males), were considered Rapamune related. In the 104-week rat study at dosages of 0, 0.05, 0.1, and 0.2 mg/kg/day (approximately 0.4 to 1 times the clinical dose adjusted for body surface area), there was a statistically significant increased incidence of testicular adenoma in the 0.2 mg/kg/day group.

There was no effect on fertility in female rats following the administration of sirolimus at dosages up to 0.5 mg/kg (approximately 1 to 3 times the clinical doses adjusted for body surface area). In male rats, there was no significant difference in fertility rate compared to controls at a dosage of 2 mg/kg (approximately 4 to 11 times the clinical doses adjusted for body surface area). Reductions in testicular weights and/or histological lesions (e.g., tubular atrophy and tubular giant cells) were observed in rats following dosages of 0.65 mg/kg (approximately 1 to 3 times the clinical doses adjusted for body surface area) and above and in a monkey study at 0.1 mg/kg (approximately 0.4 to 1 times the clinical doses adjusted for body surface area) and above. Sperm counts were reduced in male rats following the administration of sirolimus for 13 weeks at a dosage of 6 mg/kg (approximately 12 to 32 times the clinical doses adjusted for body surface area), but showed improvement by 3 months after dosing was stopped.

Pregnancy

Pregnancy Category C: Sirolimus was embryo/feto toxic in rats at dosages of 0.1 mg/kg and above (approximately 0.2 to 0.5 the clinical doses adjusted for body surface area). Embryo/feto toxicity was manifested as mortality and reduced fetal weights (with associated delays in skeletal ossification). However, no teratogenesis was evident. In combination with cyclosporine, rats had increased embryo/feto mortality compared to Rapamune alone. There were no effects on rabbit development at the maternally toxic dosage of 0.05 mg/kg (approximately 0.3 to 0.8 times the clinical doses adjusted for body surface area). There are no adequate and well controlled studies in pregnant women. Effective contraception must be initiated before Rapamune therapy, during Rapamune therapy, and for 12 weeks after Rapamune therapy has been stopped. Rapamune should be used during pregnancy only if the potential benefit outweighs the potential risk to the embryo/fetus.

Use during lactation

Sirolimus is excreted in trace amounts in milk of lactating rats. It is not known whether sirolimus is excreted in human milk. The pharmacokinetic and safety profiles of sirolimus in infants are not known. Because many drugs are excreted in human milk and because of the potential for adverse reactions in nursing infants from sirolimus, a decision should be made whether to discontinue nursing or to discontinue the drug, taking into account the importance of the drug to the mother.

Pediatric use

The safety and efficacy of Rapamune in pediatric patients below the age of 13 years have not been established.

Geriatric use

Clinical studies of Rapamune Oral Solution or Tablets did not include sufficient numbers of patients aged 65 years and over to determine whether safety and efficacy differ in this population from younger patients. Data pertaining to sirolimus trough concentrations suggest that dose adjustments based upon age in geriatric renal patients are not necessary.

ADVERSE REACTIONS

Rapamune® Oral Solution: The incidence of adverse reactions was determined in two randomized, double-blind, multicenter controlled trials in which 499 renal transplant patients received Rapamune Oral Solution 2 mg/day, 477 received Rapamune Oral Solution 5 mg/day, 160 received azathioprine, and 124 received placebo. All patients were treated with cyclosporine and corticosteroids. Data (≥12 months post-transplant) presented in the table below show the adverse reactions that occurred in any treatment group with an incidence of ≥20%.

Specific adverse reactions associated with the administration of Rapamune (sirolimus) Oral Solution occurred at a significantly higher frequency than in the respective control group. For both Rapamune Oral Solution 2 mg/day and 5 mg/day these include hypercholesterolemia, hyperlipemia, hypertension, and rash; for Rapamune Oral Solution 2 mg/day acne; and for Rapamune Oral Solution 5 mg/day anemia, arthralgia, diarrhea, hypokalemia, and thrombocytopenia. The elevations of triglycerides and cholesterol and decreases in platelets and hemoglobin occurred in a dose-related manner in patients receiving Rapamune.

Patients maintained on Rapamune Oral Solution 5 mg/day, when compared to patients on Rapamune Oral Solution 2 mg/day, demonstrated an increased incidence of the following adverse events: anemia, leukopenia, thrombocytopenia, hypokalemia, hyperlipemia, fever, and diarrhea.

In general, adverse events related to the administration of Rapamune were dependent on dose/concentration.

[See table above]

ADVERSE EVENTS OCCURRING AT A FREQUENCY OF ≥ 20% IN ANY TREATMENT GROUP IN PREVENTION OF ACUTE RENAL REJECTION TRIALS (%)[a] AT ≥ 12 MONTHS POST-TRANSPLANTATION FOR STUDIES 1 AND 2

Body System	Rapamune® Oral Solution —2 mg/day—		Rapamune® Oral Solution —5 mg/day—		Azathioprine 2–3 mg/kg/day	Placebo
Adverse Event	Study 1 (n = 281)	Study 2 (n = 218)	Study 1 (n = 269)	Study 2 (n = 208)	Study 1 (n = 160)	Study 2 (n = 124)
Body As A Whole						
Abdominal pain	28	29	30	36	29	30
Asthenia	38	22	40	28	37	28
Back pain	16	23	26	22	23	20
Chest pain	16	18	19	24	16	19
Fever	27	23	33	34	33	35
Headache	23	34	27	34	21	31
Pain	24	32	29	29	30	25
Cardiovascular System						
Hypertension	43	45	39	49	29	48
Digestive System						
Constipation	28	36	34	38	37	31
Diarrhea	32	25	42	35	28	27
Dyspepsia	17	23	23	25	24	34
Nausea	31	25	36	31	39	29
Vomiting	21	19	25	25	31	21
Hemic And Lymphatic System						
Anemia	27	23	37	33	29	21
Leukopenia	9	9	15	13	20	8
Thrombocytopenia	13	14	20	30	9	9
Metabolic And Nutritional						
Creatinine increased	35	39	37	40	28	38
Edema	24	20	16	18	23	15
Hypercholesteremia (See **WARNINGS** and **PRECAUTIONS**)	38	43	42	46	33	23
Hyperkalemia	15	17	12	14	24	27
Hyperlipemia (See **WARNINGS** and **PRECAUTIONS**)	38	45	44	57	28	23
Hypokalemia	17	11	21	17	11	9
Hypophosphatemia	20	15	23	19	20	19
Peripheral edema	60	54	64	58	58	48
Weight gain	21	11	15	8	19	15
Musculoskeletal System						
Arthralgia	25	25	27	31	21	18
Nervous System						
Insomnia	14	13	22	14	18	8
Tremor	31	21	30	22	28	19
Respiratory System						
Dyspnea	22	24	28	30	23	30
Pharyngitis	17	16	16	21	17	22
Upper respiratory infection	20	26	24	23	13	23
Skin And Appendages						
Acne	31	22	20	22	17	19
Rash	12	10	13	20	6	6
Urogenital System						
Urinary tract infection	20	26	23	33	31	26

a: Patients received cyclosporine and corticosteroids.

At 12 months, there were no significant differences in incidence rates for clinically important opportunistic or common transplant-related infections across treatment groups, with the exception of mucosal infections with *Herpes simplex*, which occurred at a significantly greater rate in patients treated with Rapamune (sirolimus) 5 mg/day than in both of the comparator groups.

Continued on next page

Rapamune—Cont.

The table below summarizes the incidence of malignancies in the two controlled trials for the prevention of acute rejection. At 12 months following transplantation, there was a very low incidence of malignancies and there were no significant differences among treatment groups.
[See table below]

Among the adverse events that were reported at a rate of ≥3% and <20%, the following were more prominent in patients maintained on Rapamune 5 mg/day, when compared to patients on Rapamune 2 mg/day: epistaxis, lymphocele, insomnia, thrombotic thrombocytopenic purpura (hemolytic-uremic syndrome), skin ulcer, increased LDH, hypotension, facial edema.

The following adverse events were reported with ≥3% and <20% incidence in patients in any Rapamune treatment group in the two controlled clinical trials for the prevention of acute rejection, BODY AS A WHOLE: abdomen enlarged, abscess, ascites, cellulitis, chills, face edema, flu syndrome, generalized edema, hernia, *Herpes zoster* infection, lymphocele, malaise, pelvic pain, peritonitis, sepsis; CARDIOVASCULAR SYSTEM: atrial fibrillation, congestive heart failure, hemorrhage, hypervolemia, hypotension, palpitation, peripheral vascular disorder, postural hypotension, syncope, tachycardia, thrombophlebitis, thrombosis, vasodilatation; DIGESTIVE SYSTEM: anorexia, dysphagia, eructation, esophagitis, flatulence, gastritis, gastroenteritis, gingivitis, gum hyperplasia, ileus, liver function tests abnormal, mouth ulceration, oral moniliasis, stomatitis; ENDOCRINE SYSTEM: Cushing's syndrome, diabetes mellitus, glycosuria; HEMIC AND LYMPHATIC SYSTEM: ecchymosis, leukocytosis, lymphadenopathy, polycythemia, thrombotic thrombocytopenic purpura (hemolytic-uremic syndrome); METABOLIC AND NUTRITIONAL: acidosis, alkaline phosphatase increased, BUN increased, creatine phosphokinase increased, dehydration, healing abnormal, hypercalcemia, hyperglycemia, hyperphosphatemia, hypocalcemia, hypoglycemia, hypomagnesemia, hyponatremia, lactic dehydrogenase increased, SGOT increased, SGPT increased, weight loss; MUSCULOSKELETAL SYSTEM: arthrosis, bone necrosis, leg cramps, myalgia, osteoporosis, tetany; NERVOUS SYSTEM: anxiety, confusion, depression, dizziness, emotional lability, hypertonia, hypesthesia, hypotonia, insomnia, neuropathy, paresthesia, somnolence; RESPIRATORY SYSTEM: asthma, atelectasis, bronchitis, cough increased, epistaxis, hypoxia, lung edema, pleural effusion, pneumonia, rhinitis, sinusitis; SKIN AND APPENDAGES: fungal dermatitis, hirsutism, pruritus, skin hypertrophy, skin ulcer, sweating; SPECIAL SENSES: abnormal vision, cataract, conjunctivitis, deafness, ear pain, otitis media, tinnitus; UROGENITAL SYSTEM: albuminuria, bladder pain, dysuria, hematuria, hydronephrosis, impotence, kidney pain, kidney tubular necrosis, nocturia, oliguria, pyelonephritis, pyuria, scrotal edema, testis disorder, toxic nephropathy, urinary frequency, urinary incontinence, urinary retention.

Less frequently occurring adverse events included: mycobacterial infections, Epstein-Barr virus infections, and pancreatitis.

Rapamune® Tablets: The safety profile of the tablet did not differ from that of the oral solution formulation. The incidence of adverse reactions up to 12 months was determined in a randomized, multicenter controlled trial (Study 3) in which 229 renal transplant patients received Rapamune Oral Solution 2 mg once daily and 228 patients received Rapamune Tablets 2 mg once daily. All patients were treated with cyclosporine and corticosteroids. The adverse reactions that occurred in either treatment group with an incidence of ≥20% in Study 3 are similar to those reported for Studies 1 & 2. There was no notable difference in the incidence of these adverse events between treatment groups (oral solution versus tablets) in Study 3, with the exception of acne, which occurred more frequently in the oral solution group, and tremor which occurred more frequently in the tablet group, particularly in Black patients. The adverse events that occurred in patients with an incidence of ≥3% and <20% in either treatment group in Study 3 were similar to those reported in Studies 1 & 2. There was no notable difference in the incidence of these adverse events between treatment groups (oral solution versus tablets) in Study 3, with the exception of hypertonia, which occurred more frequently in the oral solution group and diabetes mellitus which occurred more frequently in the tablet group. Hispanic patients in the tablet group experienced hyperglycemia more frequently than Hispanic patients in the oral solution group. In Study 3 alone, menorrhagia, metrorrhagia, and polyuria occurred with an incidence of ≥3% and <20%.

The clinically important opportunistic or common transplant-related infections were identical in all three studies and the incidences of these infections were similar in Study 3 compared with Studies 1 & 2. The incidence rates of these infections were not significantly different between the oral solution and tablet treatment groups in Study 3.

In Study 3 (at 12 months), there were two cases of lymphoma/lymphoproliferative disorder in the oral solution treatment group (0.8%) and two reported cases of lymphoma/lymphoproliferative disorder in the tablet treatment group (0.8%). These differences were not statistically significant and were similar to the incidences observed in Studies 1 & 2.

Other clinical experience: Cases of interstitial lung disease (including pneumonitis, and infrequently bronchiolitis obliterans organizing pneumonia [BOOP] and pulmonary fibrosis), some fatal, with no identified infectious etiology have occurred in patients receiving immunosuppressive regimens including Rapamune. In some cases, the interstitial lung disease has resolved upon discontinuation or dose reduction of Rapamune. The risk may be increased as the trough Rapamune level increases (see **PRECAUTIONS**).

There have been rare reports of pancytopenia.

Hepatotoxicity has been reported, including fatal hepatic necrosis with elevated sirolimus trough levels.

Abnormal healing following transplant surgery has been reported, including fascial dehiscence and anastomotic disruption (e.g., wound, vascular, airway, ureteral, biliary).

OVERDOSAGE

Reports of overdose with Rapamune have been received; however, experience has been limited. In general, the adverse effects of overdose are consistent with those listed in the **ADVERSE REACTIONS** section (see **ADVERSE REACTIONS**).

General supportive measures should be followed in all cases of overdose. Based on the poor aqueous solubility and high erythrocyte and plasma protein binding of Rapamune, it is anticipated that Rapamune is not dialyzable to any significant extent. In mice and rats, the acute oral lethal dose was greater than 800 mg/kg.

DOSAGE AND ADMINISTRATION

It is recommended that Rapamune Oral Solution and Tablets be used in a regimen with cyclosporine and corticosteroids. Two-mg Rapamune oral solution has been demonstrated to be clinically equivalent to 2-mg Rapamune oral tablets; hence, are interchangeable on a mg to mg basis. However, it is not known if higher doses of Rapamune oral solution are clinically equivalent to higher doses of tablets on a mg to mg basis. (See **CLINICAL PHARMACOLOGY: Absorption**). Rapamune is to be administered orally once daily. The initial dose of Rapamune should be administered as soon as possible after transplantation. For *de novo* transplant recipients, a loading dose of Rapamune of 3 times the maintenance dose should be given. A daily maintenance dose of 2-mg is recommended for use in renal transplant patients, with a loading dose of 6 mg. Although a daily maintenance dose of 5 mg, with a loading dose of 15 mg was used in clinical trials of the oral solution and was shown to be safe and effective, no efficacy advantage over the 2 mg dose could be established for renal transplant patients. Patients receiving 2 mg of Rapamune Oral Solution per day demonstrated an overall better safety profile than did patients receiving 5 mg of Rapamune Oral Solution per day.

To minimize the variability of exposure to Rapamune, this drug should be taken consistently with or without food. Grapefruit juice reduces CYP3A4-mediated metabolism of Rapamune and must not be administered with Rapamune or used for dilution.

It is recommended that sirolimus be taken 4 hours after administration of cyclosporine oral solution (MODIFIED) and/or cyclosporine capsules (MODIFIED).

Dosage Adjustments

The initial dosage in patients ≥13 years who weigh less than 40 kg should be adjusted, based on body surface area, to 1 mg/m²/day. The loading dose should be 3 mg/m².

It is recommended that the maintenance dose of Rapamune be reduced by approximately one third in patients with hepatic impairment. It is not necessary to modify the Rapamune loading dose. Dosage need not be adjusted because of impaired renal function.

Blood Concentration Monitoring

Routine therapeutic drug level monitoring is not required in most patients. Blood sirolimus levels should be monitored in pediatric patients, in patients with hepatic impairment, during concurrent administration of strong CYP3A4 inducers and inhibitors, and/or if cyclosporine dosing is markedly reduced or discontinued. In controlled clinical trials with concomitant cyclosporine, mean sirolimus whole blood trough levels, as measured by immunoassay, were 9 ng/mL (range 4.5–14 ng/mL [10th to 90th percentile]) for the 2 mg/day treatment group, and 17 ng/mL (range 10–28 ng/mL [10th to 90th percentile]) for the 5 mg/day dose.

Results from other assays may differ from those with an immunoassay. On average, chromatographic methods (HPLC UV or LC/MS/MS) yield results that are approximately 20% lower than the immunoassay for whole blood concentration determinations. Adjustments to the targeted range should be made according to the assay utilized to determine sirolimus trough concentrations. Therefore, comparison between concentrations in the published literature and an individual patient concentration using current assays must be made with detailed knowledge of the assay methods employed. A discussion of the different assay methods is contained in *Clinical Therapeutics*, Volume 22, Supplement B, April 2000.

Instructions for Dilution and Administration of Rapamune® Oral Solution

Bottles

The amber oral dose syringe should be used to withdraw the prescribed amount of Rapamune® Oral Solution from the bottle. Empty the correct amount of Rapamune from the syringe into only a glass or plastic container holding at least two (2) ounces (1/4 cup, 60 mL) of water or orange juice. No other liquids, including grapefruit juice, should be used for dilution. Stir vigorously and drink at once. Refill the container with an additional volume (minimum of four [4] ounces [1/2 cup, 120 mL]) of water or orange juice, stir vigorously, and drink at once.

Pouches

When using the pouch, squeeze the entire contents of the pouch into only a glass or plastic container holding at least two (2) ounces (1/4 cup, 60 mL) of water or orange juice. No other liquids, including grapefruit juice, should be used for dilution. Stir vigorously and drink at once. Refill the container with an additional volume (minimum of four [4] ounces [1/2 cup, 120 mL]) of water or orange juice, stir vigorously, and drink at once.

Handling and Disposal

Since Rapamune is not absorbed through the skin, there are no special precautions. However, if direct contact with the skin or mucous membranes occurs, wash thoroughly with soap and water; rinse eyes with plain water.

HOW SUPPLIED

Rapamune® (sirolimus) Oral Solution is supplied at a concentration of 1 mg/mL in:

1. Cartons:
   NDC # 0008-1030-06, containing a 2 oz (60 mL fill) amber glass bottle.
   NDC # 0008-1030-15, containing a 5 oz (150 mL fill) amber glass bottle.

In addition to the bottles, each carton is supplied with an oral syringe adapter for fitting into the neck of the bottle, sufficient disposable amber oral syringes and caps for daily dosing, and a carrying case.

2. Cartons:
   NDC # 0008-1030-03, containing 30 unit-of-use laminated aluminum pouches of 1 mL.
   NDC # 0008-1030-07, containing 30 unit-of-use laminated aluminum pouches of 2 mL.
   NDC # 0008-1030-08, containing 30 unit-of-use laminated aluminum pouches of 5 mL.

Rapamune® (sirolimus) Tablets are available as follows:

1 mg, white, triangular-shaped tablets marked "RAPAMUNE 1 mg" on one side.
   NDC # 0008-1031-05, bottle of 100 tablets.
   NDC # 0008-1031-10, Redipak® cartons of 100 tablets (10 blister cards of 10 tablets each).

2 mg, yellow to beige triangular-shaped tablets marked "RAPAMUNE 2 mg" on one side.
   NDC # 0008-1032-05, bottle of 100 tablets.
   NDC # 0008-1032-10, Redipak® cartons of 100 tablets (10 blister cards of 10 tablets each [2 × 5]).

Storage

Rapamune® Oral Solution bottles and pouches should be stored protected from light and refrigerated at 2°C to 8°C (36°F to 46°F). Once the bottle is opened, the contents should be used within one month. If necessary, the patient may store both the pouches and the bottles at room temperatures up to 25°C (77°F) for a short period of time (e.g., up to 24 hours for the pouches and not more than 15 days for the bottles).

An amber syringe and cap are provided for dosing and the product may be kept in the syringe for a maximum of 24 hours at room temperatures up to 25°C (77°F) or refrigerated at 2°C to 8°C (36°F to 46°F). The syringe should be discarded after one use. After dilution, the preparation should be used immediately.

Rapamune Oral Solution provided in bottles may develop a slight haze when refrigerated. If such a haze occurs allow the product to stand at room temperature and shake gently until the haze disappears. The presence of this haze does not affect the quality of the product.

Rapamune® Tablets should be stored at 20° to 25°C (USP Controlled Room Temperature) (68° to 77°F). Use cartons to protect blister cards and strips from light. Dispense in a tight, light-resistant container as defined in the USP.

℞ only

US Pat. Nos.: 5,100,899; 5,212,155; 5,308,847; 5,403,833; 5,536,729.

INCIDENCE (%) OF MALIGNANCIES IN PREVENTION OF ACUTE RENAL REJECTION TRIALS: AT 12 MONTHS POST-TRANSPLANT[a]

Malignancy	Rapamune® Oral Solution 2 mg/day (n = 511)	Rapamune® Oral Solution 5 mg/day (n = 493)	Azathioprine 2–3 mg/kg/day (n = 161)	Placebo (n = 130)
Lymphoma/lymphoproliferative disease	0.4	1.4	0.6	0
Non-melanoma skin carcinoma	0.4	1.4	1.2	3.1
Other malignancy	0.6	0.6	0	0

a: Patients received cyclosporine and corticosteroids.

PATIENT INSTRUCTIONS FOR RAPAMUNE® (SIROLIMUS) ORAL SOLUTION ADMINISTRATION
Bottles

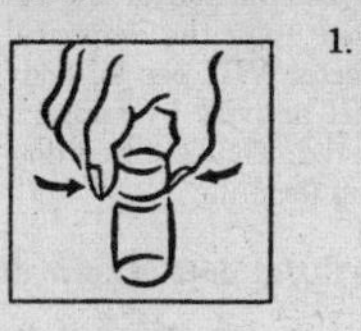

1. Open the solution bottle. Remove the safety cap by squeezing the tabs on the cap and twisting counter-clockwise.

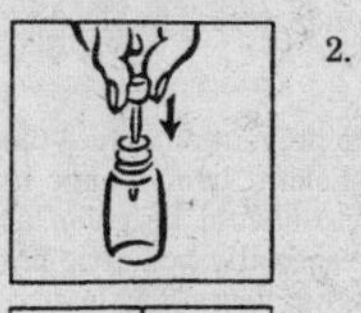

2. On first use, insert the adapter assembly (plastic tube with stopper) tightly into the bottle until it is even with the top of the bottle. Do not remove the adapter assembly from the bottle once inserted.

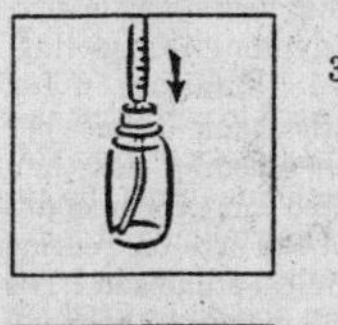

3. For each use, tightly insert one of the amber syringes with the plunger fully depressed into the opening in the adapter.

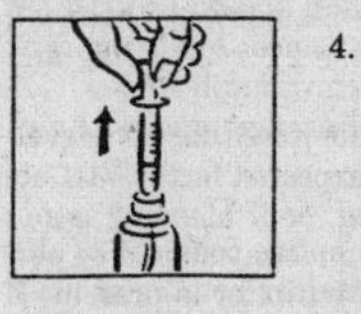

4. Withdraw the prescribed amount of Rapamune® (sirolimus) Oral Solution by gently pulling out the plunger of the syringe until the bottom of the black line of the plunger is even with the appropriate mark on the syringe. Always keep the bottle in an upright position. If bubbles form in the syringe, empty the syringe into the bottle and repeat the procedure.

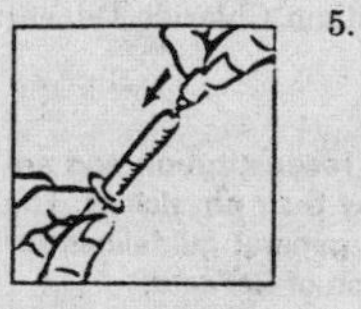

5. You may have been instructed to carry your medication with you. If it is necessary to carry the filled syringe, place a cap securely on the syringe—the cap should snap into place.

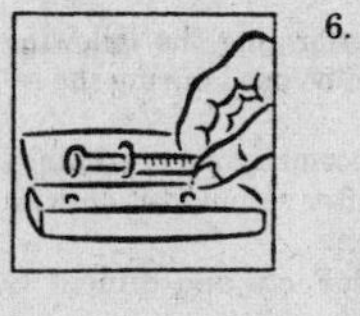

6. Then place the capped syringe in the enclosed carrying case. Once in the syringe, the medication may be kept at room temperature or refrigerated and should be used within 24 hours. Extreme temperature (below 36°F and above 86°F) should be avoided. Remember to keep this medication out of the reach of children.

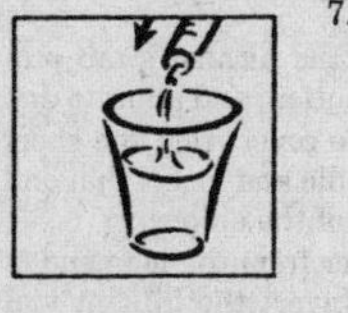

7. Empty the syringe into a glass or plastic cup containing at least 2 ounces (1/4 cup; 60 mL) of water or orange juice, stir vigorously for one (1) minute and drink immediately. Refill the container with at least 4 ounces (1/2 cup; 120 mL) of water or orange juice, stir vigorously again and drink the rinse solution. Apple juice, grapefruit juice, or other liquids are NOT to be used. Only glass or plastic cups should be used to dilute Rapamune® Oral Solution. The syringe and cap should be used once and then discarded.

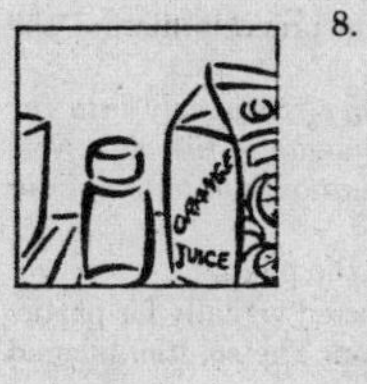

8. Always store the bottles of medication in the refrigerator. When refrigerated, a slight haze may develop in the solution. The presence of a haze does not affect the quality of the product. If this happens, bring the Rapamune® Oral Solution to room temperature and shake until the haze disappears. If it is necessary to wipe clean the mouth of the bottle before returning the product to the refrigerator, wipe with a dry cloth to avoid introducing water, or any other liquid, into the bottle.

PATIENT INSTRUCTIONS FOR RAPAMUNE® (SIROLIMUS) ORAL SOLUTION ADMINISTRATION
Pouches

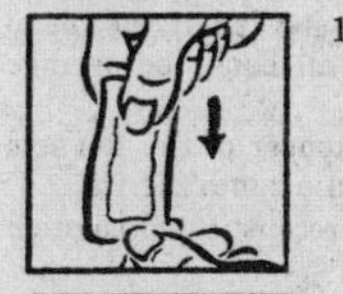

1. Before opening the pouch, squeeze the pouch from the neck area to push the contents into the lower part of the pouch.

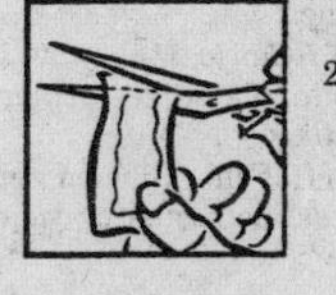

2. Carefully open the pouch by folding the marked area and then cutting with a scissors along the marked line near the top of the pouch.

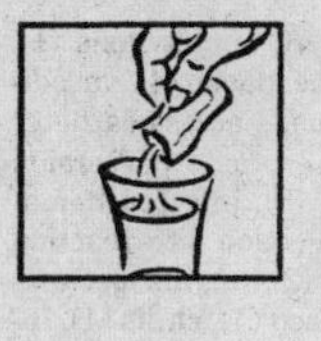

3. Squeeze the entire contents of the pouch into a glass or plastic cup containing at least 2 ounces (1/4 cup; 60 mL) of water or orange juice, stir vigorously for one (1) minute and drink immediately. Refill the container with at least 4 ounces (1/2 cup, 120 mL) of water or orange juice, stir vigorously again and drink the rinse solution. Apple juice, grapefruit juice or other liquids are NOT to be used. Only glass or plastic cups should be used to dilute Rapamune® oral solution.
4. Unused pouches should be stored in the refrigerator.

Wyeth Laboratories
Division of Wyeth-Ayerst Pharmaceuticals Inc.
Philadelphia, PA 19101 W10431C001
CI 7713-6 ET01
Rev 01/03

REFACTO® ℞
[rē-fāk'tō]
Antihemophilic Factor, Recombinant
℞ only

Prescribing information for this product, which appears on pages 3474–3476 of the 2003 PDR, has been completely revised as follows. Please write "See Supplement A" next to the product heading.

DESCRIPTION

ReFacto® Antihemophilic Factor (Recombinant) is a purified protein produced by recombinant DNA technology for use in therapy of factor VIII deficiency. ReFacto is a glycoprotein with an approximate molecular mass of 170 kDa consisting of 1438 amino acids. It has an amino acid sequence that is comparable to the 90 + 80 kDa form of factor VIII, and post-translational modifications that are similar to those of the plasma-derived molecule. ReFacto has *in vitro* functional characteristics comparable to those of endogenous factor VIII.

ReFacto is produced by a genetically engineered Chinese hamster ovary (CHO) cell line. The CHO cell line secretes B-domain deleted recombinant factor VIII into a defined cell culture medium that contains human serum albumin and recombinant insulin, but does not contain any proteins derived from animal sources. The protein is purified by a chromatography purification process that yields a high-purity, active product. The potency expressed in international units (IU) is determined using the European Pharmacopoeial chromogenic assay against the WHO standard. The specific activity of ReFacto is 11,200–15,500 IU per milligram of protein. ReFacto is not purified from human blood and contains no preservatives or added human components in the final formulation.

ReFacto is formulated as a sterile, nonpyrogenic, lyophilized powder preparation for intravenous (IV) injection. It is available in single-use vials containing the labeled amount of factor VIII activity (IU). Each vial contains nominally 250, 500, 1000 or 2000 IU of ReFacto per vial. The formulated product is a clear colorless solution upon reconstitution and contains sodium chloride, sucrose, L-histidine, calcium chloride, and polysorbate 80.

CLINICAL PHARMACOLOGY

Factor VIII is the specific clotting factor deficient in patients with hemophilia A (classical hemophilia). The administration of ReFacto® Antihemophilic Factor (Recombinant) increases plasma levels of factor VIII activity and can temporarily correct the *in vitro* coagulation defect in these patients.

Activated factor VIII acts as a cofactor for activated factor IX accelerating the conversion of factor X to activated factor X. Activated factor X converts prothrombin into thrombin. Thrombin then converts fibrinogen into fibrin and a clot is formed. Factor VIII activity is greatly reduced in patients with hemophilia A and therefore replacement therapy is necessary.

In a crossover pharmacokinetic study of eighteen (18) previously treated patients **using the chromogenic assay,** the circulating mean half-life for ReFacto was 14.5 ± 5.3 hours (ranged from 7.6–27.7 hours), which was not statistically significantly different from plasma-derived Antihemophilic Factor (Human) (pdAHF), which had a mean half-life of 13.7 ± 3.4 hours (ranged from 8.8–23.7 hours). Mean incremental recovery (K-value) of ReFacto in plasma was 2.4 ± 0.4 IU/dL per IU/kg (ranged from 1.9–3.3 IU/dL per IU/kg). This was comparable to the mean incremental recovery observed in plasma for pdAHF which was 2.3 ± 0.3 IU/dL per IU/kg (ranged from 1.7–2.9 IU/dL per IU/kg). **Results obtained from this controlled pharmacokinetic study, which used a central laboratory for the analysis of all plasma samples, showed that the one-stage factor VIII clotting assay gave results which were approximately 50% of the values obtained with the chromogenic assay** (see **DOSAGE AND ADMINISTRATION**).

In two additional clinical studies, pharmacokinetic parameters were evaluated for previously treated patients [PTPs] and previously untreated patients [PUPs]. In PTPs (n=87) ReFacto had a mean incremental recovery of 2.4 ± 0.4 IU/dL per IU/kg (ranged from 1.1–3.8 IU/dL per IU/kg) and an elimination half-life (n=67) of 10.7 ± 2.8 hours. In PUPs (n=45) ReFacto had a lower mean incremental recovery of 1.7 ± 0.4 IU/dL per IU/kg (ranged from 0.2–2.8 IU/dL per IU/kg) as compared to PTPs. Population pharmacokinetic modeling using data from 44 PUPs led to a mean estimated half-life of ReFacto in PUPs of 8.0 ± 2.2 hours. These parameters did not change over time (12 months) for PTPs or PUPs.

In clinical studies of ReFacto involving a total of 218 patients (117 PTPs including 4 who participated in the surgery study only, and 101 PUPs), more than 84 million IU were administered over a period of up to 54 months. The 117 PTPs were given a median of 230 injections (range of 4–1530 injections) over a median of 1200 days (range of 31–1640 days). The 101 PUPs were given a median of 26 injections (range of 1–490 injections) over a median of 830 days (range of 1–1298 days). One hundred thirteen PTPs and 99 PUPs were evaluated for efficacy in bleeding episodes. The 113 PTPs experienced a median of 54 bleeding episodes and the 99 PUPs experienced a median of 12 bleeding episodes. All were treated successfully on an on-demand basis or for the reduction of bleeding episodes except for one PTP and two PUPs who discontinued ReFacto treatment and switched to another product after the development of inhibitors. Bleeding episodes included hemarthroses, and bleeding in soft tissue, muscle, and other anatomical sites.

ReFacto has been studied in short-term routine prophylaxis. In uncontrolled clinical trials, an average dose of 27 ± 10 IU/kg in PTPs (n=77) and an average dose of 57 ± 20 IU/kg in PUPs (n=17) was given repeatedly at variable intervals longer than 2 weeks. In 64 patients who had both on-demand and prophylactic periods during their time on study, the mean rate of spontaneous musculoskeletal bleeding episodes was less during periods of routine prophylaxis. There were an average of 10 bleeding episodes per year during the prophylactic periods compared to an average of 37 bleeding episodes per year during the on-demand periods. The clinical trial experience with routine prophylaxis in PUPs is limited (n=17). These nonrandomized trial results should be interpreted with caution, as the investigators exercised their own discretion in deciding when and in whom prophylaxis was to be initiated and terminated.

Management of hemostasis was evaluated in the surgical setting where 28 surgical procedures have been performed in 25 patients. The average preoperative dose in PTPs was 59 IU/kg. Procedures included orthopedic procedures, inguinal hernia repair, epidural hematoma evacuation, transposition ulnar nerve, and other minor procedures (e.g., venous access catheter placement and explantation, toenail removal). Circulatory factor VIII levels targeted to restore and maintain hemostasis were achieved. While the one-stage clotting assay was used most frequently in the surgical setting (24 versus 4 surgeries), hemostasis was maintained throughout the surgical period regardless of which assay was used. Hemostatic efficacy was rated as excellent or good in all procedures.

The occurrence of neutralizing antibody (inhibitors) is well known in the treatment of patients with hemophilia A[1,2,3]. Thirty out of 101 PUPs (30%) developed an inhibitor: 16 out of 101 (16%) with a high titer (≥ 5 BU) (11 of the 16 patients had peak values ≥ 10 BU) and 14 out of 101 (14%) with a low titer (< 5 BU). In this study the incidence of inhibitor development to factor VIII using ReFacto is similar to that reported for other factor VIII products[1,2,3,5].

One of 113 (0.9%) previously treated patients (PTPs) developed a high titer inhibitor. Inhibitor development occurred in the same time frame as the development of monoclonal gammopathy of uncertain significance. The patient was noted initially to have low titer inhibitor at a local laboratory at 99 exposure days (1.2 BU) and became positive at the central laboratory at 113 exposure days, initially also with low titer inhibitor of 2 BU. After 14 months on continued treatment with ReFacto, the inhibitor level rose to nearly 13 BU and a bleeding episode failed to respond to ReFacto treatment. In this study the incidence of inhibitor development to factor VIII using ReFacto is similar to that reported for other factor VIII products[4]. Also there have been spontaneous post-marketing reports of high titer inhibitors involving previously treated patients (see also **PRECAUTIONS, General** and **ADVERSE REACTIONS**).

INDICATIONS AND USAGE

ReFacto® Antihemophilic Factor (Recombinant) is indicated for the control and prevention of hemorrhagic episodes and for surgical prophylaxis in patients with hemophilia A (congenital factor VIII deficiency or classic hemophilia).

ReFacto is indicated for short-term routine prophylaxis to reduce the frequency of spontaneous bleeding episodes. The effect of regular routine prophylaxis on long-term morbidity and mortality is unknown.

ReFacto can be of a significant therapeutic value for treatment of hemophilia A in certain patients with inhibitors to factor VIII[6]. In clinical studies of ReFacto, patients who developed inhibitors on study continued to manifest a clinical response when inhibitor titers were < 10 BU. When an inhibitor is present, the dosage requirement of factor VIII is variable. The dosage can be determined only by a clinical response and by monitoring of circulating factor VIII levels after treatment (see **DOSAGE AND ADMINISTRATION**).

ReFacto does not contain von Willebrand factor and therefore is not indicated in von Willebrand's disease.

Continued on next page

Refacto—Cont.

CONTRAINDICATIONS

Known hypersensitivity to mouse, hamster, or bovine proteins may be a contraindication to the use of ReFacto® Antihemophilic Factor (Recombinant).

WARNINGS

As with any intravenous protein product, allergic type hypersensitivity reactions are possible. Patients should be informed of the early signs of hypersensitivity reactions including hives, generalized urticaria, tightness of the chest, wheezing, hypotension, and anaphylaxis. Patients should be advised to discontinue use of the product and contact their physicians if these symptoms occur.

PRECAUTIONS

General

Activity-neutralizing antibodies (inhibitors) have been detected in patients receiving factor VIII-containing products. Low titer inhibitors are common in previously untreated patients and in previously treated patients on factor VIII products, as are high titer inhibitors in previously untreated patients. High titer inhibitors, which are generally rare in previously treated patients, have been reported in previously treated patients on ReFacto. As with all coagulation factor VIII products, patients should be monitored for the development of inhibitors that should be titrated in Bethesda Units using appropriate biological testing.

Reports of lack of effect, mainly in prophylaxis patients, have been received in the clinical trials and in the post-marketing setting. The reported lack of effect has been described as bleeding into target joints, bleeding into new joints or a subjective feeling by the patient of new onset bleeding. When switching to ReFacto it is important to individually titrate and monitor each patient's dose in order to ensure an adequate therapeutic response (see **DOSAGE AND ADMINISTRATION**).

Formation of Antibodies to Mouse and Hamster Protein

As Antihemophilic Factor (Recombinant), ReFacto contains trace amounts of mouse protein (maximum of 5 ng/1000 IU) and hamster protein (maximum of 30 ng/1000 IU), the remote possibility exists that patients treated with this product may develop hypersensitivity to these non-human mammalian proteins.

Carcinogenicity, Mutagenicity, Impairment of Fertility

ReFacto® Antihemophilic Factor (Recombinant) has been shown to be non-mutagenic in the mouse micronucleus assay. No other mutagenicity studies and no investigations on carcinogenesis or impairment of fertility have been conducted.

Pregnancy Category C

Animal reproduction and lactation studies have not been conducted with ReFacto® Antihemophilic Factor (Recombinant). It is not known whether ReFacto can affect reproductive capacity or cause fetal harm when given to pregnant women. ReFacto should be administered to pregnant and lactating women only if clearly indicated.

Pediatric Use

ReFacto® Antihemophilic Factor (Recombinant) is appropriate for use in children of all ages, including newborns. Safety and efficacy studies have been performed both in previously treated children and adolescents (N=22, ages 8-15 years) and in previously untreated neonates, infants, and children (N=101, ages 0-52 months) (see **CLINICAL PHARMACOLOGY** and **PRECAUTIONS**).

Geriatric Use

Clinical studies of ReFacto did not include sufficient numbers of subjects aged 65 and over to determine whether they respond differently from younger subjects. Other reported clinical experience has not identified differences in responses between the elderly and younger patients. As with any patient receiving ReFacto, dose selection for an elderly patient should be individualized.

ADVERSE REACTIONS

As with the intravenous administration of any protein product, the following reactions may be observed after administration: headache, fever, chills, flushing, nausea, vomiting, lethargy, or manifestations of allergic reactions. During clinical studies with ReFacto® Antihemophilic Factor (Recombinant), 77 adverse reactions in 43 of 218 patients (20%) probably or possibly-related to therapy were reported for 64,363 infusions (0.12%). These were anaphylaxis (1), dyspnea (6), urticaria (1), nausea (11), headache (4), vasodilation (5), dizziness (4), permanent venous access catheter complications (3), asthenia (3), fever (3), taste perversion [altered taste] (3), bleeding/hematoma (3), infected hematoma (1), anorexia (2), diarrhea (2), injection site reaction (2), somnolence (2), rash (2), pruritus (2), angina pectoris (1), tachycardia (1), perspiration increased (1), chills (1), increased amino transferase (1), increased bilirubin (1), pain in finger (1), muscle weakness (1), CPK increase (1), cold sensation (1), eye disorder-vision abnormal (1), coughing (1), myalgia (1), gastroenteritis (1), abdominal pain (1), acne (1), and forehead bruises (1). If any adverse reaction takes place that is thought to be related to administration of ReFacto, the rate of infusion should be decreased or stopped.

Inhibitor development is a known adverse event associated with the treatment of patients with hemophilia A. In addition to the one report of high titer inhibitors in the clinical study of PTPs (see **CLINICAL PHARMACOLOGY**), there have been reports of high titer inhibitors in PTPs in the post-marketing setting. High and low titer inhibitors have been reported in PUPs in both clinical trials and the post-marketing setting (see **PRECAUTIONS, General**).

A total of 182 adverse reactions in 54 of 218 patients (25%) who received 32,013 infusions (0.6%) were reported by the investigator to have an "unlikely" or "not assessable" relationship to ReFacto administration. The study sponsor considered that the events may be of possible or of unknown relationship to therapy because of the temporal relationship to the infusion and/or the frequency of the event for a given patient and/or because insufficient information was available to assign another causality. In this category, 25 patients experienced the following 38 events which are different from the events described above: pain (10), rhinitis (10), vomiting (4), insomnia (3), constipation (2), pharyngitis (2), flushing (1), palpitation (1), sinusitis (1), gastritis (1), dyspepsia (1), hypotension (1), and URI (1).

Other adverse experiences that were reported during the clinical trials, but which were assessed by both the investigator and the sponsor as "unlikely" to be related to ReFacto administration included: dyspnea (3), rash (2), pruritus (1), neuropathy (1), arm weakness (1), and thrombophlebitis of upper arm (1).

DOSAGE AND ADMINISTRATION

Treatment with ReFacto® Antihemophilic Factor (Recombinant) should be initiated under the supervision of a physician experienced in the treatment of hemophilia A.

The labeled potency of ReFacto is based on the European Pharmacopoeial chromogenic substrate assay, whereas other factor VIII products are labeled based on the one-stage clotting assay. With recombinant factor VIII products, the chromogenic assay typically yields results which are higher than the results obtained with the one-stage clotting assay. When switching between products it is important to individually titrate each patient's dose in order to ensure an adequate therapeutic response (see **PRECAUTIONS, General**). Results obtained from a controlled pharmacokinetic study, which used one central laboratory for the analysis of all plasma samples, showed that the one-stage factor VIII clotting assay gave results that were approximately 50% of those obtained with the chromogenic substrate assay (see **CLINICAL PHARMACOLOGY**). In addition, in clinical trials of ReFacto use in the surgical setting in which multiple laboratories were used for plasma sample analysis, the ratio of factor VIII activity results obtained by the one-stage clotting and chromogenic substrate assays ranged between 20 and 80%.

When monitoring patients' factor VIII activity levels during treatment, the available clinical data suggest that either assay may be used. Most patients in clinical trials were monitored with the one-stage clotting assay (see **CLINICAL PHARMACOLOGY**). It is necessary to adhere to the incubation/activation times and other test conditions as specified by the assay manufacturers.

Dosage and duration of treatment depend on the severity of the factor VIII deficiency, the location and extent of bleeding, and the patient's clinical condition. Doses administered should be titrated to the patient's clinical response. In the presence of an inhibitor, higher doses may be required.

Precise monitoring of the replacement therapy by means of coagulation analysis (plasma factor VIII activity) is recommended, particularly for surgical intervention.

One international unit (IU) of factor VIII activity corresponds approximately to the quantity of factor VIII in one mL of normal human plasma. The calculation of the required dosage of factor VIII is based upon the empirical finding that, on average, 1 IU of factor VIII per kg body weight raises the plasma factor VIII activity by approximately 2 IU/dL per IU/kg administered. The required dosage is determined using the following formula:

Required units = body weight (kg)
× desired factor VIII rise (IU/dL or % of normal)
× 0.5 (IU/kg per IU/dL)

The following chart can be used to guide dosing in bleeding episodes and surgery:

[See table below]

Type of Hemorrhage	Factor VIII Level Required (IU/dL or % of normal)	Frequency of Doses (h)/ Duration of Therapy (d)
Minor		
Early hemarthrosis, minor muscle or oral bleeds.	20–40	Repeat every 12 to 24 hours as necessary until resolved. At least 1 day, depending upon the severity of the hemorrage.
Moderate		
Hemorrhages into muscles. Mild trauma capitus. Minor operations including tooth extraction. Hemorrhages into the oral cavity.	30–60	Repeat infusion every 12–24 hours for 3–4 days or until adequate local hemostasis is achieved. For tooth extraction a single infusion plus oral antifibrinolytic therapy within 1 hour may be sufficient.
Major		
Gastrointestinal bleeding. Intracranial, intra-abdominal or intrathoracic hemorrhages. Fractures. Major operations.	60–100	Repeat infusion every 8–24 hours until threat is resolved or in the case of surgery, until adequate local hemostasis is achieved.

For short-term routine prophylaxis to prevent or reduce the frequency of spontaneous musculoskeletal hemorrhage in patients with hemophilia A, ReFacto should be given at least twice a week. In some cases, especially pediatric patients, shorter dosage intervals or higher doses may be necessary. Pharmacokinetic/pharmacodynamic modeling, based on pharmacokinetic data from 185 infusions in 102 PTPs, predicts that routine prophylactic dosing 3 times per week may be associated with a lower bleeding risk than with dosing twice weekly. No randomized comparison of different doses or frequency regimens of ReFacto for routine prophylaxis has been performed. In clinical studies in PTPs (ages 8–73 years) and PUPs (ages 9–52 months), the mean dose used for routine prophylaxis was 27 ± 10 IU/kg and 57 ± 20 IU/kg, respectively.

Patients using ReFacto should be monitored for the development of factor VIII inhibitors. If expected factor VIII activity plasma levels are not attained, or if bleeding is not controlled with an appropriate dose, an assay should be performed to determine if a factor VIII inhibitor is present. If the inhibitor is present at levels less than 10 Bethesda Units per mL, administration of additional antihemophilic factor may neutralize the inhibitor.

ReFacto is administered by IV infusion after reconstitution of the lyophilized powder with Sodium Chloride Diluent (provided).

INSTRUCTIONS FOR USE

Patients should follow the specific reconstitution and administration procedures provided by their physicians. The procedures below are provided as general guidelines for the reconstitution and administration of ReFacto.

Reconstitution

Always wash your hands before performing the following procedures. Aseptic technique should be used during the reconstitution procedure.

ReFacto® Antihemophilic Factor (Recombinant) is administered by intravenous (IV) infusion after reconstitution with the supplied Sodium Chloride Diluent.

1. Allow the vials of lyophilized ReFacto and diluent to reach room temperature.
2. Remove the plastic flip-top caps from the ReFacto vial and the diluent vial to expose the central portions of the rubber stoppers.
3. Wipe the tops of both vials with the alcohol swab provided, or use another antiseptic solution, and allow to dry.
4. Remove the transparent protective cover from the short end of the sterile double-ended needle and insert that end into the diluent vial at the center of the stopper.
5. Remove the colored protective cover from the long end of the sterile double-ended needle. Invert the diluent vial and, to minimize leakage, quickly insert the long end of the needle through the center of the stopper of the upright ReFacto vial.

Note: Point the double-ended needle toward the wall of the ReFacto vial to prevent excessive foaming.

6. The vacuum will draw the diluent into the ReFacto vial.
7. Once the transfer is complete, remove the double-ended needle from the ReFacto vial, and properly discard the needle with the diluent vial.

Note: If the diluent does not transfer completely into the ReFacto vial, DO NOT USE the contents of the vial. Note that it is acceptable for a small amount of fluid to remain in the solvent vial after transfer.

8. Gently rotate the vial to dissolve the powder.
9. The final solution should be inspected visually for particulate matter before administration. The solution should appear clear and colorless.

ReFacto should be administered within 3 hours after reconstitution. The reconstituted solution may be stored at room temperature prior to administration.

Administration (Intravenous Injection)

ReFacto® Antihemophilic Factor (Recombinant) should be administered using a single sterile disposable plastic syringe. In addition, the solution should be withdrawn from the vial using the sterile filter needle.

1. Using aseptic technique, attach the sterile filter needle to the sterile disposable syringe. Pull back the syringe plunger to the 5 mL mark.
2. Insert the filter needle into the stopper of the ReFacto vial. Push plunger forward to inject air into the vial.
3. Invert the vial and withdraw the reconstituted solution into the syringe.
4. Remove and discard the filter needle.

Note: If you use more than one vial of ReFacto, the contents of multiple vials may be drawn into the same syringe through a separate, unused filter needle.

5. Attach the syringe to the luer end of the infusion set tubing and perform venipuncture as instructed by your physician.

After reconstitution, ReFacto should be injected intravenously over several minutes. The rate of administration should be determined by the patient's comfort level.

Dispose of all unused solution, empty vials, and used needles and syringes in an appropriate container for throwing away waste that might hurt others if not handled properly.

Storage
Product as packaged for sale: ReFacto® Antihemophilic Factor (Recombinant) should be stored under refrigeration at a temperature of 2 to 8 °C (36 to 46 °F). ReFacto may also be stored at room temperature not to exceed 25 °C (77 °F) for up to 3 months. Freezing should be avoided to prevent damage to the diluent vial. During storage, avoid prolonged exposure of ReFacto® vial to light. Do not use ReFacto after the expiry date on the label.

Product after reconstitution: The product does not contain a preservative and should be used within 3 hours.

HOW SUPPLIED
ReFacto® Antihemophilic Factor (Recombinant) is supplied in single-use vials which contain nominally 250, 500, 1000 or 2000 IU per vial (NDC 58394-007-01, 58394-006-01, 58394-005-01, 58394-011-01, respectively) with sterile diluent, sterile double-ended needle for reconstitution, sterile filter needle for withdrawal, sterile infusion set, and two (2) alcohol swabs. Actual factor VIII activity in IU is stated on the label of each vial.

REFERENCES
1. Ehrenforth S, Kreuz W, Scharrer I, et al. Incidence of development of factor VIII and factor IX inhibitors in hemophiliacs. Lancet. 1992;339:594-598.
2. Bray GL, Gomperts ED, Courter S, et al. A multicenter study of recombinant factor VIII (Recombinate): safety, efficacy, and inhibitor risk in previously untreated patients with hemophilia A. Blood. 1994;83(9):2428-2435.
3. Lusher J, Arkin S, Abildgaard CF, Schwartz RS, Group TKPUPS. Recombinant factor VIII for the treatment of previously untreated patients with hemophilia A. N Engl J Med. 1993;328:453-459.
4. Kessler C, Sachse K. Factor VIII:C inhibitor associated with monoclonal-antibody purified FVIII concentrate. Lancet 1990; 335:1403.
5. Scharrer I, Bray G. Incidence of inhibitors in haemophilia A patients - a review of recent studies of recombinant and plasma-derived factor VIII concentrates. Hemophilia 1999; 5:145.
6. Kessler CM. An Introduction to Factor VIII Inhibitors: The Detection and Quantitation. American Journal of Medicine 91 1991, (Supplement 5A): 1S-5S.

Genetics Institute, Inc.
Cambridge MA 02140-2387, USA
Rev. 11/02 US License Number 1163
Telephone: 1-800-934-5556

750-01875
W10403C001
Rev. 11/02

ZEBETA® ℞
[zē-bā-tə]
(Bisoprolol Fumarate)
Tablets
℞ only

Prescribing information for this product, which appears on pages 3493–3495 of the 2003 PDR, has been revised as follows. Please write "See Supplement A" next to the product heading.

The **DESCRIPTION** section has been revised as follows:
Inactive ingredients include Colloidal Silicon Dioxide, Corn Starch, Crospovidone, Dibasic Calcium Phosphate, Hypromellose, Magnesium Stearate, Microcrystalline Cellulose, Polyethylene Glycol, Polysorbate 80, and Titanium Dioxide. The 5 mg tablets also contain Red and Yellow Iron Oxide.

The **CLINICAL PHARMACOLOGY** section has been revised as follows:

CLINICAL PHARMACOLOGY
ZEBETA is a beta$_1$-selective (cardioselective) adrenoceptor blocking agent without significant membrane stabilizing activity or intrinsic sympathomimetic activity in its therapeutic dosage range. Cardioselectivity is not absolute, however, and at higher doses (≥20 mg) bisoprolol fumarate also inhibits beta$_2$-adrenoceptors, chiefly located in the bronchial and vascular musculature; to retain selectivity it is therefore important to use the lowest effective dose.

In the **PRECAUTIONS** section, the **Drug Interactions** subsection has been revised as follows:

Drug Interactions
ZEBETA should not be combined with other beta-blocking agents. Patients receiving catecholamine-depleting drugs, such as reserpine or guanethidine, should be closely monitored, because the added beta-adrenergic blocking action of ZEBETA may produce excessive reduction of sympathetic activity. In patients receiving concurrent therapy with clonidine, if therapy is to be discontinued, it is suggested that ZEBETA be discontinued for several days before the withdrawal of clonidine.

ZEBETA should be used with care when myocardial depressants or inhibitors of AV conduction, such as certain calcium antagonists (particularly of the phenylalkylamine [verapamil] and benzothiazepine [diltiazem] classes), or antiarrhythmic agents, such as disopyramide, are used concurrently.

Concurrent use of rifampin increases the metabolic clearance of ZEBETA, resulting in a shortened elimination half-life of ZEBETA. However, initial dose modification is generally not necessary. Pharmacokinetic studies document no clinically relevant interactions with other agents given concomitantly, including thiazide diuretics, digoxin and cimetidine. There was no effect of ZEBETA on prothrombin time in patients on stable doses of warfarin.

Risk of Anaphylactic Reaction: While taking beta-blockers, patients with a history of severe anaphylactic reaction to a variety of allergens may be more reactive to repeated challenge, either accidental, diagnostic, or therapeutic. Such patients may be unresponsive to the usual doses of epinephrine used to treat allergic reactions.

In the **PRECAUTIONS** section, the **Carcinogenesis, Mutagenesis, Impairment of Fertility, Pregnancy Category C, Nursing Mothers, Pediatric Use,** and **Geriatric Use** subsections have been revised as follows:

Carcinogenesis, Mutagenesis, Impairment of Fertility
Long-term studies were conducted with oral bisoprolol fumarate administered in the feed of mice (20 and 24 months) and rats (26 months). No evidence of carcinogenic potential was seen in mice dosed up to 250 mg/kg/day or rats dosed up to 125 mg/kg/day. On a body weight basis, these doses are 625 and 312 times, respectively, the maximum recommended human dose (MRHD) of 20 mg, (or 0.4 mg/kg/day based on a 50 kg individual); on a body surface area basis, these doses are 59 times (mice) and 64 times (rats) the MRHD. The mutagenic potential of bisoprolol fumarate was evaluated in the microbial mutagenicity (Ames) test, the point mutation and chromosome aberration assays in Chinese hamster V79 cells, the unscheduled DNA synthesis test, the micronucleus test in mice, and the cytogenetics assay in rats. There was no evidence of mutagenic potential in these in vitro and in vivo assays.

Reproduction studies in rats did not show any impairment of fertility at doses up to 150 mg/kg/day of bisoprolol fumarate, or 375 and 77 times the MRHD on the basis of body weight and body surface area, respectively.

Pregnancy Category C
In rats, bisoprolol fumarate was not teratogenic at doses up to 150 mg/kg/day which is 375 and 77 times the MRHD on the basis of body weight and body surface area, respectively. Bisoprolol fumarate was fetotoxic (increased late resorptions) at 50 mg/kg/day and maternotoxic (decreased food intake and body weight gain) at 150 mg/kg/day. The fetotoxicity in rats occurred at 125 times the MRHD on a body weight basis and 26 times the MRHD on the basis of body surface area. The maternotoxicity occurred at 375 times the MRHD on a body weight basis and 77 times the MRHD on the basis of body surface area. In rabbits, bisoprolol fumarate was not teratogenic at doses up to 12.5 mg/kg/day, which is 31 and 12 times the MRHD based on body weight and body surface area, respectively, but was embryolethal (increased early resorptions) at 12.5 mg/kg/day.

There are no adequate and well-controlled studies in pregnant women. ZEBETA® (bisoprolol fumarate) should be used during pregnancy only if the potential benefit justifies the potential risk to the fetus.

Nursing Mothers
Small amounts of bisoprolol fumarate (< 2% of the dose) have been detected in the milk of lactating rats. It is not known whether this drug is excreted in human milk. Because many drugs are excreted in human milk caution should be exercised when bisoprolol fumarate is administered to nursing women.

Pediatric Use
Safety and effectiveness in pediatric patients have not been established.

Geriatric Use
ZEBETA has been used in elderly patients with hypertension. Response rates and mean decreases in systolic and diastolic blood pressure were similar to the decreases in younger patients in the U.S. clinical studies. Although no dose response study was conducted in elderly patients, there was a tendency for older patients to be maintained on higher doses of bisoprolol fumarate.

Observed reductions in heart rate were slightly greater in the elderly than in the young and tended to increase with increasing dose. In general, no disparity in adverse experience reports or dropouts for safety reasons was observed between older and younger patients. Dose adjustment based on age is not necessary.

The **ADVERSE REACTIONS** section has been revised as follows:

ADVERSE REACTIONS
Safety data are available in more than 30,000 patients or volunteers. Frequency estimates and rates of withdrawal of therapy for adverse events were derived from two U.S. placebo-controlled studies.

In Study A, doses of 5, 10, and 20 mg bisoprolol fumarate were administered for 4 weeks. In Study B, doses of 2.5, 10, and 40 mg of bisoprolol fumarate were administered for 12 weeks. A total of 273 patients were treated with 5-20 mg of bisoprolol fumarate; 132 received placebo.

Withdrawal of therapy for adverse events was 3.3% for patients receiving bisoprolol fumarate and 6.8% for patients on placebo. Withdrawals were less than 1% for either bradycardia or fatigue/lack of energy.

The following table presents adverse experiences, whether or not considered drug related, reported in at least 1% of patients in these studies, for all patients studied in placebo-controlled clinical trials (2.5-40 mg), as well as for a subgroup that was treated with doses within the recommended dosage range (5-20 mg). Of the adverse events listed in the table, bradycardia, diarrhea, asthenia, fatigue, and sinusitis appear to be dose related.

Body System/ Adverse Experience	All Adverse Experiences (%[a]) Bisoprolol Fumarate		
	Placebo (n=132) %	5-20 mg (n=273) %	2.5-40 mg (n=404) %
Skin			
increased sweating	1.5	0.7	1.0
Musculoskeletal			
arthralgia	2.3	2.2	2.7
Central Nervous System			
dizziness	3.8	2.9	3.5
headache	11.4	8.8	10.9
hypoaesthesia	0.8	1.1	1.5
Autonomic Nervous System			
dry mouth	1.5	0.7	1.3
Heart Rate/Rhythm			
bradycardia	0	0.4	0.5
Psychiatric			
vivid dreams	0	0	0
insomnia	2.3	1.5	2.5
depression	0.8	0	0.2
Gastrointestinal			
diarrhea	1.5	2.6	3.5
nausea	1.5	1.5	2.2
vomiting	0	1.1	1.5
Respiratory			
bronchospasm	0	0	0
cough	4.5	2.6	2.5
dyspnea	0.8	1.1	1.5
pharyngitis	2.3	2.2	2.2
rhinitis	3.0	2.9	4.0
sinusitis	1.5	2.2	2.2
URI	3.8	4.8	5.0
Body as a Whole			
asthenia	0	0.4	1.5
chest pain	0.8	1.1	1.5
fatigue	1.5	6.6	8.2
edema (peripheral)	3.8	3.7	3.0

[a] percentage of patients with event

The following is a comprehensive list of adverse experiences reported with bisoprolol fumarate in worldwide studies, or in postmarketing experience (in italics):
Central Nervous System: Dizziness, *unsteadiness*, vertigo, *syncope*, headache, paresthesia, hypoaesthesia, hyperesthesia, somnolence, *sleep disturbances*, anxiety/restlessness, decreased concentration/memory.
Autonomic Nervous System: Dry mouth.
Cardiovascular: Bradycardia, palpitations and other rhythm disturbances, cold extremities, claudication, hypotension, orthostatic hypotension, chest pain, congestive heart failure, dyspnea on exertion.
Psychiatric: Vivid dreams, insomnia, depression.
Gastrointestinal: Gastric/epigastric/abdominal pain, gastritis, dyspepsia, nausea, vomiting, diarrhea, constipation, peptic ulcer.
Musculoskeletal: Muscle/joint pain, *arthralgia*, back/neck pain, muscle cramps, twitching/tremor.
Skin: Rash, acne, eczema, *psoriasis*, skin irritation, pruritus, flushing, sweating, alopecia, *dermatitis*, *angioedema*, *exfoliative dermatitis*, cutaneous vasculitis.
Special Senses: Visual disturbances, ocular pain/pressure, abnormal lacrimation, tinnitus, *decreased hearing*, earache, taste abnormalities.
Metabolic: Gout.
Respiratory: Asthma/bronchospasm, bronchitis, coughing, dyspnea, pharyngitis, rhinitis, sinusitis, URI.
Genitourinary: Decreased libido/impotence, *Peyronie's disease*, cystitis, renal colic, polyuria.
Hematologic: Purpura.
General: Fatigue, asthenia, chest pain, malaise, edema, weight gain, angioedema.

In addition, a variety of adverse effects have been reported with other beta-adrenergic blocking agents and should be considered potential adverse effects of ZEBETA:
Central Nervous System: Reversible mental depression progressing to catatonia, hallucinations, an acute reversible syndrome characterized by disorientation to time and place, emotional lability, slightly clouded sensorium.
Allergic: Fever, combined with aching and sore throat, laryngospasm, respiratory distress.
Hematologic: Agranulocytosis, thrombocytopenia, thrombocytopenic purpura.
Gastrointestinal: Mesenteric arterial thrombosis, ischemic colitis.
Miscellaneous: The oculomucocutaneous syndrome associated with the beta-blocker practolol has not been reported with ZEBETA (bisoprolol fumarate) during investigational use or extensive foreign marketing experience.
LABORATORY ABNORMALITIES: In clinical trials, the most frequently reported laboratory change was an increase in serum triglycerides, but this was not a consistent finding. Sporadic liver test abnormalities have been reported. In the U.S. controlled trials experience with bisoprolol fumarate treatment for 4-12 weeks, the incidence of concomitant el-

Continued on next page

Zebeta—Cont.

evations in SGOT and SGPT from 1 to 2 times normal was 3.9%, compared to 2.5% for placebo. No patient had concomitant elevations greater than twice normal.
In the long-term, uncontrolled experience with bisoprolol fumarate treatment for 6-18 months, the incidence of one or more concomitant elevations in SGOT and SGPT from 1 to 2 times normal was 6.2%. The incidence of multiple occurrences was 1.9%. For concomitant elevations in SGOT and SGPT of greater than twice normal, the incidence was 1.5%. The incidence of multiple occurrences was 0.3%. In many cases these elevations were attributed to underlying disorders, or resolved during continued treatment with bisoprolol fumarate.
Other laboratory changes included small increases in uric acid, creatinine, BUN, serum potassium, glucose, and phosphorus and decreases in WBC and platelets. These were generally not of clinical importance and rarely resulted in discontinuation of bisoprolol fumarate.
As with other beta-blockers, ANA conversions have also been reported on bisoprolol fumarate. About 15% of patients in long-term studies converted to a positive titer, although about one-third of these patients subsequently reconverted to a negative titer while on continued therapy.
The **HOW SUPPLIED** *section, has been revised as follows:*
Store at controlled room temperature 20° to 25°C (68° to 77°F), protected from moisture.
Dispense in tight containers as defined in the USP.
LEDERLE PHARMACEUTICAL DIVISION
of American Cyanamid Company
Pearl River, NY 10965
Under License of E. MERCK
Darmstadt, Germany
CI 5075-4 Revised September 6, 2002

ZIAC® ℞

[*zī'ăk*]
(Bisoprolol Fumarate and Hydrochlorothiazide)
Tablets

℞ only

Prescribing information for this product, which appears on pages 3495–3498 of the 2003 PDR, has been completely revised as follows. Please write "See Supplement A" next to the product heading.

DESCRIPTION

ZIAC (bisoprolol fumarate and hydrochlorothiazide) is indicated for the treatment of hypertension. It combines two antihypertensive agents in a once-daily dosage: a synthetic beta$_1$-selective (cardioselective) adrenoceptor blocking agent (bisoprolol fumarate) and a benzothiadiazine diuretic (hydrochlorothiazide).
Bisoprolol fumarate is chemically described as (±)-1-[4-[[2-(1-methylethoxy)ethoxy]methyl]phenoxy]-3-[(1-methylethyl)amino]-2-propanol(*E*)-2-butenedioate (2:1) (salt). It possesses an asymmetric carbon atom in its structure and is provided as a racemic mixture. The S(-) enantiomer is responsible for most of the beta-blocking activity. Its empirical formula is $(C_{18}H_{31}NO_4)_2 \bullet C_4H_4O_4$ and it has a molecular weight of 766.97. Its structural formula is:

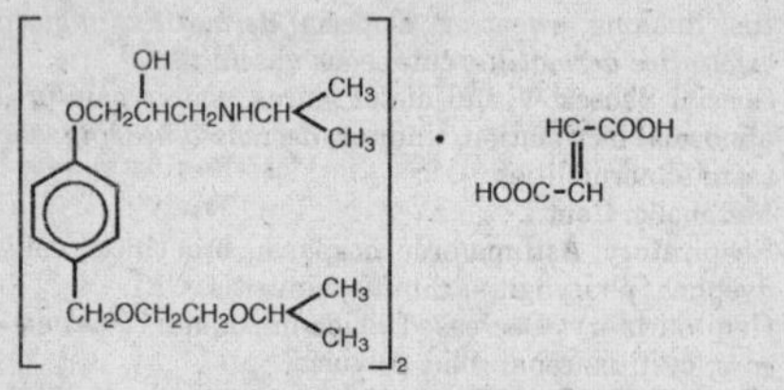

Bisoprolol fumarate is a white crystalline powder, approximately equally hydrophilic and lipophilic, and readily soluble in water, methanol, ethanol, and chloroform.
Hydrochlorothiazide (HCTZ) is 6-Chloro-3,4-dihydro-2*H*-1,2,4-benzothiadiazine-7-sulfonamide 1,1-dioxide. It is a white, or practically white, practically odorless crystalline powder. It is slightly soluble in water, sparingly soluble in dilute sodium hydroxide solution, freely soluble in n-butylamine and dimethylformamide, sparingly soluble in methanol, and insoluble in ether, chloroform, and dilute mineral acids. Its empirical formula is $C_7H_8ClN_3O_4S_2$ and it has a molecular weight of 297.73. Its structural formula is:

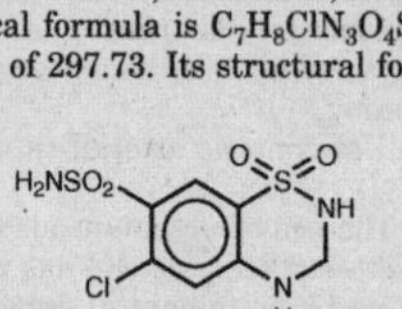

Each ZIAC®-2.5 mg/6.25 mg tablet for oral administration contains:
Bisoprolol fumarate .... 2.5 mg
Hydrochlorothiazide .... 6.25 mg
Each ZIAC®-5 mg/6.25 mg tablet for oral administration contains:
Bisoprolol fumarate .... 5 mg
Hydrochlorothiazide .... 6.25 mg
Each ZIAC®-10 mg/6.25 mg tablet for oral administration contains:
Bisoprolol fumarate .... 10 mg
Hydrochlorothiazide .... 6.25 mg
Inactive ingredients include Colloidal Silicon Dioxide, Corn Starch, Dibasic Calcium Phosphate, Hypromellose, Magnesium Stearate, Microcrystalline Cellulose, Polyethylene Glycol, Polysorbate 80, and Titanium Dioxide. The 5 mg/6.25 mg tablet also contains Red and Yellow Iron Oxide. The 2.5 mg/6.25 mg tablet also contains Crospovidone, Pregelatinized Starch, and Yellow Iron Oxide.

CLINICAL PHARMACOLOGY

Bisoprolol fumarate and HCTZ have been used individually and in combination for the treatment of hypertension. The antihypertensive effects of these agents are additive; HCTZ 6.25 mg significantly increases the antihypertensive effect of bisoprolol fumarate. The incidence of hypokalemia with the bisoprolol fumarate and HCTZ 6.25 mg combination (B/H) is significantly lower than with HCTZ 25 mg. In clinical trials of ZIAC, mean changes in serum potassium for patients treated with ZIAC 2.5/6.25 mg, 5/6.25 mg or 10/6.25 mg or placebo were less than ± 0.1 mEq/L. Mean changes in serum potassium for patients treated with any dose of bisoprolol in combination with HCTZ 25 mg ranged from -0.1 to -0.3 mEq/L.
Bisoprolol fumarate is a beta$_1$-selective (cardioselective) adrenoceptor blocking agent without significant membrane stabilizing or intrinsic sympathomimetic activities in its therapeutic dose range. At higher doses (≥20 mg) bisoprolol fumarate also inhibits beta$_2$-adrenoreceptors located in bronchial and vascular musculature. To retain relative selectivity, it is important to use the lowest effective dose.
Hydrochlorothiazide is a benzothiadiazine diuretic. Thiazides affect renal tubular mechanisms of electrolyte reabsorption and increase excretion of sodium and chloride in approximately equivalent amounts. Natriuresis causes a secondary loss of potassium.

Pharmacokinetics and Metabolism
ZIAC
In healthy volunteers, both bisoprolol fumarate and hydrochlorothiazide are well absorbed following oral administration of ZIAC. No change is observed in the bioavailability of either agent when given together in a single tablet. Absorption is not affected whether ZIAC is taken with or without food. Mean peak bisoprolol fumarate plasma concentrations of about 9.0 ng/mL, 19 ng/mL and 36 ng/mL occur approximately 3 hours after the administration of the 2.5 mg/6.25 mg, 5 mg/6.25 mg and 10 mg/6.25 mg combination tablets, respectively. Mean peak plasma hydrochlorothiazide concentrations of 30 ng/mL occur approximately 2.5 hours following the administration of the combination. Dose proportional increases in plasma bisoprolol concentrations are observed between the 2.5 and 5, as well as between the 5 and 10 mg doses. The elimination $T_{1/2}$ of bisoprolol ranges from 7 to 15 hours, and that of hydrochlorothiazide ranges from 4 to 10 hours. The percent of dose excreted unchanged in urine is about 55% for bisoprolol and about 60% for hydrochlorothiazide.
Bisoprolol Fumarate
The absolute bioavailability after a 10 mg oral dose of bisoprolol fumarate is about 80%. The first pass metabolism of bisoprolol fumarate is about 20%.
The pharmacokinetic profile of bisoprolol fumarate has been examined following single doses and at steady state. Binding to serum proteins is approximately 30%. Peak plasma concentrations occur within 2-4 hours of dosing with 2.5 to 20 mg, and mean peak values range from 9.0 ng/mL at 2.5 mg to 70 ng/mL at 20 mg. Once-daily dosing with bisoprolol fumarate results in less than twofold intersubject variation in peak plasma concentrations. Plasma concentrations are proportional to the administered dose in the range of 2.5 to 20 mg. The plasma elimination half-life is 9-12 hours and is slightly longer in elderly patients, in part because of decreased renal function. Steady state is attained within 5 days with once-daily dosing. In both young and elderly populations, plasma accumulation is low; the accumulation factor ranges from 1.1 to 1.3, and is what would be expected from the half-life and once-daily dosing. Bisoprolol is eliminated equally by renal and nonrenal pathways with about 50% of the dose appearing unchanged in the urine and the remainder in the form of inactive metabolites. In humans, the known metabolites are labile or have no known pharmacologic activity. Less than 2% of the dose is excreted in the feces. The pharmacokinetic characteristics of the two enantiomers are similar. Bisoprolol is not metabolized by cytochrome P450 II D6 (debrisoquin hydroxylase).
In subjects with creatinine clearance less than 40 mL/min, the plasma half-life is increased approximately threefold compared to healthy subjects.
In patients with liver cirrhosis, the rate of elimination of bisoprolol is more variable and significantly slower than that in healthy subjects, with a plasma half-life ranging from 8 to 22 hours.
In elderly subjects, mean plasma concentrations at steady state are increased, in part attributed to lower creatinine clearance. However, no significant differences in the degree of bisoprolol accumulation is found between young and elderly populations.
Hydrochlorothiazide
Hydrochlorothiazide is well absorbed (65%-75%) following oral administration. Absorption of hydrochlorothiazide is reduced in patients with congestive heart failure.
Peak plasma concentrations are observed within 1-5 hours of dosing, and range from 70-490 ng/mL following oral doses of 12.5-100 mg. Plasma concentrations are linearly related to the administered dose. Concentrations of hydrochlorothiazide are 1.6-1.8 times higher in whole blood than in plasma. Binding to serum proteins has been reported to be approximately 40% to 68%. The plasma elimination half-life has been reported to be 6-15 hours. Hydrochlorothiazide is eliminated primarily by renal pathways. Following oral doses of 12.5-100 mg, 55%-77% of the administered dose appears in urine and greater than 95% of the absorbed dose is excreted in urine as unchanged drug.
Plasma concentrations of hydrochlorothiazide are increased and the elimination half-life is prolonged in patients with renal disease.

Pharmacodynamics
Bisoprolol Fumarate
Findings in clinical hemodynamics studies with bisoprolol fumarate are similar to those observed with other beta-blockers. The most prominent effect is the negative chronotropic effect, giving a reduction in resting and exercise heart rate. There is a fall in resting and exercise cardiac output with little observed change in stroke volume, and only a small increase in right atrial pressure, or pulmonary capillary wedge pressure at rest or during exercise.
In normal volunteers, bisoprolol fumarate therapy resulted in a reduction of exercise- and isoproterenol-induced tachycardia. The maximal effect occurred within 1-4 hours post-dosing. Effects generally persisted for 24 hours at doses of 5 mg or greater.
In controlled clinical trials, bisoprolol fumarate given as a single daily dose has been shown to be an effective antihypertensive agent when used alone or concomitantly with thiazide diuretics (see **CLINICAL STUDIES**).
The mechanism of bisoprolol fumarate's antihypertensive effect has not been completely established. Factors that may be involved include:

1) Decreased cardiac output,
2) Inhibition of renin release by the kidneys,
3) Diminution of tonic sympathetic outflow from vasomotor centers in the brain.

Beta$_1$-selectivity of bisoprolol fumarate has been demonstrated in both animal and human studies. No effects at therapeutic doses on beta$_2$-adrenoreceptor density have been observed. Pulmonary function studies have been conducted in healthy volunteers, asthmatics, and patients with chronic obstructive pulmonary disease (COPD). Doses of bisoprolol fumarate ranged from 5 to 60 mg, atenolol from 50 to 200 mg, metoprolol from 100 to 200 mg, and propranolol from 40 to 80 mg. In some studies, slight, asymptomatic increases in airway resistance (AWR) and decreases in forced expiratory volume (FEV_1) were observed with doses of bisoprolol fumarate 20 mg and higher, similar to the small increases in AWR noted with other cardioselective beta-blocking agents. The changes induced by beta-blockade with all agents were reversed by bronchodilator therapy.
Electrophysiology studies in man have demonstrated that bisoprolol fumarate significantly decreases heart rate, increases sinus node recovery time, prolongs AV node refractory periods, and, with rapid atrial stimulation, prolongs AV nodal conduction.
Hydrochlorothiazide
Acute effects of thiazides are thought to result from a reduction in blood volume and cardiac output, secondary to a natriuretic effect, although a direct vasodilatory mechanism has also been proposed. With chronic administration, plasma volume returns toward normal, but peripheral vascular resistance is decreased.
Thiazides do not affect normal blood pressure. Onset of action occurs within 2 hours of dosing, peak effect is observed at about 4 hours, and activity persists for up to 24 hours.

CLINICAL STUDIES

In controlled clinical trials, bisoprolol fumarate/hydrochlorothiazide 6.25 mg has been shown to reduce systolic and diastolic blood pressure throughout a 24-hour period when administered once daily. The effects on systolic and diastolic blood pressure reduction of the combination of bisoprolol fumarate and hydrochlorothiazide were additive. Further, treatment effects were consistent across age groups (<60, ≥60 years), racial groups (black, nonblack), and gender (male, female).
In two randomized, double-blind, placebo-controlled trials conducted in the U.S., reductions in systolic and diastolic blood pressure and heart rate 24 hours after dosing in patients with mild-to-moderate hypertension are shown below. In both studies mean systolic/diastolic blood pressure and heart rate at baseline were approximately 151/101 mm Hg and 77 bpm.
[See table at bottom of next page]
Blood pressure responses were seen within 1 week of treatment but the maximum effect was apparent after 2 to 3 weeks of treatment. Overall, significantly greater blood pressure reductions were observed on ZIAC than on placebo. Further, blood pressure reductions were significantly greater for each of the bisoprolol fumarate plus hydrochlorothiazide combinations than for either of the components used alone regardless of race, age, or gender. There were no significant differences in response between black and nonblack patients.

INDICATIONS AND USAGE

ZIAC (bisoprolol fumarate and hydrochlorothiazide) is indicated in the management of hypertension.

CONTRAINDICATIONS

ZIAC is contraindicated in patients in cardiogenic shock, overt cardiac failure (see **WARNINGS**), second or third degree AV block, marked sinus bradycardia, anuria, and hypersensitivity to either component of this product or to other sulfonamide-derived drugs.

WARNINGS

Cardiac Failure: In general, beta-blocking agents should be avoided in patients with overt congestive failure. However, in some patients with compensated cardiac failure, it may be necessary to utilize these agents. In such situations, they must be used cautiously.

Patients Without a History of Cardiac Failure: Continued depression of the myocardium with beta-blockers can, in some patients, precipitate cardiac failure. At the first signs or symptoms of heart failure, discontinuation of ZIAC should be considered. In some cases ZIAC therapy can be continued while heart failure is treated with other drugs.

Abrupt Cessation of Therapy: Exacerbations of angina pectoris and, in some instances, myocardial infarction or ventricular arrhythmia, have been observed in patients with coronary artery disease following abrupt cessation of therapy with beta-blockers. Such patients should, therefore, be cautioned against interruption or discontinuation of therapy without the physician's advice. Even in patients without overt coronary artery disease, it may be advisable to taper therapy with ZIAC (bisoprolol fumarate and hydrochlorothiazide) over approximately 1 week with the patient under careful observation. If withdrawal symptoms occur, beta-blocking agent therapy should be reinstituted, at least temporarily.

Peripheral Vascular Disease: Beta-blockers can precipitate or aggravate symptoms of arterial insufficiency in patients with peripheral vascular disease. Caution should be exercised in such individuals.

Bronchospastic Disease: PATIENTS WITH BRONCHOSPASTIC PULMONARY DISEASE SHOULD, IN GENERAL, NOT RECEIVE BETA-BLOCKERS. Because of the relative beta$_1$-selectivity of bisoprolol fumarate, ZIAC may be used with caution in patients with bronchospastic disease who do not respond to, or who cannot tolerate other antihypertensive treatment. Since beta$_1$-selectivity is not absolute, the lowest possible dose of ZIAC should be used. A beta$_2$ agonist (bronchodilator) should be made available.

Anesthesia and Major Surgery: If ZIAC treatment is to be continued perioperatively, particular care should be taken when anesthetic agents that depress myocardial function, such as ether, cyclopropane, and trichloroethylene, are used. See **OVERDOSAGE** for information on treatment of bradycardia and hypotension.

Diabetes and Hypoglycemia: Beta-blockers may mask some of the manifestations of hypoglycemia, particularly tachycardia. Nonselective beta-blockers may potentiate insulin-induced hypoglycemia and delay recovery of serum glucose levels. Because of its beta$_1$-selectivity, this is less likely with bisoprolol fumarate. However, patients subject to spontaneous hypoglycemia, or diabetic patients receiving insulin or oral hypoglycemic agents, should be cautioned about these possibilities. Also, latent diabetes mellitus may become manifest and diabetic patients given thiazides may require adjustment of their insulin dose. Because of the very low dose of HCTZ employed, this may be less likely with ZIAC.

Thyrotoxicosis: Beta-adrenergic blockade may mask clinical signs of hyperthyroidism, such as tachycardia. Abrupt withdrawal of beta-blockade may be followed by an exacerbation of the symptoms of hyperthyroidism or may precipitate thyroid storm.

Renal Disease: Cumulative effects of the thiazides may develop in patients with impaired renal function. In such patients, thiazides may precipitate azotemia. In subjects with creatinine clearance less than 40 mL/min, the plasma half-life of bisoprolol fumarate is increased up to threefold, as compared to healthy subjects. If progressive renal impairment becomes apparent, ZIAC should be discontinued. (See **Pharmacokinetics and Metabolism.**)

Hepatic Disease: ZIAC should be used with caution in patients with impaired hepatic function or progressive liver disease. Thiazides may alter fluid and electrolyte balance, which may precipitate hepatic coma. Also, elimination of bisoprolol fumarate is significantly slower in patients with cirrhosis than in healthy subjects. (See **Pharmacokinetics and Metabolism.**)

PRECAUTIONS

General

Electrolyte and Fluid Balance Status: Although the probability of developing hypokalemia is reduced with ZIAC because of the very low dose of HCTZ employed, periodic determination of serum electrolytes should be performed, and patients should be observed for signs of fluid or electrolyte disturbances, ie, hyponatremia, hypochloremic alkalosis, hypokalemia, and hypomagnesemia. Thiazides have been shown to increase the urinary excretion of magnesium; this may result in hypomagnesemia.

Warning signs or symptoms of fluid and electrolyte imbalance include dryness of mouth, thirst, weakness, lethargy, drowsiness, restlessness, muscle pains or cramps, muscular fatigue, hypotension, oliguria, tachycardia, and gastrointestinal disturbances such as nausea and vomiting.

Hypokalemia may develop, especially with brisk diuresis when severe cirrhosis is present, during concomitant use of corticosteroids or adrenocorticotropic hormone (ACTH) or after prolonged therapy. Interference with adequate oral electrolyte intake will also contribute to hypokalemia. Hypokalemia and hypomagnesemia can provoke ventricular arrhythmias or sensitize or exaggerate the response of the heart to the toxic effects of digitalis. Hypokalemia may be avoided or treated by potassium supplementation or increased intake of potassium-rich foods.

Dilutional hyponatremia may occur in edematous patients in hot weather; appropriate therapy is water restriction rather than salt administration, except in rare instances when the hyponatremia is life-threatening. In actual salt depletion, appropriate replacement is the therapy of choice.

Parathyroid Disease: Calcium excretion is decreased by thiazides, and pathologic changes in the parathyroid glands, with hypercalcemia and hypophosphatemia, have been observed in a few patients on prolonged thiazide therapy.

Hyperuricemia: Hyperuricemia or acute gout may be precipitated in certain patients receiving thiazide diuretics. Bisoprolol fumarate, alone or in combination with HCTZ, has been associated with increases in uric acid. However, in U.S. clinical trials, the incidence of treatment-related increases in uric acid was higher during therapy with HCTZ 25 mg (25%) than with B/H 6.25 mg (10%). Because of the very low dose of HCTZ employed, hyperuricemia may be less likely with ZIAC.

Drug Interactions: ZIAC may potentiate the action of other antihypertensive agents used concomitantly. ZIAC should not be combined with other beta-blocking agents. Patients receiving catecholamine-depleting drugs, such as reserpine or guanethidine, should be closely monitored because the added beta-adrenergic blocking action of bisoprolol fumarate may produce excessive reduction of sympathetic activity. In patients receiving concurrent therapy with clonidine, if therapy is to be discontinued, it is suggested that ZIAC be discontinued for several days before the withdrawal of clonidine.

ZIAC should be used with caution when myocardial depressants or inhibitors of AV conduction, such as certain calcium antagonists (particularly of the phenylalkylamine [verapamil] and benzothiazepine [diltiazem] classes), or antiarrhythmic agents, such as disopyramide, are used concurrently.

Bisoprolol Fumarate

Concurrent use of rifampin increases the metabolic clearance of bisoprolol fumarate, shortening its elimination half-life. However, initial dose modification is generally not necessary. Pharmacokinetic studies document no clinically relevant interactions with other agents given concomitantly, including thiazide diuretics, digoxin, and cimetidine. There was no effect of bisoprolol fumarate on prothrombin times in patients on stable doses of warfarin.

Risk of Anaphylactic Reaction: While taking beta-blockers, patients with a history of severe anaphylactic reaction to a variety of allergens may be more reactive to repeated challenge, either accidental, diagnostic, or therapeutic. Such patients may be unresponsive to the usual doses of epinephrine used to treat allergic reactions.

Hydrochlorothiazide

When given concurrently the following drugs may interact with thiazide diuretics.

Alcohol, barbiturates, or narcotics—potentiation of orthostatic hypotension may occur.

Antidiabetic drugs (oral agents and insulin)—dosage adjustment of the antidiabetic drug may be required.

Other antihypertensive drugs—additive effect or potentiation.

Cholestyramine and colestipol resins—Absorption of hydrochlorothiazide is impaired in the presence of anionic exchange resins. Single doses of cholestyramine and colestipol resins bind the hydrochlorothiazide and reduce its absorption in the gastrointestinal tract by up to 85 percent and 43 percent, respectively.

Corticosteroids, ACTH—Intensified electrolyte depletion, particularly hypokalemia.

Pressor amines (eg, norepinephrine)—possible decreased response to pressor amines but not sufficient to preclude their use.

Sitting Systolic/Diastolic Pressure (BP) and Heart Rate (HR)
Mean Decrease (Δ) After 3–4 Weeks

	Study 1		Study 2			
	Placebo	B5/H6.25 mg	Placebo	H6.25 mg	B2.5/ H6.25 mg	B10/ H6.25 mg
n=	75	150	56	23	28	25
Total ΔBP (mm Hg)	-2.9/-3.9	-15.8/-12.6	-3.0/-3.7	-6.6/-5.8	-14.1/-10.5	-15.3/-14.3
Drug Effect[a]	-/-	-12.9/-8.7	-/-	-3.6/-2.1	-11.1/-6.8	-12.3/-10.6
Total ΔHR (bpm)	-0.3	-6.9	-1.6	-0.8	-3.7	-9.8
Drug Effect[a]	-	-6.6	-	+0.8	-2.1	-8.2

[a]Observed mean change from baseline minus placebo.

Skeletal muscle relaxants, nondepolarizing (eg, tubocurarine)—possible increased responsiveness to the muscle relaxant.

Lithium—generally should not be given with diuretics. Diuretic agents reduce the renal clearance of lithium and add a high risk of lithium toxicity. Refer to the package insert for lithium preparations before use of such preparations with ZIAC.

Nonsteroidal anti-inflammatory drugs—In some patients, the administration of a nonsteroidal anti-inflammatory agent can reduce the diuretic, natriuretic, and antihypertensive effects of loop, potassium sparing, and thiazide diuretics. Therefore, when ZIAC and nonsteroidal anti-inflammatory agents are used concomitantly, the patient should be observed closely to determine if the desired effect of the diuretic is obtained.

In patients receiving thiazides, sensitivity reactions may occur with or without a history of allergy or bronchial asthma. Photosensitivity reactions and possible exacerbation or activation of systemic lupus erythematosus have been reported in patients receiving thiazides. The antihypertensive effects of thiazides may be enhanced in the post-sympathectomy patient.

Laboratory Test Interactions: Based on reports involving thiazides, ZIAC (bisoprolol fumarate and hydrochlorothiazide) may decrease serum levels of protein-bound iodine without signs of thyroid disturbance.

Because it includes a thiazide, ZIAC should be discontinued before carrying out tests for parathyroid function (see **PRECAUTIONS—Parathyroid Disease**).

INFORMATION FOR PATIENTS

Patients, especially those with coronary artery disease, should be warned against discontinuing use of ZIAC without a physician's supervision. Patients should also be advised to consult a physician if any difficulty in breathing occurs, or if they develop other signs or symptoms of congestive heart failure or excessive bradycardia.

Patients subject to spontaneous hypoglycemia, or diabetic patients receiving insulin or oral hypoglycemic agents, should be cautioned that beta-blockers may mask some of the manifestations of hypoglycemia, particularly tachycardia, and bisoprolol fumarate should be used with caution.

Patients should know how they react to this medicine before they operate automobiles and machinery or engage in other tasks requiring alertness. Patients should be advised that photosensitivity reactions have been reported with thiazides.

Carcinogenesis, Mutagenesis, Impairment of Fertility

Carcinogenesis

ZIAC: Long-term studies have not been conducted with the bisoprolol fumarate/hydrochlorothiazide combination.

Bisoprolol Fumarate: Long-term studies were conducted with oral bisoprolol fumarate administered in the feed of mice (20 and 24 months) and rats (26 months). No evidence of carcinogenic potential was seen in mice dosed up to 250 mg/kg/day or rats dosed up to 125 mg/kg/day. On a body weight basis, these doses are 625 and 312 times, respectively, the maximum recommended human dose (MRHD) of 20 mg, or 0.4 mg/kg/day, based on 50 kg individuals; on a body surface area basis, these doses are 59 times (mice) and 64 times (rats) the MRHD.

Hydrochlorothiazide: Two-year feeding studies in mice and rats, conducted under the auspices of the National Toxicology Program (NTP), treated mice and rats with doses of hydrochlorothiazide up to 600 and 100 mg/kg/day, respectively. On a body weight basis, these doses are 2400 times (in mice) and 400 times (in rats) the MRHD of hydrochlorothiazide (12.5 mg/day) in ZIAC® (bisoprolol fumarate and hydrochlorothiazide). On a body surface area basis, these doses are 226 times (in mice) and 82 times (in rats) the MRHD. These studies uncovered no evidence of carcinogenic potential of hydrochlorothiazide in rats or female mice, but there was equivocal evidence of hepatocarcinogenicity in male mice.

Mutagenesis

ZIAC: The mutagenic potential of the bisoprolol fumarate/hydrochlorothiazide combination was evaluated in the microbial mutagenicity (Ames) test, the point mutation and chromosomal aberration assays in Chinese hamster V79 cells, and the micronucleus test in mice. There was no evidence of mutagenic potential in these in vitro and in vivo assays.

Bisoprolol Fumarate: The mutagenic potential of bisoprolol fumarate was evaluated in the microbial mutagenicity (Ames) test, the point mutation and chromosome aberration assays in Chinese hamster V79 cells, the unscheduled DNA synthesis test, the micronucleus test in mice, and the cytogenetics assay in rats. There was no evidence of mutagenic potential in these in vitro and in vivo assays.

Hydrochlorothiazide: Hydrochlorothiazide was not genotoxic in in vitro assays using strains TA 98, TA 100, TA 1535, TA 1537 and TA 1538 of *Salmonella typhimurium* (the Ames test); in the Chinese Hamster Ovary (CHO) test for chromosomal aberrations; or in in vivo assays using mouse germinal cell chromosomes, Chinese hamster bone marrow chromosomes, and the *Drosophila* sex-linked recessive lethal trait gene. Positive test results were obtained in the in vitro CHO Sister Chromatid Exchange (clastogenicity) test and in the mouse Lymphoma Cell (mutagenicity) assays, using concentrations of hydrochlorothiazide of 43-1300 µg/mL. Positive test results were also obtained in the *Aspergillus nidulans* nondisjunction assay, using an unspecified concentration of hydrochlorothiazide.

Continued on next page

Ziac—Cont.

Impairment of Fertility

ZIAC: Reproduction studies in rats did not show any impairment of fertility with the bisoprolol fumarate/hydrochlorothiazide combination doses containing up to 30 mg/kg/day of bisoprolol fumarate in combination with 75 mg/kg/day of hydrochlorothiazide. On a body weight basis, these doses are 75 and 300 times, respectively, the MRHD of bisoprolol fumarate and hydrochlorothiazide. On a body surface area basis, these study doses are 15 and 62 times, respectively, MRHD.

Bisoprolol Fumarate: Reproduction studies in rats did not show any impairment of fertility at doses up to 150 mg/kg/day of bisoprolol fumarate, or 375 and 77 times the MRHD on the basis of body weight and body surface area, respectively.

Hydrochlorothiazide: Hydrochlorothiazide had no adverse effects on the fertility of mice and rats of either sex in studies wherein these species were exposed, via their diet, to doses of up to 100 and 4 mg/kg/day, respectively, prior to mating and throughout gestation. Corresponding multiples of maximum recommended human doses are 400 (mice) and 16 (rats) on the basis of body weight and 38 (mice) and 3.3 (rats) on the basis of body surface area.

Pregnancy: Teratogenic Effects—Pregnancy Category C

ZIAC: In rats, the bisoprolol fumarate/hydrochlorothiazide (B/H) combination was not teratogenic at doses up to 51.4 mg/kg/day of bisoprolol fumarate in combination with 128.6 mg/kg/day of hydrochlorothiazide. Bisoprolol fumarate and hydrochlorothiazide doses used in the rat study are, as multiples of the MRHD in the combination, 129 and 514 times greater, respectively, on a body weight basis, and 26 and 106 times greater, respectively, on the basis of body surface area. The drug combination was maternotoxic (decreased body weight and food consumption) at B5.7/H14.3 (mg/kg/day) and higher, and fetotoxic (increased late resorptions) at B17.1/H42.9 (mg/kg/day) and higher. Maternotoxicity was present at 14/57 times the MRHD of B/H, respectively, on a body weight basis, and 3/12 times the MRHD of B/H doses, respectively, on the basis of body surface area. Fetotoxicity was present at 43/172 times the MRHD of B/H, respectively, on a body weight basis, and 9/35 times the MRHD of B/H doses, respectively, on the basis of body surface area. In rabbits, the B/H combination was not teratogenic at doses of B10/H25 (mg/kg/day). Bisoprolol fumarate and hydrochlorothiazide used in the rabbit study were not teratogenic at 25/100 times the B/H MRHD, respectively, on a body weight basis, and 10/40 times the B/H MRHD, respectively, on the basis of body surface area. The drug combination was maternotoxic (decreased body weight) at B1/H2.5 (mg/kg/day) and higher, and fetotoxic (increased resorptions) at B10/H25 (mg/kg/day). The multiples of the MRHD for the B/H combination that were maternotoxic are, respectively, 2.5/10 (on the basis of body weight) and 1/4 (on the basis of body surface area), and for fetotoxicity were, respectively 25/100 (on the basis of body weight) and 10/40 (on the basis of body surface area).

There are no adequate and well-controlled studies with ZIAC in pregnant women. ZIAC (bisoprolol fumarate and hydrochlorothiazide) should be used during pregnancy only if the potential benefit justifies the risk to the fetus.

Bisoprolol Fumarate: In rats, bisoprolol fumarate was not teratogenic at doses up to 150 mg/kg/day, which were 375 and 77 times the MRHD on the basis of body weight and body surface area, respectively. Bisoprolol fumarate was fetotoxic (increased late resorptions) at 50 mg/kg/day and maternotoxic (decreased food intake and body weight gain) at 150 mg/kg/day. The fetotoxicity in rats occurred at 125 times the MRHD on a body weight basis and 26 times the MRHD on the basis of body surface area. The maternotoxicity occurred at 375 times the MRHD on a body weight basis and 77 times the MRHD on the basis of body surface area. In rabbits, bisoprolol fumarate was not teratogenic at doses up to 12.5 mg/kg/day, which is 31 and 12 times the MRHD based on body weight and body surface area, respectively, but was embryolethal (increased early resorptions) at 12.5 mg/kg/day.

Hydrochlorothiazide: Hydrochlorothiazide was orally administered to pregnant mice and rats during respective periods of major organogenesis at doses up to 3000 and 1000 mg/kg/day, respectively. At these doses, which are multiples of the MRHD equal to 12,000 for mice and 4000 for rats, based on body weight, and equal to 1129 for mice and 824 for rats, based on body surface area, there was no evidence of harm to the fetus. There are, however, no adequate and well-controlled studies in pregnant women. Because animal reproduction studies are not always predictive of human response, this drug should be used during pregnancy only if clearly needed.

Nonteratogenic Effects: Thiazides cross the placental barrier and appear in the cord blood. The use of thiazides in pregnant women requires that the anticipated benefit be weighed against possible hazards to the fetus. These hazards include fetal or neonatal jaundice, pancreatitis, thrombocytopenia, and possibly other adverse reactions which have occurred in the adult.

Nursing Mothers: Bisoprolol fumarate alone or in combination with HCTZ has not been studied in nursing mothers. Thiazides are excreted in human breast milk. Small amounts of bisoprolol fumarate (<2% of the dose) have been detected in the milk of lactating rats. Because of the potential for serious adverse reactions in nursing infants, a decision should be made whether to discontinue nursing or to discontinue the drug, taking into account the importance of the drug to the mother.

Pediatric Use: Safety and effectiveness of ZIAC in pediatric patients have not been established.

Geriatric Use: In clinical trials, at least 270 patients treated with bisoprolol fumarate plus HCTZ were 60 years of age or older. HCTZ added significantly to the antihypertensive effect of bisoprolol in elderly hypertensive patients. No overall differences in effectiveness or safety were observed between these patients and younger patients. Other reported clinical experience has not identified differences in responses between the elderly and younger patients, but greater sensitivity of some older individuals cannot be ruled out.

ADVERSE REACTIONS

ZIAC

Bisoprolol fumarate/H6.25 mg is well tolerated in most patients. Most adverse effects (AEs) have been mild and transient. In more than 65,000 patients treated worldwide with bisoprolol fumarate, occurrences of bronchospasm have been rare. Discontinuation rates for AEs were similar for B/H6.25 mg and placebo-treated patients.

In the United States, 252 patients received bisoprolol fumarate (2.5, 5, 10, or 40 mg)/H6.25 mg and 144 patients received placebo in two controlled trials. In Study 1, bisoprolol fumarate 5/H6.25 mg was administered for 4 weeks. In Study 2, bisoprolol fumarate 2.5, 10, or 40/H6.25 mg was administered for 12 weeks. All adverse experiences, whether drug related or not, and drug related adverse experiences in patients treated with B2.5-10/H6.25 mg, reported during comparable, 4 week treatment periods by at least 2% of bisoprolol fumarate/H6.25 mg-treated patients (plus additional selected adverse experiences) are presented in the following table:

[See table below]

% of Patients with Adverse Experiences*

Body System/ Adverse Experience	All Adverse Experiences		Drug Related Adverse Experiences	
	Placebo† (n=144) %	B2.5-4.0/H6.25† (n=252) %	Placebo† (n=144) %	B2.5-10/H6.25† (n=221) %
Cardiovascular				
bradycardia	0.7	1.1	0.7	0.9
arrhythmia	1.4	0.4	0.0	0.0
peripheral ischemia	0.9	0.7	0.9	0.4
chest pain	0.7	1.8	0.7	0.9
Respiratory				
bronchospasm	0.0	0.0	0.0	0.0
cough	1.0	2.2	0.7	1.5
rhinitis	2.0	0.7	0.7	0.9
URI	2.3	2.1	0.0	0.0
Body as a Whole				
asthenia	0.0	0.0	0.0	0.0
fatigue	2.7	4.6	1.7	3.0
peripheral edema	0.7	1.1	0.7	0.9
Central Nervous System				
dizziness	1.8	5.1	1.8	3.2
headache	4.7	4.5	2.7	0.4
Musculoskeletal				
muscle cramps	0.7	1.2	0.7	1.1
myalgia	1.4	2.4	0.0	0.0
Psychiatric				
insomnia	2.4	1.1	2.0	1.2
somnolence	0.7	1.1	0.7	0.9
loss of libido	1.2	0.4	1.2	0.4
impotence	0.7	1.1	0.7	1.1
Gastrointestinal				
diarrhea	1.4	4.3	1.2	1.1
nausea	0.9	1.1	0.9	0.9
dyspepsia	0.7	1.2	0.7	0.9

*Averages adjusted to combine across studies

†Combined across studies.

Other adverse experiences that have been reported with the individual components are listed below.

Bisoprolol Fumarate

In clinical trials worldwide, or in postmarketing experience, a variety of other AEs, in addition to those listed above, have been reported. While in many cases it is not known whether a causal relationship exists between bisoprolol and these AEs, they are listed to alert the physician to a possible relationship.

Central Nervous System: Unsteadiness, dizziness, vertigo, headache, syncope, paresthesia, hypoesthesia, hyperesthesia, sleep disturbance/vivid dreams, insomnia, somnolence, depression, anxiety/restlessness, decreased concentration/memory.

Cardiovascular: Bradycardia, palpitations and other rhythm disturbances, cold extremities, claudication, hypotension, orthostatic hypotension, chest pain, congestive heart failure, dyspnea on exertion.

Gastrointestinal: Gastric/epigastric/abdominal pain, peptic ulcer, gastritis, dyspepsia, nausea, vomiting, diarrhea, constipation, dry mouth.

Musculoskeletal: Arthralgia, muscle/joint pain, back/neck pain, muscle cramps, twitching/tremor.

Skin: Rash, acne, eczema, psoriasis, skin irritation, pruritus, purpura, flushing, sweating, alopecia, dermatitis, exfoliative dermatitis (very rarely), cutaneous vaculitis.

Special Senses: Visual disturbances, ocular pain/pressure, abnormal lacrimation, tinnitus, decreased hearing, earache, taste abnormalities.

Metabolic: Gout.

Respiratory: Asthma, bronchospasm, bronchitis, dyspnea, pharyngitis, rhinitis, sinusitis, URI (upper respiratory infection).

Genito-urinary: Decreased libido/impotence, Peyronie's disease (very rarely), cystitis, renal colic, polyuria.

General: Fatigue, asthenia, chest pain, malaise, edema, weight gain, angioedema.

In addition, a variety of adverse effects have been reported with other betaadrenergic blocking agents and should be considered potential adverse effects:

Central Nervous System: Reversible mental depression progressing to catatonia, hallucinations, an acute reversible syndrome characterized by disorientation to time and place, emotional lability, slightly clouded sensorium.

Allergic: Fever, combined with aching and sore throat, laryngospasm, and respiratory distress.

Hematologic: Agranulocytosis, thrombocytopenia.

Gastrointestinal: Mesenteric arterial thrombosis and ischemic colitis.

Miscellaneous: The oculomucocutaneous syndrome associated with the beta-blocker practolol has not been reported with bisoprolol fumarate during investigational use or extensive foreign marketing experience.

Hydrochlorothiazide

The following adverse experiences, in addition to those listed in the above table, have been reported with hydrochlorothiazide (generally with doses of 25 mg or greater).

General: Weakness.

Central Nervous System: Vertigo, paresthesia, restlessness.

Cardiovascular: Orthostatic hypotension (may be potentiated by alcohol, barbiturates, or narcotics).

Gastrointestinal: Anorexia, gastric irritation, cramping, constipation, jaundice (intrahepatic cholestatic jaundice), pancreatitis, cholecystitis, sialadenitis, dry mouth.

Musculoskeletal: Muscle spasm.

Hypersensitive Reactions: Purpura, photosensitivity, rash, urticaria, necrotizing angiitis (vasculitis and cutaneous vasculitis), fever, respiratory distress including pneumonitis and pulmonary edema, anaphylactic reactions.

Special Senses: Transient blurred vision, xanthopsia.

Metabolic: Gout.

Genito-urinary: Sexual dysfunction, renal failure, renal dysfunction, interstitial nephritis.

LABORATORY ABNORMALITIES:

ZIAC

Because of the low dose of hydrochlorothiazide in ZIAC (bisoprolol fumarate and hydrochlorothiazide), adverse metabolic effects with B/H6.25 mg are less frequent and of smaller magnitude than with HCTZ 25 mg. Laboratory data on serum potassium from the U.S. placebo-controlled trials are shown in the following table:

[See table at top of next page]

Treatment with both beta blockers and thiazide diuretics is associated with increases in uric acid. However, the magnitude of the change in patients treated with B/H 6.25 mg was smaller than in patients treated with HCTZ 25 mg. Mean increases in serum triglycerides were observed in patients treated with bisoprolol fumarate and hydrochlorothiazide 6.25 mg. Total cholesterol was generally unaffected, but small decreases in HDL cholesterol were noted.

Other laboratory abnormalities that have been reported with the individual components are listed below.

Bisoprolol Fumarate: In clinical trials, the most frequently reported laboratory change was an increase in serum triglycerides, but this was not a consistent finding. Sporadic liver test abnormalities have been reported. In the U.S. controlled trials experience with bisoprolol fumarate treatment

Serum Potassium Data from U.S. Placebo Controlled Studies

	Placebo† (n=130*)	B2.5/ H6.25 mg (n=28*)	B5/ H6.25 mg (n=149*)	B10/ H6.25 mg (n=28*)	HCTZ25 mg† (n=142*)
Potassium					
Mean Change[a] (mEq/L)	+0.04	+0.11	-0.08	0.00	-0.30%
Hypokalemia[b]	0.0%	0.0%	0.7%	0.0%	5.5%

*Patients with normal serum potassium at baseline.
[a]Mean change from baseline at Week 4.
[b]Percentage of patients with abnomality at Week 4.
†Combined across studies.

for 4-12 weeks, the incidence of concomitant elevations in SGOT and SGPT from 1 to 2 times normal was 3.9%, compared to 2.5% for placebo. No patient had concomitant elevations greater than twice normal.
In the long-term, uncontrolled experience with bisoprolol fumarate treatment for 6-18 months, the incidence of one or more concomitant elevations in SGOT and SGPT from 1 to 2 times normal was 6.2%. The incidence of multiple occurrence was 1.9%. For concomitant elevations in SGOT and SGPT of greater than twice normal, the incidence was 1.5%. The incidence of multiple occurrences was 0.3%. In many cases these elevations were attributed to underlying disorders, or resolved during continued treatment with bisoprolol fumarate.
Other laboratory changes included small increases in uric acid, creatinine, BUN, serum potassium, glucose, and phosphorus and decreases in WBC and platelets. There have been occasional reports of eosinophilia. These were generally not of clinical importance and rarely resulted in discontinuation of bisoprolol fumarate.
As with other beta-blockers, ANA conversions have also been reported on bisoprolol fumarate. About 15% of patients in long-term studies converted to a positive titer, although about one-third of these patients subsequently reconverted to a negative titer while on continued therapy.
Hydrochlorothiazide: Hyperglycemia, glycosuria, hyperuricemia, hypokalemia and other electrolyte imbalances (see **PRECAUTIONS**), hyperlipidemia, hypercalcemia, leukopenia, agranulocytosis, thrombocytopenia, aplastic anemia, and hemolytic anemia have been associated with HCTZ therapy.

OVERDOSAGE

There are limited data on overdose with ZIAC. However, several cases of overdose with bisoprolol fumarate have been reported (maximum: 2000 mg). Bradycardia and/or hypotension were noted. Sympathomimetic agents were given in some cases, and all patients recovered.
The most frequently observed signs expected with overdosage of a beta-blocker are bradycardia and hypotension. Lethargy is also common, and with severe overdoses, delirium, coma, convulsions, and respiratory arrest have been reported to occur. Congestive heart failure, bronchospasm, and hypoglycemia may occur, particularly in patients with underlying conditions. With thiazide diuretics, acute intoxication is rare. The most prominent feature of overdose is acute loss of fluid and electrolytes. Signs and symptoms include cardiovascular (tachycardia, hypotension, shock), neuromuscular (weakness, confusion, dizziness, cramps of the calf muscles, paresthesia, fatigue, impairment of consciousness), gastrointestinal (nausea, vomiting, thirst), renal (polyuria, oliguria, or anuria [due to hemoconcentration]), and laboratory findings (hypokalemia, hyponatremia, hypochloremia, alkalosis, increased BUN [especially in patients with renal insufficiency]).
If overdosage of ZIAC (bisoprolol fumarate and hydrochlorothiazide) is suspected, therapy with ZIAC should be discontinued and the patient observed closely. Treatment is symptomatic and supportive; there is no specific antidote. Limited data suggest bisoprolol fumarate is not dialyzable; similarly, there is no indication that hydrochlorothiazide is dialyzable. Suggested general measures include induction of emesis and/or gastric lavage, administration of activated charcoal, respiratory support, correction of fluid and electrolyte imbalance, and treatment of convulsions. Based on the expected pharmacologic actions and recommendations for other betablockers and hydrochlorothiazide, the following measures should be considered when clinically warranted:
Bradycardia: Administer IV atropine. If the response is inadequate, isoproterenol or another agent with positive chronotropic properties may be given cautiously. Under some circumstances, transvenous pacemaker insertion may be necessary.
Hypotension, Shock: The patient's legs should be elevated. IV fluids should be administered and lost electrolytes (potassium, sodium) replaced. Intravenous glucagon may be useful. Vasopressors should be considered.
Heart Block (second or third degree): Patients should be carefully monitored and treated with isoproterenol infusion or transvenous cardiac pacemaker insertion, as appropriate.
Congestive Heart Failure: Initiate conventional therapy (ie, digitalis, diuretics, vasodilating agents, inotropic agents).
Bronchospasm: Administer a bronchodilator such as isoproterenol and/or aminophylline.
Hypoglycemia: Administer IV glucose.
Surveillance: Fluid and electrolyte balance (especially serum potassium) and renal function should be monitored until normalized.

DOSAGE AND ADMINISTRATION

Bisoprolol is an effective treatment of hypertension in once-daily doses of 2.5 to 40 mg, while hydrochlorothiazide is effective in doses of 12.5 to 50 mg. In clinical trials of bisoprolol/hydrochlorothiazide combination therapy using bisoprolol doses of 2.5 to 20 mg and hydrochlorothiazide doses of 6.25 to 25 mg, the antihypertensive effects increased with increasing doses of either component.
The adverse effects (see **WARNINGS**) of bisoprolol are a mixture of dose-dependent phenomena (primarily bradycardia, diarrhea, asthenia, and fatigue) and dose-independent phenomena (eg, occasional rash); those of hydrochlorothiazide are a mixture of dose-dependent phenomena (primarily hypokalemia) and dose-independent phenomena (eg, possibly pancreatitis); the dose-dependent phenomena for each being much more common than the dose-independent phenomena. The latter consist of those few that are truly idiosyncratic in nature or those that occur with such low frequency that a dose relationship may be difficult to discern. Therapy with a combination of bisoprolol and hydrochlorothiazide will be associated with both sets of dose-independent adverse effects, and to minimize these, it may be appropriate to begin combination therapy only after a patient has failed to achieve the desired effect with monotherapy. On the other hand, regimens that combine low doses of bisoprolol and hydrochlorothiazide should produce minimal dose-dependent adverse effects, eg, bradycardia, diarrhea, asthenia and fatigue, and minimal dose-dependent adverse metabolic effects, ie, decreases in serum potassium (see **CLINICAL PHARMACOLOGY**).
Therapy Guided by Clinical Effect: A patient whose blood pressure is not adequately controlled with 2.5-20 mg bisoprolol daily may instead be given ZIAC. Patients whose blood pressures are adequately controlled with 50 mg of hydrochlorothiazide daily, but who experience significant potassium loss with this regimen, may achieve similar blood pressure control without electrolyte disturbance if they are switched to ZIAC.
Initial Therapy: Antihypertensive therapy may be initiated with the lowest dose of ZIAC, one 2.5/6.25 mg tablet once daily. Subsequent titration (14 day intervals) may be carried out with ZIAC tablets up to the maximum recommended dose 20/12.5 mg (two 10/6.25 mg tablets) once daily, as appropriate.
Replacement Therapy: The combination may be substituted for the titrated individual components.
Cessation of Therapy: If withdrawal of ZIAC therapy is planned, it should be achieved gradually over a period of about 2 weeks. Patients should be carefully observed. Patients with Renal or Hepatic Impairment: As noted in the **WARNINGS** section, caution must be used in dosing/titrating patients with hepatic impairment or renal dysfunction. Since there is no indication that hydrochlorothiazide is dialyzable, and limited data suggest that bisoprolol is not dialyzable, drug replacement is not necessary in patients undergoing dialysis.
Geriatric Patients: Dosage adjustment on the basis of age is not usually necessary, unless there is also significant renal or hepatic dysfunction (see above and **WARNINGS** section).
Pediatric Patients: There is no pediatric experience with ZIAC.

HOW SUPPLIED

ZIAC®-2.5 mg/6.25 mg Tablets (bisoprolol fumarate 2.5 mg and hydrochlorothiazide 6.25 mg) are yellow, round, convex, film coated tablets, engraved with a script "LL" within an engraved heart shape on one side and "B" above "12" on the other; approximately 1/4″ in diameter, supplied as follows:
NDC 0005-3238-23—Bottle of 100
ZIAC®-5 mg/6.25 mg Tablets (bisoprolol fumarate 5 mg and hydrochlorothiazide 6.25 mg) are pink, round, convex, film coated tablets, engraved with a script "LL" within an engraved heart shape on one side and "B" above "13" on the other; approximately 9/32″ in diameter, supplied as follows:
NDC 0005-3234-23—Bottle of 100
ZIAC®-10 mg/6.25 mg Tablets (bisoprolol fumarate 10 mg and hydrochlorothiazide 6.25 mg) are white, round, convex, film coated tablets, engraved with a script "LL" within an engraved heart shape on one side and "B" above "14" on the other; approximately 9/32″ in diameter, supplied as follows:
NDC 0005-3235-38—Bottle of 30 with child resistant closure
Store at controlled room temperature 20° to 25°C (68° to 77°F).
Dispense in tight containers as defined in the USP.
LEDERLE PHARMACEUTICAL DIVISION
of American Cyanamid Company
Pearl River, NY 10965
Under License of Merck KGaA
Darmstadt, Germany
CI 6017-4 Revised September 6, 2002

ZOSYN® ℞

[zō-sĭn]
(Piperacillin and Tazobactam for Injection)
℞ Only

Prescribing information for this product, which appears on pages 3498–3502 of the 2003 PDR, has been completely revised as follows. Please write "See Supplement A" next to the product heading.

DESCRIPTION

Zosyn (piperacillin and tazobactam for injection) is an injectable antibacterial combination product consisting of the semisynthetic antibiotic piperacillin sodium and the β-lactamase inhibitor tazobactam sodium for intravenous administration.
Piperacillin sodium is derived from D(-)-α-aminobenzylpenicillin. The chemical name of piperacillin sodium is sodium (2*S*,5*R*,6*R*)-6-[(*R*)-2-(4-ethyl-2,3-dioxo-1-piperazinecarboxamido)-2-phenylacetamido]-3,3-dimethyl-7-oxo-4-thia-1-azabicyclo[3.2.0]heptane-2-carboxylate. The chemical formula is $C_{23}H_{26}N_5NaO_7S$ and the molecular weight is 539.6. The chemical structure of piperacillin sodium is:

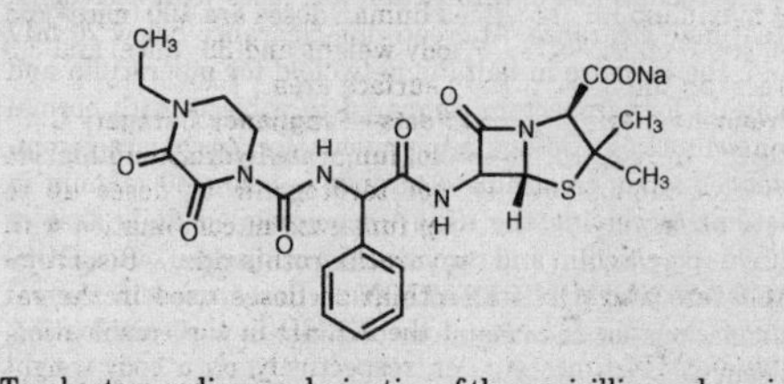

Tazobactam sodium, a derivative of the penicillin nucleus, is a penicillanic acid sulfone. Its chemical name is sodium (2*S*,3*S*,5*R*)-3-methyl-7-oxo-3-(1*H*-1,2,3-triazol-1-ylmethyl)-4-thia-1-azabicyclo[3.2.0]heptane-2-carboxylate-4,4-dioxide. The chemical formula is $C_{10}H_{11}N_4NaO_5S$ and the molecular weight is 322.3. The chemical structure of tazobactam sodium is:

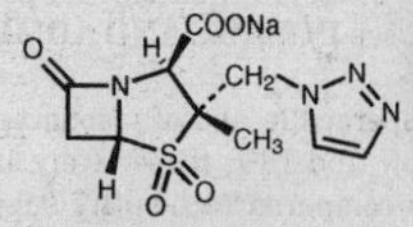

Zosyn, piperacillin/tazobactam parenteral combination, is a white to off-white sterile, cryodesiccated powder consisting of piperacillin and tazobactam as their sodium salts packaged in glass vials. The product does not contain excipients or preservatives.
Each Zosyn 2.25 g single dose vial or ADD-Vantage® vial contains an amount of drug sufficient for withdrawal of piperacillin sodium equivalent to 2 grams of piperacillin and tazobactam sodium equivalent to 0.25 g of tazobactam. Each Zosyn 3.375 g single dose vial or ADD-Vantage® vial contains an amount of drug sufficient for withdrawal of piperacillin sodium equivalent to 3 grams of piperacillin and tazobactam sodium equivalent to 0.375 g of tazobactam. Each Zosyn 4.5 g single dose vial or ADD-Vantage® vial contains an amount of drug sufficient for withdrawal of piperacillin sodium equivalent to 4 grams of piperacillin and tazobactam sodium equivalent to 0.5 g of tazobactam. Zosyn is a monosodium salt of piperacillin and a monosodium salt of tazobactam containing a total of 2.35 mEq (54 mg) of Na^+ per gram of piperacillin in the combination product.

CLINICAL PHARMACOLOGY

Peak plasma concentrations of piperacillin and tazobactam are attained immediately after completion of an intravenous infusion of Zosyn. Piperacillin plasma concentrations, following a 30-minute infusion of Zosyn, were similar to those attained when equivalent doses of piperacillin were administered alone, with mean peak plasma concentrations of approximately 134, 242 and 298 μg/mL for the 2.25 g, 3.375 g and 4.5 g Zosyn (piperacillin/tazobactam) doses, respectively. The corresponding mean peak plasma concentrations of tazobactam were 15, 24 and 34 μg/mL, respectively. Following a 30-minute I.V. infusion of 3.375 g Zosyn every 6 hours, steady-state plasma concentrations of piperacillin and tazobactam were similar to those attained after the first dose. In like manner, steady-state plasma concentrations were not different from those attained after the first dose when 2.25 g or 4.5 g doses of Zosyn (piperacillin and tazobactam for injection) were administered via 30-minute infusions every 6 hours. Steady-state plasma concentrations after 30-minute infusions every 6 hours are provided in Table 1.
Following single or multiple Zosyn doses to healthy subjects, the plasma half-life of piperacillin and of tazobactam ranged from 0.7 to 1.2 hours and was unaffected by dose or duration of infusion.
Piperacillin is metabolized to a minor microbiologically active desethyl metabolite. Tazobactam is metabolized to a single metabolite that lacks pharmacological and antibacterial activities. Both piperacillin and tazobactam are eliminated via the kidney by glomerular filtration and tubular secretion. Piperacillin is excreted rapidly as unchanged drug with 68% of the administered dose excreted in the urine. Tazobactam and its metabolite are eliminated primarily by renal excretion with 80% of the administered dose

Continued on next page

Zosyn—Cont.

excreted as unchanged drug and the remainder as the single metabolite. Piperacillin, tazobactam and desethyl piperacillin are also secreted into the bile.

Both piperacillin and tazobactam are approximately 30% bound to plasma proteins. The protein binding of either piperacillin or tazobactam is unaffected by the presence of the other compound. Protein binding of the tazobactam metabolite is negligible.

Piperacillin and tazobactam are widely distributed into tissues and body fluids including intestinal mucosa, gallbladder, lung, female reproductive tissues (uterus, ovary, and fallopian tube), interstitial fluid, and bile. Mean tissue concentrations are generally 50% to 100% of those in plasma. Distribution of piperacillin and tazobactam into cerebrospinal fluid is low in subjects with non-inflamed meninges, as with other penicillins.

After the administration of single doses of piperacillin/tazobactam to subjects with renal impairment, the half-life of piperacillin and of tazobactam increases with decreasing creatinine clearance. At creatinine clearance below 20 mL/min, the increase in half-life is twofold for piperacillin and fourfold for tazobactam compared to subjects with normal renal function. Dosage adjustments for Zosyn are recommended when creatinine clearance is below 40 mL/min in patients receiving the usual recommended daily dose of Zosyn (piperacillin and tazobactam for injection). (See **DOSAGE AND ADMINISTRATION** section for specific recommendations for the treatment of patients with renal insufficiency.)

Hemodialysis removes 30% to 40% of a piperacillin/tazobactam dose with an additional 5% of the tazobactam dose removed as the tazobactam metabolite. Peritoneal dialysis removes approximately 6% and 21% of the piperacillin and tazobactam doses, respectively, with up to 16% of the tazobactam dose removed as the tazobactam metabolite. For dosage recommendations for patients undergoing hemodialysis, see **DOSAGE AND ADMINISTRATION** section.

The half-life of piperacillin and of tazobactam increases by approximately 25% and 18%, respectively, in patients with hepatic cirrhosis compared to healthy subjects. However, this difference does not warrant dosage adjustment of Zosyn due to hepatic cirrhosis.
[See table 1 below]

Microbiology

Piperacillin sodium exerts bactericidal activity by inhibiting septum formation and cell wall synthesis. In vitro, piperacillin is active against a variety of gram-positive and gram-negative aerobic and anaerobic bacteria. Tazobactam sodium has very little intrinsic microbiologic activity due to its very low level of binding to penicillin-binding proteins; however, it is a β-lactamase inhibitor of the Richmond-Sykes class III (Bush class 2b & 2b′) penicillinases and cephalosporinases. It varies in its ability to inhibit class II and IV (2a & 4) penicillinases. Tazobactam does not induce chromosomally-mediated β-lactamases at tazobactam levels achieved with the recommended dosage regimen. Piperacillin/tazobactam has been shown to be active against most strains of the following piperacillin-resistant, β-lactamase producing microorganisms both in vitro and in clinical infections as described in the **INDICATIONS AND USAGE** section.

Gram-positive aerobes:
Staphylococcus aureus (NOT methicillin/oxacillin-resistant strains)
Gram-negative aerobes:
Escherichia coli
Haemophilus influenzae (NOT β-lactamase negative, ampicillin-resistant strains)
Gram-negative anaerobes:
Bacteroides fragilis group (*B. fragilis*, *B. ovatus*, *B. thetaiotaomicron*, or *B. vulgatus*)

The following in vitro data are available; **but their clinical significance is unknown.**

Piperacillin/tazobactam exhibits in vitro minimum inhibitory concentrations (MICs) of 16.0 μg/mL or less against most (≥90%) strains of *Enterobacteriaceae*, MICs of 1.0 μg/mL or less against most (≥90%) strains of *Haemophilus* species, MICs of 8.0 μg/mL or less against most (≥90%) strains of *Staphylococcus* species, and MICs of 16.0 μg/mL or less against most (≥90%) strains of *Bacteroides* species. Beta-lactamase negative strains should be tested against piperacillin alone; piperacillin break points should be used in evaluation of these results. However, the safety and efficacy of piperacillin/tazobactam in treating clinical infections due to these microorganisms have not been established in adequate and well-controlled clinical trials.

Gram-positive aerobes:
Enterococcus faecalis (piperacillin-susceptible)
Staphylococcus epidermidis (NOT methicillin/oxacillin-resistant strains)
Streptococcus agalactiae[†]
Streptococcus pneumoniae[†]
Streptococcus pyogenes[†]
Viridans group streptococci[†]
Gram-negative aerobes:
Klebsiella oxytoca
Klebsiella pneumoniae
Moraxella catarrhalis
Morganella morganii
Neisseria gonorrhoeae
Neisseria meningitidis[†]
Proteus mirabilis
Proteus vulgaris
Pseudomonas aeruginosa (piperacillin-susceptible)
Serratia marcescens
Gram-positive anaerobes:
Clostridium perfringens
Gram-negative anaerobes:
Bacteroides distasonis
Fusobacterium nucleatum
Prevotella melaninogenica (formerly *Bacteroides melaninogenicus*)

[†]These are not β-lactamase producing strains and, therefore, are susceptible to piperacillin alone.

Susceptibility Tests

Dilution Techniques

Quantitative methods are used to determine minimum inhibitory concentrations (MICs). These MICs provide estimates of the susceptibility of bacteria to antimicrobial compounds. The MICs should be determined using a standardized procedure. Standardized procedures are based on a dilution method (broth or agar) or equivalent with standardized inoculum concentrations and standardized concentrations of piperacillin and tazobactam powders.[1] MIC values should be determined using serial dilutions of piperacillin combined with a fixed concentration of 4 μg/mL tazobactam. The MIC values obtained should be interpreted according to the following criteria:

For *Enterobacteriaceae*:
MIC (μg/mL)	Interpretation
≤16	Susceptible (S)
32-64	Intermediate (I)
≥128	Resistant (R)

For *Haemophilus* species:
MIC (μg/mL)	Interpretation
≤1	Susceptible (S)
≥2	Resistant (R)

For *Staphylococcus* species:
MIC (μg/mL)	Interpretation
≤8	Susceptible (S)
≥16	Resistant (R)

A report of "Susceptible" indicates that the pathogen is likely to be inhibited if the antimicrobial compound in the blood reaches the concentrations usually achievable. A report of "Intermediate" indicates that the result should be considered equivocal, and, if the microorganism is not fully susceptible to alternative, clinically feasible drugs, the test should be repeated. This category implies possible clinical applicability in body sites where the drug is physiologically concentrated or in situations where high dosage of drug can be used. This category also provides a buffer zone which prevents small uncontrolled technical factors from causing major discrepancies in interpretation. A report of "Resistant" indicates that the pathogen is not likely to be inhibited if the antimicrobial compound in the blood reaches the concentrations usually achievable; other therapy should be selected.

Standardized susceptibility test procedures require the use of laboratory control microorganisms to control the technical aspects of the laboratory procedures.

Laboratory control microorganisms are specific strains of microbiological assay organisms with intrinsic biological properties relating to resistance mechanisms and their genetic expression within bacteria; the specific strains are not clinically significant in their current microbiological status. Standard piperacillin and tazobactam powders should provide the following MIC values when tested against the designated quality control strains:

Microorganism	MIC (μg/mL)
Escherichia coli ATCC 25922	1 - 4
Escherichia coli ATCC 35218	0.5 - 2
Haemophilus influenzae ATCC 49247	0.06 - 0.5
Staphylococcus aureus ATCC 29213	0.25 - 2

Anaerobic Techniques

For anaerobic bacteria, the susceptibility to piperacillin/tazobactam can be determined by the reference agar dilution method or by alternate standardized test methods.[2] For *Bacteroides* species, the dilution values should be interpreted as follows:

MIC (μg/mL)	Interpretation
≤16	Susceptible (S)
≥32	Resistant (R)

Serial dilutions of piperacillin combined with a fixed concentration of 4 μg/mL tazobactam should provide the following MIC values:

Microorganism	MIC (μg/mL)
Bacteroides fragilis ATCC 25285	0.12 - 0.5
Bacteroides thetaiotaomicron ATCC 29741	4 - 16

Diffusion Techniques

Quantitative methods that require measurement of zone diameters also provide reproducible estimates of the susceptibility of bacteria to antimicrobial compounds. One such standardized procedure requires the use of standardized inoculum concentrations.[3] This procedure uses paper disks impregnated with 100 μg of piperacillin and 10 μg of tazobactam to test the susceptibility of microorganisms to piperacillin/tazobactam. Interpretation is identical to that stated above for results using dilution techniques.

Reports from the laboratory providing results of the standard single-disk susceptibility test with a 100/10-μg piperacillin/tazobactam disk should be interpreted according to the following criteria:

For *Enterobacteriaceae*:
Zone Diameter (mm)	Interpretation
≥21	Susceptible (S)
18 - 20	Intermediate (I)
≤17	Resistant (R)

For *Staphylococcus* species:
Zone Diameter (mm)	Interpretation
≥20	Susceptible (S)
≤19	Resistant (R)

As with standardized dilution techniques, diffusion methods require the use of laboratory control microorganisms to control the technical aspects of the laboratory procedures. Laboratory control microorganisms are specific strains of microbiological assay organisms with intrinsic biological properties relating to resistance mechanisms and their genetic expression within bacteria; the specific strains are not clinically significant in their current microbiological status. For the diffusion technique, the 100/10-μg piperacillin/tazobactam disk should provide the following zone diameters in these laboratory test quality control strains:

Microorganism	Zone Diameter (mm)
Escherichia coli ATCC 25922	24 - 30
Escherichia coli ATCC 35218	24 - 30
Staphylococcus aureus ATCC 25923	27 - 36

TABLE 1
STEADY-STATE MEAN PLASMA CONCENTRATIONS IN ADULTS AFTER 30-MINUTE INTRAVENOUS INFUSION OF PIPERACILLIN/TAZOBACTAM EVERY 6 HOURS

PIPERACILLIN

| Piperacillin/Tazobactam Dose[a] | No. of Evaluable Subjects | Plasma Concentrations** (μg/mL) | | | | | | AUC** (μg·hr/mL) |
		30 min	1 hr	2 hr	3 hr	4 hr	6 hr	AUC_{0-6}
2.25 g	8	134 (14)	57 (14)	17.1 (23)	5.2 (32)	2.5 (35)	0.9 (14)[b]	131 (14)
3.375 g	6	242 (12)	106 (8)	34.6 (20)	11.5 (19)	5.1 (22)	1.0 (10)	242 (10)
4.5 g	8	298 (14)	141 (19)	46.6 (28)	16.4 (29)	6.9 (29)	1.4 (30)	322 (16)

TAZOBACTAM

| Piperacillin/Tazobactam Dose[a] | No. of Evaluable Subjects | Plasma Concentrations** (μg/mL) | | | | | | AUC** (μg·hr/mL) |
		30 min	1 hr	2 hr	3 hr	4 hr	6 hr	AUC_{0-6}
2.25 g	8	14.8 (14)	7.2 (22)	2.6 (30)	1.1 (35)	0.7 (6)[c]	<0.5	16.0 (21)
3.375 g	6	24.2 (14)	10.7 (7)	4.0 (18)	1.4 (21)	0.7 (16)[b]	<0.5	25.0 (8)
4.5 g	8	33.8 (15)	17.3 (16)	6.8 (24)	2.8 (25)	1.3 (30)	<0.5	39.8 (15)

** Numbers in parentheses are coefficients of variation (CV%).
a: Piperacillin and tazobactam were given in combination.
b: N = 4
c: N = 3

INDICATIONS AND USAGE

Zosyn (piperacillin and tazobactam for injection) is indicated for the treatment of patients with moderate to severe infections caused by piperacillin-resistant, piperacillin/tazobactam-susceptible, β-lactamase producing strains of the designated microorganisms in the specified conditions listed below:

Appendicitis (complicated by rupture or abscess) and peritonitis caused by piperacillin-resistant, β-lactamase producing strains of *Escherichia coli* or the following members of the *Bacteroides fragilis* group: *B. fragilis, B. ovatus, B. thetaiotaomicron*, or *B. vulgatus*. The individual members of this group were studied in less than 10 cases. Uncomplicated and complicated skin and skin structure infections, including cellulitis, cutaneous abscesses and ischemic/diabetic foot infections caused by piperacillin-resistant, β-lactamase producing strains of *Staphylococcus aureus*.

Postpartum endometritis or pelvic inflammatory disease caused by piperacillin-resistant, β-lactamase producing strains of *Escherichia coli*.

Community-acquired pneumonia (moderate severity only) caused by piperacillin-resistant, β-lactamase producing strains of *Haemophilus influenzae*.

Nosocomial pneumonia (moderate to severe) caused by piperacillin-resistant, β-lactamase producing strains of *Staphylococcus aureus*. (See **DOSAGE AND ADMINISTRATION**.)

As a combination product, Zosyn (piperacillin and tazobactam for injection) is indicated only for the specified conditions listed above. Infections caused by piperacillin-susceptible organisms, for which piperacillin has been shown to be effective, are also amenable to Zosyn treatment due to its piperacillin content. The tazobactam component of this combination product does not decrease the activity of the piperacillin component against piperacillin-susceptible organisms. Therefore, the treatment of mixed infections caused by piperacillin-susceptible organisms and piperacillin-resistant, β-lactamase producing organisms susceptible to Zosyn should not require the addition of another antibiotic. (See **DOSAGE AND ADMINISTRATION**.)

Zosyn is useful as presumptive therapy in the indicated conditions prior to the identification of causative organisms because of its broad spectrum of bactericidal activity against gram-positive and gram-negative aerobic and anaerobic organisms.

Appropriate cultures should usually be performed before initiating antimicrobial treatment in order to isolate and identify the organisms causing infection and to determine their susceptibility to Zosyn (piperacillin and tazobactam for injection). Antimicrobial therapy should be adjusted, if appropriate, once the results of culture(s) and antimicrobial susceptibility testing are known.

CONTRAINDICATIONS

Zosyn is contraindicated in patients with a history of allergic reactions to any of the penicillins, cephalosporins, or β-lactamase inhibitors.

WARNINGS

SERIOUS AND OCCASIONALLY FATAL HYPERSENSITIVITY (ANAPHYLACTIC/ANAPHYLACTOID) REACTIONS (INCLUDING SHOCK) HAVE BEEN REPORTED IN PATIENTS RECEIVING THERAPY WITH PENICILLINS INCLUDING ZOSYN. THESE REACTIONS ARE MORE LIKELY TO OCCUR IN INDIVIDUALS WITH A HISTORY OF PENICILLIN HYPERSENSITIVITY OR A HISTORY OF SENSITIVITY TO MULTIPLE ALLERGENS. THERE HAVE BEEN REPORTS OF INDIVIDUALS WITH A HISTORY OF PENICILLIN HYPERSENSITIVITY WHO HAVE EXPERIENCED SEVERE REACTIONS WHEN TREATED WITH CEPHALOSPORINS. BEFORE INITIATING THERAPY WITH ZOSYN, CAREFUL INQUIRY SHOULD BE MADE CONCERNING PREVIOUS HYPERSENSITIVITY REACTIONS TO PENICILLINS, CEPHALOSPORINS, OR OTHER ALLERGENS. IF AN ALLERGIC REACTION OCCURS, ZOSYN SHOULD BE DISCONTINUED AND APPROPRIATE THERAPY INSTITUTED. **SERIOUS ANAPHYLACTIC/ANAPHYLACTOID REACTIONS (INCLUDING SHOCK) REQUIRE IMMEDIATE EMERGENCY TREATMENT WITH EPINEPHRINE. OXYGEN, INTRAVENOUS STEROIDS, AND AIRWAY MANAGEMENT, INCLUDING INTUBATION, SHOULD ALSO BE ADMINISTERED AS INDICATED.**

Pseudomembranous colitis has been reported with nearly all antibacterial agents, including piperacillin/tazobactam, and may range in severity from mild to life-threatening. Therefore, it is important to consider this diagnosis in patients who present with diarrhea subsequent to the administration of antibacterial agents.

Treatment with antibacterial agents alters the normal flora of the colon and may permit overgrowth of clostridia. Studies indicate that a toxin produced by *Clostridium difficile* is one primary cause of "antibiotic-associated colitis."

After the diagnosis of pseudomembranous colitis has been established, therapeutic measures should be initiated. Mild cases of pseudomembranous colitis usually respond to drug discontinuation alone. In moderate to severe cases, consideration should be given to management with fluids and electrolytes, protein supplementation, and treatment with an antibacterial drug clinically effective against *Clostridium difficile* colitis.

PRECAUTIONS

General

Bleeding manifestations have occurred in some patients receiving β-lactam antibiotics, including piperacillin. These reactions have sometimes been associated with abnormalities of coagulation tests such as clotting time, platelet aggregation and prothrombin time, and are more likely to occur in patients with renal failure. If bleeding manifestations occur, Zosyn (piperacillin and tazobactam for injection) should be discontinued and appropriate therapy instituted.

The possibility of the emergence of resistant organisms that might cause superinfections should be kept in mind. If this occurs, appropriate measures should be taken.

As with other penicillins, patients may experience neuromuscular excitability or convulsions if higher than recommended doses are given intravenously (particularly in the presence of renal failure).

Zosyn is a monosodium salt of piperacillin and a monosodium salt of tazobactam and contains a total of 2.35 mEq (54 mg) of Na^+ per gram of piperacillin in the combination product. This should be considered when treating patients requiring restricted salt intake. Periodic electrolyte determinations should be performed in patients with low potassium reserves, and the possibility of hypokalemia should be kept in mind with patients who have potentially low potassium reserves and who are receiving cytotoxic therapy or diuretics.

As with other semisynthetic penicillins, piperacillin therapy has been associated with an increased incidence of fever and rash in cystic fibrosis patients.

In patients with renal insufficiency or in hemodialysis patients, the intravenous dose should be adjusted to the degree of renal function impairment.

Laboratory Tests

Periodic assessment of hematopoietic function should be performed, especially with prolonged therapy, ie, ≥21 days. (See **ADVERSE REACTIONS, Adverse Laboratory Events**.)

Drug Interactions

Aminoglycosides

The mixing of Zosyn with an aminoglycoside in vitro can result in substantial inactivation of the aminoglycoside. (See **DOSAGE AND ADMINISTRATION, Compatible Intravenous Diluent Solutions**.)

When Zosyn was co-administered with tobramycin, the area under the curve, renal clearance, and urinary recovery of tobramycin were decreased by 11%, 32%, and 38%, respectively. The alterations in the pharmacokinetics of tobramycin when administered in combination with piperacillin/tazobactam may be due to in vivo and in vitro inactivation of tobramycin in the presence of piperacillin/tazobactam. The inactivation of aminoglycosides in the presence of penicillin-class drugs has been recognized. It has been postulated that penicillin-aminoglycoside complexes form; these complexes are microbiologically inactive and of unknown toxicity. In patients with severe renal dysfunction (ie, chronic hemodialysis patients), the pharmacokinetics of tobramycin are significantly altered when tobramycin is administered in combination with piperacillin.[4] The alteration of tobramycin pharmacokinetics and the potential toxicity of the penicillin-aminoglycoside complexes in patients with mild to moderate renal dysfunction who are administered an aminoglycoside in combination with piperacillin/tazobactam are unknown.

Probenecid

Probenecid administered concomitantly with Zosyn prolongs the half-life of piperacillin by 21% and that of tazobactam by 71%.

Vancomycin

No pharmacokinetic interactions have been noted between Zosyn and vancomycin.

Heparin

Coagulation parameters should be tested more frequently and monitored regularly during simultaneous administration of high doses of heparin, oral anticoagulants, or other drugs that may affect the blood coagulation system or the thrombocyte function.

Vecuronium

Piperacillin when used concomitantly with vecuronium has been implicated in the prolongation of the neuromuscular blockade of vecuronium. Zosyn (piperacillin/tazobactam) could produce the same phenomenon if given along with vecuronium. Due to their similar mechanism of action, it is expected that the neuromuscular blockade produced by any of the non-depolarizing muscle relaxants could be prolonged in the presence of piperacillin. (See package insert for vecuronium bromide.)

Methotrexate

Piperacillin may reduce the excretion of methotrexate; therefore, serum levels of methotrexate should be monitored in patients to avoid drug toxicity.

Drug/Laboratory Test Interactions

As with other penicillins, the administration of Zosyn® (piperacillin and tazobactam for injection) may result in a false-positive reaction for glucose in the urine using a copper-reduction method (CLINITEST®). It is recommended that glucose tests based on enzymatic glucose oxidase reactions (such as DIASTIX® or TES-TAPE®) be used.

Carcinogenesis, Mutagenesis, Impairment of Fertility

Piperacillin/Tazobactam

Long term carcinogenicity studies in animals have not been conducted with piperacillin/tazobactam, piperacillin, or tazobactam.

Piperacillin/tazobactam was negative in microbial mutagenicity assays at concentrations up to 14.84/1.86 μg/plate. Piperacillin/tazobactam was negative in the unscheduled DNA synthesis (UDS) test at concentrations up to 5689/711 μg/mL. Piperacillin/tazobactam was negative in a mammalian point mutation (Chinese hamster ovary cell HPRT) assay at concentrations up to 8000/1000 μg/mL. Piperacillin/tazobactam was negative in a mammalian cell (BALB/c-3T3) transformation assay at concentrations up to 8/1 μg/mL. In vivo, piperacillin/tazobactam did not induce chromosomal aberrations in rats dosed I.V. with 1500/187.5 mg/kg; this dose is similar to the maximum recommended human daily dose on a body-surface-area basis (mg/m^2).

Piperacillin

Piperacillin was negative in microbial mutagenicity assays at concentrations up to 50 μg/plate. There was no DNA damage in bacteria (Rec assay) exposed to piperacillin at concentrations up to 200 μg/disk. Piperacillin was negative in the UDS test at concentrations up to 10,000 μg/mL. In a mammalian point mutation (mouse lymphoma cells) assay, piperacillin was positive at concentrations ≥2500 μg/mL. Piperacillin was negative in a cell (BALB/c-3T3) transformation assay at concentrations up to 3000 μg/mL. In vivo, piperacillin did not induce chromosomal aberrations in mice at I.V. doses up to 2000 mg/kg/day or rats at I.V. doses up to 1500 mg/kg/day. These doses are half (mice) or similar (rats) to the maximum recommended human daily dose based on body-surface area (mg/m^2). In another in vivo test, there was no dominant lethal effect when piperacillin was administered to rats at I.V. doses up to 2000 mg/kg/day, which is similar to the maximum recommended human daily dose based on body-surface area (mg/m^2). When mice were administered piperacillin at I.V. doses up to 2000 mg/kg/day, which is half the maximum recommended human daily dose based on body-surface area (mg/m^2), urine from these animals was not mutagenic when tested in a microbial mutagenicity assay. Bacteria injected into the peritoneal cavity of mice administered piperacillin at I.V. doses up to 2000 mg/kg/day did not show increased mutation frequencies.

Tazobactam

Tazobactam was negative in microbial mutagenicity assays at concentrations up to 333 μg/plate. Tazobactam was negative in the UDS test at concentrations up to 2000 μg/mL. Tazobactam was negative in a mammalian point mutation (Chinese hamster ovary cell HPRT) assay at concentrations up to 5000 μg/mL. In another mammalian point mutation (mouse lymphoma cells) assay, tazobactam was positive at concentrations ≥3000 μg/mL. Tazobactam was negative in a cell (BALB/c-3T3) transformation assay at concentrations up to 900 μg/mL. In an in vitro cytogenetics (Chinese hamster lung cells) assay, tazobactam was negative at concentrations up to 3000 μg/mL. In vivo, tazobactam did not induce chromosomal aberrations in rats at I.V. doses up to 5000 mg/kg, which is 23 times the maximum recommended human daily dose based on body-surface area (mg/m^2).

Pregnancy

Teratogenic effects—Pregnancy Category B

Piperacillin/tazobactam

Reproduction studies have been performed in rats and have revealed no evidence of impaired fertility due to piperacillin/tazobactam administered up to a dose which is similar to the maximum recommended human daily dose based on body-surface area (mg/m^2).

Teratology studies have been performed in mice and rats and have revealed no evidence of harm to the fetus due to piperacillin/tazobactam administered up to a dose which is 1 to 2 times and 2 to 3 times the human dose of piperacillin and tazobactam, respectively, based on body-surface area (mg/m^2). Piperacillin and tazobactam cross the placenta.

Piperacillin

Reproduction and teratology studies have been performed in mice and rats and have revealed no evidence of impaired fertility or harm to the fetus due to piperacillin administered up to a dose which is half (mice) or similar (rats) to the maximum recommended human daily dose based on body-surface area (mg/m^2).

Tazobactam

Reproduction studies have been performed in rats and have revealed no evidence of impaired fertility due to tazobactam administered at doses up to 3 times the maximum recommended human daily dose based on body-surface area (mg/m^2).

Teratology studies have been performed in mice and rats and have revealed no evidence of harm to the fetus due to tazobactam administered at doses up to 6 and 14 times, respectively, the human dose based on body-surface area (mg/m^2). In rats, tazobactam crosses the placenta. Concentrations in the fetus are less than or equal to 10% of those found in maternal plasma.

There are, however, no adequate and well-controlled studies with the piperacillin/tazobactam combination or with piperacillin or tazobactam alone in pregnant women. Because animal reproduction studies are not always predictive of the human response, this drug should be used during pregnancy only if clearly needed.

Nursing Mothers

Piperacillin is excreted in low concentrations in human milk; tazobactam concentrations in human milk have not been studied. Caution should be exercised when Zosyn (piperacillin and tazobactam for injection) is administered to a nursing woman.

Pediatric Use

Safety and efficacy in pediatric patients have not been established.

Continued on next page

Zosyn—Cont.

Geriatric Use
Patients over 65 years are **not** at an increased risk of developing adverse effects solely because of age. However, dosage should be adjusted in the presence of renal insufficiency. (See **DOSAGE AND ADMINISTRATION**.)

ADVERSE REACTIONS
During the initial clinical investigations, 2621 patients worldwide were treated with Zosyn (piperacillin and tazobactam for injection) in phase 3 trials. In the key North American clinical trials (n=830 patients), 90% of the adverse events reported were mild to moderate in severity and transient in nature. However, in 3.2% of the patients treated worldwide, Zosyn was discontinued because of adverse events primarily involving the skin (1.3%), including rash and pruritus; the gastrointestinal system (0.9%), including diarrhea, nausea, and vomiting; and allergic reactions (0.5%).

Adverse local reactions that were reported, irrespective of relationship to therapy with Zosyn, were phlebitis (1.3%), injection site reaction (0.5%), pain (0.2%), inflammation (0.2%), thrombophlebitis (0.2%), and edema (0.1%). In the completed study of nosocomial lower respiratory tract infections, 155 patients were treated with Zosyn in a dosing regimen of 3.375 g every 4 hours in combination with an aminoglycoside. In this trial, 88.5% of the adverse experiences reported were mild to moderate in severity and transient in nature. However, in this trial, therapy with Zosyn was discontinued in four patients (2.6%) due to adverse experiences.

Irrespective of drug relationship or degree of severity, the adverse experiences which led to the discontinuation of Zosyn (piperacillin and tazobactam for injection) in these four patients were: thrombocytopenia and pancreatitis in one patient; fever in one patient; fever and eosinophilia in another patient; and diarrhea and elevated liver enzymes in the fourth patient.

Adverse Clinical Events
Based on patients from the North American trials (n=1063), the events with the highest incidence in patients, irrespective of relationship to Zosyn therapy, were diarrhea (11.3%); headache (7.7%); constipation (7.7%); nausea (6.9%); insomnia (6.6%); rash (4.2%), including maculopapular, bullous, urticarial, and eczematoid; vomiting (3.3%); dyspepsia (3.3%); pruritus (3.1%); stool changes (2.4%); fever (2.4%); agitation (2.1%); pain (1.7%); moniliasis (1.6%); hypertension (1.6%); dizziness (1.4%); abdominal pain (1.3%); chest pain (1.3%); edema (1.2%); anxiety (1.2%); rhinitis (1.2%); and dyspnea (1.1%).

Based on patients in the completed study of nosocomial lower respiratory tract infections (n=155), using every 4 hour dosing and aminoglycoside therapy, the events with the highest incidence in patients, irrespective of relationship to Zosyn and aminoglycoside therapy, were: diarrhea (20%); constipation (8.4%); agitation (7.1%); nausea (5.8%); headache (4.5%); insomnia (4.5%); oral thrush (3.9%); erythematous rash (3.9%); anxiety (3.2%); fever (3.2%); pain (3.2%); pruritus (3.2%); hiccough (2.6%); vomiting (2.6%); dyspepsia (1.9%); edema (1.9%); fluid overload (1.9%); stool changes (1.9%); anorexia (1.3%); cardiac arrest (1.3%); confusion (1.3%); diaphoresis (1.3%); duodenal ulcer (1.3%); flatulence (1.3%); hypertension (1.3%); hypotension (1.3%); inflammation at injection site (1.3%); pleural effusion (1.3%); pneumothorax (1.3%); rash, not otherwise specified (1.3%); supraventricular tachycardia (1.3%); thrombophlebitis (1.3%); and urinary incontinence (1.3%).

Additional adverse systemic clinical events reported in 1.0% or less of the patients in the initial North American trials and/or in the patients administered Zosyn 3.375 g every 4 hours plus an aminoglycoside in the study of nosocomial lower respiratory tract infections are listed below within each body system (bracketed events occurred only in the nosocomial pneumonia trial):

Autonomic nervous system—hypotension, ileus, syncope
Body as a whole—rigors, back pain, malaise, [asthenia, chest pain]
Cardiovascular—tachycardia, including supraventricular and ventricular; bradycardia; arrhythmia, including atrial fibrillation, ventricular fibrillation, cardiac arrest, cardiac failure, circulatory failure, myocardial infarction, [angina]
Central nervous system—tremor, convulsions, vertigo, [aggressive reaction (combative)]
Gastrointestinal—melena, flatulence, hemorrhage, gastritis, hiccough, ulcerative stomatitis, [fecal incontinence, gastric ulcer, pancreatitis]

Pseudomembranous colitis was reported in one patient during the clinical trials. The onset of pseudomembranous colitis symptoms may occur during or after antibacterial treatment. (See **WARNINGS**.)

Hearing and Vestibular System—tinnitus, [deafness, earache]
Hypersensitivity—anaphylaxis
Metabolic and Nutritional—symptomatic hypoglycemia, thirst, [gout, vitamin B_{12} deficiency anemia]
Musculoskeletal—myalgia, arthralgia
Platelets, Bleeding, Clotting—mesenteric embolism, purpura, epistaxis, pulmonary embolism, [ecchymosis, hemoptysis] (See **PRECAUTIONS, General**.)
Psychiatric—confusion, hallucination, depression
Reproductive, Female—leukorrhea, vaginitis, [perineal irritation/pain]
Reproductive, Male—[balanoposthitis]
Respiratory—pharyngitis, pulmonary edema, bronchospasm, coughing, [atelectasis, dyspnea, hypoxia]
Skin and Appendages—genital pruritus, diaphoresis, [conjunctivitis, xerosis]
Special senses—taste perversion
Urinary—retention, dysuria, oliguria, hematuria, incontinence, [urinary tract infection with trichomonas, yeast in urine]
Vision—photophobia
Vascular (extracardiac)—flushing, [cerebrovascular accident]

Additional adverse events reported from worldwide marketing experience with Zosyn, occurring under circumstances where causal relationship to Zosyn is uncertain:

Gastrointestinal—hepatitis, cholestatic jaundice
Hematologic—hemolytic anemia, anemia, thrombocytosis, agranulocytosis, pancytopenia
Immune—hypersensitivity reactions, anaphylactic/anaphylactoid reactions (including shock)
Infections and Infestations—candidal superinfections
Renal—rarely, interstitial nephritis, renal failure
Skin and Appendages—erythema multiforme and Stevens-Johnson syndrome, rarely reported; toxic epidermal necrolysis

Adverse Laboratory Events (Seen During Clinical Trials)
Of the studies reported, including that of nosocomial lower respiratory tract infections in which a higher dose of Zosyn (piperacillin and tazobactam for injection) was used in combination with an aminoglycoside, changes in laboratory parameters, without regard to drug relationship, include:

Hematologic—decreases in hemoglobin and hematocrit, thrombocytopenia, increases in platelet count, eosinophilia, leukopenia, neutropenia. The leukopenia/neutropenia associated with Zosyn administration appears to be reversible and most frequently associated with prolonged administration, ie, ≥21 days of therapy. These patients were withdrawn from therapy; some had accompanying systemic symptoms (eg, fever, rigors, chills).

Coagulation—positive direct Coombs' test, prolonged prothrombin time, prolonged partial thromboplastin time
Hepatic—transient elevations of AST (SGOT), ALT (SGPT), alkaline phosphatase, bilirubin
Renal—increases in serum creatinine, blood urea nitrogen
Urinalysis—proteinuria, hematuria, pyuria

Additional laboratory events include abnormalities in electrolytes (ie, increases and decreases in sodium, potassium, and calcium), hyperglycemia, decreases in total protein or albumin, blood glucose decreased, gamma-glutamyltransferase increased, hypokalemia, and bleeding time prolonged.

The following adverse reaction has also been reported for PIPRACIL® (sterile piperacillin sodium):

Skeletal—prolonged muscle relaxation (See **PRECAUTIONS, Drug Interactions**.)

Piperacillin therapy has been associated with an increased incidence of fever and rash in cystic fibrosis patients.

OVERDOSAGE
There have been post-marketing reports of overdose with piperacillin/tazobactam. The majority of those events experienced including nausea, vomiting, and diarrhea have also been reported with the usual recommended dosages. Patients may experience neuromuscular excitability or convulsions if higher than recommended doses are given intravenously (particularly in the presence of renal failure).

Treatment should be supportive and symptomatic according to the patient's clinical presentation. Excessive serum concentrations of either piperacillin or tazobactam may be reduced by hemodialysis. (See **CLINICAL PHARMACOLOGY**.)

DOSAGE AND ADMINISTRATION
Zosyn should be administered by slow intravenous infusion over 20 to 30 minutes or slow intravenous injection (over at least 3 to 5 minutes).

Normal Renal Function (Creatinine Clearance ≥ 90 mL/min)
The usual total daily dose of Zosyn for adults is 3.375 g every six hours totalling 13.5 g (12 g piperacillin sodium/1.5 g tazobactam sodium).

Initial presumptive treatment of patients with nosocomial pneumonia should start with Zosyn at a dosage of 3.375 g every four hours plus an aminoglycoside. Treatment with the aminoglycoside should be continued in patients from whom *Pseudomonas aeruginosa* is isolated. If *Pseudomonas aeruginosa* is not isolated, the aminoglycoside may be discontinued at the discretion of the treating physician. (See **DOSAGE AND ADMINISTRATION**.)

Renal Insufficiency
In patients with renal insufficiency (Creatinine Clearance <90 mL/min), the intravenous dose of Zosyn (piperacillin and tazobactam for injection) should be adjusted to the degree of actual renal function impairment. In patients with nosocomial pneumonia receiving concomitant aminoglycoside therapy, the aminoglycoside dosage should be adjusted according to the recommendations of the manufacturer. The recommended daily doses of Zosyn for patients with renal insufficiency are as follows:

Zosyn Dosage Recommendations For All Indications Including Nosocomial Pneumonia

Creatinine Clearance (mL/min)	Recommended Dosage Regimen
>40-90	12 g/1.5 g/day in divided doses of 3.375 g q 6 h
20-40	8 g/1.0 g/day in divided doses of 2.25 g q 6 h
<20	6 g/0.75 g/day in divided doses of 2.25 g q 8 h

For patients on hemodialysis, irrespective of the condition under treatment, the maximum dose is 2.25 g Zosyn every eight hours. In addition, because hemodialysis removes 30% to 40% of a Zosyn dose in four hours, one additional dose of 0.75 g Zosyn should be administered following each dialysis period. For patients with renal failure, measurement of serum levels of piperacillin and tazobactam will provide additional guidance for adjusting dosage.

Duration of Therapy
The usual duration of Zosyn treatment is from seven to ten days. However, the recommended duration of Zosyn treatment of nosocomial pneumonia is seven to fourteen days. In all conditions, the duration of therapy should be guided by the severity of the infection and the patient's clinical and bacteriological progress.

Intravenous Administration
For conventional vials, reconstitute Zosyn per gram of piperacillin with 5 mL of a compatible reconstitution diluent from the list provided below. Shake well until dissolved. Pharmacy vials should be used immediately after reconstitution. Discard any unused portion after 24 hours if stored at room temperature (20°C to 25°C [68°F to 77°F]), or after 48 hours if stored at refrigerated temperature (2°C to 8°C [36°F to 46°F]).

Compatible Reconstitution Diluents
0.9% Sodium Chloride for Injection
Sterile Water for Injection
Dextrose 5%
Bacteriostatic Saline/Parabens
Bacteriostatic Water/Parabens
Bacteriostatic Saline/Benzyl Alcohol
Bacteriostatic Water/Benzyl Alcohol

Reconstituted Zosyn solution should be further diluted (recommended volume per dose of 50 mL to 150 mL) in a compatible intravenous diluent solution listed below. Administer by infusion over a period of at least 30 minutes. During the infusion it is desirable to discontinue the primary infusion solution.

Compatible Intravenous Diluent Solutions
0.9% Sodium Chloride for Injection
Sterile Water for Injection[‡]
Dextrose 5%
Dextran 6% in Saline

[‡]Maximum recommended volume per dose of Sterile Water for Injection is 50 mL.

ADD-Vantage® System Admixtures
Dextrose 5% in Water (50 or 100 mL)
0.9% Sodium Chloride (50 or 100 mL)

For ADD-Vantage® vials reconstitution directions, see *INSTRUCTIONS FOR USE* sheet provided in the box.

Zosyn should not be mixed with other drugs in a syringe or infusion bottle since compatibility has not been established. Because of chemical instability, Zosyn should not be used with solutions containing only sodium bicarbonate.

LACTATED RINGER'S SOLUTION IS NOT COMPATIBLE WITH ZOSYN.

Zosyn (piperacillin and tazobactam for injection) should not be added to blood products or albumin hydrolysates.

When concomitant therapy with aminoglycosides is indicated, Zosyn and the aminoglycoside should be reconstituted and administered separately, due to the in vitro inactivation of the aminoglycoside by the penicillin. (See **PRECAUTIONS, Drug Interactions**.)

Directions for Reconstitution and Dilution for Use
Intravenous
2.25 g, 3.375 g, and 4.5 g Zosyn should be reconstituted with 10 mL, 15 mL, and 20 mL, respectively. Swirl until dissolved.

Zosyn can be used in ambulatory intravenous infusion pumps.

Stability of Zosyn Following Reconstitution
Zosyn is stable in glass and plastic containers (plastic syringes, I.V. bags and tubing) when used with compatible diluents.

Pharmacy vials should be used immediately after reconstitution. Discard any unused portion after 24 hours if stored at room temperature (20°C to 25°C [68°F to 77°F]), or after 48 hours if stored at refrigerated temperature (2°C to 8°C [36°F to 46°F]). Vials should not be frozen after reconstitution.

Stability studies in the I.V. bags have demonstrated chemical stability (potency, pH of reconstituted solution and clarity of solution) for up to 24 hours at room temperature and up to one week at refrigerated temperature. Zosyn contains no preservatives. Appropriate consideration of aseptic technique should be used.

Stability of Zosyn in an ambulatory intravenous infusion pump has been demonstrated for a period of 12 hours at room temperature. Each dose was reconstituted and diluted to a volume of 37.5 mL or 25 mL. One-day supplies of dosing solution were aseptically transferred into the medication reservoir (I.V. bags or cartridge). The reservoir was fitted to a preprogrammed ambulatory intravenous infusion pump per the manufacturer's instructions. Stability of Zosyn is not affected when administered using an ambulatory intravenous infusion pump.

Stability studies with the admixed ADD-Vantage® system have demonstrated chemical stability (potency, pH and clarity) through 24 hours at room temperature. (Note: The admixed ADD-Vantage® should not be refrigerated or frozen after reconstitution.)

Parenteral drug products should be inspected visually for particulate matter or discoloration prior to administration, whenever solution and container permit.

HOW SUPPLIED

Zosyn® (piperacillin and tazobactam for injection) is supplied in the following sizes:

Each Zosyn 2.25 g vial provides piperacillin sodium equivalent to 2 grams of piperacillin and tazobactam sodium equivalent to 0.25 g of tazobactam. Each vial contains 4.69 mEq (108 mg) of sodium.

Supplied 10 per box—NDC 0206-8452-16

Each Zosyn 3.375 g vial provides piperacillin sodium equivalent to 3 grams of piperacillin and tazobactam sodium equivalent to 0.375 g of tazobactam. Each vial contains 7.04 mEq (162 mg) of sodium.

Supplied 10 per box—NDC 0206-8454-55

Each Zosyn 4.5 g vial provides piperacillin sodium equivalent to 4 grams of piperacillin and tazobactam sodium equivalent to 0.5 g of tazobactam. Each vial contains 9.39 mEq (216 mg) of sodium.

Supplied 10 per box—NDC 0206-8455-25

Each Zosyn 2.25 g ADD-Vantage® vial provides piperacillin sodium equivalent to 2 grams of piperacillin and tazobactam sodium equivalent to 0.25 g of tazobactam. Each ADD-Vantage® vial contains 4.69 mEq (108 mg) of sodium.

Supplied 10 per box—NDC 0206-8452-17.

Each Zosyn 3.375 g ADD-Vantage® vial provides piperacillin sodium equivalent to 3 grams of piperacillin and tazobactam sodium equivalent to 0.375 g of tazobactam. Each ADD-Vantage® vial contains 7.04 mEq (162 mg) of sodium.

Supplied 10 per box—NDC 0206-8454-17.

Each Zosyn 4.5 g ADD-Vantage® vial provides piperacillin sodium equivalent to 4 grams of piperacillin and tazobactam sodium equivalent to 0.5 g of tazobactam. Each ADD-Vantage® vial contains 9.39 mEq (216 mg) of sodium.

Supplied 10 per box—NDC 0206-8455-17.

Zosyn conventional and ADD-Vantage® vials should be stored at controlled room temperature (20°C to 25°C [68°F to 77°F]) prior to reconstitution.

Also Available

Zosyn is also supplied as follows:

Zosyn® (piperacillin and tazobactam for injection) in Galaxy® Container (PL 2040 Plastic) is supplied as a frozen, iso-osmotic, sterile, nonpyrogenic solution in single dose plastic containers as follows:

2.25 g (2 g piperacillin/0.25 g tazobactam) in 50 mL. Each container has 5.7 mEq (131 mg) of sodium.

Supplied 24/box—NDC 0206-8820-02

3.375 g (3 g piperacillin/0.375 g tazobactam) in 50 mL. Each container has 8.6 mEq (197 mg) of sodium.

Supplied 24/box—NDC 0206-8821-02

4.5 g (4 g piperacillin/0.5 g tazobactam) in 100 mL. Each container has 11.4 mEq (263 mg) of sodium.

Supplied 12/box—NDC 0206-8822-02

Also Available

Zosyn is also supplied as follows:

40.5 g pharmacy bulk vial containing 36 grams of piperacillin and 4.5 grams of tazobactam. Each pharmacy bulk vial contains 84.5 mEq (1,944 mg) of sodium. NDC 0206-8620-11

REFERENCES

1. National Committee for Clinical Laboratory Standards, Methods for Dilution Antimicrobial Susceptibility Tests for Bacteria that Grow Aerobically— Fourth Edition. Approved Standard NCCLS Document M7-A4, Vol. 17, No. 2, NCCLS, Wayne, PA, January, 1997.
2. National Committee for Clinical Laboratory Standards, Methods for Antimicrobial Susceptibility Testing for Anaerobic Bacteria—Third Edition. Approved Standard NCCLS Document M11-A3, Vol. 13, No. 26, NCCLS, Villanova, PA, December, 1993.
3. National Committee for Clinical Laboratory Standards, Performance Standard for Antimicrobial Disk Susceptibility Tests—Sixth Edition. Approved Standard NCCLS Document M2-A6, Vol. 17, No. 1, NCCLS, Wayne, PA, January, 1997.
4. Halstenson CE, Hirata CAI, Heim-Duthoy KL, Abraham PA, and Matzke GR. Effect of concomitant administration of piperacillin on the dispositions of netilmicin and tobramycin in patients with end-stage renal disease. Antimicrob Agents Chemother 34(1):128-133, 1990.

CLINITEST® and DIASTIX® are registered trademarks of Ames Division, Miles Laboratories, Inc.

TES-TAPE® is a registered trademark of Eli Lilly and Company.

Galaxy® is a registered trademark of Baxter International, Inc.

ADD-Vantage® is a registered trademark of Abbott Laboratories.

LEDERLE PIPERACILLIN, INC.
Carolina, Puerto Rico 00987
CI 4630-5
W10414C001
Rev 11/02

Key to Controlled Substances Categories

Products listed with the symbols shown below are subject to the Controlled Substances Act of 1970. These drugs are categorized according to their potential for abuse. The greater the potential, the more severe the limitations on their prescription.

CATEGORY	INTERPRETATION
℃_{II}	**HIGH POTENTIAL FOR ABUSE.** Use may lead to severe physical or psychological dependence. Prescriptions must be written in ink, or typewritten and signed by the practitioner. Verbal prescriptions must be confirmed in writing within 72 hours, and may be given only in a genuine emergency. No renewals are permitted.
℃_{III}	**SOME POTENTIAL FOR ABUSE.** Use may lead to low-to-moderate physical dependence or high psychological dependence. Prescriptions may be oral or written. Up to 5 renewals are permitted within 6 months.
℃_{IV}	**LOW POTENTIAL FOR ABUSE.** Use may lead to limited physical or psychological dependence. Prescriptions may be oral or written. Up to 5 renewals are permitted within 6 months.
℃_V	**SUBJECT TO STATE AND LOCAL REGULATION.** Abuse potential is low; a prescription may not be required.

Key to FDA Use-in-Pregnancy Ratings

The U.S. Food and Drug Administration's use-in-pregnancy rating system weighs the degree to which available information has ruled out risk to the fetus against the drug's potential benefit to the patient. The ratings, and their interpretation, are as follows:

CATEGORY	INTERPRETATION
A	**CONTROLLED STUDIES SHOW NO RISK.** Adequate, well-controlled studies in pregnant women have failed to demonstrate a risk to the fetus in any trimester of pregnancy.
B	**NO EVIDENCE OF RISK IN HUMANS.** Adequate, well-controlled studies in pregnant women have not shown increased risk of fetal abnormalities despite adverse findings in animals, or, in the absence of adequate human studies, animal studies show no fetal risk. The chance of fetal harm is remote, but remains a possibility.
C	**RISK CANNOT BE RULED OUT.** Adequate, well-controlled human studies are lacking, and animal studies have shown a risk to the fetus or are lacking as well. There is a chance of fetal harm if the drug is administered during pregnancy; but the potential benefits may outweigh the potential risk.
D	**POSITIVE EVIDENCE OF RISK.** Studies in humans, or investigational or post-marketing data, have demonstrated fetal risk. Nevertheless, potential benefits from the use of the drug may outweigh the potential risk. For example, the drug may be acceptable if needed in a life-threatening situation or serious disease for which safer drugs cannot be used or are ineffective.
X	**CONTRAINDICATED IN PREGNANCY.** Studies in animals or humans, or investigational or post-marketing reports, have demonstrated positive evidence of fetal abnormalities or risk which clearly outweighs any possible benefit to the patient.